ARCHIVES
OF
GENERAL PSYCHIATRY

Volume 52

January through December 1995

ARCHIVES
OF
GENERAL PSYCHIATRY

VOL 52 NO. 1, JANUARY 1995

Original Articles

Functioning and Well-being Outcomes of Patients With Depression Compared With Chronic General Medical Illnesses **11**
Ron D. Hays, PhD; Kenneth B. Wells, MD, MPH; Cathy Donald Sherbourne, PhD; William Rogers, PhD; Karen Spritzer

A Positron Emission Tomographic Study of Simple Phobic Symptom Provocation **20**
Scott L. Rauch, MD; Cary R. Savage, PhD; Nathaniel M. Alpert, PhD; Euripedes C. Miguel, MD, PhD; Lee Baer, PhD; Hans C. Breiter, MD; Alan J. Fischman MD, PhD; Peter A. Manzo; Cara Moretti; Michael A. Jenike, MD

Pharmacotherapy of Impaired Affect in Recovering Schizophrenic Patients **29**
Gerard E. Hogarty, MSW; Joseph P. McEvoy, MD; Richard F. Ulrich, MS; Ann Louise DiBarry, MSN; Partricia Bartone, MSN; Susan Cooley, MEd; Kathleen Hammill, MSN; Mary Carter, PhD; Mark R. Munetz, MD; James Perel, PhD

Adoption Study Demonstrating Two Genetic Pathways to Drug Abuse **42**
Remi J. Cadoret, MD; William R. Yates, MD; Ed Troughton; George Woodworth, PhD; Mark A. Stewart, MD

American Medical Association
Physicians dedicated to the health of America

Efficacy and Tolerability of Serotonin Transport Inhibitors in Obsessive-compulsive Disorder: A Meta-analysis 53
John H. Greist, MD; James W. Jefferson, MD; Kenneth A. Kobak, MSSW; David J. Katzelnick, MD; Ronald C. Serlin, PhD

Test-Retest Reliability of the Diagnostic Interview Schedule for Children (DISC 2.1): Parent, Child, and Combined Algorithms 61
Peter Jensen, MD; Margaret Roper, MS; Prudence Fisher, MS; John Piacentini, PhD; Glorisa Canino, PhD; John Richters, PhD; Maritza Rubio-Stipec, MA; Mina Dulcan, MD; Sherryl Goodman, PhD; Mark Davies, MPH; Donald Rae, MS; David Shaffer, MD; Hector Bird, MD; Benjamin Lahey, PhD; Mary Schwab-Stone, MD

Letters to the Editor

Treatment of Postpartum Depression With Interpersonal Psychotherapy 75
Scott Stuart, MD, Michael W. O'Hara, PhD

In Reply 76
Myrna M. Weissman, PhD, John Markowitz, MD

Relationship of Panic Disorder to Posttraumatic Stress Disorder 76
Gabriel Safadi, MD, Jacques Bradwejn, MD

In Reply 77
Steven M. Southwick, MD; John H. Krystal, MD; Dennis S. Charney, MD

Departments

Instructions for Authors 5

Classified Advertising 80

ARCHIVES OF GENERAL PSYCHIATRY

Editor:
Jack D. Barchas, MD
Department of Psychiatry
Cornell Medical Center
525 E 68th St, Box 171
New York, NY 10021
Phone: (212) 746-3771
Fax: (212) 746-3772

Assistant to Editor:
Peter M. Marzuk, MD
New York, NY

Editorial Administrator:
Angela McGregor
New York, NY

ARCHIVES OF GENERAL PSYCHIATRY

VOL 52 NO. 2, FEBRUARY 1995

News and Views

Depression in Patients With Cancer: Diagnosis, Biology, and Treatment 89
J. Stephen McDaniel, MD; Dominique L. Musselman, MD; Maryfrances R. Porter; Deborah A. Reed, RN, MSN; Charles B. Nemeroff, MD, PhD

Critical Review of Psychosocial Interventions in Cancer Care 100
Fawzy I. Fawzy, MD; Nancy W. Fawzy, RN, DNSc; Lisa A. Arndt; Robert O. Pasnau, MD

Original Articles

Switching From 'Unipolar' to Bipolar II: An 11-Year Prospective Study of Clinical and Temperamental Predictors in 559 Patients 114
Hagop S. Akiskal, MD; Jack D. Maser, PhD; Pamela J. Zeller, PhD; Jean Endicott, PhD; William Coryell, MD; Martin Keller, MD; Meredith Warshaw, MS; Paula Clayton, MD; Frederick K. Goodwin, MD

Structure and Course of Positive and Negative Symptoms in Schizophrenia 127
William W. Eaton, PhD; R. Thara, MD; Belle Federman; Beth Melton, ScM; Kung-yee Liang, PhD

Guanine Nucleotide-Binding Proteins in Bipolar Affective Disorder: Effects of Long-term Lithium Treatment 135
Husseini K. Manji, MD, FRCPC; Guang Chen, MD; Hady Shimon; John K. Hsiao, MD; William Z. Potter, MD, PhD; Robert H. Belmaker, MD

In Quest of Identifying Vulnerability Markers for Psychiatric Disorders by All-Night Polysomnography 145
Christoph J. Lauer, PhD; Wolfgang Schreiber, MD; Florian Holsboer, MD, PhD; Jürgen-Christian Krieg, MD

American Medical Association

Physicians dedicated to the health of America

James S. Todd, MD
Executive Vice President

Kenneth E. Monroe
Deputy Executive Vice President

Larry E. Joyce
Senior Vice President

George D. Lundberg, MD
Editor-in-Chief, Scientific Publications

Robert L. Kennett
Vice President, Publishing

Michael D. Springer
Publisher

Nawin Gupta, PhD
Director, Publishing Operations Division

Cheryl Iverson
Director, Editorial Processing Division

John P. Cahill
Manager, Advertising Sales

Geoffrey A. Flick
Manager, Marketing Services

Advertising Offices: East: Phillip B. Altamore, Donald M. Blatherwick, John L. Reeves, 600 Third Ave, Suite 3700, New York, NY 10016 (212) 867-6640. **Diagnostics/Devices:** M. J. Mrvica Associates, 155 S White Horse Pike, Berlin, NJ 08009; (609) 768-9360. **Midwest/Far West:** Peter L. Payerli, 515 N State St, Chicago, IL 60610 (312) 464-2551. **AMA Physician Recruitment Advertising Department:** Carri Lynch, Supervisor, 800-262-2260.

Letters to the Editor

Tryptophan Depletion in Stable Lithium-Treated Patients With Bipolar Disorder in Remission 154
Chawki Benkelfat, MD; Bernard Seletti, MD; Roberta M. Palmour, PhD; Jean Hillel, MD; Mark Ellenbogen; Simon N. Young, PhD

In Reply 155
Pedro L. Delgado, MD, Dennis S. Charney, MD

Biochemical Effects of Antidepressant Augmentation 156
Robert H. Howland, MD

Developmental Brain Abnormalities in Schizophrenia: Contributions of Genetic and Perinatal Factors 157
Antonio Vita, MD, Emilio Sacchetti, MD

In Reply 157
Tyrone D. Cannon, PhD; Sarnoff A. Mednick, PhD, DrMed; Josef Parnas, MD; Fini Schulsinger, MD; Johannes Praestholt, MD; Aage Vestergaard, MD

Reciprocal Lateralization of Frontal Lobe Functions 159
Elkhonon Goldberg, PhD, Kenneth Podell, PhD

In Reply 159
Scott L. Rauch, MD; Cary R. Savage, PhD; Lee Baer, PhD; Hans C. Breiter, MD; Nathaniel M. Alpert, PhD; Alan J. Fischman, MD, PhD; Michael A. Jenike, MD

Correction

Effect of the Menstrual Cycle on Dependent Variables in Mood Disorder Research 144
Ellen Leibenluft, MD; Patricia L. Fiero, MA; David R. Rubinow, MD

Departments

Instructions for Authors 87

Notice to Authors 134

Physician Recruitment Advertising 163

ARCHIVES OF GENERAL PSYCHIATRY

ARCHIVES OF GENERAL PSYCHIATRY

VOL 52 NO. 3, MARCH 1995

News and Views

Neuroleptic Withdrawal in Schizophrenic Patients: A Review of the Literature 173
Patricia L. Gilbert, MD; M. Jackuelyn Harris, MD; Lou Ann McAdams, PhD; Dilip V. Jeste, MD

Commentaries

Neuroleptic Withdrawal in Schizophrenic Patients 189
Ross J. Baldessarini, MD, Adele C. Viguera, MD

Why Neuroleptic Withdrawal in Schizophrenia? 192
William T. Carpenter, Jr, MD, Carol A. Tamminga, MD

Long-term Treatment for Lifetime Disorders? 197
John F. Greden, MD, Rajiv Tandon, MD

Neuroleptic Withdrawal in Schizophrenic Patients: An Idea Whose Time Has Come 200
Herbert Y. Meltzer, MD

The Early Course of Schizophrenia and Long-term Maintenance Neuroleptic Therapy 203
Keith H. Nuechterlein, PhD; Michael J. Gitlin, MD; Kenneth L. Subotnik, PhD

Risks of Withdrawing Antipsychotic Medications 205
Richard Jed Wyatt, MD

All articles published, including editorials, letters, and book reviews, represent the opinions of the authors and do not reflect the policy of the American Medical Association, the Editorial Board, or the institution with which the author is affiliated, unless this is clearly specified.

ARCHIVES
OF
GENERAL PSYCHIATRY

The ARCHIVES OF GENERAL PSYCHIATRY is a member of the consortium of AMA journals listed below. The ARCHIVES reaches more than 27 500 readers in 85 countries each month. The complete text of all AMA journals is available online from Dialog Information Services and Information Access Company.

The Journal of the American Medical Association (JAMA)
Archives of Dermatology
Archives of Family Medicine
Archives of General Psychiatry
Archives of Internal Medicine
Archives of Neurology
Archives of Ophthalmology
Archives of Otolaryngology—Head & Neck Surgery
Archives of Pediatrics & Adolescent Medicine
Archives of Surgery

The ARCHIVES OF GENERAL PSYCHIATRY (ISSN 0003-990x) is published monthly by the American Medical Association, 515 N State St, Chicago, IL 60610, and is an official publication of the Association. Second-class postage rates paid at Chicago and at additional mailing office. GST registration number: R126 255 556. Canada Post International Publications Mail (Canadian Distribution) Sales Agreement No. 318633.

Printed in the USA.

SUBSCRIPTION RATES—The subscription rates for the ARCHIVES OF GENERAL PSYCHIATRY are as follows: $95 for 1 year, $190 for 2 years in the United States and US possessions; in the Americas, 1 year $130, 2 years $260; the rest of the world, 1 year, £90, 2 years, £180. The institution rates are as follows: $110 for 1 year, $220 for 2 years in the United States and US possessions; in the Americas, 1 year, $150, 2 years, $300; the rest of the world, 1 year, £103, 2 years £206. Rates for subscriptions for delivery to Japan are available through our exclusive agent—contact the publisher. Special rates for residents and medical students in the United States and US possessions are available. Address inquiries to: Subscriber Services Center, American Medical Association, PO Box 10945, Chicago, IL 60610. Phone: (800) 262-2350. Fax: (312) 464-5831. For mailing addresses outside the US and US possessions, see International Subscription Information.

CHANGE OF ADDRESS—POSTMASTER, send all address changes to ARCHIVES OF GENERAL PSYCHIATRY, c/o Subscriber Services, American Medical Association, 515 N State St, Chicago, IL 60610. Please notify us of address change at least 6 weeks in advance to ensure uninterrupted service. Include both old and new addresses, a recent mailing label, and new ZIP code. For mailing addresses outside the US and US possessions, see International Subscription Information.

SUBSCRIBER SERVICES—For information about subscribing to any of the AMA publications, change of address, missing issues, or purchasing back issues, please contact Subscriber Services Center, American Medical Association, PO Box 10945, Chicago, IL 60610, or call (312) 670-SUBS (670-7827) between 8:30 AM and 4:30 PM CST. Fax: (312) 464-5831. For mailing addresses outside the US and US possessions, see International Subscription Information.

INTERNATIONAL SUBSCRIPTION INFORMATION—Subscriptions outside the United States and US possessions are served according to geographic region. Please address correspondence to the following two offices: 1) For delivery in North America, Central America, and South America, contact Subscriber Services Center, American Medical Association, PO Box 10945, Chicago, IL 60610, USA. Phone: 1-312-760-7827. Fax: 1-312-464-5831. 2) For delivery outside the Americas, contact JAMA & Archives Journals Reader Services Centre, PO Box 299, London, England WC1H 9TD. Phone: 44-(0)71-383 6270. Fax: 44-(0)71-383 6402.

REPRINTS—Authors place their reprint order at the time the edited typescript is reviewed and should allow 4 to 6 weeks for delivery following publication. Requests for individual reprints should be sent directly to the author at the address shown in the article.

For bulk reprint orders for commercial distribution, please contact Mark Kuhns, 600 Third Ave, New York, NY 10016. Phone: (212) 867-6640. Fax: (212) 953-2497. For reprint orders in limited quantities for educational distribution, please contact Rita Houston, 515 N State St, Chicago, IL 60610. Phone: (312) 464-2512. Fax: (312) 464-5835.

PERMISSIONS—Contact Laslo Hunyady, Permissions Assistant, 515 N State St, Chicago, IL 60610. Phone: (312) 464-2513.

ADVERTISING PRINCIPLES—Each advertisement in this issue has been reviewed and complies with the principles governing advertising in AMA scientific publications. A copy of these principles is available on request. The appearance of advertising in AMA publications is not an AMA guarantee or endorsement of the product or the claims made for the product by the manufacturer.

Reply Commentary

Considering Neuroleptic Maintenance and Taper on a Continuum: Need for Individual Rather Than Dogmatic Approach 209
Dilip V. Jeste, MD; Patricia L. Gilbert, MD; Lou Ann McAdams, PhD; M. Jackuelyn Harris, MD

Original Articles

Adrenal Gland Volume in Major Depression: Increase During the Depressive Episode and Decrease With Successful Treatment 213
Robert T. Rubin, MD, PhD; Jeffrey J. Phillips, MD; Todd F. Sadow, MD; James T. McCracken, MD

Prevalence and Correlates of Drug Use and Dependence in the United States: Results From the National Comorbidity Survey 219
Lynn A. Warner, MPP; Ronald C. Kessler, PhD; Michael Hughes, PhD; James C. Anthony, PhD; Christopher B. Nelson, MPH

Generalized Social Phobia: Reliability and Validity 230
Salvatore Mannuzza, PhD; Franklin R. Schneier, MD; Tim F. Chapman, PhD; Michael R. Liebowitz, MD; Donald F. Klein, MD; Abby J. Fyer, MD

A Trial of the Effect of a Standardized Psychiatric Consultation on Health Outcomes and Costs in Somatizing Patients 238
G. Richard Smith, Jr, MD; Kathryn Rost, PhD; T. Michael Kashner, PhD

Letter to the Editor

Clozapine Therapy and Increases in Homovanillic Acid 244
S. Craig Risch, MD, Richard R. J. Lewine, PhD

Departments

Instructions for Authors 245

Physician Recruitment Advertising 247

ARCHIVES OF GENERAL PSYCHIATRY

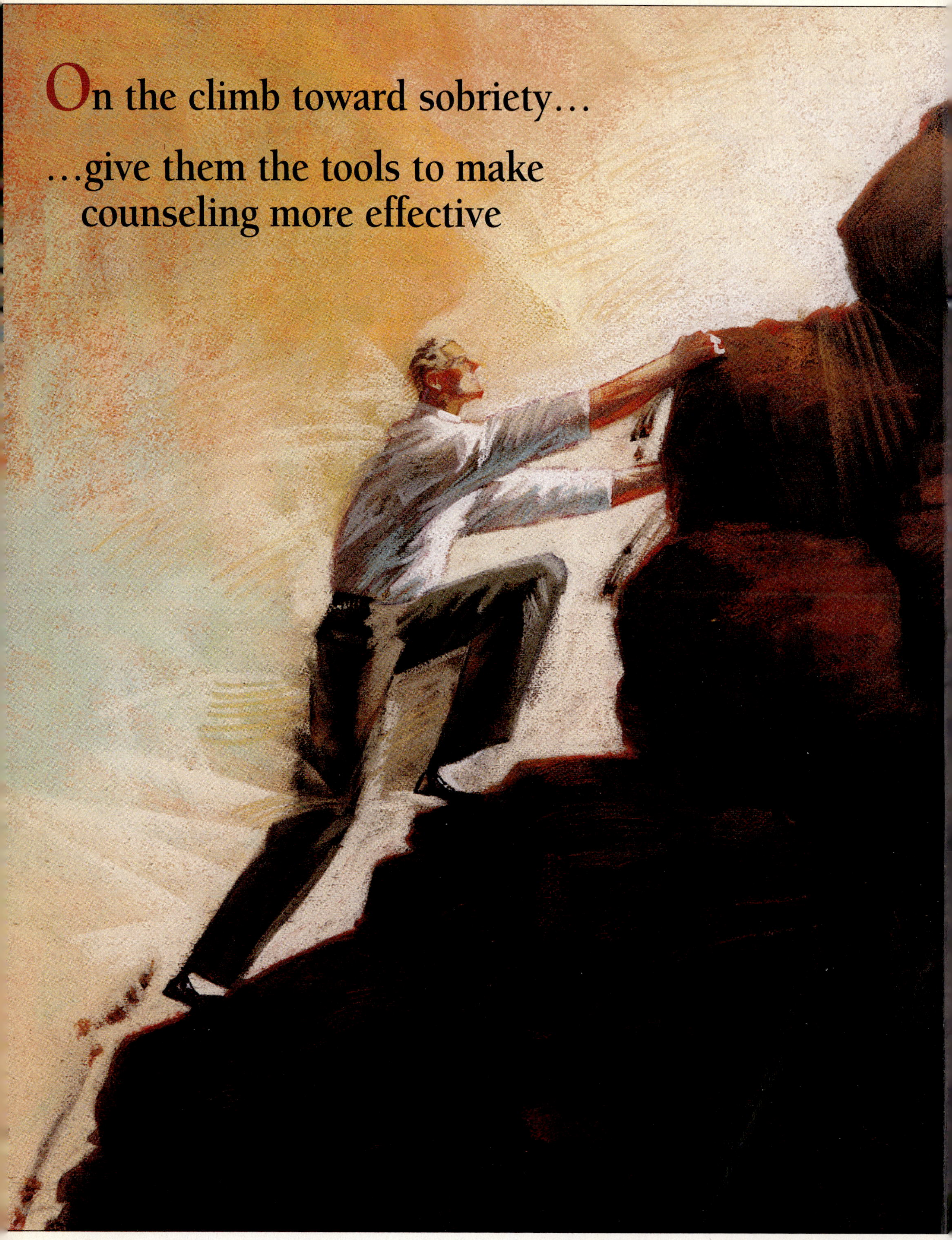
On the climb toward sobriety…
…give them the tools to make counseling more effective

ARCHIVES OF GENERAL PSYCHIATRY

VOL 52 NO. 4, APRIL 1995

Original Article

Gene Expression for Glutamic Acid Decarboxylase Is Reduced Without Loss of Neurons in Prefrontal Cortex of Schizophrenics 258
Schahram Akbarian, MD, PhD; James J. Kim; Steven G. Potkin, MD; Jennifer O. Hagman, MD; Alireza Tafazzoli; William E. Bunney, Jr, MD; Edward G. Jones, MD, PhD

Commentaries

Reduced Inhibitory Capacity in Prefrontal Cortex of Schizophrenics 267
Dennis E. Lee, Allan J. Tobin

Neural Circuitry of the Prefrontal Cortex in Schizophrenia 269
David A. Lewis, MD

In Pursuit of the Molecular Neuropathology of Schizophrenia 274
John Q. Trojanowski, MD, PhD, Steven E. Arnold, MD

In Reply 277
Scharam Akbarian, MD, PhD, Edward G. Jones, MD, PhD

Original Articles

Prefrontal Cortex and Schizophrenia: A Quantitative Magnetic Resonance Imaging Study 279
Cynthia G. Wible, PhD; Martha E. Shenton, PhD; Hiroto Hokama, MD; Ron Kikinis, MD; Ferenc A. Jolesz, MD; David Metcalf, MS; Robert W. McCarley, MD

Double-blind Parallel Comparison of Three Dosages of Sertraline and Placebo in Outpatients With Obsessive-compulsive Disorder 289
John Greist, MD; Guy Chouinard, MD; Eugene DuBoff, MD; Angelos Halaris, MD, PhD; Suck Won Kim, MD; Lorrin Koran, MD; Michael Liebowitz, MD; R. Bruce Lydiard, MD, PhD; Steven Rasmussen, MD; Kerrin White, MD; Carolyn Sikes, PhD

American Medical Association
Physicians dedicated to the health of America

All articles published, including editorials, letters, and book reviews, represent the opinions of the authors and do not reflect the policy of the American Medical Association, the Editorial Board, or the institution with which the author is affiliated, unless this is clearly specified.

Schizotypal Symptoms and Signs in the Roscommon Family Study: Their Factor Structure and Familial Relationship With Psychotic and Affective Disorders 296
Kenneth S. Kendler, MD; Mary McGuire, MB, MRCPsych; Alan M. Gruenberg, MD; Dermot Walsh, MB, FRCPI

A Prospective Study of Outcome in Bulimia Nervosa and the Long-term Effects of Three Psychological Treatments 304
Christopher G. Fairburn, DM, FRCPsych; Patricia A. Norman; Sarah L. Welch, DPhil, MRCPsych; Marianne E. O'Connor; Helen A. Doll, MSc; Robert C. Peveler, DPhil, MRCPsych

Editorial

Some Thoughts About the ARCHIVES 313
Jack D. Barchas, MD

Letters to the Editor

Risk of Alzheimer's Disease in First-Degree Relatives 317
Reinhard Heun, MD, Wolfgang Maier, MD

In Reply 318
Jeremy M. Silverman, PhD; Ge Li, MD, PhD; Richard C. Mohs, PhD; Kenneth L. Davis, MD

Low Levels of Pertussis Toxin Adenosine Diphosphate Ribosylation in the Schizophrenic Brain 319
Fumihiko Okada, MD; Takeshi Murakami, MD, PhD; Yukiko Tokumitsu, PhD

Correction

Test-Retest Reliability of the Diagnostic Interview Schedule for Children (DISC 2.1) 312
Peter Jensen, MD; Margaret Roper, MS; Prudence Fisher, MS; John Piacentini, PhD; Glorisa Canino, PhD; John Richters, PhD; Maritza Rubio-Stipec, MA; Mina Dulcan, MD; Sherryl Goodman, PhD; Mark Davies, MPH; Donald Rae, MS; David Shaffer, MD; Hector Bird, MD; Benjamin Lahey, PhD; Mary Schwab-Stone, MD

Regular Departments

This Month in the *Archives of General Psychiatry* 253

Instructions for Authors 320

Physician Recruitment Advertising 322

ARCHIVES OF GENERAL PSYCHIATRY

ARCHIVES OF GENERAL PSYCHIATRY

VOL 52 NO. 5, MAY 1995

Original Articles

Symptoms of Schizophrenia: Methods, Meanings, and Mechanisms 341
Nancy C. Andreasen, MD, PhD; Stephan Arndt, PhD; Randall Alliger, PhD; Del Miller, PharmD, MD; Michael Flaum, MD

A Longitudinal Study of Symptom Dimensions in Schizophrenia: Prediction and Patterns of Change 352
Stephan Arndt, PhD; Nancy C. Andreasen, MD, PhD; Michael Flaum, MD; Del Miller, PharmD, MD; Peg Nopoulos, MD

Commentary

Signs and Symptoms: What Can They Tell Us About the Clinical Course and Pathophysiologic Processes of Schizophrenia? 361
Jeffrey A. Lieberman, MD

Original Articles

A Family Study of Manic-Depressive (Bipolar I) Disease: Is It a Distinct Illness Separable From Primary Unipolar Depression? 367
George Winokur, MD; William Coryell, MD; Martin Keller, MD; Jean Endicott, PhD; Andrew Leon, PhD

American Medical Association

Physicians dedicated to the health of America

All articles published, including editorials, letters, and book reviews, represent the opinions of the authors and do not reflect the policy of the American Medical Association, the Editorial Board, or the institution with which the author is affiliated, unless this is clearly specified.

The Structure of the Genetic and Environmental Risk Factors for Six Major Psychiatric Disorders in Women: Phobia, Generalized Anxiety Disorder, Panic Disorder, Bulimia, Major Depression, and Alcoholism 374
Kenneth S. Kendler, MD; Ellen E. Walters, MS; Michael C. Neale, PhD; Ronald C. Kessler, PhD; Andrew C. Heath, DPhil; Lindon J. Eaves, PhD, DSc

Cingulotomy for Intractable Obsessive-compulsive Disorder: Prospective Long-term Follow-up of 18 Patients 384
Lee Baer, PhD; Scott L. Rauch, MD; H. Thomas Ballantine, Jr, MD; Robert Martuza, MD; Rees Cosgrove, MD; Edwin Cassem, MD; Ida Giriunas, RN; Peter A. Manzo; Charles Dimino, MD; Michael A. Jenike, MD

Reduced Caudate Nucleus Volume in Obsessive-compulsive Disorder 393
Delbert Robinson, MD; Houwei Wu, MD; Rafael A. Munne, MD; Manzar Ashtari, PhD; Jose Ma. J. Alvir, DrPH; Gail Lerner, MS; Amy Koreen, MD; Karyl Cole, MD; Bernhard Bogerts, MD

An In Vivo Study of the Prefrontal Cortex of Schizophrenic Patients at Different Stages of Illness via Phosphorus Magnetic Resonance Spectroscopy 399
Jeff A. Stanley, PhD; Peter C. Williamson, MD; Dick J. Drost, PhD; Tom J. Carr, MD; R. Jane Rylett, PhD; Ashok Malla, MD; R. Terry Thompson, PhD

Regular Departments

Instructions for Authors 334

This Month in the *Archives of General Psychiatry* 339

Physician Recruitment Advertising 409

ARCHIVES OF GENERAL PSYCHIATRY

ARCHIVES OF GENERAL PSYCHIATRY

VOL 52 NO. 6, JUNE 1995

Commentary

The Role of Methylphenidate in Psychiatry 429
Rachel G. Klein, PhD, Paul Wender, MD

Original Articles

A Double-blind, Crossover Comparison of Methylphenidate and Placebo in Adults With Childhood-Onset Attention-Deficit Hyperactivity Disorder 434
Thomas Spencer, MD; Timothy Wilens, MD; Joseph Biederman, MD; Stephen V. Faraone, PhD; J. Stuart Ablon; Kathleen Lapey

Efficacy of Methylphenidate for Attention-Deficit Hyperactivity Disorder in Children With Tic Disorder 444
Kenneth D. Gadow, PhD; Jeffrey Sverd, MD; Joyce Sprafkin, PhD; Edith E. Nolan, PhD; Stacy N. Ezor, MA

Is Methylphenidate Like Cocaine? Studies on Their Pharmacokinetics and Distribution in the Human Brain 456
Nora D. Volkow, MD; Yu-Shin Ding, PhD; Joanna S. Fowler, PhD; Gene-Jack Wang, MD; Jean Logan, PhD; John S. Gatley, PhD; Stephen Dewey, PhD; Charles Ashby, PhD; Jeffrey Liebermann, MD; Robert Hitzemann, PhD; Alfred P. Wolf, PhD

Family-Environment Risk Factors for Attention-Deficit Hyperactivity Disorder: A Test of Rutter's Indicators of Adversity 464
Joseph Biederman, MD; Sharon Milberger, ScD; Stephen V. Faraone, PhD; Kathleen Kiely; Jessica Guite; Eric Mick; Stuart Ablon; Rebecca Warburton; Ellen Reed

American Medical Association
Physicians dedicated to the health of America

James S. Todd, MD
Executive Vice President

Kenneth E. Monroe
Deputy Executive Vice President

Larry E. Joyce
President, Publishing and Multimedia Development

George D. Lundberg, MD
Editor-in-Chief, Scientific Publications

Robert L. Kennett
Vice President, Publishing

Michael D. Springer
Publisher

Nawin Gupta, PhD
Director, Publishing Operations Division

Cheryl Iverson
Director, Editorial Processing Division

Peter L. Payerli
Director, Advertising Sales

Geoffrey A. Flick
Manager, Marketing Services

Advertising Offices: East: Phillip B. Altamore, John L. Reeves, 119 Cherry Hill Rd, 3rd Flr, Parsippany, NJ 07054 (201) 263-9191. **Diagnostics/ Devices:** M. J. Mrvica Associates, 155 S White Horse Pike, Berlin, NJ 08009 (609) 768-9360. **Midwest/Far West:** John P. Cahill, 515 N State St, Chicago, IL 60610 (312) 464-2470. **AMA Physician Recruitment Advertising Department:** Carri Lynch, Supervisor, 800-262-2260.

All articles published, including editorials, letters, and book reviews, represent the opinions of the authors and do not reflect the policy of the American Medical Association, the Editorial Board, or the institution with which the author is affiliated, unless this is clearly specified.

In Vivo D_2 Dopamine Receptor Density in Psychotic and Nonpsychotic Patients With Bipolar Disorder 471
Godfrey D. Pearlson, MB,BS; Dean F. Wong, MD, PhD; Larry E. Tune, MD; Christopher A. Ross, MD, PhD; Gary A. Chase, PhD; Jonathan M. Links, PhD; Robert F. Dannals, PhD; Alan A. Wilson, PhD; Hayden T. Ravert, PhD; Henry N. Wagner, Jr, MD; J. Raymond DePaulo, MD

Duration of Neuroleptic Treatment and Prevalence of Tardive Dyskinesia in Late Life 478
Robert A. Sweet, MD; Benoit H. Mulsant, MD; Babu Gupta, MD; Aicha H. Rifai, MD; Rona E. Pasternak, MD; Ann McEachran, MS; George S. Zubenko, MD, PhD

Family Study of Early-Onset Dysthymia: Mood and Personality Disorders in Relatives of Outpatients With Dysthymia and Episodic Major Depression and Normal Controls 487
Daniel N. Klein, PhD; Lawrence P. Riso, PhD; Shauna K. Donaldson, PhD; Joseph E. Schwartz, PhD; Rochelle L. Anderson, PhD; Paige Crosby Ouimette, PhD; Humberto Lizardi, MA; Thomas A. Aronson, MD

The Prevalence of Dementia and Depression in the Elderly Community in a Southern European Population: The Zaragoza Study 497
Antonio Lobo, MD; Pedro Saz, MD; Guillermo Marcos, MD; José-Luis Día, MD; Concepción De-la-Cámara, MD

Letters to the Editor

Clozapine-Associated Postoperative Ileus: Case Report and Review of the Literature 507
Brenda Erickson, MD; Don M. Morris, MD; Alison Reeve, MD

The Prevalence of Schizophrenia in Ireland: Readdressing the Enigma 508
John L. Waddington, PhD, DSc; Hanafy A. Youssef, DM, FRCPsych; Anthony Kinsella, MSc

In Reply 508
Dermot Walsh, MB, FRCPI, Kenneth S. Kendler, MD

Regular Departments

This Month in *Archives of General Psychiatry* 422

Instructions for Authors 427

Physician Recruitment Advertising 510

ARCHIVES OF GENERAL PSYCHIATRY

ARCHIVES
OF
GENERAL PSYCHIATRY

VOL 52 NO. 7, JULY 1995

News and Views

Signal Transduction Pathways: Molecular Targets for Lithium's Actions 531
Husseini K. Manji, MD, FRCPC; William Z. Potter, MD, PhD; Robert H. Lenox, MD

Original Articles

Increased Rate of P300 Latency Prolongation With Age in Schizophrenia: Electrophysiological Evidence for a Neurodegenerative Process 544
Brian F. O'Donnell, PhD; Steven F. Faux, PhD; Robert W. McCarley, MD; Matthew O. Kimble; Dean F. Salisbury, PhD; Paul G. Nestor, PhD; Ron Kikinis MD; Ferenc A. Jolesz, MD; Martha E. Shenton, PhD

Impaired Mismatch Negativity Generation Reflects Widespread Dysfunction of Working Memory in Schizophrenia 550
Daniel C. Javitt, MD, PhD; Paolina Doneshka, MD, PhD; Sandra Grochowski; Walter Ritter, PhD

Commentary

Event-Related Potentials in the Study of Psychiatric Disorders 559
Adolf Pfefferbaum, MD; Walton T. Roth, MD; Judith M. Ford, PhD

Original Articles

Specificity in Familial Aggregation of Phobic Disorders 564
Abby J. Fyer, MD; Salvatore Mannuzza, PhD; Tim F. Chapman, PhD; Lynn Y. Martin, RNCS; Donald F. Klein, MD

Is the Comorbidity Between Social Phobia and Panic Disorder Due to Familial Cotransmission or Other Factors? 574
Ewald Horwath, MD, MSc; Susan I. Wolk, MD; Risë B. Goldstein, PhD, MPH; Priya Wickramaratne, PhD; Christina Sobin, PhD; Phillip Adams, PhD; Jennifer D. Lish, PhD; Myrna M. Weissman, PhD

Dose-Response Changes in Plasma Cortisol and Lymphocyte Glucocorticoid Receptors Following Dexamethasone Administration in Combat Veterans With and Without Posttraumatic Stress Disorder 583
Rachel Yehuda, PhD; David Boisoneau; Martin T. Lowy, PhD; Earl L. Giller, Jr, MD, PhD

Mental Illness and Suicide: A Case-Control Study in East Taiwan 594
Andrew T. A. Cheng, MD, PhD, MRCPsych

Letters to the Editor

Premenstrual Dysphoric Disorder and Response to Cholecystokinin-Tetrapeptide 605
Jean-Michel Le Melledo, MD; Jacques Bradwejn, MD; Diana Koszycki, PhD; Daniel Bichet, MD

Premenstrual Dysphoric Disorders, Anxiety, and Depressions: Vulnerability Traits or Comorbidity 606
Uriel Halbreich, MD

Regular Departments

This Month in *Archives of General Psychiatry* 525

Instructions for Authors 529

Physician Recruitment Advertising 607

ARCHIVES OF GENERAL PSYCHIATRY

ARCHIVES OF GENERAL PSYCHIATRY

VOL 52 NO. 8, AUGUST 1995

Original Article

Role-Relationship Models for Case Formulation 625
Mardi J. Horowitz, MD; Tracy Eells, PhD; Jerome Singer, PhD; Peter Salovey, PhD

Commentaries

Personality Theory: Clinical Practice, Social Development, and the Biology of Individual Differences 633
David Reiss, MD

Diagnosis, Assessment, and Individual Complexity 637
Robert N. Emde, MD

Progress on Case Formulation 639
Paul Crits-Christoph, Mary Beth Connolly

Between the Past and the Future of Psychotherapy Research 642
Salman Akhtar, MD, Steven Samuel, PhD

Are Case Formulations Useful for Outcomes Research? 645
John F. Clarkin, PhD

Role-Relationship Models: Are They Useful for Research and Practice? 646
Enrico E. Jones, PhD, Jennifer Dyer-Friedman, MA

'Richly Complex' but Needs an Emotion Theory 649
Hartvig Dahl, MD

Personality: Psychodynamic Perspectives 651
Theodore Shapiro, MD

Reply Commentary

Role-Relationship Model Configurations: A Summation 654
Mardi J. Horowitz, MD; Tracy Eells, PhD; Jerome Singer, PhD; Peter Salovey, PhD

American Medical Association
Physicians dedicated to the health of America

All articles published, including editorials, letters, and book reviews, represent the opinions of the authors and do not reflect the policy of the American Medical Association, the Editorial Board, or the institution with which the author is affiliated, unless this is clearly specified.

Advertising Office: J. P. Cahill & Associates, 341 S Waiola Ave, La Grange, IL 60525 (708) 352-1450. **AMA Physician Recruitment Advertising Department:** Carri Lynch, Supervisor, 800-262-2260.

Original Articles

Resting Cerebral Glucose Metabolism in First-Episode and Previously Treated Patients With Schizophrenia Relates to Clinical Features 657
Raquel E. Gur, MD, PhD; P. David Mozley, MD; Susan M. Resnick, PhD; Lyn Harper Mozley, PhD; Derri L. Shtasel, MD; Fiona Gallacher, MS; Steven E. Arnold, MD; Joel S. Karp, PhD; Abass Alavi, MD; Martin Reivich, MD; Ruben C. Gur, PhD

Mitogen-Stimulated Interleukin-2 Production in Never-Medicated, First-Episode Schizophrenic Patients: The Influence of Age at Onset and Negative Symptoms 668
Rohan Ganguli, MD; Jaspreet S. Brar, MD; K. N. R. Chengappa, MD; Marcia DeLeo, RN; Zan Wei Yang, PhD; Galina Shurin, PhD; Bruce S. Rabin, MD, PhD

Behavioral vs Biochemical Prediction of Clinical Stability Following Haloperidol Withdrawal in Schizophrenia 673
Daniel P. van Kammen, MD, PhD; Mary E. Kelley; John A. Gurklis, MD; Mark W. Gilbertson, PhD; Jeffrey K. Yao, PhD; Jeffrey L. Peters, MD

Multiple-Family Groups and Psychoeducation in the Treatment of Schizophrenia 679
William R. McFarlane, MD; Ellen Lukens, PhD; Bruce Link, PhD; Robert Dushay, PhD; Susan A. Deakins, MD; Margaret Newmark, CSW; Edward J. Dunne, PhD; Bonnie Horen, MA; Joanne Toran, MPA

Is Hyperarousal Essential to Obsessive-compulsive Disorder? Diminished Physiologic Flexibility, but Not Hyperarousal, Characterizes Patients With Obsessive-compulsive Disorder 688
Rudolf Hoehn-Saric, MD; Daniel R. McLeod, PhD; Pamela Hipsley

Quality of Care for Depressed Elderly Patients Hospitalized in the Specialty Psychiatric Units or General Medical Wards 695
Grayson Norquist, MD, MSPH; Kenneth B. Wells, MD, MPH; William H. Rogers, PhD; Lois M. Davis, PhD; Katherine Kahn, MD; Robert Brook, MD

Regular Departments

Instructions for Authors 615

This Month in *Archives of General Psychiatry* 619

Physician Recruitment Advertising 702

ARCHIVES OF GENERAL PSYCHIATRY

ARCHIVES OF GENERAL PSYCHIATRY

VOL 52 NO. 9, SEPTEMBER 1995

News and Views

Report Card on the *National Plan for Research on Child and Adolescent Mental Disorders:* The Midway Point 715
Members of the Committee for the Study of Research on Child and Adolescent Mental Disorders

Commentaries

The Report Card: Progress Report or Final Grade? 724
Gabrielle A. Carlson, MD

Comments on the Report Card From a Services Research Perspective 727
Markus J. P. Kruesi, MD, Boris Astrachan, MD

Child and Adolescent Mental Disorders Research: Current Directions, Future Needs 729
Alvin A. Rosenfeld, MD

Grading the Progress of Child and Adolescent Mental Health Research: NIMH Perspectives 732
Rex W. Cowdry, MD, Peter S. Jensen, MD

Original Articles

Meta-analyses of Studies of Ventricular Enlargement and Cortical Sulcal Prominence in Mood Disorders: Comparisons With Controls or Patients With Schizophrenia 735
Helio Elkis, MD, PhD; Lee Friedman, PhD; Alexandria Wise; Herbert Y. Meltzer, MD

Magnetic Resonance Imaging and Mood Disorders: Localization of White Matter and Other Subcortical Abnormalities 747
Renee M. Dupont, MD; Terry L. Jernigan, PhD; William Heindel, PhD; Nelson Butters, PhD; Kimberly Shafer, MS; Thomine Wilson, MA; John Hesselink, MD; J. Christian Gillin, MD

American Medical Association
Physicians dedicated to the health of America

James S. Todd, MD
Executive Vice President
Kenneth E. Monroe
Deputy Executive Vice President
George D. Lundberg, MD
Editor in Chief, Scientific Information and Multimedia
James F. Rappel
Group Vice President, Business and Management Services
Robert L. Kennett
Vice President, Publishing
Michael D. Springer
Publisher
Nawin Gupta, PhD
Director, Publishing Operations Division
Cheryl Iverson
Director, Editorial Processing Division
Peter L. Payerli
Director, Advertising Sales
Geoffrey A. Flick
Manager, Marketing Services

Advertising Office: J. P. Cahill & Associates, 341 S Waiola Ave, La Grange, IL 60525 (708) 352-1450. **AMA Physician Recruitment Advertising Department:** Carri Lynch, Supervisor, 800-262-2260.

ARCHIVES
OF
GENERAL PSYCHIATRY

The ARCHIVES OF GENERAL PSYCHIATRY is a member of the consortium of AMA journals listed below. The ARCHIVES reaches more than 27 500 readers in 85 countries each month. The complete text of all AMA journals is available on-line from Dialog Information Services and Information Access Company.

The Journal of the American Medical Association (JAMA)
Archives of Dermatology
Archives of Family Medicine
Archives of General Psychiatry
Archives of Internal Medicine
Archives of Neurology
Archives of Ophthalmology
Archives of Otolaryngology—Head & Neck Surgery
Archives of Pathology & Laboratory Medicine
Archives of Pediatrics & Adolescent Medicine
Archives of Surgery

The ARCHIVES OF GENERAL PSYCHIATRY (ISSN 0003-990x) is published monthly by the American Medical Association, 515 N State St, Chicago, IL 60610, and is an official publication of the Association. Second-class postage rates paid at Chicago and at additional mailing office. GST registration number: R126 255 556. Canada Post International Publications Mail (Canadian Distribution) Sales Agreement No. 318633.

Printed in the USA.

SUBSCRIPTION RATES—The subscription rates for the ARCHIVES OF GENERAL PSYCHIATRY are as follows: $95 for 1 year, $190 for 2 years in the United States and US possessions; in the Americas, 1 year $130, 2 years $260; the rest of the world, 1 year, £90, 2 years, £180. The institution rates are as follows: $110 for 1 year, $220 for 2 years in the United States and US possessions; in the Americas, 1 year, $150, 2 years, $300; the rest of the world, 1 year, £103, 2 years £206. Rates for subscriptions for delivery to Japan are available through our exclusive agent—contact the publisher. Special rates for residents and medical students in the United States and US possessions are available. Address inquiries to: Subscriber Services Center, American Medical Association, PO Box 10945, Chicago, IL 60610. Phone: (800) 262-2350. Fax: (312) 464-5831. For mailing addresses outside the US and US possessions, see International Subscription Information.

CHANGE OF ADDRESS—POSTMASTER, send all address changes to ARCHIVES OF GENERAL PSYCHIATRY, c/o Subscriber Services, American Medical Association, 515 N State St, Chicago, IL 60610. Please notify us of address change at least 6 weeks in advance to ensure uninterrupted service. Include both old and new addresses, a recent mailing label, and new ZIP code. For mailing addresses outside the US and US possessions, see International Subscription Information.

SUBSCRIBER SERVICES—For information about subscribing to any of the AMA publications, change of address, missing issues, or purchasing back issues, please contact Subscriber Services Center, American Medical Association, PO Box 10945, Chicago, IL 60610, or call (312) 670-SUBS (670-7827) between 8:30 AM and 4:30 PM CST. Fax: (312) 464-5831. For mailing addresses outside the US and US possessions, see International Subscription Information.

INTERNATIONAL SUBSCRIPTION INFORMATION—Subscriptions outside the United States and US possessions are served according to geographic region. Please address correspondence to the following two offices: 1) For delivery in North America, Central America, and South America, contact Subscriber Services Center, American Medical Association, PO Box 10945, Chicago, IL 60610, USA. Phone: 1-312-670-7827. Fax: 1-312-464-5831. 2) For delivery outside the Americas, contact JAMA & Archives Journals Reader Services Centre, PO Box 299, London, England WC1H 9TD. Phone: 44-(0)-171-383-6270. Fax: 44-(0)-171-383-6402.

REPRINTS—Authors place their reprint order at the time the edited typescript is reviewed and should allow 4 to 6 weeks for delivery following publication. Requests for individual reprints should be sent directly to the author at the address shown in the article.

For bulk reprint orders for distribution by commercial organizations, please contact Wanda Bartolotta, 500 Fifth Avenue #2210, New York, NY 10010. Phone: (212) 354-0050. Fax: (212) 354-1169. For reprint orders in limited quantities for distribution by educational organizations, please contact Joseph R. Rekash, 515 N State St, Chicago, IL 60610. Phone: (312) 464-2512. Fax: (312) 464-5835.

PERMISSIONS—Contact Laslo Hunyady, Permissions Assistant, 515 N State St, Chicago, IL 60610. Phone: (312) 464-2513.

Risk of Tardive Dyskinesia in Older Patients: A Prospective Longitudinal Study of 266 Outpatients 756
Dilip V. Jeste, MD; Michael P. Caligiuri, PhD; Jane S. Paulsen, PhD; Robert K. Heaton, PhD; Jonathan P. Lacro, PharmD; M. Jackuelyn Harris, MD; Anne Bailey, MS; Robert L. Fell, MS; Lou Ann McAdams, PhD

Failure of Naltrexone Hydrochloride to Reduce Self-Injurious and Autistic Behavior in Mentally Retarded Adults: Double-blind Placebo-Controlled Studies 766
Sophie H. N. Willemsen-Swinkels, MS; Jan K. Buitelaar, MD, PhD; Gerard J. Nijhof, MS; Herman van Engeland, MD, PhD

Effects of Alzheimer's Disease and Normal Aging on Cerebrospinal Fluid Norepinephrine Responses to Yohimbine and Clonidine 774
Elaine R. Peskind, MD; Dane Wingerson, MD; Sharon Murray, RN; Marcella Pascualy, MD; Dorcas J. Dobie, MD; Pascal Le Corre, PharmD, PhD; Roger Le Verge, PharmD, PhD; Richard C. Veith, MD; Murray A. Raskind, MD

Letter to the Editor

Interactions of Serotonin Reuptake Inhibitors With Tricyclic Antidepressants 783
Anne T. Harvey, PhD, Sheldon H. Preskorn, MD

In Reply 784
Anand Popli, MD; Ross J. Baldessarini, MD; Jonathan O. Cole, MD

Regular Departments

This Month in *Archives of General Psychiatry* 713

Instructions for Authors 786

Physician Recruitment Advertising 788

ARCHIVES OF GENERAL PSYCHIATRY

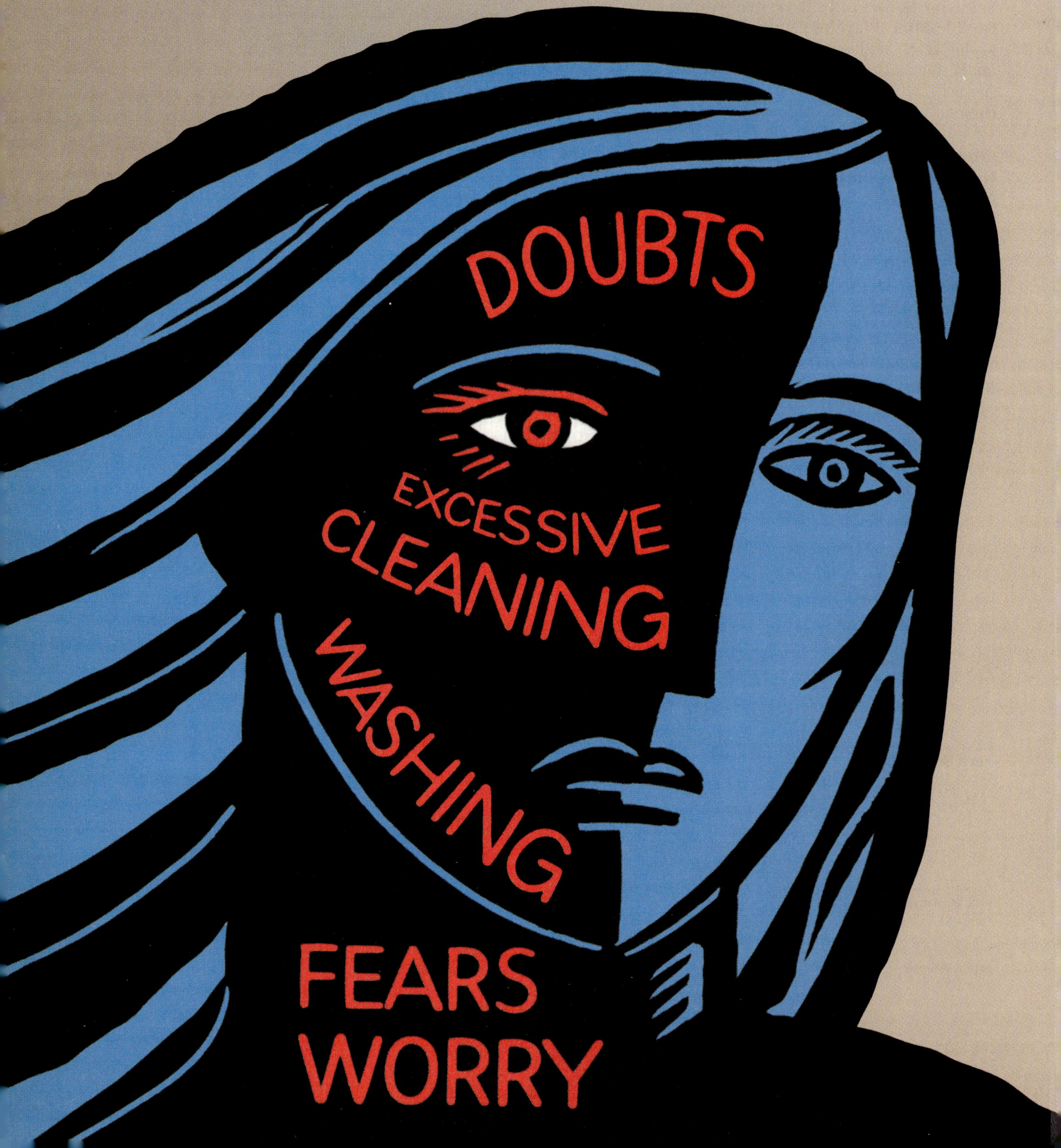
DOUBTS
EXCESSIVE
CLEANING
WASHING
FEARS
WORRY

ARCHIVES OF GENERAL PSYCHIATRY

VOL 52 NO. 10, OCTOBER 1995

Original Article

Abnormally High Neuronal Density in the Schizophrenic Cortex: A Morphometric Analysis of Prefrontal Area 9 and Occipital Area 17 805
Lynn D. Selemon, PhD; Grazyna Rajkowska, PhD; Patricia S. Goldman-Rakic, PhD

Commentary

Neocortical Abnormalities in Schizophrenia 819
Stanley J. Watson, PhD, MD, James H. Meador-Woodruff, MD

Original Articles

Spatial Working Memory Deficits in the Relatives of Schizophrenic Patients 821
Sohee Park, PhD; Philip S. Holzman, PhD; Patricia S. Goldman-Rakic, PhD

Abnormal Excitatory Neurotransmitter Metabolism in Schizophrenic Brains 829
Guochuan Tsai, MD, PhD; Lucius A. Passani, MS; Barbara S. Slusher, PhD; Ruth Carter; Lee Baer, PhD; Joel E. Kleinman, MD, PhD; Joseph T. Coyle, MD

Plasma Haloperidol Levels and Clinical Effects in Schizophrenia and Schizoaffective Disorder 837
Jan Volavka, MD, PhD; Thomas B. Cooper, MA; Pál Czobor, PhD; Morris Meisner, PhD

Suicidal Behaviors and the Tryptophan Hydroxylase Gene 846
Mocrane Abbar, MD; Philippe Courtet, MS; Stéphane Amadéo, MD; Yves Caer, MD; Jacques Mallet, PhD; Michel Baldy-Moulinier, MD; Didier Castelnau, MD; Alain Malafosse, MD, PhD

Health Care Costs of Primary Care Patients With Recognized Depression 850
Gregory E. Simon, MD, MPH; Michael VonKorff, ScD; William Barlow, PhD

American Medical Association

Physicians dedicated to the health of America

The New York High-Risk Project: Psychoses and Cluster A Personality Disorders in Offspring of Schizophrenic Parents at 23 Years of Follow-up 857
L. Erlenmeyer-Kimling, PhD; Elizabeth Squires-Wheeler, PhD; Ulla Hilldoff Adamo, MA; Anne S. Bassett, MD; Barbara A. Cornblatt, PhD; Clarice J. Kestenbaum, MD; Donald Rock, PhD; Simone A. Roberts; Irving I. Gottesman, PhD, FRCPsych(Hon)

News and Views

More Reliable Outcome Measures Can Reduce Sample Size Requirements 867
Andrew C. Leon, PhD; Peter M. Marzuk, MD; Laura Portera

Editorial

Child and Adolescent Mental Disorders and the Search for an NIMH Director: *Quo Vadis*? 873
Jack D. Barchas, MD, Peter M. Marzuk, MD

Letters to the Editor

Clozapine-Induced Increase in Plasma Levels of Soluble Interleukin-2 Receptors 877
Thomas Pollmächer, MD; Dunja Hinze-Selch, MD; Janet Mullington, PhD; Florian Holsboer, MD, PhD

In Reply 878
Rohan Ganguli, MD; Jaspreet S. Brar, MD, MPH; Bruce S. Rabin, MD, PhD

Complicating Factors in the Analysis of Acute Drug-Induced Akathisia 878
Patricia I. Rosebush, MScN, MD, FRCPC, Michael F. Mazurek, MD, FRCPC

In Reply 879
Perminder Sachdev, MD, PhD, FRANZCP

Corrections

An In Vivo Study of the Prefrontal Cortex of Schizophrenic Patients at Different Stages of Illness via Phosphorus Magnetic Resonance Spectroscopy 799
Jeff A. Stanley, PhD; Peter C. Williamson, MD; Dick J. Drost, PhD; Tom J. Carr, MD; R. Jane Rylett, PhD; Ashok Malla, MD; R. Terry Thompson, PhD

Efficacy of Methylphenidate for Attention-Deficit Hyperactivity Disorder in Children With Tic Disorder 836
Kenneth D. Gadow, PhD; Jeffrey Sverd, MD; Joyce Sprafkin, PhD; Edith E. Nolan, PhD; Stacy N. Ezor, MA

Regular Departments

Instructions for Authors 795

Index to Advertisers 797

This Month in *Archives of General Psychiatry* 798

Physician Recruitment Advertising 877

ARCHIVES OF GENERAL PSYCHIATRY

ARCHIVES OF GENERAL PSYCHIATRY

VOL 52 NO. 11, NOVEMBER 1995

Commentaries

Genetic Epidemiology in Psychiatry: Taking Both Genes and Environment Seriously 895
Kenneth S. Kendler, MD

Antisocial Behavior 900
Elliot S. Gershon, MD

Original Articles

Differential Heritability of Adult and Juvenile Antisocial Traits 906
Michael J. Lyons, PhD; William R. True, PhD; Seth A. Eisen, MD, MSc; Jack Goldberg, PhD; Joanne M. Meyer, PhD; Stephen V. Faraone, PhD; Lindon J. Eaves, PhD, DSc; Ming T. Tsuang, MD, PhD, DSc

Genetic-Environmental Interaction in the Genesis of Aggressivity and Conduct Disorders 916
Remi J. Cadoret, MD; William R. Yates, MD; Ed Troughton; George Woodworth, PhD; Mark A. Stewart, MD

Genetic Questions for Environmental Studies: Differential Parenting and Psychopathology in Adolescence 925
David Reiss, MD; E. Mavis Hetherington, PhD; Robert Plomin, PhD; George W. Howe, PhD; Samuel J. Simmens, PhD; Sandra H. Henderson, PhD; Thomas J. O'Connor, PhD; Danielle A. Bussell, PhD; Edward R. Anderson, PhD; Tracy Law, PhD

American Medical Association
Physicians dedicated to the health of America

All articles published, including editorials, letters, and book reviews, represent the opinions of the authors and do not reflect the policy of the American Medical Association, the Editorial Board, or the institution with which the author is affiliated, unless this is clearly specified.

ARCHIVES
OF
GENERAL PSYCHIATRY

The ARCHIVES OF GENERAL PSYCHIATRY is a member of the consortium of AMA journals listed below. The ARCHIVES reaches more than 27 500 readers in 85 countries each month. The complete text of all AMA journals is available online from Dialog Information Services and Information Access Company.

The Journal of the American Medical Association (JAMA)
Archives of Dermatology
Archives of Family Medicine
Archives of General Psychiatry
Archives of Internal Medicine
Archives of Neurology
Archives of Ophthalmology
Archives of Otolaryngology—Head & Neck Surgery
Archives of Pathology & Laboratory Medicine
Archives of Pediatrics & Adolescent Medicine
Archives of Surgery

The ARCHIVES OF GENERAL PSYCHIATRY (ISSN 0003-990x) is published monthly by the American Medical Association, 515 N State St, Chicago, IL 60610, and is an official publication of the Association. Second-class postage rates paid at Chicago and at additional mailing office. GST registration number: R126 255 556. Canada Post International Publications Mail (Canadian Distribution) Sales Agreement No. 318633.

Printed in the USA.

SUBSCRIPTION RATES—The subscription rates for the ARCHIVES OF GENERAL PSYCHIATRY are as follows: $95 for 1 year, $190 for 2 years in the United States and US possessions; in the Americas, 1 year $130, 2 years $260; the rest of the world, 1 year, £90, 2 years, £180. The institution rates are as follows: $110 for 1 year, $220 for 2 years in the United States and US possessions; in the Americas, 1 year, $150, 2 years, $300; the rest of the world, 1 year, £103, 2 years £206. Rates for subscriptions for delivery to Japan are available through our exclusive agent—contact the publisher. Special rates for residents and medical students in the United States and US possessions are available. Address inquiries to: Subscriber Services Center, American Medical Association, PO Box 10945, Chicago, IL 60610. Phone: (800) 262-2350. Fax: (312) 464-5831. For mailing addresses outside the US and US possessions, see International Subscription Information.

CHANGE OF ADDRESS—POSTMASTER, send all address changes to ARCHIVES OF GENERAL PSYCHIATRY, c/o Subscriber Services, American Medical Association, 515 N State St, Chicago, IL 60610. Please notify us of address change at least 6 weeks in advance to ensure uninterrupted service. Include both old and new addresses, a recent mailing label, and new ZIP code. For mailing addresses outside the US and US possessions, see International Subscription Information.

SUBSCRIBER SERVICES—For information about subscribing to any of the AMA publications, change of address, missing issues, or purchasing back issues, please contact Subscriber Services Center, American Medical Association, PO Box 10945, Chicago, IL 60610, or call (312) 670-SUBS (670-7827) between 8:30 AM and 4:30 PM CST. Fax: (312) 464-5831. For mailing addresses outside the US and US possessions, see International Subscription Information.

INTERNATIONAL SUBSCRIPTION INFORMATION—Subscriptions outside the United States and US possessions are served according to geographic region. Please address correspondence to the following two offices: 1) For delivery in North America, Central America, and South America, contact Subscriber Services Center, American Medical Association, PO Box 10945, Chicago, IL 60610, USA. Phone: 1-312-670-7827. Fax: 1-312-464-5831. 2) For delivery outside the Americas, contact JAMA & Archives Journals Reader Services Centre, PO Box 299, London, England WC1H 9TD. Phone: 44-(0)-171-383-6270. Fax: 44-(0)-171-383-6402.

REPRINTS—Authors place their reprint order at the time the edited typescript is reviewed and should allow 4 to 6 weeks for delivery following publication. Requests for individual reprints should be sent directly to the author at the address shown in the article.

For bulk reprint orders for distribution by commercial organizations, please contact Wanda Bartolotta, 500 Fifth Avenue #2210, New York, NY 10010. Phone: (212) 354-0050. Fax: (212) 354-1169. For reprint orders in limited quantities for distribution by educational organizations, please contact Joseph R. Rekash, 515 N State St, Chicago, IL 60610. Phone: (312) 464-2512. Fax: (312) 464-5835.

PERMISSIONS—Contact Laslo Hunyady, Permissions Assistant, 515 N State St, Chicago, IL 60610. Phone: (312) 464-2513.

ADVERTISING PRINCIPLES—Each advertisement in this issue has been reviewed and complies with the principles governing advertising in AMA scientific publications. A copy of these principles is available on request. The appearance of advertising in AMA publications is not an AMA guarantee or endorsement of the product or the claims made for the product by the manufacturer.

Seasonal Variation in Plasma L-Tryptophan Availability in Healthy Volunteers: Relationships to Violent Suicide Occurrence 937
Michael Maes, MD, PhD; Simon Scharpé, PhD; Robert Verkerk, RT; Peter D'Hondt, MD; Dirk Peeters, MD; Paul Cosyns, MD; Paul Thompson, PhD; Frans De Meyer, PhD; Annick Wauters, MS; Hugo Neels, PhD

Evidence of Chaotic Mood Variation in Bipolar Disorder 947
Allan Gottschalk, MD, PhD; Mark S. Bauer, MD; Peter C. Whybrow, MD

Commentary

Chaos and Complexity: Can It Help Us to Understand Mood and Behavior? 960
Cindy L. Ehlers, PhD

Editorial

Managed Care in *JAMA* and the *Archives* Journals: A Call for Papers for Coordinated Theme Issues 967
George D. Lundberg, MD

Letters to the Editor

Pindolol, 5-Hydroxytryptamine, and Antidepressant Augmentation 969
Francesc Artigas, PhD

Regular Departments

Index to Advertisers 894

This Month in *Archives of General Psychiatry* 893

Instructions for Authors 975

Physician Recruitment Advertising 979

ARCHIVES OF GENERAL PSYCHIATRY

ARCHIVES
OF
GENERAL PSYCHIATRY

VOL 52 NO. 12, DECEMBER 1995

News and Views

Glutamate Receptor Dysfunction and Schizophrenia 998
John W. Olney, MD, Nuri B. Farber, MD

Commentaries

The NMDA Receptor as a Site for Psychopathology: Primary or Secondary Role? 1008
Fritz A. Henn, PhD, MD

Constraints on Concepts of Pathogenesis: Language and the Speciation Process as the Key to the Etiology of Schizophrenia 1011
T. J. Crow, MD

Altered Glutamatergic and GABAergic Mechanisms in the Cingulate Cortex of the Schizophrenic Brain 1015
Francine M. Benes, MD, PhD

Response to Commentaries and to the Challenge of Building a Perfect Theory to Explain Schizophrenia 1019
John W. Olney, MD, Nuri B. Farber, MD

Original Articles

The Reliability and Validity of Two Structured Diagnostic Interviews for Personality Disorders 1025
Paul A. Pilkonis, PhD; Carol L. Heape, RN, MSN; Joseph M. Proietti, MS; Suzan W. Clark, MEd; Joshua D. McDavid, MD; Timothy E. Pitts, MEd

Perceived Coercion in Mental Hospital Admission: Pressures and Process 1034
Charles W. Lidz, PhD; Steven K. Hoge, MD; William Gardner, PhD; Nancy S. Bennett, MA; John Monahan, PhD; Edward P. Mulvey, PhD; Loren H. Roth, MD, MPH

American Medical Association
Physicians dedicated to the health of America

All articles published, including editorials, letters, and book reviews, represent the opinions of the authors and do not reflect the policy of the American Medical Association, the Editorial Board, or the institution with which the author is affiliated, unless this is clearly specified.

Signs of Defensive Control Locate Conflicted Topics in Discourse 1040
Mardi J. Horowitz, MD; Constance Milbrath, PhD; Charles H. Stinson, MD

Posttraumatic Stress Disorder in the National Comorbidity Survey 1048
Ronald C. Kessler, PhD; Amanda Sonnega, PhD; Evelyn Bromet, PhD; Michael Hughes, PhD; Christopher B. Nelson, MPH, PhD

Frontal and Temporal Lobe Brain Volumes in Schizophrenia: Relationship to Symptoms and Clinical Subtype 1061
Bruce Turetsky, MD; Patricia E. Cowell, PhD; Ruben C. Gur, PhD; Robert I. Grossman, MD; Derri L. Shtasel, MD; Raquel E. Gur, MD, PhD

Letters to the Editor

Conversions From Clozapine to Other Antipsychotic Drugs 1071
Ross J. Baldessarini, MD; David M. Gardner, BSPharm; David L. Garver, MD, PhD

In Memoriam

Helen Singer Kaplan, MD, PhD, February 6, 1929, to August 17, 1995 1073
Ethel Person, MD

Roland D. Ciaranello, MD, February 27, 1943, to December 14, 1994 1074
Jack D. Barchas, MD; Stanley J. Watson, MD, PhD; David A. Hamburg, MD

John Romano, MD, November 20, 1908, to June 19, 1995 1076
Robert J. Joynt, MD, PhD

Joseph Wortis, MD, October 2, 1906, to February 22, 1995 1077
Katherine Ann Halmi, MD

Samuel Wesley Perry III, MD, December 10, 1940, to March 15, 1994 1078
Judith Rabkin, PhD, Baruch Fishman, MD

Eli Robins, MD, February 22, 1921, to December 21, 1994 1080
Richard W. Hudgens, MD, George E. Murphy, MD

James W. Maas, MD, October 26, 1929, to January 14, 1995 1081
Martin M. Katz, PhD

Correction

Report Card on the *National Plan for Research on Child and Adolescent Mental Disorders: The Midway Point* 1072
Members of the Committee for the Study of Research on Child and Adolescent Mental Disorders

Regular Departments

Index to Advertisers 985

This Month in *Archives of General Psychiatry* 989

Reviewers for 1995 990

Instructions for Authors 1083

Index to Volume 52 1087

Physician Recruitment Advertising 1099

ARCHIVES OF GENERAL PSYCHIATRY

Functioning and Well-being Outcomes of Patients With Depression Compared With Chronic General Medical Illnesses

Ron D. Hays, PhD; Kenneth B. Wells, MD, MPH; Cathy Donald Sherbourne, PhD; William Rogers, PhD; Karen Spritzer

Background: Cross-sectional studies have found that depression is uniquely associated with limitations in well-being and functioning that were equal to or greater than those of chronic general medical conditions such as diabetes and arthritis. However, whether these relative limitations persist over time is not known.

Methods: We conducted a 2-year observational study of 1790 adult outpatients with depression, diabetes, hypertension, recent myocardial infarction, and/or congestive heart failure. Change in functional status and well-being was compared for depressed patients vs patients with chronic general medical illnesses, controlling statistically for medical comorbidity, sociodemographics, system, and specialty of care.

Results: Over 2 years of follow-up, limitations in functioning and well-being improved somewhat for depressed patients; even so, at the end of 2 years, these limitations were similar to or worse than those attributed to chronic medical illnesses. Similar patterns were observed for depressed patients in the mental health specialty sector and those in the general medical sector, but the patients in the mental health specialty sector improved more. More severely depressed patients improved more in functioning, but even initially depressed patients without depressive disorder had substantial persistent limitations.

Conclusion: Depressed patients have substantial and long-lasting decrements in multiple domains of functioning and well-being that equal or exceed those of patients with chronic medical illnesses.

(Arch Gen Psychiatry. 1995;52:11-19)

DEPRESSION HAS been the focus of intense clinical, research, and policy concerns in both general medical and mental health specialty practices. For example, major depression was the first psychiatric condition selected for development of clinical practice guidelines for primary care by the Agency for Health Care Policy and Research, Rockville, Md, and was one of the first selected for similar efforts in psychiatry by the American Psychiatric Association, Washington, DC. In addition, depression has been featured prominently in efforts to implement standardized methods of assessment of disease severity and functioning outcomes across a variety of general medical and mental health specialty practice settings.[1,2]

A central justification of these efforts is the notion that depression has an especially strong impact on an individual's daily functioning,[3,4] yet it often goes undetected[5] and untreated[6] in general practice. In this article, we address several important research questions about the relationship between depression and daily functioning and psychological well-being.

First, in prior cross-sectional analyses, depressive symptoms (with or without unipolar depressive disorder) were found to be uniquely associated with limitations in well-being and functioning that were equal to or greater than those of major chronic medical conditions such as diabetes and arthritis.[7] But does this conclusion hold over time? Because depression is often episodic, whereas medical conditions are persistent and progressive, it is possible that sampling patients at the time of an office visit biased the comparison of functional status toward depression at its most symptomatic point, whereas medical conditions are closer to the average level of limitation. The clinical course of depression has been shown to be associated

From RAND, Santa Monica, Calif (Drs Hays, Wells, Sherbourne, and Rogers and Ms Spritzer), and the Departments of Medicine (Dr Hays) and Psychiatry and Biobehavioral Sciences (Dr Wells), the University of California–Los Angeles; and the New England Medical Center, Boston, Mass (Dr Rogers).

See Methods on next page

METHODS

STUDY DESIGN

The MOS is an observational study of variations in physician practice styles and patient outcomes in three different systems of care: health maintenance organizations, large multispecialty groups, and solo fee-for-service practices.[14] Three study sites (Boston, Mass; Chicago, Ill; and Los Angeles, Calif) with mature forms of each system of care were chosen from standard metropolitan statistical areas. Within each system of care, a representative sample of medical specialty physicians (general internists, family physicians, cardiologists, endocrinologists, and diabetologists), psychiatrists, psychologists, and other mental health care providers was selected. In the single-specialty solo or small group practice sector, a multistage selection process was used, which consisted of stratified random sampling by national professional associations, further screening and selection, and a final enrollment offer. At the final stage, of 894 eligible clinicians, 290 refused to participate, 306 were not needed to obtain the study quota, and 298 enrolled and screened their patients. In the participating health maintenance organizations and large multispecialty groups, 225 physicians (79% of those deemed eligible) agreed to participate in the MOS. Participation did not differ by clinician specialty, average age, gender, or foreign training. Participating clinicians in health maintenance organizations had slightly lower weekly patient loads than did nonparticipants; the opposite was true for solo and large multispecialty group clinicians.

We screened all adult patients who visited any of the enrolled MOS clinicians during a 2-week period between February and October of 1986, excluding patients who were younger than 18 years, who did not speak English, or who were physically impaired in a way that would prohibit completing forms (eg, blind). Completed questionnaires were obtained for 12 571 eligible patients visiting group practices (75%) and 9828 eligible patients visiting solo practices (65%). Patients were selected for the longitudinal panel on the basis of a diagnosis of one or more of four chronic diseases (hypertension, diabetes, heart disease, or depression) and participation in baseline data collection. Depressed patients were sampled in a two-stage screening procedure.[15] A total of 5043 cases with an MOS tracer condition and 3663 cases with depressive symptoms were identified. The percentage of patients in the cross-sectional sample with each chronic condition is reported elsewhere.[16] A telephone interview was conducted with 5341 patients to collect additional information and ask eligible patients to enroll in the longitudinal panel. Ninety-one percent (n=4824) of the interviewed patients agreed to enroll in the longitudinal study. Of these, a subset of 2471 adult (ages 18 years and older), English-speaking patients was enrolled in the longitudinal study during the fall of 1986. Those excluded from the longitudinal panel tended to be healthier because priority was given to patients with more severe conditions. Patients who did not cooperate (prior to selection of the longitudinal panel) tended to have less education than those who did.

The information included in this article is based on 1790 patients in the MOS panel who completed both the enrollment and the second-year self-administered Patient Assessment Questionnaires (n=1556 from the general medical specialty sector; n=234 from the mental health specialty sector).

DEPRESSIVE DISORDER AND SYMPTOMS

Patients were defined as having depressive symptoms at the beginning of the study if they exceeded a cutoff point on an eight-item depression symptom scale that measured the intensity of symptoms of depression over the past week and periods of depressed mood over the past year.[15] This scale was selected because it had high sensitivity (over 85%) and specificity (over 90%) and an acceptable positive predictive value for identifying current major depression or dysthymia.

We assessed the presence of current depressive disorder (ie, an episode of *DSM-III* major depression in the prior 12 months with no remission since meeting full criteria or dysthymia during the prior 12 months) using an expanded version of the depression section of the Diagnostic Interview Schedule (DIS), a highly structured diagnostic interview designed to determine the presence of psychiatric disorders according to *DSM-III* criteria.[17] This instrument was administered by telephone to persons who exceeded the cutoff point on the depressive symptom screen who also met other eligibility criteria for the longitudinal study.[18] Type of depression at baseline was categorized as subthreshold (results of the screen were positive for depression but the patient had no current disorder), current major depression alone, current dysthymia alone, or current double depression (major depression and dysthymia).

This screen-based definition of subthreshold depression differs from the current symptom-based definitions used by others[19,20] by giving more weight to the duration of depression in the prior year. A comparison of subthreshold depression (using our definition) with whether or not the person had any two symptoms of major depression or dysthymia in the prior month (excluding persons who met the criteria for major depression in the prior month or had lifetime dysthymia with a period during the prior year) in the Los Angeles Epidemiologic Catchment Area Study revealed that more persons had two symptoms of depression (4%) than screened positive for depression (3%). In addition, over 60% of those who screened positive for depression did not have two current symptoms of depression, whereas 75% of those with two symptoms of depression screened positive for depression. These results suggest that our screen-based definition is more restrictive than purely symptom-based definitions because of its focus on the duration of symptoms rather than the number of symptoms.

CHRONIC MEDICAL CONDITIONS

We constructed indicators of physician-diagnosed hypertension, type I diabetes mellitus (onset before age 30 years), type II diabetes mellitus (onset at age 30 years or older), myocardial infarction within the year before the study began, and congestive heart failure based on patient and MOS clinician report. We also controlled for medical comorbidity using an unweighted count of 15 chronic and acute conditions: difficulty hearing, sinus congestion, persistent cough, chronic obstructive pulmonary disease, asthma, chronic diarrhea, constipation, diverticulitis, irritable bowel, arthritis, hip impairments, varicose veins, leg cramps while walking, anemia, and cancer. Similar analytic results were obtained when we controlled for each of the 15 comorbidities separately in sensitivity analyses (not reported herein). The comorbidity measure was available only on those who completed a medical history interview; those who did not (26% of the longitudinal panel) were assigned the sample mean on this measure to maintain an adequate sample size. A dummy variable indicating whether or not the patient had medical history data was included in the analysis. This method avoids the loss of statistical power associated with the listwise deletion of cases and provides an indication of whether or not data are missing at random.[21] Although controlling for comorbidity in this way helps account for case-mix differences, unmeasured differences in medical severity may contribute to variation in functioning and well-being.

Because of its benign impact on functioning and well-being,[7] hypertension is a relatively healthy comparison group that serves to facilitate understanding of the effects of the other chronic conditions. We also compare our estimates of functioning and well-being for patients in the MOS with estimates for a general population that were based on a separate study of 2474 adults sampled from the US general population.[22]

FUNCTIONING AND WELL-BEING MEASURES

Functioning and well-being were assessed by a 36-item short-form health survey (the SF-36) that was administered by mail at multiple waves of the study.[23] This instrument includes eight multi-item measures of functioning and well-being that represent physical and mental health status: physical functioning (10 items), role limitations due to physical health problems (four items), role limitations due to emotional health problems (three items), social functioning (two items), emotional well-being (five items), pain (two items), energy and/or fatigue (four items), and general health perceptions (five items).

The physical functioning scale assesses limitations due to health in activities that range from self-care to vigorous activities. The role-limitations scales measure the extent to which physical health (emotional problems) interfere with doing work or other regular daily activities. The extent to which health interferes with social activities with family, friends, neighbors, or groups is assessed by the social-functioning scale. The emotional–well-being scale assesses general mood or affect, including depressive symptoms, anxiety, and positive well-being. Pain frequency and extent of role interference due to pain are tapped by the pain scale. The energy and/or fatigue scale assesses perceived energy level. General health perceptions are global evaluations of health, such as feeling well or ill.

Internal consistency reliability estimates[24] were 0.78 or greater for every scale. Multitrait scaling analyses[25] supported item convergence within hypothesized scales and item discrimination across scales.[22] Additional empirical studies provide support for the construct validity of the measures.[26]

All outcome measures are scored from 0 to 100, with 100 representing optimal health and 0 representing the poorest health on the scale.

ANALYSIS PLAN

The functioning and well-being of patients with depression relative to that of patients with chronic general medical conditions was estimated by using multiple regression methods. Because patients in the study could have one or more of the chronic conditions, we estimated the unique effect of each condition. We provided separate estimates of functioning and well-being for depressed patients sampled from the medical specialty and mental health specialty sectors. For patients with chronic medical conditions, we provided estimates of functioning and well-being only in the medical specialty sector because patients with the conditions but no depression were not represented among patients in the mental health specialty sector.

Level of functioning and well-being is reported for each domain at baseline of the MOS study and 2 years later. The baseline cross-sectional data provided a point-in-time picture at the beginning of the study, and the end-point data provided a similar picture 2 years later. We did not control for baseline status in the end-point model (ie, analysis of covariance adjustment) because this variable may be positively correlated with the error term of the end point, which would be a violation of statistical assumptions. In the presence of initial differences between compared groups, an analysis of covariance adjustment for baseline level of the outcome measure often leads to biased estimates of regression coefficients.[27-29] We also conducted analyses using the difference between baseline and end status as the dependent variable. Difference scores provide appropriately conservative tests of the null hypothesis and allow each individual to serve as her or his own control.[30-32]

Covariates in each model included age, education, income, gender, ethnicity (not white vs white), site, specialty (general medical vs mental health), and system of care (prepaid vs fee for service at baseline). We recoded our continuous measure of age to four groups (17 through 44 years, 45 through 64 years, 65 through 74 years, and 75 years or older) because the effect of age on health (especially mental health) is not linear.[33] Intercepts were adjusted to reflect the scores of a patient with average sample characteristics.

We adjusted our results for design effects (eg, length of provider screening period and patient visit probability) and sample attrition (logistic regression model predicting the probability of having complete data for the analysis variables from baseline characteristics). We corrected inference statistics and SEs for the clustered sampling design using an intraclass correlation model.[34] Regression coefficients were considered significant if the probability was less than or equal to .05. Because the number of significant effects overall is inflated by chance, we interpret our results with this in mind. We also adjust for multiple comparisons using the seemingly unrelated regression analytic technique. Adjusted means represent the predicted scores for patient groups of interest, with that group having the MOS average sociodemographic characteristics and comorbidity. Because patients in the study could have one or more of the chronic conditions, these estimates represent the unique effect of each condition. Standard errors are computed from the covariance matrix of the regression estimates, using propagation of errors methods. Mean scores on the functioning and well-being scales from a sample of the US general population that were adjusted to the age and gender distribution of the MOS sample are provided for reference.

Table 1. Characteristics of Patients in and Not in the 2-Year Analytic Sample*

Patient Characteristics	Baseline Sample (n=2471)	2-y Analytic Sample (n=1790)	Not in Analytic Sample (n=681)
Age, y	55.5 (16.3)	55.9 (15.9)	54.4 (17.2)
Not white, %	20.6 (39.9)	18.7 (38.5)	25.5 (42.9)†
Male, %	39.5 (48.9)	40.4 (49.18)	37.3 (48.4)
Education, y	13.3 (2.9)	13.4 (3.0)	12.9 (2.8)†
Income (1985 adjusted household)‡	21.4 (15.5)	22.3 (15.6)	19.2 (14.9)†
Married, %	56.0 (49.0)	58.4 (48.8)	49.9 (49.3)†
Comorbidity count	2.3 (1.5)	2.3 (1.5)	2.5 (1.3)§
General medical sector (n=1556), %			
Hypertension	66.3 (46.9)	69.0 (45.9)	59.0 (48.8)†
Congestive heart failure	12.6 (32.7)	9.5 (29.3)	20.8 (40.4)†
Myocardial infarction	6.3 (24.3)	5.4 (22.6)	8.8 (28.4)†
Type I diabetes‖	2.9 (16.7)	2.9 (16.8)	2.8 (16.4)
Type II diabetes¶	23.6 (42.4)	22.8 (41.9)	25.8 (43.8)
Subthreshold depression	16.5 (37.1)	15.6 (36.3)	18.9 (39.2)
Major depression	5.6 (22.9)	4.9 (21.6)	7.4 (26.3)§
Dysthymia	3.7 (18.8)	3.1 (17.5)	5.0 (21.8)
Double depression	4.1 (19.9)	3.9 (19.4)	4.7 (21.1)
Mental health specialty sector (n=234), %			
Subthreshold depression	34.7 (47.7)	35.9 (48.1)	32.0 (46.9)
Major depression	24.9 (43.3)	25.2 (43.5)	24.3 (43.1)
Dysthymia	13.6 (34.4)	12.4 (33.0)	16.5 (37.3)
Double depression	26.7 (44.3)	26.5 (44.2)	27.2 (44.7)

**Values in parentheses represent SDs. Percentages for disease groups are calculated within the general medical and mental health specialty sectors.*
†*P*<.01 *compared with analytic sample.*
‡*Data expressed as thousands of dollars.*
§*P*<.05 *compared with analytic sample.*
‖*Onset before age 30 years.*
¶*Onset at age 30 years or older.*

with functional outcomes (disability days) in a previous study.[4] Furthermore, because of differences in disease course over the long run, medically ill patients could accumulate a greater degree of functional limitation than initially depressed patients, who may or may not be depressed at subsequent follow-up.

Second, it was reported previously that persons who exceeded a cutoff point at screening but who did not have depressive disorder had almost as much limitation in functioning and well-being as those with the disorder, especially among patients in the general medical sector.[7] But how much impact do subthreshold depressive symptoms have over time? One might expect such patients to have relatively brief and minor depression and thus to appear more like a nonpatient or asymptomatic sample at follow-up.

Third, do functioning and well-being limitations of depressed patients have a different course among patients in the general medical sector vs the mental health specialty sector? Depressed patients in the mental health specialty sector have more severe depression and somewhat greater limitations in functioning and well-being.[8] One might expect the milder depression of patients in the general medical sector to have a more favorable course over time, although this effect could be balanced in part by lower rates of detection and treatment of depression in the general medical vs the mental health specialty sector.[9]

We address these issues using 2-year follow-up data on patients who were initially sampled at the time of a visit; follow-up assessment, however, was unrelated to health care use and thus was not biased by selection of sicker patients into treatment. We do not directly examine the effect of treatment differences on outcomes because, in the nonexperimental study, there were strong selection effects, that is, sicker patients received more treatment.[8,10] Despite the current emphasis in medical effectiveness research on using nonexperimental data to draw inferences about process and outcomes links, the selection biases in the Medical Outcomes Study (MOS) severely limit this approach. Thus, our study is in the natural history tradition.[11]

In the spirit of the emerging emphasis on assessing a comprehensive set of health outcome measures,[12] we compare patients on multiple domains of functional status and well-being. An exploratory examination of an array of functioning measures is important because not enough is known about the scope of the functional impact of depression relative to chronic general medical illnesses. The little information available to date suggests that the functional decrements associated with depression are evident across multiple domains.[7,13]

RESULTS

A summary of baseline characteristics (age, ethnicity, gender, education, income, and marital status) is provided in **Table 1**. Those who were not in the analysis sample (ie, those omitted because of missing data) differed significantly from those in the analysis sample in terms of ethnicity (*P*<.001), education (*P*<.001), income (*P*<.001), marital status (*P*<.001), comorbidity (*P*=.01),

Table 2. Adjusted Physical Functioning and Well-being Measures for Depressed Patients in the MOS and MOS Patients With Chronic General Medical Conditions in the General Medical Sector*

	Physical Functioning	Role (Physical)	Freedom From Pain	General Health
Subthreshold depression (n=243)				
Baseline	71^{c,d,e} (3)	57^{c} (4)	68^{c,d} (2)	54^{c,d} (2)
2 years after baseline	71^{c,d} (3)	61^{b,c} (4)	68^{d,e} (2)	57^{b} (2)
Major depression (n=76)				
Baseline	73^{b,c,d,e} (4)	49^{c,d} (7)	64^{b,c,d,e} (5)	56^{a,b,c,d} (4)
2 years after baseline	72^{b,c,d} (3)	50^{c,d} (7)	61^{e} (4)	56^{a,b,c} (4)
Dysthymia (n=48)				
Baseline	64^{e} (4)	38^{d} (9)	59^{e} (4)	50^{c,d,e} (4)
2 years after baseline	68^{c,d} (5)	35^{d} (9)	58^{e} (6)	47^{c} (5)
Double depression (n=61)				
Baseline	67^{d,e} (5)	51^{c,d} (6)	60^{d,e} (5)	45^{e} (4)
2 years after baseline	75^{a,b,c} (4)	57^{b,c} (6)	68^{b,c,d,e} (4)	55^{b,c} (4)†
Hypertension (n=1074)				
Baseline	80^{b} (1)	69^{b} (2)	75^{a,b} (1)	64^{a} (1)
2 years after baseline	78^{a,b} (1)†	72^{a} (2)	77^{b} (2)	64^{a} (1)
Congestive heart failure (n=148)				
Baseline	64^{e} (3)	53^{c,d} (5)	71^{a,b,c,d} (3)	52^{d,e} (3)
2 years after baseline	63^{d} (3)	50^{c,d} (5)	72^{b,c,d} (3)	49^{c} (3)
Myocardial infarction (n=84)				
Baseline	79^{a,b,c} (4)	66^{b,c} (6)	79^{a} (4)	63^{a,b} (2)
2 years after baseline	82^{a} (3)	73^{a,b} (5)	84^{a} (3)	64^{a,b} (3)
Type I diabetes (n=45)				
Baseline	89^{a} (4)	86^{a} (7)	74^{a,b,c} (4)	62^{a,b,c,d} (6)
2 years after baseline	80^{a,b,c} (5)†	62^{a,b,c} (7)†	67^{c,d,e} (4)	56^{a,b,c} (8)
Type II diabetes (n=355)				
Baseline	77^{b,c,d} (2)	70^{b} (4)	74^{a,b} (2)	59^{b,c} (2)
2 years after baseline	75^{b,c} (2)	66^{a,b} (4)	75^{b,c} (2)	58^{b} (2)
General population‡	76	72	71	67

**Adjusted for comorbidity, sociodemographics, and system of care. Values in parentheses represent SEs. All measures are scored on a scale from 0 to 100, with higher scores representing better functioning and well-being. Groups sharing a superscripted letter in common in the same column (functioning or well-being measure) and time of assessment (baseline or 2 years after baseline) do not differ significantly (P>.05) from one another. MOS indicates Medical Outcomes Study.*

†Change over time for this subgroup is statistically significant (P<.05).

‡Mean scores from a sample of 2474 adults in the US general population, adjusted to the age and gender distribution of the MOS sample.

and the presence of hypertension (*P*<.001), congestive heart failure (*P*<.001), myocardial infarction (*P*=.01), and major depression (*P*=.04). Moreover, sociodemographic characteristics (age, ethnicity, gender, education, income, and marital status) accounted for between 3% and 18% of the variance in baseline measurements of functioning and well-being. Therefore, subsequent analyses are weighted for the loss of patients in the sample, and sociodemographic variables are included as covariates.

PHYSICAL FUNCTIONING AND WELL-BEING OUTCOMES FOR PATIENTS IN THE GENERAL MEDICAL SECTOR

Table 2 presents the results of adjusted baseline and 2-years-postbaseline mean physical functioning and well-being for patients in the MOS who were sampled from the general medical sector. Physical functioning scores at baseline for the depressed patients ranged from 64 to 73, and for the patients with general medical conditions, scores ranged from 64 to 89. Patients with dysthymia reported particularly poor physical functioning, which was significantly (*P*=.006 to *P*<.001) worse than that for all except one general medical condition (congestive heart failure) at baseline. Role limitations due to physical health were noteworthy for depressed patients, with baseline scores ranging from 38 to 57 compared with 53 to 86 for patients with general medical conditions. Mean levels of (freedom from) pain ranged from 59 to 68 for depressed patients and 71 to 79 for patients with general medical conditions. The mean adjusted general health perceptions score for depressed patients at baseline was 45 to 56 compared with 52 to 64 for patients with general medical conditions. Two years later, the corresponding scores tended to be similar to the baseline values, but significant improvements were obtained in general health perceptions by those with double depression (*P*=.002), and significant decrements in physical functioning occurred in patients with hypertension (*P*=.04) and type I diabetics (*P*=.02). Type I diabetics also reported significant increases in role limitations due to physical health (*P*=.006) 2 years after baseline.

The general population means in Table 2 (adjusted to the age and gender distribution of the MOS sample) are very similar to scores for patients with hypertension. Only on general health perceptions was hypertension consistently below the general population mean, and this three-point difference is consistent with previous findings from the MOS.[16]

Table 3. Adjusted Mental Functioning and Well-being Measures for Depressed Patients in the MOS and MOS Patients With Chronic General Medical Conditions in the General Medical Sector*

	Emotional Well-being	Role (Emotional)	Social Functioning	Energy or Fatigue
Subthreshold depression (n=243)				
Baseline	65[c] (2)	62[c] (4)	78[c,d] (2)	51[b] (2)
2 years after baseline	67[b] (2)	66[c] (5)	76[c,d] (3)	52[d] (2)
Major depression (n=76)				
Baseline	59[c,d] (3)	41[d] (6)	70[d,e] (5)	51[b] (4)
2 years after baseline	65[b] (3)†	62[c,d] (7)†	73[d] (4)	56[b,c,d] (4)
Dysthymia (n=48)				
Baseline	52[d,e] (4)	64[b,c] (9)	60[e,f] (4)	44[b,c] (4)
2 years after baseline	54[c] (4)	42[d] (10)†	66[d] (5)	48[c,d] (5)
Double depression (n=61)				
Baseline	43[e] (4)	32[d] (6)	56[f] (4)	38[c] (3)
2 years after baseline	54[c] (4)†	46[d] (7)†	72[d] (5)†	46[d] (4)†
Hypertension (n=1074)				
Baseline	80[b] (1)	81[a,b] (2)	91[a] (1)	61[a] (1)
2 years after baseline	81[a] (1)	84[a,b] (2)	91[a] (1)	64[a] (1)†
Congestive heart failure (n=148)				
Baseline	83[a,b] (2)	81[a,b] (5)	84[a,b,c] (4)	52[b] (3)
2 years after baseline	82[a] (2)	78[a,b,c] (5)	84[b,c] (3)	51[d] (3)
Myocardial infarction (n=84)				
Baseline	77[b] (2)	77[b] (6)	91[a,b] (3)	59[a] (2)
2 years after baseline	79[a] (2)	84[a,b] (6)	92[a,b] (4)	61[a,b] (3)
Type I diabetes (n=45)				
Baseline	88 (4)	96[a] (8)	93[a,b] (5)	64[a] (6)
2 years after baseline	81[a] (7)	93[a] (6)	88[a,b,c] (5)	75[a] (7)†
Type II diabetes (n=355)				
Baseline	80[b] (2)	83[a,b] (3)	87[b] (2)	60[a] (2)
2 years after baseline	78[a] (2)	80[b] (4)	85[b] (2)	58[b,c] (2)
General population‡	75	79	81	59

See Table 2 for explanation of footnote symbols.

MENTAL FUNCTIONING AND WELL-BEING OUTCOMES FOR PATIENTS IN THE GENERAL MEDICAL SECTOR

At baseline, depressed patients in the general medical sector tended by far to have the worst mental functioning and well-being, but those with major depression or double depression improved considerably over time (**Table 3**). These improvements were significant ($P<.001$) across the four mental functioning and well-being outcome measures after adjusting for multiple comparisons in seemingly unrelated regression models. Nevertheless, after 2 years, these patients still tended to be worse off than those with general medical conditions. In fact, means for the groups with chronic general medical illness exceeded the general population means in a majority of cases, but the depressed patients scored below the general population without exception. For example, at baseline, mean adjusted social functioning scores ranged from 56 to 78 for depressed patients compared with 84 to 93 across the general medical conditions. At 2 years, the social functioning scores for depressed groups ranged from 66 to 76 compared with 84 to 92 for the groups with general medical conditions. That is, at follow-up, depressed groups moved toward the lower (sicker) end for medical conditions rather than way below the sickest medical group (as they were at baseline). One exception to the general trends was the significant ($P=.02$) increase in role limitations due to emotional problems among patients with dysthymia.

SUBTHRESHOLD DEPRESSION VS GENERAL MEDICAL CONDITIONS

Even for patients with subthreshold depression at baseline, 2-year functioning and well-being outcomes tended to be similar to or worse than those of the groups with chronic general medical conditions. For example, at 2 years, patients with subthreshold depression in the general medical sector had significantly more limitations in physical functioning ($t=2.62$, $df=1618$, $P=.009$), had more role limitations due to physical health problems ($t=2.40$, $df=1462$, $P=.02$), reported greater bodily pain ($t=2.57$, $df=1625$, $P=.01$), and had worse general health perceptions ($t=2.36$, $df=1636$, $P=.02$) than did patients with hypertension.

GENERALIZABILITY ACROSS SPECIALTY SECTORS

As shown in **Table 4** and **Table 5**, patients with depression treated in the mental health specialty sector were initially somewhat sicker and tended to improve to a greater extent over time than did comparable patients in the medical specialty sector. In the mental health specialty sector, patients with dysthymia improved on six of the eight health status measures, patients with major depression improved significantly on four measures, and patients with double depression improved on three measures (t's ranged from 2.07 [$P=.04$] to 4.66 [$P<.001$] [df's

Table 4. Adjusted Physical Functioning and Well-being Measures for Depressed Patients in the MOS in the Mental Health Specialty Sector*

	Physical Functioning	Role (Physical)	Freedom from Pain	General Health
Subthreshold depression (n=84)				
Baseline	80[a] (2)	62[a] (5)	69[a,b] (4)	61[a] (3)
2 years after baseline	81[a] (2)	55[a,b] (6)	69[a,b] (3)	63[a] (3)
Major depression (n=59)				
Baseline	79[a,b] (3)	51[a] (6)	72[a] (4)	57[a,b] (3)
2 years after baseline	79[a,b] (3)	62[a] (6)	74[a] (3)	64[a] (3)†
Dysthymia (n=29)				
Baseline	70[b,c] (4)	23[b] (7)	52[c] (4)	47[b] (4)
2 years after baseline	72[b,c] (4)	53[a,b] (12)†	69[a,b] (7)	60[a,b] (4)†
Double depression (n=62)				
Baseline	66[c] (4)	35[b] (5)	58[b,c] (4)	48[b] (4)
2 years after baseline	68[c] (3)	44[b] (6)	64[b] (4)	50[b] (4)
General population‡	76	72	71	67

**See Table 2 for explanation of footnote symbols.*

Table 5. Adjusted Mental Functioning and Well-being Measures for Depressed Patients in the MOS in the Mental Health Specialty Sector*

	Emotional Well-being	Role (Emotional)	Social Functioning	Energy or Fatigue
Subthreshold depression (n=84)				
Baseline	62[a] (3)	40[a] (6)	69[a] (4)	50[a] (3)
2 years after baseline	61[a] (3)	54[a] (7)	74[a] (4)	57[a] (3)†
Major depression (n=59)				
Baseline	53[b] (4)	37[a] (8)	65[a] (4)	49[a,b] (4)
2 years after baseline	63[a] (3)†	58[a] (6)†	72[a,b] (4)	56[a] (3)†
Dysthymia (n=29)				
Baseline	42[c] (5)	32[a] (9)	53[b] (4)	36[b,c] (5)
2 years after baseline	61[a] (5)†	50[a] (9)†	73[a,b,c] (7)†	57[a] (4)†
Double depression (n=62)				
Baseline	39[c] (3)	25[a] (6)	48[b] (5)	31[c] (3)
2 years after baseline	49[b] (4)†	40[a] (8)	58[c] (5)†	46[b] (3)†
General population‡	75	79	81	59

**See Table 2 for explanation of footnote symbols.*

ranged from 1451 to 1636]). **Figure 1** illustrates the pattern for double depression on measures of social functioning and emotional well-being.

At the 2-year follow-up, patients with any form of depression in the mental health specialty sector tended to have worse functioning and lower well-being than did nondepressed patients in the general medical sector with chronic medical illness (**Figure 2**). For example, depressed patients in the mental health specialty sector had significantly more role limitations due to emotional problems than did patients with each of the general medical conditions (*t*'s [*df*=1451] ranging from 2.60 [*P*=.009] to 5.80 [*P*<.001])

COMMENT

This longitudinal follow-up of patients in the MOS documents the persistence of impairments in the functioning and well-being of patients with depression relative to patients with chronic medical illness. These impairments were noteworthy at baseline of the study at the time of an office visit[7] and 2 years later, unrelated to an office visit. However, on many of the outcome measures, depressed patients improved over time, which is consistent with the fact that depression is often episodic and the patients were sampled at a symptomatic point of the illness. Nevertheless, the degree of persistence in functional limitations was greater than might be expected for an episodic disorder. This general conclusion applied across types of depression, even to patients with depressive symptoms but no depressive disorder and to depressed patients in both the general medical and mental health specialty sectors. The long-term functional impairment is not surprising given that about one fourth of the patients with subthreshold depression and over one half of the patients with dysthymia at baseline had a major depressive episode during follow-up.[10]

Despite having somewhat better mental functioning and well-being at baseline than patients with depressive disorder, patients with subthreshold depressive symptoms in the general medical sector were stable over time, whereas those with depressive disorder tended to improve. The stability of functional limitations in patients with subthreshold symptoms is not due to their comorbid medical con-

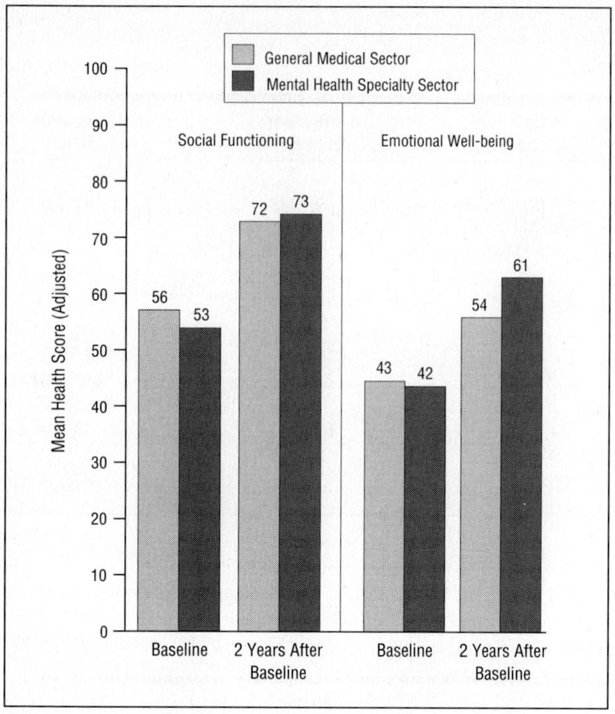

Figure 1. *Change over 2 years in social functioning and emotional well-being for patients with double depression by specialty sector.*

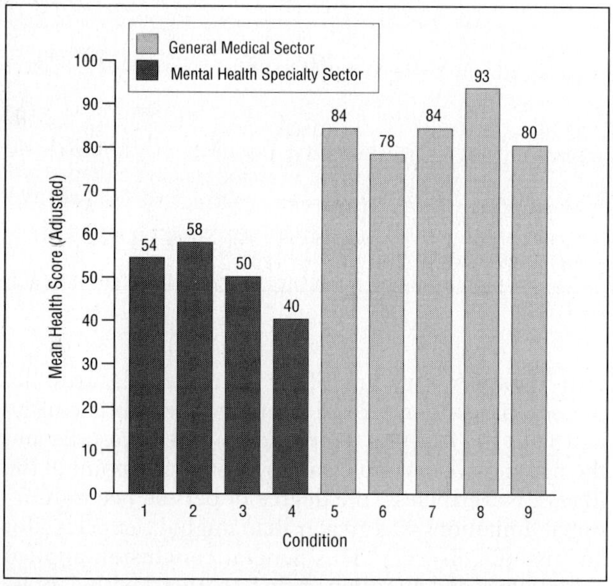

Figure 2. *Adjusted role (emotional) functioning 2 years after baseline for mental health specialty patients with depression and general medical patients with general medical conditions. Numbers indicate the following conditions: 1, subthreshold depression; 2, major depression; 3, dysthymia; 4, double depression; 5, hypertension; 6, congestive heart failure; 7, myocardial infarction; 8, type I diabetes; and 9, type II diabetes.*

ditions because these results control for the presence of medical comorbidity. Thus, this group appears to be of particular importance despite the weaker symptom presentation because of their persistent limitations, which could be due to untreated or partially treated depression.

Depressed patients in the mental health specialty sector tended to be sicker initially but also to improve more in functioning and well-being over time than did similar patients in the medical sector. These relative improvements could be due to greater recognition of depression[9] and the more appropriate and intensive mental health care provided in the mental health specialty sector. We could not directly study treatment effects on the course of depression because we observed low rates of treatment and strong selection biases.[35] Alternatively, patients in the mental health specialty sector who started at a lower scale score could have had more room to improve and regress toward the mean; the same can be said generally for more severely depressed patients in this study. Despite their relative improvements, depressed patients in the mental health specialty sector, similar to patients in the medical specialty sector, fared notably poorer than did patients with chronic medical illness 2 years after the baseline assessment.

Are the self-reports of functioning in depressed patients valid? Some have noted that depressed patients are unrealistically pessimistic,[36] and this could result in poorer scores on self-report measures than on more objective measures. This is an important issue that requires further study. The same bias may hold for all patients with serious illnesses, but in general, studies have been focused largely on depression. Our focus on self-reports emanates from the movement toward acknowledging patients' own view of their outcomes as of merit in health policy evaluations. Indeed, the results observed in this study 2 years after baseline are clinically reasonable in that depressed patients scored similarly to nondepressed patients on physical functioning, but noteworthy differences were observed on measures of mental functioning and well-being. These and other results from the MOS[26,37] provide support for the validity of the self-reports of functioning and well-being. Lastly, even if depressed patients' assessments of their functioning are to some extent unrealistic, they are associated with events such as disability days and service use.[7,38]

The depressed patients in the MOS sample are older than patients in many previous studies of mental health. The association between age and mental health is mixed. For example, there is some indication that the extent of depressive symptoms may be lowest among middle-aged patients but that rates of clinical depression may be highest.[33,39] Thus, the results of this study may not be generalizable to younger age groups.

By following up patients over a 2-year period, we have been able to document the long-lasting functional impairments associated with depression, whether defined by clinical disorder or subthreshold depressive symptoms, on the functional status and well-being of outpatients in both the medical and the mental health specialty sectors. The results of our study also make clear that appropriate caution is required in studying patients at the time of or in close proximity to an office visit for medical or mental health care. The time of a symptomatic office visit is opportune for clinical interventions, but health status measured in close proximity to this point in time may be unrepresentative of the patient's usual functional status and well-being. It is therefore critical that effectiveness studies include enough time points to separate the transitory from the long-term component of functioning and well-being.

In sum, despite substantial improvement in functional status and well-being, patients who were initially depressed at the time of a visit to their physician were for a long time afterward (ie, 2 years) still about as limited in physical health and more limited in mental health outcomes than were patients with chronic medical illnesses, regardless of whether depression was defined as depressive disorder or the broader phenomenon of depressive symptoms, and the same was true across different specialty sectors. The substantial persistence of limitations in functioning and well-being of depressed outpatients underscores the importance of efforts to improve the treatment of depressive illness in both the medical and the mental health specialty sectors, as reflected by clinical practice guidelines.

Accepted for publication August 24, 1994.

This study was supported by grant MH 42229 R01 from the National Institute of Mental Health, Rockville, Md; grants from the Robert Wood Johnson Foundation, Princeton, NJ; the Henry J. Kaiser Family Foundation, Menlo Park, Calif; the Pew Charitable Trusts, Philadelphia, Pa; the Agency for Health Care Policy and Research, Rockville, Md; and RAND, Santa Monica, Calif, out of its own research funds.

The conclusions are those of the authors and do not necessarily reflect the opinion of the sponsors or the authors' institutions.

Cooperation and assistance in recruiting physicians and patients was provided by the American College of Physicians, Philadelphia, Pa; the American Academy of Family Physicians, Kansas City, Mo; the American Academy of Pediatrics, Elk Grove Village, Ill; The American Psychiatric Association; the American Psychological Association, Washington, DC; and their local chapters in the MOS study sites. The authors gratefully acknowledge other MOS staff: John Ware, PhD; Sheldon Greenfield, MD; Sandra Berry, MA; Maureen Carney, MS; Laural Hill; Sherrie Kaplan, PhD; Elizabeth McGlynn, PhD; Lisa Meredith, PhD; Eugene Nelson, ScD; Judith Perlman; and Anita Stewart, PhD. The comments of anonymous reviewers; Richard Glass, MD; Robert Brook, MD; and Joyce Peterson, PhD, were very helpful in revising the manuscript. Thanks are due Barbara Genovese for data tabulation. We also acknowledge the cooperation of the participating health maintenance organizations: the ANCHOR Organization for Health Maintenance in Chicago (Charles Hertz, MD, and William Rollow, MD); CIGNA Healthplans of Southern California, Los Angeles (B. Ross Landess, MD); and the Harvard Community Health Plan in Boston (Stephen Schoenbaum, MD).

Correspondence to RAND, 1700 Main St, Santa Monica, CA 90407-2138 (Dr Hays).

REFERENCES

1. Tarlov AR, Ware JE Jr, Greenfield S, Nelson EC, Perrin E, Zubkoff M. Medical Outcomes Study. *JAMA.* 1989;262:925-930.
2. Rost KR, Smith GR, Burnam MA, Burns BJ. Measuring the outcomes of care for mental health problems. *Med Care.* 1992;30(suppl):MS266-MS273.
3. Broadhead WE, Blazer DG, George LK, Tse CK. Depression, disability days, and days lost from work in a prospective epidemiologic survey. *JAMA.* 1990; 264:2524-2528.
4. Von Korff M, Ormel J, Katon W, Lin EHB. Disability and depression among high utilizers of health care. *Arch Gen Psychiatry.* 1992;49:91-100.
5. Goldberg D. Identifying psychiatric illness among general medical patients. *BMJ.* 1985;291:161-162.
6. Johnson D. Study of the use of antidepressant medication in general practice. *Br J Psychiatry.* 1974;125:186-212.
7. Wells KB, Stewart A, Hays RD, Burnam MA, Rogers W, Daniels M, Berry S, Greenfield S, Ware J Jr. The functioning and well-being of depressed patients: results from the Medical Outcomes Study. *JAMA.* 1989;262:914-919.
8. Rogers WH, Wells KB, Meredith LS, Sturm R, Burnam MA. Outcomes for adult outpatients with depression under prepaid or fee-for-service financing. *Arch Gen Psychiatry.* 1993;50:517-525.
9. Wells KB, Hays RD, Burnam A, Rogers W, Greenfield S, Ware JE Jr. Detection of depressive disorders for patients receiving prepaid or fee-for-service care: results from the Medical Outcomes Study. *JAMA.* 1989;262:3298-3302.
10. Wells KB, Burnam MA, Rogers W, Hays R, Camp P. The course of depression in adult outpatients. *Arch Gen Psychiatry.* 1992;49:788-794.
11. Keller MB, Shapiro RW, Lavori PW, Wolfe N. Recovery in major depressive disorder. *Arch Gen Psychiatry.* 1982;39:905-910
12. Corrigan JM, Nielsen DM. Toward the development of uniform reporting standards for managed care organizations: the Health Plan Employer Data and Information Set (Version 2.0). *Jt Comm J Qual Improv.* 1993;19:566-575.
13. Vickrey BG, Hays RD, Rausch R, Sutherling WW, Engel J, Brook RH. Quality of life of epilepsy surgery patients as compared with outpatients with hypertension, diabetes, heart disease, and/or depressive symptoms. *Epilepsia.* 1994;35:597-607.
14. Rogers W, McGlynn E, Berry W, Nelson EC, Perrin E, Zubkoff M, Greenfield S, Wells KB, Stewart AL, Arnold SB, Ware JE Jr. Methods of sampling. In: Stewart AL, Ware JE Jr, eds. *Measuring Functional Status and Well-being: The Medical Outcomes Study Approach.* Durham, NC: Duke University Press; 1992:27-47.
15. Burnam MA, Wells KB, Leake B, Landsverk J. Development of a brief screening instrument for detecting depressive disorders. *Med Care.* 1988;26:775-789.
16. Stewart AL, Greenfield S, Hays RD, Wells K, Rogers WH, Berry SD, McGlynn EA, Ware JE Jr. Functional status and well-being of patients with chronic conditions: results from the Medical Outcomes Study. *JAMA.* 1989;262:907-913.
17. Robins LN, Helzer JE, Croughan J, Ratcliff KS. The National Institute of Mental Health Diagnostic Interview Schedule. *Arch Gen Psychiatry.* 1981;38:381-389.
18. Wells KB, Burnam MA, Leake B, Robins LN. Agreement between face-to-face and telephone administered versions of the depression section of the NIMH Diagnostic Interview Schedule. *J Psychiatr Res.* 1988;22:207-220.
19. Broadhead WE, Blazer DG, George LK, Tse CK. Depression, disability days, and days lost from work in a prospective epidemiologic survey. *JAMA.* 1990; 264:2524-2528.
20. Horwath E, Johnson J, Klerman GL, Weissman MM. Depressive symptoms as relative and attributable risk factors for first-onset major depression. *Arch Gen Psychiatry.* 1992;49:817-823.
21. Raymond MR. Missing data in evaluation research. *Eval Health Professions.* 1986;9:395-420.
22. Ware JE Jr, Snow KK, Kosinski M, Gandek B. *SF-36 Health Survey: Manual and Interpretation Guide.* Boston, Mass: The Health Institute; 1993.
23. Ware JE Jr, Sherbourne CD. The MOS 36-item short-form health survey (SF-36), I: conceptual framework and item selection. *Med Care.* 1992;30:473-483.
24. Cronbach LJ. Coefficient alpha and the internal structure of tests. *Psychometrika.* 1951;16:297-334.
25. Hays RD, Hayashi T. Beyond internal consistency reliability. *Behav Res Methods Instruments Comput.* 1990;22:167-175.
26. McHorney CA, Ware JE Jr, Rogers W, Raczek AE, Lu JFR. The validity and relative precision of MOS Short- and Long-Form Health Status Scales and Dartmouth COOP Charts. *Med Care.* 1992;30(suppl):253S-265S.
27. Kaplan RM, Berry CC. Adjusting for confounding variables. In: Sechrest L, Perrin E, Bunker J, eds. *Research Methodology.* Rockville, Md: US Dept of Health and Human Services; 1990:105-114.
28. Lord FM. A paradox in the interpretation of group comparisons. *Psychol Bull.* 1967;68:304-305.
29. Porter AC, Raudenbush SW. Analysis of covariance: its model and use in psychological research. *J Counseling Psychol.* 1987;34:383-392.
30. Allison PD. Change scores as dependent variables in regression analysis. *Sociol Methodol.* 1990;20:93-114.
31. Overall JE. Contradictions can never a paradox resolve. *Appl Psychol Meas.* 1989;13:426-428.
32. Willett JB. Questions and answers in the measurement of change. In: Rothkopf EZ, ed. *Review of Research in Education, 15.* Washington, DC: American Education Research Association; 1988:345-422.
33. Kessler RC, Foster C, Webster PS, House JS. The relationship between age and depressive symptoms in two national surveys. *Psychol Aging.* 1992;7:119-126.
34. Liang KY, Zeger SL. Longtitudinal data analysis using generalized linear models. *Biometrika.* 1986;73:13-22.
35. Wells KB, Katon W, Rogers B, Camp P. Use of minor tranquilizers and antidepressant medications by depressed outpatients: results from the Medical Outcomes Study. *Am J Psychiatry.* 1994;151:694-700.
36. Beck AT. *Cognitive Therapy and the Emotional Disorders.* New York, NY: International Universities Press Inc; 1976:116-119.
37. Hays RD, Stewart AL. The structure of self-reported health in chronic disease patients. *Psychol Assess.* 1990;2:22-30.
38. Manning WG, Wells KB. The effects of psychological distress and psychological well-being on use of medical services. *Med Care.* 1992;30:541-553.
39. Mirowsky J, Ross CE. Age and depression. *J Health Soc Behav.* 1992;33:187-205.

ORIGINAL ARTICLE

A Positron Emission Tomographic Study of Simple Phobic Symptom Provocation

Scott L. Rauch, MD; Cary R. Savage, PhD; Nathaniel M. Alpert, PhD; Euripedes C. Miguel, MD, PhD; Lee Baer, PhD; Hans C. Breiter, MD; Alan J. Fischman MD, PhD; Peter A. Manzo; Cara Moretti; Michael A. Jenike, MD

Background: The goal of this study was to determine the mediating neuroanatomy of simple phobic symptoms.

Methods: Positron emission tomography and oxygen 15 were used to measure normalized regional cerebral blood flow in seven subjects with simple phobia during control and provoked states. Stereotactic transformation and statistical parametric mapping techniques were employed to determine the locations of significant activation.

Results: Statistical parametric maps demonstrated significant increases in normalized regional blood flow for the symptomatic state compared with the control state in the anterior cingulate cortex, the insular cortex, the anterior temporal cortex, the somatosensory cortex, the posterior medial orbitofrontal cortex, and the thalamus.

Conclusions: The results suggest that anxiety associated with the simple phobic symptomatic state is mediated by paralimbic structures. Moreover, activation of somatosensory cortex may reflect tactile imagery as one component of the phobic symptomatic condition.

(Arch Gen Psychiatry. 1995;52:20-28)

THE PURPOSE of this study was to determine the mediating neuroanatomy of simple phobic (SP) symptoms. Recently, the results of an oxygen 15 (^{15}O) positron emission tomographic (PET) study of obsessive-compulsive disorder (OCD) that used a within-subject symptom-provocation paradigm were reported.[1] Briefly, the results of that study were consistent with current neurobiologic models of OCD[2-7] and were convergent with the latest PET results reported by other research groups.[4,8]

In the current study, analogous methods were employed to study the mediating neuroanatomy of SP in a cohort that met the diagnostic criteria for SP[9] of small animals. Simple phobia is a common anxiety disorder,[9,10] and subjects with small animal phobic symptoms can be reliably provoked in a manner that is logistically feasible for the PET suite setting.

Two other research teams have already performed PET symptom-provocation studies of SP, using different methods and yielding disparate results.[11,12] Mountz and colleagues[11] used a paradigm in which exposure to provocative stimuli (ie, small animals) produced significant differences in anxiety and physiologic measurements, yet they found no global or regional differences in cerebral blood flow between provoked and resting states. Fredrikson and colleagues[12] studied subjects with phobia of snakes during exposure to videotapes of snakes, control aversive stimuli, or neutral stimuli. They found significant activation within the visual association cortex during the phobic but not the aversive control or neutral states. In addition, Fredrikson's group[12] found significant correlations between thalamus and cortex activation during the phobic but not the aversive control or neutral states. They found no significant activations in the striatum or frontal cortex for the phobic state compared with other states.

In the present study, we used ^{15}O-labeled carbon dioxide (CO_2) to study normalized regional cerebral blood flow (rCBF) patterns in a control state and, a few minutes later, in a provoked SP state. In this manner, SP symptomatic-state–

See Subjects and Methods on next page

From the Departments of Psychiatry (Drs Rauch, Savage, Miguel, Baer, Breiter, and Jenike, Mr Manzo, and Ms Moretti) and Radiology (Drs Rauch, Alpert, Breiter, and Fischman) and the Division of Nuclear Medicine/Positron Emission Tomography Laboratory (Drs Rauch, Alpert, and Fischman), Massachusetts General Hospital, Harvard Medical School, Boston.

SUBJECTS AND METHODS

SUBJECTS

Inclusion criteria were the elements of the *DSM-III-R*[9] diagnosis of simple phobia as determined by clinical interview and the Structured Clinical Interview for *DSM-III-R*.[18] In addition to meeting *DSM-III-R* criteria, all subjects were specifically phobic of small animals, were at least 18 years of age, and were right-handed (as established by the Edinburgh Handedness Inventory[19]). Exclusion criteria were the presence of major medical illness or another major psychiatric disorder (eg, another anxiety disorder, schizophrenia, eating disorder, psychoactive substance use disorder, bipolar disorder, or current major depression). Meeting clinical criteria for major depression[9] or a Beck Depression Inventory[20] score of greater than 15 was grounds for exclusion. All subjects were free of all psychoactive drugs for at least 4 weeks prior to the study. Subjects were recruited by advertisement within the hospital and in local newspapers. All studies were conducted with the approval of the Subcommittee on Human Studies of the Massachusetts General Hospital, Boston. Written informed consent was obtained from each subject.

The study population comprised seven subjects, six women and one man, with a mean±SD age at study of 37.0±10.3 years (range, 22 to 55 years). Subjects had a mean±SD Beck Depression Inventory score of 3.3±3.1 (of a possible score of 63) (range, 0 to 10). Because scans were performed on subjects in both control and provoked states, subjects served as their own controls.

SP-SYMPTOM–PROVOCATION PARADIGM

The provocation paradigm that was employed was analogous to that previously described for the study of OCD.[1] After an initial habituation phase, PET scans were performed on patients with SP twice in a control state while they were responding to an innocuous control stimulus and twice again in a provoked state while they were responding to a provocative stimulus that was tailored to induce each patient's symptoms. In all cases, subjects participated in the process of identifying an appropriately provocative stimulus, including the nature of the stimulus and its required distance from the subject, so as to ensure sufficient but not overwhelming provocation of anxiety (**Table 1**).

The locations of the stimuli were matched for the provoked and control conditions in terms of distance from the subjects. For three of the subjects, this entailed actually touching the outside of the containers that housed the stimuli in both the provoked and control conditions; for the other four subjects, the stimuli were placed from less than 2 m (n=3) to approximately 6 m (n=1) away. In addition, presentations of the stimuli were counterbalanced, with one exposure on the right side and one exposure on the left side for both the control and provoked conditions. The order of left vs right was incompletely counterbalanced because of the odd number of subjects (ie, for the seven subjects, of the four possible permutations of order, three were represented twice, and one was represented once; assignment of order was random).

A counterbalanced paradigm intended to control for order effects regarding the provoked and the control conditions was considered but was deemed impractical. Pilot experience revealed that once provoked, subjects remained symptomatic for up to 1 hour, which precluded a paradigm dependent on prompt return to an asymptomatic state. Therefore, in all subjects, the control conditions preceded the provoked conditions.

A zero- to 10-point analog scale based on self-report (the Anxiety Analog Scale [AAS])[1] was used to quantify the subjective severity of each subject's anxiety during an initial habituation period as well as during each scanning period. A score of 10 was equated with the most severe symptoms ever previously experienced by the subject; a score of 0 was equated with the complete absence of symptoms. This scale provided a crude clinical measure by which to verify each subject's response to the different stimuli (innocuous vs provocative).

After being fully situated in the scanner, subjects were allowed to habituate, during which time AAS scores were obtained every 3 minutes. Sufficient habituation was operationalized as AAS scores that remained constant for two consecutive measurement periods.

Following habituation, the subjects proceeded to the control phase of the paradigm. For each of two control scans, the subjects were exposed to an innocuous stimulus that was matched to their individualized provocative stimulus in terms of primary sensory stimulation. For example, the subjects were shown an empty container, and it was identified to them as such. The empty container was then placed a predetermined distance from the subjects and remained there for approximately 2 minutes during the acquisition phase for the first control scan. Immediately after the placement of the stimulus, the subjects were instructed to close their eyes and to allow their thoughts to focus on the stimulus. Once the instructions had been given and the subjects' eyes were closed, PET acquisition commenced. At the end of each scan, vital signs, including radial pulse and respiratory rate, were monitored. The stimulus was removed, and the subjects were asked to rate the severity of their anxiety via the AAS, based on the preceding scanning period. This procedure was repeated with the stimulus placed on the contralateral side to achieve a complete set of data for each of two control scans for each subject.

Next, in the provocation phase, the procedure was repeated for two provoked scans, during which the subjects were exposed to an individualized provocative stimulus (eg, the container with the feared animal inside) (Table 1) in place of the innocuous stimulus. The interscan interval was approximately 10 minutes between successive scans in every case. In all conditions, the scans were performed with low background noise and lighting and with eyes closed and ears not plugged.

TEETH-CLENCHING CONTROL

Because a preliminary analysis of the data (n=6) indicated anterior temporal cortical activation and because extracranial muscle contraction has been reported to produce blood flow artifacts in this region,[21] a teeth-clenching control was conducted in one subject (subject 7). The subject was instructed to clench her teeth repeatedly during one scan-

Continued on next page

ning period with the innocuous stimulus on her right and during a second scan with the innocuous stimulus on her left. In this manner, a teeth-clenching condition minus control condition subtraction could be used to demonstrate the pattern of activation associated with teeth clenching.

PET FACILITIES AND PROCEDURES

The PET facilities and procedures were identical to those previously described for the OCD study.[1] A 15-slice whole-body tomograph (Scanditronix PC4096, General Electric, Milwaukee, Wis) was used in its stationary mode to acquire the PET data. A detailed report on the physical properties and reconstruction software has been published elsewhere.[22] The slice geometry consists of contiguous slices with a center-to-center distance of 6.5 mm (axial field equal to 97.5 mm) and axial resolution of 6.0 mm (full-width half maximum). Image reconstruction was performed using a measured attenuation correction and a Hanning-weighted reconstruction filter set to yield 8.0-mm in-plane spatial resolution (full-width half maximum). Additional corrections were made in the reconstruction process to account for scattered radiation, random coincidences, and counting losses due to dead time caused by the camera electronics.

SUBJECT POSITIONING

Within the PET scanner, the head was aligned relative to the canthomeatal line, using horizontal and vertical projected laser lines whose positions are known with respect to the slice positions of the scanner. An individually molded thermoplastic face mask (True Scan, Annapolis, Md) was used to minimize head motion. Once the head was in place, the patient was fitted with a nasal cannula and an overlying face mask that were attached to radiolabeled gas inflow and vacuum, respectively.

IMAGE ACQUISITION

Prior to emission scanning, several transmission measurements were made using an orbiting pin source. Each PET data acquisition run consisted of 15 periods of measurement (called frames), the first three of 10 seconds' duration each and the remaining 12 of 5 seconds' duration each. Subjects began inhaling ^{15}O-labeled CO_2 gas 30 seconds after the initiation of the scan and finished 60 seconds later. Frames 4 through 15 were summed after reconstruction to form images of relative blood flow.

The subjects were studied during a 1-minute period in which they continuously inhaled tracer quantities of ^{15}O-labeled CO_2 while breathing room air. The concentration of the delivered gas was 2960 MBq/L with a flow rate of 2 L/min, which was further diluted by free mixture with room air within the face mask, resulting in a rapidly rising count rate in the brain that reached terminal count rates of 100 000 to 200 000 events per second. An evaluation of these techniques by the Radiation Safety Committee at Massachusetts General Hospital has determined that the radiation exposure for each subject associated with participation in this study be less than a 500-mrem effective-dose equivalent. Previous work in our laboratory (N. M. Alpert, PhD, unpublished data, 1991) using radial artery cannulation has demonstrated that the integrated counts over inhalation periods of up to 90 seconds is a linear function over the flow range of 0 to 130 mL/min per 100 g. Therefore, for data to be produced with units of flow relative to whole brain, no arterialized blood and thus no arterial line was necessary.

IMAGE ANALYSES

Whole-slice tracings for each slice across conditions were compared within subjects to rule out detectable intrascan or interscan head movement. In this study, no data required exclusion on this basis.[1] The PET brain images were transformed to the standard Talairach coordinate system[23] as previously described.[1,24]

The mean concentration in each run was obtained as an area-weighted sum of the concentration of each slice and was adjusted to a nominal value of 50 mL/min per 100 g, yielding what are referred to as normalized blood flow images. The data were then rescaled and smoothed with a two-dimensional gaussian filter with a width of 20 mm (full-width half maximum).[25] These images were pooled over all subjects for each scanning condition, and pairwise subtractions were performed (within subject and between conditions) to yield images of the differences and SDs. From these data, t values were computed and converted into z values by an integral transformation that produced statistical parametric maps (SPMs) with values in z-score units (previously termed "omnibus subtraction images"[1] and sometimes called "z maps").[25]

The basic approach for statistical analysis and hypothesis testing was identical to that previously described[1] (adapted from Friston et al[25]) and allowed computation of a pixel threshold depending on image smoothness and the number of pixels in the region of interest corresponding to the hypothesis to be tested. In this manner, the threshold for statistical significance was adjusted appropriately for multiple comparisons (ie, many pixels). The parameter of image smoothness was measured as described by Friston et al and was found to be 14.2 mm.

Three types of analyses were performed once the transformations of the PET data were performed, the data were expressed in stereotactic space, and SPMs were created:

1. The entire brain was inspected for foci of activation with z scores of 3.75 or greater. Such robust activations meet the criterion for statistical significance ($P<.05$) with Bonferroni-type correction for multiple comparisons (ie, many pixels), even in the absence of any hypotheses (ie, conservatively corrected for approximately 3000 pixels per slice, which represents the number of pixels from the largest brain slice).

2. Specific regions corresponding to the a priori hypotheses were automatically and objectively outlined via a digitized mapping program[23,26] and then systematically were inspected for locations of maximal activation.

3. The whole brain was again inspected, post hoc, in search of additional regions of activation of a magnitude comparable to those achieving statistical significance by virtue of a priori hypotheses (in this case, $z\geq3.0$, which corresponds approximately to $P=.001$ uncorrected for multiple comparisons).

For all three types of analyses, SPMs of provoked minus control conditions were used.

dependent characteristics could be identified, and each patient could serve as his or her own control.

Based on neurobiologic models of anxiety,[13-17] we framed a priori hypotheses that the provocation of SP symptoms would result in increased rCBF in specific components of the limbic and paralimbic systems (ie, anterior temporal cortex, anterior cingulate cortex, parahippocampal gyrus, amygdaloid complex, and medial orbitofrontal cortex) as well as in the thalamus.

RESULTS

The study yielded usable data in the form of 11 scans rather than 14 for each of the control and provoked conditions from the seven subjects studied. For three subjects, data from one scan in each condition rather than from two were used in the analysis because anxiety was not clinically activated (n=1; AAS score was not greater than that for the control scans) and because data could not be acquired owing to the subjects' discomfort from lying flat for the necessary scanning time (n=2). Also, the study yielded two scans in the teeth-clenching condition from subject 7.

CLINICAL INDEXES

For all seven subjects, the provoked condition was associated with increased anxiety as measured by the AAS in comparison with the innocuous-stimuli condition (Table 1). Mean±SD AAS scores were 1.00±0.87 for the control and 5.14±1.49 for the provoked conditions, representing a significant mean increase in AAS of 4.1 ($t[6]=9.29$, $P<.0001$) with provocation. Autonomic indices were similarly significantly increased from the control to the provoked state; mean±SD pulse rate increased from 68.7±4.9/min to 77.1±9.4/min ($t[6]=3.42$, $P=.01$), and mean±SD respiratory rate increased from 18.6±3.6/min to 22.9±2.8/min ($t[6]=3.04$, $P=.02$).

STATISTICAL PARAMETRIC MAPS

Pertinent SPMs are shown in the **Figure**; SPMs are presented with superimposed outlines demarcating relevant regions of interest (ROIs).[23,26]

Inspection of the entire brain SPM revealed four different regional activations with maximum pixel values reflecting z scores of 3.75 or greater: in the left insular cortex, for the horizontal slice 12 mm inferior to the anterior commissure–posterior commissure (AC-PC) plane, the SPM maximum pixel value was 4.41; in anterior temporal cortex, for the horizontal slice 4 mm inferior to the AC-PC plane, the SPM maximum pixel value was 4.32 (right side only); in the anterior cingulate cortex, for the horizontal slice 12 mm superior to the AC-PC plane, the SPM maximum pixel value was 4.71; in the left somatosensory cortex, for the horizontal slice 60 mm superior to the AC-PC plane, the SPM maximum pixel value was 3.84.

Next, maximum pixel values with units in terms of z scores were identified within the boundaries of each ROI corresponding to the a priori hypotheses. These values were compared with significance thresholds that reflected an a priori criterion of $P<.05$ for one-tailed t tests and were dependent on the number of pixels for each ROI. For the anterior cingulate cortex and the anterior temporal pole, activations had already been found that met more stringent criteria for statistical significance. In the case of the medial orbitofrontal cortex, for the horizontal slice 16 mm inferior to the AC-PC plane, the SPM maximum pixel value within the ROI was 3.01, with the centroid of activation located in the left posterior medial orbitofrontal cortex. The number of pixels for the orbitofrontal cortex was 414, resulting in an adjusted significance threshold ($P<.05$) of greater than 2.85. Thus the 3.01 value reflected a probability value of $P=.03$. In the case of the thalamus, for the horizontal slice 4 mm superior to the AC-PC plane, the SPM maximum pixel value within the ROI was 3.00 (left side only). The number of pixels for the thalamus was 128 (64×2), resulting in a significance threshold ($P<.05$) of greater than 2.33. Thus the 3.00 value reflected a probability value of $P=.01$. In the case of the parahippocampal gyrus and amygdala, no foci of activation approached statistical significance (all z scores, <1.5).

Finally, in an attempt to avoid bias as a consequence of differential thresholds for statistical significance, all territories of the SPM were further inspected for any activations characterized by z scores comparable to those for the a priori hypotheses (ie, ≥3.0). No additional foci of activation achieved this more liberal criterion.

TEETH-CLENCHING CONDITION

Inspection of the mean-difference normalized rCBF map for the teeth-clenching condition minus the control condition (examined prior to stereotactic transformation) demonstrated a robust focal activation (>100%) located distinctly outside the whole brain demarcation. The Talairach coordinates of this activation centroid (determined by back transformation) were 53.0, 38.0, and −5.5 (x,y,z). Thus, the coordinates of the activation centroid were more than 23 mm anterior to the anterior temporal locus of activation. Next, the most proximal extent of activation in the teeth-clenching minus control mean-difference map was determined in an attempt to rule out the possiblity that wash from an extracranial source could be responsible for the anterior temporal activation. The most proximal pixel of positive activation that was contiguous with the teeth-clenching activation centroid was located approximately 12 mm anterolateral to the anterior temporal locus of activation. Next, at the site identified as the anterior temporal pole on Talairach transformed images, the normalized rCBF values for each of the teeth-clenching–condition scans were compared with those from the control- and provoked-condition scans: mean teeth-clenching–condition rCBF was 35.1 (individual values, 34.6 and 35.5), control-condition rCBF was 31.5 (individual values, 28.0 and 34.9), and the provoked-condition rCBF was 45.8 (only one scan was obtained). Finally, the full-cohort SPM was reinspected to determine the pattern of activation adjacent and peripheral to the identified anterior temporal locus. If this activation was attributable to wash from an extracranial source, one

Table 1. Description of Challenge Stimuli, Symptom Provoked, and Resulting Phobic Anxiety Analog Scale (AAS) Scores for Each Subject

Patient No.	Challenge Stimulus		Provoked Symptom	AAS Score	
	Innocuous	Provocative		Control*	Provoked†
1	Empty container	Container and snake	Snake phobia	1.00	6.50
2‡	Empty container	Container and rat	Rodent phobia	0	4.00
3	20×28-cm picture of horse	20×28-cm picture of snake	Snake phobia	1.50	5.50
4	Empty container	Container and bees	Stinging-insect phobia	1.00	4.00
5‡	Empty container	Container and spider	Spider phobia	1.00	7.00
6	Empty container	Container and bees	Stinging-insect phobia	2.50	6.00
7‡	Empty container	Container and spider	Spider phobia	0	3.00

*Mean±SE, 1.00±0.87.
†Mean±SE, 5.14±1.49. The increase in AAS score was significant: dependent $t(6)=9.29$, $P<.0001$.
‡The AAS scores were based on a single scan for these patients. For all other patients, scores represent mean of two scans.

would expect to see increasing z scores lateral to the identified centroid. In the relevant slice (4 mm inferior to the AC-PC plane), z scores immediately lateral to the identified anterior temporal locus of activation went from 4.32 at the centroid to 3.99 to 3.72 to 3.28 for successive pixels. Comparable patterns also were seen in the slices immediately superior and inferior to the slice of interest.

CORRELATION ANALYSES

Correlation analyses using the Pearson Product-Moment Correlation Coefficient were performed for AAS scores with rCBF for control and provoked conditions at the six sites of significant activation (ie, the sites listed in **Table 2**). For each subject in each condition, mean rCBF values were determined within circular ROIs of fixed diameter (5 pixels; 21 to 26 pixels in area). This was identical to an approach employed previously.[1] The rationale for using a ROI of fixed area deserves explanation. This approach is consistent with the analysis in stereotactic coordinates and is easily and objectively applied, facilitating the replication of the method for use in other studies. The fixed area that was selected for the ROIs reflects the heavily smoothed nature of the images and minimizes errors associated with localization. If a single pixel approach had been used, for instance, given the variability in local maxima from subject to subject, the relative magnitude of activation for each subject would likely have been misrepresented. The ROIs were positioned around the centroids of maximal statistical activation, based on the maximum pixel coordinates from the SPMs. Correlation coefficients and probability matrices were generated for all ROIs to evaluate the relationship between rCBF and AAS scores for the provoked condition or all conditions, as well as the relationship between the provoked-condition minus control-condition rCBF differences and the AAS difference scores. None of these correlations approached significance (all P's>.10).

COMMENT

In the current study, we found statistically significant normalized rCBF increases during the SP symptomatic vs control condition in left posterior medial orbitofrontal cortex, left insular cortex, left thalamus, right anterior temporal cortex, anterior cingulate cortex, and left somatosensory cortex. No statistically significant increases in rCBF were found in anterior medial orbitofrontal cortex, the parahippocampal gyrus, or the amygdaloid complex.

There exist a variety of schemes for determining significance thresholds when analyzing SPMs. Although we employed both a naturalistic and a hypothesis-driven approach with adjustment for multiple comparisons, it is important to consider how the results or interpretations might have differed had other methods been used. If a naturalistic approach alone had been taken (ie, no a priori hypotheses) and a liberal threshold had been arbitrarily adopted (ie, $z \geq 3.0$; reflecting approximately $P=.001$ without adjustment for multiple comparisons), the foci of activation identified as significant would have been identical. If a naturalistic approach alone had been taken and a conservative threshold had been adopted (ie, $z \geq 3.75$; reflecting $P<.05$ with adjustment for multiple comparisons reflecting whole-slice pixel number), the foci of activation identified as significant would have differed in that the thalamic and orbitofrontal findings would not have met this stringent criterion. If a strictly hypothesis-driven approach had been taken, insular and somatosensory cortical activations would have been missed.

The pattern of activation reported is remarkably consistent with the clinical phenomenology of SP and the known functional neuroanatomy of these paralimbic structures. The paralimbic belt comprises caudal orbitofrontal cortex, anterior temporal cortex, insular cortex, anterior cingulate cortex, and the parahippocampal gyrus.[16] This system is purported to integrate inputs from heteromodal association cortex, primary sensory cortex, and limbic structures.[16] In this way, the paralimbic system is theorized to play a critical role in the assessment of and response to the behavioral relevance of extrapersonal stimuli.[16] Studies in nonhuman primates have demonstrated that paralimbic orbitofrontal lesions result in alterations in the response to novel stimuli (eg, snakes).[27] The five paralimbic regions activated in this SP PET study also have been associated with autonomic responses when they were electrically stimulated in humans and animals.[16,28,29] Therefore, it makes sense that differential activity within this system during the provoked state should be associated with autonomic hyper-

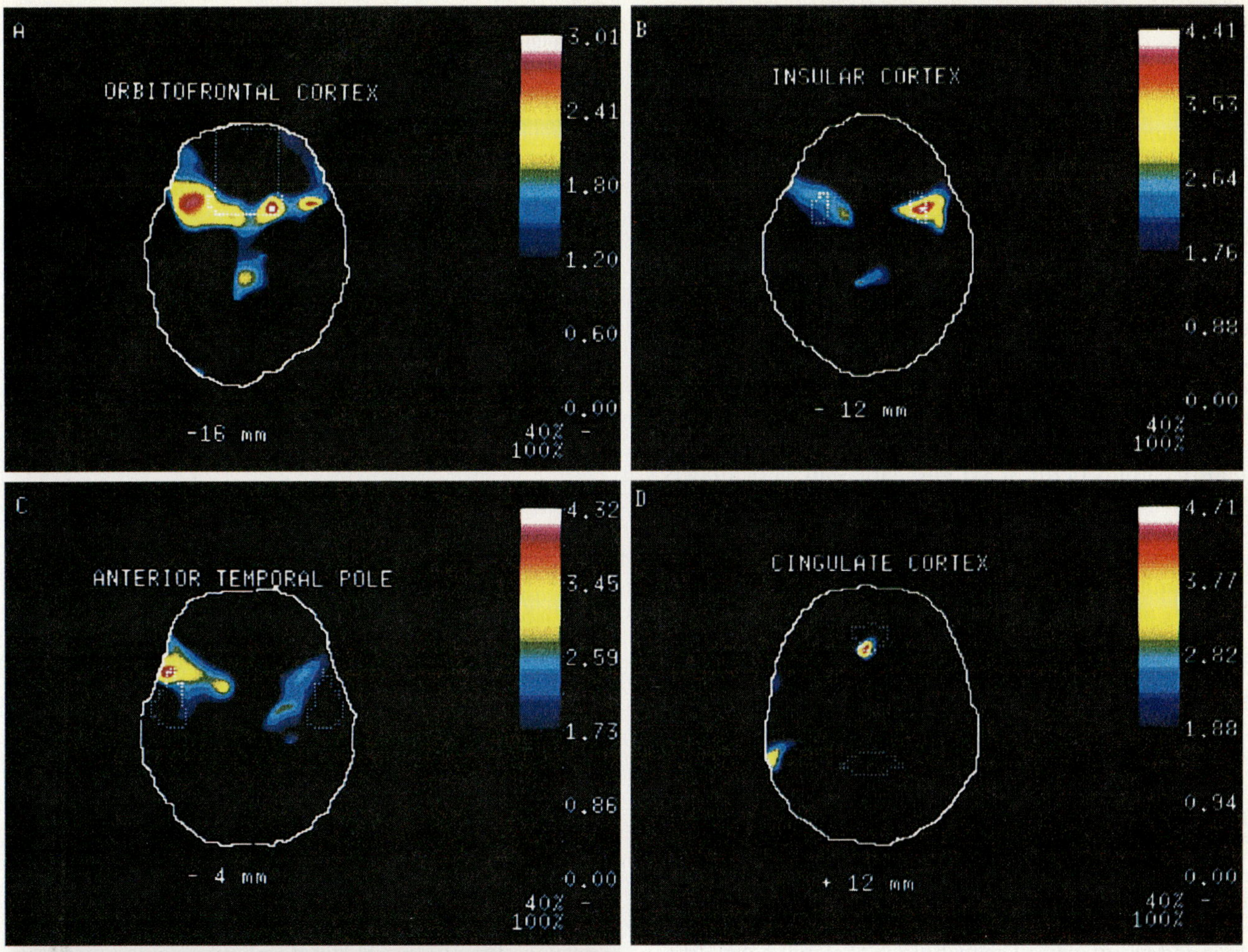

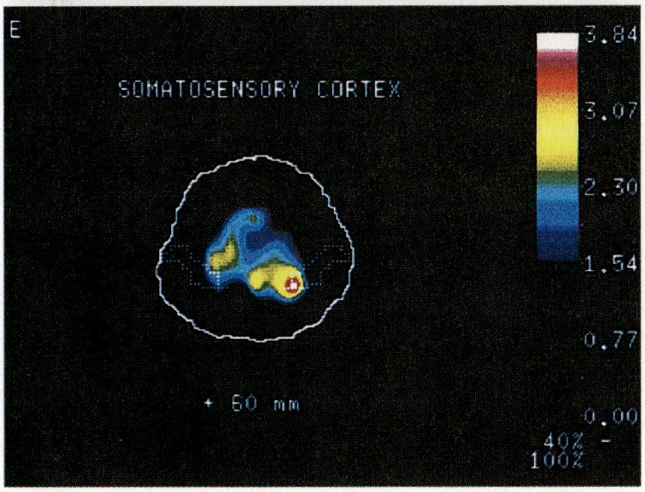

Positron emission tomographic statistical parametric maps of provoked minus control conditions for all subjects (N=7; 11 scans per condition) are displayed with a Sokoloff color scale in units of z score. White dashed outlines reflecting the boundaries of brain regions of interest, as defined via a digitized version of the Talairach atlas,[26] are superimposed for anatomical reference. Whole-brain slice outlines are demarcated with solid lines. All images are transverse sections parallel to the anterior commissure–posterior commissure (AC-PC) plane, shown in conventional neuroimaging orientation (top is anterior; bottom, posterior; right, left; and left, right). Each transverse section is labeled with its z coordinate, which denotes its position with respect to the AC-PC plane (greater than zero denotes superior). Activation is demonstrated within regions of interest. A, Left posterior medial orbitofrontal cortex (z score, 3.01). B, Left insular cortex (z score, 4.41). C, Right anterior temporal pole (z score, 4.32). D, Anterior cingulate cortex (z score, 4.71). E, Left somatosensory cortex (3.84). Activation within the left thalamus (z score, 3.00) at 4 mm superior to AC-PC plane is not shown.

activity and an exaggerated anxiety response to novel or innocuous stimuli.

Increased rCBF in somatosensory cortex was unexpected. On follow-up interviews with the subjects, all seven reported that both tactile and visual imagery were invoked during their response to the provocative stimuli; four of seven reported that tactile imagery was the most prominent sensory aspect of the phobic experience. A review of the data (not shown) demonstrated that increases in normalized rCBF during the provoked vs control condition occurred within left somatosensory cortex for all subjects and all trials (ie, during both right- and left-sided exposure to the stimulus). Moreover, it should be emphasized that four of the subjects were not touching the stimulus and that for the other three, the primary sensory stimulation was identical for the provoked and control conditions (ie, touching the outside of the same container). Therefore, because all subjects were right-handed, one interpretation of the results is that tactile imagery, as one component of the phobic symptomatic state, was mediated via dominant somatosensory cortex. Other investigators collaborating with our PET laboratory have shown that visual imagery is mediated by and topographically mapped within visual cortex.[30] Our findings are particularly interesting given that the major relay of somatosensory inflow into the limbic system is via the insular cortex.[16,31]

The reason for the observed laterality of activation foci is unclear. One possibility is that structures are involved bilaterally but that type II error acounts for unilateral findings. A second possibility is that the laterality observed reflects asymmetries that were not fully controlled in the paradigm. For instance, the preponderance of left-sided brain findings may reflect lateralized stimulation via dominant-sided imagery. A third possibility relates to functional asymmetries in the mediating neuroanatomy of the SP symptomatic state or of anxiety states in general. The right-sided anterior temporal activation, for instance, would seem to replicate previous reports by Reiman and colleagues.[32,33]

Limitations of the present study include the small number of subjects and their heterogeneity with regard to SP provocative stimuli. Replication with larger numbers could provide superior power for testing questions pertaining to interregion correlations as well as clinical measures by regional activation correlations. The finding that regional activation magnitudes did not significantly correlate with symptom severity is not surprising given the crude nature of the clinical measure used (ie, the AAS). Future studies might seek to use more refined measurements of subjective-state variables.

This study also suffers from limitations intrinsic to the methods and technologies used, which have been enumerated previously.[1] The technique of signal normalization to the whole brain, although it reduces variance and obviates the issue of whole brain P_{CO_2} correction, does not allow for the detection of changes in whole brain cerebral blood flow. In fact, it remains unclear whether changes in respiratory rate, P_{CO_2}, and whole brain cerebral blood flow might confound findings in studies such as this one that rely on normalized cerebral blood flow values. Moreover, localization of change in rCBF is constrained by the spatial resolution of PET. Head movement cannot be absolutely prevented, and there are limitations in the sensitivity of its detection and correction by the methods used in this study. Together with the technique of stereotaxic transformation, these must be acknowledged as potential sources of error in terms of precise anatomic localization. Coupled with the statistical approach of Friston et al,[25] these factors contribute to the risk of type II errors. Still, the advantages of this technique remain as follows: the capability to sum data across subjects and the superior power for identifying locations of differential activation by avoiding dependence on large arbitrary or anatomically restrictive ROIs.

Finally, an attempt was made to control for artifacts that are attributable to extracranial blood flow changes. Interpretations of the teeth-clenching control results provide additional support for the contention that the activation identified as anterior temporal in origin was not attributable to an extracranial source. Nonetheless, the limited nature of these data (n=1) do not absolutely preclude this or other confounding influences.

Table 2. Regions of Interest Exhibiting Significantly Increased Activation Associated With Provocation of Phobic Anxiety

Region of Interest	Maximum Pixel Value, *z* Score Units*	Maximum Pixel Coordinates†
Anterior cingulate cortex (right)	4.71‡	4, 31, 12
Insular cortex (left)	4.41‡	−34, 7, −12
Anterior temporal pole (right)	4.32‡	52, 15, −4
Somatosensory cortex (left)	3.84‡	−24, −41, 60
Orbitofrontal cortex (left posterior)	3.01§	−16, 10, −16
Thalamus (left)	3.00§	−15, −23, 4

*Values represent the actual maximum pixel value (in z score units) within the region of interest from the statistical parametric map.

†Coordinates defining the location of the maximum pixel values within each region of interest from the statistical parametric maps in Talairach space[23] are expressed as "x, y, z"; x>0 is right of the midsagittal plane, y>0 is anterior to the anterior commissure, and z>0 is superior to the anterior-commissure–posterior-commissure plane.*

‡Regional activations with z scores ≥3.75 corresponding to statistical significance at P<.05 for one-tailed t tests in the context of stringent Bonferroni-like correction for multiple comparisons in the absence of any a priori hypothesis (ie, approximately 3000 pixels per slice).

§Regional activations not meeting strict Bonferroni-type correction as above until the number of multiple comparisons are reduced, thereby reflecting the number of pixels in the region of interest corresponding to a priori hypotheses. z scores ≥3.0 also correspond to P=.001, uncorrected for multiple comparisons.

The power of the current findings would be enhanced by convergence with other neuroimaging studies. As noted above, two previous PET symptom-provocation studies of simple phobia yielded disparate findings, despite the application of considerable scientific rigor and the use of accepted (although different) methods.[11,12] Mountz and colleagues[11] reported negative findings altogether, whereas Fredrikson and colleagues[12] found activation of visual areas as well as frontothalamic correlations in the SP but not the control conditions. The reason for the apparent disparity in results is unknown but may be due to differences between study populations or methods. Fredrikson and colleagues studied only subjects with snake phobias, whereas we and the Mountz group studied cohorts that were representative of a variety of small animal phobias. The results of these studies are especially prone to the effects of intersubject differences because the number of subjects studied is so small.

Mountz and colleagues[11] used an ROI-based data analysis scheme that is reliant on magnetic resonance imaging templates. Depending on the placement and the size of the ROIs employed, this technique may have been less sensitive to the detection of significant activation than were the SPM techniques employed in the other two studies. The potential benefits of the SPM approach are highlighted in cases in which the structures to be inspected are large and the territories of significant activation are small, as is the case for many of the findings that we report. For instance, the activation observed in the posterior medial orbitofrontal cortex would undoubtedly have been missed in a comparison of mean cerebral blood flow averaged over the entire extent of the medial orbitofrontal cortex.

Fredrikson and colleagues[12] employed an activation paradigm that differed from the other two studies in that subjects underwent PET scanning with eyes open in the presence of ongoing affectively relevant visual stimulation. In this sense, our finding of increased rCBF in the somatosensory cortex may be conceptualized as analogous to their finding of visual cortical activation. These sensory activations may be epiphenomena that reflect the route of sensory inflow (ie, tactile imagery, visual imagery, or visual perception) from the provocative stimuli. The reason for the discrepant findings with regard to paralimbic structures is unclear. One possibility is that Fredrikson and colleagues did not analyze data from these regions (they are not mentioned with respect to a priori hypotheses or post hoc analyses). Another possibility is that subjects had their anxiety more robustly provoked in one study or the other.

Nonetheless, the findings of the current study are consonant with those of Fredrikson and colleagues[12] with respect to the implication of thalamic activation (specifically, left thalamic activation) and the absence of striatal or dorsolateral prefrontal activation in SP anxiety.

In general, to date, neuroimaging studies of anxiety have yielded many inconsistencies. For instance, early replicated findings of right temporal activation in subjects with lactate-sensitive panic disorder[32,33] were later corrected when improvements in localization techniques and the addition of control conditions suggested that the observed increased cerebral blood flow signal emanated from extracranial musculature rather than from the brain.[21] In this regard, the findings of the current study suggest that the role of anterior temporal cortex in anxiety states should be further explored and that controls for extracranial activation sources may be helpful in distinguishing brain activation from artifact. A host of other studies that examined anxiety states in normal subjects,[34-36] subjects with generalized anxiety disorder,[37] subjects with small animal phobia,[11,12] and subjects with lactate-induced panic attacks[38] have led to negative or inconsistent results. In contrast, the literature pertaining to OCD[3,5] reflects a somewhat more convergent series of findings.

As noted above, analogous methods and design were used previously to study the mediating neuroanatomy of OCD symptoms.[1] Findings of that study included a relative increase in rCBF during the OCD symptomatic state vs the control state in right caudate nucleus, left anterior cingulate cortex, as well as right posterior and left anterior medial orbitofrontal cortex.[1] Activation in the left thalamus approached but did not reach statistical significance. Those findings were consistent with previous neuroimaging studies,[4,5,8] as well as contemporary theories of OCD pathophysiology.[2-7] The OCD analog scale scores were positively correlated only with activation of left anterior medial orbitofrontal cortex.[1] Unexpected regions of activation, although only approaching statistical significance, included left angular gyrus, left visual association cortex, and bilateral dorsolateral prefrontal cortex.[1]

The data presented herein from an SP cohort may be compared with the data from the earlier OCD study[1]; however, interpretations from such a comparison must be made cautiously because the study groups are imperfectly matched (especially with regard to gender; the OCD cohort consisted of five men and three women) and the paradigms were not identical (eg, in the OCD study, all stimuli were presented to the subjects' left side). Increased normalized rCBF during the symptomatic vs control state was found for both OCD and SP cohorts in posterior medial orbitofrontal cortex, anterior cingulate cortex (both are approximately in Brodmann area 24), and the left thalamus. This overlap suggests that a system that involves these structures might mediate anxiety in a nonspecific sense. Increased normalized rCBF during only the SP symptomatic vs the control condition was found in additional paralimbic structures, including the right anterior temporal pole and left insular cortex, as well as dominant somatosensory cortex. Perhaps this reflects the more pronounced hyperautonomic aspects of the phobic state (in the OCD study,[1] there were no significant increases in pulse or respiratory rate [$P>.1$]), and that tactile imagery served as the "currency" of the phobic experience. Increased rCBF during only the OCD symptomatic vs the control state was found in the left anterior medial orbitofrontal cortex, in the right caudate nucleus, and possibly in dorsolateral prefrontal cortex along with language and visual association areas. This suggests that the obsessional state may involve a more prominent cognitive component that is mediated by heteromodal prefrontal cortex, perhaps via corticostriatal pathways. Moreover, consistent with patients' experience, the currency of obsessions typically entails internal narration and visual imagery, reflected by the observed activation of visual and language association cortex.

It must be emphasized that the liability toward type II error further mitigates against conclusions regarding the differences in activation patterns observed for these two symptomatic states. For instance, in other symptom-provocation studies of OCD, temporal[39,40] and insular[40] activations have been found. Therefore, these findings must be interpreted cautiously pending further study. Moreover, there may be substantial interindividual and intraindividual variability in the OCD as well as the SP symptomatic states, which belies composite characterization across an entire cohort.

In summary, the current study demonstrated a pattern of increased normalized rCBF that was associated with the SP symptomatic state and that included components of the paralimbic system as well as somatosensory cortex. Future studies will seek to replicate these findings as well as to explore the changes in activation patterns that accompany symptomatic improvement following treatment. Finally, rather than using a symptom-provocation approach, neuropsychological activation paradigms are being developed in the hope of probing these same neural systems in a more tightly controlled fashion (S.L.R., C.R.S., H. D. Brown, T. Curran, unpublished data, 1993).

Accepted for publication September 28, 1994.

This study was supported in part by grant 5T32CA09362-11 from the National Cancer Institute, Bethesda, Md (Dr Rauch), and by a Young Investigator Award from the National Alliance for Research on Schizophrenia and Depression, Chicago, Ill (Dr Rauch). Partial support for this project was also provided by the David Judah Research Fund, Boston.

We wish to thank Dmitry Berdichevsky, MS, Avis Loring, and Steve Weise for their technical assistance.

Reprint request to OCD Unit, 9th floor, Massachusetts General Hospital-East, 149 13th St, Charlestown, MA 02129 (Dr Rauch).

REFERENCES

1. Rauch SL, Jenike MA, Alpert NM, Baer L, Breiter HCR, Savage CR, Fischman AJ. Regional cerebral blood flow measured during symptom provocation in obsessive-compulsive disorder using oxygen 15–labeled carbon dioxide and positron emission tomography. *Arch Gen Psychiatry.* 1994;51:62-70.
2. Baxter LR, Schwartz JM, Guze BH, Bergman K, Szuba MP. Neuroimaging in obsessive-compulsive disorder: seeking the mediating neuroanatomy. In: Jenike MA, Baer L, Minichiello WE, eds. *Obsessive Compulsive Disorder: Theory and Management.* 2nd ed. St Louis, Mo: Mosby–Year Book; 1990:167-188.
3. Baxter LR. Neuroimaging studies of obsessive compulsive disorder. *Psychiatr Clin North Am.* 1992;15:871-884.
4. Baxter LR Jr, Schwartz JM, Bergman KS, Szuba MP, Guze BH, Mazziotta JC, Alazraki A, Selin CE, Ferng H-K, Munford P, Phelps ME. Caudate glucose metabolic rate changes with both drug and behavior therapy for obsessive-compulsive disorder. *Arch Gen Psychiatry.* 1992;49:681-689.
5. Insel TR. Toward a neuroanatomy of obsessive-compulsive disorder. *Arch Gen Psychiatry.* 1992;49:739-744.
6. Modell J, Mountz J, Curtis G, Greden J. Neurophysiologic dyfunction in basal ganglia/limbic striatal and thalamocortical circuits as a pathogenetic mechanism of obsessive-compulsive disorder. *J Neuropsychiatry Clin Neurosci.* 1989; 1:27-36.
7. Rauch SL, Jenike MA. Neurobiological models of obsessive compulsive disorder. *Psychosomatics.* 1993;34:20-32.
8. Swedo SE, Pietrini P, Leonard HL, Schapiro MB, Rettew DC, Goldberger EL, Rapoport SI, Rapoport JL, Grady CL. Cerebral glucose metabolism in childhood-onset obsessive-compulsive disorder: revisualization during pharmacotherapy. *Arch Gen Psychiatry.* 1992;49:690-694.
9. American Psychiatric Association. *Diagnostic and Statistical Manual of Mental Disorders, Revised Third Edition.* Washington, DC: American Psychiatric Association; 1987.
10. Robins LN, Regier DA, eds. *Psychiatric Disorders in America: the Epidemiological Catchment Area Study.* New York, NY: Free Press; 1991.
11. Mountz JM, Modell JG, Wilson MW, Curtis GC, Lee MA, Schmaltz S, Kuhl DE. Positron emission tomographic evaluation of cerebral blood flow during state anxiety in simple phobia. *Arch Gen Psychiatry.* 1989;46:501-504.
12. Fredrikson M, Wik G, Greitz T, Eriksson L, Stone-Elander S, Ericson K, Sedvall G. Regional cerebral blood flow during experimental phobic fear. *Psychophysiology.* 1993;30:126-130.
13. Charney DS, Deutch AY, Krystal JH, Southwick SM, Davis M. Psychobiologic mechanisms of posttraumatic stress disorder. *Arch Gen Psychiatry.* 1993;50: 294-305.
14. Doane BK, Livingston KF, eds. *The Limbic System: Functional Organization and Clinical Disorders.* New York, NY: Raven Press; 1986.
15. Gorman JM, Liebowitz MR, Fyer AJ, Stein J. A neuroanatomical hypothesis for panic disorder. *Am J Psychiatry.* 1989;146:148-161.
16. Mesulam M-M. Patterns in behavioral neuroanatomy: association areas, the limbic system, and hemispheric specialization. In: Mesulam M-M, ed. *Principles of Behavioral Neurology.* Philadelphia, Pa: FA Davis Co Publishers; 1985: 1-70.
17. Papez JW. Proposed mechanism of emotion. *Arch Neurol Psychiatry.* 1937; 38:725-743.
18. Spitzer RL, Williams JBW, Gibbon M, First MB. *Structured Clinical Interview for DSM-III-R: Outpatient Version.* New York, NY: Biometrics Research Department; 1988.
19. Oldfield RC. The assessment and analysis of handedness: the Edinburgh Inventory. *Neuropsychologia.* 1971;9:97-113.
20. Beck AT, Ward CH, Mendelson M, Mock J, Erbaugh J. An inventory for measuring depression. *Arch Gen Psychiatry.* 1961;4:561-571.
21. Drevets WC, Videen TO, MacLeod AK, Haller JW, Raichle ME. PET images of blood flow changes during anxiety: correction. *Science.* 1992;256:1696.
22. Kops ER, Herzog H, Schmid A, Holte S, Feinendegen LE. Performance characteristics of an eight-ring whole body PET scanner. *J Comput Assist Tomogr.* 1990;14:437-445.
23. Talairach J, Tournoux P. *Co-Planar Stereotaxic Atlas of the Human Brain.* New York, NY: Thieme Medical Publishers Inc; 1988.
24. Alpert NM, Berdichevsky D, Weise S, Tang J, Rauch SL. Stereotactic transformation of PET scans by nonlinear least squares. In: Uemura K, Lassen NA, Jones T, Kanno I, eds. *Quantification of Brain Function: Proceedings of PET '93.* Amsterdam, the Netherlands: Elsevier Science Publishers; 1993:459-463.
25. Friston K, Frith C, Liddle P, Franckowiak R. Comparing functional (PET) images: the assessment of significant change. *J Cereb Blood Flow Metab.* 1991; 11:690-699.
26. Talairach J, Szikla Z. *Atlas of Stereotactic Anatomy of the Telencephalon.* Paris, France: Masson and Cie; 1967.
27. Butter CM, Snyder DR. Alterations in aversive and aggressive behaviors following orbitofrontal lesions in rhesus monkeys. *Acta Neurobiol Exp (Warsz).* 1972;32:525-565.
28. Kaada BR. Cingulate, posterior orbital, anterior insular and temporal pole cortex. In: Magoun HW, ed. *Neurophysiology.* Baltimore, Md: Waverly Press; 1960: 1345-1372.
29. Kaada BR, Pribram KH, Epstein JA. Respiratory and vascular responses in monkeys from temporal pole, insula, orbital surface, and cingulate gyrus. *J Neurophysiol.* 1949;12:348-356.
30. Kosslyn SM, Alpert NM, Thompson WL, Maljkovic V, Weise SB, Chabris CF, Hamilton SE, Rauch SL, Buonano FS. Visual imagery activates topographically organized visual cortex: PET investigations. *J Cogn Neurosci.* 1993;5:263-287.
31. Mesulam M-M, Mufson EJ. Insula of the old world monkey, III: efferent cortical output and comments on function. *J Comp Neurol.* 1982;212:38-52.
32. Reiman EM, Rachle ME, Butler FK, Herscovitch P, Robins E. A focal brain abnormality in panic disorder, a severe form of anxiety. *Nature.* 1984;310:683-685.
33. Reiman EM, Raichle ME, Robins E, Mintun MA, Fusselman MJ, Fox PT, Price JL, Hackman KA. Neuroanatomical correlates of a lactate-induced anxiety attack. *Arch Gen Psychiatry.* 1989;46:493-500.
34. Giordani B, Boivin MJ, Berent S, Betley AT, Koeppe RA, Rothley JM, Modell JG, Hichwa RD, Kuhl DE. Anxiety and cerebral cortical metabolism in normal persons. *Psychiatry Res.* 1990;35:49-60.
35. Gottschalk LA, Buchsbaum MS, Gillin JC, Wu J, Reynolds CA, Herrera DB. The effect of anxiety and hostility in silent mentation on localized cerebral glucose metabolism. *Compr Psychiatry.* 1992;33:52-59.
36. Gur RC, Gur RE, Resnick SM, Skolnick BE, Alavi A, Reivich M. The effects of anxiety on cortical cerebral blood flow and metabolism. *J Cereb Blood Flow Metab.* 1987;7:173-177.
37. Wu JC, Buchsbaum MS, Hershey TG, Hazlett E, Sicotte N, Johnson JC. PET in generalized anxiety disorder. *Biol Psychiatry.* 1991;29:1181-1199.
38. Stewart RS, Devous MD, Rush AJ, Lane L, Bonte FJ. Cerebral blood flow changes during sodium-lactate-induced panic attacks. *Am J Psychiatry.* 1988;145:442-449.
39. Zohar J, Insel TR, Berman KF, Foa EB, Hill JL, Weinberger DR. Anxiety and cerebral blood flow during behavioral challenge: dissociation of central from peripheral and subjective measures. *Arch Gen Psychiatry.* 1989;46:505-510.
40. Breiter HC, Kwong KK, Baker JR, Stern CE, Belliveau JW, Davis TL, Baer L, O'Sullivan RL, Rauch SL, Savage CR, Cohen MS, Weisskoff RM, Brady TJ, Jenike MA, Rosen BR. Functional magnetic resonance imaging of symptom provocation in patients with obsessive-compulsive disorder versus controls. *Soc Neurosci Abstracts.* 1993;19:7. Abstract 9.2.

ORIGINAL ARTICLE

Pharmacotherapy of Impaired Affect in Recovering Schizophrenic Patients

Gerard E. Hogarty, MSW; Joseph P. McEvoy, MD; Richard F. Ulrich, MS; Ann Louise DiBarry, MSN; Partricia Bartone, MSN; Susan Cooley, MEd; Kathleen Hammill, MSN; Mary Carter, PhD; Mark R. Munetz, MD; James Perel, PhD

Background: Prominent and persistent anxiety, depression, and/or negative features characterize a substantial minority of recovered or residually psychotic schizophrenic outpatients and contribute to poor outcome. Because extrapyramidal side effects of typical neuroleptic medications often resemble such features, we first systematically studied the contribution of extrapyramidal side effects to these problems and their treatment. For patients who remained distressed, controlled trials of supplemental thymoleptics were undertaken.

Methods: In trial 1, 92 distressed (depressed and/or anxious) patients and 36 patients in a defect state (patients with negative symptoms) participated in a double-blind, intramuscular challenge that compared centrally acting benztropine mesylate with peripherally acting glycopyrrolate. In trial 2, 57 distressed patients and 22 patients in a defect state were randomly assigned to a double-blind, neuroleptic medication dose-reduction group. In trial 3, 57 chronically distressed patients who were maintained on a low dose of fluphenazine decanoate were randomly assigned to a supplemental desipramine hydrochloride, lithium carbonate, or placebo group under double-blind conditions for 12 weeks.

Results: For patients who were already maintained on antiparkinsonian medication, impaired affect was not resolved by additional benztropine. Only distressed patients with a family history of severe mental disorder (often affective) showed improvement with neuroleptic medication dose reduction. Patients in the defect-state group reported less dysphoria on a reduced neuroleptic medication dose, but negative symptoms persisted. Desipramine improved diverse aspects of mood and residual psychoticism, possibly as a prophylaxis against minor affective exacerbations. Depression improved in women only. Lithium positively affected multiple indexes of anxiety and anxious depression.

Conclusion: Most often, persistent affective impairments are neither resistant extrapyramidal side effects nor characterological traits. Thymoleptics improve the nonphasic, chronic types of anxiety and depression in contrast to the acute, episodic forms, for which little support can be found in the literature.

(Arch Gen Psychiatry. 1995;52:29-41)

ANXIETY, DEPRESSION, and defect features are frequently seen in the postpsychotic phase of schizophrenia.[1] They may contribute to handicaps in personal and social adjustment,[2-4] herald a new psychotic episode,[5] lead to noncompliance,[6] and increase the risk of suicide among recovering patients with schizophrenia.[7]

Explanations for these distressing affects in schizophrenia have ranged from theories that stress the psychological process of recovery from psychosis[8] to those that stress alterations in neurochemistry[9] or even anomalies in neuroanatomical substrates.[10] In addition, typical neuroleptic medications may produce akinesia and akathisia that mimic or at least confound the assessment of affective distress and defect features.[11,12] Defect symptoms have also been conceptualized as resulting from a hypofunctioning mesocortical dopaminergic system that may be further compromised by dopamine antagonists.[9]

Regarding treatment, controversy surrounds the role of antidepressant drug use in schizophrenia.[13-16] A successful 6-week therapeutic study of imipramine hydrochloride for postpsychotic depression[17] and a subsequent prophylactic study[18] are the most clear exceptions. Lithium carbonate (LI) enjoys a better reputation among selected schizophrenic inpatients[15,19,20] but has not been subject to controlled

See Methods on next page

From the Western Psychiatric Institute and Clinic, University of Pittsburgh (Pa) School of Medicine. Dr McEvoy is now with the Duke University Medical Center, Durham, NC, and Dr Munetz is now with the Northeastern Ohio Universities College of Medicine, Rootstown.

METHODS

Eligible patients were 18 to 55 years old, met Research Diagnostic Criteria[23] for either schizophrenia or schizoaffective disorder at the time of their last psychotic episode, and had shown persistent distress or defect features for at least 3 months prior to the study. Most often, the features were present for many years. Positive symptoms of schizophrenia either were absent or, if present, did not interfere with adjustment. All patients were maintained on FD only and, if necessary, were administered an anticholinergic antiparkinsonian drug.

Patients were first screened and selected for inclusion into a distressed (anxiety and/or depression) group based on a rating of 4 (moderate) or greater on a seven-point global judgment of personal distress. In addition, this subsample required a Raskin Depression Scale[24] score of 7 or greater (ie, an admission criterion identical to that used for depressed patients who qualify for trials of a tricyclic antidepressant) and/or a score of 7 or greater on the Covi Anxiety Scale,[25] an instrument that uses the same format as the Raskin Depression Scale. Both include three ratings (subjective report, objective appearance, and secondary neurovegetative features), each of which was scored on a scale of 1 to 5. This subsample is referred to as distressed, even though 47% also met the criteria for the defect-state sample as described below.

Patients who did not meet the distressed sample criteria required a score of 4 (moderate) or greater on a seven-point global judgment of defect state to be included, as well as a rating of severe or very severe impairment on at least two of the six negative features first scaled by Wing,[26] one of which had to be flat affect, poverty of speech, or amotivation. This subsample is referred to as the defect-state sample. By definition, no patient in the defect-state sample met Raskin Depression Scale or Covi Anxiety Scale criteria at the point of study intake, although some did have mild anxiety and/or depression.

Of the 240 potential candidates selected over 5 years, 138 entered one or more treatment trials. One hundred two patients were never admitted: 31 either could not reach stabilization criteria for positive symptoms or were rehospitalized, 50 patients refused participation, and two were jailed. Of note, 19 patients (8%) improved and no longer met the admission criteria following a change from their previous maintenance medications to FD and/or because of additional attention.

Study patients were treated in a research clinic by experienced, master's-level nurses and research psychiatrists who were trained in all measures. The same psychiatrist and nurse treated and assessed a patient throughout all relevant trials to circumvent potential rater variance because formal ongoing reliability checks were not made. Patients were assessed on a variety of self-report and clinician assessments, using standard scales as well as new scales that were specifically designed to accommodate the hypothesized outcomes. Descriptions of these methods are available from us and include questionnaires and/or structured interviews related to EPSEs, affect, psychosis, subjective responses to medication, and social adjustment. All new instruments were factor analyzed first, and existing factors or total scores from standard scales were retained. To enhance reliability and power in the face of variable subsample sizes, we further factor analyzed the derived factors or total scores that involved symptoms in a search for highly intracorrelated composite indexes, or "super factors," across rating scales and, when possible, across observers. **Table 1** lists the subscale components of the composite indexes. Most factor loadings ranged from .7 to .9, and composite scores were standardized. Global measures of social adjustment were retained as independent assessments in trial 3.

On an a priori basis, we chose to test and interpret treatment effects in a hierarchical manner. Clinical significance of main effects for anticholinergic drug (trial 1) or FD dose (trial 2) first focused on the qualifying global judgments of distress or defect state, followed by an assessment of drug main effects on the relevant composite indexes. In the absence of a drug or dose main effect on these criterion measures, we opted not to analyze individual scales and their component factors in a search for meaning. Although many independent variables were available, we tested only for the simple interaction between drug and two to six independent variables judged from the literature and our prior studies to be important to understanding drug effects in a specific trial. We ignored all higher-order interactions. When appropriate, simple *t* tests on the means of the posttreatment dependent variables were calculated first, followed by an analysis of covariance on these posttreatment means that was adjusted only for initial level. The significance of any drug or dose main effect and/or the existence of a drug interaction was further assessed by regression analyses after adjusting for the initial level of the dependent variable and the contribution of selected independent measures.

study among residually psychotic, nonmanic, schizophrenic outpatients with persistent anxiety.

Interest in the problem arose from the realization that schizophrenic patients who were successfully treated with contemporary (mid-1980s) pharmacotherapy and psychosocial interventions were often "better but not well."[21,22] Although family and individual strategies clearly delayed psychotic relapse beyond the point obtained with medication alone,[21] affective distress and defect features frequently appeared to conspire against a successful rehabilitation and led to a significant increase in relapse even though patients continued to receive depot neuroleptic medication.[22]

Because our patients had diagnoses of schizophrenia or schizoaffective disorder and were receiving maintenance doses of antipsychotic and antiparkinsonian drugs, we reasoned that little would be gained by attempting to label their distress or defect features according to traditional diagnostic systems. Rather, we simply measured the severity of apparent anxiety, depression, and defect features and determined whether and how patients changed on these measures during a series of sequential pharmacological trials.

As shown in the **Figure**, eligible patients first entered a trial that involved a double-blind challenge with a centrally acting anticholinergic drug to assess the con-

Table 1. Symptom Subscales of the Composite Indexes*

Composite Index	Symptom Subscales
Anxious depression	Affect Rating Scale:
	Depression factor†
	Anhedonia factor†
	DECS:
	Anxiety Scale
	Depression Scale
	Raskin Depression Scale (total)†
	Beck Depression Inventory (total)†
	Taylor Manifest Anxiety Scale (total)†
	Global distress judgment
	BPRS:
	Anxious depression factor†
	Minor symptoms (total)†
Defect	DECS:
	Defect Scale
	Bradykinesia Scale
	Wing Negative Symptom Scale†
	BPRS:
	Withdrawal factor†
	Global defect judgment
Akathisia and/or anxiety	Affect Rating Scale:
	Panic factor†
	Driven factor†
	DECS:
	Akathisia Scale
	Covi Anxiety Scale†
	Medical Response Questionnaire:
	Anxious mood factor
Dysthymia	Medical Response Questionnaire:
	Sluggish factor
	Dysthymia factor
	Anxious mood factor
Personal comfort	Medical Response Questionnaire:
	Feels good factor
	Energy factor

*DECS indicates Diagnostic Evaluation in Chronic Schizophrenia Scale (a structured interview for discriminating between affective disorder and extrapyramidal side effects); BPRS, Brief Psychiatric Rating Scale.
†Not included in trial 1 analyses.

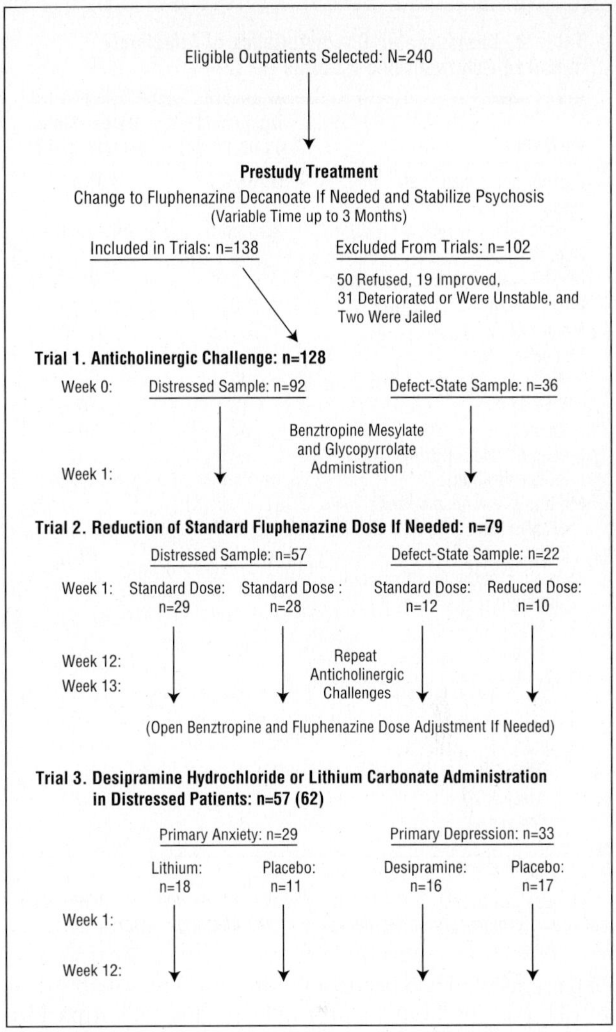

Study design.

tribution of extrapyramidal side effects (EPSEs) to distress or defect features (trial 1). Those who remained impaired and who were not already maintained on clinically determined minimum effective doses of fluphenazine decanoate (FD) then entered a 12-week double-blind dose-reduction study (trial 2). Patients who continued to be primarily depressed were next randomly assigned to a 12-week double-blind trial of supplemental desipramine hydrochloride (DMI) or its placebo (trial 3a). Primarily anxious patients entered a 12-week double-blind trial of supplemental LI or its placebo (trial 3b). Patients with mixed states were randomized to either LI- or DMI-treatment groups or to their respective placebo groups. Patients gave informed, written consent for each trial in which they participated.

RESULTS

DEMOGRAPHICS AND HISTORY CHARACTERISTICS

Table 2 describes the 92 distressed patients and 36 patients in a defect state who entered trial 1. Most striking is the chronicity of illness of the sample, in terms of both psychiatric history, including 4 to 5 years of interepisodic outpatient treatment, and long-standing social dysfunction.

CLINICAL CHARACTERISTICS

Clinical characteristics significantly discriminate between the distressed and defect-state samples (**Table 3**). Although the Raskin Depression Scale and Covi Anxiety Scale criteria clearly distinguish the distressed and defect-state samples, secondary negative features are frequently present among distressed patients, in part as a function of our selection criteria. The majority of distressed patients suffered nonphasic, persistent depression and, to a lesser extent, anxiety. This contrasts with the traditional view that depression in schizophrenia is typically of a discrete, phasic nature, a description that is increasingly challenged.[27]

TRIAL I: ANTICHOLINERGIC CHALLENGES

Patients were maintained on a prechallenge dose of FD (mean±SD, 16.5±12.3 mg every 2 weeks). Although we did not expect that the distress and negative symptoms

Table 2. Demographic Characteristics of Affectively Impaired Schizophrenic Patients (n=128)

Variable	Distressed Sample (n=92)	Defect-State Sample (n=36)
Current age (mean±SD), y	33.5±9.1	34.3±11.1
Mean±SD age at first psychotic episode, y	23.9±6.0	24.4±6.6
Gender, % M	63*	75*
Marital status, % never married	74	86
Race,* % W	79	61
Mean±SD education level†	3.29±1.0*	3.74±.95*
Residence, %		
Parental	46	56
Conjugal	17	8
Other	37	36
Mean±SD No. of prior hospitalizations	4.4±4.0	3.8±3.4
Months since hospitalized		
Mean±SD	28±36	33±43
Median	16	18
Months in outpatient treatment (lifetime)		
Mean±SD	74±73	64±57
Median	55	48
Median No. of months since wage earner's last job	30*	65*
Currently working, %	18.5	10.7
Months since adequate functioning		
Mean±SD	67±83	68±88
Median	30	27

*$P<.05$.

†*Values are based on the following scale: college degree = 2, attended college = 3, high school degree = 4, and attended high school = 5.*

of patients who had been maintained on a reasonable dose of FD (and frequently a prophylactic dose of antiparkinsonian medication) could be wholly attributed to EPSEs, it was important to determine whether a rapid,[28] additional benefit could be achieved by increasing the anticholinergic dose to the lower range of toxicity.

Patients in the distressed (n=92) and defect-state (n=36) samples were challenged on a double-blind and random basis with either the centrally acting anticholinergic drug benztropine mesylate or, as a control, the peripherally acting anticholinergic drug glycopyrrolate. Because the anticholinergic side effects of a typical antiparkinsonian medication are readily detectable at therapeutic doses, glycopyrrolate was chosen as an active placebo for benztropine. Independent evidence supported the central action of benztropine but not glycopyrrolate.[29]

On days 1 and 8, patients received either 2 mg of benztropine mesylate or 0.2 mg of glycopyrrolate in random order by intramuscular injection into the gluteal muscle. Anticholinergic effect criteria included dry mouth or a heart rate that was increased by 20 beats per minute but that did not exceed 110 beats per minute. When criteria were not met within 45 minutes, a second injection was given to approximately 60% of the patients, which is in keeping with expected individual variability.[30] One hundred four patients (81.2%) had been maintained prophylactically on an antiparkinsonian medication before the study (mean±SD, 3.54±1.96 mg/d in benztropine equivalents) without a significant difference between distressed and defect-state samples.

The analysis proceeded as described above in a search for drug main effects or selected interactions with drug. Covariates of interest included initial level of the variable being tested and the categorical variables of gender, prestudy dose of FD (>20 or <20 mg every 2 weeks), severity of EPSEs at baseline, and the number of prior hospitalizations, which was used as a compromise measure of age and chronicity, which appear to be related to persistent EPSEs.[31] The analyses compared adjusted, postinjection mean behavioral differences between the two anticholinergic drugs and ignored the order of administration. Because the same patients received both drugs on one or the other testing occasion, this subjects effect was also able to be statistically removed. Effects were tested on the entire distressed and defect-state samples separately and again after removing the 15 patients in the distressed sample and the nine patients in the defect-state sample who had not been receiving an antiparkinsonian medication before challenge. Sample size conspired against testing these 24 patients separately.

Distressed Sample Challenge Effects

Among the 92 patients, only one significant drug main effect was detected that favored benztropine once the subjects effect had been removed (composite index of personal comfort; F=4.35; df=1,182; P=.04). However, when the 15 patients who had not been receiving an antiparkinsonian medication prophylactically were removed from the analysis, the effect was no longer significant (F=2.88, P=.09).

Two drug interactions were also detected. Patients who were maintained on an FD dosage greater than 20 mg every 2 weeks before the study improved significantly following the benztropine challenge on the global judgment of defect state (F=8.84, P=.003) and the composite defect factor (F=4.18, P=.04). Not only are these variables highly intercorrelated, but the effect also diminished when the 15 patients who were not receiving an antiparkinsonian drug prophylactically were removed (P=.01 and P=.11, respectively).

Defect State Challenge Effects

No main effects of the antiparkinsonian drug were observed among the 36 patients. Two drug interactions that favored benztropine were observed among patients who received more than 20 mg of FD every 2 weeks before the study (the global judgment of distress: F=4.45; df=1,70; P=.04; and the composite anxious depression measure: F=5.21; df=1,68; P=.03). Again, these effects diminished when the nine patients who were not receiving prophylactic antiparkinsonian medication were removed from the analysis (P's=.06).

For those who might argue that our distinction between distressed and defect-state samples was arbitrary, pooling groups resulted in the same but fewer challenge results (two of three of the original findings seen among distressed patients and one of two observed among defect patients). However, results from pooling contain the error of generalizing to all patients those effects that are specific to the distressed sample or defect-state sample alone.

Comment

In contrast to the recent results of an uncontrolled study,[32] it does not appear that impairments of affect among schizophrenic patients can be easily attributed to EPSEs if the patient had been maintained prophylactically on a reasonable dose of antiparkinsonian medication before the study. Clearly, EPSEs must be viewed as a potential confounding variable of impaired affect among patients who are maintained on higher doses of a neuroleptic medication and/or who are not prescribed a prophylactic dose of antiparkinsonian medication. But affect impairments that are associated with neuroleptic medication–treated vs untreated patients[32] are more likely to be attributable to patient clinical state than to neuroleptic medications.

Among the subsample of patients who proceeded to the dose-reduction study (trial 2), a second series of anticholinergic challenges that were administered at weeks 12 and 13 were also noncontributing. Specifically, we examined the interactive effects of drug (benztropine vs glycopyrrolate) by dosage group (standard vs reduced). Hypothetically, benztropine should have had selective effects among patients who remained on a standard dose of FD compared with those whose dose was reduced. However, no dose-by-drug interactive effects were observed.

TRIAL 2: THE DOSE-REDUCTION STUDY

We next attempted to determine whether a dose reduction of maintenance FD resulted in the amelioration of distress or defect features, particularly if these symptoms reflected EPSEs that were resistant to antiparkinsonian medication. This trial was not a test of the prophylactic efficacy of a low dose of FD as a long-term maintenance strategy for schizophrenic symptoms because 1- and 2-year controlled trials had previously attested to the value of this approach.[33-35] Among the 92 distressed patients, 57 were included in the dosage analysis. Thirty-five patients were excluded: 21 patients were already maintained on the lowest maintenance dose of FD possible; six patients refused to continue; two patients clinically deteriorated; and six patients who were originally assigned to the reduced-dose condition never had a dose reduction because of their precarious clinical state. Among the 36 patients in the defect-state sample, four refused the study or were administratively terminated, and two patients who were assigned a low dose never had a subsequent dose reduction, leaving 22 patients available for the trial.

At week 1, following the anticholinergic challenges, patients were randomly assigned on a double-blind basis to their prestudy dose of FD or to a condition designed to lower their maintenance dose of FD to the minimum effective dose, which was operationally defined as the dose below which prodromal signs of psychosis appeared and, above which, more than minimal EPSEs developed. The blinded treatment team proceeded on the assumption that all study patients were to have a dose reduction. Nonblinded injection nurses were provided dose condition assignments and either maintained the same prestudy dose among standard-dose recipients (ignoring dose-reduction instructions) or lowered the dose as instructed in the reduced-dose condition. The sequential testing for drug main effects followed the strategy described earlier. Covariates included gender, prestudy dosage levels of FD that were either greater than or less than 20 mg every 2 weeks, family history of mental illness[36] (severe illness, other illness, or no illness), and current alcohol or other drug abuse, which might confound the clinical presentation of affective impairment.[37] All patients who were assigned to the reduced-dose group had at least one dose reduction. Thirty-three standard-dose recipients were maintained prophylactically on an antiparkinsonian drug (mean±SD, 3.70±1.50 mg of benztropine or equivalent) as were 36 patients who received a reduced dose (mean±SD, 3.69±2.40 mg), with no significant difference between the distressed and defect-state samples.

Distressed Sample Dose Differences

Of the 57 distressed patients, 55 completed 6 weeks of study and 50 patients completed 12 weeks. Two refused to continue, and three patients who received a standard dose and two patients who received a reduced dose clinically deteriorated. The mean±SD entry and exit dosage of FD among patients who received a standard dose and completed the 12 weeks of study was 21.7±15.4 mg every 2 weeks (mean, 23.7 mg for all 29 assignees). Among the reduced-dose group, the mean±SD entry dosage was 18.6±11.7 mg every 2 weeks (mean, 19.3 mg for all 28 assignees), and the mean±SD dose at 12 weeks was 10.7±8.2 mg. The overall reduction (mean±SD, 7.9±7.0 mg) was statistically significant (t=2.61; df=55; P=.007).

There were no dose main effects detected by t tests or analyses of covariance at either 6 or 12 weeks. Among

Table 3. Distinguishing Clinical Characteristics* of Distressed and Defect-State Samples of Schizophrenic Patients at Study Intake

Variable	Distressed Sample (n=92)	Defect-State Sample (n=36)
Raskin Depression Scale		
Mean±score	7.78±2.2	4.44±8.4
Score ≥7, %	76	0
Covi Anxiety Scale		
Mean±SD score	6.70±2.2	4.17±1.0
Score ≥7, %	54	0
Wing Negative Symptom Scale		
Mean±SD score	15.5±5.4	21.2±2.7
Two or more severe items (of 6)	47	100
Distress in last 3 months, %		
Moderate to severe and persistent	62	8
Moderate to severe and fluctuating	21	0
Moderate to severe more than 50% of time	10	3
Distinct postpsychotic depression	1	0
Distressed but more defective	6	0
Not distressed, pure defect	0	89

*$P<.001$.

the regression analyses that removed the effects of independent variables, an isolated dose effect at 12 weeks that favored reduced dose appeared on the composite index of akathisia and/or anxiety (t=2.33; df=7,49; P=.03). Regression analyses also yielded a single, interactive effect pattern at 6 weeks on the criterion measure of global distress, the composite indexes of anxious depression and personal comfort, as well as the global and composite defect variables. This effect indicated that patients who had a first-degree family member with a history of severe mental illness (n=16, 12 of whom had affective disorder) differentially improved on a reduced dose. With 7 and 49 *df*'s, *t* scores ranged from 2.25 to 3.04, and *P* values ranged from .03 to .004. At 12 weeks, the interaction between dose and family history was also observed for the composite indexes of anxious depression and personal comfort as well as the Bradykinesia Scale. Statistical trends were also apparent on the two measures of defect state but not on the global distress criterion.

Defect-State Dose Differences

All 22 patients completed 6 weeks of study, and 21 patients completed 12 weeks. At entry and termination, the 12 standard-dose assignees received a mean±SD dosage of 14.8±7.1 mg of FD every 2 weeks, and the 10 patients who received a reduced dose began the trial at a mean±SD dosage of 16.5±10.1 mg every 2 weeks and ended the trial at a dosage of 10.1±6.1 mg every 2 weeks. The mean±SD dose reduction of 6.4±5.3 mg did not reach statistical significance because of the small sample size.

Despite the small sample size, a consistent and robust dose main effect across the *t* tests, analyses of covariance, and regression analyses favored the reduced-dose group and was apparent at 6 weeks on the composite indexes that measured residual syndromes of anxious depression, dysthymia, and akathisia and/or anxiety. With 5 and 15 *df's*, *t* scores from the regression analyses ranged from 1.95 to 3.69, and *P* values ranged from .08 to .002. Except for the composite index of dysthymia, these 6-week effects were not maintained at 12 weeks, although the means were most often in the expected direction. The principal effect of dose reduction among patients in the defect-state sample appeared at the subjective level wherein patients felt less dysthymic, sluggish, and anxious on the reduced dose. However, reduced dose had little or no effect on persistent negative symptoms. A few drug interactions were observed, but small cell sizes precluded interpretation. The value in analyzing the defect-state and distressed samples separately was again reinforced because pooling samples resulted in no significant dose effects.

Table 4. Selected Characteristics of DMI- and LI-Treated Study Patients*

Variable	DMI Trial (n=33)	LI Trial (n=29)
Mean±SD age, y	31.5±7.9	35.8±9.3
Gender, %		
M	64	54
F	36	46
Race, % W	73	93
Marital status, % never married	82	71
Mean±SD Raskin Depression Scale score†	8.50±1.62	4.87±1.29
Mean±SD Covi Anxiety Scale score†	5.11±1.58	7.57±0.94
Mean±SD Wing Negative Symptom Scale Score†	15.25±4.83	12.83±4.31
Mean±SD instability of delusions†‡	2.07±1.21	2.74±1.36
Mean±SD instability of hallucinations†‡	1.89±1.20	2.52±1.27

**DMI indicates desipramine hydrochloride; LI, lithium carbonate.*
†Means are for unduplicated cases excluding five mixed-state placebo recipients.
‡Values based on a scale from 1 to 3, where 1 indicates none and 3 indicates mild.

Comment

Given the long half-life of FD, together with a history of long-term dosing before the study, we readily acknowledge that a 12-week dose-reduction trial might not have represented the best test of whether impaired affect in schizophrenia is a dose-related manifestation of EPSEs. With the data available, however, the dose of the antipsychotic drug and the attendant EPSEs do not appear to account for the severe affective impairments that are characteristic of the patients. The observation is consistent with the reported failure to observe an association between dose of FD and depression[38] and the absence of evidence from placebo-controlled trials that would support the pharmacogenesis of depression.[22] Following dose reduction in the controlled and open interstudy phase, only three patients in the distressed sample and one in the defect-state sample exited the study with significant improvement that could be attributed to dose reduction.

The single interaction with severe, first-degree familial mental disorder among distressed patients provides further evidence that the side effects of neuroleptic medications might be mediated by a family history of affective disorder.[36]

Less surprising, a dose reduction provided important subjective relief to patients in the defect-state sample. According to the long-term, well-controlled maintenance-dose studies available,[33-35] important effects accrue to low dose, including those of many patients who appeared to have been characterized by negative symptoms. Perhaps the improvement secondary to dose reduction represents relief from subtle EPSEs, which is less responsive to antiparkinsonian drugs. However, an alternative model exists as well. Negative symptoms might implicate hypodopaminergic functioning, particularly in the mesocortical track, which innervates the prefrontal cortex.[9] One could argue that higher doses of antipsychotic drugs further antagonize an already compromised dopaminergic system. Dose reduction provides relief, independent of nigrostriatal-mediated pseudoparkinsonian symptoms. Extension of the model suggests that mesocortical dopaminergic blockade by antipsychotic drugs might also be responsible for the subjective and motor signs of akathisia.[39,40] By inference, a dose reduction could thus relieve the subjective distress of subtle akathisia beyond what is possible with antiparkinsonian medication.

Table 5. Significant Effects of DMI at 12 Weeks: Main Effects*

Variable	DMI	Placebo	*t*	*P*
Covi Anxiety Scale score	4.31†	5.67	2.66	.01
BPRS				
Total score	1.61†	1.96	2.25	.03
Psychotic factor score	1.39†	1.85	2.27	.03
Global illness score	3.34†	4.02	2.23	.04
DECS				
Anxiety Scale score	1.02†	1.78	2.02	.06
Taylor Anxiety Scale score	13.24†	17.81	2.34	.03
Beck Depression Inventory score	7.21†	12.37	2.15	.04
Medical Response Questionnaire sluggish score	1.41†	1.80	2.19	.04
Heart rate (standing), beats/min	98.98	87.64†	2.30	.04

*Significant t and P values are from the multivariate regression analyses. Mean scores are posttreatment means from the analyses of covariance, adjusted for initial level. Effects are significant when all independent variables are controlled. DMI indicates desipramine hydrochloride; BPRS, Brief Psychiatric Rating Scale; and DECS, Diagnostic Evaluation in Chronic Schizophrenia Scale.

†Mean reflects treatment group with a relatively superior outcome that probably accounts for the effect.

TRIAL 3: ADJUNCTIVE THYMOLEPTIC MEDICATIONS

Fifty-seven persistently depressed and/or anxious patients received DMI, LI, or placebo, depending on presenting symptoms. Distressed patients in trial 1 who were excluded from trial 3 were characterized by interim improvement, deterioration, or administrative termination (noncompliance) in approximate proportions, with no differences that would bias testing. Sixteen patients were randomized to a DMI–treatment group, and 17, to a corresponding placebo group; 18 were randomized to a LI–treatment group, and 11, to a corresponding placebo group. (Five mixed anxious and depressed patients served as placebo controls for both the DMI and LI contrasts.) With fewer anxious patients, random assignment to LI or placebo administration was made on approximately a 2:1 ratio, which was unknown to the treating clinicians. (Anxiety, in this study, was best described as a ruminating, anguished, driven state without motor or internal restlessness.) Patients were assessed by clinician reports and self-reports at baseline and at 6 and 12 weeks. Demographic characteristics (**Table 4**) indicated more women, white subjects, and somewhat older patients in the LI trial. Clinical variables clearly demonstrate syndrome differences that are appropriate to the respective trial. The mean and the more accurate median dosages of FD were only 9.3 mg and 5.0 mg every 2 weeks among the 16 DMI recipients, 13.6 mg and 10 mg every 2 weeks among the 18 LI recipients, and 16.4 mg and 10 mg every 2 weeks among the patients who were administered placebo, respectively. The higher maintenance dose of FD among the samples that were administered LI or placebo probably reflected a lesser stability of schizophrenic symptoms (Table 4) among subjects who met Covi Anxiety Scale criteria. In keeping with their doses of FD, 65.5% of DMI recipients, 94.4% of LI recipients, and 78.2% of placebo recipients received maintenance anticholinergics (benztropine mesylate) at mean±SD daily doses of 4.1±3.2 mg, 3.4±2.2 mg, and 3.5±2.2 mg, respectively.

Plasma levels of DMI were monitored biweekly, and LI levels were measured weekly for the first month and biweekly thereafter. Treating clinicians were supplied factitious values for the subjects receiving placebo that were proportionate to the prescribed number of tablets. The DMI recipients started with a dosage of 50 mg of DMI daily, which increased weekly by 50 mg until 150 mg/d had been prescribed at 3 weeks, if it was tolerated. Four patients received 200 mg/d at some time during the last 6 weeks of treatment, and three patients were maintained on the minimum dosage of 100 mg/d. An effort was made to maintain the DMI levels of patients between 450 and 940 nmol/L.[41] Levels in two patients decreased below this range because of limiting side effects, and on rare assays, four patients exceeded the range. Mean DMI plasma levels in the first 6 weeks were 520±300 nmol/L and were 630±360 nmol/L in weeks 7 through 12. These levels were similar to those of the earlier study of Siris et al.[17]

An attempt was made to maintain the LI levels of LI recipients between 0.4 and 0.8 mmol/L, a deliberately modest level in light of our desire to avoid neurotoxic effects.[42] Most often, LI administration was initiated at 300 mg/d and was increased weekly by 300 mg until the desired level was obtained, if it was tolerated. Most patients received between 900 and 1200 mg/d. Levels in three patients exceeded 1.0 mmol/L at two testing periods, and levels in three patients decreased below 0.40 mmol/L on two testing periods during the latter 6 weeks of the study. The mean LI plasma level in the first 6 weeks was 0.474±0.14 mmol/L and was 0.586±0.21 mmol/L in the subsequent 6 weeks.

Three-Group Contrast

Drug main effects were first tested by the analysis of covariance that compared 16 DMI-treated, 18 LI-treated, and all 23 placebo-administered patients, controlling only for the initial level of the dependent variable. With the greatest *df*s available, if no robust effects were detected, our confidence in separately testing DMI, LI, and their placebos would have been reduced.

At 6 weeks, there were no drug effects on the composite or criterion variables. Isolated item differences suggested no consistent pattern of effects. The one clear find-

Table 6. Significant Effects of DMI at 12 Weeks: Interaction With Gender*

Variable	Men DMI	Men Placebo	Women DMI	Women Placebo	*t*	*P*
Global distress score	3.58	3.49	2.58†	4.42	2.28	.03
BPRS						
Total score	1.75	1.83	1.43†	2.14	2.22	.04
Nonpsychotic symptoms score	2.24	2.26	1.75†	2.99	2.47	.02
Anxious depression factor score	2.57	2.54	1.89†	3.40	2.06	.05
Medical Response Questionnaire						
Feels good factor score‡	1.62	1.63	1.95†	1.69	2.67	.02
DECS						
Depression Scale score	1.88	1.21	0.79†	1.85	2.30	.03
Beck Depression Inventory score	9.61	10.72	4.03†	15.30	2.40	.03
Heart rate (resting), beats/min	98.54	73.74†	87.44	89.62	2.03	.06

Significant t and P values are from the multivariate regression analyses. Mean scores are posttreatment means from the analyses of covariance, adjusted for initial level. Effects are significant when all independent variables are controlled. DMI indicates desipramine hydrochloride; BPRS, Brief Psychiatric Rating Scale; and DECS, Diagnostic Evaluation in Chronic Schizophrenia Scale.

†Mean reflects treatment group with a relatively superior outcome that probably accounts for the effect.

‡High score is a good outcome.

ing was an expected increased heart rate among DMI recipients.[43]

At 12 weeks, drug effects were detected. On criterion measures, the composite personal comfort index favored LI, and both LI and DMI were favored on the Covi Anxiety Scale. However, LI recipients were also observed to have somewhat elevated scores on the global defect judgment. On the Medication Response Questionnaire, LI-treated patients reported feeling better and were more comfortable and energetic, and DMI-treated patients reported feeling less sluggish. On the Taylor Anxiety Scale and Beck Depression Inventory, both LI- and DMI-treated patients were significantly improved compared with the placebo groups. The LI recipients appeared to manifest greater akathisia, however, and DMI recipients showed a continued elevation in heart rate. These observations were supported by consistent trends on many other measures that favor active medication. Thus, it appeared reasonable to explore individual contrasts between each active medication and its placebo, with the primary focus on 12-week results.

DMI vs Placebo

As suggested by the three-group analysis, there were no DMI effects at 6 weeks. An increased heart rate among DMI recipients was the sole unequivocal finding.

By 12 weeks, a circumscribed pattern of effects was observed. Clear trends across a number of criterion variables were supported by total scale or factor scores on important clinician and patient assessments. **Table 5** illustrates that clinicians reported significantly less anxiety as rated by the Covi Anxiety Scale and Diagnostic Evaluation in Chronic Schizophrenia Anxiety Scale, which was validated by the patient's self-report of anxiety (Taylor Anxiety Scale). Clinicians further observed a lower Brief Psychiatric Rating Scale total score, particularly on items that formed the psychotic factor, and this was also reflected in their global judgment of a lower degree of illness. Patients receiving DMI rated themselves as less sluggish. Again, heart rate was significantly higher among DMI recipients.

Interactions between drug and selected independent variables provided an important clarification of the DMI effect. The principal drug interaction was with gender (**Table 6**). Positive effects of DMI on distress, depression itself, and mixed anxious depression are reserved for female patients exclusively. Only the consistently observed increase in heart rate characterized the male patients. Because the one drug main effect on depression (Beck Depression Inventory) was better explained by the gender interaction, it appears that all effects of DMI on depressed mood applied to female but not to male patients. The DMI main effects that existed across gender are to be found in other domains, such as anxiety and aspects of residual schizophrenia, but not depression. Otherwise, there was no convincing evidence that DMI was a surreptitious treatment of resistant akinesia. Most often, drug interactions revealed that placebo recipients with elevated akinesia before treatment differentially improved over time. Desipramine appeared to lower withdrawal and/or retardation among patients with little or no akinesia. Furthermore, although antidepressants are reported to be selectively effective among schizophrenic patients with good premorbid adjustment,[44] interactions between drug and premorbid state revealed that only one variable, a self-report measure of "feeling good," supported this observation. However, a proclivity to increased blood pressure also appeared among these patients with good premorbid adjustment.

Regarding the possibility of psychotic exacerbation by cyclic antidepressants,[45] we found no supportive evidence of this. A low maintenance dose of an antipsychotic drug does not leave DMI-treated schizophrenic patients at risk for psychotic decompensation. Only one of 57 study patients had an unequivocal psychotic relapse, this patient being a placebo assignee. Minor psychotic episodes in the DMI trial, which were defined as an exacerbation and subsequent resolution (within 3 weeks) of positive schizophrenic symptoms, characterized one DMI-treated pa-

Table 7. Clinician Rating of Improvement*

Treatment	No. of Patients: Significant Improvement	Some Improvement	No Change	Worsening	Total
DMI	6	3	5	2	**16**
DMI placebo	4	7	3	3	**17**
LI	6	3	7	2	**18**
LI placebo	0	4	7	0	**11**

**DMI indicates desipramine hydrochloride; LI, lithium carbonate.*

Table 8. Significant Main Effects of LI at 12 Weeks*

Variable	Adjusted Means: LI	Placebo	*t*	*P*
Positive Effects				
Composite personal comfort score†	52.40‡	43.57	2.26	.03
Covi Anxiety Scale score§	5.63‡	6.91	2.00	.06
Taylor Anxiety Scale score§	12.99‡	17.75	2.56	.02
Beck Depression Inventory score	6.31‡	11.54	2.47	.02
Affect Rating Scale				
Driven factor score	1.19‡	1.51	2.11	.05
BPRS				
Nonpsychotic symptoms score	2.10‡	1.55	2.19	.04
Anxious depression factor score	2.22‡	2.95	2.38	.02
Medical Response Questionnaire				
Energy factor score†	2.10‡	1.55	2.19	.04
Feels good factor score†	2.22‡	1.80	2.32	.03
Negative Effects				
Global defect score§	2.89	2.47‡	2.10	.05
Chouinard Scale				
Akathisia score§	1.28	0.69‡	2.11	.05

**Significant* t *and* P *values are from the multivariate regression analyses. Mean scores are posttreatment means from the analyses of covariance, adjusted for the initial level. LI indicates lithium carbonate; BPRS, Brief Psychiatric Rating Scale.*

†High score is a good outcome.

‡Mean designates the treatment condition with the better outcome.

§Indicates variables that demonstrate a significant drug effect controlling for initial level but only a statistical trend ($P<.10$) when effects of gender, premorbid status, and akathisia are controlled for. Other variables are significant whether or not effects of independent variables are controlled for.

tient and one patient who was administered the placebo. Three DMI and five placebo recipients had an increase in one or more psychotic symptoms during the study. However, none of the DMI-treated patients showed evidence of increased psychotic symptoms at the termination of study. In fact, analyses indicated a resolution of residual psychoticism among DMI recipients.

Although rating scale criteria showed some value of supplemental DMI administration, the treating clinician's final global judgment of improvement for each study participant did not support the superiority of treatment with DMI. **Table 7** reveals no significant differences in global outcome between patients receiving DMI and those receiving placebo. A further evaluation of the database was made to explain this apparent discrepancy. Although only one DMI recipient and one DMI placebo recipient experienced a minor psychotic episode, seven (41.2%) of the placebo recipients but only two (12.5%) of the DMI recipients experienced a minor affective episode (χ^2=3.58, *df*=1, *P*=.06). A minor episode represented an unequivocal and severe increase in persistent affective symptoms that was subsequently aborted within 2 to 3 weeks by means of a dose adjustment of supplemental medication and/or by increased surveillance.

Although the week at which a minor affective episode first occurred was not recorded, a further evaluation of this phenomenon was attempted. First, the four most significant main effects judged by clinicians and the two most significant self-report effects identified at 12 weeks were reanalyzed for the entire sample using minor affective episode as a covariate. Only one of the six remained statistically significant (the Taylor Anxiety Scale), three became marginally significant, and two were no longer significant. Next, 12-week data were reanalyzed, eliminating all patients receiving the drug or the placebo who had experienced a minor affective episode. None of the six outcome variables remained statistically significant. (Although *df*'s were obviously lost, adjusted posttreatment means did become more similar.) Thus, we suspect that an unanticipated prophylactic effect of treatment with supplemental DMI on symptomatic "flurries" rather than a therapeutic effect across variables of persistent symptoms might

Table 9. Significant Interactive Effects of LI at 12 Weeks: LI and Gender*

	Men		Women			
Variable	LI	Placebo	LI	Placebo	*t*	*P*
Composite akathisia and/or anxiety score	50.31	49.71	40.23†	53.28	3.87	.001
Covi Anxiety Scale score	6.99	6.82	4.36†	7.08	2.63	.02
Global distress score	4.14	3.83	2.37†	4.04	2.58	.02
BPRS						
Nonpsychotic symptoms score	2.33	2.36	1.86†	3.81	3.04	.006
Anxious depression factor score	2.51	2.74	1.93†	3.32	2.01	.06
Affect Rating Scale						
Driven factor score	1.33	1.38	1.02†	1.77	2.69	.01
Panic factor score	1.42	1.36	1.09†	1.52	2.09	.05
DECS						
Anxiety Scale score	1.89	1.66	1.23†	2.25	2.19	.04

**Significant* t *and* P *values are from the multivariate regression analyses. Mean scores are posttreatment means from the analyses of covariance, adjusted for initial level. Effects are significant when all independent variables are controlled for. LI indicates lithium carbonate; BPRS, Brief Psychiatric Rating Scale; and DECS, Diagnostic Evaluation in Chronic Schizophrenia Scale.*

†Means reflect the treatment group with a relatively superior outcome that likely accounts for the interaction.

Table 10. Significant Interactive Effects of LI at 12 Weeks: LI and Premorbid Adjustment*

	Premorbid Adjustment							
	Poor		Intermediate		Good			
Variable	LI	Placebo	LI	Placebo	LI	Placebo	*t*	*P*
Composite anxious depression score	47.68	45.50	45.17	50.44	36.65†	47.02	2.25	.04
BPRS								
Anxious depression factor score	2.71	2.45	2.43	3.10	1.60†	3.12	2.71	.01
Taylor Anxiety Scale score	16.64	15.28	12.82	18.27	10.28†	19.11	3.06	.006
Beck Depression Inventory score	8.82	8.82	7.21	12.70	2.79†	12.72	2.52	.02
DECS								
Total score	1.49	1.07†	1.24	1.04	0.60	0.97	2.14	.04
Bradykinesia Scale score	0.94	0.37†	0.87	0.81	0.55	0.69	2.05	.05

**Significant* t *and* P *values are from the multivariate regression analyses. Mean scores are posttreatment means from the analyses of covariance, adjusted for initial level. Effects are significant when all independent variables are controlled for. LI indicates lithium carbonate; BPRS, Brief Psychiatric Rating Scale; and DECS, Diagnostic Evaluation in Chronic Schizophrenia Scale.*

†Means reflect the treatment group with a relatively superior outcome that likely accounts for the interaction.

better explain the DMI rating scale effect as well as the absence of clinician endorsement of significant global improvement.

Neurovegetative signs that possibly had explanatory value were also examined, but none of the six sleep, appetite, or libido measures demonstrated an effect of DMI administration. In addition, tests of a linear relationship between plasma DMI levels and clinical response revealed no association. In fact, three of six patients who were judged to have improved significantly were found among the four patients whose average DMI levels were below 380 nmol/L. Finally, there was no effect of DMI on negative symptoms, as others have noted,[46] and no effects were detected on measures of interpersonal and social adjustment derived from the Major Role Adjustment Inventory.

LI vs Placebo

As suggested by the three-group analysis, there were no main effects of LI at 6 weeks. Isolated drug interactions were ignored in the absence of a main effect.

By 12 weeks, a clear and consistent pattern of effects was observed. **Table 8** describes LI effects on various measures of anxiety and related nonpsychotic symptoms. The patients reported considerable relief and increased subjective comfort while receiving LI. A mild increase in akathisia and, we suspect, akinesia (the global defect judgment probably served as an analogue) characterizes LI recipients, although the magnitude of increase would not qualify as a neurotoxic effect. In fact, no LI-treated patient was judged to have experienced neurotoxic effects; for one patient, the judgment was "unclear."

These main effects, however, are also in need of qualification (**Table 9** and **Table 10**). Robust and consistent interactive effects with gender demonstrate that the positive effects of LI on multiple measures of anxiety as rated by clinicians, are exclusively reserved for female patients. However, no patient self-report supports this interactive effect with gender. The self-reported decrease in anxiety and associated depression, as well as the increase in personal comfort, appear valid for both sexes from the patients' perspective. Otherwise, both cli-

Table 11. Nature and Treatment of Affective Impairment (Anxiety, Depression, and Negative Symptoms) in Schizophrenia

	Phasic (Episodic) Form	Nonphasic (Persistent) Form
Acute Psychosis	Affective impairment arises in context of psychotic episode and resolves with administration of antipsychotic drug alone but resolves more slowly than do positive symptoms. Supplemental thymoleptics are of limited value or may even be harmful.	Affective impairment exists before and after psychotic episode. Antipsychotic drugs are of limited value in resolving impaired affect. There is limited evidence on the value of supplemental thymoleptics.
Remitted Psychosis	Not applicable, no persistent impairment. Maintenance with antipsychotic drug is sufficient unless a discrete affective episode develops. However, the value of supplemental thymoleptics remains undetermined.	Antipsychotic drugs are necessary for prophylaxis against psychosis but are of no added benefit regarding impaired affect. Many patients respond to supplemental thymoleptics.

nicians and patients reported a positive effect of LI on the anxious depression factors that appeared to be linearly related to good premorbid adjustment. The EPSEs of combined LI and FD were more prominent among poor premorbid patients, who, by inference, might be more likely to suffer the cost of LI without the benefit.

Unlike the DMI trial, symptomatic rating scale improvement found support in the clinician's rating of global improvement among LI recipients, as seen in Table 7. Of note, six LI recipients (all of whom had concurrent depression as well) but no placebo recipients were judged to have achieved significant improvement. However, only the less exact likelihood ratio with four *df*'s is marginally significant (P=.049); a more exact test is not (P=.06). The Mantel-Haenszel test for linear association was similarly not significant (P=.42), which suggests that there is a subsample of patients who do particularly well while receiving LI but another subgroup that does not respond or might even worsen while receiving LI.

Regarding psychotic and affective exacerbations, no patient experienced a major psychotic episode, and only one patient who received the LI placebo was judged to have had a minor psychotic episode. Clinicians believed that the study medication might have caused an increase in affective symptoms for two LI recipients. But minor affective episodes appeared to be noncontributing overall: there were two episodes among LI recipients and three among placebo recipients. A subsample of the patients in the LI trial had more psychotic symptoms present at baseline and at study termination, although absolute levels of these psychotic symptoms remained in the mild category.

Tests of the relationship between LI plasma levels and clinical improvement suggest some linearity, although the sample was too small for definitive results. For example, of the six patients judged to have significantly improved, one had an LI level below 0.36 mmol/L; two, between 0.50 and 0.69 mmol/L; and three, between 0.70 and 1.0 mmol/L. As with DMI, there was no evidence that administration of LI had a positive effect on coexisting negative symptoms or on the measures of interpersonal and social adjustment.

Comment

In our sample of anxious and/or depressed patients, 75% had suffered these distressing affects as long as clinical records existed or the referring clinicians could remember; these affects were often believed to be characterologic. For the 25% whose distress was not described as having been present "forever," the mean and median length of prestudy distress was at least 36 and 12 months, respectively. A prominent investigator in this area (S. Siris, MD, oral communication, November 1992) also indicated that the depression suffered by schizophrenic patients is often of long-standing duration.

The absence of 6-week effects in our trial might speak to a design that required 3 to 4 weeks to establish therapeutic blood levels. Conversely, for unknown reasons, patients with chronic schizophrenia who are treated with antipsychotic and anticholinergic medications might require longer trials (eg, 12 weeks) of thymoleptic medication before effects can be clearly documented. Siris et al[47] demonstrated greater effects at 9 weeks than at 6 weeks. Such a requirement could explain the negative findings of Johnson[48] in a brief (5-week) trial.

Unexpectedly, both clinicians and patients reported an antidepressant effect of DMI that was specific to schizophrenic women; other symptom areas improved for men and women, which is similar to the effects reported by Siris et al.[17] Beyond the speculation that schizophrenia might be a different disorder depending on gender[49,50] (ie, more an affective disorder in women and a neurological disorder in men), we have no plausible explanation for the treatment-resistant depression of outpatient schizophrenic men. Depression also seems more persistent among male schizophrenic inpatients who are experiencing their first episode, both at admission and at hospital discharge (G. Haas, PhD, written communication, July 1992). The outcome of schizoaffective depression is generally better for women than for men.[51]

We do not intend to demean the seemingly limited effects of DMI. Control of symptom fluctuations or "mini–affective episodes" of depression may avoid a dose increase and subsequent noncompliance with maintenance antipsychotic drug, lessen demoralization among patients and family, and lend stability and continuity to the rehabilitation plan.

Our results confirm the mediating effects of good premorbid adjustment[52-54] among responders to LI (but not to DMI) and confirm that LI efficacy extends to concurrent depression as well.[55,56] However, we find no support that LI is only useful for patients who are characterized by periodicity or good interepisodic adjustment. Our patients were socially and vocationally impaired, if not mildly psychotic, and interepisodically were persistently distressed. In this brief 12-week trial, we did not see improvement in adjustment and role performance that was associated with either drug and that a longer trial might have revealed. Concurrent negative features were unaffected as well.

The effects of DMI and LI administration cannot be explained as ameliorating EPSEs. In fact, akathisia and akinesia appear to increase slightly among LI recipients, even though the absolute levels of the antipsychotic drug and LI were low. Nonetheless, supplemental LI administration must be carefully monitored in patients who require higher doses of antipsychotic drugs and/or LI. In fact, there is only a poorly characterized subsample of anxious depressed schizophrenic patients with good premorbid adjustment that clearly responds to supplemental LI administration, a finding that is compatible with the heterogeneous response to LI among schizophrenic patients in general.[15,19,20] Reviewers of this trial must note the relatively low doses of LI and FD used, if generalizations are to be made. By contrast, we and others[17] find little or no evidence of psychotic exacerbation associated with supplemental administration of DMI, even in the context of low-dose administration of FD, although we acknowledge that poorly characterized and atypical individuals might remain at risk. However, these findings are not an endorsement of cyclic antidepressant use among schizophrenic patients with acute psychosis who appear not to benefit from these supplements.[16]

CONCLUSIONS

Following anticholinergic challenges, efforts at dose reduction of antipsychotic medication, and the statistical control of residual EPSEs in the differential treatment of study patients, we conclude that the majority of schizophrenic patients with residual and persistent impairments of affect suffer a clinical state and not a characterologic trait or resistant EPSEs. This state is often amenable to pharmacologic intervention, at least in regard to anxiety and depression. But the pathophysiologic characteristics of these impairments in recovering schizophrenic patients remain poorly understood. An abiding possibility exists that antagonism of various biogenic amine receptors by antipsychotic drugs exposes a subset of vulnerable patients to persistent affective impairment. Nonetheless, a more correct classification of these states remains to be determined. Toward this end, we offer the following speculation that there might be two possible forms of affective impairment that are better characterized by temporal course and treatment response than by cross-sectional classification (**Table 11**).

Anxiety[5] and/or depression[57-59] characterize the majority of presentations of acute schizophrenia. Given the appropriate treatment of acute schizophrenia with an antipsychotic drug, most affective impairments improve over time,[60,61] albeit more slowly than do positive symptoms. Nonetheless, among a substantial minority of patients (42% in one study[22]), these impairments of affect persist and dominate the clinical picture following recovery from psychosis. Carpenter et al[4] usefully have described a deficit and nondeficit form of negative symptoms, the former being more enduring pathophysiological aspects that are less determined, for example, by the iatrogenic effects of antipsychotic drugs or environmental understimulation. Phasic (nondeficit) forms of negative symptoms frequently respond to neuroleptic medications as positive symptoms of the illness remit,[61] but neuroleptic medications appear to provide little or no additional benefit to those with the persistent deficit form.[62] The same might be said for anxiety and depression. In the context of acute schizophrenic episodes, adequate neuroleptic treatment of positive schizophrenic symptoms frequently results in the resolution of depression and anxiety,[57,60,63] and supplemental antidepressants or LI are of little or no value.[16,63] Among the nonphasic, persistent form, typical or increased doses of neuroleptic medication provide no additional relief and may invite confounding akathisia or akinesia, whereas supplemental antidepressants or LI can be beneficial.

It is clear that much unnecessary suffering can be precluded through the rational use of supplemental thymoleptics in many nonpsychotic or residually psychotic schizophrenic patients who suffer enduring impairments of affect, particularly women. We note with some reassurance that the three interventions that are likely to improve the clinical factors most closely associated with quality of life for schizophrenic patients are control of depression, control of medication side effects (EPSEs), and provision of family psychoeducation.[64] At the least, the potential benefit for schizophrenic patients represented in the continued study of impaired affect is compelling.

Accepted for publication September 6, 1994.

This study was supported in part by grant MH 37166 from the National Institute of Mental Health, Bethesda, Md.

Princeton Pharmaceuticals, a division of Bristol-Myers Squibb, Wallingford, Conn, provided FD (Prolixin), and Smith, Kline & French Laboratories, Philadelphia, Pa, provided LI (Eskalith).

Study medications were prepared and dispensed by the Western Psychiatric Institute and Clinic Research Pharmacy, Pittsburgh, Pa, by Renee Kubacka, PharmD, and Elizabeth Grunewalder. George Alexander, MD, assisted with the clinical management of study patients. Reva Neiman, RN, and Irma Harty, RN, provided FD injections.

Reprint requests to WPIC, 3811 O'Hara St, Pittsburgh, PA 15213 (Mr Hogarty).

REFERENCES

1. Summer F, Harrow M, Westmeyer J. Neurotic symptoms in post-psychotic phase of schizophrenia. *J Nerv Ment Dis.* 1983;171:216-221.
2. Glazer W, Prusoff B, John K. Depression and social adjustment among chronic schizophrenic outpatients. *J Nerv Ment Dis.* 1981;169:712-717.
3. Knight RA, Roff JD. Affectivity in schizophrenia. In: Alpert M, ed. *Controversies in Schizophrenia.* New York, NY: Guilford Press; 1985:280-313.
4. Carpenter WT, Heinricks DW, Wagman AMI. Deficit and non-deficit forms of schizophrenia: the concept. *Am J Psychiatry.* 1988;145:578-583.
5. Herz MI. Prodromal symptoms and prevention of relapse in schizophrenia. *J Clin Psychiatry.* 1985;46:22-25.
6. VanPutten T. Why do schizophrenic patients refuse to take their drugs? *Arch Gen Psychiatry.* 1974;31:67-72.
7. Roy A. Depression, attempted suicide and suicide in patients with chronic schizophrenia. *Psychiatr Clin North Am.* 1986;9:193-206.
8. Semrad EV. Long-term therapy of schizophrenia. In: Usdin G, ed. *Psychoneurosis and Schizophrenia.* Philadelphia, Pa: JB Lippincott; 1966:155-173.
9. Davis JL, Kahn RS, Ko G, Davidson M. Dopamine in schizophrenia: a review and reconceptualization. *Am J Psychiatry.* 1991;148:1474-1486.
10. Weinberger DR. Clinical-neuropathological correlations in schizophrenia: theoretical implications. In: Alpert M, ed. *Controversies in Schizophrenia.* New York, NY: Guilford Press; 1985:92-106.
11. VanPutten T, May PRA. The many faces of akathisia. *Compr Psychiatry.* 1975; 16:43-47.
12. VanPutten T, May PRA. 'Akinetic depression' in schizophrenia. *Arch Gen Psychiatry.* 1978;35:1101-1107.
13. Siris SG, vanKammen DP, Docherty JP. Use of antidepressant drugs in schizo-

phrenia. *Arch Gen Psychiatry.* 1978;35:1368-1377.
14. Plasky P. Antidepressant usage in schizophrenia. *Schizophr Bull.* 1991;17:649-657.
15. Donaldson SR, Gelenberg AJ, Baldessarini RJ. Alternative treatments for schizophrenic psychoses. In: Arieti S, ed. *American Handbook of Psychiatry.* 2nd ed. New York, NY: Basic Books Inc; 1986:513-535.
16. Kramer MS, Vogel WH, DiJohnson C, Dewey DA, Sheves P, Cavicchia S, Little P, Schmidt R, Kimes I. Antidepressants in 'depressed' schizophrenic inpatients. *Arch Gen Psychiatry.* 1989;46:922-928.
17. Siris SG, Morgan V, Fagerstrom R, Rifkin A, Cooper TB. Adjunctive imipramine in the treatment of postpsychotic depression. *Arch Gen Psychiatry.* 1987;44:533-539.
18. Siris SG, Bermanzohn PC, Mason SE, Shuwall MA. Maintenance imipramine therapy for secondary depression in schizophrenia: a controlled trial. *Arch Gen Psychiatry.* 1994;51:109-115.
19. Atre-Vaidya N, Taylor MA. Effectiveness of lithium in schizophrenia: do we really have an answer? *J Clin Psychiatry.* 1989;50:170-173.
20. Delva NJ, Letemendia FJJ. Lithium treatment in schizophrenia and schizo-affective disorders. *Br J Psychiatry.* 1982;141:387-400.
21. Hogarty GE, Anderson CM, Reiss DJ, Kornblith SE, Greenwald DP, Javna CD, Madonia MJ. Family psychoeducation, social skills training, and maintenance chemotherapy in the aftercare treatment of schizophrenia. *Arch Gen Psychiatry.* 1986;43:633-642.
22. Hogarty GE, Munetz MR. Pharmacogenic depression among outpatient schizophrenic patients: a failure to substantiate. *J Clin Psychopharmacol.* 1984;4:17-24.
23. Spitzer RL, Endicott J, Robins E. *Research Diagnostic Criteria (RDC) for a Selected Group of Functional Disorders.* 3rd ed. New York, NY: Biometrics Research; 1978.
24. Raskin A, Schulterbrant J, Reatig N, McKeon JJ. Replication of factors of psychopathology in interview, ward behavior, and self-report ratings of hospitalized depressives. *J Nerv Ment Dis.* 1969;148:87-98.
25. Covi L, Lipman RS. Primary depression or primary anxiety? a possible psychometric approach to a diagnostic dilemma. *Clin Neuropsychopharmacol.* 1984;7:924-925.
26. Wing JK. A simple and reliable subclassification of chronic schizophrenia. *J Ment Sci.* 1961;107:862-875.
27. Bartels SJ, Drake RE. Depressive symptoms in schizophrenia: comprehensive differential diagnosis. *Compr Psychiatry.* 1988;29:467-483.
28. VanPutten T, Mutalipossi L, Malkin M. Phenothiazine induced decompensation. *Arch Gen Psychiatry.* 1974;30:102-105.
29. McEvoy JP, Freter S. The dose-response relationship for memory impairment by anticholinergic drugs. *Compr Psychiatry.* 1989;30:135-138.
30. Tune L, Coyle JT. Serum levels of anticholinergic drugs in treatment of acute extrapyramidal side effects. *Arch Gen Psychiatry.* 1980;37:293-297.
31. Moleman P, Schmitz PJM, Ladee GE. Extrapyramidal side effects and oral haloperidol: an analysis of explanatory patient and treatment characteristics. *J Clin Psychiatry.* 1982;43:492-496.
32. Harrow M, Yonan CA, Sands JR, Masengo J. Depression in schizophrenia: are neuroleptics, akinesia, or anhedonia involved? *Schizophr Bull.* 1994;20:327-338.
33. Hogarty GE, McEvoy JP, Munetz M, DiBarry AL, Bartone P, Cather R, Cooley SJ, Ulrich RF, Carter M, Madonia MJ. Dose of fluphenazine, familial expressed emotion, and outcome in schizophrenia: results of a two-year controlled study. *Arch Gen Psychiatry.* 1988;45:797-805.
34. Kane JM, Woerner M, Sarantakos S. Depot neuroleptics: a comparative review of standard, intermediate, and low dose regimens. *J Clin Psychiatry.* 1986;47(suppl):30-34.
35. Marder SR, VanPutten T, Minitz J, Leball M, McKenzie J, May PRA. Low and conventional dose maintenance therapy with fluphenazine decanoate. *Arch Gen Psychiatry.* 1987;44:518-521.
36. Galdi J, Rieder RO, Silber D, Bonato RR. Genetic factors in the response to neuroleptics in schizophrenia: a psychopharmacogenetic study. *Psychol Med.* 1981;11:713-728.
37. Siris SG, Bermanzohn PC, Mason SE, Shuwall MA. Antidepressant for substance-abusing schizophrenic patients: a mini-review. *Prog Neuropsychopharmacol Biol Psychiatry.* 1991;15:1-13.
38. Siris SG, Strahan A, Mandeli J, Cooper TB, Casey E. Fluphenazine decanoate dose and severity of depression in patients with post-psychotic depression. *Schizophr Res.* 1988;1:31-35.
39. Braude WM, Barnes TRE, Gore SM. Clinical characteristics of akathisia. *Br J Psychiatry.* 1983;143:139-150.
40. Marsden CD, Jenner P. The pathophysiology of extrapyramidal side effects of neuroleptic drugs. *Psychol Med.* 1980;10:55-72.
41. Friedel RO. Relationship of desipramine plasma levels to therapeutic response: a critical reappraisal of the data. *J Clin Psychiatry.* 1984;45:46-49.
42. Wolfe ME, Caro M, Mosnam AD. Lithium neuroleptic interactions: electroencephalographic studies. *Res Commun Psychol Psychiatry Behav.* 1991;1635-1640.
43. Janowsky DS, Byerley B. Desipramine: an overview. *J Clin Psychiatry.* 1984;45:3-7.
44. Siris SG, Rifkin A. Drug treatment of depression in patients with schizophrenia. In: Rifkin A, ed. *Schizophrenia and Affective Disorders: Biology and Drug Treatment.* Boston, Mass: John Wright-PSG Inc; 1983:291.
45. Prusoff BA, Williams DH, Weissman MM, Astrachan BM. Treatment of secondary depression in schizophrenia. *Arch Gen Psychiatry.* 1979;36:569-575.
46. Waehrens J, Gerlach J. Antidepressant drugs in anergic schizophrenia. *Acta Psychiatr Scand.* 1980;61:438-444.
47. Siris SG, Adan F, Cohen M, Mandell J, Aronson A, Fasano-Dube B. Targeted treatment of depression-like symptoms in schizophrenia. *Psychopharmacol Bull.* 1987;23:85-89.
48. Johnson DAW. Studies of depressive symptoms in schizophrenia, IV: a double-blind trial of nortriptyline for depression in chronic schizophrenia. *Br J Psychiatry.* 1981;139:97-101.
49. Hogarty GE. Resistance of schizophrenic patients to social and vocational rehabilitation. In: Dencker SJ, Kulhanek F, eds. *Treatment Resistance in Schizophrenia.* Weisbaden, Germany: Vieweg & Sohn; 1988:83-97.
50. Lewine R. Schizophrenia: an amotivational syndrome in men. *Can J Psychiatry.* 1985;30:316-318.
51. Coryell W, Grove W, van Eerdwegh M, Keller M, Endicott J. Outcome in RDC schizo-affective depression: the importance of diagnostic subtyping. *J Affect Disord.* 1987;12:47-56.
52. Carman JS, Bigelow LB, Wyatt RJ. Lithium combined with neuroleptics in chronic schizophrenia and schizo-affective patients. *J Clin Psychiatry.* 1981;42:124-128.
53. Braden W, Fink EB, Qualls B, Samuels WO. Lithium and chlorpromazine in psychotic inpatients. *Psychiatry Res.* 1982;7:69-81.
54. Hirschowitz J, Casper R, Garver DL, Chang S. Lithium response in good prognosis schizophrenia. *Am J Psychiatry.* 1980;137:916-920.
55. vanKammen DP, Alexander PE, Bunney WE. Lithium treatment in post-psychotic depression. *Br J Psychiatry.* 1980;136:479-485.
56. Lerner Y, Mintzer Y, Schestatzsky M. Lithium combined with haloperidol in schizophrenic patients. *Br J Psychiatry.* 1988;153:359-362.
57. Becker RE. Depression in schizophrenia. *Hosp Community Psychiatry.* 1988;39:1269-1274.
58. Roy A. Depression, attempted suicide and suicide in patients with chronic schizophrenia. *Psychiatr Clin North Am.* 1986;9:193-206.
59. Shanfield S, Tucker GJ, Harrow M, Detre T. The schizophrenic patient and depressive symptomatology. *J Nerv Ment Dis.* 1970;151:203-210.
60. Knights A, Hirsch SR. 'Revealed' depression and drug treatment for schizophrenia. *Arch Gen Psychiatry.* 1981;38:806-811.
61. Brier A, Wolkowitz OM, Doran AR, Roy A, Boronow J, Hommer DW, Pickar D. Neuroleptic responsivity of negative and positive symptoms in schizophrenia. *Am J Psychiatry.* 1987;144:1549-1553.
62. Angrist B, Rotrosen J, Gershon S. Differential effects of amphetamine and neuroleptics on negative and positive symptoms in schizophrenia. *Psychopharmacology.* 1980;11:1-3.
63. Garver DL, Kelly K, Fried KA, Magnusson M, Hirschowitz J. Drug response patterns as a basis of nosology for mood-incongruent psychoses (the schizophrenias). *Psychol Med.* 1988;18:873-885.
64. Sullivan G, Wells KB, Leake B. Clinical factors associated with better quality of life in a seriously mentally ill population. *Hosp Community Psychiatry.* 1992;43:794-798.

Conversions From Système International (SI) Units to Traditional Units (Modified From *The SI Manual in Health Care*)

System	Component	SI Reference Interval*	SI Unit	Conversion Factor (Divide by)	Traditional Reference Interval*	Traditional Unit
Plasma	Desipramine, therapeutic	170-700	nmol/L	3.754	50-200	ng/mL

These reference values are not intended to be definitive since each laboratory determines its own values. They are provided for illustration only.

Adoption Study Demonstrating Two Genetic Pathways to Drug Abuse

Remi J. Cadoret, MD; William R. Yates, MD; Ed Troughton; George Woodworth, PhD; Mark A. Stewart, MD

Background: Studies of adoptees have demonstrated that there are two genetic factors leading to alcohol abuse and/or dependence (abuse/dependence). In addition, environmental factors found in the adoptive family also predict alcohol abuse/dependency independently. One study has found evidence that a similar model of two genetic factors and independent adoptive family factors were involved in drug abuse. Our study was designed to test the hypothesis that genetic factors defined by alcohol abuse/dependency and antisocial personality disorder in biologic parents were etiologic in drug abuse/dependency and that psychiatric problems in adoptive parents were an additional factor associated with drug abuse/dependence.

Methods: A sample of 95 male adoptees, separated at birth from their biologic parents, were followed up as adults to determine their psychiatric diagnosis and their substance use/abuse in a structured interview administered blind to biologic parent diagnoses. A high-risk, case-control design was used wherein half of the adoptees came from biologic parents known to be alcohol abuser/dependent and/or have antisocial personalities (diagnoses from hospital or prison records). These adoptees were matched for age, sex, and adoption agency to a control group of adoptees whose biologic parents were not found in the hospital and prison record search. Adoptive home environment was assessed by structured interviews, including psychiatric assessment of both adoptive parents.

Results: Data were analyzed by log-linear modeling, which showed evidence of two genetic pathways to drug abuse/dependency. One pathway went directly from a biologic parent's alcoholism to drug abuse/dependency. The second pathway was more circuitous, and started with antisocial personality disorder in the biologic parent and proceeded through intervening variables of adoptee aggressivity, conduct disorder, antisocial personality disorder, and, eventually, ended in drug abuse/dependency. Environmental factors defined by psychiatric conditions in adoptive families independently predicted increased antisocial personality disorder in the adoptee. Adoptees born of alcohol-abusing mothers showed evidence of fetal alcohol syndrome, but controlling for this did not diminish the evidence for the direct genetic effect between an alcohol-abusing biologic parent and drug abuse/dependency in offspring.

Conclusions: This study confirms the model of two independent genetic factors involved in drug abuse/dependence and previous findings that disturbed adoptive parents are associated with adoptee drug abuse/dependency.

(Arch Gen Psychiatry. 1995;52:42-52)

Research over the past decade has suggested that there are several genetic and environmental pathways to substance abuse—as exemplified by alcoholism. In the early 1980s, Bohman et al[1] and Cloninger et al,[2] on the basis of an extensive multivariate analysis of Swedish adoption data, proposed two types of inheritance of alcoholism: type 1 was defined as a genetic diathesis for alcoholism that led to increased alcoholism in the presence of certain environmental factors; type 2, by contrast, was determined primarily by a genetic diathesis, and environmental factors showed no additional effect. Later publications from Bohman's group have associated the type 2 alcoholic with antisocial behavior because of its correlation with petty criminality.[3]

In the mid-1980s, Cadoret et al[4,5] published results of two independent adoption studies that showed several pathways to alcoholism. This empirically derived model for males is shown in **Figure 1**. These studies showed a strong

See Methods on next page

From the Departments of Psychiatry (Drs Cadoret, Yates, and Stewart and Mr Troughton), Statistics (Dr Woodworth), and Preventive Medicine (Dr Woodworth), University of Iowa, Iowa City.

METHODS

SUBJECT SELECTION

Subjects for this study were recruited from four adoption agencies in the state of Iowa: Lutheran Social Services of Iowa, Des Moines; Catholic Charities of the Archdiocese of Dubuque; Hillcrest Family Services, Cedar Rapids; and the Iowa Department of Human Services, Des Moines. Adoptees and their adoptive parents were selected on the basis of whether the adoptee had a biologic parent with alcohol abuse/dependency, antisocial personality disorder, or drug abuse/dependency (experimental group), or whether there was no evidence from available records of a biologic parent's psychopathology (control group). Controls were matched to experimental subjects for adoption agency, sex, age, and age of the biologic mother at the time of the adoptee's birth. All adoptees in the study had to have been separated from the biologic parent either at birth or within a few days after birth, placed with nonrelatives, and eventually adopted successfully by nonrelatives. Adoptees were further selected to be between 18 and 45 years of age at the time of the study. The sample of adoptees was completely different from those in previously published reports.[4,5,7,8]

Adoptive parents were initially contacted by the agency that handled the adoption. If these parents agreed to be contacted by the experimenters, then a research assistant explained the project and obtained written permission from both the adoptive parents and the adoptee to participate in the study. The contact procedure and permission request were designed to protect the confidentiality of adoptive families and were approved by the Human Subjects Internal Review Board of the University of Iowa College of Medicine.

DIAGNOSIS OF BIOLOGIC PARENTS

Psychiatric assessment of the biologic parents was carried out in the following way. Each of the four participating adoption agencies prepared lists of the names of biologic parents who had given up children for adoption at birth whose ages currently ranged from 18 to 45 years and who were adopted by nonrelatives. These lists were circulated to determine if any of the biologic parents had been hospitalized in the State Department of Human Services mental health institutions or incarcerated by the State of Iowa Department of Adult Corrections. The following hospital records were used in this search: Independence Mental Health Institute, Mt Pleasant Mental Health Institute, Clarinda Mental Health Institute, Cherokee Mental Health Institute, University of Iowa Psychiatric Hospital, and Broadlawns Hospital, Des Moines. Names of the biologic parents also were circulated through the Iowa State Department of Corrections computer databases to determine admission to the prison system. Approximately 11 700 names were circulated through each institution and the corrections system. Identification of the correct biologic parent was confirmed by comparing dates of birth of parent, place of parent's birth, names of the biologic parents, names of siblings, and other identifying data found in the institution's record with information in the adoption agency records.

When names of the biologic parents were found in hospital or prison records, the record was reproduced, deleting names and other identifying data. These copies of records were then used to diagnose the biologic parent's antisocial personality disorder, alcohol abuse/dependency, drug abuse/dependency, and other psychiatric diagnoses. By an elaborate system of coding, it was possible to connect the biologic parent's record with an adoptee without divulging the name of the biologic parent to the investigators.

Prison and hospital records of biologic parents were read independently by three psychiatrists (R.J.C., W.R.Y., and M.A.S.) to make diagnoses . The κ statistics for alcohol abuse/dependency ranged from 0.66 to 0.84 and from 0.67 to 0.79 for antisocial personality disorder. *DSM-III-R*[10] criteria were used. Adopted-away offspring of these biologic parents became the experimental group. In some cases, the biologic parent's drug abuse/dependency was found and these offspring were added to the experimental group. The κ statistics for drug abuse/dependency ranged from 0.75 to 0.88. A number of biologic parents who were antisocial or substance abusers had additional psychiatric diagnoses such as depression. The offspring of these individuals were included in the experimental group because they also had the hypothesized diatheses (a biologic parent with antisocial personality disorder and/or substance abuse) for drug abuse. *DSM-III-R* diagnostic criteria were used to determine these additional psychiatric conditions. When there was disagreement about a biologic parent's diagnosis, the three psychiatric judges met, discussed the case, and came to an agreement as to a diagnosis in most cases. When agreement was not possible, that case was not used in the study, either in the experimental or control groups.

SUBJECT ATTRITION AND SELECTION BIAS

Table 1 shows the rate of refusal encountered in the study. There was an overall refusal rate of 54.0% that varied somewhat from agency to agency, from a low of 35.8% at the Dubuque diocese to 65.6% at the Hillcrest agency. These rates are similar to those found in a previous study done with agencies from three Iowa Catholic dioceses from 1987 to 1990.[11] There is no evidence that the refusal rate is correlated with the status of the biologic parent, as can be determined by comparing column 1 with column 2 in Table 1 (χ^2=5.89, *df*=7, *P*=.55).

In this male sample, 123 adoptive families refused to participate. Reasons given for the refusal were "none" or "not interested" for 87 families (70.7%); concerns about confidentiality for 21 (17.1%); concerns about the potential upset of adoptees around adoption topics such as curiosity about biologic parents for 10 (8.1%); illness in the family for four (3.3%); and adoptee "not available" for one (0.8%). The numbers of families citing these reasons were similar across all four participating agencies. Unfortunately, there was no way to verify the illness or behavioral status of the adoptees who did not participate in the study.

STUDY INSTRUMENTS AND THEIR ADMINISTRATION

Adoptive Parent Interview

This instrument was designed to assess the parental view of the adopted child's physical health, temperament, de-

Continued on next page

velopment, school achievement, and social adjustment from infancy to the present, focusing questions on identifiable stages such as infancy, preschool, and grade school. A section of the interview also covered details about emotional or psychiatric problems in the adoptive family, including dates of problems and the amount of exposure the adoptee had to them. The questions about substance abuse and antisocial problems in the extended adoptive family were expanded from previous versions of this instrument. To do this, a family tree starting with the adoptive parents and extending to their second-degree relatives was obtained, and detailed questions about substance use and antisocial behavior were asked about each relative. The amount of contact of substance-abusing or antisocial relatives with the adoptee was also determined.

To test the hypotheses formulated in the introduction about family environmental factors that are important in drug abuse/dependency, family disturbances were especially sought after, such as separations, divorce, and stressful behavior in family members, with the dates of the disturbances specified. To clarify the types of psychiatric problems in the parents, both adoptive parents were administered the Diagnostic Interview Schedule Screening Interview, a computerized version of the Diagnostic Interview Schedule (DIS).[12] All interviews of adoptive parents were conducted in person by interviewers who were blinded to the biologic background of the adoptee. Adoptive parents and adoptees were interviewed separately and not necessarily by the same interviewer, but in no case did the interviewer know whether the adoptee was of experimental or control status.

The Adoptee Psychiatric Interview

The DIS (version 3, revised), developed by Robins and coworkers[12] was used to interview the adoptees. The DIS allows lay interviewers to assess current and lifetime prevalence of psychiatric illness by *DSM-III-R* criteria and Research Diagnostic Criteria, as well as Feighner criteria. Prior to data collection, the research assistants responsible for the interviewing attended a weeklong DIS instruction course offered by Washington University in St Louis, Mo. Grade school, high school, and medical records also were collected to verify treatment and diagnosis of psychiatric conditions or substance abuse.

Agency records containing information on the prenatal course of the birth mother, including labor and delivery, and the adoptee neonatal course were abstracted.

DIAGNOSIS OF ADOPTEE OUTCOME

DSM-III-R criteria were used to determine adoptee outcome. Diagnosis of adoptee drug abuse, drug dependence, alcohol abuse, alcohol dependence, and antisocial personality disorder were made using the computer program supplied by Washington University for the DIS interview.

Adoptees' aggressivity was measured by items in the adoptive parents' interview. These items were adapted from the aggressivity scale devised by Loney et al,[13] with the addition of five extra items (**Table 2**).

For each adoptee, a total aggressivity score was obtained by counting the number of items endorsed. An adoptee was arbitrarily determined to be aggressive if he was in the upper 25% of the total aggressivity score distribution. Adolescent conduct disorder was defined by the sum of items from Robins[9] such as truancy, school expulsion, lying, stealing, and fighting. Again, the upper 25% of the total conduct disorder score distribution were designated as having conduct disorder.

ASSESSMENT OF ENVIRONMENTAL FACTORS

Our previous adoption study[7] of drug abuse had found that marital and psychiatric problems in the adoptive parents had been associated with increased adoptee drug abuse/dependency. In the study herein, the adoptee and adop-

association between alcohol abuse and antisocial personality disorder in the adoptee (Figure 1, relationship 1). The interaction diagram shows three separate and independent pathways leading to this antisocial-alcoholic outcome. The first pathway (Figure 1, relationship 2) is a direct effect of a biologic parent with alcoholic problems increasing the risk of alcohol abuse and/or dependency (hereafter referred to as abuse/dependency) in offspring. The second pathway (Figure 1, relationship 3) is a direct (environmental) effect of alcohol problems in adoptive relatives increasing the risk of alcoholism in adoptees. The third pathway is a more complex one (Figure 1, relationship 4) and starts with a biologic parent with antisocial problems leading to an adoptee with antisocial personality disorder. The latter condition then is hypothesized as leading to alcoholism rather than the other way around. This conclusion as to the direction of effect was based on the fact that antisocial personality disorder first manifests itself in childhood and adolescence as a conduct disorder, behavior that precedes the characteristically early onset of substance use in these individuals. Adolescent conduct disorder has been known to be a precursor of adult substance abuse in addition to antisocial personality disorder, and conduct disordered behavior prior to drug abuse has been documented in a recent study.[6] Thus, the causal arrow shown in relationship 1 (Figure 1) should be construed as proceeding from antisocial personality disorder to alcoholism.

This three-pathway model of alcoholism is compatible with the hypothesis of Bohman et al[1] of two types of alcoholism, with the third pathway described above representing type 2, and the first pathway (relationship 2) representing type 1, with contributions from environmental factors as shown in relationship 3.

The place of drug abuse in this three-pathway model was described by Cadoret et al[7] and Cadoret.[8] Drug abuse showed a very strong correlation with antisocial personality disorder, even stronger than alcoholism, suggesting that one pathway to drug abuse had its origins in antisocial biologic parents. The analysis also showed a significant correlation between adoptee drug abusers who were not antisocial and a biologic parent's alcohol problems, suggesting a second, and direct, pathway to drug abuse/dependency from parental problem alcohol use. A different environmental effect was found to be associated with increased adoptee drug abuse. This factor was tive parent interview were used to assess these factors. Both the adoptee and adoptive parent interviews asked about health and behavior problems in other adoptive family members in addition to the interviewed family member. Information about the adoptee's siblings or more distant relatives such as adoptive aunts, uncles, and grandparents was obtained indirectly. Assessment of environmental factors was done blind to the adoptee's biologic background. The following environmental factors were derived from these sources: (1) alcohol problem in the adoptive parent or sibling; (2) depression in the adoptive parent or sibling; (3) anxiety diagnosis (phobia, panic disorder, general anxiety) in the adoptive parent or sibling; (4) other psychiatric diagnoses in the adoptive parent or sibling; (5) marital problems in the adoptive parent (divorce, separation); (6) serious physical health problem in the adoptive parent or sibling (eg, diabetes); and (7) rural vs urban home during childhood and adolescence of the adoptee.

STATISTICAL ANALYSIS

Because substance abuse involves a multitude of factors, multivariate statistics were chosen to determine the relationship of etiologic variables to each other and to substance abuse. Log-linear modeling was the principal analytic method used, which allows for use of nominal variables such as presence or absence of comorbid conditions such as antisocial personality disorder in the adoptee, presence or absence of evidence for genetic diatheses, and presence or absence of environmental factors.[14] Analyses were carried out using the BMDP Statistical Software, Program 4F (University of California Press, Berkeley, 1990). Variables were added together to produce models in the following general way. Adoptee outcomes of particular relevance to drug abuse/dependency such as alcohol abuse/dependency and antisocial personality disorder were first correlated together to produce a model of the outcome in the adoptee. Then, genetic factors as identified by diagnoses of the biologic parents were added to the outcome model. Using the program option of ADD=SIMPLE, variables were added to the model if they showed a significant correlation with outcome factors already in the model. Analyses were conducted separately for males and females, since previous Iowa adoption studies have shown sex differences in genetic and environmental factors.[15] Restriction of modeling to one sex limits the number of observations available to modeling. As a rule of thumb, in log-linear modeling, 15 observations per variable included in the model is desirable. In the analyses of the male sample, this restriction limits the number of variables (including outcomes) to six. With significant genetic and outcome variables in the model, gene-environment interaction was tested by using the ADD=MULTIPLE option of the statistical program. This procedure tests each combination of three factors already in the model for interaction by seeing if the correlation between any two of the factors changes significantly with changes in the third factor.

The end point of model building was determined both by limitations in the number of variables that could be added (see above) and by the goodness of fit of a model. All of the models presented here are "good" fits in that there is no significant deviation of the empiric findings from the specific model tested, as determined by both the likelihood ratio χ^2 and Pearson χ^2, which are computed by the modeling program.

Results are presented in the form of interaction diagrams that show the variables in the model and their interrelationships. The strength of association between variables is given by an odds ratio that is corrected for all of the other relationships in the model. Relationships between factors also are shown by 2×2 tables, allowing the use of percentage differences to demonstrate magnitudes of effect.

Where appropriate, *t* tests and χ^2 tests are used to test simple hypotheses. To determine diagnostic reliability for biologic parents, the κ statistic was employed.

Table 1. Biologic Parent Diagnosis by Adoptee Status in the Study

	Adoptee Status						
Biologic Parent Diagnosis	**Agreed**	**Refused**	**Adoptee Deceased**	**Parents Deceased**	**Cannot Find**	**Out of Country**	**Total**
Control	102	112	8	4	19	4	**249**
Drug abuse/dependency	5	5	0	1	0	0	**11**
ASP*	13	27	1	1	1	1	**44**
Drug abuse/dependency and ASP	7	4	0	0	1	0	**12**
Alcohol abuse/dependency	28	33	1	1	3	0	**66**
Drug and alcohol abuse/dependency	9	10	0	1	1	0	**21**
ASP and alcohol abuse/dependency	20	19	2	0	4	0	**45**
Drug abuse/dependency, ASP, and alcohol abuse/dependency	13	21	0	0	3	2	**39**
Total	**197**	**231**	**12**	**8**	**32**	**7**	**487**

**ASP indicates antisocial personality disorder.*

the presence of a "disturbed" adoptive family, defined as marital separation or divorce in adoptive parents or as adoptive parents with a psychiatric condition that required psychotropic medication. This environmental factor was different and independent from an alcohol problem in the adoptive family that continued to correlate positively with an adoptee's alcohol abuse/dependency and not with other drug abuse/dependency.

A further analysis of these adoption data uncovered another factor that was strongly predictive of drug abuse.[8]

Table 2. Aggression Variable List*

Bullies	Quarrelsome
Cruelty	Rebellious
Defiant	Resentful
Destructive	Steals
Difficult to control	Sullen
Disturbs others	Swears
Easily upset	Tantrums
Excitable	Teases
Explosive	Touchy
Fights	Uncooperative
Hard to manage	Won't mind
Irritable	Insolent†
Lies	Physically attacks adults†
Loses temper	Sets fires†
Low frustration tolerance	Threatens others†
Mean	Verbally abuses adults†
Overreacts	

*Adapted from Loney et al.[13]
†Items not in original scale of Loney et al.

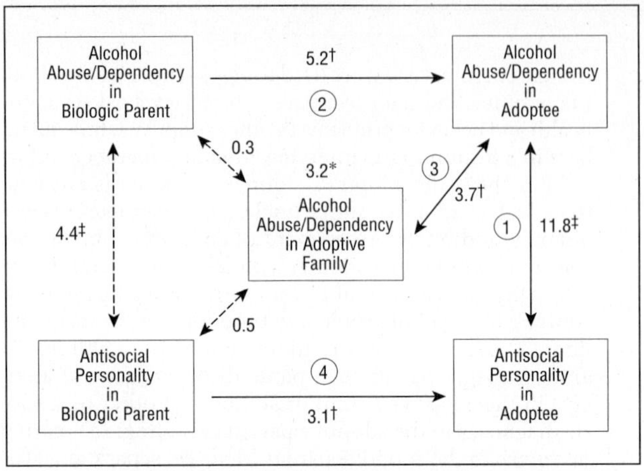

Figure 1. *Interaction diagram of etiologic factors for male adoptee's alcohol abuse and/or dependence and antisocial personality disorder. Asterisk indicates odds ratio significant at 5% level; dagger, at 1% level; and double dagger, at 0.1% level. Circled numbers refer to relationships described in the text. Solid arrows indicate relationship found in data; dashed arrows, relationship forced into the model to control for selective placement. (Modified from Cadoret et al[4].)*

This factor was aggressivity in the adoptee, which predicted change from no drug use to drug use, as well as change from drug use to abuse/dependency. Although aggressivity was strongly correlated with antisocial personality disorder, it was still independently predictive of the change from no drug use to drug use. Aggressivity was certainly a factor in pathway 4 (Figure 1) described above in showing a high correlation with antisocial personality disorder (75% of drug abusers had antisocial personality disorder contrasted with 10% who were users only or 3% who were not users). However, no correlations were found between aggressivity and a biologic parent's alcoholism, antisocial problems, or criminality, thus leaving open the answer to the question of its biologic roots. The present adoption study was designed to follow up the findings reported above and to test the following hypotheses: (1) that antisocial personality disorder and alcohol abuse in biologic parents are risk factors for drug abuse/dependency; (2) that adoptive parents' psychiatric problems would predict increased drug abuse/dependency; (3) that an adoptee's aggressivity would predict drug abuse/dependency; and, (4) in view of aggressivity being considered a basic characteristic of antisocial personality disorder,[9] that aggressivity should correlate with a biologic parent's antisocial personality disorder. This article details the findings with male adoptees.

RESULTS

The incidence of drug abuse/dependency and related outcomes vs experimental or control status of the male adoptee are shown in **Table 3**. Rates for substance abuse/dependency exceed general population rates (Epidemiologic Catchment Area data), which is in agreement with recent studies from this type of adoptee population.[11] Generally, experimental subjects who were adoptees show higher rates of substance abuse and aggressivity.

Table 3. Adoptee Outcome vs Biologic Parent Background*

Behavior Trait	Experimental Group (n=46)	Control Group (n=49)
Mean (±SD) age, y	25.5±5.8	27.4±7.7
Alcohol abuse	0	2 (4.1)
Alcohol dependence	32 (69.6)	25 (51.0)
Total	**32** (69.6)	**27** (55.1)
Drug abuse	7 (15.2)	5 (10.2)
Drug dependence	18 (39.1)	11 (22.4)
Total	**25** (54.3)	**16** (32.7)
Antisocial personality	15 (32.6)	8 (16.3)
Aggressivity	19 (41.3)	5 (10.2)
Alcohol or drug abuse/dependency	35 (76.1)	30 (61.2)

*Data are given as number (percent), except for age.

To test for a genetic effect on an adoptee's outcome, the three main clinical outcome variables of drug abuse/dependency, alcohol abuse/dependency, and antisocial personality disorder and the corresponding three main genetic factors of alcoholism, antisocial personality disorder, and drug abuse/dependency were entered into a log-linear model. The best-fitting model is shown in the interaction diagram depicted in **Figure 2**. The results show that there is a significant relationship between one genetic factor, alcohol abuse/dependency in a biologic parent and an adoptee's drug abuse/dependency. The model also shows strong correlations between antisocial personality disorder and substance abuse and between alcohol abuse/dependency and drug abuse/dependency in both parents and offspring. No other genetic factor correlated with outcome in the final model, although both antisocial personality disorder and alcohol abuse/dependency of a biologic parent showed a borderline correlation with an adoptee's antisocial personality disorder at the beginning of the log-linear analysis

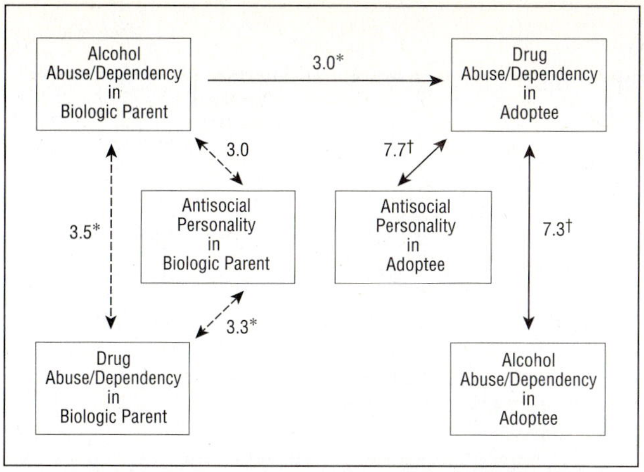

Figure 2. *Interaction diagram for male model with basic genetic and outcome variables (N=95). Asterisk indicates odds ratio significant at 5% level; dagger, at 0.1% level. Solid arrows indicate relationship found in data; dashed arrows, relationship forced into the model to control for selective placement.*

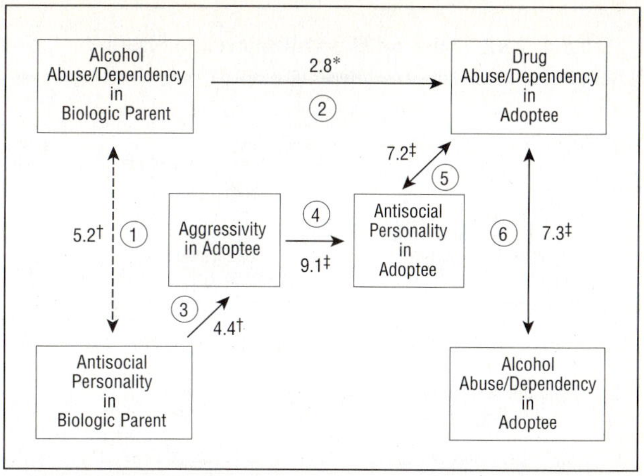

Figure 3. *Interaction diagram for male model with adoptee aggression as the intervening variable (N=95). Asterisk indicates odds ratio significant at 5% level; dagger, at 1% level; and double dagger, at 0.1% level. Circled numbers refer to 2×2 tables in Table 4. Solid arrows indicate relationship found in data; dashed arrows, relationship forced into the model to control for selective placement.*

(P=.07 and P=.05, respectively). However, when the last term enters this model, the significance of these two correlations drops to .15 and .28, respectively. One other biologic parent-adoptee correlation starts out as significant but does not enter the final model. This is the relationship between a biologic parent's drug abuse/dependency and an adoptee's alcohol abuse/dependency. This correlation is significant at .03 at the beginning but drops to .06 at the end of the modeling. Thus, the results from the log-linear modeling demonstrate a significant genetic pathway from alcohol abuse/dependency in a biologic parent to an adoptee's drug abuse/dependency, and suggest that there may be other pathways to substance abuse via a biologic parent's antisocial personality disorder (through the adoptee's antisocial personality disorder) and via a biologic parent's drug abuse/dependency (through the adoptee's alcohol abuse/dependency).

In the introduction to this article, aggressivity was discussed as a characteristic of adoptees that had in previous Iowa adoption studies predicted both drug use and abuse/dependency.[8] Aggressivity also had predicted, in the same data, antisocial personality development in attention deficit hyperactive adoptees, although in that study no genetic factor was found to account for the source of aggressivity.[16] Because of the relationship of aggressivity to both substance abuse and antisocial personality, the adoptee's outcome of aggressivity was explored by further log-linear modeling to determine its relationship to the other outcome variables and to the genetic factors. To keep the number of variables in the model as low as possible (to get better estimates of effects) the factor of a biologic parent's drug abuse/dependency was dropped in place of adoptee aggressivity, which was added as a dichotomous variable (adoptees in the upper 25th percentile of aggressivity scores were labeled "aggressive"). The resulting best-fit model is shown in **Figure 3**. This model demonstrates at least two definite pathways to drug abuse/dependency: the pathway already described from a biologic parent's alcohol abuse/dependency (Figure 2) and a new pathway from a biologic parent's antisocial personality disorder via the intermediate variables of adoptee aggression and adoptee antisocial personality disorder. The latter pathway to adoptee drug abuse/dependency occurs independent of the former direct pathway from biologic parent alcohol abuse/dependency. The 2×2 tables for the relationships in Figure 3 are shown in **Table 4**. Although the biologic parent drug abuse/dependency variable was not in the model, when it is forced into the model as one of the three biologic parent factors (drug abuse, alcohol abuse, antisocial personality disorder) it starts out with a positive correlation with adoptee alcohol abuse/dependency at a P value of .03, but drops out at the final fitting step at a P value of .06. This indicates that biologic parent drug abuse/dependency may be a starting point for an additional pathway to drug abuse via adoptee alcohol abuse/dependency, but the failure to achieve significance could well reflect the low numbers of drug-abusing biologic parents, a type II error.

Following the identification of genetic factors, a necessary step is to demonstrate that these factors are not confounded with environmental factors that could be responsible for the outcome. One environmental factor that was associated with an increased probability of drug abuse in one previous adoption study was the presence of a disturbed adoptive parent.[7] This was defined as an adoptive family in which the parents were reported to have a marital problem (divorce or separation) or a behavioral problem (antisocial behavior, alcohol abuse, or psychiatric illness). As a first step toward establishing the importance of environmental factors in the present study and of confirming the importance of a disturbed adoptive parent in the drug abuse model, we constructed a similar variable, a count of the number of the following problem types in each set of adoptive parents: (1) alcohol abuse/dependency; (2) depressive illness (major depression); (3) anxiety illness (panic disorder or generalized anxiety disorder); (4) marital problems (divorce or separation); (5) legal problems (nontraffic law prob-

Table 4. 2×2 Tables for Effects Displayed in Figure 3

			No	Yes	Corrected Odds Ratio	*P*
			Antisocial personality disorder in biologic parent			
1	Alcohol abuse/dependency in biologic parent	No	52	10	5.2	<.001
		Yes	16	17		
			Drug abuse/dependency in adoptee			
2	Alcohol abuse/dependency in biologic parent	No	41	21	2.8	.02
		Yes	13	20		
			Aggressivity in adoptee			
3	Antisocial personality disorder in biologic parent	No	57	11	4.4	.003
		Yes	14	13		
			Antisocial personality disorder in adoptee			
4	Aggressivity in adoptee	No	62	9	9.1	<.001
		Yes	10	14		
			Drug abuse/dependency in adoptee			
5	Antisocial personality disorder in adoptee	No	49	23	7.2	<.001
		Yes	5	18		
			Alcohol abuse/dependency in adoptee			
6	Drug abuse/dependency in adoptee	No	30	24	7.3	<.001
		Yes	6	35		

lems); and (6) other psychiatric illness (phobic disorders, somatization disorder, and conduct disorder).

The disturbed parent variable ranged from 0 (the modal value) to 6, with a mean of 1.5 and a median of 1. Forty-one families had two or more factors present and this group was defined as being disturbed for the log-linear analysis. The interaction diagram for this variable added to the model shown in Figure 3 appears in **Figure 4**. The disturbed adoptive parent variable is significantly correlated with adoptee antisocial personality disorder, one of the intervening variables between biologic parent antisocial personality disorder and adoptee drug abuse/dependency. This finding confirms the importance of family environmental factors demonstrated by Cadoret et al.[7] These results show that although the disturbed adoptive parent variable influences adoptee outcome, it acts independently and is not confounded with the genetic factors (Figure 4). **Table 5** shows the new 2×2 tables for the model shown in Figure 4.

To examine the separate roles of the different factors that entered into the disturbed adoptive parent variable, each of the six types of factors (parental depressive illness, anxiety illness, alcohol abuse/dependency, marital problems, legal problems, and other psychiatric problems) was correlated separately with adoptee antisocial personality disorder using 2×2 tables and χ^2 analysis to assess significance. The results for this male sample are shown in **Table 6** (data for legal problems are not shown because only three parents had this factor). Two of the six factors are significantly correlated with antisocial personality disorder: depressed and anxious parents.

COMMENT

In interpreting the results of the log-linear analyses, it is important to consider what factors are confounded with the so-called genetic variables (alcoholic, drug-abusing, or antisocial biologic parent). Interviewer bias based on the knowledge of biologic background was precluded by the blinding of the research assistants to the status of the biologic parents. One confoundthat is peculiar to adoption studies is selective placement, an adoptive placement based on the knowledge of both biologic background and adoptive environment, leading to a nonrandom assignment as would occur when an adoptee from an alcoholic background is more likely to be placed in an adoptive home with an alcoholic parent, thus confounding genetic with environmental factors. One of the advantages of the log-linear analysis is the ability to control for this type of confound by forcing into the model the correlation between a genetic factor and a possible environmental confound. This approach has been used in analyses involving the adoptive family psychiatric factors described in Table 5 and Figure 4. This technique, however, would not be effective if the selective placement were predicated on environmental factors that were not recognized or measured. The recognition of a possible confound is made difficult by the often vague placement policies practiced over the years by adoption agencies. For example, at one time childlessness due to a recognized physical problem in a parent was a requirement to adopt an infant.[17] Aside from matching adoptees with adoptive families on physical characteristics such as hair and skin color, a more prevalent but nonspecific policy has been to match the child's potential to the quality of the adoptive home. Thus, children from a biologic background of blue-collar parents might be more likely to end up in a blue-collar adoptive family, or children of parents with low IQs would be unlikely to be placed into the home of a college professor. This more subtle type of confound is difficult to control for and is a reason to measure a large number of adoptive family factors. In the present study, the psychiatric factors found in biologic families were largely predicted but they also were, for the most part, conditions that developed after an adoptee's placement so that selective placement is not a likely explanation. The log-linear control further confirms the lack of correlation between the adoptee's biologic background and the adoptive family's psychiatric conditions that correlate with drug abuse/dependency. It is the direction of effect with these environmental factors that is not clear. Whether anxiety, depression, or marital problems in an adoptive parent are causes or effects of the adoptee's drug abuse/dependency is not determined. Direction of effect could be established by consideration of temporal relationships, although it is possible that some environmental factor could cause both drug abuse in an adoptee and anxiety or depression in a parent. For example, longitudinal studies in families have shown that environmental stress (financial problems) can increase symptoms of anxiety and depression in parents and lead to increased acting out in adolescents, including substance use.[18]

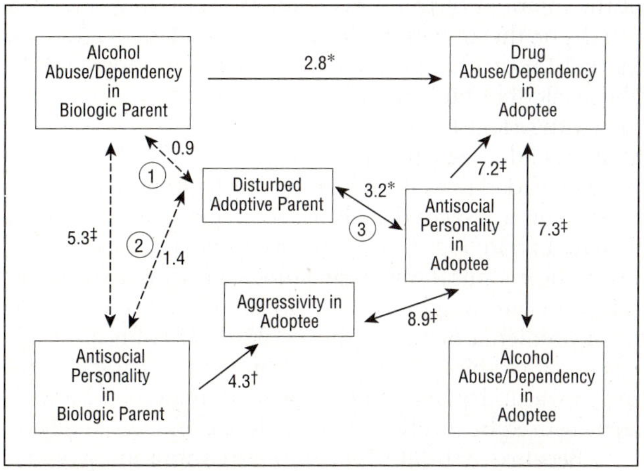

Figure 4. *Log-linear interaction diagram of male sample (N=95). Asterisk indicates odds ratio significant at 5% level; dagger, at 1% level; and double dagger, at 0.1% level. Circled numbers refer to 2×2 tables in Table 5. Solid arrows indicate relationship found in data; dashed arrows, relationship forced into the model to control for selective placement.*

There are other possible confounds with the genetic factors that need to be addressed. In women who are alcoholic, the chance of infants being born with fetal alcohol syndrome (FAS) or a milder variant, fetal alcohol effects (FAE) are high.[19,20] Children born of drinking mothers are more likely to have stigmata of FAS: dysmorphia, growth retardation, and various types of central nervous system damage.[21] The less seriously affected, those with FAE, are still described as having greater social problems in addition to milder dysmorphic signs. Increased behavior and learning problems are reported among exposed children of alcoholic mothers.[22,23] In the present study of male adoptees, there were 13 biologic mothers who were alcohol abuse/dependent and whose adopted-away offspring could have been exposed to alcohol. It is possible that alcohol exposure or other factors associ-

Table 5. 2×2 Tables for Environmental Effects Displayed in Figure 4

					Odds Ratio	*P*
			Disturbed adoptive parent			
			No	Yes		
1	Alcohol abuse/dependency in biologic parent	No	36	26	0.9	.839
		Yes	18	15		
			Disturbed adoptive parent			
			No	Yes		
2	Antisocial personality disorder in biologic parent	No	41	27	1.4	.478
		Yes	13	14		
			Antisocial personality disorder in adoptee			
			No	Yes		
3	Disturbed adoptive parent	No	46	8	3.2	.02
		Yes	26	15		

Table 6. Relationship Between Adoptee Antisocial Personality Disorder and Factors Included in Disturbed Adoptive Parent*

Disturbed Adoptive Parent Factor	Antisocial Adoptee (n=23)	Not Antisocial Adoptee (n=72)	χ^2 Difference	*P* Difference
Alcoholic parent	5 (21.7)	13 (18.1)	0.008	.93
Depressed parent	14 (60.9)	21 (29.2)	6.23	.01
Anxious parent	15 (65.2)	20 (27.8)	8.95	.003
Marital problem	8 (34.8)	17 (23.6)	0.62	.43
Other psychiatric problems	10 (43.5)	19 (26.4)	1.66	.20

*Data are given as number (percent).

ated with alcohol (eg, smoking, poor nutrition) could result in behavioral changes making for drug abuse/dependency. At present, too few children with FAS and FAE have been followed to adolescence and adulthood so that legal and substance abuse problems in clinical samples have not been evaluated. However, conduct problems such as lying and defiance occur in these individuals with FAS, raising the possibility of increased susceptibility to substance abuse/dependency.

One way to address the question of the role of FAS or FAE in the etiology of drug abuse is to eliminate the alcoholic mother from the analysis and look only at the offspring of alcoholic biologic fathers compared with the control group of adoptees whose biologic background was "clean." The contribution of alcoholic fathers, separated from alcoholic mothers to the drug abuse correlation is shown in **Table 7**. In this table 60.6% (20/33) of the male offspring from an alcoholic biologic background (totaled across sex of parent) are drug abuse/dependent, a significant contrast with the 32.7% of drug abusers in the control adoptees (χ^2=5.17, *df*=1, *P*=.02). Disregarding the one adoptee who had both an alcoholic mother and father, the individual contribution from alcoholic fathers compared with alcoholic mothers is 57.1% (12/21) vs 63.6% (7/11), a nonsignificant difference. Because of small samples, neither the male nor the female percentage is significantly different from that of the control. This failure to find significance is likely owing to a type II statistical error, but it suggests that the contributions of both parents' sex to the alcohol background–drug abuse correlation is similar. A second approach to the question of FAS confounding the genetic interpretation is to look at drinking in the biologic mothers during pregnancy. Using all available records (hospital, prison, adoption agency), it was determined that nine of the 12 alcoholic mothers were drinking during the pregnancy of the adoptee and this, combined with other factors associated with drinking such as smoking, poor nutrition, or lack of prenatal care, could have contributed to the maternal alcoholism–adoptee drug abuse correlation. Maternal drinking (and possible associated factors) did affect the adoptee as evidenced by the fact that in these data the birth weight was significantly lower in adoptees from biologic alcoholic mothers than from nonalcoholic mothers. If one omits alcoholic mothers who drank during the pregnancy from the analysis, the second column in Table 7 changes from 63.6% (7/11) drug-abusing adoptees to 33.3% (1/3), a figure indistinguishable from the control (32.7%). The sample size of three is so small as to preclude a conclusion about the effect of drinking during pregnancy on the adult adoptee outcome of drug abuse/dependency.

However, with the availability of adoptee's birth weight and other measures, such as length and gestational age, a further attempt to measure the effect of drinking apart from the genetic effect was possible. As noted above, the weight of adoptees from alcoholic mothers (nine of 12 of whom drank during pregnancy) was significantly lower than that of adoptees from nonalcoholic mothers. This difference was still found when weight was corrected for gestational age by regressing weight against gestational age in weeks. From the regression equation, standardized residuals for weight were obtained for each adoptee, and the mean±SD for the 58 adoptees from nondrinking and nonalcoholic mothers was 0.09±0.94 and for the nine adoptees from mothers who drank during pregnancy was −0.60±1.15 (*t*=1.98, *df*=65, *P*=.05). There were no significant differences in the length of the infant at birth in this comparison. Using the birth weight or the deviations from the predicted weight as a marker for drinking during pregnancy, the adoptee drug abuse–alcohol biologic parent relationship was reexamined using a logistic regression in which the dependent variable was adoptee drug abuse/dependency and the independent variables were biologic parent alcoholism and birth weight, or, in a second analysis, deviations from predicted weight. In both logistic regressions the weight variable was insignificant, but the alcohol biologic factor remained significant (with weight, *P*=.02; with standardized deviation from predicted birth weight, *P*=.008). This finding suggests that the biologic effect measured in the model (Figure 3) was independent of the effect of maternal drinking as measured by its effect on fetal development (weight).

Because of the almost complete confounding of maternal alcohol drinking during pregnancy with the biologic background of alcohol abuse/dependency in mothers and the fact that paternal alcoholism by itself is not significant in predicting an adoptee's drug abuse, there is no unequivocal answer in these data in favor of a solely genetic factor responsible for the direct effect shown in Figure 3. However, the analyses reported above strongly suggest that a genetic factor is involved.

The results are compatible with two biologic (genetic) pathways to drug abuse/dependency. The first pathway is a direct effect from an alcohol abusing/dependent biologic parent. The nature of this biologic effect is unknown but could represent some inherited physiologic mechanism making for increased liability to drug abuse/dependency in individuals exposed to substances. The number of such factors is considerable and would include the types of factors described by Schuckit et al[24-26] as present in the offspring of alcoholics, which manifest themselves as differences in body sway, subjective feelings of intoxication, and so forth in response to alcohol ingestion when compared with offspring of nonalcoholics. Similar factors could play a role in drug abuse/dependency.

The second genetic pathway to drug abuse/dependency starts with biologic antisocial parents and leads

Table 7. Comparison of Biologic Parent Alcohol Abuse/Dependence and Adoptee Drug Abuse/Dependence

		"Clean" Biologic Parent	Alcoholic Mother Only	Alcoholic Father Only	Alcoholic Mother and Father
Adoptee drug abuse/dependence	No	33	4	9	0
	Yes	16	7	12	1

to sons who are aggressive in adolescence, with the end result of both an antisocial personality diagnosis and drug abuse/dependence in the adoptee. This pathway is compatible with the hypothesis about the role of aggression in drug abuse proposed by Loney,[27] who suggested that aggressivity was an independent factor acting in hyperactive children that led to their involvement with drugs. To our knowledge, the present study demonstrates for the first time in an adoption study direct evidence for a genetic factor in aggressivity, connecting it with antisocial personality disorder in biologic parents. A family study by Mattes and Fink[28] reported that the trait of having temper outbursts was more strongly transmitted than diagnoses associated with temper outbursts, such as antisocial personality. Further family studies of heritability of aggressivity suggest stability of aggressive behavior across several generations.[29] Twin and separation studies have reported evidence of genetic inheritance of aggressivity.[30-33] Aggressivity has long been associated with substance abuse.[34-37] The present study demonstrates the linkage between biologic background, adoptee aggressivity, and drug abuse. This pathway appears to involve mechanisms of drug involvement that are different from those of the first pathway. Obviously, aggressivity and all it implies is a driving force that leads to all types of social interactions associated with substance use/abuse: "bad" company, poor social relationships, and fighting, among others. Aggressivity has been subdivided into different types by some investigators.[38] Which type of aggressivity provides the bridging behavior between the genetic factor and the antisocial personality outcome is not clear from these data.

The adolescent aggressivity factor also correlated highly with the adolescent conduct disorder measure. The latter factor was entered into the male model (Figure 3) by dropping adult antisocial personality disorder from that model and inserting the upper 25% of males in the conduct disorder distribution as a dichotomous variable. The corrected odds ratio between aggressivity and conduct disorder is 7.3 ($P<.001$). A feature of this altered model is the fact that the adolescent conduct disorder variable correlates directly with drug abuse with corrected odds ratio of 3.9 ($P<.01$). This establishes the role of conduct disorder in the genesis of drug abuse later in life and is important in suggesting that individuals need not be antisocial personality disordered as adults to develop a drug abuse problem. In these data, 20 of 25 individuals in the top 25% of the conduct disorder distribution were diagnosed as antisocial as adults while five were not, despite the circularity of the *DSM-III* diagnostic definition (which requires at least three conduct disorder behaviors prior to age 15 years).

Throughout this article we have used the term *pathway* to describe the correlational connection between variables. These connections, considered together—as, for example, from antisocial parent to adoptee aggression to conduct disorder and finally to drug abuse/dependence—are a pathway. However, it is not implied that travel down one pathway cannot involve other pathways. Obviously, an individual adoptee could (and a number did) have both an alcoholic and an antisocial parent. The interaction diagram pathways (Figures 1 through 4) show significant contributions to drug abuse vulnerability, whether genetic or environmental or both.

This study confirmed the findings of a previous report[7] that showed that a disturbed adoptive parent was a factor in drug abuse/dependency. It is unlikely that this parental factor was influenced by interviewer bias (in that the same research assistant interviewed adoptive parents and adoptees) since almost all of the information about parents used in the disturbed parent factor was obtained from the computer-administered DIS, which would minimize the opportunity for the research assistant to bias the procedure. The types of problems that correlate in this male sample with antisocial adoptee are those of depression and/or anxiety in an adoptive parent. The present findings, which are based on a structured psychiatric interview (DIS), provide more confidence in the validity of the parental psychiatric diagnoses. However, the direction of effect remains unclear—whether the adoptee misbehavior acts as a stress in the genesis of depressive and anxiety symptoms in parents or whether these psychiatric conditions affected the family interaction leading to antisocial adoptee behavior.

The multipathway model for drug abuse/dependency described by these data is remarkably similar to the model for alcohol abuse/dependency described in the introduction and depicted in Figure 1. Both models have a pathway through antisocial personality disorder starting with antisociality in a biologic parent; both feature a direct pathway to substance abuse from a substance abusing/dependent biologic parent; and both find a variety of environmental factors that act independently of the biologic factors to affect substance abuse directly or indirectly. The similarity of the models and the facts that a biologic parent's alcohol abuse predicts drug abuse outcome and a biologic parent's drug abuse and an adoptee's alcohol abuse show an almost significant relationship suggest similar biologic factors in both drug and alcohol abuse/dependency, with at least two resulting genetic pathways to abuse and additional pathways when environmental factors are considered. However, there could still be a specific genetic factor predisposition to drug abuse/dependency only. Such a factor would be obscured in our design by the fact that older biologic parents, because of low exposure decades ago to drugs, never developed a drug abuse problem and so did not receive a correct phenotypic classification.

The hypothesis of common factors leading to both

drug abuse and alcohol abuse is supported by recent studies of addiction patterns in families,[39-41] as well as by studies of biochemical and physiologic mechanisms.[42,43] The present study suggests one underlying genetically transmitted factor responsible for both alcohol and other drug abuse (the direct factor) and another genetic factor leading to substance abuse/dependency through conduct disorder, aggressivity, and antisocial personality disorder.

Accepted for publication August 24, 1994.

This work was supported by grant RO1 DA05821 from the National Institute on Drug Abuse, Rockville, Md.

We wish to acknowledge the cooperation of the following individuals and agencies in making this study possible: James Yeast, Catholic Charities of the Archdiocese of Dubuque; Craig Mosher, PhD, and Nancylee Ziese, Hillcrest Family Services; Paul Loeffelholz, MD, Iowa Department of Corrections; Marge Corkery, Iowa Department of Human Services; and Leonard Larson, PhD, Lyn Lienhard, and Louise Koch, Lutheran Social Services of Iowa.

The following individuals performed data collection: Michelle Appel, Alberta Conrad, Nancy Copeland, Donna Davis, Rebecca Hansel, Roxane Moller, Carol Moss, Scott Murray, Helen Peck, Chris Richards, Jody Speer, Sommai Ung, and Angela Wright.

Reprint requests to Department of Psychiatry, University of Iowa College of Medicine, 200 Hawkins Dr, 2887 JPP, Iowa City, IA 52242-1057 (Dr Cadoret).

REFERENCES

1. Bohman M, Cloninger CR, Sigvardsson S, von Knorring AL. Predisposition to petty criminality in Swedish adoptees, I: genetic and environmental heterogeneity. *Arch Gen Psychiatry.* 1982;39:1233-1241.
2. Cloninger CR, Bohman M, Sigvardsson S. Inheritance of alcohol abuse. *Arch Gen Psychiatry.* 1981;38:861-868.
3. von Knorring L, von Knorring AL, Smigan L. Personality traits in subtypes of alcoholics. *J Stud Alcohol.* 1987;48:523-527.
4. Cadoret RJ, O'Gorman TW, Troughton E. Alcoholism and antisocial personality: interrelationships, genetic and environmental factors. *Arch Gen Psychiatry.* 1985;42:161-167.
5. Cadoret RJ, Troughton E, O'Gorman TW. Genetic and environmental factors in alcohol abuse and antisocial personality. *J Stud Alcohol.* 1987;48:1-8.
6. Young SE, Zoccolillo MS, Mikulich TJ, Crowley TJ. Relationship between conduct disorder and adolescent substance abuse. Abstract presented at 54th Annual Scientific Meeting of the College on Problems of Drug Dependence; June 1992; Keystone, Colo.
7. Cadoret RJ, Troughton E, O'Gorman TW, Heywood E. An adoption study of genetic and environmental factors in drug abuse. *Arch Gen Psychiatry.* 1986; 43:1131-1136.
8. Cadoret RJ. Genetic and environmental factors in initiation of drug use and the transition to abuse. In: Glantz MD, Pickens RW, eds. *Vulnerability to Drug Abuse.* Washington, DC: American Psychological Association; 1992:99-113.
9. Robins LN. *Deviant Children Grown Up.* Baltimore, Md: Williams & Wilkins; 1966.
10. American Psychiatric Association. *Diagnostic and Statistical Manual of Mental Disorders, Revised Third Edition.* Washington, DC: American Psychiatric Association; 1987.
11. Cadoret RC, Troughton E, Woodworth G. Evidence of heterogeneity of genetic effect in Iowa adoption studies. *N Y Acad Sci.* 1994;708:59-71.
12. Robins L, Helzer J, Cottler L, Goldring E. NIMH Diagnostic Interview Schedule, Version 3, Revised (DIS-III-R). St Louis, Mo: Washington University School of Medicine; August 1989.
13. Loney J, Langhorne JE, Paternite CE, Whaley-Klahn MA, Blair-Broeker CT, Hacker M. The Iowa habit: hyperkinetic/aggressive boys in treatment. In: Sells SB, Crandall R, Roff, M, Strauss JS, Pollin W, eds. *Human Functioning in Longitudinal Perspective.* Baltimore, Md: Williams & Wilkins; 1980.
14. Fienberg SE. *The Analysis of Cross-Classified Categorical Data.* 2nd ed. Cambridge, Mass: The MIT Press; 1983.
15. Cadoret RJ, Cain C. Sex differences in predictors of antisocial behavior in adoptees. *Arch Gen Psychiatry.* 1980;37:1171-1175.
16. Cadoret RJ, Stewart MA. An adoption study of attention deficit/hyperactivity/aggression and their relationship to adult antisocial personality. *Compr Psychiatry.* 1991;32:73-82.
17. Cadoret RC. Adoption studies: historical and methodological critique. *J Psychol Dev.* 1986;1:45-64.
18. Conger RD, Conger KJ, Elder GH Jr, Lorenz FO, Simons RL, Whitbeck LB. A family process model of economic hardship and adjustment of early adolescent boys. *Child Dev.* 1992;63:526-541.
19. Coles CD. Prenatal alcohol exposure and human development. In: Miller M, ed. *Development of the Central Nervous System: Effects of Alcohol and Opiates.* New York, NY: Wiley-Liss; 1992:9-36.
20. Miller MW. The necessity of biomedical research on substance abuse. In: Miller M, ed. *Development of the Central Nervous System: Effects of Alcohol and Opiates.* New York, NY: Wiley-Liss; 1992:1-8.
21. Streissguth AP, Randels SP. Long-term effects of fetal alcohol syndrome. In: Robinson G, ed. *Alcohol and Child/Family Health.* Vancouver: University of British Columbia Press; 1988.
22. Shaywitz SE, Cohen DJ, Shaywitz BA. Behavioral and learning difficulties in children with normal intelligence born to alcoholic mothers. *J Pediatr.* 1980; 95:978-982.
23. Larsson G, Bohlin A-B. Fetal alcohol syndrome and preventive strategies. *Pediatrician.* 1987;14:51-56.
24. Schuckit M. Self-rating alcohol intoxication by young men with and without family histories of alcoholism. *J Stud Alcohol.* 1980;41:242-249.
25. Schuckit MA, Gold EO, Risch C. Serum prolactin levels in sons of alcoholics and control subjects. *Am J Psychiatry.* 1987;144:854-859.
26. Schuckit MA. Ethanol-induced changes in body sway seen at high alcoholism risk. *Arch Gen Psychiatry.* 1985;42:375-379.
27. Loney J. The Iowa theory of substance abuse among hyperactive adolescents. In: Lettieri DJ, Sayers M, Pearson HW, eds. *Theories on Drug Abusers: Selected Contemporary Perspectives.* Rockville, Md: National Institute on Drug Abuse; 1980. NIDA Research Monograph 30.
28. Mattes JA, Fink M. A family study of patients with temper outbursts. *J Psychiatr Res.* 1987;21:249-255.
29. Eron LD, Huessman LR. The stability of aggressive behavior—even unto the third generation. In: Lewis M, Miller SM, eds. *Handbook of Developmental Psychopathology.* New York, NY: Plenum Press; 1990:147-156.
30. Plomin R, Nitz K, Rowe D. Behavioral genetics and aggressive behavior in childhood. In: Lewis M, Miller SM, eds. *Handbook of Developmental Psychopathology.* New York, NY: Plenum Press; 1990:119-133.
31. Tellegen A, Lykken DT, Bonchara TJ, Wilcox K, Segal N, Rich S. Personality similarity in twins reared apart and together. *J Pers Soc Psychol.* 1988;54: 1031-1039.
32. Jary ML, Stewart MA. Psychiatric disorders in the parents of adopted children with aggressive conduct disorder. *Neuropsychobiology.* 1985;13:7-11.
33. Poole ED. *Relations of Aggression to Shared and Non-shared Environments of Twins.* Iowa City: University of Iowa; May 1992. Thesis.
34. Kandel DB. *Longitudinal Research on Drug Use.* Washington, DC: Hemisphere Publishing Corp; 1978.
35. Penning M, Barnes GE. Adolescent marijuana use: a review. *Int J Addict.* 1982; 17:749-791.
36. Brook JS, Cohen P, Whiteman M, Gordon AS. Psychosocial risk factors in the transition from moderate to heavy use or abuse of drugs. In: Glantz MD, Pickens RW, eds. *Vulnerability to Drug Abuse.* Washington, DC: American Psychological Association; 1992:359-388.
37. Kellam SG, Brown CH, Rubein BR, Ensminger ME. Paths leading to teenage psychiatric symptoms and substance use: developmental epidemiological studies in Woodlawn. In: Guze SB, Earle F, Barrett JE, eds. *Childhood Psychopathology and Development.* New York, NY: Raven Press; 1983.
38. Buss AH, Durkee A. An inventory for assessing different kinds of hostility. *J Consult Psychol.* 1957;21:343-349.
39. Miller NW, Gold MS, Belkin BM, Klahr AL. The diagnosis of alcohol and cannabis dependence in cocaine dependents and alcohol dependents in their families. *Br J Addict.* 1989;29:1491-1498.
40. Jacob T. Drinking, drinking styles and drug use in children of alcoholics, depressives and controls. *J Stud Alcohol.* 1989;50:427-431.
41. Smith JW, Frawley PJ. Alcoholism in relatives of primary cocaine dependent patients. *J Subst Abuse Treat.* 1992;9:153-155.
42. George FR. Is there a common biologic basis for reinforcement from alcohol and other drugs? *Behav Biochem Genders.* 1991;10:127-139.
43. Mackler SA, Eberwine JH. The molecular biology of addictive drugs. *Mol Neurobiol.* 1991;5:145-158.

ORIGINAL ARTICLE

Efficacy and Tolerability of Serotonin Transport Inhibitors in Obsessive-compulsive Disorder

A Meta-analysis

John H. Greist, MD; James W. Jefferson, MD; Kenneth A. Kobak, MSSW; David J. Katzelnick, MD; Ronald C. Serlin, PhD

Background: Questions have been raised regarding the relative efficacy and tolerability of the different serotonin transport inhibitors in the treatment of obsessive-compulsive disorder. We compared the results from four large multicenter placebo-controlled trials of the serotonin transport inhibitors clomipramine hydrochloride (N=520), fluoxetine hydrochloride (N=355), fluvoxamine maleate (N=320), and sertraline hydrochloride (N=325) for the treatment of obsessive-compulsive disorder.

Methods: Effect size was calculated by subtracting the end-point drug treatment mean change from the end-point placebo mean change and dividing by the end-point pooled change standard deviation. A test for overall differences between effect sizes was conducted, followed by all possible pairwise comparisons. The Yale-Brown Obsessive Compulsive Scale was the primary outcome measure for all four studies.

Results: All four agents were significantly more effective than placebo, with clomipramine significantly more effective than the other three treatments, which did not differ in effect size. A significantly greater percentage of patients treated with clomipramine were rated much or very much improved than were patients treated with fluoxetine, fluvoxamine, or sertraline.

Conclusion: While the results of this meta-analysis support the superiority of clomipramine, head-to-head, double-blind comparisons of these compounds would be the best test of comparative efficacy and tolerability.

(Arch Gen Psychiatry. 1995;52:53-60)

From the Dean Foundation for Health, Research and Education, Madison, Wis.

OBSESSIVE-compulsive disorder (OCD) has become the subject of substantial study in the past decade. Part of this expanded interest is owing to the availability of effective pharmacologic treatments. Agents with potent serotonin transport inhibiting properties have been shown conclusively to be effective short-[1-4] and long-term[1,5,6] treatments for this disorder. (Neuropsychopharmacologists have used "uptake" and "reuptake" to describe the mechanism of inhibition of transport of serotonin from synapse into presynaptic neuron. We appreciate the suggestion of Richard Shader, MD, that "serotonin transport inhibition" be used to describe this phenomenon.)

Proper questions have been raised regarding the relative efficacy and tolerability of the different serotonin transport inhibitors (STIs) in the treatment of OCD. This article reviews data on effectiveness and tolerability from four large multicenter, placebo-controlled trials of clomipramine hydrochloride (Anafranil),[1] fluoxetine hydrochloride (Prozac),[2,5] fluvoxamine maleate (Luvox),[3,7] and sertraline hydrochloride (Zoloft) (J.H.G. et al, unpublished data, 1993).[4]

RESULTS

EFFICACY

Figure 1 shows Y-BOCS change scores of the drug minus placebo intent-to-treat analysis for clomipramine, fluoxetine, fluvoxamine, and sertraline. There were substantial increases in placebo response over the course of time that these four studies were conducted (1986-1990). **Figure 2** shows the Y-BOCS change scores for the intent-to-treat analysis for the four drugs without subtracting placebo. **Figure 3** shows the intent-to-treat changes of patients receiving placebo in the four trials.

See Methods on next page

METHODS

THE STUDIES

All of the trials used similar, although not identical, designs, and many of the same investigators participated in more than one trial. The Yale-Brown Obsessive Compulsive Scale (Y-BOCS)[8,9] was used as a severity and change measure in all four trials and permits comparisons based on that scale. Clinical Global Impression improvement scores[10] also were available for all the studies. In addition to short-term (10- to 13-week) trials with these agents, there are more limited data available regarding extensions as long as 1 year.[1,5,6] We compared the results from these four studies with regard to short-term efficacy and side effects.

A comparison of protocol and subject characteristics is presented in **Table 1** and **Table 2**. The sample included 1520 subjects (clomipramine, N=520; fluoxetine, N=355; fluvoxamine, N=320; and sertraline, N=325) from 48 sites (clomipramine, n=21; fluoxetine, n=8; fluvoxamine, n=8; and sertraline, n=11). Subjects were a minimum age of 18 years except for those in the fluoxetine study, where the minimum age was 14 years. All the subjects met criteria for OCD as outlined in *DSM-III*[11] or *DSM-III-R*.[12] The sertraline data were from a single multicenter study (J.H.G. et al, unpublished data, 1993)[4]; the fluvoxamine data were pooled from two identical multicenter studies,[3,7] as were the fluoxetine data[2,5]; and the clomipramine data were from two multicenter studies with identical protocols,[1] with the exception that study 2 stratified patients according to Hamilton Depression Rating Scale[13] scores ($\leq$16 vs >16 on the 17-item version) and had a minimum duration of the current episode of 1 year as opposed to 2 years. The 19 subjects in clomipramine study 2 scoring above 16 on the Hamilton Depression Rating Scale were not included in the efficacy analyses but were included in the safety analyses. Three of the studies (clomipramine, fluoxetine, and fluvoxamine) began before Food and Drug Administration approval of clomipramine in December 1989, while the sertraline study was initiated in 1990. Twenty-three percent of the patients in the fluvoxamine study and 39% of the patients in the sertraline study were previously treated with an STI; data were unavailable for the fluoxetine study.

Following 1 week (fluoxetine and sertraline) or 2 weeks (clomipramine and fluvoxamine) of single-blind placebo washout, subjects were randomized to 10 weeks (clomipramine and fluvoxamine), 12 weeks (sertraline), or 13 weeks (fluoxetine) of double-blind treatment. Patients returned for biweekly evaluations in all of the studies except the clomipramine study, in which evaluations were obtained weekly. A fixed daily-dose treatment schedule was used in the fluoxetine (20, 40, and 60 mg) and sertraline (50, 100, and 200 mg) studies, while the clomipramine and fluvoxamine studies employed a flexible dose schedule. In the clomipramine study, the minimum and maximum dose range was 100 to 250 mg/d, with 300 mg/d allowable under special circumstances. For clomipramine study 1, the week 10 mean dose was 234.5 mg/d (SD, 59.47); for study 2, 218.8 mg/d. In the fluvoxamine study, the minimum and maximum doses were 100 and 300 mg/d, with a mean dose of 249 mg/d (SD, 71.27) at week 10. The clomipramine and fluvoxamine protocols contained equal numbers of subjects in the placebo and active treatment arms, while subjects in the fluoxetine and sertraline studies, as a result of the fixed-dose treatment schedule, were randomized in an approximate 3:1 ratio to active treatment or placebo.

THE ANALYSES

Effect size was calculated by subtracting the end-point drug treatment mean change from the end-point placebo treatment mean change, and dividing by the end-point pooled change SD.[14,15] Comparison of effect sizes was performed using procedures outlined by Cramer[16] and Rosenthal and Rubin.[17] The validity of calculating and comparing the significance level of the effect sizes of two or more independent (vs groups of) studies has been addressed by Rosenthal and Rubin[17,18] and others.[19-24] Because the distribution of effect sizes can be approximated by a normal distribution, Cramer's method[16] of modified minimum χ^2 was used to compare them, yielding an omnibus test statistic that is χ^2 distributed. Following the significant omnibus test, all possible pairwise comparisons among the effect sizes were performed, using the Scheffé technique.

Between-group comparisons of dropout rates and the proportion of subjects in each group rated "much improved" or "very much improved" were made using the Pearson χ^2 test for homogeneity.[25]

All analyses were performed using the mean for the fixed-dose studies (fluoxetine and sertraline), with the exception of comparisons using only the "best" dose in the fixed-dose studies (fluoxetine, 60 mg; and sertraline, 200 mg) (**Table 3**). An intent-to-treat analysis was used for all calculations.

All four agents were significantly more effective than placebo (clomipramine, $P<.001$; fluoxetine, $P<.001$; fluvoxamine, $P<.001$; and sertraline $P<.006$).

Clinical Global Impression ratings of much or very much improved for all four drugs are illustrated in **Figure 4**. A significantly greater percentage of patients treated with clomipramine were rated much or very much improved than patients treated with fluoxetine, fluvoxamine, or sertraline ($\chi^2[3]=32.60$, $P<.001$).

Effect sizes for these four medications are displayed in **Figure 5**, along with their 95% confidence intervals. All the treatments produced substantial clinical benefits, with clomipramine significantly more effective than the other three treatments, which do not differ in effect size ($\chi^2[3]=66.57$, $P<.001$).

As indicated by Amundsen et al,[26] the standardized effect size can be used to indicate the probability of a treatment subject's outperforming a control subject (**Figure 6**). Figure 6 shows the relationship between such probabilities and effect size. For example, a population effect size of 1.2 would reflect an 80% chance that a randomly selected treatment subject would outscore a randomly selected control subject. In our study, for the three groups whose effect sizes were approximately 0.5 (fluoxetine, fluvoxamine, and sertraline), the probability that patients using

Table 1. Protocol Characteristics*

Protocol Characteristic	Study: Clomipramine Hydrochloride (N=520)	Fluoxetine Hydrochloride (N=355)	Fluvoxamine Maleate (N=320)	Sertraline Hydrochloride (N=325)
Length of washout, wk	2	1	2	1
Length of double-blind treatment, wk	10	13	10	12
Diagnostic criteria	*DSM-III*	*DSM-III-R*	*DSM-III-R*	*DSM-III-R*
Minimum Y-BOCS score	16	16†	None	None
Minimum NIMH Global Severity score	7	7	7	NA‡
Maximum HAMD score	16§	None	19‖	17¶
Minimum duration of current episode, y	2#	1	1	None
Minimum age, y	18	14	18	18
Maximum age, y	None	70	68	None
No. of sites	9‖	NA	8	11
Concurrent medication	Chloral hydrate	NA	Chloral hydrate or lorazepam	Chloral hydrate
Dosing schedule	Flexible	Fixed	Flexible	Fixed
Visit interval	Weekly	Biweekly	Biweekly	Biweekly
Year initiated	1986	1987	1988	1990
Drug/placebo ratio	260/260	266/89	160/160	241/84

**Y-BOCS indicates Yale-Brown Obsessive Compulsive Scale; NA, not available; HAMD, Hamilton Depression Rating Scale; and NIMH, National Institute of Mental Health.*
†Score of 10 if obsessions or compulsions only.
‡Used Clinical Global Impression scale instead: score of 4=moderate required.
§Seventeen-item version.
‖Twelve sites in protocol 2.
¶Twenty-four–item version minus item 21 (obsessions).
#One year for protocol 2.

Table 2. Subject Characteristics*

Subject Characteristic	Study†: Clomipramine Hydrochloride (N=520)	Fluoxetine Hydrochloride (N=355)	Fluvoxamine Maleate (N=320)	Sertraline Hydrochloride (N=325)
Age, y	35.51 (10.67)	36.90 (11.71)	36.20 (11.38)	38.64 (13.00)
Sex, %				
M	44	45	49	59
F	56	55	51	41
Duration of illness, y	15.69 (6.75)	NA	15.3 (19.90)	4.98 (8.75)
Baseline Y-BOCS score	26.55 (5.16)	23.94 (5.54)	23.22 (5.56)	23.70 (5.08)
Baseline HAMD score	6.75 (3.99)	9.3 (5.72)	8.28 (4.95)	NA

**Data are given as mean (SD), except for sex. NA indicates not available; Y-BOCS, Yale-Brown Obsessive Compulsive Scale; and HAMD, Hamilton Depression Rating Scale.*
†Drug and placebo combined.

Table 3. 'Best' Dose Comparison*

	Study†: Clomipramine Hydrochloride (N=260)	Fluoxetine Hydrochloride (N=90)	Fluvoxamine Maleate (N=160)	Sertraline Hydrochloride (N=80)
Mean dose,‡ mg/d	226	60	249	200
Mean baseline Y-BOCS score	26.20	24.37	22.98	23.54
Mean terminal Y-BOCS score	16.00	17.84	18.50	17.34
Mean change in Y-BOCS score	10.2	6.5	4.5	6.2
Percent decrease	39	27	20	26
Percent much or very much improved	60	44	43	44
Effect size	1.48	0.83	0.50	0.45

**Y-BOCS indicates Yale-Brown Obsessive Compulsive Scale.*
†Drug group only.
‡End point.

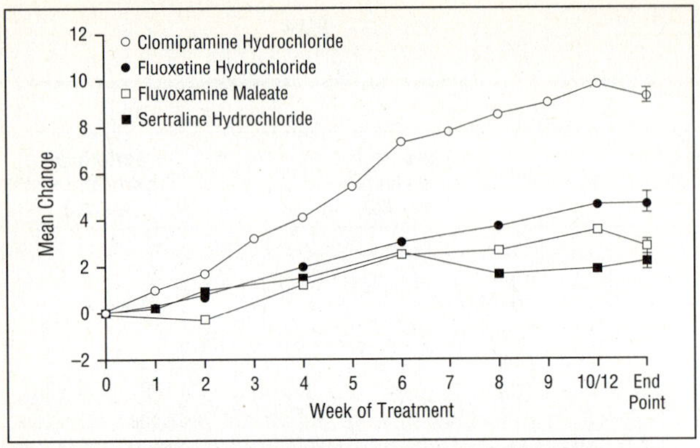

Figure 1. *Mean change in total Yale-Brown Obsessive Compulsive Scale scores for drug minus placebo intent-to-treat analysis. There were 12 weeks of treatment for the fluvoxamine and sertraline studies. Error bars indicate pooled SE of change score (available for end point only).*

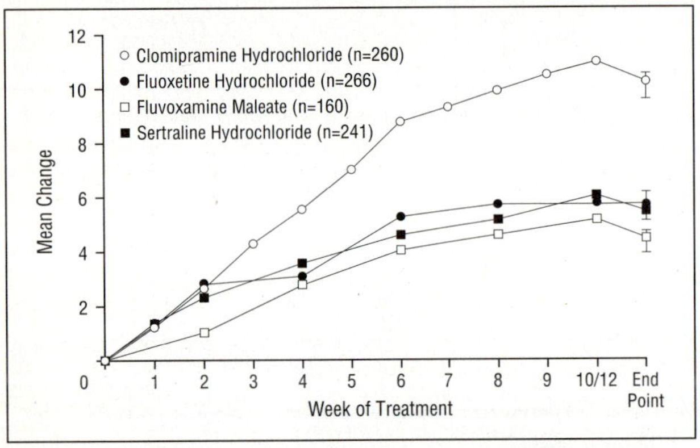

Figure 2. *Mean change in total Yale-Brown Obsessive Compulsive Scale scores for drug intent-to-treat analysis. There were 12 weeks of treatment for the fluvoxamine and sertraline studies. Error bars indicate pooled SE of change score (available for end point only).*

these treatments will show improvement compared with control subjects is approximately .63, or almost two thirds. However, with clomipramine, with an effect size of 1.48, the probability is approximately 85%, a better than 5:1 ratio that a treatment patient will show improvement compared with a control patient.

TOLERABILITY

Figure 7 shows the total dropout rate (side effects plus lack of efficacy and other causes) for each drug. Surprisingly, the total dropout rates were significantly less for clomipramine than for each of the other agents ($\chi^2[3]=40.85$, $P<.001$). There were no significant differences in dropouts because of side effects (clomipramine, 8%; fluoxetine, 12%; fluvoxamine, 15%; and sertraline, 10%).

COMMENT

The ideal is seldom captured in reality. Head-to-head, double-blind studies of these compounds would be the best tests of comparative efficacy and tolerability. However, true blinding is difficult, especially with clomipramine, which commonly has more anticholinergic and other side effects than fluoxetine,[21] fluvoxamine, and sertraline. These studies had other protocol and subject differences (Tables 1 and 2) that may have affected the results. Despite these deviations from ideality, the designs in the four multicenter trials were similar, change and outcome measures were identical, and several investigators participated in more than one trial. Thus, while recognizing some differences, to our knowledge, the present meta-analysis is the most complete and comprehensive for comparing these four compounds. While some of these data are unpublished, all of the studies have been presented at international symposia and described in posters and/or abstracts. Most meta-analysts conclude that it is appropriate to include unpublished data in primary meta-analyses.[27] Head-to-head controlled trials of some of these agents are under way or planned but we know of only one small crossover study of clomipramine and fluoxetine that has been reported.[28] The results from that crossover design trial with 11 subjects indicate a trend for clomipramine to have greater efficacy than fluoxetine. Another small (N=55) controlled comparison of these compounds also had trends and some significant differences favoring clomipramine over fluoxetine.[5]

A small double-blind study comparing clomipramine and fluvoxamine found no significant difference in efficacy. Both compounds were well tolerated with comparable dropouts because of adverse events (four [12.5%] of 32 clomipramine patients and five [14.7%] of 34 fluvoxamine patients).[29]

The short-term efficacy of all four compounds has been clearly demonstrated. Clomipramine stands out from the other three agents, which cluster closely on Y-BOCS and Clinical Global Impression change measures. Effect size calculations are consistent with other indicators of efficacy. While fluoxetine and sertraline were found to be equally effective at each dose studied, when their best-dose trend subgroups were compared with clomipramine, the superiority of clomipramine remained (Table 3).

Where studied, long-term treatment with each compound showed persistence of short-term gains[1,5,6] and, for fluoxetine[5] and clomipramine,[1] further improvement. There has been no controlled long-term study of fluvoxamine, but open-label treatments of patients from a controlled trial[30] extending to 8 years have shown durability of benefit and rapid relapse when medication was discontinued (J.H.G., oral communication, 1993). Relapse on discontinuation almost always occurs with these compounds.[31-33]

Surprisingly, there was not a higher dropout rate for clomipramine because of side effects during the short-term treatment trials. There was even a trend toward clomipramine treatment's having the lowest rate of dropouts because of side effects, despite having a higher overall rate of side effects. Overall, clomipramine treatment had a significantly lower rate of dropouts from all causes (side effects, lack of efficacy, and other causes) ($P<.001$). In part, this might be owing to the lack of other effective psychopharmacologic agents at the time the clomipramine trial was done and weekly visits in the clomipramine trial vs biweekly visits in the fluoxetine, fluvoxamine, and sertraline trials. Importantly, all of these compounds were well tolerated over their 10- to 13-week trials and the overall dropout rates for subjects receiving drug and placebo were unusually low for clinical trials in psychiatric disorders.

How can we explain and understand the apparent superiority of clomipramine efficacy and tolerability in these multicenter controlled trials? Despite marked similarities in the designs of the four studies, there are some differences (see Tables 1 and 2). The 2-week washout with the clomipramine and fluvoxamine studies might have yielded smaller placebo responses than the 1-week washout with fluoxetine and sertraline. However, all placebo response rates were low compared with pharmacologic trials in mood[34] and other anxiety disorders,[35] and there was no systematic effect favoring longer placebo washouts. The shorter 10-week trials of clomipramine and fluvoxamine may have biased against maximum benefit since clomipramine and fluvoxamine Y-BOCS scores were still decreasing between the week 8 and week 10 measurements. The Y-BOCS scores continued to decrease in the 12-week sertraline study between the last measurement points, and, while fluoxetine did not, subsequent improvement was found at the 6-month follow-up.[5] Minimum entry criteria (Y-BOCS or National Institute of Mental Health Global Obsessive Compulsive Scale) did not differ and the effect of higher Hamilton Depression Rating Scale scores, if any, could not be determined because of the small number of depressed subjects. The longer duration entry criterion in the clomipramine study may have confirmed the diagnosis more clearly but also may have correlated with the greater chronicity compared with subjects in the sertraline study (no duration entry criterion).

The fixed-dose studies (fluoxetine and sertraline) may have been disadvantaged because the dose could not be optimized for each subject. Table 3, however, shows that even the "best" doses of fluoxetine and sertraline did not approach the effectiveness of clomipramine with regard to mean change or percent decrease in Y-BOC scores, percentage of patients much or very much improved, or effect size.

There was no significant difference in the age of subjects or in gender across studies except for the sertraline study, where fewer females were included ($\chi^2[2]=20.40$, $P<.01$). Baseline Y-BOCS scores of the fluoxetine, fluvoxamine, and sertraline populations were not significantly different from each other but all three were significantly less than the baseline Y-BOCS score in the clomipramine population ($F[3,1515]=35.32$, $P<.0001$; post hoc Scheffé comparisons). Analyses of the fluvoxamine and sertraline populations showed that subjects with baseline Y-BOCS scores less than 20 had significantly higher placebo response rates than patients with baseline Y-BOCS scores greater than 20.[7,8] Less severity at baseline may have caused a ceiling effect on the amount of improvement.

Because of more frequent side effects, greater predictability of drug vs placebo condition may have occurred in the clomipramine study, and the greater proportion of patients free of side effects in the fluoxetine, fluvoxamine, and sertraline studies thereby may have increased placebo response. A recent placebo-controlled trial of fluoxetine in children and adolescents with OCD also found a large placebo response of 27%.[36]

Subjects in the clomipramine study were all STI naive, while the later studies included some subjects who had previously failed trials of clomipramine and/or fluoxetine. Patients with OCD who fail to respond to clomip-

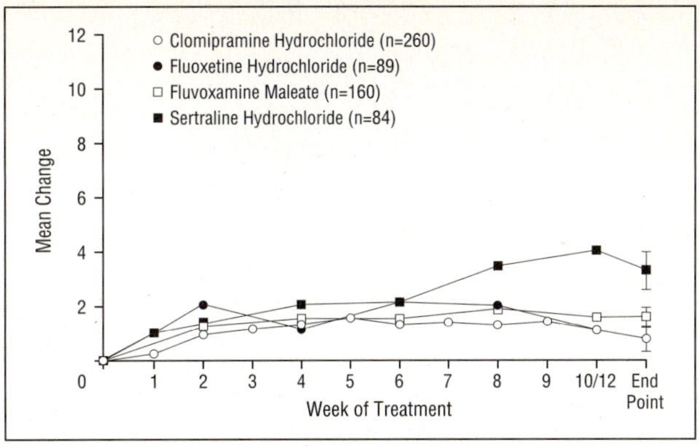

Figure 3. *Mean change in total Yale-Brown Obsessive Compulsive Scale scores for placebo intent-to-treat analysis. There were 12 weeks of treatment for the fluvoxamine and sertraline studies. Error bars indicate pooled SE of change score (available for end point only).*

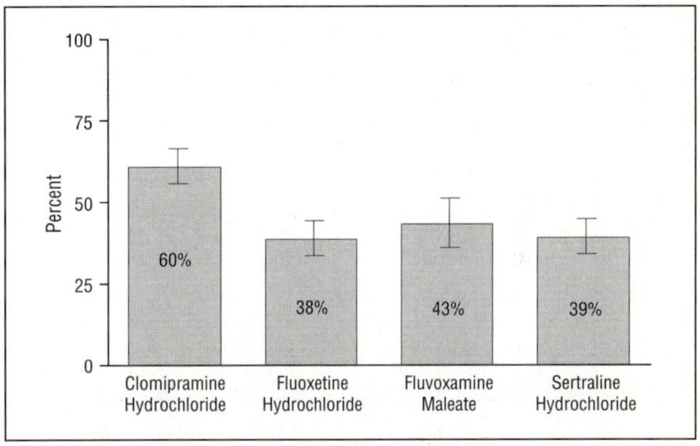

Figure 4. *Clinical Global Impression scale ratings of "much improved" or "very much improved."*

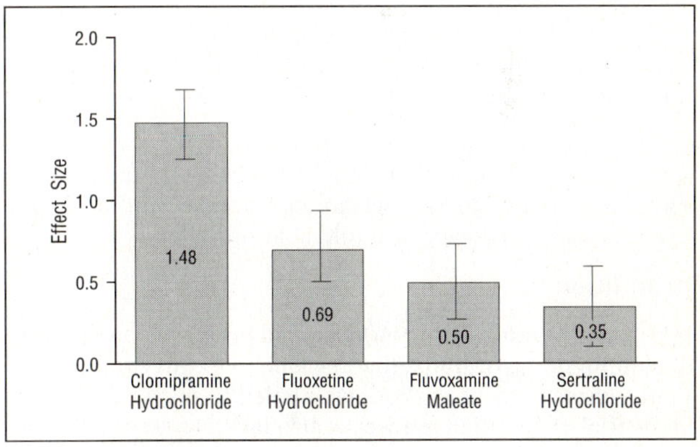

Figure 5. *Effect sizes.*

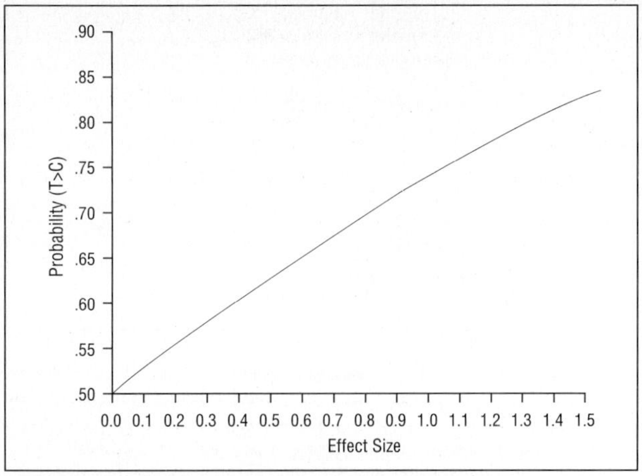

Figure 6. *Graph illustrating the probability of a treatment score (T) exceeding a control score (C) as a function of standardized effect size.*

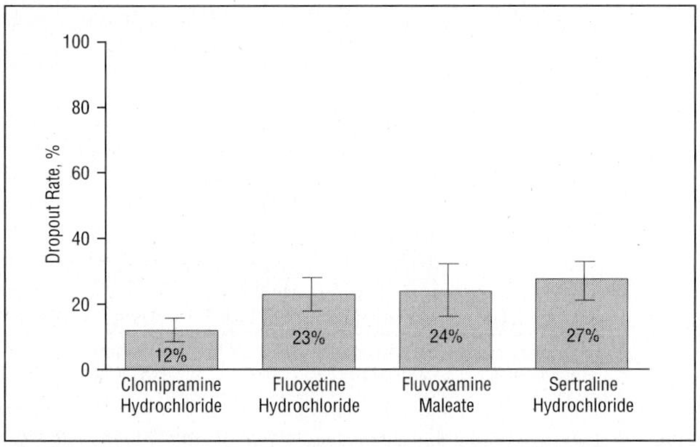

Figure 7. *Total dropout rate for each drug.*

ramine treatment often fail to respond to other STIs.[28,37,38] Thus, the later studies may have had more STI treatment failures. For example, in the fluvoxamine trial,[7]

> . . . 38 (24%) of the placebo group and 30 (19%) of the fluvoxamine group reported that they had previously failed to respond to a trial of an SRI [serotonin reuptake inhibitor], due to either lack of efficacy or intolerable side effects. . . .

In addition,

> [s]ix patients out of 31 (19%) who had previously failed trials of clomipramine or fluoxetine responded to fluvoxamine. . . . Eighty-three percent of those who failed to respond to a previous trial of an SRI at ten weeks also failed to respond to fluvoxamine in the current study, as measured by the CGI [Clinical Global Impression] compared to 50% who failed to respond to fluvoxamine who had never had a previous SRI trial.[7]

Thus, not all patients who fail to respond to clomipramine or fluoxetine fail to respond to fluvoxamine and, presumably, other serotonin selective transport inhibitors. In the only other trial where data were available (sertraline) (J.H.G. et al, unpublished data, 1993), 70 patients (22%) reported that they had failed to respond to previous treatment with an STI. We suspect that no more than this proportion of patients had failed treatment with STIs in the fluoxetine study.

In depression, side effects are usually more common and dropout rates greater for tricyclics compared with those for serotonin selective transport inhibitors. For fluoxetine vs imipramine hydrochloride, dropout rates because of side effects were 18% and 28%, respectively[39]; for fluvoxamine vs imipramine, 23% and 37%[40]; and for sertraline vs amitriptyline hydrochloride, 8.3% and 17.6% (W. Harrison, MD, oral communication, 1993). In OCD, by contrast, controlled and open trials have not found this direction of difference, despite more frequent side effects from clomipramine. For example, the only dropout from 11 patients who received clomipramine hydrochloride (mean dose of 225 mg/d) and fluoxetine hydrochloride (mean daily dose of 75 mg/d) was receiving fluoxetine.[28] In a study combining clomipramine- and fluoxetine-treated patients from two centers, dropout rates were virtually identical (clomipramine,16%; fluoxetine, 15%) despite the occurrence of side effects in more patients who received clomipramine (97%) than received fluoxetine (57%).[21] Side effects of clomipramine are more frequent in patients with OCD but they are not severe enough to affect dropout rates adversely. Patients with OCD also may tolerate side effects better than patients with other disorders.

In the end, we cannot explain fully the large differences between fluoxetine, fluvoxamine, and sertraline, which cluster closely in these multicenter controlled trials, and clomipramine. The direction of these differences is consistent with those found in controlled studies of clomipramine with other active compounds and placebo.[1]

Other meta-analyses have addressed the comparative effectiveness of STIs in OCD. Jenike et al[21] found that clomipramine (n=31) had a greater effect size than fluoxetine (n=72) and that dropout rates were identical despite a greater rate of side effects in patients receiving clomipramine. Jenike et al extended their analyses to include fluvoxamine and sertraline[41] and larger samples of clomipramine-treated patients.[1] Despite criticism,[42] their analysis found that clomipramine had the greatest effect size.[43] Davis et al[44] also found that clomipramine had the largest effect size in their meta-analyis comparing clomipramine, fluvoxamine, and sertraline. Although not comparing clomipramine with other STIs, Christenson et al[45] found an effect size of 1.7 for clomipramine, consistent with the magnitude reported in other studies. The consistency of these results by different analysts reviewing different studies at different times supports the results of the present meta-analysis of the four large multicenter controlled trials of clomipramine, fluoxetine, fluvoxamine, and sertraline in OCD. In 22 other controlled trials comparing clomipramine with placebo or other antidepressants,[1] clomipramine was better than placebo in 11 studies, better than tricyclics in five studies, and better than diphenhydramine hydrochloride in one study. In five trials there was no significant difference between clomipramine and other active comparators.

It seems that something may be missing in fluoxetine, fluvoxamine, and sertraline that clomipramine contains. Is there a salubrious combination of serotonin and noradrenergic transport inhibition that the serotonin-specific compounds lack? Would a combination of one of the serotonin-selective compounds and a selective noradrenergic transport inhibitor yield greater effectiveness? Will agents such as duloxetine hydrochloride, milnacipran, and venlafaxine hydrochloride, which have selective and potent serotonin and noradrenergic transport inhibition and a better side-effect profile than clomipramine, work well in treating OCD?

Other issues are important in the comprehensive treatment of OCD. The partial response of most patients to STIs points to the desirability of response enhancement with augmentation strategies. Combining behavior therapy with STI medications has led to greater early improvement than the use of behavior therapy alone in three trials.[46-48] In addition, some studies have shown that behavior therapy conveys protection against relapse when combined with clomipramine or fluvoxamine therapy (E. A. Hembree, PhD, et al, unpublished data, 1993). One recent study of behavior therapy using the Y-BOCS change measure found severity reductions (8 points) comparable to those seen with STIs.[49]

While theoretically attractive and supported by the results of some open trials,[50,51] serotonin augmentation strategies involving buspirone hydrochloride[52-54] and lithium carbonate[55,56] have not withstood scrutiny in controlled trials. L-tryptophan[50] and fenfluramine hydrochloride[57] augmentation also show some promise in open trials and await more thorough evaluation in controlled studies. It is probable that some individuals benefit from these augmentation approaches despite the failure to demonstrate statistically significant advantages in small population studies. Antipsychotic augmentation for patients with OCD and Gilles de la Tourette's syndrome appears effective, based on the results of one controlled trial[58] and an open trial[59] that preceded it.

For the small minority of patients with incapacitating OCD who fail to respond adequately to STIs and behavior therapy, neurosurgical treatment is often beneficial.[60]

CONCLUSION

Clomipramine, fluoxetine, fluvoxamine, and sertraline have been shown in large, carefully conducted multicenter controlled trials to be of substantial benefit for the treatment of OCD. While these large cohort studies show an apparent efficacy advantage for clomipramine, and, surprisingly, the lowest dropout rate with clomipramine as well, it is important to recognize that individual patients may obtain more benefit and/or tolerate another compound better than clomipramine. The fact that the clomipramine study contained more STI-naive patients does not fully account for its apparent efficacy advantage. Use of a potent STI in combination with behavior therapy (exposure and response prevention) is the present treatment of choice for OCD.

Accepted for publication August 1, 1994.

Correspondence to Dean Foundation for Health, Research and Education, 8000 Excelsior Dr, Madison, WI 53717 (Dr Greist).

REFERENCES

1. Clomipramine Collaborative Study Group. Clomipramine in the treatment of patients with obsessive-compulsive disorder. *Arch Gen Psychiatry.* 1991;48: 730-738.
2. Tollefson GD, Rampey AH, Potvin JH, Jenike MA, Rush AJ, Dominguez RA, Koran LM, Shear K, Goodman W, Genduso LA. A multicenter investigation of fixed-dose fluoxetine in the treatment of obsessive-compulsive disorder. *Arch Gen Psychiatry.* 1994;51:559-567.
3. Greist JH. Fluvoxamine in OCD: a multicentre parallel design double-blind placebo-controlled trial. Presented at the 18th Collegium Internationale NeuroPsychopharmacologicum Congress; June 29, 1992; Nice, France.
4. Greist JH, Chouinard G, DuBoff E, Halaris A, Kim SW, Koran L, Liebowitz M, Lydiard R, Mendels J, Rasmussen S, White K. Double-blind comparison of three doses of sertraline and placebo in the treatment of outpatients with obsessive compulsive disorder. Presented at the 18th Collegium Internationale NeuroPsychopharmacologicum Congress; June 29, 1992; Nice, France.
5. US Food and Drug Administration. Prozac/fluoxetine hydrochloride: safety and effectiveness for use in the treatment of obsessive-compulsive disorder. Presented at Psychopharmacologic Drugs Advisory Committee Meeting #40 on New Drug Application 20-187; July 20, 1993; Rockville, Md.
6. Greist J, Chouinard G, DuBoff E, Halaris A, Kim S, Koran L, Liebowitz M, Lydiard R, McElroy S, Mendels J, Rasmussen S, Flicker C. Long-term sertraline treatment of obsessive compulsive disorder: a 52-week double-blind comparative study versus placebo. Abstract from the Fifth Congress of the European College of Neuropsychopharmacology; October 19, 1992; Marbella, Spain. *Eur Neuropsychopharmacol.* 1992;2:386.
7. Rasmussen S, Goodman WK, Greist JH, Jenike MA, Kozak MJ, Liebowitz M, Robinson DG, White KL. Fluvoxamine in the treatment of obsessive-compulsive disorder: a multi-center double-blind placebo-controlled study in outpatients. *Am J Psychiatry.* In press.
8. Goodman WK, Price LH, Rasmussen SA, Mazure C, Fleischmann RL, Hill CL, Heninger GR, Charney DS. The Yale-Brown Obsessive Compulsive Scale (Y-BOCS), I: development, use, and reliability. *Arch Gen Psychiatry.* 1989;46: 1006-1011.
9. Goodman WK, Price LH, Rasmussen SA, Mazure C, Delgado P, Heninger GR, Charney DS. The Yale-Brown Obsessive Compulsive Scale (Y-BOCS), II: validity. *Arch Gen Psychiatry.* 1989;46:1012-1016.
10. Guy W. *ECDEU Assessment Manual for Psychopharmacology.* Washington, DC: US Dept of Health, Education, and Welfare; 1976:338. Publication 76.
11. American Psychiatric Association. *Diagnostic and Statistical Manual of Mental Disorders, Third Edition.* Washington, DC: American Psychiatric Association; 1980:234-235.
12. American Psychiatric Association. *Diagnostic and Statistical Manual of Mental Disorders, Revised Third Edition.* Washington, DC: American Psychiatric Association; 1987:245-247.
13. Hamilton M. A rating scale for depression. *J Neurol Neurosurg Psychiatry.* 1960;23:56-62.
14. Cohen J. *Statistical Power Analysis for the Behavioral Sciences.* New York, NY: Academic Press; 1977:19-27.
15. Glass GV, McGraw B, Smith ML. *Meta-analysis in Social Research.* Beverly Hills, Calif: Sage Publications; 1981.
16. Cramer H. *Mathematical Models of Statistics.* Princeton, NJ: Princeton University Press; 1974:506.
17. Rosenthal R, Rubin DB. Comparing effect sizes of independent studies. *Psychol Bull.* 1982;92:500-504.
18. Rosenthal R, Rubin DB. Comparing significance levels of independent studies. *Psychol Bull.* 1979;86:1165-1168.
19. Hsu LM. Tests of differences in p levels as tests of differences in effect sizes. *Psychol Bull.* 1980;88:705-708.
20. Hedges LV, Olkin I. *Statistical Methods for Meta-analysis.* Orlando, Fla: Academic Press; 1985.
21. Jenike MA, Baer L, Greist JH. Clomipramine versus fluoxetine in obsessive-compulsive disorder: a retrospective comparison of side effects and efficacy. *J Clin Psychopharmacol.* 1990;10:122-124.
22. Jenike MA, Baer L, Summergrad P, Minichiello WE, Holland A, Seymor R. Sertraline in obsessive-compulsive disorder: a double-blind comparison with placebo. *Am J Psychiatry.* 1990;147:923-928.
23. Jenike MA, Baer L. Sertraline in obsessive-compulsive disorder: a double-blind comparison with placebo [correction]. *Am J Psychiatry.* 1990;147:1393.
24. Leavitt F. *Research Methods for Behavioral Scientists.* Dubuque, Iowa: Wm Brown; 1991.
25. Gravetter FJ, Wallnau LB. *Statistics for Behavioral Sciences.* 2nd ed. St Paul, Minn: West Publishing; 1988:426-434.

26. Amundsen R, Serlin RC, Lehrer R. On the threats that do not face educational research. *Educ Res.* 1994;21:19-24.
27. Cook DJ, Guyatt GH, Ryan G, Clifton J, Buckingham L, Willan A, McIlroy W, Oxman AD. Should unpublished data be included in meta-analyses? current convictions and controversies. *JAMA.* 1993;269:2749-2753.
28. Pigott TA, Pato MT, Bernstein SE, Grover GN, Hill JL, Tolliver TJ, Murphy DL. Controlled comparisons of clomipramine and fluoxetine in the treatment of obsessive-compulsive disorder: behavioral and biological results. *Arch Gen Psychiatry.* 1990;47:926-932.
29. Freeman CPL, Trimble MR, Deakin JFW, Stokes TM, Ashford JJ. Fluvoxamine versus clomipramine in the treatment of obsessive compulsive disorder: a multicenter, randomized double-blind, parallel group comparison. *J Clin Psychiatry.* 1994;55:301-305.
30. Perse T, Greist JH, Jefferson JW, et al. Fluvoxamine treatment for obsessive-compulsive disorder. *Am J Psychiatry.* 1987;144:1543-1548.
31. Pato M, Zohar-Kadouch R, Zohar J, Murphy DL. Return of symptoms after discontinuation of clomipramine in patients with obsessive compulsive disorder. *Am J Psychiatry.* 1988;145:1521-1525.
32. Leonard HL, Swedo SE, Lenane MC, Rettew DC, Cheslow DL, Hamburger SD, Rapoport JL. A double-blind desipramine substitution during long-term clomipramine treatment in children and adolescents with obsessive-compulsive disorder. *Arch Gen Psychiatry.* 1991;48:922-927.
33. Pato MT, Murphy DL, DeVane CL. Sustained plasma concentrations of fluoxetine and/or norfluoxetine four and eight weeks after fluoxetine discontinuation. *J Clin Psychopharmacol.* 1991;11:224-225.
34. Reimherr FW, Chouinard G, Cohn CK, Cole JO, Itil TM, LaPierre YD, Masco HL, Mendels J. Antidepressant efficacy of sertraline: a double-blind, placebo- and amitriptyline-controlled, multicenter comparison study in outpatients with major depression. *J Clin Psychiatry.* 1990;51(suppl B):18-27.
35. Mavissakalian MR, Jones B, Olson S. Absence of placebo response in obsessive-compulsive disorder. *J Nerv Ment Dis.* 1990;178:268-270.
36. Riddle MA, Scahill L, King RA, Hardin MT, Anderson GM, Ort SI, Smith JC, Leckman JF, Cohen DJ. Double-blind, crossover trial of fluoxetine and placebo in children and adolescents with obsessive-compulsive disorder. *J Am Acad Child Adolesc Psychiatry.* 1992;31:1062-1069.
37. Mavissakalian M, Tamimi R, Jones B, Olson S. Are effective antiobsessional drugs interchangeable? Presented at the First International Obsessive-Compulsive Disorder Conference; March 12-13, 1993; Capri, Italy.
38. Pigott TA, L'Heureux F, Murphy DL. Pharmacological approaches to treatment-resistant OCD patients. Abstract presented at the First International Obsessive Compulsive Disorder Conference; March 12-13, 1993; Capri, Italy.
39. Stark P, Hardison CD. A review of multicenter controlled studies of fluoxetine vs imipramine and placebo in outpatients with major depressive disorder. *J Clin Psychiatry.* 1985;46:53-58.
40. Feighner JP, Boyer WF, Meredith CH, Hendrickson GG. A placebo-controlled inpatient comparison of fluvoxamine maleate and imipramine in major depression. *Int Clin Psychopharmacol.* 1989;4:239-244.
41. Jenike MA, Hyman S, Baer L, Holland A, Minichiello WE, Buttolph L, Summergrad P, Seymour R, Ricciardi J. A controlled trial of fluvoxamine in obsessive-compulsive disorder: implications for a serotonergic theory. *Am J Psychiatry.* 1990;147:1209-1215.
42. Cialdella P, Boissel JP. Serotonergic antidepressants and obsessive-compulsive disorder. *Am J Psychiatry.* 1991;148:1415-1416.
43. Baer L, Jenike MA. Serotonergic antidepressants and obsessive-compulsive disorder: Dr Baer and Dr Jenike reply. *Am J Psychiatry.* 1991;148:1416.
44. Davis J, Israni T, Janicak P, Wang Z, Holland D. A meta-analysis of drug efficacy studies in obsessive-compulsive disorder. *Biol Psychiatry.* 1991;29 (suppl):444S. Abstract.
45. Christenson H, Hadzi-Pavlovic D, Andrews G, Mattick R. Behavior therapy and tricyclic medication in the treatment of obsessive-compulsive disorder: a quantitative reveiw. *J Consult Clin Psychol.* 1987;55:701-711.
46. Marks IM, Stern RS, Mawson D, Cobb J, McDonald R. Clomipramine and exposure for obsessive-compulsive rituals. *Br J Psychiatry.* 1980;136:1-25.
47. Marks IM, Lelliott P, Basoglu M, Noshirvani H, Monteiro W, Cohen D, Kasvikis Y. Clomipramine, self-exposure and therapist-aided exposure for obsessive-compulsive rituals. *Br J Psychiatry.* 1988;152:522-534.
48. Cottraux J, Mollard E, Bouvard M, Marks I, Sluys M, Nury AM, Douge R. A controlled study of fluvoxamine and exposure in obsessive-compulsive disorder. *Int Clin Psychopharmacol.* 1990;5:17-30.
49. Fals-Stewart W, Marks AP, Schafer J. A comparison of behavioral group therapy and individual behavior therapy in treating obsessive-compulsive disorder. *J Nerv Ment Dis.* 1993;181:189-193.
50. Rasmussen SA. Lithium and tryptophan augmentation in clomipramine-resistant obsessive-compulsive disorder. *Am J Psychiatry.* 1984;141:1283-1285.
51. Markovitz PJ, Stagno SJ, Calabrese JR. Buspirone augmentation of fluoxetine in obsessive-compulsive disorder. *Am J Psychiatry.* 1990;147:798-800.
52. Pigott TA, L'Heureux F, Hill JL, Bihari K, Bernstein SE, Murphy DL. A double-blind study of adjuvant buspirone hydrochloride in clomipramine-treated OCD patients. *J Clin Psychopharmacol.* 1992;12:11-18.
53. Grady TA, Pigott TA, L'Heureux F, Hill JL, Bernstein SE, Murphy DL. Double-blind study of adjuvant buspirone for fluoxetine-treated patients with obsessive-compulsive disorder. *Am J Psychiatry.* 1993;150:819-821.
54. McDougle CJ, Goodman WK, Leckman JF, Holzer JC, Barr LC. Limited therapeutic effect of addition of buspirone in fluvoxamine-refractory obsessive-compulsive disorder. *Am J Psychiatry.* 1993;150:647-649.
55. Pigott TA, Pato MT, L'Heureux F, Hill JL, Grover GN, Bernstein SE, Murphy DL. A controlled comparison of adjuvant lithium carbonate or thyroid hormone in clomipramine-treated OCD patients. *J Clin Psychopharmacol.* 1991; 11:242-248.
56. McDougle CJ, Price LH, Goodman WK, Charney DS, Heninger GR. A controlled trial of lithium augmentation in fluvoxamine refractory obsessive-compulsive disorders lack of efficacy. *J Clin Psychopharmacol.* 1991;11:175-184.
57. Hollander E, DeCaria CM, Schneier FR, Schneier HA, Liebowitz MR, Klein DF. Fenfluramine augmentation of serotonin reuptake blockade antiobsessional treatment. *J Clin Psychiatry.* 1990;51:119-123.
58. McDougle CJ, Goodman WK, Leckman JF, Lee NC, Heninger GR, Price LH. Haloperidol addition in fluvoxamine-refractory obsessive-compulsive disorder: a double-blind, placebo-controlled study in patients with and without tics. *Arch Gen Psychiatry.* 1994;51:302-308.
59. McDougle CJ, Goodman WK, Price LH, Delgado PL, Krystal JH, Charney DS, Heninger GR. Neuroleptic addition in fluvoxamine-refractory obsessive-compulsive disorder. *Am J Psychiatry.* 1990;147:652-654.
60. Mindus P, Jenike MA. Neurosurgical treatment of malignant obsessive compulsive disorder. *Psychiatr Clin North Am.* 1992;15:921-938.

Test-Retest Reliability of the Diagnostic Interview Schedule for Children (DISC 2.1)

Parent, Child, and Combined Algorithms

Peter Jensen, MD; Margaret Roper, MS; Prudence Fisher, MS; John Piacentini, PhD; Glorisa Canino, PhD; John Richters, PhD; Maritza Rubio-Stipec, MA; Mina Dulcan, MD; Sherryl Goodman, PhD; Mark Davies, MPH; Donald Rae, MS; David Shaffer, MD; Hector Bird, MD; Benjamin Lahey, PhD; Mary Schwab-Stone, MD

Background: Previous research has not compared the psychometric properties of diagnostic interviews of community samples and clinically referred subjects within a single study. As part of a multisite cooperative agreement study funded by the National Institute of Mental Health, 97 families with clinically referred children and 278 families identified through community sampling procedures participated in a test-retest study of version 2.1 of the Diagnostic Interview Schedule for Children (DISC 2.1).

Methods: The DISC was separately administered to children and parents, and diagnoses were derived from computer algorithms keyed to *DSM-III-R* criteria. Three sets of diagnoses were obtained, based on parent information only (DISC-P), child information only (DISC-C), and information from either or both (DISC-PC).

Results: Test-retest reliabilities of the DISC-PC ranged from moderate to substantial for diagnoses in the clinical sample. Test-retest κ coefficients were higher for the clinical sample than for the community sample. The DISC-PC algorithm generally had higher reliabilities than the algorithms that relied on single informants. Unreliability was primarily due to diagnostic attenuation at time 2. Attenuation was greatest among child informants and less severe cases and in the community sample.

Conclusions: Test-retest reliability findings were consistent with or superior to those reported in previous studies. Results support the usefulness of the DISC in further clinical and epidemiologic research; however, closely spaced or repeated DISC interviews may result in significant diagnostic attenuation on retest. Further studies of the test-retest attenuation phenomena are needed, including careful examination of the child, family, and illness characteristics of diagnostic stability.

(Arch Gen Psychiatry. 1995;52:61-71)

From the National Institute of Mental Health, Rockville, Md (Drs Jensen and Richters, Ms Roper, and Mr Rae); the Division of Child and Adolescent Psychiatry, New York State Psychiatric Institute and Columbia University College of Physicians and Surgeons, New York, NY (Ms Fisher, Drs Piacentini, Shaffer, and Bird, and Mr Davies); the Department of Psychiatry, University of Puerto Rico, San Juan (Dr Canino and Ms Rubio-Stipec); the Department of Psychiatry, Emory University School of Medicine, Atlanta, Ga (Drs Dulcan and Goodman); the Department of Psychiatry, University of Miami (Fla) School of Medicine (Dr Lahey); and the Yale Child Study Center, Yale University School of Medicine, New Haven, Conn (Dr Schwab-Stone).

THE LAST decade has been a time of remarkable growth and progress in the study of child psychopathology. Despite limitations, the standardized nomenclatures[1] have enabled clinical investigators and epidemiologists to develop instruments that can be employed across clinical, laboratory, and epidemiologic settings. A number of these measures are intended to be used by trained lay interviewers, thus making possible some studies not otherwise feasible using traditional research interviews with clinically trained interviewers.[2]

Of the available diagnostic instruments for children,[3] the Diagnostic Interview Schedule for Children (DISC) has had the most extensive history of development, including four field trials. The results of the second of these trials have been recently described by Shaffer and colleagues.[4-6] Investigators have used the DISC across a range of research settings,[7-9] have examined its sensitivity with rare conditions,[10] and have evaluated its usefulness with young children.[11] In earlier versions, its criterion validity and relationships with other measures have been described[8,9] as well as the degree to which it is tolerated by subjects.[12]

The last two field trials have been conducted as part of the Cooperative Agreement for Methodologic Research for Multisite Epidemiologic Surveys of Mental Disorders in Child and Adolescent Populations (hereafter referred to as the Methodology for Epidemiology in Children and Adolescents [MECA] Study), funded by the National Institute of Mental Health, Rockville, Md. As envisioned in the original request for applications, the purpose of the MECA Study was to test the feasibility and merits of epidemiologic methods (struc-

See Methods on next page

METHODS

The data reported were obtained during the first phase of the MECA Study. The DISC 2.1 was administered as part of an extensive battery of measures being tested, including demographic characteristics, global impairment, service use, barriers to service use, potential presumed risk factors, and correlates of childhood psychopathologic conditions.

SAMPLE

The subjects were 97 clinically referred and 278 community-sampled 9- to 17-year-old children and one of their primary caretakers (usually the mother). Clinical subjects were recruited from clinical settings in three geographic areas (Atlanta, Ga; New York, NY; and Puerto Rico) involved in the MECA Study. The 278 nonclinical subjects were recruited across the three sites from community populations. For these community subjects, one site (New York) used a stratified random sampling procedure (with replacement of refusals), and two sites (Atlanta and Puerto Rico) used household probability sampling procedures (with no replacement). Data from a fourth site (Connecticut) are not presented here, since this site used different procedures and examined validity rather than reliability. The three sites' sampling procedures are described below.

New York

The New York sample was drawn from an area directly north of New York City, where there is a population with significant socioeconomic, geographic, and ethnic diversity, including sizable proportions of blacks, Hispanics, and other ethnic minorities. The aims of the New York site's sampling procedure were to achieve heterogeneity and to parallel the general population's proportions in age, sex, socioeconomic status (SES), population density, and ethnicity.

Fifty-three of the 63 subjects from the clinical sample were outpatients from school-based outpatient clinics in five counties within the designated catchment area. Ten additional participating subjects (from the same region) were currently hospitalized at a child psychiatric facility. All of the clinical subjects were active cases and had been involved with the clinical facility for a minimum of 3 months and for a maximum of 2 years. The clinical subjects were drawn from a larger sample of 123 eligible clinical subjects, resulting in a study participation rate of 51%. The community sample was obtained by using Department of Education data tapes to determine the age and ethnicity profiles of school systems, within which individual schools were selected based on their representativeness of the characteristics of the community. Within target schools, English classes (or "homeroom" classes for younger ages) were selected at random, as were students within these classes, based on the stratification target numbers. Children enrolled in classes for English as a second language and those in special education classes were excluded so that responses would not be biased by lack of language proficiency or cognitive ability. Three hundred sixty-four eligible subjects were identified, of whom the parents of 138 children indicated by letter or telephone that they did not wish to participate (38%). An additional 104 families could not be reached to secure study participation, and complete data were not available for two families. Despite these difficulties, the resulting sample (n=120; study participation rate, 33%) achieved the site's sampling aims for heterogeneity, was distributed along the socioeconomic spectrum and the age groups studied, consisted of half white and half nonwhite subjects, and paralleled the general population for urban/suburban/rural status. There was a preponderance of females in the community sample, in contrast to more males in the clinical sample (**Table 1**).

Puerto Rico

The clinical test-retest subjects were obtained from 9- to 17-year-olds consecutively admitted to an outpatient clinic (18 cases) and additional subjects (10 cases) from a substance abuse treatment center. Two thirds of subjects were male. Twenty-four of the 28 cases completed the interviews at both time points. As expected in clinical samples drawn from the public sector, children in the clinic sample were predominantly male (Table 1) and of low SES (82%). Refusal rates were not tracked, so it was not possible to examine factors that may have shaped study participation in this sample.

Community subjects were obtained from a probability sample of children ages 9 through 17 years from the San Juan metropolitan area. Sampling blocks were randomly distributed into two community subsamples of 124 subjects each to carry out two separate studies designed to measure reliability and validity of the DISC. This report concerns only one of the two samples (the reliability sample). Of these 124 families, 118 pairs (95%) agreed to participate and completed the study. This community sample resembled the 1990 census population of children in Puerto Rico ages 9 to 17 years, evenly distributed by gender, with most of low SES.

Atlanta

Twelve children being seen in a psychiatric outpatient clinic were selected for participation in the test-retest study; of these 12, one family refused (92% participation). As in the New York and Puerto Rico clinical samples, males outnumbered females. The community sample was selected from two census tracts in Georgia, one in an urban county and one in a rural county. These two census tracts were chosen so that the resultant probability sample of youths would have variation in race, urban/rural residence, and SES. A stratified multistage survey design was used to identify youths to be interviewed. Sampling regions in the urban census tract were stratified by race (mostly black, mostly white, mixed) and by SES (lower, upper). The rural census tract was stratified by race only since the SES appeared relatively homogeneous. Differential sampling rates were applied across strata to equalize the number of black and white youths and the number of lower and upper SES youths in the sample. Sample housing units were randomly selected for participation in the survey. If there was more than one child of the appropriate age living in the household, one was randomly selected using a table of random numbers. Sixty-six subjects were selected for study participation; of these, 26 refused, leaving 40 subjects and families (61%) who participated in the community test-retest study at the Atlanta site.

INSTRUMENT

The DISC 2.1, a highly structured diagnostic instrument intended for lay administration, was administered to parents and children.[6] Parent and child versions of the interview require approximately 60 to 75 minutes of the subject's time. This version of the DISC (version 2.1) differs significantly from earlier versions of the instrument,[6,8] in that items were grouped into separate diagnostic modules, each based on a set of related diagnoses. Also, the time covered by the interview was changed from 1 year to 6 months (to maintain consistency with the duration requirements in *DSM-III-R*), and questions concerning age at first episode, current impairment, treatment history, and precipitating stressors were added at the end of each diagnostic module. Further specific refinements were made based on the input of experienced clinical investigators concerning exact wording of specific questions. Also, unreliable items were deleted, based on data analyses from the earlier DISC-Revised field trials.[6]

All DISCs were administered by college or graduate level "lay" interviewers who had completed an intensive training period (usually 2 weeks, with slight site-to-site variation). The DISC interviews were monitored by experienced child interviewers and/or child clinicians through review of audiotapes. After the interview was completed, all responses from both parents and children were entered into a computer. Using computer algorithms based on *DSM-III-R* diagnostic criteria, *DSM-III-R* diagnoses were generated separately from parent information (DISC-P) and child information (DISC-C). The algorithms also generated a third set of diagnoses based on the "or" rule (DISC-PC, where PC indicates both parent and child informants). The "or" rule specifies that either informant may provide symptom information, which when combined may be used to jointly meet criteria for a particular diagnosis, even though the diagnostic criteria may not be met by any single informant. Thus, the "or" rule accepts the endorsement of a positive symptom from either the child or the adult informant, while the determination of symptom absence requires two negative responses. The application of the "or" rule generally tends to inflate prevalence but is thought to more closely approximate clinical practice.[18,19]

PROCEDURES

Clinically referred cases were generally interviewed in the clinical setting, while community subjects were interviewed in their homes. In general, retest intervals were shorter for clinical than community subjects (about 2 weeks vs 3 weeks), and sites differed significantly in test-retest intervals (Table 1). All interviews (parent, child, and test-retest) were conducted by separate interviewers who had no knowledge of the other interviews, requiring a total of four different interviewers for each parent-child pair. The use of two different interviewers for each administration introduces maximum variability of conditions and submits the instrument to a stringent test of its reliability. Parent and child interviews were conducted concurrently (at the same time but in separate rooms) for over 93% of cases. The adult who knew the selected child best (usually the mother) was chosen as the adult informant.

DATA ANALYSIS

There currently exists little empiric information that demonstrates superior validity for either parent or child information. The current standard of clinical diagnostic approaches usually involves gathering information from both the parent and the child. Accordingly, we restricted our initial analyses to the combined (DISC-PC) algorithm results. Research support for this approach is provided in several recent studies that have indicated that statistical weighting of informants' responses or exclusive reliance on single-informant algorithms does not perform as well as the simple combinatorial "or" rule against clinicians' diagnoses.[18,19]

The data analytic strategy proceeded as follows: First, reliability statistics from individual sites' data sets were compared to determine whether sites differed in reliability. This was warranted as an initial strategy given the geographic, linguistic, and sampling differences between sites. Furthermore, given the instability of κ statistics with few cases, site differences were examined only for those diagnoses for which five or more subjects met diagnostic criteria at the initial time point at two or more sites. In some instances, all three sites had sufficient cases to allow this comparison; in other instances, only two of the three sites had five or more cases; and in several instances, sites could not be compared because of insufficient numbers.

Because we found few or no site differences, further analyses of combined sites' data were undertaken. In most instances, clinical and community samples were analyzed separately. Except where noted, diagnostic reliabilities were examined for DISC-PC diagnoses. Given sufficient cases, diagnostic reliabilities were compared between males and females, younger and older children, internalizing vs externalizing disorders, clinic vs community subjects, and parent vs child informants. Some diagnoses may be more stable as a function of sex, considering the sex differences in prevalence of most childhood conditions, both before and after puberty. Similarly, some diagnoses may be more stable as a function of age, considering the age differences in prevalence of most childhood conditions.

Given the relatively small sample size and number of positive diagnoses, priority was given to examining test-retest reliability for the most common childhood conditions. There were sufficient cases of ADHD, ODD, and CD to allow for the examination of their reliabilities as separate categories. For most affective and anxiety disorders, however, too few cases were available to conduct meaningful reliability analyses across the clinical and community samples or to conduct more fine-grained analyses by age and sex. Therefore, we constructed two additional diagnostic categories: (1) Children with major depression and/or dysthymia were combined into a single depressed diagnostic group. (2) Children with any of the *DSM-III-R* anxiety disorder diagnoses (simple phobia, social phobia, separation anxiety disorder, generalized anxiety disorder, panic disorder, overanxious disorder, etc) were combined into a single group with any anxiety disorder. More detailed analyses of specific affective and anxiety disorders (eg, major depression, simple phobia, and separation anxiety disorder) are available from the authors on request.

To parallel the major conceptual distinction drawn by many investigators concerning types of childhood psychopathologic conditions, we also constructed superordinate categories of any internalizing disorder (major depressive disorder, dysthymia, and/or any anxiety disorder) and any externalizing disorder (ADHD, ODD, and CD). Reliability coefficients were computed for each of the three diagnostic algorithms (DISC-P, DISC-C, and DISC-PC).

To examine the possibility that unreliability is related to the relative oversensitivity of κ statistics to slight differences

Continued on next page

in symptom levels around the diagnostic threshold, we computed intraclass correlations based on the test-retest diagnostic criteria for all major diagnostic categories. For example, the 14 ADHD symptoms listed in the diagnostic criteria were treated as a dimensional scalar variable, and the intraclass correlation was computed between the two time points for this "scale." The criteria for most diagnoses involve some degree of summated symptoms as well as duration and age of onset items. However, because onset and duration criteria rarely can be summated for more than two items, intraclass correlations were only computed for symptom count criteria.

tured lay diagnostic interviews, multi-informant approaches, risk factor assessments, etc) in a moderate-sized survey of children and adolescents prior to mounting a full-scale nationwide study.

Further development of the DISC is forthcoming, pending analyses from the two field trials conducted during the MECA Study. The validity of the major diagnostic categories is being assessed as a part of the second MECA field trial and will form the basis of a future report. The focus of this report concerns the first MECA field trial, during which a test-retest reliability study was carried out. Information concerning the test-retest characteristics of the instrument is critical to assist field workers and clinical researchers who wish to conduct studies with this instrument.

Previous studies examining the reliability of earlier versions of the DISC reported moderate test-retest reliabilities, with the best reliabilities in the externalizing disorders (conduct disorder [CD], attention-deficit hyperactivity disorder [ADHD], oppositional defiant disorder [ODD]). These studies were carried out only in clinical settings,[4,8] an important limitation, since instruments' psychometric properties are best examined in settings similar to those where they will be used. Instruments behave quite differently in clinical vs community settings; they will likely be less reliable and less valid in the community.[4] Testing the psychometric performance of the agreed-on diagnostic interview in community settings was a central stated goal of the initial request for applications for the MECA Study. The DISC was the diagnostic instrument chosen by the MECA investigators.

Unfortunately, few systematic studies exist concerning the reliability of any child diagnostic instrument in community settings, so points of comparison are difficult to establish. Indeed, we have been unable to locate any studies that have compared the psychometric properties of diagnostic interviews for community samples and clinically referred subjects within a single study, either of children or of adults. Some relevant information bearing on this question is found in the adult literature, however. As a part of the Epidemiologic Catchment Area Study, Helzer et al[13] examined lay-clinician test-retest reliability in a community sample. They found lower reliabilities with the Diagnostic Interview Schedule (DIS) for adults than reported for clinical samples assessed with earlier versions of the instrument.[14] Similar findings have been noted by other investigators,[15-17] with low reliability, diagnostic stability, and validity in community subjects compared with clinical subjects.

Table 1. Site Characteristics

Site	No. of Parent-Child Pairs in Test-Retest	Average (SD) Age, y	M/F Ratio	Mean (SD) Retest Interval, d
		Clinic Subjects		
New York	62	12.1 (2.2)	47/15	14.7 (8.4)
Puerto Rico	24	14.3 (2.3)	16/8	10.0 (7.5)
Georgia	11	12.2 (2.8)	10/1	5.8 (6.2)
		F = .58	$\chi^2 = 2.41$	
		df = 2,94	*df* = 2	
		$P \leq .001$	*P* = 30	
		Community Subjects		
New York	120	13.4 (2.6)	51/69	19.0 (13.5)
Puerto Rico	118	12.6 (2.4)	59/59	21.3 (13.0)
Georgia	40	13.2 (2.9)	19/21	33.3 (32.3)
		F = 3.02	$\chi^2 = 1.37$	
		df = 2,275	*df* = 2	
		$P \leq .06$	*P* = .51	

If diagnostic instruments are less reliable in community settings than in clinical settings, the discrepancy may be due to several factors. First, those with severe cases may be more likely to seek out or be referred for care than those with mild cases, who may hover just above the diagnostic "threshold." Among such threshold subjects, small decreases in symptom reporting over the test-retest interval will result in decreased reliability.[13] Second, as clinical subjects and parents learn more about a diagnosis and/or its symptoms during the evaluation or treatment process, they may become more accepting of the symptoms and diagnostic process and more likely to reaffirm the presence of symptoms in a test-retest paradigm. Third, parents of children referred to clinical settings may have justifiably greater concern about their children and may respond more carefully to interview questions than parents from a community sample, whose motivation to participate is less well understood. Also, given two informants, the parent and child could confer about their interview responses between the first test and the retest. It is unclear what effects (if any) the possibility of parent-child discussions may have on retest, but some instances of attenuation may be explained by this factor.

The purpose of this report from the MECA Study is to describe the test-retest reliability of the recently revised DISC (version 2.1) in clinical settings and to extend previous research by also examining its test-retest reliability in community settings across the participating MECA sites. Factors mediating differences between clinical and community sample test-retest κ statistics are explored.

RESULTS

In Table 1 we outline the number of subjects from the clinical and community settings from each site as well

Table 2. Test-Retest Reliability by Site Using the Combined Diagnostic Algorithm

Diagnosis	κ* New York	κ* Puerto Rico	κ* Georgia	χ^2	P
Clinic Cases					
Any anxiety disorder	**.47**	**.50**	**.63**	0.25	.61
Depression and/or dysthymia	**.67**	**.73**	.56	0.06	.81
Attention-deficit hyperactivity disorder	**.72**	.38	.70	†	†
Oppositional defiant disorder	**.55**	**.59**	1.00	0.04	.84
Conduct disorder	**.67**	**.90**	−.11	0.76	.38
Community Cases					
Any anxiety disorder	**.25**	**.32**	**.47**	1.78	.18
Depression and/or dysthymia	**.38**	**.24**	**.00**	1.99	.16
Attention-deficit hyperactivity disorder	**.76**	**.53**	**.58**	3.10	.08
Oppositional defiant disorder	**.53**	**.55**	**.28**	0.06	.81
Conduct disorder	**.52**	**.82**	.79	5.54	.02

**Bold, underlined κ statistics indicate groups in which five or more cases were positive at time 1 for that site. Site comparisons were computed only between these sites.*

†Only one site had five or more cases, so comparisons were not computed.

as the mean age of subjects, male-female ratio, and test-retest intervals. Sites differed significantly in terms of age, with Puerto Rican subjects significantly older than subjects from the other two sites in the clinical setting. In contrast, Puerto Rican subjects were significantly younger than subjects from the other two sites in the community setting. Sites did not differ in proportions of males and females. There was a preponderance of males in the clinical setting, possibly reflecting the increased referral rates of young males commonly found in studies of clinical populations.[20]

Given the range of methods across sites and the differences in age noted above, in **Table 2** we considered the extent to which findings differed across sites. Given the relatively modest power to test for site differences because of the small number of cases, we did not correct for the number of comparisons in this table. Despite the methodologic, geographic, cultural, linguistic, and ethnic differences among sites and despite the fact that the DISC had been translated into Spanish for use in Puerto Rico, there was little evidence of consistent or large intersite differences in either the clinical or community setting. Therefore, data for individual sites were combined for all subsequent analyses.

Table 3 provides information on the test-retest reliability of the DISC-PC in the clinical and community settings. Extensive information is not provided on the parent and child algorithms because the DISC-PC generally yielded more stable and higher reliabilities than the DISC-P or DISC-C. Comparisons of clinical and community values indicate that, as predicted, the κ coefficients are higher in clinical than community subjects (five of five κ coefficients were higher in the clinical sample, $P \leq .05$ by one-tailed sign test). This same pattern held within each site. Further comparisons indicated that at the individual diagnostic level, clinical κ coefficients were higher than community κ coefficients for depression and/or dysthymia (.70 vs .26, $\chi^2=15.3$, $P=.0001$). A similar but nonsignificant trend was noted for any anxiety disorder (.50 vs .32, $\chi^2=2.45$, $P=.11$). Kappa coefficients for the other diagnoses did not differ between clinic and community settings (analyses available from the authors on request).

Table 4 provides further information about the test-retest reliability of the DISC-P and DISC-C. Among community subjects, four of five κ coefficients were higher for DISC-P than for DISC-C, and among clinical subjects, four of five κ coefficients were higher for DISC-P than for DISC-C.

Analyses were conducted to determine whether diagnostic reliabilities were related to the child's gender (10 comparisons, five for each major diagnostic area, with separate analyses for community and clinic subjects). These analyses yielded only one significant difference in reliability as a function of gender: within the community sample, higher test-retest reliability was found for depression and/or dysthymia among female subjects (κ=.40, N=148) than among male subjects (κ=−.01, N=126) ($\chi^2=23.5$, $P=.0001$).

To determine whether reliabilities were related to the child's age, the samples were divided into subjects 9 through 12 years and those 13 through 18 years. This split allowed the most even distribution of cases in the two age groups and is reasonably consistent with age differences in diagnoses before and after puberty. These analyses (10 comparisons, five for each major diagnostic area, with separate analyses for community and clinic subjects) yielded two significant differences as a function of age: Within the community sample, higher test-retest reliability was found for depression and/or dysthymia among older subjects (κ=.28, N=152) than among younger subjects (κ=.00, N=117). Also within the community sample, higher test-retest reliability was found for conduct disorder among older subjects (κ=.68, N=150) than among younger subjects (κ=.43, N=118) ($\chi^2=5.19$, $P=.02$). Given the small number of cases and relatively modest power to find true differences, the number of comparisons was not corrected for chance and should be viewed with caution.

To assess the possibility that unreliability is related to the sensitivity of κ statistics to slight differences in symptom or criterion levels around the diagnostic thresh-

Table 3. Test-Retest Reliability for All Sites Using the Combined Diagnostic Algorithm*

Diagnosis	No. of Diagnoses: Both Times	Time 1 Only	Time 2 Only	Neither Time	κ (SE)	Total No. for κ
Any anxiety disorder	31/35	16/61	8/14	42/166	.50 (.10)/.32 (.06)	97/276
Depression and/or dysthymia	22/5	7/23	5/2	61/244	.70 (.10)/.26 (.05)	95/274
Attention-deficit hyperactivity disorder	28/19	9/14	4/5	42/207	.68 (.11)/.62 (.06)	83/245
Oppositional defiant disorder	28/14	10/20	7/3	46/229	.61 (.11)/.51 (.06)	91/266
Conduct disorder	21/15	6/12	5/3	59/234	.71 (.11)/.64 (.06)	91/264

**All values are in the form clinic/community.*

old, intraclass correlations were computed to examine the test-retest reliability for the diagnostic criteria for all major diagnostic categories. Intraclass correlation coefficients for clinical subjects were .63 for any anxiety disorder, .68 for depression and/or dysthymia, .79 for ADHD, .76 for ODD, and .88 for CD. Similarly, community test-retest intraclass correlation coefficients were .38 for depression and/or dysthymia, .47 for any anxiety disorder, .74 for ADHD, .63 for ODD, and .68 for CD. As can be seen when these figures are compared with those in Table 3, in all instances but one the intraclass correlation coefficients were higher than the κ coefficients, and these differences were sizable, especially for community subjects. These data are supportive of the hypothesis that some difficulties with reliability occur around the diagnostic threshold, particularly in community cases. Given that the intraclass correlations themselves fell significantly short of optimal reliability estimates, however, it must be concluded that threshold cases at time 1 are not a sole or sufficient explanation for test-retest attenuation or the less-than-optimal reliabilities.

SOURCES OF UNRELIABILITY

Given the lower reliabilities found in community settings (especially for anxiety and depressive disorders), we conducted a number of post hoc analyses to further explore the sources of unreliability and attenuation. We examined the extent to which caseness unreliability might be related to symptom severity at time 1, so that cases less severely impaired at time 1 were less likely to meet diagnostic criteria on retest. We operationalized severity as a ratio of the sum of all endorsed "stem" questions (those asked of all respondents, regardless of the skip structure built into the DISC) across the five major diagnostic categories, divided by the total number of possible stem questions. As expected, in the community sample, stable cases (n=71, positive for diagnosis at both time points) endorsed an average of 43.7% of time 1 stem symptoms compared with 33.4% among attenuating cases (n=74) ($t=-4.96$, $P\leq.0001$). Similarly, in the clinical sample, stable cases (n=64) endorsed 53.4% of time 1 stem symptoms compared with 41.4% among attenuating cases (n=15) ($t=-3.04$, $P\leq.003$). Thus, attenuation at the diagnostic level is not simply a result of subjects switching to different symptom patterns at time 2 but reflects an absolute decrease in the number of symptoms.

Similarly, subjects in the community sample who had used mental health services in the past year (n=46) endorsed an average of 39.0% of time 1 stem symptoms compared with 28.7% among nonusers (n=232) ($t=-4.38$, $P\leq.0001$). Finally, we examined the proportion of community cases who used services and compared service users and nonusers on diagnostic attenuation (attenuators vs nonattenuators). Among service users, 20 (69%) of 29 cases showed diagnostic stability, while among nonusers, only 54 (47%) of 116 cases showed diagnostic stability (Fisher's Exact Test, $P\leq.04$). These findings further indicate that the lower reliabilities in community samples are related to a combination of factors, including decreased symptom severity, the presence of threshold cases, and other possible factors we did not examine (eg, mental health attitudes, stigma, burden).

MODELING UNRELIABILITY

As a final examination of the sources of unreliability, we adapted methods described by Rubio-Stipec and colleagues[21] to perform regression analyses using computed κ values as the dependent variable. Because there were five diagnostic categories, two algorithms (we used DISC-P and DISC-C only, since DISC-PC is the combination of the first two), and two settings (clinic and community) (5×2×2=20), there were 20 total κ values. In the regression analyses we entered the DISC diagnosis source (1 for child algorithm, 2 for parent algorithm), setting (1 for community, 2 for clinic), and simple ratios for the four sources of unreliability.

According to the rationale for the computation of these four ratios, under ideal circumstances and perfect reliability, the population consists of persons who are either "true cases" or "true noncases." Those who meet criteria at both time points are part of the population of true cases, while those who do not meet criteria at either time point are part of the population of true noncases. With fallible instruments administered under human conditions, however, four permutations of test-retest responses are possible: time 1 positive and time 2 positive (cell a [+/+]), time 1 positive and time 2 negative (cell b [+/−]), time 1 negative and time 2 positive (cell c [−/+]), and time 1 negative and time 2 negative (cell d [−/−]).

With these four cells, the ratio that models the error represented by persons who are from the population of true cases but fail to meet diagnostic criteria on sec-

Table 4. Test-Retest Reliability for All Sites Using the Parent vs Child Diagnostic Algorithm

	κ (N for κ)	
Diagnosis	**Parent**	**Child**
Clinic Cases		
Any anxiety disorder	.58 (97)	.39 (97)
Depression and/or dysthymia	.69 (96)	.38 (95)
Attention-deficit hyperactivity disorder	.69 (88)	.59 (88)
Oppositional defiant disorder	.67 (95)	.46 (91)
Conduct disorder	.70 (88)	.86 (90)
Community Cases		
Any anxiety disorder	.40 (278)	.30 (276)
Depression and/or dysthymia	.00 (277)	.29 (276)
Attention-deficit hyperactivity disorder	.57 (265)	.43 (261)
Oppositional defiant disorder	.65 (274)	.23 (271)
Conduct disorder	.66 (273)	.60 (270)

ond interview (for any of a variety of reasons) is b/(a+b), representing "true case attenuation." Second, a group of subjects with a tendency to impulsively overendorse symptoms in novel settings may meet caseness criteria at time 1 even though they are actually part of the population of true noncases (cell d). The ratio to approximate this error is b/(b+d), called for descriptive purposes "true noncase attenuation." Third, some true noncases might endorse and meet criteria at time 2, possibly because of measurement error, random responding, etc. The ratio to approximate this potential source of information discrepancy is c/(c+d), called for descriptive purposes "true noncase augmentation." Fourth, some subjects who are part of the population of true cases could be slow to warm up, requiring a second interview before they are fully able to disclose their symptoms (or they may have developed the disorder in the test-retest interim). The ratio to model this "error" is c/(a+c), called "true case augmentation." Of course, any number of hypotheses might be invoked to explain each of these four sources of unreliability; we have only described several of the possibilities.

These four specific ratios were entered into the regression equation along with the informant source variable (child or parent) and setting variable (clinic or community). Stepwise and hierarchical regression analyses were performed to determine the percentage variance accounted for in the κ statistics by these four sources of "error" and by the source and setting variables. As seen in **Table 5**, the regression was highly significant (as it should be, since all the variance in the κ coefficients is represented by the four ratios), and the great preponderance of decreased κ values was explained by the "true case attenuation" ratio (usually more than four times that of the other variables). A number of related analyses were run, systematically forcing each of the other variables and potential sources of unreliability first into the model; the results of these analyses were similar, in that the "true case attenuation" ratio continued to account for over 80% of the variance in κ values. The informant and setting variables did not enter into any models, as all the variance was all accounted for by three of the four ratios. Other terms did not enter into the final model, so no β weights or *t* values are noted in Table 5 for them (more extensive information is available from the authors on request).

COMMENT

Before we comment on our findings, several caveats are necessary. First, there were major differences among sites in sampling procedures and subject characteristics as well as variations in ethnicity, culture, and language. Although these differences were part of the planned, allowable site variations during the first phase of the MECA Study, they nonetheless constitute important methodologic differences and possible study limitations. Regardless, the examination of site-specific data revealed only minor variations across sites. In fact, the patterns of reliability (eg, clinic vs community and parent vs child) remained fairly stable across all sites, particularly in diagnoses for sites with at least five time 1 cases.

Furthermore, because most clinical subjects were male (whereas community subjects were equally distributed across gender) and because of the longer test-retest intervals in the community subjects, it cannot be determined whether the higher clinical test-retest reliabilities are best explained by clinical referral, male gender, or the length of the test-retest interval. However, only one difference in reliability was found as a function of gender (depression and/or dysthymia for females vs males in the community sample only), which tends to rule out gender as a major confounder in the overall pattern of results. Similarly, differences in clinical vs community test-retest intervals (2 vs 3 weeks) were small and seem unlikely to explain the clinic-community reliability differences. In contrast, post hoc analyses of community subjects indicated that a history of mental health services use was related to increased diagnostic stability, as was increased symptom severity. In our view, both of these factors are more closely related to our observed clinic-community reliability differences.

COMPARISONS WITH PREVIOUS STUDIES

In general, our reliability findings are consistent with or superior to those reported in previous studies.[4,22,23] Compared with those found using earlier versions of the DISC studied in clinical samples,[4,23] our clinical sample reliabilities are substantially better for CD, moderately better for ADHD, and equivalent or better for depressive disorders. Similarly, we found superior reliabilities for test-retest reliabilities of two anxiety disorders studied in earlier versions of the DISC,[23] .74 for separation anxiety disorder and .57 for overanxious disorder (further details of specific anxiety and depressive disorder reliabilities are available on request from the authors). Compared with test-retest studies of other diagnostic instruments, clinical sample reliabilities reported here are comparable or superior, despite the need for clinically trained interviewers for most other instruments.[23]

Unfortunately, there are few points of comparison for our community sample reliability findings. Two recent reports used a two-stage sampling design to select community subjects with a high probability of diagno-

Table 5. Modeling Sources of Diagnostic Unreliability*

Independent Variable	β	*t*	Variance Explained, %	Total Variance, %	Pearson Correlation Coefficient†
b/(a+b) (true case attenuation)	−.226	−26.79	0.885	0.885	−.941‡
c/(c+d) (true noncase augmentation)	−.066	−8.37	0.091	0.976	−.297
c/(a+c) (true case augmentation)	−.027	−3.87	0.012	0.988	−.556§
b/(b+d) (true noncase attenuation)¶					−.278
Source¶					.287
Setting¶					.436‖

*R^2=.987; R^2 (adjusted for degrees of freedom)=.985; F=422.9; P≤.0001; df, 3,16.
†Significance of zero-order correlations: ‡,P≤.001. §,P≤.01; and ‖, P≤.10.
¶These three variables did not enter the final model, so β coefficients and t values are not reported.

sis at the second stage.[11,22] However, the two-stage design of these studies makes direct comparisons of κ statistics with our data difficult, since such sampling strategies increase disorder base rates and sample heterogeneity and result in higher κ coefficients in equivalent (ie, fixed levels of sensitivity and specificity) diagnostic instruments.[24] Nonetheless, these investigators reported much lower community sample reliabilities than in previous test-retest studies in clinical samples using the same instrument.[23] Our community sample test-retest reliabilities do compare favorably (generally superior) with the reliabilities of the DIS used in the adult Epidemiologic Catchment Area studies,[13,14,25] despite the challenges entailed in obtaining and combining information from two informants in the MECA Study. However, DIS reliability data may not be directly comparable to our results, since the DIS test-retest study was conducted with two different types of interviewers (lay interviewers at time 1, clinicians at time 2).

ADEQUACY OF THE DISC

Given the lower test-retest reliability of the DISC in the community, are lay interviewers are really "up to the task" of collecting complex diagnostic data for epidemiologic studies? The κ coefficients reported in the present study must be considered in light of the fact that an instrument with acceptable characteristics (eg, sensitivity, specificity, test-retest κ coefficients) in clinical settings will demonstrate lower test-retest κ coefficients in epidemiologic (homogeneous) samples with low base rates. As others have noted,[24,26] this does not indicate a problem with κ statistics per se but reflects the true level of difficulty in obtaining agreement between two raters of less common conditions in the community. We suggest that in community samples with low disorder prevalence, "acceptable" κ values may be overly conservative, and the lower community sample reliability values reported here for the internalizing disorders (.26 to .32) should not be dismissed as too unreliable for use in epidemiologic studies.

Could clinical interviewers do better? In a recent head-to-head comparison with the DISC, clinician-generated diagnoses proved less reliable than lay interviewer–administered DISC diagnoses.[5] Large-scale epidemiologic studies with clinical interviewers are probably not logistically feasible, and clinician-generated diagnoses are likely to be quite unreliable in community settings.

It is unfortunate that our samples only included children age 9 years and older, given the relatively large proportion of younger children who come to clinical attention and are in need of services.[27,28] While previous research has indicated that problems with test-retest reliability increase as a function of younger age of the child informant, this is not necessarily the case with parental informants. In fact, evidence suggests that some diagnoses may be more reliable with the parents of younger children than with the parents of older children.[9,11,22] Certainly, more information is needed concerning the psychometric properties of diagnostic interviews for younger children.

Given the greater reliabilities among parents than their children, could one use the parent report alone for diagnostic purposes? Such a strategy is problematic because parents and children provide nonredundant information. For example, in the present report, in the community sample, most of the conduct, anxiety, and affective disorders were identified through information obtained from the DISC-C. While opposite findings were seen in the clinical sample (most cases were identified through the DISC-P), increasing evidence suggests that child-derived diagnoses in community subjects are reliable and, more important, have long-term prognostic significance.[29,30] Instead of surrendering children as potential informants, increased research is needed to determine under which circumstances (eg, clinical vs community settings) which diagnoses are best determined from which informants (parent, child, or both) for which children (eg, as a function of age and gender). Certainly, it would be dubious to fail to obtain information directly from children for internalizing diagnoses or conduct disorder, where the child often does not reveal symptoms to the parent. Even in the absence of parental endorsement, the child's report of symptoms may have meaning in terms of subthreshold conditions, other diagnostic entities, or risk for future disorder.

ATTENUATION

Collectively, our analyses indicate that test-retest changes in DISC-based diagnostic status are not just a function of random error but are significantly more likely to occur around the diagnostic threshold, occur more commonly in community than in clinic cases, and are related to symptom severity at time 1. In addition, for specific diagnoses, decreased reliability may be related to children's age (depression, CD) and gender (depression).

The level of test-retest attenuation we report here is not unique to childhood diagnostic interviews but is also a significant problem for adult diagnostic interviews, including semistructured interviews completed by clinicians and highly structured interviews conducted by lay interviewers.[13-17] This pervasiveness of test-retest attenuation has led some investigators to argue that diagnostic instability should be regarded as a phenomenon worthy of study in its own right,[15] with particular attention to personal and situational factors that are systematically related to test-retest differences in symptom reporting. It is probably too narrow a perspective to dismiss such phenomena simply as "unreliability," since systematic, measurable (and perhaps alterable) sources of variance (heretofore presumed to be "error") underlie significant amounts of test-retest attenuation.

Although test-retest attenuation in psychopathology research very much reflects a phenomenon in need of an explanation, its pervasiveness across measures, methods, and informants suggests the possibility that traditional retest strategies in this domain may constitute a poor assay of a measure's reliability. As Robins[31] has suggested, the diagnostic interview process itself appears to change subjects' response sets in ways that make a closely spaced retest interview difficult to interpret. If such a reactivity effect is operating, the comparison of two interviews over a relatively short time may be no more interpretable than retesting the effects of an acute psychological stress on heart rate immediately following an initial test. In both cases, it may be necessary to wait until a subject's reactivity to the initial stimulus condition has returned to its baseline level.

Any number of mechanisms may underlie interview-triggered changes in subjects' response sets. One possibility is that the intensive nature of diagnostic interview questions alters an individual's threshold for symptom reporting. The mere act of reporting a symptom as present may have a cathartic effect on some individuals, so that they later de-emphasize the significance of those symptoms. This hypothesis has not been examined in the literature, but it is reasonable to predict that any cathartic effect on symptom reporting would be short-lived, with subjects returning to their baseline evaluative levels following a sufficient "washout" period. Existing data (including those reported above) suggest that the catharsis hypothesis will need to be tested with test-retest durations exceeding the standard retest interval of 2 weeks.

Another source of test-retest attenuation may be a subject's conscious or unconscious desire to shorten the second interview by saying "no" to more symptom questions, having learned that "yes" responses during the initial interview result in additional questions and a longer interview. To the best of our knowledge, this hypothesis has not been tested in either the adult or child psychopathology literature. An optimal test of this hypothesis requires a design with symptom questions presented in counterbalanced order on two occasions. Support for the endorsement-avoidance hypothesis would be consistent with a significant association between likelihood of symptom endorsement and the temporal ordering of symptoms within either interview or with a negative association between the length of the first and second interviews. This hypothesis cannot be tested on our data because symptom questions were presented in a fixed order, with more severe diagnoses (and therefore lower probabilities of symptom endorsement) coming toward the end of the interview. Interestingly, Ribera and colleagues (J. Ribera, PhD, G.C., M.R.-S., et al, unpublished results, 1992) have noted that the test-retest attenuation may be lower when the subsequent interview is completed by a clinician, and they note the possibility that the interviewee continues to tell the complete story on retest, possibly because he or she may feel that the physician would notice the discrepancy between the first report and the subsequent one. These alternative explanations will be examined in more detail in subsequent reports.

THE POST HOC regression analyses do not in any sense "prove" which if any of the cells constitute the "true" cases (eg, +/+, +/–, or –/+). However, because psychopathologic conditions are not usually seen as socially desirable, because of the potential cathartic effects of the first interview, and because subjects may wish to shorten the second interview by saying no (having learned that "yes" responses result in additional questions and a lengthier interview), we tend to place greater credence on the veracity of the first interview (+/+ plus +/– subjects) rather than on the smaller number of cases who met the criteria for diagnosis in both time periods (+/+ subjects only).[31] Our analyses of the four ratios of potential unreliability (Table 5) tend to support this position, but further studies specifically examining this question are needed.

Attenuation appears to be higher in children than adults, possibly because children may be more vulnerable to cognitive distortions of the meaning of the retest. For example, children may fail to understand the meaning of the retest, thinking that they need not repeat information given earlier (assuming it is now known), or they may conclude that the interview questions are being repeated because their previous responses were incorrect. If such explanations are accurate, the actual nature of the preparation of subjects for test-retest designs is of major importance for future studies.

Other factors that may explain parent-child attenuation and reliability differences include the possibility that children are more likely to forget the details of the previous interview or attach less significance to the rereporting of all symptoms or to the diagnostic process, so that they discount symptoms more readily (resulting in greater attenuation on the second interview). Also, children are likely more impatient than adults, have a shorter attention span, and have a lower tolerance for boredom. If so, a second interview will be less novel than the first and may fail to hold their attention, with the result that they may tend to deny symptoms the second time around, attempting to rush through the interview.

A number of issues particular to child and adolescent psychopathology warrant special mention. For example, the relatively greater reliability of externalizing disorders (ADHD, ODD, and CD) than internalizing disorders (depression and/or dysthymia, any anxiety disorder) (Table 4) suggests that externalizing disorders are more "noticeable" and problematic to parents (hence remembered and recalled at time 2), while internalizing disorders are more subjective, transient, and prone to recall difficulties. Furthermore, much of the parent's and child's recall (as in studies of adult psychopathologic conditions and life stress research) may be colored by the reporter's current emotional state.[32,33] We have relatively little information about such questions, and systematic studies of these phenomena are needed.

CONCLUSIONS

In summary, the test-retest reliability data from the MECA Study range from moderate to substantial[34] in clinical settings and are comparable or superior to the reliabilities reported for other child and adolescent diagnostic instruments, despite the stringent conditions to which the DISC was submitted. However, the test-retest reliabilities from the community samples range from only fair (internalizing disorders) to substantial (externalizing disorders).[34]

Is the DISC too "unreliable" for use in field surveys? Given the ubiquitous difficulties inherent in test-retest designs (particularly in community samples with low base rates, decreased diagnostic severity, and increased attenuation), we suggest that such questions are better phrased as, "What is the validity of diagnostic information obtained at a single (first) time point?" and "Which strategies will decrease diagnostic attenuation, particularly in longitudinal studies that require repeated diagnostic assessments?" Further analyses from the second phase of the MECA studies will examine the validity of DISC diagnoses with respect to clinician interviews and external impairment criteria (eg, impairment, need for and use of mental health services). If, as expected, these data indicate robust validity correlates of time 1 DISC interviews, the DISC should provide meaningful prevalence estimates in community surveys. However, further studies of diagnostic attenuation are needed to examine variations in the DISC by reporter (parent vs child), by interviewer (layperson vs clinician), and by diagnosis. Studies of the effects of child and parent age, intelligence, attributions about symptoms, and the context in which the child and/or parent describes the child's symptoms are essential. Innovative strategies to reduce the effects of repeated assessment procedures on symptom reporting are very much needed.

Accepted for publication June 13, 1994.

The opinions and assertions contained in this article are the private views of the authors and are not to be construed as official or as reflecting the views of the Department of Health and Human Services or the National Institute of Mental Health.

The logic for the computer algorithms used to process the responses was developed by a team composed of David Shaffer, MD, Prudence Fisher, MS, and John Piacentini, PhD. The computer programming was done by Mary Rojas, PhD, Michael Parides, MS, and Mark Davies, MPH.

The MECA Program is an epidemiologic methodology study performed by four independent research teams in collaboration with staff of the Division of Clinical Research, which was reorganized in 1992 with components now in the Division of Epidemiology and Services Research and the Division of Clinical and Treatment Research of the National Institute of Mental Health (NIMH), Rockville, Md. The NIMH Principal Collaborators are Darryl A. Regier, MD, MPH, Ben Z. Locke, MSPH, Peter S. Jensen, MD, William E. Narrow, MD, MPH, and Donald S. Rae, MA; the NIMH Project Officer was William J. Huber. The Principal Investigators and Coinvestigators from the four sites are as follows: Emory University, Atlanta, Ga (UO1 MH46725): Mina K. Dulcan, MD, Benjamin B. Lahey, PhD, Donna J. Brogan, PhD, Sherryl Goodman, PhD, and Elaine Flagg, PhD; Research Foundation for Mental Hygiene at New York State Psychiatric Institute, Columbia University, New York (UO1 MH46718): Hector R. Bird, MD, David Shaffer, MD, Myrna Weissman, PhD, Patricia Cohen, PhD, Denise Kandel, PhD, Christina Hoven, PhD, Mark Davies, MPH, Madelyn S. Gould, PhD, and Agnes Whitaker, MD; Yale University, New Haven, Conn (UO1 MH46717): Mary Schwab-Stone, MD, Philip J. Leaf, PhD, Sarah Horwitz, PhD, and Judith H. Lichtman, MPH; and University of Puerto Rico, San Juan (UO1 MH46732): Glorisa Canino, PhD, Maritza Rubio-Stipec, MA, Milagros Bravo, PhD, Margarita Alegría, PhD, Julio Ribera, PhD, Sarah Huertas, MD, and Michael Woodbury, MD.

Reprint requests to Room 18C-17, Parklawn Bldg, Child and Adolescent Disorders Research Branch, National Institute of Mental Health, 5600 Fishers Ln, Rockville, MD 20857 (Dr Jensen).

REFERENCES

1. American Psychiatric Association. *Diagnostic and Statistical Manual of Mental Disorders, Revised Third Edition.* Washington, DC: American Psychiatric Association; 1987.
2. Chambers W, Puig-Antich J, Hirsch M, Paez P, Ambrosini P, Tabrizi M, Davies M. The assessment of affective disorders in children and adolescents by semistructured interview. *Arch Gen Psychiatry.* 1985;42:696-702.
3. Guttermann E, O'Brien J, Young G. Structured Diagnostic Interviews for Children and Adolescents: current status and future directions. *J Am Acad Child Adolesc Psychiatry.* 1987;26:621-630.
4. Schwab-Stone M, Fisher P, Piacentini JC, Shaffer D, Gioia P, Davies M. The Diagnostic Interview Schedule for Children–Revised Version (DISC-R), II: test-retest reliability. *J Am Acad Child Adolesc Psychiatry.* 1993;32:651-657.
5. Piacentini J, Shaffer D, Fisher P, Schwab-Stone M, Davies M, Gioia P. The Diagnostic Interview Schedule for Children–Revised Version (DISC-R), III: concurrent criterion validity. *J Am Acad Child Adolesc Psychiatry.* 1993;32:658-665.
6. Shaffer D, Schwab-Stone M, Fisher P, Cohen P, Piacentini J, Davies M, Edelbrock C, Regier D. The Diagnostic Interview Schedule for Children–Revised Version (DISC-R), I: preparation, field testing, interrater reliability, and acceptability. *J Am Acad Child Adolesc Psychiatry.* 1993;32:643-650.
7. Cohen P, O'Connor P, Lewis S, Velez N, Malachowsky B. Comparison of DISC and K-SADS-P interviews of an epidemiological sample of children. *J Am Acad Child Adolesc Psychiatry.* 1987;26:662-667.

8. Costello E, Edelbrock C, Costello A. Validity of the NIMH Diagnostic Interview Schedule for Children: a comparison between psychiatric and pediatric referrals. *J Abnorm Child Psychol.* 1985;13:579-595.
9. Edelbrock C, Costello AJ, Dulcan MK, Conover NC, Kalas R. Age differences in the reliability of the psychiatric interview of the child. *Child Dev.* 1988;56:265-275.
10. Fisher P, Shaffer D, Piacentini J, Lapkin J, Kafantaris V, Leonard H, Herzog D. Sensitivity of the Diagnostic Interview Schedule for Children, 2nd edition (DISC-2.1), for specific diagnoses of children and adolescents. *J Am Acad Child Adolesc Psychiatry.* 1993;32:666-673.
11. Schwab-Stone M, Fallon T, Briggs M, Crowther B. Reliability of diagnostic testing for children ages 6-11 years: a test-retest study of the Diagnostic Interview Schedule for Children–Revised. *Am J Psychiatry.* 1994;151:1048-1054.
12. Lewis SA. Gorsky A, Cohen P, Hartmark C. The reactions of youth to diagnostic interviews. *J Am Acad Child Adolesc Psychiatry.* 1985;24:750-755.
13. Helzer JE, Robins LN, McEvoy LT, Spitznagel EL, Stolzman RK, Farmer A, Brockington IF. A comparison of clinical and Diagnostic Interview Schedule diagnoses. *Arch Gen Psychiatry.* 1985;42:657-666.
14. Helzer J, Robins L, Croughan J, Welner A. Renard Diagnostic Interview: its reliability and procedural validity with physicians and lay interviewers. *Arch Gen Psychiatry.* 1981;38:393-398.
15. Rice JP, Rochberg N, Endicott J, Lavori PW, Miller C. Stability of psychiatric diagnoses: an application to the affective disorders. *Arch Gen Psychiatry.* 1992; 49:824-830.
16. Andreasen NC, Grove WM, Shapiro RW, Keller MB, Hirschfeld RMA, McDonald-Scott P. Reliability of lifetime diagnosis. *Arch Gen Psychiatry.* 1981;38:400-405.
17. Anthony JC, Folstein M. Comparison of the lay Diagnostic Interview Schedule and a standardized psychiatric diagnosis. *Arch Gen Psychiatry.* 1985;42:667-675.
18. Bird H, Gould M, Staghezza B. Aggregating data from multiple informants in child psychiatry epidemiological research. *J Am Acad Child Adolesc Psychiatry.* 1992;31:78-85.
19. Piacentini JC, Cohen P, Cohen J. Combining discrepant diagnostic information from multiple sources: are complex algorithms better than simple ones? *J Abnorm Child Psychol.* 1992;20:51-63.
20. Jensen PS, Bloedau L, Davis H. Children at risk, II: predictors of clinic utilization. *J Am Acad Child Adolesc Psychiatry.* 1990;29:804-812.
21. Rubio-Stipec M, Canino G, Shrout P, Dulcan M, Freeman D, Bravo M. Psychometric properties of parents and children as informants in child psychiatry epidemiology in the Spanish Diagnostic Interview Schedule for Children (DISC-2). *J Abnorm Child Psychol.* 1994;22:1-18.
22. Boyle MH, Offord DR, Racine Y, Sanford M, Szatmari P, Fleming JE, Price-Munn N. Evaluation of the Diagnostic Interview for Children and Adolescents for use in general population samples. *J Abnorm Child Psychol.* 1993;21:663-681.
23. Hodges K. Structured interviews for assessing children. *J Child Psychol Psychiatry.* 1993;34:49-68.
24. Shrout PE, Spitzer RL, Fleiss J. Quantification of agreement in psychiatric diagnosis revisited. *Arch Gen Psychiatry.* 1987;44:172-177.
25. Regier DA, Myers JK, Kramer M, Robins LN, Blazer DG, Hough RL, Eaton WW, Locke BZ. The NIMH Epidemiologic Catchment Area Program: historical context, major objectives, and study population characteristics. *Arch Gen Psychiatry.* 1984;41:934-941.
26. Kraemer HC. Charlie Brown and statistics: an exchange. *Arch Gen Psychiatry.* 1987;44:192-193.
27. Novack AH, Bromet E, Neill TK, Abramovitz RH, Storch S. Children's mental health services in an inner-city neighborhood. *Am J Public Health.* 1975;65: 133-138.
28. Offord DR, Boyle NH, Szatmari P, Rae-Grant NI, Links PS, Cadman DT, Byles JA, Crawford JW, Blum HM, Byrne C, Thomas H, Woodward CA. Ontario Child Health Study, II: six-month prevalence of disorder and rates of service utilization. *Arch Gen Psychiatry.* 1987;44:832-836.
29. McGee R, Feehan M, Williams S, Anderson J. DSM-III disorders from age 11 to age 15 years. *J Am Acad Child Adolesc Psychiatry.* 1992;31:50-59.
30. Rohde P, Lewinsohn PM, Seeley JR. Comorbidity of unipolar depression, II: comorbidity with other mental disorders in adolescents and adults. *J Abnorm Psychol.* 1991;100:214-222.
31. Robins L. Epidemiology: reflections on testing the validity of psychiatric interviews. *Arch Gen Psychiatry.* 1985;42:918-924.
32. Jenkins CD, Hurst MW, Rose RM. Life changes: do people really remember? *Arch Gen Psychiatry.* 1979;36:379-384.
33. Jensen PS, Traylor J, Xenakis SN, Davis H. Child psychopathology rating scales and interrater agreement, I: parents' gender and psychiatric symptoms. *J Am Acad Child Adolesc Psychiatry.* 1988;27:442-450.
34. Landis JR, Koch GG. The measurement of observer agreement for categorical data. *Biometrics.* 1977;33:766-771.

Notice to Our Readers

If you are unable to access AMA publications through Lexis/Nexis Research Services you may find these publications on the following online services:

Dialog Information Services, Inc
3460 Hillview Avenue
PO Box 10010
Palo Alto, CA 94303-0993
800-3-DIALOG
FAX 415-858-7069
(*JAMA*, *Archives* series)

Information Access Company
362 Lakeside Drive
Foster City, CA 94404
800-227-8431
FAX 415-378-5369
(*JAMA*, *Archives* series, *AMNews*)

CD Plus Technologies (formerly BRS-Colleague)
333 Seventh Avenue
New York, NY 10001
212-563-3006
FAX 212-563-3784
(*JAMA* only)

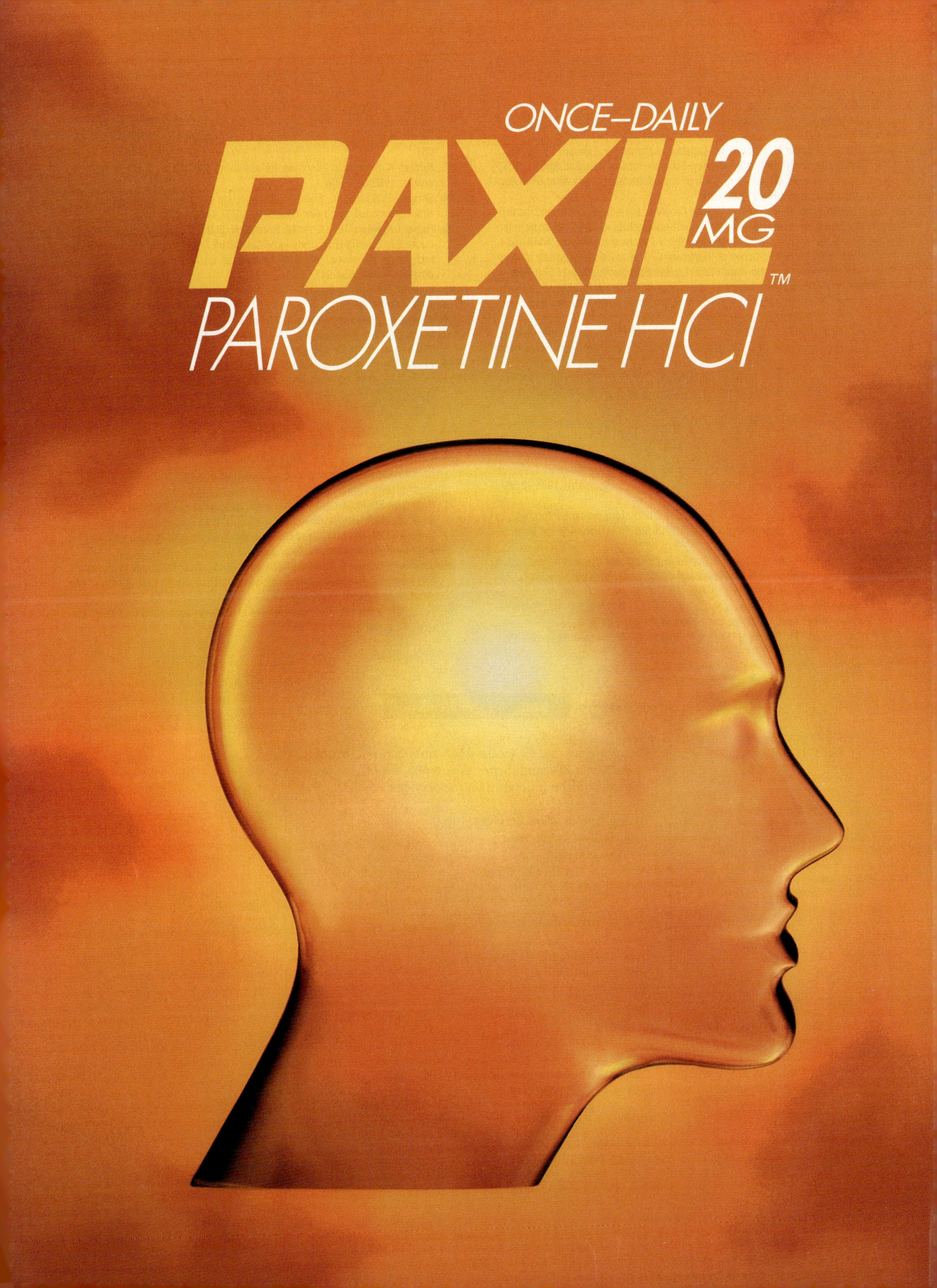
ONCE-DAILY
PAXIL 20 MG™
PAROXETINE HCl

Treatment of Postpartum Depression With Interpersonal Psychotherapy

In the past decade, psychotherapy researchers have focused on the use of short-term manualized psychosocial treatments for a number of psychiatric disorders and have emphasized empirical treatment trials that have demonstrated the efficacy of a number of psychotherapeutic treatments. There has been a growing appreciation that psychotherapeutic treatment must be tailored to specific disorders and that it must be carefully matched to the characteristics of individual patients as well.[1] Pressure to reduce health care costs and the appearance of newer psychopharmacologic agents with less toxic side effects, however, have led to an emphasis on the use of psychotherapy for conditions for which there are as yet no effective medications (eg, the use of cognitive-behavioral and interpersonal psychotherapy [IPT] for eating disorders[2,3]) or for conditions for which medication is relatively contraindicated, such as the use of IPT for conditions such as depression in geriatric patients[4,5] and in pregnant women, as outlined in the recent article by Weissman and Markowitz[6] in the ARCHIVES.

Women in the postpartum period who become depressed and who are breast-feeding are another group of patients for whom medication is relatively contraindicated.[7] The need for an effective treatment for this group of patients is quite high, as the incidence ranges from 7%[8] to 16%[9] across all childbearing women. *DSM-IV* has recognized postpartum depression as a subtype of major depression, having added the longitudinal specifier "with postpartum onset" to describe episodes of major depression that began within 4 weeks post partum.[10] At the University of Iowa, we have recently completed an open treatment trial using a modified form of IPT[11] to treat depressed postpartum women. The modifications of IPT include an emphasis on helping the patient to resolve the marital disputes and major role transitions that frequently occur after the birth of a child.[12]

Six postpartum women (average of 4.1 months post partum) who met *DSM-III-R*[13] criteria for a major depressive episode were treated for 12 weeks using IPT for postpartum depression. All of the patients were married; their ages ranged from 26 to 38 years (average age, 31.8 years). Five of the six patients were breast-feeding.

The patients had a mean Beck Depression Inventory[14] score of 27.7 (SD=5.7) and a mean Hamilton Rating Scale for Depression[15] score of 18.2 (SD=6.2). The mean termination Beck Depression Inventory score was 5.4 (SD=4.8) and the mean termination Hamilton Rating Scale for Depression score was 5.2 (SD=4.1). The changes for both measures were highly significant. None of the patients met criteria for major depressive episode at the end of treatment. In addition, the patients evidenced significant improvements in their scores on the Edinburgh Postnatal Depression Scale,[16] and the Social Adjustment Scale[17] total and marital adjustment subscale scores (**Table**).

This short-term interpersonally oriented approach to postpartum depression appears to have much potential for the treatment of a significant illness with a high degree of associated morbidity. Interpersonal psychotherapy is particularly useful in that it directly addresses issues associated with postpartum role transitions. The desire of many women to continue breast-feeding makes IPT for postpartum depression a useful alternative to the use of antidepressant medication. Before it can be considered an efficacious treatment, IPT for postpartum depression must, of course, be examined in a controlled and randomized treatment trial that compares it with standard pharmacologic treatment.

Outcome Measures for the Use of Interpersonal Psychotherapy for Postpartum Depression*

Scale	Intake Score	Termination Score	*t* (*df*=5)	*P*
Beck Depression Inventory	27.7±5.7	5.4±4.8	5.77	.002
Hamilton Rating Scale for Depression	18.2±6.2	5.2±4.1	4.29	.008
Edinburgh Postnatal Depression Scale	17.3±1.3	4.0±1.2	26.67	.001
Social Adjustment Scale (total)	2.42±0.14	1.84±0.21	17.88	.001
Social Adjustment Scale (marital)	2.56±0.54	2.00±0.46	6.14	.002

**Data are given as mean±SD.*

Scott Stuart, MD
University of Iowa
Department of Psychiatry
200 Hawkins Dr
Iowa City, IA 52242
Michael W. O'Hara, PhD
Iowa City

1. Bergin AE, Garfield SL. *Handbook of Psychotherapy and Behavior Change.* 4th ed. New York, NY: Wiley & Sons Inc; 1994:821-831.
2. Fairburn CG, Jones R, Peveler RC, Carr SJ, Solomon RA, O'Connor ME, Burton J, Hope RA. Three psychological treatments for bulimia nervosa: a comparative trial. *Arch Gen Psychiatry.* 1991;48:463-469.
3. Fairburn CG, Jones R, Peveler RC, Hope RA, O'Connor M. Psychotherapy and bulimia nervosa: longer-term effects of interpersonal psychotherapy, behavior therapy, and cognitive-behavior therapy. *Arch Gen Psychiatry.* 1993; 50:419-428.
4. Sloane RB, Stapes FR, Schneider LS. Interpersonal therapy versus nortrip-

tyline for depression in the elderly. In: Burrows GD, Norman TR, Dennerstein L, eds. *Clinical and Pharmacologic Studies in Psychiatric Disorders*. London, England: John Libbey; 1985:344-346.
5. Reynolds CF, Frank E, Perel JM, Imher SD, Cornes C, Morycz RK, Mazumdar S, Miller M, Pollock BG, Rifai AH, Stack JA, George CJ, Houck PR, Kupfer DJ. Combined pharmacotherapy and psychotherapy in the acute and continuation treatment of elderly patients with recurrent major depression: a preliminary report. *Am J Psychiatry*. 1992;149:1687-1692.
6. Weissman MM, Markowitz JC. Interpersonal psychotherapy: current status. *Arch Gen Psychiatry*. 1994;51:599-606.
7. American Academy of Pediatrics, Committee on Drugs. Transfer of drugs and other chemicals into human milk. *Pediatrics*. 1994;93:137-150.
8. Gotlib I, Whiffen VE, Mount JH. Prevalence rates and demographic characteristics associated with depression in pregnancy and the postpartum. *J Consult Clin Psychol*. 1989;57:269-274.
9. Whiffen V. Vulnerability to postpartum depression: a prospective multivariate study. *J Abnorm Psychol*. 1988;97:467-474.
10. American Psychiatric Association. *Diagnostic and Statistical Manual of Mental Disorders, Fourth Edition*. Washington, DC: American Psychiatric Association; 1994.
11. Klerman GL, Weissman MM, Rounsaville BJ, Chevron ES. *Interpersonal Psychotherapy of Depression*. New York, NY: Basic Books Inc Publishers; 1984.
12. O'Hara MW. *Postpartum Depression: Causes and Consequences*. New York, NY: Springer-Verlag. In press.
13. American Psychiatric Association. *Diagnostic and Statistical Manual of Mental Disorders, Revised Third Edition*. Washington, DC: American Psychiatric Association; 1987.
14. Beck AT, Ward CH, Mendelson M, Mock J, Erbaugh J. An inventory for measuring depression. *Arch Gen Psychiatry*. 1961;4:561-571.
15. Hamilton MA. Development of a rating scale for primary depressive illness. *Br J Soc Clin Psychol*. 1967;6:278-296.
16. Cox JL, Holden JM, Sagovsky R. Detection of postnatal depression: development of the Edinborough Postnatal Depression Scale. *Br J Psychiatry*. 1987; 150:782-786.
17. Weissman MM, Bothwell S. Assessment of social adjustment by patient self-report. *Arch Gen Psychiatry*. 1976;33:1111-1115.

In reply

We were pleased to see the testing of IPT by Stuart and O'Hara for the depression of women in the postpartum period. The modifications they have suggested dealing with marital disputes and the role transition are part of the IPT framework. We believe that psychotherapy should be available to women with depression who may not be able to take medication. Women with postpartum depression who wish to nurse may be good candidates, since drugs are secreted into the breast milk and the effect on the offspring could be problematic.

We have two comments. We would urge the investigators to undertake the controlled and randomized treatment trial comparing IPT with standard pharmacologic treatment for postpartum depression, and, if their sample size allows, compare it with another type of psychotherapy.

Stuart and O'Hara note that psychotherapy is emphasized for conditions for which there are as yet no effective treatments or for conditions for which medication is contraindicated. We hope that psychotherapy will be available for others, since some patients just do not want to take medication for any number of reasons and most patients have social and interpersonal problems that accompany their depression, either as the source or as the consequence of the illness.

Myrna M. Weissman, PhD
New York State Psychiatric Institute
722 W 168th St, Unit 14
New York, NY 10032
John Markowitz, MD
New York

Relationship of Panic Disorder to Posttraumatic Stress Disorder

We read with interest the article by Southwick et al[1] in the April 1993 issue of the ARCHIVES. Using intravenous yohimbine hydrochloride, the authors induced panic attacks in 70% and flashbacks in 40% of 20 subjects suffering from chronic posttraumatic stress disorder (PTSD). It is unclear, however, if their conclusion that panic disorder and PTSD share a common neurobiology is not, at least in part, a reflection of a lack of specificity in their assessment procedure. Furthermore, the applicability of their findings to the majority of people suffering from PTSD needs to be questioned.

Rainey et al[2] reported the effect of intravenous lactate in seven Vietnam veterans with a history of flashbacks, six of whom met *DSM-III* criteria for both PTSD and panic disorder, and one with a history of PTSD meeting *DSM-III* criteria for panic disorder at intake. All of these subjects reported flashbacks after lactate infusion. Moreover, although "anxiety states meeting *DSM-III* criteria for panic attacks" occurred in six of the seven subjects *after* the onset of flashbacks, no panic attack occurred *prior* to or in the absence of a flashback. Thus, one might wonder whether panic attacks occurring after flashbacks are qualitatively equivalent to panic attacks suffered by patients with panic disorder. It could be argued that Rainey et al simply labeled the autonomic and anxiety symptoms associated with flashbacks as being panic attacks.

Similarly, in a larger study on PTSD subjects with flashbacks, Mellman and Davis[3] suggested that a "'flashback' is a panic attack, at least insofar as it meets the *DSM-III* criteria." Of the 25 Vietnam veterans with PTSD who were assessed with a semistructured interview, none had ever experienced a panic attack unrelated to a prior flashback. Conversely, all flashbacks were accompanied by anxiety symptoms meeting *DSM-III* criteria for a panic attack.

In light of the above, more precision is required in determining the relationship between flashbacks and panic attacks and, consequently between PTSD and panic disorder. This precision is lacking from the study of Southwick et al, as the characterization of their subjects is incomplete. For example, the temporal relationship between the occurrence of the trauma and the onset of PTSD and panic disorder in these subjects is not known. The subjects are not well characterized with regard to a temporal link between spontaneous flashbacks and panic attacks or with regard to the presence of concurrent symptoms frequently associated with panic disorder, such as agoraphobia. Also, unlike the study of Rainey et al, the sequence of apparition of the symptoms of flashbacks, panic attacks, and "significant increases in core PTSD symptoms" after yohimbine infusion was not specified. Nor was it documented from their subjects' clinical history, despite prior observations by Mellman and Davis. Last but not least, it cannot be ascertained that the panic attacks observed after yohimbine induction were phenomenologically similar or identical to panic attacks induced in patients with panic disorder but free of PTSD, as no such comparative group was used. Indeed, the absence of the occurrence of panic attacks in the first-degree relatives of the subjects in the study of Southwick et al might be explained by the likelihood that these subjects did not experience true panic attacks after yohimbine infusion.

The applicability of the findings of Southwick et al in "*DSM-III-R* chronic PTSD" subjects to the majority of patients with PTSD is unclear. First, as there are no *DSM-III-R* criteria for chronic PTSD, the duration or timing criteria used for chronic PTSD should have been specified. Second, their sample consisted of inpatients with a very high lifetime rate of other *DSM-III-R* diagnoses (80% major depression, 60% panic disorder, and 85% alcohol dependence). At the time of the study, their patients' 45% current rate of *DSM-III-R* panic disorder was very high compared with that found in other reports on PTSD. For example, in a recent literature review on the epidemiology of PTSD, Davidson and Fairbanks[4] found that lifetime comorbidity of panic disorder varied from 4% to 21.2% among the five studies that assessed it. Of the only two studies that evaluated current comorbidity of panic disorder in PTSD subjects, one found an overall panic disorder rate of 8%, whereas the other found rates of 4.9% and 12.7% in men and women, respectively. Third, it is unfortunate that Southwick et al presented no data on the lifetime frequency of flashbacks in their patients. If this rate was similar to that following intravenous yohimbine (40%), it again would have seemed rather high compared with that reported in other PTSD samples. For instance, in a recent literature review by Kilpatrick and Resnick,[5] less than 15% of patients experienced flashbacks in the three study samples in which these symptoms were assessed.

To sum up, after reading the very interesting report by Southwick et al, we question whether their conclusion on the biological relationship between panic disorder and PTSD might not simply reflect a lack of precision in their approach. We also question the applicability of their findings to the majority of patients with PTSD.

Gabriel Safadi, MD
Department of Psychiatry
Charles LeMoyne Hospital
121 Taschereau Blvd
Greenfield Park, Quebec, Canada J4V 2H1
Jacques Bradwejn, MD
Montreal, Quebec

1. Southwick SM, Krystal JH, Morgan A, Johnson D, Nagy LM, Nicolaou A, Heninger GR, Charney DS. Abnormal noradrenergic function in posttraumatic stress disorder. *Arch Gen Psychiatry.* 1993;50:266-274.
2. Rainey JM, Aleem A, Ortiz A, Yeragani V, Pohl R, Berchou R. A laboratory procedure for the induction of flashbacks. *Am J Psychiatry.* 1987;144:1317-1319.
3. Mellman TA, Davis GC. Combat-related flashbacks in posttraumatic stress disorder: phenomenology and similarity to panic attacks. *J Clin Psychiatry.* 1985;46:379-382.
4. Davidson JRT, Fairbanks JA. The epidemiology of posttraumatic stress disorder. In: Davidson JRT, Foa EB, eds. *Posttraumatic Stress Disorder: DSM-IV and Beyond.* Washington, DC: American Psychiatric Press Inc; 1993:147-169.
5. Kilpatrick DG, Resnick HS. Posttraumatic stress disorder associated with exposure to criminal victimization in clinical and community populations. In: Davidson JRT, Foa EB, eds. *Posttraumatic Stress Disorder: DSM-IV and Beyond.* Washington, DC: American Psychiatric Press Inc; 1993:113-143.

In reply

As pointed out by Safadi and Bradwejn, panic attacks can be difficult to differentiate from flashbacks because flashbacks are frequently accompanied by symptoms of autonomic arousal and anxiety. Safadi and Bradwejn wonder whether the panic attacks in the intravenous lactate PTSD study by Rainey et al were mislabeled and instead "simply represented associated features of flashbacks." Further, the work of Mellman and Davis is cited, in which flashbacks are viewed as the equivalent of panic attacks.

Safadi and Bradwejn suggest that our yohimbine study,[1] like the study by Rainey et al, suffered from a lack of specificity in assessment and they wonder whether the panic attacks experienced after yohimbine infusion were "true" panic attacks. Additionally, they wonder whether yohimbine-induced panic attacks and flashbacks really differed from one another. It is not clear what they mean by true panic attacks. As detailed in the "Procedures" section of our article,[1] we used DSM-III-R *criteria for panic attack to define the presence or absence of yohimbine-induced panic attacks.* DSM-III-R *does not rely on etiology to determine the presence of panic disorder or panic attacks. As such, it is atheoretical. Panic attacks can be induced by numerous agents, including lactate, yohimbine, carbon dioxide, and caffeine. We followed the* DSM-III-R *approach and simply determined whether* DSM-III-R *panic attacks developed after yohimbine infusion. We also operationalized the definition of flashbacks. In our study there was no overlap in criteria between panic attacks and flashbacks. As described in the "Procedures" section of our article, the criteria for flashbacks were the following: (1) the patient must have reexperienced a past traumatic event during the course of drug or placebo infusion; (2) the reexperiencing must have involved one or more sensory modalities (hearing, seeing, smelling, tasting, and/or feeling); (3) for patients with a history of flashbacks, the drug-induced reexperiencing state must have been very similar to a naturally occurring flashback; and (4) there must have been consensual agreement of two research psychiatrists that a flashback had occurred.*

In the yohimbine study, 40% of patients met criteria for both panic attacks and flashbacks. Thirty percent experienced panic attacks in the absence of flashbacks. While none of the 20 patients had a yohimbine-induced flashback without a panic attack, in a subsequent study using the same criteria, three of 26 patients had a yohimbine-induced flashback without a panic attack. The above data suggest that panic attacks can be differentiated from flashbacks. The fact that flashbacks rarely occur without panic attacks may mean that flashbacks are so distressing that they frequently precipitate panic attacks (S.M.S. et al, unpublished data, 1994).

We agree with the suggestion that greater precision is required to determine the relationship between flash-

backs and panic attacks. While this was not the primary focus of our study, it is an area that needs careful attention. Of note, in a separate study, we currently are attempting to more precisely delineate the temporal sequence of symptom development after yohimbine and m-chlorophenylpiperazine infusion.

Safadi and Bradwejn also question the conclusion that PTSD and panic disorder share a common neurobiology. They are correct to point out that such conclusions cannot be drawn without the appropriate panic disorder control group. As discussed in the "Comment" section of our article,[1] comparisons with panic disorder patients were based on data from separate studies. For this reason, we were careful to use the following wording:

In fact, careful inspection of the data from the current study and from the previous work with patients with panic disorder reveals highly similar responses to yohimbine in the two patient groups, suggesting that these two disorders may share a common neurobiological abnormality that is related to altered sensitivity of the noradrenergic system.

Finally, it is important to emphasize that the patients studied were treatment-seeking combat veterans with PTSD. Clearly, they represent a subgroup of combat veterans with PTSD. The high rate of comorbid panic disorder in our patient group is probably related to their treatment-seeking status. Currently, it is not clear whether these findings are applicable to non–treatment-seeking combat veterans with PTSD.

Steven M. Southwick, MD
John H. Krystal, MD
Dennis S. Charney, MD
West Haven Veterans Affairs Medical Center
950 Campbell Ave
New Haven, CT 06516

1. Southwick SM, Krystal JH, Morgan A, Johnson D, Nagy LM, Nicolaou A, Heninger GR, Charney DS. Abnormal noradrenergic function in posttraumatic stress disorder. *Arch Gen Psychiatry*. 1993;50:266-274.

Notice to Our Readers

If you are unable to access AMA publications through Lexis/Nexis Research Services you may find these publications on the following online services:

Dialog Information Services, Inc
3460 Hillview Avenue
PO Box 10010
Palo Alto, CA 94303-0993
800-3-DIALOG
FAX 415-858-7069
(*JAMA*, *Archives* series)

Information Access Company
362 Lakeside Drive
Foster City, CA 94404
800-227-8431
FAX 415-378-5369
(*JAMA*, *Archives* series, *AMNews*)

CD Plus Technologies (formerly BRS-Colleague)
333 Seventh Avenue
New York, NY 10001
212-563-3006
FAX 212-563-3784
(*JAMA* only)

Depression in Patients With Cancer

Diagnosis, Biology, and Treatment

J. Stephen McDaniel, MD; Dominique L. Musselman, MD; Maryfrances R. Porter; Deborah A. Reed, RN, MSN; Charles B. Nemeroff, MD, PhD

This article reviews the challenge of diagnosing depression in patients with cancer. Major depression and depressive symptoms, although commonly encountered in medical populations, are frequently underdiagnosed and undertreated. This is especially true for patients with cancer in whom the diagnosis of major depression is clouded by neurovegetative symptoms that may be secondary to either cancer or depression. Well-established biological markers for major depression are proposed as diagnostic adjuncts in patients with cancer. Studies using biological markers in depressed patients with and without cancer are reviewed, and the implications of diminished immune function in depressed patients with cancer are discussed. The limited database on treatment of depression in patients with cancer also is reviewed. Treatment of depression in these patients improves their dysphoria and other signs and symptoms of depression, improves quality of life, and may improve immune function and survival time. Guidelines for future research are proposed. *(Arch Gen Psychiatry. 1995;52:89-99)*

Major depression and depressive symptoms are exceedingly common in medical populations. In fact, major depression is the most common clinical psychiatric problem seen in primary care.[1] Prevalences cited in investigations of medical outpatients that employed standardized diagnostic interviews range from 4.8% to 9.2% for major depression and from 9% to 20% for all depressive disorders.[2-7] Studies that employed structured interviews of medical inpatients have reported even higher prevalences: 8% for major depression and 15% to 36% for all depressive disorders.[8,9]

The lack of recognition of depression in the medically ill among physicians has been well documented.[10] Internists have been found to recognize depression in only one fourth to one half of their depressed medical outpatients.[4,11,12] However, recognition and treatment of depression is crucial, especially for medically ill patients, because depressive disorders may adversely affect survival,[13-17] the length of hospital stay,[17] compliance with therapy,[18] the ability to care for oneself, and quality of life.[19]

DEPRESSION AND CANCER

Studies that examined the severity of medical illness as a risk factor for depression demonstrate the prevalence of depression to be substantially higher as the severity of medical illness increases.[20-23] Only a portion of those studies that examined the prevalence of depression in patients with cancer have limited their subjects to those with specific cancer types or tumor sites, although a high rate of depression has been reported in many patients with various types of cancer.[24,25] However, interpreting differences in the prevalence of depression by tumor site is difficult because the studies vary by diagnostic method, definition of depression (syndrome vs symptom), hospitalization status, time since diagnosis, and disease stage; nonetheless, they provide important clinical information. These studies,[26-43] listed in **Table 1**, show a wide variability in prevalence categorized by cancer site, ranging from 1.5% to 50% (mean, 24%; median, 22%).

From the Department of Psychiatry and Behavioral Sciences, Emory University School of Medicine, Atlanta, Ga.

Table 1. Prevalence of Depression by Cancer Site*

Cancer Site	Source, y	No. of Subjects	Diagnostic Method	Prevalence
Pancreas	Fras et al,[26] 1967	46	Interview, MMPI, DRS	50%
	Joffe et al,[27] 1986	12	SAD-L, HSC, BDI	50%
Oropharynx	Morton et al,[28] 1984	48	Interview	40%
	Davies et al,[29] 1986	72	GHQ, LSSD	22%
	Baile et al,[30] 1992	45	Interview, MCMI	40%
Breast	Maguire et al,[31] 1978	201	Interview	26%
	Silberfarb et al,[32] 1980	146	Interview	10%, primary cancer; 15%, recurrent cancer; 4.5%, advanced cancer; 10% (mean prevalence)†
	Farber et al,[33] 1984	141	HSC	18%, severe depression; 21%, moderate depression; 19.5% (mean prevalence)†
	Grandi et al,[34] 1987	18	Interview	22%
	Fallowfield et al,[35] 1990	269	Interview	21%, mastectomy; 19%, lumpectomy; 20% (mean prevalence)†
	Hopwood et al,[36] 1991	81	HADS, RSCL	20%
	Hopwood et al,[37] 1991	222	HADS, RSCL	27%, HADS; 22%, RSCL; 24.5% (mean prevalence)†
	Goldberg et al,[38] 1992	320	RSCL	32%
	Pinder et al,[39] 1993	139	HADS, interview	13%
Colon	Fras et al,[26] 1967	64	Interview, MMPI, DRS	13%
	Koenig et al,[40] 1967	36	MMPI	25%
Gynecological‡	Evans et al,[41] 1986	83	Interview, HDRS, CRSD	23%, major depression
Lymphoma§	Devlen et al,[42] 1987	90	Interview	17%
Gastric	Joffe et al,[27] 1986	9	SADS-L, HSC, BDI	11%
Acute leukemia‖	Colon et al,[43] 1991	100	Interview	1%, major depression; 2%, organic affective syndrome; 1.5% (mean prevalence)†

**MMPI indicates Minnesota Multiphasic Personality Inventory; DRS, Depression Rating Scale; SADS-L, Schedule for Affective Disorders and Schizophrenia–Lifetime Version; HSC, Hopkins Symptom Checklist; BDI, Beck Depression Inventory; GHQ, General Health Questionnaire; LSSD, Leeds Scale for Self-Assessment of Depression; MCMI, Million Clinical Multiaxial Inventory; HADS, Hamilton Anxiety and Depression Scale; RSCL, Rotter Symptom Checklist; HDRS, Hamilton Depression Rating Scale; and CRSD, Carroll Rating Scale for Depression.*

†For the purposes of this review, a mean prevalence was determined for those individual studies that reported more than one prevalence depending on cancer disease stage,[32] depression symptom severity,[33] cancer treatment,[35] diagnostic method,[36,37] and definition.[43]

‡Gynecological refers to cervical, endometrial, or vaginal.

§Hodgkin's and non-Hodgkin's lymphoma.

‖Before bone marrow transplantation.

Less information is available with regard to whether the risk of other mood disorders (eg, psychotic depression, dysthymia, adjustment disorder, or bipolar disorder) increases with cancer severity. Some investigators[26,44-46] have measured depressive symptom severity rather than studying specific diagnoses. However, few studies have addressed the spectrum of mood disorders in their assessments of major depression. **Table 2**[33,41,43-48] reviews those investigations that have considered other mood disorders and/or depressive symptom severity. Caution must be used in interpreting these studies because, like those studies that examined depression by cancer site, they have a number of complicating variables such as hospitalization status (ie, hospitalization may or may not equate with greater cancer severity) and include a mix of cancer types and stages. Nonetheless, a clear spectrum of symptom severity is recognized in depressed patients with cancer.

In recent years, considerable research has been conducted concerning the diagnosis and management of depression in patients with cancer. A major obstacle to the study of depression in patients with cancer has been the difficulty distinguishing the depressive symptoms that are associated with syndromal depression from the symptoms that are caused by the patients' medical illnesses and/or medical treatments. The diagnostic criteria for major depression, established in the *DSM-IV*,[49] include a number of signs and symptoms that frequently are attributed to the patients' malignant neoplasms (eg, appetite loss, weight loss, insomnia, loss of interest, and loss of energy). With the extensive literature documenting neuroendocrine, neurochemical, and neuroanatomical alterations associated with depression in patients with primary mood disorders, it is evident that such biological markers may reflect the pathophysiologic characteristics of major depression in patients with complicating comorbid medical illness and, thereby, may aid in the diagnosis of depression in medically ill patients. Furthermore, it is important to recognize that pharmacological treatment of major depression in patients with cancer has been shown to treat depression effectively and to improve the quality of life of depressed patients with cancer.[50,51] Indeed, psychological treatment of patients with cancer (even those without the syndrome of major depression) has been shown to be effective in the management of a number of domains, including distress, self-concept, health locus of control, fatigue, sexual problems, anxiety, pain, and nausea.[52] Interestingly, some psychological interventions have resulted in increased survival rates in

Table 2. Prevalence Studies Utilizing Various Mood Disorder Diagnoses or Symptom Severity*

Source, y	Hospitalization Status	No. of Patients	Cancer Type	Diagnostic Method	Prevalence
Plumb and Holland,[44] 1977	Inpatient	97	Mixed	BDI	4%, severe; 19%, moderate
Bukberg et al,[45] 1984	Inpatient	67	Mixed	Interview,† HDRS, BDI	24%, severe; 18%, moderate; 14%, mild
Farber et al,[33] 1984	Outpatient	141	Breast	HSC	18%, severe; 21%, moderate
Evans et al,[41] 1986	Inpatient	83	Gynecological‡	Interview, HDRS, CRSD	23%, major depression; 24%, adjustment disorder/depressed; 14%, dysthymia
Stefanek et al,[46] 1987	Outpatient	126	Mixed	BSI	9%, severe; 24%, moderate
Kathol et al,[47] 1990	Unknown	808	Mixed	Interview,§ HDRS, BDI	25%-38%, major depression; 19% (depressive symptoms)
Razavi et al,[48] 1990	Inpatient	128	Mixed	DIS, HDRS	8%, major depression; 52%, adjustment disorder/depressed
Colon et al,[43] 1991	Inpatient	100	Acute leukemia‖	Interview	1%, major depression; 2%, organic affective syndrome; 8%, adjustment disorder/depressed

**BDI indicates Beck Depression Inventory; HDRS, Hamilton Depression Rating Scale; HSC, Hopkins Symptom Checklist; CRSD, Carroll Rating Scale for Depression; BSI, Brief Symptom Inventory; and DIS, Diagnostic Interview Schedule.*
†*Eliminated physical symptoms.*
‡*Gynecological refers to cervical, endometrial, or vaginal.*
§DSM-III-R *criteria, Research and Diagnostic Criteria, and Endicott criteria.*
‖*Before bone marrow transplantation.*

patients with cancer,[52-55] perhaps in part because of enhanced immune function.[56,57]

DIAGNOSTIC CHALLENGES IN THE DIAGNOSIS OF MAJOR DEPRESSION IN PATIENTS WITH CANCER

The psychological distress and depression that are prevalent in some patients with cancer represent complex social, psychological, and medical factors. Clinicians must take into account such issues as cancer site, clinical course, type of treatment, and presence of pain.[24] A patient's history of adjustment to illness and coping ability can offer further useful information. In their study examining factors associated with psychological distress in patients with cancer, Cassileth and colleagues[58] found those patients at greatest risk to be young, female, receiving palliative or active treatment as opposed to follow-up care, and symptomatic or not fully ambulatory. Bukberg and colleagues[45] have documented a higher prevalence of depression in patients with more advanced cancer and with a greater level of disability or discomfort. Other investigators[59] have found a direct relationship between declining physical status and psychological status. Indeed, severity of illness has been found to be the most important variable associated with depression in patients with cancer.[60-62]

Addressing some of the known risk factors may assist clinicians in diagnosing depression in patients with cancer. Weisman and Worden[63] have reported the following risk factors that may predispose patients with cancer to the development of depressive symptoms: social isolation, recent losses, a tendency toward pessimism, the presence of pain, and socioeconomic pressures. Other contributing factors that may place patients with cancer at higher risk for depression include a diagnosis of alcoholism or substance abuse and a history of mood disorders or suicide attempts.[44,64,65] Recent studies[66-69] suggest that although small numbers of cancer patients commit suicide, their relative risk of suicide is twice that of the general population. A careful review of patient medications may yield useful information because some commonly prescribed medications such as corticosteriods may produce depressive symptoms.[70]

Receiving a diagnosis of cancer may result in a cascade of emotional responses. Feelings of sadness are an expected response to painful life experiences such as being informed that one has a diagnosis of cancer. These feelings may be coupled with reactions of shock, disbelief, anxiety, and a myriad of other emotional states. However, when these symptoms are of such a magnitude and duration that they fulfill *DSM-IV* criteria for major depression, accurate diagnosis and treatment are essential. For a patient to fulfill diagnostic criteria for major depression, the patient must first have symptoms of dysphoria and/or anhedonia, which is defined as a loss of interest or pleasure, pervasively for at least a 2-week period. Patients should then have at least four of the following symptoms (or at least three of the following symptoms if they have both dysphoria and anhedonia): sleep disorder, appetite change, fatigue, psychomotor retardation and/or agitation, low self-esteem and/or guilt, poor concentration and/or indecisiveness, and thoughts of suicide and/or suicidal ideation.[49]

Diagnosing major depression in medically ill patients historically has been an area fraught with controversy. Kathol and colleagues[47,71] have reported the following problems associated with diagnosing depression in patients with medical illnesses such as cancer: first, depressive symptoms are often appropriate in the context of the stress of having a serious medical illness; second, many symptoms of depression are similar to those of the medical illness itself; and third, there have been numerous diagnostic systems proposed to diagnose depression, some of them with overlapping patient populations. Cohen-Cole et al[72] recently reviewed the conceptual approaches to the diagnosis of major depression in medically ill patients and proposed an approach to depression in these patients. They proposed two systems for diagnosis depending on whether the assessment is primarily for research (exclusive approach) or clinical (inclusive approach) purposes. The exclusive approach, which was initially proposed by researchers at the Memorial Sloan Kettering Cancer Center, New York, NY,[45] maximizes specificity by eliminating anorexia and fatigue from the list of nine depressive criteria and requires four of the remaining symptoms for a diagnosis of major depression. Anorexia and fatigue, which frequently are elements of the disease process or side effects of treatment measures, are two of the most controversial symptoms in the diagnosis of depression in patients with cancer. However, for clinical purposes, the inclusive approach to diagnosing depression maximizes sensitivity and best protects the patient from the risk of undiagnosed depression, a so-called false-negative result. This approach recommends that clinicians count each relevant depressive symptom even if there is reason to believe the symptom may not be part of a depressive syndrome but may be secondary to the disease process or its treatment.

In addition to these criteria for the inclusive approach, clinicians should generally have a lower threshold of suspicion for major depression in patients with cancer and adhere to traditional reliance on empathic, interpretative responses to clinical observations. Mermelstein and Lesko[24] recommend focusing on the psychological symptoms of persistent dysphoria, feelings of helplessness or hopelessness, loss of self-esteem, feelings of worthlessness, and wishes to die as reliable diagnostic indicators. When these symptoms overwhelm the patient or interfere with functioning, treatment is indicated.

Treatment is particularly relevant in view of recent evidence that depression in the context of physical illness is associated with increased morbidity, length of hospital stay, and overall disability.[12] Moreover, medically ill patients who have depressive symptoms may not fulfill *DSM-IV* criteria for major depression yet may experience significant improvement in quality of life with antidepressant treatment of their depressive symptoms.[51,73] For these reasons, our research team traditionally has used the inclusive approach for diagnosis and treatment of patients with cancer presenting with symptoms that are suggestive of major depression.

BIOLOGICAL MARKERS: A POTENTIAL AID IN THE DIAGNOSIS OF DEPRESSION IN THE MEDICALLY ILL

Recent advances in biological psychiatry have included the discoveries of a number of neurochemical, neuroendocrine, and neuroanatomic alterations in unipolar depression. Although few of these biological alterations have been systematically investigated in medically ill patients who often are unable to participate in a psychiatric diagnostic interview, such biological markers potentially can serve as important diagnostic adjuncts in the diagnosis of depression in those patients who experience neurovegetative symptoms that are suggestive of major depression. Furthermore, as state-dependent variables, certain markers may reflect and even portend treatment response in patients with depression.[74] To date, there have been only three studies of depression in patients with cancer that have used such biological markers. Before reviewing the findings from these studies, we briefly review the rationale underlying the use of neuroendocrine and functional and structural imaging measures in patients with psychiatric disorders.

Numerous biological markers currently are used in the diagnosis of primary depression. Alterations of the following three neuroendocrine systems have been examined: (1) the hypothalamic-pituitary-adrenal (HPA) axis (increased urinary free cortisol level, dexamethasone nonsuppression, blunted corticotropin [ACTH] response to corticotropin-releasing factor [CRF], elevated cerebrospinal fluid [CSF] CRF concentrations, and adrenal and pituitary hypertrophy); (2) the hypothalamic-pituitary-thyroid axis (blunted thyrotropin response to thyrotropin-releasing hormone (TRH) (protirelin), elevated CSF TRH concentrations, and symptomless autoimmune thyroiditis) and; (3) somatostatin neurotransmission (reduced CSF somatostatin concentrations).[25] Two other biological markers closely tied to neurotransmitter function have been studied: (1) serotonergic neurotransmission (reduced CSF 5-hydroxyindoleacetic acid concentrations, reduced brain and platelet binding to the serotonin (5-HT) transporter, and increased platelet $5\text{-}HT_2$ binding); and (2) noradrenergic neurotransmission (increased brain and lymphocyte β-adrenergic receptor binding and decreased urinary catecholamine metabolite excretion). Structural brain abnormalities (subcortical and periventricular hyperintensities and decreased volume of specific subcortical and cortical structures) and alterations in sleep architecture (reduced rapid eye movement latency, redistribution of rapid eye movement sleep, and diminished delta wave production) also remain important biological markers for primary depression.[25]

To date, only three investigations[27,41,75] have incorporated biological markers in the study of depressed patients with cancer. All three evaluated the HPA axis; one also examined the hypothalamic-pituitary-thyroid axis.[41] Although numerous biological markers are available in the study of depression, none have been validated yet in depressed patients with any comorbid medical illness. Therefore, we will limit our discussion to the most intensely scrutinized neuroendocrine axis, the HPA axis.

ALTERATIONS OF THE HPA AXIS IN DEPRESSION

Literally hundreds of reports have documented HPA axis hyperactivity in drug-free depressed patients. This is now believed at least in part to be due to central nervous system hypersecretion of CRF, which results in pituitary ACTH hypersecretion, which in turn contributes to adrenocortical glucocorticoid hypersecretion. In addition to its neuroendocrine role, CRF-containing circuits throughout the central nervous system are known to coordinate the behavioral, autonomic, and immune responses of mammals to stress. Within the hypothalamus, CRF-containing neurons that project from the paraventricular nucleus to the median eminence[76] control the secretion of ACTH and β-endorphin secretion from the anterior pituitary.[77] Extrahypothalamic CRF neurons are believed to play a preeminent role in the regulation of both affective and anxiety states. In fact, when injected directly into the central nervous system of laboratory animals, CRF produces many effects that are similar to the signs and symptoms of depression, eg, decreased appetite, decreased libido, and disrupted sleep.

Elevated CSF CRF concentrations in drug-free patients with major depression[78-82] and in depressed suicide victims[83] have been reported. The increase in CSF CRF concentrations that occurs during depression normalizes on recovery following treatment with electroconvulsive therapy[84] and antidepressants.[85] Persistently elevated CSF CRF concentrations may predict early relapse despite symptomatic improvement.[86] These elevations of CSF CRF concentrations are believed to be due to central CRF hypersecretion.[87] In normal volunteers, a reduction in CSF CRF concentrations occurs following treatment with the tricyclic antidepressant desipramine hydrochloride.[88]

One method to assess the activity of the HPA axis is by the use of the CRF stimulation test. Corticotropin-releasing factor is administered intravenously (usually in a 1-μg/kg dosage), and the ensuing ACTH (or β-endorphin) and cortisol response is measured over a 2- to 3-hour period.[89,90] In drug-free depressed patients, the ACTH and β-endorphin response to intravenously administered ovine CRF is blunted,[91-96] and this phenomenon has been shown to occur in depressed dexamethasone nonsuppressors (as explained below) but not in dexamethasone suppressors.[97]

Anatomical abnormalities associated with HPA axis dysfunction in depression, perhaps in part in response to hypersecretion of CRF, have been reported as well. Depressed patients demonstrate pituitary gland enlargement,[98] which significantly correlates with cortisol concentrations after dexamethasone administration,[99] another measure of HPA axis hyperactivity. Another morphologic change, enlargement of the adrenal gland, has been reported post mortem in suicide victims[100] and in depressed patients by the use of computed tomography.[101,102] This is most likely due to chronic ACTH hypersecretion. This adrenocortical hypertrophy may likely explain the fact that unlike the blunted ACTH and β-endorphin response to CRF, the plasma cortisol response is not different in depressed patients compared with normal controls.[91,94,95,103-105] Thus, for each release of ACTH, depressed patients with an enlarged adrenal cortex would be expected to secrete greater quantities of cortisol than would normal controls. Adrenocortical hypertrophy also could explain the heightened cortisol response to pharmacological doses of ACTH in depressed patients.[104,106-109]

The majority of the work on HPA axis activity in depression has used measures of cortisol hypersecretion, eg, elevated plasma corticosteroid concentrations[110,111] and increased levels of cortisol metabolites.[112] Thus, elevated 24-hour urinary free cortisol concentrations and nonsuppression of plasma hydroxycorticosteroid levels after the administration of dexamethasone (using the dexamethasone suppression test [DST]) have all been reported. Patients in the standard DST paradigm ingest 1 mg of dexamethasone, a synthetic glucocorticoid, by mouth at 11 PM. Blood samples for measurement of cortisol concentrations are obtained at 4 PM and 11 PM the next day. As reviewed by Schuckit,[113] one half to two thirds of depressed patients exhibit dexamethasone nonsuppression. Since Carroll's initial report[114] and subsequent claims for diagnostic utility,[115] the DST has generated considerable controversy.[116] The rate of cortisol nonsuppression after dexamethasone administration generally has been found to be correlated with the severity of the subtype of depression. Thus, nearly all patients with major depression with psychotic features exhibit dexamethasone nonsuppression.[117-120] Moreover, dexamethasone nonsuppressors have been found to have elevated CSF CRF concentrations and a blunted ACTH response to intravenously administered CRF (as explained above).[121,122] One factor that may contribute in part to dexamethasone nonsuppression is the more rapid metabolism of dexamethasone that occurs in depressed patients.[123] Therefore, the multitude of studies that report HPA hyperactivity in depressed patients could be explained by hypersecretion of CRF during and/or immediately preceding a depressive episode with secondary pituitary and adrenal gland hypertrophy and hypersecretion of ACTH and cortisol, respectively. The DST results usually normalize after recovery from depression[114,119] and may help predict early relapse.[119] Normalization of the DST results, like hypercortisolemia,[112] hypersecretion of CRF,[84] blunting of the ACTH response to CRF,[94] and adrenal gland hypertrophy,[124] appears to be state dependent.

ALTERATIONS OF THE HPA AXIS IN PATIENTS WITH CANCER

Of the three studies that have studied neuroendocrine dysfunction in patients with cancer,[27,41,75] all used the standard DST. Joffe et al[27] reported a 50% prevalence of major depression in patients with pancreatic cancer (n=9) compared with 11% in patients with gastric cancer (n=11). They also administered the DST to a subgroup of these patients (six patients with pancreatic cancer and six patients with gastric cancer). All six patients with pancreatic cancer exhibited dexamethasone nonsuppression even though only one of these six had a diagnosis of major depression. Interestingly, five of six patients with gastric cancer also exhibited dexamethasone nonsuppression when similarly tested; however, none of these six patients had a diagnosis of major depression. These findings remain difficult to interpret because of the small sample size, the absence of DST testing of the depressed patients with cancer, and the lack of dexamethasone plasma measurements in the study. Furthermore, because the DST data are so similar for the patients with pancreatic cancer and those with gastric cancer, the findings of nonsuppression in the pancreatic cancer group are less remarkable.

In our ongoing study, we are investigating not only the prevalence of depression in patients with cancer but also the underlying pathophysiologic processes of depression associated with cancer, with a focus on pancreatic cancer.[75] In comparison with other cancers, adenocarcinoma of the pancreas is associated with the highest rate of major depression (Table 1). Furthermore, case studies and clinical reports indicate that depressive symptoms in patients with pancreatic cancer may precede the onset of physical symptoms that typically are attributed to this cancer.[125] Indeed, in our study, three of five patients with pancreatic cancer reported a major depressive episode in the month prior to their diagnosis of cancer, whereas only one of 18 other patients with cancer (11 with breast cancer, six with esophageal cancer, and one with gastric cancer) reported such a phenomenon (P=.002).[75]

Furthermore, nonsuppression of plasma cortisol concentrations following dexamethasone administration occurred in two of the three patients with pancreatic cancer who were tested, whereas virtually all of the other patients with cancer (six of seven) exhibited dexamethasone suppression. As expected, the DST also discriminated between the normal controls (n=5) and the depressed controls (n=5), where all of the depressed controls exhibited DST nonsuppression in contrast to four of the five normal controls who exhibited suppression (P=.048).[75]

A large study of women with gynecological cancer (cervical, endometrial, or vaginal) was conducted by Evans and colleagues.[41] These investigators also were interested in the relationship between neuroendocrine dysfunction and depression in patients with cancer. In their study population (n=83), major depression was diagnosed in 19 (23%) of the women with cancer, and adjustment disorder with depressed mood was diagnosed in 20 (24%). Of the depressed cancer patients, eight (40%) exhibited dexamethasone nonsuppression. Interestingly, many of the women with a diagnosis of adjustment disorder with depressed mood also exhibited dexamethasone nonsuppression. These investigators[41] also conducted TRH stimulation tests on their cohort and observed a blunted thyrotropin response in six (29%) of those patients with a diagnosis of major depression and in nine (43%) of those patients who met criteria for adjustment disorder with depressed mood. These rates for DST nonsuppression and thyrotropin blunting are similar to the rates observed in depressed psychiatric inpatients without cancer. Our study[75] essentially confirms the findings of the studies of both Joffe et al[27] and Evans et al,[41] namely, that many patients with cancer exhibit a dysregulation of the HPA axis that is similar to that in depressed patients without cancer.

IMMUNE FUNCTION, DEPRESSION, AND CANCER

In recent years, a host of investigators have studied the relationship of stress and immune function, including studies assessing the influence of stress on immune function and its impact on the development and clinical outcome of cancer.[126] The plausibility of altered immune functions following exposure to stress is supported by studies that demonstrate innervation of primary and secondary immune organs,[127,128] interactions of multiple hormones with immunocyte function via hormone receptors of lymphoid cells,[129-132] and physiologic interactions between brain structures and immunological processes.[133,134]

Although laboratory animal studies have clearly documented the profound effects of stress on the immune system,[135,136] human studies have provided more conflicting data. The syndrome of depression is believed by many to be a psychological concomitant of stress, particularly stress related to the social loss and disruption seen in some patients with cancer.[137] Although numerous studies addressing the relationship of depression and immune function have appeared in the ARCHIVES in recent years,[138-143] this literature has been difficult to interpret because of complex methodological factors such as diagnostic heterogeneity, sample size, control group composition, assay techniques, and overlapping databases.[138] Furthermore, even though a recent meta-analysis[144] found substantial evidence for a relation between depression and immunity for both enumerative and functional measures of immune function, Stein et al[141] have documented the inherent complications in conducting a meta-analysis on a database with such methodologically varied studies. Although the underlying mechanism(s) of how depression has an impact on immune function and what patient subgroups are affected remain obscure, gender, age, and depression severity appear to be important variables.[139,141,143]

It also remains unclear how or whether in vitro stress-related immune alterations have a negative impact on health outcome and illness. However, recent research has illuminated psychosocial and immune interactions and outcomes in patients with cancer. One group of investigators[145] has measured natural killer (NK) cell activity (NKA) in a study of psychological factors that influence breast cancer outcomes. Using measurements of three distress indicators in women with breast cancer at the time of mastectomy and 3 months after, they found that adjustment level, lack of social support, fatigue, and depressive symptoms accounted for 30% of the NKA variance seen at 3 months. In this group, more metastatic nodes also were associated with depressive features and decreased NKA. In a subsequent study[146] that examined social support as a potential stress buffer related to NKA in patients with stage I and II breast cancer, these investigators found higher NKA could be consistently predicted by the perception of high-quality emotional support from a spouse or intimate other, perceived social support from the patient's physician, and the process of actively seeking social support as a major coping strategy.

Some investigators[147-154] have even addressed the impact of psychosocial stress and/or depression on cancer incidence and progression. Although not specifically examining immune function, seven longitudinal prospective investigations have made baseline psychological assessments of depression or depressive symptoms and then followed up the sample to examine cancer morbidity and/or mortality.[147-154] Cohort sizes have ranged from 1337[147] to 8932 subjects.[154] Although the concept of linking affective states to the onset of cancer remains controversial with conflicting study outcomes,[155] McGee and colleagues' meta-analysis[156] of these epidemiologic studies found a small but statistically significant association between depression and the later development of cancer. Such findings must be interpreted cautiously because of these studies' lack of specificity (eg, methodological differences in measurements of depression vs depressive symptoms, varying instruments, and the use of single cross-sectional measurements rather than multiple measurements over time). Moreover, the fact that the prevalence of certain behaviors such as tobacco and/or alcohol use may be increased in depressed individuals, a lack of exercise, and medical noncompliance also must be considered in evaluating studies for health outcome.[157]

In summary, numerous investigators have examined the effects of stress and depression on immune function; the most recent evidence indicates that gender, age, and symptom severity are important variables. Although the effects of stress and depression on health outcome and illness remain largely unexplored, social support appears to be an important factor in mitigating the effects of psychosocial stress and its associated immune dysfunction.[142,146] Finally, although epidemiologic studies of depressed subjects offer important information with regard to health outcome, they do not necessarily indicate a specific association between depression and immune-related morbidity and mortality.[158]

THE HPA AXIS AND IMMUNE DYSFUNCTION IN PATIENTS WITH CANCER

The long-held view that homeostatic mechanisms are integrated by the nervous and endocrine systems has been expanded by information that these systems also interact with the immune system.[159] Inhibition of neuroendocrine and immune function could conceivably influence the incidence or course of cancer by causing a loss of immune surveillance or by decreasing the production or function of tumor-rejecting NK cells.

Findings that link immune and neuroendocrine function provide explanations for the response of the HPA axis to such conditions as inflammation and infection as well as stress. Activation of the HPA axis, ie, CRF secretion, can be stimulated by elements of the immune system, which leads to glucocorticoid secretion, which results in immunosuppressive effects, including the reduction of circulating T-cell subsets.[160] In a series of elegant studies, investigators have shown that intracerebroventricular injection of CRF in rats reduces splenic and peripheral blood NKA, lymphocyte response to mitogenic stimulation, and percentage of splenic NK cell numbers.[161,162]

The activation of cytokines in the central nervous system can lead to profound changes in neural function. One such cytokine, interleukin-1, initiates a classic stress response by directly stimulating the release of hypothalamic CRF.[163] Similarly, interleukin-2, a cytokine produced mainly by T helper cells, has profound activating effects on the HPA axis.[161] Interleukin-2 activation of the HPA cascade was originally demonstrated in a preliminary report of 30 patients with cancer who received immunotherapy with interleukin-2.[164]

Whether through stress-induced (eg, infectious challenge) cytokine release or via CRF hypersecretion associated with depression, HPA hyperactivity in patients with cancer may exert untoward effects on immunological function. The diminished NKA linked to intracerebroventricular CRF administration may play a role in understanding the possible immunosuppressive influence of the HPA axis in patients with cancer. Particularly relevant to the present discussion is the observation that HPA hyperactivity induced by exposure to stress is associated with increased tumor growth in rats, particularly in the aged.[165]

Studies that examine in vitro immune changes linked to HPA dysregulation may offer important information about the possible in vivo interactions of the nervous, endocrine, and immune systems, particularly in depressed patients with cancer. The findings of Levy and colleagues[145] that psychosocial variables such as lack of social support and depressive symptoms may be linked to reduced NKA in women with breast cancer clearly illuminate the need for more research in the area, including research on neuroendocrine and immune measures in patients with cancer. From a psychoneuroimmune and endocrine standpoint, such studies may clarify the finding of Levy et al[146] that more metastatic nodes and decreased NKA were associated with depressive symptoms in their patients with breast cancer and the finding of Sapolsky and Donnelly[165] that stress-induced HPA hyperactivity is associated with increased tumor growth.

TREATMENT OF DEPRESSION IN PATIENTS WITH CANCER

Alterations in immune function in patients with cancer are of particular interest because of the potential immunoprotective effect of psychobiological interventions in patients with cancer. Spiegel et al[53] demonstrated that women with metastatic breast cancer who received weekly group psychotherapy survived an average of 18 months longer than did control patients who were randomly assigned to routine care. Richardson et al[54] reported that patients with lymphomas and leukemias who received educational in-home supportive interventions had significantly longer survival times than did patients who did not receive these interventions. Similarly, Fawzy and colleagues[55] recently evaluated recurrence in and survival of patients with malignant melanoma. For control patients who did not receive group psychotherapy, there was a statistically significant recurrence of cancer and a greater mortality rate than for patients who did receive such therapy. The patients with cancer who did receive group therapy exhibited a significant increase in the number of large granular lymphocytes and NK cells as well as indications of increased NKA.[56] Baseline NKA predicted recurrence, although the 6-month level of NKA was not predictive. This improvement in immune function persisted with significant effects 6 months following termination of the group intervention; however, the increased NKA no longer attained statistical significance at the 1-year interval. In their 18-month study of behavioral interventions (relaxation, guided imagery, and biofeedback training) in patients with stage I breast cancer, Gruber et al[57] compared immune functioning in a treatment group with that in a waiting-list control group. They found statistically significant increases in NKA, lymphocyte mitogen response, and the number of peripheral blood lymphocytes in their treatment intervention group compared with controls.

Only two research teams have investigated antidepressant drug treatment of patients with cancer in controlled studies. Costa et al[50] conducted a randomized placebo-controlled trial of mianserin hydrochloride in depressed women with cancer and found a significant treatment response with regard to both reducing the severity of depressive symptoms and improving the patients' perceived quality of life. Evans and colleagues[51] demonstrated similar results in a study of depressed patients with gynecological cancer who were treated with imipramine hydrochloride. Both a significant reduction in the Hamilton Rating Scale for Depression scores and a perceived improved quality of life were observed in the patients who received adequate doses of the tricyclic antidepressant. Unfortunately, measurements of HPA axis activity and immune function were not investigated in either study.

With the introduction of selective 5-HT reuptake inhibitors, more medically ill patients are apt to be treated without fear of complicating side effects. Because of the low affinity of 5-HT reuptake inhibitors to other neurotransmitter receptors, they diminish previously serious complications in patients with cancer that are attributed to anticholinergic, antihistaminic, antiadrenergic, sedative, and hypotensive side effects. Because of fewer potential side effects and the lack of lethality of an overdose, these agents offer significant advantages in depressed patients with cancer. Because these agents are newer than tricyclics, little systematic research on their efficacy in patients with cancer has been performed. However, our research group recently has begun a randomized, double-blind, multicenter study of paroxetine vs desipramine and placebo in patients with breast cancer (stage II, III, or IV) and major depression or adjustment disorder with depressed mood to compare efficacy and side-effect profiles in the three groups. Further studies clearly are indicated to establish safe, effective, and well-tolerated pharmacologic treatment approaches for patients with cancer and comorbid depression.

COMMENT

Three decades of research on biological alterations in unipolar depression have led to the discovery of so-called biological markers, measures that presumably reflect the underlying pathophysiologic processes of this disorder. Of all of these, none has been as intensively studied or as well characterized as the HPA axis hyperactivity in depression. Specifically, elevated CSF concentrations of CRF, a blunted ACTH response to CRF, and dexamethasone nonsuppression characterize the HPA axis hyperactivity associated with this illness. The HPA axis hyperactivity can be induced through cytokine secretion and may impair immune function. In response to stress, cytokine-mediated hypothalamic CRF secretion may induce major depression in patients with and without cancer. Hypersecretion of CRF in depressed patients (without cancer) appears to normalize following treatment with antidepressants[85] or electroconvulsive therapy.[84] Antidepressant treatment not only alleviates the signs and symptoms of unipolar depression, such as abnormal sleep, but these drugs also diminish perceived levels of pain in patients with cancer. Future investigations will determine whether normalization of HPA axis activity in patients with cancer via somatic (antidepressant or electroconvulsive therapy) treatment is associated with a bolstered immune response (eg, increasing NK cell cytotoxicity and decreasing overall tumor burden) and a normalization of HPA axis activity. Future researchers must consider the importance of using standardized methods of diagnosis (with structured interviews) and assessing the effects of age, gender, hospitalization status, tumor site, grade, stage, time since knowledge of diagnosis, pain, psychiatric history, vulnerability to mood disorders, and measures of immune status on their outcome measures.

The application of other biological markers of depression in depressed patients with comorbid medical illness, including cancer, deserves further study. Many of the current biological markers are certainly worthy of study. It is remarkable, for example, that there are no studies of platelet 5-HT transporter binding or volumetric brain magnetic resonance imaging measures in depressed patients with cancer. It is, of course, important to determine that neuroendocrine or neurochemical alterations in depressed patients with cancer are due to the depression per se and not an epiphenomenon of a single symptom, eg, pain. Moreover, it is important to determine that biological alterations in depressed patients are not secondary to altered metabolism, as for example, an increased metabolism of dexamethasone, resulting in dexamethasone nonsuppression. Illumination of the interplay between neuroendocrine and immunological processes, particularly in those patients with cancer and major depression, will undoubtedly lead to the development of new treatment modalities that will not only improve these patients' quality of life but potentially decrease their morbidity and improve long-term survival rates.

Accepted for publication November 1, 1994.

Supported by grant NIMH-1-RO1-MH49523-01 from the National Institute of Mental Health, Bethesda, Md.

Reprint requests to Department of Psychiatry and Behavioral Sciences, Emory University School of Medicine, 1639 Pierce Dr, Suite 4000, Atlanta, GA 30322 (Dr Nemeroff).

REFERENCES

1. Katon W, Sullivan MD. Depression and chronic medical illness. *J Clin Psychiatry.* 1990;51 (suppl 6):3-11.
2. Hoeper EW, Nycz GR, Cleary PD. Estimated prevalence of RDC mental disorders in primary care. *Int J Ment Health.* 1979;8:6-15.

3. Leeper J, Badger L, Milo T. Mental disorders among physical disability determination patients. *Am J Public Health.* 1985;75:78-79.
4. Schulberg HC, Saul M, McClelland M, Ganguli M, Christy W, Frank R. Assessing depression in primary medical and psychiatric practices. *Arch Gen Psychiatry.* 1985;42:1164-1170.
5. Blacker CVR, Clare AW. Depressive disorder in primary care. *Br J Psychiatry.* 1987;150:737-751.
6. Barret JE, Barret JA, Oxman TE, Gerber PD. The prevalence of psychiatric disorders in a primary care practice. *Arch Gen Psychiatry.* 1988; 45:1100-1106.
7. Von Korff M, Shapiro S, Burke JD, Teitlebaum M, Skinner EA, German P, Turner RW, Klein L, Burns B. Anxiety and depression in a primary care clinic: comparison of Diagnostic Interview Schedule, General Health Questionnaire, and practitioner assessments. *Arch Gen Psychiatry.* 1987;44:152-156.
8. Magni G, Schifano F, deLeo D. Assessment of depression in an elderly medical population. *J Affect Disord.* 1986;11:121-124.
9. Feldman E, Mayou R, Hawton K, Ardern M, Smith EB. Psychiatric disorder in medical inpatients. *Q J Med.* 1987;63:405-412.
10. Gregory RJ, Jimerson DC, Walton BE, Daley J, Paulsen RH. Pharmacotherapy of depression in the medically ill: directions for future research. *Gen Hosp Psychiatry.* 1992;14:36-42.
11. Neilsen AC, Williams TA. Depression in ambulatory medical patients: prevalence by self-report questionnaire and recognition by non-psychiatric physicians. *Arch Gen Psychiatry.* 1980;37:999-1004.
12. Wells KB, Hays RD, Burnam MA, Rogers W, Greenfield S, Ware JE. Detection of depressive disorder for patients receiving prepaid or fee-for-service care: results from the medical outcomes study. *JAMA.* 1989;262:3298-3302.
13. Abram HS, Moore GL, Westervelt FB. Suicidal behavior in chronic dialysis patients. *Am J Psychiatry.* 1971;127:1199-1204.
14. Hawton K. The long-term outcome of psychiatric morbidity detected in general medical patients. *J Psychosom Res.* 1981;25:237-243.
15. Rodin GM, Chmara J, Ennis J. Stopping life-sustaining medical treatment: psychiatric considerations in the termination of renal dialysis. *Can J Psychiatry.* 1981;26:540-544.
16. Murphy E, Smith R, Slatter J. Increased mortality rates in late-life depression. *Br J Psychiatry.* 1988;152:347-353.
17. Koenig HG, Shelp F, Goli V, Cohen HJ, Blazer DG. Survival and healthcare utilization in elderly medical inpatients with major depression. *J Am Geriatr Soc.* 1989;37:599-606.
18. Stoudemire A, Thompson TL. Medication noncompliance: systematic approaches to evaluation and intervention. *Gen Hosp Psychiatry.* 1983; 5:233-239.
19. Koenig HG, Cohen HJ, Blazer DG, Meador KG, Westlund R. A brief depression scale for use in the medically ill. *Int J Psychiatry Med.* 1992; 22:183-195.
20. Stewart MA, Drake W, Winokur G. Depression among medically ill patients. *Dis Nerv Syst.* 1968; 115:1365-1369.
21. Moffic HS, Paykel ES. Depression in medical inpatients. *Br J Psychiatry.* 1975;126:346-353.
22. Cavanaugh SA. The prevalence of emotional and cognitive dysfunction in a general medical population: using the MMSE, GHQ, and BDI. *Gen Hosp Psychiatry.* 1983;5:15-24.
23. Berkman LF, Berkman CS, Kasl S, Freeman DH Jr, Ostfeld AM, Cornoni-Huntley J, Brody JA. Depressive symptoms in relation to physical health and functioning in the elderly. *Am J Epidemiol.* 1986;124:372-388.
24. Mermelstein HT, Lesko L. Depression in patients with cancer. *Psycho-oncology.* 1992;1: 199-215.
25. McDaniel JS, Nemeroff CB. Depression in the cancer patient: diagnostic, biological and treatment aspects. In: Chapman CR, Foley KM, eds. *Current and Emerging Issues in Cancer Pain.* New York, NY: Raven Press; 1993:1-19.
26. Fras I, Litin EM, Pearson JS. Comparison of psychiatric symptoms in carcinoma of the pancreas with those in some other intra-abdominal neoplasms. *Am J Psychiatry.* 1967; 123:1553-1562.
27. Joffe RT, Rubinow DR, Denicoff KD, Maher M, Sindelar WF. Depression and carcinoma of the pancreas. *Gen Hosp Psychiatry.* 1986;8:241-245.
28. Morton RP, Davies ADM, Baker J, Baker GA, Stell PM. Quality of life in treated head and neck cancer patients: a preliminary report. *Clin Otolarnygol.* 1984;9:181-185.
29. Davies ADM, Davies C, Delpo MC. Depression and anxiety in patients undergoing diagnostic investigations for head and neck cancers. *Br J Psychiatry.* 1986;149:491-493.
30. Baile WF, Bilbertini M, Scott L, Endicott J. Depression and tumor stage in cancer of the head and neck. *Psycho-oncology.* 1992;1:15-24.
31. Maguire GP, Lee EG, Bevington DJ, Kuchemann CS, Crabtree RJ, Cornell CE. Psychiatric problems in the first year after mastectomy. *Br Med J.* 1978;1:963-965.
32. Silberfarb PM, Maurer LH, Crouthamel CS. Psychological aspects of neoplastic disease, I: functional status of breast cancer patients during different treatment regimens. *Am J Psychiatry.* 1980;137:450-455.
33. Farber JM, Weinerman BH, Kuypers JA. Psychosocial distress in oncology outpatients. *J Psychosoc Oncol.* 1984;2:109-118.
34. Grandi S, Fava GA, Cunsolo A, Ranieri G, Gozzetti G, Trombini G. Major depression associated with mastectomy. *Med Sci Res.* 1987;15:283-284.
35. Fallowfield LJ, Hall A, Maguire GP, Baum M. Psychological outcomes of different treatment policies in women with early breast cancer outside of a clinical trial. *Br Med J.* 1990;301:575-580.
36. Hopwood P, Howell A, Maguire P. Screening for psychiatric morbidity in patients with advanced breast cancer: validation of two self-report questionnaires. *Br J Cancer.* 1991;64: 353-356.
37. Hopwood P, Howell A, Maguire P. Psychiatric morbidity in patients with advanced cancer of the breast: prevalence measured by two self-ratient questionnaires. *Br J Cancer.* 1991;64: 349-352.
38. Goldberg JA, Scott RN, Davidson PM. Psychological morbidity in the first year after breast surgery. *Eur J Surg Oncol.* 1992;18:327-331.
39. Pinder KL, Ramirez M, Black E, Richards MA, Gregory WM, Rubens RD. Psychiatric disorder in patients with advanced breast cancer: prevalence and associated features. *Eur J Cancer.* 1993;29(suppl A):524-527.
40. Koenig R, Levin SM, Brennan MT. The emotional status of cancer patients as measured by a psychological test. *J Chronic Dis.* 1967;20: 923-930.
41. Evans DL, McCartney CF, Nemeroff CB, Raft D, Quade D, Golden RN, Haggerty JJ, Holmes V, Simon JS, Droba M, Mason GA, Fowler WC. Depression in women treated for gynecological cancer: clinical and neuroendocrine assessment. *Am J Psychiatry.* 1986;143:447-452.
42. Devlen J, Maguire P, Phillips P, Crowther D, Chamblers H. Psychological problems associated with diagnosis and treatment of lymphomas, I: retrospective study. *Br Med J.* 1987; 295:953-954.
43. Colon EA, Callies AL, Popkin MK, McGlave PB. Depressed mood and other variables related to bone marrow transplantation survival in acute leukemia. *Psychosomatics.* 1991;32:420-425.
44. Plumb M, Holland J. Comparative studies of psychological function in patients with advanced cancer, II: interviewer-rated current and past psychological symptoms. *Psychosom Med.* 1981;43:243-254.
45. Bukberg J, Penman D, Holland JC. Depression in hospitalized cancer patients. *Psychosom Med.* 1984;46:199-212.
46. Stefanek ME, Derogatis LP, Shaw A. Psychological distress among oncology outpatients. *Psychosomatics.* 1987;28:530-539.
47. Kathol RG, Mutgi A, Williams J, Clamon G, Noyes R. Diagnosis of major depression in cancer patients according to four sets of criteria. *Am J Psychiatry.* 1990;147:1021-1024.
48. Razavi D, Delvaux N, Bredart A, Paesmans M, Debusscher L, Bron D, Stryckmans P. Screening for psychiatric disorders in lymphoma outpatient population. *Eur J Cancer.* 1992;28 (suppl A):1869-1872.
49. American Psychiatric Association. *Diagnostic and Statistical Manual of Mental Disorders, Fourth Edition.* Washington, DC: American Psychiatric Association; 1994.
50. Costa E, Mogos I, Toma T. Efficacy and safety of mianserin in the treatment of depression of women with cancer. *Acta Psychiatr Scand.* 1985; 72:85-92.
51. Evans DL, McCartney CF, Haggerty JJ. Treatment of depression in cancer patients is associated with better life adaptation: a pilot study. *Psychosom Med.* 1988;50:72-76.
52. Trijsburg RW, Van Knippenberg FCE, Rijpma SE. Effects of psychological treatments on cancer patients: a critical review. *Psychosom Med.* 1992;54:489-517.
53. Spiegel D, Bloom JR, Kraemer HC, Gottheil E. Effect of psychosocial treatment on survival of patients with metastatic breast cancer. *Lancet.* 1989;2:888-891.
54. Richardson J, Sheldon D, Krailo M, Levine A. The effect of compliance with treatment on survival among patients with hematologic malignancies. *J Clin Oncol.* 1990;8:356-364.
55. Fawzy FI, Fawzy NW, Hyun CS, Elashoff R, Guthrie D, Fahey JL, Morton DL. Malignant melanoma: effects of an early structured psychiatric intervention, coping, and affective state on recurrence and survival 6 years later. *Arch Gen Psychiatry.* 1993;50:681-689.
56. Fawzy FI, Kemeny ME, Fawzy NW, Elashoff R, Morton D, Cousins N, Fahey JL. A structured psychiatric intervention for cancer patients, II: changes over time in immunological measures. *Arch Gen Psychiatry.* 1990;47:729-735.
57. Gruber BL, Hersh SP, Hall NRS, Waletzky LR, Kunz JF, Carpenter JK, Kverno KS, Weiss SM. Immunological responses of breast cancer patients to behavioral interventions. *Biofeedback Self Regul.* 1993;18:1-22.
58. Cassileth BR, Lusk EJ, Brown LL, Cross PA, Walsh WP, Hurwitz S. Factors assocaited with psychological distress in cancer patients. *Med Pediatr Oncol.* 1986;14:251-254.
59. Noyes R, Kathol RG, Debelius-Enemark P, Williams J, Mutgi A, Suelzer MT, Clamon GH. Distress associated with cancer as measured by the Illness Distress Scale. *Psychosomatics.* 1990; 31:321-330.
60. Cassileth BR, Lusk EJ, Strouse TB, Strouse TB, Miller DS, Brown LL, Cross PA, Tenaglia AN. Psychosocial status in chronic illness: a comparative analysis of six diagnostic groups. *N Engl J Med.* 1984;311:506-511.
61. Noyes R, Kathol RG. Depression and cancer. *Psychiatr Dev.* 1986;2:77-100.
62. Rodin G, Voshart K. Depression in the medically ill: an overview. *Am J Psychiatry.* 1986; 143:696-705.
63. Weissman A, Worden J. The existential plight in cancer: significance of the first 100 days. *Psychiatr Med.* 1976;7:1-15.
64. Massie MJ, Holland JC. The cancer patient with pain. *Med Clin North Am.* 1987;71:243-258.
65. Holland JC, Korzun AH, Tross S, Silberfarb P, Perry M, Cosmis R, Oster M. Comparative psychological disturbance in patients with pancreatic and gastric cancer. *Am J Psychiatry.* 1986; 143:982-986.

66. Breitbart W. Suicide risk and pain in cancer and AIDS patients. In: Chapman CR, Foley KM, eds. *Current and Emerging Issues in Cancer Pain.* New York, NY: Raven Press; 1993:1-19.
67. Bolund C. Suicide and cancer, II: medical and care factors in suicide by cancer patients in Sweden, 1973-1976. *J Psychosoc Oncol.* 1985;3: 17-30.
68. Fox BH, Stanek EJ, Boyd SC, Flannery JT. Suicide rates among cancer patients in Connecticut. *J Chronic Dis.* 1982;35:85-100.
69. Louhivuori KA, Hakama J. Risk of suicide among cancer patients. *Am J Epidemiol.* 1979;109:59-65.
70. Lesko L, Massie M, Holland J. Oncology. In: Stoudemire A, Fogel B, eds. *Psychiartic Care of the Medical Patient.* New York, NY: Oxford University Press; 1993:565-590.
71. Kathol RG, Noyes R, Williams J, Mutgi A, Carroll B, Perry P. Diagnosing depression in patients with medical illness. *Psychosomatics.* 1990;31:434-440.
72. Cohen-Cole SA, Brown FW, McDaniel JS. Diagnostic assessment of depression in the medically ill. In: Stoudemire A, Fogel B, eds. *Psychiatric Care of the Medical Patient,* New York, NY: Oxford University Press; 1993:53-70.
73. Quitkin FM, Stewart JW, Morison AW. Antidepressants for mild depressives. Presented at the 143rd Annual Meeting of American Psychiatric Association; May 23, 1990; New York, NY.
74. Ribeiro SCM, Tandon R, Grunhaus L, Greden JF. The DST as a predictor of outcome in depression: a meta-analysis. *Am J Psychiatry.* 1993; 150:1618-1629.
75. Musselman DL, Nemeroff CB, McDaniel JS, Reed D, Wingard J, Seelig B, Porter MF, Landry JC. Cancer and depression: diagnostic considerations and biologic markers. Presented at the 32nd Annual Meeting of the American College of Neuropsychopharmacology; December 14, 1993; Honolulu, Hawaii.
76. Swanson LW, Sawchenko PE, Rivier J, Vale W. Organization of ovine corticotropin-releasing factor immunoreactive cells and fibers in the rat brain: an immunohistochemical study. *Neuroendocrinology.* 1983;36:165-186.
77. Vale W, Spiess J, Rivier C, Rivier J. Characterization of a 41-residue ovine hypothalamic peptide that stimulates secretion of corticotropin of β-endorphin. *Science.* 1981;213:1394-1397.
78. Nemeroff CB, Evans DL. Correlation between the dexamethasone suppression test in depressed patients and clinical response. *Am J Psychiatry.* 1984;141:247-249.
79. Arato M, Banki CM, Nemeroff CB, Bissette B. Hypothalamic-pituitary-adrenal axis and suicide. *Ann N Y Acad Sci.* 1986;487:263-270.
80. Banki CM, Bissette G, Arato M, O'Connor L, Nemeroff CB. Cerebrospinal fluid corticotropin-releasing factor–like immunoreactivity in depression and schizophrenia. *Am J Psychiatry.* 1987;144:873-877.
81. France RD, Urban B, Krishnan KRR, Bissette G, Banki CM, Nemeroff CB, Spielman FJ. CSF corticotropin-releasing factor–like immunoreactivity in chronic pain patients with and without major depression. *Biol Psychiatry.* 1988; 23:86-88.
82. Risch SC, Lewine RJ, Kalin NH, Jewart RD, Risby ED, Caudle JM, Stipetic M, Turner J, Eccard MB, Pollard WE. Limbic-hypothalamic-pituitary-adrenal axis activity and ventricular-to-brain ratio studies in affective illness and schizophrenia. *Neuropsychopharmacology.* 1992;6:95-100.
83. Arato M, Banki CM, Bissette G, Nemeroff CB. Elevated CSF CRF in suicide victims. *Biol Psychiatry.* 1989;25:355-359.
84. Nemeroff CB, Bissette G, Akil H, Fin M. Neuropeptide concentrations in the cerebrospinal fluid of depressed patients treated with electroconvulsive therapy: corticotropin-releasing factor, beta-endorphin and somatostatin. *Br J Psychiatry.* 1991;158:59-63.
85. DeBellis MD, Gold PW, Geracioti TD, Listwak S, Kling MA. Fluoxetine significantly reduces CSF CRH and AVP concentrations in patients with major depression. *Am J Psychiatry.* 1993;150: 656-657.
86. Banki CB, Karmacsi L, Bissette G, Nemeroff CB. CSF corticotropin-releasing hormone and somatostatin in major depression: response to antidepressant treatment and relapse. *Eur Neuropsychopharmacol.* 1992;2:107-113.
87. Post RM, Gold P, Rubinow DR, Ballenger JC, Bunney WE, Goodwin FK. Peptides in cerebrospinal fluid of neuropsychiatric patients: an approach to central nervous system peptide function. *Life Sci.* 1982;31:1-15.
88. Veith RC, Lewis N, Langohr JI, Murburg MM, Ashleigle EA, Castillo S, Peskind ER, Pascialy M, Bissette G, Nemeroff CB, Raskind J. Effect of desipramine on cerebrospinal fluid concentrations of corticotropin-releasing factor in human subjects. *Psychiatry Res.* 1992;46:1-8.
89. Hermus AR, Pieters GF, Pesman GJ, Buys WC, Smals AG. Differential effects of ovine and human corticotropin-releasing factor in human subjects. *Clin Endocrinol (Oxf).* 1984;21:589-595.
90. Watson SJ, Lopez JF, Young EA, Vale W, Rivier J, Akil H. Effects of low-dose ovine corticotropin-releasing hormone in humans: endocrine relationships and beta-endorphin/beta-lipotropin responses. *J Clin Endocrinol Metab.* 1986;66: 10-15.
91. Gold PW, Chrousos GP, Kellner C, Post RM, Roy A, Augerinas P, Schulte H, Oldfield EH, Loriaux DL. Psychiatric implications of basic and clinical studies with corticotropin-releasing factor. *Am J Psychiatry.* 1984;141:619-627.
92. Gold PW, Loriaux DL, Roy A, Kling MA, Calabrese JR, Kellner CH, Nieman LK, Post RM, Pickar D, Gallucci W, Augerinos P, Paul S, Oldfield EH, Cutler GB, Chrousos GP. Responses to corticotropin-releasing hormone in the hypercortisolism of depression and Cushing's disease. *N Engl J Med.* 1986;314:1329-1334.
93. Holsboer F, Von Bardeleben U, Gerken A, Muler D. Blunted corticotropin and normal cortisol response to human corticotropin-releasing factor in depression. *N Engl J Med.* 1984;311: 1127.
94. Amsterdam JD, Maislin G, Winokur A, Berwish N, Kling M, Gold P. The oCRH test before and after clinical recovery from depression. *J Affect Disord.* 1988;14:213-222.
95. Kathol RG, Jaeckle RS, Lopez JR, Mullter WH. Consistent reduction of ACTH responses to stimulation with CRH, vasopressin and hypoglycaemia in patients with depression. *Br J Psychiatry.* 1989;155:468-478.
96. Young EA, Watson SJ, Kotun J, Haskett RF, Grunhaus L, Murphy-Weinberg V, Vale W, Rivier J, Akil H. β-lipotropin–β-endorphin response to low-dose ovine corticotropin releasing factor in endogenous depression. *Arch Gen Psychiatry.* 1990;47:449-457.
97. Krishnan KKR, Rayasam K, Reed D, Smith M, Clieppell P, Saunders WB, Richie JC, Carroll BJ, Nemeroff CB. The CRF corticotropin-releasing factor stimulation test in patients with major depression: relationship to dexamethasone suppression test results. *Depression.* 1993;1:133-136.
98. Krishnan KRR, Doraiswamy PM, Lurie SN, Figiel GS, Husain MM, Boyko OH, Ellinwood EH Jr, Nemeroff CB. Pituitary size in depression. *J Clin Endocrinol Metab.* 1991;72:256-259.
99. Axelson DA, Doraiswamy PM, Boyko OB, Escalona PR, McDonald WM, Ritchie JC, Ellinwood EH, Nemeroff CB, Krishnan KRR. In vivo assessment of pituitary volume using MRI and systematic sterology: relationship to dexamethasone suppression test results in patients with affective disorder. *Psychiatry Res.* 1992;46:63-70.
100. Zis KD, Zis A. Increased adrenal weight in victims of violent suicide. *Am J Psychiatry.* 1987; 144:1214-1215.
101. Amsterdam JD, Marinelli DL, Arger P, Winokur A. Assessment of adrenal gland volume by computed tomography in depressed patients and healthy volunteers: a pilot study. *Psychiatry Res.* 1987;21:189-197.
102. Nemeroff CB, Krishnan KKR, Reed D, Leder R, Beam C, Dunnick NR. Adrenal gland enlargement in major depression: a computed tomographic study. *Arch Gen Psychiatry.* 1992;49: 384-387.
103. Gold PW, Loriaux DL, Roy A, Kling MA, Calabrese JR, Kellner CH, Nieman LK, Post RM, Pickar D, Gallucci W, Augerinos P, Paul S, Oldfield EH, Cutler GB, Chrousos GP. Responses to corticotropin-releasing hormone in the hypercortisolism of depression and Cushing's disease. *N Engl J Med.* 1986;314:1329-1334.
104. Holsboer F, Haack D, Gerken A, Vecoci P. Plasma dexamethasone concentrations and different suppression response of cortisol and corticosterone in depressives and controls. *Biol Psychiatry.* 1984;19:281-291.
105. Amsterdam JD, Winokur A, Abelman E, Irwin L, Rickels K. Cosyntropin (ACTH) stimulation test in depressed patients and healthy subjects. *Am J Psychiatry.* 1983;140:907.
106. Kalin NH, Risch SC, Janowsky DS, Murphy DL. Plasma ACTH and cortisol concentrations before and after dexamethasone. *Psychiatry Res.* 1982;7:87-92.
107. Linkowski P, Mendlewicz J, LeClerq R, Brasseur M, Hubain P, Goldstein J, Copinschi G, Lauter EV. The 24-hour profile of ACTH and cortisol in major depressive illness. *J Clin Endocrinol Metab.* 1985;61:429-438.
108. Jaeckle RS, Kathol RG, Lopez JF, Meller WH, Krummel SJ. Enhanced adrenal sensitivity to exogenous ACTH stimulation in major depression. *Arch Gen Psychiatry.* 1987;44:233-240.
109. Krishnan KRR, Ritchie JC, Saunders WB, Nemeroff CB, Carroll BJ. Adrenocortical sensitivity to low-dose ACTH administration in depressed patients. *Biol Psychiatry.* 1990;27:930-933.
110. Gibbons JL, McHugh PR. Plasma cortisol in depressive illness. *J Psychiatr Res.* 1962;1:162-171.
111. Carpenter W, Bunney W. Adrenal cortical activity in depressive illness. *Am J Psychiatry.* 1971; 128:31-40.
112. Sachar E, Hellman L, Fukushima D, Gallagher T. Cortisol production in depressive illness. *Arch Gen Psychiatry.* 1970;23:289-298.
113. Schuckit MA. Trait (and state) markers of a predisposition to psychopathology. In: Michels R, Cavenar JO, Cooper AM, Guze SM, Judd LL, Klerman GL, Solnit AJ, eds. *Psychiatry.* Philadelphia, Pa: JB Lippincott Co; 1988;53:1-19.
114. Carroll BJ. Pituitary-adrenal function in depression. *Lancet.* 1968;556:1373-1374.
115. Carroll BJ. Use of the dexamethasone test in depression. *J Clin Psychiatry.* 1982;43:44-50.
116. Arana GW, Mossman D. The DST and depression: approaches to the use of a laboratory test in psychiatry. *Neurol Clin.* 1988;6:21-39.
117. Evans DL, Nemeroff CB. Use of dexamethasone suppression test using *DSM-III* criteria on an inpatient psychiatric unit. *Biol Psychiatry.* 1983;18:505-511.
118. Schatzberg AF, Rothschild AJ, Bond TC, Cole JO. The DST in psychotic depression: diagnostic and pathophysiologic implications. *Psychopharmacol Bull.* 1984;20:362-364.
119. Arana GW, Baldesarrini RJ, Ornsteen M. The dexamethasone suppression test for diagnosis and prognosis in psychiatry. *Arch Gen Psychiatry.* 1985;42:1193-204.
120. Krishnan KRR, France RD, Pelton S, McCann UD, Manepalli An, Davidson JR. What does the dexamethasone suppression test identify? *Biol Psychiatry.* 1985;20:957-964.
121. Roy A, Pickar D, Paul S, Doran A, Chrousos GP, Gold PW. CSF corticotropin-releasing hormone in depressed patients and normal control subjects. *Am J Psychiatry.* 1987;144:641-645.

122. Pitts AF, Kathol RG, Gehris TL, Samuelson SD, Carroll BT, Mehter WH, Carter J, Nemeroff CB, Bissette G. Elevated cerebrospinal fluid corticotropin-releasing hormone and arginine vasopressin in depressed patients with dexamethasone nonsuppression. *Soc Neurosci Abstr.* 1990;16:454. Abstract.
123. Ritchie JC, Belkin BM, Krishnan KRR, Nemeroff CB, Carroll BJ. Plasma dexamethasone concentrations and the dexamethasone suppression test. *Biol Psychiatry.* 1990;27:159-173.
124. Rubin RT, Phillips JJ, Sadow TF, McCracken JT. Adrenal gland volume in major depression: increase during the depressive episode and decrease with successful treatment. Presented at the 31st Annual Meeting of the American College of Neuropsychopharmacology; December 14, 1992; San Juan, Puerto Rico.
125. Green AI, Austin CP. Psychopathology of pancreatic cancer: a psychobiological probe. *Psychosomatics.* 1993;34:208-221.
126. Schulz KH, Schulz H. Overview of psychoneuroimmunological stress and intervention studies in humans with emphasis on the uses of immunological parameters. *Psycho-oncology.* 1992;1:51-70.
127. Bulloch K. Neuroanatomy of lymphoid tissue: a review. In: Guillemin R, Cohn M, Melnechuk T, eds. *Neural Modulation of Immunity.* New York, NY: Raven Press; 1985:111-141.
128. Felten DL, Felten SY, Bellinger DL, Carlson SL, Ackerman KD, Madden KS, Olschowki JA, Livnat S. Noradrenergic sympathetic neural interactions with the immune system: structure and function. *Immunol Rev.* 1987;100:225-260.
129. Plaut M. Lymphocyte hormone receptors. *Annu Rev Immunol.* 1987;5:621-669.
130. Kiess W, Hall N. Hormone im Immun-system. In: Hesch RD, ed. *Endokrinologie: Teil a Grundlagen: Innere Medizin der Gegenwart.* Munich, Germany: Urban & Schwarzernberg; 1989:346-360.
131. Blalock JE, Harbour-McMenamin D, Smith EM. Peptide hormones shared by the neuroendocrine and immunologic systems. *J Immunol.* 1985;135(suppl):858S-861S.
132. Bost KL. Hormone and neuropeptide receptors on mononuclear leukocytes. *Prog Allergy.* 1988;43:68-83.
133. Besedovsky HO, Sorkin E, Felix R, Haas H. Hypothalamic changes during the immune response. *Eur J Immunol.* 1977;7:325-328.
134. Neveu PJ. Cerebral neocortex modulation of immune functions. *Life Sci.* 1988;42:1917-1923.
135. Weiss JM, Sundar S. Effects of stress on cellular immune responses in animals. In: Tasman A, Riba MB, eds. *American Psychiatric Press Review of Psychiatry.* Washington, DC: American Psychiatric Press; 1992;11:145-168.
136. Coe CL. Psychosocial factors and immunity in nonhuman primates: a review. *Psychosom Med.* 1993;55:298-308.
137. O'Leary A. Stress, emotion, and human immune function. *Psychol Bull.* 1990;108:363-382.
138. Schleifer SJ, Keller SE, Meyerson AT, Raskin MJ, Davis KL, Stein M. Lymphocyte function in major depressive disorder. *Arch Gen Psychiatry.* 1984;41:484-486.
139. Schleifer SJ, Keller SE, Siris SG, Davis KL, Stein M. Depression and immunity. *Arch Gen Psychiatry.* 1985;42:129-133.
140. Schleifer SJ, Keller SE, Bond RN, Cohen J, Stein M. Major depressive disorder and immunity: role of age, sex, severity, and hospitalization. *Arch Gen Psychiatry.* 1989;46:81-87.
141. Stein M, Miller AH, Trestman RL. Depression, the immune system, and health and illness. *Arch Gen Psychiatry.* 1991;48:171-177.
142. Rabkin JG, Williams JB, Remien RH, Goetz R, Kertzner R, Gorman JM. Depression, distress, lymphocyte subsets, and human immunodeficiency virus symptoms on two occasions in HIV-positive homosexual men. *Arch Gen Psychiatry.* 1991;48:111-119.
143. Evans DL, Folds JD, Petitto JM, Golden RN, Pedersen CA, Corrigan M, Gilmore JH, Silva SG, Quade D, Ozer H. Circulating natural killer cell phenotypes in men and women with major depression: relation to cytotoxic activity and severity of depression. *Arch Gen Psychiatry.* 1992; 49:388-395.
144. Herbert TB, Cohen S. Depression and immunity: a meta-analytic review. *Psychol Bull.* 1993; 13:472-486.
145. Levy SM, Herberman RB, Lippman M, d'Angelo T. Correlation of stress factors with sustained depression of natural killer cell activity and predicted prognosis in patients with breast cancer. *J Clin Oncol.* 1987;5:348-353.
146. Levy SM, Herberman RB, Whitside T, Sanzo K, Lee J, Kirkwood J. Perceived social support and tumor estrogen/progesterone receptor status as predictors of natural killer cell activity in breast cancer patients. *Psychosom Med.* 1990;42:73-85.
147. Thomas CB, McCabe OL. Precursors of premature disease and death: habits of nervous tension. *Johns Hopkins Med J.* 1980;147:137.
148. Shekelle RB, Raynor WJ, Ostfeld AM, Garron DC, Bieliauskas LA, Liu SC, Maliza C, Paul O. Psychological depression and 17-year risk of death from cancer. *Psychosom Med.* 1981;43: 117-125.
149. Persky VW, Kempthorne-Rawson J, Shekelle RB. Personality and risk of cancer: 20-year follow-up of the Western Electric study. *Psychosom Med.* 1987;49:435-449.
150. Grossarth-Maticek R, Frentzel-Beyme R, Becker N. Cancer risks associated with life events and conflict solution. *Cancer Detect Prev.* 1984;7: 201-209.
151. Kaplan GA, Reynolds P. Depression and cancer mortality and morbidity: prospective evidence from the Almeda County Study. *J Behav Med.* 1988;11:1-13.
152. Zonderman AB, Costa PT, McCrae RR. Depression as a risk for cancer morbidity and mortality in a nationally representative sample. *JAMA.* 1989;262:1191-1195.
153. Linkens RW, Comstock GW. Depressed mood and the development of cancer. *Am J Epidemiol.* 1990;132:962-972.
154. Hahn RC, Petitti DB. Minnesota Multiphasic Personality Inventory–rated depression and the incidence of breast cancer. *Cancer.* 1988;61:845-848.
155. Levenson JL, Bemis C. The role of psychological factors in cancer onset and progression. *Psychosomatics.* 1991;32:124-131.
156. McGee R, Williams S, Elwood M. Depression and the development of cancer: a meta-analysis. *Soc Sci Med.* 1994;38:187-192.
157. Anderson BL, Kiecolt-Glaser JK, Glaser R. A biobehavioral model of cancer stress and disease course. *Am Psychol.* 1994;49:389-404.
158. Miller AH, Stein M. The immune system and depression. In: Tasman A, Riba MB, eds. *American Psychiatric Association Review of Psychiatry.* Washington, DC: American Psychiatric Press; 1992;11:181-201.
159. Epstein RH. Neuroendocrine-immune interactions. *N Engl J Med.* 1993;329:1246-1253.
160. Cupps TR, Fauci AS. Corticosteroid-mediated immunoregulation in man. *Immunol Rev.* 1982; 65:134-155.
161. Denicoff KD, Durkin TM, Lotze MT, Quinlan PE, Davis CL, Litwak SJ, Rosenbert SA, Rubinow DR. The neuroendocrine effects of interleukin-2 treatment. *J Clin Endocrinol Metab.* 1986; 63:1292-1299.
162. Staubaugh H, Irwin M. Central corticotropin-releasing hormone reduces cellular immunity. *Brain Behav Immun.* 1992;6:11-17.
163. Barbanel G, Ixart G, Szafarczyk A, Malaval F, Assenmacher I. Intrahypothalamic infusion of interleukin-1 beta increases the release of corticotropin-releasing hormone (CRH 41) and adrenocorticotropic hormone (ACTH) in free-moving rats bearing a push-pull cannula in the median eminence. *Brain Res.* 1990;516:31-36.
164. Irwin MR, Britton KT, Vale W. Central corticotropin releasing factor suppresses natural killer cell activity. *Brain Behav Immun.* 1987;1:81-87.
165. Sapolsky RM, Donnelly TM. Vulnerability to stress-induced tumor growth increases with age: role of glucocorticoids. *Endocrinology.* 1985; 117:662-222.

Critical Review of Psychosocial Interventions in Cancer Care

Fawzy I. Fawzy, MD; Nancy W. Fawzy, RN, DNSc; Lisa A. Arndt; Robert O. Pasnau, MD

The need for a large variety of psychosocial interventions is enhanced as increasing numbers of patients with cancer have longer survival. This article reviews the four interventions used most commonly: (1) education, (2) behavioral training, (3) individual psychotherapy, and (4) group interventions. It examines the outcomes of each type of intervention. This comprehensive review of the intervention literature reveals the availability of a wide range of options for patients with cancer and their potential psychological and physical health benefits.

(Arch Gen Psychiatry. 1995;52:100-113)

As survival rates have improved with advances in medical care, the importance of psychiatric interventions designed to assist cancer patients in dealing with diagnosis and treatment has increased.[1-3] Different intervention models have been used.[4] According to Holland,[5] the goals of these interventions are to decrease feelings of alienation by talking with others in a similar situation, to reduce anxiety about the treatments, to assist in clarifying misperceptions and misinformation, and to lessen feelings of isolation, helplessness, and being neglected by others. Interventions that are designed to help the person feel less helpless and hopeless have the added benefit of encouraging more responsibility to get well and compliance with medical regimens. Aware of the benefits of these psychosocial therapeutic interventions, today's patients often specifically request such services.

There are four major categories of interventions described most frequently in the literature. These are educational techniques, behavioral training, individual psychotherapy, and group interventions. The purpose of this article is to examine a large and diverse group of clinical research studies of these interventions. We describe and contrast these interventions, addressing the type of patient population, the research design, the details of the interventions, and the outcomes. We focus particularly on outcome measures, which include changes in coping, affective state, quality of life, knowledge regarding disease and treatment, compliance, physical status, recurrence, and survival. Because the majority of the studies used varying instruments and did not always specifically measure the outcome categories delineated above, we have used reasonable judgment in determining into which category each outcome measure falls. For example, anxiety and depression both are included in affective state. However, quality of life is only used if the research actually indicated that this was measured.

A number of researchers have shown that psychological intervention can contribute significantly to both psychological and physical health outcomes in patients with cancer.[1,6-8] This review is intended to identify the advantages and pitfalls of these interventions. It could also be used to facilitate the development of an effective model of psychosocial intervention that could be readily integrated into the comprehensive care of the cancer patient.

EDUCATION

The overall goal of education for cancer patients is to reduce the sense of helpless-

From the Department of Psychiatry and Biobehavioral Sciences, the University of California, Los Angeles, UCLA School of Medicine, (Drs F. Fawzy, N. Fawzy, and Pasnau and Ms Arndt); and the John Wayne Cancer Institute, St John's Hospital and Health Center, Santa Monica, Calif (Dr N. Fawzy).

ness and inadequacy due to uncertainty and lack of knowledge. This intervention seeks to replace helplessness with a sense of mastery and control. Education for cancer patients may cover technical disease and treatment information, and it may also include information about coping, emotional issues, and much more. This article reviews only those studies that primarily educated about the disease and its treatment (**Table 1**).

Jacobs et al[9] employed a purely educational intervention in a randomized study of patients with Hodgkin's disease. Twenty-one patients in an experimental group received a 27-page booklet with disease-related information as well as a newsletter. Three months later, the intervention group had increased their knowledge levels compared with the 26 control patients. On the "Cancer Patient Behavior Scale," the intervention group also showed decreased anxiety and treatment problems. They not only showed a trend for decreased depression and life disruption but also, interestingly, a decrease in social competency. These authors suggested that increased knowledge led to more self-awareness and therefore more self-consciousness in social situations.

Rainey[10] tested 30 sequential patients undergoing radiation therapy for knowledge and emotional status using the state component of the State-Trait Anxiety Scale and the Profile of Mood States (POMS) Total Mood Disturbance score. The next 30 patients were provided with a 12-minute educational slide presentation about radiation therapy prior to testing. Both groups were then retested at the end of radiation therapy approximately 4 to 6 weeks later. The intervention group scored higher on the initial knowledge test but there was no difference between groups for anxiety or total mood disturbance. By the follow-up point, both groups demonstrated equally high levels of knowledge, but the intervention group had lower levels of state anxiety and total mood disturbance.

Ali and Khalil[11] conducted a 30- to 60-minute preoperative intervention for 30 patients with bladder cancer who were about to have a urinary diversion. This consisted of providing information about the procedure, the site and appearance of the stoma, and external collection devices, and a visit from a well-functioning ostomate patient. In addition, patients were encouraged to express their fears and anxieties. The outcome measure used was state anxiety, which they found to be decreased on the third and 12th days postoperatively.

Richardson et al[12] randomly assigned 94 patients with newly diagnosed hematological malignant cancer to a control group or one of three educational intervention groups. The purpose of the intervention was to increase compliance in taking the medications allopurinol and prednisone. The intervention consisted of a 1-hour educational session with a nurse who discussed the disease and treatment plus one of the following: (1) a four-level pill-shaping component carried out in the hospital prior to discharge; (2) a home visit to organize a "cueing" system for pill taking; or (3) a combination of the two. Compliance was measured by obtaining blood levels of two drugs and a record of whether patients kept the monthly clinic appointment during 6 months. Survival was measured in days from enrollment in the study to death within the 6 months. Compliance was accomplished equally by all three of the educational interventions for allopurinol but not for prednisone. Appointment keeping was positively enhanced by all three interventions. Using regression analysis, it was concluded that low severity of disease, assignment to an educational program (any one), plus high compliance with allopurinol therapy were predictive of increased survival in patients with newly diagnosed hematological malignant cancer.

Pruitt et al[13] randomized 31 patients with mixed diagnoses receiving radiation therapy to either a three-session intervention (1 hour each session) or a standard control group. The education consisted of information about radiation therapy and cancer, coping strategies, and communication skills. Knowledge using an author-constructed instrument, psychological distress using the Brief Symptom Inventory, and current concerns using the Inventory of Current Concerns were measured at baseline and at 1 and 3 months after the intervention. Knowledge levels were unchanged in both groups. This finding was attributed to the older age of the patients and their high anxiety levels. Depression was the only measure of affective state to improve. Health concerns, existential concerns, and self-appraisal were the areas of concern that showed the greatest correlation with affective state measures. Although coping strategies and communication skills were taught, they were not directly measured.

Several researchers have stressed the importance of educational interventions for cancer patients. Many patients have inadequate levels of information and desire more.[14] Patient education not only offers diagnosis- and treatment-specific information to patients who may have misconceptions, no conceptions at all, and who may be hesitant to ask for such information, but may also enhance coping skills.[15] Yet, of the five educational studies, only two actually measured knowledge outcomes. The one study[13] that added coping and communication to the disease and treatment education also failed to measure changes in these specific areas.

Future educational interventions should carefully delineate the topic of education and measure outcomes within a clearly defined theoretical framework. This should include changes in actual levels of knowledge and resultant changes in behavior and/or affective state. Subsequent changes in physiological status should also be considered.

BEHAVIORAL TRAINING

Behavioral training has been used in many cancer interventions to help reduce psychological stress as well as the physical complications that often stem from cancer treatment (eg, chemotherapy and radiation therapy). It is a wide category of interventions that encompasses a variety of techniques. Some of these techniques are progressive muscle relaxation (PMR), hypnosis (self-hypnosis or therapist-induced hyp-

Table 1. Educational Studies*

Study, Year	Patient Population: Diagnosis	N/M	M/F	Design, No. of Groups: R/NR	Experimental (n)	Control (n)	Intervention: Duration	Content
Jacobs et al,[9] 1983	Hodgkin's disease	N	32/16	R	1 (21)	1 (26)	Patient determined	Information booklet and newsletters
Rainey,[10] 1985	Mixed, RTx	N and M	30/30	NR	1 (30)	1 (30)	1 × 12 min	RTx slide presentation
Ali and Khalil,[11] 1989	Bladder cancer	N	23/7	R	1 (15)	1 (15)	1 × 30-60 min	Preoperative information
Richardson et al,[12] 1990	Mixed hematological cancer	N	59/35	R	1 (22) 2 (23) 3 (24)	1 (25)	1, 1 h + home visit; 2, 1 h + hospital; 3, 1 h + hospital + home visit	1, education + "cueing"; 2, education + shaping; 3, education + cueing + shaping
Pruitt et al,[13] 1993	Mixed, RTx	N	22/9	R	1 (15)	1 (16)	3 × 1 h over 3 wk	RTx information, common concerns, coping, and communication

N/M indicates newly diagnosed vs metastatic/recurrence; R/NR, randomized/nonrandomized; RTx, radiation therapy; affect, affective state; QOL, quality of life; know, knowledge; comp, compliance; phys, physical health; immune, immune system; R/S, recurrence/survival; plus sign, an improvement in intervention group(s); minus sign, a decrease in intervention group(s); X, change over time occurred but no difference between groups at end point; and NC, no changes.

nosis), deep breathing, meditation, biofeedback, passive relaxation, and guided imagery (GI) (also called visualization). This last technique includes both the "imagine a pleasant scene" and the "imagine one's immune system destroying cancer cells" types. All of these techniques are used in the reviewed studies in various combinations or alone.

This article examines 10 studies that used behavioral training as the key component in their intervention. These studies varied in their specific techniques and measured outcomes. The first six articles that we reviewed were of interventions intended to reduce the biological and psychological effects of chemotherapy. The final four articles addressed the more general use of behavioral training as a way of reducing psychological distress and enhancing the immune system (**Table 2**).

Behavioral Training to Reduce Chemotherapy Effects

Chemotherapy is usually a physically and psychologically difficult process for the patient to endure. Each patient faces a number of possible physical side effects, ranging from drug-induced symptoms to conditioned side effects, particularly nausea and vomiting. Increased levels of negative affective states ranging from depression to anxiety are experienced as well. Although medications are often administered to control such side effects, they have not been completely effective.[16] These limitations have persuaded researchers to find other methods of supportive chemotherapy care, including behavioral training.

In the first article reviewed, Burish and Lyles[17] used PMR training combined with GI as a means of reducing both the emotional distress and the physical toll on patients undergoing chemotherapy. They randomly assigned 14 females and two males to either a PMR/GI intervention group or a control group. All of the subjects in this study experienced anticipatory anxiety, nausea, and/or vomiting that did not respond to antiemetic medication. Pretreatment, treatment, and posttreatment progress was measured using physiological methods (blood pressure and pulse rate) and patient-reported and nurse-reported indices of negative affect. The results suggested that PMR and GI instructions were effective tools in reducing the adverse side effects of chemotherapy.

Morrow and Morrell[18] looked at the effects of systematic desensitization as a way of reducing the anticipated nausea and vomiting induced by chemotherapy. Randomly assigning 60 cancer patients undergoing chemotherapy to one of three groups (no treatment control, counseling only, and desensitization with PMR), the researchers carefully ensured stable baseline measurements as well as two follow-up assessments. The experimental group were taught counterconditioning responses to the stimuli (such as PMR) that would have normally elicited the negative response (nausea and vomiting). The counseling group was used to control for potential placebo effects of the patients' expectation of change. This consisted of several 1-hour counseling sessions during which patients discussed their own methods of reducing anticipatory nausea. The patients who had received systematic desensitization had significant reductions in the frequency, severity, and duration of their anticipatory side effects.

Lyles et al[19] divided subjects into three possible interventions. The first offered patients both PMR and GI training before, during, and after chemotherapy treatments; the second group was presented with a therapist who provided support and encouragement but no actual behavioral training; and the third was a control group of subjects who received standard medical treatment. Measured by self-reports and attending nurses' observations, a total of 50 subjects participated in this randomized experiment. The results confirmed previous reports that PMR and GI instruction improve the chemotherapy patient's physical and emotional reaction to treatment, but showed only slight differences between the nonintervention control condition and the therapist-controlled condition. The data were supported again during the follow-up session, making it clear that

	Outcomes of Intervention							
Follow-up	Coping	Affect	QOL	Know	Comp	Phys	Immune	R/S
3 mo	+ −	+		+				
4-6 wk		+		+ X				
12 d		+						
6 mo					+			+
3 mo		+		NC				

PMR and GI may be effective for helping chemotherapy patients cope with common side effects.

Cotanch[20] collected measures of 12 subjects' physiological arousal, state-trait anxiety levels, food-fluid intake, degree and frequency of vomiting, change in total body weight, and quantity of antiemetic therapy following drug infusion at pretraining and posttraining periods. Despite antiemetic therapy, all 12 patients continued to experience nausea and vomiting. Once PMR training was added to their chemotherapy course, nine of the 12 patients had a decrease in nausea and vomiting.

Carey and Burish[21] assessed 45 patients using self-reports, physiological tests, and nurse observation measures during a sequence of five chemotherapy sessions. The patients were randomly assigned to one of four conditions: (1) a professionally trained therapist who taught PMR and GI to the patients; (2) a trained volunteer (paraprofessional) who taught both PMR and GI to the patients; (3) a set of audiotapes that explained PMR and GI to the patients; or (4) a standard treatment design (control group) with no behavioral training. The outcome of the study suggested that professionally administered PMR and GI training significantly reduced emotional distress and physiological arousal (allowing for an increased food intake) in chemotherapy patients. Although the patients seemed comfortable with the use of audiotapes for private use of the PMR and GI techniques once they had gone through the live sessions, live sessions were seen as superior over the audiotape sessions. This alternative intervention showed that behavioral training had significant benefits for patients (as compared with a control group) and that specific implementations of such techniques (a live professional vs an audiotape) may work even better.

The sixth study, by Burish et al,[22] also assigned 60 chemotherapy patients to a general coping preparation package, known as PREP. Designed by the authors, the PREP was a 90-minute intervention administered before the subject's first chemotherapy session. The PREP group received PMR and GI training, a tour of the oncology clinic, a presentation about chemotherapy, an information booklet, and an educational session regarding chemotherapy. The two other groups consisted of a control group (with no additional treatment) and a group in which subjects received only PMR and GI instruction (not a PREP session). Assessed with self-reports, nurse observations, family observations, and physiological instruments, the subjects were followed through five sequential chemotherapy courses. The results of this study found that the PREP intervention reduced patient distress more than PMR and GI treatment alone. The control group showed the lowest reductions in emotional and physical complaints. The authors suggested that one-time educational interventions (such as PREP) may actually prove more effective than the often-used PMR and GI procedures alone.

Behavioral Training to Reduce General Distress

The following four studies demonstrated the usefulness of behavioral training interventions in reducing general cancer-related distress (Table 2).

Davis[23] measured the ability of biofeedback and cognitive therapy to reduce multilevel stress in 25 women newly diagnosed as having breast cancer. All of the patients participated in a psychosocial intervention, and of the 19 who completed the trial, the subjects were further divided into one of three groups: biofeedback treatment (experimental); cognitive therapy (experimental); or no further treatment (control). Urinary cortisol levels and state anxiety were used as dependent variables, and the data of both experimental conditions were compared with those of the nontreated group. The correlations between subjects' ages and cortisol levels were not significant and no patient received chemotherapy during the study. As expected, the results of this randomized study showed an overall significant improvement in the anxiety levels in the 12 patients in the experimental groups. Moreover, the cortisol levels among these patients were reduced relative to those of the control patients.

Gruber et al[24] studied the effect of behavioral training on the immune systems of 10 adult patients with metastatic cancer. Over a period of 1 year, subjects who had no prior experience with either technique used imagery and relaxation, while monthly samples of blood were drawn for examination in a laboratory, blind to their identity or specific conditions. Compared with their own baseline data, several measures of immune system function were found to be significantly elevated over the course of 1 year. The subjects' psychological states were

Table 2. Behavioral Training Studies*

Study, Year	Patient Population: Diagnosis	N/M	M/F	Design, No. of Groups: R/NR	Experimental (n)	Control (n)	Intervention: Duration	Content
Burish and Lyles,[17] 1981	Mixed, chemotherapy	M	2/14	R	1 (8)	1 (8)	5 × 1 h over 60 d	PMR, GI
Morrow and Morrell,[18] 1982	Mixed, chemotherapy	M	18/42	R	1 (20) 2 (20)	1 (20)	2 × 1 h over 2 wk	1, SD (PMR); 2, talking
Lyles et al,[19] 1982	Mixed, chemotherapy	M	19/31	R	1 (18) 2 (14)	1 (18)	5 × 1 h over 60 d	1, PMR, GI; 2, talking
Cotanch,[20] 1983	Mixed, chemotherapy	M	7/5	NR	1 (12)	None	1 × 1 h	PMR
Carey and Burish,[21] 1987	Mixed, chemotherapy	M	20/25	R	3 (NS)	1 (NS)	5 × ~1 h over 60 d	PMR, GI: 1, professional; 2, paraprofessional; 3, audiotape
Burish et al,[22] 1991	Mixed, chemotherapy	N	31/29	R	1 (15) 2 (15) 3 (15)	1 (15)	1, 45 min 2, 90 min 3, 135 min	1, PMR, GI; 2, PREP; 3, PREP, PMR, GI
Davis,[23] 1986	Breast cancer	N	0/25	R	1 (7) 2 (5)	1 (7)	13 × 45 min over 8 wk	1, PMR, B; 2, PMR, CT
Gruber et al,[24] 1988	Mixed	M	5/5	NR	1 (10)	Crossover-B	12 × ? h over 1 y	PMR, GI, B
Gruber et al,[25] 1993	Breast cancer	N	0/13	R	1 (7) Crossover	2 (6)	9 wk + monthly follow-up	PMR, letting go, GI, B
Baider et al,[26] 1994	Mixed	N and M	25/98	NR	1 (123)	None	6 × 1.5 h over 6 wk	PMR, GI

**PMR indicates progressive muscle relaxation; GI, guided imagery; SD, systemic desensitization; B, biofeedback; CT, cognitive therapy; PREP, a general coping preparation package; and NS, not specified. See Table 1 for explanation of other abbreviations.*

also examined, revealing increased aggression and internal locus of control. Both immune and emotional changes paralleled the use of relaxation and imagery.

In another study, Gruber et al[25] randomly assigned 13 patients with breast cancer to either an immediate treatment group that received PMR, GI, and biofeedback training or a delayed treatment control group. Pretreatment and posttreatment measures included blood samples, psychological testing, and a computerized psychophysiological stress evaluation. The results showed that the only psychological difference was in anxiety levels, which were reduced shortly after each group began the intervention. Immune system parameters (such as natural killer cell activity, mixed lymphocyte responsiveness, and the number of peripheral blood lymphocytes) were significantly improved and directly correlated with the behavioral interventions.

Finally, Baider and coworkers[26] studied the immediate and long-term effects of a six-session PMR and GI training intervention on 86 cancer patients. The patients were assessed using three self-report instruments: the Multiple Locus of Control, the Brief Symptom Inventory, and the Impact of Events Scale. This study found notable improvement on the Brief Symptom Inventory and the Impact of Events Scale for all 86 patients who completed the behavioral intervention. This improvement was maintained up to the 6-month follow-up. This finding supports the findings of other investigators who showed that psychological improvement was maintained long after the interventions were completed.[6,27,28]

INDIVIDUAL PSYCHOTHERAPY

Individual psychotherapy is a long-established method used to ease the distress and disruption that accompany the diagnosis of cancer. Support, compassion, and empathy form the cornerstone of successful individual psychotherapy. A major problem, however, is that the exact format of the psychotherapy employed in different studies is not explained. "Therapy," "psychotherapy," and "counseling" are the terms most commonly used, without any clear definition or attempt to differentiate them. It appears from all the studies reviewed that the critical component of these interventions was the support and emotional engagement of the patient regardless of which term was used. Thirteen studies describing the use of individual psychotherapy as a primary modality in helping cancer patients cope with their disease were examined. In some of the studies, additional techniques were employed, such as education, but these were also provided on an individual basis (ie, not in a group). The other components of the intervention, if used, were noted (**Table 3**).

Capone et al[29] investigated the effectiveness of in-hospital, individual therapy for patients newly diagnosed as having gynecological cancers. Ninety-seven subjects were randomly assigned regardless of age, race, or prognosis to one of two conditions. In the experimental condition, 56 subjects underwent psychological counseling before, during, and after primary medical treatment during which they remained hospitalized. They were reassessed on returning for their 3-, 6-, and 12-month posttreatment examinations using the Self-Rating Symptom Scale, the POMS, and the Tennessee Self-Concept Scale. Forty-one patient controls were assessed

Follow-up	Outcomes of Intervention							
	Coping	Affect	QOL	Know	Comp	Phys	Immune	R/S
75 d	+	+				+		
60 d	+	NC	+			+		
75 d	+	+	+			+	+	+
48 h	+	+				+	+	
2 wk	+	+				+	+	
90 d	+	+						
8 mo	+	+					+	+
1 y	+		+			+	+	
15 mo	+	NC				+	+	
8 mo	+		+					

using the same set of instruments, but they did not receive any individual counseling. The results suggested that all of the subjects had similar levels of psychological distress at the start of the study (pretreatment). However, at 3 months after treatment, the counseled patients reported significantly less emotional upset, confusion, and social isolation than the control patients. The results of this study indicated that individual counseling interventions during the initial hospitalization had a significant effect in reducing sexual dysfunction specifically related to the diagnosis and treatment of genital cancer. Follow-up results suggested that patients in the intervention group were more likely to return to normal vocational and sexual functions after the first year of treatment.

Gordon et al[30] collected five different types of data to determine the efficacy of counseling interventions for cancer patients: medical, demographic, behavioral, psychosocial, and a personal interview. They administered a systematic program of rehabilitation that included education regarding living with an illness, consultation with health care personnel, referral services, and professional counseling to their experimental group of 138 patients. A total of 131 control subjects were evaluated but not offered any form of psychosocial intervention. With little difference between the demographic or medical status of subjects in both conditions, the results showed that the intervention group had a more rapid decline of negative affect, a more active use of time, a higher proportion of vocational return, and a more realistic outlook on life than the control patients. Most important, the individual counseling, education, and personnel consultations provided to the experimental group appeared to help them deal more effectively with some of their psychosocial problems.

Maguire et al[31] conducted a study to determine if counseling by a specialist nurse would prevent the psychiatric morbidity associated with mastectomy in patients with breast cancer. Seventy-five women were randomized to a counseling intervention condition during their stay on a surgical unit and 77 women, to a control condition. The experimental condition consisted of individual sessions with a specialist nurse before and after surgery, as well as follow-up home and clinic visits to monitor their progress. The results of this design failed to show any significant prevention in psychiatric morbidity. However, with regular individual assessment, the nurse was able to refer those patients who needed further psychiatric help. In the absence of close personal contact, only a few control subjects were recognized as being in need of referral. Thus, some individuals who might have benefited from psychiatric care did not receive it. On the other hand, distressed patients in the experimental condition were readily identified and referred for appropriate psychiatric care. As a result, the experimental group showed a reduced level of morbidity 12 to 18 months after the mastectomy. Overall, this study indicated that the recognition and early detection of psychiatric morbidity and subsequent referral service are successful in reducing the high levels of distress and morbidity in patients with breast cancer.

Linn et al[32] randomly assigned 120 patients with late-stage cancer to either an experimental or a control condition to study the effects of individual counseling on stress reduction. During a 12-month period, patients were assessed on their quality of life and functional status. The patients in the experimental group were seen regularly several times a week by a professional counselor trained in hospice work. Counseling was intended to reduce denial but maintain hope, encourage patients to participate in meaningful activities, help patients complete any unfinished business, and provide increased self-esteem and life satisfaction. Although functional status and survival did not differ between the two conditions, there were significant improvements for the experimental group in terms of quality of life after 3 months. While it may not be possible to improve physical functioning or survival in patients with late-stage cancer, counseling interventions helped to enhance the quality of life of patients with end-stage cancer.

Examining a completely different oncology population, Worden and Weisman[33] studied the effec-

Table 3. Individual Psychotherapy Studies*

Study, Year	Patient Population: Diagnosis	N/M	M/F	Design, No. of Groups: R/NR	Experimental (n)	Control (n)	Intervention: Duration	Content
Capone et al,[29] 1980	Gynecological cancer	N	0/97	R	1 (56)	1 (41)	4 × ? h over ? wk	IP
Gordon et al,[30] 1980	Breast cancer, lung, cancer, malignant melanoma	N	70/147	NR	1 (157)	1 (151)	~24 × ? h over 6 mo	IP, E, C
Maguire et al,[31] 1980	Breast cancer	N	0/152	R	1 (75)	1 (77)	4 × ? h over ? wk	IP
Linn et al,[32] 1982	Mixed	M	120/0	R	1 (62)	1 (58)	3 × wk × ? h over 12 mo	IP
Worden and Weisman,[33] 1984	Mixed	N	NS	R	1 (59)	1 (58)	~4 × ? h over 1 mo	IP
Grossarth-Maticek et al,[34] 1984	Breast cancer	M	0/179	R	1 (24) 2 (12) 3 (14) 4 (49)	1 (17) 1 (49)	1, 30 h 2, 30 h 3, 30 h 4, 20 h	1, IP; 2, BT; 3 and 4, creative novation therapy
Forester et al,[39] 1985	Mixed, RTx	N and M	50/50	R	1 (48)	1 (52)	10 × 30 min over 10 wk	IP
Houts et al,[40] 1986	Gynecological cancer	N	0/32	R	1 (14)	1 (18)	3 calls over 12 wk	IP
McCorkle et al,[41] 1989	Lung cancer	N and M	105/61	R	2 (NS)	1 (NS)	? × weekly × over 6 mo	1, IP, oncology nurse; 2, IP, regular nurse
Mermelstein and Holland,[42] 1991	Lymphoma, ovarian cancer	M	0/2	NR	1 (2)	None	? calls over 3-6 mo	IP (via telephone)
Edgar et al,[43] 1992	Mixed	N and M	52/153	R	1 (103) Crossover	2 (102)	5 × 1 h over 5? wk	IP, E: 1, early intervention; 2, late intervention
Greer et al,[28] 1992†	Mixed	M	32/124	R	1 (72)	1 (84)	6 × 1 h over 8 wk	IP, C, BT
Moorey, et al,[44] 1994†	Mixed	N and M	32/124	R	1 (72)	1 (84)	6 × 1 h over 8 wk	IP, C, BT

**IP indicates individual psychotherapy; E, education; C, coping strategies; BT; behavioral training; and NS, not specified. See Table 1 for explanation of other abbreviations.*

†Same study with 1-year follow-up.

tiveness of preventive psychosocial interventions in 381 patients newly diagnosed as having cancer. Prescreened and approached if at a high risk of emotional distress and poor coping, subjects were randomly divided into one of two identical short-term interventions or a control condition. The month-long interventions following the initial diagnosis were aimed at lowering distress and improving coping skills among the participants. Each intervention consisted of individual sessions with a psychologist and a follow-up meeting with a social worker at 2, 4, 6, and 12 months after the therapist-patient relationship was terminated. Using the POMS, Index of Vulnerability, and Inventory of Current Concerns, they reported a significant lowering of emotional distress as well as an increase in coping skills in the intervention group. Although the number of problems experienced by both groups were similar, the patients who received counseling had a significant increase in their level of problem resolution.

Grossarth-Maticek et al[34] performed two studies that attempted to modify negative psychosocial factors using psychotherapy. The authors were also interested in the interaction between psychosocial and organic risk factors in cancerogenesis. In the first study, 50 women with breast cancer were randomly assigned to 30 hours of one of three psychotherapies: behavior therapy, intensive psychotherapy, or "creative novation therapy," developed by the authors. The behavior therapy option made use of imagery and desensitization techniques to modify "undesirable" behaviors. Intensive psychotherapy focused on traumatic experiences in early childhood as a primary cause of psychosocial maladjustment. During these sessions, the patients explored the origin of their behaviors with therapists trained in exploring early trauma. The final option, creative novation therapy, was described as a form of cognitive behavior therapy that attempted to substitute an undesirable behavior with a new one. The primary assumption in creative novation therapy was that a change in perception and interpretation of social constructs can bring new cognitive resolutions. The results concluded that all three forms of psychotherapy increased survival by 3.64 months. When combined with chemotherapy, survival increased to a mean of 22.40 months. Among the three types of psychotherapies, creative novation therapy had the highest increase in survival, with behavior therapy following, and intensive psychotherapy providing the weakest results.

In the second study, Grossarth-Maticek et al[34] further explored the relation between survival and creative novation therapy. Ninety-eight patients with regional lymph node metastases agreed to receive 20 hours of creative novation therapy during radiotherapy. The results suggested that patients given therapy

	Outcomes of Intervention							
Follow-up	Coping	Affect	QOL	Know	Comp	Phys	Immune	R/S
12 mo	+	+						
6-12 mo	+	+						
18 mo	NC	NC						
12 mo			+			+		NC
12 mo	+	+						
15 mo							+	+
10 wk	+	+				+		
12 wk	NC	NC						
35 wk	+	+				−		
4 mo	+	+		+−				
1 y	+	+		+				
4 mo	+	+−						
1 y	+	+						

lived an average of 9.4 months longer than their paired controls. While it appeared that psychotherapeutic interventions may increase survival, the authors stressed that therapy should only be administered in a multidisciplinary fashion, with careful assessment of medical, clinical, immunological, and psychosocial aspects.

Given the rather remarkable results and conclusions made by the authors of these two studies, it is important to note that they have been severely criticized as having numerous and serious methodological flaws. An entire issue of the *Journal of Psychological Inquiry* was devoted to discussing these issues.[35] Specifically, Van der Ploeg[36] cited inadequacies regarding patient demographics and how the control sample was obtained and matched on several variables. He also states that the specific nature of the interventions is never clearly spelled out and, in fact, differs among several publications with one even including an exercise program, changes in diet, vitamin supplementation, and the medications imipramine or phenobarbital. Further, Spiegel[37] states "the amount of work required for the intervention studies (5500 hours of psychotherapy) delivered entirely by Dr Grossarth-Maticek seems to defy the available resources." It also raises questions regarding the feasibility of such an intervention and whether the results are a function of the therapy or the therapist. Finally, Fox[38] advises the reader to be cautious about drawing conclusions from the reported results in view of the considerable number of inconsistencies, differences in reporting, inaccuracies, and the highly unlikely numbers.

Forester and colleagues[39] set out to determine the effects of ongoing individual psychotherapy for patients receiving radiotherapy. Fifty-two randomly assigned subjects served as controls while 48 subjects received weekly counseling sessions for 10 weeks, 4 weeks beyond the period of radiotherapy. A significant reduction in physical and emotional distress was found in the patients receiving psychotherapy. Within the experimental group there were further differences. For example, even though men seemed to suffer more distress than women, they demonstrated a better therapeutic response to psychotherapy.

Houts et al[40] randomly assigned 32 patients newly diagnosed as having gynecological cancer to either extra counseling services or regular support services. They created four possible coping strategies within the experimental condition. These were to maintain normal relations with family and friends, to make positive plans for the future, to ask the medical staff any and all questions, and to keep up normal routines whenever possible. These four coping skills were presented to the patients in the experimental condition in two separate interventions: the first group was introduced to the coping skills by experienced social workers who had once had cancer themselves, and the second group was simply given a notebook and audiocassette that explained the coping strategies. Measured with the POMS questionnaire at baseline, 6 weeks, and 12 weeks, this study found no statistically significant data to support the authors' hypothesis that former cancer patients would serve as better counselors to newly diagnosed patients than other therapists.

In a randomized clinical trial of patients with progressive lung cancer, McCorkle and associates[41] assigned 166 male and female patients with metastatic disease to one of three conditions: home care from oncology nurses; home care from regular nurses; or standard health care with no home care services. The two experimental conditions, receiving home care, provided patients with physical assessments, symptom management care, psychosocial assessments, grief and mourning care, and community resource information during their in-home visits. The study took place over a period of 6 months, with assessment interviews held every 6 weeks. Measured with the Symptom Distress Scale, the POMS, the Inventory of Current Concerns, and the Enforced Social Dependency Scale, the 166 participants showed no significant differences in pain or mood disturbance and concerns regardless of their assigned condition. The results indicated that patients in the two home care conditions had greater independence, less distress, but worse health perceptions over time. Remarkably, the non–home care condition suggested more distress and dependency, but improved health perceptions. The authors concluded that home care assists patients in forestalling distress and maintaining independence, while still allowing them to acknowledge the reality of their illness.

Another problem facing some cancer patients is the physical inability to go to a therapist's office on a regular basis to receive much needed help in dealing with their disease. Mermelstein and Holland[42] addressed this issue in a case study of two patients, one with lymphoma and the other with ovarian cancer, who benefited highly from telephone therapy. The authors suggested that the anonymity, accessibility, and formality brought on by telephone counseling actually permitted this method to be a more effective psychotherapeutic tool for patients who were seriously ill. In using the telephone, both patients were able to establish a genuine patient-therapist bond and sense of hope despite their physical limitations. The notable negative features of telephone therapy are the loss of visual and nonverbal cues that often provide therapists with a good deal of information about the patient's emotional state. However, in this study, the parameters of the patient's tone, inflection, volume, rate, and progression of voice did assist in a therapeutic connection that proved successful. With advancing technology and the invention of the videophone, the researchers hope to expand and improve the already positive results of telephone therapy.

Edgar et al[43] evaluated the emotional coping skills of 205 newly diagnosed cancer patients throughout a 1-year period using 4-month assessments. Two interventions were tested: an early intervention condition that began immediately after diagnosis and a later intervention that began after a 4-month delay. Both conditions included five individual sessions with a nurse, with each one addressing a specific issue: goal setting, cognitive reappraisal, problem-solving techniques, effective use of resources, and relaxation training. At the 8-month assessment, the later intervention group was found to be less depressed, anxious, and worried than the early intervention participants. During the course of the yearlong study, the later intervention group continued to have less anxiety, although all of the subjects improved in emotional coping skills by the end of the year. The authors suggested that patients with low ego strength pose a higher risk for psychological complications and may benefit from a psychosocial intervention.

Cancer patients with confirmed malignant disease were selected to participate in a randomized controlled trial to determine the effects of adjuvant psychological therapy. Greer and colleagues[28] measured 174 patients on hospital anxiety and depression scales, the Rotterdam Symptom Checklist, Mental Adjustment to Cancer Scale, and the Psychosocial Adjustment to Illness Scale (PAIS) over a period of 8 weeks. The experimental condition included a brief, problem-focused, cognitive-behavioral program specifically designed to meet the needs of individual cancer patients, while the control condition received no therapy. At 8 weeks, the therapy group had statistically significant lower scores than control patients on helplessness, fatalism, anxiety, psychological symptoms, and they had higher scores on fighting spirit. During a follow-up assessment 4 months later, patients receiving therapy continued to have lower scores than control subjects on anxiety, psychological symptoms, and psychological distress. The authors concluded that the adjuvant psychological therapy approach, geared toward assisting cancer patients, produced significant improvement in dealing with their serious illnesses.

In 1993, Moorey and colleagues[44] completed a 1-year follow-up study of the previous study. The experimental group continued to exhibit less anxiety and depression than controls, justifying further investigation of the benefits and efficacy of brief, adjuvant psychological therapy interventions for newly diagnosed cancer patients.

GROUP INTERVENTIONS

In the late 1970s, reports began appearing in the literature of group interventions for cancer patients (**Table 4**). Wood et al[45] reported on a pilot study with 15 patients with cancer of various diagnoses. Eight weekly 1½-hour sessions were held. The groups were co-led by a psychiatrist, a registered nurse, and a social worker. The focus of the discussions was on issues of living and coping with cancer. A survey using a Likert scale and covering 20 areas of changed experience was used to evaluate effectiveness. The authors reported difficulty in keeping the group focused, although the patients reported that the intervention was useful in helping them to talk about and face fears and anxieties, to get information, to feel less isolated, and to feel supported in general.

Ferlic et al[46] provided 30 newly diagnosed cancer patients with six 1½-hour group counseling sessions over 2 weeks. The content consisted of the following: (1) patient education; (2) team presentations (nursing perspectives, medical and psychological aspects, religion, sexuality, and nutrition); and (3) group support. A social worker co-led the session each week with the help of one other team member (ie, one of three nurses, two physicians, two chaplains, an occupational therapist, and a dietitian). Group members were compared with a similar group of patients who did not attend the sessions. It was not clear how patients were assigned to groups. The Patient Perception Test and Self-Concept Questionnaire were administered before and after intervention and 6 months later by mail. However, not enough tests were returned to provide valid 6-month data. The intervention proved useful in improving patients' scores in group attitude, hospital adjustment, relationship strength, cancer knowledge, and perceptions about death. It also served to enhance self-concept.

The Omega Project[47] used a structured intervention that addressed common questions and concerns of cancer patients, provided education, and taught relaxation techniques. The program used four audiotapes and 10 sets of illustrated "problem" cards to focus discussions, and consisted of four group sessions during a 6-week period. Fifty-nine subjects with mixed cancer sites participated in the intervention while 58 were in the control condition. Screened for variables such as religion, socioeconomic status, race, and demographics, the assessment instruments, including the POMS, the Index of Vulnerability, Therapist Rating Form, Patient Evaluation of Psychosocial Intervention, and the Inventory of Current Concerns, demonstrated the positive psychological impact that the intervention had on patients. The results showed that this intervention increased communication and coping skills in subjects when compared with controls after 6 months. In 1982, Sobel and Worden[48] published the *Practitioner's Manual* to guide other professionals in implementing their intervention program for cancer patients.

Spiegel et al[6,49] performed a prospective intervention study of patients with metastatic breast cancer. The patients in the experimental group met weekly in psychological support groups for 1 year. Meetings were informal and consisted of heuristic interpersonal exploration, as well as discussions of death and dying, family problems, communication problems, and living as richly as possible with a terminal illness. Emphasis was placed on group cohesion, support, sharing of mutual fears, self-disclosure, and interaction between patients outside the weekly meeting. At 12 months, the experimental patients showed significantly less tension, fatigue, and confusion and more vigor than the control group. In addition, there was a significant reduction in levels of pain. A trend toward having less depression, fewer maladjusted coping responses, and fewer phobias was also apparent. A 10-year follow-up of these patients showed that of the original 86, only three were alive and death records were obtained for the remaining 83. Survival was significantly different, with a mean of 36.3 months in the intervention group compared with 18.9 months in the control group. Lower mood disturbance and higher ratings of vigor on the POMS at the end of the intervention period were significantly associated with greater longevity.

Johnson[50] paired then randomized 52 patients with newly diagnosed or recurrent cancer to either a 4-week, eight-session structured psychoeducational group intervention, titled "I Can Cope," or a control group. The patients were measured before and after intervention for anxiety, knowledge about cancer, and perceived purpose and meaningfulness in life (ie, cognitive coping). The structured intervention positively affected all three dependent variables.

Vachon et al[51] compared 64 women with breast cancer who resided at a hospital lodge while going through approximately 3 weeks of radiation therapy with 104 women who went through their therapy while living at home. Patients stayed in the lodge because they lived too far from the hospital to commute for their radiation therapy treatments. The lodge provided "coping with cancer" support groups. In these groups, the patients were given disease information, opportunities to vent emotions, taught coping skills, and met with patients who had completed therapy and were doing well. It was not clear how many group sessions were held during the 3 weeks. Affective state was assessed via the General Health Questionnaire. Residence in the lodge with attendance in the groups was associated with a decreased chance of change for the worse in affective state and an increased chance of change for the better.

Heinrich and Schag[52] compared 26 patients with various cancer diagnoses who participated in a "stress and activity management" (SAM) group with 25 patients who were in a "current available care" control group. The patients were not randomized but were recruited in sequential groups of about 10 to whatever condition was open at the time they were recruited. Twelve spouses in the treatment group and 13 in the control group also participated. The SAM was a comprehensive, structured 6-week group intervention that consisted of education, exercise, and coping, including problem solving and stress management techniques such as relaxation exercises. The patients were assessed before treatment, after treatment, and 2 and 4 months later using the Karnofsky Performance Status Scale, the Cancer Information Test, the PAIS, the Depression, Anxiety, and Global Severity Index from the Hopkins 90-Item Symptom Checklist, Revised, the Quality of Life Scale, and a daily activity diary. The patients and spouses in the SAM group all showed an increase in knowledge even though most of the patients had been dealing with their cancer for more than 2 years. Patients and spouses in the SAM group also reported being able to cope better and had a better attitude toward treatment. There was no difference between groups in psychosocial adjustment to illness. This may have been a function of the instrument used (PAIS), which may not have been sensitive enough to pick up differences in this population even though it is very useful in extremely ill patients.

Cain et al[53] randomly assigned 80 women with gynecological cancer to a no-treatment control group or to an individual or group thematic counseling intervention. Coping and adjustment were measured by the PAIS, and affective state was measured with the Hamilton Depression Rating Scale. The eight weekly sessions of thematic counseling (individual or group) were provided by social workers, aided at times by an oncology nurse and fellow, a radiologist, and a dietitian. The themes included the nature of cancer; causes; impact of treatment, particularly on body image and sexuality; relaxation; diet and exercise; relating to caregivers; talking with family and friends; and goal

Table 4. Group Intervention Studies*

Study, Year	Patient Population: Diagnosis	N/M	M/F	Design, No. of Groups: R/NR	Experimental (n)	Control (n)	Intervention: Duration	Content
Wood et al,[45] 1978	Mixed	N and M	M and F	NR	1 (15)	None	8 ×1.5 h over 8 wk	C
Ferlic et al,[46] 1979	Mixed	N and M	30/30	NR	1 (30)	1 (30)	6 × 1.5 h over 2 wk	E, C, ES
Weisman et al,[47] 1980	Mixed	NS	41/74	R	1 (59)	1 (58)	4 × ? h over 6 wk	C, SM, BT
Spiegel et al,[6,49] 1981 and 1989	Breast cancer	M	0/58	R	1 (34)	1 (24)	52 ×1.5 h over 1 y	E, C, BT, ES
Johnson,[50] 1982	Mixed	N and M	NS	R	1 (26)	1 (26)	8 ×1.5 h over 4 wk	E, C, ES
Vachon et al,[51] 1982	Breast cancer, RTx	N	0/168	NR	1 (64)	1 (104)	? × ? h over 3 wk	E, C, ES
Heinrich and Schag,[52] 1985	Mixed	M	35/16	NR	1 (26)	1 (25)	6 × 2 h over 6 wk	E, C, SM, BT, ES
Cain et al,[53] 1986	Gynecological cancer	N	0/80	R	1 (21) 2 (28)	1 (31)	8 × 2 h over 8 wk	E, C, BT, ES: 1, individual; 2, group
Telch and Telch,[54] 1986	Mixed	N and M	14/27	R	1 (13) 2 (14)	1 (14)	6 × 1.5 h over 6 wk	1, C, SM, BT; 2, ES
Cunningham and Tocco,[55] 1989	Mixed	N and M	14/39	R NR	1 (28) 2 (25) 3 (39)	1 (18)	6 × 2 h over 6 wk	1, E, C, ES; 2 and 3, E, C, SM, BT, ES
Cunningham et al,[56] 1993	Mixed	N and M	95/307	NR	1 (402)	None	7 × 2 h over 7 wk	E, C, BT, ES
Cella et al,[57] 1993	Mixed	N and M	14/63	NR	1 (77)	None	8 × ? h over 8 wk	E, C, ES
Berglund et al,[58] 1994	Mixed	N and M	7/192	R	1 (98)	1 (101)	11 × 2 h over 7 wk	E, C, SM, physical training
Fawzy et al,[27,60] 1990	Malignant melanoma	N	47%/53%	R	1 (38)	1 (28)	6 ×1.5 h over 6 wk	E, C, SM, BT, ES
Fawzy et a,[1] 1993	Malignant melanoma	N	33/35	R	1 (34)	1 (34)	6 × 1.5 h over 6 wk	E, C, SM, BT, ES

**E indicates education; C, coping strategies; SM, stress management; BT, behavioral training; ES, emotional support; and NS, not specified. See Table 1 for explanation of other abbreviations.*

setting. It was concluded that the individual and group counseling were equally effective in decreasing anxiety and depression and increasing adjustment to the illness up to 6 months later. The authors also claimed that the intervention group subjects were significantly more knowledgeable about their illness and treatment, but there was no objective measurement of knowledge included in the design.

Forty-one cancer patients with different diagnoses and stages of disease who were exhibiting marked levels of psychosocial distress were randomized by Telch and Telch[54] to a coping skills instruction group, an emotional support group, or a no-treatment control group. The two group interventions met once a week for 6 weeks for about 90 minutes each session. The emotional support group was unstructured and geared toward encouraging patients to express feelings and emotions. The coping skills groups had a set agenda that emphasized the teaching and rehearsal of cognitive, behavioral, and affective coping strategies. Patients were assessed before group assignment and immediately after the 6-week groups. The primary instruments used were the POMS to assess affective state and the Cancer Inventory of Problem Situations. The coping skills group showed consistent improvement in affective state, satisfaction related to work, social activities, physical appearance, sexual intimacy, physical and social activities, cognitive distress, communications, and coping with medical procedures. Patients in the emotional support group showed little or no improvement, while the control patients actually deteriorated in their psychological functioning.

Cunningham and Tocco[55] randomly assigned 60 cancer patients with mixed diagnoses to one of two group treatments: a supportive discussion group with education in coping skills or a supportive discussion group alone. The psychoeducational intervention consisted of supportive discussion, venting of feelings, general problem solving and information sharing, PMR, self-hypnosis, GI, goal setting, and general lifestyle management that included diet, exercise, work, recreation, and discussion of spiritual issues. The authors referred to the second group as the control intervention, which consisted of just the supportive discussion, venting of feelings, general problem solving, and information sharing. Another group of 18 patients who delayed starting the intervention for 6 weeks were also tested and they served as a nonrandomized control group. These three groups were all tested before and immediately after group assignment, and 2 to 3 weeks later. Furthermore, a fourth group of 39 patients, who were also nonrandomized, participated in the psychoeducational intervention and were fol-

Follow-up	Outcomes of Intervention: Coping	Affect	QOL	Know	Comp	Phys	Immune	R/S
8 wk	+	+		+				
6 mo	+			+				
6 mo	+	+						
1 y	+	+				+		+
4 wk	+	+		+				
3 wk		+						
4 mo	+	+	+	+		NC		
6 mo	+	+						
3 mo	+	+						
3 mo		+						
5 mo	+	+						
8 wk	+	+	+					
12 wk	+		+	+		+		
6 mo	+	+	+				+	
6 y								+

lowed up for 3 months. Assessments were done with the POMS and the Hopkins 90-Item Symptom Checklist, Revised, both measures of affective state. Both intervention groups showed a significant improvement in affective state compared with the no treatment control group. The psychoeducational group showed a greater gain. The 39 patients in the fourth group demonstrated a sustained improvement to the 3-month follow-up.

Cunningham et al[56] used the POMS, the Functional Living Index for Cancer, and the Stanford Inventory of Cancer Patient Adjustment to assess improvements in the quality of life among 400 cancer patients who completed a brief support group program intended to train patients in coping skills. The results showed that subgroups based on religious status, gender, education level, marital status, and previous experience with mental self-help techniques did not vary significantly, but the overall program increased coping skills and enhanced mood states for most of the subjects involved. The seven-session intervention appeared to benefit younger patients somewhat more than older ones, and at the 3-month follow-up, positive improvements remained. There was no random selection or a control group used in this study.

Cella and associates[57] detailed an 8-week support group for 77 cancer patients in a local community. There was no random selection or a control group in this study. As expected, self-reported quality of life improved significantly by the final session, compared with reports completed at the start of the intervention. Community and peer support was noted by participants as the most helpful aspect of the program and the group evaluations showed high satisfaction levels in all areas.

Berglund et al[58] established a prospective randomized study with 98 cancer patients who took part in a rehabilitation program and 101 patients who served as controls. The intervention, which focused on "starting again," consisted of 11 structured, 2-hour group sessions that were led by an oncology nurse during a period of 7 weeks. Physical training, coping skills, and information were the primary goals of the program, while assessments were made using the Cancer Inventory of Problem Situations, the Quality of Life (two global items) Scale, and the Mental Adjustment to Cancer Scale. The subjects in the experimental condition improved significantly in physical training, physical strength, fighting spirit, body image, sufficient information, and sleeping when compared with the control patients. All three goals of the intervention were met, and results indicated that the "Starting Again" program has many beneficial effects for cancer patients.

Finally, Fawzy et al[59] recognized that each of the categories of therapies resulted in some positive effects but that the variance accounted for by each of these alone was small. Therefore, specific portions of those interventions that were found to be effective and appropriate were combined in a 6-week structured group intervention that was tailored to encompass health education, stress management, coping skills, and supportive group psychotherapy.

Health care information specific to the particular type of cancer was provided. The stress management component was divided into two main sections. First, the patients were taught about stress awareness, which was defined as identifying the sources of stress and their personal reactions to it. The second component was the actual management of stress. Patients were taught simple relaxation exercises, including PMR followed by GI or self-hypnosis. In the coping skills component of the intervention, patients were first taught the components of problem-solving and were then introduced to the concept of coping methods. The final part of the coping skills component involved integrating the stress management and problem-solving techniques with the information on coping methods and applying these to specific situations. The method used was modeled after the Omega Project.[47,48] New pictures illustrating 10 common problems and/or situations encountered by cancer patients were developed.[27] Psychological support was inherent throughout the intervention. The interaction of patients within the group provided a significant source of emotional support.

This intervention was used for a group of patients with newly diagnosed malignant melanoma who had undergone standard surgical treatment. The patients were randomly assigned to either a control group that received routine medical care or an experimental group that received the same kind of routine medical care plus the intervention described above.

All the patients reported moderate to high levels of psychological distress at baseline comparable to other cancer patients. However, at the end of the 6-week structured group intervention, the experimental subjects exhibited significantly lower levels of distress than the control subjects. Six months following the intervention, the group differences were even more pronounced. The experimental group reported significantly lower levels of confusion, depression, fatigue, and total mood disturbance, and higher levels of vigor on the POMS.

Immediately following the 6-week structured intervention, the experimental subjects showed significantly greater use of active-behavioral coping methods than the control subjects. In addition, the experimental subjects used significantly more active-positive, active-expressive, active-reliance, cognitive-positive, and distraction coping strategies. Six months following the intervention, patients in the experimental group continued to use significantly more active-behavioral coping methods as well as more active-cognitive coping methods than the controls.

At the end of the 6-week intervention, there was a significant increase in the percentage of large granular lymphocytes (defined as CD57 with Leu-7). Six months following the intervention, there continued to be an increase in the percentage of large granular lymphocytes (defined as CD57 with Leu-7) as well as increases in natural killer cells (defined as CD16 with Leu-11 and CD56 with Leu-19) and interferon α–augmented natural killer cell cytotoxicity.

In both experimental and control subjects combined, quality of life was strongly negatively correlated with anxiety (P=.0001), depression (P=.0001), anger (P=.007), confusion (P=.0001), and total mood disturbance (P=.0001) at 6 months' follow-up. As negative affective state decreased through lower levels of anxiety, depression, anger, confusion, and total mood disturbance, the quality of life of these patients increased.

At the 6-year follow-up, recurrence and survival were assessed. For the control group, there was a trend for recurrence (13 of 34) and statistically significant greater rate of death (10 of 34) than for the experimental patients (seven of 34 and three of 34, respectively).[1,60]

CONCLUSIONS

The psychological and medical problems encountered by cancer patients are numerous and unique. Based on a review of the literature and our clinical and research experience, cancer patients may benefit from a variety of psychological intervention programs. A structured, psychiatric intervention consisting of health education, stress management and behavioral training, coping including problem-solving techniques, and psychosocial group support offers the greatest potential benefit for patients who are newly diagnosed or in the early stages of their treatment. Patients are usually distressed, anxious, and unable to effectively utilize their normal coping styles. A structured intervention offered early on during the course of cancer diagnosis and treatment may be less stigmatizing and more readily accepted by both patients and staff and easily integrated into the comprehensive medical care of patients with cancer. The advantages of such a program include easy implementation and replication, promotion of important illness-related problem-solving skills, and increased participation in decision making and active coping. A short-term, structured, psychoeducational group intervention is the model that we propose to be used for newly diagnosed patients and/or patients with good prognoses. The focus is on learning how to live with cancer. We also encourage the development of ongoing weekly group support programs for patients with advanced metastatic disease, based on the studies of Spiegel et al,[6,49] that focus on daily coping, pain management, and dealing with the existential issues related to death and dying. Psychiatric interventions should be used as an integral part of competent, comprehensive medical care and not as an independent treatment modality for cancer.

Accepted for publication December 14, 1994.

Reprint requests to UCLA Neuropsychiatric Institute, 760 Westwood Plaza, Los Angeles, CA 90024-1759 (Dr F. Fawzy).

REFERENCES

1. Fawzy FI, Fawzy NW, Hyun CS, Elashoff R, Guthrie D, Fahey JL, Morton D. Malignant melanoma: effects of an early structured psychiatric intervention, coping, and affective state on recurrence and survival 6 years later. *Arch Gen Psychiatry.* 1993;50:681-689.
2. Cohen J, Cullen J, Martin L. *Psychosocial Aspects of Cancer.* New York, NY: Raven Press; 1982.
3. Fawzy FI, Fawzy NW. Psychosocial aspects of cancer. *Diagnosis and Management of Cancer.* Menlo Park, Calif: Addison-Wesley Publishing Co; 1982.
4. Bloom JR, Ross RD, Burnell GM. The effect of social support on patient adjustment following breast surgery. *Patient Counseling Health Educ.* 1978;1:50-59.
5. Holland J. The current concepts and challenges in psychosocial oncology. *Current Concepts in Psychosocial Oncology: Syllabus of Postgraduate Course.* New York, NY: Memorial Sloan-Kettering Cancer Center; 1982.
6. Spiegel D, Bloom JR, Kraemer HC, Gottheil E. Effect of psychosocial treatment on survival of patients with metastatic breast cancer. *Lancet.* 1989;2:888-891.
7. Ornish D, Brown SE, Scherwitz LW, Billings JH, Armstrong WT, Ports TA, McLanahan SM, Kirkeeide RL, Brand RJ, Gould KL. Can lifestyle changes reverse coronary heart disease? *Lancet.* 1992;336:129-133.
8. Greer S. Psychological response to cancer and survival. *Psychol Med.* 1991;21:43-49.
9. Jacobs C, Ross RD, Walker IM, Stockdale FE.

Behavior of cancer patients: a randomized study of the effects of education and peer support groups. *Am J Clin Oncol.* 1983;6:347-353.
10. Rainey LC. Effects of preparatory patient education for radiation oncology patients. *Cancer.* 1985;56:1056-1061.
11. Ali NS, Khalil HZ. Effect of psychoeducational intervention on anxiety among Egyptian bladder cancer patients. *Cancer Nurs.* 1989;12:236-242.
12. Richardson JL, Shelton DR, Krailo M, Levine AM. The effect of compliance with treatment on survival among patients with hematologic malignancies. *J Clin Oncol.* 1990;8:356-364.
13. Pruitt BT, Waligora-Serafin B, McMahon T, Byrd G, Besselman L, Kelly GM, Drake DA, Cuellar D. An educational intervention for newly-diagnosed cancer patients undergoing radiotherapy. *Psycho-oncology.* 1993;2:55-62.
14. Cassileth B, Volckmar D, Goodman RL. The effect of experience on radiation therapy patients desire for information. *Int J Radiat Oncol Biol Phys.* 1980;6:493-496.
15. Massie MJ, Holland JC, Straker N. Psychotherapeutic interventions. *Handbook of Psychooncology.* New York, NY: Oxford Univeristy Press; 1989: 455-469.
16. Laszlo J. *Antiemetics and Cancer Chemotherapy.* Baltimore, Md: Williams & Wilkins; 1983.
17. Burish TG, Lyles JN. Effectiveness of relaxation training in reducing adverse reactions to cancer chemotherapy. *J Behav Med.* 1981;4:65-78.
18. Morrow GR, Morrell C. Behavioral treatment for the anticipatory nausea and vomiting induced by cancer chemotherapy. *N Engl J Med.* 1982;307: 1476-1480.
19. Lyles JN, Burish TG, Krozely MG, Oldham RK. Efficacy of relaxation training and guided imagery in reducing the aversiveness of cancer chemotherapy. *J Consult Clin Psychol.* 1982;50: 509-524.
20. Cotanch PH. Relaxation training for control of nausea and vomiting in patients receiving chemotherapy. *Cancer Nurs.* 1983;6:277-283.
21. Carey MP, Burish TG. Providing relaxation training to cancer chemotherapy patients: a comparison of three delivery techniques. *J Consult Clin Psychol.* 1987;55:732-737.
22. Burish TG, Snyder SL, Jenkins RA. Preparing patients for cancer chemotherapy: effect of coping preparation and relaxation interventions. *J Consult Clin Psychol.* 1991;59:518-525.
23. Davis H-IV. Effects of biofeedback and cognitive therapy on stress in patients with breast cancer. *Psychol Rep.* 1986;59:967-974.
24. Gruber BL, Hall NR, Hersh SP, Dubois P. Immune system and psychological changes in metastatic cancer patients using relaxation and guided imagery: a pilot study. *Scand J Behav Ther.* 1988; 17:25-46.
25. Gruber BL, Hersh SP, Hall NRS, Waletzky LR, Kunz JF, Carpenter JK, Kverno KS, Weiss SM. Immunological responses of breast cancer patients to behavioral interventions. *Biofeedback Self Regul.* 1993;18:1-21.
26. Baider L, Uziely B, De-Nour AK. Progressive muscle relaxation and guided imagery in cancer patients. *Gen Hosp Psychiatry.* 1994;16:340-347.
27. Fawzy FI, Cousins N, Fawzy NW, Kennedy ME, Elashoff R, Morton D. A structured psychiatric intervention for cancer patients, I: changes over time in methods of coping and affective disturbance. *Arch Gen Psychiatry.* 1990;47:720-725.
28. Greer S, Moorey S, Baruch JDR. Adjuvant psychological therapy for patients with cancer: a prospective randomised trial. *BMJ.* 1992;304:675-680.
29. Capone MA, Good RS, Westie KS, Jacobson AF. Psychosocial rehabilitation of gynecologic oncology patients. *Arch Phys Med Rehabil.* 1980; 61:128-132.
30. Gordon WA, Freidenbergs I, Diller L, Hibbard M, Wolf C, Levine L, Lipkins R, Ezrachi O, Lucido D. Efficacy of psychosocial intervention with cancer patients. *J Consult Clin Psychol.* 1980;48: 743-759.
31. Maguire P, Tait A, Brooke M, Thomas C, Sellwood R. Effect of counseling on the psychiatric morbidity associated with mastectomy. *BMJ.* 1980; 281:1454-1456.
32. Linn MW, Linn BS, Harris R. Effects of counseling for late-stage cancer patients. *Cancer.* 1982; 49:1048-1055.
33. Worden JW, Weisman AD. Preventive psychosocial intervention with newly diagnosed cancer patients. *Gen Hosp Psychiatry.* 1984;6:243-249.
34. Grossarth-Maticek R, Schmidt P, Vetter H, Arndt S. Psychotherapy research in oncology. In: Steptoe A, Mathews A, eds. *Health Care and Human Behavior.* London, England: Academic Press; 1984: 325-341.
35. Pervin LA. *Psychological Inquiry: An International Journal of Peer Commentary and Review.* Hillsdale, NJ: Lawrence Erlbaum Associates; 1991; 2(no. 3).
36. Van der Ploeg HM. What a wonderful world it would be: a reanalysis of some of the work of Grossarth-Maticek. *Psychol Inquiry.* 1991;2:280-285.
37. Spiegel D. Second thoughts on personality, stress, and disease. *Psychol Inquiry.* 1991;2:266-268.
38. Fox BH. Quandaries created by unlikely numbers in some of Grossarth-Maticek's studies. *Psychol Inquiry.* 1991;2:242-247.
39. Forester B, Kornfeld DS, Fleiss JL. Psychotherapy during radiotherapy: effects on emotional and physical distress. *Am J Psychiatry.* 1985;142:22-27.
40. Houts PS, Whitney CW, Mortel R, Bartholomew MJ. Former cancer patients as counselors of newly diagnosed cancer patients. *J Natl Cancer Inst.* 1986;76:793-796.
41. McCorkle R, Benoliel JQ, Donaldson G, Georgiadou F, Moinpour C, Goodell B. A randomized clinical trial of home nursing care for lung cancer patients. *Cancer.* 1989;64:1375-1382.
42. Mermelstein HT, Holland JC. Psychotherapy by telephone. *Psychosomatics.* 1991;32:407-412.
43. Edgar L, Rosberger Z, Nowlis D. Coping with cancer during the first year after diagnosis. *Cancer.* 1992;69:817-828.
44. Moorey S, Greer S, Watson M, Baruch JDR, Robertson BM, Mason A, Rowden L, Tunmore R, Law M, Bliss JM. Adjuvant psychological therapy for patients with cancer: outcome at one year. *Psycho-oncology.* 1994;3:39-46.
45. Wood PE, Milligan M, Christ D, Liff D. Group counseling for cancer patients in a community hospital. *Psychosomatics.* 1978;19:555-561.
46. Ferlic M, Goldman A, Kennedy BJ. Group counseling in adult patients with advanced cancer. *Cancer.* 1979;43:760-766.
47. Weisman AD, Worden JW, Sobel HJ. *Psychosocial Screening and Intervention With Cancer Patients: Research Report.* Cambridge, Mass: Shea Bros; 1980.
48. Sobel HJ, Worden JW. *Practitioner's Manual: Helping Cancer Patients Cope.* New York, NY: Guilford Publications; 1982:1-32.
49. Spiegel D, Bloom JR, Yalom I. Group support for patients with metastatic cancer. *Arch Gen Psychiatry.* 1981;38:527-533.
50. Johnson J. The effects of a patient education course on persons with a chronic illness. *Cancer Nurs.* 1982;April:117-123.
51. Vachon MLS, Lyall WAL, Rogers J, Cochrane J, Freeman SJJ. The effectiveness of psychosocial support during post-surgical treatment of breast cancer. *Int J Psychiatry Med.* 1982; 11:365-372.
52. Heinrich RL, Schag CC. Stress and activity management: group treatment for cancer patients and spouses. *J Consult Clin Psychol.* 1985;33:439-446.
53. Cain EN, Kohorn EI, Quinland DM, Latimer K, Schwartz PE. Psychosocial benefits of a cancer support group. *Cancer.* 1986;57:183-189.
54. Telch CF, Telch MJ. Group coping skills instruction and supportive group therapy for cancer patients: a comparison of strategies. *J Consult Clin Psychol.* 1986;54:802-808.
55. Cunningham AJ, Tocco EK. A randomized trial of group psychoeducational therapy for cancer patients. *Patient Educ Counsel.* 1989;14:101-114.
56. Cunningham AJ, Lockwood GA, Edmonds CVI. Which cancer patients benefit most from a brief, group, coping skills program? *Int J Psychiatry Med.* 1993;23:383-398.
57. Cella DF, Sarafian B, Snider PR, Yellen SB, Winicour P. Evaluation of a community-based cancer support group. *Psycho-oncology.* 1993;2: 123-132.
58. Berglund G, Bolund C, Gustafsson U, Sjoden P. A randomized study of a rehabilitation program for cancer patients: the 'starting again' group. *Psycho-oncology.* 1994;3:109-120.
59. Fawzy FI, Fawzy NW, Hyun CS. Short-term psychiatric intervention for patients with malignant melanoma: effects on psychological state, coping, and the immune system. The Psychoimmunology of Cancer. New York, NY: Oxford University Press; 1994:292-319.
60. Fawzy FI, Kemeny ME, Fawzy N, Elashoff R, Morton D, Cousins N, Fahey JL. A structured psychiatric intervention for cancer patients, II: changes over time in immunological measures. *Arch Gen Psychiatry.* 1990;47:729-735.

ORIGINAL ARTICLE

Switching From 'Unipolar' to Bipolar II

An 11-Year Prospective Study of Clinical and Temperamental Predictors in 559 Patients

Hagop S. Akiskal, MD; Jack D. Maser, PhD; Pamela J. Zeller, PhD; Jean Endicott, PhD; William Coryell, MD; Martin Keller, MD; Meredith Warshaw, MS; Paula Clayton, MD; Frederick Goodwin, MD

Background: Given the therapeutic and prognostic importance of the unipolar-bipolar dichotomy, predicting which patients will become bipolar subsequent to index diagnosis of major depressive disorder (MDD) is of paramount clinical significance. We sought to characterize the profile of patients with MDD who would convert to the more subtle bipolar subtype (known as BPII) on the basis of clinical and personality variables obtained during MDD episodes.

Methods: A total of 559 patients, comprehensively evaluated with the Schedule of Affective Disorders and Schizophrenia and "unipolar" MDD at entry, were administered 17 self-report personality measures. Hypomanic and manic episodes were systematically recorded over a prospective observation period of up to 11 years. We compared 48 converters to BPII (8.6%) with 22 converters to bipolar I (BPI) (3.9%) and the remaining larger group of unipolar patients.

Results: Except for greater acuteness, severity, and psychotic symptomatology, BPI converters were essentially similar to MDD nonconverters. By contrast, BPII converters were robustly distinguished from those with MDD who remained unipolar on the basis of self-report measures along the newly derived factors of Mood Lability, Energy-Activity, and Daydreaming. This profile was associated with early age at onset of MDD and pleomorphic psychopathology beyond the usual affective realm, high rates of substance abuse, as well as educational, marital, and occupational disruption and minor antisocial acts prior to discrete hypomanic episodes. Overall, BPII switchers had a more protracted and tempestuous course with shorter well intervals. "Habitual self" descriptions of temperamental instability during MDD episodes provided useful clinical information for predicting which depressed patients will switch to BPII, attaining a sensitivity of 91% for all three factors combined (23 items); Mood Lability alone (nine items) was the most specific predictor (86%), though of lower sensitivity (42%).

Conclusions: The BPII subtype is best understood by such lability intruding into, and possibly its accentuation during, depressive episodes, thereby creating an intimate interweaving of trait and state. Clinicians must note that the foregoing temperamental profile appears more fundamental in defining the affective dysregulation of the BPII subtype than hypomanic episodes emphasized in *DSM-IV*.

(Arch Gen Psychiatry. 1995;52:114-123)

From the National Institute of Mental Health (NIMH) Collaborative Program on the Psychobiology of Depression (Clinical Studies) (Drs Akiskal, Maser, Endicott, Coryell, Keller, Clayton, and Goodwin and Ms Warshaw) and DataMax, Inc, Rockville, Md (Dr Zeller). For other members of the NIMH Collaborative Program on the Psychobiology of Depression, see box at the end of the article.

THE SWITCH process (ie, hypomanic or manic shifts in clinically depressed patients) and the broader phenomenon of bipolar conversion over the course of major depressive disorder (MDD) are fascinating from a psychobiologic perspective.[1,2] Given the therapeutic and prognostic significance of the unipolar-bipolar dichotomy, predicting which patients will become bipolar subsequent to an index diagnosis of MDD is of considerable clinical significance. Much past research has focused on conversions of MDD to full-blown manic depressive or bipolar I (BPI) disorders.[3-8] Rates have varied from 0%[8] to 37.5%[4] (median, 9.7%). Bipolar family history in consecutive generations, adolescent or early adult age at onset, and acute onset of episodes with stupor or psychotic features have been reported to distinguish converters from nonconverters.[5,6] These variables, which were tested more recently by Coryell et al,[9] were found to be of relatively modest clinical utility because of their very low sensitivity; moreover, their main relevance is for BPI conversion.

Because of the difficulties of ascertaining hypomania by history,[10-13] conversion to bipolar II (BPII) disorder presents the greater challenge for the clinician. This

See Methods on next page

METHODS

THE COLLABORATIVE DEPRESSION STUDY

The data reported are drawn from the National Institute of Mental Health (NIMH) Collaborative Depression Study (CDS), a longitudinal, prospective investigation of the phenomenology, nosology, familial aggregation, and course in 955 moderately to severely ill affective probands seeking treatment at one of five university centers. As described elsewhere,[19-21] the probands were predominantly inpatients (79.7%); all were white, English speaking, at least 17 years old, knowledgeable about both biological parents, had an IQ of at least 70, and were without evidence of concurrent organic mental disorder or terminal illness.

The subjects were comprehensively evaluated for current and past history of mental disorders using the Research Diagnostic Criteria (RDC),[22] based on the Schedule of Affective Disorders and Schizophrenia (SADS).[23] Prospective data were gathered at 6-month intervals for 5 years and yearly thereafter, through 11 years at this writing, via the Longitudinal Interval Follow-up Evaluation[21] or variations of that form designed for less frequent follow-up. Information from psychiatric records was routinely incorporated into the patients' intake and follow-up interviews, thereby ensuring a record of hypomania (and/or mania) if or when it occurred.

PERSONALITY BATTERY

Patients and controls completed a 436-item self-report personality battery[24] that consisted of 17 conventional personality scales thought to be relevant to affective disorders: the General Activity, Restraint, Ascendance, Sociability, Emotional Stability, Objectivity, and Thoughtfulness scales of the Guilford-Zimmerman Temperament Survey (GZTS)[25]; the Emotional Reliance on Another Person, Lack of Social Self-confidence, and Assertion of Autonomy scales of the Interpersonal Dependency Inventory[26]; the Orality, Obsessionality, and Hysterical Pattern scales of the short form of the Lazare-Klerman-Armor Personality Inventory[27]; the Neuroticism and Extraversion-Introversion scales of the Maudsley Personality Inventory[28]; and the Ego Resiliency and Ego Control-5 scales of the Minnesota Multiphasic Personality Inventory (MMPI).[29]

Previous reports from the CDS[30-32] have reported personality measures organized into groups of scales based on their theoretical similarities (eg, emotional strength, interpersonal dependency). For the present article, the 17 scales have been organized into five groups according to their factorial structure (using principal components factor analysis with varimax rotations). By this new analysis (P.J.Z. et al, unpublished data, 1993), seven scales constitute the first group: Neuroticism, Objectivity, Ego Resiliency, Emotional Stability, Orality, Emotional Reliance on Another Person, and Lack of Social Self-confidence. A second group consists of Extraversion, Sociability, and Ascendance. A third group consists of Thoughtfulness and Restraint and a fourth subsumes Ego Control-5 and Obsessionality. Scales measuring Hysterical Pattern, Assertion of Autonomy, and General Activity did not share common variance with any other scales and so are considered alone. The first four of these factors are reminiscent of similar factors in two new widely acclaimed and empirically derived personality systems.[33,34]

IDENTIFICATION OF BIPOLAR CONVERSION IN MDD PATIENTS

Of the 955 patients who entered the CDS (**Table 1**), 730 had definite MDD at intake with no evidence of schizophrenia or schizoaffective disorder (at any time during follow-up). Ninety-six patients with mania prior to intake (BPI) and 75 with hypomania but no mania prior to intake (BPII) were further excluded.

For the remaining 559 patients with MDD defined as having unipolar illness ("unipolar") as of their entry into the study, all available follow-up data were examined to identify those whose first lifetime RDC diagnosis of mania or hypomania developed during the course of prospective follow-up. Mania developed in 22 patients (3.9%) and they were reclassified as BPI converters; hypomania developed first in eight of these 22 and then mania. Hypomania, but no mania, developed in 48 (8.6%) during follow-up (BPII converters). This left 489 index patients with unipolar MDD (87.5%) who remained unipolar throughout follow-up, and provide a comparison to the two groups of converters considered in this article. Because of our focus on BPII, schizoaffective cases were excluded, which is the main reason

Continued on next page

disorder is characterized by severe depressions, typically recurrent, and milder hypomanias of at least a few days' duration. As a result, unless expertly questioned about hypomania, the bipolar nature of these depressions can be missed.

Coryell et al[9] reported that 7.2% of patients with nonbipolar MDD converted to BPII; young age and protracted depressive episodes were the main predictors. The present article focuses on prospective predictors of BPII switching from the vantage of a broader array of clinical, anamnestic, and personality parameters, most of which have not been tested in previous research; data on BPI conversion are presented primarily for comparison. Most important, we undertook these analyses in an effort to characterize self-report trait measures by which depressed patients, who might ultimately be classified as BPII, describe themselves. Such self-description is particularly relevant in that the BPII subtype is often considered to have lifelong instability with cyclothymic and/or labile mood shifts but without necessarily meeting discrete criteria for hypomanic episodes.[14,15] We specifically set out to characterize such temperamental factors that clinical observation[16-18] has linked to "soft" bipolar expressions. Finally, we wished to examine the predictive power of such self-rated temperamental measures relative to observer-rated variables.

RESULTS

COURSE AND EPISODE CHARACTERISTICS OF BIPOLAR CONVERSION

Although 20 of 48 onsets of first BPII disorder (41.7%), compared with six of 22 onsets of first BPI disorder for minor variation in the rates of bipolar conversion compared with an earlier CDS anaysis by Coryell et al[9] (8.6% vs 7.2%).

A high percentage (32.9%) of bipolar converters, eight of 22 BPI and 15 of 48 BPII, began their first lifetime hypomanic or manic episodes during the first 6 months of prospective follow-up. Thereafter, conversion to bipolarity was spread as follows: five cases between 6 months and 1 year of follow-up (7.1%), 10 in the second year of follow-up (14.3%), 23 in the third to fifth years (32.9%), and nine in the sixth to ninth years of follow-up (12.9%). Thus, in line with previous data,[6,9] much of bipolar conversion took place in the first 5 years.

ANALYSIS OF DEMOGRAPHIC AND CLINICAL VARIABLES

Because past research[5,6,9] has shown that different variables would distinguish bipolar converters from the group who remained unipolar, separate χ^2 comparisons to MDD were performed for each of the two converting groups on gender, age, marital status, and education, total number of lifetime episodes of MDD and nonaffective diagnoses, indices of severity of the intake episode, SADS items and scores describing the index MDD episode, and SADS items pertaining to occupational-educational adjustment since age 15 years. To complement clinician-evaluated psychopathology, self-reported symptoms for the week preceding intake and standard scores from the 90-item Hopkins Symptom Checklist-90 (SCL-90)[35] were subjected to analyses of variance, covarying for age and gender.

ANALYSIS OF PERSONALITY VARIABLES

This article goes beyond an analysis of the scores of published scales[24] to delineate the personality profile of bipolar converters based on a regrouping of 436 individual items of the self-report battery. To minimize the state effects of depression on personality,[30] (1) subjects were instructed to ignore their current affective disorder and describe their usual or "habitual self," and (2) the personality battery was administered at the index episode after severe symptoms had abated. Seven additional patients were eliminated from further analyses because their personality assessment was subsequent to their bipolar conversion leaving 20 BPI and 43 BPII converters as the focus of our analyses.

Because past research[16-18] has related certain temperamental traits to soft bipolar disorder such as BPII, we hypothesized that item analyses of certain hypomanic or hyperthymic traits might shed additional light beyond scale score differences. To do so, we first identified those overall scale scores significantly differentiating BPII converters from unipolar patients; items were included if the difference in adjusted means between the groups (after covarying for age and gender) was statistically significant ($P<.05$). Perusal of many items from various scales of the separate instruments in the battery suggested greater commonality than is represented by the conventional names of the scales. For instance, "I have had periods when I felt so full of pep that sleep did not seem necessary for days at a time" is an MMPI Ego Resiliency scale item, yet it has face validity as a measure of Activity-Energy (GZTS), with distinct hypomanic flavor.

To identify the dimensions most relevant to bipolar conversion, principal components factor analyses were performed on 86 items of the personality battery that significantly differentiated BPII from BPI converters. All patients' index personality batteries were used in the factor analysis, regardless of their psychiatric status at the time of personality assessment. Five-factor and 14-factor solutions were selected based on examination of the eigenvalues; factors were rotated by the varimax method, which yields maximally independent factors. Factor scores were generated, based on factor weights for the 86 items, and analyses of variance were performed on the resulting factor scores to compare BPI and BPII converters and unipolar subjects, covarying for age and gender.

To examine the power of index clinical and self-report variables to predict conversion to BPII, logistic regression analyses were performed (SAS LOGISTIC procedure, SAS Institute Inc, Cary, NC) on those variables that had discriminated BPII from unipolar subjects at $P<.05$ by covariate analysis of variance or χ^2 test. The sensitivity and specificity of each of the three most powerful sets of discriminators then were computed for determining their utility as clinical "test" predictors of BPII switching. In this context, sensitivity refers to the percentage of MDD patients with the variable who have switched to BPII, and specificity to the percentage of nonswitchers without the variable.

(27.3%), occurred when the subjects had not yet recovered from the intake episode, this difference was not statistically significant. However, BPI converters recovered from their intake episodes in significantly less than half the time (mean, 24.3 weeks) than did BPII or unipolar patients (mean, 52.5 and 59.3 weeks, respectively; $P<.05$ by generalized Wilcoxon test of Kaplan-Meier product-limit estimates of the survivorship functions). Thus, the index BPI depressive episode was more acute in nature.

Because much of bipolar conversion occurred during the first 5 years, we were interested in comparing the duration of ill vs well periods for the three affective groups. The two converting groups each had a significantly higher number of episodes during this period (mean, 4.0 and 3.5 episodes for BPI and BPII converters, respectively) than the unipolar group (mean, 2.2 episodes; overall $F=27.41$, $df=2$, $P<.001$). Furthermore, BPII converters were ill significantly more than unipolar patients (mean±SD, 119.6±69.0 vs 90.0±87.0 weeks; $t=2.1$, $P<.05$), which means well interepisodic intervals were curtailed in BPII patients.

We next sought to examine whether treatment with heterocyclic antidepressants could account for bipolar conversion. This possibility is unlikely because during the month prior to switching, fewer BPI and BPII converters received heterocyclic antidepressants compared with unipolar probands in a comparable period, ie, their first month of prospective follow-up (40.9%, 28.9%, and 67.7%, respectively).

Bipolar I converters had more severe index episodes than unipolar patients as indicated by the greater likelihood of their being hospitalized (95.4% vs 76.9%, $\chi^2=4.19$, $P=.041$). They also had significantly lower Global Assess-

Table 1. Subject Selection and Rates of Conversion to Bipolar Disorder for 559 Patients With Major Depressive Disorder (MDD) With No History of Mania or Hypomania Followed Up 2 to 11 Years

	No. (%)
Patients entering Collaborative Depression Study	955 (100)
Definite MDD, never schizophrenic or schizoaffective	730 (76.4)
Prior mania (bipolar I)	96 (13.2)
Prior hypomania (bipolar II)	75 (10.3)
Nonbipolar as of index intake	559 (76.6)
Mania during follow-up (bipolar I converters)	22 (3.9)
Hypomania (and no mania) during follow-up (bipolar II converters)	48 (8.6)
No mania or hypomania during follow-up (unipolar MDD)	489 (87.5)

ment Scale scores (indicative of more impaired functioning) in the week prior to the index assessment (36.9±8.7 vs 43.4±11.5, t=3.30, P<.001). Bipolar I converters were rated by clinicians as being significantly worse than unipolar patients on individual SADS items that pertained to feelings of inadequacy and discouragement, psychic anxiety, inability to concentrate, social withdrawal, and impaired functioning, as well as delusions and/or hallucinations (all P<.05). No SCL-90 scores differentiated BPI converters from those who remained unipolar. The same was true for all 17 of the personality scales.

CLINICAL CORRELATES OF BPII CONVERSION

Bipolar II converters and unipolar probands were similar in terms of gender (68.8% and 59.1% female, respectively). However, they were significantly younger than subjects who remained unipolar (average age of 33.7 vs 40.1 years, t=2.84, P=.005). Converters were less likely to be married or living with a partner at the time of admission to the study (31.2% vs 50.9%) and were more likely to be separated, widowed, or divorced (33.3% vs 20.9%) or never married (35.4% vs 28.1%) (overall χ^2=7.29, P=.03). To control for the possible effect of age, marital status was examined among those subjects who were at least 25 years old at admission, and the risk of marital disruption remained 1.7 times higher for BPII converters than for unipolar patients.

Bipolar II converters also had a significantly earlier age of onset at first MDD episode (mean±SD, 25.4±10.2 vs 31.3±14.3 years, t=2.79, P=.006). In terms of overall characteristics of their index MDD episode, subjects who converted to BPII disorder had a significantly longer period of illness prior to entry into the study (median duration of 142 vs 57 weeks; χ^2 test for difference of medians, P=.04). However, converters did not differ significantly from unipolar patients on primary/secondary MDD, inpatient/outpatient status, level of overall functioning during the index episode (by Global Assessment Scale), or on the highest level of overall functioning during the 5 years before admission.

Rates of lifetime RDC diagnoses of nonaffective disorders were similar for BPII converters and unipolar patients, except that converters were more likely to be rated as ever having RDC cyclothymic personality (8.3% vs 2.9%, χ^2=4.04, P=.04) or drug use disorder other than alcohol (22.9% vs 11.4%, χ^2=5.26, P=.022). Lifetime rates of alcoholism were similar for the two groups (BPII, 31.2%; unipolar, 29.2%), and the same was true for anxiety-related diagnoses (BPII, 18.8%; MDD, 15.1%).

Bipolar II converters were compared with patients who remained unipolar on individual SADS items and scores describing the index episode. Converters were significantly more socially withdrawn than unipolar patients (52.1% vs 35.4%, χ^2=5.24, P=.02). Furthermore, converters were more than twice as likely to have been rated by the clinician as currently or recently engaging at least occasionally in minor antisocial acts of a clinically significant nature (14.6% vs 6.1%; χ^2=4.86, P=.03), but they were still well below the diagnostic threshold for antisocial personality. Significantly more BPII converters than unipolar patients (37.5% vs 23.9%) were rated as having shown evidence of poor long-term occupational or educational adjustment (χ^2=4.28, P=.04), based on frequent job changes, long periods of unemployment, frequent absences from work, or poor academic performance.

This unstable profile is further reflected in pleomorphic symptomatology beyond typical affective boundaries. Thus, subjects who became BPII during follow-up scored significantly worse than unipolar subjects on summary SADS scores on Miscellaneous Psychopathology (mean±SD, 26.2±6.4 vs 24.2±5.8, t=2.06, P=.04) during the index episode. Among nonpsychotic patients, this last score summarizes responses to SADS items on obsessions-compulsions, somatic preoccupation, depersonalization, subjective anger, suspiciousness, ideas of reference, self-pity, and demandingness. The foregoing clinician-rated complex psychopathology was paralleled by significantly higher self-reported Interpersonal Sensitivity, Depression, Phobic Anxiety, and Psychoticism scores on the SCL-90 (**Table 2**) in BPII converters compared with those subjects who remained unipolar.

PERSONALITY AND BPII CONVERSION

Compared with patients who remained unipolar, BPII converters scored significantly higher during their index episode on scales measuring Neuroticism, Orality, Emotional Reliance on Another Person, and Lack of Social Self-confidence, while being significantly lower on scales measuring Ego Resiliency and Emotional Stability (**Table 3**). Objectivity was marginally lower for the BPII converters (P=.05). The rest of the personality scales were comparable in the two groups.

We next describe four newly derived personality factors that differentiated the BPII converters from patients who remained unipolar (**Table 4**).

Mood Lability, combining items from the GZTS Emotional Stability and MMPI Neuroticism scales, emerged as the unique discriminating trait of BPII. Thus, the average weighted factor score for BPII converters was +0.69, which is dramatically higher than the +0.11 for unipolar subjects. Curiously, BPI converters' weighted score on this factor (+0.12) was similar to that of patients with unipolar MDD.

Table 2. Hopkins Symptom Checklist-90 (SCL-90) Significant Scores and Items for Patients With Major Depressive Disorder at Index Who Converted to Bipolar II During Follow-up vs Those Who Remained Unipolar*

SCL-90 Score and Items†	Bipolar II Converters (N=47)‡	Unipolar (N=475)‡	*P*
Interpersonal Sensitivity (two of nine items significant)	27.0 (8.5)	24.4 (9.2)	.051
61. Feeling uneasy when people are watching or talking about you	3.1 (1.6)	2.6 (1.4)	.025
69. Feeling very self-conscious with others	3.4 (1.4)	2.8 (1.4)	.004
Depression (four of 13 items significant)	35.1 (8.3)	32.4 (9.2)	.049
9. Feeling lonely	4.0 (1.3)	3.4 (1.4)	.006
54. Feeling hopeless about the future	4.0 (1.2)	3.5 (1.4)	.011
71. Feeling everything is an effort	3.9 (1.2)	3.1 (1.4)	.001
79. Feelings of worthlessness	3.9 (1.5)	3.3 (1.5)	.007
Phobic Anxiety (five of seven items significant)	23.2 (1.2)	19.2 (8.5)	.002
13. Feeling afraid in open spaces or on the street	2.1 (1.4)	1.6 (1.1)	.010
25. Feeling afraid to go out of your house alone	2.1 (1.4)	1.6 (1.1)	.006
47. Feeling afraid to travel on buses, subways, or trains	2.1 (1.5)	1.6 (1.2)	.012
70. Feeling uneasy in crowds, such as shopping or at a movie	3.0 (1.5)	2.3 (1.5)	.003
75. Feeling nervous when you are left alone	3.1 (1.5)	2.3 (1.4)	.0004
Psychoticism (three of 10 items significant)	21.6 (7.1)	19.4 (6.6)	.031
77. Feeling lonely even when you are with people	3.5 (1.3)	2.9 (1.4)	.005
88. Never feeling close to another person	3.0 (1.3)	2.4 (1.5)	.007
90. The idea that something is wrong with your mind	3.4 (1.4)	2.9 (1.5)	.014

Analysis of variance, covarying for age and sex. Data are given as adjusted mean (SD).

†Scores based on response to items describing how much symptom bothered or distressed the patient during the past week or so, with response opinions as follows: 1=not at all; 2=a little bit; 3=moderately; 4=quite a bit; and 5=extremely.

‡One bipolar II converter and 14 unipolar patients did not complete an intake SCL-90.

The second factor that distinguished BPII converters from unipolar MDD subjects is Energy-Activity. Five items of the GZTS General Activity scale define this factor, which also includes items from three other personality instruments. It is noteworthy that the GZTS General Activity scale did not significantly differentiate the two groups, yet the new factor indicating hyperenergetic involvement in activities did (average factor score of +0.32 for BPII vs −0.20 for unipolar). Bipolar I converters' average score of −0.01 on this factor indicates neither high nor low energy.

Items pertaining to the third factor, Daydreaming, come from three different GZTS scales, plus the Maudsley Personality Inventory Neuroticism and MMPI Ego Resiliency scales. Together they comprise a set of items that significantly differentiated BPII converters from unipolar subjects (mean factor scores of +0.34 and −0.07, respectively). Bipolar I converters had a low positive score on this factor (+0.09).

The fourth factor that differentiated BPII converters from unipolar subjects is related to insecurity concerning social encounters (Social Anxiety), and is defined by several items from the Interpersonal Dependency Inventory Lack of Social Self-confidence scale, with additional items from four other scales within the personality battery. Bipolar II converters averaged +0.35 on the weighted factor score for this dimension, compared with −0.01 for unipolar patients, and −0.16 for BPI converters.

RELATIVE PREDICTIVE POWER OF CLINICAL VS PERSONALITY VARIABLES

The unique predictive power of each variable, statistically controlling for all the other variables, was determined by a logistic regression that considered all the variables together. Of the different types of predictors analyzed herein, three of four of the newly derived measures of self-reported usual personality (Mood Lability, Energy-Activity, and Daydreaming) each had stronger predictive power for identifying BPII converters than any other variable considered. Three of the SCL-90 scores, reflecting self-reported Phobic Anxiety, Depression, and Interpersonal Sensitivity, were the next best predictors of BPII conversion; these were followed by the newly derived personality factor of Social Anxiety, and the SCL-90 Psychoticism score.

The power of each set of the foregoing predictors was further evaluated through separate logistic regression analyses using the three subsets of variables: clinical descriptors, self-reported symptoms, and self-reported personality (**Table 5**). Among the clinical predictors, age and the SADS score summarizing Miscellaneous Psychopathology were the only two that entered the model, indicating that the predictive power of all other clinical descriptors was captured in these two variables. In an analysis based on self-reported symptoms alone, the SCL-90 scores representing Phobic Anxiety and Depression entered the model, with Interpersonal Sensitivity and Psychoticism contributing no further prediction to BPII conversion. In the analysis based on self-reported usual personality, the three scores measuring Mood Lability, Energy-Activity, and Daydreaming significantly predicted BPII switching; Social Anxiety did not contribute further to the prediction of BPII conversion. The agreement (concordance) between rank-ordered predicted vs actual outcome (switching to BPII disorder) was 79.6% for the three personality factor scores, compared with 67.0% for the two self-reported symptom scores and 64.4% for the two strongest clinical predictors.

In addition to overall goodness of fit, the logistic regression models can be evaluated in terms of their sensitivity or ability to correctly identify BPII converters (true positives) vs their specificity or ability to correctly iden-

Table 3. Index Personality Scores of Patients With Unipolar Major Depression Disorder Who Switched to Bipolar II During Follow-up vs Those Who Remained Unipolar*

Personality Scale†	Bipolar II Converters (N=43)‡	Unipolar (N=447)	Significance
Neuroticism (MPI)	37.9 (8.6)	32.5 (11.3)	F=9.18, *P*=.003
Objectivity (GZTS)	12.0 (5.0)	13.7 (5.6)	F=3.72, *P*=.054
Ego Resiliency (MMPI)	16.7 (4.1)	18.4 (5.3)	F=4.30, *P*=.039
Emotional Stability (GZTS)	8.2 (5.4)	10.7 (6.4)	F=6.22, *P*=.013
Orality (LKA)	10.4 (4.3)	8.7 (4.4)	F=6.36, *P*=.012
Emotional Reliance on Another Person (IDI)	54.4 (9.2)	48.9 (9.7)	F=12.29, *P*=.0005
Lack of Social Self-confidence	40.9 (9.9)	37.0 (9.0)	F=7.16, *P*=.008
Extraversion (MPI)	20.6 (10.1)	21.0 (10.5)	F=0.06, *P*=.81
Sociability (GZTS)	15.1 (7.0)	14.3 (7.2)	F=0.53, *P*=.47
Ascendance (GZTS)	12.0 (6.1)	12.3 (6.4)	F=0.13, *P*=.72
Thoughtfulness (GZTS)	18.7 (4.3)	18.3 (5.0)	F=0.25, *P*=.61
Restraint (GZTS)	17.4 (5.2)	17.9 (4.6)	F=0.47, *P*=.49
Ego Control-5 (MMPI)	16.2 (4.9)	17.1 (4.8)	F=1.57, *P*=.21
Obsessionality (LKA)	11.9 (3.5)	11.9 (3.6)	F=0.00, *P*=.99
Hysterical Pattern (LKA)	6.6 (4.0)	6.2 (3.9)	F=0.34, *P*=.56
Assertion of Autonomy (IDI)	29.1 (8.4)	28.2 (7.3)	F=2.8, *P*=.01
General Activity (GZTS)	16.9 (6.9)	15.1 (6.7)	F=2.8, *P*=.01

**Analysis of variance, covarying for age and sex. Data are given as adjusted mean (SD).*

†MPI indicates Maudsley Personality Inventory[28]; GZTS, Guilford-Zimmerman Temperament Survey[25]; MMPI, Minnesota Multiphasic Personality Inventory[29]; LKA, Lazare-Klerman-Armor Personality Inventory (short form)[27]; and IDI, Interpersonal Dependency Inventory.[26]

‡Personality was assessed late in the index episode; cases are omitted if switching occurred prior to such assessment (48−5=43).

tify patients with MDD who remain unipolar (true negatives) at different thresholds or cut points of predicted value. At a high level of sensitivity (81.0%), the two best clinical predictors and the two best self-described symptom scores each had low specificity (32.7% and 38.8%, respectively). By comparison, prediction based on the three new personality factor scores of Mood Lability, Energy-Activity, and Daydreaming attained a sensitivity level of 90.7%, with a specificity of 44.9%. This high sensitivity was achieved at the expense of a high rate of false positives (55.1%). Given the low probability of BPII conversion in this sample (8.6%), the high sensitivity of prediction from the newly derived personality self-report measures provides a promising approach in identifiying persons at risk for converting to BPII disorder. The highest specificity (86.2%) was achieved with Mood Lability (all nine items), albeit with low sensitivity (41.9%).

COMMENT

Consistent with previous studies,[5,6] including a more recent definitive report from the CDS,[9] BPI conversion was more likely from an acute, severe, psychotic depression (even though the present analyses had excluded schizoaffective patients), while BPII converters tended to pursue a course characterized by protracted depressive episodes with shorter well intervals.[36] The present analyses sought to characterize the temperamental instability predictive of the latter course pattern.

Our major finding is the differential impact of "habitual self" descriptions by clinically depressed patients in predicting those who will ultimately switch to BPII. Conceivably contaminated by state depression, these descriptors of presumably long-term trait characteristics—Mood Lability, Energy-Activity, and Daydreaming—nonetheless robustly distinguished them from both BPI converters and those who remained unipolar for up to 11 years of prospective observation. The discussion that follows addresses various methodologic, conceptual, and clinical issues relevant to BPII conversion.

Although family history for mania is a risk factor for the development of BPI disorder,[5,6,9] it makes relatively little contribution in defining the BPII subtype.[37] The Family History-RDC procedure[38] used with each patient in the CDS has no provision for recording periods of hypomania or even making inquiry for them. This is considered problematic for the proband's personal history, let alone for family members. Accordingly, the present analyses did not examine this variable for BPII conversion.

The diagnosis of BPII is generally considered to be unreliable,[10] principally because hypomanic episodes can easily be missed if the clinical interview is conducted by nonexperts[13,39] and when the patient is the sole source of information. The first question, then, is whether some or many patients characterized by these traits were already BPII, but were misclassified at the index interview. This is plausible, given that some of the items describing these traits have a hypomanic or cyclothymic ring to them (Table 4, factors 1 and 2). Although more of the BPII converters met RDC criteria for cyclothymia—which suggests that hypomaniclike features perhaps were experienced prior to prospectively observed switching—they did not meet RDC criteria for BPII, which, by the conventions of the state-of-the-art instrument we used (ie, the SADS), requires major depressive and discrete hypomanic episodes. Nonetheless, because RDC cyclothymia occurred in only 8.3% of the BPII converters in the present study, it cannot account for the personality measures reported here. Cyclothymia according to RDC refers to alternating subsyndromal mood swings, lasting for at least a few days in one or the other direction[16] that are often disruptive because of their intermittent chronicity. The personality items reported in the present study seem to fall below that threshold, both in terms of intensity and duration, perhaps occupying a position between cyclothymia and normality. These considerations suggest that the conservative SADS conventions for the diagnosis of BPII should be changed, permitting the diagnosis of this affective subtype on the basis of temperamental dysregulation. Indeed, Cassano et al[39] have recently published data that support such liberalization of the diagnostic threshold for this prevalent affective subtype. Ultimately, it must be conceded that clinicians experienced in diagnosing BPII will outperform research assistants generating instrument-based diagnoses.[12,13]

Previously, the CDS has demonstrated state dependency for many personality measures.[30] While some col-

Table 4. Personality Factors That Differentiate Bipolar II (BPII) Converters From Patients Who Remained Unipolar (UP)*

Personality Scale and Item Number†	
Factor 1: Mood Lability (BPII>UP, *P*<.001)	
GZTS 75	Mood often changes, happiness to sadness, without my knowing why‡
GZTS 55	Have frequent ups and downs in mood, with and without apparent cause
GZTS 45	Often feel guilty without a very good reason for it
MPI 23	Feelings are rather easily hurt
GZTS 60	There are times when my future looks very dark
MPI 39	Ideas run through my head so that I cannot sleep
GZTS 105 (neg§)	I keep in fairly uniform spirits
GZTS 25	Often find it difficult to go to sleep because of thinking what happened during day
MPI 45	Often feel disgruntled
Factor 2: Energy-Activity (BPII>UP, *P*<.01)	
GZTS 86	Inclined to rush from one activity to another without pausing for enough rest
LKA 31	I am a horse for work; I am seldom exhausted
GZTS 42	I am the kind of person who is "on the go" all the time
GZTS 71	I am able to work unusually long hours without feeling tired
GZTS 16	I am often so much on the go that sooner or later I wear myself out
GZTS 51	I am quick in my actions
MPI 01	Happiest when involved in a project that calls for rapid action
MMPI 65	Period so full of pep that sleep didn't seem necessary for days at a time
Factor 3: Daydreaming (BPII>UP, *P*<.01)	
GZTS 50	I daydream a great deal
MPI 31	Like to indulge in a reverie (daydreaming)
MMPI 26 (neg)	I daydream very little
GZTS 198	I frequently find myself in a meditative state
GZTS 167	I am inclined to think about myself much of the time
MPI 13	My daydreams frequently are about things that can never come true
Factor 4: Social Anxiety (BPII>UP, *P*<.05)	
IDI 17	It is hard for me to ask someone for a favor
IDI 39	When I meet new people, am afraid I won't do the right thing
IDI 38	Feel that I never really get all that I need from people
IDI 36	Don't like to buy clothes for myself
IDI 41	Would rather stay free of involvements with others than risk disappointments
MMPI 60 (neg)	While in trains, buses, etc, often talk to strangers
LKA 27	Hope only brings disappointment
MPI 30	I am inclined to be shy in the presence of opposite sex

Based on factor analysis and analysis of variance on factor scores, covarying for age and sex.

†See Table 3 for explanations of abbreviations.

‡For the sake of consistency, all pronouns were changed to the first person.

§False response adds +1.0 to factor.

oring of self-report by clinical depression is unavoidable, it is unlikely to be the main explanation for the findings reported herein. The self-report measures that typified BPII converters (ie, Mood Lability, Energy Activity, and Daydreaming) were, in aggregate, uncharacteristic of BPI converters and the majority of patients with MDD who did not change polarity. If state influences were strongly operative, moodiness and hyperenergetic activity should have been blunted during BPII depression as well. Moreover, the self-report temperamental traits in BPII converters clustered in clinically meaningful ways—as predicted from past research[40]—thereby suggesting that they do not represent spurious statistical findings.

We submit that BPII patients are unstable precisely because their depressions are contaminated with their special temperament. In other words, the temperamental instability does not seem to go away during depressive episodes.[41] Observer-evaluated clinical data in this article in support of such instability include the significantly higher rate of antisocial behavior during the index episode and history of educational and occupational maladjustment, drug use, and marital disruption in BPII converters as opposed to nonconverters. Finally, self-reported traits indicative of Social Anxiety and Daydreaming are cross-validated by clinician-observed social withdrawal and self-rated symptom scores of interpersonal sensitivity and phobic anxiety. Again, this clinical corroboration of the instability in BPII probands is itself strong evidence that the personality items that characterized them are not spurious statistical artifacts of a large number of analyses. Overall, these data explain why BPII psychopathology and course have been found to be highly variable, pleomorphic, and tempestuous.[14,36,42]

We next examine the question of whether switching to BPII is related to unstable temperament or to some specific consequence of it (eg, drug abuse, turmoil due to marital disruption). Stepwise logistic regression analysis (data not shown) failed to reveal any predictive value of drug use for BPII switching beyond that of marital disruption. In a past contribution on cyclothymia, Akiskal et al[16] found that repeated romantic and marital failure were characteristic; one third of their cyclothymic cohort developed MDD during prospective course. Given past NIMH research on the possible role of catecholaminergic excess and that of morning rapid eye movement sleep in the switch out of depression,[1,2] it has been hypothesized that sleep loss might be one of the mediating mechanisms in this process.[43,44] Thus, the emotional turmoil and arousal associated with unstable object relationships might represent one of the putative factors favoring switching to BPII and the generally tempestuous life course of this subtype.

Whether treatment with heterocyclic antidepressants favors a switch into hypomania or mania in vulnerable individuals with bipolar diathesis[5,6,16,45] cannot be answered definitively with the methods of the present study. A case-control study and, ideally, a prospective controlled trial of antidepressants vs placebo in BPII are needed to resolve this question. The ideal study may never be done because of ethical considerations regard-

Table 5. Summary of Logistic Regression Analyses to Predict Conversion to Bypolar II Disorder During Follow-up From Clinical Measures, Self-Reported Symptom Scores, and Self-Reported Usual Personality*

Variables Significant From Univariate Test†	Unique Contribution of Each Variable‡ χ^2	P	Predictive Power of Key Variables Within Each Set‡ Log-Likelihood χ^2	P	Concordance Statistic, %
Clinical variables					
Index age, y	8.12	.004	12.90	.0016	64.4
Miscellaneous psychopathology (SADS score 12)	7.02	.008			
Ever RDC drug use disorder	7.16	.008			
Age at onset of first affective disorder	5.02	.025			
Ever RDC cyclothymia	4.54	.033			
Married or living together as of entry	4.10	.043			
Poor performance at job or school since age 15 y	3.73	.053			
Social withdrawal	3.29	.070			
Impaired functioning (SADS score 9)	3.06	.080			
At least minor antisocial acts	2.91	.088			
Inpatient status at entry	1.97	.160			
Duration of index episode >1 y at entry	1.87	.171			
SCL-90 self-reported symptom scores for index episode					
Phobic Anxiety (SCL-90 score 7)	13.48	.0002	14.7	.0005	67.0
Depression (SCL-90 score 9)	12.40	.0004			
Interpersonal Sensitivity (SCL-90 score 3)	11.59	.0007			
Psychoticism (SCL-90 score 9)	10.55	.0012			
Morbid personality scores describing usual personality					
Mood Lability	19.92	.0001	46.18	.0001	79.6
Energy-Activity	17.75	.0001			
Daydreaming	16.40	.0001			
Social Anxiety	10.90	.0010			

*SADS indicates Schedule of Affective Disorders and Schizophrenia; RDC, Research Diagnostic Criteria; and SCL-90, Hopkins Symptom Checklist-90.
†Significant at $P<.05$.
‡Within each set of variables, no other predictor was added to the separation of groups once the braced predictors were entered into the regression models.

ing the induction of or acceleration into hypomania in temperamentally unstable depressive patients. This factor is probably operative in the present sample: Clinicians must have judged that heterocyclic antidepressants were unsuitable for some patients—that indeed they were at risk for switching—because only 28.9% of the switchers as opposed to 67.7% of the nonswitcher unipolar patients had received antidepressants. The fact that many conversions, both into BPI and BPII, occurred during intake episodes or shortly thereafter is compatible with the hypothesis that preswitching depressive patients are more unstable and hence more likely to present for treatment and that the emotional turmoil surrounding affective episodes, interacting in unknown ways with treatment parameters, could have facilitated switching.

It is striking that the temperamental profile of Mood Lability described for BPII converters was absent in BPI converters and those who remained unipolar. That these habitual self measures were taken prior (often years before) the actual conversion was observed, suggests "traitness." Mood Lability itself might represent the very mechanism that underlies the ease with which switching into hypomania occurs. "Switching," which connotes suddenness, explains our terminologic preference for the process of BPII conversion. Hyperenergetic behavior (Energy-Activity) has obvious hypomanic elements, while a rich mental life (Daydreaming) captures the intense self-absorption and active fantasy so characteristic of the depressive dips of cyclothymia.[16] We submit that daydreaming is an active process that represents the mental counterpart of hyperenergetic behavior, which is even observed during depression. Thus, temperament and subaffective manifestations seem to merge in a continuum of trait and state.[40] The reported temperamental data on switching supplement earlier CDS findings[37,46] and those by others[47] on the distinctness of BPII.

The difficulties in the cross-sectional diagnosis of BPII prior to switching appear to reflect their antecedent temperamental instability. Our data raise the possibility that such instability is so woven into the fluctuating affective course of BPII that it constitutes a core defining characteristic of this disorder, possibly sharing the same pathophysiologic mechanisms.[40] In other words, Mood Lability appears to be an integral part of the affective dysregulation that underlies BPII. Temperamental excesses along these lines probably precede the onset of full-blown affective disorder by a decade or longer; actually, they have been identified in adolescents and children in clinical,[48] epidemiologic,[49] and high-risk[50,51] bipolar samples.

Mood Lability then appears as a stable trait across the life span well into adulthood. Other investigators too have commented on the tempestuous histories of BPII patients compared with those with the BPI subtype.[36,42,52] In the present study, this tempestuous affective course was associated with significant interpersonal and vocational instability. These factors might account for the relative unreliability (temporal instability),[53] as well as the low sensitivity of current diagnostic criteria for hypomania and BPII (leading to underdiagnosis).[12,13] Our newly derived personality factors (Mood Lability, Energy-Activity, and Daydreaming) raise the sensitivity of predicting who will switch to a respectable rate of 91%. If specificity is the desired goal of the clinician, patient endorsement of all nine traits consituting Mood Lability provides a figure of 86%; however, such specificity tends to drop the diagnostic sensitivity rate to 42%.

With respect to Interpersonal Sensitivity, Phobic Tendencies, Daydreaming, and Miscellaneous Psychopathology beyond the usual affective realm, and especially for its propensity to Mood Lability, BPII overlaps considerably with the constructs of hysteroid dysphoria and atypical depression.[54,55] This is of great therapeutic relevance, since both atypical depressive and BPII patients respond to monoamine oxidase inhibitors and, in at least two studies,[56,57] have been found to do significantly less well with tricyclic antidepressants.

The most important clinical implication of our data, however, resides in the fact that the unstable temperamental profile that presaged switching to BPII was obtained during antecedent clinical depression, ie, at a time when practitioners normally have access to personality data. Our findings are difficult to translate to *DSM-IV*'s Axis II.[58] However, judging from Axis II diagnoses given to cyclothymic and BPII patients,[16,59] patients with MDD who meet erratic or cluster B criteria (especially borderline and histrionic) at the trait level—*concurrently* with shy-sensitive traits of the avoidant type from cluster C—should be suspected as belonging to the BPII subtype.

We submit that it is the combined restless emotionality of cluster B and the introverted neuroticism of cluster C that contributes to the special instability of BPII. This combination seems to be an incompatible alignment of temperamental traits that often proves highly distressing to the sufferer (and significant others). That may be why patients with MDD having such features are liable to switching. Actually, emotional lability and hyperenergetic activity during a major depressive episode suggest that BPII is, in a certain measure, a mixed episode.[41] On a more hypothetical level, the emotional storms of these patients might teleologically represent attempts for self-cure from depressive inertia, affect, and self-absorption; hence, their erratic behavior, which might even be misconstrued as psychopathic.[14,60] Temperamental instability, coupled with the miscellaneous psychopathologic symptoms beyond that which is considered typical of depression, explains why such patients often are diagnosed as borderline, thereby obscuring the affective origin of the psychopathology.

Bipolar II represents the most fascinating interface between affective episodes and temperamental instability. Indeed, it might be the most common phenotype of bipolar disorder.[12,39,43,61] Although there is some possibility that it might breed true[37] in terms of family morbidity rates for full-blown bipolar illness, it is intermediate between BPI and strict unipolar disorder.[47,39] Despite some division of opinion in the research literature,[62] earlier suggestions by Dunner et al,[42] supported by us and others,[43,46,63,64] have finally led to its inclusion into *DSM-IV*[58] as a bipolar subtype. Given that it responds to treatment with lithium salts,[65,66] clinicians will now have to struggle to make sense of this interface between soft bipolarity and Axis II. As documented elsewhere,[16-18] temperamentality along cyclothymic and hyperthymic lines—examined longitudinally—constitutes genuine affective dysregulation distinct from psychopathy. In particular, switching to hypomania does not occur in the antisocial personality spectrum (including Briquet's disorder).[16] In a subsequent article, we will examine to what extent the temperamental traits predictive of BPII switching match the temperamental profile of an unselected sample of patients with BPII disorder.

Accepted for publication September 9, 1994.

Donald Vena provided database development and statistical programming.

This article has been endorsed by the Publication Committee of the Collaborative Depression Study.

Reprint requests to Department of Psychiatry, University of California, San Diego, 9500 Gilman Dr, La Jolla, CA 92093-0603 (Dr Akiskal).

REFERENCES

1. Bunney WE Jr, Goodwin FK, Murphy DL, House KM, Gordon EK. The 'switch process' in manic-depressive illness, II: relationship to catecholamines, REM sleep, and drugs. *Arch Gen Psychiatry.* 1972;27:304-309.
2. Sitaram N, Gillin JG, Bunney WE Jr. Circadian variation in time of switch and sleep and manic ratings before and after switch. *Acta Psychiatr Scand.* 1978; 58:267-278.
3. Dunner DL, Fleiss JL, Fieve RR. The course of development of mania in patients with recurrent depression. *Am J Psychiatry.* 1976;133:905-908.
4. Rao AV, Nammalvar N. The course and outcome in depressive illness: a follow-up study of 122 cases in Madurai, India. *Br J Psychiatry.* 1977;130:392-396.
5. Strober M, Carlson G. Bipolar illness in adolescents with major depression: clinical, genetic, and psychopharmacologic predictors in a three- to four-year prospective follow-up investigation. *Arch Gen Psychiatry.* 1982;39:549-555.
6. Akiskal HS, Walker P, Puzantian VR, King D, Rosenthal TL, Dranon M. Bipolar outcome in the course of depressive illness: phenomenologic, familial, and pharmacologic predictors. *J Affect Disord.* 1983;5:115-128.
7. Winokur G, Wesner R. From unipolar depression to bipolar illness: 29 who changed. *Acta Psychiatr Scand.* 1987;76:59-63.
8. Lehmann HE, Fenton FR, Deutsch M, Feldman S, Engelsmann F. An 11-year follow-up study of 110 depressed patients. *Acta Psychiatr Scand.* 1988;78: 57-65.
9. Coryell W, Endicott J, Maser JD, Keller MB, Leon AC, Akiskal HS. Polarity and diagnostic confidence. *Am J Psychiatry.* In press.
10. Andreasen NC, Grove WM, Shapiro RW, Keller MB, Hirschfeld RM, McDonald-Scott P. Reliability of lifetime diagnosis: a multicenter collaborative perspective. *Arch Gen Psychiatry.* 1981;38:400-405.
11. Coryell W, Keller M, Endicott J, Andreasen N, Clayton P, Hirschfeld R. Bipolar II illness: course and outcome over a five-year period. *Psychol Med.* 1989;19: 129-141.
12. Akiskal HS, Mallya G. Criteria for the 'soft' bipolar spectrum: treatment implications. *Psychopharmacol Bull.* 1987;23:68-73.
13. Dunner DL, Kai Tay L. Diagnostic reliability of the history of hypomania in bipolar II patients and patients with major depression. *Compr Psychiatry.* 1993; 34:303-307.
14. Akiskal HS. Subaffective disorders: dysthymic, cyclothymic and bipolar II disorders in the 'borderline' realm. *Psychiatr Clin North Am.* 1981;4:25-46.
15. Endicott NA. Psychophysiological correlates of 'bipolarity.' *J Affect Disord.* 1989; 17:47-56.
16. Akiskal HS, Djenderedjian AM, Rosenthal RH, Khani MK. Cyclothymic disorder: validating criteria for inclusion in the bipolar affective group. *Am J Psychiatry.* 1977;134:1227-1233.
17. Depue RA, Slater JF, Wolfstetter-Kausch H, Klein D, Goplerud E, Farr D. A behavioral paradigm for identifying persons at risk for bipolar depressive disorder: a conceptual framework and five validation studies. *J Abnorm Psychol.* 1981;90:381-437.
18. Akiskal HS. Delineating irritable and hyperthymic variants of the cyclothymic temperament. *J Pers Disord.* 1992;6:326-342.
19. Katz MM, Secunda SK, Hirschfeld RM, Koslow SH. NIMH Clinical Research

Branch Collaborative Program on the Psychobiology of Depression. *Arch Gen Psychiatry.* 1979;36:765-771.
20. Andreasen NC, Rice J, Endicott J, Coryell W, Grove WM, Reich T. Familial rates of affective disorder: a report from the National Institute of Mental Health Collaborative Study. *Arch Gen Psychiatry.* 1987;44:461-469.
21. Keller MB, Lavori PW, Friedman B, Nielsen E, Endicott J, McDonald-Scott P, Andreasen NC. The Longitudinal Interval Follow-up Evaluation: a comprehensive method for assessing outcome in prospective longitudinal studies. *Arch Gen Psychiatry.* 1987;44:540-548.
22. Spitzer RL, Endicott J, Robins E. *Research Diagnostic Criteria for a Selected Group of Functional Disorders.* New York: New York State Psychiatric Institute, Biometrics Research Division; 1977.
23. Spitzer RL, Endicott J. *Schedule for Affective Disorders and Schizophrenia (SADS).* 3rd ed. New York: New York State Psychiatric Institute, Biometrics Research Division; 1979.
24. Hirschfeld RMA, Cross CK. Psychosocial aspects of depression: personality. In: Marsella AJ, Hirschfeld RMA, Katz MM, eds. *The Measurement of Depression: Clinical, Biological, Psychological, and Psychosocial Perspectives.* New York, NY: Guilford Publications; 1985.
25. Guilford JP, Zimmerman WS. *The Guilford-Zimmerman Temperament Survey Manual.* Beverly Hills, Calif: Sheridan Supply Co; 1949.
26. Hirschfeld RM, Klerman GL, Gough HG, Barrett J, Korchin SJ, Chodoff P. A measure of interpersonal dependency. *J Pers Assess.* 1977;41:610-618.
27. Lazare A, Klerman GL, Armor DJ. Oral, obsessive, and hysterical personality patterns: an investigation of psychoanalytic concepts by means of factor analysis. *Arch Gen Psychiatry.* 1966;14:624-630.
28. Eysenck HJ. *The Maudsley Personality Inventory.* San Diego, Calif: Educational & Industrial Testing Service; 1962.
29. Hathaway SR, McKinley JC. *The Minnesota Multiphasic Personality Inventory, Revised.* New York, NY: Psychological Corporation; 1951.
30. Hirschfeld RM, Klerman GL, Clayton PJ, Keller MB, McDonald-Scott P, Larkin BH. Assessing personality: effects of the depressive state on trait measurement. *Am J Psychiatry.* 1983;140:695-699.
31. Hirschfeld RM, Klerman GL, Clayton PJ, Keller MB. Personality and depression: empirical findings. *Arch Gen Psychiatry.* 1983;40:993-998.
32. Hirschfeld RM, Klerman GL, Lavori P, Keller MB, Griffith P, Coryell W. Premorbid personality assessments of first onset of major depression. *Arch Gen Psychiatry.* 1989;46:345-350.
33. Costa PT, Widiger TA, eds. *Personality Disorders and the Five-Factor Model.* Hyattsville, Md: American Psychological Association; 1993.
34. Cloninger CR, Svrakic DM, Przybeck TR. A psychobiological model of temperament and character. *Arch Gen Psychiatry.* 1993;50:975-990.
35. Derogatis LR, Lipman RS, Covi L. SCL-90: an outpatient psychiatric rating scale—preliminary report. *Psychopharmacol Bull.* 1973;9:13-28.
36. Ayuso-Gutierrez JL, Ramos-Brieva JA. The course of manic-depressive illness: a comparative study of bipolar I and bipolar II patients. *J Affect Disord.* 1982;4:9-14.
37. Coryell W, Endicott J, Reich T, Andreasen N, Keller M. A family study of bipolar II disorder. *Br J Psychiatry.* 1984;145:49-54.
38. Andreasen NC, Endicott J, Spitzer RL, Winokur G. The family history method using diagnostic criteria: reliability and validity. *Arch Gen Psychiatry.* 1977; 34:1229-1235.
39. Cassano GB, Akiskal HS, Savino M, Musetti L, Perugi G. Proposed subtypes of bipolar II and related disorders: with hypomanic episodes (or cyclothymia) and with hyperthymic temperament. *J Affect Disord.* 1992;26:127-140.
40. Akiskal HS, Akiskal K. Cyclothymic, hyperthymic and depressive temperaments as subaffective variants of mood disorders. In: Tasman A, Riba MB, eds. *American Psychiatric Association Review.* Washington, DC: American Psychiatric Press; 1992:43-62.
41. Akiskal HS. The distinctive mixed states of bipolar I, II, and III. *Clin Neuropharmacol.* 1992;15:632A-633A. Abstract.
42. Dunner DL, Gershon ES, Goodwin FK. Heritable factors in the severity of affective illness. *Biol Psychiatry.* 1976;11:31-42.
43. Akiskal HS. The bipolar spectrum: new concepts in classification and diagnosis. In: Grinspoon L, ed. *Psychiatry Update: The American Psychiatric Association Annual Review.* Washington, DC: American Psychiatric Press; 1983: 271-292.
44. Wehr TA, Sack DA, Rosenthal NE. Sleep reduction as a final common pathway in the genesis of mania. *Am J Psychiatry.* 1987;144:201-204.
45. Wehr TA, Goodwin FK. Can antidepressants cause mania and worsen the course of affective illness? *Am J Psychiatry.* 1987;144:1403-1411.
46. Endicott J, Nee J, Andreasen N, Clayton P, Keller M, Coryell W. Bipolar II: combine or keep separate? *J Affect Disord.* 1985;8:17-28.
47. Heun R, Maier W. The distinction of bipolar II disorder from bipolar I and recurrent unipolar depression: results of a controlled family study. *Acta Psychiatr Scand.* 1993;87:279-284.
48. Costello EJ, Benjamin R, Angold A, Silver D. Mood variability in adolescents: a study of depressed, nondepressed and comorbid patients. *J Affect Disord.* 1991;23:199-212.
49. Carlson GA, Kashani JH. Manic symptoms in a non-referred adolescent population. *J Affect Disord.* 1988;15:219-226.
50. Zahn-Waxler C, Cummings EM, McKnew DH, Radke-Yarrow M. Altruism, aggression, and social interactions in young children with a manic-depressive parent. *Child Dev.* 1984;55:112-122.
51. Akiskal HS, Downs J, Jordan P, Watson S, Daugherty D, Pruitt DB. Affective disorders in referred children and younger siblings of manic-depressives: mode of onset and prospective course. *Arch Gen Psychiatry.* 1985;42:996-1003.
52. Angst J. The course of affective disorders, II: typology of bipolar manic-depressive illness. *Arch Psychiatr Nervenkr.* 1978;226:65-73.
53. Rice JP, McDonald-Scott P, Endicott J, Coryell W, Grove WM, Keller MB, Altis D. The stability of diagnosis with an application to bipolar II disorder. *Psychiatry Res.* 1986;19:285-296.
54. Liebowitz MR, Klein DF. Hysteroid dysphoria. *Psychiatr Clin North Am.* 1979; 2:555-575.
55. Davidson JR, Miller RD, Turnbull CD, Sullivan JL. Atypical depression. *Arch Gen Psychiatry.* 1982;39:527-534.
56. Liebowitz MR, Quitkin FM, Stewart JW, McGrath PJ, Harrison WM, Markowitz JS, Rabkin JG, Tricamo E, Goetz DM, Klein DF. Antidepressant specificity in atypical depression. *Arch Gen Psychiatry.* 1988;45:129-137.
57. Himmelhoch JM, Thase ME, Mallinger AG, Houck P. Tranylcypromine versus imipramine in anergic bipolar depression. *Am J Psychiatry.* 1991;148:910-916.
58. American Psychiatric Association. *Diagnostic and Statistical Manual of Mental Disorders, Fourth Edition.* Washington, DC: American Psychiatric Association; 1994.
59. Levitt AJ, Joffe RT, Ennis J, MacDonald C, Kutcher SP. The prevalence of cyclothymia in borderline personality disorder. *J Clin Psychiatry.* 1990;51:335-339.
60. Coid JW. An affective syndrome in psychopaths with borderline personality disorder? *Br J Psychiatry.* 1993;162:641-650.
61. Simpson SG, Folstein SE, Meyers DA, McMahon FJ, Brusco DM, DePaulo JR Jr. Bipolar II: the most common bipolar phenotype. *Am J Psychiatry.* 1993; 150:901-903.
62. Kupfer DJ, Carpenter LL, Frank E. Is bipolar II a unique disorder? *Compr Psychiatry.* 1988;29:228-236.
63. Fieve RR, Dunner DL. Unipolar and bipolar affective states. In: Flach FF, Draghi SC, eds. *The Nature and Treatment of Depression.* New York, NY: John Wiley & Sons; 1975:145-160.
64. Gershon ES, Hamovit J, Guroff JJ, Dibble E, Leckman JF, Sceery W, Targum SD, Nurnberger JI Jr, Goldin LR, Bunney WE Jr. A family study of schizoaffective, bipolar I, bipolar II, unipolar, and normal control probands. *Arch Gen Psychiatry.* 1982;39:1157-1167.
65. Kane JM, Quitkin FM, Rifkin A, Ramos-Lorenzi JR, Nayak DD, Howard A. Lithium carbonate and imipramine in the prophylaxis of unipolar and bipolar II illness: a prospective, placebo-controlled comparison. *Arch Gen Psychiatry.* 1982;39: 1065-1069.
66. Peselow ED, Dunner DL, Fieve RR, Lautin A. Lithium prophylaxis of depression in unipolar, bipolar II, and cyclothymic patients. *Am J Psychiatry.* 1982; 139:747-752.

The NIMH Collaborative Program on the Psychobiology of Depression—Clinical Studies

Investigators

M. B. Keller, MD (chairperson), Providence, RI; W. Coryell, MD (cochairperson), Iowa City, Iowa; H. S. Akiskal, MD, J. D. Maser, PhD, Washington, DC; P. W. Lavori, PhD, T. I. Mueller, MD, M. T. Shea, PhD, Meredith Warshaw, MSS, Providence; J. Fawcett, MD, W. A. Scheftner, MD, Chicago, Ill; J. Haley, Iowa City; J. Endicott, PhD, A. Leon, PhD, J. Loth, MSW, New York, NY; and J. Rice, PhD, T. Reich, MD, St Louis, Mo.

Other or Past Contributors

N. C. Andreasen, MD, PhD; P. J. Clayton, MD; J. Croughan, MD; G. L. Klerman, MD (deceased); R. M. A. Hirschfeld, MD; M. M. Katz, PhD; E. Robins, MD; R. W. Shapiro, MD (deceased); R. L. Spitzer, MD; G. Winokur, MD; and M. A. Young, PhD.

Because o

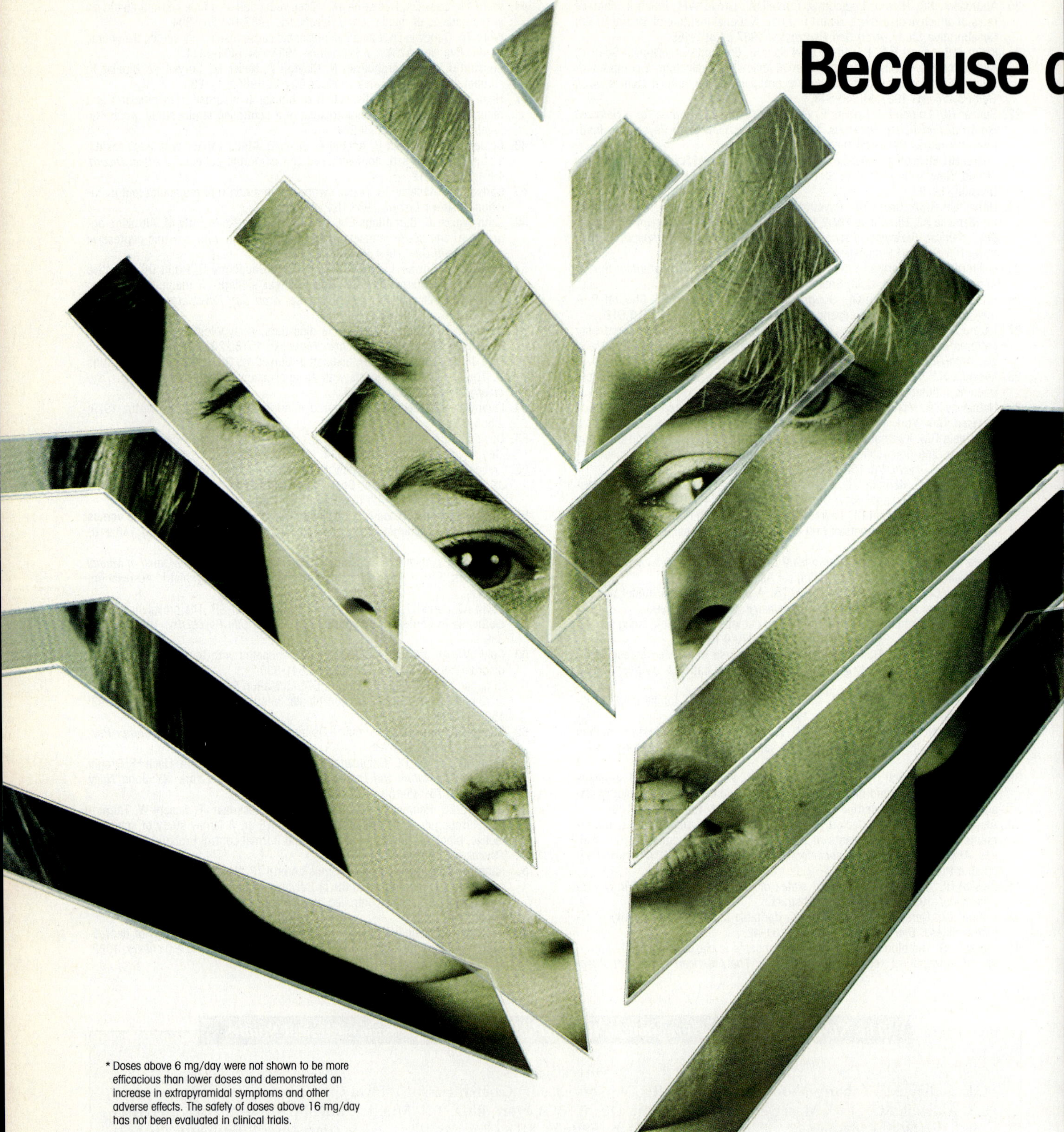

* Doses above 6 mg/day were not shown to be more efficacious than lower doses and demonstrated an increase in extrapyramidal symptoms and other adverse effects. The safety of doses above 16 mg/day has not been evaluated in clinical trials.

† Antipsychotic activity is presumed to be mediated through a combination of dopamine D_2 and serotonin 5-HT_2 antagonism, although the exact mechanism of action is unknown.

Please see brief summary of Prescribing Information at the end of this advertisement.

 JPI-RS-084

SB SmithKline Beecham
Pharmaceuticals

For additional medical information, please call
1-800-JANSSEN,
(1-800-526-7736),
Monday through Friday,
9AM to 5PM, Eastern Time.

JANSSEN · PHARMACEUTICA · · RESEARCH FOUNDATION ·

Structure and Course of Positive and Negative Symptoms in Schizophrenia

William W. Eaton, PhD; R. Thara, MD; Belle Federman; Beth Melton, ScM; Kung-yee Liang, PhD

Background: This article focuses on the underlying structure and temporal course of the symptoms of schizophrenia.

Methods: Ratings of symptoms in 90 schizophrenic patients were made each month for 10 years following the first hospitalization. The analytic methods consisted of cross-tabulation, dichotomous factor analysis, and bivariate dichotomous time series.

Results: The factor analyses revealed positive and negative factors with a slight tendency to merge over time. The prevalence of positive and negative symptoms declined in the year following first hospitalization and was stable thereafter. Positive and negative symptoms in 1 month were highly predictive of the same type of symptoms in the next month. Neither type of symptom was strongly associated with the other type in the following month when both types were included in the model. The predictability of the process increased with time.

Conclusions: With a few minor caveats, the results suggest that the positive and negative symptom clusters are independent, both cross-sectionally and longitudinally.

(Arch Gen Psychiatry. 1995;52:127-134)

THE EXTRAORDINARY range of symptoms included in the clinical picture of schizophrenia was brought together into one disorder primarily because the course of the disorder was hypothesized to be relatively uniform and distinct from other psychoses. Over the last 100 years, the homogeneity of the nosologic category of schizophrenia has been challenged repeatedly by subcategories that can be recognized by the clinician and purportedly have been connected to other aspects of the disorder, such as its etiology, pathophysiology, course, or outcome. In general, these subcategories have not proved useful in anything other than description.

In the last two decades the division into positive and negative schizophrenia has been a subject of intense interest.[1,2] Positive symptoms have been characterized by delusions, hallucinations, formal thought disorder, and bizarre behavior; negative symptoms by flat affect, alogia, asociality, apathy, and attentional impairment. In the past decade there have been many attempts to validate the two types. Many latent variable analyses have been conducted on the covariation of symptoms of schizophrenia (termed *internal construct validity* by Young[3] in 1982), revealing a pattern of factors, constructs, or classes similar to that originally hypothesized.[4-9] Hallucinations and delusions are found in a single factor in almost all studies; and flat affect, alogia, social withdrawal, and apathy on a distinct factor are found in almost all studies. Thought disorder and bizarre behavior sometimes load on the positive symptom factor and sometimes on a third distinct factor. In some studies the third factor has included cognitive impairment of various types. The studies of factor structure have been conducted on cross-sectional data from samples usually defined by an index admission relatively early in the course. We know of only one study that has focused on the stability of the factor structure, conducting the analyses at index admission[6] and 18 to 30 months later.[10]

Other research on the positive-negative distinction has focused on the association of the symptom groups with etiology, pathophysiology, treatment

From the Departments of Mental Hygiene (Dr Eaton and Ms Federman) and Biostatistics (Dr Liang and Ms Melton), School of Hygiene and Public Health, The Johns Hopkins Universtity, Baltimore, Md; and the Schizophrenia Research Foundation, Madras, India (Dr Thara).

See Methods on next page

METHODS

SAMPLE

The sample consisted of 90 schizophrenic patients admitted to the Government General Hospital in Madras, India, from 1981 to 1982. To be included in the study, subjects had to meet *International Classification of Diseases, Ninth Revision*[22] and Feighner criteria[23] for schizophrenia. On the basis of the original data, it has been determined that 72 of the 90 patients met *DSM-III-R*[24] criteria for schizophrenia. These were first-onset cases, drawn from a slightly larger sample of consecutive admissions to the hospital as part of a 5-year three-center collaborative study of prognosis funded by the India Medical Research Council.[25] There were 45 males and 45 females, and 33 of the subjects were younger than 20 years of age. The range of socioeconomic status included lower and middle classes, with only 19% completing secondary school. After funding ended, the principal investigator in Madras (R.T.) continued the follow-up without further government funds. At about the 10th year, funding from the US National Institute of Mental Health supported an intensive effort to locate and examine all subjects. Of the 90 initial subjects, there were 75 for whom symptom ratings were made every month or nearly so, and including the final month. Nine subjects had died, four could not be located, one refused to cooperate with the study, and one completed all but the final month. Sociodemographic and clinical differences between the 75 who completed the study and the original 90 enrolled were insignificant. The 10-year completion rate for surviving subjects is thus 75 of 81, or 93%. Roughly consistent with some other samples from less developed countries, about 25% of this sample has had a single episode, with about 75% having had one or more repeated episodes, with or without full remissions.

MEASURES

At the beginning of the study, the Present State Exam (PSE)[26] was completed for every subject by the principal investigator, who had been trained at the India site of the International Pilot Study of Schizophrenia sponsored by the World Health Organization.[27] A PSE-based form for the collection of data on a monthly basis for 12 symptoms was designed: the Interim Followup Schedule (IFS). Aside from the 12 symptoms, data on the use of medication, hospitalization, and other treatment also were obtained.

The reliability and validity of the IFS were not tested explicitly in this study. However, a workshop conducted at the beginning of the project by the Indian investigators for the International Pilot Study of Schizophrenia included reliability exercises in Madras on the first 20 patients, and every 10th thereafter, yielding a κ value of 0.85 for PSE-based diagnosis. Almost all the IFS ratings were made by the senior psychiatrist (R.T.); in a few instances ratings were made by a psychiatric social worker. The raters had no particular biases about the nature of the course of schizophrenia and attempted to rate each month's symptoms independently. The fact that almost all the measurements were made by a single individual probably enhances reliability but may threaten validity since after the first episode is over, the effect of repeated testing may bias toward heightened continuity of psychopathologic symptoms. Use of the PSE as the basis for the IFS has the advantage of providing a standard terminology and glossary of definition, which may counteract this problem somewhat.

To gain maximum information from the data, values were coded without face-to-face interviews with the pa-

response, and course ("external construct validity" of Young[3]). For example, Crow[11] proposed that individuals with negative schizophrenia had structural abnormalities in the brain, were less responsive to treatment, and had poor outcome relative to positive schizophrenics, who had normal brain structures, good response to treatment, and better outcome. The etiology of the two syndromes remains obscure, but there are some indications of different neurologic structures in the two subtypes.[12] Concerning course and outcome, a recent review concluded that, although the evidence was not conclusive, neither positive nor negative symptoms, measured at onset or index admission, predicted the early course; negative symptoms predicted poor long-term outcome.[13]

Much research on the course and outcome of positive and negative symptoms is retrospective; available prospective studies, on the other hand, have limited duration.[14] Samples in most studies are not defined by their first onset but rather by an episode later in the course—a crucial limit to generalizability.[15] To our knowledge, there are no published studies of first-onset samples with measures of positive and negative symptoms collected in a true prospective fashion over a relatively long period.

This report concerns 90 schizophrenic patients with monthly symptom data collected in a standardized fashion for 10 years, starting with the first hospital episode. A prior article presents details of methodology and analyses on predictors of course.[16] One important goal of the analysis reported herein was to replicate prior research, including one study in the Indian culture,[6] on the factor structure of positive and negative symptoms. A second goal was to explore the temporal stability of the latent structure that defines the positive and negative syndromes. Here, the null hypothesis is that the factor structure is stable, in effect, confirming the work of others who have not had the advantage of longitudinal data. A third goal was to estimate the prevalence of individual positive and negative symptoms over 10 years after first onset. Some have suggested a gradual increase in the prevalence of negative symptoms, but not positive symptoms, after the first episode subsides,[17-20] ie, in the latter half of the 10-year period studied here. A fourth goal was to determine whether the process becomes more predictable from month to month, as the years pass, and whether this possible increase in stability is different for the positive vs negative symptoms.[20,21] The third and fourth goals are both related to the concept of "progressive deteriotient in some instances. If the subject did not appear for the monthly appointment, the investigator made a special effort to determine if medication was being taken by talking with a relative as agreed on by all three collaborating centers. Case notes made during the conversation often indicated the presence or absence of delusions, hallucinations, or thought disorder, since these symptoms were used in deciding about medication. Data analyses were performed with and without these imputations. Although they required a good deal of effort, in the end the imputations had trivial effects on the data analyses and results.

ANALYTIC TECHNIQUES

These data are very rich and stretch the ability of currently available statistical techniques. For the first research question, factor analysis has been used extensively in prior investigations by others. But the PSE-type response values generate highly skew data for which normal factor analysis is inappropriate. Normal factor analysis is particularly in jeopardy when factor structures are to be compared across observations that differ in their skewness, as we suspected would be the case here (ie, declining prevalence of symptoms after the first episode, for example, as found by McCreadie et al[28]). Therefore, the PSE-based response values were dichotomized into present (scale values of 1 or 2) vs absent (scale value of 0), and the technique of dichotomous factor analysis was employed.[29,30] To avoid attrition bias, the factor analyses, were conducted on the sample of 75 individuals who completed all 10 years of the study.

Statistical inference for advanced latent variable techniques, such as dichotomous factor analysis, is still in its infancy. There is no statistical method to choose how many factors to extract, for example, or to compare the goodness of fit of factor structures from the same subjects at different points in time. Therefore, like other investigators, we rely on the interpretation of relative sizes of eigenvalues and patterns of factor loadings. To stabilize the factor structures in the dichotomous factor analyses, we collapsed as many as 12 monthly observations to present analyses for the first, sixth, and 10th years. This procedure violates the statistical assumption of independence, in effect, inflating the sample size. Unfortunately, we know of no statistical procedure to compare dichotomous factor structures in the same individuals at one or more points in time. It is also true that our conclusions are based more on the pattern of coefficients than on measures related to statistical inference. To check, factor structures also were estimated for the first, 61st, and 109th month, with latent structures not remarkably different.

For the fourth and fifth research questions, multiple time series analysis was the technique of choice for data such as these, with up to 120 monthly observations on each subject. A form of longitudinal data analysis for dichotomous data recently has been developed, called "generalized estimating equations" (GEE).[31,32] In this situation we used an adaptation of the GEE method suitable to our interest in simultaneously estimating cross-lagged effects for two dependent variables.[33] For the time series, we formed triplets of adjacent months to estimate a second-order process. The focus is on the month-to-month stability of the symptom groups, and the sample of interest is all individuals still in the study at the time the triplet is formed. Therefore, these analyses were estimated, taking advantage of every triplet that could be created without missing data (ie, forming and including triplets from the early part of the follow-up on individuals who later dropped out of the study or died). The GEE adaptation corrects for the over time, within-subject correlation by estimating it and adjusting for it.

ration," which has been a controversial issue. Finally, a fifth goal was to assess the temporal independence of the positive and negative syndromes. The research question in this case addresses the nosologic issue of the homogeneity of the construct of schizophrenia.

RESULTS

The prevalence of the symptoms changes distinctly from the first to later years. **Table 1** presents the first-, sixth-, and 10th-year prevalences for the 10 most frequent of the 12 symptoms assessed. To be consistent with the later factor analyses, these data collapse all available monthly observations within the year for the 75 subjects on whom measures were made throughout the follow-up. The pattern for years 2 through 5 and 7 through 9 is not shown for reasons of efficiency of presentation; these years strongly resemble years 6 and 10. Data on the prevalence for individual months do not differ substantially from these collapsed data. The prevalence for any given individual symptom is about 20% in the first year, which includes the episode of first hospitalization. The prevalence of any given symptom declines to about 10% by the sixth year, and remains roughly stable through year 10. The prevalence of either positive or negative symptoms (ie, the sum of the three lowest rows) is about 60% in the first year, but declines to about 20% to 25% in years 6 and 10.

Dichotomous factor analyses, with varimax rotation, at years 1, 6, and 10 reveal distinct positive and negative factors. The year 1 analysis reveals four factors with latent roots greater than the traditional threshold value of 1.0, but there is little change in the size of the factors after the third factor (eigenvalues of 6.4, 1.4, 1.2, and 1.2, respectively). For years 6 and 10, the eigenvalues for the third factor are less than 1.0. An intriguing aspect of the three factor analyses is the increase in importance of the first factor from the first (eigenvalue of 4.4) to the sixth (7.3) and the 10th year (7.4). After the first episode is over, the first factor explains a larger portion of the variance. To maximize comparability and not lose any possible informative factor, loadings for three factors are reported below for each of the three periods.

In the first year, the positive symptoms of delusions, hallucinations, and thought disorder are highly associated with the second factor (loadings of 0.63, 0.89, and 0.68, respectively, as shown in boldface in **Table 2**). Other symptoms have low loadings on this factor. Fac-

Table 1. Prevalence of 10 Symptoms in the Madras Longitudinal Study of Schizophrenia, 12 Monthly Observations*

Symptom	Year 1	Year 6	Year 10
Delusions	25.4	9.7	12.6
Hallucinations	41.1	11.2	13.3
Thought disorder	30.1	11.6	11.5
Psychomotor problems	29.2	13.0	12.0
Flat affect	22.6	5.8	8.1
Apathy	15.6	6.0	7.3
Social withdrawal	17.4	10.8	14.6
Odd behavior	19.0	14.7	16.6
Self-neglect	4.4	10.4	11.1
Anxiety	3.7	1.8	1.3
Any symptom	66.0	26.6	30.5
No positive or negative	40.1	76.6	74.1
Positive only†	29.3	10.4	9.0
Negative only†	7.0	4.6	4.6
Both positive and negative	23.6	8.4	12.3

**For each symptom, subjects with missing values for that disorder were excluded from the denominator.*

†For positive and negative syndromes, if one symptom had a valid value but the other had a missing value, then the missing one was considered as absent. Subjects with both symptoms missing were excluded from the denominator.

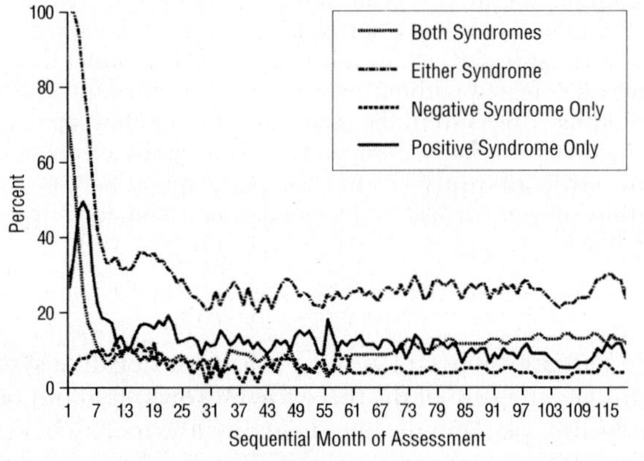

Prevalence of positive and negative syndromes for the follow-up cohort of 75 subjects in the Madras Longitudinal Study. After the first year, the relative stability of syndrome prevalence is demonstrated by month-to-month data.

tor one is the negative factor, with high loadings of flat affect, social withdrawal, and apathy (0.90, 0.87, and 0.59, respectively, in boldface in Table 2). Psychomotor problems also load strongly on this factor. The third factor consists of odd behavior, self-neglect, and psychomotor problems. These findings are broadly consistent with the early descriptions of the two symptom groups[2] and with empirical studies that followed, except that in many studies thought disorder and bizarre behavior formed a distinct third factor. These findings are also consistent with other research in India,[6] confirming again the existence of the two syndromes in the Indian culture.

In the sixth and 10th years, a dominant factor emerges that is associated with *both* positive and negative symptoms. There is no precise comparison to this finding in the longitudinal studies in the literature that focus on the latent structure of positive and negative symptoms, but the available data do not contradict this result. Kay et al[34] studied three separate samples of patients with acute, chronic, and long-term chronic illness and found internally consistent and distinct positive and negative factors in all three groups. Our findings are consistent with theirs, but because they did not report a factor analysis, the presence of a third, "growing" factor cannot be confirmed by their data. Kulhara et al[6] report principal components analysis for the index admission (not necessarily first) and for a follow-up measurement taken 18 to 30 months later.[10] At intake there were clear positive and negative factors, as well as a factor involving thought disorder and bizarre behavior. At the follow-up, there was a clear negative factor and a clear factor involving thought disorder and bizarre behavior; but, as with these data from Madras, the positive factor had become mixed with negative symptoms such as avolition, anhedonia, and attentional impairment.

In years 6 and 10, the second factor includes symptoms that are neither positive nor negative (thought disorder, psychomotor problems, withdrawal, odd behavior, and anxiety); the highest loadings on this factor are anxiety (1.10 and 1.13, respectively). Factor loadings greater than 1.0 sometimes occur in dichotomous factor analysis, when the matrix is not strictly positive definite. This situation occurs when some of the items are rare, as is the case for anxiety in years 6 (9 person-months with anxiety present) and 10 (12 person-months with anxiety present).

The results of the factor analyses supported the formation of symptom indices for positive and negative symptoms. Consistent with our view of the nature of the psychopathology, a positive symptom was recorded as present if a PSE-type value of 1 or 2 was present for delusions, hallucinations, or thought disorder. A negative symptom was recorded as present if a value of 1 or 2 was present for apathy, social withdrawal, or flat affect. The present-absent distinction is not as tenable for negative symptoms, which might be better regarded as more or less intense or severe. We use it here because it is consistent with the present-absent orientation of the IFS and its parent PSE and to avoid unnecessarily complicating the time series analysis.

There is a steep decline in the prevalence of positive and negative syndromes during the first year and then relative stability of syndrome prevalence, as shown in month-to-month data for the follow-up cohort of 75 subjects, presented in the **Figure**. As reported in a shorter series by McCreadie et al,[28] the prevalence of positive and negative syndromes is high at onset, dropping to 20% to 40% thereafter, and remaining stable. At the onset, 70% of patients had both positive and negative symptoms, and fully 100% had either one or the other. Less than 10% had only the negative symptoms present, and 30% had only the positive symptoms present. These data are consistent with the prevalence of individual symptoms for years 1, 6, and 10, as shown in Table 1, except that the clustering into syndromes has led to higher prevalences in the early part of the course (in effect, counting *any* symptom in the syndrome group). The month-to-

Table 2. Dichotomous Factor Analysis of 10 Symptoms in Three Groups of 12 Person-Months for 75 First-Onset Schizophrenics*

	Year 1			Year 6			Year 10		
Symptom	1	2	3	1	2	3	1	2	3
Delusions	0.13	**0.63**	0.33	0.57	−0.03	**0.54**	**0.64**	0.05	0.38
Hallucinations	0.18	**0.89**	0.16	0.73	0.19	**0.59**	**0.98**	0.21	0.31
Thought disorder	0.19	**0.68**	0.04	0.44	0.68	**0.62**	**0.59**	0.77	0.32
Psychomotor problems	0.54	0.19	0.50	0.42	0.62	0.69	0.61	0.77	0.30
Flat affect	**0.90**	0.20	0.04	**0.71**	0.01	0.39	0.36	0.13	**0.95**
Apathy	**0.87**	0.19	0.23	**0.95**	0.14	0.33	0.62	0.19	**0.59**
Withdrawal	**0.59**	0.24	0.27	**0.82**	0.61	0.20	0.39	0.73	**0.64**
Odd behavior	0.24	0.30	0.55	0.53	0.63	0.58	0.55	0.75	0.39
Self-neglect	0.15	0.15	0.99	0.39	0.03	0.97	0.71	0.18	0.65
Anxiety	0.09	0.14	0.08	−0.10	1.10	−0.09	−0.24	1.13	−0.12

**Entries in the table are factor loadings for three factors for each year. Symptoms loading highly on positive and negative factors are in boldface. Data are based on person-months of 809 for year 1, 844 for year 6, and 887 for year 10.*

Table 3. Prevalence of Positive and Negative Symptoms by Prior Month's Symptoms, Madras Longitudinal Study*

	Year 1		Year 6		Year 10	
Prior Month's Symptoms	**Positive**	**Negative**	**Positive**	**Negative**	**Positive**	**Negative**
No symptoms	7.4	4.9	2.2	0.3	1.5	0.3
Other, alone	14.3	12.5	0.0	1.3	2.6	0.0
Same, alone	74.5	66.7	90.0	87.5	91.1	97.4
Both	80.7	66.0	88.6	82.9	96.7	97.5

**Entries in the table are percents. Data are based on person-months of 658 for year 1, 462 for year 6, and 896 for year 10.*

month data show that the decline takes place during the first half of the first year.

There is little evidence of an increase in negative symptoms in the later part of the course. The Figure contrasts those with negative symptoms only to those with positive symptoms only; both lines reveal prevalence at about 5% to 10%, and they do not show any trend upward. The trend is also flat for negative symptoms, with or without positive symptoms (about 15% to 20% prevalence, data not shown); and flat for positive symptoms, with or without negative symptoms (15% to 20% prevalence, data not shown). The prevalence of subjects with *either* positive or negative symptoms stabilizes at about 20% to 25% prevalence after about 2 years. Two years has been one standard threshold of chronicity since before the era of community mental health care.[35] The stable prevalence of about 20% to 25% is roughly consistent with the literature on symptom outcome in long-term course.[36] There does appear to be a slight upward trend for the prevalence of both positive and negative symptoms, which reaches its nadir of only 2% prevalence after about 30 months and gradually rises to nearly 15% during the 10th year (Figure).

The positive and negative symptoms are relatively stable over time. **Table 3** shows the prevalence of symptoms in years 1, 6, and 10, according to the prior months' symptoms. The number of observations (person-months with complete data) is low during the sixth year because more subjects were missing visits during that period. The number of observations is lower in the first year because the first 2 months' observations must necessarily be omitted in the formation of triplets. For efficiency of presentation and to facilitate appropriate comparisons, the titles of the rows are designed to be in reference to the columns. For example, in the left-most column in year 1, the figure of 14.3% for "other, alone" refers to the prevalence of positive symptoms in a given month (t), when in the prior month (t−1) there were negative symptoms only; the adjacent figure of 12.5% refers to the prevalence of negative symptoms in a given month (t) when there were positive symptoms only in the prior month (t−1). This design of the table allows presentation of syndrome-specific stability and crossover effects, which are tested statistically below.

For subjects with neither positive nor negative symptoms present, the prevalence in the following month is only 7.4% for positive symptoms and 4.9% for negative symptoms; in years 6 and 10, the analogous prevalences are even lower (Table 3). For those with the complementary symptom (second row in Table 3), the prevalence is slightly higher: 14.3% for positive symptoms and 12.5% prevalence of negative symptoms as noted above. Prevalences in later years decline for this configuration at t−1, down to almost nothing. The stability of the two symptom groups is shown in the third row of the table: 74.5% prevalence of positive symptoms in month t, when only positive symptoms are present; 66.7% prevalence of negative symptoms, when only negative symptoms are present at t−1. The addition of the complementary symptom at t−1 changes the prevalence at t only a little, eg, 80.7% prevalence of positive symptoms at t for those with both symptoms at t−1, compared with 74.5%

Table 4. Time Series Model for Positive and Negative Symptoms, Madras Longitudinal Study*

Characteristic	Odds Ratio in a Given Month: Positive Symptoms	Negative Symptoms
Sex		
M	1.0	1.0
F	0.6†	0.9
Age at onset, y		
>25	1.0	1.0
20-24	0.5†	1.1
<20	0.8	1.5†
Type of onset		
Acute	1.0	1.0
Insidious	1.4†	1.4†
Neuroleptic use (t−1)		
None	1.0	1.0
Irregular	0.9	1.5†
Regular	0.7†	0.8
Positive symptoms		
Absent (t−1)	1.0	1.0
Present (t−1)	76.1†	2.1
Absent (t−2)	1.0	...
Present (t−2)	2.7†	...
Negative symptoms		
Absent (t−1)	1.0	1.0
Present (t−1)	2.6†	104.2†
Absent (t−2)	...	1.0
Present (t−2)	...	3.8†
Intercept	0.04	0.01

**N=7148 person-months. t−1 indicates prior month; t−2, 2 months prior.*

†Value exceeds 95% confidence interval.

prevalence for those with positive symptoms only; for negative symptoms there is actually a small decrement in prevalence at t when both symptoms are present.

The prevalence at t for subjects with the same symptom at t−1 suggests a temporal increase in the stability of the symptoms (Table 3). For positive symptoms, the prevalence rises from 74.5% in year 1, to 90.0% in year 6, to 91.1% in year 10. For negative symptoms, the prevalence rises from 66.7% in year 1, to 87.5% in year 5, to 97.4% in year 10.

The values in Table 3 are informative but do not adjust for prior individual characteristics and medication, which have been shown to affect the course of schizophrenia. Also, the presentation in Table 3 does not permit statistical inference. Issues of stability, independence, and temporal changes can be addressed more precisely with a single multivariate binary time series model, as shown in **Table 4**. The presence of positive or negative symptoms is predicted from a combination of time-invariant subject characteristics (sex, age at onset, and type of onset), time-dependent covariates (use of medication in the prior month), and the positive and negative symptoms themselves in the prior month and the month before (t−2). The model was estimated using the GEE program with 7148 person-months as data. Table 4 displays odds ratios (ORs), denoting ORs for which the 95% confidence interval excluded the value of 1.0, which indicates no association.

Prior research studies are not consistent on the association of gender and age at onset with positive and negative symptoms (as concluded by McGlashan and Fenton[13]). In the Madras data, female subjects are less likely to have positive symptoms than males over the course of the follow-up (OR of 0.6), but there is little difference in negative symptoms for males vs females. Subjects with later onset are likely to have more positive symptoms and less negative symptoms. Insidious onset is associated with the presence of both positive and negative symptoms over the course of the follow-up, as might be expected. Regular use of medications is protective against positive symptoms, as should be expected: over 10 years, there is 70% the chance of having a positive symptom in any given month, if medication use was recorded as "regular" in the prior month. The effect is in the same (protective) direction, but not significant, for negative symptoms. When medication use is recorded as "irregular," there is an increased chance of a negative symptom in the following month (OR of 1.5).

The stability of the positive and negative syndromes is displayed by the high ORs for month-to-month prediction: 76.1 for positive symptoms, and 104.2 for the negative symptoms. The complementary syndrome adds comparatively little in the way of predictability: ORs of 2.6 predicting positive from negative and of 2.1 predicting negative from positive. Thus, the results suggest high stability of the positive and negative symptoms and a moderate degree of independence from each other.

The small effects of the second-order lag contributed to our decision not to estimate a third-order process. The identical symptoms at month t−2 added comparatively little (OR of 2.7 for predicting positive symptoms at month t from positive symptoms at month t−2, adjusting for other covariates, including the positive symptoms at t−1; OR of 3.8 for predicting negative symptoms at t from negative symptoms at t−2, after adjusting for other covariates, including negative symptoms at month t−1). The complementary symptoms at t−2 made only trivial contributions to the equation and thus were omitted.

It has been hypothesized that there is an increase in the stability of the process over time, and the cross-classificatory analysis in Table 3 suggests such an increase. Interaction terms were entered into the model to test the hypothesis statistically. The interaction models were formed by creating two time-indicator variables for each triplet at month t: one taking the value of 1.0 when the "t" person-month was during the first 24 months, and 0 for other person-months; and a second time-indicator variable taking the value of 1.0 when the "t" person-month was in the third, fourth, or fifth year, and 0 for other person-months. These terms were positive and highly significant in the model, consistent with the decline in syndrome prevalences shown in the Figure. Interaction terms were created by multiplying the time-indicator variables by the t−1 and t−2 symptom variables. When the interaction terms were entered into the model, effects of other covariates reported in Table 4 did not change in direction, strength, or significance, except that the effects of regular medication use dropped below barely significant. Therefore, results for the model including interaction terms, reported below, are not shown.

There were strong and significant temporal increases in predictability. After adjusting for the main effects of time and the other covariates, subjects with negative symptoms at t−1 during the first 2 years were only 36% (OR of 0.36) as likely to have negative symptoms at time t compared with subjects with negative symptoms at time t−1 during years 6 through 10. The effect was in the same direction for years 3 through 5 compared with years 6 through 10 (OR of 0.48). Subjects with positive symptoms at t−1 during the first 2 years were 74% as likely to have positive symptoms at t compared with subjects with positive symptoms at t−1 during years 6 through 10. The OR comparing stability of positive symptoms in years 3 through 5 vs years 6 through 10 was 0.87.

The time-by-symptom interactions give statistical tests of the increase in the stability of the process over time. The increase in the stability of negative symptoms at time t−1, predicting negative symptoms at time t, is highly significant comparing years 1 through 2 with years 6 through 10 (logistic regression coefficient of 3.58 and robust SE of 0.65; $P<.0000$) and comparing years 3 through 5 with years 6 through 10 (coefficient of 2.23 and robust SE of 0.75; $P<.02$). For positive symptoms at t−1, predicting positive symptoms at t, the comparison of stability for years 1 through 2 vs 6 through 10 is highly significant also (coefficient of 1.46 and robust SE of 0.36; $P<.0005$), but the comparison of stability for comparing years 3 through 5 with years 6 through 10 is not (coefficient of 0.37 and robust SE of 0.50; $P\leq.23$). These findings indicate a statistically significant increase in the stability of the process of symptom evolution that is stronger and more enduring for negative than for positive symptoms.

COMMENT

The prevalences of positive and negative syndromes drop sharply in the 6 months following first hospitalization and remain low thereafter. For the cohort as a whole, and on the basis of simple trends in prevalence, there is no evidence in support of the idea of an increase in negative symptoms after the first 2 years. On the other hand, there is a small tendency for an increase in the proportion of the cohort with *both* positive and negative syndromes simultaneously present, from sometime in the third year through the 10th year. Also, there is strong evidence that the process becomes more stable over time, especially with regard to negative symptoms.

The data suggest the utility of the constructs of positive and negative syndromes throughout the 10-year course. But there was evidence that the latent structure evolves over time, with an increase in the importance of a single factor including both positive and negative symptoms. This evolution is consistent with the slight increase, from years 3 through 10, in prevalence of the cooccurrence of the two syndromes.

Each syndrome strongly predicted its presence from month to month, with relatively weak predictability from one syndrome to the other and relatively weak evidence of substitutability between positive and negative symptoms. From the point of view of the natural history, it may be more useful to think of positive and negative symptoms as independent syndromes rather than parcels of the overall disorder called schizophrenia.

The results have important limitations. The cohort studied was based on a hospital sample and not drawn from the general population. All measurements were made by just a few clinicians, whose intuitions or hypotheses may have subtly affected the results, in spite of research training and deliberate attempts to avoid biases. The ability to compare factor structures over time is limited by the available techniques of statistical inference. The deaths of 10% of the cohort may have generated a bias toward better prognosis if those who died were more severely ill in ways we were unable to detect. Other studies of the natural history of schizophrenia have these limitations.

The most important limit to generalizability of these results is that the sample is entirely from south India, which may be distinctive. Early studies from the World Health Organization[37] and studies summarized above[4-9] repeatedly demonstrate that the cross-sectional picture of schizophrenia is remarkably similar in many cultures around the world. But longitudinal studies from the World Health Organization[27] and elsewhere[36] repeatedly show that the long-term course of schizophrenia is more benign in developing countries like India than in developed countries like the United States. Longitudinal studies under way now may be able to replicate these findings in the near future.

Accepted for publication November 1, 1994.

This article was supported by the Indian Medical Research Council, the Schizophrenia Research Foundation, Madras, and grant 44653 from the National Institute of Mental Health, Rockville, Md.

Reprint requests to The Johns Hopkins University, Department of Mental Hygiene, 624 N Broadway, Room 880, Baltimore, MD 21205 (Dr Eaton).

REFERENCES

1. Strauss JS, Carpenter WT, Bartko JJ. The diagnosis and understanding of schizophrenia, part III: speculations on the processes that underlie schizophrenic symptoms and signs. *Schizophr Bull.* 1974;11:61-79.
2. Andreasen NC, Olsen S. Negative vs positive schizophrenia. *Arch Gen Psychiatry.* 1982;39:789-794.
3. Young MA. Evaluating diagnostic criteria: a latent class paradigm. *J Psychiatr Res.* 1982;17:285-296.
4. Arndt S, Alliger RJ, Andreasen NC. The distinction of positive and negative symptoms: the failure of a two-dimensional model. *Br J Psychiatry.* 1991;158:317-322.
5. Gur RE, Mozley PD, Resnick SM, Levick S, Erwin R, Saykin AJ, Gur RC. Relations among clinical scales in schizophrenia. *Am J Psychiatry.* 1991;148:472-478.
6. Kulhara P, Kota SK, Joseph S. Positive and negative subtypes of schizophrenia. *Acta Psychiatr Scand.* 1986;74:353-359.
7. Liddle PF. The symptoms of chronic schizophrenia: a re-examination of the positive-negative dichotomy. *Br J Psychiatry.* 1987;151:145-151.
8. Liddle PF, Barnes TRE. Syndromes of chronic schizophrenia. *Br J Psychiatry.* 1990;157:558-561.
9. Moscarelli M, Maffei C, Cesana BM, Boato P, Farma T, Grilli A, Lingiardi V, Cazzullo CL. An international perspective on assessment of negative and positive symptoms in schizophrenia. *Am J Psychiatry.* 1987;144:1595-1598.

10. Kulhara K, Chandiramani K. Positive and negative subtypes of schizophrenia: a follow-up study from India. *Schizophr Res.* 1990;3:107-116.
11. Crow TJ. Molecular pathology of schizophrenia: more than one disease process? *BMJ.* 1980;280:66-68.
12. Andreasen NC, Flaum M, Swayze VW, Tyrrell G, Arndt S. Positive and negative symptoms in schizophrenia. *Arch Gen Psychiatry.* 1990;47:615-621.
13. McGlashan TH, Fenton WS. The positive-negative distinction in schizophrenia. *Arch Gen Psychiatry.* 1992;49:63-72.
14. Fenton WS, McGlashan TH. Natural history of schizophrenia subtypes. *Arch Gen Psychiatry.* 1991;48:978-986.
15. Ram R, Bromet EJ, Eaton WW, Pato C, Schwartz JE. The natural course of schizophrenia: a review of first admission studies. *Schizophr Bull.* 1992;18: 185-207.
16. Thara R, Henrietta M, Joseph A, Rajkumar S, Eaton WW. Ten-year course of schizophrenia—The Madras Longitudinal Study. *Acta Psychiatr Scand.* In press.
17. Pogue-Geile MF, Harrow M. Negative symptoms in schizophrenia: their longitudinal course and prognostic importance. *Schizophr Bull.* 1985;11:427-439.
18. Biehl H, Maurer K, Jung E, Krumm B. The WHO psychological impairments rating schedule (WHO/PIRS), II: impairments in cross-sectional and longitudinal perspective-the Mannheim experience in two independent samples. *Br J Psychiatry.* 1989;155(suppl 7):71-77.
19. Lindenmayer J-P, Kay SR, Friedman C. Negative and positive schizophrenic syndromes after the acute phase: a prospective follow-up. *Compr Psychiatry.* 1986;27:276-286.
20. Pfohl B, Winokur G. The evolution of symptoms in institutionalized schizophrenics. *Br J Psychiatry.* 1982;141:567-572.
21. Johnstone EC, Owens DGC, Frith CD, Crow TJ. The relative stability of positive and negative features in chronic schizophrenia. *Br J Psychiatry.* 1986;150:60-64.
22. World Health Organization. *Manual of the International Statistical Classification of Diseases, Injuries, and Causes of Death, Based on the Recommendations of the Ninth Revision Conference, 1975.* Geneva, Switzerland: World Health Organization; 1977.
23. Feighner JP, Robins E, Guze SB, Woodruff RA, Winokur G, Munoz R. Diagnostic criteria for use in psychiatric research. *Arch Gen Psychiatry.* 1972;26: 57-63.
24. American Psychiatric Association. *Diagnostic and Statistical Manual of Mental Disorders, Revised Third Edition.* Washington, DC: American Psychiatric Association; 1987.
25. Verghese A, John JK, Rajkumar S, Richard J, Sethi BB, Trivedi JK. Factors associated with the course and outcome of schizophrenia in India: results of a two-year multi-centre follow-up study. *Br J Psychiatry.* 1989;154:499-503.
26. Wing JK, Cooper JE, Satorius N. *Measurement and Classification of Psychiatric Symptoms.* 9th ed. London, England: Cambridge University Press; 1974.
27. Leff J, Sartorius N, Jablensky A, Anker M, Korten A, Gulbinat W, Ernberg G. The International Pilot Study of Schizophrenia: five-year follow-up findings. In: Hafner H, Gattaz WF, eds. *Search for the Causes of Schizophrenia-Volume II.* Berlin, Germany: Springer-Verlag; 1991:57-66.
28. McCreadie RG, Wiles D, Grant S, Crockett GT, Mahmood Z, Livingston MG, Watt JAG, Greene JG, Kershaw PW, Todd NA, Scott AM, Loudon J, Dyer JAT, Philip AE, Batchelor D. The Scottish First Episode Schizophrenia Study, VII: two-year follow-up. *Acta Psychiatr Scand.* 1989;80:597-602.
29. Muthen B. Contributions to factor analysis of dichotomous variables. *Psychometrika.* 1978;43:551-560.
30. Muthen BO. *LISCOMP: Analysis of Linear Structural Equations With a Comprehensive Measurement Model.* 2nd ed. [computer program]. Mooresville, Ind: Scientific Software Inc; 1988.
31. Liang K-Y, Zeger SL. Longitudinal data analysis using generalized linear models. *Biometrika.* 1986;73:13-22.
32. Zeger SL, Liang KY. Longitudinal data analysis for discrete and continuous outcomes. *Biometrics.* 1986;42:121-130.
33. Liang K-Y, Zeger SL. A class of logistic regression models for multivariate binary time series. *J Am Stat Assoc.* 1989;84:447-451.
34. Kay SR, Fiszbein A, Lindenmayer JP, Opler LA. Positive and negative syndromes in schizophrenia as a function of chronicity. *Acta Psychiatr Scand.* 1986;74:507-518.
35. Brown GW. Length of hospital stay and schizophrenia: a review of statistical studies. *Acta Psychiatr Neurol Scand.* 1960;35:414-430.
36. Eaton WW. Update on the epidemiology of schizophrenia. *Epidemiol Rev.* 1991; 13:320-328.
37. World Health Organization. *Schizophrenia: A Multinational Study.* Geneva, Switzerland: World Health Organization; 1975.

Notice to Authors

Length of Text. Ideally, the text of manuscripts (not including abstract, tables, figures, and references) should be under 5000 words. Include a word count on the title page.

Title. The title should be short, specific, and descriptive, emphasizing the main point of the article. Avoid two-part titles, if at all possible. Do not number titles, eg, "I" or "Part I." Title length, including punctuation and spaces, ideally should be under 100 characters and must not exceed 200 characters.

Abstract. The abstract should be structured into four parts and be no longer than 250 words.

Tables and Figures. Material should provide substantive data and not merely illustrate the text. While the main finding of a table or figure may be discussed in the narrative, the table or figure should not duplicate the text. Although no specific guideline applies to all articles, the number and length of tables and figures should be considered carefully and kept to a minimum.

References. All references should be selected carefully to acknowledge previous work or to document a specific point. They should not be exhaustive.

Please consult the "Instructions to Authors" on page 87 of this issue for other details regarding manuscript preparation.

ORIGINAL ARTICLE

Guanine Nucleotide-Binding Proteins in Bipolar Affective Disorder

Effects of Long-term Lithium Treatment

Husseini K. Manji, MD, FRCPC; Guang Chen, MD; Hady Shimon; John K. Hsiao, MD; William Z. Potter, MD, PhD; Robert H. Belmaker, MD

Background: This study examines recent suggestions from a number of investigators that signal-transducing guanine nucleotide-binding (G) proteins may be involved in the pathophysiology of bipolar affective disorder and may represent molecular targets for lithium's mood-stabilizing actions.

Methods: We used selective antibodies to quantitate the levels of the G protein α subunits that regulate adenylate cyclase activity ($G\alpha_s$ and $G\alpha_{i2}$) and phosphoinositide turnover ($G\alpha_{q/11}$). We also quantitated levels of pertussis toxin–catalyzed phosphate 32–labeled adenosine diphosphate ([^{32}P]ADP) ribosylation in platelet and leukocyte membranes from a group of 14 untreated (predominantly manic) patients with bipolar affective disorder, 20 lithium-treated euthymic patients with bipolar affective disorder, and 11 healthy controls.

Results: In both tissues, the immunolabeling of the 45-kd form of $G\alpha_s$ was higher in the bipolar affective disorder group considered as a whole (treated or untreated) compared with controls, effects that reached statistical significance in the leukocyte membranes. There were no significant differences in the immunolabeling of $G\alpha_{i1/2}$, $G\alpha_{q/11}$, or pertussis toxin–catalyzed [^{32}P]ADP ribosylation in either tissue in the untreated bipolar affective disorder group compared with controls. In both tissues, lithium-treated subjects demonstrated lower levels of $G\alpha_{q/11}$ and higher levels of pertussis toxin–catalyzed [^{32}P]ADP-ribosylation, which reached significance in the platelet membranes.

Conclusions: Our results are complementary to the previously reported findings of elevated $G\alpha_s$ levels in postmortem brain tissue from patients with bipolar affective disorder and in mononuclear leukocytes obtained from depressed patients with bipolar (but not unipolar) affective disorder. The significantly higher levels of pertussis toxin–catalyzed [^{32}P]ADP ribosylation in the subjects receiving long-term lithium-treatment replicates our findings in rat cortex and in healthy volunteers and adds to the growing body of evidence implicating $G\alpha_i$ as a target of lithium's actions.

(Arch Gen Psychiatry. 1995;52:135-144)

BIPOLAR AFFECTIVE disorder is a common (lifetime prevalence, 1.2%[1]), severe, chronic, and life-threatening disease.[2] Despite a well-established genetic diathesis[2,3] and extensive research, the biochemical abnormalities underlying the predisposition to and the pathophysiology of bipolar affective disorder remain to be clearly established. Early theories regarding the etiology of bipolar affective disorder have focused on various neurotransmitters, in particular, the biogenic amines.[2,4-6] In recent years, however, advances in our understanding of the molecular mechanisms underlying neuronal communication have focused research on the role of receptor and postreceptor sites, and indeed, numerous findings from both clinical and preclinical studies suggest that abnormalities in receptor-effector responsiveness may be involved in the pathophysiology of bipolar affective disorder.[7-11]

Data from a complementary line of research on the cellular mechanism(s) of action of mood-stabilizing agents have also been used to provide clues about the biochemical processes involved in the pathogenesis of bipolar affective disorder. There has been a growing appreciation that neurotransmitter function might be altered indirectly through alterations in intracellular signaling, and mood-stabilizing agents such as lithium might be effective not because they are catecholaminergic or cholinergic agents per se but because they alter the postsynaptic signal generated in

From the Experimental Therapeutics Branch, National Institute of Mental Health, Bethesda, Md (Drs Manji, Chen, Hsiao, and Potter), and Ben-Gurion University of the Negev, Beersheva, Israel (Ms Shimon and Dr Belmaker).

See Methods on next page

METHODS

PATIENTS

The group of untreated inpatients with bipolar affective disorder consisted of 10 male and four female subjects (mean±SD age, 47±13 years), 11 of whom were manic; two, depressed; and one, euthymic. Patients' conditions were diagnosed by clinical history and behavioral observations according to *DSM-III-R*[52] criteria by a research psychiatrist. All but one of the patients had not received any psychotropic medications other than lithium for at least 1 month (as determined by personal and family interviewing by a research psychiatrist) and had not received lithium treatment for a mean±SD of 11±12 months (range, 0.5 to 36 months). With the exception of one patient with bipolar affective disorder (a diabetic woman whose glucose levels were adequately controlled by an oral hypoglycemic agent at the time of the study), all subjects were established to be free of significant medical illness by medical history, a complete physical examination, a complete blood cell count and differential cell count, serum electrolyte measures, hepatic and renal function tests, thyroid function tests, and urinalysis.

The lithium-treated group consisted of eight male and 12 female patients (mean±SD age, 42±15 years). All of the lithium-treated patients were outpatients who were euthymic at the time of the blood drawing and who had been maintained on regular lithium treatment for a mean±SD of 17±15 months (range, 3 to 60 months). Lithium levels were obtained at the time of platelet and leukocyte collection and averaged 0.65±0.22 mmol/L (mean±SD). All patients' conditions were diagnosed according to *DSM-III-R* criteria by a research psychiatrist, and all patients consented to the blood drawing. The healthy control group consisted of seven men and four women (mean±SD age, 39±12 years) from the medical staff of the Beersheva (Israel) Mental Health Centre. Control subjects were free of all medications for at least 2 weeks prior to entry into the study, had no active medical problems, and had no personal or family history of psychiatric disorders, alcoholism, or drug abuse as determined by clinical interview.

BLOOD CELL ISOLATION AND MEMBRANE PREPARATION

Blood samples (50 mL) were obtained by venipuncture. The MNLs and platelets were isolated from the fresh blood (with heparin sodium as the anticoagulant) using a Ficoll (Histo-Paque, Sigma Chemical Co, St Louis, Mo) gradient, with minor modification of the procedure of Boyum.[53] The buffy coat that remained after the removal of the platelet-rich plasma was then removed with a Pasteur pipette, was diluted 1:1 with phosphate-buffered saline solution, and was layered carefully onto Ficoll gradient and subjected to gradient centrifugation. The leukocyte band was carefully removed, washed with phosphate-buffered saline solution, and centrifuged, and the pellet was frozen at −80°C until use. Ten milliliters of blood routinely yielded 1×10^6 to 2×10^6 mononuclear cells that consisted of over 90% clear MNLs. Cells were homogenized, washed in ice-cold isotonic buffer that contained ethylenediaminetetraacetic acid (2 mmol/l), egtazic acid (5 mmol/L), dithiothreitol (1 mmol/L), leupeptin (1 mg/mL), phenylmethylsulfonyl fluoride (2 mmol/L), and benzamidine (100 mmol/L), pH 7.5. The suspension was sonicated with 4×10-second pulses, and intact cells were removed by centrifugation at 1500g. The leukocyte lysate was then centrifuged in an ultracentrifuge (Beckman TL-100, Beckman Instruments, Fullerton, Calif) at 45 000g for 1 hour at 4°C to obtain a crude plasma membrane fraction. Following resuspension in TRIS hydrochloride (10 mmol/L, pH 7.5), the membrane protein concentrations were determined in triplicate according to the method of Bradford,[54] and the samples were frozen in appropriate aliquots at −80°C until use.

After removal of the platelet-rich plasma, the platelet pellet was obtained by centrifugation of the platelet-rich plasma at 1200g for 15 minutes, and the pellet was rinsed with phosphate-buffered saline solution and then frozen at −80°C until subsequent use. Pellets were resuspended in ice-cold TRIS hydrochloride buffer that contained ethylenediaminetetraacetic acid (2 mmol/l), egtazic acid (5 mmol/L), dithiothreitol (1 mmol/L), leupeptin (1 mg/mL), phenylmethylsulfonyl fluoride (2 mmol/L), and benzamidine (100 mmol/L), pH 7.5. The suspension was sonicated with 4×10-second pulses, and intact platelets were removed by cen-

response to multiple, endogenous neurotransmitters. In this context, signal transduction pathways are in a pivotal position in the central nervous system (CNS), are able to affect the functional balance between neurotransmitter systems, and have been postulated to explain lithium's efficacy in treating multiple aspects of the illness. It is thus not suprising that over the past several years, research aimed at the elucidation of the molecular mechanisms underlying lithium's therapeutic effects have focused on signal transduction pathways.

Of particular interest, several independent laboratories have shown that lithium, on long-term administration at therapeutically relevant doses, unequivocally affects second-messenger–generating systems,[7,9-16] and indeed, lithium inhibition of vasopressin-sensitive[17] or thyrotropin-sensitive[18] adenylate cyclase is thought to underlie (at least in part) the commonly observed side effects of nephrogenic diabetes insipidus and subclinical hypothyroidism, respectively. Because lithium has been demonstrated to affect both phosphoinositide turnover[19-21] and adenylate cyclase activity,[22-25] recent research has focused on mechanisms shared in common by these two major second-messenger–generating systems, namely, the signal-transducing guanine nucleotide-binding (G) proteins.[7,9,26-30] A brief overview of the role of G proteins in the regulation of transmembrane signal transduction is presented before proceeding to a discussion of the evidence supporting a role for G proteins in human diseases.

In recent years, there have been significant advances in the elucidation of the molecular mechanisms underlying neuronal communication, particularly with respect to defining the obligatory role of G proteins in the transduction of a vast array of extracellular, receptor-detected signals across cell membranes to intracellular effectors. Most of the neurotransmitters and neuromodulators that initiate cellular signaling cannot penetrate the hydrophobic plasma membrane lipid bilayer but rather trifugation at 1500g. The platelet lysate was then centrifuged in an ultracentrifuge (Beckman TL-100) at 45 000g for 1 hour at 4°C to obtain a crude plasma membrane fraction. Following resuspension in TRIS hydrochloride (10 mmol/L, pH 7.5), the membrane protein concentrations were determined in triplicate according to the method of Bradford,[54] and the samples were then frozen in appropriate aliquots at −80°C until use.

IMMUNOBLOT ANALYSIS

The linearity of the plasma membrane protein concentration for Western blotting was ascertained by resolution of selected quantities of protein (between 10 and 200 μg). Subsequent studies were performed using a protein concentration known to be within the linear range for immunolabeling of the G protein α subtypes. Western blotting was performed on all samples in duplicate using previously described procedures, with selective antibodies directed against synthetic decapeptides that corresponded to the carboxy-termini of the respective $G\alpha_s$, $G\alpha_{q/11}$, and $G\alpha_{i1/2}$ subunits (Dupont, Wilmington, Del).[55,56] In brief, 25 to 50 μg of membrane protein were solubilized in denaturing buffer,[50] and proteins were resolved by sodium dodecyl sulfate–polyacrylamide gel electrophoresis on 10% polyacrylamide gels. Proteins thus resolved were electrophoretically transferred onto nitrocellulose paper. Protein binding sites on the nitrocellulose were blocked with low detergent (Blotto, Advanced Biotechnologies Inc, Columbia, Mo) containing 5% nonfat dry milk. After a thorough washing with distilled water, the blots were incubated at room temperature overnight with specific polyclonal anti-$G\alpha_s$ (RM), anti-$G\alpha_{i1/2}$ (AS), and anti-$G\alpha_{q/11}$ (QL) antiserum (all 1:5000 dilution) and, after appropriate washing, were incubated with iodine 125–labeled protein A (Amersham, Arlington Heights, Ill) for 2 hours at room temperature. The labeled blots were then washed, dried, and exposed to roentgenographic film with intensifying screens at −80°C. Quantitation of the immunoblots was performed by densitometric scanning of the autoradiograms using an image analysis system (NIH Image 1•47, National Institutes of Health, Bethesda, Md). An aliquot of pooled standard platelet or MNL membranes was run on one lane of every gel, and the immunolabeling was calculated relative to this standard. Data were normalized against pooled platelet or leukocyte membrane fractions, which were run on all blots to minimize between-blot variability.

PERTUSSIS TOXIN–CATALYZED [^{32}P]ADP RIBOSYLATION

Pertussis toxin–catalyzed labeling of platelet and leukocyte G_i was performed using previously described methods.[28,57] There was insufficient material to perform cholera toxin–catalyzed [^{32}P]ADP-ribosylation of G_s. In brief, the frozen membranes were thawed and resuspended in potassium phosphate buffer (pH 7.5, 1.5 mg of protein per milliliter), then were incubated at 37°C for 60 minutes in a final volume of 0.2 mL, containing potassium phosphate buffer (100 mmol/L, pH 7.5), thymidine (100 mmol/L), arginine (10 mmol/L), adenosine triphosphate (0.5 mmol/L), GTP (50 μmol/L), and α-^{32}P-labeled nicotinamide adenine dinucleotide (10 μmol/L) (92.5×10^{10} Bq/mmol) (New England Nuclear, Boston, Mass) with and without activated toxin. Prior to incubation, pertussis toxin (5 μg per tube) (List Biological Laboratories, Campbell, Calif) was activated with dithiothreitol (10 mmol/L) for 30 minutes at 37°C. The linearity of the plasma membrane protein concentration for pertussis toxin–catalyzed ^{32}P labeling was ascertained by resolution of selected quantities of membrane protein (between 20 and 400 μg). Subsequent studies were performed using protein concentrations (50 to 100 μg) that were known to be within the linear range for toxin-catalyzed ^{32}P labeling. Pertussis toxin–catalyzed [^{32}P]ADP ribosylation of all samples was performed in duplicate. Labeled membranes were washed in ice cold buffer, and proteins were solubilized and subjected to sodium dodecyl sulfate–polyacrylamide gel electrophoresis on 10% polyacrylamide gels using the method of Laemmli.[50] The gels were dried and exposed to a roentgenographic film (Kodak X-omat, Eastman Kodak, Rochester, NY) with an intensifying screen at −80°C. Estimation of the molecular weights of labeled protein bands was made by comparison with molecular weight standards. An aliquot of pooled standard platelet or MNL membranes were run on one lane of every gel, and the quantitation of ^{32}P incorporation was calculated relative to this standard. Values are expressed as means±SDs.

transmit their message via cell-surface receptors. It has been estimated that about 80% of all known hormones, neurotransmitters, and neuromodulators (numbering over 200) elicit cellular responses through G proteins coupled to a variety of intracellular effectors.

Guanine nucleotide-binding proteins are a ubiquitous family of proteins that play the critical role of tranducers of information across the plasma membrane, coupling receptors to various effectors.[7,31-33] The G proteins are heterotrimers that are localized to the inner surface of the plasma membrane and consist of an α subunit, which binds and hydrolyzes guanosine triphosphate (GTP), and β and γ subunits, which form a tightly but noncovalently linked dimer.[31-33] The α subunits have generally been assumed to confer receptor and effector specificity to the G protein, but recent evidence has also demonstrated critical roles for β and γ subunits in signal transduction pathways.[34-36]

Information traverses catalytically across a G protein–coupled system in a guanosine triphosphatase (GTPase) cycle, resulting in a several-thousand–fold amplification of the original signal. The G proteins that coordinate receptor-effector activity are derived from a large gene family, and recent cloning and sequencing of complementary DNAs that encode the α subunits have defined four major classes (G_s, G_i, G_q, and G_{12}) with at least 16 isotypes.[31-33] The G protein cycle, which is at the center of receptor-effector communication, has been described as a carefully timed molecular switch that allows the cell to respond rapidly to low stimulus concentration and that produces a major amplification of the original neurotransmitter signal.[31,37]

Given the variety of functions subserved by G protein–coupled signal transduction, it is not suprising that abnormalities in G protein–coupled pathways have been implicated in a variety of human diseases.[7,32,38-42] For example, an inherited form of generalized hormone resistance, Albright's hereditary osteodystrophy (also called pseudohypoparathyroidism Ia) is associated with a 50% deficiency of $G\alpha_s$ in all tissues.[32,40,42] Multiple distinct heterozygous mutations in the $G\alpha_s$ gene, most of which lead to reduced messenger RNA (mRNA) formation and/or stability, have been found in affected family members.[32,40,42] Although one might intuitively expect that such dramatic reductions in the levels of this key protein necessarily would be associated with severe clinical manifestations, it is noteworthy that a 50% reduction in $G\alpha_s$ levels has also been observed in family members without overt clinical disease (pseudopseudohypoparathyroidism). This suggests that similar to a number of neuropsychiatric diseases, additional factors (eg, environmental factors) must determine clinical expression of the disease. In contrast to this hypofunctional disease, a mutation in the $G\alpha_s$ gene that results in constitutive activation of G_s in affected tissues has been demonstrated to underlie the pathophysiology of McCune-Albright syndrome. McCune-Albright syndrome is a sporadic disorder in which the subjects manifest heterogeneous symptoms such as polyostotic fibrous dysplasia, café au lait skin pigmentation, and autonomous hyperfunctioning of one or more endocrine glands (gonad, adrenal cortex, thyroid, or pituitary somatotrophs).[32,41]

These examples highlight the diverse range of clinical manifestations that arise from alterations in the levels and/or functioning of these key signal transducers. Indeed, the G proteins that coordinate receptor-effector activity are especially important in the CNS, where they play widespread critical roles in the regulation of neuronal function, maintain the functional balance between neurotransmitter systems,[7,43-46] and represent attractive putative molecular sites underlying the pathophysiology of bipolar affective disorder and/or where they serve as targets for lithium's efficacy in treating multiple aspects of the illness.

Three previous studies[47-49] have examined G proteins in patients with bipolar affective disorder. Schreiber and colleagues[47] reported hyperfunctional G protein function in the leukocytes of untreated manic patients by demonstrating that agonist-stimulated binding of tritiated guanyl imidodiphosphate (a stable, nonhydrolyzable analogue of GTP) was enhanced in leukocyte membranes of untreated manic patients compared with those of controls. These findings suggest the presence of increased levels of G proteins and/or enhanced receptor-mediated activation of G proteins in leukocytes from untreated manic subjects. Complementary to these findings, Young and associates[48,49] have reported increased levels of $G\alpha_s$ in patients with bipolar affective disorder in two separate studies. They observed increased levels of $G\alpha_s$ in cerebral cortex but not cerebellum in postmortem brain tissue from patients with bipolar affective disorder.[48] More recently, the same group of investigators observed significantly higher levels of $G\alpha_s$ in mononuclear leukocytes (MNLs) from depressed patients with bipolar affective disorder but not in those from depressed patients with unipolar affective disorder[49]; the latter study did not examine euthymic patients with bipolar affective disorder, leaving open the question of the role of the illness state on the levels of $G\alpha_s$ in peripheral cells. These studies, although preliminary, suggest that alterations in the levels and/or function of certain G proteins may underlie the pathophysiology of bipolar affective disorder.

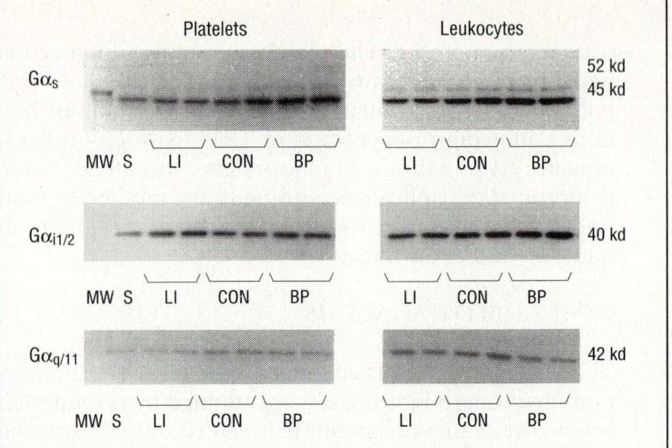

Figure 1. *Representative Western blots of guanine nucleotide-binding (G) protein α subunits. Western blotting was performed on platelet and leukocyte membranes, which were prepared according to the methods described in the text. Blots were incubated overnight with specific polyclonal anti-$G\alpha_s$ (top), anti-$G\alpha_{i1-2}$ (center), and anti-$G\alpha_{q/11}$ (bottom) antiserum (all 1:5000 dilution) and, after appropriate washing, were incubated with iodine 125–labeled protein A for 2 hours at room temperature. The labeled blots were then washed, dried, and exposed to roentgenographic film with intensifying screens at −80°C. An aliquot of pooled standard platelet or mononuclear leukocyte membranes was run on one lane of every gel to reduce interblot variability, and the quantitation of the appropriate band was calculated relative to this standard. MW, indicates molecular weight standards; S, standard platelet or leukocyte membranes; LI, lithium-treated subjects; CON, control subjects; and BP, untreated subjects with bipolar affective disorder.*

In the present study, we have sought to directly examine the levels of G protein α subunits in both platelets and leukocytes from a group of untreated (predominantly manic) patients with bipolar affective disorder, a group of lithium-treated euthymic patients with bipolar affective disorder, and age- and sex-matched controls. Using specific antibodies, we quantitate the levels of the G protein α subunits that mediate stimulation and inhibition of adenylate cyclase ($G\alpha_s$ and $G\alpha_{i2}$, respectively) and stimulation of phosphoinositide turnover ($G\alpha_{q/11}$). Additionally, we have examined pertussis toxin–catalyzed phosphate 32–labeled adenosine diphosphate ([^{32}P]ADP) ribosylation because we previously demonstrated effects of long-term lithium administration on this variable both in rat cortex and in platelets from healthy volunteers.[24,50,51]

RESULTS

Figure 1 shows representative immunoblots of G protein α subunit immunoreactivity in platelet and leukocyte membranes from untreated (predominantly manic) patients with bipolar affective disorder, euthymic lithium-treated patients, and healthy controls. All three polyclonal G protein antisera used in the present study selectively recognized distinct G protein α subunits as has been previously described.[55,56] Thus, the $G\alpha_s$ antisera recognized a major band that was migrating with an apparent molecular mass of 45 kd and a minor band that was migrating at 52 kd in both leukocyte and platelet membranes. The $G\alpha_{i1/2}$ antisera recognized a single band

G Proteins in Bipolar Affective Disorder*

	All Patients With Bipolar Affective Disorder (n=34)	Untreated Patients (n=14)	LI-Treated Patients (n=20)	Controls (n=11)
		Leukocyte		
$G\alpha_s$ (52 kd)	124±46	140±46	113±39	101±44
$G\alpha_s$ (45 kd)	125±37†	129±35	123±38	98±41
$G\alpha_{i1/2}$	94±48	99±24	89±59	94±28
$G\alpha_{q/11}$	78±36	93±44	68±25†	90±39
Pertussis toxin [^{32}P]ADPR	103±73	90±48	114±90	70±65
		Platelet		
$G\alpha_s$ (52 kd)	212±71	184±72	230±67	209±69
$G\alpha_s$ (45 kd)	119±24	121±30	119±20	104±20
$G\alpha_{i1/2}$	124±46	141±46	113±43	130±41
$G\alpha_{q/11}$	123±26	139±22	112±23†	142±28
Pertussis toxin [^{32}P]ADPR	130±57	111±35	141±42†	96±32

*Values are expressed as standardized densitometry units. LI indicates lithium; [^{32}P]ADPR, phosphate 32–labeled adenosine diphosphate ribosylation.
†P<.05 compared with controls.

(known to be predominantly α_{i2} in human platelets) with an apparent molecular mass of of 40 kd, and the $G\alpha_{q/11}$ antisera recognized a single band with an apparent molecular mass of of 42 kd in both leukocyte and platelet membranes. Quantitation of the immunoblots was performed by densitometric scanning of the autoradiograms, and the data were normalized against pooled platelet or leukocyte membranes, which were run on all blots to minimize between-blot variability. There were no significant age effects as determined by analysis of variance, and we did not find any significant effects of red blood cell contamination or pellet size on either immunolabeling or [^{32}P]ADP ribosylation. The **Table** summarizes the results of the densitometric analysis.

LEUKOCYTE AND PLATELET $G\alpha_s$ IN BIPOLAR AFFECTIVE DISORDER

$G\alpha_s$ (45 kd)

When the untreated bipolar affective disorder group and the lithium-treated group were considered separately, analysis of variance revealed trends toward statistically significant differences in both leukocytes ($F[2,42]=2.27$; $P=.12$) and platelets ($F[2,43]=2.25$; $P=.12$). In view of these trends and the previously reported findings,[48] we also analyzed the data considering the bipolar affective disorder group as a whole (treated or untreated). In both platelets and leukocytes, the bipolar affective disorder group considered as a whole (untreated or treated) showed a greater immunolabeling of the major (45-kd) form of $G\alpha_s$ compared with controls. The approximately 25% greater immunolabeling of the 45-kd form of leukocyte $G\alpha_s$ in the bipolar group reached statistical significance (bipolar affective disorder group, 125±37 optical density units, standardized (OD U/STD); control group, 98±41 OD U/STD; $t=2.15$; $df=43$; $P<.05$). The levels of leukocyte $G\alpha_s$ (45 kd) in the lithium-treated bipolar affective disorder group was not significantly different from the untreated bipolar affective disorder group (untreated patients, 129±35 OD U/STD; lithium-treated patients, 123±38 OD U/STD; $t=0.14$; $P=.88$). Analysis of the manic subset of patients revealed similar results to those of the bipolar affective disorder group as a whole.

In platelet membranes, the bipolar affective disorder group also exhibited an approximately 20% greater immunolabeling of 45-kd $G\alpha_s$ compared with controls (bipolar affective disorder group vs control group: $t=1.95$, $df=41$, $P=.06$).The levels of 45-kd $G\alpha_s$ in the lithium-treated bipolar affective disorder group was not significantly different from those in the untreated bipolar affective disorder group.

There were no significant correlations between the levels of 45-kd $G\alpha_s$ in either platelets or leukocytes and plasma lithium levels or duration of time receiving and not receiving lithium.

$G\alpha_s$ (52 kd)

In leukocytes, the immunolabeling of the long (52-kd) form of $G\alpha_s$ in the bipolar affective disorder group considered as a whole (untreated or treated) was approximately 20% higher than that of the control subjects, although this did not reach statistical significance. When only the manic subjects (n=11) from the overall bipolar group were examined, the higher immunolabeling of the 52-kd form of $G\alpha_s$ showed a trend toward statistical significance (manic patients vs controls: $t=1.81$, $df=17$, $P=.08$). By contrast, in platelet membranes, the immunolabeling of the 52-kd form of $G\alpha_s$ in the overall bipolar group was almost identical to that of the control group. The levels of platelet $G\alpha_s$ (52 kd) in the manic subgroup of patients was not significantly different from those of controls.

LEUKOCYTE AND PLATELET $G\alpha_{i1/2}$ IN BIPOLAR AFFECTIVE DISORDER

In leukocytes, there were no statistically significant differences in the immunolabeling of $G\alpha_{i1/2}$ in the three groups (untreated patients with bipolar affective disorder, 99±24 OD U/STD; lithium-treated patients, 89±59 OD U/STD; controls, 94±28 OD U/STD; $F[2,42]=0.25$; $P=.78$). When only the manic subjects (n=11) from the overall bipolar group were examined, similar results were observed. Similarly, there were no statistically significant differences in the levels of $G\alpha_{i1/2}$ in platelet membranes from the three groups, although the lithium-treated group had modestly lower levels than did the untreated bipolar affective disorder group (untreated patients with bipolar affective disorder, 141±46 OD U/STD; lithium-treated patients, 113±43 OD U/STD; P was not significant [$P=.32$]).

LEUKOCYTE AND PLATELET $G\alpha_{q/11}$ IN BIPOLAR AFFECTIVE DISORDER

In both leukocyte and platelet membranes, there were no significant differences in the immunolabeling of $G\alpha_{q/11}$ in the untreated bipolar affective disorder group compared

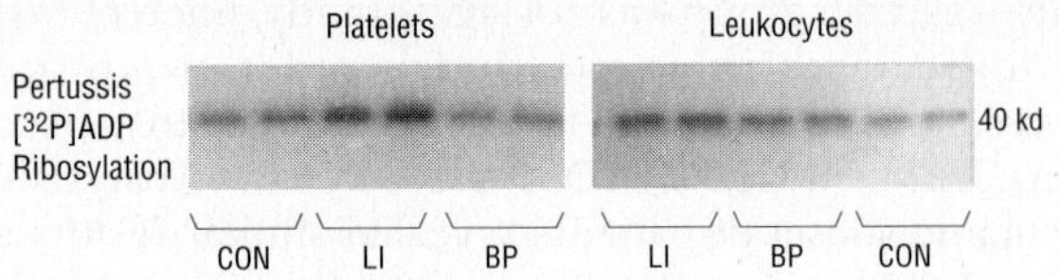

Figure 2. *Representative autoradiogram of pertussis toxin–catalyzed phosphate 32–labeled adenosine diphosphate ([^{32}P]ADP) ribosylation. Platelet and leukocyte membranes were subjected to pertussis toxin–catalyzed labeling with α-^{32}P–labeled nicotinamide adenine dinucleotide (10 μmol/L) (92.5×10 Bq/mmol) and activated toxin as described in the "Methods" section. Labeled membranes were washed in ice-cold buffer, and proteins were solubilized and subjected to sodium dodecyl sulfate–polyacrylamide gel electrophoresis. An aliquot of pooled standard platelet or mononuclear leukocyte membranes was run on one lane of every gel to reduce inter-blot variability, and the quantitation of [^{32}P] incorporation was calculated relative to this standard. CON indicates control subjects; LI, lithium-treated subjects; and BP, untreated subjects with bipolar affective disorder.*

with the control group. In both tissues, the lithium-treated euthymic group exhibited lower levels of $G\alpha_{q/11}$. Thus, in leukocytes, the levels of $G\alpha_{q/11}$ were approximately 20% lower in the lithium-treated group (untreated patients with bipolar affective disorder, 93±44 OD U/STD; lithium-treated patients, 68±25 OD U/STD; controls, 90±39 OD U/STD; $F[2,41]=3.35$; $P<0.05$); these effects were statistically significant when the lithium-treated group was compared with the untreated bipolar affective disorder group (lithium-treated vs untreated patients with bipolar affective disorder: $t=2.48$, $df=27$, $P<.05$; lithium-treated patients vs controls: $t=2.03$, $df=18$, $P=.06$). The levels of $G\alpha_{q/11}$ were also lower in platelets in the lithium-treated group compared with the other two groups (untreated patients with bipolar affective disorder, 139±22 OD U/STD; lithium-treated patients, 112±3 OD U/STD; controls, 142±28 OD U/STD; $F[2,42]=4.45$; $P<.05$).

PERTUSSIS TOXIN–CATALYZED [^{32}P]ADP-RIBOSYLATION OF LEUKOCYTE AND PLATELET MEMBRANES IN BIPOLAR AFFECTIVE DISORDER

Figure 2 shows a representative blot of pertussis toxin–catalyzed [^{32}P]ADP ribosylation in platelet and leukocyte membranes from untreated patients with bipolar affective disorder, euthymic lithium-treated patients, and healthy controls. Similar to the immunolabeling of $G\alpha_{i1/2}$, pertussis toxin catalyzed the [^{32}P]ADP ribosylation of a single major band with an apparent molecular mass of 40 kd in both tissues. In both leukocyte and platelet membranes, the pertussis toxin–catalyzed ^{32}P labeling of $G\alpha_{i1/2}$ was approximately 25% to 30% higher in the lithium-treated group compared with the control group; in both tissues, the ^{32}P labeling was nonsignificantly higher in the untreated bipolar group compared with the control groups. The increased ^{32}P labeling of the lithium-treated group showed a trend toward statistical significance in the platelet membranes (platelet membranes: untreated patients with bipolar affective disorder, 111±35 OD U/STD; lithium-treated patients, 141±42 OD U/STD; controls, 96±32 OD U/STD; $F(2,40)=2.23$; $P=.12$), largely because of the increased ^{32}P labeling in the lithium-treated group compared with the control group (lithium-treated group vs control group: $t=2.88$, $df=22$, $P<.05$).

COMMENT

This study is the first that we are aware of to directly quantitate the levels of the major G protein α subunits in leukocytes and platelets from both untreated (predominantly manic) and lithium-treated euthymic patients with bipolar affective disorder. We did not observe significant differences in the levels of $G\alpha_{i1/2}$ or $G\alpha_{q/11}$ or in the levels of pertussis toxin–catalyzed [^{32}P]ADP ribosylation in either tissue from the untreated patients with bipolar affective disorder compared with control subjects. The stimulatory G protein, $G\alpha_s$, is present in both a long (52-kd) and a short (45-kd) form in most tissues, with the latter being the predominant form in both leukocytes and platelets.[58,59] There were no significant differences in the levels of the long form of $G\alpha_s$ (52 kd) in the untreated bipolar affective disorder group compared with controls. However, in both platelet and leukocyte membranes, we observed higher levels of the 45-kd form of $G\alpha_s$ in the overall group of patients with bipolar affective disorder (treated or untreated) compared with controls. Similar to our previous findings in platelets from healthy volunteers,[13,28] the lithium-treated group exhibited higher pertussis toxin–catalyzed [^{32}P]ADP-ribosylation.

The elevated levels of $G\alpha_s$ (45 kd) that we have observed in both platelets and leukocytes is consistent with the previous studies of G proteins in bipolar affective disorder. Young and associates[49] observed elevated levels of $G\alpha_s$ (45 kd) in leukocytes obtained from bipolar (but not unipolar) depressed patients. Interestingly, they observed a positive correlation between the levels of leukocyte $G\alpha_s$ and Hamilton Depression Rating Scale scores. We did not use any standardized rating instruments in our study, but our findings of similarly elevated levels of $G\alpha_s$ in the group of lithium-treated euthymic patients suggests that it is not simply a function of illness state.

In a postmortem study of bipolar affective disorder, increased levels of $G\alpha_s$ were observed in cerebral cortex but not in cerebellum.[48] It should be noted that in that study, levels of both the short (45-kd) and long (52-kd) form of $G\alpha_s$ were elevated, although only the latter significantly so in prefrontal cortex. It is now well established that these different forms of $G\alpha_s$ arise as a result of alternative splicing of a single gene, resulting in a differential relative expression of the subtypes in various tissues. Interestingly, in most brain regions, the 52-kd form predominates, whereas in circulating blood cells, the 45-kd form is much more abundant.[58,59] Thus, in both the present study and the studies by Young and associates,[48,49] elevations were observed in the levels of the predominant subspecies of $G\alpha_s$ present in the tissues examined. Moreover, because both forms arise from a single gene,[58,59] abnormalities in this key component of signal transduction represent a potential molecular basis underlying the predisposition to bipolar affective disorder and is worthy of further study (as discussed below).

The other major previous study of G proteins in bipolar affective disorder reported enhanced G protein activation in leukocytes of untreated manic patients.[47] Schreiber and associates[47] reported that isoproterenol-stimulated binding of tritiated guanyl imidodiphosphate (a stable, nonhydrolyzable analogue of GTP) was enhanced in leukocyte membranes of untreated manic patients compared with controls. These findings suggested the presence of elevated levels of G_s and/or enhanced receptor-mediated activation of G_s in leukocytes from untreated manic subjects. Although these results are consistent with the findings of the present study, it should be noted that the two studies used markedly different methods, making a direct comparison of the results difficult. We did not observe any significant differences in the levels of $G\alpha_s$ between the untreated bipolar affective disorder group and the lithium-treated group, but the cross-sectional design of our study does not allow us to completely rule out possible effects of lithium treatment on the levels of $G\alpha_s$ in peripheral cells. Although our laboratory has not observed any significant effects of long-term lithium treatment on the levels of $G\alpha_s$ in rat frontal cortex,[27] abundant evidence has shown that long-term treatment with lithium attenuates receptor-G_s coupling.[7,9,13-15,22-25] Taken together, the results suggest that long-term lithium administration may attenuate receptor-G_s function[7,9,13-15,22-25] by a process that does not involve alterations in the amount of $G\alpha_s$ per se.

THE RELEVANCE of our findings to the pathophysiology of bipolar affective disorder is presently unclear. To begin with, considerable caution is obviously necessary when extrapolating from the findings obtained in peripheral blood cells to signal transduction systems in the CNS. The major limitation of these peripheral models is that the blood cells are exposed to a potentially completely different environment (including circulating catecholamines and hormones)[51,60,61] from that of brain tissue, which may lead to marked differences in G protein–coupled signal transduction pathways.[62,63] Although one might intuitively expect desensitized, hypofunctional leukocyte β-adrenergic–G_s responses in untreated manics due to exposure to elevated levels of circulating catecholamines,[2,4] recent physiological data show that regulation of leukocyte β-adrenergic sensitivity is a complex, multifaceted process.[51,60,61] In this context, it is noteworthy that short-term activation of the sympathetic nervous system produces increased leukocyte β-adrenergic sensitivity[51,60,61] because of a release of activated leukocyte subsets from the spleen into the circulation. Because we did not measure the relative leukocyte subpopulations in the present study, it remains a possibility that the observed elevations in levels of $G\alpha_s$ (45 kd) in subjects with bipolar affective disorder are due, at least in part, to differences in leukocyte subpopulations, and additional studies will be necessary to address this potentially confounding variable. However, the demonstration of elevated levels of $G\alpha_s$ in areas of brain obtained at post mortem from patients with bipolar affective disorder[48] suggests that the alterations observed in peripheral blood cells may not be simply due to alterations in the circulating environment.

Additional issues worth addressing are the fact that the magnitude of the elevations in levels of $G\alpha_s$ are relatively modest and that $G\alpha_s$ is a ubiquitously expressed protein. As discussed in the introduction, the G proteins that coordinate and regulate receptor-effector coupling also serve as major signal amplifiers,[7,31-33] which results in a several-thousand–fold amplification of the original signal[31,37]; thus, even a 25% alteration in the levels of $G\alpha_s$ may significantly affect physiological processes. Additionally, there is already precedence for clinical disorders that arise from abnormalities in the levels of $G\alpha_s$, presenting with relatively limited clinical manifestations despite the ubiquitous expression of $G\alpha_s$. Patients with pseudopseudohypoparathyroidism show relatively limited clinical symptoms (eg, they exhibit no cardiac dysfunction) despite a 50% reduction in the levels of $G\alpha_s$ in all cells.[30,40,42] In pseudohypoparathyroidism Ia, the 50% reduction in the levels of $G\alpha_s$ is associated with a somewhat more generalized reduction in end-organ responsiveness.[30,40,42] Even in this disorder, despite a 50% reduction in the levels of $G\alpha_s$, some tissues from these patients show no abnormality in the levels of basal or receptor-stimulated cyclic adenosine monophosphate. These heterogeneous effects have been postulated to arise from differences in receptor, G protein, and effector stoichiometries in different tissues and to differences in the ability of different cells to compensate (eg, by the alteration in the activities of different phosphodiesterases) for the primary alteration in the levels of $G\alpha_s$.[30,40,42]

Given the complexities in the regulation of CNS function, it is possible that the elevations in the levels of $G\alpha_s$ in bipolar affective disorder may be manifest primarily as psychiatric symptoms. It should be emphasized, however, that there is at present no evidence to suggest that the alterations in the levels of $G\alpha_s$ are due to a mutation in the $G\alpha_s$ gene itself. Indeed, there are numerous transcriptional and posttranscriptional mechanisms that regulate the levels of G protein α subunits,[29,30,62-65] and the elevated levels of $G\alpha_s$ could potentially represent the sequelae of alterations in any one of these other biochemical pathways. Thus, the elucidation of the mechanism(s) underlying the elevations in the levels of $G\alpha_s$ both in the brain and in peripheral cells may provide important clues regarding the complex biochemical changes in this disorder.

We did not observe any differences in the levels of pertussis toxin–catalyzed [^{32}P]ADP ribosylation in the untreated bipolar affective disorder group compared with control subjects. However, the lithium-treated euthymic patients demonstrated higher [^{32}P]ADP-ribosylation compared with control subjects, which reached statistical significance in the platelets. Pertussis toxin is known to selectively catalyze the [^{32}P]ADP ribosylation of the inactive (αβγ) conformation of selected G proteins (G_t, G_o, and G_i).[66] In platelets and leukocytes, however, G_i is the only pertussis toxin substrate present; thus, when used in conjunction with methods to quantitate the levels of $G\alpha_i$ (eg, enzyme-linked immunosorbent assay or immunolabeling), the [^{32}P]ADP ribosylation can provide useful information about the conformational state of G_i. Given the cross-sectional nature of our study, we cannot definitively conclude that the higher levels of pertussis toxin–catalyzed [^{32}P]ADP ribosylation are due to lithium treatment. Nevertheless, we have observed strikingly similar results in both platelet membranes from healthy volunteers[13,28] and in rat prefrontal cortex[27] after long-term lithium administration, which suggests that our present results do not simply reflect the secondary sequelae of alterations in mood-state–dependent variables that are associated with the lithium treatment of patients.

At present, the precise mechanism(s) underlying the lithium-induced increases in pertussis toxin–catalyzed [^{32}P]ADP ribosylation remain to be fully established. We have not observed any significant differences in the levels of $G\alpha_{i1/2}$ in peripheral tissues from lithium-treated patients with bipolar affective disorder compared with control subjects (present study) and have not observed any lithium-induced alterations in healthy volunteers[13,28] or rat cortex.[27] Similar to our findings, one independent laboratory has observed no changes in the levels of $G\alpha_{i1/2}$ in rat cortex[29] after long-term lithium administration, in contrast to the findings of Colin and associates[30] (who have observed small decreases in the levels of $G\alpha_{i1/2}$ in rat cortex). However, both of these laboratories have observed small decreases in the levels of $G\alpha_{i2}$ mRNA in rat cortex,[29,30] which suggests that lithium exerts complex transcriptional and/or posttranscriptional effects on these G proteins.[39,40,64]

There is much more agreement about the effects of lithium on G_i function, and several independent laboratories have now demonstrated that long-term lithium administration attenuates G_i function (as assessed by adenylate cyclase activity) in humans and in rodents.[15] In previous studies in both humans and rodents,[13,15,27,28] the attenuation of G_i function was accompanied by significant increases in pertussis toxin–catalyzed [^{32}P]ADP ribosylation. Because pertussis toxin selectively ADP-ribosylates the undissociated, inactive $\alpha\beta\gamma$ heterotrimeric form of G_i,[66] these results suggest that lithium inactivates G_i via a stabilization of the inactive conformation.[13,67]

A novel finding to emerge from the present study is the significantly lower levels of $G\alpha_{q/11}$ in both platelets and leukocytes from the the lithium-treated euthymic group. $G\alpha_q$ and $G\alpha_{11}$ are the G protein α subunits that couple receptors to stimulation of phosphoinositide turnover in most tissues, including brain and peripheral cells.[68,69] The phosphoinositide second-messenger–generating system has been the focus of extensive recent research[16,19-21] following the demonstration that lithium (at therapeutically relevant concentrations) is a potent inhibitor of inositol-1-monophosphatase.[70,71] Interestingly, increasing evidence has suggested that reduced agonist-stimulated phosphoinositide hydrolysis following long-term lithium administration is not simply the consequence of inositol depletion as originally proposed[70,71] but likely involves complex posttranslational effects on components of the receptor-mediated phosphoinositide-generating system.[12,64,67] In this context, a recent elegant study has demonstrated a reduction in agonist- and GTPγS-stimulated phosphoinositide hydrolysis following long-term lithium treatment of rats, even when tritiated phosphoinositide was exogenously supplied as the substrate (which should bypass any putative depletion of inositol).[21] However, neither our laboratory (H.K.M., G.C., W.Z.P., unpublished data, July 1994) nor Li et al[72] have observed alterations in the immunolabeling of $G\alpha_{q/11}$ in rat frontal cortex after long-term lithium treatment. It should be noted, however, that the relative abundances of $G\alpha_q$ and $G\alpha_{11}$ in human platelets and rat frontal cortex likely differ markedly, making a direct comparison of the results in these two tissues using an antibody that recognizes both $G\alpha_q$ and $G\alpha_{11}$ difficult. Nevertheless, the results do raise the possibility that the reduced levels of $G\alpha_{q/11}$ that we have observed in platelets and leukocytes in the lithium-treated group may be due to alterations in the circulating environment and/or in the rate of protein turnover in peripheral cells, which may not occur in the CNS.

It is beyond the scope of this article to discuss in detail all the potential transcriptional and posttranscriptional mechanisms by which lithium may affect the levels of G protein α subunits and/or the G protein α subunit mRNA levels.[29,30,62-65] However, it is noteworthy that lithium has marked effects on protein kinase C[11,64,67,73-76] and that protein kinase C has been demonstrated to inhibit G_i function,[46,77-81] to decrease the levels of $G\alpha_{i2}$ mRNA,[65] and to increase levels of pertussis toxin–catalyzed [^{32}P]ADP ribosylation[78-80] and may be involved in the regulation of the levels of $G\alpha_{q/11}$[82]—effects that are all strikingly similar to those we and other laboratories have observed following long-term lithium treatment.

To summarize then, the present study demonstrates modest, but significant elevations in the levels of $G\alpha_s$ (45 kd) in peripheral cells from patients with bipolar affective disorder and adds to the growing body of evidence that demonstrates alterations in G protein function by long-term administration of lithium at therapeutic levels. Given the pivotal roles of the G proteins in the amplification and integration of signals in the CNS, a longitudinal study of these components of signal transduction in a well-characterized, "pure" population of patients with bipolar affective disorder during various illness and treatment stages is warranted and may serve to facilitate our understanding of the molecular mechanisms involved in the pathophysiology of the disorder. Additionally, molecular scanning studies currently under way (P. V. Gejman, MD, oral communication, August 1994) should serve to delineate the role(s) of signal-transducing G proteins as possible factors in the predisposition to bipolar affective illness.

Accepted for publication November 15, 1994.

Reprint requests to Section on Clinical Pharmacology, NIMH, Bldg 10, Room 2D46, 9000 Rockville Pike, Bethesda, MD 20892 (Dr Manji).

REFERENCES

1. Weissman MM, Leaf PJ, Tischler GL, DG Blazer, Karno M, Bruce ML, Florio LP. Affective disorders in five United States communities. *Psychol Med.* 1988;18:141-153.
2. Goodwin FK, Jamison KR. *Manic-Depressive Illness.* New York, NY: Oxford University Press; 1990.
3. McGuffin P, Katz R. The genetics of depression and manic-depressive illness. *Br J Psychiatry.* 1989;155:294-304.

4. Potter WZ, Rudorfer MV, Goodwin FK. Biological findings in bipolar disorders. In: Hales RE, Frances AJ, eds. *APA Annual Review*. Washington, DC: American Psychiatric Press Inc; 1987;6:32-60.
5. Schildkraut JJ. The catecholamine hypothesis of affective disorders: a review of the supporting evidence. *Am J Psychiatry*. 1965;122:56-62.
6. Janowsky DS, El-Yousef MK, Davis JM, Sekerke HJ. A cholinergic-adrenergic hypothesis of mania and depression. *Lancet*. 1972;2:632-635.
7. Manji HK. G proteins: implications for psychiatry. *Am J Psychiatry*. 1992;149: 746-760.
8. Lachman HM, Papolos DF. Abnormal signal transduction: a hypothetical model for bipolar affective disorder. *Life Sci*. 1991;45:1413-1426.
9. Hudson CJ, Young LT, Li PP, Warsh JJ. CNS signal transduction in the pathophysiology and pharmacotherapy of affective disorders and schizophrenia. *Synapse*. 1993;13:278-293.
10. Dubovsky SL, Murphy J, Christiano J, Lee C. The calcium second messenger system in bipolar disorders: data supporting new research directions. *J Neuropsychiatry Clin Neurosci*. 1992;4:3-14.
11. Friedman E, Hoau YW, Levinson D, Connell TA, Singh H. Altered platelet protein kinase C activity in bipolar affective disorder: manic episode. *Biol Psychiatry*. 1993;33:520-525.
12. Jope RS, Williams MB. Lithium and brain signal transduction systems. *Biochem Pharmacol*. 1994;77:429-441.
13. Manji HK, Bitran JA, Masana MI, Chen GA, Hsiao JK, Risby ED, Rudorfer MV, Potter WZ. Signal transduction modulation by lithium: cell culture, cerebral microdialysis and human studies. *Psychopharmacol Bull*. 1991;27:199-208.
14. Mork A, Geisler A, Hollund P. Effects of lithium on second messenger systems in the brain. *Pharmacol Toxicol*. 1992;71(suppl 1):4-17.
15. Risby ED, Hsiao JK, Manji HK, Bitran J, Moses F, Zhou DF, Potter WZ. The mechanisms of action of lithium, II: effects on adenylate cyclase activity and beta-adrenergic receptor binding in normal subjects. *Arch Gen Psychiatry*. 1991; 48:513-524.
16. Baraban JM, Worley PF, Snyder SH. Second messenger and psychoactive drug action: focus on the phosphoinositide system and lithium. *Am J Psychiatry*. 1989;146:1251-1260.
17. Dousa TP. Interaction of lithium with vasopressin-sensitive cyclic AMP system of human renal medulla. *Endocrinology*. 1974;95:1359-1366.
18. Tseng FY, Pasquali D, Field JB. Effects of lithium on stimulated metabolic parameters in dog thyroid slices. *Acta Endocrinol (Copenh)*. 1989;121:615-620.
19. Godfrey PP, McClue SJ, White AM, Wood AJ, Grahame SD. Subacute and chronic in vivo lithium treatment inhibits agonist- and sodium fluoride-stimulated inositol phosphate production in rat cortex. *J Neurochem*. 1989;52:498-506.
20. Whitworth P, Kendall DA. Lithium selectively inhibits muscarinic receptor-stimulated inositol tetrakisphosphate accumulation in mouse cerebral cortex slices. *J Neurochem*. 1988;51:258-265.
21. Song L, Jope RS. Chronic lithium treatment impairs phosphatidylinositol hydrolysis in membranes from rat brain regions. *J Neurochem*. 1992;58:2200-2206.
22. Belmaker RH. Receptors, adenylate cyclase, depression, and lithium. *Biol Psychiatry*. 1981;16:333-350.
23. Dousa T, Hechter O. Lithium and brain adenyl cyclase. *Lancet*. 1970;1:834-835.
24. Ebstein RP, Moscovich D, Zeevi S, Amiri Z, Lerer B. Effect of lithium in vitro and after chronic treatment on human platelet adenylate cyclase activity: post-receptor modification of second messenger signal amplification. *Psychiatry Res*. 1987;21:221-228.
25. Mork A, Geisler A. The effects of lithium in vitro and ex vivo on adenylate cyclase in brain are exerted by distinct mechanisms. *Neuropharmacology*. 1989; 28:307-311.
26. Manji HK, Hsiao JK, Risby ED, Oliver J, Rudorfer MV, Potter WZ. The mechanisms of action of lithium, I: effects on serotoninergic and noradrenergic systems in normal subjects. *Arch Gen Psychiatry*. 1991;48:505-512.
27. Masana MI, Bitran JA, Hsiao JK, Potter WZ. In-vivo evidence that lithium inactivates Gi modulation of adenylate cyclase activity in brain. *J Neurochem*. 1992;59:200-205.
28. Hsiao JK, Manji HK, Chen GA, Bitran JA, Risby ED, Potter WZ. Lithium administration modulates platelet Gi in humans. *Life Sci*. 1992;50:227-233.
29. Li PP, Tam YK, Young LT, Warsh JJ. Lithium decreases Gs, Gi-1 and Gi-2 alpha-subunit mRNA levels in rat cortex. *Eur J Pharmacol*. 1991;206:165-166.
30. Colin SF, Chang HC, Mollner S, Pfeuffer T, Reed RR, Duman RS, Nestler EJ. Chronic lithium regulates the expression of adenylate cyclase and Gi-protein alpha subunit in rat cerebral cortex. *Proc Natl Acad Sci U S A*. 1991;88:10634-10637.
31. Gilman AG. G proteins: transducers of receptor-generated signals. *Annu Rev Biochem*. 1987;56:615-649.
32. Spiegel AM, Shenker A, Weinstein LS. Receptor-effector coupling by G proteins: implications for normal and abnormal signal transduction. *Endocrinol Rev*. 1992;13:536-565.
33. Taylor CW. The role of G proteins in transmembrane signalling. *Biochem J*. 1990;272:1-13.
34. Federman AD, Conklin BR, Schrader KA, Reed RR, Bourne HR. Hormonal stimulation of adenylyl cyclase through Gi-protein beta gamma subunits. *Nature*. 1992;356:159-161.
35. Birnbaumer L. Receptor-to-effector signaling through G proteins: roles for beta gamma dimers as well as alpha subunits. *Cell*. 1993;71:1069-1072.
36. Simonds WF, Manji HK, Lupas A, Garritsen A. G proteins and βARK: a new twist for the coiled-coil. *Trends Biochem Sci*. 1993;18:315-317.
37. Levitzki A. From epinephrine to cyclic AMP. *Science*. 1988;241:800-806.
38. Milligan G, Wakelman M. *G Proteins: Signal Transduction and Disease*. New York, NY: Academic Press; 1992.
39. Lyons J, Landis CA, Harsh G, Vallar L, Grunewald K, Feichtinger H, Duh QY, Clark OH, Kawasaki E, Bourne HR. Two G protein oncogenes in human endocrine tumors. *Science*. 1990;249:655-659.
40. Patten JL, Johns DR, Valle D, Eil C, Gruppuso PA, Steele G, Smallwood PM, Levine MA. Mutation in the gene encoding the stimulatory G protein of adenylate cyclase in Albright's hereditary osteodystrophy. *N Engl J Med*. 1990;322: 1412-1419.
41. Weinstein LS, Shenker A, Gejman PV, Merino MJ, Friedman E, Spiegel AM. Activating mutations of the stimulatory G protein in the McCune-Albright syndrome. *N Engl J Med*. 1991;325:1688-1695.
42. Weinstein LS, Gejman PV, Friedman E, Kadowaki T, Collins RM, Gershon ES, Spiegel AM. Mutations of the Gs alpha-subunit gene in Albright hereditary osteodystrophy detected by denaturing gradient gel electrophoresis. *Proc Natl Acad Sci U S A*. 1990;87:8287-8290.
43. Bourne HR, Nicoll R. Molecular machines integrate coincident synaptic signals. *Cell*. 1993;72:65-75.
44. Freissmuth M, Casey PJ, Gilman AG. G proteins control diverse pathways of transmembrane signaling. *FASEB J*. 1989;3:2125-2131.
45. Ross EM. Signal sorting and amplification through G protein-coupled receptors. *Neuron*. 1989;3:141-152.
46. Swartz KJ. Modulation of $Ca2+$ channels by Protein kinase C in Rat central and peripheral neurons: disruption of G protein-mediated inhibition. *Neuron*. 1993;11:305-320.
47. Schreiber G, Avissar S, Danon A, Belmaker RH. Hyperfunctional G proteins in mononuclear leukocytes of patients with mania. *Biol Psychiatry*. 1991;29:273-280.
48. Young LT, Li PP, Kish SJ, KP Siu, Warsh JJ. Postmortem cerebral cortex Gs α-subunit levels are elevated in bipolar affective disorder. *Brain Res*. 1991; 553:323-326.
49. Young LT, Li PP, Kamble A, Siu KP, Warsh JJ. Mononuclear leukocyte levels of G proteins in depressed patients with bipolar disorder or major depressive disorder. *Am J Psychiatry*. 1994;151:594-596.
50. Laemmli UK. Cleavage of structural proteins during the assembly of the head of the bacteriophage. *Nature*. 1970;227:680-685.
51. Van Tits LJ, Michel MC, Grosse-Wilde H, Happel M, Eigler FW, Soliman A, Brodde OE. Catecholamines increase lymphocyte beta 2-adrenergic receptors via a beta 2-adrenergic, spleen-dependent process. *Am J Physiol*. 1990;258: E191-E202.
52. American Psychiatric Association. *Diagnostic and Statistical Manual of Mental Disorders, Revised Third Edition*. Washington, DC: American Psychiatric Association; 1987.
53. Boyum A. Isolation of mononuclear cells and granulocytes from blood, II: isolation of mononuclear cells by one centrifugation and sedimentation at 1 g. *Scand J Clin Lab Invest*. 1968;21:77-89.
54. Bradford MM. A rapid and sensitive method for the quantitation of microgram quantities of protein utilizing the principle of protein-dye binding. *Anal Biochem*. 1968;72:248-254.
55. Simonds WF, Goldsmith PK, Woodward CJ, Unson CG, Spiegel AM. Receptor and effector interactions of Gs: functional studies with antibodies generated to the alpha s carboxyl-terminal decapeptide. *FEBS Lett*. 1993;249:189-194.
56. Mumby SM, Kahn RA, Manning DR, Gilman AG. Antisera of designed specificity for subunits of guanine nucleotide-binding regulatory proteins. *Proc Natl Acad Sci U S A*. 1986;83:265-269.
57. Odagki Y, Koyama T, Yamashita I. Quantitative determination of pertussis-sensitive G proteins using [^{32}P]ADP-ribosylation in human platelet membranes: negative correlations with ages. *Life Sci*. 1992;50:1851-1857.
58. Bray P, Simons C, Guo B, Puckett C, Kamholz J, Spiegel A, Nirenberg M. Human cDNA clones for four species of $G\alpha_s$ signal transduction protein. *Proc Natl Acad Sci U S A*. 1986;83:8893-8897.
59. Robishaw JD, Smigel MD, Gilman AG. Molecular basis for two forms of the G protein that stimulates adenylate cyclase. *J Biol Chem*. 1986;261:9587-9590.

60. Maisel AS, Knowlton KU, Fowler P, Rearden A, Ziegler MG, Motulsky HJ, Insel PA, Michel MC. Adrenergic control of circulating lymphocyte subpopulations: effects of congestive heart failure, dynamic exercise, and terbutaline treatment. *J Clin Invest.* 1990;85:462-467.
61. Werstiuk ES, Steiner M, Burns T. Studies on leukocyte β-adrenergic receptors in depression: a critical appraisal. *Life Sci.* 1990;47:85-105.
62. Milligan G, Green A. Agonist control of G-protein levels. *Trends Pharmacol Sci.* 1991;12:207-209.
63. Hadcock JR, Malbon CC. Agonist regulation of gene expression of adrenergic receptors and G proteins. *J Neurochem.* 1993;60:1-9.
64. Manji HK, Lenox RH. Long-term action of lithium: a role for transcriptional and posttranscriptional factors regulated by PKC. *Synapse.* 1994;16:11-28.
65. Thiele EA, Eipper BA. Effect of secretagogues on components of the secretory system in AtT-20 cells. *Endocrinology.* 1990;126:809-817.
66. Moss J, Vaughn M. *ADP-Ribosylation Toxins and G Proteins: Insights Into Signal Transduction.* Washington, DC: American Society for Microbiology; 1990.
67. Lenox RH, Manji HK. Lithium. In: Nemeroff CB, Schatzberg AF, eds. *American Psychiatric Press Textbook of Psychopharmacology.* Washington, DC: American Psychiatric Press Inc. In press.
68. Mitchell FM, Mullaney I, Godfrey PP, Arkinstall SJ, Wakelam MJ, Milligan G. Widespread distribution of Gq alpha/G11 alpha detected immunologically by an antipeptide antiserum directed against the predicted C-terminal decapeptide. *FEBS Lett.* 1991;287:171-174.
69. Smrcka AV, Hepler JR, Brown KO, Sternweis PC. Regulation of polyphosphoinositide-specific phospholipase C activity by purified Gq. *Science.* 1991;251: 804-807.
70. Allison JH, Stewart MA. Reduced brain inositol in lithium-treated rats. *Nature New Biol.* 1971;233:267-268.
71. Berridge MJ, Downes CP, Hanley MR. Neural and developmental actions of lithium: a unifying hypothesis. *Cell.* 1989;59:411-419.
72. Li PP, Sibony D, Green MA, Warsh JJ. Lithium modulation of phosphoinositide signaling system in rat cortex: selective effect on phorbol ester binding. *J Neurochem.* 1993;61:1722-1730.
73. Lenox RH, Watson DG, J Patel, Ellis J. Chronic lithium administration alters a prominent PKC substrate in rat hippocampus. *Brain Res.* 1992;570:333-340.
74. Manji HK, Etcheberrigaray R, Chen G, Olds JL. Lithium decreases membrane-associated protein kinase C in hippocampus: selectivity for the α isozyme. *J Neurochem.* 1993;61:2303-2310.
75. Wang HY, Friedman E. Lithium inhibition of protein kinase C activation-induced serotonin release. *Psychopharmacology.* 1989;99:213-218.
76. Casebolt TL, Jope RS. Effects of chronic lithium treatment on protein kinase C and cyclic AMP-dependent protein phosphorylation. *Biol Psychiatry.* 1991;29: 233-243.
77. Garcia-Sainz JA, Gutierrez VG. Activation of protein kinase C alters the interaction of alpha 2-adrenoceptors and the inhibitory GTP-binding protein (Gi) in human platelets. *FEBS Lett.* 1989;257:427-430.
78. Halenda SP, Volpi M, Zavoico GB, Shaafi RI, Feinstein MB. Effects of thrombin, phorbol myristate acetate, and prostaglandin D2 on 40-41 kDa protein that is ADP ribosylated by pertussis toxin in platelets. *FEBS Lett.* 1986;204: 341-346.
79. Houslay MD. 'Crosstalk': a pivotal role for protein kinase C in modulating relationships between signal transduction pathways. *Eur J Biochem.* 1991;195:9-27.
80. Olianas MC, Onali P. Phorbol esters increase GTP-dependent adenylate cyclase activity in rat brain striatal membranes. *J Neurochem.* 1986;47:890-897.
81. Yatomi Y, Arata Y, Tada S, Kume S, Ui M. Phosphorylation of the inhibitory guanine-nucleotide-binding protein as a possible mechanism of inhibition by protein kinase C of agonist-induced Ca2+ mobilization in human platelet. *Eur J Biochem.* 1992;205:1003-1009.
82. Mitchell FM, Buckley NJ, Milligan G. Enhanced degradation of the phosphoinositidase C-linked guanine-nucleotide-binding protein Gq alpha/G11 alpha following activation of the human M1 muscarinic acetylcholine receptor expressed in CHO cells. *Biochem J.* 1993;293:495-499.

Conversions From Système International (SI) Units to Traditional Units (Modified From *The SI Manual in Health Care*)

System	Component	SI Reference Interval*	SI Unit	Conversion Factor (Divide by)	Traditional Reference Interval*	Traditional Unit
Serum	Lithium ion, therapeutic	0.50-1.50	mmol/L	0.001441	350-1050	μg/dL
		0.50-1.50	mmol/L	1.441	0.35-1.05	mg/dL

These reference values are not intended to be definitive since each laboratory determines its own values. They are provided for illustration only.

Correction

Incomplete Reference Citation. In the article titled "Effect of the Menstrual Cycle on Dependent Variables in Mood Disorder Research," published in the October issue of the ARCHIVES (1994;51:761-781), a portion of reference 94 was accidentally omitted. The correct reference citation is as follows: Seki K, Nagata I. Effects of a dopamine antagonist (metoclopramide) on the release of LH, FSH, TSH and PRL in normal women throughout the menstrual cycle. *Acta Endocrinol (Copenh).* 1990;122:211-216.

ORIGINAL ARTICLE

In Quest of Identifying Vulnerability Markers for Psychiatric Disorders by All-Night Polysomnography

Christoph J. Lauer, PhD; Wolfgang Schreiber, MD; Florian Holsboer, MD, PhD; Jürgen-Christian Krieg, MD

Background: The persistence of a depressionlike sleep pattern in fully remitted depressed patients suggests that the pattern is a trait characteristic of sleep measurements. However, in the past, subjects have undergone investigation only after the onset of the disorder, and, therefore, the altered sleep pattern may merely represent a biological scar.

Methods: We polysomnographically investigated 54 healthy subjects who had no lifetime or current diagnosis of a psychiatric disorder but had at least one first-degree relative with major depression or a bipolar disorder and at least one further close relative with major depression, a bipolar disorder, or a schizophrenic disorder. Twenty unrelated control probands without a personal and family history of psychiatric disorders and 18 unrelated inpatients with major depression served as reference groups. Prior to investigation, all healthy subjects had been free of any prescription and nonprescription drug for at least 3 months. The depressed patients were free of drugs for at least 1 week. All subjects slept for 2 nights in the sleep research unit. The sleep of the second night was recorded and visually scored.

Results: Analysis of the individual sleep cycles in these subjects revealed both a reduced amount of slow wave sleep and increased rapid eye movement density in the first sleep cycle. Discriminant analysis showed that 10 subjects (18%) had sleep patterns similar to those of depressed patients.

Conclusions: According to our observations, one fifth of the healthy subjects with a high genetic load for psychiatric disorders showed a conspicuous (depressionlike) sleep pattern. The follow-up will determine whether this sleep pattern indeed represents a trait marker indicating vulnerability.

(Arch Gen Psychiatry. 1995;52:145-153)

IN THE majority of depressed patients (DPs), a disturbed sleep maintenance, a deficit of slow wave sleep (SWS) especially during the first sleep cycle, an earlier onset of the first rapid eye movement (REM) sleep period, and an increased REM density during REM sleep are well-established findings.[1-3] However, the issue of whether these alterations are merely state dependent or persist during remission is still unresolved. Several authors have studied the same and mainly unipolar DPs in both the symptomatic and remitted states. Some have claimed a disappearance of the depressionlike electroencephalographic (EEG) sleep alterations in remission,[4,5] but others have described a persistence, even when the patients were clinically fully recovered.[6,7] Extending the latter findings, Giles and colleagues[8] found the continuance of shortened REM latencies during remission to be associated with an increased risk for relapses or recurrence. These findings suggest a trait characteristic of at least some of the depressionlike EEG sleep alterations. However, all these studies of DPs,whether conducted during the acute illness or in remission, were performed *after* the onset of the disorder. Therefore, neurobiological alterations (scars) acquired sometime during the course of the illness may account for the persistence of the depressionlike EEG sleep pattern, rather than the pattern being a true trait marker of depression.

The answer to the question "trait or scar?" lies in the investigation of potential patients *before* the onset of the disorder. In this regard, one strategy is to perform field studies. This, of course, is an

See Methods on next page

From the Department of Psychiatry, Max Planck Institute of Psychiatry, Clinical Institute, Munich, Germany.

METHODS

GENERAL PROCEDURE

An HRP is defined as a first-degree relative of an "index patient," the latter being an inpatient with major depression, a bipolar disorder, or a bipolar II disorder (bipolar disorder not otherwise specified [NOS] with at least one major depressive episode and one hypomanic episode) diagnosed according to *DSM-III-R*[17] and verified by the Structured Clinical Interview for *DSM-III-R* (SCID, German version).[18] Patients with the diagnosis of dysthymia, a depressive disorder NOS, or a bipolar disorder NOS other than specified above were not accepted as index patients. In addition, index patients had to have at least one first-degree relative with the diagnosis of an affective disorder or a schizophrenic or a schizoaffective disorder (relatives with the diagnosis of a dysthymia, a depressive disorder NOS, or a bipolar disorder NOS other than specified above were not accepted; the respective diagnosis was verified by the SCID or by the Munich Diagnostic Checklist for *DSM-III-R*[19] [MDCL]) to ensure the sampling of families highly loaded with psychiatric disorders. Furthermore, it had to be guaranteed that the HRP did not have *any* current or lifetime *DSM-III-R* psychiatric disorder (verified by the SCID). We limited the age range of the HRPs to 18 and 45 years because the likelihood of the first occurrence of an affective disorder is drastically reduced after about 50 years of age.[20] (In addition, this age range well ensures the possibility of long-term follow-up.) Finally, the HRP had to be a resident of the local vicinity to increase the likelihood of participation in the follow-up study.

HIGH-RISK PROBANDS

During the study period (July 1988 to July 1992), a total of 431 newly admitted inpatients with an affective disorder underwent screening (**Figure 1**). The family history of 290 patients (67%) was negative, and 69 patients (16%) had no first-degree relatives meeting the inclusion criteria (no lifetime or current psychiatric disorder, aged 18 to 45 years, living in the vicinity).

Of the remaining 72 patients who met all inclusion criteria, 37 patients refused to let their relatives participate in the study. Thus, the final sample of index patients consisted of 35 subjects.

The families of these index patients provided 66 HRPs meeting the inclusion criteria and 54 of them (24 women and 30 men; age range, 18 to 45 years) agreed to participate in the study (21 families provided one HRP; 10 families, two HRPs; three families, three HRPs; and one family, four HRPs).

The *DSM-III-R* diagnoses of the index patients' conditions were bipolar disorder (n=13; one patient showed psychotic features; 21 HRPs were recruited from these families), a recurrent episode of major depression (n=15; two patients showed psychotic features; 21 HRPs were recruited from these families), and a single episode of major depression (n=7; one patient showed psychotic features; 12 HRPs were recruited from these families). The affected first-degree relatives of the index patients had the following *DSM-III-R* diagnoses: bipolar disorder (n=5), a recurrent episode of major depression (n=11), a single episode of major depression (n=14), and schizophrenic disorder (n=5).

Thirty-two HRPs were offspring of the respective index patients; the remaining 22 HRPs were siblings. Of the 22 siblings, 17 had at least one parent with an affective disorder (second ill relative). Thus, the study sample of HRPs consisted of 49 subjects with and five subjects without a parental affective disorder (33 vs two families).

CONTROL PROBANDS

Twenty healthy volunteers (nine women and 11 men; age range, 18 to 42 years) from 20 different families served as the CPs. They underwent careful screening to exclude any personal history (using the SCID) or family history (clinical interview applying specific *DSM-III-R* diagnostic criteria) of psychiatric disorders. In case of doubt, the relatives of CPs were contacted personally to confirm the complete absence of psychiatric disorders in their families. If any question remained, the CP did not enter the study.

DEPRESSED PATIENTS

Eighteen unrelated inpatients with major depression (ie, DPs, n=11, all without psychotic features) or a depressed subtype of bipolar disorder (n=7, all without psychotic features) served as a reference group (nine women and nine

extremely time-consuming and uneconomical approach. An alternative strategy is to investigate healthy subjects who, due to their genetic load, bear a high risk for development of a psychiatric disorder. Identification of a vulnerability marker would be of great interest because strategies could then be developed to minimize the risk for onset of a psychiatric disorder in individuals with this trait.

Studies investigating this issue in healthy first-degree relatives of patients with an affective disorder are extremely scanty and limited by the fact that relatives with and without a personal history of a psychiatric disorder were intermingled.[9,10] Hence, it is difficult to draw any firm and conclusive estimations from these studies.

In the present study, we have extended this approach by examining subjects who had no lifetime or current diagnosis of a psychiatric disorder but who, owing to their family history, are at high risk of development of one. We have already reported preliminary findings based on 12 such subjects, whom we term high-risk probands (HRPs).[11] In addition, we have investigated the specific effects of a cholinergic stimulus (RS-86) on sleep regulation in a separate subsample of 21 HRPs.[12] Briefly, we found the basal sleep of the HRPs to be shallower (eg, containing less SWS) than that of control probands (CPs), but without alterations of the REM sleep patterns. The administration of RS-86 resulted in a hastened onset of REM sleep in the HRPs but not in the CPs. Both observations parallel the findings in young DPs[13-16] and point to a depressionlike EEG sleep pattern dysregulation in a certain percentage of the HRPs.

The present report contains the detailed description of the EEG sleep pattern in our final study sample, consisting of 54 HRPs (including the subjects of previmen; age range, 20 to 45 years). Diagnoses were confirmed by the SCID. All patients were moderately to severely depressed (mean [±SD] 21-Item Hamilton Depression Rating Scale score, 21.8±7.2). Patients who had been treated with tricyclic antidepressants (patients receiving other kinds of psychoactive medication were not included) were free of such medication for at least 1 week prior to the study, which is a sufficient washout period to exclude confounding effects of prior psychoactive medication on the EEG sleep pattern.[21]

POLYSOMNOGRAPHY

All HRPs and CPs had been free of any prescription or nonprescription drug (including antihistamines and salicylates) for at least 3 months. On the 2 days before polysomnography, no intake of caffeine (apart from a cup of coffee in the morning) or alcohol was allowed. The absence of insomnia, sleep apnea, and periodic movements in sleep syndrome were confirmed by clinical exploration and the visual inspection of the polysomnograms. In case of doubt, the protocol required exclusion from the study. Possible concurrent medical disorders and drug abuse were ruled out by a thorough medical examination and laboratory tests (including electrocardiogram, blood analysis, and urinary screening for drugs [amphetamines, barbiturates, benzodiazepines, cannabinoids, cocaine, and opiates] by means of a commercially available detection method [Du Pont, Willmington, Del]). Furthermore, none of the participants had been subjected to sleep deprivation, excessive alcohol (>25 g/d) or coffee (>500 mL/d) intake, shift work, or time shifts 3 hours or longer during the 3 months prior to the study period. During the 2 weeks preceding the polysomnography, both the HRPs and CPs were instructed to go to bed between 10:30 and 11:30 PM. This was to habituate the subjects to the lights-off time point prescribed in the study protocol. They also had to fill in a sleep log during this time span. The tolerated latitude in deviation from the requested lights-off time was 30 minutes and was monitored via the sleep log and a personal interview.

All subjects slept in the sleep research unit for two consecutive nights. After one night of adaptation, sleep was recorded between 11 PM and 7 AM using standard procedures (EEG, positions C_3-A_2, C_4-A_1 [time constant, 0.3 seconds; low-pass filtering, 70 Hz]; horizontal electrooculogram; submental electromyogram). The sleep records were scored visually according to standard criteria[22] by a trained technician without knowledge of the subjects' group membership. Definitions of most of the EEG sleep parameters calculated are described in detail elsewhere.[23] Sleep onset latency was defined as the time span between lights off (11 PM) and the first occurrence of stage II sleep. Slow wave sleep latency was defined as the time span between sleep onset (first occurrence of stage II sleep) and the first occurrence of stage III or stage IV sleep. Rapid eye movement sleep latency T (traditional) was defined as the time span between sleep onset and the onset of the first REM period (first occurrence of REM sleep; although 30 seconds of REM sleep were sufficient for us to accept the first REM period, the alternative requirement of at least 3 consecutive minutes of REM sleep was also met by all subjects). Rapid eye movement sleep latency C (conservative) was defined as the REM latency T minus the time awake during the first non-REM period. Mean REM density index was defined as the average ratio of 3-second miniepochs of REM sleep, including REMs, to the total amount of 3-second miniepochs of REM sleep. The REM density index of each single REM period indicates the ratio of 3-second miniepochs of REM sleep per REM period, including REMs, to the total amount of 3-second miniepochs of REM sleep per REM period.

STATISTICAL METHODS

Group means were compared using MANOVA. If there was a significant main group effect, univariate F tests were calculated within the MANOVA to identfy those variables contributing to the overall group difference. After such variables had been determined, their subeffects on group differences were analyzed over parameter estimates for contrasts (HRPs vs CPs, HRPs vs DPs, and CPs vs DPs) using Student's *t* test for independent samples (method: modified least significant tests to control for the increase in type I error rate). To test for differences between observed and expected frequencies (eg, gender), χ^2 tests were performed. In addition, linear canonical discriminant analysis (method: minimizing Wilks' lambda) was performed to determine which subjects in the HRP group belonged to the DP group and which to the CP group on the basis of their EEG sleep patterns.

ous reports[11,12]). We hypothesized that some of the probands would exhibit a depressionlike EEG sleep pattern during basal conditions. For this reason, we used both a group-oriented (multivariate analysis of variance [MANOVA]) and an individual-oriented (discriminant analysis) approach. Furthermore, we addressed the question of whether there are differences between HRPs from families highly loaded with unipolar depression and those from families highly loaded with bipolar disorders.

RESULTS

TOTAL SAMPLE OF 54 HRPs

The HRPs, CPs, and DPs were of similar age, and the ratio of women to men in the three groups did not differ significantly (**Table 1**).

Multivariate analysis of variance applied to the sleep parameters under investigation revealed a significant main group effect (Wilks' lambda=2.17; $P<.001$). The univariate F tests within the MANOVA showed that the following variables contributed significantly to this effect (Table 1): SWS latency, relative amount of REM sleep, REM latencies T and C, mean REM density, duration of the first REM period, amount of SWS during the first and second non-REM periods, and REM density of the first and second REM periods. Finally, the relative amount of stage II sleep and the REM density of the third REM period (stage II sleep: $F[2,89]=3.46$, $P<.04$; third REM density: $F[2,89]=31.60$, $P<.001$) contributed significantly to the main group effect.

No effects were found regarding the following variables: sleep continuity measures (sleep period time, sleep efficiency index, sleep onset latency, wake time after sleep

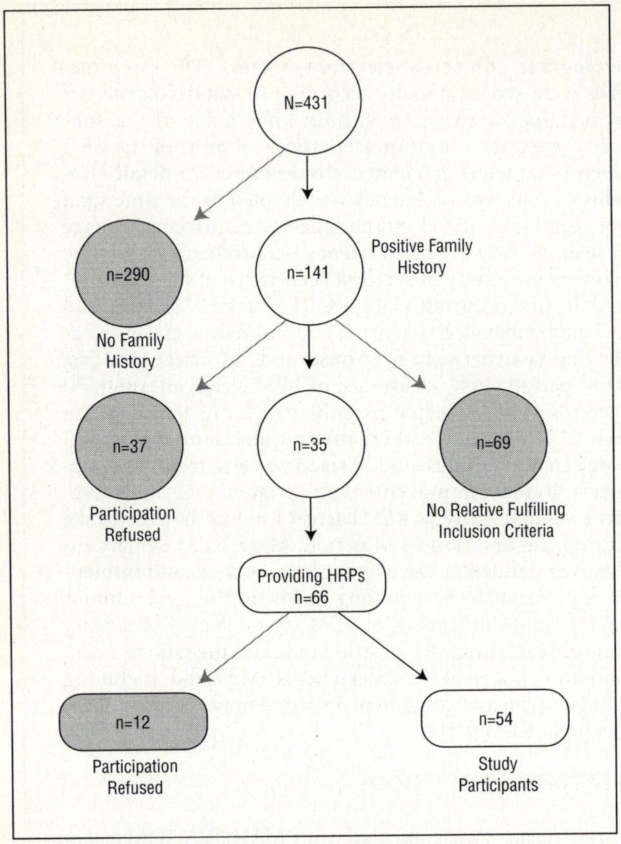

Figure 1. *Procedure for selecting the study sample of probands at high risk of psychiatric disorders (HRPs). Positive family history indicates at least one first-degree relative with a psychiatric disorder.*

onset, and early morning awakening), wake time during the first, second, and third non-REM periods, and the amount of SWS for the total night and during the third non-REM period.

To locate the significant differences, contrasts were applied and tested within the MANOVA. Compared with the DPs, both the HRPs and CPs had a shorter SWS latency, less REM sleep, a shorter duration of the first REM period, and a lower REM density both in the first three REM periods and averaged for the total night. Furthermore, both the REM latency T and C were longer in the HRPs and CPs than in the DPs (none of the HRPs and CPs, but four DPs [22%] showed a sleep onset REM period [REM latency, <20 minutes]). On the other hand, the HRPs as well as the DPs spent less time in SWS during the first non-REM period than the CPs (**Figure 2**), and their REM density during the first REM period was increased (whereas it was significantly higher in the DPs than in the HRPs) (**Figure 3**). Finally, the HRPs had less SWS during the second non-REM period than the CPs and the DPs.

DISCRIMINANT ANALYSIS

To identify those HRPs who exhibited a depressionlike EEG sleep pattern, we first calculated four different discriminant functions (DFs) based on the work of Gillin et al,[24] Feinberg et al,[25] Kerkhofs et al,[26] and Lauer et al[27] to distinguish best between the CPs and DPs. Subsequently, we used the respective DFs to determine which HRPs belonged to the group of CPs and which to the group of DPs.

Table 2 summarizes the EEG sleep parameters used for each DF, with the parameters necessary for the best discrimination between CPs and DPs in the present study indicated. Table 2 also gives the classification results.

Using the set of EEG sleep parameters proposed by Gillin et al[24] (but only 11 of the original 12 EEG sleep parameters were included, because REM index is not routinely calculated by our computer program for EEG sleep analysis), we were able to correctly classify 94.7% (36/38) of the grouped subjects (CPs, 100% [20/20]; DPs, 89% [16/18]). With this equation, 91% (40/54) of HRPs were correctly classified as CPs and 9% (5/54) as DPs. The same classification results were obtained when the DF was computed according to Kerkhofs et al[26] (the number of stage shifts, which was a part of the original equation, was not included in our analysis). With the five EEG sleep parameters used by Feinberg et al,[25] the overall percentage of correct classification dropped to 63.2% (CPs, 55% [11/20]; DPs, 72% [13/18]); this DF assigned 74% (40/54) of HRPs to the group of CPs and 26% (14/54) to the group of DPs.

Finally, we performed a discriminant analysis with an equation by Lauer et al[27] initially based on data from 13 CPs and 11 DPs (these subjects were also part of the present study sample). This DF included three EEG sleep parameters not used in the other DFs and all describing the first sleep cycle: SWS latency, wake time during the first non-REM period, and duration of the first REM period. With this DF, mean REM density contributed most to the best discrimination, followed by the amount of REM sleep, sleep onset latency, SWS latency, wake time during the first non-REM period, duration of the first REM period, and REM latency T. With this equation, 97% (37/38) of grouped subjects were correctly classified (CPs, 100% [20/20]; DPs, 94% [17/18]); 81% (44/54) of HRPs were classified as CPs and the remaining 19% (10/54) as DPs. These two HRP subsamples did not differ in age or in the type of affective disorder of the index patient. There was, however, a slight trend toward a difference in gender distribution, with more women than expected being classified as conspicuous (P=.07) (**Table 3**). Finally, it is important to note that the 10 HRPs with conspicuous EEG sleep patterns were members of 10 different families, and all had at least one parent with an affective disorder.

SUBSAMPLES OF HRPs

Splitting the sample of 54 HRPs according to whether they were relatives of patients with unipolar (n=22) or bipolar (n=13) disorders resulted in two subgroups (n=33 and n=21, respectively) of similar age (30.2±8.3 and 30.6±8.2 years, respectively) ($F[1,52]$=0.02; P=.89) and similar gender ratio (female-male, 17:16 and 7:14, respectively) (χ^2=1.72; P=19). The EEG sleep parameters of the subgroups were identical except for REM latency C, which tended to be shorter in the relatives of the patients with bipolar disorders (77.5±28.4 minutes vs 92.0±36.1 minutes) ($F[1,52]$=3.16; P=.08), but for the relatives of these

Table 1. Electroencephalogram Sleep Parameters of the Total Sample*

Characteristics and Parameters	Control Probands (n=20)	High-Risk Probands (n=54)	Nonrelated Depressed Patients (n=18)	MANOVA F (2,89)	MANOVA P
Mean (±SD) age, y	29.1±6.8	30.4±8.2	31.1±7.7	0.35	.71
Sex, F/M	9/11	24/30	9/9	0.17†	.92
Overall sleep structure					
SPT, min	445.2±26.3	437.5±34.3	437.2±22.9	0.50	.60
Sleep efficiency index, %	90.9±8.1	87.4±9.7	87.7±9.6	1.06	.35
Sleep onset latency, min	23.8±12.7	25.8±28.6	22.4±14.4	0.16	.85
WASO, min	21.9±27.7	30.7±29.2	37.3±42.1	1.13	.33
Early morning awakening, min	2.9±6.8	7.2±19.8	7.5±10.2	0.56	.58
Slow wave sleep latency, min	16.0±9.6‡	18.1±12.3‡	35.3±31.3	7.76	.001
Slow wave sleep, % of SPT	15.9±5.6	12.4±7.2	13.3±8.0	1.70	.19
REM sleep, % of SPT	18.3±4.8‡	17.6±5.2‡	22.2±7.1	4.65	.01
REM latency T, min	80.8±33.8‡	97.7±46.0‡	54.0±33.2	7.68	.001
REM latency C, min	77.7±29.8‡	86.3±33.8‡	48.0±28.0	9.76	<.001
Mean REM density index	2.09±0.63‡	2.17±0.80‡	4.13±0.93	45.42	<.001
First sleep cycle					
REM period, min	14.9±12.6‡	15.8±12.0‡	29.8±19.2	7.77	<.001
Wake time, % of NREMP	2.8±4.8	8.0±12.1	6.1±15.7	1.40	.25
Slow wave sleep, % of NREMP	41.6±18.2‡	31.2±22.3§	22.3±27.0	3.53	.03
REM density index, first REMP	1.37±0.52‡	1.74±1.04‡§	3.66±1.41	27.58	<.001
Second sleep cycle					
NREMP, min	81.5±13.3	85.4±23.3	81.0±21.8	0.41	.67
REMP, min	24.2±12.9	23.8±12.8	23.4±15.5	0.02	.98
Wake time, % of NREMP	5.4±11.2	4.4±7.4	2.1±2.2	0.97	.38
Slow wave sleep, % of NREMP	31.9±17.9	21.1±16.8‡§	33.9±20.4	4.77	.01
REM density index, second REMP	1.87±0.79‡	2.02±0.91‡	4.01±1.15	33.70	<.001

**MANOVA indicates multivariate analysis of variance; SPT, sleep period time; WASO, wake time after sleep onset; REM, rapid eye movement; REM latency T, time between sleep onset and first epoch of REM sleep; REM latency C, REM latency T minus wake time; REMP, REM period; and NREMP, non-REMP. Unless otherwise indicated, data are presented as mean±SD.*

†Determined by χ^2 test.

‡Indicates significant difference between high-risk probands and depressed patients or control probands and depressed patients by modified least significant tests.

§Indicates significant difference between high-risk probands and control probands by modified least significant tests.

patients it was similar to that of the CPs. With our DF, the rate of HRPs classified as DPs was similar in the relatives of patients with unipolar and bipolar disorders (6/33 [18%] and 4/21 [19%], respectively) (χ^2=0.01; *P*=.99).

As already mentioned, the 54 HRPs were from 35 families. We, therefore, reanalyzed the data, including only those from HRPs who entered the study protocol as the first family member (n=35). Statistical evaluation of this reduced database (not shown) yielded results identical to those for the total sample. Moreover, in this subsample, the percentages of HRPs classified as DPs with the four DFs were about the same as in the total sample (according to Gillin et al[24] and Kerkhofs et al,[26] 11% [4/35]; according to Feinberg et al,[25] 26% [9/35]; according to Lauer et al,[27] 17% [6/35]). Identical results emerged when considering only those HRPs of this subgroup in whom a parental affective disorder had been verified (n=33).

COMMENT

The EEG sleep patterns of the subjects without a personal history but with a strong family history of an affective disorder (HRPs) differed from those of the CPs without any personal history or family history of psychiatric disorders in the following two ways: (1) the HRPs spent less time in SWS during the first non-REM period, and (2) their REM density index for the first REM period was increased. The EEG sleep patterns showed no other features characteristic of depression, such as a prolonged SWS latency, a shortened REM latency, a prolonged duration of the first REM period, or an increased mean REM density. Application of several DFs reported in the literature classified from 9% to 26% of HRPs as being conspicuous, indicating that their EEG sleep patterns resembled those of the DPs. With our DF, which focuses especially on the first sleep cycle and discriminated best between CPs and DPs, 18% of the HRPs were classified as having a conspicuous (depressionlike) EEG sleep pattern.

In the present study, the EEG sleep patterns of the healthy CPs and of the DPs as well as the differences between them closely resemble those usually reported in the literature.[1-3] Thus, both samples can be regarded as valid reference groups. Moreover, the present analysis, like previous ones,[23,28] provides clear evidence that the SWS deficit in DPs, if it exists at all, is restricted to the first sleep cycle and is compensated for during the subsequent sleep cycles.

The finding of no major changes in the overall sleep structure of the HRPs but of alterations within the individual sleep cycles in general confirms our earlier findings.[11,12] To our knowledge, only two other polysomnographic studies have yet addressed a similar issue.[9,10] In these investigations, however, either symptom-free sub-

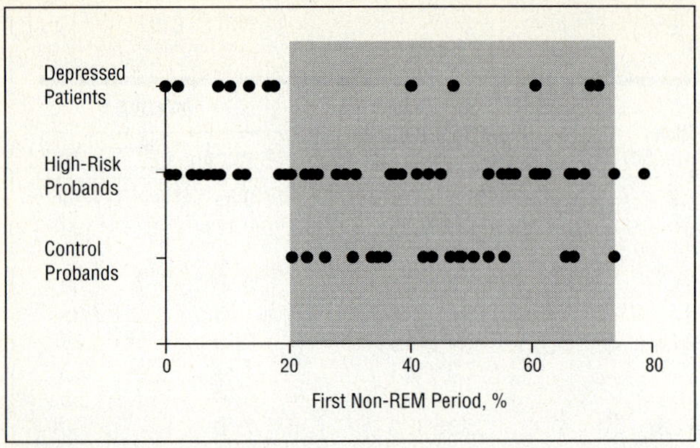

Figure 2. *Relative amount of slow wave sleep during the first non–rapid eye movement (REM) period in 54 probands at high risk of psychiatric disorders, 20 control probands, and 18 depressed inpatients. The shaded area indicates the data range for the control probands. Subjects are described in the "Methods" section of the text.*

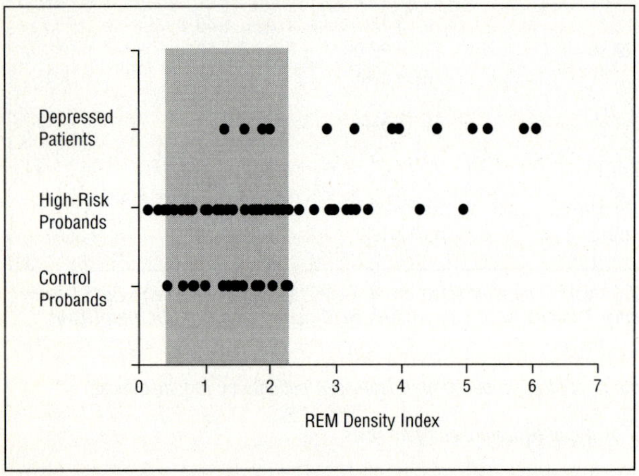

Figure 3. *Rapid eye movement (REM) density index of the first REM period in 54 probands at high risk of psychiatric disorders, 20 control probands, and 18 depressed inpatients. The shaded area indicates the data range for the control probands. Subjects are described in the "Methods" section of the text.*

jects with a previous episode of an affective disorder (ie, patients with remitted depression) were intermingled with HRPs in our sense, or the subjects were subdivided according to a REM latency cutoff score of 65 minutes. (This value is alleged to discriminate best between patients with unipolar depression and controls as well as between patients with endogenous and nonendogenous depression.[10] In the present study, however, this cutoff score would be of minor value, since a considerable percentage of CPs [8/20, or 40%] but only less than two thirds of the DPs [11/18, or 61%] had a REM latency shorter than 65 minutes, without DPs with unipolar or bipolar disorders showing any differences in this respect.) Furthermore, neither study included a control group of healthy subjects without a personal history or family history of psychiatric disorders. Therefore, a comparison of these reports with ours is difficult. Nevertheless, Giles and coworkers[10] found a similar overall EEG sleep pattern in their "short–REM-latency subjects" with a personal history of unipolar depression and in "short–REM-latency HRPs" without such a history. Given the reports of recovered sleep patterns in patients with fully remitted depression,[4,5] these findings suggest an undisturbed *overall sleep structure* in HRPs, which indeed is the case in the present study.

On the other hand, there are also studies in which the persistence of a depressionlike EEG sleep pattern during remission was observed.[6,7] On the basis of these findings, one would assume that the similarity of EEG sleep patterns in patients with remitted depression and HRPs reported by Giles et al[10] points toward a depressionlike polysomnogram in HRPs. Our sample of subjects at high risk did not show depressionlike features in the overall sleep structure (eg, a shortened REM latency), but did show significant changes in the *individual sleep cycles,* ie, a reduced amount of SWS during the first non-REM period and an increased REM density during the first REM period. These changes, and especially the latter one, are reported to be more stable and reliable findings than a shortening of REM latency in young to middle-aged patients with major depression.[3,23,29] Furthermore, in a recent study,[12] we found that the response pattern of the HRPs to a cholinergic stimulus was similar to that of young depressed inpatients: no disturbance of REM sleep regulation (normal REM latency) under baseline conditions, but a significantly hastened onset of the first REM period after the administration of the cholinergic agent RS-86. These observations suggest an increased susceptibility of the REM sleep–regulating system to cholinergic stimulation in a subgroup of HRPs that parallels that seen in DPs.[9,16,30-32] Thus, one may conclude that healthy first-degree relatives of patients with an affective disorder show changes in EEG sleep patterns in part resembling those observable in patients with major depression.

When dealing with the issue of biological alterations in HRPs, however, a group-oriented approach as presented above is not sufficient because conservative estimates indicate that a psychiatric disorder will develop in only 20% to 30% of the first-degree relatives of patients with affective disorders.[33,34] At the time of investigation, however, it is not known which of the HRPs are indeed at true risk. Consequently, the study sample is a heterogeneous one in which true-risk subjects (carriers of the trait marker[s]) are intermingled with those who are not at risk (not carriers of the trait marker[s]). Thus, if there are indeed trait markers for psychiatric disorders that are detectable by EEG sleep recording, they will be present only in a subgroup of the HRPs and, hence, may be concealed if one looks only at the total group. This renders an individual-oriented approach necessary to identify HRPs with a conspicuous sleep pattern.

Based on the assumption that the hypothesized trait marker (or set of trait markers) is mirrored by an altered EEG sleep pattern in DPs, one should be able to discriminate such patients from healthy volunteers using a set of polysomnographic measures. So far, Gillin et al,[24] Feinberg et al,[25] and Kerkhofs et al[26] have addressed this issue. By computing DFs, they were able to classify correctly 83%, 67%, and 69%, of their subjects, respectively. In the discriminant analyses performed with the sets of EEG sleep variables intro duced by these authors, we were able to classify correctly 55% to 100% of our CPs and 72% to 89% of our

Table 2. Classification of Subjects Based on Four Different Discriminant Equations*

Discriminant Equations, Reference (EEG Sleep Parameters Used)†	Subjects	Group Membership, Predicted, % (No. of Patients): CP	DP	Subjects Correctly Classified, %
Gillin et al[24] (TIB; TST; SEI; SOL; WASO; EMA; SWS, %; REM, %; *REM, min; REM latency T; mean REM density*)	CPs	100 (20)	0	94.7
	DPs	11 (2)	89 (16)	
	HRPs	91 (49)	9 (5)	. . .
Feinberg et al[25] (TIB; SEI; WASO; EMA; *REM latency C*)	CPs	55 (11)	45 (9)	63.2
	DPs	28 (5)	72 (13)	
	HRPs	74 (40)	26 (14)	. . .
Kerkhofs et al[26] (*SOL*; WASO; SWS, %; *REM latency T; mean REM density*)	CPs	100 (20)	0	94.7
	DPs	11 (2)	89 (16)	
	HRPs	91 (49)	9 (5)	. . .
Lauer et al[27] (*SOL; SWS latency; REM, %; REM latency T; mean REM density index; first REMP duration; wake time, % of first NREMP*)	CPs	100 (20)	0	97.4
	DPs	6 (1)	94 (17)	
	HRPs	81 (44)	19 (10)	. . .

**EEG indicates electroencephalographic; CP, control proband; DP, nonrelated depressed patient; HRP, high-risk proband; TIB, time in bed; TST, total sleep time; SEI, sleep efficiency index; SOL, sleep onset latency; WASO, wake time after sleep onset; EMA, early morning awakening; SWS, slow wave sleep; REM, rapid eye movement; REM latency T, time between sleep onset and first epoch of REM sleep; REM latency C, REM latency T minus wake time; REMP, REM period; and NREMP, non-REMP.*

†The parameters in italics are those necessary for the best discrimination between the CPs and DPs in the present study.

Table 3. Characteristics of HRP Classified as CPs and DPs*

Characteristics	Predicted Group Membership: CPs (n=44)	DPs (n=10)	F and/or χ^2 Test	P
Mean (±SD) age, y	29.8±7.8	32.9±10.0	F (1,52)=1.17	.28
Sex, F/M	17/27	7/3	χ^2 (1)=3.24	.07
Member of families loaded with unipolar/bipolar disorder, No.	27/17	6/4	χ^2 (1)=0.01	.94
HRPs with/without parental affective disorder, No.	39/5	10/0	χ^2 (1)=1.25	.26

**CPs indicates control probands; DPs, depressed patients; and HRPs, high-risk probands.*

DPs; 74% to 91% of the HRPs were assigned to the group of CPs and 9% to 26% to the group of DPs. (It should be mentioned, however, that in the present study not all of the original parameters were necessary for the best discrimination between CPs and DPs [Table 2]). With our own DF, we correctly classified 100% of CPs and 95% of DPs. In our opinion, this DF is more sensitive than the others because it mainly describes the initial hours of polysomnography and, thus, that part of the night that is most disturbed in DPs.[2,23,28] With this DF, 82% of HRPs were classified as CPs. The remaining 18% (10/54, including five HRPs who were identified as being conspicuous by *all* of the discriminant equations) were classified as DPs and thus as having a conspicuous (depressionlike) EEG sleep pattern. Interestingly, the two samples of conspicuous and nonconspicuous HRPs did not differ regarding various clinical and demographic data (eg, age and the type of affective disorder of the respective index patient [unipolar depression or bipolar disorder]). The only exception was a slight trend toward more women than expected being classified as conspicuous.

Before drawing any conclusions, we need to consider several factors that are likely to influence or limit our observations. First, some family studies indicate a higher prevalence of affective diseases in relatives of patients with bipolar disorders than in those of patients with unipolar depression.[35,36] Although Lauer et al[37] and others[25,38-41] demonstrated similar EEG sleep patterns in inpatients with unipolar and bipolar disorders, the differing prevalence rates may result in an increased frequency of depressionlike EEG sleep patterns in relatives of patients with bipolar disorders (and thus in a higher rate of HRPs classified as conspicuous), a stronger impairment of sleep, or both. The results of the present study, however, do not confirm these suggestions. Neither the frequency of HRPs assigned to the DP group between relatives of patients with unipolar and bipolar disorders (18% and 19%, respectively) nor the EEG sleep pattern of these two subgroups differed. The only exception was a shorter REM latency C (conservative definition of REM latency) in the HRPs from families with bipolar disorders, which, however, was quite similar to that of the CPs.

Second, in some families, more than one HRP participated in the study, and hence there may have been genetic influences affecting our observations. Three preliminary studies[42-44] reported controversial evidence about genetic determination of the timing of the cyclic structure of sleep (duration of the REM and non-REM periods), the architectural aspects of sleep (amount of each sleep stage), or the cholinergic REM induction response. More recently, Linkowski and colleagues[45,46] found strong genetic effects on wake time, stage II sleep, and SWS in monozygotic but not in dizygotic twins. On the other hand, REM sleep measures (except the REM density) showed no such genetic influences. To control at least indirectly for genetic effects, we reanalyzed the data, including only those HRPs who entered the study as the first members of their families. The results obtained were identical to those observed for the total group of HRPs (EEG sleep parameters, percentage of subjects assigned to the CPs and the DPs, and membership in families with unipolar vs bipolar disorders). In addition, in all families with more than one HRP, no more than one HRP was classified as being conspicuous. Therefore, hereditary determinants (with respect to HRPs recruited from the same family) and membership in families with unipolar or bipolar disorders are unlikely to have affected the present findings.

Third, one might argue that our strategy not to assess the EEG sleep pattern of the index patients limits the power of the present observations. For example, Giles and colleagues[47] reported that relatives of patients with unipolar disorders who exhibit a REM latency of less than 65 minutes also tend to have a reduced REM latency. This observation was independent of whether the relatives were asymptomatic (former patients) or had no personal history of depression. In a preliminary report, these authors found that major depression was more likely to develop in "short REM latency" relatives of "short REM latency" DPs.[48] These findings appear to favor the strategy of a parallel investigation of index patients and their relatives. However, with our procedure of recruiting newly admitted patients, such a strategy would create a difficult situation: a substantial number of our index patients were in need of immediate psychopharmacological treatment, making a polysomnographic investigation unreasonable (due to the well-documented effects of psychoactive medication on sleep). Furthermore, several of the patients fulfilling the inclusion criteria were admitted while receiving medication, which would necessitate a sufficiently long washout period prior to the investigation without, however, knowing in advance whether the respective HRP would and could in fact participate in the study. Therefore, we decided not to investigate the index patients but instead DPs unrelated to the HRPs. Such an apparent limitation of the study is, however, well compensated for by the introduction of a DF consisting of a set of weighted sleep measures instead of focusing on only a single sleep measure (eg, REM latency). The advantage of this strategy is that if a DP lacks depressionlike values in some sleep parameters (eg, a shortened REM latency) but shows true depressionlike values in others (eg, increased REM density), he or she is still likely to be correctly identified by the DF. Based on the classification result of 95% correctly identified DPs in the present study, the probability that the sleep pattern of a given index patient would also be correctly classified is very high. Furthermore, by introducing an age-matched reference group of DPs, age-confounding effects on sleep measures (which are known to differ between DPs and healthy subjects[3] and would emerge when comparing the EEG sleep pattern of HRPs and their parents) were excluded. Therefore, the power of our observations is limited only slightly, if at all, by not assessing the EEG sleep patterns of the index patients.

In conclusion, the HRPs as a group of healthy first-degree relatives—and in the majority offspring—of patients with an affective disorder showed some features of a depressionlike EEG sleep pattern: a reduced amount of SWS during the first non-REM period and an increased REM density index during the first REM period. However, since a psychiatric disorder indeed will develop in only 20% to 30% of these HRPs, an individual-oriented approach is needed when searching for neurobiological measures indicating vulnerability. By means of a discriminant analysis, we found that 18% of HRPs exhibited a sleep pattern resembling that of DPs and, thus, were classified as conspicuous. We are now following up the HRPs to determine whether a conspicuous EEG sleep pattern remains stable over time in a given individual (a major prerequisite for a trait marker) and whether discrete EEG sleep pattern changes indicate an increased risk for the development of psychiatric disorders.

Accepted for publication November 1, 1994.

Reprint requests to Department of Psychiatry, Max Planck Institute of Psychiatry, Clinical Institute, Kraepelinstrasse 10, 80804 Munich, Germany (Dr Lauer).

REFERENCES

1. Gillin JC, Sitaram N, Wehr T, Duncan W, Post R, Murphy DL, Mendelson WB, Wyatt RJ, Bunney WE. Sleep and affective illness. In: Post RM, Ballenger JC, eds. *Neurobiology of Mood Disorders.* Baltimore, Md: Williams & Wilkins; 1984: 157-189.
2. Reynolds CF, Kupfer DJ. Sleep research in affective illness: state of the art circa 1987. *Sleep.* 1987;10:199-215.
3. Lauer CJ, Riemann D, Wiegand M, Berger M. From early to late adulthood: changes in EEG sleep of depressed patients and healthy volunteers. *Biol Psychiatry.* 1991;29:979-993.
4. Schulz H. Sleep in affective disorders: an experimental study in depressed and remitted patients. In: Smirne S, Franceschi M, Ferini-Strambi L, eds. *Sleep in Medical and Neuropsychiatric Disorders.* New York, NY: Masson Publishing USA Inc; 1988:75-86.
5. Riemann D, Berger M. EEG sleep in depression and in remission and the REM sleep response to the cholinergic agonist RS-86. *Neuropsychopharmacology.* 1989;2:145-152.
6. Rush AJ, Erman MK, Giles DE, Schlesser MA, Carpenter G, Vasavada N, Roffwarg HP. Polysomnographic findings in recently drug-free and clinically remitted depressed patients. *Arch Gen Psychiatry.* 1986;43:878-884.
7. Steiger A, von Bardeleben U, Herth T, Holsboer F. Sleep-EEG and nocturnal secretion of cortisol and human growth hormone in male patients with endogenous depression before treatment and after recovery. *J Affect Disord.* 1989; 16:189-195.
8. Giles DE, Jarrett RB, Roffwarg HP, Rush AJ. Reduced rapid eye movement latency: a predictor of recurrence in depression. *Neuropsychopharmacology.* 1987;1:33-39.
9. Sitaram N, Dube S, Keshavan M, Davies A, Reynal P. The association of supersensitive cholinergic REM-induction and affective illness within pedigrees. *J Psychiatry Res.* 1987;21:487-497.
10. Giles DE, Kupfer DJ, Roffwarg HP, Rush AJ, Biggs MM, Etzel BA. Polysomnographic parameters in first-degree relatives of unipolar probands. *Psychiatry Res.* 1989;27:127-136.
11. Krieg J-C, Lauer CJ, Hermle L, von Bardeleben U, Pollmächer T, Holsboer F. Psychometric, polysomnographic, and neuroendocrine measures in subjects at high risk for psychiatric disorders: preliminary results. *Neuropsychobiology.* 1990;23:57-67.
12. Schreiber W, Lauer CJ, Krumrey K, Holsboer F, Krieg J-C. Cholinergic REM sleep induction test in subjects at high risk for psychiatric disorders. *Biol Psychiatry.* 1992;32:79-90.
13. Goetz RR, Puig-Antich J, Ryan N, Rabinovich H, Ambrosini PJ, Nelson B,

Krawiec V. Electroencephalographic sleep of adolescents with major depression and normal controls. *Arch Gen Psychiatry.* 1987;44:61-68.
14. Appelboom-Fondu J, Kerkhofs M, Mendlewicz J. Depression in adolescents and young adults: polysomnographic and neuroendocrine aspects. *J Affect Disord.* 1988;14:35-40.
15. Kupfer DJ, Frank E, Ehlers CL. EEG sleep in young depressives: first and second night effects. *Biol Psychiatry.* 1989;25:87-97.
16. Lauer CJ, Krieg J-C, Riemann D, Zulley J, Berger M. A polysomnographic study in young psychiatric inpatients: major depression, anorexia nervosa, bulimia nervosa. *J Affect Disord.* 1990;18:235-245.
17. American Psychiatric Association. *Diagnostic and Statistical Manual of Mental Disorders, Revised Third Edition.* Washington, DC: American Psychiatric Association; 1987.
18. Wittchen H-U, Zaudig M, Schramm E, Spengler P, Mombour W, Klug J, Horn R. *SKID: Strukturiertes Klinisches Interview für DSM-III-R.* Weinheim, Germany: Beltz; 1990.
19. Hiller W, Zaudig M, Mombour W. Development of diagnostic checklists for use in routine clinical care: a guideline designed to assess *DSM-III-R* diagnoses. *Arch Gen Psychiatry.* 1990;47:782-784.
20. Cross-National Collaborative Group. The changing rate of major depression: cross-national comparisons. *JAMA.* 1992;268:3098-3105.
21. Lauer CJ, Pollmächer T. On the issue of drug washout prior to polysomnographic studies in depressed patients. *Neuropsychopharmacology.* 1992;6:11-16.
22. Rechtschaffen A, Kales A. *A Manual of Standardized Terminology: Techniques and Scoring System for Sleep Stages of Human Subjects.* Washington, DC: National Institute of Health Publications; 1968.
23. Lauer CJ, Krieg J-C, Garcia-Borreguero D, Özdaglar A, Holsboer F. Panic disorder and major depression: a comparative electroencephalographic sleep study. *Psychiatry Res.* 1992;44:41-54.
24. Gillin JC, Duncan W, Pettigrew KD, Frankel BL, Snyder F. Successful separation of depressed, normal, and insomniac subjects by EEG sleep data. *Arch Gen Psychiatry.* 1979;36:85-90.
25. Feinberg M, Gillin JC, Carroll BJ, Greden JF, Zis AP. EEG studies of sleep in the diagnosis of depression. *Biol Psychiatry.* 1982;17:305-316.
26. Kerkhofs M, Hoffmann G, De Martelaere V, Linkowski P, Mendlewicz J. Sleep EEG recordings in depressive disorders. *J Affect Disord.* 1985;9:47-53.
27. Lauer CJ, Hermle L, Pollmächer T, Krieg J-C, Holsboer F. A polysomnographic study in subjects at high risk for psychiatric disorders. Presented at the 10th Congress of European Sleep Research Society; March 20, 1990; Strasbourg, France.
28. Kupfer DJ, Ulrich RF, Coble PA, Jarrett DB, Grochocinski VJ, Doman J, Matthews G, Borbély AA. Application of automated REM and slow wave sleep analysis, II: testing the assumption of the two-process model of sleep regulation in normal and depressed patients. *Psychiatry Res.* 1984;13:335-343.
29. Cashman MA, Coble P, McCann BS, Taska L, Reynolds CF, Kupfer DJ. Sleep markers of major depressive disorder in adolescent patients. *Sleep Res.* 1986;15:91.
30. Sitaram N, Gillin JC, Bunney WE. Cholinergic and catecholaminergic receptor sensitivity in affective illness. In: Post RM, Ballenger JC, eds. *Neurobiology of Mood Disorders.* Baltimore, Md: Williams & Wilkins; 1984:629-651.
31. Berger M, Riemann D, Höchli D, Spiegel R. The cholinergic rapid eye movement sleep induction test with RS-86: state or trait marker of depression? *Arch Gen Psychiatry.* 1989;46:421-428.
32. Gillin JC, Sutton L, Ruiz C, Kelsoe J, Dupont RM, Darko D, Risch SC, Golshan S, Janowsky D. The cholinergic rapid eye movement induction test with arecoline in depression. *Arch Gen Psychiatry.* 1991;48:264-270.
33. Weissman MM, Gershon ES, Kidd KK, Prusoff BA, Leckman JF, Dibble E, Hamovit J, Thompson WD, Pauls DL, Guroff J. Psychiatric disorders in the relatives of probands with affective disorders. *Arch Gen Psychiatry.* 1984;41:13-21.
34. McGuffin P, Katz R. Nature, nurture and affective disorders. In: Deakin JFW, ed. *The Biology of Affective Disorders.* London, England: Gaskell Press; 1986.
35. Gershon ES, Hamovit J, Guroff JJ, Dibble E, Leckamn JF, Schery W, Targum SD, Nurnberger JI, Goldin RL, Bunney WE Jr. A family study of schizoaffective, bipolar I, bipolar II, unipolar and normal control probands. *Arch Gen Psychiatry.* 1982;39:1157-1167.
36. Rice J, Reich T, Andreasen NC, Endicott J, Van Eerdewegh M, Fishman R, Hirschfeld RMA, Klerman GL. Familial transmission of bipolar illness. *Arch Gen Psychiatry.* 1987;44:441-447.
37. Lauer CJ, Wiegand M, Krieg J-C. All-night electroencephalographic sleep and cranial computed tomography in depression: a study of unipolar and bipolar patients. *Eur Arch Psychiatry Clin Neurosci.* 1992;242:59-68.
38. Duncan WC, Pettigrew KD, Gillin JC. REM architecture changes in bipolar and unipolar depression. *Am J Psychiatry.* 1979;136:1424-1427.
39. Giles DE, Rush AJ, Roffwarg HP. Sleep parameters in bipolar I, bipolar II, and unipolar depression. *Biol Psychiatry.* 1986;21:1340-1343.
40. de Maertelaer V, Hoffmann G, Lemaiere M, Mendlewicz J. Sleep spindle activity changes in patients with affective disorder. *Sleep.* 1987;10:443-451.
41. Kerkhofs M, Kempenaers C, Linkowski P, de Maertelaer V, Mendlewicz J. Multivariate study of sleep EEG in depression. *Acta Psychiatr Scand.* 1988;77:463-468.
42. Webb WB, Campbell SS. Relationship in sleep characteristics of identical and fraternal twins. *Arch Gen Psychiatry.* 1983;40:1093-1095.
43. Nurnberger J, Sitaram N, Gershon ES, Gillin JC. A twin study of cholinergic REM induction. *Biol Psychiatry.* 1983;18:1161-1165.
44. Hori A. Sleep characteristics in twins. *Jpn J Psychiatry Neurol.* 1986;40:35-46.
45. Linkowski P, Kerkhofs M, Hauspie R, Susanne C, Mendlewicz J. EEG sleep patterns in man: a twin study. *Electroencephalogr Clin Neurophysiol.* 1989;73:279-284.
46. Linkowski P, Kerkhofs M, Hauspie R, Mendlewicz J. Genetic determinants of EEG sleep: a study in twins living apart. *Electroencephalogr Clin Neurophysiol.* 1991;79:114-118.
47. Giles DE, Biggs MM, Rush AJ, Roffwarg HP. Risk factors in families of unipolar depression, I: incidence of illness and reduced REM latency. *J Affect Disord.* 1988;14:51-59.
48. Giles DE, Kupfer DJ, Roffwarg RP. EEG sleep before and after the first episode of depression. *Sleep Res.* 1990;19:161.

Tryptophan Depletion in Stable Lithium-Treated Patients With Bipolar Disorder in Remission

Delgado et al[1] have reported that acute tryptophan depletion reversed antidepressant-induced remission in patients with major depression; the reappearance of depressive symptoms was more often observed in depressed patients treated with serotonergic antidepressants. In their study, five of the 21 patients investigated were treated with a combination of antidepressant (desipramine hydrochloride, fluvoxamine) and lithium carbonate. We adopted a similar paradigm to investigate the extent to which the same effect would be seen in patients with affective disorder who were treated with lithium only. Clinically, lithium displays a unique pharmacological profile: weak intrinsic antidepressant properties, useful as an augmenting agent to potentiate the effectiveness of other antidepressants, antimanic, and mood stabilizer. The molecular effects mediating these various pharmacological properties are complex and almost certainly involve multiple neurotransmitters, transduction mechanisms, and/or second messenger systems. One current theory is that lithium exerts some of its therapeutic effects, ie, potentiation of antidepressant treatments, by enhancing central serotonergic neurotransmission (for review, see deMontigny et al[2]). In the study presented herein, we tested the hypothesis that acute tryptophan depletion would transiently reverse some of the therapeutic effects of lithium in stable, remitted patients with bipolar disorder. The subjects were 10 men (mean±SD age, 39±15 years) who fulfilled the *DSM-III-R* criteria for bipolar disorder as determined by the Structured Clinical Interview for *DSM-III-R* (patient version).[3] They were all in remission, and the duration (mean±SD) of their illness was 14±11 years. All patients had been euthymic for the past year (mean duration of remission, 4±11 years; range, 1 to 15 years), and they were all treated solely with lithium carbonate (mean [±SD] daily dose, 930±386 mg/d). The study used a double-blind, counterbalanced, placebo-controlled design. Each subject consumed a low-protein diet during the day preceding test days, which were 1 to 2 weeks apart. The mood scales used by the raters were the Hamilton Depression Rating Scale[4] and the Beigel and Murphy Manic-State Rating Scale,[5] while the Zung Depression Scale[6] and the Visual Analog Mood Scale[7] were completed by the patients. The scales were administered before and 5 hours after ingestion of a balanced amino acid load or a similar amino acid load devoid of tryptophan. Blood was drawn at the same time points for the determination of plasma tryptophan concentrations. Lithium plasma levels did not differ significantly between treatment groups. Plasma tryptophan concentrations were elevated by 39% at 5 hours after ingestion of the control mixture, while the tryptophan-deficient amino acid load resulted in an 85% reduction in total plasma tryptophan levels. Despite this marked decrease in tryptophan plasma concentrations, tryptophan depletion in patients with bipolar disorder who were stable with lithium therapy did not induce any measurable change in affective symptoms. There were no significant effects of condition (balanced or tryptophan-deficient amino acid loads), or time (0 or 5 hours), or condition × time interactions on Hamilton Depression Rating Scale

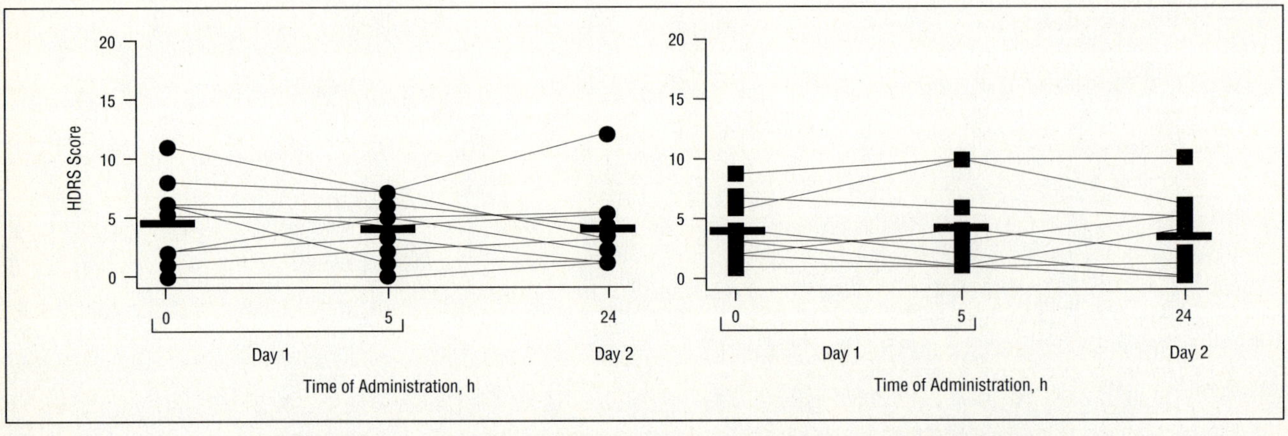

Individual mood ratings on the Hamilton Depression Rating Scale (HDRS) in patients with bipolar disorder (n=10) stable with lithium carbonate therapy following the ingestion of a balanced (left) and tryptophan-deficient (right) amino acid load. No significant differences between the two treatment groups were found (two-way, treatment × time repeated measures analysis of variance).

scores (**Figure**), or in any other of the mood scales used (data not shown). These negative results are in sharp contrast with those reported by Delgado et al[1] in 1990 on the reversal of the therapeutic effect of antidepressant treatments by tryptophan depletion. Differences in the results between the two studies may be accounted for not only by the intrinsic differences in the pharmacological properties of antidepressants and lithium, but also by other methodological differences, such as differences in the clinical sample characteristics (percentage of patients with bipolar disorder in each study sample, 25% vs 100% in the present study; male-female ratio, 38% vs 100%) or in the time frame defining the period of remission/stability (2 weeks vs 1 year). It is also conceivable that the effects of tryptophan depletion may be too brief (hours) to affect mood stability in patients in remission for a year or more. These negative results are consistent with a relatively modest contribution of serotonin (5-HT) vs other neurotransmitter systems in the mechanism of action of long-term lithium treatment. They suggest that the therapeutic effects of long-term treatment with lithium do not depend primarily on 5-HT availability in the central nervous system.

Chawki Benkelfat, MD
Bernard Seletti, MD
Roberta M. Palmour, PhD
Jean Hillel, MD
Mark Ellenbogen
Simon N. Young, PhD
Department of Psychiatry
McGill University
1033 Pine Ave W
Montreal, Quebec, Canada H3A 1A1

Reprint requests to Dr Benkelfat.

1. Delgado PL, Charney DS, Price LH, Aghajanian GK, Landis H, Heninger GR. Serotonin function and the mechanism of antidepressant action: reversal of antidepressant-induced remission by rapid depletion of plasma tryptophan. *Arch Gen Psychiatry.* 1990;47:411-418.
2. deMontigny C, Chaput Y, Blier P. Lithium augmentation of antidepressant treatments: evidence for the involvement of the 5HT system? In: Briley M, Fillion G, eds. *New Concepts in Depression.* London, England: The MacMillan Press; 1988:144-160.
3. Spitzer RL. *Structured Clinical Interview for DSM-III-R.* New York, NY: Biometrics Research Department, New York State Psychiatric Institute; 1987.
4. Hamilton M. Rating depressive patients. *J Clin Psychiatry.* 1960;41:21-24.
5. Beigel A, Murphy DL, Bunney WE. The Manic-State Rating Scale: scale construction, reliability, and validity. *Arch Gen Psychiatry.* 1971;25:256-262.
6. Zung WWK. A self-rating depression scale. *Arch Gen Psychiatry.* 1965;21:63-70.
7. Bond A, Lader M. The use of analogue scales in rating subjective feelings. *Br J Med Psychol.* 1974;47:211-218.

In reply

Benkelfat and colleagues report the lack of behavioral effect of tryptophan depletion in stable bipolar patients in clinical remission (1 to 4 years) receiving lithium monotherapy. The authors contrast their results to our first report of tryptophan depletion in recently remitted (2 to 4 weeks) depressed patients. They point out significant differences between our studies: the differing lengths of remission, the lithium monotherapy, and the differences in diagnosis and gender, as well as the possibility that the duration of plasma tryptophan depletion may be too brief to affect mood stability in these patients. The authors conclude that the therapeutic effects of long-term lithium therapy may not depend primarily on 5-HT availability in the central nervous system.

We generally agree with the explanations suggested by Benkelfat et al, and especially concur with the conclusion that short-term fluctuations in 5-HT availability may not disrupt affective state in euthymic, stable, lithium-maintained patients with bipolar disorder. In our own work to date, gender and diagnosis have not correlated with behavioral response to tryptophan depletion (P.L.D. et al, unpublished data, 1994).[1,2] *The most important factors in determining behavioral response to tryptophan depletion in depressed patients are the pharmacological effects of the antidepressant drug to which they recently have responded. The greatest likelihood of change in affective state is in patients having responded to selective 5-HT reuptake inhibitors, while those having responded to norepinephrine reuptake inhibitors have the least likelihood of change (P.L.D. et al, unpublished data, 1994).*[2,3]

While the antidepressant effects of lithium augmentation in depression are well established and are hypothesized to be due to increased presynaptic release of 5-HT,[4] *this pharmacological property is unlikely to account for the mood-stabilizing effect of lithium in patients with bipolar disorder. Serotonin uptake inhibitors, monoamine oxidase inhibitors, and 5-HT releasing agents are not generally effective in stabilizing mood in patients with bipolar disorder and frequently induce mania.*[5] *Further, lithium monotherapy is not an effective antidepressant treatment in the majority of depressed patients.*[4] *The therapeutic effects of lithium as a mood-stabilizing agent have been hypothesized to involve changes in intracellular mechanisms rather than changes in monoamine release.*[6,7]

The data presented by Benkelfat et al are consistent with these hypotheses and highlight our own thinking that drugs with therapeutic effects in patients with affective disorders have multiple mechanisms of action.[3] *These data also indirectly support the developing hypothesis that affective disorders may not be directly caused by dysfunction of the monoamine systems but rather involve dysfunction in brain regions postsynaptic to and modulated by the monoamine systems.*[8]

Pedro L. Delgado, MD
Department of Psychiatry
University of Arizona College of Medicine
1501 N Campbell Ave
Tucson, AZ 85724
Dennis S. Charney, MD
West Haven, Conn

1. Delgado PL, Charney DS, Price LH, Aghajanian GK, Landis H, Heninger GR. Serotonin function and the mechanism of antidepressant action: reversal of antidepressant-induced remission by rapid depletion of plasma tryptophan. *Arch Gen Psychiatry.* 1990;47:411-418.
2. Delgado PL, Price LH, Miller HL, Salomon RM, Licinio J, Krystal JH, Heninger GR, Charney DS. Rapid serotonin depletion as a provocative challenge test for patients with major depression: relevance to antidepressant action and the neurobiology of depression. *Psychopharmacol Bull.* 1991;27:321-330.
3. Delgado PL, Miller HM, Salomon RM, Licinio J, Gelenberg AJ, Charney DS.

Monoamines and the mechanism of antidepressant action: effects of catecholamine depletion on mood in patients treated with antidepressants. *Psychopharmacol Bull.* 1993;29:389-396.
4. Price LH, Heninger GR. Lithium in the treatment of mood disorders. *N Engl J Med.* 1994;331:591-598.
5. Sachs GS. Adjuncts and alternatives to lithium therapy for bipolar affective disorder. *J Clin Psychiatry.* 1989;50(12 suppl):31-39.
6. Avissar S, Schreiber G. Interaction of antibipolar and antidepressant treatments with receptor-coupled G proteins. *Pharmacopsychiatry.* 1992;25:44-50.
7. Nahorski SR, Ragan CI, Challiss RAJ. Lithium and the phosphoinositide cycle: an example of uncompetitive inhibition and its pharmacological consequences. *Trends Pharmacol Sci.* 1991;12:297-303.
8. Delgado PL, Price LH, Miller HM, Salomon RM, Aghajanian GK, Heninger GR, Charney DS. Serotonin and the neurobiology of depression: effects of tryptophan depletion in drug-free depressed patients. *Arch Gen Psychiatry.* 1994; 51:865-874.

Biochemical Effects of Antidepressant Augmentation

In their report on the use of pindolol to augment selective serotonin (5-HT) reuptake inhibitors and monoamine oxidase inhibitors, Artigas et al[1] suggest that this may be mediated by presynaptic 5-HT_{1A} antagonism, resulting in enhanced serotonergic function. Buspirone, a 5-HT_{1A} agonist, also may be effective in augmenting selective 5-HT reuptake inhibitors in refractory depression.[2-5] Because pindolol and buspirone have opposite effects on 5-HT_{1A} function, their efficacy is therefore difficult to reconcile on this basis. Furthermore, it is not clear how 5-HT_{1A} antagonism could account for the effect of pindolol, because reduced sensitivity of presynaptic 5-HT_{1A} receptors is found in major depression.[6,7]

A major metabolite of buspirone is the α_2-adrenergic antagonist 1-(2-pyrimidinyl)-piperazine.[8,9] α_2-Adrenergic antagonism by 1-(2-pyrimidinyl)-piperazine could enhance the release of norepinephrine and result in mood elevation,[10] which is consistent with the mechanism of antidepressants such as mianserin[11] and similar to the hypomania reported after abrupt discontinuation of treatment with the α_2-adrenergic agonist clonidine.[12] Pindolol also has significant intrinsic β-adrenergic agonist activity.[13] β-Adrenergic down-regulation, a common characteristic of antidepressants, including selective 5-HT reuptake inhibitors,[14,15] depends on adequate serotonergic function.[16] Although this has been criticized,[17] the combination of fluoxetine and desipramine down-regulates β-adrenergic receptors more rapidly,[18] with an accelerated antidepressant response.[19] The combination of mianserin and imipramine also down-regulates β-adrenergic receptors more rapidly,[20] and the combination of mianserin and isocarboxazid induces a rapid remission of major depression.[21] Similarly, in patients treated with selective 5-HT reuptake inhibitors and monoamine oxidase inhibitors, pindolol and buspirone both may potentiate β-adrenergic down-regulation through their adrenergic rather than serotonergic effects.[10]

Antidepressant augmentation is presumed to enhance serotonergic function, but this is not well supported.[22] Moreover, impaired β-adrenergic function is found in refractory depression.[23] Thus, additional research on the adrenergic and serotonergic effects of buspirone and pindolol augmentation is clearly needed.[7,22] Also, comparing the efficacy of β-blockers that are 5-HT_{1A} antagonists but have different intrinsic adrenergic agonist effects or that have similar intrinsic adrenergic effects but different 5-HT_{1A} activity would be interesting.[24]

Robert H. Howland, MD
Western Psychiatric Institute and Clinic
3811 O'Hara St
Pittsburgh, PA 15213

1. Artigas F, Perez V, Alvarez E. Pindolol induces a rapid improvement of depressed patients treated with serotonin reuptake inhibitors. *Arch Gen Psychiatry.* 1994;51:248-251.
2. Bakish D. Fluoxetine potentiation by buspirone: three case histories. *Can J Psychiatry.* 1991;36:749-750.
3. Jacobsen FM. Possible augmentation of antidepressant response by buspirone. *J Clin Psychiatry.* 1991;52:217-220.
4. Joffe RT, Schuller DR. An open study of buspirone augmentation of serotonin reuptake inhibitors in refractory depression. *J Clin Psychiatry.* 1993;54: 269-271.
5. Lebert F, Pasquier F, Goudemand M, Petit H. Euphoria with buspirone after fluoxetine treatment. *Am J Psychiatry.* 1993;150:167.
6. Lesch KP, Mayer S, Disselkamp-Tietze J, Hoh A, Schoellnhammer G, Schulte HM. Subsensitivity of the 5-hydroxytryptamine$_{1A}$ (5-HT_{1A}) receptor-mediated hypothermic response to ipsapirone in unipolar depression. *Life Sci.* 1990;46:1271-1277.
7. Cowen PJ, Power AC, Ware CJ, Anderson IM. 5-HT_{1A} receptor sensitivity in major depression: a neuroendocrine study with buspirone. *Br J Psychiatry.* 1994;164:372-379.
8. Bianchi G, Garattini S. Blockade of alpha$_2$-adrenoceptors by 1-(2-pyrimidinyl)-piperazine (PmP) in vivo and its relation to the activity of buspirone. *Eur J Pharmacol.* 1988;147:343-350.
9. Gower AJ, Tricklebank MD. Alpha$_2$-adrenoceptor antagonist activity may account for the effects of buspirone in an anticonflict test in the rat. *Eur J Pharmacol.* 1988;155:129-137.
10. Howland RH. Biochemical and clinical effects of buspirone augmentation. *J Clin Psychiatry.* 1994;55:264.
11. Rose A, McCulloch MW, Sarantos-Laska C, Rand MJ. Effects of mianserin on noradrenergic mechanisms. *J Psychiatr Res.* 1984;18:79-88.
12. Tollefson GD. Hyperadrenergic hypomania consequent to the abrupt cessation of clonidine. *J Clin Psychopharmacol.* 1981;1:93-95.
13. Weiner N. Drugs that inhibit adrenergic nerves and block adrenergic receptors. In: Gilman AG, Goodman LS, Gilman A, eds. *The Pharmacological Basis of Therapeutics.* 6th ed. New York, NY: Macmillan Publishing Co Inc; 1980:176-210.
14. Byerly WF, McConnell EJ, McCabe RT, Dawson TM, Grosser BI, Wamsley JK. Decreased beta-adrenergic receptors in rat brain after chronic administration of the selective serotonin uptake inhibitor fluoxetine. *Psychopharmacology.* 1988;94:141-143.
15. O'Flynn K, O'Keane V, Lucey JV, Dinan TG. Effect of fluoxetine on noradrenergic mediated growth hormone release: a double blind, placebo-controlled study. *Biol Psychiatry.* 1991;30:377-382.
16. Sulser F. Serotonin-norepinephrine receptor interactions in the brain: implications for the pharmacology and pathophysiology of affective disorders. *J Clin Psychiatry.* 1987;48(suppl):12-18.
17. Hensler JG, Ordway GA, Gambarana C, Areso P, Frazer A. Serotonergic neurons do not influence the regulation of beta adrenoceptors induced by either desipramine or isoproterenol. *J Pharmacol Exp Ther.* 1991;256:656-664.
18. Baron BM, Ogden AM, Siegel BW, Stegeman J, Ursillo RC, Dudley MW. Rapid down regulation of beta-adrenoceptors by co-administration of desipramine and fluoxetine. *Eur J Pharmacol.* 1988;154:125-134.
19. Nelson JC, Mazure CM, Bowers MB, Jatlow PI. A preliminary, open study of the combination of fluoxetine and desipramine for rapid treatment of major depression. *Arch Gen Psychiatry.* 1991;48:303-307.
20. Klysner R, Geisler A. Rapid downregulation of cerebral beta-adrenoceptors by combined treatment with imipramine and mianserin. In: Amsterdam JD, ed. *Refractory Depression.* New York, NY: Raven Press; 1991:109-113.
21. Riise IS, Holm P. Concomitant isocarboxazid/mianserin treatment of major depressive disorder. *J Affect Disord.* 1984;6:175-179.
22. Cowen PJ, McCance SL, Ware CJ, Cohen PR, Chalmers JS, Julier DL. Lithium in tricyclic-resistant depression: correlation of increased brain 5-HT function with clinical outcome. *Br J Psychiatry.* 1991;159:341-346.
23. Howland RH. Thyroid dysfunction in refractory depression: implications for pathophysiology and treatment. *J Clin Psychiatry.* 1993;54:47-54.
24. Tang SW, Remington G, Persad E, Rosenblat R. Coadministration of a beta-adrenergic antagonist and a tricyclic antidepressant: a pilot study. *Psychiatry Res.* 1990;33:101-106.

Developmental Brain Abnormalities in Schizophrenia: Contributions of Genetic and Perinatal Factors

In the progress of their pivotal work on individuals from the Copenhagen Schizophrenia High-risk Project, Cannon et al[1] found linearly increasing measures of the cerebral ventricular system to be a function of the level of genetic risk for schizophrenia and the presence of obstetric complications (OCs) in the offspring of normal and schizophrenic parents. They discuss these results as being suggestive of the "neurodevelopmental nature of brain abnormalities in schizophrenia."

However, whether results obtained in a cohort of mainly nonschizophrenic subjects may be transferred *tout court* to schizophrenia is not obvious.

The controversial literature on the association between family history (FH) of schizophrenia and ventricular size in schizophrenia is more compatible with an inverse rather than a direct relationship between the two variables.[2,3]

Further, twin studies recognize a genetic control of ventricular size but indicate also a disease effect, with the schizophrenic twins showing consistently larger ventricles than their healthy co-twins.[4]

As for OCs, there have been negative reports concerning their possible enlarging effect on ventricular size in schizophrenia.[5]

Finally, when the combined effect of OCs and FH on ventricular size has been analyzed in schizophrenic samples, OC and FH have been found to have opposite effects.[6]

It may be not without relevance that, when the 15 schizophrenic offspring were excluded from the cohort analyzed by Cannon et al,[1] the statistical significance of the interaction between genetic risk and OCs increased (from $P<.05$ to $P<.03$), suggesting that the effect that was detected mainly pertained to healthy individuals.

Further suggesting that data from the high-risk cohort may not be completely representative in the case of schizophrenia are the results obtained in a computed tomographic study performed on a sample of 125 males and 68 females, aged 16 to 45 years (mean age, 26.1 ± 6.7 years), who fulfilled the *DSM-III-R* criteria for schizophrenia. A multifactor analysis of variance with ventricle-brain ratio as the dependent variable and FH of schizophrenia in first-degree relatives and history of OCs as the independent variables demonstrated a trend for positive FH to be associated with lower ventricle-brain ratios ($F=2.69$; $df=1,189$; $P=.10$), no effect of OCs on ventricular size ($F=1.85$; $df=1,189$; $P=.18$), and no interaction between OCs and FH ($F=0.35$; $df=1$; $P=.56$). The retrospective assessment of OCs by means of a questionnaire applied to the patient's mother, and in few exceptions to a close reliable relative, and the all-or-nothing classification of positive and negative FH and OCs obviously limit the possibility of drawing firm and definitive conclusions from these results.

However, the absolute lack of fit between our results and those of Cannon et al[1] with respect to the relationship between ventricular size and both FH and OCs and their interaction argues against the possibility of applying the findings obtained in a sample of mainly nonschizophrenic subjects sharing genetic and environmental factors with schizophrenic parents (such as in the Copenhagen cohort) to samples of unselected and unrelated schizophrenics.

Antonio Vita, MD
First Psychiatric Clinic
University of Milan
Policlinico, Pad Guardia II
via F Sforza 35
20122 Milan, Italy
Emilio Sacchetti, MD
Brescia, Italy

Carried out within the activities of the Italian Research Group for Affective and Schizophrenic Disorders, under the auspices of the Janssen Research Council and Fondazione Italiana per la Schizofrenia, Rome, Italy.

1. Cannon TD, Mednick SA, Parnas J, Schulsinger F, Praestholm J, Vestergaard A. Developmental brain abnormalities in the offspring of schizophrenic mothers, I: contributions of genetic and perinatal factors. *Arch Gen Psychiatry*. 1993;50:551-564.
2. Murray RM, Reveley AM, Lewis SW. Family history, obstetric complications and cerebral abnormality in schizophrenia. In: Tsuang MT, Simpson JC, eds. *Handbook of Schizophrenia: Nosology, Epidemiology and Genetics*. New York, NY: Elsevier Science Publishing Co Inc; 1988;3:563-577.
3. Vita A, Deici M, Giobbio GM, Garbarini M, Morganti C, Braga M, Internizzi G. A reconsideration of the relationship between cerebral structrual abnormalities and family history of schizophrenia. *Psychiatry Res*. 1994;53:41-55.
4. Suddath RL, Christison GW, Torrey EF, Casanova MF, Weinberger DR. Anatomical abnormalities in the brains of monozygotic twins discordant for schizophrenia. *N Engl J Med*. 1990;332:789-794.
5. Reddy R, Mukherjee S, Schnur DB, Chin J, Degreef G. History of obstetric complications, family history, and CT scan findings in schizophrenic patients. *Schizophr Res*. 1990;3:311-314.
6. Lewis SW, Murray RM. Obstetric complications, neurodevelopmental deviance and risk of schizophrenia. *J Psychiatr Res*. 1987;21:413-422.

In reply

Drs Vita and Sacchetti raise a number of interesting issues with respect to the generalizability of our findings of familial and obstetric influences on ventricular and sulcal enlargement in the Copenhagen High-risk Project sample.[1] Their central concern appears to be that associations between these variables in a group of affected and unaffected individuals with schizophrenic first-degree relatives are not necessarily representative of their associations in the population of schizophrenic patients as a whole. While we certainly agree that generalizability in this context is an important issue that remains to be quantified, we disagree with these authors' interpretation of the findings that are cited in favor of nonrepresentativeness.

First, it is important to note that most of the previous studies that have investigated associations between familial risk for schizophrenia and ventricular enlargement have compared morphologic measures among patients with and without a positive FH of the disorder. The results of these studies are not at all consistent, and despite a few reports of an inverse relationship, the majority failed to detect a significant association.[2] As we have argued in detail elsewhere,[1,2] the inconsistent results of these studies are likely to be explained by the vulnerability of the FH method to a high rate of false-negative classifications, particularly in view of the relatively high probability that genotypic risk for schizophrenia is present but nevertheless fails to manifest itself phenotypically in many first-degree relatives of affected probands. This point can be appreciated by considering that the morbid risks for schizophrenia are elevated to an equivalent degree in the offspring of affected and unaffected monozygotic (MZ) co-twins.[3,4] *Thus, the genetic transmission of schizophrenia does not depend on the presence of an affected individual among first-degree relatives, which clearly undermines the logic of the FH approach. Moreover, it is not possible at present to determine whether any given schizophrenic represents a "nongenetic" case. Estimates of the degree of heritability of schizophrenia based on concordance rates in MZ and dizygotic twins are in the range of 70% to 80%,*[5] *despite the fact that only 5% to 10% of schizophrenics in the population as a whole have an affected first-degree relative. Environmental factors may account for 20% to 30% of the variance in manifestation of schizophrenia, but not necessarily for 20% to 30% of schizophrenic patients (ie, such factors might act additively or interactively with genetic predisposition in every case). In principle, the generalizability of findings on genetic determinants of biological markers of schizophrenia from high-risk studies will be limited to the extent that purely environmentally determined cases of schizophrenia exist. Since such cases are unlikely to constitute more than a small minority of the total population of schizophrenics, their possible existence does not pose a serious threat to the generalizability of findings from high-risk studies.*

Second, while it is true that twin studies have shown a disease-specific effect on ventricular enlargement, such that schizophrenic members of discordant twin pairs are consistently observed to have greater degrees of ventricular enlargement than their unaffected co-twins, this form of analysis does not address the question of the genetic contribution to ventricular size. In particular, the study of Suddath et al[6] *did not compare the morphologic values of the unaffected co-twins of schizophrenics with those of unrelated normal controls. All four of the published studies that have directly compared measures of ventricular enlargement between unaffected relatives of schizophrenics and normal controls, including our report on the Danish High-risk Project sample,*[1,7-9] *found significant or nearly significant increases in ventricular size among the healthy relatives of schizophrenics. The consistent results of these studies suggest strongly that there is a positive relationship between the risk for carrying a genotype that predisposes to schizophrenia and structural abnormalities on a brain scan. Further, in the Copenhagen study, the relationship between ventricular enlargment and familial risk was postively sloping and dose-dependent* across three levels of genotypic risk.[1] *It is difficult to imagine how such an effect could be observed if the true population correlation between these variables was even slightly negative.*

Third, Drs Vita and Sacchetti question the generalizability of our findings with respect to the interaction of genetic risk and OCs in the prediction of ventricular enlargement in schizophrenia, citing studies in which there was no correlation between OCs and ventricular size and an inverse relationship between FH and OCs in some patient samples.[10,11] *These latter findings are limited by the inherent fallibility of the FH approach in defining genotypic risk for the disorder. Further, in our view, findings in studies that determined OCs by asking the patients' mothers to remember events that may or may not have occurred 20 to 30 years previously should not be taken to represent the true relationship between OCs and structural abnormalities in the general population of schizophrenics. In particular, why results based on maternal recall are to be preferred over our findings based on objective perinatal records completed at the time of the delivery by attending midwives is not immediately obvious. That the statistical significance of the interaction between genetic risk for schizophrenia and OCs increased slightly (from* $P<.05$ *to* $P<.03$*) when schizophrenics were excluded from our analyses is not a threat to the generalizability of these findings; the change in significance was itself not significant. A minor fluctuation in significance might be expected after removing the schizophrenics because there is greater variability in exposure to OCs in these individuals than among unaffected high-risk individuals.*[12]

In summary, the direct examination of affected and unaffected high-risk individuals is a method of proven sensitivity in assessing genetic and perinatal influences on biological markers in schizophrenia. While the extent to which findings in such samples generalize to the population of patients as a whole remains to be quantified (ie, based on the prevalence of cases in which genetic factors do not play a role), there is as yet no compelling empirical or theoretical basis for doubting their representativeness.

Tyrone D. Cannon, PhD
Department of Psychology
University of Pennsylvania
3815 Walnut St
Philadelphia, PA 19104
Sarnoff A. Mednick, PhD, DrMed
Los Angeles, Calif
Josef Parnas, MD
Fini Schulsinger, MD
Johannes Praesthold, MD
Aage Vestergaard MD
Copenhagen, Denmark

1. Cannon TD, Mednick SA, Parnas J, Schulsinger F, Praestholm J, Vestergaard A. Developmental brain abnormalities in the offspring of schizophrenic mothers, I: contributions of genetic and perinatal factors. *Arch Gen Psychiatry.* 1993;50:551-564.
2. Cannon TD, Marco EJ. Structural brain abnormalities as indicators of vulnerability to schizophrenia. *Schizophr Bull.* 1994;20:89-102.
3. Fischer M. Psychoses in the offspring of schizophrenic monozyotic twins and their normal co-twins. *Br J Psychiatry.* 1971;118:43-52.
4. Gottesman II, Bertelsen A. Confirming unexpressed genotypes for schizophrenia: risks in the offspring of Fischer's Danish identical and discordant twins. *Arch Gen Psychiatry.* 1989;46:867-872.
5. Kendler KS. Overview: a current perspective on twin studies of schizophrenia. *Am J Psychiatry.* 1983;140:1413-1425.
6. Suddath RL, Christison GW, Torrey EF, Casanova MF, Weinberger DR. Anatomical abnormalities in the brains of monozygotic twins discordant for schizophrenia. *New Engl J Med.* 1990;332:789-794.
7. Weinberger DR, DeLisi LE, Neophytides AN, Wyatt RJ. Familial aspects of CT scan abnormalities in chronic schizophrenic patients. *Psychiatry Res.* 1981; 4:65-71.
8. Reveley AM, Reveley MA, Clifford CA, Murray RM. Cerebral ventricular size in twins discordant for schizophrenia. *Lancet.* 1982;1:540-541.
9. DeLisi LE, Goldin LR, Hamovit JR, Maxwell ME, Kurtz D, Gershon ES. A family study of the association of increased ventricular size with schizophre-

nia. *Arch Gen Psychiatry*. 1986;43:148-153.
10. Reddy R, Mukherjee S, Schnur DB, Chin J, Degreef G. History of obstetric complications, family history, and CT scan findings in schizophrenic patients. *Schizophr Res*. 1990;3:311-314.
11. Lewis SW, Murray RM. Obstetric complications, neurodevelopmental deviance and risk of schizophrenia. *J Psychiatr Res*. 1987;21:413-422.
12. Cannon TD, Mednick SA, Parnas J. Antecedents of predominantly negative- and predominantly positive-symptom schizophrenia in a high-risk population. *Arch Gen Psychiatry*. 1990;47:622-632.

Reciprocal Lateralization of Frontal Lobe Functions

In the January 1994 issue of the ARCHIVES, Rauch et al[1] report the relationship between regional cerebral blood flow (rCBF) and obsessive-compulsive symptoms measured by the Obsessive-Compulsive Disorder [OCD] Analogue Scale (OCDAS). In a provoked OCD state, OCDAS scores were positively correlated with left orbitofrontal rCBF and negatively correlated with right orbitofrontal rCBF. Rauch et al conclude that "... these two regions may play opposing roles in mediating and suppressing OCD symptoms respectively."

These OCD findings strongly resonate with our own findings in patients with lateralized focal frontal lesions.[2] We have designed an inherently ambiguous cognitive activation procedure, the Cognitive Bias Task (CBT). A high CBT score indicates a context-dependent, internally driven behavior; and a low score, context-independent, externally driven behavior. The CBT scores of healthy controls are in the middle of the scale, suggesting a balanced response selection strategy. Lateralized frontal lesions produced extreme deviations of CBT scores, and in opposite directions: toward extreme context dependence following right prefrontal lesions and toward extreme context independence following left prefrontal lesions. When the task ambiguity is removed in the control conditions, the lesion effects disappear, despite the fact that all the other cognitive task demands remain unchanged.

Both our data and those of Rauch et al, suggest a synergistic relationship between the two frontal systems and a dynamic balance between them under normal conditions. Furthermore, they suggest that certain frontal and neostriatal syndromes are best understood as functional imbalance rather than as absolute deficiency.

The CBT may provide a useful quantitative measure of the degree of such an imbalance between the two frontal systems, to be correlated with clinical scales and neuroimaging measures of dysfunctional lateralization. The CBT score also may prove to be a useful marker for the treatment efficacy of the syndromes affecting the frontal-cingulate-neostriatal circuitry.

Rauch et al studied a sample of five males and three females, but apparently they were not concerned with gender differences. Our lesion data suggest a strong sexual dimorphism in the degree of lateralization of frontal lobe functions: enhanced in males and virtually nonexistent in females. In females, both left-frontal and right-frontal lesion effects were similar to the right-frontal lesion effects in males. If established, a similar pattern of interaction between gender and rCBF could help account for the gender differences in the epidemiology and clinical expression of OCD and the closely related Tourette's syndrome.

An intimate anatomical and functional relationship exists between prefrontal cortex and neostriatum, and between the frontal and striatal syndromes. Tourette's syndrome takes different forms along a continuum defined at its extremes by iterations and perseverations—the "stereotypic" variant and incessant exploration and environmental dependency—the "phantasmagoric" variant.[3] It is possible that these Tourette's subtypes reflect subtle lateralization of neostriatal dysfunction to one hemisphere or the other, or a subtle imbalance between the control exerted by left and right frontostriatal systems.

Elkhonon Goldberg, PhD
Department of Psychiatry
New York University Medical Center
550 First Ave
New York, NY 10016
Kenneth Podell, PhD
Philadelphia, Pa

Reprint requests to Dr Goldberg.

1. Rauch SL, Jenike MA, Alpert NM, Baer L, Breiter HCR, Savage CR, Fischman AJ. Regional cerebral blood flow measured during symptom provocation in obsessive-compulsive disorder using oxygen 15–labeled carbon dioxide and positron emission tomography. *Arch Gen Psychiatry*. 1994;51:62-70.
2. Goldberg E, Podell K, Harner R, Lovell M, Riggio S. Cognitive bias, functional cortical geometry, and the frontal lobes: laterality, sex, and handedness. *J Cog Neurosci*. 1994;6:274-294.
3. Sacks O. Tourette's syndrome and creativity. *BMJ*. 1992;305:1515-1516.

In reply

We read with interest the letter of Goldberg and Podell commenting on our positron emission tomography symptom provocation study of OCD.[1] Goldberg et al[2] have developed a measure (CBT) of a parameter they call context dependence. Based on natural lesion experiments, they have inferred a tentative functional neuroanatomy of this behavioral bias (context dependence vs context independence) that is lateralized and gender dimorphic. Goldberg and Podell suggest that their findings resonate with our report of positive correlation of left anterior medial orbitofrontal relative rCBF with OCDAS and negative correlation of right posterior medial orbitofrontal rCBF with OCDAS. They propose that the CBT could provide a behavioral measure to be correlated with rCBF in future studies. They assume that we were not concerned with gender differences because we studied a cohort of five males and three females. Finally, they hypothesize that a pattern of gender-dimorphic lateralized frontal rCBF could help account for gender differences in OCD and Tourette's syndrome.

First, we were intentionally cautious when interpreting our finding of reciprocal lateralized correlations between medial orbitofrontal rCBF and OCDAS scores. The OCDAS is a crude measure of symptom severity, especially when applied between subjects. Moreover, the provocative stimuli in our study were presented on the left in all cases, thereby mitigating our ability to interpret lateralized findings conclusively.

With the above caveats in mind, we found the comments of Goldberg and Podell most intriguing. Obsessive-compulsive disorder is characterized by unwanted thoughts and/or repetitive behaviors that are internally driven and persistent despite changing external environmental cues. Therefore, within the scheme of context dependence vs independence, the obsessive-compulsive symptomatic state could be conceptualized as highly context dependent.

It is noteworthy that although functional neuroimaging studies of OCD to date have yielded generally convergent results, there has been great inconsistency with regard to laterality.[3] There are several possible explanations for the variability in laterality reported to date, and apropos of the above comments, differences in the gender composition of the study cohorts is one possible contributing factor. Because functional neuroimaging research is typically conducted using small sample sizes, the benefits of study population homogeneity must be weighed against the benefits of broader, more representative samples that provide for greater generalizability of findings. The point is well taken that the issue of gender composition always must be considered in neuroimaging research, and especially so when the object of study is thought to be gender dimorphic.

The proposed mediating neuroanatomy of the CBT reflects theoretical considerations and results from natural lesion experiments. We would suggest that Goldberg and colleagues consider testing these hypotheses more directly via a functional neuroimaging paradigm. As we understand the CBT, it could be modified for use as a cognitive activation probe in conjunction with positron emission tomography and oxygen 15.

As for the findings of their natural lesion experiments, although frontal cortex is implicated in the manner that they suggest, only a minority of their cases involved lesions of medial orbitofrontal cortex. Therefore, we would caution against drawing any parallels that rely on the treatment of frontal cortex as functionally monolithic. As we previously have emphasized, frontal cortex, even orbitofrontal cortex, is composed of functionally distinct subterritories.[4]

Finally, with respect to their speculations surrounding the role of laterality, gender, and Tourette's syndrome, we believe that there is an emerging neuroimaging literature that speaks to these issues. There has been independent replication of findings in Tourette's syndrome that points to an attenuation of the normal left-greater-than-right asymmetry in lenticulate nucleus.[5] Recently, we have completed a morphometric study of patients with OCD that suggests analogous findings in the caudate rather than the lenticulate (M.A.J. et al, unpublished data, 1994). Together, these results support the theory of Baxter et al[6] that the OCD–Tourette's syndrome clinical spectrum may reflect the topography of dysfunction within the striatum. It has been proposed that, whereas the caudate (implicated in cognitive functional systems) mediates the obsessions of OCD, the putamen (involved in sensorimotor systems) mediates the tics of Tourette's syndrome.

Scott L. Rauch, MD
Cary R. Savage, PhD
Lee Baer, PhD
Hans C. Breiter, MD
Nathaniel M. Alpert, PhD
Alan J. Fischman, MD, PhD
Michael A. Jenike, MD
Obsessive Compulsive Disorders Unit
Massachusetts General Hospital–East
149 13th Street, CNY-9130
Charlestown, MA 02129

1. Rauch SL, Jenike MA, Alpert NM, Baer L, Breiter HCR, Savage CR, Fischman AJ. Regional cerebral blood flow measured during symptom provocation in obsessive-compulsive disorder using oxygen 15–labeled carbon dioxide and positron emission tomography. *Arch Gen Psychiatry*. 1994;51:62-70.
2. Goldberg E, Podell K, Harner R, Lovell M, Riggio S. Cognitive bias, functional cortical geometry, and the frontal lobes: laterality, sex, and handedness. *J Cog Neurosci*. 1994;6:274-294.
3. Insel TR. Toward a neuroanatomy of obsessive-compulsive disorder. *Arch Gen Psychiatry*. 1992;49:739-744.
4. Rauch SL, Savage CR, Alpert NM. Self-induced dysphoria and neural correlates. *Am J Psychiatry*. 1994;151:784-785.
5. Witelson SF. Clinical neurology as data for basic neuroscience: Tourette's syndrome and the human motor system. *Neurology*. 1993;43:859-861.
6. Baxter LR, Schwartz JM, Guze BH, Bergman K, Szuba MP. Neuroimaging in obsessive-compulsive disorder: seeking the mediating neuroanatomy. In: Jenike MA, Baer L, Minichiello WE, eds. *Obsessive-Compulsive Disorders: Theory and Management*. 2nd ed. Chicago, Ill: Year Book Medical Publishers Inc; 1990: 167-188.

Neuroleptic Withdrawal in Schizophrenic Patients

A Review of the Literature

Patricia L. Gilbert, MD; M. Jackuelyn Harris, MD; Lou Ann McAdams, PhD; Dilip V. Jeste, MD

In the treatment of chronic schizophrenia, there are risks associated with both neuroleptic maintenance (eg, tardive dyskinesia) and neuroleptic withdrawal (eg, psychotic exacerbation or relapse). We reviewed 66 studies on neuroleptic withdrawal involving 4365 patients with schizophrenia. The mean cumulative relapse rate was 53% in patients withdrawn from neuroleptic therapy and 16% in those maintained on neuroleptic therapy over a mean follow-up period of 9.7 months. The relapse rate was positively associated with length of follow-up. Predictors of relapse reported in individual studies included younger age, higher baseline neuroleptic dosage, and shorter length of hospitalization. Adverse effects of neuroleptic withdrawal other than relapse were usually mild and transient. The risk-benefit ratio of neuroleptic maintenance vs withdrawal should be assessed carefully in individual patients. A slow taper to the lowest effective dosage may be the preferred strategy in many patients. *(Arch Gen Psychiatry. 1995;52:173-188)*

Neuroleptic or antipsychotic drugs are the mainstay of treatment for patients with schizophrenia. The efficacy of these medications in reducing both the severity of psychotic symptoms and the risk of psychotic relapse has been well documented.[1-3] It has been suggested that early treatment with neuroleptic medication reduces morbidity in some patients with schizophrenia.[4] Many patients with chronic schizophrenia need to be maintained on neuroleptic therapy for prolonged periods. In a recent review, Schooler[5] concluded that alternatives to continuous long-term neuroleptic treatment (eg, targeted medication strategies) may be feasible in some patients, yet they also carry significant risks and should be studied further. At the same time, continued treatment with neuroleptic drugs is also associated with an increased risk of serious side effects, such as orthostatic hypotension, extrapyramidal symptoms, and, of particular concern, persistent tardive dyskinesia (TD).[6-8] Kane et al[9] reported an annual incidence of TD of 4% to 5% in neuroleptic-treated young adults. Saltz et al[10] as well as Jeste and Caligiuri[11] reported an incidence of TD that was at least six times greater in older psychiatric patients.

The issue of prolonged neuroleptic treatment in a patient with chronic schizophrenia places the clinician on the horns of a dilemma. Since neuroleptic treatment does not cure schizophrenia, a large majority of such patients need long-term treatment. At the same time, prolonged use of these drugs carries a high risk of adverse effects, including TD. It is therefore recommended that continued prescription of antipsychotic drugs over a long period not be undertaken without adequate justification for both clinical and medicolegal purposes.[1,7,11] This may imply attempts at neuroleptic withdrawal. Drug withdrawal, however, is associated with a risk of psychotic relapse. To complicate matters further, a number of patients withdrawn from antipsychotic therapy do not experience relapse, at least over a short period, while some patients maintained on therapy do experience relapse. Thus, the clinician and the patient have to choose between two unwelcome risks: relapse and adverse effects of continued treatment.

Neuroleptic withdrawal is also important yet problematic from a research

From the Department of Psychiatry, University of California–San Diego, and the San Diego Veterans Affairs Medical Center.

perspective. Neuroleptic use is frequently a confounding factor in interpreting neurochemical and other findings in schizophrenia. It would be ideal to keep patients off neuroleptic drugs for as long as is possible, provided they can be maintained in a clinically stable state, ie, without relapse. Unfortunately, there is no clear guidance in the available literature about what type of patients can be withdrawn from antipsychotic drug therapy and for how long, as well as the optimal way of stopping drug therapy. To our knowledge, there has been no recent, comprehensive review of this important but controversial topic. Hence, we undertook the following review.

We asked the following questions: What is the risk of relapse in patients with schizophrenia after neuroleptic therapy has been stopped; in other words, what proportion of patients can be withdrawn from neuroleptic therapy without precipitating a relapse? Similarly, what is the likelihood of relapse in patients maintained on antipsychotic therapy over a comparable period? What are the other consequences of stopping neuroleptic therapy? Finally, what patient-related and treatment-related factors are associated with an increased or decreased danger of relapse and other adverse effects of stopping neuroleptic therapy?

METHODS

SELECTION OF STUDIES

We performed a computerized search of the literature on the MELVYL MEDLINE system using the following key words: *schizophrenia, antipsychotic, neuroleptic, withdrawal, discontinuation,* and *taper.* Cross-references were obtained from the bibliographies of the retrieved articles. We included English- and foreign-language articles about a minimum of 10 subjects with a diagnosis of schizophrenia or schizoaffective disorder. We included only articles with new data; review articles, such as that by Davis,[12] were thus excluded from our analyses. Because of unspecified or small sample sizes (fewer than 10 subjects each), we excluded from our analyses reports by Spivak et al,[13] Melamed et al,[14] Kushnir,[15] and Calev et al.[16] (We will, however, refer to these studies in discussing various adverse effects of neuroleptic withdrawal.) We included seven studies[17-23] that contained mixed diagnostic groups, but we excluded nonschizophrenic subjects in those studies from our analyses. Twenty-nine (44%) of the 66 studies included patients maintained on neuroleptic therapy who served as matched control groups for the neuroleptic withdrawal groups. The neuroleptic withdrawal groups from these 29 studies will be referred to in this review as "matched neuroleptic withdrawal groups." The term *matched* is used here for lack of a more suitable alternative. In a majority of these studies, the "control" groups were obtained by random assignment,[17,19,23-45] whereas five studies[46-50] specifically selected controls matched for age, diagnosis, duration of illness, and other variables.

A few research groups have published several sequential studies on neuroleptic withdrawal. Hence, data on individual subjects might have been used in more than one publication. We went through each article carefully and excluded the earlier publications from which data had been reused in later studies by the same group of investigators. Occasionally, however, it was not possible to weed out overlapping data. We cannot therefore exclude the possibility of a small bias resulting from the individual subjects' data being represented more than once in the cumulative data analysis. This was, however, not a major problem in our review, which involved more than 4000 patients.

SELECTION OF VARIABLES

For each study we examined the rate of relapse as well as possible predictors of relapse, such as age, gender, duration of illness, length of hospitalization, neuroleptic type and dose, length of neuroleptic taper, and length of follow-up. For the data analysis we selected those relevant variables on which at least 30 out of the 66 studies reviewed had provided usable information. (The only exception was percentage of patients receiving anticholinergic therapy, for which data were available in only 20 studies; we thought it to be too important a variable to be excluded.) We also reviewed other clinical or neurochemical effects of neuroleptic withdrawal in both the neuroleptic withdrawal and neuroleptic maintenance groups (when present).

STATISTICAL ANALYSIS

For each study we extracted the following descriptive summary statistics for both the neuroleptic withdrawal group and the neuroleptic maintenance (control) group, if present: the "average" values for age, duration of illness, length of hospitalization, baseline neuroleptic dose in milligram chlorpromazine equivalents (mg CPZE),[6] length of taper, and length of follow-up period. The means of the variables were utilized if these had been provided by the authors, but the midpoint of the range was substituted (as "averages") if the authors had provided that information instead of the mean. Study characteristics were noted, and the percentage of studies specifying diagnostic criteria as well as the percentage of studies with different designs (open, nonblind, single blind, or double blind) were determined.

To summarize the information in these studies, we computed unweighted means and SDs across studies from the individual study averages (means or midpoints), percentages, or sample sizes for the neuroleptic withdrawal groups and for the neuroleptic maintenance groups.

The matched neuroleptic withdrawal groups were compared with the matched neuroleptic maintenance groups by paired *t* tests. We used Bonferroni-corrected criterion α levels to limit the chance of a type I error from multiple comparisons. The matched neuroleptic withdrawal groups were also compared with the unmatched neuroleptic withdrawal groups on each of the listed variables using *t* tests, Mann-Whitney *U* Tests, or χ^2 analyses as appropriate, using Bonferroni-corrected criterion α levels.

Since the average length of follow-up varied considerably from study to study, we attempted to relate the relapse rate of a study to its average length of follow-up. Because the follow-up time was positively skewed, a common logarithm was taken of the sum of the length of follow-up (in months) plus 1 for each group (neuroleptic withdrawal and neuroleptic maintenance) in each study that had both groups before this variable was related to others. This transformation also improved the linearity of any associations. A linear regression of relapse rate on the log transformation of the average length of follow-up was performed separately for all the neuroleptic withdrawal groups, the unmatched and the matched neuroleptic withdrawal groups, and the matched neuroleptic maintenance groups. Because the matched pairs of groups had the same average length of follow-up, we were also able to regress the difference in relapse rates between the matched groups on the log-transformed average length of follow-up.[51]

We also attempted to improve on the linear association between the relapse rate and the logarithm of the average length of follow-up and between the differences in relapse rates and the logarithm of the average length of follow-up by employing the empirical unweighted logit transformation of the relapse rate and the difference in logits, respectively. Occasional studies had relapse rates of zero; since one cannot take the logarithm of zero, we added 0.5 to each cell count.[52]

Finally, we attempted to improve the prediction of the relapse rate or logarithmic odds of the relapse rate or their respective differences between the matched withdrawal and matched maintenance groups by substituting or adding any of the other potential predictors in the data by means of a stepwise multiple regression analysis.

RESULTS

In the literature reviewed, 64 articles containing 66 studies* (each of two articles[47,56] reported two separate studies) including a total of 4365 subjects (3141 subjects withdrawn from neuroleptic therapy and 1224 comparison subjects maintained on neuroleptic therapy) met our inclusion criterion, ie, a minimum of 10 subjects with schizophrenia or schizoaffective disorder. **Table 1** summarizes descriptive features of the 66 studies reviewed.[86,87]

We derived summary data from the 66 studies, including the relapse rate. The descriptive statistics based on the summary data are shown in **Table 2**.

METHODOLOGICAL ASPECTS OF THE STUDIES REVIEWED

Sample Size

The sample sizes ranged from 10 to 519, with the average number of subjects in the neuroleptic withdrawal groups being 47.6.

Amount of Other Information Available

In general, the amount of information provided by the individual studies varied greatly. For example, in terms of age, 28 studies gave mean age only, nine reported age range only, 22 reported both mean age and range, while seven studies did not specify age at all.

Diagnostic Criteria

None of the 30 articles prior to 1981 defined or utilized specific diagnostic criteria for schizophrenia. If any reference was made to diagnosis, it was only noted that the subjects were "diagnosed by two psychiatrists."[19,24,26,30] Beginning in 1981, however, all of the studies reviewed except for one[62] employed specific diagnostic criteria, such as Research Diagnostic Criteria (RDC), *DSM-III, International Classification of Diseases, Ninth Revision, Clinical Modification* (*ICD-9-CM*), and *DSM-III-R*.

Study Design

Thirty-seven of the 66 withdrawal studies (n=38) were double blind. Twenty-nine studies utilized a control group, ie, patients maintained on neuroleptic therapy. (Double-blind studies without control groups used placebo during neuroleptic withdrawal and had both patients and raters "blind" to the medication status.)

Medication Type and Dose

The neuroleptic medication used varied from study to study in terms of specific type and daily dosage. Phenothiazines and haloperidol were the most commonly prescribed neuroleptic agents. The average daily dosages, where stated, ranged from 228 to 1736 mg/d CPZE, with an average of 630.0 mg/d CPZE.

Of the 20 studies that specified concurrent medications, only one study specifically excluded patients receiving anticholinergic medication.[69]

Length of Neuroleptic Taper

Neuroleptic therapy was withdrawn acutely over 1 day in 42 of the studies where information about taper was given. The remaining studies used taper periods ranging from 2 to 60 days.

Length of Follow-up

The follow-up period after neuroleptic withdrawal ranged from 0.5 to 24 months, with an average of 6.3 months for all 66 studies and 9.7 months for the 29 studies with control groups. Since most studies did not specify the exact time of relapse in individual patients, we used the mean follow-up period. The matched withdrawal groups had a significantly longer average length of follow-up (Mann-Whitney *U* Test, $P=.0001$) and logarithmic follow-up ($t=5.47$, $df=64$, $P<.0001$) than the unmatched withdrawal groups.

Definition of Relapse

Twenty-two studies did not provide any definition of relapse.† *Relapse* was defined as a "return to active medication" in 11 studies.‡ The

*References 17-34, 37-43, 45-50, 53-85.

†References 17, 19-22, 25, 47, 53-57, 61, 62, 69, 71, 73, 76, 79, 80, 85.

‡References 18, 24, 26, 27, 30, 41, 60, 63, 72, 75, 81.

Table 1. Literature Review on Neuroleptic Withdrawal*

Source, y	No./Sex	Mean (Range) Age, y	Mean (Range) Duration of Illness, y	Mean (Range) Length of Hospitalization, y	Diagnostic Criteria	Study Design
Good et al,[53] 1958	112/M	(22-50)	NS	(0.2-?)	NS	DB
Brooks,[54] 1959	28/F	40.4 (19-53)	NS (chronic)	(1-25)	NS	SB
Diamond and Marks,[46] 1960	E: 20 C: 20	46.3	NS	E: 11.4 C: 11.6	NS	DB with control group
Rothstein,[55] 1960	17	45.2	NS (chronic)	8.4	NS	SB
Blackburn and Allen,[27] 1961	E: 28/M C: 25/M	(20-40)	Chronic	(0.3-10.8)	NS	Open with control group
Judah et al,[56] 1961 (two studies)	87	NS	NS (chronic)	(2-5)	NS	SB
	519	NS	NS	NS	NS	SB
Gross and Reeves,[57] 1961	E: 70 C: 36	41.8 (19-66)	NS	4.6 (0.5-10)	NS	DB with control group
Freeman and Alson,[17] 1962	E: 46/M (42 with SZ) C: 44/M	E: 41.1 C: 46.2	NS	E: 13.2 C: 11.3	NS	DB with control group
Olson and Peterson,[47] 1962 (two studies)	E: 60 C: 30	51 (21-78)	NS (chronic)	(>1.5)	NS	DB with control group
	E: 30 C: 30	51 (21-78)	NS (chronic)	(>1.5)	NS	DB
Whitaker and Hoy,[30] 1963	E: 26/M C: 13/M	E: 50 (27-66) C: 51.8	NS	E: 15.5 C: 19.9	NS (2 psychiatrists agreed)	DB with control group
Caffey et al,[32] 1964	E: 171/M C: 88/M	40	NS	10	NS	DB with control group
Marjerrison et al,[58] 1964	31 (15/M, 16/F)	47	(13-21)	(13-20)	NS	DB
Garfield et al,[33] 1966	E: 18/F C: 9/F	E: 42.4 (22-59) C: 42.6	NS	E: 11.4 C: 11.2	NS	DB with control group
Melnyk et al,[59] 1966	E: 20 (7/M, 13/F) C: 20	NS	12.8 (3-32)	1.5 (0.3-3)	NS	DB with control group
Hughes and Little,[18] 1967	21/F (12 with SZ)	57 (26-74)	NS (chronic)	10	NS	SB
Morton,[24] 1968	E: 20/M C: 20/M	(25-55)	NS	(≥2)	NS (2 psychiatrists agreed)	DB with control group
Prien et al,[60] 1968	210 (30 each at 7 hospitals)	41.6 (61% >40)	NS	14.5	NS	DB
Prien et al,[37] 1969	E: 120 C: 240	41.8	NS (chronic)	15 (2-33)	NS	DB with control group
Gleser et al,[65] 1970	74 (35/M, 39/F)	42.9 (24-54)	NS	11	NS	DB
Rassidakis et al,[19] 1970	E: 43 (36/M, 7/F) (33 with SZ) C: 28	E: 49.3 (26-74) C: 42.8 (33-60)	E: 23.5 (4-45) C: 18.1 (3-38)	NS	NS (2 psychiatrists agreed)	Open with control groups
Baro et al,[38] 1970	E: 26 C: 12	(24-71)	NS	NS	NS	DB with control group
Leff and Wing,[39] 1971	E: 15 C: 20	(16-55)	NS	NS	NS	DB with control group
Hershon et al,[50] 1972	E: 32 (17/M, 15/F) C: 30 (15/M, 15/F)	E: 53.6 (M), 60.4 (F) C: 57.3	NS (chronic)	NS	NS	DB with control group
Hirsch et al,[40] 1973	E: 41 (27/M, 14/F) C: 40 (25/M, 15/F)	E: 44.3±10.0† C: 42.6±10.5†	NS	NS	NS (case records)	DB with control group
Andrews et al,[26] 1976	E: 17/M C: 14/M	(50-63)	NS	6	Psychiatrist confirmed	DB with control group

Neuroleptic Type/Mean (Range) Dosage, mg/d	Mean (Range) Length of Taper, d	Mean (Range) Length of Follow-up, mo	Definition of Relapse	Relapse Rate, %	Predictors of Relapse
CPZ/(200-800)	1 (Acute)	6	NS	NS	NS
CPZ/(150-600), reserpine/(1.5-4)	1 (Acute)	0.5	NS	NS	NS
CPZ/400 (300-800), trifluopromazine/150 (50-300)	1 (Acute)	6	Worsening clinical condition	E: 70 C: 25	NS
CPZ	1 (Acute)	3	NS	6	NS
Phenothiazines	1 (Acute)	4	(1) Rating score decreased by 1 SE from baseline (2) Emergent resumption of medications (3) Transfer to closed ward	E: 46 C: 12	NS
CPZ, other phenothiazines	1 (Acute)	5	NS	60	NS
CPZ/(300-600)	1 (Acute)	3	Hyperactive, mute, threatening behavior	72	NS
Mainly CPZ	60 (28-150)	6	NS	E: 75.7 C: 13.9	NS
CPZ/228	1 (Acute)	6	NS	E: 31 C: 13	NS
CPZ, thioridazine	1 (Acute)	6	NS	29 (with placebo)	None
CPZ, thioridazine	1 (Acute)	6	NS	85 (without placebo)	NS
Perphenazine	1 (Acute)	2.5	Major relapse, return to medications	E: 39 C: 7.7	NS
CPZ/400, thioridazine/350	4	4	Withdrawal agitation, thinking disturbance	45	None
Trifluoperazine, chlorprothixene	1 (Acute)	7	Behavioral worsening	NS	NS
CPZ/610, other phenothiazines	7	5	Difference of ±2 on IMPS[86] factor scores and of ±4 on morbidity scores indicated positive or negative change	E: 31 C: 13	NS
CPZ, thioridazine	1 (Acute)	1.5	Return of symptoms similar to before drug treatment	E: 50 C: 0	NS
CPZ/(75-450)	1 (Acute)	18	Return to medications	19	NS
Trifluoperazine, CPZ	1 (Acute)	6	Return to medications	E: 70 C: 25	NS
CPZ	1 (Acute)	6	Regressed, returned to neuroleptic medication before end of 6 mo	40	(1) Higher prior dose of medications (2) Younger patients (<40 y)
Trifluoperazine/(15-80)	1 (Acute)	6	Deteriorated behavior	E: 45 C: 20	Longer hospitalization, type of phenothiazine medication
Phenothiazines	1 (Acute)	1	Assaultive or suicidal	5.4	NS
Thioridazine, haloperidol, CPZ	1 (Acute)	9	NS	E: 58.1 C: 34.1	Younger age at onset, younger current age, and nonparanoid subtype
R16341/20 (10-40)	1 (Acute)	2.5	Disorganization, agitation, abnormal thought process	E: 100 C: 0	NS
CPZ/(100-300), trifluoperazine/(5-15)	1 (Acute)	12	Return to SZ symptoms	E: 80 C: 35	Younger age, male, situational anxiety
Trifluoperazine/17	1 (Acute)	4	Delusions, hallucinations, aggression, regressed behavior	E: 28.1 C: 6.7	Younger current age, longer duration of neuroleptic treatment, higher prior medication dose
Fluphenazine decanoate/25 mg/mo	1 (Acute)	9	Deteriorated condition	E: 66 C: 8	NS
CPZ/(50-450)	1 (Acute)	10.5	Deteriorated behavior and return to medications	E: 35 C: 7	Higher prior medication dose

(*continued*)

Table 1. Literature Review on Neuroleptic Withdrawal* (cont)

Source, y	No./Sex	Mean (Range) Age, y	Mean (Range) Duration of Illness, y	Mean (Range) Length of Hospitalization, y	Diagnostic Criteria	Study Design
Rifkin et al,[34] 1977	E: 51 (34/M, 17/F) C: 22 (16/M, 6/F)	E: 23.7 (17-38) C: (17-30)	NS NS	NS NS	Kraepelinian signs of SZ	DB with control group
Lacoursiere et al,[61] 1976	48	37	NS	6	NS	DB
Hogarty and Goldberg,[41] 1973	E: 182 C: 192	34.4 (18-55)	NS	NS	Confirmed by research psychiatrist	DB with control group
Levine et al,[42] 1980	E: 50 C: 17	NS	NS	NS	NS	DB with control group
Zander et al,[62] 1981	13 (8/M, 5/F)	45.2±6.5‡	22	13.6	NS	NS
Brown and Laughren,[63] 1981	28/M	(28-66)	NS	NS	RDC	Open
Branchey et al,[49] 1981	E: 21 (13/M, 8/F) C: 11 (6/M, 5/F)	E: 51.4±9.6† (27-62) C: 52.2±8.9† (33-62)	NS	E: 25.4±8.6† (7-40) C: 25.9±10.3† (10-39)	RDC	DB with control group
Herz et al,[64] 1982	13 (6/M, 7/F)	43.5	NS	NS	*DSM-III*	Open
Kane et al,[23] 1982	E: 17 C: 11	E: 22.1±3.6† C: 21.5±5.4†	NS	NS	RDC	DB with control group
Kirch et al,[20] 1983	19 (13/M, 6/F) (12 with SZ)	19-56	NS	NS	*DSM-III*	Open
Johnson et al,[48] 1983	E: 60 (group A: 20, group B: 20, group C: 20) C: 56 (group A: 20, group B: 20, group C: 16)	E: 31.97 (group A: 29.4, group B: 31.4, group C: 35.1) C: 33.8 (group A: 31.1, group B: 32.7, group C: 37.6)	NS	NS	First-rank symptoms of Schneider	Open with control group
Naber et al,[66] 1985	36/M	46±11† (27-60)	17	16	*ICD-9-CM*	SB
Pietzcker et al,[25] 1986	E: 34 (17/M, 17/F) C: 14 (7/M, 7/F)	E: 41 C: 34	E: 9.9 C: 8.6	NS	*ICD-9* and RDC	Randomized, open with control group
Pickar et al,[67] 1986	11 (7/M, 4/F)	28±2.8§	NS	NS	*DSM-III*	DB
Crow et al,[43] 1986	E: 66 (39/M, 27/F) C: 54 (35/M, 19/F)	E: 24.3 (16-56) C: 28.2 (17-59)	E: (0.1-7.7) C: (0.1-8.4)	NS	RDC	DB with control group
Lieberman et al,[68] 1987	29	29.1±2.5† (18-50)	7.2	NS	RDC	DB

Neuroleptic Type/Mean (Range) Dosage, mg/d	Mean (Range) Length of Taper, d	Mean (Range) Length of Follow-up, mo	Definition of Relapse	Relapse Rate, %	Predictors of Relapse
Oral fluphenazine/(5-30), fluphenazine decanoate/12.5 mg biweekly	1 (Acute)	12	Substantial clinical deterioration	E: 68 C: 10	NS
CPZE/800	1 (Acute)	1	NS	NS	NS
CPZ	1 (Acute)	12	Return to medications	E: 67.5 C: 30.9	Younger age, earlier onset of illness
NS	1 (Acute)	12	Rehospitalization or deterioration of clinical condition	E: 46 C: 24	NS
CPZE/(273-396)	1 (Acute)	4.8	NS	61.5	Early relapsers: younger age, shortest duration of psychosis, shortest duration of medical therapy and hospitalization
CPZE/(75-1250)	14	10	Development of symptoms requiring return to medications	29	NS
E: Loxapine/70.9±44.7 (10-130), Loxapine/66.4±44.3 (20-160)	28	6	Development of new or worsening of preexisting symptoms	E: 76 C: 18	Higher baseline neuroleptic dose
CPZE/340 (100-690)	56	8	Low rating on GAS	23	Younger age at onset, recent hospitalization, higher medication doses
Oral fluphenazine or fluphenazine decanoate	1 (Acute)	12	Clinical deterioration	E: 41.2 C: 0	Poorer social adjustment
CPZE/807	1 (Acute)	0.5	NS	NS	NS
Depot neuroleptics: fluphenazine decanoate, flupenthixol decanoate	NS	E: 12 C: 18	Worsening of previous psychotic symptoms causing a 20% increase in the BPRS score and the Krawiecka Scale[87] or appearance of new SZ symptoms	E (12 mo): 65 (group A: 70, group B: 65, group C: 60) E (18 mo): 80 group A: 80, group B: 90, group C: 70) C (12 mo): 16 (group A: 25, group B: 10, group C: 13) C (18 mo): 23 (group A: 35, group B: 15, group C: 19)	NS
CPZE/560	1 (Acute)	0.5	Increase in total BPRS score ≥7 points or ≥5 points on subscales	11	NS
NS	Gradual	6	NS	E: 21 C: 0	NS
Fluphenazine	1 (Acute)	1.3	Worsening of symptoms or increase in pHVA level	NS	Increase in pHVA level
CPZ	30	24	Readmission to psychiatric care	62 46	Duration of illness prior to starting medication
NS	20 (oral medications), 42 (fluphenazine decanoate)	12	(1) Increase of 10 points on BPRS factors III, IV, V (2) Increase of 2 points on SADS Psychosis and Disorganization items	70.6	(1) Patients with TD relapsed sooner (2) Positive responders to Ritalin (methylphenidate hydrochloride) relapsed sooner

(continued)

Table 1. Literature Review on Neuroleptic Withdrawal* (cont)

Source, y	No./Sex	Mean (Range) Age, y	Mean (Range) Duration of Illness, y	Mean (Range) Length of Hospitalization, y	Diagnostic Criteria	Study Design
Dufresne and Wagner,[69] 1988	27 (13/M, 14/F)	32.7±9.9† (M) 33.1±11.2† (F)	12.0	NS	*DSM-III*	Open
Kirch et al,[70] 1988	22 (14/M, 8/F)	27 (18-41)	8	NS	*DSM-III*	DB
Kuhs and Eikelmann,[71] 1988	21 (11/M, 10/F)	25±6†	1.9	NS	*ICD-9-CM*	Open
Baron et al,[21] 1989	22 (18/M, 4/F) (17 with SZ)	46 (21-83)	NS	NS	*DSM-III*	Open
Glazer et al,[72] 1989	19	51	27	4.8	RDC	SB
Thaker et al,[73] 1989	10	28±5.3†	NS	NS	RDC	Open
van Kammen et al,[74] 1989	32/M	34.2±7.61†	11.2 (SD, 6.6)	NS	*DSM-III*	DB
Jolley et al,[44] 1990	E: 27 (10/M, 17/F) C: 27 (13/M, 14/F)	E: 41 C: 42	E: 12 C: 13	NS	*DSM-III*	DB with control group
Glazer et al,[22] 1990	49 (15/M, 34/F) (10 with SZ)	54±13†	32	0.5	RDC	Open
Green et al,[75] 1990	22/M	(22-66)	(4-25)	NS	RDC	Open
Khan et al,[76] 1990	32/M	39.1±11.4	22.8±4.7	NS	*DSM-III*	Open
Singh et al,[77] 1990	10	40.5	(11-32)	NS	*DSM-III-R* and SSP	DB
Carpenter et al,[29] 1990	E: 57 (34/M, 23/F) C: 59 (37/M, 22/F)	E: 28.4 C: 27.8	5.5 4.6	NS	RDC	SB with control group
Davidson et al,[78] 1991	23	38.5±11.2†	16.4±10.5	8.0±6.4	RDC and *DSM-III-R*	Open
Harvey et al,[79] 1991	24/M	36±10†	(22-23)	(3-10)	*DSM-III* and RDC	SB
Ruskin and Nyman,[31] 1991	E: 10 C: 8	60.1	NS	NS	*DSM-III*	DB with control group
Wolf et al,[80] 1991	20	(33-37)	NS	7	*DSM-III*	Open
Herz et al,[45] 1991	E: 50 (28/M, 22/F) C: 51 (26/M, 25/F)	E: 34.6±10.8† C: 37.4±11.7†	NS	NS	RDC	DB with control group
Glovinsky et al,[81] 1992	45 (28/M, 17/F)	29.5 (18-45)	9.5	NS	*DSM-III* and *DSM-III-R*	DB
Neylan et al,[82] 1992	18/M	35±6† (26-45)	10.7±6.7	NS	*DSM-III-R*	DB

Neuroleptic Type/Mean (Range) Dosage, mg/d	Mean (Range) Length of Taper, d	Mean (Range) Length of Follow-up, mo	Definition of Relapse	Relapse Rate, %	Predictors of Relapse
Haloperidol/(5-40), thioridazine, molindone	2	0.5	NS	NS	NS
Mostly haloperidol, CPZE/1736	1 (Acute)	1.5	Increase of 36% in BPRS score	NS	Increase in pMHPG level, increase in pHVA level
Mostly haloperidol/(10-30)	1 (Acute)	1	NS	NS	NS
Phenothiazines or haloperidol, CPZE/(1.4-285.4)	NS	2	NS	NS	NS
CPZE/326	(7-10)	0.5	Required return to medications (behavioral changes, psychosis)	26	Increase in pHVA level after withdrawal, lower baseline pHVA level, higher prior medication dose, higher BPRS score during withdrawal, longer neuroleptic exposure
Mostly haloperidol/(5-40)	1 (Acute)	0.5	NS	NS	NS
Haloperidol/12.8±9.5	7	1.5	Increase of 10 points on BPRS psychosis subscale and 3 points on Bunney-Hamburg psychosis item	43.8	Increase in CSF NE level
	NS	24	Reemergence of severe psychiatric symptoms	E: 50 C: 12	NS
CPZE/255	30	12	NS	NS	NS
CPZE/(50-1350)	21	10	Developed symptoms requiring return to neuroleptic medication	NS	Low prolactin level during neuroleptic treatment
NS	1 (Acute)	1.5	NS	NS	NS
CPZE/(413-930)	1 (Acute)	0.5	Any increase from baseline BPRS score	None	NS
NS	1 (Acute)	24	Hospitalization	E: 53 C: 36	NS
NS	1 (Acute)	1.5	Increase of ≥2 points on BPRS psychosis items for 2 wk	39.1	pHVA level was higher in decompensated group
CPZE/500	1 (Acute)	1.5	NS	50 (nonkraepelinian)	NS
Haloperidol, CPZE/324.7	14	6	Significant clinical decline per research psychiatrist (new psychotic symptoms, increase in old psychotic symptoms, or prodromal symptoms with anxiety/insomnia)	E: 50 C: 12.5	Younger age, higher prior medication dose, higher baseline BPRS score, recent psychiatric hospitalization
CPZE/(2000-2600)	42	1.5	NS	NS	NS
E: CPZE/322.8±270.0 C: CPZE/259.0±150.1	42	24	Increase in certain psychotic symptoms	E: 30 C: 16	NS
NS	NS	2	Symptom worsening, return to medications	NS	NS
Haloperidol	1 (Acute)	1.5	Mean increase ≥3 points on global psychosis item of Bunney-Hamburg Scale	50	None found

(continued)

Table 1. Literature Review on Neuroleptic Withdrawal* (cont)

Source, y	No./Sex	Mean (Range) Age, y	Mean (Range) Duration of Illness, y	Mean (Range) Length of Hospitalization, y	Diagnostic Criteria	Study Design
Kirkpatrick et al,[83] 1992	18/M	30 (18-39)	9.5	NS	RDC	Open
Jeste et al,[84] 1993	20/M	48.4 (33-68)	21.3 (1-37)	4.6 (0-20)	*DSM-III-R*	SB
Arndt et al,[85] 1993	43 (30/M, 13/F)	32.7±9.7† (22-56)	NS	NS	*DSM-III-R*	Open

**NS indicates not specified; DB, double blind; CPZ, chlorpromazine; SB, single blind; E, experimental; C, control; SZ, schizophrenia; IMPS, Inpatient Multidimensional Psychiatric Scale; CPZE, chlorpromazine equivalent; RDC, Research Diagnostic Criteria; GAS, Global Assessment Scale; BPRS, Brief Psychiatric Rating Scale;* ICD-9-CM, International Classification of Diseases, Ninth Revision, Clinical Modification; ICD-9, International Statistical Classification of Diseases, Injuries, and Causes of Death, Based on the Recommendations of the Ninth Revision Conference; *pHVA, plasma homovanillic acid; TD, tardive dyskinesia; pMHPG, plasma methoxyhydroxyphenylglycol; SADS, Schedule for Affective Disorders and Schizophrenia; CSF, cerebrospinal fluid; NE, norepinephrine; SSP, supersensitivity psychosis; and CGI, Clinical Global Impression.*

†*Value is mean±SD.*

‡*Meaning of plus-or-minus value not specified.*

§*Value is mean±SEM.*

remaining 33 studies defined *relapse* as either emergence of "behavioral worsening" (with agitation, aggression, insomnia, anxiety, hallucinations, delusions, or assaultive or suicidal behavior) or a specified change seen on clinical rating scales, such as the Brief Psychiatric Rating Scale (BPRS).[88]

RATE OF RELAPSE

Relationship of Relapse Rate to Neuroleptic Withdrawal

The rate of relapse in the 66 studies of neuroleptic withdrawal groups ranged from 0% to 100%. We found a significant difference (t=10.64, df=28, P<.0001) in the mean rate of relapse for the matched withdrawal groups (53.2%) vs matched maintenance groups (15.6%) in the 29 studies that included control groups. The mean rate of relapse in the neuroleptic withdrawal groups from all the 66 studies was 46.6%. There was an outlier study[38] with a relapse rate of 100% in the neuroleptic withdrawal patients and 0% in the neuroleptic maintenance patients (n=13 each) at 2.5 months of follow-up. This difference in the percentage relapse rate was more than 3 SDs from the mean difference for all 29 studies. With this group excluded, the mean relapse rates for the withdrawal and maintenance groups were 51.5% and 16.2%, respectively (paired t=12.48, df=27, P=.0001).

Relationship of Relapse Rate to Length of Follow-up

With the outlier study[38] removed and with percentage relapse expressed as a natural logarithm (odds) and follow-up time expressed as logarithmic follow-up, there was a significant association between relapse and follow-up for all the withdrawal groups (r=.500, df=45, P=.001), for the unmatched withdrawal groups (r=.493, df=17, P=.032), and for the matched maintenance groups (r=.503, df=26, P<.006). The matched withdrawal groups exhibited a nonsignificant positive association (r=.231, df=26, P=.237). The two regression lines for the matched withdrawal and matched maintenance groups were, however, converging with significantly different slopes, as indicated by the significant regression of the natural logarithm (odds ratio) on logarithmic follow-up (r=−.383, df=26, P=.044): ln (odds ratio) = ln (odds for withdrawal groups) − ln (odds for maintenance groups), where ln indicates natural logarithm. The negative correlation indicated that the differences in ln (odds) were diminishing over follow-up time (**Figure**).

Other Predictors of Relapse

Even without Bonferroni corrections, other study characteristics (eg, average duration of illness, use of specific diagnostic criteria for schizophrenia) made no significant contributions to the prediction of the logit transform of the relapse rate beyond that of the logarithm of the length of follow-up. Individual studies, however, reported that certain individual characteristics were predictors of relapse after neuroleptic therapy was stopped. These included younger current age,[19,31,39,50,60,62] earlier age of onset of illness,[19,64] higher baseline neuroleptic dose,[26,31,49,50,60,64,72] nonparanoid subtype of schizophrenia,[19] recent psychiatric hospitalization,[31,64] poor social adjustment,[23] male gender,[39] and nonpiperazine type of phenothiazine medication.[37]

Response to Reinstitution of Neuroleptics

Patients who experienced relapse after neuroleptic withdrawal were usually found to have a rapid return to baseline when neuroleptic therapy was reinstituted.[31,53,55,81] Recompensation was observed within 3 days to 3 weeks after neuroleptic treatment was restarted.

Neuroleptic Type/Mean (Range) Dosage, mg/d	Mean (Range) Length of Taper, d	Mean (Range) Length of Follow-up, mo	Definition of Relapse	Relapse Rate, %	Predictors of Relapse
Fluphenazine, haloperidol, trifluoperazine	NS	1	Increase in or reappearance of psychotic symptoms	NS	No relationship between prolactin concentration and time to subsequent relapse
Variable, CPZE/(379±533)	7	0.5	Increase ≥2 points on BPRS or CGI Scale, or dangerousness to self or others	0	Not applicable
Variable	3.2 (2-4)	1	NS	NS	NS

OTHER CLINICAL EFFECTS OF NEUROLEPTIC WITHDRAWAL

Cholinergic Rebound

In the first 2 weeks after neuroleptic therapy was stopped, patients were reported to experience a variety of symptoms consistent with cholinergic rebound, including nausea, malaise, diaphoresis, vomiting, and insomnia.[54,61,89,90] These effects were generally mild and transient and did not require treatment.

Withdrawal-Emergent Dyskinesia

Dufresne and Wagner[69] reported the occurrence of withdrawal-emergent dyskinesia 2 weeks after neuroleptic therapy was stopped. Maintaining patients with withdrawal-emergent dyskinesia or TD off neuroleptic drugs for long periods tended to improve the dyskinesia,[20] especially in younger patients.[72]

Other Adverse Effects

There have been anecdotal case reports of neuroleptic malignant syndrome,[13] tardive akathisia,[69] progressive parkinsonism,[14] and even hematemesis[20] following neuroleptic withdrawal. Such untoward reactions must be very rare, however.

Neuropsychological Effects

Orzak et al[91] and Spohn et al[92] compared patients with schizophrenia maintained on neuroleptic therapy with those withdrawn from neuroleptic therapy and found improved performance on tests of attention and information processing in the neuroleptic maintenance group. Simon,[93] however, found no significant difference between the neuroleptic maintenance and withdrawal groups on the Trail Making Test, while Depue et al[94] observed no change in Wechsler Adult Intelligence Scale (WAIS) IQ score after neuroleptic withdrawal.

Changes in Sleep Architecture

Thaker et al[73] reported decreased total sleep time, decreased rapid eye movement sleep, and decreased rapid eye movement latency after neuroleptic withdrawal. Neylan et al[82] found similar changes but also noted that relapsers had greater decreases than nonrelapsers in total sleep time, in non–rapid eye movement sleep, and in stage 2 sleep.

Neurochemical Effects

The following neurochemical changes were reported after neuroleptic withdrawal, although not all studies yielded consistent results: increased concentrations of plasma homovanillic acid, a metabolite of dopamine[20,67,72,76]; increased concentrations of plasma 3-methoxy-4-hydroxyphenylglycol (MHPG), a metabolite of norepinephrine[70]; initial decrease followed by an increase in plasma prolactin concentrations[73,75,95]; decreased plasma prolactin concentrations during neuroleptic treatment associated with earlier relapse[75]; lower baseline plasma prolactin concentrations associated with earlier relapse[63]; decreased plasma norepinephrine concentrations[62,66]; and increased cerebrospinal fluid norepinephrine concentrations in relapsers.[74] Finally, some investigators reported increased plasma cortisol concentrations,[66] increased plasma β-endorphin concentrations,[66] and increased density of striatal dopamine D_2 receptors on positron emission tomography scan after neuroleptic withdrawal.[21]

COMMENT

The limitations of this report stem in part from methodologic aspects of the studies reviewed, such as differences in methods and materials, variable and sometimes small sample sizes, a lack of specific diagnostic cri-

Table 2. Summary Characteristics

Variable	All Neuroleptic Withdrawal Groups (N=66)	Unmatched Neuroleptic Withdrawal Groups (N=37)	Matched Neuroleptic Withdrawal Groups (N=29)	Matched Neuroleptic Maintenance Groups (N=29)
	Unweighted Mean (SD) [Sample Size*]			
Sample size, No. of subjects†	47.6 (70.6) [N=66]	48.5 (87.4) [N=37]	46.4 (41.8) [N=29]	42.2 (51.5) [N=29]
Male, %	69.1 (29.7) [n=43]	69.7 (31.0) [n=25]	68.2 (28.6) [n=18]	69.8 (27.0) [n=18]
Average‡ age, y	40.0 (9.0) [n=62]	39.5 (8.2) [n=35]	40.4 (10.4) [n=25]	40.8 (10.4) [n=25]
Average‡ duration of illness, y	14.9 (7.5) [n=25]	16.0 (7.6) [n=19]	11.4 (7.1) [n=6]	10.0 (5.3) [n=6]
Average‡ length of hospitalization, y	8.7 (5.9) [n=31]	8.1 (5.2) [n=18]	9.5 (6.9) [n=13]	9.7 (7.4) [n=13]
% Specifying diagnostic criteria§	34 (52) [n=65]	25 (68) [N=37]	9 (35) [n=26]	9 (35) [n=26]
Study design, No. (%)§				
Open	18 (28) [n=65]	14 (39) [n=36]	4 (14) [N=29]	4 (14) [N=29]
Single blind	9 (14) [n=65]	8 (22) [n=36]	1 (3) [N=29]	1 (3) [N=29]
Double blind	38 (58) [n=65]	14 (39) [n=36]	24 (83) [N=29]	24 (83) [N=29]
Average‡ baseline neuroleptic dose, mg/d (chlorpromazine equivalent)	630.0 (453.7) [n=32]	713.7 (506.4) [n=22]	445.8 (236.4) [n=10]	439.2 (234.7) [n=10]
Average‡ length of taper, d	7.5 (14.0) [n=60]	7.2 (13.3) [n=34]	7.9 (15.1) [n=26]	NA‖
Patients receiving anticholinergic therapy, %	75.0 [n=20]	75.0 [n=16]	75.0 [n=4]	75.0 [n=4]
Average‡ length of follow-up, mo	6.3 (6.3) [N=66]	3.7 (4.2) [N=37]	9.7 (6.9) [N=29]	9.7 (6.9) [N=29]
Definition of relapse, No. (%)§				
No definition	22 (3.3)	15 (41)	5 (17)	5 (17)
Returned to neuroleptic medication	11 (17)	4 (11)	4 (14)	4 (14)
Other definition	33 (50) [N=66]	18 (49) [N=37]	20 (69) [N=29]	20 (69) [N=29]
Relapse rate, ¶	46.6 (23.5) [n=48]	36.7 (25.9) [n=19]	53.2 (19.6) [N=29]	15.6 (12.4) [N=29]

*In each cell, the sample size is the number of studies that provided the specific information. For the two matched groups, both groups needed to have the data for the variable to be included in the summary statistic for that variable.

†The matched neuroleptic withdrawal groups had a significantly larger log-transformed sample size than the matched neuroleptic maintenance groups ($t=2.95$, $df=28$, $P<.01$), but the difference was not significant after the Bonferroni correction.

§These values are numbers and percentages of studies rather than unweighted means and SDs.

‡Average indicates study mean or midpoint of range.

‖NA indicates not applicable.

¶The matched neuroleptic withdrawal groups had a significantly larger relapse rate ($t=10.64$, $df=28$, $P<.0001$) that was still significant after the Bonferroni correction.

teria for schizophrenia in earlier studies, and incomplete presentation of information. One particularly vexing problem relates to the variable definitions of *relapse;* better terms might be *symptom recurrence* or *exacerbation*. Moreover, not all the work undertaken has been published. Thus, there may be a bias; studies with negative results may not see print. Furthermore, in spite of our best efforts, we may not have accessed every available article on the subject of neuroleptic withdrawal. Another limitation is inherent in our attempt to infer relationships in individuals from the aggregate data provided by a literature review. Finally, it is conceivable that relapse rates in research settings may differ from those in "the real world" because of patient-related as well as methodological biases.

Nevertheless, we attempted to perform and present a search of the literature on neuroleptic withdrawal that was as extensive and complete as possible. Next, in an attempt to overcome the difficulties noted in some of the studies, we reanalyzed the data in different ways. Although only 29 of the 66 studies reviewed used neuroleptic maintenance (control) groups, the overall results of neuroleptic withdrawal in these 29 studies were generally similar to those in the total group of 66 studies, indicating generalizability of their findings.

Of all the variables examined, only the mean relapse rate was significantly different between the groups of patients withdrawn from neuroleptic therapy and those maintained on neuroleptic therapy. Groups of patients with schizophrenia withdrawn from neuroleptic therapy had a relapse rate more than three times higher than the rate of those maintained on neuroleptic therapy. On the other hand, approximately half of all the patients withdrawn from neuroleptic therapy remained stable without relapse over

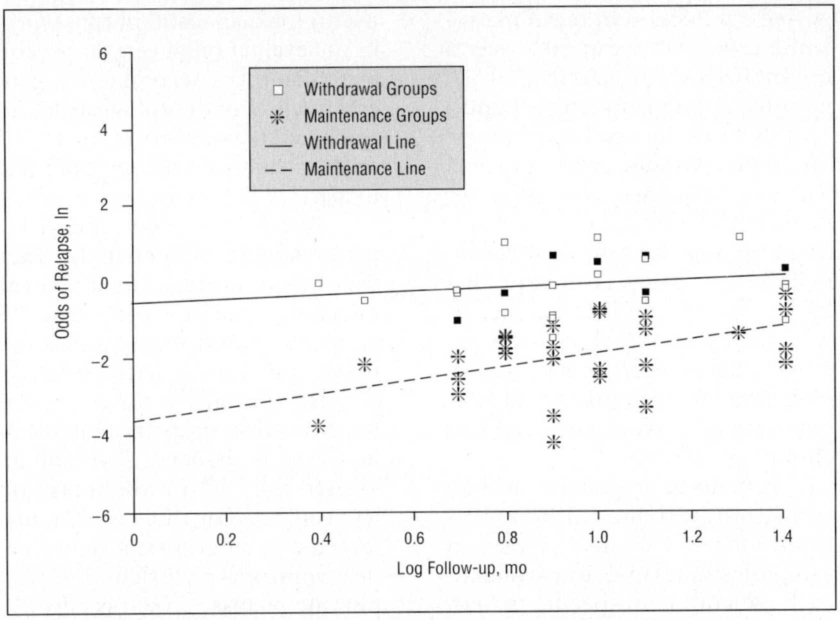

The natural logarithm of the relapse rate vs the logarithmic average length of follow-up in the matched withdrawal and maintenance groups (N=28).[38] A study of an outlier pair of matched withdrawal and maintenance groups was omitted. (See the text for details.)

average follow-up periods of 6.3 to 9.7 months, while, despite neuroleptic maintenance, 15.6% patients relapsed over an average follow-up period of 7.9 months. The rate of relapse was associated positively with the length of follow-up.

Individual studies have reported predictors of relapse such as younger age, earlier age of onset of illness, higher neuroleptic dose at baseline, and recent psychiatric hospitalization. In our aggregate data analysis, however, we did not find any specific predictors of relapse except for average length of follow-up. This may be caused in part by reduced sample sizes because of missing data as well as by the expected insensitivity resulting from the use of aggregate data; our analysis used summary measures from each study in lieu of the ranges of values within individual studies. Perhaps, however, there are few across-the-board predictors of schizophrenic relapse just as there are few consistent predictors of long-term prognosis of schizophrenia (except for chronicity).[96,97]

Patients who underwent decompensation after neuroleptic therapy was stopped were seen to recompensate quickly when treatment was restarted.[31,53,55,81] This suggests that even when patients experience psychotic symptoms after neuroleptic withdrawal, they are generally not subjected to any prolonged exacerbation if neuroleptic therapy is restarted soon.

Finally, concerning other adverse effects of neuroleptic withdrawal, some of the serious symptoms described in the case reports, such as hematemesis or neuroleptic malignant syndrome, were not common and might be associated only with abrupt neuroleptic withdrawal. Other side effects (eg, insomnia, vomiting) were usually mild and transient.

RESEARCH RECOMMENDATIONS

A proposed study of neuroleptic withdrawal should have clinically justifiable criteria for selection of patients; a proper consenting procedure; an adequate sample size based on power analysis; specific diagnostic criteria for schizophrenia, such as *DSM-IV*[98]; an appropriate comparison group maintained on neuroleptic therapy; quantitative double-blind assessments using standardized rating scales that have significant and high interrater reliability; neurochemical determinations of possible antecedents of relapse, such as changes in plasma homovanillic acid concentrations[72]; and suitable statistical analyses, such as survival analysis with covariates. A comprehensive baseline evaluation of patients is necessary for a better delineation of patients who can tolerate maintenance off neuroleptic therapy without relapsing. Certain measures should perhaps be assessed at regular intervals after baseline, eg, indicators of movement disorder. Neurological, neuropsychological, and brain imaging assessments have rarely been done in such studies and may be useful. For example, it is not known whether patients with neurological "soft" signs, cognitive impairment, and structural brain abnormalities on magnetic resonance imaging are more or less likely to relapse after neuroleptic withdrawal, although such patients are known to be less responsive to neuroleptic therapy.[99] Close monitoring of the patients is necessary throughout the study period to detect and treat any early unacceptable exacerbation or recurrence of psychotic symptoms to avoid a full-blown relapse. Different taper schedules (eg, acute vs gradual withdrawal of neuroleptic therapy) have not been systematically compared, except in isolated instances,[100] and this should be done. Special populations, such as first-break patients or the elderly, need to be studied from the viewpoint of the relative risks and benefits of neuroleptic withdrawal. Given that the risk of relapse is lower in the first few days or weeks after neuroleptic therapy is stopped, short-term withdrawal, such as that entailed in placebo-controlled studies of the acute efficacy of new antipsychotic drugs, would appear to be less hazardous. Whether still-persisting small amounts of neuroleptic agents from previous therapy delay relapse in early stages should also be tested.

CLINICAL RECOMMENDATIONS

It is possible to make divergent clinical recommendations based on our findings. On the one hand, it could be argued that neuroleptic withdrawal is extremely risky, with the chances of relapse more than three times greater than with neuroleptic maintenance. Psychotic relapse is associated with a possibility of patients harming themselves and/or others; it is certainly likely to disrupt the patient's and family's lives and may result in hospitalization, with the attendant psychosocial and financial costs. On the other hand, our results show that nearly half of the patients do not relapse when kept off neuroleptic therapy over a 10-month period. Maintaining medication would seem unnecessary, especially considering the risk of persistent TD. This is a clinical as well as a medicolegal dilemma. A physician may be held liable either for withdrawing neuroleptic therapy and "precipitating" a relapse or for maintaining neuroleptic therapy and "predisposing" to TD. The optimal solution in a substantial proportion of cases would probably be to slowly taper the neuroleptic therapy to the lowest dose that would control the symptoms of schizophrenia to a satisfactory degree. In some patients, the lowest dose may be zero—stopping neuroleptic therapy. Relative contraindications to attempting a complete stop in neuroleptic therapy in outpatients may include severe active psychopathologic symptoms; a history of relapse with dangerousness to self or others or requiring psychiatric hospitalization following neuroleptic withdrawal; or refusal by the patient, caregiver, or treating clinician to comply with the proposed medication withdrawal.

We believe that neuroleptic taper (dosage reduction) should be attempted very gradually to prevent unpleasant and even potentially dangerous withdrawal effects. A report by Green et al[100] demonstrated that slow neuroleptic withdrawal (over an 8-week period) was preferable to rapid withdrawal (over 2 weeks) because the rapid reduction group had a higher relapse rate (50%) than the slow reduction group (8%) over a follow-up period of 6 months. Recently, Smith[101] used a strategy of very slow reduction of dosage (by one fifth to one third of the current dose every 1 or 2 months if the patient's clinical condition did not worsen appreciably) in 16 chronically psychotic schizophrenic or schizoaffective patients who had been hospitalized continuously for a mean of 11.5 years. The author reported a reduction in mean neuroleptic dosage of about 60% over a mean follow-up period of 10 months, accompanied by a significant decrease in psychopathologic symptoms. In patients being treated with anticholinergic medications for neuroleptic-induced extrapyramidal symptoms, the withdrawal of anticholinergic drugs is an issue that has not been properly researched. It is probably preferable to stop administering these drugs at least a few days *after* neuroleptic therapy is withdrawn to avoid symptoms of cholinergic rebound.

Patients undergoing neuroleptic withdrawal should be monitored closely for early signs and symptoms of relapse. In particular, each patient's own specific pattern of relapse, ie, signs and symptoms that in the past heralded relapse, should be documented. If there is a clinically significant worsening of psychotic symptoms, the dosage may have to be increased until the patient's clinical condition is restabilized, and the value and strategy of subsequent taper will have to be reassessed. In the event of a relapse, patients may need to be hospitalized, and in general, steps should be taken to prevent harm to the patient or to others as a consequence of psychotic relapse.

The risk-benefit ratio of neuroleptic withdrawal vs maintenance should be assessed carefully in individual patients. Thus, a patient with a recurrent history of psychotic relapse on neuroleptic withdrawal (initiated by the physician or by the patient) is very likely to need continued neuroleptic treatment. In contrast, an elderly patient (who has a far greater risk of persistent TD than younger adults[11]) with new onset of a relatively mild psychotic episode and who has an adequate social network may be considered for neuroleptic taper after the acute symptoms have been controlled. Older patients with recently developed TD may deserve special consideration for taper, since studies suggest that the risk of persistence of dyskinesia with neuroleptic continuation is much higher in older patients than in younger patients.[102-104] Stopping neuroleptic therapy, or at least dosage reduction, may also be useful for diagnostic purposes, eg, in the evaluation of certain psychiatric disorders secondary to general medical or neurological conditions, such as delirium, or in the differentiation of agitation from akathisia.

We do not recommend repeated lengthy (several months at a time) drug holidays as a routine means of preventing persistent TD. Studies by us and others have shown that frequent and lengthy periods of stopped neuroleptic therapy either have no effect on persistent TD or may even be associated with an increased risk.[105,106] Furthermore, Jolley et al[28] and Carpenter et al[29] found targeted or intermittent neuroleptic treatment of early signs of schizophrenic relapse to be less effective than continuous neuroleptic therapy in preventing relapse.

There is a critical need for further research in this area, especially to identify patients who do not need long-term neuroleptic maintenance therapy and to optimize strategies for neuroleptic taper that minimize the danger of relapse. We should also intensify efforts to develop new antipsychotic agents that do not carry the risk of TD or other serious side effects.

Accepted for publication July 8, 1994.

This work was supported in part by the Department of Veterans Affairs and by grants MH45131, MH43693, and MH49671-01 from the National Institute of Mental Health, Rockville, Md.

The authors thank Anne Bailey for help with data analysis.

Reprint requests to Geriatric Psychiatry Clinical Research Center, San Diego VA Medical Center, 116A, 3350 La Jolla Village Dr, San Diego, CA 92161 (Dr Jeste).

REFERENCES

1. Baldessarini RJ, Cole JO, Davis JM, Gardos G, Preskorn SH, Tarsy D. *Tardive Dyskinesia: A Task Force Report of the American Psychiatric Association.* Washington, DC: American Psychiatric Association; 1980.
2. Davis JM, Baxter JT, Kane JM. Antipsychotic drugs. In: Kaplan HI, Sadock BJ, eds. *Comprehensive Textbook of Psychiatry.* 5th ed. Baltimore, Md: Williams & Wilkins; 1989;2:1591-1626.
3. Marder SR, Wirshing WC, Van Putten T. Drug

treatment of schizophrenia: overview of recent research. *Schizophr Res.* 1991;4:81-90.

4. Wyatt RJ. Neuroleptics and the natural course of schizophrenia. *Schizophr Bull.* 1991;17:325-351.
5. Schooler NR. Maintenance medication for schizophrenia: strategies for dose reduction. *Schizophr Bull.* 1991;17:311-324.
6. Jeste DV, Wyatt RJ. *Understanding and Treating Tardive Dyskinesia.* New York, NY: Guilford Press Inc; 1982.
7. Kane JM, Jeste DV, Barnes TRE, Casey DE, Cole JO, Davis JM, Gualtieri CT, Schooler NR, Sprague RL, Wettstein RM. *Tardive Dyskinesia: A Task Force Report of the American Psychiatric Association.* Washington, DC: American Psychiatric Association; 1992.
8. Casey DE. Neuroleptic drug-induced extrapyramidal syndromes and tardive dyskinesia. *Schizophr Res.* 1991;4:109-120.
9. Kane JM, Woerner M, Lieberman J. Tardive dyskinesia: prevalence, incidence, and risk factors. *J Clin Psychopharmacol.* 1988;8:52S-56S.
10. Saltz BL, Woerner MG, Kane JM, Lieberman JA, Alvir JMJ, Bergmann KJ, Blank K, Koblenzer J, Kahaner K. Prospective study of tardive dyskinesia incidence in the elderly. *JAMA.* 1991;266:2402-2406.
11. Jeste DV, Caligiuri MP. Tardive dyskinesia. *Schizophr Bull.* 1993;19:303-315.
12. Davis JM. Overview: maintenance therapy in psychiatry, I: schizophrenia. *Am J Psychiatry.* 1975;132:1237-1245.
13. Spivak B, Weizman A, Wolovick L, Hermesh H, Tyano S, Munitz H. Neuroleptic malignant syndrome during abrupt reduction of neuroleptic treatment. *Acta Psychiatr Scand.* 1990;81:168-169.
14. Melamed E, Achiron A, Shapira A, Davidovicz S. Persistent and progressive parkinsonism after discontinuation of chronic neuroleptic therapy: an additional tardive syndrome? *Clin Neuropharmacol.* 1991;14:273-278.
15. Kushnir SL. Hematemesis following discontinuation of psychoactive drugs in geriatric patients. *J Am Geriatr Soc.* 1988;36:1045-1046.
16. Calev A, Nigal D, Kugelmass S, Weller M, Lerer B. Performance of long-stay schizophrenics after drug withdrawal on matched immediate and delayed recall tasks. *Br J Clin Psychol.* 1991;30:241-245.
17. Freeman LS, Alson E. Prolonged withdrawal of chlorpromazine in chronic patients. *Dis Nerv Syst.* 1962;23:522-525.
18. Hughes JS, Little JC. An appraisal of the continuing practice of prescribing tranquillizing drugs for long-stay psychiatric patients. *Br J Psychiatry.* 1967;113:867-873.
19. Rassidakis NC, Kondakis X, Papanastassiou A, Michalakeas A. Withdrawal of antipsychotic drugs from chronic psychiatric patients. *Bull Menninger Clin.* 1970;34:216-222.
20. Kirch D, Hattox S, Bell J, Murphy R, Freedman R. Plasma homovanillic acid and tardive dyskinesia during neuroleptic maintenance and withdrawal. *Psychiatry Res.* 1983;9:217-223.
21. Baron JC, Martinot JL, Cambon H, Boulenger JP, Poirier MF, Caillard V, Blin J, Huret JD, Loc'h C, Maziere B. Striatal dopamine receptor occupancy during and following withdrawal from neuroleptic treatment: correlative evaluation by positron emission tomography and plasma prolactin levels. *Psychopharmacology.* 1989;99:463-472.
22. Glazer WM, Morgenstern H, Schooler N, Berkman CS, Moore DC. Predictors of improvement in tardive dyskinesia following discontinuation of neuroleptic medication. *Br J Psychiatry.* 1990;157:585-592.
23. Kane JM, Rifkin A, Quitkin F, Nayak D, Ramos-Lorenzi J. Fluphenazine vs placebo in patients with remitted, acute first-episode schizophrenia. *Arch Gen Psychiatry.* 1982;39:70-73.
24. Morton MR. A study of the withdrawal of chlorpromazine or trifluoperazine in chronic schizophrenia. *Am J Psychiatry.* 1968;124:1585-1588.
25. Pietzcker A, Gaebel W, Kopcke W, Linden M, Muller P, Muller-Spohn F, Schussler G, Tegeler J. A German multi-center study on the neuroleptic long-term therapy of schizophrenic patients: preliminary report. *Pharmacopsychiatry.* 1986;19:161-166.
26. Andrews P, Hall JN, Snaith RP. A controlled trial of phenothiazine withdrawal in chronic schizophrenic patients. *Br J Psychiatry.* 1976;128:451-455.
27. Blackburn HL, Allen JL. Behavioral effects of interrupting and resuming tranquilizing medication among schizophrenics. *J Nerv Ment Dis.* 1961;133:303-308.
28. Jolley AG, Hirsch SR, McRink A, Manchanda R. Trial of brief intermittent neuroleptic prophylaxis for selected schizophrenic outpatients: clinical outcome at one year. *BMJ.* 1989;298:985-990.
29. Carpenter WT, Hanlon TE, Heinrichs DW, Summerfelt AT, Kirkpatrick B, Levine J, Buchanan RW. Continuous versus targeted medication in schizophrenic outpatients: outcome results. *Am J Psychiatry.* 1990;147:1138-1163.
30. Whittaker CB, Hoy RM. Withdrawal of perphenazine in chronic schizophrenia. *Br J Psychiatry.* 1963;109:422-427.
31. Ruskin PE, Nyman G. Discontinuation of neuroleptic medication in older, outpatient schizophrenics: a placebo-controlled, double-blind trial. *J Nerv Ment Dis.* 1991;179:212-214.
32. Caffey EM, Diamond LS, Frank TV, Grasberger JC, Herman L, Klett CJ, Rothstein C. Discontinuation or reduction of chemotherapy in chronic schizophrenics. *J Chronic Disord.* 1964;17:347-358.
33. Garfield SL, Gershon S, Sletten I, Neubauer H, Ferrel E. Withdrawal of ataractic medication in schizophrenic patients. *Dis Nerv Syst.* 1966;27:321-325.
34. Rifkin A, Quitkin F, Rabiner CJ, Klein DF. Fluphenazine decanoate, fluphenazine hydrochloride given orally, and placebo in remitted schizophrenics. *Arch Gen Psychiatry.* 1977;34:43-47.
35. Keck PE, Pope HG, Cohen BM, McElroy SL, Nierenber AA. Risk factors for neuroleptic malignant syndrome. *Arch Gen Psychiatry.* 1989;46:914-918.
36. Jeste DV, ed. *Neuropsychiatric Dementias: Current Perspectives.* Washington, DC: American Psychiatric Press; 1986.
37. Prien RF, Levine J, Cole JO. High dose trifluoperazine therapy in chronic schizophrenia. *Am J Psychiatry.* 1969;126:305-313.
38. Baro F, Brugmans J, Dom R, Lommel RV. Maintenance therapy of chronic psychotic patients with a weekly oral dose of R 16 341: a controlled double-blind study. *J Clin Pharmacol.* 1970;10:330-341.
39. Leff JP, Wing JK. Trial of maintenance therapy in schizophrenia. *BMJ.* 1971;3:559-604.
40. Hirsch R, Gaind R, Rohde PD, Stevens BC, Wing JK. Outpatient maintenance of chronic schizophrenic patients with long-acting fluphenazine: double-blind placebo trial. *BMJ.* 1973;1:633-637.
41. Hogarty GE, Goldberg SC. Drug and sociotherapy in the aftercare of schizophrenic patients. *Arch Gen Psychiatry.* 1973;28:54-64.
42. Levine J, Schooler NR, Severe J, Escobar J, Gelenberg A, Mandel M, Sovner R, Steinbook R. Discontinuation of oral and depot fluphenazine in schizophrenic patients after one year of continuous medication: a controlled study. *Adv Biochem Psychopharmacol.* 1980;24:483-493.
43. Crow TJ, MacMillan JF, Johnson AL, Johnstone EC. A randomised controlled trial of prophylactic neuroleptic treatment. *Br J Psychiatry.* 1986;148:120-127.
44. Jolley AG, Hirsch SR, Morrison E, McRink A, Wilson L. Trial of brief intermittent neuroleptic prophylaxis for selected schizophrenic outpatients: clinical and social outcome at two years. *BMJ.* 1990;301:837-842.
45. Herz MI, Glazer WM, Mostert MA, Sheard MA, Szymanski HV, Hafez H, Mirza M, Vana J. Intermittent vs maintenance medication in schizophrenia. *Arch Gen Psychiatry.* 1991;48:333-339.
46. Diamond LS, Marks JB. Discontinuance of tranquilizers among chronic schizophrenic patients receiving maintenance dosage. *J Nerv Ment Dis.* 1960;131:247-251.
47. Olson GW, Peterson DB. Intermittent chemotherapy for chronic psychiatric inpatients. *J Nerv Ment Dis.* 1962;134:145-149.
48. Johnson DAW, Pasterski G, Ludlow JM, Street K, Taylor RDW. The discontinuance of maintenance neuroleptic therapy in chronic schizophrenic patients: drug and social consequences. *Acta Psychiatr Scand.* 1983;67:339-352.
49. Branchey MH, Branchey LB, Richardson MA. Effects of neuroleptic adjustment on clinical condition and tardive dyskinesia in schizophrenic patients. *Am J Psychiatry.* 1981;138:608-612.
50. Hershon HI, Kennedy PF, McGuire RJ. Persistence of extra-pyramidal disorders and psychiatric relapse after withdrawal of long-term phenothiazine therapy. *Br J Psychiatry.* 1972;120:41-50.
51. Smith PJ, Choi SC. Simple tests to compare two dependent regression lines. *Technometrics.* 1982;24:123-126.
52. Cox DR. *The Analysis of Binary Data.* London, England: Chapman & Hall Ltd; 1970.
53. Good WW, Sterling M, Holtzman WH. Termination of chlorpromazine with schizophrenic patients. *Am J Psychiatry.* 1958;115:433-448.
54. Brooks GW. Withdrawal from neuroleptic drugs. *Am J Psychiatry.* 1959;115:931-932.
55. Rothstein C. An evaluation of the effects of discontinuation of chlorpromazine. *N Engl J Med.* 1960;262:67-69.
56. Judah LN, Josephs ZM, Murphree OD. Results of simultaneous abrupt withdrawal of ataraxics in 500 chronic psychotic patients. *Am J Psychiatry.* 1961;118:156-158.
57. Gross M, Reeves WP. Relapses after withdrawal of ataractic drugs: an interim report. In: Greenblatt M, ed. *Mental Patients in Transition.* Springfield, Ill: Charles C Thomas Publisher; 1961:313-321.
58. Marjerrison G, Irvine D, Stewart CN, Williams R, Matheu H, Demay M. Withdrawal of long-

term phenothiazines from chronically hospitalized psychiatric patients. *Can Psychiatr Assoc J.* 1964;9:290-298.

59. Melnyk WT, Worthington AG, Laverty SG. Abrupt withdrawal of chlorpromazine and thioridazine from schizophrenic patients. *Can Psychiatr Assoc J.* 1966;11:410-412.
60. Prien RF, Cole JO, Belkin NF. Relapse in chronic schizophrenics following abrupt withdrawal of tranquillizing medication. *Br J Psychiatry.* 1968; 115:679-686.
61. Lacoursiere RB, Spohn HE, Thompson K. Medical effects of abrupt neuroleptic withdrawal. *Compr Psychiatry.* 1976;17:285-294.
62. Zander KJ, Fischer B, Zimmer R, Ackenheil M. Long-term neuroleptic treatment of chronic schizophrenic patients: clinical and biochemical effects of withdrawal. *Psychopharmacology.* 1981;73:43-47.
63. Brown WA, Laughren T. Low serum prolactin and early relapse following neuroleptic withdrawal. *Am J Psychiatry.* 1981;138:237-239.
64. Herz MI, Szymanski HV, Simon JC. Intermittent medication for stable schizophrenic outpatients: an alternative to maintenance medication. *Am J Psychiatry.* 1982;139:918-922.
65. Gleser GC, Gottschalk LA, Stone WN, Cleghorn J. Changes in the severity of social alienation-personal disorganization in chronic schizophrenic patients: psychometric and psychopharmacological factors: phenothiazine withdrawal in chronic schizophrenics. *Compr Psychiatry.* 1970;11:123-140.
66. Naber D, Albus M, Burke H, Muller-Spahn F, Munch U, Reinertshofer T, Wissmann J, Ackenheil M. Neuroleptic withdrawal in chronic schizophrenia: CT and endocrine variables relating to psychopathology. *Psychiatry Res.* 1985; 16:207-219.
67. Pickar D, Labarca R, Doran AR, Wolkowitz OM, Roy A, Breier A, Linnoila M, Paul SM. Longitudinal measurement of plasma homovanillic acid levels in schizophrenic patients. *Arch Gen Psychiatry.* 1986;43:669-676.
68. Lieberman JA, Kane JM, Sarantakos S, Gadaleta D, Woerner M, Alvir J, Ramos-Lorenzi J. Prediction of relapse in schizophrenia. *Arch Gen Psychiatry.* 1987;44:597-603.
69. Dufresne RL, Wagner RL. Antipsychotic-withdrawal akathisia versus antipsychotic-induced akathisia: further evidence for the existence of tardive akathisia. *J Clin Psychiatry.* 1988;49:435-438.
70. Kirch DG, Jaskiw G, Linnoila M, Weinberger DR, Wyatt RJ. Plasma amine metabolites before and after withdrawal from neuroleptic treatment in chronic schizophrenic inpatients. *Psychiatry Res.* 1988;25:233-242.
71. Kuhs H, Eikelmann B. Suspension of neuroleptic therapy in acute schizophrenia. *Pharmacopsychiatry.* 1988;21:197-202.
72. Glazer WM, Bowers MB, Charney DS, Heninger GR. The effect of neuroleptic discontinuation on psychopathology, involuntary movements, and biochemical measures in patients with persistent tardive dyskinesia. *Biol Psychiatry.* 1989; 26:224-233.
73. Thaker GK, Wagman AM, Kirkpatrick B, Tamminga CA. Alterations in sleep polygraphy after neuroleptic withdrawal: a putative supersensitive dopaminergic mechanism. *Biol Psychiatry.* 1989;25:75-86.
74. van Kammen DP, Peters J, van Kammen WB, Nugent A, Goetz KL, Yao J, Linnoila M. CSF norepinephrine in schizophrenia is elevated prior to relapse after haloperidol withdrawal. *Biol Psychiatry.* 1989;26:176-188.
75. Green AI, Faraone SV, Brown WA. Prolactin shifts after neuroleptic withdrawal. *Psychiatry Res.* 1990;32:213-219.
76. Khan RS, Amin F, Powchik P, Knott P, Goldstein M, Apter S, Kerman B, Jaff S, Davidson M. Increments in plasma homovanillic acid concentrations after neuroleptic discontinuation are associated with worsening of schizophrenic symptoms. *Prog Neuropsychopharmacol Biol Psychiatry.* 1990;14:879-884.
77. Singh H, Hunt JI, Vitiello B, Simpson GM. Neuroleptic withdrawal in patients meeting criteria for supersensitivity psychosis. *J Clin Psychiatry.* 1990;51:319-321.
78. Davidson M, Kahn RS, Powchik P, Warne P, Losonezy MF, Kaminsky R, Spter S, Jaff S, Davis KL. Changes in plasma homovanillic acid concentrations in schizophrenic patients following neuroleptic discontinuation. *Arch Gen Psychiatry.* 1991;48:73-76.
79. Harvey PD, Putnam KM, Davidson M, Kahn RS, Powchik P, McQueeney R, Keefe RSE, Davis KL. Brief neuroleptic discontinuation and clinical symptoms in kraepelinian and nonkraepelinian chronic schizophrenic patients. *Psychiatry Res.* 1991;38:285-292.
80. Wolf MA, Bailly L, Diener JM, Martinet JP, Peretti S, Garneau Y. Sevrage neuroleptique complet chez des patients schizophrènes présentant une symptomatologie intense et résistant au traitement. *Encephale.* 1991;17:255-261.
81. Glovinsky D, Kirch DG, Wyatt RJ. Early antipsychotic response to resumption of neuroleptics in drug-free chronic schizophrenic patients. *Biol Psychiatry.* 1992;31:968-970.
82. Neylan TC, van Kammen DP, Kelley ME, Peters JL. Sleep in schizophrenic patients on and off haloperidol therapy. *Arch Gen Psychiatry.* 1992;49:643-649.
83. Kirkpatrick B, Carpenter WT, Buchanan RW, Breier A, Tamminga CA. Plasma prolactin as a predictor of relapse in drug-free schizophrenic outpatients. *Biol Psychiatry.* 1992;32:1049-1054.
84. Jeste DV, Lacro JP, Gilbert PL, Kline J, Kline N. Treatment of late-life schizophrenia with neuroleptics. *Schizophr Bull.* 1993;19:817-830.
85. Arndt SE, Davis CS, Miller DD, Andreasen NC. Effect of antipsychotic withdrawl on extrapyramidal symptoms: statistical methods for analyzing single-sample repeated-measures data. *Neuropsychopharmacology.* 1993;8:67-75.
86. Lorr M. *Manual: Inpatient Multidimensional Psychiatric Scale (IMPS).* Washington, DC: Veterans Administration; 1962.
87. Krawiecka M, Goldberg D, Vaughan M. A standard psychiatric assessment scale for chronic psychiatric patients. *Acta Psychiatr Scand.* 1977; 55:299-308.
88. Overall JE, Gorham DR. The Brief Psychiatric Rating Scale. *Psychol Rep.* 1962;10:799-812.
89. Luchins DJ, Freed WJ, Wyatt RJ. The role of cholinergic supersensitivity in the medical symptoms associated with withdrawal of antipsychotic drugs. *Am J Psychiatry.* 1980;137:1395-1398.
90. Hunt JI, Singh H, Simpson GM. Neuroleptic-induced supersensitivity psychosis: retrospective study of schizophrenic inpatients. *J Clin Psychiatry.* 1988;49:258-261.
91. Orzak MH, Kornetsky C, Freeman H. The effects of daily administration of carphenazine on attention in the schizophrenic patient. *Psychopharmacologia.* 1967;11:31-38.
92. Spohn H, Lacoursiere R, Thompson K, Coyne L. Phenothiazine effects on psychological and psychophysiological dysfunction in chronic schizophrenia. *Arch Gen Psychiatry.* 1977;34: 633-644.
93. Simon SH. Effect of tranquilizers on the Trail Making Test with chronic schizophrenics. *J Consult Psychol.* 1967;31:322-323.
94. Depue RA, Dubicki MD, McCarthy T. Differential recovery of intellectual, associational, and psychophysiological functioning in withdrawn and active schizophrenics. *J Abnorm Psychol.* 1975;84:325-330.
95. Kirkpatrick B, Buchanan RW, Maeda K, Carpenter WT, Jauch D, Tamminga CA. Effect of neuroleptic withdrawal on plasma prolactin: a possible marker of receptor adaptation. *Biol Psychiatry.* 1989;26:131-138.
96. Yassa R, Uhr S, Jeste DV. Gender differences in chronic schizophrenia: need for further research. In: Light E, Lebowitz B, eds. *The Elderly With Chronic Mental Illness.* New York, NY: Springer-Verlag NY Inc; 1991:16-31.
97. McGlashan TH. A selective review of recent North American long-term follow-up studies of schizophrenia. *Schizophr Bull.* 1988;14:515-542.
98. American Psychiatric Association. *Diagnostic and Statistical Manual of Mental Disorders, Fourth Edition.* Washington, DC: American Psychiatric Association; 1994.
99. Jeste DV, Kleinman JE, Potkin SG, Luchins DJ, Weinberger DR. Ex uno multi: subtyping the schizophrenia syndrome. *Biol Psychiatry.* 1982; 17:199-222.
100. Green AI, Faraone SV, Brown WA, Guttierez J, Tsuang MT. Neuroleptic dose reduction studies: clinical and neuroendocrine effects. Presented at the 31st annual meeting of the American College of Neuropsychopharmacology; December 14-18, 1992; San Juan, Puerto Rico.
101. Smith RC. Lower-dose therapy with traditional neuroleptics in chronically hospitalized schizophrenic patients. *Arch Gen Psychiatry.* 1994; 51:427-429.
102. Lacro JP, Gilbert PL, Paulsen JS, Fell R, Bailey A, Juels C, Caligiuri M, McAdams LA, Harris MJ, Jeste DV. Course of new-onset tardive dyskinesia in older patients. *Psychopharmacol Bull.* In press.
103. Nair V. Course and prognosis of tardive dyskinesia: a meta-analysis. In: *APA Annual Meeting Syllabus and Proceedings Summary.* Washington, DC: American Psychiatric Press Inc; 1994: 135. Abstract.
104. Casey DE. The long-term natural course of tardive dyskinesia. In: *APA Annual Meeting Syllabus and Proceedings Summary.* Washington, DC: American Psychiatric Press Inc; 1993: 139. Abstract.
105. Jeste DV, Potkin SG, Sinha S, Feder SL, Wyatt RJ. Tardive dyskinesia: reversible and persistent. *Arch Gen Psychiatry.* 1979;36:585-590.
106. Goldman MB, Luchins DJ. Intermittent neuroleptic therapy and tardive dyskinesia: a literature review. *Hosp Community Psychiatry.* 1984; 35:1215-1219.

Neuroleptic Withdrawal in Schizophrenic Patients

In this issue of the Archives, Gilbert and her colleagues[1] provide a scholarly, comprehensive meta-analysis of research concerning the discontinuation of neuroleptic treatment. We find that additional information can be obtained from their analyses, which adds to an emerging impression that abrupt withdrawal of neuroleptic drugs and other maintenance medications is associated with a high risk for early recurrence of acute illness. Their analysis involves a total of nearly 5600 psychotic patient-subjects in 66 studies reported between 1958 and 1993, including 29 paired comparisons with cohorts continued on treatment with medication. The results strongly indicate that the discontinuation of maintenance neuroleptic medication carries a significant early risk for severe exacerbation of illness ("relapse"), averaging 53% within 9.7 months after discontinuation vs 15.6% with continued medication. These results accord closely with a similar analysis of this literature up to the early 1980s, in which the risk after stopping neuroleptic treatment or treatment with a placebo averaged 58.0% compared with 16.4% with continued treatment in a total of 28 paired cohorts.[2]

See also pages 173, 192, 197, 200, 203, 205, and 209

Detailed analysis and interpretation of this important body of research are made difficult by several factors, many of which are considered by Gilbert and colleagues.[1] They include a lack of diagnostic details in about one third of the studies; diverse criteria to define "relapse"; and inclusion of conditions that might not be diagnosed as schizophrenia by contemporary criteria, particularly in the 45% of studies reported before the 1980s. Other limitations are uncertain duration and dosing of the preceding treatment, unstated proximity of drug discontinuation to an acute episode of illness, the basis of selection for continued vs interrupted treatment, and the generally short duration of follow-up provided in most studies (averaging 9.7 months, but as short as 2 weeks in several reports). Furthermore, doses of neuroleptics typically were uncontrolled, often involved more than one agent, and sometimes mixed oral and injected long-acting depot preparations. The overall average mean (±SD) daily equivalent of 610±430 mg of oral chlorpromazine was used in 34 of the studies providing dosage data. Risks for the abrupt discontinuation of treatment with such doses may not be equivalent to the risks associated with gradual discontinuation of lower doses now often employed.[3] Such uncertainties severely limit the conclusions that can be extracted from this broad assortment of studies arising over virtually the entire five-decade lifetime of neuroleptic therapy.

FURTHER ANALYSIS OF DISCONTINUED NEUROLEPTIC TREATMENT

The studies cited by Gilbert and colleagues[1] provide relapse rates in 29 paired cohorts involving discontinued vs continued treatment that showed a threefold difference in mean (±SD) relapse rates (54.8%±12.3% vs 16.6%±12.1%; paired t=10.5, P<.0001). This difference is even greater if the mean ratio of relapse risk within pairs is considered (5.78±7.12, weighted by number of subjects per study; **Table**). However, the risk ranged from 0% to 100% among patients taken off neuroleptic treatment.[1] This high variance may reflect the heterogeneity of the clinical samples, variation in methods of diagnosis and assessment, or differences in the duration of follow-up. When relapse risk was compared for similar periods of follow-up (9 to 12 months), there was again a threefold difference in risk (54.1%±18.6% vs 18.3%±13.1%; 19 df; t=5.2, P<.001). There was no apparent change in relapse risk or its variance across the years, as might reflect recent changes in diagnostic criteria (52.5%±22.4% [N=25; coefficient of variation (SD/mean)=42.7%] before 1980 vs 44.5%±20.8% [N=23; coefficient of variation=46.7%] in or since 1980).

An extraordinarily large (13-fold) excess of relapse risk arose within the first 3 months after discontinuing neuroleptic treatment (50% vs 3.8%). The cumulative relapse risk rose moderately for those continued on maintenance medication to an average of 28.5% by 2 years. In contrast, there was little additional gain of risk after the first 3 months after drug discontinuation, with a maximal risk of 54% to 62% by 12 months. The relative risk fell over time to less than twofold (Table). These findings indicate that risk was *nonlinearly* distributed over time and that much of the excess risk after stopping treatment arose early.

Data from studies of treatment discontinuation can be further characterized for risk over time by the application of survival analysis. We reported a preliminary survival analysis for discontinuing treatment with oral neuroleptic medication in comparison with interrupting lithium maintenance monotherapy in bipolar disorder,[4] and we recently extended this analy-

Cumulative Relapse Risk in Schizophrenia After Continued vs Discontinued Neuroleptic Treatment*

Time at Risk, mo	Continued Treatment	Discontinued Treatment	Ratio
0-3	3.8±2.7 (26)	49.5±1.2 (173)	12.9
3-6	17.4±4.0 (402)	55.8±7.4 (1254)	3.2
6.5-12	22.6±3.5 (450)	62.1±4.5 (639)	2.7
18-24	28.5±3.6 (247)	54.0±6.1 (281)	1.9

Data are given as relapse risk± SD (total number of subjects studied), weighted by the number of subjects per study based on data of Gilbert et al.[1] The overall weighted mean ratio of the within-study difference in relapse risk was 5.78± 7.12.

sis, comparing oral vs injected neuroleptic preparations.[5] We found that the mean (±SE) time to 50% risk for reccurrence of illness was 4.0±0.1 months after discontinuing oral neuroleptic treatment (N=984 cases)[5] compared with a value of approximately 3.0 months based on data provided by Gilbert et al[1] (Table; N=199). These times are remarkably similar to the value of 3.2±0.2 months found in patients with bipolar I disorder (N=101) after stopping lithium treatment.[4] In contrast, reaching 50% risk was significantly delayed after stopping treatment with long-acting injected neuroleptics (6.7±0.3 months; N=83).[5] At 3 months, the risk for relapse was 39% after stopping treatment with oral medication vs only 18% for depot neuroleptics.[5] The latter timing is consistent with observations indicating the requirement of 8 to 10 months to clear detectable plasma levels of the drug, and 6 to 7 months for elevated plasma prolactin levels to subside to normal values following discontinuation of long-term treatment with injections of fluphenazine decanoate or other depot agents.[6,7] Such washout times are substantially longer than those following discontinuation of oral neuroleptic treatment even after prolonged administration.[8] It is particularly interesting that relapse risk following the discontinuation of depot injections remained lower than that after stopping treatment with oral neuroleptics into the second year (60% to 65% vs 85% to 90%), suggesting that very slow elimination of medication may actually have prevented some of the risk of relapsing and not merely delayed it.[5]

SIGNIFICANCE OF NEUROLEPTIC WITHDRAWAL–ASSOCIATED PSYCHOTIC EXACERBATIONS

An interpretation conventionally ascribed to these and similar findings is that continued or maintained neuroleptic treatment is clinically superior to discontinued treatment in schizophrenia. While this conclusion is secure, it may be too limited, as the findings have implications for the design, conduct, and interpretation of experimental therapeutic trials as well as for clinical practice. Underlying most research on maintenance therapies is an implicit assumption of similarity of risk following interruption of treatment to that associated with no treatment. Such studies typically involve the treatment of acute illness, clinical stabilization, and later random assignment to interrupted vs continued treatment. However, findings with manic-depressive patients indicate that the state following the interruption of maintenance treatment may not be clinically or psychobiologically identical to that reflected in the natural history of the untreated illness.[4]

Meta-analyses involving bipolar disorders suggest that pharmacologic stress factors may operate following the interruption of maintenance psychopharmacologic treatment, particularly abrupt interruption.[4,5,9,10] That is, relapse risk and suicidal risk, at least temporarily, may be greater than would be predicted by the course of untreated manic-depressive illness.[4,9,11] It seems consistent with this proposal that 50% relapse risk in schizophrenia following the interruption of oral neuroleptic therapy came within the first 12 to 16 weeks[5] (Table). However, it is not easy to distinguish between a proposed iatrogenic-pharmacologic stress effect and the reemergence of symptoms of more-or-less chronic illness. The hypothesis that drug discontinuation–associated stress contributes to early relapse is particularly difficult to test in the complex disorders considered as "schizophrenia" in studies reported over the past five decades. The course of schizophrenia, even as diagnosed by contemporary criteria, usually involves fluctuation of symptom severity, not necessarily with discrete episodes of illness, and the natural history is poorly defined and probably variable and heterogeneous.[12-14] The lack of clear predictability and timing of discrete major exacerbations, as well as a lack of data on the course of illness in the same subjects before and after discontinuing neuroleptic treatment, limit the possibility of testing the hypothesis of treatment withdrawal–associated relapse risk in schizophrenia.

In contrast, the shortest time to a major recurrence in subjects with bipolar I disorder before starting lithium treatment averaged 11.6±2.9 months, while that following its discontinuation in the same persons averaged only 1.7±0.5 months, or nearly seven times sooner.[9] Additional evidence that pharmacologic withdrawal stress factors may occur in bipolar disorders is that gradual withdrawal carried much lower risk for early recurrence than did rapid interruption of lithium maintenance treatment.[10] Even abrupt reduction of the dose or blood levels of lithium or of imipramine in major mood disorders may carry an excess risk for early relapse.[4,15,16] For schizophrenia, the sustained reduction in relapse risk after the interruption of slowly eliminated injected vs oral neuroleptics[5] also suggests that the presence of a pharmacologic stressor was at work whose effect may be minimized by very slow removal of the drug. Additional suggestive evidence on this point is provided by Green and his colleagues (in a 1993 article[4] as well as an earlier written communication, December 1992), who found a much higher risk for exacerbation in a small group of chronically psychotic patients in the 6 months following a major dose reduction of oral neuroleptics (by an average of 85%) over 2 weeks vs 2 months (four of eight patients vs one of 13; Fisher's Exact Test $P=.045$).

Another important consideration is that the risk for treatment withdrawal–associated relapse evidently is not eliminated by prolonged periods of clinical stabilization in psychotic disorders. In studies of bipolar disorder, even subjects free of major episodes for several years continued to manifest a high risk for early relapse after the abrupt removal of lithium maintenance treatment.[4,9,10] In schizophrenia, too, there is evidence from a meta-analysis of a large series of research subjects for whom relapse risk within the first year after recovery from an index episode of psychosis (68%) was very similar to that found after a year of stabilization prior to the removal of antipsychotic maintenance treatment (65%).[17]

PREDICTIVE RISK FACTORS IN SUSCEPTIBILITY TO NEUROLEPTIC WITHDRAWAL

Gilbert and colleagues[1] explored several potential factors that may predict relapse risk after interrupting maintenance neuroleptic therapy and rejected most of these. On reanalysis, we found some evidence that the rate of discontinuing the neuroleptic drug may matter. Among 46 studies,[1] 33 involved abrupt discontinuation (less than 14 days, and usually 1 day) and 13 involved more gradual discontinuation (2 weeks to 2 months) or use of long-acting depot injections in many or all of the subjects. The mean daily dose of neuroleptic drug did not differ significantly by the rate of discontinuation (400 ± 165 vs 566 ± 334 mg chlorpromazine equivalents, or somewhat lower with rapid interruption). The proportion of patients relapsing per month was threefold greater after abrupt discontinuation of treatment ($14.5\%\pm11.7\%$ vs $5.31\%\pm2.92\%$; $F[1,44]=7.6$, $P=.008$). This finding is consistent with previous observations concerning abrupt vs gradual discontinuation of lithium treatment in bipolar I and II manic-depressive disorders.[10]

The San Diego group[1] found support in some studies for the hypothesis that the preceding dose of neuroleptic also may predict risk for exacerbation in schizophrenia after stopping treatment, and such a relationship was found earlier.[18] In studies involving mainly oral neuroleptic drugs with a defined chlorpromazine equivalent daily dose,[1] there was a weak relationship between higher doses (or log dose) and higher relapse risk ($N=22$; $r=.208$, $P=.35$). In studies involving relatively high (≥600 mg) vs low (<500 mg) daily chlorpromazine equivalent doses, there also was a weakly greater risk after stopping a higher-dose treatment ($49.8\%\pm21.4\%$ vs $38.4\%\pm22.2\%$; $F[1,16]=1.0$, $P=.34$). Finding any evidence of such a relationship is remarkable since dose was almost never controlled for in the studies reviewed, but assigned on a clinical basis. Because dosing may covary with illness severity, a relationship of risk and dose may not represent a pharmacologic stress factor, but may have clinical value for predicting risks of interrupting neuroleptic therapy. In addition to the rate of drug discontinuation and perhaps neuroleptic dose, other plausible risk factors may include interruption of treatment early in psychotic illnesses or in geriatric age groups, as well as a severe history of psychotic illness in individual patients.[1]

CONCLUSIONS

We propose that, in chronic idiopathic psychoses and other severe psychiatric disorders, the sudden removal of much or all of a maintenance psychopharmacologic treatment carries an excess risk for severe symptomatic exacerbation or relapse within several months.[1,4,19,20] The timing or degree of this risk may vary with the pharmacokinetic or physiologic half-life of the agents involved, which can be more prolonged, even with oral neuroleptics, than is predicted by their nominal plasma half-life.[8,21] An excess of relapse following rapid drug withdrawal may inflate drug vs nodrug comparisons, as can arise in controlled trials that involve the removal of ongoing treatment or use of a placebo for more than a few weeks. Moreover, the clinical risks for morbidity or even mortality involved might sometimes exceed those associated with the natural history of the untreated illness.[4,9,11] In short, discontinuing treatment may not be equivalent to not treating. If these impressions are valid, then caution is required in the design, management, and interpretation of maintenance studies in many disorders.[4] It seems reasonable to expect that *gradual* lowering of moderate but effective doses of antipsychotic agents should delay and may reduce the risk for symptomatic exacerbation, but this proposal requires experimental verification and optimization. In general, the full clinical and research implications of the hypothesized phenomenon of postneuroleptic withdrawal exacerbation in schizophrenia remain to be clarified. Further specification of the risks associated with the discontinuation of neuroleptic treatment should ideally include controlled and randomly assigned drug doses and rates of discontinuation so that scientifically and clinically sound research protocols can be devised and implemented.

Ross J. Baldessarini, MD
Adele C. Viguera, MD
Bipolar and Psychotic Disorders Program and Laboratories for Psychiatric Research
Mailman Research Center 316
McLean Hospital
115 Mill St
Belmont, MA 02178

Supported in part by grants MH-31154 and MH-47370 from the National Institute of Mental Health, Rockville, Md, and awards from the Bruce J. Anderson Foundation and Vivian M. Temte Psychiatric Research Fund.

Gianni L. Faedda, MD; David L. Garver, MD; Trisha Suppes, MD, PhD; Leonardo Tondo, MD; Daniel van Kammen, MD, PhD; Richard J. Wyatt, MD; and David M. Gardner provided valuable discussions.

Correspondence to Dr Baldessarini.

REFERENCES

1. Gilbert PL, Harris MJ, Jeste DV. Neuroleptic withdrawal in schizophrenic patients: a review of the literature. *Arch Gen Psychiatry.* 1995;52:173-188.
2. Baldessarini RJ. *Chemotherapy in Psychiatry: Principles and Practice.* Cambridge, Mass: Harvard University Press; 1985:14-92.
3. Baldessarini RJ, Cohen BM, Teicher MH. Significance of neuroleptic dose and plasma level in the pharmacological treatment of psychoses. *Arch Gen Psychiatry.* 1988;45:79-91.
4. Suppes T, Baldessarini RJ, Faedda GL, Tondo, L, Tohen M. Discontinuing maintenance treatment in bipolar manic-depression: risks and implications. *Harvard Rev Psychiatry.* 1993;1:131-144.
5. Viguera AC, Baldessarini RJ, van Kammen D, Suppes T. Clinical survival following discontinuation of maintenance treatment with oral or long-acting, injected neuroleptics or lithium. In: Proceedings of the Annual Meeting of the American Psychiatric Association; 1995; Miami, Fla. In press.
6. Wistedt B, Wiles D, Kolakowska T. Slow decline of plasma drug and prolactin levels after discontinuation of chronic treatment with depot neuroleptics. *Lancet.* 1981;1:1163.
7. Sampath G, Shah A, Krska J, Soni SD. Neuroleptic discontinuation in the very stable schizophrenic patient: relapse rates and serum neuroleptic levels. *Hum Psychopharmacol.* 1992;7:255-264.
8. Sramek J, Herrera J, Costa J, Heh C. Persistence of plasma neuroleptic levels after drug discontinuation. *J Clin Psychopharmacol.* 1987;7:436-437.
9. Suppes T, Baldessarini RJ, Faedda GL, Tohen M. Risk of recurrence following discontinuation of lithium treatment in bipolar disorder. *Arch Gen Psychiatry.* 1991;48:1082-1088.
10. Faedda GL, Tondo L, Baldessarini RJ, Suppes T, Tohen M. Outcome after rapid vs gradual discontinuation of lithium treatment in bipolar mood disorders. *Arch Gen Psychiatry.* 1993;50:448-455.
11. Tondo L, Baldessarini RJ, Silvetti F, Tohen M, Rudas N. Suicidal behavior in manic-depressive patients with and without lithium maintenance treatment. In: Proceedings of the International Aretaeus Association Symposium on Prophylaxis in Manic-Depressive Illness. December 1994; Rome, Italy. Abstract.
12. Fenton WS, McGlashan TH. Natural history of schizophrenia subtypes. *Arch Gen Psychiatry.* 1991;48:969-977.
13. Wyatt RJ. Neuroleptics and the natural course of schizophrenia. *Schizophr Bull.* 1992;17:325-351.
14. Ram R, Bromet EJ, Eaton WW, Pato C, Schwartz JE. The natural course of schizophrenia: a review of first admission studies. *Schizophr Bull.* 1992;18:185-207.
15. Rosenbaum JF, Sachs GS, Lafer B, Kane JM, Keller MB, Gelenberg AJ. High rates of relapse in bipolar patients abruptly changed from standard to low plasma lithium levels in a double-blind, controlled trial. In: Proceedings of the Annual Meeting of New Clinical Drug Evaluation Unit. Washington, DC: National Institute of Mental Health; 1992.
16. Frank E, Kupfer DJ, Perel JM, Cornes C, Mallinger AG, Thase ME, McEachran AB, Grochocinski VJ. Comparison of full-dose vs half-dose pharmacotherapy in the maintenance treatment of recurrent depression. *J Affect Disord.* 1993;27:139-145.
17. Hogarty GE. Depot neuroleptics: the relevance of psychosocial factors—a United States perspective. *J Clin Psychiatry.* 1984;45(suppl):36-42.
18. Prien RF, Cole JO, Belkin, NF. Relapse in chronic schizophrenics following abrupt withdrawal of tranquilizing medication. *Br J Psychiatry.* 1968;115:679-686.
19. Kupfer DJ, Frank E, Perel JM, Cornes C, Mallinger AG, Thase ME, McEachran AB, Grochocinski VJ. Five-year outcome for maintenance therapies in recurrent depression. *Arch Gen Psychiatry.* 1992;49:769-773.
20. Lader M. Benzodiazepines: a risk-benefit profile. *CNS Drugs.* 1994;1:377-387.
21. Cohen BM, Tsuneizumi T, Baldessarini RJ, Campbell A, Babb S. Differences between antipsychotic drugs in persistence of brain levels and behavioral effects. *Psychopharmacology.* 1992;108:338-344.

Why Neuroleptic Withdrawal in Schizophrenia?

In this issue of the Archives, the analysis of Gilbert and colleagues[1] of the extensive literature on neuroleptic withdrawal makes clear that all treatment approaches to schizophrenia have significant risk. Years of a narrow treatment focus on psychosis and rehospitalization (rather than broad psychopathologic and quality-of-life assessment), apprehension regarding litigation, and the false hope that increasing drug dose will increase efficacy have led to excessive medication for most patients despite adverse effects, high rates of noncompliance, and patient dissatisfaction. Dose-reduction strategies are feasible, advantageous, and effective for many patients[2] but do not necessarily require complete drug withdrawal. What, then, are the circumstances appropriate for neuroleptic drug withdrawal? Consider the following: (1) a clinically stable patient who refuses to comply with a continuous medication strategy; (2) emerging evidence of tardive dyskinesia, dystonia, neuroleptic malignant syndrome, water intoxication, or

See also pages 173, 189, 197, 200, 203, 205, and 209

severe cardiac effects; (3) a stable patient of advancing years with increased risk for adverse effects and decreased risk for psychosis; (4) a single-episode patient with lengthy stability who may not have a recurrent psychotic illness; (5) a new approach to drug treatment that requires a neuroleptic washout period for safety and/or clearer interpretation of treatment response; (6) pregnancy; and (7) clinical investigations requiring medication-free observation or placebo-controlled evaluation of an experimental treatment.

These considerations suggest that clinician-recommended drug withdrawal should be considered with some frequency. Gilbert et al provide extensive reassurance that this can be accomplished at modest risk. In clinical practice, risk can be further reduced. Patients can be selected who are at low risk for exacerbation and/or who are quickly responsive at treatment initiation. Clinicians can gradually decrease medication, avoiding full withdrawal in patients who become symptomatic. Clinicians can monitor the medication-free patient closely and engage the patient and others in the recognition of early warning signs of exacerbation, with a shared plan for implementing effective relapse prevention. High-risk patients with a history of abrupt and difficult-to-treat relapses can be excluded. Drug withdrawal is sometimes necessary in higher-risk circumstances based on patient refusal of medication or emerging side effects. In these cases, the same strategy for detecting early warning signs and initiating drug treatment is required. A collaborative approach between patient and clinician is far safer than unmonitored noncompliance. We do not deny that some patients are at more substantial risk during medication-free periods, but clinical considerations can minimize off-medication risk in the complex clinical context, where many aspects of treatment are imperfect and risk-benefit analysis must be specifically applicable to each situation.

Clinical investigators may also decrease risk by excluding very-high-risk subjects, by maintaining placebo or medication-free status for the minimum time required to answer study questions, and by establishing effective procedures for rapid intervention to minimize exacerbation. Research settings often enhance other aspects of clinical care and treatment to offset risks involved in drug withdrawal. That this is an effective strategy was borne out in a study at the Maryland Psychiatric Research Center, Baltimore, in which patients were safely withdrawn from medication[3] and randomly assigned to continuous drugs with standard care or to an experimental noncontinuous targeted drug approach. In this 2-year study, courses of illness, including rehospitalization rates, were similar for the two groups, suggesting that the enhanced care compensated for the increased risk of relapse associated with medication withdrawal.[4] This view was verified in a second, independent study that provided the enriched psychosocial clinical care and early-intervention program to a continuous medication group and thereby achieved superiority for relapse prevention compared with targeted medication.[5]

The issue of medication withdrawal is now in public debate. Wyatt[6] speculates that psychosis exacerbation causes structural damage to the brain. Katz,[7] who argues that physician-initiated medication withdrawal in schizophrenia is unethical, includes toxic effects in the brain in his rationale. However, Wyatt cites no evidence documenting a cause-and-effect relationship between time psychotic and any brain finding, and he notes the presence of brain structure abnormalities at the first episode. Nonetheless, he proposes that the more severe course associated with insidious onset and prolonged psychosis is caused by psychosis-induced toxic effects in the brain rather than representing the natural course of schizophrenia with a poor prognosis. In his review, particularly of contemporaneous controlled studies, he finds a complex situation in which some patients appear to do better under a strategy that limits neuroleptic treatment, and he finds that the overall course is not clearly different over the long term. Contrary to Wyatt's hypothesis, Curson et al[8] found no symptoms or social disadvantages at 7-year follow-up of patients originally randomly assigned to placebo (66% relapse rate) compared with fluphenazine decanoate (8% relapse rate).

Although adverse events, such as suicide, dissatisfied patients or relatives, loss of job, deteriorating course, and brain abnormalities, can all be observed during drug withdrawal, each of these is also commonly encountered in the clinical care of medicated patients! There are very cogent clinical reasons why symptom reduction and reduced rate of relapse are achieved with neuroleptic drug therapy in most patients most of the time, and the explanation need not be based on frightening speculations of brain tissue destruction. In an illness that tends toward chronicity, dysfunction, and recurrent symptom exacerbation during neuroleptic treatment, it is crucial to discern whether long-lasting adverse effects are associated with drug withdrawal. Gilbert and colleagues' report of rapid return to baseline in most cases is very reassuring in this regard, as is the extensive similarity of most measures over the long term in prospective studies that randomly assign patients to continuous vs noncontinuous medication. As with Wyatt's review, most of the data are derived from research studies conducted before rapid-intervention targeted drug treatment was documented as effective. Neuroleptic treatment is now ubiquitous in schizophrenia because the therapeutic gap between drug and nondrug treatment is wide and compelling. However, the gap between continuous medication and purposeful and careful noncontinuous drug treatment is more narrow, and there are advantages and disadvantages associated with each. The several circumstances in which patients may prudently experience a drug-withdrawal phase constitute a crucial component of clinical care and research, and the reassuring data reviewed by Gilbert and colleagues are welcome.

William T. Carpenter, Jr, MD
Carol A. Tamminga, MD
Maryland Psychiatric Research Center
PO Box 21247
Baltimore, MD 21228

REFERENCES

1. Gilbert PL, Harris MJ, McAdams LA, Jeste DV. Neuroleptic withdrawal in schizophrenic patients: a review of the literature. *Arch Gen Psychiatry.* 1995;52:173-188.
2. Kane JM, Marder SR. Psychopharmacologic treatment of schizophrenia. *Schizophr Bull.* 1993;19:287-302.
3. Heinrichs DW, Carpenter WT Jr. Experience with a drug-free month in schizophrenic outpatients. *Psychopharmacol Bull.* 1985;21:117-119.
4. Carpenter WT Jr, Heinrichs DW, Hanlon TE. A comparative trial of pharmacologic strategies in schizophrenia. *Am J Psychiatry.* 1987;144:1466-1470.
5. Carpenter WT Jr, Hanlon TE, Heinrichs DW, Summerfelt A, Kirkpatrick B, Levine J, Buchanan RW. Continuous versus targeted medication in schizophrenic outpatients: outcome results. *Am J Psychiatry.* 1990;147:1138-1148.
6. Wyatt RJ. Neuroleptics and the natural course of schizophrenia. *Schizophr Bull.* 1991;17:325-351.
7. Katz J. Human experimentation and human rights. *St Louis Univ Law J.* Fall 1993;38:7-54.
8. Curson DA, Hirsch SR, Platt SD, Bamber RW, Barnes TR. Does short-term placebo treatment of chronic schizophrenia produce long-term harm? *BMJ.* 1986;293:726-728.

Because a

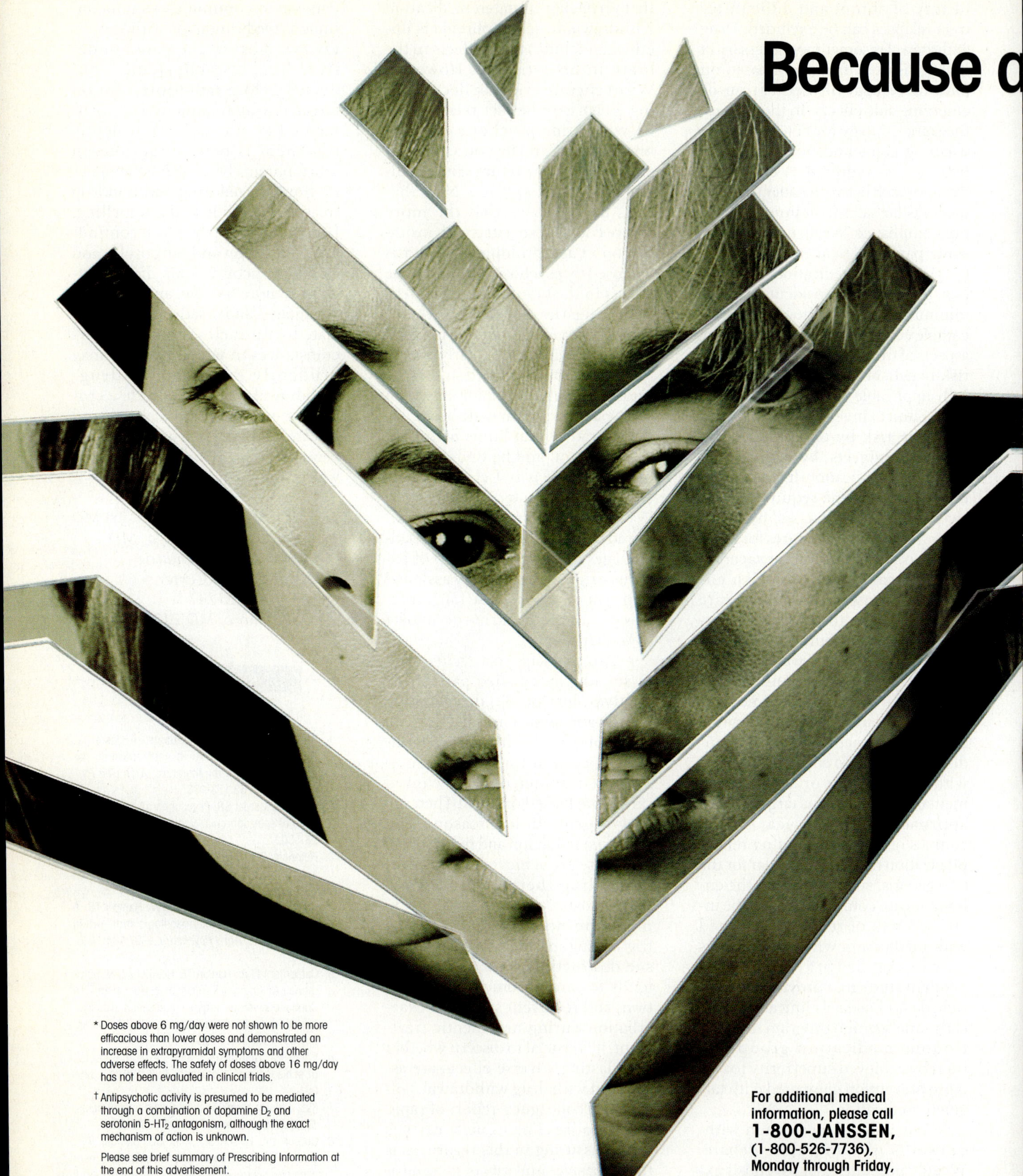

Long-term Treatment for Lifetime Disorders?

MAJOR psychiatric disorders characteristically are lifetime in duration. Some, such as mood or panic disorders, tend to be episodic and recurrent; others, exemplified best by schizophrenia, typically have more chronic, persistent courses punctuated with exacerbations. When confronted with long-term disorders, clinicians must consider a sequence of questions that pertain to long-term maintenance treatment: (1) What medications are available to help prevent relapse, and at what dosage must they be given to be efficacious? (2) What is the risk of relapse if long-term treatment is stopped, and how does this compare with the risk when treatment is sustained? (3) How severe are the risks or side effects associated with maintenance regimens? (4) Are there clinical or laboratory predictors that might foretell when a relapse might be expected so that risky treatments could be withheld until signs of impending relapse appear? (5) What are the safety, side-effect, and financial cost-benefit ratios associated with maintenance treatments, especially if administered over years or decades? (6) When do risks of stopping treatment outweigh those of continuing and vice versa?

See also pages 173, 189, 192, 200, 203, 205, and 209

Despite four decades of studying treatments known to be moderately efficacious in altering the acute symptoms of schizophrenia or mood disorders, most of these important questions about long-term maintenance treatment remain enigmatic. As a result, costs and consequences of repeated relapses in schizophrenia and mood disorders remain truly staggering, characterized by multiple episodes, chronicity, treatment refractoriness, repeated hospitalizations, job losses, financial deterioration, marital dysfunction, secondary medical complications, progressive morbidity, and even occasional death. Our knowledge gaps about long-term maintenance treatment may be the most important issue faced by psychiatry today.

When addressing long-term treatment of schizophrenia, we can learn from data already collected and from experience with other lifetime psychiatric syndromes, especially bipolar and unipolar mood disorders. Gilbert and associates,[1] in the accompanying article, have compiled a scholarly review of studies assessing the impact of neuroleptic withdrawal in patients with schizophrenia. Their report catalyzed us to rethink and perhaps challenge the wisdom of psychiatry's traditional maintenance treatment approach for schizophrenia and, for that matter, for recurrent mood disorders.

Gilbert et al identified 66 discrete studies of neuroleptic withdrawal; 29 included a control group of schizophrenic patients maintained on neuroleptic medication. When followed up for an average of 10 months (a relatively short duration in a lifetime disorder), the mean relapse rate in patients withdrawn from neuroleptics was 53% compared with 16% for those receiving maintenance neuroleptic treatment. The only consistent predictor of relapse was duration of follow-up. Other than relapse, adverse effects of neuroleptic withdrawal were found to be relatively minor. Gilbert and associates interpret these results as supporting the current clinical practice in the maintenance treatment of schizophrenia, ie, a slow taper of neuroleptic medication to the lowest effective dose.

We suggest that the detailed withdrawal data actually challenge the currently accepted emphasis on searching for how and when to withdraw or how to seek the *lowest* possible doses, particularly in the context of the availability of newer antipsychotic and antidepressant agents with more favorable safety and side-effect profiles. The remainder of this Commentary will reflect on this position, emphasizing patients with schizophrenia but comparing patients with mood disorders whenever parallels seem informative.

NEUROLEPTIC WITHDRAWAL, NEUROLEPTIC SIDE EFFECTS, AND RELAPSE PREVENTION IN SCHIZOPHRENIA

The essential finding of the review by Gilbert et al is fairly basic: there is a significantly greater risk of relapse in schizophrenic patients not receiving neuroleptic medication than in patients receiving neuroleptic medication. The authors summarize the adverse effects of continued neuroleptic use, particularly tardive dyskinesia, and suggest the need for a careful risk-benefit assessment of neuroleptic maintenance therapy vs withdrawal in each patient with schizophrenia. While there is no simple way to assess this equation, a psychotic relapse with increased paranoia, disorganization, and agitation is accompanied by major short-term negative consequences, especially impaired self-care, increased risk of aggressive behavior and harm to others, increased likelihood of hospitalization or legal confinement with attendant psychosocial and financial costs, increased risk of suicide, and severe disruption of the lives of the patient and family.

Repetitive psychotic relapses also are associated with major long-term negative consequences and progressive deterioration.[2-4] Gilbert and associates note that patients who de-compensate following neuroleptic withdrawal often recompensate quickly when treatment is restarted; this statement must be juxtaposed with the following conclusion of Wyatt[2] in his review of the impact of neuroleptic treatment on the natural course of schizophrenia: "There is evidence that stable schizophrenic patients whose neuroleptics are discontinued and have relapses may have a difficult time returning to their previous level of function." While data remain insufficient, there is a distinct probability that the greater the number of psychotic episodes in those with schizophrenia, the greater the risk of treatment refractoriness; ie, with each relapse, the illness becomes more difficult to treat. In this regard, parallels to unipolar and especially bipolar mood disorders might encourage caution. Recent studies have revealed that for perhaps the majority of patients with unipolar and bipolar mood disorders, the risk of additional episodes increases with each successive episode[5-7] and that some patients become refractory to treatment if maintenance therapy is stopped and a relapse occurs.[7,8] Various mechanisms have been postulated to explain this hypothesis, and all are fertile areas for future research.

SINCE REPEATED withdrawals of pharmacologic treatments *do* contribute to more relapses with the full range of accompanying costs and consequences and *might* contribute to the development of treatment nonresponsiveness, it is critical that clinicians seek to minimize relapse potential to the extent possible. Medication status is the best predictor of relapse in schizophrenia, with a threefold greater risk of relapse in neuroleptic-free patients than in neuroleptic-treated patients.

Gilbert and colleagues noted what may seem obvious, ie, some patients receiving neuroleptic treatment relapse while some without neuroleptic treatment do not. The authors chose to emphasize that "nearly half of the patients do not relapse when kept off neuroleptic therapy over a 10-month period. Maintaining medication would seem unnecessary, especially considering the risk of TD [tardive dyskinesia]." Conversely, we are impressed that more than half the neuroleptic-free patients with a chronic (generally lifelong) illness such as schizophrenia did relapse in just 10 months. The percentage of relapsers in the neuroleptic-free group increased to over 80% over a 2-year follow-up period. This contrasts with a 15% risk of relapse over 10 months and approximately 30% over a 2-year period in neuroleptic-treated patients. The data collected by the authors convincingly document the benefits of neuroleptic treatment in reducing the risk of relapse; this point cannot be overemphasized.

Considering these data and the painful consequences of continued clinical turmoil, it would seem contraindicated to ever stop treatment were it not for the fact that some deleterious side effects are associated with ongoing treatment. These include an increased risk of tardive dyskinesia, extrapyramidal symptoms, akathisia, sexual impairment, and other side effects. The presence of these negative consequences probably helps explain our propensities to stop treatment, administer intermittently, employ drug holidays, or implement a slow taper to the lowest effective dose. Since these approaches have been tried during the past decades, it should be noted that strategies of intermittent neuroleptic treatment (targeted treatment and drug holidays)[9-12] have been found to be inferior to continuous neuroleptic prophylaxis in the maintenance treatment of schizophrenia. When considering the current prevalent guideline for maintenance treatment in schizophrenia, ie, continuous treatment using the lowest effective dose, a parallel observation emerges: the lower the dose of maintenance medication, the higher the risk of relapse.[13,14] Efforts to lower maintenance doses to the lowest effective dose (by first finding the highest dose at which symptoms occur!) are almost certainly associated with greater risk of relapse, especially since there are no currently available approaches for determining beforehand what that dose is likely to be.

Are there alternative strategies for minimizing risks and side effects, such as tardive dyskinesia, other than engaging in the perilous courses of stopping or interrupting treatments or of progressively reducing treatment dosage while seeking the lowest effective dose? Data remain incomplete, but there is some basis for optimism: atypical antipsychotic agents, such as clozapine[15] and risperidone,[16] appear to have different and usually more favorable side-effect profiles. Clozapine, in studies to date, is associated with a much lower risk of tardive dyskinesia, the side effect of greatest concern, and there is a possibility that risperidone and the various atypical antipsychotic agents in development may share this property. Most of the studies reported by Gilbert et al were conducted before these newer neuroleptic agents were available. If newer antipsychotic agents have equal or enhanced benefit in reducing risk of relapse while lowering severe side effects, this would provide further momentum for abandoning the risky traditions of stopping treatment, administering it intermittently, or seeking the lowest effective dose.

A second strategy for minimizing unnecessary long-term antipsychotic use would be to use standardized criteria in the diagnosis of schizophrenia and to avoid diagnosing it loosely.

Another strategy for minimizing risk would be to avoid megadoses during the acute phase of treatment,[17,18] with no attempt to progressively taper this modest "acute treatment" dose downward in maintenance treatment.

A fourth strategy would be to develop predictors of relapse or nonrelapse so that we might know when treatments could be safely stopped. Both clinical[19,20] and laboratory[21-23] predictors of relapse in schizophrenia have been studied; sadly, no consistent predictors are identifiable, but we must not cease searching. However, it appears that clinical (severity of positive and negative symptoms)[20] or neurobiological (eg, abnormal neuroendocrine or sleep findings)[21,22] evidence of active disease is associated with an increased risk of relapse. A rather obvious maintenance treatment axiom appears to emerge: Ongoing pathophysiologic conditions mandate ongoing treatment. Most clinicians accept and adhere to this philosophy. However, the inverse proposition does not seem to be supportable: the resolution of symptoms or abnormal laboratory findings does not imply that neuroleptic treatment can be withdrawn with relative safety. However, this is the pattern often followed in clinical practice.

There are several parallels between schizophrenia and recurrent mood disorders. With regard to dosage, the pattern for years was to seek the lowest effective dose when treating mood disorders, whether using antidepressant agents or lithium. Assessments now reveal, however, that lower doses of antidepressant agents are less effective than standard doses in preventing relapses in recurrent depression,[24] that reduction of dosage—which would occur through seeking the "lowest effective dose"—is associated with considerably higher risks of relapse,[25] and that lower doses of lithium are less effective than standard doses in preventing relapses in those with bipolar disorder.[26] A story is developing: until new data emerge to show something different, the maintenance treatment dosage for patients with schizophrenia or bipolar or unipolar disorder should probably be the same as the acute treatment dosage if relapses are to be avoided. Another, parallel lesson may apply when considering side-effect profiles of antidepressant agents, since the newer agents make it easier for patients and clinicians to choose maintenance treatment. The introduction of the selective serotonin reuptake inhibitors (SSRIs) and venlafaxine, with their more favorable side-effect profiles but probably equal efficacy in relapse prevention in recurrent depression,[27,28] has helped shift the balance in favor of long-term antidepressant prophylaxis. A final parallel with mood disorders is that ongoing indications of pathophysiologic conditions in patients with mood disorders, such as persistent symptoms or laboratory abnormalities (eg, an abnormal dexamethasone suppression test result[29]), are associated with a higher risk of relapse, just as in schizophrenia, but the "absence" of symptoms does not indicate that medications can be safely withdrawn.

CONCLUSIONS

When dealing with severe lifetime disorders, the primary objective should be the prevention of relapses, chronicity, and deterioration. Our research priorities have not reflected this, perhaps because long-term maintenance studies are complicated, frustrating, expensive, relatively neglected by funding agencies, and hardly conducive to rapid academic advancement. While there is a clear need to alter our research priorities, we can take some consolation in the fact that after four decades, long-term databases have grown to meaningful sizes, enabling us to make some clinical judgments for both schizophrenia and mood disorders. The review by Gilbert and colleagues adds to this momentum.

While much research remains to be done, a relatively convincing case can be made for the following: (1) Maintenance treatments have been shown to help prevent relapse for schizophrenia. (2) There is a high risk of relapse if ongoing treatment is stopped, so high that relapse is essentially predictable for most patients within 2 years. (3) This risk is considerably lower if treatment is sustained, but to be effective, such treatment probably must be given at the same dosage that resolved the acute psychotic state, a pattern similar to that seen with mood disorders. (4) Since we cannot pinpoint which patients will not relapse despite being neuroleptic-free, the conventional practice of taking all patients off medications in an effort to see if they might belong to the small minority of schizophrenic patients (approximately 10%) who may not relapse despite being neuroleptic-free is highly questionable. (5) Risks and side effects have been identified with maintenance neuroleptic regimens; however, the most disturbing—tardive dyskinesia—may be less of a problem with the newer antipsychotic agents. (6) There are still no clinical or laboratory predictors that foretell when a relapse might be expected so that maintenance treatments can be withheld until signs of impending relapse appear. (7) Treatment probably should never be stopped if active clinical or laboratory signs of pathophysiologic conditions are still identifiable. (8) The absence of acute symptoms or laboratory tests does not indicate that withdrawal is safe. (9) There is reason to hope that newer medications, because of their more favorable side-effect profiles, may make it easier to adhere to a long-term or lifetime course of maintenance treatment. (10) While the recommendation to "taper the neuroleptic to the lowest effective dose" appears at first glance to be safe and reasonable, identifying this lowest effective dose for a given patient in the clinical setting is difficult and not achievable without risk.

As with recurrent mood disorders, perhaps the data compiled by Gilbert et al should prompt us to adopt a new standard of decision making for those with schizophrenia, ie, that treatment withdrawal or lowering of dosage needs to be justified rather than expected and should occur infrequently rather than regularly.

John F. Greden, MD
Rajiv Tandon, MD
Schizophrenia Program and Department of Psychiatry
University of Michigan Medical Center
Ann Arbor, MI 48109-0704

REFERENCES

1. Gilbert PL, Harris MJ, McAdams LA, Jeste DV. Neuroleptic withdrawal in schizophrenic patients: a review of the literature. *Arch Gen Psychiatry.* 1995;52:173-188.
2. Wyatt RJ. Neuroleptics and the natural course of schizophrenia. *Schizophr Bull.* 1991;17:325-351.
3. Crow TJ, Macmillan JF, Johnson AL, Johnstone EC. A randomized controlled trial of prophylactic neuroleptic treatment. *Br J Psychiatry.* 1986;148:120-127.
4. May PRA, Tuma AH, Dixon WJ. Schizophrenia: a follow-up study of results of five forms of treatment. *Arch Gen Psychiatry.* 1981;38:776-784.
5. NIMH/NIH Consensus Development Panel. Mood disorders: pharmacologic prevention of recurrences (NIMH/NIH consensus development conference statement). *Am J Psychiatry.* 1985;142:469-476.
6. Thase ME. Relapse and recurrence in unipolar major depression: short-term and long-term approaches. *J Clin Psychiatry.* 1990;51(suppl 6):51-57.
7. Post RM. Mechanisms underlying the evolution of affective disorders: implications for long-term treatment. In: Grunhaus L, Greden JF, eds. *Severe Depressive Disorders.* Washington, DC: American Psychiatric Press; 1994:23-65.
8. Post RM, Rubinow DR, Ballenger JC. Condition-

ing and sensitization in the longitudinal course of affective illness. *Br J Psychiatry.* 1986;149: 191-201.
9. Jolley AG, Hirsch SR, Morrison E, McRink A, Wilson L. Trial of brief intermittent prophylaxis for selected schizophrenic outpatients: clinical and social outcome at two years. *BMJ.* 1990;301:837-842.
10. Carpenter WT Jr, Hanlon TE, Heinrichs DW, Summerfelt A, Kirkpatrick B, Levine J, Buchanan RW. Continuous vs targeted medication in schizophrenic outpatients: outcome results. *Am J Psychiatry.* 1990;147:1138-1148.
11. Herz MI, Glazer WM, Mostert MA, Sheard MA, Szymanski HV, Hafez H, Mizra M, Vana J. Intermittent vs maintenance medication in schizophrenia: two-year results. *Am J Psychiatry.* 1991; 48:333-339.
12. Pietzcker A, Gaebel W, Kopcke W, Linden M, Muller P, Muller-Spahn F, Tegeler J. Intermittent versus maintenance neuroleptic long-term treatment in schizophrenia: 2-year results of a German multicenter study. *J Psychiatr Res.* 1993; 27:321-339.
13. Kane JM, Rifkin A, Woerner MG, Reardon GT, Sarantakos S, Schiebel D, Ramos-Lorenzi J. Low-dose neuroleptic treatment of outpatient schizophrenics. *Arch Gen Psychiatry.* 1983;40:893-896.
14. Johnson DAW, Ludlow JM, Street K, Taylor RDW. Double-blind comparison of half-dose and standard flupenthixol decanoate in the maintenance treatment of stabilized outpatients with schizophrenia. *Br J Psychiatry.* 1987;151:634-638.
15. Kane JM, Honigfeld G, Singer J, Meltzer HY. Clozapine for the treatment-resistant schizophrenic: a double-blind comparison with chlorpromazine. *Arch Gen Psychiatry.* 1988;45:789-796.
16. Marder SR, Meibach RC. Risperidone in the treatment of schizophrenia. *Am J Psychiatry.* 1994; 151:825-835.
17. Neborsky R, Janowsky D, Munson E, Depry D. Rapid treatment of acute psychotic symptoms with high and low dose haloperidol. *Arch Gen Psychiatry.* 1981;38:195-199.
18. Rifkin A, Doddi S, Karagi B, Borenstein M, Wachpress M. Dosage of haloperidol for schizophrenia. *Arch Gen Psychiatry.* 1991;48:166-170.
19. Breier A, Schreiber JL, Dyer J, Pickar D. National Institute of Mental Health longitudinal study of chronic schizophrenia: prognosis and predictors of outcome. *Arch Gen Psychiatry.* 1991;48: 239-246.
20. Ribeiro S, Ricoy R, Tandon R, Goodson J, Craig K, Mazarra C. Clinical predictors of one-year outcome in schizophrenia. *Psychopathology.* 1992; 25:331-334.
21. Tandon R, Mazzara C, DeQuardo J, Craig KA, Meador-Woodruff JH, Goldman R, Greden JF. Dexamethasone suppression test in schizophrenia: relationship to symptomatology, ventricular enlargement, and outcome. *Biol Psychiatry.* 1991;29:953-964.
22. Taylor S, Tandon R, Shipley JE, Eiser A, Goodson J. Sleep onset REM periods in schizophrenic patients. *Biol Psychiatry.* 1991;30:205-209.
23. Lieberman JA, Kane JM, Sarantakos S, Gadaleta D, Woerner M, Alvir J, Ramos-Lorenzi J. Prediction of relapse in schizophrenia. *Arch Gen Psychiatry.* 1987;44:597-603.
24. Frank E, Kupfer DJ, Perel JM, Cornes C, Jarrett DB, Mallinger AG, Thase ME, McEachran AB, Grochocinski VJ. Three-year outcomes for maintenance therapies in recurrent depression. *Arch Gen Psychiatry.* 1990;47:1093-1099.
25. Greden JF. Antidepressant maintenance medications: when to discontinue and how to stop? *J Clin Psychiatry.* 1993;54(suppl 8):39-45.
26. Gelenberg AJ, Kane JM, Keller MB, Lavori P, Rosenbaum JF, Cole K, Lavelle J. Comparison of standard and low serum levels of lithium for maintenance treatment of bipolar disorder. *N Engl J Med.* 1989;321:1489-1493.
27. Montgomery SA, Dufour H, Brion S, Gailledreau J, Laqueille X, Ferrey G, Moron P, Parant-Lucena N, Singer L, Danion JM, Beuzen JN, Pierredon MA. The prophylactic efficacy of fluoxetine in unipolar depression. *Br J Psychiatry.* 1988; 153(suppl 3):69-76.
28. Doogan DP, Caillard V. Sertraline in the prevention of depression. *Br J Psychiatry.* 1992;160:217-222.
29. Ribeiro SCM, Tandon R, Grunhaus L, Greden JF. Course of illness and biological measures in affective disorders: a critical review of the DST literature. *Am J Psychiatry.* 1993;150:1618-1629.

Neuroleptic Withdrawal in Schizophrenic Patients

An Idea Whose Time Has Come

GILBERT and colleagues[1] have provided a much needed review of the risk of relapse following neuroleptic withdrawal compared with neuroleptic maintenance in patients with schizophrenia. They also have provided some sensible recommendations for clinicians and guidelines for further research concerning neuroleptic maintenance treatment vs withdrawal. This review comes at a time of increased public and professional concern about the ethics of research concerning neuroleptic withdrawal in schizophrenia, stimulated in part by national attention to complaints from the families of patients who participated in a neuroleptic withdrawal study at the University of California–Los Angeles. However, there is another issue that this review can provide the basis for further consideration of, ie, the desirability of indefinite maintenance treatment with neuroleptic drugs in patients with schizophrenia. This is the course recommended by Gilbert et al, albeit at the lowest possible dose to prevent relapse, as compared with the substitution of clozapine or risperidone, or, eventually, other novel antipsychotic drugs. To my surprise, I found no consideration of the latter issue at any point in the review. This possibility should not be ignored when making clinical and research recommendations about maintenance treatment, as happened here. A new era in the pharmacotherapy of schizophrenia began with the approval of these two novel antipsychotics, clozapine and risperidone, and the possible introduction of four others in the next 2 to 4 years: olanzapine; ICI 204,636; sertindole; and ziprasidone. Gilbert et al, in my view, at least should have considered whether the neuroleptics as a class should be withdrawn altogether from clinical use as maintenance treatment in schizophrenia in favor of the newer agents, much as the sulfonamides were withdrawn as treatment for bacterial infections after the development of penicillin, tetracycline, and others.

See also pages 173, 189, 192, 197, 203, 205, and 209

Before discussing the latter issue, comments on the methodology of the review by Gilbert et al that bear on how much can be learned from it are in order. The method of identifying the relevant literature and criteria for inclusion and rejection is clearly stated and is entirely reasonable. However, three decisions with regard to data analysis are questionable: (1) the decision to use classic methods of analyzing data from multiple studies rather than conduct a meta-analysis[2]; (2) the use of unweighted means and SDs of relapse rates, time to relapse, etc, across studies; and (3) the midpoint of the range for any variable for which means were not provided. A meta-analysis would have dealt with the last two problems by providing a means of adjusting for sample size and the rigorous criteria for inclusion. Weighting based on sample size provides a more reliable estimate of the effect of neuroleptic withdrawal vs continued maintenance and permits more appropriate testing of the influence of factors such as age and gender than that which was done here by multiple regression and unweighted measures. The conclusion that age, gender, duration of illness, or neuroleptic dose do not predict relapse when all available data are combined, based on no weighting of studies, may not be valid. Gilbert et al also might have considered factors such as psychosocial treatment, community support, expressed emotion, and type and severity of symptoms while taking medication (to be discussed below) as potential influences on relapse rates. The interval between the last relapse and the beginning withdrawal also would influence the rate and timing of subsequent relapse and this should have been considered. Finally, the rate of relapse was presented only as a function of the log of the duration of the follow-up period. Since duration of withdrawal clearly influenced the proportion of relapsed cases, it would have been a real service to clinicians to also provide the rate as a function of time, without log transformation.

As just mentioned, a key factor influencing relapse rate during maintenance treatment or withdrawal that would have been useful to examine is neuroleptic resistance vs neuroleptic responsivity, a distinction that has become more important because of the availability of clozapine. Differential relapse rates during withdrawal are to be expected in these two groups. Patients who show moderate to severe positive symptoms despite adequate doses of neuroleptics are, after withdrawal, likely to show smaller percentage changes in psychopathologic symptoms than those who have minimal psychopathologic symptoms while taking typical neuroleptic drugs. However, the time course of change could be more rapid in the neuroleptic-resistant patients and severity might be worse. The effect of increased symptoms in both groups is likely to be different and so should be considered separately.

Despite these caveats, it appears that Gilbert et al have provided a reasonable ballpark estimate of the probability of relapse over a 0.5- to 24- month period in an unselected population of patients with schizophrenia. Their most important finding is that the mean relapse rates for the withdrawal and maintenance groups were 51.5% and 16.2%, respectively (P=.0001), over a mean (±SD) follow-up of 9.7±6.9 months (median, 6 months). These figures can provide a meaningful basis for clinical decisions, current policy, and formulating future research regarding neuroleptic maintenance. They also provide benchmarks for evaluating the results of maintenance treatment and withdrawal from the novel antipsychotic drugs that are being introduced into the mainstream of treatment.

The authors note as problems with indefinite neuroleptic maintenance treatment that 16% of patients will relapse despite continued treatment with these drugs and that 4% to 5% per year in the younger group will develop tardive dyskinesia. The rate may be five times higher in older patients. One can also add the limited ability of neuroleptics to ameliorate the cognitive deficits in schizophrenia, the adverse influence of extrapyramidal side effects on volitional behavior, and the generally poor quality of life and social function that is the fate of most patients with schizophrenia as reasons for considering withdrawal of neuroleptic treatment rather than automatically assuming they are desirable. Their ability to cause anhedonia[3] and so-called secondary negative symptoms[4] are also reasons for considering withdrawal.[3,5] These disadvantages of current treatment together with the fact that 56% of schizophrenic patients did not relapse in a 9-month follow-up further make the case for more frequent attempts at withdrawal of neuroleptic drugs with maintenance of active psychosocial support and efforts to improve the early detection of impending relapse, by both clinical and laboratory means, in selected patients. As Gilbert et al note, this view, if it were implemented, should take into account the particular history of each patient with regard to prior withdrawal.

Clearly, patients who need drug treatment to prevent relapse in weeks or several months should receive some drug treatment. However, the alternative to maintenance treatment with neuroleptics is no longer just no drug treatment. Maintenance treatment with atypical antipsychotic drugs is a real alternative. The possibility that the time has come, or is near at hand, for neuroleptics as a class to be withdrawn entirely in all patients with schizophrenia because of their risks and limited benefits compared with other therapies now available must be given serious consideration. Specifically, clinicians should be asking themselves whether patients with schizophrenia should remain on treatment with typical neuroleptics or whether they should be treated with clozapine or risperidone, both of which have been shown to be more effective and to have fewer side effects in groups of schizophrenic patients than typical neuroleptics. Reliable data demonstrating these advantages are available for clozapine for both neuroleptic-resistant and -responsive patients,[6,7] and for risperidone for neuroleptic-responsive patients.[8,9] These advantages, at least for clozapine, include superior efficacy for disorganization, positive and negative symptoms,[10] improvement in cognitive function,[11] essentially complete freedom of risk of tardive dyskinesia[12] and very little extrapyramidal symptoms, no prolactin level elevations,[13] reduced risk of suicide,[14] decreased need for hospitalization,[15] and lower overall cost, if hospitalization had been required at least 15 to 30 days per year.[15] It is not yet clear how many of these advantages are shared by risperidone, olanzapine, and other novel drugs, but it is likely that many are. Of course, these drugs have their own risks, especially clozapine, and not all patients will actually have a better response to these drugs than they would to typical neuroleptics. It is not my intention to overvalue the benefits of clozapine and its successors as much as it is to make the point that satisfaction with and complacency about maintenance treatment with typical neuroleptics is usually unwarranted. As that view becomes more widespread, efforts to find alternatives to neuroleptic maintenance will increase and be accepted.

Future research on maintenance treatment, therefore, should include effectiveness studies of clozapine, risperidone, or other novel drugs vs low doses of neuroleptics, given orally or parenterally (long-acting forms). It is my prediction that some, if not all, of the atypical antipsychotic drugs will show better efficacy, fewer relapses, better compliance, and less tardive dyskinesia. A drug-free group should be included as well to provide an estimate of the effect of drug treatment per se in these studies. Substitution of clozapine, risperidone, and their congeners, if the advantages noted above are established, then would be the recommended approach to maintenance treatment. Development of a long-acting atypical drug for biweekly or monthly use would be particularly advantageous.

Finally, Gilbert et al correctly point out that neuroleptic withdrawal may be essential to permit biological and cognitive research in schizophrenia to go forward, independent of the influence of neuroleptics or other psychoactive drugs. Implicit in this view is the idea that drug-free research should be done in patients who have shown a wide range of psychopathology, from virtual remission to a florid level, although cooperation of the latter group will likely be quite limited. Some patients and families do appreciate the need for encouraging patient participation in this endeavor and will sometimes sanction it depending on their own view of the consequences of a relapse or slightly prolonged symptomatology. The evidence provided by this review that response to reinstitution of neuroleptics is usually robust and rapid (3 days to 3 weeks) should add to the likelihood that patients and families will consent to research-driven neuroleptic withdrawal. The delay in treatment of noncompliant and, thus, already neuroleptic-free, newly hospitalized schizophrenic patients who are experiencing an acute exacerbation as a means to assemble a group of drug-free patients for research is fading fast in this era of managed care with minimal lengths of stay and the decline of state- or Veterans Affairs–funded research units. Therefore, the antipsychotic withdrawal protocol may be the sole means possible for the study of drug-free schizophrenic patients. If neuroleptic withdrawal is the only means by which significant progress can be made in understanding this illness so that more effective treatments can be developed, few would argue against permitting voluntary withdrawal studies, but with due safeguards for informed consent and patient welfare, including close surveillance and a low threshold for restarting treatment. Withdrawal may be most ethical in patients who have little or no demonstrable response to neuroleptic drugs, ie, the type of patients who were included in the US Clozaril Multicenter Trial, but it is essential that the full range of patients with schizophrenia be permitted to participate in such research.

In conclusion, Gilbert et al have provided reliable estimates of the limited value of maintenance treatment with neuroleptics and the risks associated with its termination. They have shown that withdrawal will cause about 60% of patients to relapse in a 6- to 9-month period, but that response to their reinstitution is fairly rapid. I believe that the goal with regard to maintenance treatment with neuroleptic drugs should be ending it for most patients with schizophrenia, with the substitution of clozapine or risperidone. Further research on neuroleptic withdrawal should include atypical antipsychotic drugs as an alternative strategy for long-term maintenance treatment.

Herbert Y. Meltzer, MD
Laboratory of Biological Psychiatry
Case Western Reserve
University School of Medicine
Cleveland, Ohio

The research reported was supported in part by US Public Health Service (USPHS) grants MH 41684 and GCRC MO1RR00080 and the National Alliance for Research on Schizophrenia and Depression as well as grants from the Elisabeth Severance Prentiss and John Pascal Sawyer Foundations and Stanley Foundation. Dr Meltzer is the recipient of a USPHS Research Career Scientist Award MH 47808.

The secretarial assistance of Lee Mason is greatly appreciated.

Reprint requests to Department of Psychiatry, University Hospitals of Cleveland, 2040 University Hospital Dr, Cleveland, OH 44106 (Dr Meltzer).

REFERENCES

1. Gilbert PL, Harris MJ, McAdams LA, Jeste DV. Neuroleptic withdrawal in schizophrenic patients: a review of the literature. *Arch Gen Psychiatry.* 1995;52:173-188.
2. Hedges LV, Olkin I. *Statistical Methods for Meta-Analysis.* San Diego, Calif: Academic Press Inc; 1985.
3. Elomaa E. Long-term 'treatment of schizophrenics with typical neuroleptics': a crime against humanity. *Med Hypotheses.* 1993;41:434.
4. Carpenter WT, Heinrichs DW, Alphs LD. Treatment of negative symptoms. *Schizophr Bull.* 1985; 11:440-452.
5. Carpenter WT Jr, Stephens JH, Rey AC, Hanlon TE, Heinrichs DW. Early intervention versus continuous pharmacotherapy of schizophrenia. *Psychopharmacol Bull.* 1982;18:21-23.
6. Kane J, Honigfeld G, Singer J, Meltzer HY, Clozaril Collaborative Study Group, 1988. Clozapine for the treatment-resistant schizophrenic: a double-blind comparison with chlorpromazine. *Arch Gen Psychiatry.* 1988;45:789-796.
7. Meltzer HY. Treatment of the neuroleptic nonresponsive schizophrenic patient. *Schizophr Bull.* 1992;18:515-542.
8. Meltzer HY. Dimensions of outcome with clozapine. *Br J Psychiatry.* 1992;160(suppl 17):46-53.
9. Chouinard G, Jones B, Remington G, Bloom D, Addington D, MacEwan GW, Labelle A, Beauclair L, Arnott W. A Canadian multicenter placebo-controlled study of risperidone and haloperidol in the treatment of chronic schizophrenic patients. *J Clin Psychopharmacol.* 1993;13:25-40.
10. Marder SR, Meibach RC. Risperidone in the treatment of schizophrenia. *Am J Psychiatry.* 1991; 151:825-835.
11. Hagger C, Buckley P, Kenny JT, Friedman L, Ubogy D, Meltzer HY. Improvement in cognitive functions and psychiatric symptoms in treatment-refractory schizophrenic patients receiving clozapine. *Biol Psychiatry.* 1993;34:702-712.
12. Lieberman JA, Johns C, Cooper T. Clozapine pharmacology and tardive dyskinesia. *Psychopharmacology.* 1989;99(suppl):S118-S121.
13. Meltzer HY, Goode DJ, Schyve PM, Young M, Fang VS. Effect of clozapine on human serum prolactin levels. *Am J Psychiatry.* 1979;136: 1550-1555.
14. Meltzer HY, Okayli G. The reduction of suicidality during clozapine treatment in neuroleptic-resistant schizophrenia: effect on risk-benefit considerations. *Am J Psychiatry.* In press.
15. Meltzer HY, Cola P, Way L, Thompson PA, Bastani B, Davies MA, Snitz B. Cost-effectiveness of clozapine in neuroleptic-resistant schizophrenia. *Am J Psychiatry.* 1993;150:1630-1638.

The Early Course of Schizophrenia and Long-term Maintenance Neuroleptic Therapy

IN THEIR computation of results across studies, Gilbert et al[1] find a mean relapse rate of 53% for patients with schizophrenia participating in neuroleptic withdrawal periods in 29 studies that included matched neuroleptic withdrawal and neuroleptic maintenance groups, with average follow-up of about 10 months. The relapse rate for the matched medication maintenance groups is significantly lower, although 16% of these patients relapsed within the average follow-up period of 10 months despite continuous medication. These studies have in

See also pages 173, 189, 192, 197, 200, 205, and 209

almost all cases involved patients who have been ill for many years, leaving unanswered many critical questions about continuous maintenance medication in the early course of a schizophrenic or schizophreniform illness. Because typical neuroleptic medications have substantial side effects, including the increasing possibility of persistent and potentially irreversible tardive dyskinesia with continued use, clinicians, patients, and their families often face very difficult decisions about long-term continuous maintenance medication in the initial years after onset of schizophrenia or schizophreniform disorder. These difficult decisions about risks vs benefits would be greatly aided by the development of reliable predictors that would identify patients, particularly in the years following initial diagnosis, who have relatively low short-term risk of relapse after stopping maintenance neuroleptic medication. As Gilbert et al point out, we currently lack reliable predictors that successfully generalize across studies to allow such identification.

DIVERSITY OF OUTCOME DEFINITIONS

Attempts to reach conclusions about the risks and benefits of medication-free periods for patients with schizophrenia are currently greatly hampered by the lack of a consistent definition of relapse and other clinical outcomes. Indeed, one third of the studies reviewed by Gilbert et al provided no definition of relapse at all, and another one sixth used resumption of active medication as the definition. Thus, in half of the reviewed studies, we simply do not know how much symptomatic change occurred before it was decreed that the patients had "relapsed." In those studies that did give operational relapse criteria, the criteria varied all the way from a 2-point increase in the ratings for Brief Psychiatric Rating Scale psychosis items to rehospitalization.

The definition of *relapse* is important when considering the findings from studies of medication-free periods. Studies using small changes in symptom ratings as a criterion will likely report higher rates of such relapses, only some of which are comparable to clinically judged relapses. For example, in a recent study of a medication-free period that we and our colleagues conducted (K.H.N., M.J.G., et al, unpublished results, 1994), we used a small change in symptom ratings as the definition of psychotic exacerbation. The use of such a criterion resulted in a relatively high rate of such outcomes, while the number of hospitalizations was correspondingly very low. Future research should distinguish among small changes in symptoms (psychotic exacerbations), return of high levels of psychotic symptoms (symptomatic relapses), and clinical consequences (eg, rehospitalization), so that separate conclusions regarding the frequency and predictors of the different outcomes and the efficacy of reinstituting medications can be better assessed.

STUDIES OF THE EARLY COURSE OF ILLNESS

Turning to controlled studies of medication-free periods among patients who have only recently developed schizophrenia or schizophreniform disorder, only two[2,3] of the 66 reviewed studies examined this initial period. Kane et al[2] found a 1-year relapse rate of 41% (seven of 17) among recently recovered first-episode schizophrenic patients randomly assigned to placebo, compared with none of 11 patients assigned to continuous medication for 1 year. In this study, relapse was defined as "substantial clinical deterioration with a potential for marked social impairment."[2(p71)] This initial study, while limited by its small sample size, suggested that an initial year of maintenance medication after a first episode may play a role in reducing the relapse rate.

In a later, larger placebo-controlled study, Crow et al[3] also found that an initial period of maintenance medication after a first schizophrenic episode may reduce the likelihood of relapse, with relapse observed within 2 years in 62% (41/66) of patients assigned to placebo vs 46% (25/54) of patients assigned to active maintenance medication. Relapse was defined as a point at which the responsible clinician considered rehospitalization to be necessary or resumption of active antipsychotic medication to be essential. Thus, in the study by Crow et al, continuous maintenance antipsychotic medication after an initial diagnosis of schizophrenia did significantly reduce the relapse rate across all patients, but even maintenance medication did not prevent a relapse within 2 years in a substantial percentage of these patients. While our traditional neuroleptic medications are apparently helpful in reducing the chances of relapse in the initial period after onset of schizophrenia, they are far from totally effective.

Equally important is that a closer examination of the curves for the actuarial percentage of patients who are relapse free in the report of Crow et al[3] reveals that the subgroup of patients who remained relapse free after 1 year on placebo had a relatively low risk for relapse in the second year on placebo. Specifically, the actuarial percentage of patients who were relapse free only dropped from 37% at the end of 1 year to 30% at the end of 2 years. Thus, there may be a subgroup of patients in the initial years after illness onset who are at relatively low risk for relapse and who may not need continuous antipsychotic medication.

More recent analyses of occupational outcome data for patients in the study by Crow et al highlight the continuing importance of finding predictors early in the illness to identify those patients who have low short-term risk of relapse when not receiving continuous medication.[4] In patients with less than 1 year of illness duration before antipsychotic medication began, occupational outcome was significantly better while receiving placebo than while receiving antipsychotic medication. Considering these additional findings from the study by Crow et al, Johnstone et al[4(p188)] conclude, "It suggests the disquieting conclusion that the benefits of active neuroleptics in reducing relapse may exact a price in occupational terms. This emphasises the need to find more effective means of predicting which patients derive benefit from maintenance neuroleptics and which do not." Thus, in the initial years of illness, lowered occupational functioning may need to be added as a possible risk of continuous antipsychotic medication and may need to be weighed against the potential benefit of a reduced relapse rate.

We recently completed a study of the initial years after onset of schizophrenia (K.H.N., M.J.G., et al, unpublished results, 1994), in which medication-free periods were offered to clinically stable patients after at least 1 year of antipsychotic medication, in the context of a battery of potential predictors of outcome and course. Potential predictors included variables measuring premorbid functioning, family history of psychiatric disorder, psychophysiological factors, information processing, medication plasma levels, life stressors, and living environment. We monitored symptom ratings for small changes along psychotic dimensions (psychotic exacerbations) to allow medication to be recommended as clinically needed, well before rehospitalization would be considered. Until these data and those of similar studies by others are fully analyzed and published, it remains unclear whether such predictors can help to identify a subgroup of recent-onset patients whose short-term risk of return of psychotic symptoms is lower than that of other patients and who might be best treated through reintroduction of antipsychotic medication when symptoms return.

The need for course predictors to allow better evaluation of individual risk-benefit ratios of short-term vs long-term maintenance neuroleptic therapy in the initial period after onset of schizophrenia is heightened by the limited validity of nonpsychotic prodromal symptoms as more immediate predictors of psychotic exacerbations. Marder and colleagues[5] recently reported that for schizophrenic patients treated with a low maintenance dose of a neuroleptic drug (5 to 10 mg of fluphenazine decanoate every 2 weeks), psychotic exacerbation was preceded by prodromal symptoms only 37% of the time. Furthermore, 52% (17/33) of prodromes were not followed by a psychotic exacerbation even if no pharmacological intervention occurred. Thus, while we clearly endorse recent efforts to try to develop better ways to detect prodromal symptoms that precede psychotic exacerbations, our current understanding of the clinical significance of prodromal symptoms and of optimal treatment strategies when prodromal symptoms occur remains limited.

DISTINGUISHING TYPES OF STUDIES

An additional consideration when medication-free periods are considered is that the functional consequences of a return of psychotic symptoms are highly variable. In his reinterpretation of some past studies, Wyatt[6] suggested that prolonged periods of untreated psychotic symptoms might increase long-term morbidity for patients. This conclusion was primarily based on two kinds of studies: (1) studies of first-episode patients who were given neuroleptic medication soon after onset of the first psychotic episode compared with many months after first onset and (2) studies of schizophrenic patients in which full-blown psychotic episodes were treated with or without antipsychotic medication. On the other hand, Gilbert et al[1] review studies[7-10] that suggest that patients who experienced relapse and were then treated "were usually found to have rapid return to baseline when neuroleptic therapy was reinstituted." Thus, it is critical to distinguish among three different types of studies: (1) studies of the effects of immediate use vs much later use of neuroleptic medication for resolving the first episode, (2) studies that examined whether full-blown psychotic episodes could be successfully treated with treatments other than neuroleptic medication, and (3) studies in which neuroleptic-free periods were followed by reinstatement of antipsychotic medication when psychotic symptoms returned. The functional outcomes of the three types of studies appear to be quite different.

RISK-BENEFIT CONSIDERATIONS

The higher relapse rates when schizophrenic patients are withdrawn from maintenance neuroleptic therapy, along with the difficulties inherent in interpreting prodromal symptoms, might suggest the desirability of long-term maintenance treatment for all schizophrenic patients. However, as noted by Gilbert et al,[1] the risks of not treating with continuous neuroleptics (symptomatic exacerbation or relapse, etc) must be weighed against the risks of such neuroleptic use (acute side effects, tardive dyskinesia with continued use, possible occupational disadvantage in early illness course, etc). An additional important factor, particularly in the initial years after onset of a schizophrenic or schizophreniform disorder, is that patients will often not agree to continue antipsychotic medication unless a drug-free period is attempted. Each clinician needs to determine whether to recommend a drug-free period based on an assessment of the risk-benefit ratio and consideration of the particular clinical situation.

Given all these variables—the many definitions of relapse, the paucity of studies examining recent-onset or first-break schizophrenic patients, the adverse side effects of traditional neuroleptics, and the uncertain clinical significance of prodromal symptoms—we believe that the conclusions reached by Gilbert et al[1] point to the need for additional carefully conceived and focused research. For recent-onset patients, important issues, as noted by Gilbert et al, include identification of predictors of the likelihood of exacerbation, relapse, and clinical deterioration. Consideration should also be given to evaluating the implications of shifts in risk-benefit ratios associated with newer antipsychotic medications that may have fewer side effects. Results of such research would allow clinicians, patients, and their families to consider individualized risks and benefits of long-term continuous neuroleptic treatment.

Keith H. Nuechterlein, PhD
Michael J. Gitlin, MD
Kenneth L. Subotnik, PhD
Department of Psychiatry and Biobehavioral Sciences
University of California, Los Angeles
Room 2240
300 UCLA Medical Plaza
Los Angeles, CA 90024-6968

Reprints are available from Dr Nuechterlein at the above address.

REFERENCES

1. Gilbert PL, Harris MJ, McAdams LA, Jeste DV. Neuroleptic withdrawal in schizophrenic patients: a review of the literature. *Arch Gen Psychiatry.* 1995;52:173-188.
2. Kane JM, Rifkin A, Quitkin F, Nayak D, Ramos-Lorenzi J. Fluphenazine vs placebo in patients with remitted, acute first-episode schizophrenia. *Arch Gen Psychiatry.* 1982;39:70-73.
3. Crow TJ, MacMillan JF, Johnson AL, Johnstone EC. The Northwick Park Study of First Episodes of Schizophrenia, II: a randomised controlled trial of prophylactic neuroleptic treatment. *Br J Psychiatry.* 1986;148:120-127.
4. Johnstone EC, MacMillan JF, Frith CD, Benn DK, Crow TJ. Further investigation of the predictors of outcome following first schizophrenic episodes. *Br J Psychiatry.* 1990;157:182-189.
5. Marder SR, Wirshing WC, Van Putten T, Mintz J, McKenzie J, Johnston-Cronk K, Lebell M, Liberman RP. Fluphenazine vs placebo supplementation for prodromal signs of relapse in schizophrenia. *Arch Gen Psychiatry.* 1994;51:280-287.
6. Wyatt RJ. Neuroleptics and the natural course of schizophrenia. *Schizophr Bull.* 1991;17:325-351.
7. Glovinsky D, Kirch DG, Wyatt RJ. Early antipsychotic response to resumption of neuroleptics in drug-free chronic schizophrenic patients. *Biol Psychiatry.* 1992;31:968-970.
8. Good WW, Sterling M, Holtzman WH. Termination of chlorpromazine with schizophrenic patients. *Am J Psychiatry.* 1958;115:443-448.
9. Rothstein C. An evaluation of the effects of discontinuation of chlorpromazine. *N Engl J Med.* 1960;262:67-69.
10. Ruskin PE, Nyman G. Discontinuation of neuroleptic medication in older, outpatient schizophrenics: a placebo-controlled, double-blind trial. *J Nerv Ment Dis.* 1991;179:212-214.

Risks of Withdrawing Antipsychotic Medications

In an excellent meta-analysis of 66 studies involving more than 4000 patients, Gilbert and colleagues[1] found a cumulative relapse rate of 51.5% in patients who had stopped taking antipsychotic medications. Of patients who were maintained on antipsychotic medications, however, only 16.2% relapsed. The study by Gilbert et al raises important and provocative questions. For instance, what are the arguments for and against maintenance medication in schizophrenic patients? What clinical circumstances warrant stopping medications? Might the relapse rate of patients off antipsychotic medications be even higher than Gilbert et al suggest in their review?

UNDER WHAT CIRCUMSTANCES SHOULD ANTIPSYCHOTIC MEDICATIONS BE WITHDRAWN?

Reasons to Take Patients off Medications

The risk of tardive dyskinesia is one of the reasons to minimize a patient's time receiving antipsychotic medications. As noted by Gilbert et al, recent studies have found 1-year incidence rates of tardive dyskinesia in elderly schizophrenic patients to be greater than 50%. While this is extremely worrisome, the mean age of the patients in the review of Gilbert et al was 40 years. Patients closer to age 40 years have been found to have a 4% to 5% per year incidence of tardive dyskinesia[2]; although still troubling, these much lower rates may not adequately reflect the true risk to patients. For example, one recent study found a 15% prevalence of definite oral/facial or tardive dyskinesia–like movements in a group of relatively young patients with chronic schizophrenia who had never been given antipsychotic medications,[3] indicating that some of the movements attributed to antipsychotic medications are either part of the illness or otherwise independent of medication.[4] Furthermore, we do not have incidence data on the severity of tardive dyskinesia in terms of loss of function, disfigurement, and discomfort. For instance, what percentage of those patients developing tardive dyskinesia at a rate of 4% to 5% per year[2] were embarrassed or incapacitated by their abnormal movements? Such knowledge is imperative in making informed decisions about withdrawing antipsychotic medications for the purpose of decreasing the risk of tardive dyskinesia.

See also pages 173, 189, 192, 197, 200, 203, and 209

Other side effects, such as dysphoria, dulling of senses, and anticholinergic effects, are also reasons to lower dosage or withdraw antipsychotic medications.

Reasons for Patients to Remain on Medications

There are a number of potential dangers in stopping antipsychotic medications. These potential dangers include a greater number of high-risk behaviors, increased psychosocial risks, a greater risk of tardive dyskinesia, and an increase in the long-term morbidity of the illness. Surprisingly, there has been little investigation into these areas despite the large number of withdrawal studies. Unfortunately, many of my comments in this section are necessarily speculative.

High-Risk Behaviors. High-risk behaviors almost certainly increase in those schizophrenic patients withdrawn from antipsychotic medications. Johnson et al[5] (1983) found that patients whose antipsychotic medications were withdrawn had seven times as many incidents of antisocial behavior, such as assault, criminal and property damage, arson, and stealing, as patients who were maintained on medications. The same patients had about 2½ times as many incidents of self-injury, including wrist cutting, poisoning, and attempted hanging. There is a disconcerting lack of information about the risk of suicide in patients who stop taking medications.

Psychosocial Risks. Individuals with schizophrenia whose bizarre behavior increases because their antipsychotic medications have been withdrawn may be less welcome in their homes or community. The question remains whether relapses triggered by the withdrawal of antipsychotic medications contribute to stigmatization specifically because prejudices are confirmed by reality.

The effect of a schizophrenic individual on family structure and the family's effect on a schizophrenic family member is a complex interaction that can cause stress for both parties. It seems probable that the degree to which a disruptive schizophrenic family member can disrupt or destroy a family system depends on the patient's psychiatric status.

Intermittent Use of Antipsychotic Medications May Increase the Risk of Tardive Dyskinesia. There is increasing evidence that intermittent use of antipsychotic medications may well constitute a risk factor for tardive dyskinesia[6,7]; starting and stopping medications may ultimately prove to be a greater hazard than uninterrupted use for those patients who must be maintained on them. Unfortunately, medical practices designed to prevent tardive dyskinesia may, in the long run, prove responsible for increasing its risk.

The Effects of Antipsychotic Medication on Long-term Morbidity. There is now considerable evidence that not treating schizophrenia with antipsychotic medications early in its course increases the long-term morbidity of the disorder.[8-11] It is less clear if stopping antipsychotic medications in stabilized patients also increases long-term morbidity.

In the "Results" section of their article, Gilbert et al state, "Patients who experienced relapse after neuroleptic withdrawal were usually found to have a rapid return to baseline when neuroleptic therapy was reinstituted." Later, in the "Comment" section, they are somewhat more cautious, stating that patients "are generally not subjected to any prolonged exacerbation if neuroleptic therapy is restarted soon." They cite four studies[12-15] that, unfortunately, provide little guidance.

In the 1958 study by Good et al,[12] either patients were not free of medication long enough to relapse (3 months), or, if they were (6 months), no information was provided about their progress after antipsychotic therapy was restarted. In the 1960 study by Rothstein,[13] patients with schizophrenia who had been treated with antipsychotic medications on a long-term basis as inpatients received placebo for 3 months. One patient regressed 1 month into the placebo trial and returned to his prestudy adjustment within 1 week after treatment with antipsychotic medications was restarted. Ruskin and Nyman[14] (1991) studied 18 schizophrenic outpatients whose average age was 60 years and whose last hospitalization was almost 13 years earlier. Eight of the patients were randomly assigned to a haloperidol treatment group and 10 to placebo. Over a 6-month period, only one of the eight patients treated with medications relapsed, while five of 10 placebo-treated patients relapsed. The patients who relapsed did so slowly, and caregivers were aware of the changes. Only one patient (treated with placebo) required hospitalization, and he returned to baseline quickly and completely. The fourth study (Glovinsky et al[15]) was one in which I participated. Patients with chronic, relatively treatment-refractory schizophrenia received first placebo, then a standard dose of antipsychotic medication. At the end of 28 days of treatment with antipsychotic medication, most but not all patients had improved, and half of that improvement occurred within 3 days. No attempt was made, however, to determine if the 28-day response was equivalent to the preplacebo level.

Taken as a whole, these results do not inspire overwhelming confidence that withdrawing antipsychotic medications in schizophrenic patients is harmless, especially since relapses during these four studies were relatively brief and occurred while the patients were closely monitored. Two other relevant studies provide a less optimistic picture. In a study referred to above, Johnson et al[5] (1983) looked at 56 patients with chronic but psychiatrically stable schizophrenia whose antipsychotic medication was withdrawn after they had lived in the community for 12 to 48 months. These patients were matched with another group of 60 schizophrenics who continued taking their antipsychotic medications. In those patients who relapsed when off antipsychotic medications, both social and work functions were adversely affected for some months after antipsychotic medications were reinstituted.

Curson et al[16] (1985) followed up a group of outpatients with chronic schizophrenia for 7 years after all had been initially stabilized on depot antipsychotic medications for at least 8 weeks. Patients who had more relapses had the worst social adjustment. The authors noted that, while maintenance depot medication does not eliminate relapses, it does seem to postpone them. Although the study points out that the relationship between relapse rates, drug treatment, and social disability is complex, it also suggests that, for the majority of patients, frequent relapse may inhibit improvement in social performance long after florid symptoms have been controlled by medications. Of concern, in over half of these cases, the treatment agency was not aware that patients had relapsed. This study as well as clinical experience suggests that when antipsychotic medications are withdrawn, close monitoring of patients is not always possible; this, in turn, often results in severe consequences.

I have elsewhere proposed that some aspects of psychosis may in themselves be toxic.[9,11] The best evidence for this notion is the relationship between delayed intervention early in the treatment of schizophrenia and poor long-term outcome. A similar relationship may exist later in the illness, so that prolonged severe psychosis would make recovery to baseline slower or even less likely. Clinically, I have noted that schizophrenic patients who have been stable and then develop psychotic symptoms appear to respond much more quickly if their antipsychotic medications are raised in dosage or restarted as soon as the symptoms are noted. In fact, this appears to be cause to watch for and aggressively treat prodromal symptoms.[17,18] Empirical studies in this area are badly needed, as is evidence that putative biological changes occur during psychosis.

WHEN SHOULD ANTIPSYCHOTIC MEDICATIONS BE WITHDRAWN?

Chronic vs First Break Schizophrenia

In practice, most patients with chronic schizophrenia have been taken off antipsychotic medications at one time or another—either deciding to stop taking the medications themselves or at the instigation of their physician—and the clinical consequences are well known. One practical issue not addressed in Gilbert and colleagues' review is how long to keep patients with first-break schizophrenia on antipsychotic medications; in fact, I know of no studies that address this question in a rigorous manner. In lieu of experimental data, a consensus committee has recommended maintaining first-episode patients on antipsychotic medications for at least 1 to 2 years.[19]

Length of Follow-up

Gilbert and colleagues found that the only specific predictor of relapse was average length of follow-up. Approximately half of the patients withdrawn from antipsychotic medications relapsed within an average follow-up period of 10 months. However, studies of patients with first-episode schizophrenia withdrawn from their medication indicate that between 60% and 90% relapse within 2 years.[20] Other studies have suggested that relapses are more likely to occur during the second year of neuroleptic withdrawal.[21] Therefore, the average follow-up in the review by Gilbert et al (10 months) is relatively short; the relapse rate is likely to be much higher when patients are followed up for longer periods.

HOW SHOULD ANTIPSYCHOTIC MEDICATIONS BE WITHDRAWN?

Gilbert et al recommend that clinicians slowly taper antipsychotic medications, and, presumably, watch carefully for prodromal signs of a relapse. Their basic conclusion is that schizophrenic patients can, in many cases, be safely and completely withdrawn from their antipsychotic medications. The evidence that a slow taper is better than abrupt withdrawal is sparse,[22] but until such evidence becomes available, the course of action they endorse is sensible. Abrupt withdrawal of medications that affect both normal and abnormal systems is likely to disrupt these systems, produce internal stress, and perhaps in itself cause a relapse.[23] The majority of patients in the studies reviewed by Gilbert et al experienced a relatively abrupt withdrawal of their medications; a large portion of these patients would ultimately relapse, but many had not done so at 10 months. If medications were tapered over months to years, I predict that breakthroughs would be less severe and relapses more easily treated. Furthermore, clinical experience suggests that some of the most severe cases of tardive dyskinesia have occurred in patients whose antipsychotic medications have suddenly been stopped. Nevertheless, the speed at which medications should be tapered is another question requiring careful study.

Under all circumstances, careful monitoring of patients taken off antipsychotic medications must go on for an extended period because of the continued high risk of relapse in the second year following withdrawal of medications.

The vast majority of schizophrenic patients will almost certainly need to remain on antipsychotic medications indefinitely. Even when patients remain free of relapse on medication, the evidence suggests that their need for antipsychotic medications is not diminished.[21,24-28] There is ample evidence, however, that many patients can do as well on lower doses of antipsychotic medication, as long as psychosocial treatments are provided in addition to those medications.[29] It is clear that any medication withdrawal effort should incorporate psychosocial treatments; similarly, if the patient is living at home or interacts with his or her family regularly, the family needs to be involved, educated, and informed.

Any decision to decrease or withdraw antipsychotic medications should be an individual decision, one that carefully weighs the risks associated with relapse against the risks of tardive dyskinesia and other side effects.

Richard Jed Wyatt, MD
Neuropsychiatry Branch
National Institute of Mental Health
Neuroscience Center at St Elizabeth's
2700 Martin Luther King Jr Ave
Washington, DC 20032

I thank Ioline Henter for her invaluable editorial and organizational assistance in the preparation of the manuscript.

REFERENCES

1. Gilbert PL, Harris MJ, McAdams LA, Jeste DV. Neuroleptic withdrawal in schizophrenic patients: a review of the literature. *Arch Gen Psychiatry.* 1995;52:173-188.
2. Kane JM, Jeste DV, Barnes TRE, Casey DE, Cole JO, Davis JM, Gualtieri CT. *Tardive Dyskinesia: A Task Force Report of the American Psychiatric Association.* Washington, DC: American Psychiatric Press; 1992.
3. Fenton WS, Wyatt RJ, McGlashan TH. Risk factors for spontaneous dyskinesia in schizophrenia. *Arch Gen Psychiatry.* 1994;51:643-650.
4. Khot V, Wyatt RJ. Not all that moves is tardive dyskinesia. *Am J Psychiatry.* 1991;148:661-666.
5. Johnson DAW, Pasterski G, Ludlow JM, Street K, Taylor RDW. The discontinuance of maintenance neuroleptic therapy in chronic schizophrenic patients: drug and social consequences. *Acta Psychiatr Scand.* 1983;67:339-352.
6. Jeste DV, Wyatt RJ. Therapeutic strategies against tardive dyskinesia: two decades of experience. *Arch Gen Psychiatry.* 1982;39:803-816.
7. Kane JM. Incidence and prevalence of tardive dyskinesia. Presented at the 150th Annual Meeting of the American Psychiatric Association; May 25, 1994; Philadelphia, Pa.
8. Crow TJ, Macmillan JF, Johnson AL, Johnstone EC. A randomized controlled trial of prophylactic neuroleptic treatment. *Br J Psychiatry.* 1986; 148:120-127.
9. Wyatt RJ. Neuroleptics and the natural course of schizophrenia. *Schizophr Bull.* 1991;17:325-351.
10. Loebel AD, Lieberman JA, Alvir JM, Mayerhoff DI, Geisler SH, Symanski SR. Duration of psychosis and outcome in first-episode schizophrenia. *Am J Psychiatry.* 1992;149:1183-1188.
11. Wyatt RJ. Antipsychotic medication and the long-term course of schizophrenia: therapeutic and theoretical implications. In: Shriqui C, Nasrallah H, eds. *Contemporary Issues in the Treatment of Schizophrenia.* Washington, DC: American Psychiatric Press. In press.
12. Good WW, Sterling M, Holtzman WH. Termination of chlorpromazine with schizophrenic patients. *Am J Psychiatry.* 1958;115:433-448.
13. Rothstein C. An evaluation of the effects of discontinuation of chlorpromazine. *N Engl J Med.* 1960;262:67-69.
14. Ruskin PE, Nyman G. Discontinuation of neuroleptic medication in older, outpatient schizophrenics: a placebo-controlled, double-blind trial. *J Nerv Ment Dis.* 1991;179:212-214.
15. Glovinsky D, Kirch DG, Wyatt RJ. Early antipsychotic response to resumption of neuroleptics in drug-free chronic schizophrenic patients. *Biol Psychiatry.* 1992;31:968-970.
16. Curson DA, Barnes TRE, Bamber RW, Platt SD, Hirsch SR, Duffy JC. Long-term depot maintenance of chronic schizophrenic out-patients: the seven-year follow-up of the Medical Research Council fluphenazine/placebo trial. *Br J Psychiatry.* 1985;146:464-480.
17. Herz MI, Glazer W, Mirza M, Mostert M, Hafez H. Treating prodromal episodes to prevent relapse in schizophrenia. *Br J Psychiatry Suppl.* July 1989:123-127.
18. Carpenter WT Jr, Hanlon TE, Heinrichs DW, Summerfelt AT, Kirkpatrick B, Levine J, Buchanan RW. Continuous versus targeted medication in schizophrenic outpatients: outcome results. *Am J Psychiatry.* 1990;147:1138-1148.
19. Kissling W, ed. *Guidelines for Neuroleptic Relapse Prevention in Schizophrenia.* New York, NY: Springer-Verlag NY Inc; 1991.
20. Ram R, Bromet EJ, Eaton WW, Pato C, Schwartz JE. The natural course of schizophrenia: a review of first-admission studies. *Schizophr Bull.* 1992;18:185-207.
21. Dencker SJ, Lapp M, Malm U. Do schizophrenics well-adapted in the community need neuroleptics? a depot neuroleptic withdrawal study. *Acta Psychiatr Scand Suppl.* 1980;279:64-76.
22. Green AI, Faraone SV, Brown WA. Prolactin shifts after neuroleptic withdrawal. *Psychiatry Res.* 1990; 32:213-219.
23. Faedda GL, Tondo L, Baldessarini RJ, Suppes T, Tohen M. Outcome after rapid vs gradual discontinuation of lithium treatment in bipolar disorders. *Arch Gen Psychiatry.* 1993;50:448-455.
24. Hogarty GE, Ulrichs RF, Mussare F, Aristigueta N. Drug discontinuation among long-term successfully maintained schizophrenic outpatients. *Dis Nerv Syst.* 1976;37:494-500.
25. Johnson DAW. The duration of maintenance therapy in chronic schizophrenia. *Acta Psychiatr Scand.* 1976;53:298-301.
26. Johnson DAW. Further observations on the duration of depot neuroleptic maintenance therapy in schizophrenia. *Br J Psychiatry.* 1979;119:267-276.
27. Cheung HK. Schizophrenics fully remitted on neuroleptics for 3-5 years: to stop or continue drugs? *Br J Psychiatry.* 1981;138:490-494.
28. Wistedt B. A depot neuroleptic withdrawal study. *Acta Psychiatr Scand.* 1981;64:65-84.
29. Bellack AS, Mueser KT. Psychosocial treatment for schizophrenia. *Schizophr Bull.* 1993;19:317-336.

REPLY COMMENTARY

Considering Neuroleptic Maintenance and Taper on a Continuum

Need for Individual Rather Than Dogmatic Approach

What is the nature of the bioelectrical and biochemical perturbations . . . which constitute the physical ground of psychotic states? How do our drugs act on these perturbations? It is difficult at present to take a stand, since later on it might be absolutely senseless on a more refined plane.

Henri Laborit (1960)[1]

THE ABOVE statement by the French surgeon who discovered the psychotropic effects of chlorpromazine is still valid 35 years later. While we know a lot more today about the pathophysiology of schizophrenia and other psychoses and about the mechanism of action of neuroleptic drugs than we did in 1960, there is yet much more that is unknown. Our lack of adequate understanding in these areas is reflected clinically in the history of wide fluctuations in the practice of neuroleptic use over the past four decades. In the years following the introduction of neuroleptic drugs into psychiatric practice, these drugs were prescribed for a growing number of indications and in increasing dosages. Subsequently, as persistent tardive dyskinesia came to be recognized as a serious problem with the long-term use of neuroleptics, regular "drug holidays" were recommended and, in some cases, even legally mandated. Now the pendulum may be swinging to the other side, with the suggestion being that any attempt at reducing neuroleptic dose in a patient with schizophrenia must be avoided because of the risk of relapse. Yet, throughout these debates three facts have remained unchanged: (1) schizophrenia is a heterogeneous syndrome, clinically as well as pathophysiologically; (2) neuroleptics are highly potent drugs that constitute the most effective available therapy for treating and preventing psychotic relapse; and (3) neuroleptics carry a clear risk of serious adverse effects, especially when given in high doses or for prolonged periods. A rational policy for the long-term use of the antipsychotic medications in schizophrenic patients must take into account all three of these factors.

See also pages 173, 189, 192, 197, 200, 203, and 205

We want to thank Baldessarini and Viguera,[2] Carpenter and Tamminga,[3] Greden and Tandon,[4] Meltzer,[5] Nuechterlein et al,[6] and Wyatt[7] for their thoughtful and thought-provoking commentaries on our article.[8] It is noteworthy that there are important differences in the clinical recommendations for neuroleptic maintenance vs withdrawal made by these expert psychopharmacologists, in spite of the fact that they have unanimity of opinion about the need to prevent psychotic relapse and to minimize the incidence of adverse effects of neuroleptic treatment. These differences in the suggested practice reflect understandable variations in the long-term use of neuroleptics in patients with chronic schizophrenia. One may, therefore, conclude that there is no single "100% correct way" that can be recommended dogmatically for treating all chronic schizophrenic patients. In other words, treatment must be individualized. Furthermore, as a given patient's level of psychopathological symptoms and the overall clinical situation change with time, so would his or her needs for neuroleptic therapy and other treatment (eg, psychosocial support).

DATA ANALYSIS STRATEGY

We want to take this opportunity to elaborate on some aspects of our review.[8] Our goal was to conduct a thorough review of the literature with the inclusion of a large number of studies with sample sizes of 10 or more. Our analysis may or may not be called a meta-analysis. We analyzed the results of other analyses—in that sense, we conducted a meta-analysis. We did not conduct a weighted estimation of relapse percent or a weighted regression analysis, although weighting is a commonly employed tool of meta-analysis. If that is the criterion, then we did not conduct a meta-analysis. Our choice of analytic strategy was deliberate.

Weighting data by sample size has both potential benefits and risks. In the analysis of data from a large number of studies, weighting estimates of values of continuous variables by sample size is based on the assumption that sample size (*precision*) is more important than other aspects of methodology that could introduce *bias*, eg, diagnostic criteria used, definition of relapse, age and gender distribution, and especially rates of dropout. Because a larger sample size yields more precision of estimate but not necessarily less bias, and in view of the large differences among the studies reviewed on these and other important methodological aspects, we do not believe that larger studies were necessarily better ones. In addition, because of the longitudinal nature of these studies, there were variable (and usually unstated) dropout rates. Hence, sample sizes at the beginning of the study were different from those at various follow-up periods, making it difficult to calculate effective sample sizes. Weighting by initial sample sizes in long-term follow-up studies without data on dropouts is hazardous.

The use of the midpoint of range when the mean was not provided did not seem to make much difference in any of the values. For example, the mean age for the 52 neuroleptic withdrawal groups for which this information was available was 39.9 years, while the "average" age for all the 62 neuroleptic withdrawal groups was 40.0 years.

RELAPSE RATE AS A FUNCTION OF TIME

The cumulative proportion of relapse in the neuroleptic withdrawal and neuroleptic maintenance groups as a function of time without log-transformation was as follows:

Time, mo	Neuroleptic Withdrawal	Neuroleptic Maintenance
3	44%	6%
6	49%	11%
9	52%	14%
12	54%	17%
15	55%	20%
18	57%	22%
21	58%	25%
24	59%	27%

Thus, the relative likelihood of relapse was higher in the initial rather than the later phases of follow-up in the neuroleptic withdrawal group. Weighting by sample size (inverse of variance) did not greatly alter these figures: the individual percentages differed by no more than 6% for any comparable time period, and differences between the experimental and control groups amounted at most to three percentage points. We must, however, stress the limitations in extrapolating proportions based on aggregate data to individual patients.

There are numerous potentially important predictors of relapse that we would have liked to examine in the data reviewed, eg, psychosocial treatment, community support, history of treatment resistance vs responsiveness, and interval between last relapse and beginning withdrawal of medication. Unfortunately, too few studies provided information on these variables to undertake their meaningful analysis.

NEUROLEPTIC MAINTENANCE

Neuroleptic drugs are invaluable in the prevention of psychotic relapse. As our literature review[8] showed, 53% of the schizophrenic patients withdrawn from neuroleptic treatment relapsed in contrast to only 16% of those maintained on neuroleptic treatment over a mean follow-up period of 9.7 months. In view of the serious physical and psychosocial consequences of relapse, neuroleptic withdrawal in chronic schizophrenic patients would, therefore, need strong justification. Not surprisingly, a majority of the patients with chronic schizophrenia would presently be expected to require maintenance treatment with neuroleptic medications (either the conventional ones or the newer serotonin-dopamine antagonists) for many years. This does not mean, though, that every schizophrenic patient must continue for lifetime receiving the same high doses of antipsychotic drugs that were used to control his or her acute psychotic episode. There is a long list of acute, subacute, and chronic side effects with different neuroleptic drugs. Not surprisingly, medication noncompliance is common in chronic schizophrenic patients. In a review of 17 studies of "drug deviation" in various psychiatric conditions but primarily focusing on schizophrenia, Blackwell[9] found a noncompliance rate of 25% to 50% in outpatients.

It is most appropriate to consider neuroleptic maintenance and withdrawal on a continuum rather than as two distinct and diametrically opposite strategies. At one end of the continuum is uninterrupted use of high-dose neuroleptic drugs for lifetime. Extremely sick patients whose psychopathological symptoms worsen with even a small reduction in antipsychotic dosage would be candidates for such treatment. These patients definitely deserve a trial of clozapine, risperidone, and/or one of the newer antipsychotic agents.

NEUROLEPTIC WITHDRAWAL

At the other extreme of the continuum is an older patient (with a high risk of persistent or severe tardive dyskinesia) who has a first-break late-onset acute schizophreniform episode with the various reported indicators of good prognosis (eg, short duration of psychopathological symptoms, few negative symptoms, rapid response to a low dose of an antipsychotic drug, excellent premorbid adjustment, absence of a family history of schizophrenia, and high level of psychosocial support). After maintaining such a patient on neuroleptic therapy for a number of months (eg, 1 to 2 years), an attempt may be made to very slowly begin to reduce the dose. If there is no exacerbation of symptoms, it may be possible to withdraw the medication entirely at some point. Obviously, the patient *must* be monitored closely throughout the course of medication use and observed subsequently, with an eye to detecting any early signs of exacerbation.

GRADUAL DOSE REDUCTION

Most chronic schizophrenic patients would fall between the two extremes described above. We *do not* recommend neuroleptic withdrawal for a majority of the chronic schizophrenic patients; we *do* recommend a gradual reduction of the neuroleptic dose to the lowest effective level.[8] Also, we do not believe that the determination of the lowest effective dosage involves first finding the amount that precipitates relapse and then increasing the dose to a higher level. A relapse is not likely to occur suddenly during a gradual taper of medication. An advantage of a slow reduction in dosage is that the patient, caregiver, or clinician may decide at any time that the dose needs to be increased. Even relatively small fluctuations in symptoms (which, by the way, occur commonly in patients maintained on neuroleptic treatment too) may lead to a decision to increase dosage.

Two recent studies[10,11] show that well-monitored gradual taper of neuroleptic dosage in chronic schizophrenic patients is not only feasible but can also be therapeutically beneficial. In one report,[10] the neuroleptic dose was reduced very slowly, by about 60% over a 10-month period, in 16 chronically hospitalized schizophrenic or schizoaffective patients; this resulted in a significant improvement in psychopathological symptoms. In the other study, Inderbitzin et al[11] evaluated, in a double-blind fashion, the effects of reducing relatively high doses of fluphenazine decanoate by 50% over 5 months in 23 chronic unstable schizophrenic patients and compared them with a control group of 20 patients who were maintained on treatment with a fixed dose. The two groups experienced a similar decrease in the rate of hospitalization over a year; the reduced-dose group also had lower severity of extrapyramidal symptoms and of tardive dyskinesia than the control group.

ABRUPT WITHDRAWAL

Baldessarini and Viguera[2] make an excellent point regarding the relapse rate being three times greater following abrupt withdrawal compared with gradual discontinuation. This finding reinforces our clinical recommendation for the medication taper to be very slow. The situations that may necessitate rapid withdrawal of antipsychotic medications include severe allergic or other serious idiosyncratic reactions to the drug (eg, agranulocytosis), development of an acute medical emergency requiring neuroleptic discontinuation, neuroleptic malignant syndrome, and possibly pregnancy. Investigations of experimental or newly approved drugs, and occasionally, clinical decisions to switch to therapy with different neuroleptic drugs also require abrupt withdrawal of antipsychotic medications. Because of the heightened risk of psychotic relapse following sudden discontinuation, patients would usually need to be hospitalized or otherwise very closely monitored for some time.

DRUG HOLIDAYS

There seems to be very little, if any, justification for repeated lengthy drug withdrawals. We had previously reported that the number of drug-free periods of 3 months or longer (typically a result of the patient's noncompliance) was positively associated with an increased frequency of persistent tardive dyskinesia.[12] A recently completed, well-designed multicenter study of three medication strategies for schizophrenia (continuous moderate dose, continuous low dose, and targeted early intervention) found that the targeted treatment was associated with the highest rate of relapses and rehospitalizations (N. R. Schooler, PhD, written communication, December 12, 1994). The continuous low-dose medication strategy was associated with a higher relapse rate than (but a similar number of rehospitalizations as) continuous moderate dose treatment, suggesting to us that a fixed low-dose strategy is less satisfactory than one employing necessary adjustments in dosage according to a patient's varying clinical needs at different times.

SPECIFIC SUBPOPULATIONS

The risk-benefit ratio for neuroleptic use varies in different subsets of the schizophrenic population, such as the elderly. Just as children are not smaller adults, the elderly are not merely older adults. There is a greater biological heterogeneity among the geriatric population than in younger subjects. With aging, patients' requirement for neuroleptic amount decreases mainly because of pharmacokinetic factors such as hepatic and renal dysfunction. Additionally, the severity of positive symptoms tends to decrease, and a small but sizable minority of patients remit,[13] ie, return to their premorbid level of functioning and do not need therapy with antipsychotic drugs. Continuing to treat these patients with neuroleptic drugs is not only unnecessary but also dangerous because of a markedly heightened risk of tardive dyskinesia. We found an annual incidence of tardive dyskinesia of 26% in outpatients over age 45 years, most of whom were being treated with relatively low neuroleptic doses.[14] The incidence of most other adverse effects increases with aging too. Common problems in the aged, including sensory deficits, other physical comorbidity, polypharmacy, and cognitive impairment, expose the elderly to greater risks with the long-term use of any potent drugs. Furthermore, the consequences of miscompliance (which includes not only forgetting to take medications but also mistakenly taking excessive amounts) are likely to be more serious in this age group. It is important that the risk-benefit ratio of neuroleptic maintenance vs withdrawal be considered separately for every patient.

BRAIN DAMAGE DUE TO PSYCHOTIC RELAPSE AND NEUROLEPTICS

A psychotic relapse is a very serious event and every effort must be made to prevent it. We do not know of any satisfactory evidence, however, that demonstrates irreversible structural brain damage as a direct result of psychotic exacerbation. On the other hand, there are at least some suggestive data indicating microscopic and electron microscopic alterations in nigrostriatal neurons with the prolonged use of neuroleptic drugs in animals.[15,16] The clinical implications of the animal findings are unclear. Studies by us as well as others have found no significant relationship of chronicity of schizophrenia or its long-term treatment with neuroleptic drugs to neuropsychological or brain imaging abnormalities.[17,18] If either repeated relapses or long-term neuroleptic treatments typically produced irreversible and clinically significant structural brain abnormalities and cognitive deterioration, most of the chronic schizophrenic patients who have lived into old age would be expected to have greater functional impairments than at any earlier point in their lives. Yet, Belitsky and McGlashan,[19] who reviewed the limited literature on the course of schizophrenia in old age, concluded that deterioration in schizophrenia seemed to be restricted primarily to the first 5 to 10 years of illness, and that subsequently, there was a tendency for functioning to become stable or to improve. In one of the longest (30 to 40 years) catamnestic studies involving 289 formerly hospitalized schizophrenic patients, most of whom were over age 65 years at the last follow-up, Ciompi[20] reported that 49% of the patients were considered to have a favorable prognosis and 27% achieved complete social remission, some after many years of severe illness.

During the course of their disease, many of the chronic schizophrenic patients experience one or more psychotic exacerbations (occurring either spontaneously or due to noncompliance with medication therapy). Yet, neither the exacerbation(s) nor the prolonged use of neuroleptics has been shown to directly produce clinically significant and irreversible structural brain abnormalities in patients with chronic schizophrenia. (The neuropathological basis of persistent tardive dyskinesia is still unclear.) This fact should be stressed in discussions with the patients and their family members about the pros and cons of neuroleptic maintenance.

NEWER NEUROLEPTICS

We concluded our review[8] by stressing the need for intensifying efforts to develop new antipsychotic agents without the risk of tardive dyskinesia or other serious side effects. There is now excellent evidence showing that clozapine has unique therapeutic efficacy and also a lower risk for tardive dyskinesia than the conventional antipsychotic drugs. Because of its various other adverse effects and especially because of the requirement for weekly blood monitoring, however, it is unlikely that clozapine itself will be widely used. The recently approved risperidone[21] as well as the other serotonin-dopamine antagonists, such as olanzapine, sertindole, and others that are in the pipeline, may indeed come to entirely replace the "typical" neuroleptic agents in the next few years. It is, however, too early to predict with certainty that this is about to happen shortly. As we and other investigators continue to gather data on the long-term safety as well as effectiveness of these exciting and potentially revolutionary compounds, a clearer picture of the neuroleptic drugs of the future will emerge. At this time, it is best to be cautiously optimistic about the new drugs and to continue research in this field with renewed vigor.

INFORMED CONSENT

A full understanding by the patient, the caregiver, and the clinician of the possibility of a relapse is critical before contemplating neuroleptic withdrawal. The Office for Protection from Research Risks at the National Institutes of Health has recently issued some guidelines about informed consent. It stresses that

> the basic elements of the legally effective informed consent include a description of the procedures to be followed and identification of any experimental procedures, a description of reasonably foreseeable risks, and the disclosure of alternative procedures or courses of treatment.

CONCLUSION

Neuroleptics do not cure schizophrenia, and they should be considered as a part (although a very important part) of the overall management of the schizophrenic patient. Psychosocial aspects of the supportive treatment are integral to patient care. The use of neuroleptic therapy must be individualized. Withdrawal of treatment with antipsychotic medications, especially an abrupt one, carries a high risk of psychotic relapse in schizophrenic patients. There is little justification for repeated prolonged withdrawals of medications in chronic schizophrenic patients. A majority of these patients need maintenance treatment with neuroleptics for many years, although the dosage should be adjusted according to the patient's needs at different times. A very gradual and well-monitored reduction in neuroleptic dosage to the lowest effective maintenance level can be achieved in a substantial proportion of patients without precipitating relapse. The newer serotonin-dopamine antagonists such as risperidone seem quite promising at this time, although more experience is required before predicting their long-term impact on the treatment of schizophrenia.

Dilip V. Jeste, MD
Patricia L. Gilbert, MD
Lou Ann McAdams, PhD
M. Jackuelyn Harris, MD
Department of Psychiatry
University of California, San Diego
San Diego Veterans Affairs
Medical Center 116A
3350 La Jolla Village Dr
San Diego, CA 92161

This work was supported, in part, by the Department of Veterans Affairs and by grants MH45131, MH43693, MH49671-01, and MH51459 from the National Institute of Mental Health.

We thank Nina Schooler, PhD, and George Simpson, MD, for helpful discussions prior to the preparation of the manuscript.

Reprint requests to Dr Jeste.

REFERENCES

1. Caldwell AE. *Origins of Psychopharmacology: From CPZ to LSD.* Springfield, IL: Charles C Thomas Publisher; 1970.
2. Baldessarini RJ, Viguera AC. Neuroleptic withdrawal in schizophrenic patients. *Arch Gen Psychiatry.* 1995;52:189-192.
3. Carpenter WT, Tamminga SA. Why neuroleptic withdrawal in schizophrenia? *Arch Gen Psychiatry.* 1995;52:192-193.
4. Greden JF, Tandon R. Long-term treatment for lifetime disorders? *Arch Gen Psychiatry.* 1995; 52:197-200.
5. Meltzer HY. Neuroleptic withdrawal in schizophrenic patients. *Arch Gen Psychiatry.* 1995;52: 200-202.
6. Nuechterlein KH, Gitlin MJ, Subotnik KL. The early course of schizophrenia and long-term maintenance neuroleptic therapy. *Arch Gen Psychiatry.* 1995;52:203-205.
7. Wyatt RJ. The risks of withdrawing antipsychotic medications. *Arch Gen Psychiatry.* 1995; 52:205-208.
8. Gilbert PL, Harris MJ, McAdams LA, Jeste DV. Neuroleptic withdrawal in schizophrenic patients: a review of the literature. *Arch Gen Psychiatry.* 1995;52:173-188.
9. Blackwell B. Drug deviation in psychiatric patients. In: Ayd FJ, ed. *The Future of Pharmacotherapy: New Drug Delivery Systems.* Baltimore, Md: International Drug Therapy Newsletter; 1973:17-31.
10. Smith RC. Lower-dose therapy with traditional neuroleptics in chronically hospitalized schizophrenic patients. *Arch Gen Psychiatry.* 1994;51: 427-429.
11. Inderbitzin LB, Lewine RR, Scheller-Gilkey G, Swofford CD, Egan GJ, Gloersen BA, Vidanagama BP, Waternaux C. A double-blind dose-reduction trial of fluphenazine decanoate for chronic, unstable schizophrenic patients. *Am J Psychiatry.* 1994;151:1753-1759.
12. Jeste DV, Potkin SG, Sinha S, Feder SL, Wyatt RJ. Tardive dyskinesia: reversible and persistent. *Arch Gen Psychiatry.* 1979;36:585-590.
13. McGlashan TH. A selective review of recent North American long-term followup studies of schizophrenia. *Schizophr Bull.* 1988;14:515-542.
14. Jeste DV, Lacro JP, Gilbert PL, Kline J, Kline N. Treatment of late-life schizophrenia with neuroleptics. *Schizophr Bull.* 1993;19:817-830.
15. Jeste DV, Lohr JB, Manley M. Study of neuropathologic changes in the striatum following four, eight and twelve months of treatment with fluphenazine in rats. *Psychopharmacology.* 1992; 106:154-160.
16. Benes FM, Paskevich PA, Domesick V. Haloperidol-induced plasticity of axon terminals in rat substantia nigra. *Science.* 1983;221:969-971.
17. Heaton R, Paulsen J, McAdams LA, Kuck J, Zisook S, Braff D, Harris MJ, Jeste DV. Neuropsychological deficits in schizophrenia: relationship to age, chronicity, and dementia. *Arch Gen Psychiatry.* 1994;51:469-476.
18. Weinberger DR, Jeste DV, Wyatt RJ, Teychenne PF. Cerebral atrophy in elderly schizophrenic patients: effects of aging and of long-term institutionalization and neuroleptic therapy. In: Miller NE, Cohen GD, eds. *Schizophrenia and Aging: Schizophrenia, Paranoid and Schizophreniform Disorders in Later Life.* New York, NY: Guilford Press; 1987:109-118.
19. Belitsky R, McGlashan TH. At issue: the manifestations of schizophrenia in late life, a dearth of data. *Schizophr Bull.* 1993;19:683-685.
20. Ciompi L. Catamnestic long-term study on the course of life and aging of schizophrenics. *Schizophr Bull.* 1980;6:606-618.
21. Marder SR, Meibach RC. Risperidone in the treatment of schizophrenia. *Am J Psychiatry.* 1994; 151:825-835.

ORIGINAL ARTICLE

Adrenal Gland Volume in Major Depression

Increase During the Depressive Episode and Decrease With Successful Treatment

Robert T. Rubin, MD, PhD; Jeffrey J. Phillips, MD; Todd F. Sadow, MD; James T. McCracken, MD

Background: Hyperactivity of the pituitary-adrenocortical axis is the most prominent neuroendocrine abnormality in major depression. It is state-related, returning to normal with resolution of the depressive episode. Adrenal gland enlargement also has been reported in patients with major depression and has been hypothesized as an index of cumulative lifetime depression. However, whether or not adrenal enlargement decreases with successful treatment of depression has not yet been studied, to our knowledge. We, therefore, determined adrenal gland volume in patients with major depression before and after treatment and in matched normal controls, and compared adrenal size with functional indexes of pituitary-adrenocortical activity.

Methods: Adrenal volumes were measured by magnetic resonance imaging in nine adult and two adolescent patients with major depression during their illness and during full remission when medication had been stopped for at least 1 month, and in nine adult and two adolescent normal control subjects individually matched to the patients. Basal, 4 to 7 PM plasma corticotropin 1-39 and cortisol levels, and corticotropin 1-39 and cortisol responses to administration of ovine corticorelin and low-dose cosyntropin also were measured.

Results: Mean adrenal gland volume was significantly larger, by about 70%, in the patients while depressed than after successful treatment, and it also was significantly larger, again by about 70%, than the mean adrenal gland volume of their matched controls. After treatment, the mean adrenal volume of the patients decreased and was no longer significantly different from that of their controls at baseline. The magnitude of the decrease was significantly positively correlated with the duration of the depressive episode. Basal, late-afternoon plasma corticotropin 1-39 levels were significantly lower in the patients while depressed than in their matched controls, but basal plasma cortisol levels did not differ significantly among the three groups, nor did the corticotropin 1-39 and cortisol responses to corticorelin or the cortisol response to cosyntropin. Correlations between adrenal gland volume and basal corticotropin and cortisol levels, and the corticotropin and cortisol responses to hormone challenge, were not consistently in the expected direction in any of the three groups of subjects.

Conclusions: Adrenal gland enlargement occurring during an episode of major depression appears to be state-dependent, in that it reverts to the normal size range during remission after treatment. It thus does not appear to be an index of cumulative lifetime depression. The lack of a discernible relationship between adrenal volume and pituitary-adrenocortical activity remains to be explained and might be related to noncorticotropin influences on the adrenal gland, including other trophic hormones and/or neural mechanisms.

(Arch Gen Psychiatry. 1995;52:213-218)

From the Neurosciences Research Center, Allegheny Campus of the Medical College of Pennsylvania and Hahnemann University, Pittsburgh (Dr Rubin); and Departments of Radiology (Dr Phillips) and Psychiatry (Drs Sadow and McCracken), Harbor–UCLA Medical Center, Torrance, Calif.

SEVERAL ABNORMALITIES of anterior pituitary and target endocrine gland hormone secretion patterns have been reported in patients with the endogenous subtype of major depression. The most prominent and well studied of these abnormalities is hyperactivity of the hypothalamopituitary-adrenocortical (HPA) axis.[1-5] Because hypertrophy of the adrenal glands can occur after long-term stimulation by corticotropin,[6] adrenal gland volume and weight have been measured in a few studies of patients with major depression or victims of violent suicide in whom depression before death was inferred.[7-11] Increases in volume and weight have been found in most studies, and it has been hypothesized that enlargement of the adrenal glands may be a measure of cumulative lifetime depression.[8]

See Subjects and Methods on next page

SUBJECTS AND METHODS

SUBJECTS

As part of a larger study of HPA axis function in 38 patients with major depression, nine adult and two adolescent depressed patients who responded fully to treatment were studied twice in the Clinical Research Center of the Harbor–UCLA Medical Center, Torrance, Calif, once while the patients were ill, before any treatment had been initiated, and again after recovery and discontinuation of antidepressant medication (where used). Nine adult and two adolescent normal control subjects, individually matched to each patient by age, sex, race, Tanner stage, height and weight, and menstrual status for the women, were studied once. Power analysis, based on previous reports of adrenal size differences between depressive patients and controls,[7,8] was used to determine sample sizes, with $\alpha=.01$ (two tailed) and $\beta=.90$.[12]

The patients were referred from the hospital psychiatric emergency and crisis clinics, from community psychiatric facilities and psychiatrists in private practice, and through public service announcements. The control subjects were recruited from hospital employees, their families and friends, and newspaper announcements.

Each patient and control was initially interviewed by the research coordinator. If the subject was suitable for study, the experimental protocol was explained in detail, and written informed consent was obtained. For the adolescents, written informed consent also was obtained from a parent or legal guardian.

Based on the Structured Clinical Interview for *DSM-III-R*,[13] conducted by a psychiatrist (R.T.R, T.F.S., or J.T.M.), each patient was classified according to *DSM-III-R*.[14] The Hamilton Depression Rating Scale[15] also was completed for each subject; only patients with *DSM-III-R* primary, major depression with a Hamilton score of 17 or greater (first 21 items) were included. The controls had no past or present psychiatric illness, as assessed with the nonpatient version of the Structured Clinical Interview for *DSM-III*, and their Hamilton scores were all 2 or less.

After the first testing, the patients were sent back to their referring physicians or to the psychiatric outpatient clinic for treatment. Their second testing occurred when they were recovered from their depressive episode (Hamilton scores ≤ 6) and, if medicated, to have had antidepressants discontinued for at least 1 month by their treating psychiatrists. (One patient never sought treatment and had an apparent spontaneous remission.) An average ($\pm$SD) of 11.4 ± 3.3 months elapsed between the first and second testings (range, 9 to 18 months). As mentioned, the controls were tested only once. Both groups of subjects were studied without regard to the season of the year.

A physical examination, urinalysis and urine screen for common drugs of abuse, M-300 blood chemistry panel, chest radiograph, and electrocardiogram (for the subjects older than 40 years) were obtained on each subject. Anyone with a history of concomitant psychiatric illness, such as schizophrenia, alcohol abuse, or drug abuse; with a history of major medical illness, such as hypertension, diabetes, or other endocrinopathy; with abnormal physical or laboratory findings; or who was taking any medication that might interfere with the endocrine testing was excluded.

Most of the patients had received little or no psychotropic medication in the weeks before the study. Those who had been treated underwent a 2- to 3-week drug washout period, under close clinical supervision, before neuroendocrine testing. For these patients, the depression rating scales were completed again, just before testing. These scores were used to meet the inclusion criteria specified above, and as the baseline values.

MR IMAGING OF THE ADRENAL GLANDS

Before any neuroendocrine testing, adrenal MR images were obtained with a 0.5-T superconducting magnet (Picker International, Highland Heights, Ohio). In all subjects, nongated spin-echo images were obtained in the axial plane, with 5-mm section thickness and no intersection gap. Relative T_1 weighting was achieved with a repetition time of 600 milliseconds and an echo time of 20 milliseconds, four signal averages, and a 256×192-pixel matrix. A field size of 46 cm was photographed at $\times2$ magnification to facilitate adrenal measurement. The same technician obtained all scans.

In the present study, we used magnetic resonance (MR) imaging to measure adrenal volumes in 11 patients with carefully diagnosed, unmedicated, major depression during their illness and while free of medication for at least 1 month after successful treatment, and in 11 normal control subjects individually matched to the patients by age, sex, race, height and weight, and menstrual status for the women. To relate functional measures of HPA axis activity to adrenal size, we also measured basal, late-afternoon circulating concentrations of corticotropin 1-39 and cortisol, and corticotropin 1-39 and cortisol responses to ovine corticorelin and cosyntropin administration, in these patients and controls. Our hypothesis was that these measures, including adrenal gland size, would reflect HPA axis hyperactivity in patients during the depressive episode and would return to control values after successful treatment.

RESULTS

The nine adult depressive patients had a median age of 46.0 years (range, 30 to 62 years), and eight were female. The two adolescent depressive patients were aged 14 and 15 years, both Tanner stage 4, and both were male. Ten patients had unipolar illness; one adult had bipolar illness. Of the eight women, three were premenopausal, one was postmenopausal with no hormonal replacement therapy, one had had a panhysterectomy and had no replacement therapy, and three either had had a panhysterectomy or were postmenopausal and were being treated with hormone replacement therapy, which was the same at the times of both studies. This consisted of conjugated estrogens, 1.25 to 3.0 mg/d, and for one postmenopausal patient and control, medroxyprogesterone

Contact prints were made of the adrenal gland images. In those sections in which the glands appeared, the left and right gland borders were traced by a radiologist (J.J.P.) with a cross-hair mouse on a graphics tablet (Kurta IS/ADB, Kurta Corp, Phoenix, Ariz) connected to a computer (Macintosh, Apple Corp, Cupertino, Calif). Software (MiniCad+ CAD, Graphsoft Inc, Ellicott City, Md) was used to calculate the area of each tracing in square centimeters. For precision, each section was traced five times; the five areas were averaged, summed across sections, and divided by two (sections 5 mm thick) to yield the volume of each gland in milliliters.[16] We previously showed that adrenal volumes determined with MR imaging correlate extremely well with those determined by computed tomography (CT) and that, with the scanners we used, MR imaging yielded volumes of phantoms closer to their physically measured volumes than did CT.[16] The radiologist was unaware of diagnosis (patient or control), and patient and control adrenal glands were assessed in random order.

NEUROENDOCRINE PROTOCOL

Each subject was admitted to the Clinical Research Center at 2 PM on two separate days about a week apart. Shortly after admission, indwelling 21-gauge "butterfly" needles were inserted into a vein in each arm. All subjects were ambulatory. A standard hospital dinner was served at 5 PM. Blood sampling, 7 mL every 30 minutes, was begun at 4 PM and continued for 3 hours. At 7 PM, either ovine corticorelin, 1.0 μg/kg, or cosyntropin (Cortrosyn, Organon Inc, West Orange, NJ), 0.1 μg/kg, was given intravenously as a bolus. The low dose of cosyntropin was used to test adrenal sensitivity, rather than maximal secretory capacity as with the usual 250-μg dose. The order of testing was randomized. Blood sampling was continued from the other arm every 15 minutes until 8 PM and then every 30 minutes until 11 PM. Each sample was drawn into a chilled syringe, placed into chilled plastic tubes containing 100 μL of 15% edetic acid and 50 μL of 20% sodium azide, and centrifuged under refrigeration for 15 minutes at 500g. Aliquots of plasma were pipetted into 1.5-mL conical polypropylene tubes, capped, and frozen until analysis for corticotropin 1-39 and cortisol.

HORMONE ASSAYS

All samples from each patient's first study and his or her matched control were analyzed in duplicate in the same assay. The samples from the patients' second studies, which were done many months later, also were analyzed in duplicate, but in separate assays. Control serum was analyzed in each assay for the determination of interassay variability. Cortisol was analyzed by radioimmunoassay, the details of which (characteristics of tracer and antibody, assay sensitivity, interassay and intra-assay variability) have been given earlier.[4] Corticotropin 1-39 was analyzed by a highly specific immunoradiometric assay (Nichols Institute, San Juan Capistrano, Calif). Interassay and intra-assay coefficients of variation were 7% and 3%, respectively, and assay sensitivity was 1.0 pg/mL. All hormone values were computed by means of log-logit transformation and a noniterated, unweighted regression of the standard curve, followed by dose interpolation of the samples.[17]

STATISTICAL ANALYSIS

The seven blood samples taken between 4 and 7 PM, before corticorelin or cosyntropin administration, were averaged across both sessions and used as the measure of baseline hormone secretion. Intersession coefficients of variation averaged 17% for cortisol and 23% for corticotropin 1-39. For cortisol, we have shown that the 4 to 7 PM baseline is an estimator of cortisol secretion comparable with the 24-hour average value or the 16-hour postdexamethasone value.[18] The area under the curve for the blood samples taken between 7:15 and 11 PM, after corticorelin or cosyntropin administration, was calculated by the trapezoidal rule and used as the measure of the hormone response to challenge.

Some of the adrenal volume, corticotropin 1-39, and cortisol data were log-distributed across the depressive patients and the controls. Therefore, median values and first and third quartiles are presented. Because the controls were individually matched to the patients, repeated-measures analyses of variance were used as the initial test, and paired t tests were used for multiple comparisons when significant F ratios were present. All reported significance levels are two tailed.

as well. One premenopausal and one postmenopausal patient also were receiving low-dose thyroid replacement, which was the same at both studies.

The depressive patients were all outpatients at the time of the first study. None met criteria for *DSM-III-R* melancholia, and none had psychotic features. They had had a median of two depressive episodes during their lives (range, two to four), and the median length of their present episode was 3.2 months (range, 2 to 72 months). The mean (±SD) 21-item Hamilton Depression Rating Scale total score for the patients was 25.4±4.6 (median, 27) at the time of the first testing, before treatment, and 2.5±2.5 (median, 2) at the second testing, after successful treatment.

As mentioned above, 11.3±3.3 months elapsed between the first and the second testing in the patients. During this time they had no major illnesses, but they did have occasional upper respiratory tract and other minor illnesses. Their long-term medication regimen was similar at both times, eg, thyroid or estrogen replacement, as noted above. As also mentioned above, the control subjects were chosen on a post hoc basis to be matched individually to the patients, thereby controlling for the diversity of the patients in age, sex, menstrual status in the women, and body surface area (a measure derived from height and weight). The mean Hamilton scale total score for the controls was less than 1 (median, 0).

The **Table** presents values for Hamilton scale total score, body surface area, adrenal gland total volume, and basal, corticorelin-stimulated, and cosyntropin-stimulated pituitary-adrenocortical hormone measures for the depressive patients before and after treatment and for their matched controls. Also given in the Table are the re-

Subject Characteristics and Physiologic Measures in 11 Patients With Major Depression Compared With Matched Normal Controls*

	Patients				
	Pretreatment (N=11)	Posttreatment (N=11)	Controls (N=11)	Repeated-Measures ANOVA	*P*, by Multiple Comparisons Paired *t* Tests
Hamilton Depression Scale (24-item), total score	27 (21-28)	2 (0-6)	0 (0-1)	...	...
Body surface area, m²	1.77±0.28	1.80±0.30	1.73±0.16	F=0.96; *P*<.50	...
Adrenal gland total volume, mL	5.7 (3.6-6.2)	2.9 (2.5-5.7)	3.4 (3.2-3.6)	F=5.44; *P*<.02	Pretreatment>posttreatment (<.008); pretreatment>control (<.02)
4-7 PM corticotropin 1-39, pmol/L	0.71 (0.28-1.57)	1.15 (0.91-1.51)	1.73 (0.98-2.28)	F=4.41; *P*<.03	Pretreatment<control (<.03)
4-7 PM cortisol, nmol/L	148 (42-190)	113 (81-178)	131 (123-174)	F=0.19; *P*<.90	...
Corticotropin 1-39 AUC† after corticorelin, 10³ pmol/L × min	0.52 (0.36-1.72)	1.51 (0.84-2.24)	1.16 (0.87-1.70)	F=1.66; *P*<.25	...
Cortisol AUC† after corticorelin, 10³ nmol/L × min	92 (14-114)	98 (70-133)	82 (72-121)	F=1.40; *P*<.30	...
Cortisol AUC† after cosyntropin, 10³ nmol/L × min	103 (21-116)	94 (80-132)	98 (89-121)	F=2.04; *P*<.20	...

*Values are given as mean±SD or as median (first and third quartiles) where data were not gaussian-distributed across subjects. ANOVA indicates analysis of variance.

†AUC indicates area under the curve during the 4 hours of sampling (7 to 11 PM).

sults of the repeated-measures analyses of variance and multiple comparisons performed for the analyses of variance that were significant. The Hamilton scale total score fell markedly between illness and recovery in the patients (a criterion for retesting). Body surface area was not significantly different between the patients at either testing and their controls, indicating good matching on this variable. (Body surface area of the patients during illness and recovery correlated at .99; at these two times it correlated at .72 and .67, respectively, with the body surface area of the controls, another indication of the strength of matching on this variable.) Similarly, height and weight, the two variables used in the calculation of body surface area, were not significantly different between the patients at either testing and their controls (data not shown).

Adrenal gland total volume was significantly greater, by about 70%, in the patients while depressed than after successful treatment (*P*<.008), and it also was significantly larger, again by about 70%, than the adrenal gland volume of their matched controls (*P*<.013). During remission, the adrenal volume of the patients was not significantly different from that of their controls (*P*<.60), indicating a reduction in adrenal gland volume with resolution of the depressive episode. The correlations between body surface area and adrenal volume ranged between .45 and .62 for all three groups, consistent with our previous findings in normal subjects.[16]

There was no significant effect of the order of testing (ie, the first vs the second day of the challenge tests) on any of the baseline hormone values. Basal plasma corticotropin 1-39 levels were significantly lower in the patients while depressed than in their matched controls (*P*<.025), but basal plasma cortisol levels did not differ significantly among the three groups (*P*<.90). The corticotropin 1-39 response to corticorelin in the patients while depressed was less than half that after recovery, but the differences across the three groups were not significant (*P*<.25). Neither the cortisol response to corticorelin nor its response to cosyntropin differed significantly among the three groups (*P*<.30 and <.20, respectively).

The correlations between adrenal gland volume and basal corticotropin 1-39 and cortisol levels, and the corticotropin 1-39 and cortisol responses to hormone challenge, were not consistently in the expected direction in any of the three groups of subjects. In the patients while depressed, adrenal volume correlated nonsignificantly with Hamilton total score, duration of the present episode, and number of episodes (*r*=−.03, .23, and −.44, respectively). With body surface area partialed out, these correlations remained nonsignificant (.18, .32, and −.28). In the patients, the correlation between the magnitude of the decrease in adrenal volume between depression and recovery and the number of depressive episodes was nonsignificant (*r*=.34, and .19 with body surface area partialed out). However, the decrease in adrenal volume between depression and recovery was significantly positively correlated with the duration of the present depressive episode before treatment (*r*=.63; with body surface area partialed out, *r*=.66; both *P*<.05).

COMMENT

The most striking finding of this study was the approximately 70% larger adrenal gland volume (median, 5.7 mL), as determined by MR imaging, in the depressed patients while they were ill compared with both their adrenal volume after successful treatment (median, 2.9 mL) and the adrenal gland volume of their matched normal controls (median, 3.4 mL) studied once at baseline. Larger adrenal glands in patients before treatment compared with controls have been noted in the few previous studies of adrenal volume in depression. Amsterdam et al,[7] using CT, reported a mean (±SD) total adrenal gland volume of 4.5±1.9 mL for 13 female and three male patients with major depression compared with 3.5±0.45 mL for seven female and four male normal control subjects, a nonsignificant 28% difference. In contrast, Nemeroff et al,[8] also using CT, reported a significant ($P<.008$) 57% greater mean total adrenal volume of 14.0±5.9 mL for 16 female and 20 male patients with major depression, compared with a mean volume of 8.9±2.5 mL for four female and seven male controls. Dorovini-Zis and Zis[9] reported the mean (±SD) total adrenal gland weight of 16 persons who committed violent suicide as 9.77±1.74 g, vs 7.74±0.82 g for 10 persons who died suddenly of traumatic or natural causes, a 26% difference that was highly significant ($P<.001$). By inference, the suicide victims had psychiatric illnesses, of which about 50% were most likely depressive. Similarly, Szigethy et al[11] reported a significantly greater ($P<.02$) mean (±SEM) total adrenal weight of 11.3±0.9 g for 12 suicide victims compared with 9.3±0.4 g for 22 controls with sudden death. However, Stein et al[10] did not find a significant difference in adrenal weights between 21 violent suicide victims and 88 controls with sudden death (the mean total adrenal weights of both groups were the largest of all the studies to date, being 14 to 16 g).

THE RESULTS among these studies, including the present one, are reasonably consistent, but there are important methodologic differences in type of subjects studied (patients with major depression, suicide victims), age and sex of the patients (we included adult and adolescent depressive patients), technique of gland measurement (CT, MR imaging, autopsy), sample size, degree of matching of controls to patients, and method of statistical analysis. These issues have been addressed in detail elsewhere.[19] With regard to the present study, an important methodologic issue was our inability, for logistic reasons, to study the controls a second time, close to the retesting of the patients to whom they were matched. We thus do not have direct information concerning MR imaging test-retest variability in the controls, as background for the changes in the patients. However, several factors militate against our findings' being primarily the result of measurement or other error: (1) the large decrease in adrenal volume in the patients after treatment; (2) the fact that pretreatment and posttreatment patient and control MR images and tracings were intermixed, with no general trend, either upward or downward, in adrenal size measurements from the start to the end of the study; and (3) the significant, positive correlation between the magnitude of the decrease in adrenal volume between depression and recovery and the duration of the preceding depressive episode, suggesting by inference that there was an original increase in adrenal size from preepisode baseline that was related to episode duration.

An important issue that concerns the Amsterdam et al,[7] Nemeroff et al,[8] and present studies is the reported lack of relationship between adrenal gland size and several indexes of pituitary-adrenocortical function. Amsterdam et al[7] found no significant correlation between adrenal volume and either baseline 9 AM serum cortisol levels or 4 PM postdexamethasone serum cortisol levels in their depressed patients. Similarly, Nemeroff et al[8] found no significant correlation between adrenal volume and 3 or 10 PM postdexamethasone cortisol values in their depressive patients. Finally, as mentioned above, in our subjects the correlations between adrenal volume and baseline plasma corticotropin 1-39 and cortisol levels, and corticotropin 1-39 and cortisol responses to corticorelin and cosyntropin administration, were not consistently in the expected direction. This lack of a significant relationship between increased adrenal gland size and functional indexes of pituitary-adrenocortical activity is of interest, in view of the well-established fact that increased stimulation of the adrenal gland by corticotropin ultimately leads to increased steroid output and glandular hypertrophy. The different measures of HPA axis activity used in the three studies, the potential time lag between changes in trophic hormone levels and reactive changes in gland size, and the need to control for other determinants of adrenal size, such as body surface area and season of the year, make inferences from these studies difficult. In the present study, the lack of a significant positive correlation between adrenal volume and the cortisol response to cosyntropin also may have been related to the low cosyntropin dose used; a supramaximal stimulatory dose, eg, 250 μg, which tests adrenal secretory capacity, might have yielded a different result.

Factors other than corticotropin also might have been responsible for the alterations in adrenal gland size, without necessarily having influenced corticosteroid output to a similar degree. Two categories of potential stimuli are neurochemical and neurohormonal and neural.[6,20] With regard to the former, the NH_2 terminal fragment of proopiomelanocortin, epidermal and fibroblast growth factors, insulinlike growth factor I (somatomedin C), and angiotensin II all have been implicated.[6,20] Although increased plasma, cerebrospinal fluid, and urinary epinephrine concentrations have been found in patients with major depression,[21,22] it is unlikely that adrenal medullary changes underlie the increased gland size; the medulla represents only about 10% of adrenal mass.[23,24] Also, adrenal medullary volume in rats is unchanged after long-term corticotropin stimulation, in contrast to the hypertrophy that occurs in all layers of the cortex.[25]

With regard to neural influences, there is autonomic innervation of the adrenal cortex in humans as well as in other species: postganglionic unmyelinated fibers with vesicle-containing terminal boutons have been demonstrated in proximity to endocrine cells in the human zona fasciculata.[26] In rats, unilateral adrenalectomy results an approximately 25% increase in the weight of the remaining adrenal gland within 3 days, which is sustained for 10 days.[27] This compensatory hypertrophy is abolished by hypothalamic lesions on the ipsilateral, but not the contralateral, side of the remaining gland, indicating that it is neurally mediated. We currently have no evidence of the function of any non-corticotropin–mediated mechanisms in the adrenal enlargement that occurs in depressed patients, but their possible role must be kept in mind.

Finally, the return of adrenal volume to control values with remission of the depressive episode in our patients, and the lack of a significant positive correlation between the number of depressive episodes and either adrenal gland volume during depression or the decrease in adrenal volume between depression and recovery, argue against the hypothesis of Nemeroff et al[8] that adrenal gland enlargement may be a measure of cumulative lifetime depression.

Accepted for publication December 13, 1994.

This study was supported by research grant MH28380 (Dr Rubin), Research Scientist Award MH47363 (Dr Rubin), and Physician Scientist Award MH00722 (Dr McCracken) from the National Institute of Mental Health, Rockville, Md, and grant RR00425 from the National Institutes of Health, Bethesda, Md (to the Harbor–UCLA Clinical Research Center).

Sylvia Williams, PA, and Scott McGeoy provided valuable technical assistance.

Reprint requests to Neurosciences Research Center, Allegheny Campus, Medical College of Pennsylvania and Hahnemann University, 320 E North Ave, Pittsburgh, PA 15212-4772 (Dr Rubin).

REFERENCES

1. Carroll BJ, Feinberg M, Greden JF, Tarika J, Albala AA, Haskett RF, James NM, Kronfol Z, Lohr N, Steiner M, de Vigne JP, Young E. A specific laboratory test for the diagnosis of melancholia: standardization, validation, and clinical utility. *Arch Gen Psychiatry.* 1981;38:15-22.
2. Gold PW, Chrousos G, Kellner C, Post R, Roy A, Augerinos P, Schulte H, Oldfield E, Loriaux DL. Psychiatric implications of basic and clinical studies with corticotropin-releasing factor. *Am J Psychiatry.* 1984;141:619-627.
3. Arana GW, Baldessarini RJ, Ornsteen M. The dexamethasone suppression test for diagnosis and prognosis in psychiatry: commentary and review. *Arch Gen Psychiatry.* 1985;42:1193-1204.
4. Rubin RT, Poland RE, Lesser IM, Winston RA, Blodgett ALN. Neuroendocrine aspects of primary endogenous depression, I: cortisol secretory dynamics in patients and matched control subjects. *Arch Gen Psychiatry.* 1987;44:329-336.
5. Rubin RT. Pharmacoendocrinology of major depression. *Eur Arch Psychiatr Neurol Sci.* 1989;238:259-267.
6. Orth DN, Kovacs WJ, DeBold CR. The adrenal cortex. In: Wilson JD, Foster DW, eds. *Williams Textbook of Endocrinology.* 8th ed. Philadelphia, Pa: WB Saunders Co; 1992:489-619.
7. Amsterdam JD, Marinelli DL, Arger P, Winokur A. Assessment of adrenal gland volume by computed tomography in depressed patients and healthy volunteers: a pilot study. *Psychiatry Res.* 1987;21:189-197.
8. Nemeroff CB, Krishnan KRR, Reed D, Leder R, Beam C, Dunnick NR. Adrenal gland enlargement in major depression: a computed tomographic study. *Arch Gen Psychiatry.* 1992;49:384-387.
9. Dorovini-Zis K, Zis AP. Increased adrenal weight in victims of violent suicide. *Am J Psychiatry.* 1987;144:1214-1215.
10. Stein E, McCrank E, Schaeffer B, Goyer R. Adrenal gland weight and suicide. *Can J Psychiatry* 1993;38:563-566.
11. Szigethy E, Conwell Y, Forbes NT, Cox C, Caine ED. Adrenal weight and morphology in victims of completed suicide. *Biol Psychiatry.* 1994;36:374-380.
12. Cohen J. *Statistical Power Analysis for the Behavioral Sciences.* 2nd ed. Hillsdale, NJ: Lawrence Erlbaum Associates; 1988.
13. Spitzer RL, Williams JBW, Gibbon M, First MB. *Structured Clinical Interview for DSM-III-R.* Washington, DC: American Psychiatric Press; 1990.
14. American Psychiatric Association. *Diagnostic and Statistical Manual of Mental Disorders, Revised Third Edition.* Washington, DC: American Psychiatric Press; 1987.
15. Hamilton M. Development of a rating scale for primary depressive illness. *Br J Soc Clin Psychol.* 1967;6:278-296.
16. Rubin RT, Phillips JJ. Adrenal gland volume determination by computed tomography and magnetic resonance imaging in normal subjects. *Invest Radiol.* 1991;26:465-469.
17. Chang PC, Rubin RT, Yu M. Optimal statistical design of radioimmunoassays and competitive protein binding assays. *Endocrinology.* 1975;96:973-981.
18. Thompson LM, Rubin RT, McCracken JT. Neuroendocrine aspects of primary endogenous depression, XII: receiver operating characteristic and kappa analyses of serum and urine cortisol measures in patients and matched controls. *Psychoneuroendocrinology.* 1992;17:507-515.
19. Rubin RT, Phillips JJ. Adrenal gland volume in major depressives. *Arch Gen Psychiatry.* 1993;50:833-834.
20. Hornsby PJ. The regulation of adrenocortical function by control of growth and structure. In: Anderson DC, Winter JSD, eds. *Adrenal Cortex.* London, England: Butterworths; 1985:1-31.
21. Wyatt RJ, Portnoy B, Kupfer DJ, Snyder F, Engelman K. Resting plasma catecholamine concentrations in patients with depression and anxiety. *Arch Gen Psychiatry.* 1971;24:65-70.
22. Davis JM, Koslow SH, Gibbons RD, Maas JW, Bowden CL, Casper R, Hanin I, Javaid JI, Chang SS, Stokes PE. Cerebrospinal fluid and urinary biogenic amines in depressed patients and healthy controls. *Arch Gen Psychiatry.* 1988;45:705-717.
23. Neville AM, O'Hare MJ. *The Human Adrenal Cortex.* Berlin, Germany: Springer-Verlag; 1982:16.
24. Landsberg L, Young JB. Catecholamines and the adrenal medulla. In: Wilson JD, Foster DW, eds. *Williams Textbook of Endocrinology.* 8th ed. Philadelphia, Pa: WB Saunders Co; 1992:621-705.
25. Malendowicz K. A correlated stereological and functional studies on the long-term effects of ACTH on rat adrenal cortex. *Folia Hist Cytobiol.* 1986;24:203-212.
26. Dorovini-Zis K, Zis AP. Innervation of the zona fasciculata of the adult human adrenal cortex: a light and electron microscopic study. *J Neural Transm.* 1991;84:75-84.
27. Engeland WC, Dallman MF. Compensatory adrenal growth is neurally mediated. *Neuroendocrinology.* 1975;19:352-362.

ORIGINAL ARTICLE

Prevalence and Correlates of Drug Use and Dependence in the United States

Results From the National Comorbidity Survey

Lynn A. Warner, MPP; Ronald C. Kessler, PhD; Michael Hughes, PhD; James C. Anthony, PhD; Christopher B. Nelson, MPH

Objectives: To analyze nationally representative data on the lifetime and 12-month prevalences of use of and dependence on illegal drugs (marijuana/hashish, cocaine/crack, heroin, hallucinogens), nonmedical prescription psychotropic drugs (sedatives, tranquilizers, stimulants, analgesics), and inhalants; and to examine data on the sociodemographic correlates of use and dependence.

Methods: The data come from the National Comorbidity Survey, a structured diagnostic interview administered to persons aged 15 to 54 years that generates reliable diagnoses according to the definitions and criteria of *DSM-III-R*.

Results: Of the respondents, 51.0% used one of the above drugs at some time in their lives, and 15.4% did so in the past 12 months. These estimates are similar to those obtained in the 1991 National Household Survey of Drug Abuse, where lifetime prevalence was 45.2% and 12-month prevalence was 16.7% among respondents in the age range 15 to 54 years. Of National Comorbidity Survey respondents, 7.5% (14.7% of lifetime users) were dependent at some time in their lives and 1.8% were dependent in the past 12 months. The prevalence estimate for lifetime dependence was reduced to 5.3% when calculated the percentage of respondents in the age range of 28 to 54 years who reported an onset of dependence as of 10 years earlier (ie, when they were 18 to 44 years old) was computed. This is similar to the Epidemiologic Catchment Area Study estimate of 5.1% among respondents in the age range 18 to 44 years, a comparison that matches the two studies on year of assessment, age of risk, and cohort. Males were significantly more likely to report both lifetime and 12-month use and dependence. Use and dependence were found to be more common in cohorts born after World War II than those born before the end of the war. The demographic predictors of lifetime use differed from the predictors of lifetime dependence among users, and these, in turn, differed from the predictors of recent dependence among people with a lifetime history of dependence.

Conclusions: Drug use and dependence are highly prevalent in the general population. The fact that there are differences in the correlates of first use, dependence among users, and persistence of dependence means that future research aimed at pinpointing modifiable risk factors must be based on disaggregated analyses of separate stages of progression.

(Arch Gen Psychiatry. 1995;52:219-229)

SEVERAL ONGOING national data collection systems are currently in place to gauge drug use levels and trends.[1] These include the Drug Abuse Warning Network,[2] which tracks the prevalence of drug mentions in emergency department admissions and medical examiners' death records; the National Household Survey on Drug Abuse,[3] which tracks the prevalence of drug use in the total national household population aged 12 years and over; and the High School Senior Survey,[4] which tracks the prevalence of drug use among junior high, high school, college, and young adult populations and, beginning in 1993, school dropouts. While all of these systems include some information about problems caused by drug use, they have been criticized because none produces accurate estimates of the prevalence of drug abuse or drug dependence.[5,6] Without such information, it is difficult to assess the full magnitude of the nation's drug problem.

Although a number of surveys have reported estimates of drug abuse or dependence in particular communities and regions,[7,8] the landmark Epidemiologic Catchment Area (ECA) Study is the only large-scale general population survey to have produced national esti-

From the Institute for Social Research (Ms Warner, Dr Kessler, and Mr Nelson) and the Department of Sociology (Dr Kessler), The University of Michigan, Ann Arbor; Department of Sociology, Virginia Polytechnic Institute and State University, Blacksburg (Dr Hughes); and Department of Mental Hygiene, The Johns Hopkins University, Baltimore, Md (Dr Anthony).

See Materials and Methods on next page

MATERIALS AND METHODS

SAMPLE

The NCS is based on a stratified, multistage area probability sample of persons aged 15 to 54 years in the noninstitutionalized civilian population in the 48 coterminous states as well as a representative supplemental sample of students living in campus group housing. Fieldwork was carried out by the staff of the Survey Research Center at the University of Michigan, Ann Arbor, between September 14, 1990, and February 6, 1992. Interviewers were carefully trained and closely monitored throughout the data collection period. The response rate was 82.4%, with a total of 8098 participants. A more detailed discussion of the NCS sampling design is presented elsewhere.[11]

Because of previous evidence that survey nonrespondents have more psychiatric disorders than respondents,[12,13] a supplemental nonresponse survey was conducted in tandem with the main NCS survey. A financial incentive was offered to a random sample of initial nonrespondents to complete a short form of the diagnostic interview. The 353 completed short forms disclosed higher rates of both lifetime and current psychiatric disorders among initial nonrespondents than among initial respondents. These results were used to construct a nonresponse adjustment weight for the main survey data to compensate for this systematic nonresponse. A second weight was used to adjust for variation in probabilities of selection both within and between households. A third weight, finally, was used to poststratify the data to approximate the national population distribution of the cross-classification of age, sex, race/ethnicity, marital status, education, living arrangement, region, and urbanicity as defined by the 1989 US National Health Interview Survey.[14] Comparisons between the NCS and National Health Interview Survey results are presented in **Table 1**.

DIAGNOSTIC ASSESSMENT

The NCS questions on illicit drug use and nonmedical use of prescription drugs were based on those asked in the National Household Survey on Drug Abuse (NHSDA).[3] The question series began by defining nonmedical use as use (1) without a physician's prescription, (2) in greater amounts than prescribed, or (3) more frequently than prescribed. Respondents were then asked about their lifetime and recent nonmedical use of each of four categories of prescription drugs (sedatives, tranquilizers, stimulants, and analgesics). This was followed by questions concerning the use of four categories of illicit drugs (marijuana/hashish, cocaine/crack, hallucinogens, and heroin) and inhalants. The procedures of the NHSDA were followed in providing a detailed verbal definition and illustrative list of qualifying drugs in each category before inquiring about use.

The NCS deviated from the procedures of the NHSDA in three major respects. First, questions were interviewer-administered rather than self-administered. This change in procedures was dictated by the requirement that the interviewer know about the respondent's drug use to administer subsequent questions about dependence. Second, we did not use the colored pill card employed in the NHSDA in asking about use of prescription psychotropic drugs. Third, we included a screening question that does not exist in the NHSDA concerning dependence in the absence of nonmedical use of prescription drugs, namely, whether persons who used prescription drugs under the supervision of a physician ever believed that they could not stop or that they were dependent even though they were following the physician's directions concerning amount and frequency of use.

Lifetime use of a drug, for purposes of this article, was defined as having tried at least one of the above drugs at least one time, excluding medical use that did not lead to feelings of dependence. As in the ECA Study, further questions that assess dependence were asked only of lifetime users. Our NCS definition of use, however, was more inclusive than the ECA definition in two ways. First, the ECA did not include people who were using a prescription drug under the supervision of a physician even if the patient felt dependent. Second, the ECA assessed dependence only among those who had used a drug more than five times in their lives, while the NCS considered a respondent a user even if he or she had used only one time.

Dependence was defined according to the definitions and criteria of *DSM-III-R*.[15] The NCS questions used to generate this diagnosis are based on the Composite International Diagnostic Interview,[16] a state-of-the-art structured diagnostic instrument designed for use by trained

mates of the prevalence of these disorders.[9] Unfortunately, representativeness of these estimates can be called into question because the five community samples that made up the ECA were not nationally representative.[10] Furthermore, the ECA estimates are now more than a decade old.

This article presents updated estimates of the prevalence of drug use and dependence in the US household population on the basis of the National Comorbidity Survey (NCS). The NCS was designed to take the next step beyond the ECA by administering a structured psychiatric diagnostic interview to a nationally representative sample of the noninstitutionalized population and using these data to calculate the prevalence of and risk factors for psychiatric disorders in the United States.

RESULTS

THE PREVALENCE OF LIFETIME AND 12-MONTH USE

The NCS estimates of lifetime and 12-month prevalence of drug use are presented in **Table 2** separately by age and sex of respondents. Overall, somewhat more than half of respondents (51.0%) reported using an illegal drug or nonmedically using a prescription drug at least once in their lives, and 15.4% reported having done so in the past 12 months. Males were significantly more likely than females to have used a controlled substance both in their lifetimes (55.8% vs 46.4%, t=4.7, P<.001) and in the past 12 months interviewers who are not clinicians.[17] World Health Organization field trials of the Composite International Diagnostic Interview have documented high interrater reliability,[18,19] test-retest reliability,[20,21] and validity of the diagnosis of psychoactive substance dependence.[22-28]

A lifetime diagnosis of dependence, generated by the Composite International Diagnostic Interview diagnostic computer program,[29] requires the respondent to have at least three of nine *DSM-III-R* criterion A symptoms at some time in his or her life (eg, developing tolerance; experiencing withdrawal; unsuccessfully attempting to control use; continuing use despite the recognition that it is related to social, psychological, or physical problems) and to fulfill the requirements of criterion B by endorsing two or more Composite International Diagnostic Interview questions concerning duration of symptoms over a period of at least 1 month or repeatedly over a longer period. Consistent with *DSM-III-R*, no requirement is imposed for the criterion A symptoms to cluster in time for a diagnosis of lifetime dependence. Our definition of 12-month prevalence, in comparison, required a clustering of three or more criterion A symptoms in the 12 months before the interview in the subsample of respondents who qualified for lifetime diagnosis.

ANALYSIS PROCEDURES

Data analyses included the estimation of lifetime and 12-month prevalences, the estimation of cohort-specific cumulative age-at-onset prevalence curves, and the estimation of demographic correlates of use and dependence. Prevalence analyses were stratified by sex on the basis of well-documented evidence of a sex difference in drug use and disorder rates.[3,9,30-35]

Because of the complex sample design and weighting, SEs of the estimates could not be based on conventional methods. In the case of the lifetime and 12-month prevalences, SEs were obtained by means of the Taylor series linearization method.[36] The PSRATIO program in the OSIRIS IV software package[37] was used to make these calculations. We calculated *t* tests for sex differences in proportions of use and dependence on the basis of these SEs.

Cumulative age-at-onset curves were generated by means of the survival analysis methods operationalized in the SURVIVAL program in the SPSS-X software package.[38] Prevalences were estimated within 10-year cohorts for 5-year age intervals (eg, cumulative lifetime prevalences by the ages of 4, 9, 14, 19, and 24 years among respondents in the age range 15 to 24 years at the time of the interview). Cumulative prevalences for ages that exceeded the current ages of some cohort members (eg, cumulative prevalence by age 24 years in the cohort currently between the ages of 15 and 24 years) were based on the at-risk subsample of the cohort at the beginning of the 5-year interval (eg, the subsample of the 15- to 24-year-old cohort currently between the ages of 19 and 24 years). Individuals in this subsample were assumed to have experienced half of the year in which they were censored. Among those with a first onset in the interval, this meant assuming that they had an onset in the middle of the year of their reported age at onset, while among those with no lifetime history, it meant assuming that they were in the middle of the year of risk corresponding to their age at interview. Discrete-time (person-year) survival files[39] were analyzed to generate z statistics to assess significant intercohort differences in the slopes of the cumulative onset curves. The survival models were conceptualized as nested logistic regression equations,[40] in which age, cohort, and age-by-cohort interactions were treated as predictors. Design-based estimates of the SEs were obtained by the method of balanced repeated replications in 44 balanced subsamples.[41,42] The balanced repeated replication estimates take into account the clustering and weighting of the data without the linearization constraint required in the Taylor series method, yielding somewhat less biased estimates of SEs and confidence intervals in nonlinear models, such as logistic regression.[43] The LOGISTIC module in SAS-UNIX (version 6.07) was used to make these calculations, while a SAS macro was used to compute the SEs on the basis of comparison of estimates across the replicates.

Odds ratios for the demographic correlates of use and dependence were derived by exponentiating the logistic regression coefficients, and design-based estimates of the confidence intervals were generated by the same balanced repeated replication methods described above. An odds ratio of 1.0, or indistinguishable from 1.0 as bounded by the 95% confidence interval, was considered insignificant. Significance tests were made without adjustments for multiple tests.

(18.4% vs 12.4%, t=4.9, P<.001). There was also a powerful inverse relationship between age and 12-month use, from a high of 23.8% among respondents in the age range 15 to 24 years to a low of 5.5% among respondents in the age range 45 to 54 years.

The association between age and lifetime use was complicated by the fact that there was both a positive association between age and years of risk and a negative association between cohort and age-specific risk. A disaggregation of this complex pattern is presented in **Figure 1**, where respondent reports on their age of first use are presented in curves for the age-specific cumulative probabilities of lifetime use separately for each of the four 10-year birth cohorts in the NCS. Cohort 1 (born in 1966 to 1975) includes the youngest NCS respondents, while cohort 4 (born in 1936 to 1945) includes the oldest. It is useful to recognize, in studying Figure 1, that respondents in cohort 4, the only NCS respondents born before the end of World War II, would normally have completed high school by the mid-1960s, before the widespread introduction of marijuana and subsequently other illicit drugs into youth culture.[30,44-46] Cohort 3 went through adolescence in the early years of the youth drug culture, cohort 2 at its height, and cohort 1 during the years of downturn in drug use that has taken place during the last decade.

These differences in cohort experience are reflected in the cohort-specific age trends in Figure 1. The age-at-onset curve in cohort 4 shows that cumulative prevalence of drug use did not begin to rise until middle adolescence (15- to 19-year age range), at the end of which only about 7% of the cohort had any experience with drugs. Cumulative prevalence increased to approximately 13% by the end of late adolescence (20- to 24-year age range) and continued in roughly linear fashion through the present. The curves in the three more recent cohorts, in comparison, show uniform evidence of a dramatic rise in first use between early adolescence (10- to 14-year age range) and late adolescence, at which time 48% of cohort 3, 63% of cohort 2, and 57% of cohort 1 had used drugs at least once. The slopes of the onset curves become flatter after late adolescence. Consistent with the fact that respondents in cohort 2 were adolescents during the height of the youth drug culture, the onset curve is consistently higher in cohort 2 than in either cohort 1 or cohort 3 beginning in the age range 15 to 19 years.

Significance tests for intercohort differences in the slope of the onset curve between early adolescence and late adolescence (10- to 24-year age range) documented a significantly less steep slope among respondents in cohort 4 than in the three more recent cohorts (z=3.2, P=.001) as well as a significant difference between the two most recent cohorts, with the slope for cohort 2 significantly more steep than that for cohort 1 (z=2.4, P=.004). Contrasts between cohorts 1 and 3 and cohorts 2 and 3 in the survival models failed to show significant differences. An evaluation of differences in the cumulative probability of use as of the end of late adolescence (ages 20 to 24 years) showed that differences were significant between all pairs of cohorts (z tests between 2.1 and 22.4 for pairwise comparisons, with P between .009 and .001). This means that the lower cumulative probability of use in cohort 1 compared with cohort 2 at this age likely represents a genuine decrease rather than a sampling artifact. There are also significant differences in the survival models in the slopes of the onset curves in the years after late adolescence (cohort 2 vs cohort 4, z=2.1, P=.009; cohort 3 vs cohort 4, z=3.6, P<.001; cohort 2 vs cohort 3, z=1.3, P=.05), showing that first use after late adolescence was more common in cohort 4 than the more recent cohorts.

Sex-specific cohort differences in drug use are presented in **Table 3**. For both males and females the probability of use by age 24 years was lower in the youngest cohort (cohort 1) than cohort 2 (63% vs 68% for males; 51% vs 58% for females). The table also indicates that for both sexes in the three youngest cohorts, most first use occurred in the age range 15 to 19 years, with little initiation after the age of 20 years. For members of the oldest cohort, initiation was less dramatic in the 15- to 19-year age range and continued through the age of 34 years.

THE PREVALENCE OF LIFETIME DEPENDENCE

The results in **Table 4** show that 7.5% of NCS respondents had a lifetime history of psychoactive substance dependence. Males were significantly more likely than females to have a lifetime history of dependence (9.2% vs 5.9%, t=3.8, P<.001). This is not merely because males were more likely to use drugs. They were also signifi-

Table 1. Characteristics of National Comorbidity Survey (NCS) Respondents Compared With Total US Population

	US Population, % (N=65 244)*	NCS, % (N=8098) Weighted	NCS, % (N=8098) Unweighted
Sex			
M	49.1	49.5	47.5
F	50.9	50.5	52.5
Race			
White	75.0	75.3	75.1
Black	11.9	11.5	12.5
Hispanic	8.6	9.7	9.1
Other	4.5	3.5	3.3
Education, y			
0-11	22.5	22.3	18.2
12	36.8	37.4	33.1
13-15	21.2	21.7	26.3
≥16	19.5	18.6	22.4
Marital status			
Married	59.8	62.9	54.4
Separated, widowed, divorced	10.1	10.0	15.5
Never married	30.1	27.1	30.1
Region			
Northeast	20.0	20.2	19.2
Midwest	24.6	23.8	25.6
South	33.7	36.4	35.6
West	21.7	19.6	19.6
Age, y			
15-24	25.5	24.7	21.8
25-34	30.8	30.1	32.4
35-44	25.9	27.1	27.7
45-54	17.8	18.1	18.1
Urbanicity			
Metropolitan	71.2	67.8	68.9
Other urban	8.1	7.5	6.5
Nonurban	20.7	24.7	24.6

The US population characteristics are based on results from the 1989 US National Health Interview Survey.

Table 2. Lifetime and 12-Month (1990 to 1992) Drug Use, by Sex and Age

	%±SE					
	Males		Females		Total	
Age, y	Lifetime Use	12-mo Use	Lifetime Use	12-mo Use	Lifetime Use	12-mo Use
15-24	46.4±2.3	29.5±2.2	38.9±2.8	17.6±1.8	42.8±1.8	23.8±1.4
25-34	69.8±2.3	21.8±1.8	60.4±1.9	14.4±1.3	64.7±1.7	17.8±1.2
35-44	64.1±2.4	13.5±1.8	48.6±2.3	9.7±1.3	56.4±1.6	11.6±1.0
45-54	35.5±3.0	5.4±1.3	27.4±2.7	5.6±1.3	31.5±1.8	5.5±0.8
Total	55.8±1.3	18.4±1.0	46.4±1.5	12.4±0.7	51.0±1.0	15.4±0.6

cantly more likely than females to be dependent in the subsample of lifetime users (16.4% vs 12.6%, t=2.4, P=.004).

There was also an age-cohort effect in Table 4. In the sample as a whole, respondents in cohort 4 were significantly less likely to report a lifetime history of dependence than those in more recent cohorts (2.9% vs 7.3% to 9.5% in more recent cohorts, t tests between 3.2 and 5.5 for pairwise comparisons, all of them significant at P<.001). Among females, this lower prevalence resulted entirely from respondents in cohort 4 being much less likely than younger respondents to have ever used a drug, as shown by the fact that there was no significant association between age and lifetime dependence in the subsample of females who ever used a drug (cohort-specific prevalences between 11.7% and 14.1%, t tests between 0.1 and 0.5 for pairwise comparisons, with .15<P<.23). The situation was different for males, though, among whom prevalence of lifetime dependence was substantially lower for cohort 4 than more recent cohorts in the subsample of lifetime users (5.8% vs 16.7% to 19.7%, t=3.2 to 3.8 for pairwise comparisons, P<.001).

A disaggregated analysis of age and cohort effects is presented in **Figure 2**, where we show the cohort-specific cumulative probabilities of lifetime dependence among respondents who used drugs by specified ages. There was a consistent trend for higher prevalence of dependence among users in successively more recent cohorts. For example, whereas only 2.1%±1.2% (SE) of those respondents in cohort 4 who reported using drugs by the age of 24 years had a lifetime history of dependence by that age, the comparable percentages in more recent cohorts increased consistently to 10.0%±1.2% in cohort 3, 12.3%±1.4% in cohort 2, and 17.3%2.3% in cohort 1. Not only was this trend significant (z=6.3, P<.001) but, equally important for current policy purposes, the percentage was significantly larger in the most recent cohort (cohort 1) than the second most recent cohort (cohort 2; 17.3% vs 12.3%, z=1.9, P=.01), suggesting either a continuation of the trend among respondents currently in the age range 15 to 24 years or a systematic association between age and recall bias concerning age at first onset.

A disaggregation of these cohort differences by sex is presented in **Table 5**. Three intriguing patterns can be seen in this table. First, there was a consistent trend for the probability of lifetime dependence to be higher among female than male users at all ages in the oldest cohort. Second, there was an equally consistent trend for the probability of lifetime dependence to be higher among males than females in more recent cohorts. Third, there was a consistent sex difference in the age range at first onset of dependence. Among males, the vast majority of dependence occurred by the age of 24 years. Among females, in comparison, dependence had a later age at onset, with more than a doubling of the number of females who became dependent between the ages of 25 and 34 years compared with those with a history of dependence as of age 24 years. It is important to note that this sex difference in the age distribution of onset appears consistently across all cohorts.

THE PREVALENCE OF 12-MONTH DEPENDENCE

The results in **Table 6** show that 1.8% of NCS respondents were drug dependent during the 12 months before the interview. This represents 3.5% of lifetime users and 23.8% of persons with a lifetime history of dependence. It is worth repeating that our definition of 12-month dependence requires the respondent to meet full *DSM-III-R* A criteria within the past 12 months. If we relax this requirement and include persons with a lifetime history of dependence and at least one dependence

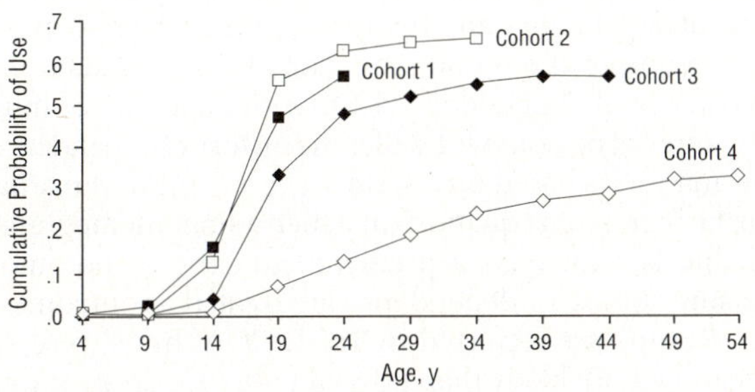

		Age, y										
		4	9	14	19	24	29	34	39	44	49	54
Cohort 1	CP	0	.02	.16	.47	.57						
	SE	0	0	.01	.02	.02						
Cohort 2	CP	0	0	.13	.56	.63	.65	.66				
	SE	0	0	.01	.02	.02	.02	.02				
Cohort 3	CP	0	0	.04	.33	.48	.52	.55	.57	.57		
	SE	0	0	.01	.01	.02	.02	.02	.02	.02		
Cohort 4	CP	0	0	.01	.07	.13	.19	.24	.27	.29	.32	.33
	SE	0	0	0	.01	.01	.01	.02	.02	.02	.02	.02

Figure 1. *Cumulative probability (CP) of drug use, by cohort.*

Table 3. Cumulative Probability of Drug Use, by Sex and Cohort

		Cumulative Probability±SE by Age Category, y								
Sex	**Cohort**	**10-14**	**15-19**	**20-24**	**25-29**	**30-34**	**35-39**	**40-44**	**45-49**	**50-54**
M	1	.19±.02	.51±.02	.63±.02	...	...	...	...	...	...
	2	.16±.02	.62±.02	.68±.02	.70±.02	.71±.02	...	...	...	...
	3	.05±.01	.43±.02	.58±.02	.62±.03	.64±.02	.64±.02	.64±.02	...	...
	4	.01±.01	.09±.02	.15±.02	.22±.02	.27±.03	.31±.03	.34±.03	.36±.03	.36±.03
F	1	.13±.02	.43±.03	.51±.03	...	...	...	...	...	...
	2	.10±.01	.51±.02	.58±.02	.61±.02	.62±.02	...	...	...	.
	3	.02±.01	.24±.02	.37±.02	.42±.02	.47±.02	.49±.02	.50±.02	...	...
	4	.01±.01	.05±.01	.10±.01	.16±.02	.20±.02	.23±.02	.25±.02	.28±.03	.29±.03

Table 4. Lifetime Drug Dependence in the Total Sample and Among Lifetime Users, by Sex and Age

	%±SE					
	Males		Females		Total	
Age, y	Total Sample	Lifetime Users	Total Sample	Lifetime Users	Total Sample	Lifetime Users
15-24	9.1±1.5	19.7±2.8	5.5±1.1	14.1±2.7	7.3±1.1	17.3±2.3
25-34	12.4±1.3	17.8±1.5	7.1±1.0	11.7±1.5	9.5±0.9	14.7±1.2
35-44	10.8±1.6	16.7±2.4	6.1±0.8	12.5±1.3	8.5±0.9	14.9±1.5
45-54	2.1±0.9	5.8±2.4	3.8±1.2	13.8±3.8	2.9±0.8	9.2±2.5
Total	9.2±0.7	16.4±1.2	5.9±0.5	12.6±1.0	7.5±0.4	14.7±0.7

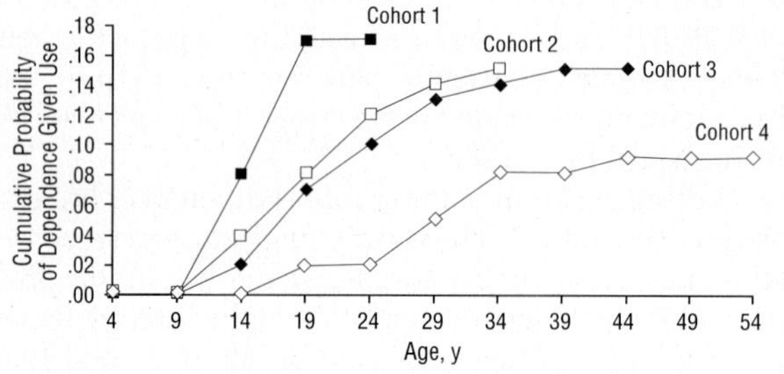

		Age, y										
		4	9	14	19	24	29	34	39	44	49	54
Cohort 1	CP	.00	.00	.08	.17	.17						
	SE	0	0	.02	.02	.02						
Cohort 2	CP	.00	.00	.04	.08	.12	.14	.15				
	SE	0	0	.01	.01	.01	.01	.01				
Cohort 3	CP	.00	.00	.02	.07	.10	.13	.14	.15	.15		
	SE	0	0	.01	.01	.01	.01	.02	.02	.02		
Cohort 4	CP	.00	.00	.00	.02	.02	.05	.08	.08	.09	.09	.09
	SE	0	0	0	.01	.02	.02	.02	.02	.02	.03	.03

Figure 2. *Cumulative probability (CP) of drug dependence, given use, by cohort.*

symptom in the past 12 months, the prevalence increases to 2.8%±0.2%, equivalent to 5.4%±0.5% of lifetime users and 37.9%±3.2% of persons with a lifetime history of dependence.

As in earlier tables, the overall proportion of respondents with 12-month dependence shown in Table 6 is significantly greater among males than females (2.3% vs 1.3%, *t*=2.2, *P*=.007). This is because males are both more likely than females to use drugs at some time in their lives and more likely to become dependent once they use them. In comparison, there was no significant sex difference in 12-month dependence in the subsample of persons with a lifetime history of dependence (24.9% vs 22.2%, *t*=0.5, *P*=.15).

Table 6 shows that 12-month dependence was significantly more prevalent among respondents in the 15- to 24-year age range (3.3%) than among those who were 25 to 34 years old (1.6%, *t*=2.2, *P*=.007), 35 to 44 years old (1.3%, *t*=2.6, *P*=.002), or 45 to 54 years old (0.7%, *t*=3.2, *P*<.001). A less obvious result captured in the last two columns of the table is that this association largely results from young people being more likely to be recent users. That is, there was no meaningful association between age and 12-month dependence in the subsample of 12-month users (eg, 13.0% among 15- to 24-year-old males vs 11.9% among 45- to 54-year-old males, *t*=0.1, *P*=.23).

DEMOGRAPHIC CORRELATES OF USE AND DEPENDENCE

The prevalence estimates reported above document the existence of significant age and sex differences in both drug use and dependence. A broader set of demographic correlates is considered in this section of the article. While a number of different contrasts are of potential interest, we focus on three stages of progression: (1) the predictors of first use (lifetime use in the total sample); (2) the predictors of first onset of dependence among users (lifetime dependence in the subsample of lifetime users); and (3) the predictors of persistence of dependence (12-month dependence in the subsample of persons with a lifetime history of dependence). The analysis is based on a series of three sets of univariate logistic regression equations in which a single demographic variable is treated as a predictor and the dichotomous measures of use or dependence are treated as outcomes.

Results are reported in **Table 7**. Whites were significantly more likely than nonwhites to use drugs at some time in their lives. Among lifetime users, there was no significant association between race and dependence. Among respondents with a lifetime history of dependence, blacks were significantly more likely than whites to have 12-month dependence. Respondents in the "other" (largely Asian) racial category, finally, had the lowest odds ratios (ORs) in all the contrasts.

There was a generally positive association between education and lifetime use of drugs. This pattern reversed, though, in predicting progression to dependence, where the ORs for respondents with 0 to 11 (OR, 2.30) or 12 (OR, 1.69) years of education were significantly greater than 1.0. The ORs of recent dependence among respondents with a lifetime history of dependence were also elevated in the subsamples with 0 to 11 and 12 years of education, although these coefficients were not statistically significant.

There was no association between family income and lifetime use in the NCS. Among users, however, there was a negative relationship between income and lifetime dependence. This was particularly pronounced among respondents in the lowest income category.

Lifetime probability of drug use was significantly higher in the Northeast and West than the Midwest or South. Given use, respondents in regions other than the Midwest had a higher odds of lifetime dependence, but

Table 5. Cumulative Probability of Drug Dependence Given Use, by Cohort and Sex

Sex	Cohort	Cumulative Probability±SE by Age Category, y: 10-14	15-19	20-24	25-29	30-34	35-39	40-44	45-49	50-54
M	1	.06±.02	.19±.03	.20±.03	...	...	...	...	...	...
	2	.03±.01	.11±.01	.16±.02	.18±.02	.19±.02	...	...	...	...
	3	.00±.0	.09±.02	.12±.02	.15±.02	.16±.02	.17±.02	.17±.02	...	...
	4	.00±.0	.01±.01	.01±.01	.02±.01	.05±.03	.05±.02	.06±.03	.06±.03	.06±.02
F	1	.11±.04	.14±.03	.14±.03	...	...	...	...	...	...
	2	.05±.01	.06±.02	.09±.02	.11±.02	.12±.02	...	...	...	
	3	.03±.01	.03±.01	.06±.02	.10±.01	.12±.01	.13±.01	.13±.01	...	...
	4	.00±.0	.04±.02	.04±.02	.10±.05	.10±.04	.10±.04	.13±.04	.14±.04	.14±.04

Table 6. Twelve-Month (1990 to 1992) Drug Dependence in the Total Sample, Among Lifetime Users, Among Respondents With Lifetime Dependence, and Among 12-Month Users, by Sex and Age

Sex	Age, y	%±SE: Total Sample	Lifetime Users	Lifetime Dependent	12-mo Users
M	15-24	4.5±1.1	9.6±2.2	48.8±8.7	13.0±3.0
	25-34	2.2±0.5	3.2±0.7	17.8±4.1	9.9±2.2
	35-44	1.4±0.4	2.0±0.7	13.3±3.7	9.7±3.0
	45-54	0.6±0.5	1.8±1.4	30.6±21.1	11.9±8.8*
	Total	2.3±0.4	4.0±0.6	24.9±3.9	11.3±1.9
F	15-24	2.1±0.5	5.4±1.4	38.1±7.7	10.6±2.5
	25-34	1.2±0.3	1.9±0.6	16.6±4.5	8.1±2.1
	35-44	1.1±0.4	2.2±0.8	17.8±6.4	11.1±4.3
	45-54	0.8±0.7	2.9±2.5	21.3±15.8	0.4±0.4*
	Total	1.3±0.2	2.8±0.5	22.2±3.8	9.0±1.4
Total	15-24	3.3±0.7	7.8±1.5	45.0±6.1	12.2±2.3
	25-34	1.6±0.3	2.5±0.5	17.3±3.1	9.1±1.6
	35-44	1.3±0.3	2.1±0.5	14.9±3.3	10.3±2.6
	45-54	0.7±0.4	2.3±1.4	24.7±11.7	6.1±4.4
	Total	1.8±0.2	3.5±0.5	23.8±3.1	10.3±1.4

**Low precision.*

residents of the West comprised the only group for whom this difference was significant. There were no significant regional differences in the persistence of dependence.

Urbanicity was examined at the county level by distinguishing major metropolitan counties (metropolitan), urbanized counties that are not in major metropolitan areas (urban), and rural counties. There was a significant positive association between urbanicity and lifetime drug use. Given use, however, urbanicity was not significantly related to either lifetime dependence or persistence of dependence. Readers who are interested in the effect of a particular demographic correlate when the others are controlled for may request multivariate analysis results from us.

COMMENT

PREVALENCE ESTIMATES

The NCS drug use prevalence estimates are generally similar to those obtained in the 1991 NHSDA.[1] The NHSDA lifetime prevalence estimate among respondents in the age range of 15 to 54 years is 45.2% compared with the NCS estimate of 51.0%, whereas the NHSDA 12-month prevalence estimate is 16.7% compared to the NCS estimate of 15.4%.

Methodologic studies carried out by NHSDA staff show that willingness to admit drug use is reduced in the NHSDA when questions are administered by interviewers, as they are in the NCS, rather than self-administered.[47] On the basis of this evidence, the 1991 NHSDA drug use questions were self-administered. It is somewhat surprising, in light of this methodologic research, that the NCS estimate (based on interviewer-administered questions rather than self-administered questionnaires) is higher than the NHSDA estimate for lifetime use and only slightly lower than the NHSDA estimate for 12-month use. We have no way of investigating the reasons for this with our data, but we suspect that it has something to do with the fact that the NCS was a health survey rather than a drug survey. Because of our focus on health, the NCS asked about drug use in the context of other health-relevant behaviors, such as exercise and diet, and it is possible that this difference in context led to a reduction in respondent hesitation to admit drug use.

It is difficult to make direct comparisons to assess the consistency of the NCS estimates of the prevalence

Table 7. Demographic Correlates of Lifetime Drug Use in the Total Sample, Lifetime Dependence Among Users, and 12-Month Dependence Among Those With Lifetime Dependence*

	Lifetime Use (Total Sample)		Lifetime Dependence (User Subsample)		12-mo Dependence (Lifetime Dependent Subsample)	
	OR	95% CI	OR	95% CI	OR	95% CI
Race						
White	1.00	. . .	1.00	. . .	1.00	. . .
Black	0.62†	0.51-0.74	0.69	0.46-1.03	3.05†	1.05-8.84
Hispanic	0.70†	0.50-0.98	1.05	0.65-1.69	2.38	0.77-7.33
Other	0.37†	0.25-0.56	0.97	0.39-2.42	0.22	0.04-1.05
Education, y						
0-11	0.53†	0.45-0.63	2.30†	1.60-3.29	2.25	0.74-6.85
12	0.81†	0.70-0.93	1.69†	1.21-2.37	2.11	0.80-5.62
13-15	1.07	0.91-1.26	1.30	0.88-1.91	1.27	0.46-3.52
≥16	1.00	. . .	1.00	. . .	1.00	. . .
Income, ×$1000						
0-19	1.00	0.80-1.26	2.24†	1.43-3.52	1.81	0.57-5.80
20-34	0.96	0.78-1.19	1.51	0.90-2.54	1.00	0.33-3.03
35-69	0.91	0.74-1.12	1.29	0.76-2.21	0.84	0.27-2.69
≥70	1.00	. . .	1.00	. . .	1.00	. . .
Region						
Northeast	1.47†	1.17-1.84	1.22	0.86-1.71	1.16	0.40-3.35
Midwest	1.00	. . .	1.00	. . .	1.00	. . .
South	0.93	0.78-1.12	1.24	0.89-1.73	1.57	0.68-3.62
West	1.76†	1.34-2.32	1.64†	1.23-2.19	1.39	0.59-3.25
Urbanicity						
Metropolitan	1.85†	1.46-2.35	1.40	0.98-2.00	1.17	0.47-2.90
Other urban	1.54†	1.13-2.11	1.38	0.92-2.08	1.28	0.56-2.91
Nonurban	1.00	. . .	1.00	. . .	1.00	. . .

*OR indicates odds ratio; CI, confidence interval.
†An odds ratio with a confidence interval that does not include 1.0 is statistically significant.

of drug dependence with those of previous surveys because the latter have usually been based on either health maintenance organization or treatment samples[8,48] and have often used measures of dependence that are not comparable with the *DSM-III-R* criteria used in the NCS.[49] It is possible, however, to compare the NCS estimate of dependence with that of the ECA Study. Before the NCS, the ECA Study provided the most up-to-date estimate of the national prevalence of drug dependence. The NCS estimate of 7.5% lifetime dependence is somewhat higher than the 5.1% estimate obtained in the ECA Study for lifetime prevalence of *DSM-III* drug dependence among respondents in the age range of 18 to 44 years.[9] However, when we focus on NCS respondents who are currently in the age range of 28 to 54 years and compute the percentage who reported an onset of dependence as of 10 years earlier (ie, when they were 18 to 44 years old)—a comparison that matches NCS data with ECA Study data on year of assessment, age of risk, and cohort—the NCS prevalence estimate for lifetime dependence is reduced to 5.3%±0.6%, very similar to the ECA Study estimate of 5.1%.

SEX, AGE, AND COHORT EFFECTS

The NCS finding that males are more likely than females to use and to be dependent on drugs is consistent with previous research.[3,9,30-32] The finding that male drug users are more likely than female users to become dependent is inconsistent with the ECA Study finding that lifetime drug use disorders are equally prevalent among male and female extramedical drug users.[9] Additionally, our finding of no sex difference in 12-month dependence among respondents with a lifetime history of dependence is at odds with the ECA Study finding that men are significantly more likely than women to experience current problems associated with lifetime abuse or dependence.[9]

Our finding of an inverse relationship between age and use has been repeatedly found in previous research,[3,46] as has our finding that use and dependence are both much more common in cohorts born after World War II.[9,30,44-46,50] The decrease in the cumulative probability of use by age 24 years in cohort 1 compared with cohort 2 is consistent with recent trends from the data that show decreases in use over the last several years for 12th graders.[51]

The interaction found in the NCS between sex and cohort in predicting lifetime dependence was also found in weaker form in the ECA Study, where women in the 45- to 64-year age range were slightly more likely than men to qualify for lifetime dependence (0.4% vs 0.2%, $t=.07$, $P=.24$), while men had higher lifetime dependence than women in other age groups.[9] Males in the NCS had a higher lifetime prevalence of dependence than females among respondents in the cohorts born after the end of World War II but a lower prevalence than females in the cohort born in the decade before the end of

World War II, despite the fact that older males are more likely than older females to have a history of drug use. This result may be related to a finding in previous studies that females predominate among people who are dependent on psychotherapeutic medicines, while males predominate among people who are dependent on other drugs.[52-54] The former would be expected to be responsible for a larger proportion of drug dependence among persons in cohort 4, as they are the only NCS cohort to go through adolescence before the introduction of marijuana and other drugs into youth culture. Consistent with this possibility, disaggregated cohort-specific analyses of NCS dependence data by type of drug reported elsewhere shows that men are more likely than women to use psychotherapeutic drugs but female users are more likely than male users to become dependent.[55] More complex analyses are needed to determine whether this accounts for the sex-by-cohort interaction in dependence among users found here. Another plausible interpretation is that the interaction between sex and cohort comes about because of greater selection bias among males than females with a history of dependence, possibly because of a stronger association between dependence and early mortality among males than females.

We are unaware of any previous research documenting that the conditional probability of dependence among users has increased among respondents who are currently in the age range 15 to 24 years (cohort 1) compared with earlier cohorts (Figure 2), despite the fact that the probability of lifetime use is lower in cohort 1 than cohort 2 (Figure 1). A methodologic interpretation of this increased probability of dependence among users is possible, emphasizing some combination of differential recall bias, differential willingness to admit use, and differential sample selection bias in cohort 1 compared with earlier cohorts. A substantive interpretation is also possible, emphasizing the possibility that the people who are selected into use of drugs during a time when use is becoming less prevalent are likely to be more vulnerable (eg, more likely to have a history of psychopathology) and, as a result, more likely to become dependent.[56,57] It would be possible to evaluate this interpretation in more detailed analyses by studying cohort differences in retrospective reports concerning history of other disorders before the onset of drug use.

The findings regarding a significantly higher prevalence of 12-month dependence among the youngest respondents but no cohort difference in 12-month dependence among 12-month users is somewhat surprising in light of evidence that use is more likely to be experimental during the teenage years[51] and the likelihood that younger users are less likely to be using drugs associated with a high risk of dependence.[58] However, it has been argued that early age at onset contributes to an increased likelihood of dependence.[46] We also found a sex difference in the relationship between cohort and prevalence of lifetime dependence. The lower prevalence among females born before vs after the end of World War II results entirely from their lower probability of ever using a drug, whereas the lower prevalence of lifetime dependence among males born before vs after World War II results from a combination of lower probability of ever using a drug and lower probability of dependence among users. This might reflect a sex difference in drug of choice or in the changing centrality of drug use to other aspects of male and female life-styles across cohorts.

A sex difference in drug of choice could also help explain our finding that the curves for age at onset of dependence differ for males and females, with the lifetime prevalence of dependence among females doubling in the age range of 25 to 34 years, while virtually all dependence among males occurred by the age of 24 years. This difference is consistent with evidence that prescription drugs are responsible for a larger part of female than male dependence.[44] It also suggests the possibility that there may be a longer time between first use and onset of dependence among females than males.

OTHER DEMOGRAPHIC CORRELATES OF USE AND DEPENDENCE

Our results concerning other demographic correlates are broadly consistent with previous research in finding that drug use is positively associated with being white rather than nonwhite,[4,59] well educated rather than poorly educated,[30,60] urban rather than rural,[30,32] and a resident of the Northeast or West rather than the South or Midwest.[30,32]

We also documented that the predictive power of demographic variables often differs from one stage of disorder to the next. For example, whites are significantly more likely than blacks ever to use one of the drugs considered here, indistinguishable from blacks in their probability of lifetime dependence after first use, and significantly less likely than blacks to have persistent dependence. These results are consistent with Kandel's finding[61] that blacks are less likely than whites to experiment with most drugs but more likely than whites to persist in their use. Results such as these underscore the complexity of the issues surrounding substance use disorders and support the argument made nearly two decades ago by Robins[62] that an adequate understanding of risk factors for substance use disorders requires a decomposition of risk factors into stages.

LIMITATIONS

The NCS prevalence estimates probably underestimate the true prevalence of drug use and dependence in the total population because the sampling frame (the household population) excludes the homeless and residents of institutional settings and group housing and because reporting errors among respondents are likely to be in the direction of underreporting rather than overreporting these experiences.

Many results hinge on respondent recall of ages when use first occurred or they first became dependent. Recall bias in reporting these dates could lead to errors in the age-at-onset analyses. If these errors differ by current age, they could distort intercohort comparisons. This, in turn, could lead to the impression that there are substantive cohort differences when, in fact, these differences result from differential recall bias.[63] As a result, caution is needed in interpreting results concerning cohort differences.

Finally, the results concerning demographic correlates should be taken as descriptive rather than as evidence concerning risk factors because these results are all based on univariate prediction equations. It is likely that some of the significant associations would disappear in more complex multivariate analyses. Anthony,[64] for example, showed no significant association between being black and drug dependence when a control was introduced for neighborhood. Even when results hold up after the introduction of controls, the causal order of associations is not always clear. For example, the significant association between low educational attainment and lifetime dependence in the subsample of lifetime users could result from an effect of educational failure on subsequent onset of dependence, an effect of dependence on subsequent school dropout, an effect of other variables on both education and dependence, or some combination of these effects. Future analyses of the NCS data will rely on survival models in which age at onset of use and disorder are treated as outcome variables, and predictors that may be reciprocally related to the outcomes are treated as time-varying covariates to clarify this temporal uncertainty in the predictors of the progression from first use to dependence.

Accepted for publication November 15, 1994.

The NCS is a collaborative epidemiologic investigation of the prevalence, causes, and consequences of psychiatric morbidity and comorbidity in the United States supported by the US Alcohol, Drug Abuse, and Mental Health Administration (grant 5 R01 MH46376) with supplemental support from the W. T. Grant Foundation (grant 90135190), Ronald C. Kessler, principal investigator. Preparation for this report was also supported by Research Scientist Development Award 1 K01 MH00507 (Dr Kessler).

The Addiction Research Foundation, Toronto, Ontario (Robin Room, PhD), Duke University Medical Center, Durham, NC (Dan Blazer, MD, and Marvin Swartz, MD), The Johns Hopkins University, Baltimore, Md (James Anthony, PhD, William Eaton, PhD, and Philip Leaf, PhD), Max Planck Institute of Psychiatry, Munich, Germany (Hans-Ulrich Wittchen, PhD), the Medical College of Virginia, Richmond (Kenneth Kendler, MD), The University of Michigan, Ann Arbor (Lloyd Johnston, PhD, and Ronald Kessler, PhD), the National Institute of Mental Health, Bethesda, Md, (Darrell Kirch, MD, and Darrel Regier, MD), New York (NY) University (Patrick Shrout, PhD), State University of New York, Stony Brook (Evelyn Bromet, PhD), The University of Toronto (Ontario) (R. Jay Turner, PhD), and Washington University School of Medicine, St Louis, Mo (Linda Cottler, PhD). A complete list of NCS publications can be obtained from the NCS Study Coordinator, Room 1006, Institute for Social Research, The University of Michigan, Box 1248, Ann Arbor, MI 48106-1248.

We appreciate the helpful comments of Lloyd Johnston, PhD, and Denise Kandel, PhD.

Reprints not available.

REFERENCES

1. Kozel NJ. Epidemiology of drug abuse in the United States: a summary of methods and findings. *Bull Pan Am Health Organ.* 1990;24:53-62.
2. US Dept of Health and Human Services. *Annual Emergency Room Data, 1990.* Rockville, Md: National Institute on Drug Abuse; 1991b.
3. US Dept of Health and Human Services. *National Household Survey on Drug Abuse, Population Estimates 1991.* Rockville, Md: National Institute on Drug Abuse; 1991a.
4. Johnston LD, O'Malley PM, Bachman JG. *Smoking, Drinking, and Illicit Drug Use Among American Secondary School Students, College Students, and Young Adults, 1975-1991: Volume 1, Secondary School Students.* Rockville, Md: US Dept of Health and Human Services; 1992.
5. Harrison LD. Trends in illicit drug use in the United States: conflicting results from national surveys. *Int J Addict.* 1992;27:817-847.
6. Kozel NJ, Adams EH. Epidemiology of drug abuse: an overview. *Science.* 1986; 234:970-974.
7. Kandel DB, Davies M. Decline in the use of illicit drugs by high school students in New York State: a comparison with national data. *Am J Public Health.* 1991;81:1064-1067.
8. Kilbey MM, Breslau N, Andreski P. Cocaine use and dependence in young adults: associated psychiatric disorders and personality traits. *Drug Alcohol Depend.* 1992;29:283-290.
9. Anthony JC, Helzer JE. Syndromes of drug abuse and dependence. In: Robins LN, Regier DA, eds. *Psychiatric Disorders in America: The Epidemiologic Catchment Area Study.* New York, NY: Free Press; 1991:116-154.
10. Robins LN, Regier DA, eds. *Psychiatric Disorders in America: The Epidemiologic Catchment Area Study.* New York: Free Press; 1991.
11. Kessler RC, McGonagle KA, Zhao S, Nelson CB, Hughes M, Eshleman S, Wittchen H-U, Kendler KS. Lifetime and 12-month prevalence of *DSM-III-R* psychiatric disorders in the United States: Results from the National Comorbidity Survey. *Arch Gen Psychiatry.* 1994;51:8-19.
12. Allgulander C. Psychoactive drug use in a general population sample, Sweden: correlates with perceived health, psychiatric diagnoses, and mortality in an automated record-linkage study. *Am J Public Health.* 1989;79:1006-1010.
13. Eaton WW, Anthony JC, Tepper S, Dryman, A. Psychopathology and attrition in the Epidemiologic Catchment Area Study. *Am J Epidemiol.* 1992;135:1051-1059.
14. US Dept of Health and Human Services. *National Health Interview Survey, 1989.* Hyattsville, Md: National Center for Health Statistics; 1992. Computer file.
15. American Psychiatric Association. *Diagnostic and Statistical Manual of Mental Disorders, Revised Third Edition.* Washington, DC: American Psychiatric Association; 1987.
16. World Health Organization. *Composite International Diagnostic Interview (CIDI, Version 1.0).* Geneva, Switzerland: World Health Organization; 1990.
17. Robins LN, Wing J, Wittchen H-U, Helzer JE. The Composite International Diagnostic Interview: an epidemiologic instrument suitable for use in conjunction with different diagnostic systems and in different cultures. *Arch Gen Psychiatry.* 1988;45:1069-1077.
18. Wittchen H-U, Robins LN, Cottler LB, Sartorius N, Burke JD, Regier DA, participants in the Multicenter WHO/ADAMHA Field Trials. Cross-cultural feasibility, reliability and sources of variance in the Composite International Diagnostic Interview (CIDI). *Br J Psychiatry.* 1991;159:645-653.
19. Cottler LB, Robins LN, Grant BF, Blaine J, Towle LH, Wittchen H-U, Sartorius N, participants in the WHO/ADAMHA Field Trials. The CIDI-core substance abuse and dependence questions: cross-cultural and nosological issues. *Br J Psychiatry.* 1991;159:653-658.
20. Semler G, von Cranach M, Wittchen H-U, eds. *Comparison Between the Composite International Diagnostic Interview and the Present State Examination: Report to the WHO/ADAMHA Task Force on Instrument Development.* Geneva, Switzerland; World Health Organization; February 1987.
21. Wacker HR, Battegay R, Mullejans R, Schlosser C. Using the CIDI-C in the general population. In: Stefanis CN, Rabavilas AD, Soldatos CR, eds. *Psychiatry: A World Perspective.* Amsterdam, the Netherlands: Elsevier Science Publishers BV; 1990:138-143.
22. Semler G, ed. *Reliabilitat und Validitat des Composite International Diagnostic Interview: Inaugural-Dissertation zur Erlangung des akademischen Grades eines Doktors der Philosophie.* Mannheim, Germany: Universitat Mannheim; 1989.
23. Spengler P, Wittchen H-U. Procedural validity of standardized symptom questions for the assessment of psychotic symptoms: a comparison of the CIDI with two clinical methods. *Compr Psychiatry.* 1989;29:309-322.
24. Janca A, Robins LN, Cottler LB, Early TS. Clinical observation of CIDI assessments: an analysis of the CIDI field trials—wave II at the St. Louis site. *Br J Psychiatry.* 1992;160:815-818.

25. Leitmeyer P, ed. *Zur Symptomerfassung mit dem standarisierten Interview CIDI-C in der Allgemeinpraxis: Inaugural dissertation zur Erlangung des medizinischen Doktorgrades fur Klinische Medizin.* Mannheim, Germany: Universitat Mannheim; 1990.
26. Farmer AE, Katz R, McGuffin P, Bebbington P. A comparison between the Present State Examination and the Composite International Diagnostic Interview. *Arch Gen Psychiatry.* 1987;44:1064-1068.
27. Farmer AE, Jenkins PL, Katz R, Ryder L. Comparison of CATEGO-derived *ICD-8* and *DSM-III* classifications using the Composite International Diagnostic Interview in severely ill subjects. *Br J Psychiatry.* 1991;158:177-182.
28. Wittchen H-U, Burke JD, Semler G, Pfister H. Recall and dating of psychiatric symptoms: test-retest reliability of time-related symptom questions in a standardized psychiatric interview. *Arch Gen Psychiatry.* 1989;46:437-443.
29. World Health Organization. *Composite International Diagnostic Interview.* Geneva, Switzerland: World Health Organization; 1991. Computer program.
30. Abelson HI, Miller JD. A decade of trends in cocaine use in the household population. In: Kozel NJ, Adams EH, eds. *Cocaine Use in America, Epidemiologic and Clinical Perspectives.* Washington, DC: National Institute on Drug Abuse; 1985:35-49. Research monograph 61.
31. Kandel DB, Yamaguchi K. Developmental patterns of the use of legal, illegal, and medically prescribed psychotropic drugs from adolescence to young adulthood. In: Jones CL, Battjes RJ, eds. *Etiology of Drug Abuse: Implications for Prevention.* Washington, DC: National Institute on Drug Abuse; 1985:193-235. Research monograph 56.
32. O'Malley PM, Johnston LD, Bachman JG. Quantitative and qualitative changes in cocaine use among American high school seniors, college students, and young adults. In: Schober S, Schade C, eds. *The Epidemiology of Cocaine Use and Abuse.* Washington, DC: National Institute on Drug Abuse; 1991:19-43. Research monograph 110.
33. Boyd CJ, Blow F, Orgain LS. Gender differences among African-American substance users. *J Psychoactive Drugs.* 1993;25:301-305.
34. Lex BW. Some gender differences in alcohol and polysubstance users. *Health Psychol.* 1991;10:121-132.
35. Thomas SM, Fick AC, Henderson J, Doherty K. Tobacco, alcohol, and marijuana use among black adolescents: a comparison across gender, grade, and school environment. *J La State Med Soc.* 1990;142:37-42.
36. Woodruff RS, Causey BD. Computerized method for approximating the variance of a complicated estimate. *J Am Stat Assoc.* 1976;71:315-321.
37. University of Michigan. *OSIRIS VII.* Ann Arbor, Mich: Institute for Social Research, University of Michigan; 1981.
38. Norusis MJ, ed. *SPSS/PC+ Advanced Statistics 4.0 for the IBM PC/XT/AT and PS/2.* Chicago, Ill: SPSS Inc; 1990.
39. Kalbfleisch JD. *The Statistical Analysis of Failure Time Data.* New York, NY: John Wiley & Sons Inc; 1980.
40. Willett JB, Singer JD. Investigating onset, cessation, relapse and recovery: why you should, and how you can, use discrete-time survival analysis to examine event occurrence. *J Consult Clin Psychol.* 1993;61:952-965.
41. Kish L, Frankel MR. Balanced repeated replications for standard errors. *J Am Stat Assoc.* 1970;65:1071-1094.
42. Koch GG, Lemeshow S. An application of multivariate analysis to complex sample survey data. *J Am Stat Assoc.* 1972;67:780-782.
43. Kalton G. Practical methods for estimating survey sampling errors. *Bull Int Stat Inst.* 1977;47:495-514.
44. Clayton RR, Voss HL, Robbins C, Skinner WF. Gender differences in drug use: an epidemiological perspective. In: Ray BA, Braude MC, eds. *Women and Drugs: A New Era for Research.* Washington, DC: National Institute on Drug Abuse; 1986:80-99. Research monograph 65.
45. Johnston LD. The etiology and prevention of substance use: what can we learn from recent historical changes? In: Jones CL, Battjes RJ, eds. *Etiology of Drug Abuse: Implications for Prevention.* Washington, DC: National Institute on Drug Abuse; 1985:155-177. Research monograph 56.
46. Robins LN, Przybeck TR. Age of onset of drug use as a factor in drug and other disorders. In: Jones CL, Battjes RJ, eds. *Etiology of Drug Abuse: Implications for Prevention.* Washington, DC: National Institute on Drug Abuse; 1985: 178-192. Research monograph 56.
47. Turner CF, Lessler JT, Gfroerer JC. Future directions for research and practice. In: Turner CF, Lessler JT, Gfroerer JC, eds. *Survey Measurement of Drug Use: Methodological Studies.* Washington, DC: National Institute on Drug Abuse; 1992:299-306.
48. Rapaport MH, Tipp JE, Schuckit MA. A comparison of *ICD-10* and *DSM-III-R* criteria for substance abuse and dependence. *Am J Drug Alcohol Abuse.* 1993; 19:143-151.
49. Anglin MD, Hser Y-I, McGlothlin WH. Sex differences in addict careers, 2: becoming addicted. *Am J Drug Alcohol Abuse.* 1987;13:59-71.
50. Burke KC, Burke JD, Rae DS, Regier DA. Comparing age at onset of major depression and other psychiatric disorders by birth cohorts in five U.S. community populations. *Arch Gen Psychiatry.* 1991;48:789-795.
51. Johnston LD, O'Malley PM, Bachman JG. *Smoking, Drinking, and Illicit Drug Use Among American Secondary School Students, College Students, and Young Adults, 1975-1991.* Rockville, Md: US Dept of Health and Human Services; 1992.
52. Almog YJ, Anglin MD, Fisher DG. Alcohol and heroin use patterns of narcotics addicts: gender and ethnic differences. *Am J Drug Alcohol Abuse.* 1993;19: 219-238.
53. Bell DS. Dependence on psychotropic drugs and analgesics in men and women. In: Kalant OJ, ed. *Alcohol and Drug Problems in Women.* New York, NY: Plenum Press; 1980;5:423-463.
54. Cooperstock R, Parnell P. Research on psychotropic drug use: a review of findings and methods. *Soc Sci Med.* 1982;16:1179-1196.
55. Anthony JC, Warner LA, Kessler RC. Comparative epidemiology of dependence on tobacco, alcohol, controlled substances, and inhalants: basic findings from the National Comorbidity Survey. *Exp Clin Psychopharmacol.* 1994; 2:244-268.
56. Weiss RD, Mirin SM, Griffin ML, Michael JL. Psychopathology in cocaine abusers: changing trends. *J Nerv Ment Dis.* 1988;176:719-725.
57. Kessler RC. The epidemiology of psychiatric comorbidity. In: Tsaung M, Tohan M, Zahner G, eds. *Textbook of Psychiatric Epidemiology.* New York, NY: John Wiley & Sons Inc; 1995:179-197.
58. Kandel DB, Faust R. Sequences and stages in patterns of adolescent drug use. *Arch Gen Psychiatry.* 1975;32:923-932.
59. US Dept of Health and Human Services. *National Household Survey on Drug Abuse, Population Estimates 1992.* Rockville, Md: National Institute on Drug Abuse; 1993.
60. Adams EH, Gfroerer JC, Rouse BA. Epidemiology of substance abuse including alcohol and cigarette smoking. *Ann N Y Acad Sci.* 1989;562:14-20.
61. Kandel DB. The social demography of drug use. In: Bayer R, Oppenheimer GM, eds. *Confronting Drug Policy: Illicit Drugs in a Free Society.* New York, NY: Cambridge University Press; 1993:24-77.
62. Robins LN. Estimating addiction rates and locating target populations: how decomposition into stages helps. In: Rittenhouse JD, ed. *The Epidemiology of Heroin and Other Narcotics.* Washington, DC: National Institute on Drug Abuse; 1977:78-559. Research monograph series 16. Dept of Health, Education, and Welfare publication 1 (ADM).
63. Simon GE, VonKorff M. Reevaluation of secular trends in depression rates. *Am J Epidemiol.* 1992;135:1411-1422.
64. Anthony JC. The epidemiology of drug addiction. In: Miller NS, ed. *Comprehensive Handbook of Drug and Alcohol Addiction.* New York, NY: Marcel Dekker Inc; 1991:55-86.

ORIGINAL ARTICLE

Generalized Social Phobia

Reliability and Validity

Salvatore Mannuzza, PhD; Franklin R. Schneier, MD; Tim F. Chapman, PhD; Michael R. Liebowitz, MD; Donald F. Klein, MD; Abby J. Fyer, MD

Objective: To investigate the reliability and validity of *DSM-III-R* "generalized" social phobia by examining interrater agreement and comparing patients with generalized and "nongeneralized" social phobia on demographic characteristics, clinical variables, and familial social phobia.

Design: Two senior clinicians classified 129 patients attending an anxiety clinic as having *DSM-III-R* social phobia that is generalized (fears most social situations) or nongeneralized (less than most) based on independent narrative review.

Results: Good reliability was achieved (κ=0.69). Patients with generalized social phobia were more often single, had earlier onsets of social phobia, had more interactional fears, and had higher rates of atypical depression and alcoholism. Familial social phobia was more common among patients with generalized social phobia than patients with nongeneralized social phobia and controls, with no difference between the latter two groups.

Conclusions: Generalized social phobia (1) can be distinguished reliably from nongeneralized social phobia, (2) is a valid subtype, and (3) may characterize a familial form of the disorder.

(Arch Gen Psychiatry. 1995;52:230-237)

THIS STUDY investigates the reliability and validity of "generalized" social phobia by (1) examining interrater agreement of two clinicians (S.M. and F.R.S.), and (2) comparing patients with generalized and "nongeneralized" social phobia on demographic characteristics, clinical variables, and familial psychopathologic conditions. Social phobia is a common disorder affecting 2% to 7% of the general population. More than two thirds of individuals with the syndrome have had at least one other mental disorder at some time in their lives. Even in its uncomplicated form (ie, no lifetime comorbid disorder), social phobia is associated with increased rates of suicidal ideation, financial dependency, and help-seeking.[1]

Social phobia first became an officially recognized diagnosis in 1980.[2] In 1985, Liebowitz et al[3] referred to social phobia as "a neglected anxiety disorder." Since then, numerous articles on the syndrome have been published.[4] However, although there is ample evidence that social phobia can be differentiated from other anxiety disorders,[5-7] the syndrome remains poorly understood with respect to homogeneous subtypes.

Heterogeneity of social phobia has been addressed systematically only recently.[8] It has long been known that there is a broad spectrum of fears, avoidance, and functional impact within social phobia, ranging from circumscribed performance concerns to all social situations. Moreover, "subtypes" may be more valid than social phobia as a whole (compare *DSM-II* anxiety neurosis reclassified as panic disorder and generalized anxiety disorder in *DSM-III*). Providing convincing evidence of a homogeneous subtype within social phobia would stimulate additional etiologic, treatment, and prognostic studies.

The generalized type was introduced in 1987 in the revised edition of *DSM-III*[9] following recognition[3] that *DSM-III* had been too restrictive in defining social phobia primarily as performance anxiety. The *DSM-III-R* stated that, in generalized social phobia, "the phobic situation includes most social situations."[9(p243)] No additional guidelines or criteria were provided.

See Subjects and Methods on next page

From the Department of Psychiatry, Columbia University, College of Physicians and Surgeons, and the Anxiety Disorders Clinic, Department of Therapeutics, New York State Psychiatric Institute, New York, NY.

SUBJECTS AND METHODS

Patients were consecutive admissions to the Columbia University College of Physicians and Surgeons/New York State Psychiatric Institute Anxiety Disorders Clinic (New York, NY) between 1983 and 1988 and during the last 6 months of 1989. The clinic recruits patients for treatment or biologic studies through news media and by word-of-mouth referral.

Patients meeting the following criteria were accepted irrespective of the anxiety disorder for which they sought treatment: (1) ongoing diagnosis of social phobia based on semistructured interview assessment (described below); (2) no lifetime psychotic disorder; and (3) no major depression or substance use disorder (including alcoholism) during the past 3 months. Exclusion criteria were those stipulated by treatment or biologic study protocols.

There were 129 patients ranging in age from 19 to 58 years (mean±SD, 34.5±8.6 years). Most (84%) were white and about half (55%) were college graduates.

SAMPLE REPRESENTATIVENESS

The present sample is comparable to patients described in the social phobia literature regarding sex ratio, marital status, and age at onset. Studies of clinic samples reported that 46% to 60% of patients with social phobia were male.[11,13,17-21] In the present study, 56% were male.

In studies of clinic samples, 30% to 57% of patients with social phobia never married,[17,18,20,22] compared with 51% of patients in the present study. Most studies reported mean age at onset in the midteens, with two thirds to three quarters developing the disorder by age 19 years.[13,21,23-25] However, social phobia can begin at any age, with reported onsets as early as ages 4 or 5 years[17,25] and as late as ages 39 and 40 years.[24,25] In the present sample, mean (±SD) age at onset was 13.8±7.2 years, with three quarters of patients developing the disorder by age 18 years (range, 4 to 44 years).

DIAGNOSIS OF SOCIAL PHOBIA

Patients were administered the Schedule for Affective Disorders and Schizophrenia–Lifetime Anxiety version (SADS-LA)[26,27] by doctoral level clinical psychologists and psychiatric social workers trained in differential diagnosis. The κ for social phobia was 0.71 based on test-retest SADS-LA interviews of 104 patients in the anxiety clinic.[28] About half of these patients were included in the present sample.

All patients fulfilled 1985 working draft *DSM-III-R* criteria for social phobia.[29] We are confident that all patients also met finalized *DSM-III-R* criteria,[9] not available when the SADS-LA was developed. Both require the following: a persistent fear of one or more social situations and concerns of humiliation or embarrassment; an immediate anxiety response on exposure to the phobic stimulus; avoidance or endurance with intense anxiety; interference with functioning or marked distress about having the fear; and recognition that the fear is excessive or unreasonable.

Two criteria in the finalized *DSM-III-R* were not included in the 1985 working draft: (1) "If an Axis III or another Axis I disorder is present, the [social phobic] fear is unrelated to it." Our interviewers were trained to follow this criterion, eg, by *not* diagnosing social phobia in a patient with panic disorder who avoided crowded gatherings for fear of having a panic attack. (2) "If the person is under 18, the disturbance does not meet the criteria for Avoidant Disorder of Childhood or Adolescence." None of our patients were younger than 18 years.

Two criteria in the 1985 working draft were not included in the finalized *DSM-III-R*: (1) "The phobic stimulus [or stimuli] is unrelated to the content of the obsessions of Obsessive Compulsive Disorder or to a Sexual Dysfunction." This criterion is simply a special case of criterion 1 above. (2) "What the individual fears will happen occurs only when he or she is the focus of others' attention; or if it occurs while alone, causes little or no distress." This criterion simply underscores the importance of concerns about scrutiny. It is not inconsistent with any of the finalized *DSM-III-R* criteria. We conclude that all patients of the present study fulfilled finalized *DSM-III-R* criteria for social phobia.

We are also confident that all patients fulfilled *DSM-IV*[15] criteria for social phobia since there were no major changes between *DSM-III-R* and *DSM-IV* for this diagnosis. Specifically, the following apply: (1) *DSM-IV* social phobia subsumes *DSM-III-R* avoidant disorder of childhood; (2) *DSM-IV* requires a "marked and persistent" [vs *DSM-III-R* "persistent"] fear of one or more situations; (3) *DSM-IV* requires a 6-month duration if the individual is younger than 18 years; and (4) *DSM-IV* includes an organic exclusion criterion. None of these differences affected social phobia diagnoses in the present study.

The SADS-LA interviewers wrote comprehensive narratives describing lifetime psychiatric history and documenting all anxiety, mood, and substance use diagnoses. One of us (A.J.F.) reviewed all narratives for diagnostic accuracy and completeness.

SOCIAL PHOBIC SITUATIONS IN THE SADS-LA

The SADS-LA includes assessment of fear and avoidance in 10 social situations: speaking, eating, writing, and performing in public; test taking; using public lavatories; asking directions; speaking to strangers; attending social affairs; and dealing with authority figures. Each of these 10 situations was assessed independently, for each patient, and discussed separately in the narrative summary. If all *DSM-III-R* criteria were met for a particular situation, then the diagnosis was made. For example, if a patient feared and avoided speaking before an audience, experienced palpitations and sweating when approaching the podium, and was refused job promotions because of inability to supervise small groups, then social phobia of public speaking was diagnosed. Thus, a patient could be given a social phobia diagnosis involving one to 10 situations on the SADS-LA.

Interviewers probed the full range of social stimuli and were not limited to the above 10 situations. For example, if a patient was extremely nervous on dates, had difficulty initiating conversations, avoided speaking on the telephone, and so on, these also were discussed in the narrative.

CATEGORIZATION OF PATIENTS AS HAVING GENERALIZED AND NONGENERALIZED SOCIAL PHOBIA

Two of us (S.M. and F.R.S.) independently reviewed the SADS-LA narratives of the 129 patients and classified each patient as fearing or avoiding most (generalized) or less than most (nongeneralized) social situations. In addition, since

Continued on next page

certain studies have supported the utility of more qualitative distinctions such as performanace vs interactional fears (see Heimberg et al[8]), patients were also rated on whether they feared or avoided the following: at least one performance situation, and none, one or two, or at least three interactional situations. "Performance situations" were those involving activities that could be engaged in comfortably when alone (eg, writing, eating, speaking). "Interactional situations" were those involving interpersonal interactions (eg, attending formal affairs, dating, speaking on the telephone).

Following independent review, the clinical raters discussed each case and made consensus judgments. Of 129 patients, 67 (52%) were judged as fearing or avoiding most social situations (generalized) and 62 (48%) as less than most (nongeneralized).

Table 1 shows the relationship among most vs less than most, performance, and interactional consensus judgments. The following rules governed independent and consensus ratings: (1) A situation was "counted" as phobic if the patient *avoided* it (eg, refused to attend parties), experienced significant *distress* when in the situation (eg, disturbing autonomic hyperactivity when giving a speech), or reported at least moderate anxiety in *anticipation* of it (eg, apprehensive expectation days before meeting with an employer). (2) Most vs less-than-most judgments were not limited to the 10 specific social stimuli included in the SADS-LA. For example, several patients described fear and avoidance of dating and of initiating conversation in general. All social situations were considered in the clinical narrative review. However, a non–SADS-LA feared social stimulus was never the deciding factor of most vs less than most. (3) Most vs less-than-most judgments were made independent of performance and interactional ratings. As shown in Table 1, among patients rated as fearing or avoiding most social situations, three feared or avoided only one or two interactional situations, and three other patients did not fear or avoid any performance situations. The terms *generalized* (ie, fear or avoidance of most social situations) and *nongeneralized* (ie, less than most) will be used throughout the remainder of this article.

BEST ESTIMATE DIAGNOSES OF RELATIVES OF PATIENTS

Direct (SADS-LA[26]) and informant (Family Informant Schedule and Criteria[30]) interviews were available for 96 first-degree relatives of 33 patients with generalized social phobia and 88 first-degree relatives of 30 patients with nongeneralized social phobia. For purposes of comparison, data from relatives of "never mentally ill" (NMI) control probands included in our family studies are also presented. The NMI probands were recruited using an extension of the acquaintanceship procedure.[31] They were judged as having no lifetime mental disorder based on SADS-LA evaluation.

This article reports *DSM-III-R* best-estimate diagnoses for relatives of patients and NMI controls. In this procedure, clinical narrative summaries based on the direct interview of each relative (SADS-LA) and informant interviews with family members asked about that relative (Family Informant Schedule and Criteria) were combined, and they were reviewed blindly and independently by two senior staff members (S.M., a psychiatric social worker, a clinical psychologist, and/or a psychiatric nurse). Subsequently, the two reviewers met to discuss each case and arrived at lifetime *DSM-III-R* best-estimate consensus diagnoses.

Six senior staff members of the Anxiety Disorders Clinic (four who reviewed cases from the present study) blindly and independently reviewed 18 cases to assess best-estimate interrater reliability. The κ for social phobia was 0.83.

Family study findings on a subset of the present sample were previously published.[16] However, in that report, (1) patient probands were limited to those with social phobia *but no other lifetime anxiety disorder*, and (2) relative diagnoses were based on direct SADS-LA interviews.

DATA ANALYSES

Interrater agreement of patient classifications based on narrative reviews was assessed with unweighted κ, a chance-corrected reliability statistic. In general, κ values greater than 0.75 suggest excellent agreement, values less than 0.40 suggest poor agreement, and values in between suggest fair to good agreement beyond chance.[32]

An uncorrected χ^2 test was used to compare nominal variables (eg, gender, marital status, and presence or absence of comorbid disorders) and Student's *t* test was used to compare interval and ratio variables (eg, age at interview). All reported probabilities are two tailed. Significance is stipulated as $P \leq .05$.

Dunn's Test[33] was used to correct for multiple statistical tests by limiting the type I error rate. Specifically, for a 5% α level and X contrasts, the error rate per comparison would be set at 0.05/X (X signifies number of contrasts).

STUDY OBJECTIVES

This study systematically addresses the following questions: (1) Can generalized social phobia be distinguished reliably from nongeneralized social phobia (as measured by the κ statistic)? (2) Is generalized social phobia a valid concept as inferred from differences between patients with generalized and nongeneralized social phobia on the following variables: demographic characteristics such as gender and marital status; clinical features such as symptoms and lifetime comorbidity for other mental disorders; and family history of social phobia?

Differences between patients with generalized and other (discrete, specific, nongeneralized, etc) social phobias have been reported on demographic characteristics,[10] type and severity of symptoms,[7,10-13] level of functioning,[10] onset of social phobia,[13] and self-reported, observer-rated, and physiologic responses to behavioral challenges.[10,14] However, definitions of subtypes have been applied inconsistently, in part, owing to a lack of agreement on the essential feature(s) of generalized social phobia. Whereas most studies defined generalized social phobia as fear of most social situations, one study[11] required that patients with generalized social phobias fear parties or initiating or maintaining conversations. Assigning special significance to these social stimuli (parties and conversations) departs substantially from the *DSM-III-R* definition of the subtype. In addition, comparison groups have

Table 1. Relationship Between Patient Classifications Based on Narrative Reviews*

Category of Social Situation/ No. of Situations Feared or Avoided	Fears or Avoids Most Social Situations (n=67)	Fears or Avoids Less-Than-Most Social Situations (n=62)
Performance		
None	3 (4)	4 (6)
At least 1	64 (96)	58 (94)
Interactional		
None	0 (0)	18 (29)
1 or 2	3 (4)	40 (65)
At least 3	64 (96)	4 (6)

*Classifications are based on the consensual agreements of two clinicians who independently reviewed each of the 129 narrative summaries of patients with social phobia. Data are expressed as number (percent).

Table 2. Interrater Reliability of Patient Classifications Based on Narrative Reviews*

Patient Classification†	κ
Most ("generalized") vs less-than-most ("nongeneralized")	0.69 (0.57-0.81)
Performance situations	
None vs at least 1	0.76 (0.50-1.00)
Interactional situations	
None vs 1 or 2 vs at least 3‡	0.65 (0.53-0.77)
None vs at least 1	0.78 (0.62-0.94)
None, 1, or 2 vs at least 3	0.67 (0.54-0.80)

*Two clinicians independently reviewed 129 narrative summaries of patients with social phobia. Numbers in parentheses show the 95% confidence intervals for each κ.

†Classifications refer to the proportion (most vs less-than-most), type (performance, interactional), and number (none, 1 or 2, etc) of social situations that were feared or avoided.

‡3×3 κ (all other κ statistics are 2×2).

varied widely. One was limited to patients with public speaking social phobia[10]; one included patients who feared only one or two situations[7]; some defined "discrete" or "circumscribed" in terms of performance fears[11,14]; whereas others compared patients with generalized social phobias with patients with nongeneralized social phobias (ie, all other).[12,13]

The present study systematically addresses reliability and validity of the generalized subtype, as defined in *DSM-III-R*, in the largest clinic sample of patients with social phobia studied to date (to our knowledge). Establishing that a subtype can be identified consistently is a necessary first step toward investigating its validity. Patients with generalized social phobia (ie, those who fear most social situations) are compared with patients with nongeneralized social phobia (ie, those who fear less than most social situations) on several measures as a preliminary assessment of validity. If the generalized vs nongeneralized distinction is unreliable or if no differences are found, then this would suggest that the subtype may not be useful. Since *DSM-IV* has retained the *DSM-III-R* definition of generalized social phobia,[15] this study is particularly relevant to current research and practice.

Comparison variables in the present study represent multiple domains: demographic characteristics (gender, education, marital status); clinical features (symptoms, age at onset of social phobia, age at first treatment, lifetime comorbidity for other disorders); and familial social phobia. Family study results based on a subset of the present sample (ie, probands with social phobia with no additional lifetime anxiety diagnosis) were previously reported.[16]

RESULTS

RELIABILITY

Clinician agreements based on independent reviews of SADS-LA narratives were good to excellent for judgments concerning fear or avoidance of most vs less-than-most social situations (κ=0.69), and for performance and interactional concerns (κs=0.65 to 0.78; **Table 2**).

Of the 20 most vs less-than-most disagreements, consensus judgments were "most" for 10 cases and "less than most" for 10 cases. Therefore, ambiguous cases did not tend to be classified in one particular category.

There were multiple sources of disagreement. In some cases, the most vs less-than-most judgment was complicated by a coexisting episode of panic disorder (eg, it was not clear if avoidance of "social" [and nonsocial] situations was due to fear of having a panic attack and therefore not to be counted). In other cases, comorbid major depression created difficulties (eg, social withdrawal during a dysphoric period in which the "focus of fear" was unclear). Cases with fluctuating course also led to disagreements since it was not clear whether all periods (including those that were brief, relative to a chronic episode) should be given equal weight. Then there were cases in which certain "situations" were discounted by one clinician and counted by the other (eg, avoidance of a single authority figure who made the subject feel uncomfortable and intimidated).

On a more basic level, the question of what constitutes a situation (and, in turn, "most situations") arose. For example, is "attending social affairs" one situation or many (weddings, business luncheons, parties, etc)? Similarly, should each encounter be considered in the most vs less-than-most judgment or should a situation be counted only once? These issues are discussed further in the "Comment" section. Despite these ambiguities and interpretive differences, good reliability on the most (generalized) vs less-than-most (nongeneralized) distinction was achieved (κ=0.69).

DEMOGRAPHIC CHARACTERISTICS

About two thirds of patients with generalized social phobia vs one third of patients with nongeneralized social phobia had never married (64% vs 37%) (P=.01). There were no significant differences in gender, ethnicity, education, or age when seen at the clinic (**Table 3**).

CLINICAL CHARACTERISTICS

Patients with generalized social phobia had significantly earlier onsets of social phobia than did patients with nongeneralized social phobia (means=10.9 vs 16.9)

Table 3. Demographic Characteristics of Patients With Generalized and Nongeneralized Social Phobia*

Variable	Generalized (n=67)	Nongeneralized (n=62)	P
Sex, No. (%)			
F	28 (42)	29 (47)	.99
Race, No. (%)			
White	56 (84)	52 (84)	.99
Black	5 (7)	5 (8)	
Hispanic	3 (4)	2 (3)	
Other	3 (4)	3 (5)	
Age at interview, y			
Mean±SD	32.8±8.3	36.3±9.0	.54
Range	19-54	22-58	
Education, No. (%)			
College graduate	32 (48)	39 (63)	.42
Marital status, No. (%)			
Single (never married)	43 (64)	23 (37)	.01

**Patients were classified as having generalized or nongeneralized social phobia based on consensual agreement of two senior clinicians who independently reviewed narratives of trained interviewers.*

Table 4. Clinical Characteristics of Patients With Generalized and Nongeneralized Social Phobia*

Variable	Generalized (n=67)	Nongeneralized (n=62)	P
Onset of social phobia, y			
Mean±SD	10.9±5.8	16.9±9.3	.001
Median	9.5	15.5	
Range	4-29	5-44	
Age at first treatment for social phobia, y†			
Mean±SD	26.8±9.8	30.5±9.5	.83
Social phobia by situation, No. (%)‡			
Attending social affairs	63 (94)	23 (37)	.001
Public speaking	59 (88)	49 (79)	.99
Dealing with authority figures	40 (60)	17 (27)	.001
Performing in public	39 (58)	23 (37)	.20
Speaking to strangers	25 (37)	6 (10)	.001
Eating in public	22 (33)	12 (19)	.82
Asking directions	18 (27)	0 (0)	.001
Writing in public	12 (18)	9 (15)	.99
Taking a test	11 (16)	6 (10)	.99
Using public lavatories	2 (3)	5 (8)	.99

**Patients were classified as having generalized or nongeneralized social phobia based on consensual agreement of two senior clinicians who independently reviewed narratives of trained interviewers.*

†Forty-eight patients with generalized (72%) and 39 patients with nongeneralized (63%) social phobia were treated for social phobia at some time in their lives.

‡Ordered from highest to lowest prevalence among patients with generalized social phobia.

(P=.001), with half of the former developing the full syndrome before age 10 years (**Table 4**).

Table 4 shows lifetime prevalences of the 10 non-mutually exclusive social phobic situations included in the SADS-LA, based on *interviewer* diagnoses. Nearly 90% of patients with generalized social phobia and 79% of patients with nongeneralized social phobia were diagnosed as having a public speaking phobia. Also, all of the social situations generally categorized as "interactional" were significantly more prevalent among patients with generalized social phobia (attending social affairs, dealing with authority figures, speaking to strangers, and asking directions). Furthermore, these were the only situations that distinguished the two patient groups. These results are consistent with the clinical narrative review ratings (Table 1) that showed the following: (1) nearly all patients in both groups feared or avoided at least one performance situation; (2) about two thirds of patients with nongeneralized social phobia (vs all patients with generalized social phobia) feared or avoided at least one interactional situation; and (3) nearly all patients with generalized social phobia (vs only 6% of patients with nongeneralized social phobia) feared or avoided at least three interactional situations.

DISTRIBUTION OF NUMBER OF FEARS

There are 10 specific social situations (shown in Table 4) included in the SADS-LA. Interviewers systematically rated each of these 10 situations on a seven-point scale ranging from 1 being no fear or discomfort, to 5 being definite irrational fear resulting in some behavioral change (eg, partial avoidance), to 7 being irrational fear plus considerable avoidance.

The **Figure** shows the distribution of number of situations rated 5 or greater for patients with generalized and nongeneralized social phobia. They are based on the SADS-LA ratings of specially trained, experienced interviewers (clinical psychologists and psychiatric social workers). These distributions were *not* derived from the senior clinician's judgments, which were strictly based on narrative reviews, and which were not limited to SADS-LA social phobia types.

Patient groups are clearly distinguished, with modes of five and two for generalized and nongeneralized, respectively. However, there is considerable overlap, primarily for three and four social phobic fears.

LIFETIME COMORBIDITY FOR OTHER DISORDERS

The only disorders that differentiated groups, both more prevalent among patients with generalized social phobia, were atypical depression (36% vs 13%) and alcoholism (25% vs 6%) (**Table 5**). Nearly two thirds of patients with generalized social phobia with major depression (24/38) suffered from the atypical depressive subtype, characterized by mood reactivity plus at least two associated features (hypersomnia, anergia, weight gain or increased appetite, rejection sensitivity). Moreover, the excess of major depression among patients with generalized social phobia (57% vs 37%) is entirely accounted for by the atypical subtype.

FAMILIAL PSYCHOPATHOLOGY

Preliminary analyses of the subset of patients who participated in our family study[16] suggest that generalized social phobia may represent a familial form of the disorder. Rate of social phobia was as follows: (1) significantly greater among relatives of patients with general-

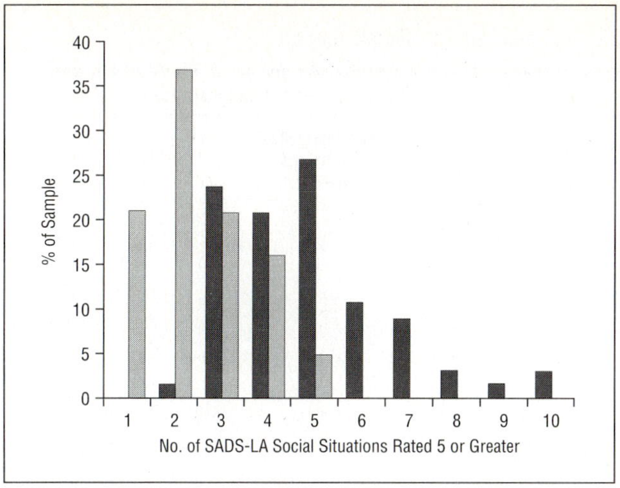

The distribution of number of social fears for patients with generalized (darker bars) and nongeneralized (lighter bars) social phobia. SADS-LA indicates Schedule for Affective Disorders and Schizophrenia–Lifetime Anxiety version.

Table 5. Lifetime Comorbidity for Other Disorders in Patients With Generalized and Nongeneralized Social Phobia*

Diagnosis	Generalized (n=67)	Nongeneralized (n=62)	*P*
Anxiety disorders			
Panic disorder	10 (15)	21 (34)	.13
Obsessive-compulsive disorder	7 (10)	3 (5)	.99
Simple phobia	14 (21)	16 (26)	.99
Generalized anxiety disorder	4 (6)	7 (11)	.99
Any anxiety	26 (39)	32 (52)	.99
Mood disorders			
Major depression	38 (57)	23 (37)	.99
Atypical type†	24 (36)	8 (13)	.03
Any mood	43 (64)	33 (53)	.99
Substance use disorders (SUD)			
Alcohol	17 (25)	4 (6)	.04
Other	8 (12)	3 (5)	.99
Any SUD	22 (33)	6 (10)	.01

**Patients were classified as having generalized or nongeneralized social phobia based on consensual agreement of two senior clinicians who independently reviewed narratives of trained interviewers. Data are given as number (percent).*

†Mood reactivity plus at least two of the following four symptoms: hypersomnia, anergia, weight gain/increased appetite, and rejection sensitivity.

ized vs nongeneralized social phobia (16% vs 6%) ($P<.05$); (2) significantly greater among relatives of patients with generalized social phobia vs NMI controls (16% vs 6%) ($P<.05$); and (3) identical for relatives of patients with nongeneralized social phobia and controls (6%).

The same pattern of results emerged when families rather than first-degree relatives were counted. Considering families in which at least one relative had social phobia, the following was observed: (1) patients with generalized vs nongeneralized social phobia, 36% vs 13%, $P<.05$; (2) patients with generalized social phobia vs controls, 36% vs 19%; $P<.05$; and (3) patients with nongeneralized social phobia vs controls, 13% vs 19%; P=not significant.

There was no evidence that patients with generalized social phobia were more likely to transmit the generalized form of the syndrome. Regardless of proband group, nearly all relatives with social phobia feared or avoided only one or two social situations. Of the 15 relatives of patients with generalized social phobia who, themselves, had social phobia, 7, 6, 1, and 1 relative had social phobia involving 1, 2, 3, and 4 SADS-LA situations, respectively. Of the five relatives of patients with nongeneralized social phobia who, themselves, had social phobia, 2, 2, and 1 relative had social phobia involving 1, 2, and 3 SADS-LA situations, respectively. However, these samples are too small to allow for a meaningful assessment of whether these subtypes breed true.

COMMENT

RELIABILITY

The present study found that generalized social phobia, as defined in *DSM-III-R*, can be distinguished reliably from nongeneralized social phobia. Although encouraging, this finding should be viewed as preliminary for the following reasons.

First, subjects were patients seen in an anxiety clinic. It is not known whether these results would generalize to other populations (eg, community samples, mood disorder clinic attendees).

Second, although certain classification rules were stipulated prior to narrative review (see "Categorization of Patients as Having Generalized and Nongeneralized Social Phobia"), certain basic issues were never resolved. Most salient among these was how situation should be operationalized. For example, should "speaking to strangers" be counted as one situation or many (speaking to strangers while on the job, attending a party, on the telephone, etc)? During our consensus meetings, we usually split, rather than lumped situations when in doubt. For example, a teacher who "barely muddled through" his or her classes because of nervousness, made up excuses to avoid presentations before his or her peers, and often "called in sick" when it was his or her turn to host lodge meetings was counted as fearing or avoiding multiple (public speaking) situations. We believed that representing the pervasiveness of the patient's syndrome more accurately reflected the clinical reality of the case. However, other clinicians might disagree. The point is that, unless criteria are formulated, patients with generalized social phobia at one site might be very different from those at another, *despite* good within-site reliabilities.

This dilemma is even more apparent when psychiatric interview schedules are used to classify subjects. The original SADS-LA includes 10 specific social situations, six performance and four interactional. The revised version of the schedule[34] includes 13—talking on the telephone and dating were added, and attending social affairs was split into large gatherings and small or intimate social affairs. The Anxiety Disorders Interview Schedule–Revised[35] includes 11. The Liebowitz Social Anxiety Scale[36] includes 24. These scales differ in descriptions (and numbers) of situations and in how each situation is rated (four-

Table 6. Within-Group Comparisons of Patients With 'Generalized' and 'Nongeneralized' Social Phobia*

Variable†	Generalized: Most Situations (n=67)	Generalized: ≥5 Situations (n=38)	Nongeneralized: Less-Than-Most Situations (n=62)	Nongeneralized: 1 or 2 Situations (n=37)
Single (never married), %	64	55	37	30
Mean onset of social phobia, y	10.9	10.8	16.9	18.5
Social phobia by situation, %				
Attending social affairs	94	95	37	24
Dealing with authority figures	60	68	27	30
Speaking to strangers	37	45	10	8
Asking directions	27	29	0	0
Lifetime comorbidity, %				
Major depression, atypical type	36	32	13	14
Alcoholism	25	26	6	8
Families with social phobia,‡ %	36	40	13	0

**The second columns in each group ("5 or more" and "1 or 2") represent subsamples of the first columns ("most" and "less-than-most," respectively).*
†Only variables that differed significantly between "most" and "less-than-most" groups are shown.
‡Total number of families = 33, 10, 30, 7, for columns 1, 2, 3, and 4, respectively.

vs seven-point scale; separately, for fear and avoidance or some combination of both, etc). Obviously, if only ratings are used to determine which subjects fear or avoid most social situations, samples could vary considerably depending on which scale and conventions are used.

In summary, our findings suggest that good reliability on the generalized and nongeneralized distinction does not require complete operationalizing of these subtypes. This is consistent with the results of the MacArthur data reanalysis for *DSM-IV*[37] that included about half of the patients in the present study for its New York site analyses. In that report, a completely operationalized system did not perform substantially better than the most vs less-than-most clinical review procedure used in the present study, ie, both performed well.

As for operationalizing situation, this may be an impossible task since there are an infinite number of conceivable social encounters that an individual may experience. In practice, perhaps the best that one can do is rigorously explore multiple interpersonal domains in judging pervasiveness of social impairment and concerns.

VALIDITY

Collectively, differences between patients with generalized and nongeneralized social phobia support the validity of this distinction. Compared with patients with nongeneralized social phobia, patients with generalized social phobia were more often single (about two thirds had never married), had earlier onsets of social phobia (mean age, 10.9 years), were more often characterized by fears of interpersonal interactions, and had higher rates of atypical depression and alcoholism.

These differences have been inconsistent across studies. Whereas three studies[10,11,13] reported that patients with generalized social phobia scored significantly higher on the Beck Depression Inventory, one study[38] found no difference in rates of major depression among patients with generalized (37%) and nongeneralized social phobia (30%). (However, to our knowledge, the atypical subtype was never studied.) Whereas one study[13] reported significantly earlier onsets of social phobia for patients with generalized social phobia, another[12] found no onset difference. Whereas one study[10] found that patients with generalized social phobia tended to be single, another[12] did not. These inconsistencies are difficult to reconcile given differences in subtype definitions and comparison groups across studies.

Perhaps the most convincing support for the validity of generalized social phobia is provided by the blind best-estimate consensus diagnoses of relatives. More than one third of the families of patients with generalized social phobia had social phobia, whereas prevalence of the disorder among relatives of patients with nongeneralized social phobia did not differ from relatives of controls. These findings suggest that generalized social phobia (different from other forms of the disorder) may characterize a familial form of the syndrome.

Our findings that nearly two thirds of patients with generalized social phobia with major depression had the atypical form of the syndrome, and that all depressive excess was due to the atypical subtype, are consistent with the dopaminergic model of generalized social phobia of Liebowitz et al.[39] Briefly, patients with atypical depression and generalized social phobia are characterized by hypersensitivity to criticism and rejection; both respond well to monoamine oxidase inhibitors and are less often helped by tricyclic antidepressants; also, monoamine oxidase inhibitors have a greater dopaminergic effect than do tricyclic antidepressants. Liebowitz et al[39] review other literature supporting their view that dopaminergic mechanisms may partially account for the successful monoamine oxidase inhibitor treatment of both of these conditions.

DOES GENERALIZED SOCIAL PHOBIA REPRESENT A DISTINCT CLINICAL ENTITY?

The present findings suggest that generalized social phobia is a useful concept. However, they do not directly address whether it is a distinct clinical syndrome or simply a severe form of the disorder. Perhaps degree of pervasiveness of social fears accounts for group differences. As shown in the Figure, although two positively skewed distributions emerge when clinically derived groups are portrayed as a function of number of feared situations (based on SADS-LA ratings), there is considerable overlap.

If group differences are associated with quantitative rather than qualitative distinctions, then "extreme" groups (defined by number of feared situations) should differ more markedly. As shown in the Figure, there was essentially no overlap between patients with clinically derived generalized and nongeneralized social phobia who feared five or more and one or two situations. **Table 6** compares these extreme groups with the entire groups of patients with clinically derived social phobia from which each was drawn. There are few within-group differences on any of these variables (compare most vs five or more, and less-than-most vs one or two); and by and large, extreme groups do not differ more markedly than clinically derived groups (compare five or more vs one or two, and most vs less-than-most).

These comparisons are limited by the number and specific types of situations included in the SADS-LA. However, taken together with our findings of differences on demographic and clinical characteristics, onset, comorbidity of other disorders, and familial psychopathologic condition, they suggest that generalized social phobia may represent a distinct clinical syndrome.

Accepted for publication November 7, 1994.

This investigation was supported in part by grants MH-21411, MH-23864, and MH-37592 and Mental Health Clinic Research Center grant MH-30906, all from the National Institute of Mental Health, Rockville, Md.

Reprints not available.

REFERENCES

1. Schneier FR, Johnson J, Hornig CD, Liebowitz MR, Weissman MM. Social phobia: comorbidity and morbidity in an epidemiologic sample. *Arch Gen Psychiatry.* 1992;49:282-288.
2. American Psychiatric Association. *Diagnostic and Statistical Manual of Mental Disorders, Third Edition.* Washington, DC: American Psychiatric Association; 1980.
3. Liebowitz MR, Gorman JM, Fyer AJ, Klein DF. Social phobia: review of a neglected anxiety disorder. *Arch Gen Psychiatry.* 1985;42:729-736.
4. Heimberg RG, ed. Social phobia. *Clin Psychol Rev.* 1989;9(special issue):1-140.
5. Mannuzza S, Fyer AJ, Liebowitz MR, Klein DF. Delineating the boundary of social phobia: its relationship to panic disorder and agoraphobia. *J Anxiety Dis.* 1990;4:41-59.
6. Turner SM, Beidel DC. Social phobia: clinical syndrome, diagnosis, and comorbidity. *Clin Psychol Rev.* 1989;9:3-18.
7. Gelernter CS, Stein MB, Tancer ME, Uhde TW. An examination of syndromal validity and diagnostic subtypes in social phobia and panic disorder. *J Clin Psychiatry.* 1992;53:23-27.
8. Heimberg RG, Holt CS, Schneier FR, Spitzer RL, Liebowitz MR. The issue of subtypes in the diagnosis of social phobia. *J Anxiety Dis.* 1993;7:249-269.
9. American Psychiatric Association. *Diagnostic and Statistical Manual of Mental Disorders, Revised Third Edition.* Washington, DC: American Psychiatric Association; 1987.
10. Heimberg RG, Hope DA, Dodge CS, Becker RE. *DSM-III-R* subtypes of social phobia. *J Nerv Ment Dis.* 1990;178:172-179.
11. Turner SM, Beidel DC, Townsley RM. Social phobia: a comparison of specific and generalized subtypes and avoidant personality disorder. *J Abnorm Psychol.* 1992;101:326-331.
12. Schneier FR, Spitzer RL, Gibbon M, Fyer AJ, Liebowitz MR. The relationship of social phobia subtypes and avoidant personality disorder. *Compr Psychiatry.* 1991;32:496-502.
13. Holt CS, Heimberg RG, Hope DA. Avoidant personality disorder and the generalized subtype of social phobia. *J Abnorm Psychol.* 1992;101:318-325.
14. Levin AP, Saoud JB, Strauman T, Gorman JM, Fyer AJ, Crawford R, Liebowitz MR. Responses of 'generalized' and 'discrete' social phobics during public speaking. *J Anxiety Dis.* 1993;7:207-221.
15. American Psychiatric Association. *Diagnostic and Statistical Manual of Mental Disorders, Fourth Edition.* Washington, DC: American Psychiatric Association; 1994.
16. Fyer AJ, Mannuzza S, Chapman TF, Liebowitz MR, Klein DF. A direct interview family study of social phobia. *Arch Gen Psychiatry.* 1993;50:286-293.
17. Amies PL, Gelder MG, Shaw PM. Social phobia: a comparative clinical study. *Br J Psychiatry.* 1983;142:174-179.
18. Herbert JD, Hope DA, Bellack AS. Validity of the distinction between generalized social phobia and avoidant personality disorder. *J Abnorm Psychol.* 1992;101:332-339.
19. Marks IM. The classification of phobic disorders. *Br J Psychiatry.* 1970;116:377-386.
20. Solyom L, Ledwidge B, Solyom C. Delineating social phobia. *Br J Psychiatry.* 1986;149:464-470.
21. Thyer BA, Parrish RT, Curtis GC, Nesse RM, Cameron OG. Ages of onset of *DSM-III* anxiety disorders. *Compr Psychiatry.* 1985;26:113-121.
22. Marks IM. *Fears and Phobias.* New York, NY: Academic Press Inc; 1969.
23. Cameron OG, Thyer BA, Nesse RM, Curtis GC. Symptom profiles of patients with *DSM-III* anxiety disorders. *Am J Psychiatry.* 1986;143:1132-1137.
24. Ost LG. Age of onset in different phobias. *J Abnorm Psychol.* 1987;96:223-229.
25. Turner SM, Beidel DC, Dancu CV, Keys DJ. Psychopathology of social phobia and comparison to avoidant personality disorder. *J Abnorm Psychol.* 1986;95:389-394.
26. Fyer AJ, Endicott J, Mannuzza S, Klein DF. *Schedule for Affective Disorders and Schizophrenia—Lifetime Anxiety Version.* New York, NY: Anxiety Disorders Clinic, New York State Psychiatric Institute; 1985.
27. Mannuzza S, Fyer AJ, Klein DF, Endicott J. Schedule for Affective Disorders and Schizophrenia—Lifetime Anxiety Version: rationale and conceptual development. *J Psychiatr Res.* 1986;20:317-325.
28. Mannuzza S, Fyer AJ, Martin LY, Gallops MS, Endicott J, Gorman JM, Liebowitz MR, Klein DF. Reliability of anxiety assessment, I: diagnostic agreement. *Arch Gen Psychiatry.* 1989;46:1093-1101.
29. American Psychiatric Association, Work Group to Revise *DSM-III. DSM-III-R in Development.* Washington, DC: American Psychiatric Association; 1985.
30. Mannuzza S, Fyer AJ, Endicott J, Klein DF. *Family Informant Schedule and Criteria.* New York, NY: Anxiety Disorders Clinic, New York State Psychiatric Institute; 1985.
31. Mannuzza S, Fyer AJ, Endicott J, Gallops MS, Martin LY, Reich T, Klein DF. An extension of the acquaintanceship procedure in family studies of mental disorder. *J Psychiatr Res.* 1992;26:45-57.
32. Shrout PE, Spitzer RL, Fleiss JL. Quantification of agreement in psychiatric diagnosis revisited. *Arch Gen Psychiatry.* 1987;44:172-177.
33. Klockars AJ, Sax G. *Quantitative Applications in the Social Sciences: Multiple Comparisons.* Beverly Hills, Calif: Sage Publications; 1986.
34. Schleyer B, Aaronson C, Mannuzza S, Martin LY, Fyer AJ. *Schedule for Affective Disorders and Schizophrenia—Lifetime Anxiety Version, Revised.* New York, NY: Anxiety Disorders Clinic, New York State Psychiatric Institute; 1990.
35. DiNardo PA, Moras K, Barlow DH, Rapee RM, Brown TA. Reliability of *DSM-III-R* anxiety disorder categories using the Anxiety Disorders Interview Schedule-Revised (ADIS-R). *Arch Gen Psychiatry.* 1993;50:251-256.
36. Liebowitz MR. Social phobia. *Mod Probl Pharmacopsychiatry.* 1987;22:141-173.
37. Schneier FR, Liebowitz MR, Beidel DC, Garfinkel R, Heimberg R, Juster H, Mannuzza S, Oberlander E, Turner SM, Law K, Mattia J, Orsillo S. MacArthur data reanalysis for social phobia. In: Widiger TA, Frances AJ, Pincus HA, First MB, Ross R, Davis W, eds. *DSM-IV Source Book (vol 2).* Washington, DC: American Psychiatric Press. In press.
38. Stein MB, Tancer ME, Gelernter CS, Vittone BJ, Uhde TW. Major depression in patients with social phobia. *Am J Psychiatry.* 1990;147:637-639.
39. Liebowitz MR, Schneier FR, Campeas R, Hollander E, Hatterer J, Fyer AJ, Gorman J, Papp L, Davies S, Gully R, Klein DF. Phenelzine vs atenolol in social phobia: a placebo-controlled comparison. *Arch Gen Psychiatry.* 1992;49:290-300.

ORIGINAL ARTICLE

A Trial of the Effect of a Standardized Psychiatric Consultation on Health Outcomes and Costs in Somatizing Patients

G. Richard Smith, Jr, MD; Kathryn Rost, PhD; T. Michael Kashner, PhD

Background: Patients who somatize but who do not meet criteria for somatization disorder are common in the community. Virtually no research has been conducted to determine how to treat these patients.

Methods: We conducted a randomized controlled clinical trial of a psychiatric consultation intervention we had previously shown to improve the management of somatization disorder. The study population included 51 physicians treating 56 somatizing patients who had a history of seeking help for six to 12 lifetime unexplained physical symptoms. At the onset of the experiment, physicians randomized to the treatment condition received a consultation letter recommending a specific management approach; physicians randomized to the control/crossover condition received the consultation letter after 12 months. Data on health outcomes and charges were collected every 4 months for 2 years after randomization for 96% of subjects who entered the study.

Results: Patients of physicians who received the intervention reported significantly increased physical functioning, an improvement that remained stable during the year after the intervention. The intervention reduced annual medical care charges by $289 (95% confidence interval, $40 to $464) in 1990 constant dollars, which equates to a 32.9% reduction in the annual median cost of their medical care.

Conclusions: Somatizing patients with a lifetime history of six to 12 unexplained physical symptoms reported better physical functioning after their primary care physician was provided appropriate treatment recommendations via a psychiatric consultation. Such a consultation is cost-effective because it reduces subsequent charges for medical care, while improving health outcomes in a chronically impaired population.

(Arch Gen Psychiatry. 1995;52:238-243)

From the Department of Psychiatry and Behavioral Sciences, University of Arkansas for Medical Sciences, National Institute of Mental Health Center for Rural Mental Healthcare Research, and Veterans Affairs Health Services Research and Development Field Program for Mental Health, Little Rock (Drs Smith and Rost); and Department of Psychiatry, University of Texas Southwestern Medical School, Dallas, and Research Service, Dallas Veterans Affairs Medical Center (Dr Kashner).

CLINICAL STUDIES estimate that 20% to 84% of patients in general medical settings present somatic complaints for which no organic cause can be found.[1-4] Unfortunately, there is little research to guide physicians about treatment for patients who somatize but do not meet the diagnostic criteria for somatization disorder. To address this problem, we tested a psychiatric consultation intervention, which had previously improved the management of somatization disorder, in a group of patients with somatization syndrome. Using an experimental design, we demonstrate that this intervention improved physical functioning and reduced medical charges in somatizing patients.

Somatization syndrome (defined as a lifetime history of at least six of 37 somatization symptoms in females, or at least four in males[5]) is a common and well-described chronic condition associated with considerable impairment and substantial health care utilization.[6-10] In the Epidemiologic Catchment Area Study, 11.6% of community respondents met criteria for lifetime somatization syndrome. Only 9% of subjects with lifetime somatization syndrome reported no unexplained physical symptoms in the past year.[6] Of those studied with five or more current unexplained somatic symptoms, 63% reported current psychological symptoms and 50% met criteria for a current psychiatric disorder.[10] Somatizers report considerably more impairment in physical, social, and role functioning than patients whose physical problems can be medically diagnosed, spending between 1.3 and 4.9 days in bed each month on average.[11-13] In contrast, patients with most major medical problems average 1 day or less in bed each month.[13]

Of particular concern to both clini-

See Subjects and Methods on next page

SUBJECTS AND METHODS

RECRUITMENT AND DATA COLLECTION

State and county medical society membership lists and state licensing boards were used to identify all general practitioners, family physicians, and general internists in a seven-county area surrounding Little Rock, Ark. These primary care physicians in central Arkansas were asked in a letter to refer "patients who had a history of multiple unexplained somatic complaints" to the study. Advertisements were also placed in the local media seeking volunteers who suffered from "multiple unexplained medical problems for which no cause could be found." To be eligible for the study, patients had to have a lifetime history of six to 12 unexplained medical symptoms. These symptoms must have been severe enough to cause subjects to take medicine, see a physician, or change their lifestyle. This operational definition of somatization syndrome has been used extensively.[6-9] The number of unexplained medical symptoms was determined by a research psychiatrist by means of a checklist that contained the 37 items that make up the diagnostic criteria for somatization disorder according to *DSM-III-R* criteria.[5] Patients were excluded from the study if they did not have a primary care physician who agreed to allow the research team to see the patient; if they lacked transportation to the medical center; if they indicated they would be moving from the area during the course of the study; or if their physician had participated in one of our previous studies. Extensive review of the patients' completed medical records (see "Measurement of Health Care Utilization" below) by the research psychiatrist excluded all patients with documented physical disorders, such as systemic lupus erythematosus, which could account for the symptoms or impairment.

The university's Institutional Review Board approved the study's protocol. After the research project was explained, all patients gave informed consent. After the initial interview, patients from both groups were visited in their homes every 4 months for 2 years by research assistants who were masked to randomization. At these home visits, the patients' health outcomes and health care utilization for the intervening 4 months were assessed.

RESEARCH DESIGN AND INTERVENTION

The study design was a prospective randomized controlled trial with a one-way crossover from the control condition to the intervention (**Figure**). Physicians were randomly assigned to receive the intervention at the onset of the experiment or 1 year later. In our sample all patients' physicians referred who met the criteria for our study. We assigned all patients a particular physician referred to the group in which the physician had originally been randomized. Patients of physicians randomized to receive the intervention at the onset are referred to as treatment patients. Patients of physicians randomized to receive the intervention at 1-year follow-up are referred to as control/crossover patients.

Immediately after initial data had been collected at the beginning of the study, physicians assigned to receive the intervention at the onset received the same psychiatric consultation letter tested in the previous studies with patients with somatization disorder.[15,17] The letter told the physician that the patient met criteria for somatization syndrome and described the chronic, relapsing course and low morbidity and mortality associated with somatization.[18] In addition, the letter suggested regularly scheduled brief appointments with the primary care physician for the patient, possibly every 4 to 6 weeks, and that "as-needed" appointments be avoided. We further suggested that a brief physical examination be performed at each visit, especially concentrating on the organ system or body part where the patient had complaints. We recommended that, during the examination, the physician look for signs of disease rather than taking symptoms at face value. We also suggested that physicians avoid hospitalization, diagnostic procedures, surgery, and laboratory evaluations unless clearly indicated. Finally, the physician was encouraged not to tell the patient that the disorder was "all in your head" but was instead encouraged to view the development of symptoms as an unconscious process.

Physicians in the control/crossover group assigned to receive the intervention at 1-year follow-up were sent letters immediately after the psychiatric evaluation thanking them for allowing us to study their patient and telling them that our research assistants would follow them up. At the end of the 1-year follow-up period, these physicians were sent the same psychiatric consultation letter.

MEASUREMENT OF HEALTH OUTCOMES

Health outcomes were assessed by means of the RAND Health Status Measures developed for the Health Insurance Experiment.[19] These patient self-report measures assessed physical functioning (Physical Functioning Index), mental health (Mental Health Index), social functioning (Social Well-Being Index), and general health (General Health Ratings Index). Scores on all scales were standardized on a scale of 0 to 100, with 100 representing

Continued on next page

cians and health policymakers are the extensive and questionably effective medical services somatizing patients use. Although the prevalence of somatization syndrome in clinical settings and the associated health care costs have not been rigorously estimated, available data indicate that somatizing patients use hospital services extensively. More than a quarter of somatizing respondents in the Epidemiologic Catchment Area Study reported hospitalization in the last year, compared with 12% of nonsomatizers.[6] Primary care patients with somatization syndrome averaged 2.2 days in the hospital annually,[11] compared with the national average of 0.9 day.[14] Complex and costly inpatient procedures to diagnose physical problems may often be inappropriate since the illness is a psychiatric syndrome. Such procedures may even be counterproductive if they reinforce the patient's belief that the symptoms have an elusive physical cause.

Standard clinical practice for the last three decades has been for consultation/liaison psychiatrists to recommend that primary care physicians limit the number of different physicians a somatizing patient sees, to see the patient frequently, and to avoid surgery and invasive procedures. During the

the best possible functioning. Days in bed during the past month were also measured.

MEASUREMENT OF HEALTH CARE UTILIZATION

Health care utilization was quantified for 2½ years retrospectively and for a 2-year period prospectively after randomization. Utilization before study entry was determined retrospectively by asking patients to provide consent for release of information from all providers and payers of health care for the preceding 2½ years. This strategy, which estimates utilization and charges from medical and billing records rather than from the subject's memory, has been accepted as a reasonable method for measuring utilization retrospectively over long periods.[15] We chose to measure utilization during a 2½-year period because it provided a better estimate of the subject's use of services before the intervention than the standard 6-month interval, given the highly episodic nature of somatic symptoms. Prospective health care utilization was obtained in a similar manner except that patients were interviewed every 4 months to obtain sources of care for the intervening period.

Providers and payers were contacted multiple times by writing, by telephone, or in person until all essential medical and billing records were obtained. All records were reviewed by clinicians for other sources of care that were not included in the subject's initial list. The new sources were then contacted and records obtained. This process was repeated until the records were complete. Data from various sources were compared to prevent duplication, before they were double entered and corrected for errors.

The actual charge for each service the patient received was recorded; if that was not obtainable, the "usual, customary, and reasonable" charge of the Arkansas Blue Cross–Blue Shield organization was used. Although no actual charge was made for the consultation, it was valued at $150 in calculating the cost-effectiveness of the intervention. Charges were divided into medical charges and psychiatric charges. A charge was considered medical if the patient had an outpatient procedure other than psychiatric (psychiatric *Current Procedural Terminology 4* codes ranging from 90801 to 90899) or was admitted to the hospital for a condition other than psychiatric (psychiatric *International Classification of Diseases, Ninth Revision* codes ranging from 290 to 319). All charges were inflated at an annual compounded rate of 7.3% to 1990 dollars.

DATA ANALYSIS

Data from pilot studies we conducted to inform the design of this study indicated that the large variance of our dependent variables in somatizing patients would make it difficult to judge whether the intervention had a clinically significant effect by examining differences between the two groups in how means changed over time. After reviewing multiple analytic methods for panel data, we selected cross-sectional time-series analysis as an efficient and theory-driven method of evaluating the intervention.[20] A more extensive discussion of the rationale for and application of this analytic strategy to the evaluation of psychiatric interventions has previously been described.[17]

A set of maximum likelihood regression models were fit simultaneously. There were two types of models in this set of regression equations. The first type modeled the relationship between the outcome measured at a specific point in time and patient characteristics. The second type modeled the relationship between change in outcome measured at two specific successive time points and patient characteristics, correcting for correlation from the repeated assessment of patients. The effect of the intervention was estimated by including an intervention indicator variable in each model that assumed the value of one if the patient's physician had received the intervention during that period or any previous period, and zero otherwise. This approach allows the simultaneous estimation of the difference in outcome between treatment and control/crossover patients, and the difference in outcome over time resulting from the intervention in each group. Although randomization produced two groups that did not have significantly different sociodemographic characteristics on health status, we estimated the effects of the intervention from models correcting for the effect of differences between the two groups in sociodemographic and initial health status characteristics on the outcomes of interest to rule out that these factors explained the differences we observed.

The same analytic strategy was used to determine whether there were differences in health care charges between treatment and control/crossover patients. To estimate conservatively any reductions in expenditures given the skewed distribution of charges, we calculated the effect of the intervention on health care expenditures for all patients by standardizing expenditure data with the use of median charges, which more accurately reflected health care charges for the typical somatizing patient in our sample. We then used a log transformation to normalize the error term in the model.

Cross-sectional time series analysis did not prove to be a useful method for examining between-group differences in utilization because key constructs, such as hospital days per quarter, were bimodally distributed. To understand better the intervention's effect on utilization, we used linear regressions to model between group differences in the number of hospital days, emergency department visits, and physician visits during the first year of the study, controlling for patient age, gender, race, education, and marital status.

past decade, this approach has been demonstrated to be cost-effective in the treatment of patients with somatization disorder, the most extreme form of somatization.[15,16] We, therefore, reasoned that this intervention may also be effective in patients with somatization syndrome. Thus, to allow better-informed clinical decisions about how aggressively to manage the problems these patients present, we tailored a psychiatric consultation directed toward the primary care physician treating somatizing subjects and tested it in a randomized controlled clinical trial for its effect on health outcomes and charges. Based on our previous work[15] at the time of this trial, we hypothesized that patients who received the intervention would have decreased health care charges.

RESULTS

One hundred fifty-one patients were studied in person by the research team. Fifty-six patients met criteria to partici-

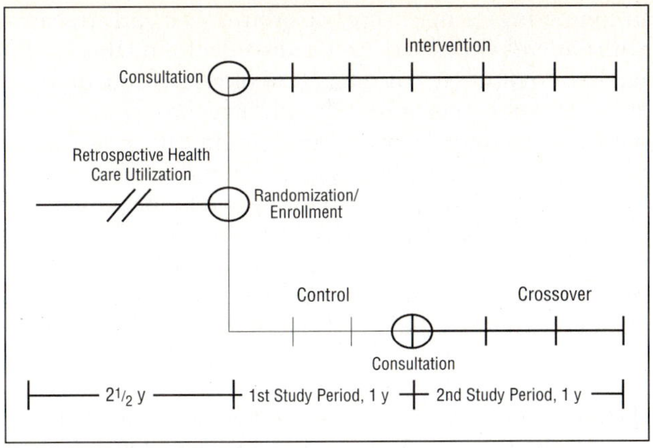

Study design.

Table 1. Sociodemographic and Health Status Characteristics of Somatizers Whose Physicians Were Randomized to Treatment and Control/Crossover Conditions at the Onset of the Experiment

	Treatment (n=27)	Control/ Crossover (n=29)
Sociodemographic characteristics		
Female, %	81.5	69.0
White, %	88.9	79.3
Currently married, %	63.0	62.1
Age, y (mean±SD)	42.2±12.3	43.9±12.5
Education, y (mean±SD)	12.6±2.1	11.3±4.0
Health status characteristics at onset of experiment (mean±SD)		
Physical functioning	33.3±35.1	26.4±28.8
Mental health	52.7±18.9	54.7±25.5
General health	33.7±12.9	34.2±15.6
Social functioning	40.2±18.2	38.2±18.8
Health insurance status,*%		
Medicare	11.1	13.8
Medicaid	3.7	3.4
Other health insurance	66.7	62.1
Health maintenance organization	0	0
No health coverage	18.6	17.2

**One subject in the control/crossover group refused to provide this information.*

pate in the study; all 56 patients agreed to participate. The vast majority of the 95 patients who did not meet entry criteria for this study had somatization disorder and are the subject of other reports.[16] The subjects in this study were predominantly female (75.0%), white (83.9%), currently married (62.5%), and not on Medicare or Medicaid (87.5%), with a mean age of 43.1 years and a mean education of 11.9 years. Fifty-one physicians provided primary care to these patients, who averaged 9.4±2.0 (SD) medically unexplained physical problems during their lifetime. Median annual charges for medical care during the year before entry into the study were $878 (mean±SD, $3185±$7026). Median annual charges for psychiatric care during the same period for the 26% of patients who received any mental health services were $715. There were no significant sociodemographic, health, or health insurance status differences at the onset of the experiment between the 27 patients randomized to the treatment condition and the 29 patients randomized to the control/crossover condition (**Table 1**). Nor were there significant differences between the two groups in the percentage who came from physician referral or via advertisement.

These patients had a high prevalence of comorbid psychiatric disorders[21,22] (**Table 2**). There were no statistically significant differences between the treatment and control/crossover groups for any of the 11 conditions assessed.

Fifty-four (96%) of 56 patients who entered the study completed all four follow-up interviews during the 2-year investigation. The analytic strategy allowed us to maintain all subjects in the analysis because no subject was missing data from more than two follow-up periods.

Examination of health status data showed differences in functioning as a result of the intervention 1 year after physicians received the psychiatric consultation letter. As **Table 3** demonstrates, after the intervention, patients reported significantly better physical functioning. Specifically, patients' physical functioning improved 6.87 units on the physical functioning scale during the year after the intervention (P=.002). Statistical models examining change over time indicated that this improvement in physical functioning remained stable for the 2 years after the intervention. The intervention had no statistically significant effect on emotional health or social functioning. While the general health ratings patients reported had a tendency to decline after the intervention (P=.06), this difference was most likely not clinically significant.[13] Patients reported 0.85 fewer bed day per month after the intervention, although this difference was not statistically significant (P=.07).

Examination of utilization data indicated that no treatment or control/crossover patient had visits to the referring physician at the frequency recommended by the psychiatric consultation letter during the first year of the study. Treatment patients averaged 2.6±2.7 visits to the referring physician, as opposed to control/crossover patients, who averaged 2.1±3.1 visits during the first 4 months (P=.50). Treatment patients had 0.5 fewer hospital day, 0.7 more emergency department visit, and 0.2 more outpatient visits than control/crossover patients, adjusting for sociodemographic characteristics in the year after the intervention. None of these utilization differences was statistically significant, as Table 3 demonstrates.

During the year after the intervention, annual medical care charges decreased $289 (95% confidence interval, $40 to $464), which equates to a 32.9% reduction in annual median charges for medical care. This reduction in charges also remained stable for the 2 years during which we observed subjects after the intervention, and it appears to be a function of fewer hospital days a year. Charges for psychiatric care remained virtually unchanged.

COMMENT

This study provides the first evidence, to our knowledge, that any intervention can improve the physical functioning of somatizing patients. At the same time, charges for medical care were also decreased by $289 in the first year, making the psychiatric consultation tested in this study cost-effective compared with usual care.

The seven-point improvement associated with the in-

Table 2. Lifetime Axis I* Comorbidity for the Treatment Group, the Control/Crossover Group, and the Total Sample

	No. (%)		
Disorder	Treatment (n=27)	Control/Crossover (n=29)	Total (N=56)
Agoraphobia	1 (3.7)	2 (6.9)	**3** (5.4)
Alcohol abuse or dependence	2 (7.4)	7 (24.1)	**9** (16.1)
Bipolar	1 (3.7)	2 (6.9)	**3** (5.4)
Bulimia	0 (0.0)	2 (6.9)	**2** (3.6)
Drug abuse	2 (7.4)	3 (10.4)	**5** (8.9)
Dysthymia	9 (33.3)	8 (27.6)	**17** (30.4)
Generalized anxiety	10 (37.0)	11 (37.9)	**21** (37.5)
Major depression	13 (48.2)	13 (44.8)	**26** (46.4)
Obsessive-compulsive	3 (11.1)	6 (20.7)	**9** (16.1)
Panic	3 (11.1)	8 (27.6)	**11** (19.4)
Phobia	5 (18.5)	5 (17.2)	**10** (17.9)

**Diagnostic Interview Schedule*[21] *and* DSM-III[22] *diagnoses.*

Table 3. Effect of a Psychiatric Consultation Letter on Health Status, Health Care Utilization, and Health Care Costs 1 Year After the Consultation*

Domain	Change	*P*
Physical functioning	6.87	.002
General health	−2.23	.06
Mental health	−0.79	.33
Social functioning	−0.97	.26
Bed days	−0.85	.07
Hospital days	−0.5	.88
Emergency department visits	−0.7	.50
Outpatient visits	0.2	.95
Annual savings in medical costs, $	289.11	.02
Annual savings in psychiatric costs, $	51.93	.15

**All results reported have been adjusted for between-group differences in patient age, race, sex, education, and marital status. Health status and cost comparisons were derived from cross-sectional times series analysis. Utilization differences were derived from linear regression. Positive scores on physical functioning, general health, mental health, and social functioning indicate improvement associated with the intervention. Negative scores on bed days indicate improvement associated with the intervention. Health status change scores are scores for the RAND Health Status Measures standardized on 100-point scale. Positive scores on all utilization variables indicate greater use of services in the treatment group.*

tervention was clinically significant, even given the substantial variation in physical functioning in our subjects. Previous research indicates that seven- to 10-point differences in physical functioning are equivalent to the impairment associated with gastrointestinal tract disorders (−6.7), diabetes (−7.6), arthritis (−9.3), and back problems (−9.5).[23,24] For example, arthritic patients who report ever having acute or chronic pain, swelling, or stiffness in the fingers, hips, or knees report an average of nine points more impairment in physical functioning than do patients with no chronic conditions. Thus, the intervention improves the physical functioning of somatizing patients nearly as much as the improvement a patient with mild arthritis would experience if his or her condition went into complete remission. Our statistical model could both estimate how the between-group difference in physical functioning at the beginning of the study affected its change over time and control for such differences in comparing change in the two groups. Our early research with patients with somatization disorder found that the intervention resulted in no change in physical functioning.[15] However, subsequent research with larger groups of patients with somatization disorder found significant and substantial improvements in physical functioning with a similar intervention.[15] These findings add support to the present observation of enhanced physical functioning.

The cost of the "treatment" resulting in this improvement can be easily recovered by the reduction in medical charges we observed when physicians received the consultation letter. Using a conservative method of calculating the savings associated with the intervention, we estimate that the intervention saves $289 a year for somatizing patients with median baseline health care charges, or 32.9% of their annual median expenditures for medical care.

The cost reductions associated with the intervention with somatizing patients replicates parallel research we conducted that demonstrated that consultation letters to primary care physicians treating patients with somatization disorder result in a 34% reduction in health care charges and improve patients' physical capacity.[16,17] We attribute the smaller cost savings that both of these studies demonstrated in comparison with the initial test of this intervention[15] to the institution of diagnosis related groups in the interim, which drastically reduced hospital stays for somatization.[1]

The intervention produced a smaller improvement in physical functioning in patients with somatization syndrome than it did in patients who meet criteria for somatization disorder.[16,17] This difference can be most easily explained by noting that with no intervention, patients with somatization disorder report greater levels of physical impairment than do subthreshold somatizers, as would be expected with a more severe form of any disorder. These findings, which show that somatizers improve in response to the same treatment as do patients with somatization disorder, also make an important contribution to psychiatric nosology,[25] supporting the argument that the two groups share a similar psychiatric condition.

We observed no statistically or clinically significant change in measures of general health, mental health, and social functioning of these patients. This is similar to our findings with patients with somatization disorder[15-17] with a similar intervention. However, in patients with somatization disorder, a more elaborate intervention, group treatment, resulted in improvement in the mental health measure.[26] These earlier findings suggest that one reason for our observing no change in these measures is the sparseness of the intervention. An alternative explanation is that the sample provided limited power to find a difference if in fact one existed in several of the outcomes measures with large variances.

The internal validity of our findings can be challenged because some physicians treated more than one patient in the same experimental condition. This clustering, involving only four physicians in our sample, occurred too infrequently to estimate any inadvertent contribution of this feature of the design to the effect size of the intervention. We expect that the contribution is too minimal to change the clinical significance of our findings. Because the analytic strategy estimates the effect of the intervention by a combination of a randomized trial and a preintervention-postintervention comparison, it is possible that pressures for physicians to lower costs and limit tests for all patients may explain part of the 32% reduction in median costs we discovered with the intervention. Since these findings are similar to our previous work, it is unlikely that these time-related trends explain the entire cost savings or the improvement in physical functioning we observed with the intervention.

Although patients in this study were recruited directly by advertisements, the vast majority (86%) were referred by their primary care physicians. The seven subjects who responded to the advertisements all had primary care physicians; however, these patients may be somewhat different from the referred patients in unknown ways. It is unlikely that these possible differences affected the results, since they were relatively balanced between the treatment and the control/crossover groups.

Since these patients were recruited from 51 diverse practices across central Arkansas, the results of our study have substantial external validity to other practices. Future research should attempt to replicate our findings in a larger random (case finding) vs referred sample of patients with six to 12 lifetime unexplained physical symptoms and control for the possibility of type I errors given multiple comparisons. This replication is necessary to determine whether physicians will change their practice patterns to incorporate the management recommendations we propose in treating all somatizing patients within their practice who meet the criteria, not just those they label as problematic. With the current research design, we cannot rule out the possibility that the change in physician practice patterns we observed reflected physicians' willingness to limit care only after they had exhausted the usefulness of more traditional medical approaches. Finally, further work is needed to develop other complementary interventions, such as short-term group therapy, to improve important patient outcomes, including mental health, which this intervention did not influence.

As described in this research, somatization syndrome is a subthreshold disorder, meaning that it does not meet diagnostic criteria as defined in *DSM-IV*.[27] This is similar to "minor depression"[28] and "depressive symptoms,"[13] which have also been found to lead to substantial disability and impaired functioning. It is becoming increasingly clear that primary care clinicians should be watchful for these subthreshold conditions and attentive to their treatment.

This intervention is for patients with *unexplained* somatic complaints, not simply patients with multiple symptoms. The clinician should first be satisfied that the symptoms do not represent an undiagnosed condition before embarking on this management strategy.

Thus, this study contributes to the literature by describing a successful test of a psychiatric consultation intervention for patients who somatize but who do not meet diagnostic criteria for somatization disorder. If subsequent studies replicate our findings, consultations to physicians treating somatizing patients hold substantial promise to improve physical functioning while simultaneously reducing costs of medical care.

Accepted for publication December 6, 1994.

This research was supported by grants R01 MH46090 and P50 MH48197 from the National Institute of Mental Health, grant 12142 from the Robert Wood Johnson Foundation, the Veterans Affairs Health Services Research and Development Field Program for Mental Health, and Research Scientist Development Award K02MH00843, Level II, from the National Institute of Mental Health (Dr Smith).

We thank Debbie Hodges, Martha Mobbs, Carla Williams, and Cindy Mosley for their dedicated work on this project.

Reprint requests to Department of Psychiatry, Slot 554, University of Arkansas for Medical Sciences, 4301 W Markham, Little Rock, AR 72205 (Dr Smith).

REFERENCES

1. Kellner R. Functional somatic symptoms in hypochondriasis. *Arch Gen Psychiatry.* 1985;42:821-833.
2. Kellner R. Neurosis in general practice. *Br J Clin Practice.* 1965;19:681-682.
3. Mayou R. Chest pain in the cardiac clinic. *J Psychosom Res.* 1978;17:353-357.
4. Mayou R. The nature of bodily symptoms. *Br J Psychiatry.* 1976;129:55-60.
5. American Psychiatric Association. *Diagnostic and Statistical Manual of Mental Disorders, Revised Third Edition.* Washington, DC: American Psychiatric Association; 1987.
6. Swartz M, Landerman R, George L, Blazer D, Escobar J. Somatization disorder. In: Robins LN, Regier D, eds. *Psychiatric Disorders in America.* New York, NY: Free Press; 1990:228.
7. Escobar JI, Burnham A, Karno M, Forsythe A, Golding JM. Somatization in the community. *Arch Gen Psychiatry.* 1987;44:713-718.
8. Escobar JI, Golding JM, Hough RL, Karno M, Burnam MA, Wells KB. Somatization in the community: relationship to disability and use of services. *Am J Public Health.* 1987;77:837-840.
9. Escobar JI, Rubio-Stipec M, Canino G, Karno M. Somatic symptom index (SSI): a new and abridged somatization construct. *J Nerv Ment Dis.* 1989;177:140-146.
10. Simon GE, VonKorff M. Somatization and psychiatric disorder in the NIMH epidemiologic catchment area study. *Am J Psychiatry.* 1991;148:1494-1500.
11. Rost KM, Smith GR, Kashner TM. Clinical differentiation between somatization disorder patients and somatizers: a test of two hypotheses. Presented at the Fourth Annual NIMH International Conference on the Classification and Treatment of Mental Disorders in General Medical Settings, Washington, DC, June 13, 1990.
12. Katon W, Lin E, Von Korff M, Russo J, Lipscomb P, Bush T. Somatization: a spectrum of severity. *Am J Psychiatry.* 1991;148:34-40.
13. Wells KB, Stewart A, Hays RD, Burnam MA, Rogers W, Daniels M, Berry S, Greenfield S, Ware J. The functioning and well-being of depressed patients: results from the medical outcomes study. *JAMA.* 1989;262:914-919.
14. Lefkowitz D, Monheit AC. *National Medical Expenditure Research Findings: Health Insurance, Use of Health Services, and Health Care Expenditures.* Rockville, Md: Center for General Health Services Intramural Research, Agency for Health Care Policy and Research; 1991.
15. Smith GR Jr, Monson RA, Ray DC. Psychiatric consultation in somatization disorder: a randomized, controlled study. *N Engl J Med.* 1986;314:1407-1413.
16. Rost K, Kashner TM, Smith GR Jr. Effectiveness of psychiatric intervention with somatization disorder patients: improved outcomes at reduced costs. *Gen Hosp Psychiatry.* 1994;16:381-387.
17. Kashner TM, Rost K, Smith GR, Lewis S. An analysis of panel data: the impact of a psychiatric consultation letter on the expenditures and outcomes of care for patients with somatization disorder. *Med Care.* 1992;30:811-821.
18. Coryell W. Diagnosis-specific mortality. *Arch Gen Psychiatry.* 1981;38:939-942.
19. Brook RH, Ware JE Jr, Davies-Avery A, Stewart AL, Donald CA, Rogers WH, Williams KN, Johnston SA. *Conceptualization and Measurement of Health for Adults in the Health Insurance Study, Vol VII: Overview.* Santa Monica, Calif: RAND Corp; 1979.
20. Kmenta J. *Elements of Econometrics.* New York, NY: Macmillan Publishing Co Inc; 1971.
21. Robins LN, Helzer JE, Croughan J, Ratcliff KS. National Institute of Mental Health Diagnostic Interview Schedule: history, characteristics, and validity. *Arch Gen Psychiatry.* 1981;38:381-389.
22. American Psychiatric Association. *Diagnostic and Statistical Manual of Mental Disorders, Third Edition.* Washington, DC: American Psychiatric Association; 1980.
23. Stewart AL, Greenfield S, Hays RD, Wells K, Rogers WH, Berry SD, McGlynn EA, Ware JE. Functional status and well-being of patients with chronic conditions: results from the medical outcomes study. *JAMA.* 1989;262:907-913.
24. Ware JE Jr, Snow KK, Kosinski M, Gandek B. *SF-36 Health Survey Manual and Interpretation Guide.* Boston, Mass: Health Institute, New England Medical Center; 1993.
25. Robins LN, Barrett JE. *The Validity of Psychiatric Diagnosis.* New York, NY: Raven Press; 1989.
26. Kashner TM, Rost K, Cohen B, Anderson M, Smith GR. Enhancing the health of somatization disorder patients: the cost effectiveness of short term group therapy. *Psychosomatics.* In press.
27. American Psychiatric Association. *Diagnostic and Statistical Manual of Mental Disorders, Fourth Edition.* Washington, DC: American Psychiatric Association; 1994.
28. Broadhead WE, Blazer DG, George LK, Tse CK. Depression, disability days, and days lost from work in a prospective epidemiologic survey. *JAMA.* 1990; 264:2524-2528.

Clozapine Therapy and Increases in Homovanillic Acid

Kahn and colleagues[1] reported that increases in the cerebrospinal fluid (CSF) homovanillic acid (HVA) to 5-hydroxyindoleacetic acid (5-HIAA) ratio (HVA/HIAA ratio) are correlated with antipsychotic response to haloperidol treatment in patients with schizophrenia or schizoaffective disorder. In their study, haloperidol treatment was associated with significant increases in both CSF HVA concentrations and the CSF HVA/5-HIAA ratio, while CSF 5-HIAA concentrations were unchanged. Of interest, only the increase in the CSF HVA/5-HIAA ratio was correlated with antipsychotic response.

We have been studying the relationship of CSF HVA and 5-HIAA concentrations to antipsychotic response with the "atypical" neuroleptic clozapine. We[2] and Szymanski et al[3] previously have reported the replication of the original findings of Pickar et al[4] that showed a low pretreatment CSF HVA/5-HIAA ratio is more likely to be associated with clinical response to clozapine in patients unresponsive to "typical" neuroleptics.

We now report preliminary data, paralleling the data of Kahn et al,[1] that suggest that antipsychotic improvement with clozapine is also accompanied by increases in the CSF HVA/5-HIAA ratio. Eight medication-free patients meeting *DSM-III-R* and Research Diagnostic Criteria criteria for schizophrenia received research lumbar punctures prior to the initiation of clozapine therapy and after approximately 42 weeks of clozapine therapy. The patients were rated by experienced and trained clinicians blind to the CSF neurotransmitter metabolite concentrations at each of the two time points. Clozapine was titrated into the range of approximately 450 to 600 mg/d based on the treating physician's judgment of the individual patient's optimal treatment response. The CSF HVA and 5-HIAA concentrations were determined by validated high-power liquid chromatography-electrochemical detection methods previously described.[5]

Clozapine therapy was accompanied by no significant group mean (±SD) change in CSF 5-HIAA concentrations (change in [Δ] 5-HIAA=−0.02±22.4 pg/mL; t=−0.003, P=.998); HVA concentrations (ΔHVA=−17.9±50.9 pg/mL; t=−0.996, P=.35), or the HVA/5-HIAA ratio (Δratio=−0.17±0.62; t=0.79, P=.46). However, in three of the eight subjects who experienced a very significant clinical improvement with clozapine pharmacotherapy (ΔBrief Psychiatric Rating Scale [BPRS] scores=−14 to −29), there was a substantial increase in the CSF HVA concentrations (Δ[+]26 pg/mL-[+]109 pg/mL) and the CSF HVA/5-HIAA ratio (Δratio=[+]0.43−[+]1.37). In the remaining five patients who showed no improvement or significant worsening with clozapine pharmacotherapy, there was only a very small increase, no change, or a significant decrease in the HVA/5-HIAA ratio (Δratio=[+]0.04−[−]0.40). Clozapine associated changes in BPRS scores were negatively correlated with changes in the CSF HVA/5-HIAA ratio (r=−.62, P=.06) and with changes in CSF HVA (r=−.69, P=.05). The CSF 5-HIAA changes were not correlated with antipsychotic response to clozapine (r=.06, P=.897). H. Y. Meltzer, MD (written communication, June 24, 1994), has observed that clozapine response as measured by BPRS Total and Positive Symptoms scores at 6 months is inversely related to duration of illness in neuroleptic-resistant schizophrenic patients treated with clozapine. Thus, length-of-illness differences among patients need to be considered in any reports of predictors of clozapine response. In our small study, there was not a significant correlation between length of illness and clozapine response, and this did not therefore confound the measures reported in this study.

Of particular note, Szymanski and colleagues[3] sampled CSF prior to and 3 weeks subsequent to the initiation of clozapine therapy in 19 neuroleptic-refractory and -intolerant schizophrenic patients. They also observed that increases in the "change ratio" (ΔCSF HVA/ΔCSF 5-HIAA) were greater in clozapine responders than in clozapine nonresponders, although the difference did not reach statistical significance.

These preliminary results that clozapine-associated increases in the CSF HVA/5-HIAA ratio are correlated with clinical improvement are remarkably consistent with the pattern of response reported by Kahn et al[1] for haloperidol pharmacotherapy and by Szymanski and colleagues[3] for clozapine pharmacotherapy. However, our results differ from these reports in that improvement with clozapine as measured after 42 weeks of clozapine pharmacotherapy was also correlated with increases in CSF HVA. Our results add further credence to the proposals by Meltzer[6] and others that central nervous system dopaminergic-serotonergic interactions may be mechanistically important in understanding antipsychotic pharmacotherapy.

S. Craig Risch, MD
Medical University of South Carolina
171 Ashley Ave
Charleston, SC 29425-0742
Richard R. J. Lewine, PhD
Atlanta, Ga

1. Kahn RS, Davidson M, Knott P, Stern RG, Apter S, Davis KL. Effect of neuroleptic medication on cerebrospinal fluid monoamine metabolite concentrations in schizophrenia: serotonin-dopamine interactions as a target for treatment. *Arch Gen Psychiatry.* 1993;50:599-605.
2. Risch SC, Lewine RRJ. Low cerebrospinal fluid homovanillic acid-5-hydroxyindoleacetic acid ratio predicts clozapine efficacy: a replication. *Arch Gen Psychiatry.* 1993;50:670.
3. Szymanski S, Lieberman J, Pollack S, Munne R, Saferman A, Kane J, Kronig M, Cooper T. The dopamine-serotonin relationship in clozapine response. *Psychopharmacology.* 1993;112(suppl):S85-S89.
4. Pickar D, Owen RR, Littman RE, Konicki PE, Guitierrez R, Rapaport MH. Clinical and biological response to clozapine in patients with schizophrenia: crossover comparison with fluphenazine. *Arch Gen Psychiatry.* 1992;49:345-353.
5. Risch SC, Lewine RH, Kalin NH, Jewart RD, Risby ED, Caudle JM, Stipetic M, Turner J, Eccard MB, Pollard WE. Limbic-hypothalamic-pituitary-adrenal axis activity and ventricular-to-brain ratio studies in affective illness and schizophrenia. *Neuropsychopharmacology.* 1992;6:95-100.
6. Meltzer HY. Clinical studies on the mechanism of action of clozapine: the dopamine-serotonin hypothesis of schizophrenia. *Psychopharmacology.* 1989;99:518-527.

MANUSCRIPT CRITERIA AND INFORMATION

Submit manuscripts to Jack D. Barchas, MD, Editor, ***Archives of General Psychiatry*, Cornell Medical Center, Dept of Psychiatry, Box 171, 525 E 68th St, Room F2315, New York, NY 10021.** Manuscripts are received with the understanding that they are not under simultaneous consideration by another publication, have not been published previously, and have the approval of each author. Accepted manuscripts become the permanent property of the ARCHIVES. They may not be republished without permission from the publisher (AMA).

Editing. Copyediting follows AMA style and requires corresponding author approval. The authors are responsible for all statements made in their work, including changes made by the copy editor and authorized by the corresponding author.

Reprints. Forms for ordering are included with the edited typescript sent for approval. Reprints are shipped 6 to 8 weeks after publication.

Cover Letter

- In the cover letter, designate one author as correspondent and provide a complete address and telephone and fax numbers.

- For a manuscript to be reviewed, considered, or edited, the following statement must be signed by *all* authors:

"I have been sufficiently involved in this work to take public responsibility for its validity and final presentation as an original publication. I can and will provide documentation of my work upon reasonable request and I have fulfilled the obligations for full disclosure and authorship as described by *Archives of General Psychiatry*. . . ." This signed statement must conclude with *one* of the two following sentences: "Accordingly, I hereby transfer, assign, or otherwise convey all copyright ownership to the AMA in the event such work is published by the AMA." [OR] "No copyright ownership can be transferred since this work was produced in the course of my official duties as a US government officer or employee."

Manuscript Preparation[1,2]

- Submit an original double-spaced typescript and 7 copies.
- **Manuscripts will not be returned after the review process.** Unpublished manuscripts will be destroyed.
- Type—double-spaced throughout (including references)—on one side only of 8½ × 11-in white bond paper. Number all pages. Do not justify right-hand margins. Use a printer of at least letter quality.
- Titles cannot exceed 200 characters, including punctuation and spaces, and should be as brief as possible.
- The title page should list full names, degrees, academic affiliations and their locations, and the name and address to whom reprint requests should be sent. If the paper was presented at a meeting, include the organization, place, and date of presentation. Acknowledgment of grant or drug company support should also be made on this page. Include a word count of the text only (excluding the abstract, references, and tables).
- Include a structured abstract of 250 words or less that states in defined sections the Background, Methods, Results, and Conclusions.
- Use Système International (SI) measurements throughout the manuscript.
- Use generic names of drugs, unless the specific trade name is directly relevant to the study design or discussion.
- Do not use abbreviations in the title or abstract. Limit their use in the text.
- *Do not use footnotes or appendixes.* Such materials should either be incorporated into the text or offered to interested readers on request.
- Include a statistical analysis section under *Methods* that fully describes the application of each statistical procedure used. If a test is used that is not commonly presented in the ARCHIVES, briefly describe its purpose and how it is to be interpreted. Results should report the test statistic (eg, χ^2, F or *t* value), degrees of freedom, and *P* value. Measures of central tendency (eg, means) should be accompanied by measures of variability (eg, standard deviations). In the cover letter, state the name of your statistical consultant, if appropriate.
- Acknowledge fully any material taken from other publications, and submit written permission from the owner to reprint in any language or form without limitation.

Tables. Double-space on separate sheets of 8½ × 11-in white bond paper. Title each one and number them in the order of their citation in the text. If a table must be continued, repeat the title on a second sheet, followed by "(cont)." Any explanatory notes to be printed with the table must be typed single-spaced beneath the table.

Figures. Once manuscripts are accepted, two sets of professionally prepared, high-contrast glossy prints (preferably in a proportion of 5 × 7 in) are required. If full-color figures are necessary, the ARCHIVES may pay part of the expense with the balance to be borne by the author.

- Number figures according to their order in the text. Type the figure number, proper orientation (eg, top), name of the senior author, and an abbreviated title on a gummed label; affix it to the back of the print.

- Double-space legends (maximum length, 40 words) on a separate sheet of 8½ × 11-in paper.

References. Number references in the order they are mentioned in the text; do *not* alphabetize. In text, tables, and legends, identify references with superscript arabic numbers. In listing references, follow AMA style and abbreviate names of journals according to *Index Medicus.* List all authors and/or editors. Citation accuracy is the responsibility of the author.

Examples:

1. DuBois RN, Lazenby AJ, Yardley JH, Hendrix TR, Bayless TM, Giardiello FM. Lymphocytic enterocolitis in patients with 'refractory sprue.' *JAMA*. 1989;262:935-937.

2. Ritchie JM, Greene NM. Local anesthetics. In: Gilman AG, Goodman LS, Rall TW, Murad F, eds. *The Pharmacological Basis of Therapeutics*. 7th ed. New York, NY: Macmillan Publishing Co Inc; 1985:309-310.

Informed Consent and Confidentiality. A statement of informed consent for human investigation should be made. Authors must ensure that patient confidentiality is in no way breached. Do not use real names, initials, or disclose information that might identify a particular subject.

Obligations for Full Disclosure and Authorship[3,4]

Previous Publications. Manuscripts that are submitted must not have been previously published in *whole* or *substantial part* and must not be simultaneously under consideration elsewhere. This policy applies to the essential contents, tables, or figures, but does not apply to abstracts. Authors must disclose in their cover letters if the submitted manuscript contains any data or material that have already been published or are in press, submitted, or nearly submitted. Copies of closely related manuscripts should be submitted to the Editor for examination.

Financial Disclosure. At the time of initial submission, each author should disclose any financial arrangement he or she has with companies who either have products featured in the manuscript or with companies that produce competing products. These arrangements include, but are not limited to, company support, consultantships, patent rights, stock ownership, or other equity interests. Such arrangements do not constitute grounds for automatic rejection of the manuscript. Financial information will be held in confidence. If the manuscript is accepted for publication, the Editor and the author(s) will confer about the way this information will be communicated to the readers. Reviewers are also expected to notify the Editor of their own financial arrangements involving companies whose products (or competing products) are featured in the manuscripts they agree to review.

Other Disclosures. Authors should disclose to the Editor at the time of submission any special circumstances, vested interests, or sources of bias that might affect the integrity of the reported information. These disclosures also apply to referees.

Authorship does not require expertise in every aspect of the work. It does mean that each author within his or her own limits has exerted sufficient reasonable effort to vouch for the validity of the entire work and to bear public accountability for maintaining the integrity of the scientific information communicated. Each author must have had enough substantial involvement in generating and formulating the published product to bear such accountability. More than six authors requires a statement of justification in the cover letter.

Letters to the Editor

Letters to the Editor will be considered for publication if they are accompanied by a cover letter stating they are "for publication." Their purpose should be to comment on articles published in the ARCHIVES or to provide significant news that can be conveyed in a short format. The Editor reserves the right to edit the material prior to publication.

Letters intended for publication *must* follow manuscript preparation guidelines (eg, double-spaced, copyright transfer). They generally should not exceed 750 words. Include 3 copies. Illustrative material is not usually accepted; brief tables may occasionally be considered. Authors will receive only a brief acknowledgment of acceptance or rejection.

Review Process

A submitted manuscript will be acknowledged by postcard and assigned a manuscript number, which is to be used in all further correspondence. Manuscripts are reviewed and given a priority based upon their originality, scientific merit, appropriateness of statistical analyses, importance of their findings, significance for the field, lucidity, interest to readers, suitability for publication, and the journal's current portfolio. All reviewers remain anonymous and are expected to maintain the curtain of strict confidentiality. After the review process has been completed, authors will be informed by mail of the Editor's decision.

References

1. Iverson CI, Dan BB, Glitman P, et al. *American Medical Association Manual of Style*. 8th ed. Baltimore, Md: Williams & Wilkins; 1988.

2. International Committee of Medical Journal Editors. Uniform requirements for manuscripts submitted to biomedical journals. *Ann Intern Med*. 1988;108:258-265.

3. Freedman DX. The meaning of full disclosure. *Arch Gen Psychiatry*. 1988;45:689-691.

4. Freedman DX. Megamultiple authorship. *Arch Gen Psychiatry*. 1982;39:351.

Checklist

____ (1) Cover letter including all information deemed necessary for the editor's review.

____ (2) Statement on copyright and authorial responsibility, signed by *all* authors.

____ (3) Corresponding author identified and address and telephone and fax numbers provided.

____ (4) Original manuscript (including structured abstract, references, legends, tables, and figures) plus 7 copies.

____ (5) Right-hand margin unjustified.

____ (6) Copies of publications considered to be helpful for the review process or that bear on any possible overlap of published data.

THIS MONTH IN

ARCHIVES OF GENERAL PSYCHIATRY

Disturbances of orderly brain development are thought to contribute to the reported alterations in inhibitory, GABAergic transmission in the prefrontal cortex of schizophrenics. **Akbarian et al** (page 258) show that a gene for glutamic acid decarboxylase (GAD), the key enzyme for GABA synthesis, was expressed at lower levels in the prefrontal cortex of schizophrenics, in comparison with matched controls. Neuronal numbers and prefrontal volume did not differ between the schizophrenics and the controls, indicating a functional down-regulation in GAD gene expression, without loss of GABAergic neurons in the prefrontal cortex of schizophrenics. Defective brain development in schizophrenia probably does not affect the overall structure of the prefrontal cortex. However, it is likely to compromise the formation of cortical connections, leading to prefrontal hypoactivity and a decrease in gene expression for neurotransmitter-related molecules such as GAD. Three commentaries regarding this article are included in this issue.

Prefrontal cortex abnormalities have been thought to underlie deficits in attention, working memory, and judgment in schizophrenic patients. However, structural studies of this region, using magnetic resonance imaging (MRI) to measure volume, have yielded mixed results. **Wible et al** (page 279) measured the volume of a larger area of prefrontal cortex, with higher resolution volume elements (1.3 mm^3) and used more sophisticated gray/white segmentation methods than any study to date. The schizophrenic subjects had previously been shown to have volume reductions in several areas of the temporal lobe, mostly on the left side. The volumes of left and right prefrontal gray and white matter in schizophrenic patients were not statistically different from that of carefully matched control subjects. However, in schizophrenics, unlike controls, the volume of left prefrontal gray matter was highly correlated with the volume of several left temporal lobe areas that were previously shown to be abnormal. These results suggest a pathological process that is common to both temporal and frontal areas, but one that produces only subtle abnormalities in the prefrontal cortex that are below the threshold for MRI detection.

The optimal dosing strategy for sertraline in patients with obsessive-compulsive disorder was examined. **Greist et al** (page 289) found that doses of 50 mg, 100 mg, and 200 mg of sertraline were significantly more effective than placebo in reducing obsessions and compulsions. A dose of 50 mg was as effective as the larger doses and produced fewer side effects. Results support the safety and efficacy of all three doses in the short-term treatment of patients with obsessive-compulsive disorder.

Although schizotypal personality disorder aggregates in families of individuals with schizophrenia, the current criteria for this disorder may not be optimal either in describing the dimensions of schizotypal phenomena or in identifying those with a high familial liability to schizophrenia. In relatives from the Roscommon Family Study, **Kendler et al** (page 296) found seven meaningful schizotypal factors: negative schizotypy, positive schizotypy, borderline symptoms, social dysfunction, avoidant symptoms, odd speech, and suspicious behavior. Compared with relatives of matched controls, relatives of schizophrenic probands were best characterized by odd or digressive speech, negative schizotypal signs such as poor rapport and odd behavior, social dysfunction such as poor occupational achievement, and social avoidance or isolation. Schizotypy appears to be a complex, multidimensional clinical construct, whose various dimensions differ widely both in the degree and specificity with which they reflect the familial liability to schizophrenia.

Little is known about the outcome of the eating disorder bulimia nervosa. **Fairburn et al** (page 304) followed up patients from two psychotherapy trials for an average of 6 years. They report that almost half still had an eating disorder of clinical severity. Long-term outcome was related to the type of treatment received, with those patients who had received cognitive behavior therapy or focal interpersonal therapy doing much better than those who had received behavior therapy. These findings underscore the serious nature of bulimia nervosa and the value of these particular treatments.

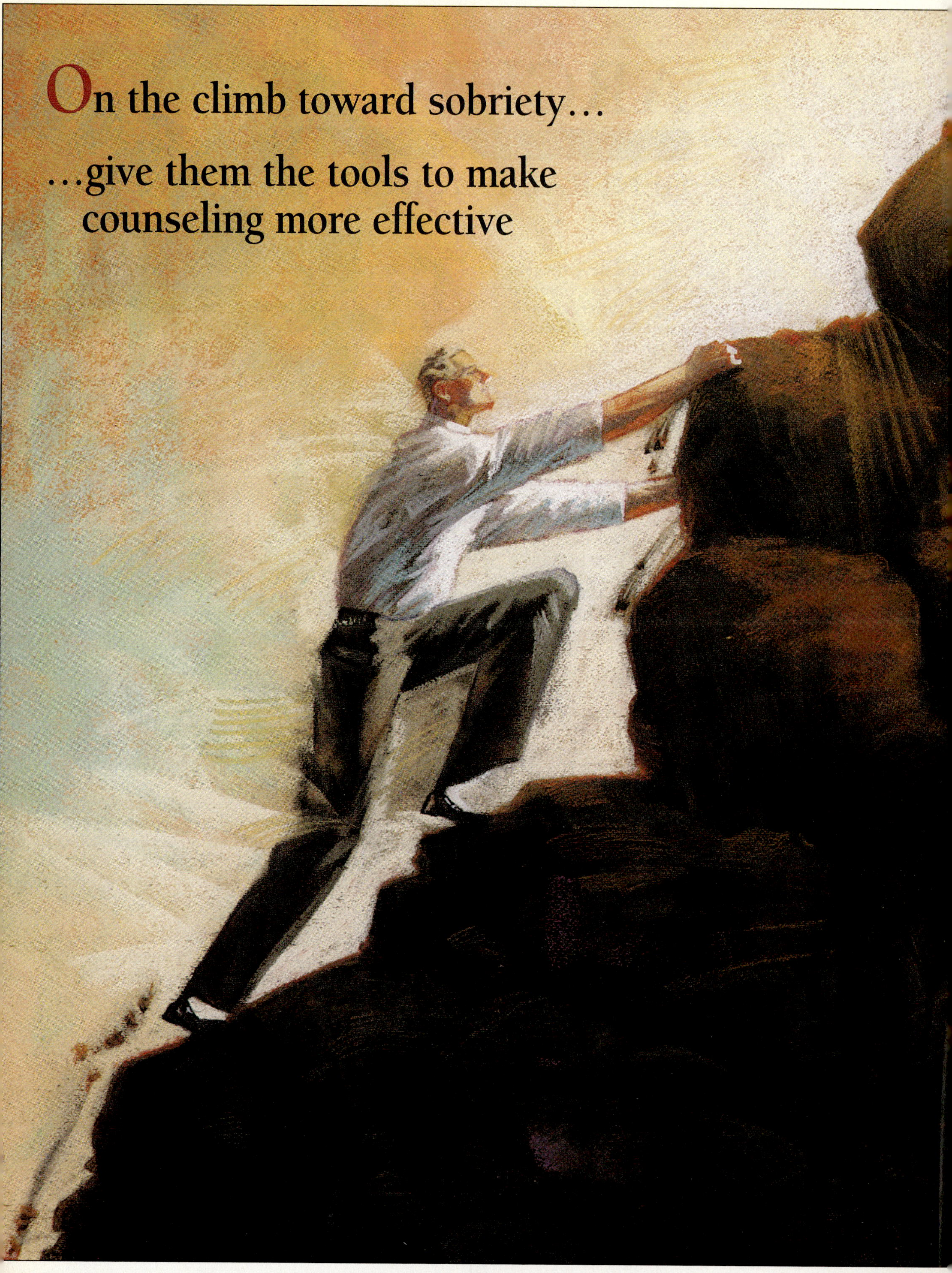
On the climb toward sobriety…
…give them the tools to make counseling more effective

follows enumerates adverse events that occurred at an incidence of 1% or more, and were more frequent than in the placebo group, among SERZONE-treated patients who participated in short-term (6- to 8-week) placebo-controlled trials in which patients were dosed with SERZONE to ranges of 300 to 600 mg/day. This table shows the percentage of patients in each group who had at least one episode of an event at some time during their treatment. Reported adverse events were classified using a standard COSTART-based Dictionary terminology.

The prescriber should be aware that these figures cannot be used to predict the incidence of side effects in the course of usual medical practice where patient characteristics and other factors differ from those which prevailed in the clinical trials. Similarly, the cited frequencies cannot be compared with figures obtained from other clinical investigations involving different treatments, uses, and investigators. The cited figures, however, do provide the prescribing physician with some basis for estimating the relative contribution of drug and nondrug factors to the side-effect incidence rate in the population studied.

Treatment-Emergent Adverse Experience Incidence in 6- to 8-Week Placebo-Controlled Clinical Trials[1]
SERZONE 300 to 600 mg/day Dose Range

Body System	Preferred Term	SERZONE (n=393)	Placebo (n=394)
Body as a Whole	Headache	36%	33%
	Asthenia	11%	5%
	Infection	8%	6%
	Flu syndrome	3%	2%
	Chills	2%	1%
	Fever	2%	1%
	Neck rigidity	1%	0%
Cardiovascular	Postural hypotension	4%	1%
	Hypotension	2%	1%
Dermatological	Pruritus	2%	1%
	Rash	2%	1%
Gastrointestinal	Dry mouth	25%	13%
	Nausea	22%	12%
	Constipation	14%	8%
	Dyspepsia	9%	7%
	Diarrhea	8%	7%
	Increased appetite	5%	3%
	Nausea & Vomiting	2%	1%
Metabolic	Peripheral edema	3%	2%
	Thirst	1%	<1%
Musculoskeletal	Arthralgia	1%	<1%
Nervous	Somnolence	25%	14%
	Dizziness	17%	5%
	Insomnia	11%	9%
	Lightheadedness	10%	3%
	Confusion	7%	2%
	Memory impairment	4%	2%
	Paresthesia	4%	2%
	Vasodilatation[2]	4%	2%
	Abnormal dreams	3%	2%
	Concentration decreased	3%	1%
	Ataxia	2%	0%
	Incoordination	2%	1%
	Psychomotor retardation	2%	1%
	Tremor	2%	1%
	Hypertonia	1%	0%
	Libido decreased	1%	<1%
Respiratory	Pharyngitis	6%	5%
	Cough increased	3%	1%
Special Senses	Blurred vision	9%	3%
	Abnormal vision[3]	7%	1%
	Tinnitus	2%	1%
	Taste perversion	2%	1%
	Visual field defect	2%	0%
Urogenital	Urinary frequency	2%	1%
	Urinary tract infection	2%	1%
	Urinary retention	2%	1%
	Vaginitis[4]	2%	1%
	Breast pain[4]	1%	<1%

1 Events reported by at least 1% of patients treated with SERZONE and more frequent than the placebo group are included; incidence is rounded to the nearest 1% (<1% indicates an incidence less than 0.5%). Events for which the SERZONE incidence was equal to or less than placebo are not listed in the table, but included the following: abdominal pain, pain, back pain, accidental injury, chest pain, neck pain, palpitation, migraine, sweating, flatulence, vomiting, anorexia, tooth disorder, weight gain, edema, myalgia, cramp, agitation, anxiety, depression, hypesthesia, CNS stimulation, dysphoria, emotional lability, sinusitis, rhinitis, dysmenorrhea,[4] dysuria.

2 Vasodilatation—flushing, feeling warm.

3 Abnormal vision—scotoma, visual trails.

4 Incidence adjusted for gender.

Dose Dependency of Adverse Events: The table that follows enumerates adverse events that were more frequent in the SERZONE (nefazodone hydrochloride) dose range of 300 to 600 mg/day than in the SERZONE dose range of up to 300 mg/day. This table shows only those adverse events for which there was a statistically significant difference ($p \le 0.05$) in incidence between the SERZONE dose ranges as well as a difference between the high dose range and placebo.

Dose Dependency of Adverse Events in Placebo-Controlled Trials[1]

Body System	Preferred Term	SERZONE 300-600 mg/day (n = 209)	SERZONE ≤300 mg/day (n = 211)	Placebo (n = 212)
Gastrointestinal	Nausea	23%	14%	12%
	Constipation	17%	10%	9%
Nervous	Somnolence	28%	16%	13%
	Dizziness	22%	11%	4%
	Confusion	8%	2%	1%
Special Senses	Abnormal vision	10%	0%	2%
	Blurred vision	9%	3%	2%
	Tinnitus	3%	0%	1%

1 Events for which there was a statistically significant difference ($p \le 0.05$) between the nefazodone dose groups.

Vital Sign Changes: (See PRECAUTIONS Section, Postural Hypotension Subsection.)

Weight Changes: In a pooled analysis of placebo-controlled premarketing studies, there were no differences between nefazodone and placebo groups in the proportions of patients meeting criteria for potentially important increases or decreases in body weight (a change of ≥7%).

Laboratory Changes: Of the serum chemistry, serum hematology, and urinalysis parameters monitored during placebo-controlled premarketing studies with nefazodone, a pooled analysis revealed a statistical trend between nefazodone and placebo for hematocrit, i.e., 2.8% of nefazodone patients met criteria for a potentially important decrease in hematocrit (≤37% male or ≤32% female) compared to 1.5% of placebo patients ($0.05 < p \le 0.10$). Decreases in hematocrit, presumably dilutional, have been reported with many other drugs that block $alpha_1$-adrenergic receptors. There was no apparent clinical significance of the observed changes in the few patients meeting these criteria.

ECG Changes: Of the ECG parameters monitored during placebo-controlled premarketing studies with nefazodone, a pooled analysis revealed a statistically significant difference between nefazodone and placebo for sinus bradycardia, i.e., 1.5% of nefazodone patients met criteria for a potentially important decrease in heart rate (≤50 bpm and a decrease of ≥15 bpm) compared to 0.4% of placebo patients ($p < 0.05$). There was no obvious clinical significance of the observed changes in the few patients meeting these criteria.

Other Events Observed During the Premarketing Evaluation of SERZONE

During its premarketing assessment, multiple doses of SERZONE were administered to 3496 patients in clinical studies, including more than 250 patients treated for at least one year. The conditions and duration of exposure to SERZONE varied greatly, and included (in overlapping categories) open and double-blind studies, uncontrolled and controlled studies, inpatient and outpatient studies, fixed-dose and titration studies. Untoward events associated with this exposure were recorded by clinical investigators using terminology of their own choosing. Consequently, it is not possible to provide a meaningful estimate of the proportion of individuals experiencing adverse events without first grouping similar types of untoward events into a smaller number of standardized event categories.

In the tabulations that follow, reported adverse events were classified using a standard COSTART-based Dictionary terminology. The frequencies presented, therefore, represent the proportion of the 3496 patients exposed to multiple doses of SERZONE who experienced an event of the type cited on at least one occasion while receiving SERZONE. All reported events are included except those already listed in the Treatment-Emergent Adverse Experience Incidence table, those events listed in other safety-related sections of this insert, those adverse experiences subsumed under COSTART terms that are either overly general or excessively specific so as to be uninformative, those events for which a drug cause was very remote, and those events which were not serious and occurred in fewer than two patients.

It is important to emphasize that, although the events reported occurred during treatment with SERZONE (nefazodone hydrochloride), they were not necessarily caused by it.

Events are further categorized by body system and listed in order of decreasing frequency according to the following definitions: frequent adverse events are those occurring on one or more occasions in at least 1/100 patients (only those not already listed in the tabulated results from placebo-controlled trials appear in this listing); infrequent adverse events are those occurring in 1/100 to 1/1000 patients; rare events are those occurring in fewer than 1/1000 patients.

Body as a Whole—*Infrequent:* allergic reaction, malaise, photosensitivity reaction, face edema, hangover effect, abdomen enlarged, hernia, pelvic pain, and halitosis. *Rare:* cellulitis.

Cardiovascular System—*Infrequent:* tachycardia, hypertension, syncope, ventricular extrasystoles, and angina pectoris. *Rare:* AV block, congestive heart failure, hemorrhage, pallor, and varicose vein.

Dermatological System—*Infrequent:* dry skin, acne, alopecia, urticaria, maculopapular rash, vesiculobullous rash, and eczema.

Gastrointestinal System—*Frequent:* gastroenteritis. *Infrequent:* eructation, periodontal abscess, abnormal liver function tests, gingivitis, colitis, gastritis, mouth ulceration, stomatitis, esophagitis, peptic ulcer, and rectal hemorrhage. *Rare:* glossitis, hepatitis, dysphagia, gastrointestinal hemorrhage, oral moniliasis, and ulcerative colitis.

Hemic and Lymphatic System—*Infrequent:* ecchymosis, anemia, leukopenia, and lymphadenopathy.

Metabolic and Nutritional System—*Infrequent:* weight loss, gout, dehydration, lactic dehydrogenase increased, SGOT increased, and SGPT increased. *Rare:* hypercholesteremia and hypoglycemia.

Musculoskeletal System—*Infrequent:* arthritis, tenosynovitis, muscle stiffness, and bursitis. *Rare:* tendinous contracture.

Nervous System—*Infrequent:* vertigo, twitching, depersonalization, hallucinations, suicide attempt, apathy, euphoria, hostility, suicidal thoughts, abnormal gait, thinking abnormal, attention decreased, derealization, neuralgia, paranoid reaction, dysarthria, increased libido, suicide, and myoclonus. *Rare:* hyperkinesia, increased salivation, cerebrovascular accident, hyperesthesia, hypotonia, ptosis, and neuroleptic malignant syndrome.

Respiratory System—*Frequent:* dyspnea and bronchitis. *Infrequent:* asthma, pneumonia, laryngitis, voice alteration, epistaxis, hiccup. *Rare:* hyperventilation and yawn.

Special Senses—*Frequent:* eye pain. *Infrequent:* dry eye, ear pain, abnormality of accommodation, diplopia, conjunctivitis, mydriasis, keratoconjunctivitis, hyperacusis, and photophobia. *Rare:* deafness, glaucoma, night blindness, and taste loss.

Urogenital System—*Frequent:* impotence.[a] *Infrequent:* cystitis, urinary urgency, metrorrhagia,[a] amenorrhea,[a] polyuria, vaginal hemorrhage,[a] breast enlargement,[a] menorrhagia,[a] urinary incontinence, abnormal ejaculation,[a] hematuria, nocturia, and kidney calculus. *Rare:* uterine fibroids enlarged,[a] uterine hemorrhage,[a] anorgasmia, and oliguria.

[a]Adjusted for gender.

DRUG ABUSE AND DEPENDENCE

Controlled Substance Class

SERZONE (nefazodone hydrochloride) is not a controlled substance.

Physical and Psychological Dependence

In animal studies, nefazodone did not act as a reinforcer for intravenous self-administration in monkeys trained to self-administer cocaine, suggesting no abuse liability. In a controlled study of abuse liability in human subjects, nefazodone showed no potential for abuse.

Nefazodone has not been systematically studied in humans for its potential for tolerance, physical dependence, or withdrawal. While the premarketing clinical experience with nefazodone did not reveal any tendency for a withdrawal syndrome or any drug-seeking behavior, it is not possible to predict on the basis of this limited experience the extent to which a CNS-active drug will be misused, diverted, and/or abused once marketed. Consequently, physicians should carefully evaluate patients for a history of drug abuse and follow such patients closely, observing them for signs of misuse or abuse of SERZONE (e.g., development of tolerance, dose escalation, drug-seeking behavior).

OVERDOSAGE

Human Experience

There is very limited experience with nefazodone overdose. In premarketing clinical studies, there were seven reports of nefazodone overdose alone or in combination with other pharmacological agents. The amount of nefazodone ingested ranged from 1000 mg to 11,200 mg. Commonly reported symptoms from overdose of nefazodone included nausea, vomiting, and somnolence. One nonstudy participant took 2000–3000 mg of nefazodone with methocarbamol and alcohol; this person reportedly experienced a convulsion (type not documented). None of the patients died.

Overdose Management

Overdosage may cause an increase in incidence or severity of any of the reported adverse reactions (see ADVERSE REACTIONS Section).

There is no specific antidote for SERZONE (nefazodone hydrochloride). Treatment should be symptomatic and supportive in the case of hypotension or excessive sedation. Any patient suspected of having taken an overdose should have the stomach emptied by gastric lavage.

In managing overdosage, consider the possibility of multiple drug involvement. The physician should consider contacting a poison control center on the treatment of any overdose.

DOSAGE AND ADMINISTRATION

Initial Treatment

The recommended starting dose for SERZONE (nefazodone hydrochloride) is 200 mg/day, administered in two divided doses (BID). In the controlled clinical trials establishing the antidepressant efficacy of SERZONE, the effective dose range was generally 300 to 600 mg/day. Consequently, most patients, depending on tolerability and the need for further clinical effect, should have dose increased. Dose increases should occur in increments of 100 mg/day to 200 mg/day, again on a BID schedule, at intervals of no less than 1 week. As with all antidepressants, several weeks on treatment may be required to obtain a full antidepressant response.

Dosage for Elderly or Debilitated Patients

The recommended initial dose for elderly or debilitated patients is 100 mg/day on a BID schedule. These patients often have reduced nefazodone clearance and/or increased sensitivity to the side effects of CNS-active drugs. It may also be appropriate to modify the rate of subsequent dose titration. As steady-state plasma levels do not change with age, the final target dose based on a careful assessment of the patient's clinical response may be similar in healthy younger and older patients.

Maintenance/Continuation/Extended Treatment

There is no body of evidence available from controlled trials to indicate how long the depressed patient should be treated with SERZONE. It is generally agreed, however, that pharmacological treatment for acute episodes of depression should continue for up to six months or longer. Whether the dose of antidepressant needed to induce remission is identical to the dose needed to maintain euthymia is unknown. Although there are no efficacy data that specifically address maintenance antidepressant treatment with SERZONE, the safety of nefazodone in long-term use is supported by data from both double-blind and open-label trials involving more than 250 patients treated for at least one year.

Switching Patients to or from a Monoamine Oxidase Inhibitor

At least 14 days should elapse between discontinuation of an MAOI and initiation of therapy with SERZONE. In addition, at least 7 days should be allowed after stopping SERZONE before starting an MAOI.

HOW SUPPLIED

SERZONE® (nefazodone hydrochloride) tablets are hexagonal tablets imprinted with BMS and the strength (i.e., 100 mg) on one side and the identification code number on the other. The 100 mg (white) and 150 mg (peach) tablets are bisect scored on both tablet faces. The 200 mg (light yellow) and 250 mg (white) tablets are unscored.

Store at room temperature, below 40° C (104° F) and dispense in a tight container.

References: 1. Data on file, Medical Affairs Department, Bristol-Myers Squibb Company. **2.** Fontaine R, Ontiveros A, Elie R, et al. A double-blind comparison of nefazodone, imipramine, and placebo in major depression. *J Clin Psychiatry.* 1994;55:234-241. **3.** Rickels K, Schweizer E, Clary C, Fox I, Weise C. Nefazodone and imipramine in major depression: a placebo-controlled trial. *Br J Psychiatry.* 1994;164:802-805. **4.** Mendels J, Reimherr F, Roberts D, et al. A double-blind comparison of high-dose nefazodone, low-dose nefazodone, and placebo in the treatment of depressed outpatients. Presented at the annual meeting of the ECNP: October 6-9, 1991. **5.** Armitage R, Rush AJ, Trivedi M, Cain J, Roffwarg HP. The effects of nefazodone on sleep architecture in depression. *Neuropsychopharmacology.* 1994;10:123-127. **6.** Ware JC, Rose FV, McBrayer RH. The acute effects of nefazodone, trazodone and buspirone on sleep and sleep-related penile tumescence in normal subjects. *Sleep.* 1994;17:544-550.

Bristol-Myers Squibb Company
Princeton, New Jersey 08543, U.S.A.

P8375-00 Issued: December 1994 Printed in U.S.A.

ORIGINAL ARTICLE

Gene Expression for Glutamic Acid Decarboxylase Is Reduced Without Loss of Neurons in Prefrontal Cortex of Schizophrenics

Schahram Akbarian, MD, PhD; James J. Kim; Steven G. Potkin, MD; Jennifer O. Hagman, MD; Alireza Tafazzoli; William E. Bunney, Jr, MD; Edward G. Jones, MD, PhD

Background: Up-regulation of γ-aminobutyric $acid_A$ ($GABA_A$) receptors and decreased GABA uptake in the cerebral cortex of schizophrenics suggest altered GABAergic transmission, which could be caused by primary disturbance of GABA synapses or by decreased production of the transmitter. Decreased production could be due to a shutdown in GABA production or to loss of GABA neurons caused by cell death or their failure to migrate to the cortex during brain development.

Methods: To discriminate between these possibilities, we quantified levels of messenger RNA (mRNA) for the 67-kd isoform of glutamic acid decarboxylase (GAD), the key enzyme in GABA synthesis, and the number and laminar distribution of GAD mRNA–expressing neurons in the dorsolateral prefrontal cortex (DLPFC) of schizophrenics and matched controls, using in situ hybridization-histochemistry, densitometry, and cell-counting methods. These data were compared with the total number of neurons, the number of small, round or ovoid neurons 8 to 15 μm in diameter, and overall frontal lobe volume. As a control, mRNA levels for type II calcium-calmodulin–dependent protein kinase (CamIIK) were quantified.

Results: Schizophrenics showed a pronounced decrease in GAD mRNA levels in neurons of layer I (40%) and layer II (48%) and an overall 30% decrease in layers III to VI. There were also strong overall reductions in GAD mRNA levels. The CamIIK mRNA levels showed no significant differences between samples. No differences were found in the total number of neurons nor in small, round or ovoid neurons, which should include a majority of the GABA cells. Prefrontal gray and white matter volume did not differ significantly between controls and schizophrenics.

Conclusions: The prefrontal cortex of schizophrenics shows reduced expression for GAD in the absence of significant cell loss. This may be brought about by an activity-dependent down-regulation associated with the functional hypoactivity of the DLPFC. The lack of significant alterations in cell numbers in the DLPFC and frontal lobe volume in schizophrenics also implies that overall cortical neuronal migration had not been compromised in development. Previous reports of altered neuronal distribution in the subcortical white matter of schizophrenic brains in comparison with that of controls may indicate disturbances of migration or programmed cell death in the cortical subplate, leading to altered connection formation in the overlying cortex of schizophrenics and activity-dependent down-regulation of neurotransmitter-related gene expression.

(Arch Gen Psychiatry. 1995;52:258-266)

DISTURBANCES OF early brain development are thought to play a contributory role in the origins of schizophrenia.[1] These include environmental factors such as viral illness during the second trimester of pregnancy,[2-6] malnutrition during the first trimester,[7] and obstetrical complications,[8] all of which increase the incidence of schizophrenia in offspring at risk.

A number of putative morphological abnormalities found in the brains of schizophrenics have been suggested to be indications of disordered neuronal development. These include abnormal orientation of hippocampal neurons[9-11] and alterations of cytoarchitecture in the parahippocampal gyrus,[12-14] although the cytoarchitectonic heterogeneity of this cortical region[15] requires further investigations. These morphological alterations of the medial temporal cortext of schizophrenics were interpreted as resulting from a disturbance in the normal pattern of neuronal migration, during which young neurons generated in the neuroepithelium that lines the ventricular walls traverse the intermediate

From the Departments of Anatomy and Neurobiology (Drs Akbarian and Jones and Messrs Kim and Tafazzoli) and Psychiatry and Human Behavior (Drs Potkin, Hagman, and Bunney), University of California–Irvine.

See Materials and Methods on next page

MATERIALS AND METHODS

Tissue from the brains of 10 chronic schizophrenos[35] and 10 controls matched for age, gender, and autolysis time (**Table 1**) was used in the present study. The matching process was done prior to all experimental procedures and quantitative analyses. Brain tissue used in this study came from a brain bank at the University of California–Irvine that contained the brains of 20 schizophrenics and 70 controls. Specimens in this brain bank were obtained from the Orange County (California) and Ventura County (California) coroners' offices and a number of southern California general hospitals. All brains were removed and processed in a standard manner by the same autopsy technician. For each schizophrenic and control subject used in this study, a complete medical history until death was available. Schizophrenic and control subjects who had incomplete medical histories or prolonged agonal state or for whom time of death and postmortem autolysis interval were not exactly known were excluded. Slices of the brains had been fresh-frozen under controlled conditions.[36] The diagnosis of schizophrenia, according to *DSM-III-R*[35] criteria, was made by prospective or retrospective analysis. All diagnoses were finalized prior to postmortem studies. At the time of death, nine of the 10 schizophrenics were receiving neuroleptics. The remaining schizophrenic had received no neuroleptics for 10 years prior to death. Control and schizophrenic subjects with a history of substance abuse and neurological illness or control subjects with a history of other psychiatric illness were excluded. No gross neuropathological features were evident. The absence of a chronic degenerative process was confirmed by the absence of plaques and tangles in thioflavine S–stained sections. Small blocks, 2 cm^3 in size (two per brain), were cut out from the middle thirds of the left superior frontal gyrus (Brodmann's area 9), thaw fixed,[37] and sectioned on a freezing microtome. Series of 20-μm thick, slide-mounted sections were processed for in situ hybridization histochemistry analysis with UTP ^{35}S (uridine triphosphate attached to sulfur 35)–labeled, 365-nucleotide sense and antisense complementary RNA (cRNA) probes derived from a monkey cDNA clone complementary to an mRNA coding for the 67-kd form of GAD[38,39] or with UTP ^{35}S–labeled, 373-nucleotide sense and antisense cRNA probes derived from a monkey cDNA clone complementary to the alpha subunit of type II calcium-calmodulin–dependent protein kinase (CamIIK).[38,39] Selected tissue sections were pretreated withribonuclease A (RNase A) (1 μg/mL) and 0.25% Triton X-100 in phosphate buffer (0.1 mol/L). Sections were incubated in glycine (0.1 mol/L) in phosphate buffer (0.1 mol/L) (3 minutes) and in phosphate buffer (0.1 mol/L) alone (15 minutes), followed by treatment with proteinase K (10 μg/mL, 30 minutes at 37°C, pH 8) and incubation in 0.25% acetic anhydride per 0.1 mol of triethanolamine per liter (10 minutes) and two washes in 2× saline sodium citrate (SSC) that contained sodium thiosulfate (0.16 g per 100 mL). Sections were dehydrated in alcohols, and lipid was extracted in chloroform (5 minutes), rehydrated to 85% ethanol, and air dried. Three hundred microliters of hybridization buffer per section (50% deionized formamide, 10% dextran sulfate, 0.7% Ficoll [Sigma Chemical Co, St Louis, Mo], 0.7% polyvinyl pyrolidone, bovine serum albumin [10 mg/mL], denaturated herring sperm [0.35 mg/mL], yeast t-RNA [0.12 mg/mL], dithiothreitol [40 mol/L], and ^{35}S-riboprobe [10 000 or 13 000 cpm/μL]) was placed on the slides with a pipette. A coverslip was placed over the drop of fluid and sealed with DPX (BDH Laboratory Supplies, Poole, England), and the slides were incubated in a wet chamber at 60°C for 48 hours. After removal of the coverslip, sections were washed twice in 4×SSC at 60°C, treated with RNase A (20 μg/mL) (30 minutes at 45°C, pH 8), washed twice in 2×SSC (30 minutes at room temperature), twice in 0.5×SSC, and twice in 0.1×SSC (30 minutes each at 60°C), and, after an overnight wash in 0.1×SSC, air dried and exposed to Beta Max film (Amersham, Arlington Heights, Ill) for 3 days at room temperature. After development of the film, the slides were dehydrated in alcohol, lipid was extracted again in chloroform (20 minutes), and the slides were rehydrated and air dried. Sections of blocks taken from each pair of brains were hybridized using riboprobe concentrations of 10 000 and 13 000 cpm/μL. Sections were dipped in Kodak NTB-2 emulsion (Eastman Kodak, New Haven, Conn), exposed for 14 to 28 days at 4°C, developed, fixed, and stained with cresyl violet. Unprocessed, parallel series of sections were stained with thioflavine-S or thionin. Tissue from schizophrenics and controls with identical gender and similar autolysis time and age were always processed together, using identical solutions and incubation times.

In all cases, the histological quality of the tissue was comparable to that shown in **Figure 1** and **Figure 2**.[18,19] None of the brains suffered from freezing artifacts at this

Continued on next page

zone of the developing cerebral hemisphere to reach their definitive positions in the cortical plate.[16,17] In previous investigations, we showed that a particular population of cortical neurons was displaced in the prefrontal and lateral

See also pages 267, 269, 274, and 277

temporal cortex of schizophrenics.[18,19] This group of neurons that normally expresses the enzyme nicotinamide adenine dinucleotide phosphate diaphorase (NADPH-d) were decreased in the cortex proper and the immediately subjacent white matter, but they were increased in white matter more than 2 mm deep to the cortex. Those that are normally found in relatively large numbers in the subcortical white matter of the adult brain are remnants of the cortical subplate,[20,21] a transitory zone of early-generated neurons and synaptic neuropil that is thought to play a substantial role in the development and maturation of the overlying cortex.[22] The cells that normally remain in the white matter of the adult brain are thought to have escaped the developmentally regulated program of cell death that causes the disappearance of most of the subplate cells.[22]

The maldistributions of subplate-derived cells in schizophrenic brains could reflect a primary disturbance of neuronal migration that might, therefore, be expected to affect all cortical neurons. However, other interpretations are also possible. An alteration in the normal level of resolution, which is in accordance with previous publications that used similar freezing and fixation procedures.[18,19,37]

QUANTITATIVE ANALYSIS

All cell counting and other procedures were performed under blind conditions. For each brain, the total number of GAD mRNA–expressing neurons, identified by localized concentrations of silver grains at least 4× density of the background in the emulsion autoradiographs (Figures 1 and 2), was counted in each cortical layer. Camera lucida drawings were made at ×15 magnification, showing the cortex and boundaries of the six cortical layers. Twenty vertical strips through the thickness of the cortex of each brain were identified on the camera lucida drawings obtained from 10 sections per brain. These were each 3000 μm long and 250 μm wide and were selected so that thicknesses of cortical layers I through VI were in the proportions of 1:1:4:1:2:3. Variations in thickness ratios and vertical depth were tolerated to a limited degree (±25% for a particular layer or total strip). The delineated strips of cortex were then examined under the compound microscope at ×400 magnification, and cells labeled with the cRNA probe and sectioned through the nucleus were counted within successive steps, which were outlined by an eyepiece reticule covering an area 62 500 μm^2 in extent. The eyepiece reticule was also used for measuring the exact vertical extent (±10 μm) of each of the six cortical layers of a particular cortical strip. The cell counts were subsequently normalized to the size of a 3000×250-μm standard strip in which the ratios of layer thickness were fixed as above. Using an identical counting method in strips of the same dimensions in parallel Nissl-stained sections, and again counting only cells sectioned through the nucleus, the total number of neurons and the subtotal of small neurons with round or ovoid somata (diameter 8 to 15 μm) were counted through the thickness of the cortex. The diameter of individual neurons was directly measured using reference lines in the counting grid that were 12.5 and 15 μm apart. The distinction between glial cells and small neurons was made as described by Benes et al.[25] For each brain, the diameter of 30 GAD mRNA–expressing neurons (five neurons per layer) was measured in emulsion autoradiograms, using the reference lines of the counting grid as described above.

Optical densities on the film autoradiograms from each brain were measured in 10 to 15 sample areas of each cortical layer by computer-controlled densitometry (MCID/M4, IMAGING Research Inc, St Catherine, Ontario). The GAD and CamIIK mRNA levels were expressed as nanocuries per gram (100 nCi equals 3.7×10^3 Bq) of tissue by reference to radioactive standards (carbon 14–labeled polymer microscales, Amersham) exposed on the same piece of film after performing background subtraction on each section. Background was defined as the optical density of deep white matter regions. Total GAD and CamIIK mRNA through the thickness of the cortex was determined by normalizing the layer-specific values to a standard strip of the same size, with the ratios of layer thickness as above.

POSTMORTEM VOLUMETRIC MEASUREMENTS

For each brain, the total volume of the portion of the frontal lobe extending from the frontal pole to the posterior surface of the genu of the corpus callosum was determined, along with the volumes of the following two regions of interest within it: PFG and PFW, excluding basal ganglia and ventricles. Volumetric measurements were performed using ×2 original magnification of the photographs taken of each coronal slice at the time of brain processing. Magnification was determined from the image of the metric scale placed next to each slice when photographed. Total areas and the areas of PFG and PFW were measured using a digitizing pad and SigmaScan software (Jandel Scientific, Corte Madera, Calif) for each of the five to six frontal slices per brain. The thickness of each slice was measured with a caliper gauge. Volumes were determined by multiplying area by thickness of the slice.

STATISTICAL ANALYSIS

For each brain and cortical layer, the mean values of neuronal cell densities and GAD and CamIIK mRNA levels were calculated, and the mean value and SEM for each of the two cohorts was calculated from the 20 single mean values. Statistical significance between the mean values of schizophrenics and controls was determined by using BMDP software (BMDP Statistical Software, Inc, Los Angeles, Calif) and multivariate analysis of variance (MANOVA),[40] using the two cohorts as groups and cortical layers as variates. In addition, univariate analysis of variance was used to determine significance of differences between the two cohorts for each cortical layer separately. Significance of differences of frontal lobe volumes was measured by a two-tailed, pooled *t* test.

pattern of physiological cell death in the subplate could account for the maldistribution of NADPH-d cells, especially in the absence of changes in other cortical cell populations. Disturbance of the program of physiological cell death could have consequences for the establishment of a normal pattern of connections in the overlying cortex. When stressed, an imperfectly ordered set of cortical connections could show functional decompensation, leading to symptoms of psychosis.

One potential indicator of functional decompensation in schizophrenia is the hypoactivity of the dorsolateral prefrontal cortex (DLPFC).[23,24] Alterations in the balance of intracortical excitation and inhibition could underlie this dysfunction, but it is not known if these could result from cell death, from the failure of neurons to migrate to their definitive cortical loci during brain development, or from disturbed connection formation secondary to a disturbance of the embryonic subplate. A loss of small neurons has been reported in cortical layer II, especially in brains of schizophrenic patients with affective disturbances,[25] and increased γ-aminobutyric $acid_A$ ($GABA_A$) receptor binding has been reported in layers I and II of the adjacent cingulate cortex in schizophrenics.[26] These findings suggest that the superficial cortical layers, which are important for associative information processing,[27] may be compromised in this disease, and inhibitory GABAergic cells are among those affected. Other findings in schizophrenic cortex, eg, reduced GABA uptake[28,29] and defective GABA release,[30] also imply that GABA transmission may be affected.

Table 1. Characteristics of Matched Pairs

	Schizophrenics					Controls		
Subject Number	*DMS-III-R** Diagnosis	Age at Onset, y	Sex/Age, y	Cause of Death	Autolysis Time, h	Sex/Age, y	Cause of Death	Autolysis Time, h
1	Chronic paranoid schizophrenia	15	F/47	Suicide	30.2	F/51	Myocardial infarction	26.5
2	Chronic undifferentiated schizophrenia	19	M/72	Heart failure	9.0	M/75	Heart failure	7.5
3	Chronic undifferentiated schizophrenia	25	F/70	Myocardial infarction	11.2	F/68	Respiratory insufficiency	7.0
4	Chronic paranoid schizophrenia	28	M/79	Heart failure	5.5	M/81	Respiratory insufficiency	8.0
5	Chronic disorganized schizophrenia	22	M/71	Heart failure	24.5	M/61	Heart failure	25.5
6	Schizophrenia, residual type	25	M/79	Pneumonitis, respiratory arrest	5.0	M/84	Heart failure	6.0
7	Chronic paranoid schizophrenia	22	M/60	Cardiac arrest	26.0	M/63	Pulmonary thromboembolism	23.5
8	Chronic paranoid schizophrenia	18	F/69	Metastatic cancer, respiratory failure	7.30	F/69	Cardiovascular, failed mitral valve	7.25
9	Chronic undifferentiated schizophrenia	20	M/55	Lung cancer, respiratory failure	21.15	M/51	Myocardial infarction	21.5
10	Chronic paranoid schizophrenia	14	M/32	Acute peritonitis	26.5	M/39	Work accident hemorrhage	27.75

*From the American Psychiatric Association.[35]

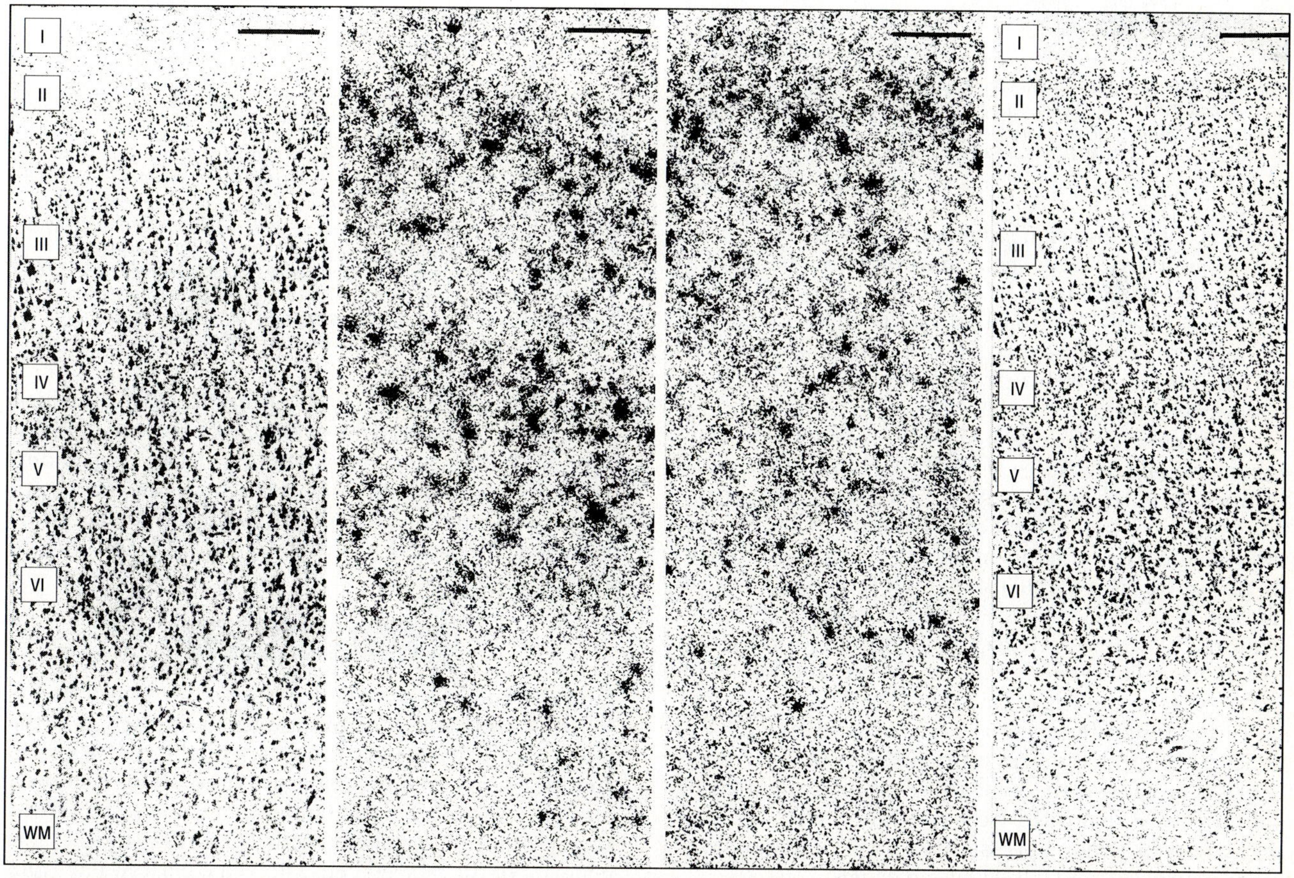

Figure 1. *Photomicrographs of thionin-stained sections (far left and far right) and film autoradiograms of adjacent sections (left center and right center) showing hybridization of the radioactive cRNA probe to glutamic acid decarboxylase (GAD)–expressing cells through the thickness of the superior frontal gyrus. Far left and center left sections are from normal control 4; center right and far right sections, matched schizophrenic 4. Note reduction in GAD-expressing cells in the center right section. Far left and center right sections are representative of histological quality of all material used. Roman numerals indicate cortical layers; WM, white matter; and bar, 500 μm. Schizophrenics and controls are described in Table 1.*

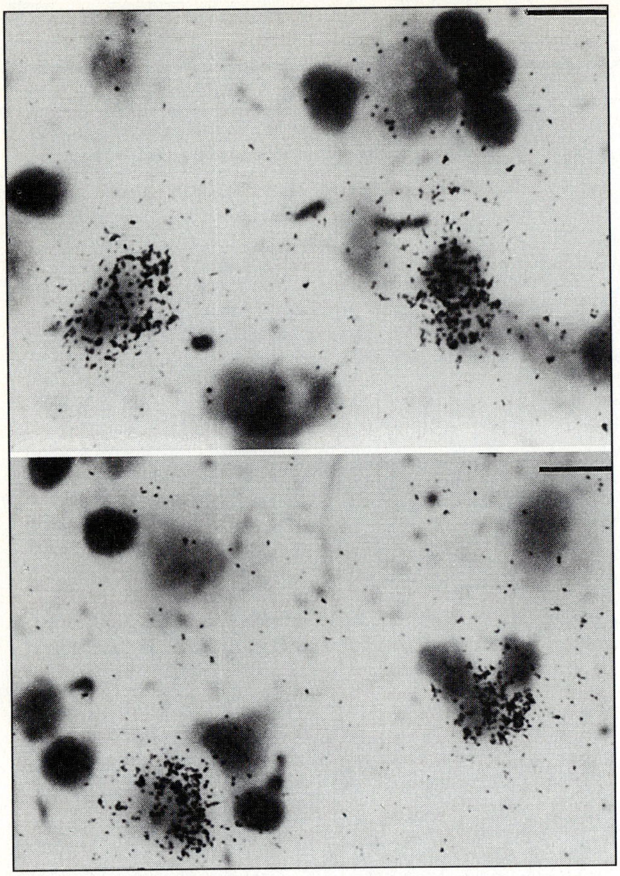

Figure 2. *Photomicrographs from cortical layer II in emulsion autoradiographs showing glutamic acid decarboxylase mRNA–expressing neurons in schizophrenic 1 (top) and control 1 (bottom). Bars indicate 10 μm. Schizophrenics and controls are described in Table 1.*

It is not yet known if reductions in numbers of small cells in an individual cortex can be directly related to a migratory disturbance. It is also not known if the increased ligand binding that has been reported[26,31] implies receptor up-regulation in response to reduced GABA release or reduced biosynthesis of GABA in inhibitory neurons.

Glutamic acid decarboxylase (GAD) is the key enzyme in the synthesis of GABA in inhibitory interneurons. It is regulated in an activity-dependent manner in the cerebral cortex of nonhuman primates. In the visual cortex of adult monkeys, conduction block in the optic nerve causes reversible reductions in immunoreactive GAD and GABA levels in local circuit neurons.[32,33] These decreases in GABA immunoreactivity are associated over time with decreased levels of GAD messenger RNA (mRNA),[34] suggesting that activity-dependent regulation of cortical GABA depends in the long-term on regulation of GAD gene expression. Hence, the hypoactive prefrontal cortex of schizophrenics could be associated with down-regulation of gene expression for GAD and possibly other neurotransmitter-related molecules.

Using the in situ hybridization technique, cell-counting methods, and computerized densitometry in postmortem material from a schizophrenic sample and matched controls, the present study measured levels of GAD mRNA in the six layers of the DLPFC, calculated the number and laminar distribution of neurons expressing GAD mRNA, and compared these data with the number and laminar distribution of all neurons and small, putatively nonpyramidal neurons in adjacent Nissl-stained sections and prefrontal gray (PFG) and white matter (PFW) volumes.

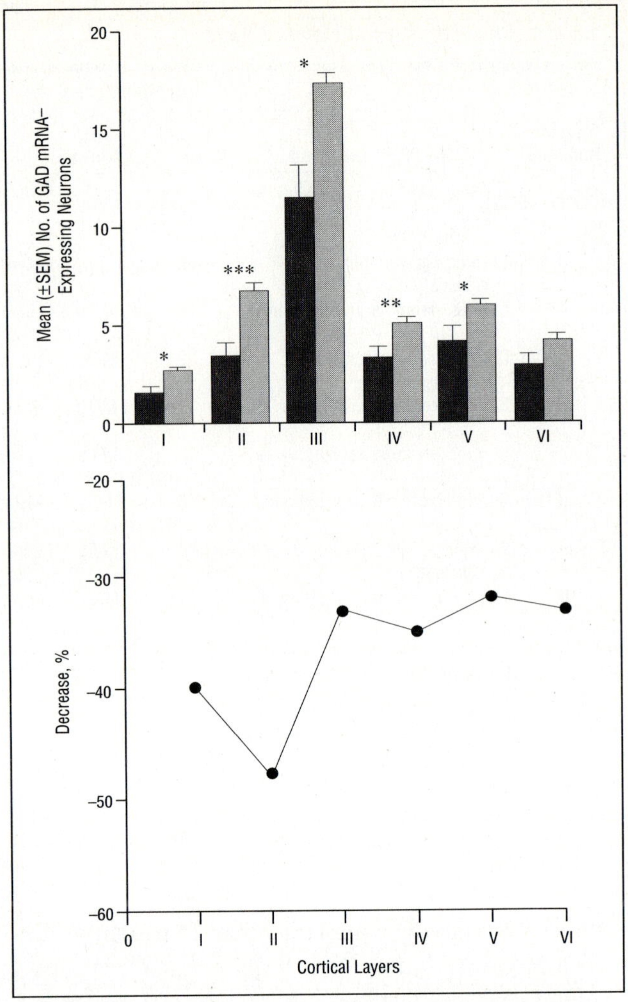

Figure 3. *Top, Mean (±SEM) number of glutamic acid decarboxylase mRNA (GAD mRNA)–expressing neurons in cortical layers I through VI of the schizophrenic (dark-shaded bars) and control (light-shaded bars) cohorts. Bottom, Percentage of decrease of GAD mRNA–expressing neurons in cortical layers I through VI of the schizophrenic cohort. Asterisk indicates* $P<.05$; *double asterisk,* $P<.01$; *and triple asterisk,* $P<.001$. *Schizophrenics and controls are described in Table 1.*

RESULTS

Film and emulsion autoradiographs of sections from the schizophrenic and control samples hybridized with the high concentration of GAD antisense riboprobe (13 000 cpm/μL), after 14 days' exposure time, showed numerous, intensely labeled cell bodies that could easily be distinguished from unlabeled cells (Figures 1 and 2). The majority of the labeled cells showed a pericellular grain density 10- to 20-fold above average background grain density, which was two to five grains per 300 μm^2. Cells showing the weakest labeling still showed a pericellular grain density of fourfold to fivefold above background grain density. Sections hybridized with the lower probe concentration (10 000 cpm/μL) and all sections after the longer exposure time (28 days) invariably showed a lower signal-to-noise ratio. Hence, only material hybridized with the 13 000-cpm/μL probe and exposed for 14 days was used for counting GAD mRNA–labeled cells. Only film autoradiograms of these sections were used for densitometry. Control hybridizations with either 10 000 or 13 000 cpm/μL of the sense riboprobe or tissue sections that had been pretreated with RNase A caused weak background labeling only, with two to five grains per 300 μm^2 in emulsion-dipped sections. Sections that had been pretreated with Triton X-100 did not show superior labeling in comparison with untreated sections.

Sections from both the schizophrenic and control samples showed numerous neurons expressing GAD mRNA throughout the thickness of the cortex. In schizophrenics, the number of GAD mRNA–expressing neurons was significantly decreased through the full thickness of the cortex (MANOVA, F[6,13]=4.14 [*P*=.015]). Layer-by-layer analysis revealed a significant decrease of GAD mRNA–expressing neurons in layers I, II, III, IV, and V of schizophrenics (*P*<.001 to *P*<.05) (**Figure 3**, top), while the decrease in layer VI was not significant (*P*=.11). Changes were pronounced in layers I and II (40% decrease in layer I, 48% decrease in layer II). In layers III to VI, there was an overall 30% to 35% decrease (Figure 3, bottom). The diameter of GAD mRNA–expressing cells measured in emulsion autoradiographs was similar in both cohorts. In the control cohort, 83%±1.3% had a diameter from 8 through 15 μm, and 17%±1.3% had a diameter larger than 15 μm. In schizophrenics, 86%±1.4% of all GAD mRNA–expressing neurons had a diameter from 8 to 15 μm, and 14%±1.4% had a diameter larger than 15 μm. These differences did not reach the level of significance (*P*>.1).

The concentration of GAD mRNA in the cortex, as determined by optical density measurements on film autoradiograms, was highest in layers II and IV. In the schizophrenic cohort, GAD mRNA levels were reduced throughout all cortical layers (MANOVA, F[6,13]=4.19 [*P*=.014]). The percentage decrease was greatest in layer II (37%). Layer-by-layer comparison between schizophrenics and controls revealed significant differences in layers II, III, IV, and V (*P*<.05) (**Figure 4**, top).

The average number of GAD mRNA–expressing neurons per standard strip in the one patient who had not received neuroleptics in the 10 years prior to death (patient 3) was 11.4 cells, compared with the average of 27.2 labeled cells in the nine patients who had received medication and the average of 40.1 labeled cells in the controls. The levels of GAD mRNA, as measured by optical density, were also lower in the schizophrenic receiving no neuroleptics than in the nine other patients (107.7 vs 184.6 nCi/g, respectively, vs 259.0 nCi/g in the controls).

The total number of Nissl-stained neurons and subpopulation of small, round or ovoid neurons through the full thickness of the cortex did not show any significant difference between the schizophrenic and control cohorts (total number of neurons, MANOVA, F[6,13]=1.58 [*P*=.23]; small, round or ovoid neurons, MANOVA, F[6,13]=1.51 [*P*=.25]). Layer-by-layer comparison revealed no significant differences between schizophrenics and controls (**Table 2**). There were no significant differences in numbers of cells per standard strip between the schizophrenic and control cohorts. In layer II, where GAD-expressing cells and mRNA levels showed the greatest reduction, schizophrenics showed a tendency for higher variability (F test, *P*<.1) in the numbers of small round or ovoid cells, but the mean values (Table 2) for layer II were only slightly different between the cohorts.

Layers II to VI in sections hybridized with antisense CamIIK riboprobes showed numerous labeled neurons. Labeling was heaviest over large neurons (diameter, >15 μm) in layers III, V, and VI. The CamIIK mRNA labeling was not restricted to somata but included dense labeling of the neuropil, reflecting the large concentrations of CamIIK mRNA found in dendrites.[38,39,41] By contrast with the significant changes in GAD mRNA levels in the schizophrenic DLPFC, CamIIK mRNA levels throughout the full thickness of the cortex did not dif-

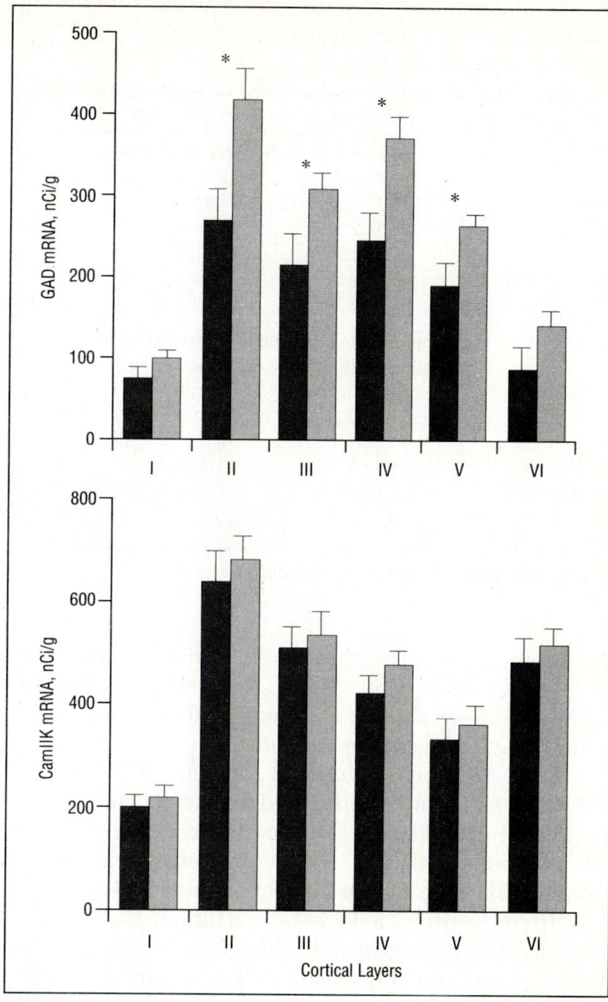

Figure 4. *Top, Levels of glutamic acid decarboxylase mRNA (GAD mRNA), and bottom, levels of calcium-calmodulin–dependent protein kinase (CamIIK) mRNA, as measured by optical densitometry, across the six cortical layers (100 nCi equals 3.7×10³ Bq). Data are shown as mean±SEM. Light-shaded bars indicate controls; dark-shaded bars, schizophrenics; and asterisk,* P<.05. *Schizophrenics and controls are described in Table 1.*

Table 2. Layer-by-Layer Comparison of Cortex in Schizophrenics and Controls*

Cortical Layer	Controls	Schizophrenics	P
Total Neurons per Standard Strip, Mean (±SEM) No.			
I	3.3±0.4	3.4±0.5	.66
II	41.3±1.9	42.4±1.4	.73
III	82.6±2.5	81.8±3.3	.88
IV	36.8±1.2	33.4±2.3	.20
V	42.6±0.9	44.1±2.1	.73
VI	47.9±0.94	50.5±2.6	.33
Total Small, Round or Ovoid Neurons per Standard Strip, Mean (±SEM) No.			
I	3.5±0.3	3.4±0.4	.42
II	24.8±0.9	24.5±1.4	.74
III	14.9±1.5	16.5±1.9	.90
IV	23.4±1.3	21.9±1.6	.30
V	7.6±0.5	8.4±0.9	.78
VI	5.9±0.5	5.8±0.6	.85

**Schizophrenics and controls are described in Table 1.*

fer significantly between the schizophrenics and controls (MANOVA, $F[6,13]=0.21$ [$P=.96$]). Layer-by-layer comparison showed a nonsignificant decrease in the schizophrenics (Figure 4, bottom).

Total prefrontal volume in the control cohort was 132.4±3.9 cm^3 and in the schizophrenic cohort was 121.6±6.1 cm^3. The percentage difference was 8%, but this was not significant ($P>.1$). Prefrontal gray matter volume was 65.2±2.8 cm^3 in controls and 58.4±3.0 cm^3 in schizophrenics, a 10% reduction in the schizophrenic cohort. Prefrontal white matter volume was 61.9±2.2 cm^3 in controls and 59.8±3.5 cm^3 in schizophrenics, a 3% difference in volume. None of these differences reached the level of significance.

COMMENT

The present study demonstrated an overall reduction in 67-kd GAD expression in cortical neurons, without evidence of significant cell loss, in the DLPFC of schizophrenics. That is, GABA cells showed reduced GAD mRNA expression but did not die. Levels of GAD mRNA, as measured by densitometry, were decreased overall in the schizophrenic cohort. Therefore, the decline in GAD mRNA expression in cortical GABAergic neurons is not counterbalanced by an overexpression of GAD mRNA in the remaining GABAergic neurons. It is not known if the reduced expression of GAD mRNA could be a secondary effect due to neuroleptics, although a direct neuroleptic effect seems unlikely because the one schizophrenic receiving no medication in the sample had the lowest levels of GAD mRNA. However, a controlled experimental study to confirm this would be desirable. At present, it is not known if gene expression for the 65-kd form of GAD[42] is similarly affected.

The schizophrenic and control samples did not differ significantly in the total number of neurons nor in the subpopulation of small, round or ovoid neurons. The observed decrease in GAD mRNA levels in the schizophrenic sample is therefore unlikely to be due to a general loss of cells or a specific loss of GABAergic cells. Although it is difficult in Nissl stains to distinguish pyramidal from nonpyramidal cells, most of the GABAergic, inhibitory interneurons from previous quantitative studies in other primates[43] would tend to be included in the small, round or ovoid neuronal population that showed no reduction in numbers. The largest GABA cells, particularly the large basket cells,[44] would be excluded from the counts of small cells because their somata tend to exceed 15 μm in diameter. However, the large basket cells are absent from layer II, in which the greatest changes in GAD mRNA expression were found, and, in any case, neuronal numbers were unchanged throughout the cortex. The present results are not in agreement with those reporting a selective loss of small neurons in layer II of the DLPFC in certain schizophrenics, especially those with mood disturbances.[25] We have no explanation for this difference, except that none of the schizophrenics of the present study showed evidence of major depression, schizoaffective disorder, or bipolar affective psychosis. The relationship of symptoms in individual schizophrenics to neuropathological features needs to be pursued further.

Given the fact that GAD gene expression is activity dependent,[33,34] a likely explanation of the present results is that GAD gene expression has been decreased as the result of changes in the functional activity of neural circuits in the DLPFC of the present schizophrenic sample. The observed changes in GAD mRNA expression were most pronounced in layers I and II. In conjunction with a recent report showing a selective increase in $GABA_A$ receptor binding in layers I through III of the cingulate cortex in schizophrenia,[26] these findings suggest that cortical GABA-mediated transmission is compromised in the superficial layers of the neocortex in this condition. The superficial layers are important for corticocortical associative information processing.[27] Thus, the disturbance of frontal lobe–specific associative functions in schizophrenia[23,24,45-47] could potentially be explained by a breakdown of GABAergic signal transmission in the upper cortical layers.[26] Other transmitter-specific pathways may be compromised as well[48-53] because it is doubtful that a loss of GABA activity alone would predispose to functional hypoactivity of the DLPFC. Other neuronal pathological features found in the schizophrenic brain, eg, disturbances in cytoskeletal proteins,[54] also may contribute to these functional alterations.

The results of the present study suggest that changes at cortical GABAergic synapses in schizophrenia[26,28-31] are associated with decreased production of GABA due to reduced production of GAD. The GAD synthesis takes place in the cell body of inhibitory neurons. The observed decrease in the amount of GAD mRNA in these cells in the DLPFC of schizophrenics suggests that the causative mechanism acts at the level of gene transcription, although a reduction in mRNA stability is not ruled out. The reduced gene expression for GAD could be directly related to a genetic defect[55] or the influence of a pathogenic agent.[56] In light of the present results, however, a pathogenic effect would have to be unaccompanied by cortical cell death. Down-regulation of GAD expression also could be the outcome of developmental alterations of the cerebral cortex that cause defective patterns in cell settling and altered circuit development, which may lead to functional hypoactivity of the DLPFC in schizophrenia.[23,24,46,47]

The present results, showing a lack of significant changes in frontal volumes and overall numbers of cells in the DLPFC of schizophrenics, make it unlikely that a generalized disturbance of neuronal migration during brain development has substantially affected all neuronal populations of the DLPFC. Our earlier findings on the distorted distribution of NADPH-d neurons in the schizophrenic cerebral cortex in comparison with the cerebral cortex of controls[18,19] may therefore more specifically reflect a primary disturbance of the developmentally regulated cortical subplate. This in turn may mark the timing of an environmental insult in schizophrenics, since the subplate normally reaches its peak of development in the second trimester. Whether there is a migratory disturbance of the early generated subplate cells or an alteration in their pattern of programmed cell death awaits further investigation. A primary disturbance of the subplate, however, from experimental evidence in animals, can have major consequences for the formation of a normal pattern of cortical connections.[57,58] Any compromise in the establishment of this pattern could affect the balance of excitation and inhibition in the DLPFC of schizophrenics and thus lead to activity-dependent alterations in gene expression for transmitter-related molecules such as GAD.

Accepted for publication September 22, 1994.

Supported by grant MH44188 from the National Institute of Mental Health, Rockville, Md (Dr Jones), grant NS21377 from the National Institutes of Health, Bethesda, Md (Dr Jones), the National Alliance For Research on Schizophrenia and Depression, Chicago, Ill (Dr Akbarian), and the Stanley Foundation (Research Award from the National Alliance of the Mentally Ill), Arlington, Va (Dr Jones).

Resources for processing brains were provided by W. W. Tourtellotte, MD, PhD, and I. Rosario, RN, at the National Neurological Research Specimen Bank, West Los Angeles (Calif) Veterans Affairs Hospital. The authors thank Curt Sandman, PhD, and Bill Hettrick, PhD, for statistical advice; Madhu Reddy and Joyce Fairshter for administrative assistance; the families of patients who participated in these studies; the California Alliance for the Mentally Ill, Tustin; J. Beisner, W. King, and B. Lyles of the Orange County Sheriff/Coroner's Office; M. Wingate and L. Hierholzer of the Orange County Eye and Tissue Bank; W. Lovell, MD, Ventura County Medical Examiner/ Coroner; and the residents and staff of Harbor View House, Costa Mesa, Calif.

Reprint requests to Department of Anatomy and Neurobiology, University of California–Irvine, Irvine, CA 92717 (Dr Jones).

REFERENCES

1. Waddington JL. Schizophrenia: developmental neuroscience and pathobiology. *Lancet.* 1993;341:531-536.
2. Mednick SA, Machon RA, Huttunen MO, Bonett D. Adult schizophrenia following prenatal exposure to an influenza epidemic. *Arch Gen Psychiatry.* 1988; 45:189-192.
3. Kendell RE, Kemp IW. Maternal influenza in the etiology of schizophrenia. *Arch Gen Psychiatry.* 1989;46:878-882.
4. Barr CE, Mednick SA, Munk-Jorgensen P. Exposure to influenza epidemics during gestation and adult schizophrenia. *Arch Gen Psychiatry.* 1990;47:869-874.
5. O'Callaghan E, Sham P, Takei N, Glover G, Murray RM. Schizophrenia after prenatal exposure to 1957 A2 influenza epidemic. *Lancet.* 1991;337:1248-1250.
6. Sham PC, O'Callaghan E, Takei N, Murray GK, Hare H, Murray RM. Schizophrenia following prenatal exposure to influenza epidemics between 1939 and 1960. *Br J Psychiatry.* 1992;160:461-466.
7. Susser ES, Lin SP. Schizophrenia after prenatal exposure to the Dutch hunger winter of 1944-1945. *Arch Gen Psychiatry.* 1992;49:983-988.
8. Mednick SA, Cannon TD. Fetal development, birth and the syndromes of adult schizophrenia. In: Mednick SA, Cannon TD, Barr CE, Lyon M, eds. *Fetal Neural Development and Adult Schizophrenia.* New York, NY: Cambridge University Press; 1991:3-13.
9. Scheibel AB, Kovelman JA. Disorientation of the hippocampal pyramidal cell and its processes in the schizophrenic patient. *Biol Psychiatry.* 1981;16:101-102.
10. Kovelman JA, Scheibel AB. A neurohistological correlate of schizophrenia. *Biol Psychiatry.* 1984;19:1601-1621.
11. Conrad AJ, Abebe T, Austin R, Forsythe S, Scheibel AB. Hippocampal pyramidal cell disarray in schizophrenia as a bilateral phenomenon. *Arch Gen Psychiatry.* 1991;48:413-417.
12. Jakob H, Beckmann H. Prenatal developmental disturbances in the limbic allocortex of schizophrenics. *J Neural Transm.* 1986;65:303-326.
13. Jakob H, Beckmann H. Gross and histological criteria for developmental disorders in brains of schizophrenics. *J R Soc Med.* 1989;82:466-469.
14. Arnold SE, Hyman BT, Van Hoesen GW, Damasio AR. Some cytoarchitectural abnormalities of the entorhinal cortex in schizophrenia. *Arch Gen Psychiatry.* 1991;48:625-632.
15. Beall MJ, Lewis DA. Heterogeneity of layer II neurons in human entorhinal cortex. *J Comp Neurol.* 1992;321:241-266.
16. Rakic P. Mode of cell migration to the superficial layers of the fetal monkey neocortex. *J Comp Neurol.* 1972;145:61-84.
17. Rakic P. Neurons in rhesus monkey visual cortex: systematic relationship between time of origin and eventual disposition. *J Comp Neurol.* 1974;183:425-427.
18. Akbarian S, Bunney WE Jr, Potkin SG, Wigal SB, Hagman JO, Sandman CA, Jones EG. Altered distribution of nicotinamide-adenine dinucleotide phosphate–diaphorase cells in frontal lobe of schizophrenics implies disturbances of cortical development. *Arch Gen Psychiatry.* 1993;50:169-177.
19. Akbarian S, Viñuela A, Kim JJ, Potkin SG, Bunney WE Jr, Jones EG. Distorted distribution of nicotinamide-adenine dinucleotide phosphate–diaphorase neurons in temporal lobe of schizophrenics implies anomalous cortical development. *Arch Gen Psychiatry.* 1993;50:178-187.
20. Kostovic I, Rakic P. Developmental history of the transient subplate zone in the visual and somatosensory cortex of the macaque monkey and human brain. *J Comp Neurol.* 1990;297:441-470.
21. Chun JJM, Shatz CJ. Interstitial cells of the adult neocortical white matter are the remnant of the early generated subplate population. *J Comp Neurol.* 1989; 282:555-569.
22. Shatz CJ, Gosh A, McConnell SK, Allendoerfer KL, Friauf E, Antonini A. Pioneer neurons and target selection in cerebral cortical development. In: *Cold Spring Harbor Symposia on Quantitative Biology: The Brain.* 1990;55:469-480.
23. Buchsbaum MS, DeLisi LE, Holcomb HH, Cappalletti J, King AC, Johnson J, Hazlett E, Dowling-Zimmerman S, Post RM, Morihisa J, Carpenter W, Cohen R, Pickar D, Weinberger DR, Margolin R, Kessler RM. Anteroposterior gradients in cerebral glucose use in schizophrenia and affective disorders. *Arch Gen Psychiatry.* 1984;41:1159-1166.
24. Weinberger DR, Berman KF, Zec RF. Physiologic dysfunction of dorsolateral prefrontal cortex in schizophrenia, I: regional cerebral blood flow evidence. *Arch Gen Psychiatry.* 1986;43:114-124.
25. Benes FM, McSparren J, Bird ED, SanGiovanni JP, Vincent SL. Deficits in small interneurons in prefrontal and cingulate cortices of schizophrenic and schizoaffective patients. *Arch Gen Psychiatry.* 1991;48:996-1001.
26. Benes FM, Vincent SL, Alsterberg G, Bird ED, SanGiovanni JP. Increased $GABA_A$ receptor binding in superficial layers of cingulate cortex in schizophrenics. *J Neurosci.* 1992;12:924-929.
27. Jones EG. Laminar distribution of cortical efferent cells. In: Peters A, Jones EG, eds. *Cerebral Cortex: Cellular Components of the Cerebral Cortex.* New York, NY: Plenum Press; 1984;1:521-553.

28. Simpson MDC, Slater P, Deakin JFW, Royston MC, Skan WJ. Reduced GABA uptake in the temporal lobe in schizophrenia. *Neurosci Lett.* 1989;107:211-215.
29. Simpson MDC, Slater P, Royston MC, Deakin JFW. Regionally selective deficits in uptake sites for glutamate and γ-aminobutyric acid in the basal ganglia in schizophrenia. *Psychiatry Res.* 1992;42:273-282.
30. Sherman AD, Davidson AT, Baruah S, Hegwood TS, Waziri R. Evidence of glutamatergic deficiency in schizophrenia. *Neurosci Lett.* 1991;121:77-80.
31. Hanada S, Mita T, Nishinok N, Tanaka C. ^{3}H-muscimol binding sites increased in autopsied brains of chronic schizophrenics. *Life Sci.* 1987;40:259-266.
32. Hendry SHC, Jones EG. Reduction in number of immunostained GABAergic neurons in deprived-eye dominance columns of monkey area 17. *Nature.* 1986; 320:750-753.
33. Hendry SHC, Jones EG. Activity-dependent regulation of GABA expression in the visual cortex of adult monkeys. *Neuron.* 1988;1:701-712.
34. Benson DL, Huntsman MM, Jones EG. Activity-dependent changes in GAD and preprotachykinin mRNAs in visual cortex of adult monkeys. *Cereb Cortex.* 1994; 4:40-51.
35. American Psychiatric Association. *Diagnostic and Statistical Manual of Mental Disorders, Revised Third Edition.* Washington, DC: American Psychiatric Association; 1987.
36. Tourtellotte WW, Berman K. Brain banking. In: Adelman G, ed. *Encyclopedia of Neuroscience.* Boston, Mass: Birkhaeuser; 1981;1:156-158.
37. Jones EG, Hendry SHC, Liu XB, Potkin SG, Tourtellotte WW. A method for fixation of previously fresh frozen human adult and fetal brains that preserves histological quality and immunoreactivity. *J Neurosci Methods.* 1992;44:133-144.
38. Benson DL, Isackson PJ, Gall CM, Jones EG. Differential effects of monocular deprivation on glutamic acid decarboxylase and type II calcium-calmodulin–dependent protein kinase gene expression in the adult monkey visual cortex. *J Neurosci.* 1991;11:31-47.
39. Benson DL, Isackson PJ, Hendry SHC, Jones EG. Differential gene expression for glutamic acid decarboxylase and type II calcium-calmodulin–dependent protein kinase in basal ganglia, thalamus and hypothalamus of the monkey. *J Neurosci.* 1991;11:1540-1564.
40. Tatsuoka M. *Multivariate Analysis of Variance: Technique for Educational and Psychological Research.* 2nd ed. New York, NY: MacMillan Publishing Co Inc; 1988:85-86.
41. Burgin KE, Waxham MN, Rickling S, Westgate SA, Mobley WC, Kelly PT. In situ hybridization histochemistry of Ca^{2+}/calmodulin-dependent protein kinase in developing rat brain. *J Neurosci.* 1990;10:1788-1798.
42. Erlander MG, Tillakaratne NJ, Feldblum S, Patel N, Tobin AJ. Two genes encode distinct glutamate decarboxylases. *Neuron.* 1991;7:91-100.
43. Hendry SHC, Schwark HD, Jones EG, Yan J. Numbers and proportions of GABA-immunoreactive neurons in different areas of monkey cerebral cortex. *J Neurosci.* 1987;7:1503-1519.
44. Jones EG, Hendry SHC. Basket cells. In: Peters A, Jones EG, eds. *Cerebral Cortex: Cellular Components of the Cerebral Cortex.* New York, NY: Plenum Press; 1984:309-336.
45. Volkow ND, Wolf AP, Gelder PV, Brodie JO, Overall JE, Cancro R, Gomez-Mont F. Phenomenological correlates of metabolic activity in 18 patients with chronic schizophrenia. *Am J Psychiatry.* 1987;144:151-158.
46. Cohen RM, Semple WE, Gross M, Nordahl TE, DeLisi LE, Holcomb HH, King AC, Morihisa JM, Pikar D. Dysfunction in a prefrontal substrate of sustained attention in schizophrenia. *Life Sci.* 1987;40:2031-2039.
47. Paulman RG, Devous MD Sr, Gregory RR, Herman JH, Jennings L, Bonte FJ, Nasrallah HA, Raese JD. Hypofrontality and cognitive impairment in schizophrenia: dynamic single-photon tomography and neuropsychological assessment of schizophrenic brain function. *Biol Psychiatry.* 1990;27:377-399.
48. Kleinman JE, Karoum F, Rosenblatt J, Gillin JC, Hong J, Bridge TP, Zalcman S, Storch F, Delcarmen R, Wyatt RJ. Catecholamines and peptides in postmortem schizophrenic brains. In: Perris C, Struwe G, Jannonson B, eds. *Biological Psychiatry.* Amsterdam, the Netherlands: Elsevier Science Publishers; 1981:711-714.
49. Reynolds GP. Postmortem neurochemistry of schizophrenia. *Psychol Med.* 1988; 18:793-797.
50. Deakin JFW, Simpson MDC, Gilchrist AC, Skan WJ, Royston MC, Reynolds GP, Cross AJ. Frontal cortical and left temporal glutamatergic dysfunction in schizophrenia. *J Neurochem.* 1989;52:1781-1786.
51. Nakai T, Kitamura N, Hashimoto T, Kajmoto Y, Nishino N, Mita T, Tanaka C. Decreased histamine H_1 receptors in the frontal cortex of brains from patients with chronic schizophrenia. *Biol Psychiatry.* 1991;30:349-356.
52. Arora RC, Meltzer HY. Serotonin ($5\text{-}HT_2$) receptor binding in the frontal cortex of schizophrenic patients. *J Neural Transm.* 1991;85:19-29.
53. Kurumaji A, Ishimaru M, Toru M. α-[^{3}H]Amino-3-hydroxy-5-methylisoxazole-4-propionic acid binding to human cerebral cortical membranes: minimal changes in postmortem brains of chronic schizophrenics. *J Neurochem.* 1992;59:829-837.
54. Arnold SE, Lee VM, Gur RE, Trojanowski JQ. Abnormal expression of two microtubule-associated proteins (MAP-2 and MAP-5) in specific subfields of the hippocampal formation in schizophrenia. *Proc Natl Acad Sci U S A.* 1991;88: 10 850-10 854.
55. Kendler KS, Diehl SR. The genetics of schizophrenia: a current, genetic-epidemiologic perspective. *Schizophr Bull.* 1993;19:261-285.
56. Stevens JR. Neuropathology of schizophrenia. *Arch Gen Psychiatry.* 1982;39: 1131-1139.
57. Gosh A, Antonini A, McConnell SK, Shatz CJ. Requirement for subplate neurons in the formation of thalamocortical connections. *Nature.* 1990;347:179-181.
58. Gosh A, Shatz CJ. Involvement of subplate neurons in the formation of ocular dominance columns. *Science.* 1992;255:1441-1443.

COMMENTARY

Reduced Inhibitory Capacity in Prefrontal Cortex of Schizophrenics

UNDERSTANDING the neural substrates of schizophrenia has long been a goal of psychiatrists and neurobiologists. For the clinician, more precise understanding could translate into advances in diagnosis and treatment. For the neurobiologist, such knowledge could provide general insights into the mechanisms of higher cognitive function.

Much recent work has focused on the prefrontal cortex (PFC), especially the dorsolateral PFC (DLPFC), which roughly corresponds to Brodmann's area 9. While changes in other brain regions have been reported,[1,2] a growing body of converging evidence suggests that disruptions of the DLPFC play a particularly important role in the origins and course of the illness. Positron emission tomography studies,[3] regional cerebral blood flow studies in patients performing the Wisconsin Card Sort,[4] and cytoarchitectonic studies[1] have revealed abnormalities in the DLPFC. These studies suggest that in schizophrenics, the DLPFC is hypoactive relative to other brain regions.

See also pages 258, 269, 274, and 277

The neuronal substrates underlying DLPFC hypoactivity therefore assume considerable importance. Several explanations are possible, including reduction of cell numbers in the DLPFC, disrupted connections between DLPFC neurons and other neurons as a result of abnormal cell migration during early neuronal development, and deficits in the cellular machinery within DLPFC neurons. The resolution of this issue could help to guide research into therapeutic options.

ALTERED GENE EXPRESSION IN INHIBITORY NEURONS

The present work of Akbarian et al[5] suggests that an important correlate of DLPFC hypoactivity occurs at the cellular level. While they found no difference in the number of DLPFC neurons in the brains of schizophrenics vs controls, they report a reduction in the level of messenger RNA (mRNA) for glutamic acid decarboxylase$_{67}$ (GAD$_{67}$), which is present in the 20% to 30% of DLPFC neurons that use γ-aminobutyric acid (GABA) as a neurotransmitter. This decrease occurred in all six layers of the DLPFC, but especially in the superficial layers.

Glutamic acid decarboxylase$_{67}$ is one of two forms of glutamate decarboxylase, the enzyme that catalyzes the synthesis of GABA, the most prominent inhibitory neurotransmitter in the central nervous system.[6] The GAD$_{67}$ isoform is present in both the cell bodies and the axon terminals of GABA neurons throughout the central nervous system; the other GAD isoform, GAD$_{65}$, is present primarily in axon terminals.[7] The two GAD isoenyzmes, which derive from homologous unlinked genes, differ primarily in the sequences near their amino terminal ends. The distinct intracellular distributions of the two GADs suggest that they may subserve distinct GABA pools.[7] A reduction in GAD$_{67}$ mRNA levels would be expected to result in reduced GABA synthesis in DLPFC neurons and perhaps a corresponding change in neural activity in areas to which DLPFC neurons project.

Previous work has documented alterations in GABAergic function in other cortical and subcortical regions. The report by Akbarian et al[5] suggests that these changes may be secondary to the reduction of GAD-catalyzed GABA synthesis in the DLPFC. For example, previously reported increases in ligand binding to GABA$_A$ receptors in the cingulate cortex[8] and caudate nucleus,[9] both of which receive inputs from the DLPFC,[10] could be compensatory responses to functional reduction of DLPFC GABA neurotransmission. Similarly, decreases in GABA reuptake seen in various subcortical[11] and non–frontal-cortical sites,[12] such as the polar temporal cortex, could also be compensatory responses to decreased GABA production in the DLPFC.

The pronounced reduction of GAD$_{67}$ mRNA in the superficial cortical layers may account for the intense disruptions of higher cognitive function in schizophrenics, since the superficial layers are particularly important in associative, integrative processing, with corticocortical connections particularly prominent in the superficial layers. Previously reported increases in ligand-binding to GABA$_A$ receptors in subcortical areas, as well as the reduced GABA reuptake in these areas, may be connected to the reduced expression of GAD$_{67}$ mRNA in the deeper layers of DLPFC.

CLINICAL IMPLICATIONS

The heterogeneity locations of DLPFC projections may account for the seemingly intractable problem of negative symptoms. It has long been known that neuroleptics are more effective in treating the positive rather than the negative symptoms of schizophrenia.[13] Because hypoactivity of the DLPFC disrupts connections to a broad spectrum of brain areas, both cortical and subcortical, different symptoms may result from disrupted DLPFC projections to different brain regions.

The positive symptoms of schizophrenia, for example, may result from dopaminergic overactivity in the basal ganglia,[4] which could be secondary to the DLPFC GABA deficits and a corresponding alteration in the input to subcortical nuclei. In contrast, negative symptoms may result from altered DLPFC projections to either brain region, involving nondopaminergic systems, thereby explaining the limited spectrum of action of current neuroleptics. A tantalizing hypothesis is that DLPFC GABA deficits result in alterations in function of other cortical regions, as opposed to subcortical regions, resulting in complex cognitive deficits.

These possibilities, implicit in the study by Akbarian et al,[5] provide some new suggestions for rational pharmacological research and drug design. It is possible that increased GABA production in the DLPFC, rather than dopamine receptor blockade in basal ganglia, would produce more global improvements in both positive and negative symptoms of schizophrenics. The use of GABA agonists selectively targeted to the DLPFC might be worth further examination in schizophrenia. For example, the GABA-mimetic agents γ-vinyl GABA and 4,5,6,7-tetrahydroisoxazolo-(5,4-c)pyridine-3-ol have been shown to increase cerebrospinal GABA levels and decrease neuroleptic-induced dyskinesias in schizophrenic patients.[14] A possible approach might be to use such GABA-mimetic agents before neuroleptic treatment is initiated, since the latter might produce functional GABAergic changes that are not easily reversible. Indeed, neuroleptic-treated schizophrenics have shown reduced cerebrospinal fluid GABA levels, compared with untreated patients.[14]

NEUROBIOLOGICAL IMPLICATIONS

The work of Akbarian et al[5] raises questions that can only be clarified by future research. For example, the finding that DLPFC cell numbers are not decreased is inconsistent with the work of Benes et al,[1] who found decreased interneuron levels in DLPFC. It is possible that patient heterogeneity accounts for this discrepancy, since the neuron loss in the sample studied by Benes et al[1] was more pronounced in those patients suffering from comorbid affective disorders. Future research segregating patients according to population subtypes might clarify this issue and might provide more insight into the rich complexity of the disorder.

One discrepancy remains, however: the 1986 article by Hanada et al,[9] who reported no loss of GAD activity in the PFC of schizophrenics. The reason for this discrepancy is not readily apparent. Many of their patients died suddenly, and these deaths may have been suicides (no details were provided in the article). Patients dying of prolonged terminal illness "often with coma" showed lower GAD activity than controls, while patients with sudden death showed no differences. In the article by Akbarian et al,[5] the causes of death are not listed. It is possible that suicidal schizophrenic patients are less likely to have decreased GAD activity. Results of autopsies of brains of successful suicides have suggested various neurochemical deficits different from those in the brains of nonsuicides,[15] raising the possibility that variability in impulse control may be another source of heterogeneity in schizophrenic patients.

An important issue that has plagued research in this area has been the extensive use of neuroleptics in most of the schizophrenic patients whose brains have been examined. Only one patient of the sample examined by Akbarian et al[5] had not been treated with neuroleptics, a sample size too small to rule out the possibility that neuroleptics are involved in some of the observed abnormalities. The effects of neuroleptic treatment will remain a difficult problem to circumvent because of the ethical issues involved. The development of a noninvasive measure of GABA levels in the brains of living patients at intake, before they receive medication, would certainly be useful.

CONCLUSION

Akbarian et al[5] provide important evidence for intracellular neuronal dysfunction in schizophrenics rather than gross morphological abnormalities. These findings should stimulate further questions and research and have important implications for psychiatry and neurobiology.

Dennis E. Lee
Interdepartmental Program for Neuroscience
University of California, Los Angeles
Los Angeles, CA 90095
Allan J. Tobin
Los Angeles

Correspondence to Life Sciences Building, University of California, Los Angeles, Los Angeles, CA 90024-1606 (Dr Tobin).

REFERENCES

1. Benes FM, McSparren J, Bird ED, SanGiovanni JP, Vincent SL. Deficits in small interneurons in prefrontal and cingulate cortices of schizophrenic and schizoaffective patients. *Arch Gen Psychiatry.* 1991;48:996-1001.
2. Scheibel AB, Kovelman JA. Disorientation of the hippocampal pyramidal cell and its processes in the schizophrenic patient. *Biol Psychiatry.* 1981; 16:101-102.
3. Buchsbaum MS, DeLisi LE, Holcomb HH, et al. Anteroposterior gradients in cerebral glucose use in schizophrenia and affective disorders. *Arch Gen Psychiatry.* 1984;41:1159-1166.
4. Weinberger DR, Berman KF, Zec RF. Physiologic dysfunction of dorsolateral prefrontal cortex in schizophrenia, I. *Arch Gen Psychiatry.* 1986;43:114-124.
5. Akbarian S, Kim JJ, Potkin SG, et al. Gene expression for glutamic acid decarboxylase is reduced without loss of neurons in prefrontal cortex of schizophrenics. *Arch Gen Psychiatry.* 1995;52:258-266.
6. Erlander MO, Tobin M. The structural and functional heterogeneity of glutamic acid decarboxylase: a review. *Neurochem Res.* 1991;16:215-226.
7. Erlander MO, Tillakaratne NJK, Feldblum S, Patel N, Tobin M. Two genes encode distinct glutamate decarboxylases. *Neuron.* 1991;7:91-100.
8. Benes FM, Vincent SL, Alsterberg O, Bird ED, SanGiovanni JP. Increased $GABA_A$ receptor binding in superficial layers of cingulate cortex in schizophrenics. *J Neurosci.* 1992;12:924-929.
9. Hanada S, Mita T, Nishinio N, Tanaka C. [^{3}H]Muscimol binding sites increased in autopsied brains of chronic schizophrenics. *Life Sci.* 1986;40: 259-266.
10. Fuster J. *The Preftontal Cortex.* New York, NY: Raven Press; 1980.
11. Simpson MDC, Slater P, Royston MC, Deakin JFW. Regionally selective deficits in uptake sites for glutamate and gamma-aminobutyric acid in the basal ganglia of schizophrenics. *Psychiatry Res.* 1992;42:273-282.
12. Simpson MDC, Slater P, Deakin JFW, Roysteon MC, Skan WJ. Reduced GABA uptake sites in the temporal lobe in schizophrenia. *Neurosci Lett.* 1989;107:211-215.
13. Bannon MJ, Roth RH. Pharmacology of mesocortical dopamine neurons. *Pharmacol Rev.* 1983; 35:53-68.
14. Thaker GK, Tamminga CA, Alphs LD, Lafferman J, Ferraro TN, Hare TA. Brain γ-aminobutyric acid abnormality in tardive dyskinesia: reduction in cerebrospinal fluid GABA levels and therapeutic response to GABA agonist treatment. *Arch Gen Psychiatry.* 1987;44:522-529.
15. Crow TJ, Cross AJ, Cooper SJ, et al. Neuotransmitter receptors and monoamine metabolites in the brains of patients with Alzheimer-type dementias and depression, and suicides. *Neuropharmacology.* 1984;23:1561-1569.

COMMENTARY

Neural Circuitry of the Prefrontal Cortex in Schizophrenia

THE FINDINGS of an increasing number and variety of studies have implicated the prefrontal cortex (PFC), especially the dorsolateral region, as a site of dysfunction in schizophrenia. For example, schizophrenic patients perform poorly on cognitive tasks that are subserved by neural systems involving PFC circuitry.[1,2] In addition, functional imaging studies have demonstrated reduced blood flow or metabolic activity in this region of the cerebral cortex in many schizophrenic patients.[3-7]

See also pages 258, 267, and 274

However, despite the accumulating evidence of PFC dysfunction in schizophrenia, major challenges for research in this area continue to include (1) the identification of specific alterations of PFC circuitry in schizophrenia and (2) the development of a rational pathophysiological accounting, based on our current understanding of the structure and operation of cortical neural systems, for the relation between altered PFC circuitry and disturbed PFC function in schizophrenia.

Although relegated to the graveyard two decades ago,[8] investigations of postmortem brain specimens from schizophrenic patients have been resurrected and shown to be a viable and valuable tool for addressing these difficult but critical challenges in schizophrenia research. Postmortem studies are likely to remain a vital component of these research efforts for a variety of reasons,[9] perhaps the most notable one being that postmortem studies are the only currently available avenue of investigation that provides the resolution necessary at the anatomical level to identify the types of relatively subtle alterations in PFC circuitry that may be present in schizophrenia. The report by Akbarian and colleagues[10] in this issue of the ARCHIVES provides a compelling example of the usefulness of postmortem studies not only in revealing evidence of such abnormalities of PFC circuitry in schizophrenia, but also in providing insights into the possible mechanisms that may have produced those abnormalities. Despite the inherent limitations of postmortem studies,[9] Akbarian and colleagues have employed several important features in their study that reduce the impact of those limitations. For example, the experimental design, which involves the pairwise matching of schizophrenic and control subjects, helps to minimize the influence of factors such as sex, age, and autolysis time that can seriously confound the results of postmortem studies. In addition, although the relative merits of the specific measures employed may be debated, the use of a combination of several different experimental procedures in the same cases produced a more complete and convincing story regarding the nature of PFC abnormalities than would have been obtained with one approach alone.

In this study, Akbarian and colleagues used in situ hybridization techniques to determine the number of neurons that expressed the messenger RNA (mRNA) for glutamic acid decarboxylase (GAD), the synthesizing enzyme for the inhibitory neurotransmitter γ-aminobutyric acid (GABA), in postmortem brain specimens of PFC (area 9) from 10 pairs of schizophrenic and matched control subjects. They also determined the number of neurons in the same cortical region, as well as the volume of the PFC. Their findings reveal a significant decrease in the number of neurons with detectable levels of GAD mRNA and in the total amount of this mRNA in the PFC of schizophrenic subjects. These changes were observed in the absence of any differences in the number of PFC neurons between schizophrenics and controls, suggesting that the observed decrease in GAD mRNA was not attributable to a loss of GABA neurons. In concert with the results of other studies,[11-15] these findings provide converging support for the hypothesis that GABA neurotransmission is altered in the PFC of schizophrenic patients, and they suggest that this impairment is the consequence of reduced GABA biosynthesis in the inhibitory local circuit neurons of the PFC.

Clearly, understanding both the possible etiological and pathophysiological significance of these findings depends on knowing what factors contributed to the decrease in GAD mRNA levels. Although a decrease in the number of small, presumably local-circuit GABA neurons in the superficial layers of PFC from schizophrenic and schizoaffective subjects has been reported,[13] the present study by Akbarian et al[10] as well as several other recent studies[16,17] failed to find evidence of a decrease in cortical neuron number in schizophrenics. Consequently, it seems unlikely that the decrease in number of GAD mRNA-positive neurons is the consequence of a loss of GABA neurons. However, the decreased GAD mRNA levels in schizophrenia could reflect a decrease in GAD expression in all PFC GABA neurons, with GAD mRNA levels dropping below detectability in only a subset. Alternatively, GAD expression might be reduced in only a subpopulation of neurons with normal GAD mRNA levels, with presumably normal levels of GABA retained in the remainder. Determining which of these alternatives is the case might be accomplished by counting the density of silver grains deposited over each labeled neuron (a direct correlate of the amount of mRNA) and comparing the distribution of grains per neuron in schizophrenics and controls. Substantial overlap between schizophrenics and controls in the distributions of grains per neuron would suggest that the decrease in GAD mRNA expression was restricted to a subpopulation of GABA neurons.

Distinguishing between these two alternatives is important for understanding the possible pathophysiological significance of a reduction in GAD mRNA levels because separate subpopulations of cortical GABA neurons appear to be specialized for substantially different roles in PFC circuitry. Although GABA neurons, which constitute 25% to 30% of all neurons in the primate neocortex,[18] share a number of characteristics that distinguish them from the excitatory pyramidal neurons of the cortex,[19] they constitute a variety of distinct subtypes. Based on differences in axonal features and synaptic targets, at least 10 different morphological subclasses of local circuit neurons have been identified in the primate neocortex,[19-21] and most of these subtypes have been found in both monkey and human PFC.[22-24] In addition, GABA neurons are chemically heterogeneous, and separate subpopulations can be identified by the presence of specific neuropeptides or calcium-binding proteins.[25] For example, the calcium-binding proteins calbindin, calretinin, and parvalbumin are expressed in distinct subgroups of GABA neurons with different laminar distributions in monkey PFC.[26] Together, these morphological and chemical features define subpopulations of GABA neurons that appear to have different roles in PFC circuitry. The GABA neurons of the chandelier class, which may also express either the neuropeptide corticotropin-releasing factor[27] or the calcium-binding parvalbumin,[28,29] are found primarily in cortical layers II to V in monkey PFC.[22,28] The distinctive axon terminals of these neurons are arrayed as cartridges that provide symmetric, inhibitory synapses to the axonal initial segment of pyramidal neurons,[21,30-34] the site of action potential generation. Each chandelier cell may contact up to 300 pyramidal neurons within a radius of 150 to 200 μm from its cell body.[35] Thus, chandelier cells exert critical inhibitory control over the activity of a localized group of pyramidal neurons and as a consequence appear to be specialized to regulate the output of a cortical column. In contrast, the axons of wide-arbor (basket) neurons, which form symmetric inhibitory synapses with the cell bodies of pyramidal neurons,[36] spread horizontally for considerable distances (up to 1.0 mm) within the PFC.[22] These neurons may be specialized to provide inhibitory constraints on the patterns of intra-areal excitation propagated by horizontally oriented axon collaterals of PFC pyramidal neurons.[37,38] Given these types of differences among GABA cells, it is clear that understanding the functional consequences of a decrease in GAD mRNA expression will ultimately depend on knowledge of which group(s) of GABA neurons are affected.

In addition to having different synaptic targets and functional roles in PFC circuitry, separate classes of GABA neurons appear to be regulated by specific types of afferent input. For example, about 30% of the synapses formed by dopamine axon terminals in the superficial layers of monkey PFC are on the dendrites of GABA neurons.[39,40] In addition, this input appears to target a specific population of GABA neurons, since local circuit neurons that contain the calcium-binding protein calretinin do not form synapses with dopamine axon terminals.[41] The specificity of this connectivity between dopamine afferents and GABA local circuit neurons may have functional implications for the interaction between dopamine and GABA in the PFC of schizophrenic patients. In addition, it may also be of relevance for determining the extent to which the observed decrease in GAD mRNA levels in the PFC of schizophrenics might be influenced by neuroleptic administration.

THE TYPES and nature of afferent drives to PFC GABA neurons are also important in considering future studies to test the hypothesis, proposed by Akbarian and colleagues,[10] that the decreased GAD mRNA levels in the PFC of schizophrenics reflects an activity-dependent down-regulation of GAD gene expression. What types of events might lead to this down-regulation? Although the available data do not permit us to distinguish among them, there are at least several options. For example, the axons of pyramidal neurons in the superficial layers, the location of the greatest decline in GAD mRNA,[10] furnish excitatory projections to other cortical regions[42,43] and are a major source of horizontally spreading intra-areal excitatory connections in the primate PFC.[37] The local axon collaterals of these pyramidal neurons also furnish excitatory inputs to GABA neurons, which in turn supply inhibitory control over pyramidal cell activity. Thus, a decrease in GAD expression could reflect a compensation for decreased activity in PFC pyramidal cells by diminishing the magnitude of feedback inhibition to these pyramidal neurons. Consequently, a down-regulation of GAD expression and GABA neurotransmission might contribute to some degree of normalization in the function of PFC intrinsic circuitry, at least under tonic conditions. Although there is no direct evidence of a decrease in PFC pyramidal cell activity in schizophrenia, the preliminary results of some recent postmortem investigations, which have shown a loss of dendritic spines,[44] a decrease in synaptic markers,[45] and a decrease in cortical neuropil[16] in the PFC of schizophrenics, may be consistent with a loss of afferent drive to pyramidal neurons. In this regard, it may also be of interest to note that the adolescence-related decline in PFC synaptic density[46] involves primarily the loss of asymmetric synapses on dendritic spines,[47,48] the principal source of excitatory drive to PFC pyramidal neurons.

A decrease in GABA mRNA expression could also be related to changes in afferent drive to the PFC from the thalamus. Although most thalamocortical inputs terminate on spines and thus pyramidal neurons, GABA neurons also receive synaptic input from the thalamus.[49,50] The primary thalamic input to the PFC arises from the dorsomedial thalamic nucleus and terminates in the deep portion of layer III and in layer IV.[51] Although the decrease in GAD mRNA in the schizophrenic subjects was not restricted to these layers, in other cortical regions such as primary sensory areas, decreased activity in thalamic inputs has produced a decrease in GAD expression that was not restricted to the cortical laminae receiving the thalamic input, although it was less marked in other layers.[52,53] A decrease in thalamic drive to the PFC in schizophrenia may not be unreasonable to postulate, given the reports that the size of the thalamus is diminished in schizophrenics[54] and that the number of neurons in the dorsomedial thalamic nucleus is reduced.[55] However, the impact on cortical GABA neurons of activity-related changes in thalamic input have all been studied in sensory and motor regions of cortex.[56] Consequently, the extrapolation of this phenomena to higher-order association areas such as the PFC, which may be relatively more influenced by corticocortical than thalamocortical input, has to be made with caution.

Finally, if the decreased GAD mRNA levels do reflect a decrease in afferent drive to the PFC in schizophrenia, how does this arise? Akbarian and colleagues[10] have previously reported that the distribution of a small population of white matter neurons, identified by nicotinamide-adenine dinucleotide phosphate–diaphorase (NADPH-d) histochemical analysis, was altered in the frontal and temporal lobes of schizophrenic subjects.[57,58] Although these observations could be due to a disturbance in the prenatal migration of cortical neurons, based on their present finding of a normal complement of neurons in the PFC grey matter of schizophrenics, the authors suggest that the altered patterns of NADPH-d labeling reflect an abnormality in the cortical subplate, a transient but critical structure in cortical development.

AT THE earliest stage of development, the cerebral wall is composed of an outer cell-free marginal zone and an inner ventricular zone, a single layer of pseudostratified epithelium from which all neurons are eventually generated. The first postmitotic cells migrate from the ventricular zone to form the preplate, a group of loosely packed cells located below the marginal zone. The continuing processes of neurogenesis and migration subsequently produce a cell-dense zone, the cortical plate, which splits the preplate cells into two populations, a superficial group in the marginal zone (which later becomes layer I of the cerebral cortex) and a deeper zone termed the subplate. Additional waves of neurons continue to be generated and to migrate through the subplate and into the cortical plate, which eventually forms layers II to VI of the adult cerebral cortex.

Subplate neurons are not only the first neurons generated in the cortex, they are also the earliest to mature.[59] Their axons pioneer descending pathways to the thalamus and other subcortical structures,[60,61] project into the cortical plate,[62] and furnish collateral branches within the subplate.[62-64] Subplate neurons also appear to be the initial synaptic targets for many afferents to the cerebral cortex, including projections from the thalamus[59] and the contralateral cortex.[65] Both thalamic and callosal axons accumulate within the subplate for extended periods of time, especially in primates, before invading the cortical plate.[66-68] The interactions between subplate neurons and cortical afferents during this waiting period[66] appear to be critical for the subsequent formation of proper connections with cortical neurons. For example, following lesions of the subplate, axons from the lateral geniculate nucleus continue to grow past the visual cortex, suggesting that subplate neurons are required for these thalamic axons to recognize their appropriate cortical target.[69] In addition, subplate neurons appear to be essential for the final patterning (the formation of ocular dominance columns) of thalamocortical afferents within layer IV of the visual cortex.[70,71] Following the completion of these maturational processes, the majority of subplate neurons die, leaving as a remnant the interstitial neurons of the adult white matter.[72-74]

Thus, as indicated by Akbarian and colleagues,[10] the characteristics of subplate neurons suggest that abnormalities in these neurons could underlie the alterations in PFC circuitry in schizophrenia. For example, due to their early maturation, subplate neurons might be particularly sensitive to prenatal or perinatal insults,[59] the types of events that have been implicated as etiological factors in at least some cases of schizophrenia.[75] Given their importance in the formation of cortical circuitry, even a restricted lesion of the subplate during prenatal development could result in extensive errors in axon targeting and connectivity during later development.[59] It is also important to note that the number of subplate neurons, the relative size of the subplate to the cortical plate, and the length of time during which subplate neurons persist are all much greater in humans[23,76] than in the other species in which most studies of the subplate have been conducted. Consequently, the role of subplate neurons in the development of the human cerebral cortex may be even more complex than is currently understood from animal studies.

Does the white matter of postmortem brain specimens from schizophrenic patients contain the residual evidence of a prenatal developmental abnormality in the cortical subplate? Does such a disturbance lead to altered patterns of PFC circuitry that are manifest as a downregulation of GABA neurotransmission much later in life? Do the consequences of these prenatal deficits in PFC circuitry remain relatively quiescent until the postnatal refinements of PFC circuitry are completed during adolescence? The answers to these questions await the replication and extension of the exciting study of Akbarian and colleagues.[10] However, the pursuit of these answers, using experimental designs and data interpretations that are informed by the findings of basic neuroscience research, hold great promise for the continued advancement of knowledge regarding the etiological and pathophysiological factors that contribute to PFC dysfunction in schizophrenia.

David A. Lewis, MD
Western Psychiatric Institute and Clinic
Departments of Psychiatry and Neuroscience
University of Pittsburgh
3811 O'Hara St
Biomedical Science Tower W1651
Pittsburgh, PA 15213-2593

REFERENCES

1. Park S, Holzman PS. Schizophrenics show spatial working memory deficits. *Arch Gen Psychiatry.* 1992;49:975-982.
2. Weinberger DR, Berman KF, Zec RF. Physiological dysfunction of dorsolateral prefrontal cortex in schizophrenia, I: regional cerebral blood flow (rCBF) evidence. *Arch Gen Psychiatry.* 1986;43:114-125.
3. Rubin P, Holm S, Friberg L, Videbech P, Anderson HS, Bendsen BB, Strømsø N, Larsen JK, Lassen NA, Hemmingsen R. Altered modulation of prefrontal and subcortical brain activity in newly diagnosed schizophrenia and schizophreniform disorder. *Arch Gen Psychiatry.* 1991;48:987-995.
4. Andreasen NC, Rezai R, Alliger R, Swayze VW II, Flaum M, Kirchner P, Cohen G, O'Leary DS. Hypofrontality in neuroleptic-naive patients and in patients with chronic schizophrenia: assessment with xenon 133 single-photon emission computed tomography and the Tower of London. *Arch Gen Psychiatry.* 1992;49:943-958.
5. Berman KF, Torrey EF, Daniel DG, Weinberger DR. Regional cerebral blood flow in monozygotic twins discordant and concordant for schizophrenia. *Arch Gen Psychiatry.* 1992;49:927-934.
6. Buchsbaum MS, Haier RJ, Potkin SG, Neuchterlein K, Bracha HS, Katz M, Lohr J, Wu J, Lottenberg S, Jerabek PA, Trenary M, Tafalla R, Reynolds C, Bunney WE Jr. Frontostriatal disorder of cerebral metabolism in never-medicated schizophrenics. *Arch Gen Psychiatry.* 1992;49:935-942.
7. Wolkin A, Sanfilipo M, Wolf AP, Angrist B, Brodie JD, Rotrosen J. Negative symptoms and hypofrontality in chronic schizophrenia. *Arch Gen Psychiatry.* 1992;49:959-965.
8. Plum F. Neuropathological findings. In: Kety SS, Malthysse SM, eds. *Prospects for Research on Schizophrenia.* Cambridge, Mass: Massachusetts Institute of Technology Press; 1972:385-388.
9. Kleinman JE, Hyde TM, Herman MM. Methodological issues in the neuropathology of mental illness. In: Bloom FE, Kupfer DJ, eds. *Psychopharmacology: A Third Generation of Progress.* New York, NY: Raven Press. In press.
10. Akbarian S, Kim JJ, Potkin SG, Hagman JO, Tafazzoli A, Bunney WE Jr, Jones EG. Gene expression for glutamic acid decarboxylase is reduced without loss of neurons in prefrontal cortex of schizophrenics. *Arch Gen Psychiatry.* 1995;52:258-266.
11. Benes FM, Vincent SL, Alsterberg G, Bird ED, SanGiovanni JP. Increased $GABA_A$ receptor binding in superficial layers of cingulate cortex in schizophrenics. *J Neurosci.* 1992;12:924-929.
12. Benes FM, Snyder-Marie A, Vincent S, Khan Y. Upregulation of $GABA_A$ receptor binding activity in prefrontal cortex of schizophrenic brain. *Soc Neurosci Abstr.* 1993;19:8.
13. Benes FM, McSparren J, Bird ED, SanGiovanni JP, Vincent SL. Deficits in small interneurons in prefrontal and cingulate cortices of schizophrenic and schizoaffective patients. *Arch Gen Psychiatry.* 1991;48:996-1001.
14. Sherman AD, Davidson AT, Baruah S, Hegwood TS, Waziri R. Evidence of glutamateric deficiency in schizophrenia. *Neurosci Lett.* 1991;121:77-80.
15. Simpson MDC, Slater P, Deakin JFW, Royston MC, Skan WJ. Reduced GABA uptake sites in the temporal lobe in schizophrenia. *Neurosci Lett.* 1989;107:211-215.
16. Selemon LD, Rajkowska G, Goldman-Rakic PS. Cytologic abnormalities in area 9 of the schizophrenic cortex. *Soc Neurosci Abstr.* 1993;19:200.
17. Pakkenberg B. Total nerve cell number in neocortex in chronic schizophrenics and controls estimated using optical disectors. *Biol Psychiatry.* 1993;34:768-772.
18. Hendry SHC, Schwark EG, Jones EG, Yan J. Numbers and proportions of GABA-immunoreactive neurons in different areas of monkey cerebral cortex. *J Neurosci.* 1987;7:1503-1519.
19. Fairen A, DeFelipe J, Regidon J. Nonpyramidal neurons, general account. In: Peters A, Jones EG, eds. *Cerebral Cortex: Cellular Components of the Cerebral Cortex.* New York, NY: Plenum Press; 1984;1:201-245.
20. Lund JS. Organization of neurons in the visual cortex, area 17, of the monkey (*Macaca mulatta*). *J Comp Neurol.* 1973;147:455-496.
21. Jones EG. Varieties and distribution of nonpyramidal cells in the somatic sensory cortex of the squirrel monkey. *J Comp Neurol.* 1975;160:205-268.
22. Lund JS, Lewis DA. Local circuit neurons of developing and mature macaque prefrontal cortex: Golgi and immunocytochemical characteristics. *J Comp Neurol.* 1993;328:282-312.
23. Mrzljak L, Uylings HBM, Kostovic I, Van Eden CG. Prenatal development of neurons in the human prefrontal cortex, I: a qualitative Golgi study. *J Comp Neurol.* 1988;271:355-386.
24. Mrzljak L, Uylings HBM, Kostovic I, Van Eden CG. Prenatal development of neurons in the human prefrontal cortex, II: a quantitative Golgi study. *J Comp Neurol.* 1992;316:485-496.
25. DeFelipe J. Neocortical neuronal diversity: chemical heterogeneity revealed by colocalization studies of classic neurotransmitters, neuropeptides, calcium-binding proteins, and cell surface molecules. *Cereb Cortex.* 1993;3:273-289.
26. Condé F, Lund JS, Jacobowitz DM, Baimbridge KG, Lewis DA. Local circuit neurons immunoreactive for calretinin, calbindin D-28k, or parvalbumin in monkey prefrontal cortex: distribution and morphology. *J Comp Neurol.* 1994;341:95-116.
27. Lewis DA, Foote SL, Cha CI. Corticotropin-releasing factor immunoreactivity in monkey neocortex: an immunohistochemical analysis. *J Comp Neurol.* 1989;290:599-613.
28. Lewis DA, Lund JS. Heterogeneity of chandelier neurons in monkey neocortex: corticotropin-releasing factor and parvalbumin immunoreactive populations. *J Comp Neurol.* 1990;293:599-615.
29. DeFelipe J, Hendry SHC, Jones EG. Visualization of chandelier cell axons by parvalbumin immunoreactivity in monkey cerebral cortex. *Proc Natl Acad Sci U S A.* 1989;86:2093-2097.
30. DeFelipe J, Hendry SHC, Jones EG, Schmechel D. Variability in the terminations of GABAergic chandelier cell axons on initial segments of pyramidal cell axons in the monkey sensory-motor cortex. *J Comp Neurol.* 1985;231:364-384.
31. Fairen A, Valverde F. A specialized type of neuron in the visual cortex of cat: a Golgi and electron microscope study of chandelier cells. *J Comp Neurol.* 1980;194:761-779.
32. Peters A, Proskauer CC, Ribak CE. Chandelier neurons in rat visual cortex. *J Comp Neurol.* 1982;206:397-416.
33. Somogyi P. A specific axo-axonal interneuron in the visual cortex of the rat. *Brain Res.* 1977;136:345-350.
34. Szentagothai J, Arbib M. Conceptual models of neural organization. *Neurosci Res Program Bull.* 1974;12:307-510.
35. Peters A. Chandelier cells. In: Jones EG, Peters A, eds. *Cerebral Cortex: Cellular Components of the Cerebral Cortex.* New York, NY: Plenum Press; 1984;1:361-380.
36. Jones EG, Hendry SHC. Basket cells. In: Jones EG, Peters A, eds. *Cerebral Cortex: Cellular Components of the Cerebral Cortex.* New York, NY: Plenum Press; 1984;1:309-336.
37. Levitt JB, Lewis DA, Yoshioka T, Lund JS. Topography of pyramidal neuron intrinsic connections in macaque monkey prefrontal cortex (areas 9 & 46). *J Comp Neurol.* 1993;338:360-376.

38. Lund JS, Yoshioka T, Levitt JB. Comparison of intrinsic connectivity in different areas of macaque monkey cerebral cortex. *Cereb Cortex.* 1993; 3:148-162.
39. Smiley JF, Goldman-Rakic PS. Heterogeneous targets of dopamine synapses in monkey prefrontal cortex demonstrated by serial section electron microscopy: a laminar analysis using the silver-enhanced diaminobenzidine sulfide (SEDS) immunolabeling technique. *Cereb Cortex.* 1993; 3:223-238.
40. Sesack SR, Snyder CL, Lewis DA. Synaptic associations between dopamine terminals and GABA interneuroms in rat and monkey cortex. *Soc Neurosci Abstr.* 1993;19:927.
41. Lewis DA, Snyder CL, Sesack SR. Calretinin-immunoreactive neurons in monkey prefrontal cortex: ultrastructure and associations with dopamine afferents. *Soc Neurosci Abstr.* 1994;20: 1416.
42. Barbas H. Architecture and cortical connections of the prefrontal cortex in the rhesus monkey. *Adv Neurol.* 1992;57:91-115.
43. Jones EG. Laminar distribution of cortical efferent cells. In: Peters A, Jones EG, eds. *Cerebral Cortex: Cellular Components of the Cerebral Cortex.* New York, NY: Plenum Press; 1984;1:521-553.
44. Garey LJ, Patel T, Ong WY. Loss of dendritic spines from cortical pyramidal cells in schizophrenia. *Schizophr Res.* 1994;11:137.
45. Glantz LA, Lewis DA. Decreased synaptophysin immunoreactivity in prefrontal cortex of schizophrenics. *Biol Psychiatry.* 1994;35:717.
46. Huttenlocher PR. Synaptic density in human frontal cortex: developmental changes and effects of aging. *Brain Res.* 1979;163:195-205.
47. Bourgeois J-P, Goldman-Rakic PS, Rakic P. Synaptogenesis in the prefrontal cortex of rhesus monkeys. *Cereb Cortex.* 1994;4:78-96.
48. Anderson SA, Classey JD, Condé F, Lund JS, Lewis DA. Synchronous development of pyramidal neuron dendritic spines and parvalbumin-immunoreactive chandelier neuron axon terminals in layer III of monkey prefrontal cortex. *Neuroscience.* In press.
49. Freund TF, Martin CAC, Soltescz I, Somogyi P, Whitteridge DI. Arborization pattern and postsynaptic targets of physiologically identified thalamocortical afferents in striate cortex of the macaque monkey. *J Comp Neurol.* 1989;289:315-356.
50. Kisvárday ZF, Cowey A, Somogyi P. Synaptic relationships of a type of GABA-immunoreactive neuron (clutch cell), spiny stellate cells and lateral geniculate nucleus afferents in layer IVC of the monkey striate cortex. *Neuroscience.* 1986; 19:741-761.
51. Giguere M, Goldman-Rakic PS. Mediodorsal nucleus: areal, laminar, and tangential distribution of afferents and efferents in the frontal lobe of rhesus monkeys. *J Comp Neurol.* 1988;277: 195-213.
52. Hendry SHC, Jones EG. Reduction in number of GABA immunostained neurons in deprived-eye dominance columns of monkey area 17. *Nature.* 1986;320:750-753.
53. Hendry SHC, Jones EG. Activity-dependent regulation of GABA expression in the visual cortex of adult monkeys. *Neuron.* 1988;1:701-712.
54. Andreasen NC, Arndt S, Swayze V II, Cizadlo T, Flaum M, O'Leary D, Ehrhardt JC, Yuh WTC. Thalamic abnormalities in schizophrenia visualized through magnetic resonance image averaging. *Science.* 1994;266:294-298.
55. Pakkenberg B. Stereological quantitation of human brains from normal and schizophrenic individuals. *Acta Neurol Scand Suppl.* 1992;137: 20-33.
56. Jones EG. GABAergic neurons and their role in cortical plasticity in primates. *Cereb Cortex.* 1993; 3:361-372.
57. Akbarian S, Bunney WE Jr, Potkin SG, Wigal SB, Hagman JO, Sandman CA, Jones EG. Altered distribution of nicotinamide-adenine dinucleotide phosphate–diaphorase cells in frontal lobe of schizophrenics implies disturbances of cortical development. *Arch Gen Psychiatry.* 1993;50:169-177.
58. Akbarian S, Viñuela A, Kim JJ, Potkin SG, Bunney WE Jr, Jones EG. Distorted distribution of nicotinamide-adenine dinucleotide phosphate–diaphorase neurons in temporal lobe of schizophrenics implies anomalous cortical development. *Arch Gen Psychiatry.* 1993;50:178-187.
59. Allendoerfer KL, Shatz CJ. The subplate, a transient neocortical structure: its role in the development of connections between thalamus and cortex. In: Cowan WM, Shooter EM, Stevens CF, Thompson RF, eds. *Annual Review of Neuroscience.* Palo Alto, Calif: Annual Reviews Inc; 1994; 185-218.
60. McConnell SK, Ghosh A, Shatz CJ. Subplate pioneers and the formation of descending connections from cerebral cortex. *J Neurosci.* 1994;14: 1892-1907.
61. McConnell SK, Ghosh A, Shatz CJ. Subplate neurons pioneer the first axon pathway from the cerebral cortex. *Science.* 1989;245:978-982.
62. Friauf E, McConnell SK, Shatz CJ. Functional synaptic circuits in the subplate during fetal and early postnatal development of cat visual cortex. *J Neurosci.* 1990;10:2601-2613.
63. Wahle P, Meyer G. Morphology and quantitative changes of transient NPY-ir neuronal populations during early postnatal development of the cat visual cortex. *J Comp Neurol.* 1987;261:165-192.
64. Chun JJM, Shatz CJ. The earliest-generated neurons of the cat cerebral cortex: characterization by MAP2 and neurotransmitter immunohistochemistry during fetal life. *J Neurosci.* 1989;9: 1648-1657.
65. Innocenti GM. Growth and reshaping of axons in the establishment of visual callosal connections. *Science.* 1991;212:824-827.
66. Rakic P. Prenatal development of the visual system in rhesus monkey. *Philos Trans R Soc London Ser B.* 1977;278:245-260.
67. Lund RD, Mustari MJ. Development of the geniculocortical pathway in rats. *J Comp Neurol.* 1977;173:289-306.
68. Shatz CJ, Luskin MB. The relationship between the geniculocortical afferents and their cortical target cells during development of the cat's primary visual cortex. *J Neurosci.* 1986;6:3655-3668.
69. Ghosh A, Antonini A, McConnell SK, Shatz CJ. Requirement for subplate neurons in the formation of thalamocortical connections. *Nature.* 1990; 347:179-181.
70. Ghosh A, Shatz CJ. Involvement of subplate neurons in the formation of ocular dominance columns. *Science.* 1992;255:1441-1443.
71. Ghosh A, Shatz CJ. Segregation of geniculocortical afferents during the critical period: a role for subplate neurons. *J Neurosci.* 1994;14:3862-3880.
72. Kostovic I, Rakic P. Cytology and the time of origin of interstitial neurons in the white matter in infant and adult human and monkey telencephalon. *J Neurocytol.* 1980;9:219-242.
73. Chun JJM, Shatz CJ. Interstitial cells of the adult neocortical white matter are the remnant of the early generated subplate neuron population. *J Comp Neurol.* 1989;282:555-569.
74. Woo TU, Beale JM, Finlay BL. Dual fate of subplate neurons in a rodent. *Cereb Cortex.* 1991; 1:433-443.
75. Waddington JL. Schizophrenia: developmental neuroscience and pathobiology. *Lancet.* 1993; 341:531-536.
76. Kostovic I, Rakic P. Developmental history of the transient subplate zone in the visual and somatosensory cortex of the macaque monkey and human brain. *J Comp Neurol.* 1990;297:441-470.

COMMENTARY

In Pursuit of the Molecular Neuropathology of Schizophrenia

THE SEARCH for the defining neuropathological features of schizophrenia continues to be one of the highest priority areas of research on this severely debilitating and very common neuropsychiatric disorder (for recent updates and comprehensive reviews of previous studies of the regional neuropathology of schizophrenia as well as an extensive compilation of the pertinent more general literature on this subject, see Carpenter and Buchanan,[1] Kerwin,[2] Shapiro,[3] and Winn[4]). There are a number of compelling reasons that justify intense research efforts to delineate the central nervous system (CNS) lesions that constitute a primary "cause" of schizophrenia as well as those secondary events that underlie the varied behavioral symptoms of this highly complex disease. Specifically, the identification of such lesions would markedly enhance the pace of research on schizophrenia by enabling investigators to (1) generate testable hypotheses about the cause and molecular pathogenesis of this disorder; (2) develop specific neuropathological criteria for the postmortem diagnosis of schizophrenia similar to those that exist for many other brain disorders; (3) establish experimental model systems for studies of the neurobiological basis of schizophrenia; (4) understand the structure/function relations of the human CNS that are altered in schizophrenia; and (5) identify potential molecular targets for the development of innovative interventions to prevent schizophrenia or to ameliorate the behavioral sequelae of this illness.

See also pages 258, 267, 269, and 277

Contemporary research and earlier studies of the neuropathology of schizophrenia dating back to the end of the 19th century have enumerated many intriguing findings in the brains of patients with schizophrenia, but the identification and characterization of specific brain lesions that may be considered "diagnostic" of schizophrenia have so far eluded the determined efforts of a host of clinical investigators and basic neuroscientists.[1-4] In part, this undoubtedly reflects the considerable heterogeneity in the clinical phenotypes that are grouped together and included in the diagnosis of schizophrenia. Indeed, it is highly likely that schizophrenia is a syndrome that encompasses a group of etiologically diverse diseases of the CNS that share common clinical features.[1] Further, the conceptual basis for the nosology or classification of schizophrenia has evolved considerably even over the last three decades as understanding of at least some aspects of this disease has improved.[1]

This notwithstanding, accumulating data from a number of clinical, neuroimaging, and postmortem studies of the brains of patients with schizophrenia suggest that the emergence of this disease may reflect the occurrence of prenatal or early postnatal "insults" that alter or disrupt normal neurodevelopmental events in the human CNS.[1-3] For example, the presence of rather static or fixed focal abnormalities in brain imaging studies at the onset of the illness in schizophrenic patients coupled with the absence of prominent or stereotypical reactive neuropathological changes (eg, gliosis) in the postmortem brains of schizophrenics are all consistent with the notion that schizophrenia has its origins early in the developing or maturing CNS.[1-3] Unfortunately, however, there is no definitive proof of this and there are no straightforward strategies to test the validity of this hypothesis in an unequivocal manner.[1-3] Nonetheless, the mechanisms that lead to chronic schizophrenia and the progressive behavioral symptoms associated therewith are likely to be quite distinct from those that induce the behavioral and structural brain abnormalities that are hallmarks of some forms of mental retardation or well-known neurodegenerative disorders.

On the basis of clinical and neuroimaging data, two primary brain regions have been implicated as sites of potential pathological abnormalities in schizophrenia, ie, the temporal lobe and the frontal lobe.[1-4] Certain hallmark clinical features of schizophrenia, such as hallucinations and delusions, are common in other CNS diseases that affect the hippocampal region of the temporal lobe (eg, temporal lobe epilepsy, tumors, Alzheimer's disease[5,6]), and neuropsychological studies have demonstrated prominent memory impairments in patients with schizophrenia,[7-9] which also is consistent with hippocampal dysfunction. Neuroimaging studies have consistently demonstrated a reduction in the volume of the temporal lobe in patients with schizophrenia even at the earliest symptomatic stages, and metabolic abnormalities have likewise been identified in the temporal lobe.[1-3,10-12] Further, qualitative and quantitative postmortem histopathological studies of the temporal lobe have revealed a variety of hippocampal abnormalities in the brains of patients with schizophrenia (reviewed in Carpenter and Buchanan,[1] Kerwin,[2] and Shapiro,[3] but see also Arnold et al[13] for a more recent update on postmortem studies of the hippocampal formation in schizophrenics and additional data on this subject). Included among these abnormalities are (1) a decrease in the area or whole volume of the hippocampus or parahippocampal gyrus; (2) a decrease in the number of hippocampal neurons; (3) abnormalities in the orientation of hippocampal neurons; (4) a decrease in the size of hippocampal neurons; and (5) alterations in the expression of neuronal cytoskeletal proteins in selected subfields of the hippocampus and entorhinal cortex. Remarkably, the neuronal cytoskeletal abnormalities seen in the hippocampal formation of elderly schizophrenic patients, including those with obvious dementia, are quite distinct from those seen in Alzheimer's disease or other neurodegenerative conditions; and the hippocampus as well as other brain regions of elderly patients with schizophrenia is remarkably free of the neuronal cytoskeletal lesions that accumulate with normal aging.[14-16] However, many of the morphological, architechtonic, and neuropathological abnormalities ascribed specifically to schizophrenia by one or more groups of investigators have not always been detected in the hippocampus of all patients with schizophrenia.[1,3]

Considerable attention also has been focused on the dorsolateral prefrontal cortex (DLPFC) as a potential locus of disease in schizophrenia.[1-4] Certain clinical features of schizophrenia, particularly the negative symptom complex, would be consistent with frontal lobe dysfunction, and some (although not all) neuropsychological studies find impairments in the performance of frontal lobe–mediated tasks.[1-4] Functional neuroimaging studies have found abnormalities in the frontal neocortex, the presence of which has been related to the behavioral symptoms and the neuropsychological performance in patients with schizophrenia. Compared with the temporal lobe, there have been fewer postmortem investigations focusing on the frontal neocortex, and the findings (including alterations in neuron density, neuron size, and synapse-related protein densities) have been more controversial (see Shapiro[3] and Arnold et al[13] for further citations and additional details). Notably, as in the case of data obtained from research conducted on the hippocampus and other regions of the schizophrenic brain, postmortem studies of the DLPFC have not yet led to the identification of neuropathological lesions that are specific for or diagnostic of schizophrenia.[1,3] Accordingly, it is entirely possible that structural brain abnormalities that are detectable by conventional neuropathological methods for the diagnostic assessment of the postmortem brain may not turn out to be the most prominent or constant hallmarks of schizophrenia. This realization has prompted many investigators to pursue alternative neuroscience research strategies to identify neurochemical or molecular abnormalities that are unique to the brains of patients with schizophrenia.

The report by Akbarian et al[17] in this issue of the Archives is an example of this kind of approach. The authors of that article describe in situ hybridization studies of glutamic acid decarboxylase (GAD) messenger RNA (mRNA) levels in neurons of the DLPFC of schizophrenic patients and controls. Furthermore, morphometric studies also were conducted to assess neuron density and cortical volume in the same regions of the DLPFC in schizophrenic patients and controls. The postmortem brain samples studied here were carefully and systematically collected and also were examined for evidence of confounding brain abnormalities, but not all of the patients were followed up prospectively. Notably, variations in the clinical assessment and follow-up of psychiatric patients as well differences in the procedures for retrospective chart reviews may account for some of the contradictory data on the neuropathology of schizophrenia.[1,3,13,14,18] Nonetheless, Akbarian et al demonstrated a pronounced reduction in the expression of GAD mRNA containing neurons of the DLPFC in the brains of schizophrenics. One obvious interpretation of these data is that they indicate a loss of or a failure to generate a subpopulation of GAD-expressing neurons in the DLPFC. However, this seems unlikely because complementary morphometric analyses by these investigators did not provide direct evidence for a reduction in the number of DLPFC neurons. Further, there also were no changes in the cortical volume of the DLPFC in the schizophrenic patients. Significantly, the in situ data on mRNA levels did not appear to reflect a generalized failure of transcription in the brains of the schizophrenic patients since there were no reductions in the levels of another unrelated mRNA species, and the degree of reduced GAD mRNA expression varied throughout the DLPFC in a cortical lamina-specific manner. Another control experiment that would have been helpful in assessing the regional specificity of the GAD mRNA data from the DLPFC would have been to run parallel studies of another brain region that is not implicated in the pathobiology of schizophrenia, such as primary visual or motor cortex. Nevertheless, the important hypothesis that emerges from these novel studies is that the DLPFC in patients with schizophrenia is populated by an appropriate number of neurons but that a significant subpopulation of these neurons fail to acquire or retain a specific neurotransmitter phenotype, the molecular "signature" of which is the expression of GAD mRNA.

Given the notable absence of "hard" or consistent structural, pharmacological, or morphological abnormalities in the brains of schizophrenic patients, at least as determined by traditional neuropathological or pharmacological methods, one might anticipate that the CNS substrates of schizophrenia will correspond to subtle changes in the expression of neuronal mRNAs or proteins. Although subtle, the effects of these changes could profoundly disrupt the normal function of neurons, thereby leading to the behavioral symptoms of schizophrenia, but without necessarily compromising the survival of the affected neurons or perhaps even their basic morphological features. As thoughtfully discussed by Akbarian et al,[17] the reduced expression of GAD could have profound consequences on GABAergic synaptic transmission by neurons in the DLPFC of schizophrenic patients since GAD is the key enzyme involved in γ-aminobutyric acid (GABA) synthesis. Indeed, the findings described here could explain observations reported in earlier studies that $GABA_A$ receptors are upregulated and that GABA uptake is decreased in the cerebral cortex of the schizophrenic brain.[1-3,17] Thus, if it is plausible to think that alterations in GABAergic synaptic transmission by populations of dysfunctional DLPFC neurons may be relevant to some of the behavioral symptoms of schizophrenia, then the work of Akbarian et al[17] provides new insights into the potential mechanisms whereby synaptic transmission by GABAergic neurons might be perturbed.

These findings do not contradict other leading hypotheses about the pharmacological basis of schizophrenia (eg, the dopamine or serotonin hypotheses), but they also do not provide an unambiguous conceptual framework for understanding the relationship of a number of neuropathological abnormalities that have been described throughout many disparate regions of the brains of patients with schizophrenia. Further, they do not clarify whether schizophrenia ultimately is due to the occurrence of abnormal neurodevelopmental events in the late gestational prenatal or young postnatal brain. If schizophrenia is indeed a heterogeneous disorder, or if the cause of schizophrenia is multifactorial, involving several different genetic abnormalities or susceptibility genes that render affected individuals more vulnerable to epigenetic insults, it may not be possible to explain schizophrenia on the basis of a single pathogenetic mechanism or one final common pathway. Alternatively, it would be possible to link many of the disparate observations obtained from studies of the postmortem brains of schizophrenics if fundamental neurodevelopmental processes such as neurogenesis, neuronal migration, or the establishment of neuronal polarity are root causes of schizophrenia. Additional studies like those described here by Akbarian et al[17] will be needed to distinguish between these possibilities and to fully elucidate the molecular neuropathology of schizophrenia.

John Q. Trojanowski, MD, PhD
Steven E. Arnold, MD
Departments of Pathology and Laboratory Medicine and Psychiatry
University of Pennsylvania School of Medicine
HUP/Maloney, Room A009
36th and Spruce streets
Philadelphia, PA 19104-4283

REFERENCES

1. Carpenter WT, Buchanan RW. Schizophrenia. *N Engl J Med.* 1994;330:681-690.
2. Kerwin RW. Glutamate receptors, microtubule associated proteins and developmental anomaly in schizophrenia: an hypothesis. *Psychol Med.* 1993; 23:547-551.
3. Shapiro RM. Regional neuropathology in schizophrenia: where are we? where are we going? *Schizophr Res.* 1993;10:187-239.
4. Winn P. Schizophrenia research moves to the prefrontal cortex. *Trends Neurosci.* 1994;17:265-268.
5. Davison K. Schizophrenia-like psychoses associated with organic cerebral disorder: a review. *Psychiatr Dev.* 1983;1:1-34.
6. Flor-Henry P. Psychosis and temporal lobe epilepsy. *Epilepsia.* 1969;10:363-395.
7. Saykin AJ, Gur RC, Gur RE, Mozley D, Mozley LH, Resnick SM, Kester B, Stafiniak P. Neuropsychological function in schizophrenia: selective impairment in memory and learning. *Arch Gen Psychiatry.* 1991;48:618-624.
8. Gold JM, Randolph C, Carpenter CJ, Goldberg TE, Weinberger DR. Forms of memory failure in schizophrenia. *J Abnorm Psychol.* 1992;101: 487-494.
9. Saykin AJ, Shtasel DL, Gur RE, Kester DB, Mozley LH, Stafiniak P, Gur RC. Neuropsychological deficits in neuroleptic naive patients with first-episode schizophrenia. *Arch Gen Psychiatry.* 1994;51:124-131.
10. Breier A, Buchanan RW, Elkashef A, Munson RC, Kirkpatrick B, Gellad F. Brain morphology and schizophrenia: a magnetic resonance imaging study of limbic, prefrontal cortex, and caudate structures. *Arch Gen Psychiatry.* 1992;49:921-926.
11. Weinberger DR, Berman KF, Torrey EF. Correlations between abnormal hippocampal morphology and prefrontal physiology in schizophrenia. *Clin Neuropharmacol.* 1992;15:393A-394A. Abstract.
12. Friston KJ, Liddle PF, Frith CD, Hirsch SR, Frackowiak RS. The left medial temporal region and schizophrenia: a PET study. *Brain.* 1992; 115:367-382.
13. Arnold SE, Franz BR, Gur RC, Gur RE, Shapiro RM, Moberg PJ, Trojanowski JQ. Decreased neuron size in schizophrenia for hippocampal subfields that mediate cortical-hippocampal interactions. *Am J Psychiatry.* In press.
14. Arnold SE, Franz BR, Trojanowski JQ. Elderly patients with schizophrenia exhibit infrequent neurodegenerative lesions. *Neurobiol Aging.* 1994; 15:299-303.
15. Arnold SE, Lee VMY, Gur RE, Trojanowski JQ. Abnormal expression of two microtubule-associated proteins (MAP2 and MAP5) in specific subfields of the hippocampal formation in schizophrenia. *Proc Natl Acad Sci U S A.* 1991; 88:10850-10854.
16. Purohit DP, Davidson M, Perl DP, Powchik P, Haroutunian VH, Bierer LM, McCrystal J, Losonsczy M, Davis KL. Severe cognitive impairment in elderly schizophrenic patients: a clinicopathological study. *Biol Psychiatry.* 1993;33: 255-260.
17. Akbarian S, Kim JJ, Potkin SG, Hagman JO, Tafazzoli A, Bunney WE Jr, Jones EG. Gene expression for glutamic acid decarboxylase is reduced without loss of neurons in prefrontal cortex of schizophrenics. *Arch Gen Psychiatry.* 1995; 52:258-266.
18. Arnold SE, Gur RE, Shapiro RM, Fisher KR, Moberg PJ, Gibney MR, Gur RC, Blackwell P, Trojanowski JQ. Prospective clinicopathologic studies of schizophrenia: accrual and assessment. *Am J Psychiatry.* In press.

In Reply

EACH OF THE three commentaries on our article[1] raises important issues for discussion.

Lee and Tobin[2] claim a discrepancy between our findings of reduced glutamic acid decarboxylase messenger RNA (GAD mRNA) levels in the prefrontal cortex of schizophrenics and the lack of similar changes in GAD enzyme activity reported by Hanada et al.[3] This is not surprising, given the fact that GAD enzyme is unstable and its activity is influenced by confounding factors such as autolysis time[4] and cause of death.[3,5] Two other studies reported decreased GAD activity in schizophrenics,[6,7] but one only found decreased GAD activity in schizophrenics who did not die a sudden death.[5]

See also pages 258, 267, 269, and 274

The GAD mRNA is far more resistant to autolysis, and localization by in situ hybridization was successful in all patients and controls included in this study. In the same specimens, staining of GAD enzyme by means of immunohistochemistry proved to be very difficult, again indicating that GAD enzyme is not well preserved in postmortem tissue. Levels of GAD enzyme in the primate cerebral cortex are regulated by gene expression,[8] so GAD mRNA appears to be a reliable and valid marker for the assessment of GAD production in the human brain.

We agree with Lee and Tobin[2] that GAD activity and GAD gene expression in brains of schizophrenics who committed suicide could potentially be different in comparison with those in brains of schizophrenics who died of other causes. As indicated in Table 1 of our article,[1] only one patient in our study committed suicide. Therefore, it remains open if GAD mRNA levels are influenced by sudden death and suicide. However, both schizophrenics and controls died of a variety of causes, and it is unlikely that the decreased levels of GAD mRNA in the schizophrenic cohort are due to a specific cause of death.

Lewis[9] and also Lee and Tobin[2] ask about the potential influence of neuroleptics. Experimental studies, using microdialysis, report either a decrease[10-12] or an increase[13] of extracellular γ-aminobutyric acid (GABA) in the cerebral cortex and basal ganglia of neuroleptic-treated animals. Release of GABA in synaptosome preparations obtained from the cerebral cortex is increased on acute exposure to neuroleptics.[7] Studies conducted in rodents report that blockade of dopamine receptors leads to *increased* mRNA levels for the 67- and the 65-kd isoforms of GAD in the cerebral cortex and in the striatum.[14,15] Based on these findings, the *decreased* GAD mRNA levels in the schizophrenic sample of our study[1] are probably not due to neuroleptics.

Lewis[9] mentions that it is important to find out if specific subpopulations of GABAergic neurons selectively show the reduction in GAD gene expression that might give further insight into the pathophysiological basis of prefrontal dysfunction in schizophrenia. Future studies that combine immunohistochemical staining for neuropeptides or other markers such as calcium-binding proteins that are selectively expressed in subpopulations of cortical GABAergic neurons with in situ hybridization for GAD mRNA could provide the answer to this question. Lewis[9] also suggests that three different but possibly interrelated factors could mediate the activity-dependent down-regulation of GAD gene expression in the prefrontal cortex of schizophrenics: (1) a direct dopaminergic input on the dendrites of GABA neurons; (2) a compensatory decrease in local, inhibitory feedback activity due to dysfunction of excitatory pyramidal neurons; and (3) decreased afferent input from the mediodorsal and other thalamic nuclei. In individual schizophrenics, each of these three factors could independently cause down-regulation of GAD gene expression but might differentially affect cortical function.

Trojanowski and Arnold[16] mention the structural alterations reported in the hippocampal region of brains of schizophrenics. In vivo imaging studies also present evidence for involvement of the lateral temporal cortex, particularly the superior temporal gyrus.[17-19] It is of note that the reported reduction in volume of the superior temporal gyrus is linked to psychopathological symptoms such as hallucinations and thought disturbances[17,18] and is often associated with alterations in auditory-evoked potentials.[19] These abnormalities, along with those in the hippocampal region and prefrontal cortex, demonstrate the diverse nature of schizophrenic pathology.

Trojanowski and Arnold[16] may be right in stating that "it is entirely possible that structural brain abnormalities that are detectable by conventional neuropathological methods for the diagnostic assessment of the postmortem brain may not turn out to be the most prominent or constant hallmarks of schizophrenia." What is now necessary is to develop theories that are able to explain why widespread regions of the cerebral cortex are functionally affected but show only rather subtle structural alterations. Epidemiological studies and prospective studies in children at risk for schizophrenia suggest that disturbances of brain development may be involved in the origins of schizophrenia.[20,21] Therefore, it is possible that the malfunction of the cerebral cortex in adult schizophrenics results from a defect in brain development.[22,23] As mentioned by Lewis,[9] evidence has been presented that the embryonic subplate, a transitory neuronal structure located underneath the developing cerebral cortex, may have been affected in the prefrontal and lateral temporal regions of the brains of schizophrenics.[24,25] Studies in developing cat visual cortex have demonstrated that disturbances of the embryonic subplate potentially cause profound alterations in the establishment of thalamocortical connections without alterations in cytoarchitecture of the visual cortex.[26,27] Therefore, the prefrontal cortex and other cortical regions of schizophrenics may have alterations in thalamocortical and corticocortical connectivity without overt changes in gross shape, cortical gyration, or cortical cell density. Trojanowski and Arnold[16] are concerned that the findings reported in our present article[1]

do not provide an unambigous conceptual framework for understanding the relationship of a number of neuropathological abnormalities that have been described throughout many disparate regions of the brains of patients with schizophrenia.

However, when these findings are integrated into theories based on developmental defects of cortical connectivity that lead to activity-dependent changes in gene expression for molecules involved in the neurotransmission process, they may provide a valuable pathophysiological model for at least some cases of schizophrenia.

Scharam Akbarian, MD, PhD
Edward G. Jones, MD, PhD
Department of Anatomy and Neurobiology
University of California, Irvine
Irvine, CA 92717

Reprint requests to Dr Jones.

REFERENCES

1. Akbarian S, Kim JJ, Potkin SG, Hagman JO, Tafazzoki A, Bunney WE Jr, Jones EG. Gene expression for glutamic acid decarboxylase is reduced without loss of neurons in prefrontal cortex of schizophrenics. *Arch Gen Psychiatry.* 1995; 52:258-266.
2. Lee DE, Tobin AJ. Reduced inhibitory capacity in prefrontal cortex of schizophrenics. *Arch Gen Psychiatry.* 1995;52:267-268.
3. Hanada S, Mita T, Nishino N, Tanaka C. [^{3}H]Muscimol binding sites increased in autopsied brains of chronic schizophrenics. *Life Sci.* 1987;40: 259-266.
4. Spokes EGS. An analysis of factors influencing measurements of dopamine, noradrenaline, glutamate decarboxylase and choline acetylase in human post-mortem brain tissue. *Brain.* 1979; 102:333-346.
5. Bird ED, Spokes EGS, Iversen LL. Increased dopamine concentration in limbic areas of brain from patients dying with schizophrenia. *Brain.* 1979; 102:347-360.
6. McGeer PL, McGeer E. Possible changes in striatal and limbic cholinergic systems in schizophrenia. *Arch Gen Psychiatry.* 1977;34:1319-1323.
7. Sherman AD, Davidson AT, Baruah S, Hegwood TS, Waziri R. Evidence of glutamatergic deficiency in schizophrenia. *Neurosci Lett.* 1991; 121:77-80.
8. Benson DL, Huntsman MM, Jones EG. Activity-dependent changes in GAD and preprotachykinin mRNAs in visual cortex of adult monkeys. *Cereb Cortex.* 1994;4:40-51.
9. Lewis DA. Neural circuitry of the prefrontal cortex in schizophrenia. *Arch Gen Psychiatry.* 1995; 52:269-273.
10. Fuxe K, O'Connor WT, Antonelli T, Osborne PG, Tanganelli S, Agnati LF, Ungerstedt U. Evidence for a substrate of neuronal plasticity based on pre- and postsynaptic neurotensin-dopamine receptor interactions in the neostriatum. *Proc Natl Acad Sci U S A.* 1992;89:5591-5595.
11. See RE, Chapman MA, Klitenick MA. Chronic neuroleptic administration decreases extracellular GABA in the nucleus accumbens but not in the caudate-putamen of rats. *Brain Res.* 1992;588: 177-180.
12. Bourdelais AJ, Deutch AY. The effects of haloperidol and clozapine on extracellular GABA levels in the prefrontal cortex of the rat: an in vivo microdialysis study. *Cereb Cortex.* 1994;4:69-77.
13. Drew KL, O'Connor WT, Kehr J, Ungerstedt U. Regional specific effects of clozapine and haloperidol on GABA and dopamine release in rat basal ganglia. *Eur J Pharmacol.* 1990;187:385-397.
14. Lindefors N. Dopaminergic regulation of glutamic acid decarboxylase mRNA expression and GABA release in the striatum: a review. *Prog Neuropsychopharmacol Biol Psychiatry.* 1993;17: 887-903.
15. Qin Z-H, Zhang S-P, Weiss B. Dopaminergic and glutamatergic drugs differentially regulate glutamic acid decarboxylase mRNA in mouse brain. *Mol Brain Res.* 1994;21:293-302.
16. Trojanowski JQ, Arnold SE. In pursuit of the molecular neuropathology of schizophrenia. *Arch Gen Psychiatry.* 1995;52:274-276.
17. Barta PE, Pearlson GD, Powers RE, Richards SS, Tune LE. Auditory hallucinations and smaller superior temporal gyral volume in schizophrenia. *Am J Psychiatry.* 1990;147:1457-1462.
18. Shenton ME, Kikinis R, Jolesz FA, Pollak SD, LeMay M, Wible CG, Hokama H, Martin J, Coleman M, McCarley RW. Abnormalities of the left temporal lobe and thought disorder in schizophrenia: a quantitative magnetic resonance imaging study. *N Engl J Med.* 1992;327:604-612.
19. McCarley RW, Shenton ME, O'Donnell BF, Faux SF, Kikinis R, Nestor G, Jolesz FA. Auditory P300 abnormalities and left superior temporal gyrus volume reduction in schizophrenia. *Arch Gen Psychiatry.* 1993;50:190-197.
20. Mednick SA, Cannon TD. Fetal development, birth and the syndromes of adult schizophrenia. In: Mednick SA, Cannon TD, Barr CE, Lyon M, eds. *Fetal Neural Development and Adult Schizophrenia.* New York, NY: Cambridge University Press; 1991:3-13.
21. Fish B, Marcus J, Hans SL, Auerbach JG, Perdue S. Infants at risk for schizophrenia: sequelae of a genetic neurointegrative defect: a review and replication analysis of pandysmaturation in the Jerusalem Infant Development Study. *Arch Gen Psychiatry.* 1992;49:221-235.
22. Scheibel AB, Conrad AS. Hippocampal dysgenesis in mutant mouse and schizophrenic man: is there a relationship? *Schizophr Bull.* 1993;19: 21-33.
23. Hyde TM, Ziegler JC, Weinberger DR. Psychiatric disturbances in metachromatic leukodystrophy: insights into the neurobiology of psychosis. *Arch Neurol.* 1992;49:401-406.
24. Akbarian S, Bunney WE Jr, Potkin SG, Wigal SB, Hagman JO, Sandman CA, Jones EG. Altered distribution of nicotinamide-adenine dinucleotide phosphate–diaphorase cells in frontal lobe of schizophrenics implies disturbances of cortical development. *Arch Gen Psychiatry.* 1993;50:169-177.
25. Akbarian S, Viñuela A, Kim JJ, Potkin SG, Bunney WE Jr, Jones EG. Distorted distribution of nicotinamide-adenine dinucleotide phosphate–diaphorase neurons in temporal lobe of schizophrenics implies anomalous cortical development. *Arch Gen Psychiatry.* 1993;50:178-187.
26. Ghosh A, Antonini A, McConnell SK, Shatz CJ. Requirement for subplate neurons in the formation of thalamocortical connections. *Nature.* 1990; 347:179-181.
27. Ghosh A, Shatz CJ. Involvement of subplate neurons in the formation of ocular dominance columns. *Science.* 1992;255:1441-1443.

ORIGINAL ARTICLE

Prefrontal Cortex and Schizophrenia

A Quantitative Magnetic Resonance Imaging Study

Cynthia G. Wible, PhD; Martha E. Shenton, PhD; Hiroto Hokama, MD; Ron Kikinis, MD; Ferenc A. Jolesz, MD; David Metcalf, MS; Robert W. McCarley, MD

Objective: To measure prefrontal cortical volume in a group of schizophrenic subjects who presented with mainly positive symptoms and who were previously shown to have volume reductions in left temporal lobe structures.

Method: Fourteen men with chronic schizophrenia and 15 male control subjects were matched for age, IQ, handedness, and parental socioeconomic status. Magnetic resonance images were obtained by means of a 1.5-T magnet, and contiguous 1.5-mm slices of the entire brain were obtained.

Results: No significant differences were found between schizophrenic and control subjects in mean values for prefrontal white or gray matter on either the right or the left side. However, within the schizophrenic group, there was evidence of a relationship between the volumes of left prefrontal gray matter and left temporal lobe structures that was not present in the control group.

Conclusions: At least in this group of schizophrenic subjects with mainly positive symptoms, temporal lobe abnormalities can exist in conjunction with no gross volumetric abnormalities of the prefrontal cortex.

(Arch Gen Psychiatry. 1995;52:279-288)

STUDIES OF schizophrenia that have used neuropsychological tests and measures of physiologic function have found abnormalities putatively localized to the prefrontal portion of the frontal lobe. Schizophrenic subjects show cognitive and behavioral deficits that are frequently associated with frontal lobe damage, such as deficits in performance of the Wisconsin Card Sort Test,[1,2] abnormalities in eye movement,[3] deficits in performance of a spatial working memory task known to be impaired by prefrontal lesions in monkeys,[4] and defect symptoms, such as impairments in planning abilities, abstract reasoning, attention, insight, judgment, and decreased drive.[5]

Prefrontal cortical function in schizophrenic subjects has also been measured by means of such physiologic indexes as cerebral blood flow and glucose utilization, as measured by xenon 133, positron emission tomography, and single-photon emission computed tomography[6,7] (see Andreasen et al[8] for a review). The literature has been inconsistent, with some studies reporting hypofrontality,[7,9-13] some reporting no frontal abnormalities, and at least one report showing hyperfrontality in never-medicated schizophrenics.[14] It has been suggested that hypofrontality can only be detected during performance of a task, such as the Wisconsin Card Sort Test, that activates prefrontal cortex.[15]

Magnetic resonance (MR) imaging studies have found reduced volume in the frontal lobe,[16-22] with one study finding reduced white matter but not gray matter volume.[23] However, abnormalities in frontal lobe structures have not been consistently demonstrated. Several studies that used MR imaging reported no volumetric differences in the frontal lobe between schizophrenic and control subjects.[24-28]

What might account for the inconsistent findings with regard to the frontal lobe? One contributing factor to the differences among prefrontal structural studies could be the large variation in MR imaging methods. Measurements of brain volume have ranged from the use of one 10-mm-thick slice to manually delineate cortical volume, to one study that used several 3-mm-thick slices through a large portion of the frontal lobe in conjunction with an automated

See Subjects and Methods on next page

From the Department of Psychiatry, Harvard Medical School, Boston, the Brockton (Mass) Veterans Affairs Medical Center, Massachusetts Mental Health Center, Boston, and McLean Hospital, Belmont, Mass (Drs Wible, Shenton, Hokama, and McCarley); and the Department of Radiology, Harvard Medical School, and MRI Division, Surgical Planning Laboratory, Brigham and Women's Hospital, Boston (Drs Kikinis and Jolesz and Mr Metcalf).

SUBJECTS AND METHODS

SUBJECTS

Magnetic resonance images were obtained for a previous study[33] from 15 schizophrenic subjects and 15 control subjects, all right-handed men. The frontal lobe portion of the scans for one subject was unusable because of artifact, resulting in 14 schizophrenic subjects. Schizophrenic subjects were recruited from the Brockton (Mass) Veterans Affairs Medical Center; 12 were hospitalized and two were in Veterans Affairs foster homes. All were receiving neuroleptic medication, and the mean (±SD) time in the hospital was 7.1±4.6 years. Control subjects were recruited through newspaper advertisements. Patient diagnoses were made in accord with *DSM-III-R,* on the basis of chart review, and from information obtained from administration of the Schedule for Affective Disorders and Schizophrenia.[41] Subjects were required to be between the ages of 20 and 55 years and have no history of electroconvulsive shock treatment, neurologic illness, or steroid use, and no lifetime history of alcohol or other drug addiction or abuse (*DSM-III-R*) within the past 5 years. Control subjects were also excluded if they or their first-degree relatives had a history of psychiatric illness.

The two groups of subjects were matched for age and handedness, and there were no statistically significant differences between the two groups in height, weight, head circumference, socioeconomic status of the family of origin, or scores on the Wechsler Adult Intelligence Scale–Revised information subscale.[42] There was a difference between groups in education level. However, matching for education level may lead to groups that are unmatched in terms of premorbid ability levels, because schizophrenic subjects may start to show symptoms at the time when they would normally be finishing high school and going on to college. We therefore matched subjects on parental socioeconomic status and Wechsler Adult Intelligence Scale–Revised information subscale, both of which are likely to correspond better with premorbid functioning.

CLINICAL EVALUATIONS

Three instruments were used to assess symptoms: the Scale for the Assessment of Positive Symptoms,[43] the Scale for Assessment of Negative Symptoms,[44] and the Thought Disorder Index.[45] In the Andreasen classification, 11 of the 14 patients were assessed as having mainly positive symptoms, and three patients were characterized as having mixed symptoms. None of the patients had predominately negative symptoms, but some negative symptoms were present (mean Scale for Assessment of Negative Symptoms score of 9.1 vs mean Scale for the Assessment of Positive Symptoms score of 10.9). The average score on the Thought Disorder Index was 65, with a range of 1.7 to 212.5. Normal subjects score less than 5.

MR IMAGING METHOD

All MR images were acquired at the Brigham and Women's Hospital, Boston, Mass, with a 1.5-T system (Signa, General Electric Medical Systems, Milwaukee, Wis). The MR imaging method is described in detail elsewhere[33] and will be briefly described here. For the measurement of specific ROIs, a three-dimensional Fourier transform spoiled gradient-recalled acquisition in steady state (SPGR) was used to obtain images throughout the entire brain that were reformatted into 124 contiguous 1.5-mm coronal slices. This protocol creates images with good gray-white matter contrast. The SPGR images were obtained with the following parameters: echo time, 5 milliseconds; repetition time, 35 milliseconds; one repetition; nutation angle, 45°; field of view, 24 cm; acquisition matrix, 256×256×124; voxel dimensions, 0.9375×0.9375×1.5 mm.

For the measurement of the intracranial contents, 108 (54 for each echo) contiguous double-echo spin-echo 3-mm axial slices were obtained throughout the extent of the brain. Imaging parameters were as follows: echo time, 30 milliseconds; repetition time, 3000 milliseconds; field of view, 24 cm; acquisition matrix, 256×256; voxel dimensions, 0.9375×0.9375×3 mm. No gross abnormalities were found in the scans when they were evaluated by a clinical neuroradiologist.

IMAGE PROCESSING

The image processing stages were different for the whole brain and the individual ROI measurements. The image processing for the ROI measurements on the SPGR images proceeded in five stages. (1) The SPGR images were filtered to reduce noise.[46] (2) The intracranial cavity was extracted from the image in several stages. First an image was produced for each slice in which the brain, bone marrow, skin, muscle, and connective tissue were assigned to one tissue class, and the cerebrospinal fluid (CSF) and skull between the brain and skin were assigned to a second class (both the CSF and skull give little signal in these images and appear dark, like the background). This procedure resulted in a segmentation in which the brain was separated from the skull and other associated tissue except for a few connective tissue bridges across the CSF. These connective bridges were then erased by manual editing, and then a connectivity algorithm[47-49] was used to assign brain and extraneous tissue to different classes. The part of the image that contained the brain was used in conjunction with the SPGR image to mask out the skull and other extraneous tissue from the SPGR image. (3) The SPGR image that included only the brain and surrounding CSF was segmented into white matter, gray matter, and CSF by means of an algorithm in which the user selected sample points from those tissue classes, and each voxel in the image was then automatically assigned to one of the three tissue classes.[48-51] (4) The results of the segmentation were then superimposed on the original SPGR image and edited with an image editing program, slice by slice, on the computer workstation to improve the tissue classifications. The slice editor contained algorithms to perform manual drawing of ROIs, connectivity, island removal, erosion, and dilation of tissue classes, a color editor to assign colors to different ROIs, and a magnifier to magnify the image to a user-chosen level of magnification. These slice editor tools were used to reassign pixels that were misclassified by the automated algorithms. (5) A dividing cubes algorithm was used to reconstruct the segmentation to allow for a three-dimensional view of each tissue class.[48,49] The voxels for each tissue class were summed to compute the volume for each slice and the cumulative volume.

The image processing procedures for the measurement of intracranial content (used to compute the relative volume measurements) were described in detail in a previous study.[33] The 3-mm double-echo axial images were used for this measurement, and the image processing required some of the same algorithms as those used in measurement of the specific prefrontal ROIs, including a preprocessing filter, and algorithms for segmentation, connectivity, three-dimensional reconstruction, and visualization, and an algorithm for calculating volume.

SPECIFIC BRAIN ROI

The gray matter of the prefrontal cortex was measured starting anteriorly from the first slice that contained brain tissue. The posterior landmark was determined by first locating the most anterior slice that contained the temporal stem (the white matter tract connecting the temporal and frontal lobes), then moving anteriorly three slices. This landmark was chosen because it was reliable and it controlled for any difference between schizophrenics and controls in lateral asymmetries (reliability for all anterior-posterior landmarks is discussed in the next section). The posterior boundary coincided with the separation of frontal and temporal lobe areas. As illustrated in **Figure 1**, left, the region of prefrontal cortex gray matter measured stopped a few slices anterior to the most inferior aspect of the precentral sulcus, and the posterior bound differed slightly on the left and right, reflecting the different anteroposterior onset of left and right temporal stems. Thus, the gray matter volume compared in this study excluded Brodmann's area 4 (motor cortex) and at least parts of area 6 (supplementary and premotor cortexes).

To ensure a high degree of reliability, different anteroposterior landmarks were used for the prefrontal white matter volume than for the gray matter. Anteriorly, the white matter was measured beginning with the first slice that contained white matter and extended posteriorly to the slice immediately anterior to the slice that contained the lateral ventricles. The extent of the white matter measurement is marked by a blue line on the surface of the brain in Figure 1, left. A reconstruction of the white matter is shown in relationship to the ventricles in Figure 1, right. These landmarks were chosen for the white matter because it is invaded posteriorly by the gray matter structures of basal ganglia and the claustrum, both of which were not accurately segmented by the present semiautomated segmentation procedures and would have required extensive manual editing. Reliability for the gray and white matter volumes will be discussed below.

RELIABILITY OF IMAGE PROCESSING TECHNIQUES

Interrater Reliability for the Frontal Lobe Volumetric Measures

The 29 cases were first segmented by two different raters, each working on half of the cases. Interrater reliability was assessed by having each rater segment a randomly chosen case that was initially processed by the other rater. A third rater also segmented the two cases, resulting in three estimates of volume (from three raters) for the two cases (one control and one schizophrenic patient). The intraclass correlation for three raters (C.G.W., H.H., and Ihan Chou) was r_i=.98. The interrater reliability of the first two raters was of interest, since they performed the segmentations. The average percentage error for the first two raters was computed by subtracting the volumes obtained on the same case by the two raters for each category of tissue measured (ie, white and gray matter on the left and right) and dividing the difference by the first rater's volume score; the average percentage difference between raters was 1.75% for the schizophrenic case and 3.63% for the control case. Pearson correlations between volumetric scores for the two original raters for the two cases were also calculated by performing a correlation between the volume for each tissue class on each slice for the same case segmented by two different raters; the correlation between tissue volumes for the two raters for the schizophrenic case was r=.99, and that for the control case was r=.99.

Intrarater Reliability for the Volumetric Measures

Intrarater reliability was obtained for the two raters who segmented each of the brains for the study (C.G.W., H.H.). After the segmentation was completed for all cases, intrarater reliability was determined by having each of the two raters reapply the image processing stages to a randomly selected case that this rater had previously segmented. Since each rater originally segmented half of the cases, one rater's case was randomly chosen from the 15 cases that the rater had originally segmented, and the other rater's case was randomly chosen from the subset of cases that he or she had originally segmented. This procedure produced two estimates of all four prefrontal ROIs (left and right gray and white matter) for two cases. The average percentage difference between the first and second segmentations of the case was 3.25% for rater C.G.W., with a correlation between volumes of segmented tissue for each slice between the first and second segmentations of r=.98 (see above paragraph for information on how summary statistics were calculated). For rater H.H., the percentage difference was 4.25% and the correlation between segmentations was r=.99.

Reliability for the Identification of Landmark Boundaries

Intrarater and interrater reliability for the identification of the landmarks used to delineate gray and white matter boundaries was also assessed. Three cases for each of the two raters were chosen randomly from those initially processed by that rater, resulting in a total of six cases that were used for landmark reliability. The landmarks for gray and white matter on the left and right were judged blindly for all six cases by the two raters, resulting in landmark values for each case from the original segmentation, a second judgment from the original rater, and a third judgment from the rater who had not originally processed the case. The intraclass correlation for landmark reliability over six cases each rated three times was r_i=.99.

Comparison of Semiautomated and Manually Drawn Segmentation

The semiautomated image processing techniques used in segmentation were directly compared with manual

Continued on next page

delineation of ROIs, the technique that is traditionally used in the literature to obtain volumetric brain measurements. A case was chosen randomly from the two cases already designated for the measurement of interrater reliability, and the two raters used a computer mouse to outline manually the gray and white matter on the same five slices of the case. The segmentation for one of the slices with the two methods for one rater is shown in **Figure 2**. The two methods resulted in similar volume measurements, with an average difference of only 2% between estimates of the different tissue classes.

STATISTICAL ANALYSES

Left and right volumes of prefrontal gray and white matter were analyzed by means of a multivariate analysis of variance that used the variables group (schizophrenic vs control), tissue class (white or gray matter), and side (right or left). An analysis of covariance was also used, and the factors analyzed in the multivariate analysis of variance were covaried with age. The correlation between age and gray matter volume was assessed separately for the two groups of subjects. Analyses were computed separately for absolute volumes and for relative volumes, which corrected for head size by dividing the absolute volume by the volume of the intracranial contents and multiplying by 100.

Volumetric data were available for several temporal lobe structures for the subjects used in this study. The hypotheses guiding the examination of the relationship between volumes of prefrontal and temporal ROIs in patients with left-lateralized temporal lobe abnormalities were that prefrontal-temporal correlations would be (1) maximal for schizophrenics (compared with controls); (2) maximal on the left; and (3) maximal in the schizophrenic group for the temporal lobe ROI with greatest volume reduction (in the temporal lobe study, anterior hippocampal-amygdala complex showed the greatest volume reduction, while anterior-posterior superior temporal gyrus and the parahippocampal gyrus showed slightly lesser amounts and the posterior hippocampus showed no statistically significant reduction).

For evaluation of these predictions, we performed two stepwise multiple regressions in each subject group, one using left prefrontal gray matter as the dependent variable and the other using left prefrontal white matter. For both regressions, the six predictor (independent) variables were the six temporal lobe ROIs described above. Because the number of subjects was relatively small for this number of predictor variables, we conservatively term these analyses "exploratory," although they were prediction-driven and results were consistent with our predictions. (These analyses and statistical characterizations were primarily based on the guidelines of Kleinbaum et al.[52]) The regressions were performed on both absolute and relative volumes, and the results of the analyses with absolute volumes are reported if they met the criterion that the two measures showed consistent results (ie, both showed P values $<.05$). Univariate correlation coefficients were also computed for these variables, and also, for comparison, for right temporal lobe structures and right prefrontal gray and white matter.

Correlations were also performed, for schizophrenic patients only, between clinical measures and prefrontal left and right, gray and white matter, to assess the degree of association between symptoms and prefrontal volume measurements.

thresholding procedure to define gray-white matter boundaries.[23] Currently, most of the studies are based on volumetric observations taken from only a few brain slices for each subject. In addition, some studies measured the entire frontal cortex, while others restricted measurements to the prefrontal cortex (see Raine et al[19] for discussion).

Differences between studies in subject matching procedures could also create inconsistencies; the studies are generally heterogeneous in their subject matching procedures. In one study, subject matching procedures affected whether or not the schizophrenic group showed decreased prefrontal volume as measured with MR imaging.[24]

A set of more complex theoretical issues may also be contributing to the inconsistencies in findings. Abnormalities in areas other than the prefrontal cortex have also been reported in schizophrenic brains. Temporal lobe structures, such as the amygdala, hippocampus, entorhinal cortex, parahippocampal gyrus, and superior temporal gyrus, have been relatively consistently shown to be abnormal in schizophrenic subjects, especially on the left side.[29-38] These temporal lobe structures are highly interconnected with the prefrontal cortex.[39,40]

Findings of abnormalities in both frontal and temporal lobe areas allow for several theoretical possibilities for the correspondence between brain abnormalities and schizophrenic symptoms. Abnormalities in a single brain area (either the prefrontal cortex or temporal lobe structures) may account for both negative and positive symptoms, or, alternatively, a single area may contribute to producing only a subset of the symptoms. For example, prefrontal abnormalities have been suggested to contribute to negative as opposed to positive symptoms.[8] If this is the case, then schizophrenic subject heterogeneity across studies might contribute to inconsistent findings with a different mix of subjects with predominantly positive symptoms and predominantly negative symptoms showing different MR imaging and/or functional alterations (see Andreasen et al[8] for a discussion). Given the extent and complexity of prefrontal interconnectivity with temporal lobe structures, it is also possible that functional and/or structural abnormalities within either region are secondary to a more severe or primary dysfunction of the other region.

Careful, quantitative structural evaluations of frontal and temporal lobe regions in schizophrenic patients become critical in resolving these issues. The present study measured prefrontal gray and white matter in closely matched groups of schizophrenic subjects (previously shown to have volume reductions in several left temporal lobe regions of interest [ROIs][33]) and normal controls by means of quantitative volumetric techniques on

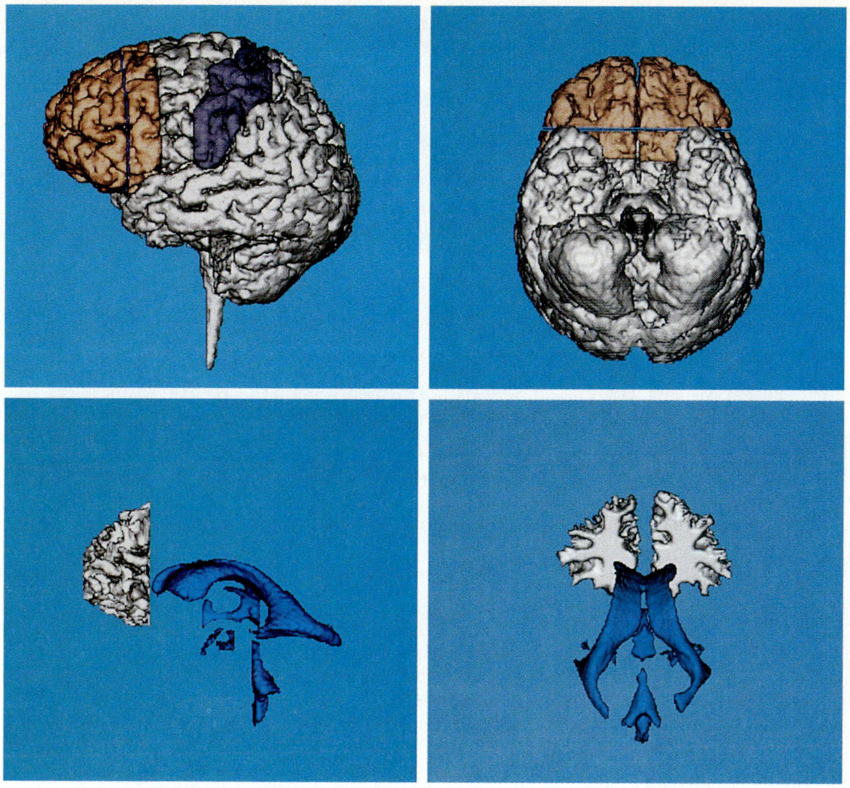

Figure 1. *Three-dimensional reconstructions of prefrontal gray and white matter measured in relationship to the cortex and the ventricles. Top, Prefrontal gray matter. Top left, Left lateral view shows gray matter (in peach) in relationship to the precentral and postcentral gyri (in purple). The slice corresponding to the posterior landmark for the measurement of the white matter is contained within the prefrontal gray matter area (the slice is blue). Top right, Ventral view of the same brain as in top left. Bottom, Prefrontal white matter. Bottom left, Left lateral view shows white matter in relation to the ventricles. Bottom right, Posterior view of the same white matter and ventricles as in top right.*

high-resolution MR images with 1.5×0.937×0.937-mm voxels. Prefrontal cortex was measured with an average span of 36 slices for gray and 25 slices for white matter measurement. In addition, the gray-white segmentation was edited carefully on each slice, resulting in very accurate separation.

RESULTS

PREFRONTAL VOLUME MEASURES

Control and schizophrenic subjects had similar mean values for both gray (**Figure 3**) and white (**Figure 4**) matter volume. No significant differences were found between schizophrenic and control subjects in prefrontal cortex volume using either the absolute or the relative brain volumes. For brevity, only the results of the absolute measures will be reported in the text (relative and absolute volumes are reported in the **Table**). The multivariate analysis of variance showed no main effect of subject group (control vs schizophrenic) (F=0.17, *df*=1,28, $P<.68$), and there were no differences either in total or in right or left gray or white matter, as shown by an absence of a two-way interaction between group and tissue (F=0.57, *df*=1,27, $P<.46$) and the absence of a three-way interaction between group, tissue type (white or gray matter), and side (right or left) (F=0.10, *df*=1,28, $P<.76$). An analysis of covariance, performed with age as a covariate, also failed to show significant effects. The Table shows the mean absolute and relative gray and white matter volumes for schizophrenic and control subjects, and the mean numbers of slices used to measure the volumes. The mean numbers of slices used to measure volumes were almost identical in schizophrenic patients and controls.

PREFRONTAL-TEMPORAL REGRESSION ANALYSES

Schizophrenic Subjects

When the volumes of left anterior and posterior portions of the amygdala-hippocampal complex, parahippocampal gyrus, and superior temporal gyrus were entered in a stepwise regression analysis, left anterior hippocampal-amygdala complex volume accounted for a significant proportion of the variance of left prefrontal cortical gray matter volume, with adjusted R^2=.47 (adjusted for number of variables and subjects) (F=12.65, P=.004); the other five ROI variables did not significantly add to the magnitude of this R^2.

Exactly the same results were obtained with prefrontal white matter volume as the dependent variable, with the adjusted R^2=.46 (F=12.23, P=.004). Significant values were also obtained with the use of relative volumes. It is important to note that the regression used ROI volumes of anterior temporal lobe areas that were highly intercorrelated in the schizophrenic group (**Figure 5**). This high degree of intercorrelation between the three anterior temporal lobe areas precludes making inferences about which of these three left anterior temporal lobe structures accounted for the most variance of left prefrontal areas.

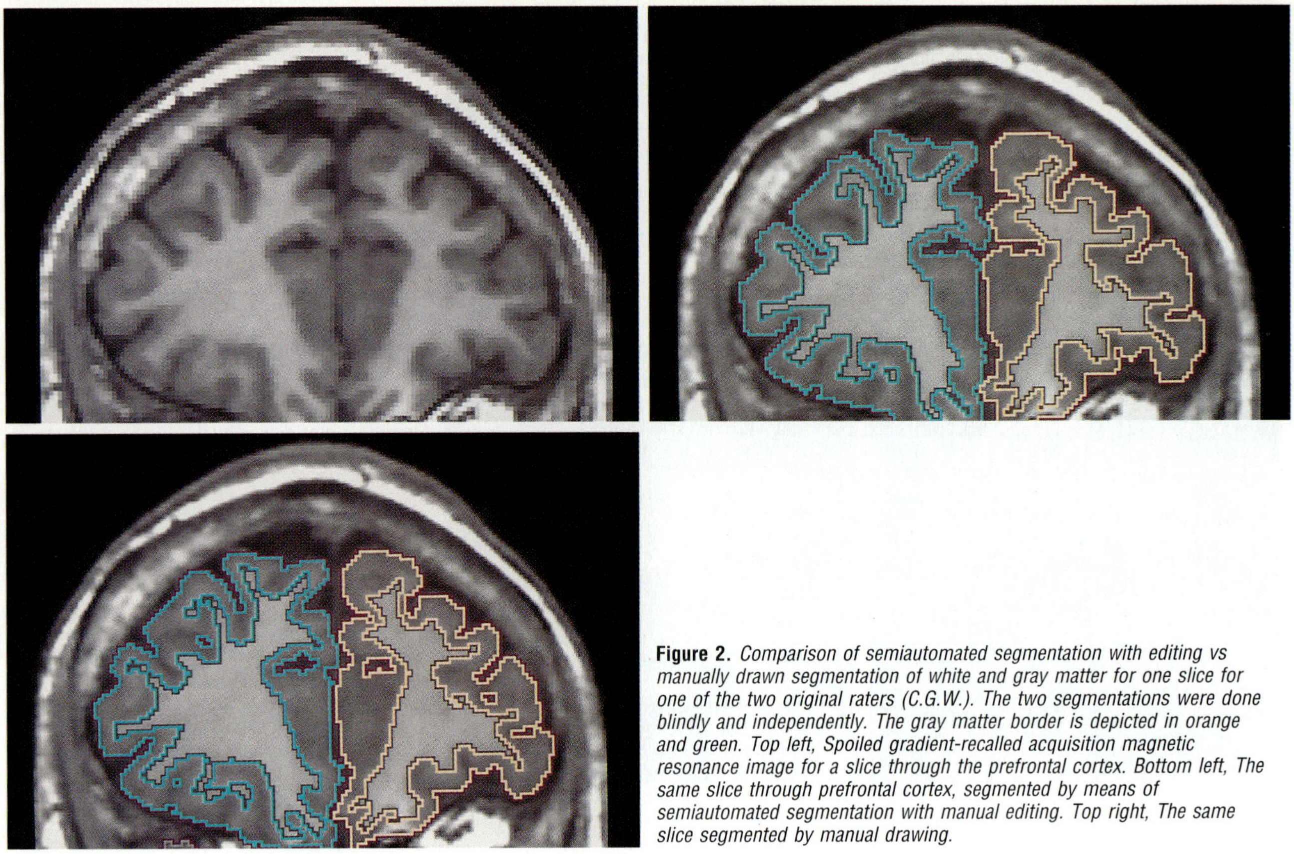

Figure 2. *Comparison of semiautomated segmentation with editing vs manually drawn segmentation of white and gray matter for one slice for one of the two original raters (C.G.W.). The two segmentations were done blindly and independently. The gray matter border is depicted in orange and green. Top left, Spoiled gradient-recalled acquisition magnetic resonance image for a slice through the prefrontal cortex. Bottom left, The same slice through prefrontal cortex, segmented by means of semiautomated segmentation with manual editing. Top right, The same slice segmented by manual drawing.*

Control Group

The control group did not show consistent statistically significant results between absolute and relative measures on the regression analyses for prefrontal gray or white matter volume and temporal lobe ROI.

PREFRONTAL-TEMPORAL UNIVARIATE PEARSON PRODUCT-MOMENT CORRELATIONS

Schizophrenic Group

There were high correlations between left prefrontal gray and white matter volumes and all three anterior temporal areas (Figure 5). These are exploratory analyses, and significance levels are not reported, but the correlations reported in Figure 5 that have $r > .50$ would be statistically significant at the $P < .05$ level in single planned comparisons. Figure 5 shows all correlations greater than .5 on at least one of the volume measures (either the absolute or relative volume). In contrast, the highest correlation for the posterior temporal areas and prefrontal lobe was the posterior superior temporal gyrus (absolute volume, $r = .33$; relative volume, $r = .36$ with prefrontal gray matter volume), which was still small compared with the r values for anterior temporal lobe ROIs.

Control Group

None of the left anterior temporal lobe areas showed high correlations with left prefrontal gray matter, but the left anterior hippocampal-amygdala complex and parahippocampal gyrus did show high correlations with left prefrontal white matter volume. The left *posterior* hippocampal-amygdala complex showed a high correlation with left prefrontal gray matter, a result not evident in the schizophrenic group. All correlations between temporal and prefrontal structures not shown in Figure 5 for the control subjects were $r \leq .20$.

PREFRONTAL-TEMPORAL CORRELATIONS ON THE RIGHT SIDE

Exploratory correlations were done separately for the two subject groups between right prefrontal white and gray matter volumes and the volumes of right anterior and posterior temporal lobe structures used in the regression analyses described above. The only high correlation (ie, with an uncorrected $P < .05$) was in the schizophrenic group between right posterior amygdala-hippocampal complex and right prefrontal white matter (n=14, $r = .53$ for absolute and n=14, $r = .58$ for the relative measure).

PREFRONTAL ROI-CLINICAL CORRELATIONS

Scores on the Scale for the Assessment of Negative Symptoms were negatively correlated with left prefrontal white matter volume (n=14, $r = -.63$) in the schizophrenic group. Neither the Scale for the Assessment of Positive Symptoms nor the Thought Disorder Index scores were correlated with any measure of prefrontal cortex volume.

Finally, the sensitivity of the segmentation procedures was assessed by correlating gray matter volume with

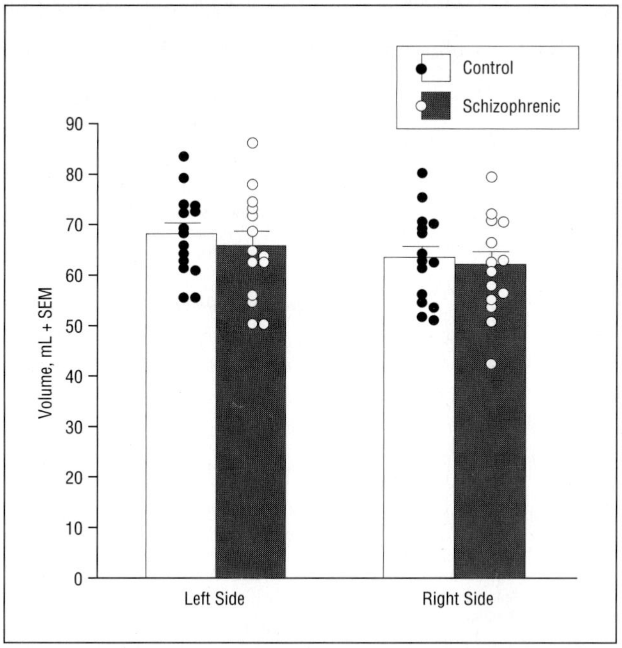

Figure 3. *Prefrontal gray matter volumes (+SEM) for controls and schizophrenics shown separately for the left and right sides.*

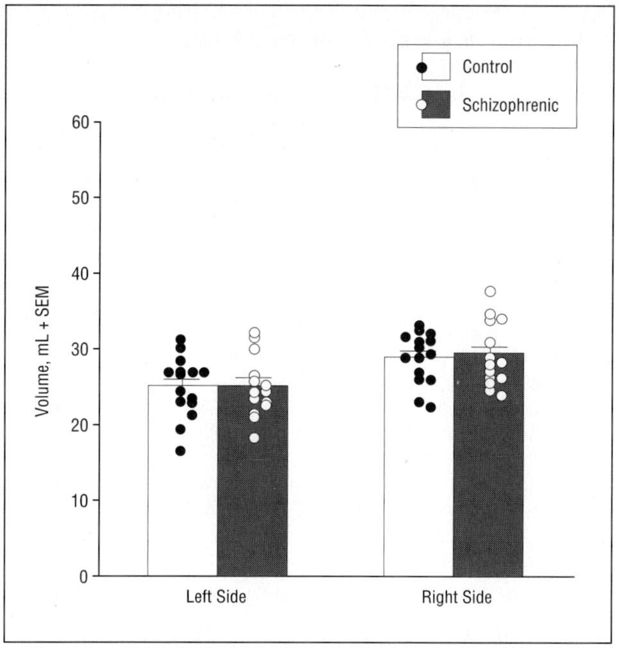

Figure 4. *Prefrontal white matter volumes (+SEM) for controls and schizophrenics shown separately for the left and right sides.*

age.[37,39] Gray matter on the left and right was significantly correlated with age for the entire group of subjects; the Pearson Product Moment Correlation between age and prefrontal gray matter on the left was $r=-.49$ (n=29, $P<.01$), and that on the right, $r=-.46$ (n=29, $P<.01$). These correlations were also significant when analyzed within each group of subjects.

COMMENT

The present study used high-resolution MR imaging in conjunction with semiautomated image processing procedures to measure whole prefrontal cortical gray and prefrontal white matter volume in schizophrenic and control subjects. No significant differences were found between the two groups in either right or left white or gray matter volume. The validity of our volumetric measurements is supported by the high correlation between age and gray matter volume in our study, and by previous data on the segmentation of a phantom.[50] These results are in agreement with several studies that have found no volumetric differences in this area between schizophrenic and control subjects.[24-28]

Prefrontal cortex abnormalities have been found in schizophrenic patients by means of MR imaging.[16-22] Methodologic differences in MR imaging procedures could account for the conflicting results. A few of the studies that showed differences measured volume throughout the entire prefrontal region, with one study using contiguous 3-mm slices,[23] two using 5-mm slices with 2.5-mm gaps between slices,[18,22] and a third using 10-mm slices.[19] The remaining studies measured volume with the use of one or two slices. In the present study, prefrontal white and gray matter volume was measured with a mean of 25 and 36 slices 1.5 mm thick, respectively, for each subject, and may be expected to differ from data obtained with methods that use a few slices to measure volume. Breier et al[23] used 3-mm slices, and their study is most comparable with the present study in terms of method. Breier et al also found no gray matter volume reductions in schizophrenic subjects, but they did report white matter volume reduction on both sides of the brain.

The schizophrenic subjects in the present study were previously shown to have volume reductions in several temporal lobe structures, including the left anterior portions of the hippocampal-amygdala complex, parahippocampal gyrus, and superior temporal gyrus.[33] The volume of these left temporal lobe areas was also highly intercorrelated in schizophrenic subjects, but not controls (Figure 5). Temporal lobe abnormalities have been demonstrated in schizophrenic subjects by means of both MR imaging and postmortem histologic studies.[36-38]

Exploratory analyses examined the relationship between volumes of temporal and prefrontal areas. In the schizophrenic group, but not the control group, the anterior portion of the left hippocampal-amygdala complex accounted for a significant proportion of the variance of prefrontal gray and white matter volume with both absolute and relative volume measures. However, the high intercorrelations among left anterior temporal lobe areas in schizophrenic subjects precluded absolute identification of the specific anterior temporal lobe area that was accounting for the variance of prefrontal volume. Univariate correlations showed preliminary evidence of a relationship between anterior portions of the hippocampal-amygdala complex, parahippocampal gyrus, and superior temporal gyrus and prefrontal white and gray volume on the left side in schizophrenic subjects (Figure 5). For control subjects, a consistent result was not found between absolute and relative measures on the regression analyses. However, control subjects did show high correlations between anterior portions of the hippocampal-amygdala complex and parahippocampal gyrus and prefrontal white matter on the left. A previous study also found a significant cor-

Prefrontal Gray and White Matter Volumes for Control and Schizophrenic Subjects

	Absolute Volume, mL*	No. of Slices	Relative Volume, mL*
Gray matter			
Left			
Control	68.1±8.2	37.5	4.3±0.46
Schizophrenic	65.6±10.8	37.6	4.0±0.58
Right			
Control	63.5±8.9	35.8	4.0±0.51
Schizophrenic	61.9±9.8	35.2	3.8±0.53
White matter			
Left			
Control	25.0±3.9	25.3	1.6±0.18
Schizophrenic	25.6±4.0	25.3	1.6±0.21
Right			
Control	29.3±3.4	25.5	1.9±0.14
Schizophrenic	29.8±4.2	25.4	1.8±0.23

*Values are mean±SD.

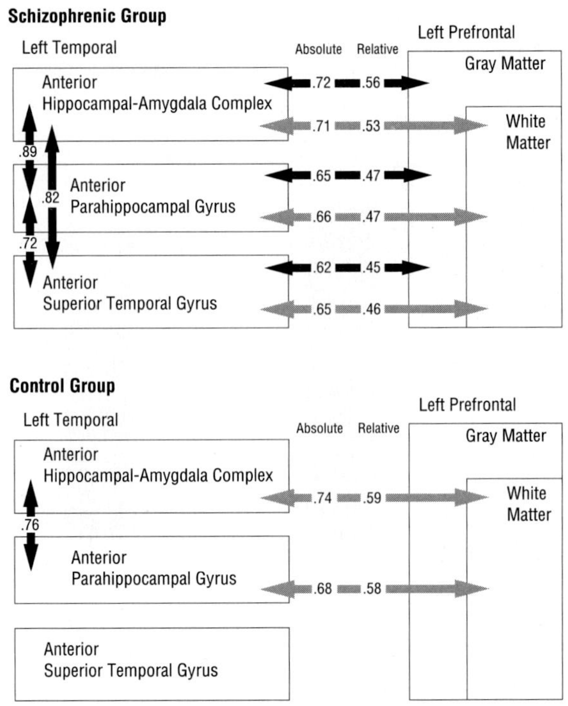

Figure 5. *Correlations between the volumes of temporal lobe structures and prefrontal cortical gray matter (black arrows) and white matter (gray arrows). The Pearson correlation coefficients for absolute and relative volume measures for structures are shown within the arrows.*

relation between the right hippocampal-amygdala complex and right prefrontal white matter [23] in schizophrenic subjects. Although the correlational data are tentative and should be interpreted with caution until larger subject groups are examined, one interpretation of these data is that these temporal and prefrontal structures form a tightly linked functional system in both control and schizophrenic subjects. A (use-dependent[37] and/or developmental) pathologic process that affects temporal lobe structures may also be affecting prefrontal cortical areas in a parallel manner, resulting in stronger than normal relationships between volumes in these areas.

The finding of no prefrontal volume reductions in schizophrenic subjects may appear to contradict evidence of prefrontal dysfunction from neuropsychological tests[1-5] and functional activation studies.[7-14] However, these data may be consistent when functional interactions between brain areas are taken into account. When the role of prefrontal vs temporal cortex abnormalities in schizophrenia is assessed, it is important to be clear about the role of evidence from neuropsychological tests, physiologic activation measures, and morphologic measures, and their implications for brain function. Structural abnormalities, including cell loss, in the temporal lobe may lead to a disconnection between temporal and frontal areas, with both structural and functional consequences in the prefrontal cortex. It is also possible that structural abnormalities in the temporal lobe could lead to functional abnormalities in the prefrontal cortex without any functionally significant structural and/or chemical defects in the prefrontal cortex. For example, during the performance of tasks that include a memory component, and thus presumably activate medial temporal areas, it is possible that a failure or dysfunction of temporal lobe structures could cause a failure to activate, or aberrant activation, in prefrontal areas.

The hippocampus and related temporal lobe structures are thought to be important in the storage, retrieval, and consolidation of memory in cortical areas.[53,54] The dorsolateral portion of the prefrontal cortex is thought to be involved in the maintenance of working memory representations.[55] Working memory may rely on memory representations established and processed by the hippocampal system (ie, the hippocampus and related structures), and hence a failure or dysfunction of the hippocampal system could result in a lack of normal activation of the prefrontal cortex during task performance.

In a study that used twin pairs that were discordant for schizophrenia, decreased hippocampal volume was correlated with low prefrontal activation during the Wisconsin Card Sort Test in schizophrenic subjects.[56] Performance of both the Wisconsin Card Sort Test and delayed response task, two tasks often used to assess prefrontal cortical function, is also impaired by lesions of the temporal lobe.[57,58] In addition, hippocampal single-unit activity was correlated with aspects of the delayed response task during performance by monkeys.[59] Thus, it is important to distinguish between functional abnormalities that arise from intrinsic physiologic defects and those that arise from an earlier failure of information processing in other brain areas. The left temporal lobe structures that have been reported to be abnormal in schizophrenic subjects (hippocampus, amygdala, parahippocampal gyrus, and superior temporal gyrus) are thought to be involved in verbal memory and language processing.[53,60-63] A dysfunction of the verbal memory system in the form of aberrant activation or overactivation of representations could lead to such symptoms as thought disorder and verbal hallucinations.[64] Although schizophrenic patients show generalized impairments when compared with controls, disproportionate deficits in learning and memory were found when patients were given a battery of neuropsychological tests,[65] and these types of deficits were associated with MR imaging volume reductions in left temporal lobe structures in a different study.[66]

What do the current findings suggest in terms of the correspondence between brain areas and symptoms? There are several possible interpretations of the main findings, and further studies are needed to make firm conclusions or to exclude alternative hypotheses. However, one possibility that should be considered is that frontal lobe functional and/or structural abnormalities may be secondary to structural abnormalities in temporal lobe areas in patients who present with positive symptoms, and that positive symptoms stem primarily from temporal lobe abnormalities. At least two patterns of results are consistent with this possibility; the first is no volume reduction in the prefrontal cortex in conjunction with reductions in temporal lobe structures. The second is a lesser degree of volume reduction in the prefrontal cortex than in temporal lobe structures, because of the deafferentation of, or excitotoxic damage to, the prefrontal cortex, in conjunction with a pattern of high correlations between the volume of prefrontal lobe and the volume of temporal lobe structures. The present study found no volume reductions in prefrontal cortex but did find high correlations between abnormal temporal lobe areas and prefrontal cortex, suggesting, but not conclusively demonstrating, a link between positive symptoms and temporal lobe areas.

In conjunction with this view, there are at least two possibilities for the cause of negative symptoms. They could stem from prefrontal cortical dysfunction, or alternatively, at least some negative symptoms could be a secondary consequence of positive symptoms; there is no evidence that negative symptoms stem directly from temporal lobe abnormality.

Prefrontal abnormalities have been hypothesized to be the source of negative symptoms in patients. For example, there is evidence that prefrontal activation deficits are seen only in patients with negative symptoms.[8] The lack of prefrontal volume reduction in patients with predominantly positive symptoms is consistent with this hypothesis. In addition, we found preliminary evidence of a negative correlation between negative symptoms and left prefrontal white matter volume.

A preliminary conclusion based on the current findings is that positive symptoms arise from a dysfunction of temporal lobe structures. This conclusion is tentative for two reasons. First, although we found no global differences in prefrontal cortex, it is possible that small circumscribed areas of prefrontal cortex have reduced volume. For example, in a previous study in our laboratory, even though schizophrenic subjects showed volume reductions in several left temporal structures, the volume of the whole temporal lobe was not different between schizophrenic and control subjects.[33] The possibility of small areas showing abnormalities is currently being investigated.

A second caution concerns the nature of what is measured by MR imaging. Abnormalities in cellular orientation, connectivity, receptor distribution and sensitivity, and neurotransmitter distribution, among other factors, are not detectible by MR imaging. Cellular and neurotransmitter abnormalities have been reported in the prefrontal cortex of schizophrenic patients. For example, reduced neuronal density was found in prefrontal cortex in schizophrenic patients and was reported to be due to a reduction in small interneurons.[67,68] Thus, the prefrontal cortex could have small circumscribed volume reductions, cellular abnormalities, or neurotransmitter abnormalities that were undetected in the present study.

The results of the current study suggest that if abnormalities of prefrontal cortex exist in schizophrenic patients who present with mainly positive symptoms, then they are not as severe, circumscribed to a small area, or of a different type than those found in temporal lobe structures.

Accepted for publication January 23, 1995.

This research was supported by the National Institute of Mental Health, Bethesda, Md (grant 40 799), the Department of Veterans Affairs Schizophrenia Center, Washington, DC, the National Alliance for Research in Schizophrenia and Depression, Chicago, Ill, and the Commonwealth of Massachusetts Research Center, Boston (Dr McCarley); the Clinical Research Training Program, Bethesda, Md (T32MH16259-13), and a Health and Education Fund Award from the Massachusetts Mental Health Center, Boston (Dr Wible); K02-MH-0111-01 and the Scottish Rite Foundation, Lexington, Mass (Dr Shenton); the Stanley Foundation, Arlington, Va (Drs Shenton and Kikinis); a National Institute of Health Career Development Award, Bethesda, Md (Dr Jolesz); and the Swiss National Foundation, Bern (Dr Kikinis).

Reprint requests to Department of Psychiatry—116A, 940 Belmont St, Brockton, MA 02401 (Dr McCarley).

REFERENCES

1. Goldberg TE, Weinberger DR, Berman KF, Pliskin NH, Podd M. Further evidence for dementia of the prefrontal type in schizophrenia? *Arch Gen Psychiatry.* 1987;44:1008-1014.
2. Gruzelier J, Seymour K, Wilson L, Jolley A, Hirsch S. Impairments on neuropsychologic tests of temporohippocampal and frontohippocampal functions and word fluency in remitting schizophrenia and affective disorders. *Arch Gen Psychiatry.* 1988;45:623-629.
3. Holzman PS. Eye movement dysfunction and psychosis. *Int Rev Neurobiol.* 1985;27:197-205.
4. Park S, Holzman PS. Schizophrenics show spatial working memory deficits. *Arch Gen Psychiatry.* 1992;49:975-982.
5. Weinberger DS. Schizophrenia and the frontal lobe. *Trends Neurosci.* 1988:11:367-370.
6. Buchsbaum MS, Haier RJ, Potkin SG, Nuechteriein K, Bracha HS, Katz M, Lohr J, Wu J, Lottenberg S, Jerabek PA, Trenary M, Tafalla R, Reynolds C, Bunney WE. Frontostriatal disorder of cerebral metabolism in never-medicated schizophrenics. *Arch Gen Psychiatry.* 1992;49:935-942.
7. Berman KF, Torrey EF, Daniel DG, Weinberger DR. Regional cerebral blood flow in monozygotic twins discordant and concordant for schizophrenia. *Arch Gen Psychiatry.* 1992;49:927-934.
8. Andreasen NC, Rezai K, Alliger R, Swayze VW, Flaum M, Kirchner P, Cohen G, O'Leary DS. Hypofrontality in neuroleptic-naive patients and in patients with chronic schizophrenia. *Arch Gen Psychiatry.* 1992;49:943-958.
9. Buchsbaum MS, Ingvar DH, Kessler R, Waters RN, Cappelletti J, van Kammen DP, King AC, Johnson JJ, Manning RG, Flynn RM, Mann LS, Bunney WE Jr, Sokoloff L. Cerebral glucography with positron tomography in normals and in patients with schizophrenia. *Arch Gen Psychiatry.* 1982;39:251-259.
10. Ingvar DH, Franzen G. Abnormalities of cerebral blood flow distribution in patients with chronic schizophrenia. *Acta Psychiatr Scand.* 1974;50:425-462.
11. Paulman RG, Devous MD, Gregory RR, Herman JH, Jennings L, Bonte FJ, Nasrallah HA, Raese JD. Hypofrontality and cognitive impairment in schizophrenia: dynamic single-photon tomography and neuropsychological assessment of schizophrenic brain function. *Biol Psychiatry.* 1990;27:377-399.
12. Weinberger DR, Berman BF, Illowsky B. Physiological dysfunction of dorsolateral prefrontal cortex in schizophrenia, III: a new cohort and evidence for a monoaminergic mechanism. *Arch Gen Psychiatry.* 1988;45:609-615.
13. Wolkin A, Angrist B, Wolf A, Bodie JD, Wolkin B, Jaeger J, Cancro R, Rotrosen J. Low frontal glucose utilization in chronic schizophrenia: a replication study. *Am J Psychiatry.* 1988;145:251-253.
14. Cleghorn JM, Garnett ES, Nahmias C, Firnau G, Brown GM, Kaplan R, Szecht-

man H, Szechtman B. Increased frontal and reduced parietal glucose metabolism in acute untreated schizophrenia. *Psychiatry Res.* 1989;28:119-133.
15. Weinberger DR, Berman KF. Speculation on the meaning of cerebral metabolic hypofrontality in schizophrenia. *Schizophr Bull.* 1988;14:157-168.
16. Andreasen N, Nasrallah HA, Dunn V, Olson SC, Grove WM, Eharhardt JC, Coffman JA, Crossett JHW. Structural abnormalities in the frontal system in schizophrenia. *Arch Gen Psychiatry.* 1986;43:136-144.
17. DeMyer MK, Gilmor RL, Hendrie HC, DeMyer WE, Augustyn GT, Jackson RK. Magnetic resonance brain images in schizophrenic and normal subjects: influence of diagnosis and education. *Schizophr Bull.* 1988;14:21-32.
18. Jernigan TL, Zisook S, Heaton RK, Moranville JT, Hesselink JR, Braff DL. Magnetic resonance imaging abnormalities in lenticular nuclei and cerebral cortex in schizophrenia. *Arch Gen Psychiatry.* 1991;48:881-890.
19. Raine A, Lencz T, Reynolds GP, Harrison G, Sheard C, Medley I, Reynolds LM, Cooper JE. An evaluation of structural and functional prefrontal deficits in schizophrenia: MRI and neuropsychological measures. *Psychiatry Res.* 1992;45:123-137.
20. Stratta P, Rossi A, Gallucci M, Amicarelli I, Passariello R, Casacchia M. Hemispheric asymmetries and schizophrenia: a preliminary magnetic resonance imaging study. *Biol Psychiatry.* 1989;25:275-284.
21. Williamson P, Pelz D, Merskey H, Morrison S, Conlon P. Correlation of negative symptoms in schizophrenia with frontal lobe parameters on magnetic resonance imaging. *Br J Psychiatry.* 1991;159:130-134.
22. Zipursky RB, Lim KO, Sullivan EV. Widespread cerebral gray matter volume deficits in schizophrenia. *Arch Gen Psychiatry.* 1992;49:195-205.
23. Breier A, Buchanan RW, Elkashef A, Munson RC, Kirkpatrick B, Gellad F. Brain morphology and schizophrenia: a magnetic resonance imaging study of limbic, prefrontal cortex, and caudate structures. *Arch Gen Psychiatry.* 1992;49:921-926.
24. Andreasen NC, Ehrhardt JC, Swayze VW, Alliger RJ, Yuh WTC, Cohen G, Ziebell S. Magnetic resonance imaging of the brain in schizophrenia. *Arch Gen Psychiatry.* 1990;47:35-44.
25. Kelsoe JR, Cadet JL, Pickar D, Weinberger DR. Quantitative neuroanatomy in schizophrenia: a controlled magnetic resonance imaging study. *Arch Gen Psychiatry.* 1988;45:533-541.
26. Smith RC, Baumgartner R, Calderon M. Magnetic resonance imaging studies of the brains of schizophrenic patients. *Psychiatry Res.* 1987;20:33-46.
27. Suddath RL, Casanova MF, Goldberg TE, Daniel DG, Kelsoe JR, Weinberger DR. Temporal lobe pathology in schizophrenia: a quantitative magnetic resonance imaging study. *Am J Psychiatry.* 1989;146:464-472.
28. Uematsu M, Kaiya H. Midsagittal cortical pathomorphology of schizophrenia: a magnetic resonance imaging study. *Psychiatry Res.* 1989;30:11-20.
29. Barta PE, Pearlson GD, Powers RE, Richards SS, Tune LE. Auditory hallucinations and smaller superior temporal gyral volume in schizophrenia. *Am J Psychiatry.* 1990;147:1457-1462.
30. Bogerts B, Ashtari M, Degreef G, Alvir JM, Bilder RM, Lieberman JA. Reduced temporal limbic structure volumes on magnetic resonance images in first episode schizophrenia. *Psychiatry Res Neuroimaging.* 1990;35:1-13.
31. Dauphinias D, DeLisi LE, Crow TJ, Alexandropoulos K, Colter N, Tuma I, Gershon ES. Reduction in temporal lobe size in siblings with schizophrenia: a magnetic resonance imaging study. *Psychiatry Res Neuroimaging.* 1990;35:137-147.
32. DeLisi LE, Hoff AL, Schwartz JE, Shields GW, Halthore SN, Gupta SN, Henn FA, Anand AK. Brain morphology in first-episode schizophrenic-like psychotic patients: a quantitative magnetic resonance imaging study. *Biol Psychiatry.* 1991;29:159-175.
33. Shenton ME, Kikinis R, Jolesz FA, Pollak SD, LeMay M, Wible CG, Hokama H, Martin J, Metcalf D, Coleman M, McCarley M. Abnormalities of the left temporal lobe and thought disorder in schizophrenia: a quantitative magnetic resonance imaging study. *N Engl J Med.* 1992;327:604-612.
34. Suddath RL, Christison GW, Torrey EF, Casanova MF, Weinberger DR. Anatomical abnormalities in the brains of monozygotic twins discordant for schizophrenia. *N Engl J Med.* 1990;322:789-794.
35. Young AH, Blackwood DHR, Roxborough H, McQueen JK, Martin MJ, Kean D. A magnetic resonance imaging study of schizophrenia: brain structure and clinical symptoms. *Br J Psychiatry.* 1991;158:158-164.
36. Crow TJ. Temporal lobe asymmetry as the key to the etiology of schizophrenia. *Schizophr Bull.* 1990;16:433-443.
37. McCarley RW, Shenton ME, O'Donnell BF, Nestor PG. Uniting Kraepelin and Bleuler: the psychology of schizophrenia and the biology of temporal lobe abnormalities. *Harvard Rev Psychiatry.* 1993;1:36-56.
38. Roberts GW, Bruton CJ. Annotation notes from the graveyard: neuropathology and schizophrenia. *Neuropathol Appl Neurobiol.* 1990;16:3-16.
39. Goldman-Rakic PS, Selemon LD, Schwartz ML. Dual pathways connecting the dorsolateral prefrontal cortex with the hippocampal formation and the parahippocampal cortex in the rhesus monkey. *Neuroscience.* 1984;12:719-743.
40. Pandya DN, Yeterian EH. Prefrontal cortex in relation to other cortical areas in rhesus monkey: architecture and connections. *Prog Brain Res.* 1990;85:63-94.
41. Spitzer RL, Endicott J. *Schedule for Affective Disorders and Schizophrenia–Life Time Version.* New York, NY: Biometrics Research Division, New York State Psychiatric Institute; 1978.
42. Wechsler D. *Wechsler Adult Intelligence Scale–Revised.* New York, NY: Harcourt Brace Jovanovich Inc; 1981.
43. Andreasen NC. *Scale for the Assessment of Positive Symptoms (SAPS).* Iowa City, Iowa: Dept of Psychiatry, University of Iowa College of Medicine; 1984.
44. Andreasen NC. *Scale for the Assessment of Negative Symptoms (SANS).* Iowa City, Iowa: Dept of Psychiatry, University of Iowa College of Medicine; 1981.
45. Johnston MH, Holzman PS. *Assessing Schizophrenic Thinking.* San Francisco, Calif: Jossey-Bass Inc Publishers; 1979.
46. Gerig G, Kikinis R, Kubler O. *Significant Improvement of MR Image Data Quality Using Anisotropic Diffusion Filtering.* Zurich, Switzerland: Communication Technology Laboratory, Image Science Division; 1990. Technical Report BIWI-TR-124.
47. Cline HE, Dumoulin CL, Hart HR, Lorensen W, Ludke S. 3D reconstruction of the brain from magnetic resonance images using a connectivity algorithm. *Magn Reson Imag.* 1987;5:345-352.
48. Cline HE, Lorensen WE, Ludke S, Crawford CR, Teeter BC. Two algorithms for the three-dimensional reconstruction of tomograms. *Med Physiol.* 1988;15:320-327.
49. Cline HE, Lorensen WE, Kikinis R, Jolesz F. Three-dimensional segmentation of MR images of the head using probability and connectivity. *J Comput Assist Tomogr.* 1990;14:1037-1045.
50. Cline HE, Lorensen WE, Souza SP, Jolesz FA, Kikinis R, Geric G, Kennedy TE. 3D surface rendering: MR images of the brain and its vasculature. *J Comput Assist Tomogr.* 1991;15:344-355.
51. Kikinis R, Shenton ME, Jolesz FA, Gerig G, Martin J, Anderson M, Metcalf D, Guttman C, McCarley RW, Lorensen W, Cline H. Routine quantitative analysis of brain and cerebrospinal spaces with MR imaging. *J Magn Reson Imag.* 1992;2:619-629.
52. Kleinbaum DG, Kupper LL, Miller KE. *Applied Regression Analysis and Other Multivariate Methods.* 2nd ed. Belmont, Calif: Duxbury Press; 1987:718.
53. Squire LR, Zola-Morgan S. The medial temporal lobe memory system. *Science.* 1991;253:1380-1386.
54. Eichenbaum H, Cohen NJ, Otto T, Wible CG. Memory representation in the hippocampus: functional domain and functional organization. In: Squire LR, Lynch G, Weinberger NM, McGaugh JL, eds. *Memory: Organization and Locus of Change.* New York, NY: Oxford University Press; 1992:163-204.
55. Goldman-Rakic PS, Friedman HR. The circuitry of working memory revealed by anatomy and metabolic imaging. In: Levin HS, Eisenberg HM, Benton AL, eds. *Frontal Lobe Function and Dysfunction.* New York, NY: Oxford University Press, 1991:72-91.
56. Weinberger DR. Anteromedial temporal-prefrontal connectivity: a functional neuroanatomical system implicated in schizophrenia. In: Carroll BJ, Barrett JE, eds. *Psychopathology and the Brain.* New York, NY: Raven Press; 1991:25-43.
57. Anderson SW, Damasio H, Jones RD, Tranel D. Wisconsin Card Sorting Test performance as a measure of frontal lobe damage. *J Clin Exp Neuropsychol.* 1991;13:909-922.
58. Zola-Morgan S, Squire LR. Medial temporal lesions in monkeys impair memory in a variety of tasks sensitive to human amnesia. *Behav Neurosci.* 1985;99:22-34.
59. Watanabe T, Niki H. Hippocampal unit activity and delayed response in the monkey. *Brain Res.* 1985;325:241-254.
60. Ojemann GA, Creutzfeldt O, Lettich E, Haglund M. Neuronal activity in human lateral temporal cortex related to short-term verbal memory, naming and reading. *Brain.* 1988;111:1383-1403.
61. Ojemann GA. Cortical organization of language. *J Neurosci.* 1991;11:2281-2287.
62. Penfield W, Perot P. The brain's record of auditory and visual experience: a final summary and discussion. *Brain.* 1963;86:596-695.
63. Frisk V, Milner B. The role of the left hippocampal region in the acquisition and retention of story content. *Neuropsychologia.* 1990;28:349-359.
64. Wible CG, Shenton ME, McCarley RW. Do positive symptoms in schizophrenia result from abnormalities of functionally linked temporal lobe structures? a new theory. Read before the Society of Biological Psychiatry Annual Meeting; May 2, 1992; Washington, DC.
65. Saykin AJ, Gur RC, Gur RE, Mozley PD, Mozley LH, Resnick SM, Kestor DB, Stafiniak P. Neuropsychological function in schizophrenia: selective impairment in memory and learning. *Arch Gen Psychiatry.* 1991;48:618-624.
66. Nestor PG, Shenton ME, McCarley RW, Haimson J, Smith SR, O'Donnell B, Kimble M, Kikinis R, Jolesz FA. Neuropsychological correlates of MRI temporal lobe abnormalities in schizophrenia. *Am J Psychiatry.* 1993;150:1849-1855.
67. Benes FM, Davidson J, Bird ED. Quantitative cytoarchitectural studies of the cerebral cortex of schizophrenics. *Arch Gen Psychiatry.* 1986;43:31-35.
68. Benes FM, McSparren J, Bird ED, SanGiovanni JP, Vincent SL. Deficits in small interneurons in prefrontal and cingulate cortex of schizophrenic and schizoaffective patients. *Arch Gen Psychiatry.* 1991;48:996-1001.

ORIGINAL ARTICLE

Double-blind Parallel Comparison of Three Dosages of Sertraline and Placebo in Outpatients With Obsessive-compulsive Disorder

John Greist, MD; Guy Chouinard, MD; Eugene DuBoff, MD; Angelos Halaris, MD, PhD; Suck Won Kim, MD; Lorrin Koran, MD; Michael Liebowitz, MD; R. Bruce Lydiard, MD, PhD; Steven Rasmussen, MD; Kerrin White, MD; Carolyn Sikes, PhD

Background: Anecdotal evidence suggests patients with obsessive-compulsive disorder (OCD) are treated with selective serotonin uptake inhibitors at dosages significantly higher than those used with depressed patients. The current study examined the efficacy, safety, and optimal dosing strategy of sertraline in patients with OCD.

Methods: Three hundred twenty-four nondepressed outpatients with OCD from 11 sites followed identical protocols using a double-blind parallel design. Following 1 week of single-blind placebo, patients were randomly assigned to 12 weeks of treatment with one of three fixed dosages of sertraline (50, 100, or 200 mg/d) or placebo.

Results: Sertraline patients exhibited significantly greater improvement ($P<.05$) at end point than placebo patients on all three main efficacy measures in the 50-mg/d and 200-mg/d groups and on one measure in the 100-mg/d group. The placebo response was larger in this population of subjects with OCD than in those previously studied. Adverse experiences were common in the sertraline and placebo groups and appeared to be dose-related in the sertraline-treated patients.

Conclusions: Results support the safety and efficacy of daily dosages of 50, 100, and 200 mg of sertraline in the short-term treatment of patients with OCD.

(Arch Gen Psychiatry. 1995;52:289-295)

OBSESSIVE-COMPULSIVE disorder (OCD) is a common condition[1,2] with an early onset[3] and chronic course.[4] Now recognized to be generally unresponsive to dynamic psychotherapies,[5] OCD does respond to behavior therapy[6,7] with exposure and response prevention and to pharmacological treatment (with clomipramine,[8-17] fluoxetine,[11] fluvoxamine [S.R., M. Jenike, MD, J.G., D. Robinson, MD, unpublished results, 1994],[18-21] and sertraline[22]). These potent serotonin uptake inhibitors convey benefit where agents lacking prominent serotonin uptake inhibition have not been systematically useful.[12,16,20] Sertraline is a potent and selective serotonin uptake inhibitor with established efficacy in the treatment of depression[23] and the prevention of depression relapse.[24] The neuropharmacologic specificity and the freedom from anticholinergic or cardiotoxic effects of sertraline constitute possible therapeutic advantages over clomipramine.[23]

The objective of the present study was to assess the efficacy and safety of sertraline in an 11-center, random-assignment, fixed-dose, placebo-controlled study of 325 patients with OCD. This is the largest population of patients with OCD whose treatment in a single clinical trial has been reported to date. As a fixed-dose study, the results provide valuable evidence with regard to the optimal dosing strategy for patients with OCD. Anecdotal evidence suggests that these patients are commonly treated at dosage levels that are significantly higher than those used in depressed patients. The sertraline dosage range examined in the present study, 50 to 200 mg/d, was the same as that used in the treatment of depression.

From the Dean Foundation for Health, Research, and Education, Madison, Wis (Dr Greist); Allan Memorial Institute, Montreal, Quebec (Dr Chouinard); Center for Behavioral Medicine, Denver, Colo (Dr DuBoff); Metro Health Medical Center, Jackson, Miss (Dr Halaris); Hennepin County Medical Center, Minneapolis, Minn (Dr Kim); Stanford (Calif) University School of Medicine (Dr Koran); New York State Psychiatric Institute, New York (Dr Liebowitz); Medical University of South Carolina, Charleston (Dr Lydiard); Butler Hospital, Providence, RI (Dr Rasmussen); St Elizabeth's Medical Center, Boston, Mass (Dr White); and Pfizer Inc, New York, NY (Dr Sikes).

RESULTS

DEMOGRAPHIC CHARACTERISTICS

No group differences in sex distribution, baseline weight, ethnicity, or duration of illness were found among the treatment conditions (**Table 1**). However, the pooled sertraline group was significantly older (39.6 years) than the placebo group

See Subjects and Methods on next page

SUBJECTS AND METHODS

DESIGN

A 1-week placebo lead-in period was employed to eliminate early placebo responders and to allow for washout of any prior psychotropic medications. Patients were evaluated on day 1 of the washout period; 1 week later at the end of the washout period (baseline); and at the end of 1, 2, 4, 6, 8, 10, and 12 weeks of double-blind treatment. Treatment responders (moderate or marked improvement on the Clinical Global Impression [CGI] Scale Efficacy Index at the end of week 12) were offered an additional 40 weeks of double-blind treatment; nonresponders underwent downtitration over a 2-week period, and treatment was discontinued.

Efficacy measures included the Yale-Brown Obsessive Compulsive Scale (Y-BOCS),[25,26] the National Institute of Mental Health (NIMH) Global Obsessive-Compulsive Scale,[27] and the CGI Scale.[28] These scales were completed by the investigator at baseline (the end of the single-blind placebo washout week) and at the end of weeks 1, 2, 4, 6, 8, 10, and 12. Blood for drug plasma level determinations was collected on day 1 of the washout period and after 10 weeks of double-blind therapy (or at discontinuation), 10 to 24 hours after the last dose of medication. Routine hematology, biochemistry profile, and urinalysis tests were performed on day 1 of the washout period and after 2, 6, and 10 weeks of double-blind treatment. Thyroid function was measured at the beginning of the washout period. Vital signs were obtained at each visit; a 12-lead electrocardiogram was completed on day 1 of the washout period and after 2 and 10 weeks of double-blind therapy (or at discontinuation); and a physical examination was performed during the baseline washout period and on discontinuation. All adverse experiences volunteered by the patient or observed by the investigator were recorded at each visit.

SUBJECTS

Participants were male or female outpatients, 18 years of age or older, who met the *DSM-III-R*[29] criteria for OCD and had a baseline score of 7 or more on the NIMH Scale.[27] Patients were free of significant depression, as determined by a total score of 17 or less on the 24-item Hamilton Depression Rating Scale (excluding item 21, Obsessions) at baseline and a score of 1 or less on item 1 (Depression item).

Pregnant or nursing women or women of childbearing potential not using adequate contraceptive measures were excluded, as were patients with organic mental disorders, patients with organic brain syndromes, and patients with a primary *DSM-III-R* diagnosis of major depression; bipolar disorder (depressed or atypical); schizophrenic disorder, paranoid disorder, or psychotic disorder not elsewhere classified (currently or by history); anxiety states (including panic disorder, phobic disorder, and severe generalized anxiety state); or obvious personality disorders of sufficient magnitude to interfere with the patient's ability to participate in the study. Patients who were known to have abused or to have been dependent on any drug (including alcohol) within the past 6 months were excluded. Other reasons for exclusion were medical contraindications to therapy with antidepressants; known allergy or hypersensitivity to sertraline or to other antidepressants; evidence or history of significant hepatic (liver function test results twice the upper limit of normal), hematologic, endocrine, cardiovascular, renal, gastrointestinal, or neurological disease (including childhood febrile convulsions and all forms of epilepsy); concomitant therapy with another investigational drug at study entry or within 1 month prior to entering the study; concomitant therapy with any psychotropic drug (or any drug with a psychotropic component) except chloral hydrate for sleep; behavior therapy while in the study; anticoagulant therapy; use of a monoamine oxidase inhibitor (MAOI) within 2 weeks prior to the administration of double-blind study medication; treatment with any depot neuroleptic within 6 months or any regular daily neuroleptic, anxiolytic, or antidepressant medication within 2 weeks prior to the administration of double-blind study medication.

Each site obtained study approval from its institutional review board, and written informed consent was obtained from all patients prior to participation.

DRUG ADMINISTRATION

Patients who continued to meet study entry criteria at the end of the placebo washout period were randomly assigned to treatment either with one of three fixed dosages of sertraline (50, 100, or 200 mg/d) or with placebo. All patients were instructed to take four capsules each day in a single dose with the evening meal. The study drug was packaged so that the appropriate dosage was received by each subject. Subjects receiving more than 50 mg/d underwent upward titration so that 100 mg was reached by day 5 and 200 mg by day 14.

Treatment responders who entered the 40-week continuation phase remained on their same dose of double-blind medication; nonresponders underwent titration to 0 mg/d by taking one capsule fewer every 3 days during weeks 13 and 14. Chloral hydrate, in a maximum daily dose of 1 g, was permitted on an intermittent basis if required for sleep. Patients were asked to abstain from alcohol while in the study.

DATA ANALYSIS

Treatment response was measured by the change from baseline to final value within the 12-week comparative phase of the study. During weeks 13 and 14, dosages were downtitrated to 0 mg for nonresponders, so these data points were not included. The efficacy variables, except for the CGI Improvement Scale, were analyzed by analysis of covariance, with the effects of baseline, site, and treatment in the model, and baseline as the covariate. The CGI Improvement Scale, which has no baseline, was analyzed by analysis of variance with the effects of treatment and site in the model. Since there were no significant treatment-by-site or treatment-by-baseline interactions in the end-point analyses, these interaction terms were dropped from the analyses. Between-group differences in the incidence of adverse experiences, laboratory abnormalities, and changes in vital signs were analyzed by Fisher's Exact Test or the χ^2 test.

(35.9 years) (t=2.28, df=323, P=.02). Average duration of illness since psychiatric diagnosis did not differ significantly among the four treatment groups, with means ranging from 4.6 years for placebo to 5.8 years for sertraline, 200 mg/d. There were eight nonwhites in the study, evenly distributed among the four groups. Approximately two thirds of the patients came from middle-class (Hollingshead Index III) and upper-middle-class (I and II) backgrounds.

PATIENT DISPOSITION

Three hundred twenty-five patients entered the double-blind phase of the study and received at least one dose of double-blind study medication. One patient was excluded from efficacy analyses because no on-medication efficacy ratings had been obtained. Eighty-four patients were randomized to placebo treatment and 241 to sertraline treatment (80 to 50 mg/d, 81 to 100 mg/d, and 80 to 200 mg/d). Seventy-three percent of sertraline-treated patients (79% [63/80] receiving 50 mg/d, 67% [54/81] receiving 100 mg/d, and 74% [59/80] receiving 200 mg/d) completed the 12-week comparative phase of the study, as did 71% (60/84) of placebo-treated patients. The reasons patients were dropped from the study are listed in **Table 2**. The most frequent reasons for noncompletion were insufficient clinical response (8% receiving sertraline vs 13% receiving placebo) and adverse experiences (10% receiving sertraline vs 6% receiving placebo).

Table 1. Baseline Comparison of Demographic Variables

Variable	Sertraline 50 mg/d (n=80)	Sertraline 100 mg/d (n=81)	Sertraline 200 mg/d (n=80)	Placebo (n=84)
Sex, % M	45	45	50	51
Weight, kg*	166.1 (13)	165.0 (39)	167.7 (34)	160.3 (27)
Age, y*	39.6 (13)	40.1 (12)	39.1 (13)	35.9 (13)
Duration of illness, y*	5.0 (9)	4.7 (7)	5.8 (12)	4.6 (8)

Values are mean (SD).

Table 2. Reasons for Patients Dropped From the Study

Reason	No. of Patients Dropped: Sertraline 50 mg/d (n=80)	Sertraline 100 mg/d (n=81)	Sertraline 200 mg/d (n=80)	Placebo (n=84)
Insufficient clinical response	5	7	7	11
Adverse experience	6	11	6	5
Other (relocated, pregnancy, unavailable for follow-up, noncompliant)	2	4	1	4
Intercurrent illness	1	1	4	2
Refusal to continue	2	2	2	1
Protocol violation	0	2	1	1
Administrative reasons	1	0	0	0
Total	**17**	**27**	**21**	**24**

EFFICACY

Differences for the efficacy measures at baseline between the pooled sertraline groups and the placebo group were small and neither clinically nor statistically significant (**Table 3**). As illustrated in **Figure 1** through **Figure 4**, clinical improvement was significantly greater in both the 50-mg/d (Y-BOCS, P=.007; NIMH, P=.02; CGI Severity, P=.007; and CGI Improvement, P=.01) and 200-mg/d (Y-BOCS, P=.005; NIMH, P=.005, CGI Severity, P=.05; and CGI Improvement, P=.02) sertraline dosage groups than in the placebo group on all efficacy measures; the 100-mg/d sertraline group showed significantly greater improvement than the placebo group on the NIMH Scale only (P=.03). Comparisons among the three sertraline dosage groups showed no significant differences; thus, pooled data from the three treatment groups provided the best estimate of the overall effect of sertraline. **Table 4** shows that the pooled sertraline group (n=240) exhibited significantly greater improvement than the placebo group (n=84) on all efficacy measures: Y-BOCS, P=.006; NIMH, P=.002; CGI Severity, P=.02; and CGI Improvement, P=.01. Weekly analyses revealed that greater treatment effects for sertraline were evident throughout the study, and statistically significant differences emerged either at week 2 (Y-BOCS, P=.05) or at week 4 (NIMH, P=.003; CGI Improvement, P=.009; and CGI Severity, P=.01) of double-blind treatment. The Y-BOCS score decreased a mean of 23.4% from baseline to week 12 in sertraline-treated patients compared with 14.6% in placebo-treated patients.

The general pattern of improvement in the four treatment groups is depicted in the figures, which illustrate the observed mean change in efficacy scores across the 12 weeks of treatment. On the Y-BOCS (Figure 1), all three sertraline treatment groups exhibited greater improvement from baseline than the placebo group, beginning at 1 week of double-blind treatment and continuing to the end of the study. A similar pattern of change is observed for the other outcome measures (Figures 2 through 4).

Table 3. Baseline Comparison of Efficacy Variables in Patients With Obsessive-Compulsive Disorder*

Scale†	Sertraline 50 mg/d (n=79)	Sertraline 100 mg/d (n=81)	Sertraline 200 mg/d (n=80)	Sertraline Pooled (n=240)	Placebo (n=84)	Pooled Sertraline vs Placebo: F	df	P
Y-BOCS	23.2 (5.9)	24.7 (5.6)	23.5 (4.3)	23.8 (5.3)	23.4 (4.9)	0.47	1, 312	.50
NIMH	9.2 (1.7)	9.7 (1.7)	9.1 (1.4)	9.3 (1.6)	9.2 (1.5)	0.53	1, 312	.47
CGI Severity	4.7 (0.8)	4.9 (0.8)	4.6 (0.7)	4.8 (0.8)	4.7 (0.8)	0.36	1, 312	.55

Values are group mean (SD).
†*Y-BOCS indicates Yale-Brown Obsessive-Compulsive Scale; NIMH, National Institute of Mental Health; and CGI, Clinical Global Impression.*

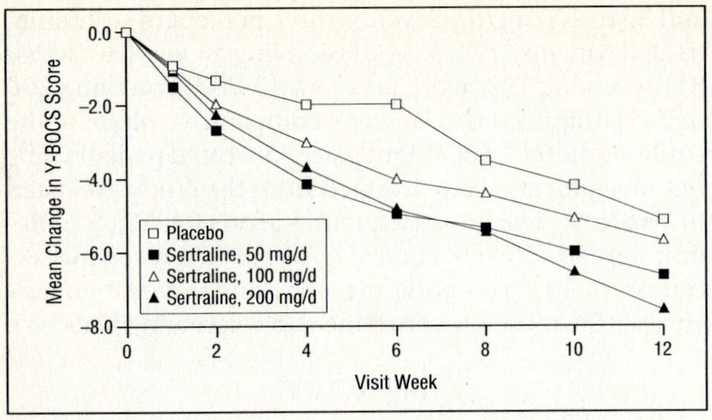

Figure 1. *Change in Yale-Brown Obsessive-Compulsive Scale (Y-BOCS) scores by visit.*

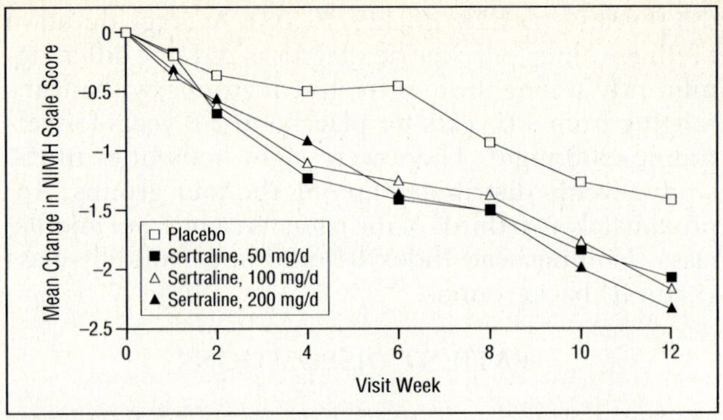

Figure 2. *Change in National Institute of Mental Health (NIMH) Global Obsessive-Compulsive Scale scores by visit.*

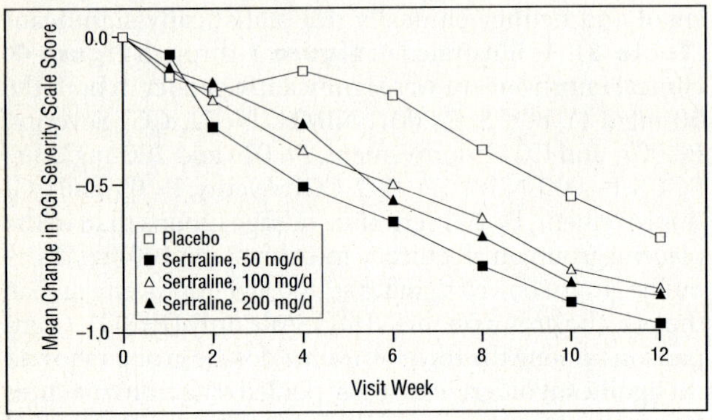

Figure 3. *Change in Clinical Global Impression (CGI) Severity Scale scores by visit.*

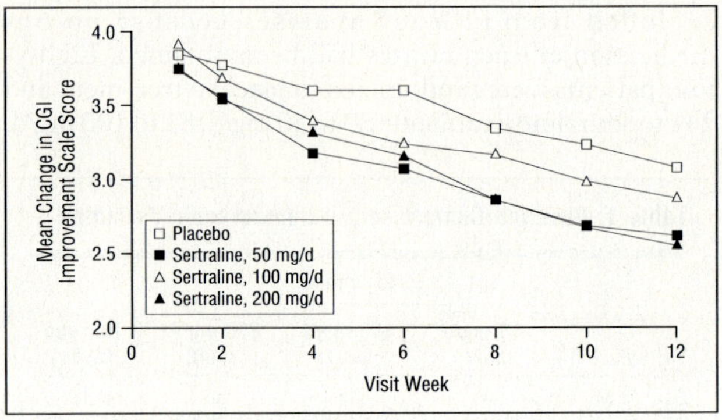

Figure 4. *Change in Clinical Global Impression (CGI) Improvement Scale scores by visit.*

When treatment response on the CGI improvement scale is defined as a rating of "much improved" or "very much improved" at end point, 38.9% of sertraline-treated patients were improved over the course of treatment, whereas 30% of the placebo-treated patients improved (**Table 5**). The main severity criterion for entry to the study was an NIMH score of 7 or more. At end point, 35.4% (85/240) of the sertraline-treated patients had scores of 6 or lower compared with 24% (20/84) of the placebo-treated patients.

Table 6 shows the mean baseline clinical rating scores for all treatment responders (ie, moderate or marked improvement on the CGI Efficacy Index) and nonresponders at week 12. Patients entering the continuation phase had significantly lower mean scores at baseline than patients not entering the continuation phase on the three investigator-rated instruments (Y-BOCS, CGI Severity, and NIMH). This effect was most pronounced in the placebo group (eg, baseline Y-BOCS score was 20.7 for placebo responders vs 24.3 for placebo nonresponders; t=3.27, df=41, P=.002), although a nonsignificant trend was observed in the sertraline treatment groups as well.

ADVERSE EXPERIENCES

All reported adverse experiences were categorized by the *World Health Organization Dictionary–Preferred Terminology*. Multiple episodes of the same complaint were counted only once but rated at the greatest level of severity. Overall, adverse experiences were reported by 77% (65/84) of patients given placebo compared with 93% (223/241) of patients receiving sertraline (Fisher's Exact Test, P<.001).

Table 7 shows the most common adverse experiences in the pooled sertraline and placebo treatment groups in order of frequency in the sertraline group. A significantly higher incidence of patients with the following adverse events was reported for sertraline than for placebo (placebo-adjusted): diarrhea (difference of 19%), insomnia (16%), decreased libido (15%), nausea (13%), anorexia (11%), ejaculation failure (8%), tremor (7%), increased sweating (7%), and increased weight (5%).

As the sertraline dosage increased, so did the number of side effects experienced at a significantly higher rate than in the placebo group. At 50 mg/d, there were three statistically significant side effects (decreased libido, diarrhea, and anorexia); at 100 mg/d, five (decreased libido, diarrhea, anorexia, nausea, and increased sweating); and at 200 mg/d, 12 (decreased libido, diarrhea, anorexia, nausea, increased sweating, insomnia, ejaculation failure, tremor, weight increase, yawning, dyspepsia, and headache). Thus, any adverse experience with an incidence significantly greater in the 50-mg/d sertraline group than in the placebo group also occurred with an incidence significantly greater in the 100-mg/d and 200-mg/d groups than in the placebo group. The majority of adverse experiences were characterized as either mild or moderate, but approximately 6% of the adverse experiences reported in both the sertraline and the placebo groups were characterized as severe.

PATIENTS DROPPED FROM THE STUDY

Twenty-seven percent of sertraline-treated patients (n=65) discontinued participation compared with 29% of placebo-treated patients (n=24). Ten percent (23/241) of patients receiving sertraline and 6% (5/84) of patients receiving placebo discontinued participation because of adverse experiences (two-tailed Fisher's Exact Test, $P=.37$). Among sertraline-treated patients, discontinuing participation because of adverse experiences did not appear to be dose dependent: 8% (6/80) in the 50-mg/d group, 14% (11/81) in the 100-mg/d group, and 8% (6/80) in the 200-mg/d group ($\chi^2=4.03$, $df=2$, $P=.13$). Two percent (6/241) of sertraline-treated patients and 2% (2/84) of placebo-treated patients (Fisher's Exact Test, $P>.99$) were dropped from the study because of intercurrent illness. Two patients receiving sertraline, 100 mg/d, were dropped for other medical reasons: one because of a laboratory abnormality (an asymptomatic drop in white blood cell count from 4.17×10^9/L at baseline to 3.09×10^9/L at the end of week 4) and one because of pregnancy. There were no statistically significant treatment effects on the number of patients dropped from the study because of adverse experiences or other medical reasons (Fisher's Exact Test, $P=.33$). Nonmedical reasons for patients dropped from the study included insufficient clinical response (8% [19/241] in the sertraline group vs 13% [11/84] in the placebo group; Fisher's Exact Test, $P=.19$), refusal to continue (3% [6/241] in the sertraline group vs 1% [1/84] in the placebo group; Fisher's Exact Test, $P=.68$), protocol violation (1% [3/241] in the sertraline group vs 1% [1/84] in the placebo group; Fisher's Exact Test, $P>.99$), and administrative reasons (0.4% [1/241] in the sertraline group vs none in the placebo group; Fisher's Exact Test, $P>.99$).

OTHER SAFETY MEASURES

Fifty-two clinically significant laboratory abnormalities were reported, 39 among 34 (14%) sertraline-treated patients and 13 among 12 (14%) placebo-treated patients. One sertraline-treated patient was dropped from the study because of a white blood cell count decrease. There were no statistically significant differences in the incidence of clinically significant laboratory abnormalities for any parameter between sertraline- and placebo-treated patients. Two patients developed clinically significant increases in alanine and aspartate aminotransferase levels, but in both cases, values returned to normal while patients continued receiving sertraline.

No serious adverse events associated with vital sign changes were seen in any subjects in the study, and none of the changes observed was clinically significant or warranted dropping patients from the study. No clinically significant treatment-emergent electrocardiographic abnormalities were recorded during the study in any patient.

The incidence of intercurrent illnesses in the sertraline and placebo groups was similar and in exact proportion to randomization; six sertraline-treated patients and two placebo-treated patients were dropped from the study because of intercurrent illness.

MONITORING OF PLASMA DRUG CONCENTRATIONS

For technical reasons, satisfactory samples were available for only 95 sertraline-treated subjects (39 receiving 50 mg/d, 25 receiving 100 mg/d, and 31 receiving 200 mg/d). Mean plasma sertraline concentrations were 59, 146, and 278 nmol/L (18.1, 44.7, and 85.3 ng/mL), respectively. Since sertraline has a terminal elimination half-life of approximately 1 day, these concentrations at week 10 may be assumed to represent steady-state values. Regression analysis indicates a linear relationship, with no significant *y*-intercept, between the dosage of sertraline administered and the plasma sertraline concentration.

No significant correlations were found between the sertraline concentration and change from baseline in Y-BOCS rating for the pooled sertraline group, for any of the three sertraline groups, for the group of responding patients only, or for the group of responding patients in any of the three sertraline groups.

Table 4. End-Point Analysis for 324 Patients With Obsessive-Compulsive Disorder

Scale*	Sertraline (n=240)	Placebo (n=84)	S†	$F_{1,31}$ for Treatment Effect	Main Effect *P*
Y-BOCS	−5.57‡	−3.41‡	6.19	7.57	.006
NIMH	−1.79‡	−1.01‡	2.01	9.45	.002
CGI Severity	−0.76‡	−0.46‡	0.98	5.82	.02
CGI Improvement	2.96§	3.34§	1.21	6.26	.01

*Y-BOCS indicates Yale-Brown Obsessive-Compulsive Scale; NIMH, National Institute of Mental Health; and CGI, Clinical Global Impression.
†The residual error term obtained from the statistical model; this can be interpreted as the pooled SD of the individual changes.
‡Mean change from baseline, adjusted for site and baseline.
§Mean, adjusted for site.

Table 5. Distribution of Clinical Global Impression Improvement Scale Scores at End Point

	Pooled Sertraline, No. (Cumulative %) of Patients	Placebo, No. (Cumulative %) of Patients
Very much improved	33 (13.9)	4 (5)
Much improved	60 (38.9)	21 (30)
Minimally improved	52 (60.4)	16 (49)
No change	76 (92.1)	31 (86)
Minimally worse	17 (99.2)	9 (96)
Much worse	1 (99.6)	3 (100)
Very much worse	1 (100.0)	0 (100)
Total	**240**	**84**

COMMENT

Patients in the pooled sertraline group showed significantly greater improvement than patients in the placebo group on all efficacy measures, based on intent-to-treat end-point analyses. Onset of therapeutic effect was detectable by week 2 for the Y-BOCS and by week 4 for the NIMH and CGI scales. Pairwise comparisons of individual sertraline dosage groups with the placebo group resulted in *P* values less than .05 on all outcome measures for the 50-mg/d and 200-mg/d groups and on the NIMH Scale only for the 100-mg/d group. The less pronounced improvement in the 100-mg/d group may be partly attributable to the greater number of patients in this group who were dropped from the study early. The largest mean treatment effect on the Y-BOCS and NIMH ratings was observed in the 200-mg/d group, although differences among sertraline treatment groups were not statistically sig-

Table 6. Baseline Comparison of Efficacy Variables for Treatment Responders* and Nonresponders at Week 12 (All Patients)

Scale†	Treatment Responders (n=118)‡	Treatment Nonresponders (n=206)‡	P	t	df
Y-BOCS	22.4 (4.9)	24.4 (5.2)	<.001	3.35	322
NIMH	8.94 (1.4)	9.46 (1.7)	.005	2.80	322
CGI Severity	4.56 (0.63)	4.83 (0.84)	.002	3.10	322
MOC	15.0 (5.0)§	15.8 (5.6)‖	.20	1.27	280

*Treatment responders are patients who were moderately or markedly improved on the Clinical Global Impression (CGI) Efficacy Index and who entered the continuation phase.

†Y-BOCS indicates Yale-Brown Obsessive-Compulsive Scale; NIMH, National Institute of Mental Health; and MOC, Maudsley Obsessive-Compulsive Inventory.

‡Values are mean (SD).

§n=103.

‖n=179.

Table 7. Adverse Experiences Occurring in 10% or More of Patients With Obsessive-Compulsive Disorder Treated With Sertraline

Adverse Experience	Sertraline Patients, %	Placebo Patients, %	Difference, Percentage Points	Fisher's Exact Test, P*
Headache	38	26	12	.06
Insomnia	34	18	16	.008
Nausea	29	16	13	.02
Diarrhea	29	10	19	<.001
Fatigue	17	13	4	.40
Dizziness	17	13	4	.49
Somnolence	15	14	1	<.99
Decreased libido	15	0	15	<.001
Dry mouth	13	11	2	.70
Anorexia	13	2	11	.005
Dyspepsia	10	6	4	.37

*NS indicates not significant.

nificant. Based on CGI Improvement ratings of "much improved" or "very much improved," 38.9% of the sertraline-treated patients were improved compared with 30% of the placebo-treated patients.

While adverse experiences were reported by 93% of patients receiving sertraline and 77% of patients given placebo, only 10% of sertraline-treated patients were dropped from the study prematurely because of adverse experiences, compared with 6% of placebo-treated patients. The number of adverse experiences with an incidence significantly greater than in the placebo group increased in a dose-dependent manner: three at 50 mg/d, five at 100 mg/d, and 12 at 200 mg/d. Most adverse experiences were characterized as mild or moderate in severity, and there was little difference in severity between treatment groups.

Analyses show that plasma sertraline levels increase with dosage, and there is dosage proportionality over the range of 50 to 200 mg/d. However, no apparent relationship between clinical improvement and plasma sertraline levels was found.

Placebo response was substantially greater than reported in some[8,19] but not all[18,30] serotonin uptake inhibitor trials in patients with OCD. In the present study, the less severely ill patients in the placebo group tended to show a better treatment response than the more severely ill patients at week 12; this in part accounts for the comparatively large placebo response in this sertraline trial. There has been a trend for greater placebo response in more recent studies compared with earlier studies. Subjects with OCD studied in recent controlled trials of pharmaceutical agents apparently differ from those who participated in early trials. Baseline Y-BOCS scores are lower (eg, 24 in this multicenter sertraline trial vs 27 in the multicenter clomipramine trial[31]), and patients with shorter durations from disorder onset have been allowed to participate in the recent trials (eg, no minimum duration in this sertraline trial vs 2 years in the clomipramine trial).

Other possible changes over time in the samples of patients with OCD participating in clinical trials are less easily quantified. Some placebo patients may be benefiting from covert behavior therapies (homework exposure and response prevention) as these effective treatment techniques have become more widely available to patients with OCD through such sources as the *Obsessive Compulsive Foundation Newsletter* and patient self-help guides.[32-35] Patients are increasingly aware of the availability of effective medications for the treatment of OCD symptoms, and this added positive expectation probably contributes to the magnitude of the placebo response. Furthermore, side effects experienced by patients in the clomipramine trials were those typical of the tricyclic antidepressants, including constipation, sedation, dry mouth, blurred vision, tremor, dizziness, and weight gain. The adverse events in the sertraline-treated patients were mainly gastrointestinal disturbances, and the predominant (>10%) adverse events in the sertraline and placebo groups were similar. This qualitative difference in side-effect profiles may have diminished the ability of patients and clinicians to predict drug or placebo conditions in the sertraline study, and patients without side effects could no longer be assumed to be receiving placebo, as in the clomipramine trial. Better blinding of patients and clinicians may have increased placebo response. Finally, patients who had failed to benefit from their participation in other trials may have viewed this as their "last chance" to improve. A shorter placebo washout period (1 week in this sertraline trial vs 2 weeks in the clomipramine trial) may also have contributed to a higher placebo response rate. The design requirement that sertraline responders be "much" or "very much" improved to enter the extension phase of the study (vs "minimally" improved in the clomipramine trial) may have added to the placebo response rate.

Clinically, it appears wise to continue with a 50-mg/d dosage of sertraline for at least 4 weeks before increasing the dosage because this small dosage was as effective as the larger dosages and produced fewer side effects. In a disorder that has been present for a decade or more, one may be tempted to push dosages to the maximum limit in a few days or weeks, overshooting an optimal level at which patients would both respond and have fewer side effects.

While studies of potent serotonin uptake–inhibiting agents have shown consistent benefit in OCD (S.R., M. Jenike, MD, J.G., D. Robinson, MD, unpublished results, 1994),[8-22] the amount of improvement is limited and the durability of response is dependent on continued medication.[36-38] Combinations of behavior therapy and serotonin uptake inhibitors have increased the amount and durability of improvement.[6,10,21] Behavior therapy alone is an effective treatment for many patients.[7] For patients with incapacitating OCD in whom treatment with serotonin uptake inhibitors and behavior therapy fail, neurosurgical treatment has sometimes proven helpful.[39]

In summary, the results of this double-blind, placebo-controlled, multicenter study indicate that sertraline, in daily dosages of 50, 100, and 200 mg/d, is safe, effective, and well tolerated in the treatment of OCD.

Accepted for publication January 23, 1995.

This research was supported by a grant from Pfizer Inc, New York, NY.

The authors have received support from Pfizer Pharmaceuticals in the form of research grants (Drs Greist, Chouinard, DuBoff, Halaris, Kim, Koran, Liebowitz, Lydiard, and Rasmussen), consultantships (Drs Greist, Chouinard, Halaris, Liebowitz, Lydiard, and Rasmussen), and lecture fees (Drs Greist, Chouinard, DuBoff, Halaris, Kim, Koran, Liebowitz, Lydiard, and Rasmussen). Dr Sikes is employed as an Associate Director for New Drug Development at the sponsor company. Pfizer Inc; as such, she has financial holdings in the company. The authors have received similar support from Bristol-Myers Squibb Co, Evansville, Ind (Dr Koran); Ciba-Geigy Corp, Summit, NJ (Drs Greist, Chouinard, DuBoff, Halaris, Kim, Liebowitz, and Rasmussen); CoCensys Inc, Irvine, Calif (Drs Greist and Rasmussen); Glaxo Inc, Research Triangle Park, NC (Dr Kim); Eli Lilly & Co, Indianapolis, Ind (Drs Greist, Chouinard, DuBoff, Halaris, Koran, Liebowitz, Lydiard, and Rasmussen); Parke-Davis, Morris Plains, NJ (Dr Lydiard); Smith-Kline Beecham Pharmaceuticals, Philadelphia, Pa (Drs DuBoff, Kim, Koran, and Liebowitz); Solvay Pharmaceuticals, Marietta, Ga (Drs Greist, Koran, and Rasmussen); and The Upjohn Co, Kalamazoo, Mich (Dr Kim), pharmaceutical companies that produce competing products. The authors own no stock in any pharmaceutical companies, except possibly through retirement programs over which they have no control.

Correspondence to Dean Foundation for Health, Research, and Education, Suite 302, 8000 Excelsior Dr, Madison, WI 53717-1914 (Dr Greist).

REFERENCES

1. Myers JK, Weissman MM, Tischler GL, Holzer CE, Leaf PJ, Orvaschel H, Anthony JC, Boyd JH, Burke JC, Kramer M, Stoltzman R. Six-month prevalence of psychiatric disorders in three sites. *Arch Gen Psychiatry.* 1984;41:959-967.
2. Karno M, Golding JM, Sorenson SB, Burnam MA. The epidemiology of obsessive-compulsive disorder in five US communities. *Arch Gen Psychiatry.* 1988;45: 1094-1099.
3. Black A. The natural history of obsessional neurosis. In: Beech HR, ed. *Obsessional States.* New York, NY: Methuen Inc; 1974:19-54.
4. Rasmussen SA, Eisen JL. Clinical and epidemiologic findings of significance to neuropharmacologic trials in OCD. *Psychopharmacol Bull.* 1988;24:466-470.
5. Malan D. *Individual Psychotherapy and the Science of Psychodynanics.* Stoneham, Mass: Butterworths-Heinemann; 1979:218-219.
6. Marks IM, Stern RS, Mawson D, Cobb J, McDonald R. Clomipramine and exposure for obsessive-compulsive rituals, I. *Br J Psychiatry.* 1980;136:1-25.
7. Christensen, H, Hadzi-Pavlovi, P, Andrews, G, Mattick, R. Behavior therapy and tricyclic medication in the treatment of obsessive-compulsive disorder. *J Consult Clin Psychol.* 1987;55:701-711.
8. The Clomipramine Collaborative Study Group. Clomipramine in the treatment of patients with obsessive-compulsive disorder. *Arch Gen Psychiatry.* 1991; 48:730-738.
9. Jenike MA, Baer L, Greist JH. Clomipramine versus fluoxetine in obsessive-compulsive disorder: a retrospective comparison of side effects and efficacy. *J Clin Psychopharmacol.* 1990;10:122-124.
10. Marks IM, Lelliott P, Basoglu M, Noshirvani H, Monteiro W, Cohen D, Kasvikis Y. Clomipramine, self-exposure and therapist-aided exposure in obsessive-compulsive rituals. *Br J Psychiatry.* 1988;152:522-534.
11. Pigott TA, Pato MT, Bernstein SE, Grover GN, Hill JL, Tolliver TJ, Murphy DL. Controlled comparisons of clomipramine and fluoxetine in the treatment of obsessive-compulsive disorder: behavioral and biological results. *Arch Gen Psychiatry.* 1990;47:926-932.
12. Leonard HL, Swedo SE, Rapoport JL, Koby EV, Lenane MC, Cheslow DL, Hamburger SD. Treatment of obsessive-compulsive disorder with clomipramine and desipramine in children and adolescents: a double-blind crossover comparison. *Arch Gen Psychiatry.* 1989;46:1088-1092.
13. Volavka J, Neziroglu F, Yaryura-Tobias JA. Clomipramine and imipramine in obsessive-compulsive disorder. *Psychiatry Res.* 1985;14:85-93.
14. Montgomery SA. Clomipramine in obsessional neurosis: a placebo-controlled trial. *Pharm Med.* 1980;1:189-192.
15. Flament MF, Rapoport JL, Berg CJ, Sceery W, Kilts C, Mellstrom B, Linnoila M. Clomipramine treatment of childhood obsessive-compulsive disorder: a double-blind controlled study. *Arch Gen Psychiatry.* 1985;42:977-983.
16. Thoren P, Asberg M, Cronholm B, Jornestedt L, Traskman L. Clomipramine treatment of obsessive-compulsive disorder, I: a controlled clinical trial. *Arch Gen Psychiatry.* 1980;37:1281-1285.
17. Insel TR, Murphy DL, Cohen RM, Alterman I, Kilts C, Linnoila M. Obsessive-compulsive disorder: a double-blind trial of clomipramine and clorgyline. *Arch Gen Psychiatry.* 1983;40:605-612.
18. Perse T, Greist JH, Jefferson JW, Rosenfeld R, Dar R. Fluvoxamine treatment for obsessive-compulsive disorder. *Am J Psychiatry.* 1987;144:1543-1548.
19. Goodman WK, Price LH, Rasmussen SA, Delgado PL, Heninger GR, Charney DS. Efficacy of fluvoxamine in obsessive-compulsive disorder: a double-blind comparison with placebo. *Arch Gen Psychiatry.* 1989;46:36-44.
20. Goodman WK, Price LH, Delgado PL, Palumbo J, Krystal JH, Nagy LM, Rasmussen SA, Heninger GR, Charney DS. Specificity of serotonin reuptake inhibitors in the treatment of obsessive-compulsive disorder: comparison of fluvoxamine and desipramine. *Arch Gen Psychiatry.* 1990;47:577-585.
21. Cottraux J, Mollard E, Bouvard M, Marks I, Sluys M, Nury AM, Douge R, Cialdella P. A controlled study of fluvoxamine and exposure in obsessive-compulsive disorder. *Int Clin Psychopharmacol.* 1990;5:17-30.
22. Chouinard G, Goodman W, Greist JH, Jenike M, Rasmussen S, White K, Hackett E, Gaffney M, Bick PA. Results of a double-blind placebo controlled trial of a new serotonin uptake inhibitor, sertraline, in the treatment of obsessive-compulsive disorder. *Psychopharmacol Bull.* 1990;26:279-284.
23. Reimherr FW, Byerley WF, Ward MF, Lebegue BJ, Wender PH. Sertraline, a selective inhibitor of serotonin uptake, for the treatment of outpatients with major depressive disorder. *Psychopharmacol Bull.* 1988;24:200-205.
24. Doogan DP, Caillard V. Sertraline in the prevention of depression. *Br J Psychiatry.* 1992;160:217-222.
25. Goodman WK, Price LH, Rasmussen SA, Mazure C, Fleischmann RL, Hill CL, Heninger GR, Charney DS. The Yale-Brown Obsessive-Compulsive Scale, I: development, use, and reliability. *Arch Gen Psychiatry.* 1989;46:1006-1011.
26. Goodman WK, Price LH, Rasmussen SA, Mazure C, Delgado P, Heninger GR, Charney DS. The Yale-Brown Obsessive-Compulsive Scale, II: validity. *Arch Gen Psychiatry.* 1989;46:1012-1016.
27. Murphy DL, Pickar D, Alterman IS. Methods for the quantitative assessment of depressive and manic behavior. In: Burdock EI, Sudilovsky A, Gershon S, eds. *The Behavior of Psychiatric Patients.* New York, NY: Marcel Dekker Inc; 1982:355-391.
28. Guy W. *ECDEU Assessment Manual for Psychopharmacology.* Washington, DC: US Dept of Health and Human Services; 1987. Publication ABM 76-338.
29. American Psychiatric Association. *Diagnostic and Statistical Manual of Mental Disorders, Revised Third Edition.* Washington, DC: American Psychiatric Association; 1987.
30. Riddle MA, Scahill L, King RA, Hardin MT, Anderson GM, Ort SI, Smith JC, Leckman JF, Cohen DJ. Double-blind, crossover trial of fluoxetine and placebo in children and adolescents with obsessive-compulsive disorder. *J Am Acad Child Adolesc Psychiatry.* 1992;31:1062-1069.
31. The Clomipramine Collaborative Study Group. Clomipramine in the treatment of patients with obsessive-compulsive disorder. *Arch Gen Psychiatry.* 1991; 48:730-738.
32. Greist JH, Jefferson JW, Marks IM. *Anxiety and Its Treatment: Help Is Available.* Washington, DC: American Psychiatric Press; 1986.
33. Marks IM. *Living With Fear.* New York, NY: McGraw-Hill International Book Co; 1978.
34. Baer L. *Getting Control.* Boston, Mass: Little Brown & Co Inc; 1991.
35. Foa EB, Wilson R. *Stop Obsessing: How to Overcome Your Obsessions and Compulsions.* New York, NY: Bantam Books; 1991.
36. Pato MT, Zohar-Kadouch R, Zohar J, Murphy DL. Returns of symptoms after discontinuation of clomiprarnine in patients with obsessive-compulsive disorder. *Am J Psychiatry.* 1988;145:1521-1525.
37. Pato MT, Murphy DL, DeVane CL. Sustained plasma concentrations of fluoxetine and/or norfluoxetine 4 and 8 weeks after fluoxetine discontinuation. *J Clin Psychopharmacol.* 1991;11:224-225.
38. Leonard HL, Swedo SE, Lenone MC, Rettew DC, Cheslow DL, Hamburger SO, Rapport JL. A double-blind desipramine substitution during long-term clomipramine treatment in children and adolescents with obsessive-compulsive disorder. *Arch Gen Psychiatry.* 1991;48:922-926.
39. Mindus P. Neurosurgical treatment of malignant obsessive compulsive disorder. *Psychiatr Clin North Am.* 1992;15:921-938.

ORIGINAL ARTICLE

Schizotypal Symptoms and Signs in the Roscommon Family Study

Their Factor Structure and Familial Relationship With Psychotic and Affective Disorders

Kenneth S. Kendler, MD; Mary McGuire, MB, MRCPsych; Alan M. Gruenberg, MD; Dermot Walsh, MB, FRCPI

Background: Although schizotypal personality disorder aggregates in relatives of schizophrenic probands, the criteria for this disorder may not be optimal either in describing the dimensions of schizotypal phenomena or in identifying those with a high familial liability to schizophrenia.

Methods: In the Roscommon Family Study, an epidemiologically based family study of major psychiatric disorders conducted in the west of Ireland, we examined 25 individual schizotypal symptoms and signs, assessed by structured personal interview, in 1544 first-degree relatives (without chronic psychosis or mental retardation) of five proband groups: schizophrenia; other nonaffective psychoses; psychotic affective illness; nonpsychotic affective illness; and matched, unscreened controls.

Results: We obtained seven meaningful schizotypal factors: negative schizotypy, positive schizotypy, borderline symptoms, social dysfunction, avoidant symptoms, odd speech, and suspicious behavior. Taken individually, all of these factors, except borderline symptoms, significantly discriminated relatives of schizophrenic probands from relatives of controls; in descending order of the odds ratios, they were odd speech, social dysfunction, suspicious behavior, negative schizotypy, avoidant symptoms, and positive schizotypy. In a multivariate analysis, four of these factors remained significant: odd speech, negative symptoms, social dysfunction, and avoidant symptoms. These schizotypal factors differed in their specificity. Three of the four most predictive schizotypal factors also significantly discriminated relatives of probands with other nonaffective psychoses from relatives of controls.

Conclusion: "Schizotypy" is a complex, multidimensional clinical construct, whose various dimensions differ widely both in the degree and specificity with which they reflect the familial liability to schizophrenia. Subpsychotic thought disorder; negative schizotypal signs, such as poor rapport and odd behavior; deficient occupational functioning; and social isolation/avoidance best characterized relatives of schizophrenic probands compared with relatives of matched controls.

(Arch Gen Psychiatry. 1995;52:296-303)

From the Departments of Psychiatry and Human Genetics, Medical College of Virginia/Virginia Commonwealth University, Richmond (Dr Kendler); St Patrick's Hospital and the Western Health Board, Castlerea, Ireland (Dr McGuire); Dave Garroway Laboratory for the Study of Depression, Pennsylvania Hospital, and Department of Psychiatry, University of Pennsylvania School of Medicine, Philadelphia (Dr Gruenberg); and The Health Research Board and St Loman's Hospital, Dublin, Ireland (Dr Walsh).

Clinicians and researchers have long noted that some close relatives of patients with schizophrenia, though never psychotic, displayed symptoms and signs reminiscent of schizophrenia.[1-5] Increasingly, rigorous attempts have recently been made to document this observation and to accurately define this "schizophrenia-like" personality, herein called schizotypy.[6]

In 1979, Spitzer et al[7] proposed a new diagnostic category, "schizotypal personality disorder" (SPD). The criteria were developed from interviews with relatives from the Danish Adoption Study of Schizophrenia[8] who were diagnosed as having borderline or uncertain schizophrenia.[7] These interviews were rereviewed and 17 possible schizotypal clinical features were identified, the eight most common of which were then incorporated into the SPD diagnosis in *DSM-III*.[7,9] One more criterion (odd or eccentric behavior) was added in *DSM-III-R*,[10] with little additional change in *DSM-IV*.[11]

Clinicians and researchers have debated about the structure of schizotypy—whether it represents one or several psychopathologic dimensions. Several authors have suggested a two-dimensional construct, termed *positive* and *negative*[12] or *cognitive-perceptual* and *social-interpersonal*.[3] Large-scale multivariate studies of schizotypy have, to our knowledge, only

See Methods on next page

METHODS

SAMPLE

The Roscommon Family Study, an epidemiologic family study of major mental illness, was based in a rural county in western Ireland.[25] Three proband groups were ascertained: (1) "schizophrenic"—all cases with a diagnosis of schizophrenia from the Roscommon County Case Register[26] (n=303); (2) "affective"—a randomly chosen 75% subsample of cases from the register with a diagnosis of major affective disorder (n=99); and (3) control—age- and sex-matched controls chosen from the electoral registry (n=150). We attempted to personally and blindly interview all probands and their first-degree relatives aged 16 years and older residing in Ireland, Northern Ireland, and central and eastern England. All available psychiatric hospital records for probands and relatives were obtained and abstracted.

While an adaptation of the Structured Clinical Interview for *DSM-III-R*[27] diagnoses was used for the Axis I conditions in probands and relatives, the interview-based assessment for Axis II disorders was performed using versions 1.0 or 1.1 of the Structured Interview for Schizotypy (SIS).[28] The SIS was designed to assess those schizotypal symptoms and signs considered to be both potentially relevant in identifying the deviant but nonpsychotic relatives of individuals with schizophrenia and practical to collect in a rural, traditional Catholic population. By "symptoms," we mean items evaluated by respondent report. By "signs," we mean items based on interviewer's observation of respondent behavior. Version 1.1 contained 14 schizotypal symptoms and 11 schizotypal signs (**Table 1**). Symptoms were scored on four- or five-point scales by trained interviewers on the basis of responses to semistructured interview questions. Signs were all scored on a scale of 1 to 4 (not present, mild, moderate, marked). Interrater reliability of these symptoms and signs was assessed by 100 joint interviews. Adequate variance was available to meaningfully assess reliability for 22 of the items by intraclass correlation,[29] which ranged from +0.41 (for anxiety) to +0.88 (for ideas of reference) with a mean (±SD) of +0.76±0.13 (Table 1). Reliability was higher for schizotypal symptoms (n=13, +0.82±0.06) than for signs (n=9, +0.68±0.16). Blind, best-estimate diagnoses were made by one of us (K.S.K. or A.M.G.) for probands and relatives using all available information with personal interviews and/or hospital records using *DSM-III-R* criteria[10] with high interrater reliability.[25,30,31]

As outlined previously,[25] a number of individuals and families in the Roscommon Family Study were ascertained more than once. To obtain the correct risk in relatives, we used the "general proband method" in which all individuals are counted once for each time they were independently ascertained.[32] All counts of relatives in this report refer to numbers of ascertained relatives.

In this study, we examined the interviewed relatives of four proband groups selected from the original patient probands and the relatives of the original control probands. The four proband groups, defined hierarchically, are schizophrenia, ONAP (including schizoaffective, schizophreniform or delusional disorder, or psychosis not otherwise specified), PAI, and NPAI. Of the 1753 personally interviewed relatives (85.8% of all living and traceable relatives of probands), 10 were eliminated because they were missing all relevant data and 124 were eliminated (from all but the factor analyses) because the proband to whom they were related did not belong to one of the five specified groups. In addition, we excluded from all analyses relatives with a diagnosis of schizophrenia (n=41), schizoaffective disorder (n=19), or mental retardation (n=15). Relatives with schizophrenia and schizoaffective disorder were excluded because with these disorders it is difficult to determine whether schizotypal symptoms and/or signs reflect personality or the sequelae of the illness. Exclusion of these relatives is conservative in that we thereby eliminate individuals with a high liability to schizophrenia, whom we already know are more common in relatives of schizophrenia spectrum vs control probands.[25,33] Relatives with mental retardation were excluded because it was sometimes difficult to discriminate whether schizotypal signs reflected personality or mental retardation.

Total sample sizes of the relatives by proband group used in this report (along with, respectively, the number eliminated from analysis because of the diagnosis of schizophrenia or schizoaffective disorder and mental retardation) were as follows: schizophrenia, 314 (23, 4); ONAP, 268 (14, 2); PAI, 204 (14, 2); NPAI, 183 (4, 6); and control, 575 (5, 1). A total of 1272 relatives had complete data on *all* 25 schizotypal symptoms and signs and served as the sample for factor analysis.

Continued on next page

used self-report questionnaires, which may sample only a limited range of schizotypal phenomena. Nonetheless, these studies demonstrate multiple dimensions of schizotypy.[13-17]

If schizotypy is multidimensional, it is important to understand how different schizotypal dimensions relate to the familial liability to schizophrenia. For example, negative or social-interpersonal schizotypy may reflect the familial vulnerability to schizophrenia more closely than positive or cognitive-perceptual schizotypy.[3,18] We are aware of four studies[18-21] examining the prevalence of individual schizotypal symptoms and signs in relatives of schizophrenic vs control probands. All four found wide differences among signs and symptoms in their ability to differentiate the two groups of relatives.

Nearly all family studies have examined schizotypy only in relatives of schizophrenic vs control probands.[22] We are aware of three studies[20,23,24] that have also examined the diagnosis of SPD in relatives of probands with affective illness. Of these, one[20] found evidence for elevated rates of SPD in relatives of probands with affective disorder, while two did not.[23,24] Overall, we know relatively little about the specificity of the dimensions of schizotypal traits. Do the individual schizotypal dimensions reflect the familial vulnerability specifically to schizophrenia or more broadly to all nonaffective psychosis? Might some dimensions of schizotypy be nonspecific, reflecting the predisposition to all forms of psychosis or even to all forms of major mental illness?

STATISTICAL ANALYSIS

Orthogonal and oblique factor analyses were conducted using the VARIMAX and PROMAX routines in SAS[34] applied to a Pearson product-moment correlation matrix of the 25 schizotypal symptoms and signs. The number of factors extracted was chosen using eigenvalue criterion of 1.00 or greater. Because of the nonnormal distributions of most schizotypal symptoms and signs, the results of the factor analyses are only approximate, although adequate for our goal of constructing factor-derived scales. We examined a polychoric correlation matrix to assess the stability of the factor solutions obtained, but the endorsement frequency of several items was too low to obtain stable estimates.

On the basis of the VARIMAX analysis, factor-derived scales were formed by assigning each item to the factor on which it loaded most strongly. In the formation of factor-derived scale scores for individuals, we took the following steps. First, individuals missing more than 50% of the items were excluded from analysis. This occurred in fewer than 2% of the sample for six of the seven factors. However, no borderline symptoms were included in SIS version 1.0, so analyses with this factor required the exclusion of 24% of the sample. Second, for 13.7% of the remaining person-scale scores, the respondent answered 50% or more but fewer than 100% of all the scale items. For these individuals, we imputed missing values from the standardized scores on the items to which they responded. Third, because the scales differed in the number of items, for these imputed scores, as well as for the remaining 86.3% of the person-scale scores that contained complete data, we divided the total scale score by the number of items to obtain a mean item score that would be directly comparable across all scales.

Because both individual items and factor-derived scales were significantly predicted by gender, age, and the relationship of the relative to the proband, we controlled for these covariates in all major analyses. Schizotypal symptoms were ordinal variables with a highly skewed distribution so that parametric approaches were inappropriate.

The conventional approach to analysis would be to predict schizotypy in relatives from the proband's diagnosis. However, in most research contexts, investigators use schizotypal symptoms and signs to *infer* familial/genetic loading for schizophrenia. Therefore, we employed logistic regression, as operationalized in the LOGISTIC procedure in SAS[34] to predict the diagnostic group of the proband from the schizotypal factor scores of the relatives. We examined two groups of relatives at a time, first comparing relatives of schizophrenic and control probands. This analytic approach yields a useful odds ratio (OR) estimate. When comparing relatives of schizophrenic and control probands, this OR reflects the increasing odds that the relative is related to a schizophrenic proband (rather than a control proband) for each unit increase in the average schizotypal symptom score. Thus, an OR of 2 means that for an increase of one unit of the mean scale score, the odds that that relative was related to a schizophrenic vs control proband increases twofold. Since being related to a schizophrenic vs control proband is a proxy for a high familial/genetic vulnerability to schizophrenia, this OR can be seen as reflecting the degree of association between the schizotypal symptom and the familial liability to schizophrenia. Because of concerns about the possible effect of including covariates, we repeated these analyses using a simple χ^2 test, where each individual's average factor score was rounded to the nearest integer. These results were very similar to those obtained by logistic regression.

Because schizotypal factors are likely to be intercorrelated, we investigated the *unique* predictive power of each factor by a stepwise logistic regression,[34] using an entry and exit criterion of 0.10. Stepwise multivariate logistic regression has been shown to compare favorably with a stepwise discriminant analysis in the selection of variables.[35] Stepwise regression excludes subjects who are missing data on any variable. The initial stepwise regression therefore lost over 20% of the sample who were not assessed for borderline symptoms. If borderline symptoms were not included in the final solution in these initial analyses, we repeated the stepwise regression excluding that factor, thereby maximizing our sample size and statistical power.

To test the specificity of schizotypal factors, we examined their ability to identify relatives of control probands vs relatives of probands with ONAP, PAI, or NPAI. Finally, we performed two additional tests. As another, more rigorous, test of specificity, we examined the ability of these individual schizotypal factors to differentiate between relatives of schizophrenic probands and relatives of probands with NPAI and relatives of probands with PAI.

P values are reported two tailed, with statistical significance restricted to *P* values of .05 or less and .10 or less in the univariate and multivariate analyses, respectively.

In this report, we empirically evaluate a broadly defined diagnostic construct of schizotypy in the Roscommon Family Study,[25] addressing three questions: (1) What is the structure of schizotypy as assessed at personal interview in a large nonclinical sample of relatives? (2) Given that schizotypy is multidimensional, do the individual schizotypal factors differ in their ability to identify relatives of schizophrenic vs control probands? And, taken together, what combination of factors optimally differentiates the relatives of schizophrenic probands? and (3) When examined in relatives of probands with other nonaffective psychoses (ONAP) and psychotic (PAI) and nonpsychotic affective illness (NPAI), do the individual schizotypal dimensions differ in the specificity with which they reflect the familial liability to schizophrenia, psychosis, or major mental illness?

RESULTS

FACTOR ANALYSIS

A factor analysis of the 25 assessed schizotypal symptoms and signs identified seven factors accounting for 53.7% of the total variance (Table 1). After VARIMAX rotation, these factors were readily interpretable as negative schizotypy, positive schizotypy, borderline symptoms, social dysfunction, avoidant symptoms, odd speech, and suspicious behavior. An oblique rotation, performed using PROMAX, yielded an identical factor pattern and very similar factor loadings. Of

Table 1. Factor Loadings From a VARIMAX Factor Analysis of 25 Schizotypal Symptoms and Signs in 1272 Relatives, With Complete Information, From the Roscommon Family Study*

Schizotypal Item	Interrater Intraclass Correlation	Negative Schizotypy	Positive Schizotypy	Borderline Symptoms	Social Dysfunction	Avoidant Symptoms	Odd Speech	Suspicious Behavior
Poor rapport†	.46	**87**	−3	0	4	9	9	10
Aloofness/coldness†	.60	**86**	0	2	5	6	−2	12
Guardedness†	.71	**61**	10	−2	3	1	1	46
Odd behavior†	.77	**54**	10	−10	23	19	27	−8
Illusions	.87	−2	**73**	−1	1	1	−2	−1
Ideas of reference	.88	2	**64**	7	9	28	0	9
Magical thinking	.80	6	**63**	14	−2	13	15	2
Depersonalization	.87	7	**50**	15	16	−22	−9	−23
Suspiciousness	.80	9	**47**	23	−4	30	−2	19
Recurrent suicidal threats	‡	−15	**35**	24	3	15	13	16
Inappropriate anger	.81	−6	−1	**70**	−2	3	3	11
Affective instability	.80	0	20	**61**	11	18	0	3
Jealousy	.87	4	2	**56**	0	10	−4	−6
Impulsivity	.76	−5	26	**53**	8	−21	−7	−4
Chronic boredom	.67	4	30	**40**	2	24	8	24
General lack of motivation†§	.76	10	7	4	**89**	9	5	1
Occupation functioning below expected†‖	.78	8	4	9	**87**	7	3	14
Social isolation	.88	9	6	−7	13	**68**	16	6
Social anxiety	.87	6	20	22	2	**64**	−11	−11
Hypersensitivity	.81	4	18	35	−10	**55**	−8	−10
Anxiety†	.41	11	4	−1	23	**37**	1	21
Cognitive slippage†	‡	5	−3	1	7	0	**84**	−3
Odd speech†	.83	11	12	−3	−1	1	**83**	5
Hypervigilance†	‡	4	13	−6	27	7	−3	**75**
Irritability†	.81	31	−5	17	−9	−7	5	**66**
Variance, %	. . .	9.5	9.1	8.0	7.4	7.2	6.4	6.1

*From the Structured Interview for Schizotypy.[28] Highest factor loading for each item is in boldface.
†Schizotypal sign; otherwise item is a self-report symptom.
‡Insufficient variation to calculate being rated as present by either rater on three or fewer of the 100 interviews.
§General lack of motivation for occupational, educational, and social endeavors.
‖Given educational and social background and not resulting from physical illness or overall economic conditions over which the person has no control.

the 21 interfactor correlations, 19 were small (−0.10 to +0.20). Positive schizotypy was modestly correlated with borderline (+0.34) and avoidant symptoms (+0.29).

Individual items from the SIS could, with rare exception, be unambiguously assigned to one factor, thereby creating seven factor-derived scales. All items assigned to the seven scales had apparent face validity with two exceptions—neither suicidal threats nor suspiciousness would probably have, a priori, been considered positive schizotypal symptoms.

Of these seven factor-derived scales, four (negative schizotypy, social dysfunction, odd speech, and suspicious behavior) consisted entirely of signs, two (positive schizotypy and borderline symptoms) consisted entirely of symptoms, and one (avoidant symptoms) contained both signs and symptoms.

DISCRIMINATING RELATIVES OF SCHIZOPHRENIC VS CONTROL PROBANDS

Factor-Derived Scales, Taken One at a Time, Predicting Proband Diagnosis in Relatives of Schizophrenic vs Control Probands

Table 2 presents the mean (±SEM) standardized score on each of the seven schizotypal factors and the proportion of relatives rated at least mild on one or more items for relatives of our five proband classes. Three of the factors (positive schizotypy, borderline features, and avoidant symptoms) were commonly endorsed. Negative schizotypy was intermediate in frequency, and social dysfunction, odd speech, and suspicious behavior were considerably rarer.

We began by examining the ability of scores on each of the seven schizotypal factor-derived scales to predict whether a relative was related to a schizophrenic or a control proband. We report two measures of this relationship: the OR, reflecting the magnitude of the association, and the χ^2 test (all with df=1), which reflects both the magnitude of the association *and* the frequency of the schizotypal symptoms. Only the level of borderline symptoms did not significantly distinguish relatives of schizophrenic probands from relatives of control probands (**Table 3**, leftmost column) (OR=0.86; χ^2=0.31, P=.58). In descending order of OR, a proband diagnosis of schizophrenia was most strongly predicted by the level of odd speech (OR=5.69; χ^2=8.91, P=.003), social dysfunction (OR=3.40; χ^2=11.21, P=.0008), negative schizotypy (OR=3.08; χ^2=30.18, P=.0000), suspicious behavior (OR=2.47; χ^2=8.40, P=.004), positive schizotypy (OR=1.93; χ^2=7.96, P=.005), and avoidant symptoms (OR=1.62; χ^2=13.12, P=.0003).

Although odd speech more highly discriminated relatives of schizophrenic vs control probands (as reflected by

Table 2. Scores* for Relatives and Percentage of Relatives Scoring at Least Mild on One or More Items on the Seven Factor-Derived Schizotypy Scales by Proband Diagnosis

	Score, Mean±SEM (% >1.00)				
Schizotypy Scale	Schizophrenia	Other Nonaffective Psychoses	Psychotic Affective Illness	Nonpsychotic Affective Illness	Control
Negative schizotypy	1.28±0.03 (36.4)	1.23±0.03 (35.1)	1.22±0.03 (32.4)	1.16±0.02 (25.8)	1.11±0.01 (19.3)
Positive schizotypy	1.30±0.02 (70.2)	1.24±0.02 (63.0)	1.24±0.02 (58.2)	1.28±0.03 (68.5)	1.25±0.01 (65.3)
Borderline features	1.22±0.02 (55.6)	1.31±0.03 (64.1)	1.24±0.02 (54.6)	1.26±0.02 (65.0)	1.28±0.02 (60.5)
Social dysfunction	1.09±0.02 (7.4)	1.10±0.02 (8.6)	1.05±0.02 (5.4)	1.03±0.01 (3.8)	1.02±0.01 (1.6)
Avoidant symptoms	1.63±0.04 (80.0)	1.54±0.03 (75.9)	1.47±0.04 (67.0)	1.48±0.04 (76.1)	1.48±0.02 (71.8)
Odd speech	1.05±0.01 (6.7)	1.05±0.01 (6.7)	1.05±0.01 (6.4)	1.05±0.02 (3.8)	1.01±0.01 (1.6)
Suspicious behavior	1.10±0.02 (10.5)	1.06±0.01 (7.8)	1.04±0.01 (5.4)	1.02±0.01 (3.8)	1.03±0.01 (3.5)

**Scores are standardized, so the mean varies from 1 to 4. A score of 1.00 means the individual was given a rating of absent for all scale items.*

the high OR), negative schizotypy was much more statistically significant as a predictor of proband status. As seen in Table 2, this pattern of results stems from large differences in the baseline frequency of the individual schizotypal factors. While 36.4% of relatives of schizophrenics vs 19.3% of relatives of controls were rated at least mild on one or more negative schizotypal item, the parallel figures for odd speech were 6.7% and 1.6%.

Stepwise Analysis of the Factor-Derived Scales

In the initial stepwise logistic regression analysis on the reduced sample, borderline symptoms were not predictive of proband status and were not included in the final best model. Therefore, to maximize sample size, these analyses were repeated on the entire sample using only the remaining six schizotypal factor-derived scales. These multivariate analyses found that four of these factor-derived scales continued to predict proband diagnosis, which, in order of their retention, were as follows: negative schizotypy (OR=2.35; χ^2=14.61, *df*=1, *P*=.0001), social dysfunction (OR=2.21; χ^2=4.23, *df*=1, *P*=.04), avoidant symptoms (OR=1.33; χ^2=3.99, *df*=1, *P*=.05), and odd speech (OR=3.14; χ^2=3.40, *df*=1, *P*=.07). In the presence of these four factors, neither positive schizotypy nor suspicious behavior significantly predicted proband diagnosis.

Specificity of Relationship of Factor-Derived Scales in Relatives to Diagnosis in Proband

In addition to reporting our results for schizophrenic vs control probands, Table 3 also outlines the association between the individual schizotypal scales and proband diagnosis. When comparing relatives of control probands with relatives of probands with ONAP, PAI, and NPAI, four basic patterns are seen. First, positive symptom schizotypy, avoidant symptoms, and suspicious behavior did not significantly distinguish relatives of ONAP, PAI, or NPAI probands from relatives of controls. Second, social dysfunction significantly differentiated relatives of controls from relatives of probands with ONAP but not from relatives of PAI or NPAI probands. Third, both negative schizotypy and odd speech distinguished relatives of probands with ONAP or PAI from relatives of controls. In addition, at a marginal level of significance (χ^2=3.88, *df*=1, *P*=.05), odd speech was the only schizotypal factor to distinguish relatives of NPAI probands from relatives of controls. Finally, borderline symptoms did not differentiate relatives from any of the ill proband groups from relatives of controls.

Another rigorous test of specificity was to predict proband diagnosis from schizotypal factors in relatives of schizophrenic probands compared with relatives of probands with NPAI. Relatives of NPAI probands were chosen because, although they lacked a familial predisposition to schizophrenia or psychosis, they had an elevated familial liability to affective illness, another major psychiatric disorder. Scores on three schizotypal factors significantly predicted whether a relative was related to a schizophrenic vs an NPAI proband: negative schizotypy (OR=1.86; χ^2=5.23, *P*=.02), avoidant symptoms (OR=1.90; χ^2=10.28, *P*=.001), and suspicious behavior (OR=4.86; χ^2=5.37, *P*=.02).

Finally, to attempt to further separate schizotypal features associated with schizophrenia specifically vs psychosis more generally, we examined the ability of schizotypal factors to predict proband diagnosis in relatives of schizophrenic probands compared with relatives of probands with PAI. While only one symptom factor distinguished between these two groups of relatives at traditional levels of significance (avoidant symptoms: OR=1.54; χ^2=6.41, *P*=.01), two further symptoms produced suggestive results (suspicious behavior: OR=2.24; χ^2=3.58, *P*=.06, and negative schizotypy: OR=1.46; χ^2=2.96, *P*=.09).

COMMENT

THE STRUCTURE OF SCHIZOTYPY

The historical literature contains a large number of symptoms and signs that have been considered reflections of schizotypy.[4] Several previous investigators have suggested that schizotypy is not a unitary construct, but incorporated at least two separate psychopathologic dimensions.[3,12] A number of studies that administered self-report questionnaires designed to measure schizotypy[13-17] have repeatedly found evidence for more than one factor. We know of only one study[12] that examined the factor structure of schizotypy as assessed by face-to-face interview. In a small sample study of twins from a population-based registry assessed with the SIS,[28] factor analysis yielded two factors reflecting positive and negative symptom schizotypy.[12]

Table 3. Odds Ratios of Factor-Derived Schizotypal Scales for Identifying Relatives of Probands With Schizophrenia, Other Nonaffective Psychoses, Psychotic Affective Illness, and Nonpsychotic Affective Illness vs Relatives of Controls

Schizotypy Scale	Odds Ratio of Proband Diagnosis			
	Schizophrenia	Other Nonaffective Psychoses	Psychotic Affective Illness	Nonpsychotic Affective Illness
Negative schizotypy	3.08*	2.39*	2.15†	1.58
Positive schizotypy	1.93†	1.00	0.90	1.15
Borderline symptoms	0.86	1.53	0.86	0.77
Social dysfunction	3.40‡	4.02‡	2.32	1.58
Avoidant symptoms	1.62‡	1.28	0.92	0.96
Odd speech	5.69†	6.50†	5.53†	3.18§
Suspicious behavior	2.47†	1.71	0.93	0.53

*$P \leq .0001$.
†$P \leq .01$.
‡$P \leq .001$.
§$P \leq .05$.

In the report herein, which used a large, epidemiologically ascertained sample of relatives, including a subset with a high familial liability to schizophrenia, we found the structure of schizotypy to be more complex than previously suggested. Orthogonal factor analysis revealed seven distinct and readily interpretable factors.

While initially skeptical of this complex structure, two sets of findings supported this interpretation. First, the same factor structure was obtained by oblique rotation with low interfactor correlations, suggesting the existence of seven relatively independent symptom dimensions. Second, these symptom dimensions differed meaningfully in their distribution in relatives of the various proband classes.

In this factor analysis, schizotypal symptoms and schizotypal signs formed nearly independent groupings. Six of the seven factors consisted entirely of either symptoms or signs. Only the factor reflecting avoidant traits included three symptoms (social isolation, social anxiety, and hypersensitivity) and one sign (anxiety, as rated on interview). These results suggest that schizotypal symptoms and signs may reflect fundamentally different psychopathologic domains. This result, consistent with our previous small-sample study,[12] suggests that attempts to measure schizotypy by self-report questionnaire (of necessity limited to the symptoms) may have significant inherent limitations.

SCHIZOTYPAL FACTORS IN RELATIVES OF SCHIZOPHRENIC VS CONTROL PROBANDS

Univariate Analyses

The original descriptions of schizotypy were attempts to characterize the deviant but nonpsychotic relatives of schizophrenic patients.[4] Therefore, given our schizotypal factors, a key question is the degree to which these factors reflect the underlying familial vulnerability to schizophrenia. We assessed this by determining the ability of factor scores in a relative to predict whether that relative was related to a schizophrenic vs a control proband. Initially, we analyzed one schizotypal factor-derived scale at a time.

As indices of the familial liability to schizophrenia, the seven schizotypal factors differed widely. Features of borderline personality disorder in the SIS did not predict proband diagnosis. Congruent with other family, twin, and adoption studies that have addressed this question,[23,36-40] our results suggest no familial relationship between borderline personality traits and schizophrenia. (Of note, the borderline symptoms in the SIS, in forming a relatively discrete factor, supported prior evidence for the distinction between "borderline" and "schizotypal" symptoms.[7])

Of the remaining six factors, three (odd speech, social dysfunction, and negative schizotypy) strongly distinguished relatives of schizophrenic probands from relatives of control probands, while three (suspicious behavior, positive schizotypy, and avoidant symptoms) were weaker, but still significant discriminators. We are aware of four previous studies[18-21] with which our results can be compared. Symptoms indicative of negative schizotypy, as defined herein, were found to significantly characterize relatives of schizophrenics in all four reports: "poor rapport,"[18] "eccentricity and detachment,"[19] "inappropriate affect and odd behavior,"[20] and "negative symptoms."[21] Both studies that specifically examined odd speech found that it was significantly more common in the relatives of schizophrenic vs control probands.[18,20] Only one study specifically examined "social adaptation" and found it to be one of the most powerful discriminators of their borderline schizophrenic cases.[19] Suspiciousness and avoidant symptoms were explicitly examined in only two studies.[18,20] Suspiciousness was substantially more common in relatives of schizophrenic probands in both, reaching statistical significance in one[18] and at the trend level in the other.[20] In one study,[20] the avoidant symptoms of social isolation and social anxiety did not distinguish relatives of schizophrenic and control probands. In the other,[18] social isolation was significantly more common in relatives of schizophrenic probands, while social anxiety was not.

Positive schizotypal symptoms did not strongly distinguish relatives of schizophrenic probands in these studies. Two studies[18,20] examined the three core positive schizotypal symptoms of magical thinking, ideas of reference, and illusions. In one study,[18] none of these symptoms significantly differentiated relatives of schizophrenic probands, while in the other[20] only illusions did. In another[19] of the studies, psychoticlike cognitive and perceptual symptoms did not identify borderline schizophrenic cases. Finally, the fourth study[21] found that the rates of subclinical levels of positive psychotic symptoms were similar in relatives of schizophrenic and depressed probands.

Although the previous studies of this question all had significant methodologic problems, including small sample size,[19-21] absence of a normal control group,[21] and lack of an assessment instrument focused on schizotypal symptoms,[18,20,21] a reasonably consistent picture emerges. The three schizotypal factors that strongly identified relatives of schizophrenic probands in this study (negative symptoms, odd speech, and social dysfunction), when examined, consistently performed similarly in previous studies. The three schizotypal factors that were weaker discriminators of relatives of schizophrenics in the Roscommon Family Study (suspicious behavior, positive schizotypy, and avoidant symptoms) also produced less consistent findings in the preceding studies.

Multivariate Stepwise Analyses

The individual schizotypal factors identified in this study were, on average, weakly and positively correlated with one another. It is therefore of interest to control for the effect of the other schizotypal factors by a stepwise regression, thereby examining each factor's *unique* relationship with the familial vulnerability to schizophrenia. Of the six schizotypal factors that, taken one at a time, significantly predicted proband diagnosis in relatives of schizophrenics and controls, four remained predictive when examined together: negative schizotypy, social dysfunction, avoidant symptoms, and odd speech. Of the 12 items contained in these four scales, nine were signs and only three were symptoms. Compared with self-report symptoms, signs observed by trained interviewers in these data are more powerful at detecting personality traits reflecting the familial vulnerability to schizophrenia.

To our knowledge, no previous study has used multivariate methods to assess the ability of schizotypal symptoms and signs to discriminate relatives of schizophrenic and control probands. However, Gunderson et al[19] did perform a discriminant function analysis to assess what set of 45 symptoms and signs from the Danish Adoption Study interviews distinguished cases diagnosed as having borderline schizophrenia from a group of mixed "control" relatives. The most discriminating symptoms (poor social adaptivity, eccentricity, detached and flat affect, and the absence of impulsivity and psychoticlike phenomena) bear some resemblance to the results obtained herein.

These findings reinforce concerns that *DSM-III-R* and *DSM-IV* criteria for SPD may not optimally define the deviant but nonpsychotic relatives of schizophrenic probands.[3,4] Social dysfunction is not included in the SPD criteria, and *DSM-IV* criteria contain several items that, according to our analysis, have little or no unique predictive ability to identify relatives of schizophrenic probands.

SPECIFICITY OF SCHIZOTYPAL TRAITS

If schizotypal traits discriminate relatives of schizophrenics and relatives of controls, this could be because they reflect the familial vulnerability to schizophrenia, nonaffective psychotic illness, psychosis, and all major mental illness.

Our current knowledge of the validity of these four hypotheses is limited. In two studies on the same cohort, Squires-Wheeler et al[20,41] found results supportive of the final "nonspecific" hypothesis: neither individual schizotypal symptoms nor the diagnosis of SPD distinguished offspring of parents with schizophrenia and affective disorder, although both groups differed from relatives of controls. In our examination of schizophrenia-related personality disorders in the Roscommon Family Study,[24] we found that, compared with relatives of controls, SPD was significantly more common in relatives of probands with schizophrenia and ONAP. However, the rate of SPD was not significantly elevated in relatives of probands with affective disorder. These results generally favor the second hypothesis (that schizotypal traits reflect vulnerability to nonaffective psychoses). Two other studies provide evidence against the final nonspecific hypothesis, reporting higher levels of either SPD[23] or of negative symptoms[21] in relatives of probands with schizophrenia vs affective disorder.

Our results suggest variable specificity for individual schizotypal factors. While of considerable interest, these results merit replication before serving as the basis for extensive theorizing about the nature of the familial vulnerability to schizophrenia and related disorders. Probably the most important trend observed was that only one (avoidant symptoms) of the four factors that reflected the familial liability to schizophrenia in the multivariate analysis was specific only to relatives of schizophrenic probands. Compared with relatives of controls, relatives of probands with ONAP had significantly higher levels of the other three factors (negative schizotypy, social dysfunction, and odd speech). These results argue strongly against the first "highly specific" hypothesis (that schizotypal traits reflect vulnerability *only* to schizophrenia).

However, we also found three schizotypal factors that significantly distinguished relatives of schizophrenics from relatives of NPAI probands, two (negative schizotypy and avoidant symptoms) of which also differentiated, in multivariate analyses, relatives of schizophrenic probands from relatives of controls. Thus, our results also argue against the final nonspecific hypothesis. Overall, our findings about the specificity of individual schizotypal factors bear considerable resemblance to the conclusions we have previously reached with regard to the nature of the familial vulnerability to schizophrenia[22]: it is neither highly specific nor highly nonspecific.

IMPLICATIONS

A number of eminent psychiatrists of previous generations, including Kraepelin,[42] Kretschmer,[43] and Schneider,[44] postulated a close etiologic relationship between personality and the vulnerability to major psychiatric disorders. The present results suggest that personality traits assessed in relatives on the basis of a single face-to-face interview can indeed be meaningfully and highly significantly related to the diagnosis in their proband relative.

Although replication is required, these results suggest that further refinement of the personality "substrates" for the major psychoses might hold promise for increasing the power of several key research paradigms in psychiatry. A reliable method of assessing the familial/genetic vulnerability to schizophrenia in a nonpsychotic population could substantially aid research aimed at clarifying the underlying familial/genetic, neurobiologic, developmental, or neuropsychologic substrates of the major psychoses.

LIMITATIONS

These results should be considered in the context of four methodologic limitations. First, while designed to assess schizophrenialike personality traits, the SIS did not examine all possibly relevant schizotypal symptoms and signs. The inclusion of other items might have resulted in a different factor pattern and a consequent different performance of the schizotypal factors.

Second, our covariates (age, gender, and relationship with proband) might be considered inadequate. It might be argued that we should control for social class (which significantly predicted several schizotypal factors) or the presence of other psychiatric disorders in relatives. We repeated the analyses controlling for the social class of the relative and then controlling for the diagnosis of affective illness. The results changed little, although when controlling for either of these additional covariates, odd speech no longer significantly differentiated relatives of NPAI probands from relatives of controls.

Third, our factor and logistic regression analysis did not correct for the correlated nature of observations in relatives. While this should affect neither our factor structure nor our estimated regression coefficients (and the ORs derived therefrom), it does mean that our SEs and *P* values are probably modestly underestimated.

Fourth, although statistically appropriate, perhaps our use of the general proband method "overweighted" results from multiply ascertained families. However, none of the four scales that predicted proband status for relatives of all schizophrenic vs control relatives in a multivariate analysis significantly differentiated between relatives in families with one vs more than one ill proband. Our findings did not result from a few multiply ascertained families containing relatives with very deviant schizotypal symptoms.

Accepted for publication January 30, 1995.

This project was largely supported by grant MH41953 from the National Institute of Mental Health, Rockville, Md. Additional support came from the Scottish Rite Benevolent Foundation's Schizophrenia Research Program, Northern Masonic Jurisdiction, United States.

We gratefully acknowledge the assistance of Aileen O'Hare, MSocSci, Mary Spellman, MB, and the staffs of the Roscommon Family Study, St Patrick's Hospital, Castlerea, Ireland, the Roscommon Case Register, and the Health Research Board. John Myers, MS, and Leroy Thacker, MS, assisted in the statistical analyses.

Reprint requests to Department of Psychiatry, Virginia Commonwealth University, Psychiatric Genetics Research Program, Box 980710, Richmond, VA 23298-0710 (Dr Kendler).

REFERENCES

1. Essen-Möller E. The concept of schizoidia. *Psychiatrie und Neurologie.* 1946;112:258-271.
2. Planansky K. Conceptual boundaries of schizoidness: suggestions for epidemiological and genetic research. *J Nerv Ment Dis.* 1966;142:318-331.
3. Siever LJ, Gunderson J. The search for a schizotypal personality disorder: historical origins and current status. *Compr Psychiatry.* 1983;24:199-212.
4. Kendler KS. Diagnostic approaches to schizotypal personality disorder: a historical perspective. *Schizophr Bull.* 1985;11:538-553.
5. Lencz T, Raine A. Schizotypal personality: synthesis and future directions. In: Raine A, Lencz T, Mednick SA, eds. *Schizotypal Personality.* New York, NY: Cambridge University Press. In press.
6. Rado S. Dynamics and classification of disordered behavior. *Am J Psychiatry.* 1953;110:406-416.
7. Spitzer RL, Endicott J, Gibbon M. Crossing the border into borderline personality and borderline schizophrenia. *Arch Gen Psychiatry.* 1979;36:17-24.
8. Kety SS, Rosenthal D, Wender PH, Schulsinger F, Jacobsen B. Mental illness in the biological and adoptive families of adopted individuals who have become schizophrenic: a preliminary report based on psychiatric interviews. In: Fieve R, Rosenthal D, Brill H, eds. *Genetic Research in Psychiatry.* Baltimore, Md: Johns Hopkins Press; 1975:147-165.
9. American Psychiatric Association. *Diagnostic and Statistical Manual of Mental Disorders, Third Edition.* Washington, DC: American Psychiatric Association; 1980.
10. American Psychiatric Association. *Diagnostic and Statistical Manual of Mental Disorders, Revised Third Edition.* Washington, DC: American Psychiatric Association; 1987.
11. American Psychiatric Association. *Diagnostic and Statistical Manual of Mental Disorders, Fourth Edition.* Washington, DC: American Psychiatric Association; 1994.
12. Kendler KS, Ochs AL, Gorman AM, Hewitt JK, Ross DE, Mirsky AF. The structure of schizotypy: a pilot multitrait twin study. *Psychiatry Res.* 1991;36:19-36.
13. Hewitt JK, Claridge G. The factor structure of schizotypy in a normal population. *Pers Individual Differences.* 1989;10:323-329.
14. Bentall RP, Claridge GS, Slade PD. The multidimensional nature of schizotypal traits: a factor analytic study with normal subjects. *Br J Clin Psychol.* 1989;28:363-375.
15. Kendler KS, Hewitt JK. The structure of self-report schizotypy in twins. *J Pers Disord.* 1992;6:1-17.
16. Raine A, Allbutt J. Factors of schizoid personality. *Br J Clin Psychol.* 1989;28:31-40.
17. Muntaner C, Garcia-Sevilla L, Fernandez A, Torrubia R. Personality dimensions, schizotypal and borderline personality traits and psychosis proneness. *Pers Individual Differences.* 1988;9:257-268.
18. Kendler KS, Gruenberg AM, Tsuang MT. The specificity of *DSM-III* schizotypal symptoms. In: *Abstracts of the Annual Meeting of the American Psychiatric Association.* 1983;140.
19. Gunderson JG, Siever LJ, Spaulding E. The search for a schizotype: crossing the border again. *Arch Gen Psychiatry.* 1983;40:15-22.
20. Squires-Wheeler E, Skodol AE, Bassett A, Erlenmeyer-Kimling L. *DSM-III-R* schizotypal personality traits in offspring of schizophrenic disorder, affective disorder, and normal control parents. *J Psychiatr Res.* 1989;23:229-239.
21. Tsuang MT, Gilbertson MW, Faraone SV. Genetic transmission of negative and positive symptoms in the biological relatives of schizophrenics. In: Marneros A, Andreasen NC, Tsuang MT, eds. *Negative Versus Positive Schizophrenia.* Berlin, Germany: Springer-Verlag; 1991:265-291.
22. Kendler KS, Diehl SR. The genetics of schizophrenia: a current, genetic-epidemiologic perspective. *Schizophr Bull.* 1993;19:261-285.
23. Onstad S, Skre I, Edvardsen J, Torgersen S, Kringlen E. Mental disorders in first-degree relatives of schizophrenics. *Acta Psychiatr Scand.* 1991;83:463-467.
24. Kendler KS, McGuire M, Gruenberg AM, O'Hare A, Spellman M, Walsh D. The Roscommon Family Study, III: schizophrenia-related personality disorders in relatives. *Arch Gen Psychiatry.* 1993;50:781-788.
25. Kendler KS, McGuire M, Gruenberg AM, O'Hare A, Spellman M, Walsh D. The Roscommon Family Study, I: methods, diagnosis of probands, and risk of schizophrenia in relatives. *Arch Gen Psychiatry.* 1993;50:527-540.
26. Walsh D, O'Hare A, Blake B, Halpenny JV, O'Brien PF. The treated prevalence of mental illness in the Republic of Ireland. *Psychol Med.* 1980;10:465-470.
27. Spitzer RL, Williams JB, Gibbon M. *Structured Clinical Interview for DSM-III-R.* New York, NY: Biometrics Research Department, New York State Psychiatric Institute; 1987.
28. Kendler KS, Lieberman JA, Walsh D. The Structured Interview for Schizotypy (SIS): a preliminary report. *Schizophr Bull.* 1989;15:559-571.
29. Bartko JJ. The intraclass correlation coefficient as a measure of reliability. *Psychological Rep.* 1966;19:3-11.
30. Kendler KS, Gruenberg AM. An independent analysis of the Copenhagen sample of the Danish Adoption Study of Schizophrenia, VI. *Arch Gen Psychiatry.* 1984;41:555-564.
31. Kendler KS, Gruenberg AM, Tsuang MT. Psychiatric illness in first-degree relatives of schizophrenic and surgical control patients: a family study using *DSM-III* criteria. *Arch Gen Psychiatry.* 1985;42:770-779.
32. Crow JF. Problems of ascertainment in the analysis of family data. In: Neel JV, Shaw MW, Schull WJ, eds. *Genetics and the Epidemiology of Chronic Diseases.* Washington, DC: US Dept of Health, Education, and Welfare; 1965:23-44.
33. Kendler KS, McGuire M, Gruenberg AM, Spellman M, O'Hare A, Walsh D. The Roscommon Family Study, II: the risk of nonschizophrenic nonaffective psychoses in relatives. *Arch Gen Psychiatry.* 1993;50:645-652.
34. SAS Institute. *SAS/STAT User's Guide, Version 6.* 4th ed. Cary, NC: SAS Institute Inc; 1990;1-2.
35. O'Gorman TW, Woolson RF. Variable selection to discriminate between two groups. *Am Statistician.* 1991;45:187-193.
36. Lowing PA, Mirsky AF, Pereira R. The inheritance of schizophrenia spectrum disorders. *Am J Psychiatry.* 1983;140:1167-1171.
37. Baron M, Gruen R, Rainer JD, Kane J, Asnis L, Lord A. A family study of schizophrenia and normal control probands. *Am J Psychiatry.* 1985;142:447-455.
38. Frangos E, Athanassenas G, Tsitourides S, Katsanou N, Alexandrakou P. Prevalence of *DSM-III* schizophrenia among the first-degree relatives of schizophrenic probands. *Acta Psychiatr Scand.* 1985;72:382-386.
39. Baron M, Gruen R, Asnis L, Lord S. Familial transmission of schizotypal and borderline personality disorders. *Am J Psychiatry.* 1985;142:927-934.
40. Torgersen S. Genetic and nosologic aspects of schizotypal and borderline personality disorders: a twin study. *Arch Gen Psychiatry.* 1983;41:546-554.
41. Squires-Wheeler E, Skodol AE, Friedman D, Erlenmeyer-Kimling L. The specificity of *DSM-III* schizotypal personality traits. *Psychol Med.* 1988;18:757-765.
42. Kraepelin E. *Clinical Psychiatry: A Text-Book for Students and Physicians.* (Abstracted and adapted from the sixth German edition of Kraepelin's "Lehrbuch der Psychiatrie" by A. Ross Diefendorf, MD). New York, NY: The Macmillan Company; 1904.
43. Kretschmer E. *Physique and Character.* London, England: Kegan Paul, Trench Trubner; 1936.
44. Schneider K. *Psychopathic Personalities.* London, England: Cassell; 1958.

A Prospective Study of Outcome in Bulimia Nervosa and the Long-term Effects of Three Psychological Treatments

Christopher G. Fairburn, DM, FRCPsych; Patricia A. Norman, BA; Sarah L. Welch, DPhil, MRCPsych; Marianne E. O'Connor, BA; Helen A. Doll, MSc; Robert C. Peveler, DPhil, MRCPsych

Background: Little is known about the longer-term outcome of bulimia nervosa and the distal effects of treatment.

Methods: Prospective follow-up of subjects from two randomized controlled trials, involving a comparison of cognitive behavior therapy, behavior therapy, and focal interpersonal therapy.

Results: Ninety percent (89/99) underwent reassessment by interview (mean [±SD] length of follow-up, 5.8±2.0 years). Almost half (46%) had a *DSM-IV* eating disorder; 19%, bulimia nervosa; 3%, anorexia nervosa; and 24%, eating disorder not otherwise specified. There was a low rate of other psychiatric disorders. Premorbid and paternal obesity predicted a poor outcome. While the three treatments did not differ with respect to the proportion of subjects with anorexia nervosa or bulimia nervosa at follow-up, they did differ once all forms of *DSM-IV* eating disorder were considered together. Those who had received cognitive behavior therapy or focal interpersonal therapy were doing markedly better than those who had received behavior therapy.

Conclusions: The longer-term outcome of bulimia nervosa depends on the nature of the treatment received. Patients who receive a treatment such as behavior therapy, which only has a short-lived effect, tend to do badly, whereas those who receive treatments such as cognitive behavior therapy or focal interpersonal therapy have a better prognosis.

(Arch Gen Psychiatry. 1995;52:304-312)

From the Department of Psychiatry, University of Oxford (England), Warneford Hospital.

SINCE BULIMIA nervosa has only recently been described, little is known about its course or the long-term effects of treatment. The first formal descriptions of the disorder were by Russell[1] in 1979 and the American Psychiatric Association[2] in 1980. Both were pessimistic about outcome. Russell described the disorder as "intractable" and "an ominous variant of anorexia nervosa," and, in *DSM-III*,[2] the course was said to be "chronic and intermittent over a period of many years." Since then, opinions have been divided. For example, Keller and colleagues[3] have described "extraordinarily high rates of chronicity, relapse, recurrence, and psychosocial morbidity," whereas others have reported a more favorable outcome.[4-9]

The first aim of the present study was to obtain a detailed and comprehensive description of the longer-term outcome of bulimia nervosa using standardized assessment measures. The second aim was to identify predictors of outcome. To date, no consistent predictors of longer-term outcome have been identified. The third aim was to investigate the distal effects of three leading treatments for bulimia nervosa, cognitive behavior therapy (CBT), behavior therapy (BT), and focal interpersonal therapy (FIT). Knowledge of the relative long-term effects of different treatments is needed, since bulimia nervosa can run a chronic course. We were able to compare the distal effects of CBT, BT, and FIT, since we had a cohort of subjects who had participated in two complementary psychotherapy trials.[10-12]

RESULTS

THE SAMPLE

Follow-up information was obtained on 91 (92%) of the original 99 subjects. Of the remaining eight subjects, two could not be traced, three did not reply to the invitation to take part, and three

See Subjects and Methods on next page

SUBJECTS AND METHODS

SUBJECTS

The subjects were patients in one or the other of two psychotherapy trials conducted in Oxford, England, during the 1980s. These trials were similar in design. Each recruited secondary referrals of patients with bulimia nervosa from general practitioners and psychiatrists in the county of Oxfordshire (England). The trials consisted of a treatment phase in which the patients received a short-term psychological treatment administered in 19 sessions over 18 weeks. This was followed by a 1-year "closed" follow-up phase during which they received no further psychiatric treatment. The findings have been described in four main publications.[10-13]

The 24 patients in the first trial were recruited between 1982 and 1984. They were randomized to one of two forms of treatment. One was a form of CBT designed specifically for bulimia nervosa.[14,15] The comparison treatment was a form of focal psychotherapy therapy in which the emphasis was on current interpersonal problems rather than the eating disorder itself. Further details are provided in the original report.[10]

The 75 patients in the second trial were recruited between 1985 and 1988. They were randomized to one of three treatments. One was the form of CBT studied in the first trial. The second was a "dismantled" form of this treatment (BT), which consisted solely of its behavioral procedures, with the exception of those directed at concerns about shape and weight. The third treatment was a modified form of interpersonal psychotherapy, the extensively studied focal psychotherapy for depression.[16] This treatment was chosen in place of the original interpersonal treatment since it was similar to it in style and focus, with the advantages of being better established and having a detailed treatment manual. Like the former treatment, the focus of interpersonal psychotherapy was on current interpersonal problems rather than the eating disorder.[17] Thus, the patients in the two trials had one of the following three forms of treatment: CBT, BT, or FIT.

RECRUITMENT FOR THE FOLLOW-UP STUDY

The 99 patients entered into the two treatment trials formed the target sample, whether or not they had subsequently dropped out of treatment or had been withdrawn on clinical grounds. A letter was sent to each patient's last known address. If no reply was received, a second letter was sent. If there was no reply to this letter, the address was checked through various means, including National Health Service general practitioner patient records and the United Kingdom Family Health Services Network.

After being fully informed about the study, those subjects who consented to be interviewed were assessed by one of two interviewers (P.A.N. or S.L.W.), both of whom were blind to the subjects' original treatment condition.

OUTCOME MEASURES

Specific Psychopathology

The Eating Disorder Examination (EDE)[18,19] was used both to measure eating disorder psychopathology and to generate eating disorder diagnoses. The EDE provides full operational definitions of the *DSM-IV*[20] eating disorder diagnoses anorexia nervosa and bulimia nervosa.[19] Diagnoses of the third *DSM-IV* eating disorder, eating disorder not otherwise specified (EDNOS),[20] were made by two experienced clinicians (including C.G.F.) after being briefed in detail about eligible subjects' clinical state. These judgments were made independently, with the clinicians blind to the subject's identity and treatment group. There were three disagreements between the two clinicians (3/40 [8%]), and all were easily resolved on discussion.

General Psychopathology and Social Adjustment

Sections from the Structured Clinical Interview for *DSM-III-R*[21,22] were used to identify mood disorders, anxiety

Continued on next page

declined. Eighty-nine subjects were assessed by interview, 85 by face-to-face interview and four by telephone (three of whom were abroad at the time). One was only willing to undergo assessment by self-report questionnaire. The other subject had died 3 years after completing treatment. This report focuses on the 89 subjects (90% of the original sample) who were interviewed, since this is the preferred method for assessing eating disorders.[35]

The mean (±SD) age of the sample at follow-up was 29.6±5.5 years, and the mean (±SD) length of follow-up was 5.8±2.0 years. The majority of the subjects (62/89 [70%]) were followed up for 4 to 6 years. Twenty-seven (30%) were single, 61 (69%) were married or living as married, and one (1%) was divorced. Sixty-three (71%) were in paid employment, eight (9%) were students, 13 (15%) were at home with children, four (4%) were unemployed, and one (1%) was declared unfit for work owing to psychiatric illness. The distribution of occupations using the standard United Kingdom classificatory scheme[36] was as follows: nine (14%) were class I (professional); 22 (35%), class II (intermediate); 18 (29%), class IIINM (skilled nonmanual occupation); three (5%), class IIIM (skilled manual occupation); seven (11%), class IV (partly skilled occupation); and four (6%), class V (unskilled occupation).

Fifty-five subjects (62%) had received psychiatric treatment prior to their original referral, and the mean (±SD) duration of eating disorder at presentation was 6.7±5.1 years. **Table 1** shows the subjects' characteristics at recruitment. It can be seen that, with the exception of the frequency of purging, which was higher in the first trial, the two samples were very similar. The mean (±SD) duration of follow-up for the subjects in the two trials was 9.0±1.0 (range, 8 to 11) years and 4.8±0.9 (range, 3 to 7) years, respectively (t_{87}=17.1; P<.0001).

disorders, and psychoactive substance use disorders. A continuous measure of the severity of general psychiatric symptoms was provided by the Brief Symptom Inventory.[23]

Social functioning was assessed using an investigator-based interview based in part on the Adult Personality Functioning Assessment interview.[24] The time period considered was the preceding 12 months, and the following five domains of functioning were evaluated: work, friendships, confidants, relationship with partner, and relationships with family of origin.

Physical Health

Subjects were questioned in detail about their current physical health and medical history. They were also weighed.

INDICES OF OUTCOME

Two outcome indices were used for the predictive analyses. Outcome index 1 was whether or not the subject was classified as having either one of the two major *DSM-IV* eating disorders, anorexia nervosa or bulimia nervosa.[20] Outcome index 2 was the proportionate degree of change in the severity of eating disorder psychopathology (as measured by the global EDE score[19]) from recruitment to follow-up.

PREDICTORS OF OUTCOME

Potential predictor variables were chosen either on the basis of existing research on factors predictive of short-term outcome or on a priori grounds. They belonged to two main categories. The first consisted of the following parental and personal history variables: parental and personal histories of affective disorder, alcoholism, eating disorder, and obesity[25,26]; parental style, as measured by the Parental Bonding Instrument[27,28]; age at onset of disturbed eating; and history of sexual abuse prior to that age. Parental obesity was regarded as present when the subject reported that their parent's highest ever weight was equivalent to a body mass index (BMI) of 30 or more. The family history information was obtained using the family history method,[29] that is, from the subjects themselves, and the focus was on first-degree relatives only. The method for assessing sexual abuse has been described in a separate publication.[30]

The second group of predictor variables consisted of the following indices of the severity or character of the eating disorder and associated symptoms at presentation: frequency of objective bulimic episodes (the EDE term for *DSM-IV* binges),[19,31] presence of "purging" (vomiting or laxative misuse), and severity of concerns about shape and weight, all measured using the EDE; BMI; severity of general psychiatric symptoms, measured using the Index of Definition of the Present State Examination[32]; self-esteem, as measured by the Rosenberg Self-esteem Scale[33]; social functioning, as measured by a modified version of the Social Adjustment Scale[34]; duration of the eating disorder; and histories of anorexia nervosa and excessive drinking.

STATISTICAL METHODS

Parametric and nonparametric tests, as appropriate, were used to assess the univariate significance of differences in means, medians, and proportions. To identify which variables were most independently predictive of outcome (likelihood ratio test, $P<.05$), forward stepwise regression analyses were performed on the variables that were significantly associated with outcome on univariate analysis. The analyses were performed while controlling for the duration of follow-up and type of treatment received.

To examine the relative long-term effects of the three treatments, a 3×4 (treatment group multiplied by time before treatment, end of treatment, 12-month follow-up, and 6-year follow-up) repeated measures analysis of variance was performed on the global EDE scores. In addition, to describe variations in the proportions of subjects who no longer had an eating disorder of clinical severity and who were abstinent from the key behavioral features of the disorder, log-odds models of treatment and time were fitted.

AIM 1—OUTCOME AT FOLLOW-UP

Eating Disorder Diagnoses

At follow-up, 17 subjects (19%) met operational *DSM-IV* diagnostic criteria for bulimia nervosa and three (3%) met criteria for anorexia nervosa. Twenty-one subjects (24%) were judged by the two independent clinical assessors to meet criteria for EDNOS[20]; that is, they had an eating disorder of clinical severity, but it did not meet the criteria for anorexia nervosa or bulimia nervosa. Thirteen of these subjects had what may be termed a "subthreshold eating disorder."[37] In nine cases, the disorder resembled bulimia nervosa, except that the frequency of objective bulimic episodes was below the threshold level or the amount eaten was not large; in four cases, the disorder resembled anorexia nervosa, except that body weight was not sufficiently low. The other eight subjects had a "partial syndrome"[37] in that one or more of the essential diagnostic features of anorexia nervosa or bulimia nervosa was missing. Four subjects had repeated objective bulimic episodes accompanied by self-induced vomiting, but there was no overconcern about shape or weight. In these cases, the binge eating and vomiting seemed to be a habitual response to stress. In three subjects, the only feature was frequent self-induced vomiting, and one subject had recurrent episodes of binge eating in the absence of extreme weight-control behavior (binge eating disorder).[20] The remaining 48 subjects (54%) did not have an eating disorder.

A thorough review of each subject's history, with the assistance of questionnaires that had been completed at annual intervals, indicated that in the great majority (74/89 [83%]), there had been virtually no change in their eating disorder over the previous 3 years, whereas the eating disorder features of the remainder had fluctuated in severity.

Table 2 shows how the subjects' diagnostic status had changed since completing treatment. Of those in remission at the end of treatment (ie, those who did not have a *DSM-IV* eating disorder), 82% (31/38) were still in remission at 12-month follow-up, and 71%

Table 1. Recruitment Characteristics of the Follow-up Sample*

Characteristics	Trial 1 (n=20)	Trial 2 (n=69)	*P*
Age, y	22.5±3.8	24.3±6.0	.12
Duration of eating disorder, y	5.3±3.9	7.0±5.3	.18
Age at onset of eating disorder, y	17.2±3.3	17.2±4.5	.99
No. of objective bulimic episodes per 28 days (median No. of episodes)†	31.0±22.6 (26)	23.0±16.9 (20)	.091
No. of purging episodes per 28 days (median No. of episodes)†‡	66.7±58.7 (39)	27.0±23.6 (20)	<.001
Psychiatric symptom score§	23.0±7.3	22.0±10.5	.71
Body mass index‖	21.0±2.4	22.3±3.3	.121

*Data are given as mean±SD, unless otherwise indicated.
†Determined by the Eating Disorder Examination, described by Fairburn and Cooper.[19]
‡Indicated by frequency of self-induced vomiting or laxative misuse.
§Determined by total symptom score on the Present State Examination.[32]
‖Indicated by weight in kilograms divided by height in square meters.

Table 2. Change in Diagnostic Status Over Time*

End of Treatment	12-mo Follow-up	6-y Follow-up
Negative (38/89[43])	Negative (31/38[82])	Negative (23/31[74])
		Positive (8/31[26])
	Positive (7/38[18])	Negative (4/7[57])
		Positive (3/7[43])
Positive (51/89[57])	Negative (12/51[24])	Negative (10/12[83])
		Positive (2/12[17])
	Positive (39/51[76])	Negative (11/39[28])
		Positive (28/39[72])

*Data are given as No. (%) of subjects. Mean (±SD) length of follow-up was 5.8±2.0 years. Negative and positive status refer to the proportion of subjects at each time point who did not and did meet DSM-IV diagnostic criteria for an eating disorder (ie, anorexia nervosa, bulimia nervosa, or an eating disorder not otherwise specified), respectively.

(27/38) were in remission at longer-term follow-up. There was somewhat less stability among those who had an eating disorder at the end of treatment in that 24% (12/51) and 41% (21/51) were in remission at 12-month and longer-term follow-ups, respectively.

Eating Disorder Features

The eating disorder features at recruitment and follow-up are shown in **Table 3**. There was a marked reduction in their overall severity as measured by the global EDE score (mean [±SD] reduction, 1.7±1.3; t_{66}=11.2; *P*<.0001). Fifty subjects (56%) had a global EDE score within 1 SD of the mean of young women from the same geographical area (ie, 1.53).[38]

Overeating and Purging. Fifty-five subjects (62%) reported having had no objective bulimic episodes over the preceding 3 months. Among the remainder, the mean (±SD) frequency of binge eating was 11.9±16.0 episodes per month (median, 6.3; range, 0.33 to 76.00). Between initial presentation and follow-up, the frequency of objective bulimic episodes fell by an average of 82% (Wilcoxon matched pairs, *z*=−7.36; *P*<.0001).

Of the 72 subjects who practiced self-induced vomiting at presentation, 33 (46%) had not vomited over the previous 3 months. Five subjects who reported vomiting at follow-up had not done so beforehand. Among those who vomited at follow-up, the mean (±SD) frequency was 16.0±50.0 episodes per month (median, 2.33; range, 0.33 to 330). Between presentation and follow-up, there was an overall mean reduction of 75% in the frequency of vomiting (Wilcoxon matched pairs, *z*=−6.57; *P*<.0001).

Of the 28 subjects who misused laxatives at presentation, 20 (71%) had not done so over the previous 3 months. There were three new cases of laxative misuse. Among those who misused laxatives at follow-up, the mean (±SD) frequency of use was 8.55±11.65 times per month (median, 3.33; range, 0.33 to 33). Between presentation and follow-up, there was an overall mean reduction of 68% in the frequency of laxative misuse (Wilcoxon matched pairs, *z*=−4.01; *P*<.0001). None of the subjects misused diuretics.

Thirty-six (42%) of 85 subjects were classified as fully "abstinent" at follow-up; ie, they reported that over the preceding months, they had experienced no objective bulimic episodes, no vomiting, and no misuse of laxatives or diuretics.

Dietary Restraint. This was measured using the Restraint subscale of the EDE. As shown in Table 3, there was a marked decrease in the degree of dietary restraint from presentation to follow-up (t_{66}=11.23; *P*<.0001). Among those subjects who did not meet *DSM-IV* criteria for an eating disorder, the level of dietary restraint was 1.17±1.29, compared with 0.94±1.09 for subjects in the community (differences were not significant).[38]

Attitudes to Shape and Weight. The disturbed attitudes to shape and weight characteristic of patients with eating disorders were measured using the Shape Concern and Weight Concern subscales of the EDE. As shown in Table 3, the scores on these subscales also decreased markedly from presentation to follow-up (t_{66}=8.57 and t_{66}=9.42, respectively; *P*<.0001 for both subscales). Among those subjects who did not meet *DSM-IV* criteria for an eating disorder, the levels of concern about shape and weight were 1.48±1.18 and 1.19±1.00, respectively, compared with 1.34±1.09 and 1.18±0.93 for subjects in the community (both differences were not significant).[38]

Table 3. Clinical Characteristics at Recruitment and Follow-up*

Characteristics	Recruitment	Follow-up	P
No. of objective bulimic episodes per 28 days (median No. of episodes)†	24.8±18.5 (20.0)	4.5±11.4 (0)	<.0001
No. of self-induced vomiting episodes per 28 days (median No. of episodes)†	31.9±38.8 (24.0)	7.9±35.9 (0)	<.0001
No. of laxative misuse episodes per 28 days (median No. of episodes)†	4.3±10.0 (0)	1.1±4.9 (0)	<.0001
Dietary Restraint score†‡	3.5±1.3	2.2±1.7	<.0001
Overeating score†‡	3.1±0.6	1.2±1.3	<.0001
Eating Concern score†‡	2.9±1.4	1.1±1.4	<.0001
Shape Concern score†‡	3.9±1.3	2.2±1.6	<.0001
Weight Concern score†‡	4.0±1.4	2.0±1.5	<.0001
Global Eating Disorder Examination score†‡	3.5±0.9	1.7±1.3	<.0001
Psychiatric symptom score‡§	1.4±0.8	0.7±0.7	<.0001
Body weight, kg	60.6±10.1	62.1±11.8	.018
Body mass index‖	22.0±3.1	22.5±3.6	.053

*Data are given as mean±SD, unless otherwise indicated.
†Determined by the Eating Disorder Examination, described by Fairburn and Cooper.[19]
‡Data are from the second trial only.
§Determined by the Brief Symptom Inventory (Global Severity Index).[23]
‖Indicated by weight in kilograms divided by height in square meters.

General Psychiatric Symptoms and Substance Abuse

Table 3 shows that the level of general psychiatric symptoms decreased from presentation to follow-up, as measured by the Global Symptom Index of the Brief Symptom Inventory (t_{62}=7.89; $P<.0001$). Twenty-five (28%) subjects met *DSM-III-R*[39] criteria for a general psychiatric disorder: eight had major depressive disorder; 16 had an anxiety disorder, of whom five had panic disorder, two had generalized anxiety disorder, two had social phobia, six had specific phobia, and one had obsessive-compulsive disorder; and one had sexual aversion disorder. Those subjects with a general psychiatric disorder at follow-up had higher levels of psychiatric disturbance at recruitment than those who did not (mean [±SD] Present State Examination total symptom score, 27.1±9.8 and 20.3±9.2, respectively) (t_{83}=3.01; P=.002). The rates of general psychiatric disorders among those with and without bulimia nervosa or anorexia nervosa were 60% (12/20) and 19% (13/69), respectively (χ^2_1=13.00; $P<.001$).

Few subjects had problems with substance abuse. Three met *DSM-III-R* criteria for a psychoactive substance use disorder. There was one case of alcohol dependence (severe) combined with diazepam abuse, one case of alcohol abuse, and one case of combined opioid and temazepam abuse. Among the full sample, two subjects (2%) drank on average more than 35 U of alcohol per week, and 13 (15%) drank between 14 and 35 U weekly. The rates of drinking 14 U or more per week among those with and without bulimia nervosa or anorexia nervosa were 25% (5/20) and 15% (10/67), respectively (differences were not significant).

Social Functioning

The majority of the sample reported no significant interpersonal problems. Forty-nine percent (44/89) were in full-time employment; 75% (63/84) had a current partner, of whom 59% (37/63) reported that the relationship was excellent or good; 85% (73/86) had a good relationship with their family of origin; and 54% (46/85) had at least three confiding relationships.

There were no significant differences between those who had bulimia nervosa or anorexia nervosa and those who did not with respect both to the proportion in full-time employment (8/20 [40%] and 36/69 [52%], respectively) and the proportion with a current partner (16/20 [80%] and 47/64 [73%], respectively). However, those with bulimia nervosa or anorexia nervosa were less likely than the remainder to report a good relationship with their partner (5/15, [33%] and 32/48 [68%], respectively) (χ^2_1=4.35; P=.037) and with their family of origin (14/20 [70%] and 59/65 [91%], respectively) (Fisher's Exact Test, P=.03).

Physical Health

Systematic inquiry about the physical health of the subjects revealed few findings of note other than the presence of nonspecific gastrointestinal complaints. These were reported by 47% (8/17) of those who continued to meet diagnostic criteria for bulimia nervosa, compared with 43% (20/46) of those who did not meet *DSM-IV* criteria for an eating disorder (differences were not significant).

Inquiry about the development of medical conditions since the onset of the eating disorder revealed two cases each of hypothyroidism, peptic ulcer disease, and osteoporosis. Both the subjects in whom osteoporosis developed had a history of anorexia nervosa. One subject had had a pituitary tumor successfully removed, one had multiple sclerosis, and one had had a repair to a hiatus hernia (secondary to a crush injury). None of these conditions seemed to have influenced the eating disorder. The one subject who had died had a long history of epilepsy. She died during a grand mal seizure 3 years after completing treatment.

In the group as a whole, there was a modest increase in body weight from presentation to follow-up (mean increase [±SD], 1.57±6.14 kg) (t_{88}=2.42; P=.02).

Table 4. Univariate Associations Between Paternal and Premorbid Obesity and Outcome

Obesity	Outcome Index 1 Current Anorexia Nervosa or Bulimia Nervosa, No. (%) of Subjects	P	Outcome Index 2 Proportionate Global Eating Disorder Examination Change, Mean±SD (No. of Subjects)*	P
Paternal				
Absent	11/66 (17)	<.001†	0.56±0.34 (52)	.007§
Moderate	4/13 (31)		0.37±0.29 (10)	
Severe	4/4 (100)		−0.02±0.10 (3)	
Premorbid				
Absent	11/64 (17)	.013‡	0.56±0.35 (48)	.034‖
Moderate	6/14 (43)		0.37±0.32 (12)	
Severe	3/6 (50)		0.34±0.27 (6)	

*Described in Fairburn and Cooper.[19]
†χ^2_1 linear trend=12.22.
‡χ^2_1 linear trend=6.14.
§$F_{2,62}$=5.44.
‖t_{64}=2.16. Statistical test refers to absent vs moderate or severe.

However, there was considerable variability between subjects, with 27 (30%) subjects gaining 5 kg or more and 13 (15%) losing 5 kg or more. The mean (±SD) increase in BMI was 0.47±2.28 (t_{87}=1.96; *P*=.05). Seven subjects (8%) met accepted criteria for being overweight (BMI ≥27), compared with six (7%) at presentation, and 18 (20%) were underweight (BMI <20), compared with 23 (26%) at presentation. There was little movement between these categories: of the seven subjects who were overweight at follow-up, five (71%) had been overweight at presentation; and of the 18 who were underweight, 11 (61%) had been underweight at presentation (χ^2_4=64.1; *P*<.0001).

AIM 2—PREDICTORS OF OUTCOME

On univariate analysis, only two variables were significantly associated with both outcome indexes. These were paternal and premorbid obesity, each of which was associated with a poor outcome (**Table 4**). Although based on small numbers, there were significant linear trends for both variables. The only other variable significantly associated with outcome index 1 was paternal overprotection, as measured by the Parental Bonding Instrument, but the relationship was nonlinear and therefore difficult to interpret. Two variables were significantly associated with outcome index 2. They were both self-esteem, as measured by the Rosenberg Self-esteem Scale and BMI. These relationships were also nonlinear. Maternal obesity was not significantly related to either outcome index.

After adjusting for type of treatment received and duration of follow-up on multivariate analysis, paternal and premorbid obesity (both considered as binary variables because of the small numbers) remained significantly and independently associated with outcome (outcome index 1, χ^2_1 for improvement, 7.21 [*P*=.007] and 6.15 [*P*=.01], respectively; outcome index 2, R^2=.08 [*P*=.007] and R^2=.09 [*P*=.005], respectively). Subjects with a history of paternal obesity were almost six times as likely to meet criteria for anorexia nervosa or bulimia nervosa at follow-up as those without such a history (odds ratio [OR], 5.73; 95% confidence limits [CL], 1.56, 21.1), and those with premorbid obesity were more than four times as likely to meet these criteria (OR, 4.31; 95% CL, 1.35, 13.7). No other variable had a consistent and interpretable association with outcome.

AIM 3—LONG-TERM EFFECTS OF THE THREE TREATMENTS

Of the 89 subjects who were interviewed at follow-up, 35 (39%) had received CBT; 22 (25%), BT; and 32 (36%), FIT. Although the subjects who received the two forms of FIT were followed-up for different lengths of time (mean [±SD] times, 8.9±0.9 [range, 8 to 11] years and 4.9±0.9 [range, 3 to 7] years, respectively) (t_{30}=12.0; *P*<.001), there were no statistically significant differences in outcome between the two groups, thereby justifying their amalgamation. Thirty-four subjects (38%) subsequently received additional psychiatric treatment (for any problem): 13 (37%) from the CBT group, nine (41%) from the BT group, and 12 (38%) from the FIT group (differences were not significant). There was no difference between the treatment groups in the amount or form of treatment received. Of those who had bulimia nervosa or anorexia nervosa at follow-up, two thirds (13/20 [65%]) had received additional psychiatric treatment, compared with less than one third of the remainder (20/67 [30%]) (χ^2_1=8.07; *P*=.005).

There was no significant difference between the three treatment conditions in the proportion with bulimia nervosa or anorexia nervosa at follow-up (CBT, n=7 [20%]; BT, n=6 [27%]; FIT, n=7 [22%]), although there was a significant difference when all forms of *DSM-IV* eating disorder were considered together (CBT, n=13 [37%]; BT, n=19 [86%]; FIT, n=9 [28%]) (χ^2_2=19.65; *P*<.0001). This difference is due to the large proportion of subjects who had received BT (n=13 [59%]) who were classified as having an EDNOS. The **Figure** shows the proportion of subjects in the three treatment conditions who were in remission (ie, did not have a *DSM-IV* eating disorder) at the end of treatment, at 12-month follow-up, and at longer-term follow-up. This proportion differed across

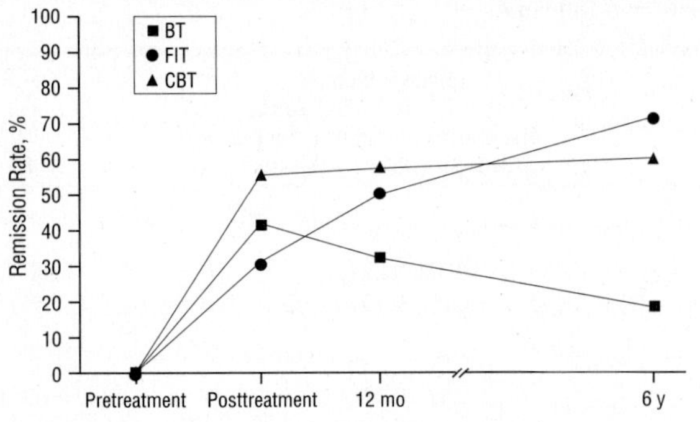

Remission rates (ie, proportion not meeting DSM-IV *criteria for an eating disorder) in patients who received cognitive behavior therapy (CBT) (n=35), behavior therapy (BT) (n=22), or focal interpersonal therapy (FIT) (n=32). Mean (±SD) length of follow-up was 5.8±2.0 years.*

the treatments (χ^2_2=14.90; P<.001), with subjects who had received FIT and CBT doing better than those who had received BT; subjects who received FIT were twice as likely to be in remission (OR, 2.58; 95% CL, 1.32, 5.02), while those who received CBT were more than three times as likely to be in remission (OR, 3.43; 95% CL, 1.77, 6.63). There was no significant difference between those who had received CBT or FIT. As illustrated in the Figure, there was deterioration among those in the BT group (the effect of time differed among the treatments) (χ^2_4=13.49; P=.01), while there was little change among those who received CBT or FIT. The comparatively poor outcome of the patients who received BT cannot be attributed to differences in the characteristics of the patients allocated to the three treatments. The treatment groups did not differ significantly in their recruitment characteristics or in their personal or family histories, nor can the poor showing of BT be attributed to differences in the duration of follow-up. There was no significant difference between the treatment conditions in their length of follow-up, and after adjusting for length of follow-up, treatment type remained significantly associated with outcome, with those patients who had received BT doing worse than those who had received CBT or FIT.

All three treatments had a substantial and sustained effect on the global EDE score (for effect of time, $F_{3,132}$=64.12; P<.001). The mean (±SD) reductions from recruitment to follow-up were 2.22±1.00, 1.36±1.32, and 1.51±1.00 for those who received CBT, BT, and FIT, respectively ($F_{2,64}$=3.71; P=.04). At follow-up, those who had received CBT had a lower overall level of symptoms than those who had received BT or FIT (1.27±1.12, compared with 2.08±1.27 [t_{54}=2.51; P=.015] and 1.50±1.20 [t_{64}=0.82; P=.049], respectively) ($F_{2,84}$=3.14; P=.049). Twenty-six (74%) of those who had received CBT had global EDE scores within 1 SD of the mean for young women.[38] The comparable figures for BT and FIT were seven (33%) and 17 (55%), respectively (χ^2_1 for linear trend from BT to CBT, 9.03; P=.003).

The outcome of bulimia nervosa may also be measured in terms of "abstinence" from key behavioral features (ie, no objective bulimic episodes, no vomiting, and no laxative or diuretic misuse). While there was no significant overall effect of treatment on the proportion of abstinent subjects and no differential effect of treatment over time, at follow-up a significantly smaller proportion of those who received BT were abstinent (4/22 [18%]) than were those who received CBT or FIT (16/32 [50%] and 16/31 [52%], respectively) (χ^2_2=6.87; P=.044).

COMMENT

Three strengths of this study merit comment. First, the two original samples are likely to be representative of secondary referrals with the disorder. They were recruited from consecutive referrals from a defined geographical area in which there were no competing treatment facilities and, of these, almost all who had a sufficiently severe eating disorder were included. Second, 90% of the original cohort were reassessed by interview. A high response rate is essential in studies of this type, since nonresponders may represent an atypical group, and their absence may therefore significantly bias the findings. Third, eating disorder features were measured using the EDE,[18,19] an interview that is widely regarded as the assessment method of choice for studying the outcome of eating disorders.[35,40,41] Since the EDE was used at each time point, it was possible to make a detailed assessment of changes in symptoms and diagnoses over the whole time period, and since normative EDE data were available on women of the same age and from the same geographical area,[38] it was possible to evaluate the severity of any residual symptoms.

Two limitations of the study are also of note. First, the length of follow-up varied. Whereas the majority of subjects were followed up for 4 to 6 years, the range was from 3 to 11 years. On the other hand, the fact that outcome was not related to length of follow-up indicates that by this point, the subjects' clinical state was relatively stable, a finding confirmed on interview. The second limitation applies to the comparison of the three forms of treatment. This involved combining data from patients randomized to two separate treatment trials and amalgamating two forms of FIT. While this is not ideal, it can be justified, since there was no difference in outcome between these two very similar treatments.

The first aim of the study was to assess the longer-term outcome of bulimia nervosa. There were three main findings: first, one in five patients still had bulimia nervosa; second, the subsequent development of anorexia nervosa was most unusual; and third, a quarter of the sample met criteria for EDNOS. Although it is problematic to compare findings across studies, it is of note that these figures are broadly similar to those obtained by three other studies.[5,6,42] In contrast, they are better than those reported by Fallon and colleagues[43] in their follow-up study of inpatients and rather worse than those from the 10-year follow-up study of Collings and King.[9] The findings indicate that bulimia nervosa is far from "intractable," as originally suggested by Russell.[1] On the other hand, if account is taken of the development of atypical eating disorders (ie, cases of EDNOS),[37] then a less positive picture emerges, since almost half the sample had a *DSM-IV* eating disorder at follow-up.

We found that a quarter of the subjects had a general psychiatric disorder, the presence of such a disorder being significantly associated with the continued presence of an eating disorder. In common with other investigators, we found no evidence that bulimia nervosa evolves into other psychiatric disorders over time, nor was there evidence of any persistent impairment in social functioning. The majority of subjects were functioning well in most domains, although those who met criteria for bulimia nervosa or in whom anorexia nervosa developed had more interpersonal problems than those who did not have an eating disorder. There was no tendency for subjects to become obese or for other adverse physical sequelae to develop.

The second aim of the study was to identify predictors of longer-term outcome. To this end, variables of putative etiological significance were studied in addition to measures of the severity of the disorder at presentation. The only variables to have robust relationships with outcome were premorbid and paternal obesity, both of which showed linear trends in which there was a worse outcome with increasing obesity. To our knowledge, this is the first time that the predictive power of these variables has been studied. One possible explanation for their association with outcome is that, given social pressures to be slim, it is more difficult for those vulnerable to obesity to cease to diet, and, as a result, they remain prone to episodes of binge eating. On the other hand, this explanation is not consistent with the absence of a significant relationship between maternal obesity and outcome. Since both variables were assessed indirectly and applied only to about a quarter of the sample, this finding requires confirmation.

The third aim of the study was to investigate the long-term effects of the treatments that the subjects had received as participants in the two trials. There have been no previous studies of this type. Perhaps surprisingly, given the length of follow-up and the fact that over one third of the sample had received subsequent treatment, differential treatment effects were observed. Those subjects who had received BT fared much the worst: at follow-up, 86% had a *DSM-IV* eating disorder, compared with 37% and 28% for those who had received CBT and FIT, respectively. This difference was due to the large number of subjects who had received BT who met criteria for EDNOS. There was no difference between the three treatments in the proportion of subjects who met criteria for bulimia nervosa or anorexia nervosa, with about a fifth fulfilling diagnostic criteria for one or other of these disorders (bulimia nervosa in the great majority). Since two thirds of these particular subjects had received additional psychiatric treatment in the interim, it seems that they were a particularly refractory group.

It is unlikely that BT was actually harmful to the patients, since it contained many of the ingredients of CBT and since it was comparable to CBT in short-term outcome.[11] Rather, it seems to have had a short-lived effect, with its effects subsequently tending to deteriorate. The poor outcome of the patients who received BT resembles the outcomes reported in early descriptions of the disorder[1,2] and the findings of Keller and colleagues,[3] who have been conducting an open study of a clinical cohort. It also resembles the course of most of these patients' eating disorder prior to referral. Perhaps, therefore, it represents the natural outcome of clinical cases.

Accepted for publication January 20, 1995.

This study was funded by grant 8921076 from the United Kingdom Medical Research Council, London (Drs Fairburn and Peveler). The original treatment studies were supported by grant 8008656 from the Medical Research Council, and grant 13961 from the Wellcome Trust, London. Dr Fairburn holds a Wellcome Trust Senior Lectureship (13123), and Drs Welch and Mss Doll and O'Connor were also supported by grants 13123, 018157, and 030583, from the Wellcome Trust.

Correspondence to University of Oxford, Department of Psychiatry, Warneford Hospital, Oxford OX3 7JX, England (Dr Fairburn).

REFERENCES

1. Russell GFM. Bulimia nervosa: an ominous variant of anorexia nervosa. *Psychol Med.* 1979;9:429-448.
2. American Psychiatric Association. *Diagnostic and Statistical Manual of Mental Disorders, Third Edition.* Washington, DC: American Psychiatric Association; 1980.
3. Keller MB, Herzog DB, Lavori PW, Bradburn IS, Mahoney EM. The naturalistic history of bulimia nervosa: extraordinarily high rates of chronicity, relapse, recurrence, and psychosocial morbidity. *Int J Eat Disord.* 1992;12:1-10.
4. Mitchell JE, Pyle RL, Hatsukami D, Goff G, Glotter D, Harper J. A 2-5 year follow-up study of patients treated for bulimia. *Int J Eat Disord.* 1989;8:157-165.
5. Hsu LKG, Sobkiewicz TA. Bulimia nervosa: a four to six-year follow-up study. *Psychol Med.* 1989;19:1035-1038.
6. Johnson-Sabine E, Reiss D, Dayson D. Bulimia nervosa: a 5-year follow-up study. *Psychol Med.* 1992;22:951-959.
7. Fichter MM, Quadflieg N, Rief W. The German Longitudinal Bulimia Nervosa Study, I. In: Herzog W, Deter H-C, Vandereycken W, eds. *The Course of Eating Disorders.* New York, NY: Springer-Verlag NY Inc; 1991:133-149.
8. Lacey JH. Long-term follow-up of bulimic patients treated in integrated behavioural and psychodynamic treatment programmes. In: Herzog W, Deter H-C, Vandereycken W, eds. *The Course of Eating Disorders.* New York, NY: Springer-Verlag NY Inc; 1991:150-173.
9. Collings S, King M. Ten-year follow-up of 50 patients with bulimia nervosa. *Br J Psychiatry.* 1994;164:80-87.
10. Fairburn CG, Kirk J, O'Connor M, Cooper PJ. A comparison of two psychological treatments for bulimia nervosa. *Behav Res Ther.* 1986;24:629-643.
11. Fairburn CG, Jones R, Peveler RC, Carr SJ, Solomon RA, O'Connor ME, Burton J, Hope RA. Three psychological treatments for bulimia nervosa: a comparative trial. *Arch Gen Psychiatry.* 1991;48:463-469.
12. Fairburn CG, Jones R, Peveler RC, Hope RA, O'Connor M. Psychotherapy and bulimia nervosa: the longer-term effects of interpersonal psychotherapy, behavior therapy, and cognitive behavior therapy. *Arch Gen Psychiatry.* 1993; 50:419-428.
13. Fairburn CG, Peveler RC, Jones R, Hope RA, Doll HA. Predictors of twelve-month outcome in bulimia nervosa and the influence of attitudes to shape and weight. *J Consult Clin Psychol.* 1993;61:696-698.
14. Fairburn CG. A cognitive behavioural approach to the management of bulimia. *Psychol Med.* 1981;11:707-711.
15. Fairburn CG, Marcus MD, Wilson GT. Cognitive-behavioral therapy for binge eating and bulimia nervosa: a comprehensive treatment manual. In: Fairburn CG, Wilson GT, eds. *Binge Eating: Nature, Assessment and Treatment.* New York, NY: Guilford Press; 1993:361-404.
16. Klerman GL, Weissman MM, Rounsaville BJ, Chevron ES. *Interpersonal Psychotherapy of Depression.* New York, NY: Basic Books Inc Publishers; 1984.
17. Fairburn CG. Interpersonal psychotherapy for bulimia nervosa. In: Klerman GL,

Weissman MM, eds. *New Applications of Interpersonal Psychotherapy.* Washington, DC: American Psychiatric Press; 1992:353-378.
18. Cooper Z, Fairburn CG. The Eating Disorder Examination: a semi-structured interview for the assessment of the specific psychopathology of eating disorders. *Int J Eat Disord.* 1987;6:1-8.
19. Fairburn CG, Cooper Z. The Eating Disorder Examination (12th edition). In: Fairburn CG, Wilson GT, eds. *Binge Eating: Nature, Assessment and Treatment.* New York, NY: Guilford Press; 1993:317-360.
20. American Psychiatric Association. *Diagnostic and Statistical Manual of Mental Disorders, Fourth Edition.* Washington, DC: American Psychiatric Association; 1994.
21. Spitzer RL, Williams JBW, Gibbon M, First MB. The Structured Clinical Interview for *DSM-III-R* (SCID), I: history, rationale, and description. *Arch Gen Psychiatry.* 1992;49:624-629.
22. Williams JBW, Gibbon M, First MB, Spitzer RL, Davis M, Borus J, Howes MJ, Kane J, Pope HG, Rounsaville B, Wittchen HU. The Structured Clinical Interview for *DSM-III-R* (SCID), II: multisite test-retest reliability. *Arch Gen Psychiatry.* 1992;49:630-636.
23. Derogatis LR, Spencer PM. *The Brief Symptom Inventory: Administration, Scoring and Procedures Manual.* Baltimore, Md: Clinical Psychometric Research; 1982.
24. Hill J, Harrington R, Fudge H, Rutter M, Pickles A. Adult Personality Functioning Assessment (APFA): an investigator-based standardised interview. *Br J Psychiatry.* 1989;155:24-35.
25. Spitzer RL, Endicott J. *Schedule for Affective Disorders and Schizophrenia—Lifetime Version.* New York, NY: Biometrics Research; 1975.
26. Endicott J, Andreasen N, Spitzer R. *Family History-Research Diagnostic Criteria (FH-RDC) 7/18/78.* New York, NY: Biometrics Research, New York State Psychiatric Institute; 1978.
27. Parker G, Tupling H, Brown LB. A Parental Bonding Instrument. *Br J Med Psychol.* 1979;52:1-10.
28. Parker G. The Parental Bonding Instrument: psychometric properties reviewed. *Psychiatr Dev.* 1989;4:317-335.
29. Thompson WD, Orvaschel H, Prusoff BA, Kidd KK. An evaluation of the family history method for ascertaining psychiatric disorders. *Arch Gen Psychiatry.* 1982;39:53-58.
30. Welch SL, Fairburn CG. Sexual abuse and bulimia nervosa: three integrated case control comparisons. *Am J Psychiatry.* 1994;151:402-407.
31. Fairburn CG, Wilson GT. Binge eating: definition and classification. In: Fairburn CG, Wilson GT, eds. *Binge Eating: Nature, Assessment and Treatment.* New York, NY: Guilford Press; 1993:3-14.
32. Wing JK, Cooper JE, Sartorius N. *The Measurement and Classification of Psychiatric Symptoms.* New York, NY: Cambridge University Press; 1974.
33. Rosenberg M. *Society and the Adolescent Self-Image.* Princeton, NJ: Princeton University Press; 1965.
34. Cooper PJ, Osborn M, Gath D, Feggetter G. Evaluation of a modified self-report measure of social adjustment. *Br J Psychiatry.* 1982;141:68-75.
35. Garner DM. Assessment of eating disorder psychopathology. In: Brownell KD, Fairburn CG, eds. *Eating Disorders and Obesity.* New York, NY: Guilford Press. In press.
36. Office of Population Censuses and Surveys. *Classification of Occupations.* London, England: Her Majesty's Stationery Office; 1980.
37. Fairburn CG, Walsh BT. Atypical eating disorders. In: Brownell KD, Fairburn CG, eds. *Eating Disorders and Obesity.* New York, NY: Guilford Press. In press.
38. Beglin SJ. *Eating Disorders in Young Adult Women.* Oxford, England: University of Oxford; 1990. Thesis.
39. American Psychiatric Association. *Diagnostic and Statistical Manual of Mental Disorders, Revised Third Edition.* Washington, DC: American Psychiatric Association; 1987.
40. Wilson GT. Assessment of binge eating. In: Fairburn CG, Wilson GT, eds. *Binge Eating: Nature, Assessment and Treatment.* New York, NY: Guilford Press; 1993: 227-249.
41. Rosen JC, Srebnik D. The assessment of eating disorders. In: McReynolds P, Rosen JC, Chelune G, eds. *Advances in Psychological Assessment.* New York, NY: Plenum Press; 1991:229-259.
42. Fichter MM, Quadflieg N, Rief W. Longer-term (6-year) course of bulimia nervosa. *Neuropsychopharmacology.* 1994;10(suppl 3):772S.
43. Fallon BA, Walsh BT, Sadik C, Saoud JB, Lukasik V. Outcome and clinical course in inpatient bulimic women: a 2- to 9-year follow-up study. *J Clin Psychiatry.* 1991;52:272-278.

Correction

Error in Table. In the article titled "Test-Retest Reliability of the Diagnostic Interview Schedule for Children (DISC 2.1)," which appeared in the January 1995 issue of the ARCHIVES (1995;52:61-71), an error occurred in Table 1 on page 64. Under the table heading, "M/F Ratio," for clinic subjects, the probability value should be *P*=.30, not *P*=30. The Journal apologizes for its error.

EDITORIAL

Some Thoughts About the ARCHIVES

DURING THE past year, I have begun the daunting task of editing the ARCHIVES. The journal has had three editors. My predecessors, Roy R. Grinker, Sr, MD (1959-1969), and Daniel X. Freedman, MD (1970-1993), were men I knew and revered.

Some have asked how the journal acquired its name. In 1959, when the *Archives of Neurology and Psychiatry* was split into two separate journals for each specialty, Roy Grinker decided that the title of the psychiatry journal must contain the word "general" because he fervently believed that the role of the ARCHIVES was to cover all areas of psychiatry. In that spirit we will continue—and attempt to broaden—the coverage of the ARCHIVES to include all perspectives of our field: biological, psychological, and social. Our principal focus has been and always will be human studies, but we expect to continue the tradition of publishing some studies in basic science that are particularly relevant for the behavioral sciences. At a time when psychiatry is undergoing major changes in its practice and reimbursement, we are also committed to publishing the data that add to our knowledge in evaluation and outcomes research. All of these areas, from biology to psychosocial research, play a critical role in the understanding of the science, technology, and art of our field.

The ARCHIVES has never backed down from health policy debates. Indeed, both former editors, as witnessed by their editorials, were deeply involved in the politics of research and clinical practice. At a time when health care and scientific investigation are undergoing extraordinary change, the ARCHIVES must continue to illuminate these issues, focus the discussion, and provide a lively forum where health policy issues can be aired and debated. To accomplish this aim, we will seek commentaries on some of these controversial issues from a broad range of scholars. Many of these may take off from reports by the Institute of Medicine and its board on Biobehavioral Science and Mental Disorders, which is frequently presented with questions of pressing national interest. We hope the dialogues within our pages will enhance the quality of debate about where our field is going and where it should go.

The ARCHIVES must continue to be a journal where the best and most important work in psychiatry can be presented. It has always had a consistent approach to evaluating submissions. We ask: Is this study interesting? important? hypothesis-driven or generating? carefully and correctly done? definitive? (or if not, does it at least set the stage for the next step?). In short, we intend to continue the tradition of asking: Is this study *Archival*?

These high standards could never have been achieved without the contributions of thousands of different expert reviewers over the years. Dan Freedman believed that all of our contributors were educated by the review process. Collectively, our reviewers and author-scholars compose an "international university" for our field and continue to be a powerful force underlying scientific advances in behavioral science. The prodigious numbers of critiques he solicited for each reviewed submission were legendary, but in the end, of course, our readers benefit from the multiple and often sharply different visions of the reviewers. We hope to preserve this tradition—albeit sparing our authors from having to "diagnose" quite so many reviews!

Psychiatric research—from imaging to psychodynamics—is becoming more specialized, technical, and perhaps inherently difficult to grasp. In light of this, we are asking our authors to place a greater emphasis on clearer, more concise presentation so that our readership can more readily appreciate the science and significance behind the articles in our pages. Furthermore, publishing shorter articles will allow us to accept more of the papers that are submitted. Also in deference to our contributors, we are striving to complete our initial evaluation of each manuscript within 8 to 12 weeks and have reduced the time between final acceptance and publication.

Various members of the editorial board and our readership have suggested a number of new features that, with some trepidation, we will add. To have loved Dan was to have known his pain with format changes. Dan would be happy to know that these additions will not decrease the overall space in the journal, because the American Medical Association (AMA) has agreed to add pages to permit these new features.

Both Roy and Dan thrived on the controversy sparked by new ideas and approaches to scientific inquiry. In that spirit, we intend to publish one or more "go with" commentaries with selected articles to create a roundtable discussion in print. These commentaries may further explain the studies, highlight the scientific or clinical importance of results, place the findings in a different context, outline the next needed step in the research, or even provide a vastly different way of interpreting the data.

Three new features will be added to the journal. A single, monthly page titled "This Month in *Archives of General Psychiatry*" will provide our readers with an overview of the contents of that issue. A book review section will feature critiques of recent publications about research advances or health policy, which members of the Editorial Board believe are particularly noteworthy. Finally, we will publish a few obituaries of individuals whose contributions reflected the goals and ideals of this journal.

The members of the Editorial Board of the ARCHIVES have been extraordinarily helpful throughout the life of this journal, and especially during the recent transitional period between editors. Their conscientious and detailed manuscript reviews are renowned throughout the field. Recently, there have been some turnover and expansion on the Board. We give heartfelt thanks to departing board members Jonathan O. Cole, MD, Roger E. Meyer, MD, Donald J. Scherl, MD, and Joel Yager, MD, for their service. We particularly wish to congratulate our colleague, Floyd Bloom, MD, a reviewer who can look at almost any paper with extraordinary clarity of thought, who is leaving the Board to assume the editorship of *Science*. New members include Huda Akil, PhD, William Carpenter, MD, Glen Elliott, MD, Eric Nestler, MD, Charles O'Brien, MD, PhD, Alan Schatzberg, MD, and Gary Tischler, MD. They bring a new depth and breadth in such areas as psychobiology, schizophrenia, childhood disorders, neurobiology, substance abuse and alcoholism, clinical research and health care provision, and economics. In addition, the ARCHIVES board now includes a statistical editor, Helena Kraemer, PhD, of Stanford University's Department of Psychiatry. She is a top expert on a wide range of statistical and methodological issues and has a particular interest in clinical applications.

We are also indebted to Grayson Norquist, MD, MSPH, for overseeing the editorial office after Dan's death. Without his characteristic calm and diligence during those often traumatic 10 months, the journal—and Dan Freedman's vision for it—may not have survived. Upon Dan's death, Grayson was offered the title of "Acting Editor" or "Interim Editor" by the AMA. He adamantly refused these in favor of his usual listing on the masthead as "Assistant to the Chief Editor," and during the transitional period Dan's name was kept on the masthead as Chief Editor. Grayson's job, as he saw it, was to tend what Dan called his "factory" (the ARCHIVES' editorial office) in keeping with Dan's spirit and vision. It is doubtful any better Assistant to the Chief could have been found. We continue to benefit from Grayson's wise counsel as he serves on the Editorial Board.

The new Assistant to the Editor is Peter M. Marzuk, MD. A member of the Cornell University faculty where he is Assistant Professor of Psychiatry, Dr Marzuk has interests in epidemiology and the psychosocial aspects of psychiatry. His research centers on suicide and violence. He has already brought wit, a keen respect for deadlines, and an awareness of the feelings of both authors and readers to all of our actions.

It was a major coup for us to have Angela McGregor make the transition from Los Angeles to New York. She had worked closely with Dan as Editorial Administrator of the ARCHIVES for 3 years prior to his death and with Grayson Norquist during the transition period. Angela has such a superb sense of the inner workings of the journal, its constituencies and its traditions, that she has proved invaluable.

We are deeply grateful to George Lundberg, MD, the Editor in Chief of the AMA scientific publications and of *JAMA*, Michael Springer, Publisher, and Richard Glass, MD, an ARCHIVES board member and *JAMA*'s Deputy Editor for Scientific Research. As they were during the transition, they continue to be extraordinarily helpful and supportive of our mission and endeavors.

Finally, it is with a great sense of humility that I have taken the title Editor. For me, Dan will always be the Editor in Chief.

Jack D. Barchas, MD
Editor

Notice to Authors

Length of Text. Ideally, the text of manuscripts (not including abstract, tables, figures, and references) should be under 5000 words. Include a word count on the title page.

Title. The title should be short, specific, and descriptive, emphasizing the main point of the article. Avoid two-part titles, if at all possible. Do not number titles, eg, "I" or "Part I." Title length, including punctuation and spaces, ideally should be under 100 characters and must not exceed 200 characters.

Abstract. The abstract should be structured into four parts and be no longer than 250 words.

Tables and Figures. Material should provide substantive data and not merely illustrate the text. While the main finding of a table or figure may be discussed in the narrative, the table or figure should not duplicate the text. Although no specific guideline applies to all articles, the number and length of tables and figures should be considered carefully and kept to a minimum.

References. All references should be selected carefully to acknowledge previous work or to document a specific point. They should not be exhaustive.

Please consult the "Instructions to Authors" on page 87 of this issue for other details regarding manuscript preparation.

Risk of Alzheimer's Disease in First-Degree Relatives

In an article published in the July 1994 issue of the ARCHIVES, Silverman et al[1] reported on the risks of first-degree relatives of patients with Alzheimer's disease for primary progressive dementia (PPD). They used the family history method for the evaluation of relatives and survival analysis for statistical calculations. The most remarkable finding was a reduction of the hazard rates in the 85- to 89-year age interval in the patient sample and, consequently, the reduction of the familial contribution to the risk for PPD compared with relatives of controls in this age range.

The study had two important shortcomings: first, relatives had not been interviewed personally; second, different informants provided family history information (ie, one or two relatives in the patient group and in the first control group and the index proband in the second control group). When using family history information, it might be that an age-dependent variation of the criteria of the informants for cognitive impairment and deviant behavior among their relevant others biases the age-specific hazard rates. The sensitivity of the family history method to detect PPD might be reduced with the increasing age of the subject. In addition, the sensitivity might be reduced if informants have less experience with relatives with dementia. This bias becomes more pronounced when fewer informants provide data on patients' histories, as was the case in the second control group in the study by Silverman et al.[1]

We had the opportunity to test the sensitivity of the family history method[2] in an ongoing family study, using direct examination and the best-estimate diagnosis[3] for comparison. In this study, all available relatives of 49 patients with Alzheimer's disease and 40 controls from the general population were examined using the Composite International Diagnostic Interview[4] and the Structured Interview for the Diagnosis of Dementia of the Alzheimer-type, Multi-infarct Dementia, and Dementia of Other Etiology.[5] Characteristics of patients (n=49; mean±SD age, 77.5±8.5 years; 14.3% male), controls (n=40; mean±SD age, 69.4±9.4 years; 27.5% male) and their relatives (patients' relatives: n=437; mean±SD age, 60.8±19.1 years; 49.5% male; and controls' relatives: n=345; mean±SD age, 58.7±19.1 years; 46.9% male) were comparable. Two hundred twenty-eight (58.3%) of 391 living relatives could be personally interviewed.

Interviewers were kept blind to other relatives' diagnoses. In addition, a family history concerning psychiatric disorders and dementia was received for all living and deceased relatives (n=782) using the Family History Questionnaire[6] and the Dementia Questionnaire.[2] For each relative, a family history was received from 2.4±1.7 (mean±SD) other family members. Final diagnoses were made by two experienced psychiatrists using the best-estimate procedure.[3]

Among the 228 relatives who were directly examined by clinical means and structured interviews (including 92 subjects who were older than 60 years), 12 relatives were found to suffer from PPD. Personal examinations and interviews of these relatives in their usual environment provided consistent evidence for dementia, but in only three cases had other family members provided a positive family history of PPD. In nine cases, the family (two to four relatives per subject) had not been aware of the disorder of the subject with dementia. Thus, the sensitivity of the family history method in relation to direct examination in this small sample was only 25%. Not a single subject of all those who were personally examined and who did not have dementia was reported to have dementia by other family members. Consequently, the family history method seems to underestimate the hazard rates for PPD. These limitations demonstrate the need to reaffirm the major results of Silverman et al[1] in an independent sample using the family study method. This was intended in the present ongoing study. Statistical methods of survival analysis were equivalent to those of Silverman et al.[1] As mentioned, 12 relatives with PPD were found by personal examination. In addition, 32 other relatives (29 were dead and three were living but unavailable for examination) received a diagnosis of PPD by family history. The **Table** presents the cumulative risk for PPD and the age-specific hazard rates for relatives of patients and controls. In accordance with Silverman et al,[1] the hazard rate in relatives of patients with Alzheimer's disease in the age group between 85 and 89 years was reduced compared with relatives aged 80 to 84 years and compared with relatives of con-

Cumulative Lifetime Risks and Age-Specific Hazard Rates in Relatives of 49 Patients With Alzheimer's Disease and 40 Controls*

	Relatives of Patients With Alzheimer's Disease		Relatives of Controls	
Age Interval, y	Cumulative Risks, %	Hazard Rates, %	Cumulative Risks, %	Hazard Rates, %
50-54	0.42±0.42	0.08±0.08	0	0
55-59	0.90±0.64	0.10±0.10	1.14±0.08	0.23±0.16
60-64	2.55±1.13	0.34±0.19	1.14±0.08	0
65-69	2.55±1.13	0	1.14±0.08	0
70-74	8.66±2.35	1.30±0.46	2.41±1.49	0.26±0.26
75-79	17.75±3.66	2.34±0.74	12.07±4.32	2.08±0.93
80-84	31.89±5.24	3.52±1.24	17.84±5.64	1.36±0.96
85-89	36.58±6.66	1.43±1.43	26.72±7.78	2.29±1.61

*Values are means±SEMs.

trols aged 85 to 89 years. Even though our data are preliminary, they provide further support for the results and conclusions of Silverman et al.[1] Our results should be less biased by retrospective evaluation and by group differences during data collection.

Reinhard Heun, MD
Wolfgang Maier, MD
Department of Psychiatry
University of Mainz
Untere Zahlbacher St 8
Mainz, Germany D-55131

1. Silverman JM, Li G, Zaccario ML, Smith CJ, Schmeidler J, Mohs RC, Davis KL. Patterns of risk in first-degree relatives of patients with Alzheimer's disease. *Arch Gen Psychiatry.* 1994;51:577-586.
2. Silverman JM, Breitner JCS, Mohs RC, Davis KL. Reliability of the family history method in genetic studies of alzheimer's disease and related dementias. *Am J Psychiatry.* 1986;143:1279-1282.
3. Leckman JF, Sholomskas D, Thompson WD, Belanger A, Weissman MM. Best estimate of lifetime psychiatric diagnosis. *Arch Gen Psychiatry.* 1982;39:879-883.
4. World Health Organization. *Composite International Diagnostic Interview.* Geneva, Switzerland: Division of Mental Health, World Health Organization; 1990.
5. Zaudig M, Mittelhammer J, Hiller W, Pauls A, Thora C, Morinigo A, Mombour W. SIDAM: a structured interview for the diagnosis of dementia of the Alzheimer type, multi-infarct dementia and dementias of other aetiology according to *ICD-10* and *DSM-III-R. Psychol Med.* 1991;21:225-236.
6. Andreasen NC, Endicott J, Spitzer RL, Winokur G. The family history method using diagnostic criteria: reliability and validity. *Arch Gen Psychiatry.* 1977; 34:1229-1235.

In reply

The reliance on informants for information on the relatives of an index subject is an inherent limitation of the family history method. However, in contrast to the weak sensitivity observed by Huen and Maier, a recent study of the validity of this method suggests that, despite this limitation, highly accurate information can be obtained.[1] Although the Dementia Questionnaire[2] was used to finally diagnose PPD in relatives, Huen and Maier's use of the Family History Questionnaire[3] as a screening tool may have contributed to the poor sensitivity observed because that instrument was not primarily designed to screen for dementia. Our approach has been to apply the Dementia Questionnaire when there was even a slight indication of memory or other cognitive problems as elicited by the Alzheimer's Disease Risk Questionnaire.[4] Furthermore, as noted in our article,[5] for investigations of late-onset diseases such as Alzheimer's disease (AD), there is often no realistic alternative to the family history method because most of the relatives of greatest interest will already be dead. A good example of this is Huen and Maier's ongoing study; despite their efforts to evaluate relatives directly, close to three quarters of the relatives with PPD were either dead or unavailable for interview and thus had to be identified through family informants.

A weakness of our study was the use of only one informant in our second control group (although the average number of informants in the first control group was virtually identical to that of the proband group with AD). However, our concerns about a possible decreased level of accurate ascertainment of the relatives in this group were mitigated by the strong similarity in the risk curves and age-specific hazard rates in the two control groups and by the similar percentages of persons with PPD between families assessed with two informants vs those assessed with one informant in both the proband group with AD and the first group of control families.[5]

Huen and Maier suggest two plausible sources of bias in family history studies of probands with AD and controls. They suggest that informants in general may be more likely to recognize and report dementia in younger relatives and that informants of controls, in particular, having had less exposure to dementia, may be less sensitive to it when it may have emerged in their families compared with those of probands with AD. Although we know of no study that has investigated the sensitivity of PPD diagnoses in relatives of cases vs controls, in our study of interinformant reliability, we found good and comparable levels of agreement between independent family informants for relatives of controls and probands.[2] However, if we assume that these biases were present and influenced the results in our article, then it is interesting to consider how our findings would change if these biases could be eliminated, ie, if we could identify the patients with PPD that were missed because they were older or because they were relatives of controls. These biases would be operating in concert only in the assessment of the older relatives of the control families. That group would be disproportionately underascertained, and the diminishing proportion of risk with increasing age that is attributable to a relationship with a proband with AD would be even stronger than was, in fact, observed.

As Huen and Maier note, the reduced age-specific hazard rate in the 85- to 89-year age interval offers further support for a diminishing role of familial factors in AD associated with increasing age. However, in contrast to their assertion that the reduction of the hazard rate for relatives of probands with AD who were in their late 80s was the most noteworthy finding in our study, we would argue that specific comparisons of rates at any single interval is less important than the overall pattern of rates as they change across the late lifespan. This is particularly true for the very late age intervals for which age-specific estimates are inevitably derived from the smallest samples and hence are the most unstable. In this regard, it is interesting to note that, using Huen and Maier's preliminary results, the attributable proportion of risk associated with being related to a proband with AD drops from 0.80 at the 70- to 74-year age interval to 0.11 in the 75- to 79-year age interval, rises to 0.61 in the 80- to 84-year age interval, and then finally drops sharply to −0.60 in the 85- to 89-year age interval. Although the rates did not decline steadily from one interval to the next, perhaps owing to the small number of relatives in their two groups, the overall trend toward decreasing familial risk with increasing age also supports the conclusions of our study.

Jeremy M. Silverman, PhD
Ge Li, MD, PhD
Richard C. Mohs, PhD
Kenneth L. Davis, MD
Department of Psychiatry
Mount Sinai School of Medicine
1 Gustave L. Levy Pl
New York, NY 10029

1. Kawas C, Segal J, Stewart WF, Corrado M, Thal L. A validation study of the Dementia Questionnaire. *Arch Neurol.* 1994;51:901-906.
2. Silverman JM, Breitner JCS, Mohs RC, Davis KL. Reliability of the family history method in genetic studies of Alzheimer's disease and related dementias. *Am J Psychiatry.* 1986;143:1279-1282.
3. Andreasen NC, Endicott J, Spitzer RL, Winokur G. The family history method using diagnostic criteria: reliability and validity. *Arch Gen Psychiatry.* 1977;34:1229-1235.
4. Breitner JCS, Folstein MF. Familial Alzheimer's disease: a prevalent disorder with specific clinical features. *Psychol Med.* 1984;14:63-80.
5. Silverman JM, Li G, Zaccario ML, Smith CJ, Schmeidler J, Mohs RC, Davis KL. Patterns of risk in first-degree relatives of patients with Alzheimer's disease. *Arch Gen Psychiatry.* 1994;51:577-586.

Low Levels of Pertussis Toxin Adenosine Diphosphate Ribosylation in the Schizophrenic Brain

The family of guanosine triphosphate–binding proteins (G proteins) plays a key role in the transmembrane signaling pathway in a variety of cells: Gs and Gi stimulate and inhibit adenylate cyclase, respectively; Gp activates polyphosphoinositide phosphodiesterase; Gk activates K^+ channels; and Go inhibits the voltage-dependent Ca^{2+} channel.[1] Recently, Hepler and Gilman[2] reviewed further advances of G protein research; they described how the task of unraveling the complexity of the G protein–regulated cellular switchboard expands exponentially as the number of identified G protein subunits continues to grow.

Measurements of the level of Gi/Go in the schizophrenic brain utilizing pertussis toxin (islet-activating protein)–catalyzed adenosine diphosphate (ADP) ribosylation showed that the amount of Gi/Go was significantly decreased in the putamen[3] and hippocampus[4] of the left hemisphere in schizophrenic patients compared with controls. Unfortunately, these experiments with islet-activating protein could not distinguish multiple species of subunits of pertussis toxin–sensitive G proteins. On the other hand, when we investigated the α-subunit of G proteins (Gαo and $G\alpha i_2$) using the highly sensitive enzyme immunoassay method, there were no significant differences in Gαo in the hippocampus and putamen of the left hemisphere in schizophrenic patients compared with controls, while there was a significant decrease in Gαo in the hippocampus and caudate head of the right hemisphere in schizophrenic patients.[5] The concentrations of $G\alpha i_2$ did not differ significantly in any area.[5]

Our study[5] could not determine concentrations of $G\alpha i_1$ for methodological reasons; however, Asano et al[6] have reported that the amounts of $G\alpha i_1$ and $G\alpha i_2$ were about 36% and 8%, respectively, of that of Gαo in hippocampus of rats. Therefore, the amounts of ADP-ribosylated products reported previously in hippocampus or putamen were mainly those of the heterotrimeric structures of Go and Gi_1; the level of ADP ribosylation of Gi_2 can be disregarded in this case.

The discrepancies between ADP ribosylation and immunoassay would be explained by the hypothesis of Seeman et al[7,8] that dopamine receptors in schizophrenic subjects are locked in a high-affinity state; this hypothesis was introduced by Taubes[9] in the Research News section of *Science*. On the basis of their studies of dopamine receptors, Seeman et al[7,8] explained that, normally, G proteins rapidly switch dopamine receptors back and forth between states of high and low affinity but that in schizophrenic subjects, the receptor ceases to function. It is only in schizophrenia that something is wrong with the receptors' ability to switch.[9]

When receptors couple with G proteins (or in the case of the dopamine system, when D_2 or D_4 dopamine receptors couple with Gi), the subunit equilibrium of heterotrimeric Gi ($\alpha\beta\gamma \rightleftarrows \alpha + \beta\gamma$) shifts to the right. Since ADP ribosylation by pertussis toxin occurs only when the α-subunit has combined with the βγ subunit in the tight trimeric structure,[10] this reaction cannot be induced during dissociation of α from βγ. Therefore, when locked in a high-affinity state, ADP ribosylation is suppressed owing to the dissociation of α from βγ. It would follow, then, that the total amount of Gi/Go would be decreased to about three quarters, since Gi probably accounts for one quarter of the amount of ADP ribosylation. Meanwhile, the trimeric structure is not necessary for reaction of the anti-Gαo antibodies against Gαo.

Therefore, the hypothesis of Seeman et al[7,8] explains the hitherto puzzling contradiction between our results using ADP ribosylation and those using the immunoassay. In turn, our results appear to support their hypothesis.

Fumihiko Okada, MD
Health Administration Center
Hokkaido University
Sapporo, Japan
Takeshi Murakami, MD, PhD
Yukiko Tokumitsu, PhD
Sapporo

1. Graziano MP, Gilman AG. Guanine nucleotide-binding regulatory proteins: mediators of transmembrane signaling. *Trends Pharmacol Sci.* 1987;8:478-481.
2. Hepler JR, Gilman AG. G proteins. *Trends Biochem Sci.* 1992;17:383-387.
3. Okada F, Crow TJ, Roberts GW. G-proteins (Gi, Go) in the basal ganglia of control and schizophrenic brain. *J Neural Transm.* 1990;79:227-234.
4. Okada F, Crow TJ, Roberts GW. G proteins (Gi, Go) in the medial temporal lobe in schizophrenia: preliminary report of a neurochemical correlate of structural change. *J Neural Transm.* 1991;84:147-153.
5. Okada F, Tokumitsu Y, Takahashi N, Crow TJ, Roberts GW. Reduced concentrations of the α-subunit of GTP-binding protein Go in schizophrenic brain. *J Neural Transm.* 1994;95:95-104.
6. Asano T, Shinohara H, Morishita R, Kato K. Immunochemical and immunohistochemical localization of the G protein Gi 1 in rat central nervous tissues. *J Biochem.* 1990;108:988-994.
7. Seeman P, Niznik HB, Guan H-C, Booth G, Ulpian C. Link between D_1 and D_2 dopamine receptors is reduced in schizophrenia and Huntington diseased brain. *Proc Natl Acad Sci U S A.* 1989;86:10156-10160.
8. Seeman P, Guan H-C, Van Tol HHM. Dopamine D_4 receptors elevated in schizophrenia. *Nature.* 1993;365:441-445.
9. Taubes G. Will new dopamine receptors offer a key to schizophrenia? *Science.* 1994;265:1034-1035.
10. Katada T, Ui M. Direct modification of the membrane adenylate cyclase system by islet-activating protein due to ADP-ribosylation of a membrane protein. *Proc Natl Acad Sci U S A.* 1982;79:3129-3133.

MANUSCRIPT CRITERIA AND INFORMATION

Submit manuscripts to Jack D. Barchas, MD, Editor, ***Archives of General Psychiatry*, Cornell Medical Center, Dept of Psychiatry, Box 171, 525 E 68th St, Room F2315, New York, NY 10021.** Manuscripts are received with the understanding that they are not under simultaneous consideration by another publication, have not been published previously, and have the approval of each author. Accepted manuscripts become the permanent property of the ARCHIVES. They may not be republished without permission from the publisher (AMA).

Editing. Copyediting follows AMA style and requires corresponding author approval. The authors are responsible for all statements made in their work, including changes made by the copy editor and authorized by the corresponding author.

Reprints. Forms for ordering are included with the edited typescript sent for approval. Reprints are shipped 6 to 8 weeks after publication.

Cover Letter

- In the cover letter, designate one author as correspondent and provide a complete address and telephone and fax numbers.

- For a manuscript to be reviewed, considered, or edited, the following statement must be signed by *all* authors:

"I have been sufficiently involved in this work to take public responsibility for its validity and final presentation as an original publication. I can and will provide documentation of my work upon reasonable request and I have fulfilled the obligations for full disclosure and authorship as described by *Archives of General Psychiatry*. . . ." This signed statement must conclude with *one* of the two following sentences: "Accordingly, I hereby transfer, assign, or otherwise convey all copyright ownership to the AMA in the event such work is published by the AMA." [OR] "No copyright ownership can be transferred since this work was produced in the course of my official duties as a US government officer or employee."

Manuscript Preparation[1,2]

- Submit an original double-spaced typescript and 7 copies.
- **Manuscripts will not be returned after the review process.** Unpublished manuscripts will be destroyed.
- Type—double-spaced throughout (including references)—on one side only of 8½ × 11-in white bond paper. Number all pages. Do not justify right-hand margins. Use a printer of at least letter quality.
- Titles cannot exceed 200 characters, including punctuation and spaces, and should be as brief as possible.
- The title page should list full names, degrees, academic affiliations and their locations, and the name and address to whom reprint requests should be sent. If the paper was presented at a meeting, include the organization, place, and date of presentation. Acknowledgment of grant or drug company support should also be made on this page. Include a word count of the text only (excluding the abstract, references, and tables).
- Include a structured abstract of 250 words or less that states in defined sections the Background, Methods, Results, and Conclusions.
- Use Système International (SI) measurements throughout the manuscript.
- Use generic names of drugs, unless the specific trade name is directly relevant to the study design or discussion.
- Do not use abbreviations in the title or abstract. Limit their use in the text.
- *Do not use footnotes or appendixes.* Such materials should either be incorporated into the text or offered to interested readers on request.
- Include a statistical analysis section under *Methods* that fully describes the application of each statistical procedure used. If a test is used that is not commonly presented in the ARCHIVES, briefly describe its purpose and how it is to be interpreted. Results should report the test statistic (eg, χ^2, F or t value), degrees of freedom, and P value. Measures of central tendency (eg, means) should be accompanied by measures of variability (eg, standard deviations). In the cover letter, state the name of your statistical consultant, if appropriate.
- Acknowledge fully any material taken from other publications, and submit written permission from the owner to reprint in any language or form without limitation.

Tables. Double-space on separate sheets of 8½ × 11-in white bond paper. Title each one and number them in the order of their citation in the text. If a table must be continued, repeat the title on a second sheet, followed by "(cont)." Any explanatory notes to be printed with the table must be typed single-spaced beneath the table.

Figures. Once manuscripts are accepted, two sets of professionally prepared, high-contrast glossy prints (preferably in a proportion of 5 × 7 in) are required. If full-color figures are necessary, the ARCHIVES may pay part of the expense with the balance to be borne by the author.

- Number figures according to their order in the text. Type the figure number, proper orientation (eg, top), name of the senior author, and an abbreviated title on a gummed label; affix it to the back of the print.
- Double-space legends (maximum length, 40 words) on a separate sheet of 8½ × 11-in paper.

References. Number references in the order they are mentioned in the text; do *not* alphabetize. In text, tables, and legends, identify references with superscript arabic numbers. In listing references, follow AMA style and abbreviate names of journals according to *Index Medicus*. List all authors and/or editors. Citation accuracy is the responsibility of the author.

THIS MONTH IN

ARCHIVES OF GENERAL PSYCHIATRY

Although most patients with obsessive-compulsive disorder (OCD) can now be successfully treated, some remain incapacitated by their symptoms. For a subset of these unresponsive patients who are severely incapacitated by OCD, cingulotomy, a neurosurgical operation, has been reported to be effective and safe. **Baer et al** (page 384) followed up a group of patients who had undergone cingulotomy. At average follow-up of 2 years, five of the 18 patients (28%) had responded, and another three (16%) had partially responded. Most showed large improvements in quality of life and no evidence of serious side effects. This study, although not placebo controlled, suggests that more than a quarter of patients with untreatable OCD become, and remain, much improved after this treatment of last resort.

Magnetic resonance spectroscopy (MRS) offers a new approach in schizophrenia research through its ability to assess the biochemistry of a defined brain region in living patients. **Stanley et al** (page 399) report a study in which the prefrontal cortex of patients with schizophrenia at different stages of illness were investigated using in vivo phosphorus MRS. At the early stage of illness, prior to any neuroleptic medication, significant increases in the breakdown products of cell membranes and significant decreases in precursors of cell membranes were observed. In the chronic stage only, significant decreases in precursors were observed. These alterations in the membrane phospholipids may point to specific metabolic abnormalities in schizophrenia.

Patients with schizophrenia suffer from a diverse and sometimes confusing array of symptoms. **Andreasen et al** (page 341) use statistical techniques to examine the correlations between symptoms and find that they fall naturally into three dimensions: psychoticism, disorganization, and negative symptoms. Examining serious mental illnesses using these three dimensions may assist in identifying underlying biological mechanisms that are common across disorders or in measuring the effects of treatment.

Very few outcome studies have been completed using newer dimensional approaches, which divide the symptoms of schizophrenia into two positive dimensions (psychoticism and disorganization) and a third negative dimension. **Arndt et al** (page 352) examined these dimensions in a group of patients with schizophrenia, most of whom had not received previous antipsychotic treatment. All three dimensions were prominent during the initial acute episode, but the two positive dimensions tended to decline during the 2-year follow-up period, whereas the negative symptoms tended to persist. In addition, changes in each of the dimensions tended to occur independently of one another over the 2-year period, indicating these dimensions may have differences in neural and cognitive mechanisms, psychosocial correlates, and responses to treatment.

There is controversy whether manic depressive illness (bipolar) should be considered a separate disease from the larger group of depressions that occur unassociated with mania. **Winokur et al** (page 367) found that mania is more frequent in families of patients with bipolar illness than in controls or families of depressed patients and that the latter two groups did not differ in the frequency of mania. Also, patients who had a more severe mania associated with psychotic symptoms did not differ from nonpsychotic manic patients in the risks for familial mania or depression. These distinct familial patterns suggest that bipolar illness is a separate illness from those disorders that manifest depression only.

Little is known about the interrelationship between the genetic and the environmental risk factors for a range of psychiatric disorders. In an epidemiologic sample of female-female twin pairs, **Kendler et al** (page 374) found evidence for two main genetic factors—one influencing the risk for major depression and generalized anxiety disorder and the other, the risk for phobia, panic disorder, and bulimia nervosa. Genetic influences on alcoholism appear largely unique to alcoholism alone. Familial environmental influences impacted significantly only on bulimia. These results begin to clarify the complex relationship between current psychiatric diagnostic categories and the relevant genetic and environmental risk factors.

Abnormal functioning in brain circuits linking the cortex, striatum, and thalamus has been hypothesized to cause obsessive-compulsive disorder (OCD). Using MRI, **Robinson et al** (page 393) found that patients with OCD have smaller (possibly abnormal) caudates than do healthy control subjects. This underscores the need to study other structures within the cortical-striatal-thalamic circuits for anatomical abnormalities in OCD.

ORIGINAL ARTICLE

Symptoms of Schizophrenia

Methods, Meanings, and Mechanisms

Nancy C. Andreasen, MD, PhD; Stephan Arndt, PhD; Randall Alliger, PhD; Del Miller, PharmD, MD; Michael Flaum, MD

Background: The "group of schizophrenias," normally referred to with a single nominative, is phenomenologically heterogeneous. Its symptoms represent multiple psychological domains, including perception, inferential thinking, language, attention, social interaction, emotion expression, and volition. Studies of psychopathology have simplified this complex array in several ways, one of which is a subdivision into positive and negative symptoms.

Methods: This study examined the positive vs negative distinction in a sample of 243 patients with schizophrenia or schizophreniform disorder who were evaluated with the Scale for the Assessment of Negative Symptoms and the Scale for the Assessment of Positive Symptoms. A two-stage factor analysis was applied, beginning with a principal components analysis applying varimax rotation, followed by an extension analysis. The purpose of these analyses was to evaluate the correlational relationships of the various symptoms of schizophrenia.

Results: The results confirmed previous reports by our group and others suggesting that the symptoms of schizophrenia fall into three natural dimensions, as assessed by the correlational interrelationships: positive symptoms subdivide into psychotic and disorganized dimensions, while a third negative dimension also emerges.

Conclusion: Because these dimensions have impressive consistency across studies, future work must examine their relationship to clinically relevant concepts such as prognosis or etiology and examine four different aspects: longitudinal course, neural mechanisms, relationship to treatment, and interrelationships in other pathological conditions.

(Arch Gen Psychiatry. 1995;52:341-351)

From the The Mental Health Clinical Research Center (Drs Andreasen, Arndt, Alliger, Miller, and Flaum), Department of Psychiatry (Drs Andreasen, Miller, and Flaum), and Department of Preventive Medicine and Environmental Health (Dr Arndt), The University of Iowa Hospitals and Clinics, College of Medicine, Iowa City.

THE GROUP of illnesses that we conventionally refer to as "schizophrenia," typically using a single nominative for simple verbal convenience (and perhaps out of intellectual laziness), is diverse in nature and covers a broad range of cognitive, emotional, and behavioral domains.[1-3] The symptoms used to define schizophrenia in standard nomenclatures, such as *DSM-IV*[4] or *International Classification of Diseases, 10th Revision*,[5] include various forms of delusions, hallucinations, thought disorders, and abnormalities in emotional expression, social interaction, attention, and volition and drive. From the perspective of cognitive psychology, these symptoms represent a variety of systems, including inferential and abstract thinking; language; appetitive drives; auditory, visual, and tactile perception; and a host of others. This situation presents us with several paradoxes that make it difficult for both novices and experienced professionals to "get their minds around" the concept of schizophrenia. First, we typically use a single word to refer to a disorder that may be etiologically and pathophysiologically heterogeneous and therefore constitutes multiple illnesses that should properly be referred to as "the schizophrenias." Second, this disorder is also cross-sectionally and symptomatically heterogeneous; that is, two patients given this diagnosis may have totally different and nonoverlapping symptom patterns, if the current *DSM-IV* diagnostic criteria are applied. Stated succinctly, these paradoxes reduce to: the *schizophrenias* are a polythetic construct.

Investigators have used a variety of mental mechanisms and intellectual strategies to cope with the confusion and chaos

See Methods on next page

METHODS

SUBJECTS

Subjects in this study consisted of 243 patients with either schizophrenia or schizophreniform disorder who were consecutively admitted to the Mental Health Clinical Research Center (MHCRC) at The University of Iowa Hospitals and Clinics in Iowa City. All patients admitted to the MHCRC receive a comprehensive evaluation that includes the CASH as well as weekly ratings using the SANS and SAPS. All the patients were diagnosed using *DSM-III-R* diagnostic criteria. Diagnoses were established using two consensus conferences, one occurring shortly after admission and the second occurring at the time of discharge. Senior MHCRC medical staff participated in these consensus diagnostic sessions, which involved integration of cross-sectional interview data with repeated longitudinal assessments and information obtained from family members and previous treating physicians. The subjects in this study consisted of 229 patients having a diagnosis of core schizophrenia and 14, schizophreniform disorder. Patients also received a comprehensive general medical evaluation (history and physical examination) and were excluded if they suffered from a general medical or neurological disorder. The clinical and demographic characteristics of these patients are summarized in **Table 2**. Seventy-four patients were female and 169 were male.

RATINGS

The ratings of positive and negative symptoms used for analysis in this particular study were taken from the SANS and SAPS scales in the "Current Condition" section of the CASH. These particular ratings were selected for analysis because they were considered to provide the purest and most accurate measure of core or trait symptoms in this group of patients. As administered in the MHCRC, the CASH involves repeated evaluations and assessments throughout the hospital stay, including a 3-week medication washout period for most patients. Ratings of positive and negative symptoms for the current condition assess each sign or symptom at its worst during the past month; for those patients (particularly first-episode patients) who have been ill for longer than a month, but with clearly defined onset, the symptom is rated at its worst during the entire episode. These rating instructions are designed to permit investigators to capture the manifestation of each symptom in a way that will reflect the underlying pathophysiology to the greatest extent possible. Because nearly all the patients were evaluated in a medication-free state, we were able to observe positive symptoms emerge that might otherwise have been covered over through treatment effects. Further, we also were able to evaluate negative symptoms independent of drug side effects. The reliability of the various SANS and SAPS items has been assessed repeatedly and has been found to be good to excellent for most items, using both interrater and test-retest reliability measures.[2,30,58]

RATERS

The SANS and SAPS ratings used in these analyses were completed at the consensus conference conducted at the time of discharge by the research team; they are based on an agreement between the research psychiatrist who has cared for the patient throughout the hospital stay, nursing personnel who have observed the patient on a daily basis, and a research assistant assigned to follow each patient. Thus, they represent longitudinal rather than cross-sectional ratings. All the raters participated in weekly training and calibration meetings to ensure that ratings remained stable over time and that rater drift did not occur.

DATA ANALYSIS

Data analysis was conducted in two stages. An initial principal components analysis was used to validate the previous three-dimensional results and to provide structural definition for an extension analysis. Based on our earlier work,[97,98] we selected delusions, hallucinations, bizarre/disorganized behavior, positive formal thought disorder, inappropriate affect, affective flattening, anhedonia/asociality, and avolition/apathy as the symptoms for the initial analysis. Alogia and attentional impairment were withheld for the extension analysis because the specific purpose of this part of the study was to determine the interrelationships between items on these subscales to guide decisions concerning future revisions. Our previous analyses suggested that these two symptoms might be factorially complex. In the principal components analysis, the criterion used to select the number of factors was eigenvalues greater than unity. A maximum likelihood factor solution verified the number of factors. The initial factor solution then was rotated to simple structure using the varimax procedure.

To study the dimensional nature of the individual items in the SANS and SAPS as well as the global items excluded from the preliminary principal components analysis, an extension analysis of the principal components factor structure was explored.[107] This statistical procedure requires calculating factor scores from the principal components analysis and correlating them with the item scores. Correlations also were computed for the alogia and attentional impairment items that were not included in the principal components analysis. Statistical tests of these correlations are appropriate because the items that were not included in the factor solution are free to vary. However, because there are 50 items correlated across three factors, finding significant correlations capitalizes on chance. Therefore, a Bonferroni correction was applied to the statistical tests. A significance level of .001 was used to test the correlations.

Finally, multiple R^2 values were calculated between the individual items of a given symptom and its global rating. The purpose here was to provide a measure of internal consistency between a global rating and individual items of a symptom. A large R^2 suggests that the item ratings, taken together, differentiate subjects in a manner similar to the global rating. This lends support to the validity of the global rating. The global rating should reflect symptom severity as a function of the observable behavioral characteristics sampled by the item ratings.

produced by that observation. One strategy has been to identify core symptoms that are either highly specific or pathognomonic. Examples include the Bleulerian four A's, or more properly six A's (associations, affective, ambivalence, autism, attention, and avolition).[6] Kraepelin concurred with Bleuler in that if any symptoms could be considered fundamental or core, they would be "a weakening of those emotional activities which promptly form the mainspring of volition and the loss of the inner unity of activities, intellect, emotion, and volition."[7] Schneiderian first-rank symptoms represented an alternative approach to identifying pathognomonic symptoms.[8-10] The Bleulerian-Kraepelinian emphasis ran aground because of concerns about both specificity and reliability, while the Schneiderian influence has been reduced because of nonspecificity.[11-24] In the turbulent conceptual waters that were produced in the absence of a single clear guideline as to the essence of the group of schizophrenias, the concept of positive and negative symptoms emerged for a time as a calming influence.[25-52] This approach to discussing the symptoms of schizophrenia has dominated the past decade.

See also pages 352 and 361

The earliest comprehensive discussion of positive and negative symptoms was presented by Hughlings-Jackson, a 19th-century neurologist, although Reynolds had made an earlier, less extensive presentation.[25-27] Jackson was writing in a era when evolutionary theory provided the prevailing worldview, and he developed a model of brain function that reflected it: the brain was organized like an onion, with deeper primitive layers to which higher, more civilizing layers were added. Jackson applied this model to the understanding of various syndromes, including the psychoses. He suggested that positive symptoms, such as delusions or hallucinations, represented release phenomena; they were symptoms arising when a higher cortical regulator or organizer had been lost and the activity from a lower level therefore emerged unchecked. Negative symptoms, such as avolition or emotional blunting, were due to "dissolution"; that is, they represented a diffuse or generalized loss of higher centers.

While Fish[53] and others[54] in Britain had echoed Jacksonian concepts, Strauss et al[28] were the first to write a comprehensive discussion of Jacksonian ideas in relation to the group of schizophrenias in recent times. They proposed that three kinds of manifestations of schizophrenia could be used to evaluate prognosis and outcome: positive symptoms, negative symptoms, and disordered relationships. They suggested that positive symptoms were relatively nonspecific and prone to fluctuate, while negative symptoms and disorders of personal relationships were more fundamental and likely to have greater prognostic significance. They also proposed that this conceptualization be largely descriptive, rather than rooted in a Jacksonian model of brain function. Although forward-looking, this set of ideas did not capture the collective imagination of psychiatric investigators to the same extent as Crow's[29] formulation of the two-syndrome hypothesis in 1980. Crow's two-syndrome model of schizophrenia has been widely discussed and studied, largely because it combined within a single theoretical model methods for thinking about onset, cross-sectional symptoms, outcome, treatment, and underlying neural mechanisms.[43-52] Crow proposed that a positive type of schizophrenia was characterized by acute onset, prominent positive symptoms, normal brain structure and function, a biochemical disorder involving dopaminergic transmission, good response to neuroleptics, and better outcome, while the negative type was characterized by an opposite pattern and most important by underlying structural abnormalities that were irreversible and led to poor neuroleptic response. While the Strauss formulation was purely descriptive, the Crow formulation returned the positive/negative distinction to a Jacksonian tradition in form, if not content, by rooting thinking about positive and negative symptoms in brain-behavior relationships.

One elemental component in discussions of positive and negative symptoms during the past decade has involved discussions about the best methods for defining and rating these symptoms. Two scales, the Scale for the Assessment of Negative Symptoms (SANS) and the Scale for the Assessment of Positive Symptoms (SAPS) were developed in 1982 to permit exploration of the clinical and neural correlates of these symptoms in schizophrenia and related psychotic illnesses, with the recognition that they would be relevant to the study of various affective disorders as well.[30-42]

These scales draw on constructs of cognitive psychology and identify domains that are relevant to the study of schizophrenia: perception, inference, language, behavioral monitoring, behavioral activity, emotional expression, conceptual and verbal fluency, pleasure drives, volition, and attention.[55-57] Early versions of the SANS and SAPS identified 10 symptoms that corresponded to these domains, five of which were positive and five of which were negative: hallucinations, delusions, positive thought disorder, bizarre/disorganized behavior, catatonic motor behavior, affective blunting, alogia, anhedonia, avolition, and attentional impairment.[30-33] Following Jacksonian thinking, the first five of these symptoms were considered to be positive because they represented distortions in normal functions that could be due to injury at a higher cortical level, while the five negative symptoms simply represented a loss of a function.[55] A principal components analysis of the first sample to be studied with these scales revealed a first factor that accounted for 42% of the variance and that had large positive loadings on affective flattening, alogia, avolition, anhedonia, attentional impairment, and catatonic motor behavior, with negative loadings on delusions and hallucinations.[31] A second factor had large positive loadings on positive thought disorder and bizarre behavior. Because catatonic motor behavior was in fact extremely rare, it was subsequently dropped from the positive symptom list in early versions of the SAPS, although methods for rating it remain in the more extensive structured interview that contains the SANS and SAPS scales, the Comprehensive Assessment of Symptoms and History (CASH).[58]

Since that early study, many subsequent investigations have explored the concept of positive and negative symptoms, and the terms have achieved widespread use at the clinical level, suggesting that they may meet an important conceptual need by simplifying or clarifying thinking about the nature of the symptoms of schizophrenia.[34-52,59-96] Discussions of the distinction between positive and negative symptoms have also produced many questions and problems, however. Two of the most basic questions have echoed conceptual history as it has moved from Jackson to Strauss to Crow. Why should a symptom be classified as negative or positive? Should it be based on some hypothesized brain-behavior relationship, as it was for Jackson and Crow? Is it sufficient to show a relationship at a descriptive level, using correlational and factor analytic techniques and demonstrating predictive validity using measures such as onset, outcome, or response to treatment? Can these symptoms be assessed cross-sectionally, or must longitudinal or repeated measures be added as well? If one postulates related groups of symptoms, how are they related to one another, ie, must they be independent, or do they have some type of interactive influence on one another? What effects do other confounding factors have on the assessment of positive and negative symptoms, such as neuroleptic medication or coexisting depressive symptoms? Are any of these symptoms specific to schizophrenia, or do they occur in other disorders?

One large body of literature has adopted the descriptive strategy and applied correlational and factor analytic techniques to examine the interrelationships between positive and negative symptoms. A total of four have been completed to date within our own center,[31,36,97,98] while we know of 10 others that have been completed in other centers.[46,96,99-106] A review of these studies suggests a surprising convergence of results and indicates that, at a descriptive level, three dimensions rather than two are required to account for the interrelationships among the symptoms of schizophrenia. The positive symptoms subdivide into two dimensions, one of which is typically composed of delusions and hallucinations and represents a psychosis dimension, while the other is typically composed of disorganized speech, disorganized behavior, and inappropriate affect and represents a "disorganization dimension." The negative symptoms remain robust as originally conceptualized, apart from attention, which sometimes loads with other negative symptoms but occasionally shows a relationship to the two positive symptom dimensions. As noted in a recent review by Minas et al,[104] even our original 1982 study[31] supports the existence of three dimensions, since a varimax rotation produces a three-factor solution. The various factor analytic studies are summarized in **Table 1**. Given that they represent samples collected from all over the world (England, India, Italy, Australia, Spain, and the United States), that many are based on small samples, and that they have used a variety of different factor analytic techniques, the convergence of results is striking.

Because of the convergence, and because the SANS and SAPS are widely used throughout the world in research investigations to explore the effects of treatment and neurobiological correlates of schizophrenia, we have conducted a fifth analysis of the SANS and SAPS in their current incarnation to guide us toward revisions that can be used in the future to explore these three dimensions. We report herein on a factor analysis of a sample of 243 patients. To answer some specific psychometric questions raised by our earlier work, we have conducted the factor analysis in two stages, using an initial principal components analysis to provide a firm structural definition of the dimensions, followed by an extension analysis to examine two of the negative symptom scales (alogia and attention) in more detail. This analysis was delayed until we were able to amass a sample of adequate size. Samples of 10 to 20 subjects per variable in a multivariate analysis are normally recommended, suggesting that 100 to 200 subjects would be desirable for a study analyzing 10 symptoms. A minimum sample of 200 has been recommended for stable estimates in factor analysis.[107]

RESULTS

Means and SDs of global ratings on the SANS and SAPS are shown below.

Symptom	Mean (SD)
Avolition	3.59 (1.16)
Anhedonia	3.89 (0.92)
Affective flattening	2.78 (1.23)
Inappropriate affect	1.67 (1.62)
Positive formal thought disorder	2.13 (1.45)
Bizarre behavior	2.43 (1.34)
Delusions	3.50 (1.25)
Hallucinations	2.81 (1.73)

Pearson correlations among the SANS and SAPS items are shown in **Table 3**.

The principal components analysis of the eight items yielded a three-factor solution. The three factors accounted for 66.59% of the total variance. The maximum likelihood analysis agreed with the prinicipal components estimate of the number of factors. The test for two common factors produced a significant lack of fit (maximum likelihood χ^2=27.296, *df*=13, *P*<.012), while the three-factor solution fit the data well (χ^2=2.292, *df*=7, *P*<.927). Furthermore, the third factor provided a significant contribution (χ^2=25.004, *df*=6, *P*<.005) to the solution.

Table 4 shows the principal components factor structure after the factors were rotated to simple structure using the varimax rotation procedure. The first factor reflects a negative symptom dimension and accounts for 27.94% of the variance. Avolition, anhedonia, and affective flattening all load highly with this factor. All three of these negative symptoms have a correlation greater than 0.80 with the first factor. The second factor, accounting for 20.65% of the variance, reflects a disorganization dimension. Inappropriate affect and positive formal thought disorder have strong loadings with this factor. Bizarre behavior loads on the disorganization factor, although it also loads on the negative factor. The third factor reflects a dimension indicative of psychosis that accounts for 18.00% of the variance. Delusions and hallucinations load highly with this third factor.

Table 1. Studies of Schizophrenia Using Factor Analysis Techniques*

Source, y	N	Technique	No. of Factors	Comment
Andreasen et al,[31] 1982	52	PCA	2 or 3	Original PCA (unrotated) showed one large bipolar factor (positive and negative factors); later analysis using varimax shows three, corresponding to psychotic, disorganized, and negative factors
Bilder et al,[99] 1985	32	PCA, varimax rotation	3	Factor 1 combines alogia, attention, thought disorder, and bizarre behavior; factor 2, negative symptoms; factor 3, psychotic symptoms
Andreasen et al,[36] 1986	117	PCA	3, possibly 4	First two factors represented negative symptoms; factor 3, delusions and hallucinations; factor 4, bizarre behavior
Kulhara et al,[100] 1986	98	PCA	3	Negative symptoms, psychoticism, and disorganization
Moscarelli et al,[96] 1987	59	PCA	2 or 3	Clear negative factor; positive factors less cohesive
Liddle,[86] 1987	40	PCA, rotation	3	"Psychomotor poverty, disorganization, and reality distortion"; based on only a subset of SANS and SAPS items
Lenzenweger et al,[101] 1989	302	Confirmatory factor analysis using maximum likelihood techniques to compare several models	2, possibly more	Retrospective reanalysis of twin data; positive and negative factors
Schuldberg et al,[102] 1990	370	PCA, varimax rotation	2	Clear negative factor, positive factor mainly psychoticism
Arndt et al,[97] 1991	207	PCA, varimax rotation, maximum likelihood techniques	3	Negative symptoms, psychoticism, and disorganization
Gur et al,[103] 1991	47	PCA, rotation	3	Negative symptoms, psychoticism, and disorganization
Minas et al,[104] 1992	114	Multidimensional scaling	3	Negative symptoms, psychoticism, and thought disorder; based on item analysis rather than global ratings
Peralta et al,[106] 1992	115	PCA, varimax rotation	4	Negative symptoms, psychoticism, and thought disorder; loadings on bizarre behavior not reported
Brown and White,[105] 1992	139	PCA, varimax rotation	3	Cross-sectional ratings using SANS and Manchester Scale; negative symptoms, psychoticism, inattentiveness, and inappropriate affect
Miller et al,[98] 1993	90	PCA, varimax rotation	3	Negative symptoms, psychoticism, and disorganization

**PCA indicates principal components analysis; SANS, Scale for the Assessment of Negative Symptoms; and SAPS, Scale for the Assessment of Positive Symptoms.*

EXTENSION ANALYSIS OF ALOGIA AND ATTENTION

The analysis of alogia and attentional impairment is reported in **Table 5**. The alogia and attentional impairment items, as well as the global ratings, do not consistently correlate significantly with a single factor. The item correlations for alogia load with either the negative factor or the disorganization factor. The global rating for alogia correlates most highly with negative symptoms. Similarly, the items and global rating for attentional impairment correlate most strongly with the negative factor, but also show correlations with the disorganization factor.

EXTENSION ANALYSIS OF THE SANS AND SAPS ITEMS

Table 6 reports the results of the extension analysis performed on the individual items that constitute the various global ratings. The factor loadings for the global ratings are shown again for comparison. The items constituting avolition, anhedonia, and affective flattening all correlated significantly with the negative factor. Uniformly, the highest correlations for these items with the three factors occurred on the negative factor. None of the items correlated with the psychotic factor, although three of the items (grooming and hygiene, ability to feel intimacy and closeness, and decreased spontaneous move-

Table 2. Demographic and Clinical Characteristics of Subjects

Characteristic	Mean	SD
Age, y	31.98	10.57
Education, y	12.59	2.25
Age at onset, y	20.97	5.75
Global Assessment Scale score at admission	32.07	8.38
Total duration of previous hospitalizations, mo	23.14	40.42
No. of previous hospitalizations	5.70	4.97

Table 3. Pearson Correlations Among SANS and SAPS Global Ratings*

Symptom	Avolition	Anhedonia	Affective Flattening	Inappropriate Affect	Thought Disorder	Bizarre Behavior	Delusions
Avolition	1.000						
Anhedonia	0.646	1.000					
Affective flattening	0.517	0.486	1.000				
Inappropriate affect	0.122	0.140	0.010	1.000			
Thought disorder	0.112	0.146	−0.023	0.336	1.000		
Bizarre behavior	0.412	0.400	0.247	0.315	0.378	1.000	
Delusions	0.239	0.201	0.078	0.058	0.292	0.311	1.000
Hallucinations	0.230	0.197	0.184	0.113	0.132	0.214	0.347

**SANS indicates Scale for the Assessment of Negative Symptoms; SAPS, Scale for the Assessment of Positive Symptoms.*

ment) had modest but significant correlations with the disorganization factor.

The items constituting positive formal thought disorder all correlated significantly with the disorganization factor. Except for the derailment item's significant correlation with the psychotic factor, none of the items correlated with either the negative or the psychotic factor.

The items constituting bizarre behavior, however, did not show as distinctive factor loadings as positive formal thought disorder on the disorganization factor. Although three of the four items had their highest correlations with the disorganization factor, many of the items also correlated significantly with the negative factor. This mirrors the split loading of the global rating of bizarre behavior with the negative factor and disorganization factor in the principal components analysis.

The items constituting delusions and hallucinations clearly correlated with the psychotic factor. All these correlations were the highest for the psychotic factor. Only grandiose delusions correlated significantly with another factor. Because of a low base rate (mean item rating=0.21, SD=0.71), the delusions of jealousy item failed to correlate significantly with any factor.

The multiple R^2 values for all global ratings with their respective scale items were all greater than 0.70 and most were greater than 0.80. Thus, the individual items demonstrate good internal consistency.

COMMENT

A fifth factor analysis study from our group has again shown that positive and negative symptoms do not subdivide neatly into two categories. These results are quite similar to four previous studies completed at Iowa. The first study,[31] reported in 1982, was interpreted at the time as suggesting the possibility of only two dimensions, but this finding is primarily the result of not subjecting the data to varimax rotation; after rotation, the factor structure appears similar to that observed in the study herein.[104] Our second study,[36] reported in 1986, suggested the possibility of four factors, with the first and second representing two different aspects of negative symptoms; the third, psychoticism; and the fourth, thought disorder. Our third study,[97] reported in 1991, again suggested that the symptoms might be best described by the dimensions of psychoticism, disorganization, and negative symptoms. A fourth study,[98] reported in 1993, had similar results. Most of these studies also have reported correlation matrices, and most have commented on the fact that indices of internal consistency within the positive symptom scale, usually as measured by Cronbach's α, have been low, suggesting that positive symptoms are not a homogeneous concept. Thus, recent reports from other centers suggesting the nonhomogeneity of positive symptoms are not a surprise and are consistent with observations that we have made since the original description of rating scales for positive and negative symptoms in 1982. Cronbach's α for positive symptoms as reported in 1982 was .397 compared with .849 for negative symptoms.[31] Taken as a group, these studies conducted over the past decade comprise more than 500 patients and represent the largest repeated and systematic study of the correlational relationships between the symptoms of schizophrenia that has been completed to date.

At the descriptive level, the conclusions seem clear. Like schizophrenia itself, the symptoms are heterogeneous when assessed using the correlational methods of factor analysis. Such a consistency of results within a single group and from other groups throughout the world is quite reassuring, given the difficulties in replicating findings that often occur in the study of schizophrenia.

Nevertheless, we should also remind ourselves what factor analysis can and cannot tell us. Factor analysis is essentially a data reduction method. It demonstrates which items in a group are highly correlated with one another, indicating that they co-occur together. Demonstrating that they co-occur does not necessarily prove a conceptual relationship or an etiological relationship, however. The relationship is simply descriptive until other methods are used to demonstrate that the relationship has conceptual, diagnostic, clinical, or biological meaning. Extensive additional study is needed before inferences can be made concerning these aspects of the interrelationships between the symptoms of schizophrenia. One cannot infer that these symptoms are likely to have a common mechanism or etiology, nor can one infer that they have important prognostic significance. This must be demonstrated through empirical research. The robustness of the findings across various groups does suggest good generalizability, but at this point the generalizability is limited to core schizophrenia, since most studies have been limited to samples composed of patients given that *DSM* diagnosis. The applicability of these relationships to other patients within the schizophrenia spectrum or to other diagnostic groups (eg, psychotic mania or depression) is still an open question.

Table 4. Varimax Rotated Factor Structure for SANS and SAPS Global Ratings*

Symptom	Factor		
	Negative	Disorganized	Psychotic
Avolition	**0.832**	0.131	0.172
Anhedonia	**0.818**	0.179	0.110
Affective flattening	**0.809**	−0.105	0.036
Inappropriate affect	0.057	**0.796**	−0.114
Thought disorder	−0.050	**0.754**	0.267
Bizarre behavior	**0.426**	**0.598**	0.249
Delusions	0.071	0.175	**0.821**
Hallucinations	0.168	0.012	**0.759**
Variance explained	2.235	1.652	1.440
Percentage	27.938	20.650	18.000

**SANS indicates Scale for the Assessment of Negative Symptoms; SAPS, Scale for the Assessment of Positive Symptoms. The highest correlations (r>0.4) on a factor for a given item is boldfaced.*

Table 5. Correlation of Factor Scores With Alogia and Attention*

Symptom	Factor		
	Negative	Disorganized	Psychotic
Alogia			
Poverty of speech	**0.589**†	−0.010	−0.123
Poverty of content of speech	0.115	**0.467**†	0.075
Blocking	0.135	**0.193**	0.110
Increased latency of response	**0.458**†	0.132	0.064
Perseveration	0.022	**0.218**‡	0.009
Global rating	**0.574**†	0.216‡	−0.029
R^2=0.739			
Attention			
Social inattentiveness	**0.477**†	0.327†	0.133
Inattentive during mental testing (n=232)	0.259†	**0.295**†	0.164
Global rating	**0.454**†	0.335†	0.153
R^2=0.848			

**The highest correlation on a factor for a given item is boldfaced.*
†$P<.0001$.
‡$P<.001$.

Should the vocabulary used to discuss the symptoms of schizophrenia be changed and references to positive and negative symptoms be dropped altogether? Changes in usage will no doubt evolve naturally. A terminology that speaks of positive and negative symptoms using the words descriptively to refer to exaggerations of normal functions vs loss of normal functions seems to have found a comfortable linguistic niche in clinical usage, since it provides a modest conceptual simplification to clinicians grappling with the complex symptomatology of schizophrenia. Positive symptoms are readily understood as those that are more florid and that tend to be more associated with exacerbations of the illness, while negative symptoms tend to have a basic underlying persistence. Looked at in a more fine-grained way, positive symptoms subdivide into two dimensions: psychoticism (delusions and hallucinations) and disorganization (positive formal thought disorder, bizarre behavior, and inappropriate affect). As we move toward discussing these three dimensions of psychopathology, we must keep in mind that they are dimensions and not subtypes. That is, although a factor analysis can pull them apart statistically, these dimensions often overlap within given individuals. Unitary categorization without overlap defines a subtype, while dimensions have magnitude, may overlap, and can be additive.

These results suggest specific future directions for the use of the SANS and SAPS. Because of their wide use, they have not been subjected to extensive revisions to date, since such tinkering can be confusing and disruptive for the investigators who use them. Work on revised versions of the scales currently is under way; however, this work will emphasize designing the scales so they can be used more efficiently to explore the three dimensions, will involve a more detailed description of various aspects of attention so their components and correlates can be examined, and will involve more work on other subitems such as poverty of content of speech. As of now, we believe the current results suggest that in dimensional analyses, negative symptoms may include alogia, affective blunting, anhedonia, avolition, and attention. Attention should only be considered a negative symptom at a provisional level, however, because it has the least robust correlation and may ultimately be heterogeneous. Alogia may be better assessed if the current poverty of content item is revised and defined differently. Poverty of speech and poverty of content are linked conceptually and yet currently defined in such a way that they cannot be correlated with one another; the definitions specify that poverty of speech involves limited speech, while poverty of content involves speech that is adequate in amount but empty in content. Thus, one or the other of these possible components of alogia can be present but both cannot occur together. Because factor analysis separates uncorrelated items, it pulls apart two symptoms that are associated conceptually through sharing the fundamental characteristic of intellectual emptiness. In factor analysis studies, poverty of content tends to spill over to positive thought disorder, which also is characterized by abundant speech that is difficult to understand. Thus, definitional changes may be needed for poverty of content as its relationship to alogia is evaluated in future studies.

Future directions in the study of the symptoms of schizophrenia should emphasize efforts to link clinical description with models, meanings, and mechanisms. Techniques such as factor analysis will take us only part of the way to understanding the symptoms of this illness and its interrelationships. Empirical description alone will lead to intellectual bankruptcy. Until symptoms are linked to clinically relevant concepts such as prognosis or etiology, no firm conclusions can be reached about the best way to divide or group the symptoms of schizophrenia. The ultimate level of understanding will be based on learning how these symptoms are produced at the level of brain mechanisms. Future studies also should pursue at least four different aspects of these dimensions: their neural mechanisms, longitudinal course, relationship to treatment, and interrelationships in other pathological conditions apart from schizophrenia.

The robustness of these three dimensions suggests that they are a launching platform for exploring neural correlates. Our ability to build models will be limited necessarily by our relatively limited understanding about how cog-

Table 6. Correlation of Factor Scores With SANS and SAPS Ratings*

Symptom	Negative	Disorganized	Psychotic
Avolition/apathy			
Grooming and hygiene	**0.568†**	0.216‡	0.158
Impersistence at work or school	**0.735†**	0.173	0.177
Physical anergia	**0.643†**	−0.088	0.108
Global rating	**0.832**	0.131	0.172
R^2=0.840			
Anhedonia/asociality			
Recreational interests and acts	**0.675†**	0.176	0.151
Sexual interests and activity	**0.435†**	0.004	0.066
Ability to feel intimacy/closeness	**0.367†**	0.260†	0.120
Relationships with friends/peers	**0.667†**	0.192	0.109
Global rating	**0.818**	0.179	0.110
R^2=0.820			
Affective flattening			
Unchanging facial expression	**0.751†**	−0.153	0.049
Decreased spontaneous movement	**0.481†**	−0.225§	−0.077
Paucity of expressive gestures	**0.595†**	−0.077	−0.065
Poor eye contact	**0.526†**	0.132	0.088
Affective nonresponsivity	**0.588†**	0.004	0.174
Lack of vocal inflection	**0.563†**	−0.027	−0.035
Global rating	**0.809**	−0.105	0.036
R^2=0.894			
Inappropriate affect			
Global rating	0.057	**0.796**	−0.114
Positive formal thought disorder			
Derailment	−0.007	**0.732†**	0.238§
Tangentiality	−0.017	**0.709†**	0.183
Incoherence	0.055	**0.427†**	0.003
Illogicality	−0.075	**0.415†**	0.002
Circumstantiality	−0.178	**0.340†**	0.182
Pressure of speech	−0.182	**0.355†**	0.154
Distractible speech	−0.005	**0.320†**	0.185
Clanging	−0.051	**0.304†**	−0.029
Global rating	−0.050	**0.754**	0.267
R^2=0.868			
Bizarre behavior			
Clothing and appearance	0.132	**0.268†**	0.104
Social and sexual behavior	0.329†	**0.539†**	0.160
Aggressive and agitated behavior	0.232§	**0.479†**	0.288†
Ritualistic or stereotyped behavior	**0.252†**	0.130	−0.035
Global rating	0.426	**0.598**	0.249
R^2=0.770			
Delusions			
Persecutory delusions	0.072	0.164	**0.635†**
Delusions of jealousy	−0.039	0.028	**0.120**
Delusions of sin or guilt	0.160	−0.034	**0.258†**
Grandiose delusions	−0.001	0.265†	**0.327†**
Religious delusions	0.064	0.163	**0.329†**
Somatic delusions	−0.026	0.034	**0.296†**
Ideas and delusions of reference	0.092	0.082	**0.479†**
Delusions of being controlled	0.060	−0.025	**0.334†**
Delusions of mind reading	0.030	−0.021	**0.418†**
Thought broadcasting	0.045	−0.048	**0.262†**
Thought insertion	0.005	−0.042	**0.334†**
Thought withdrawal	0.025	−0.028	**0.257†**
Global rating	0.071	0.175	**0.821**
R^2=0.704			
Hallucinations			
Auditory hallucinations	0.151	0.016	**0.684†**
Somatic/tactile hallucinations	0.004	0.083	**0.392†**
Olfactory hallucinations	0.027	−0.014	**0.216‡**
Visual hallucinations	0.174	0.083	**0.404†**
Global rating	0.168	0.012	**0.759**
R^2=0.874			

*SANS indicates Scale for the Assessment of Negative Symptoms; SAPS, Scale for the Assessment of Positive Symptoms. The highest correlation on a factor for a given item is boldfaced.
†P<.0001.
‡P<.001.
§P<.0005.

nitive functions such as attention or language are mediated in the normal brain. A consensus has clearly emerged that simple localization models (ie, localization of language in the left hemisphere perisylvian area) are not sufficient, that language may be bilaterally represented, and that it is based on distributed parallel processing. The distributed processing models of brain function currently proposed in cognitive neuroscience almost certainly reflect a more real view of how the brain works, but they also complicate building models that will link the understanding of psychopathology to neural mechanisms. Nevertheless, we will be unable to understand what these various symptoms mean until we can define them at the neural level. Thus, future explorations of these dimensions will use the techniques of experimental cognitive psychology, neuropsychology, and neuroimaging to examine interrelationships between them and their underlying neural mechanisms.

A second way in which these three dimensions should be explored is an examination of their longitudinal course. Past and current wisdom suggest that negative symptoms are likely to be more persistent and fundamental, while psychotic symptoms are associated more with exacerbations. The disorganization dimension is conceptually newer, less studied, and less clear. To some extent, the meaning of these dimensions may be disorder specific; disorganized speech tends to remit in mania, while it tends to persist in schizophrenia.[108] Investigation of the longitudinal course of symptoms has important implications for understanding neural mechanisms, since symptoms that wax and wane are probably produced by mechanisms different from those of symptoms that remain more persistent. Identification of different patterns of course across disorders also may lead to identifying different mechanisms for a given symptom within a

Table 7. Dimensional-Diagnostic Crosswalk

Factor	Core Schizophrenia	Schizophreniform Disorder	Schizotypal Personality Disorder	Simple Schizophrenia	Schizoaffective Disorder	Mania	Depression
Psychotic	X	X			X	X	X
Disorganized	X	X			X	X	
Negative	X	?	X	X	?		X

Table 8. The Symptom Spectrum

Symptom	Core Schizophrenia	Schizophreniform Disorder	Schizotypal Personality Disorder	Simple Schizophrenia	Schizoaffective Disorder	Mania	Depression
Delusions	X	X			X	X	X
Hallucinations	X	X			X	X	X
Disorganized speech	X	X			X	X	
Disorganized behavior	X	X		?	X	X	
Inappropriate affect	X	X			X		
Attention	X	X			X	X	X
Alogia	X	?	X	X	X		X
Affective blunting	X	?	X	X			X
Anhedonia	X	?	X	X			X
Avolition	X	?	X	X			X

given disorder. For example, although hallucinations occur in schizophrenia, delirium, mania, and lysergic acid diethylamide–induced psychosis, the time pattern is different in all four disorders. The first stage in examining the course of symptoms must, however, establish a solid empirical base. The companion article in this issue of the ARCHIVES[109] on the longitudinal course of these three dimensions provides an example of one preliminary effort at empirical description of the course of symptoms and dimensions.

Examination of these three dimensions in other pathological conditions is another important avenue for exploration. Both the three dimensions and the individual symptoms discussed in this report also occur in other disorders. **Table 7** and **Table 8** provide an illustrative crosswalk. To the extent that there is a commonality of symptoms or dimensions across disorders and that evidence from other validators suggests a commonality of mechanism, we may be able to obtain additional leverage on building models to explain dimensions or symptoms. For example, "hypofrontality" has been repeatedly reported in schizophrenia and, using techniques from neuroimaging, has sometimes been found to be associated with negative symptoms.[110-112] Hypofrontality also has been observed relatively consistently in depression, using both neuroimaging techniques and lesion methods.[113-115] Obvious conceptual links exist between negative symptoms and depressive symptoms. Although students of psychopathology in the past have often emphasized specificity and attempted to identify pathognomonic symptoms, it may be that identifying commonalities among symptoms across disorders is a more helpful strategy for identifying underlying neural mechanisms. Again, the first step must be descriptive. Only a modest literature currently exists that applies standardized rating techniques to the study of mania, depression, the dementias, and other disorders that share many of the symptoms of schizophrenia.[37,116,117]

A final strategy must involve the study of these dimensions in relation to treatment. Again, clinical lore indicates that some symptoms and dimensions are more amenable to treatment than others. Psychotic symptoms in affective disorders tend to respond well to neuroleptics and also respond well, although less robustly, in schizophrenia. Observations such as these are powerful for generating hypotheses about the underlying mechanisms of symptoms and dimensions. As the therapeutic armamentarium grows to include medications that affect various components of individual transmitter systems (eg, the various classes of dopamine receptors), as well as other transmitter systems (eg, serotonin, norepinephrine, glutamate, γ-aminobutyric acid), our understanding of the neural mechanisms of these symptoms will grow. Much work also needs to be done at the simple descriptive level. For example, nearly all factor analysis studies completed to date have evaluated treated patients with variable levels of chronicity. It should be interesting to determine whether the same dimensions are found in first-episode patients or in untreated patients.

As these explorations progress, we should be prepared to entertain the possibility that each of the various individual symptoms may have somewhat different mechanisms and that our correlational observations suggesting three dimensions may begin to fall apart. For example, delusions and hallucinations are correlated consistently in almost all studies completed to date. At the neural level, however, they very likely are produced by different mechanisms. Thus, future explorations of the mechanisms and meanings of the three dimensions of psychopathology consistently noted in studies to date should not assume that the matter is prematurely closed and that three dimensions are sufficient. Alternately, it is also possible that these apparently separate and uncorrelated dimensions could be due to a single mechanism.

Accepted for publication August 1, 1994.

This research was supported in part by grants MH31593, MH40856, and MHCRC 43271 and Research Scientist Award MH00625 from the National Institute of Mental Health, Rockville, Md, and The Nellie Ball Trust Fund, Iowa State Bank and Trust Company, Iowa City, trustee.

Reprint requests to Department of Psychiatry, Mental Health Clinical Research Center, University of Iowa Hospitals and Clinics, 200 Hawkins Dr, 2911 JPP, Iowa City, IA 52242 (Dr Andreasen).

REFERENCES

1. Andreasen NC. The diagnosis of schizophrenia. *Schizophr Bull.* 1987;13:9-22.
2. Andreasen NC, Flaum M. Schizophrenia: the characteristic symptoms. *Schizophr Bull.* 1991;17:27-49.
3. Andreasen NC, Carpenter WT. Diagnosis and classification of schizophrenia. *Schizophr Bull.* 1993;19:199-214.
4. American Psychiatric Association. *Diagnostic and Statistical Manual of Mental Disorders, Fourth Edition.* Washington, DC: American Psychiatric Association; 1994.
5. World Psychiatric Association. *International Classification and Diagnosis-10.* Geneva, Switzerland: World Health Organization; 1993.
6. Bleuler E; Zinkin J, trans. *Dementia Praecox of the Group of Schizophrenias (1911).* New York, NY: International Universities Press; 1950.
7. Kraepelin E, Barclay RM, Robertson GM. *Dementia Praecox and Paraphrenia.* Edinburgh, Scotland: E & S Livingstone; 1919.
8. Mellor CS. First-rank symptoms of schizophrenia. *Br J Psychiatry.* 1970;117:15-23.
9. Schneider K; Hamilton MW, trans. *Clinical Psychopathology.* New York, NY: Grune & Stratton Inc; 1959.
10. Schneider K. Primary and secondary symptoms in schizophrenia. In: Hirsch SR, Sheperds M, eds. *Themes and Variations in European Psychiatry.* Bristol, England: John Wright & Sons Ltd; 1974:40-46.
11. Taylor MA. Schneiderian first-rank symptoms and clinical prognostic features in schizophrenia. *Arch Gen Psychiatry.* 1972;26:64-67.
12. Abrams R, Taylor M. First-rank symptoms, severity of illness, and treatment response in schizophrenia. *Compr Psychiatry.* 1973;14:353-355.
13. Carpenter WT Jr, Strauss JS, Muleh S. Are there pathognomonic symptoms in schizophrenia? an empirical investigation of Schneider's first-rank symptoms. *Arch Gen Psychiatry.* 1973;28:847-852.
14. Carpenter WT Jr, Heinrichs DW, Alphs LD. Treatment of negative symptoms. *Schizophr Bull.* 1985;11:440-452.
15. Andreasen NC, Akiskal HS. The specificity of Bleulerian and Schneiderian symptoms: a critical reevaluation. *Psychiatr Clin North Am.* 1983;6:41-54.
16. Kendell RE, Cooper JE, Gourlay AG. Diagnostic criteria of American and British psychiatrists. *Arch Gen Psychiatry.* 1971;25:123-130.
17. Wing JK, Cooper JE, Sartorius N. *The Measurement and Classification of Psychiatric Symptoms.* Cambridge, England: Cambridge University Press; 1974.
18. Wing J, Nixon J. Discriminating symptoms in schizophrenia: a report from the international pilot study of schizophrenia. *Arch Gen Psychiatry.* 1975;32:853-859.
19. Pope HG Jr, Lipinski JF Jr. Diagnosis in schizophrenia and manic-depressive illness: a reassessment of the specificity of 'schizophrenic' symptoms in the light of current research. *Arch Gen Psychiatry.* 1978;35:811-828.
20. Andreasen NC. Thought, language, and communication disorders, I: clinical assessment, definition of terms, and evaluation of their reliability. *Arch Gen Psychiatry.* 1979;36:1315-1321.
21. Andreasen NC. Thought, language, and communication disorders, II: diagnostic significance. *Arch Gen Psychiatry.* 1979;36:1325-1330.
22. Lewine R, Renders R, Kirchhofer M, Monsour A, Watt N. The empirical heterogeneity of first-rank symptoms in schizophrenia. *Br J Psychiatry.* 1982;140:498-502.
23. Harrow M, Grinker RR Sr, Silverstein ML, Holzman P. Is modern-day schizophrenic outcome still negative. *Am J Psychiatry.* 1978;135:1156-1162.
24. Andreasen NC. Affective flattening and the criteria for schizophrenia. *Am J Psychiatry.* 1979;136:944-947.
25. Reynolds JR. *Essays and Addresses.* London, England: Macmillan Publishing Co; 1896.
26. Jackson JH. *Selected Writings of J. H. Jackson.* London, England: Hodder & Stoughton; 1931.
27. Berrios GE. Positive and negative signals: a conceptual history. In: Marneros A, Andreasen NC, Tsuang MT, eds. *Negative Versus Positive Schizophrenia.* Berlin, Germany: Springer-Verlag Berlin; 1991:8-27.
28. Strauss JS, Carpenter WT, Bartko JJ. The diagnosis and understanding of schizophrenia, III: speculations on the processes that underlie schizophrenia symptoms and signs. *Schizophr Bull.* 1974;1:61-69.
29. Crow TJ. Molecular pathology of schizophrenia: more than one disease process? *BMJ.* 1980;280:66-68.
30. Andreasen NC. Negative symptoms in schizophrenia: definition and reliability. *Arch Gen Psychiatry.* 1982;39:784-788.
31. Andreasen NC, Olsen S. Negative vs positive schizophrenia: definition and validation. *Arch Gen Psychiatry.* 1982;39:789-794.
32. Andreasen NC. *The Scale for the Assessment of Negative Symptoms (SANS).* Iowa City: The University of Iowa; 1983.
33. Andreasen NC. *The Scale for the Assessment of Positive Symptoms (SAPS).* Iowa City: The University of Iowa; 1984.
34. Andreasen NC. Positive vs negative schizophrenia: a critical evaluation. *Schizophr Bull.* 1985;11:380-389.
35. Andreasen NC. Negative syndrome in schizophrenia: strategies for long-term management. *Adv Biochem Psychopharmacol.* 1985;40:1-7.
36. Andreasen NC, Grove WM. Evaluation of positive and negative symptoms in schizophrenia. *Psychiatr Psychobiol.* 1986;2:108-121.
37. Andreasen NC. The concept of negative symptoms: definition, specificity, and significance. *Psychiatr Psychobiol.* 1987;4:240-251.
38. Andreasen NC. The Scale for the Assessment of Negative Symptoms (SANS): conceptual and theoretical foundations. *Br J Psychiatry.* 1989;155(suppl 7):49-52.
39. Andreasen NC. Methods for assessing positive and negative symptoms. In: Andreasen NC, ed. *Schizophrenia: Positive and Negative Symptoms and Syndromes. Modern Problems in Pharmacopsychiatry.* Basel, Switzerland: Karger; 1990:73-88.
40. Andreasen NC. Positive and negative symptoms: historical and conceptual aspects. In: Andreasen NC, ed. *Schizophrenia: Positive and Negative Symptoms and Syndromes. Modern Problems of Pharmacopsychiatry.* Basel, Switzerland: Karger; 1990:1-42.
41. Andreasen NC, Flaum M, Swayze VW, Tyrrell G, Arndt S. Positive and negative symptoms in schizophrenia: a critical reappraisal. *Arch Gen Psychiatry.* 1990;47:615-621.
42. Andreasen NC, Flaum M, Arndt S, Alliger R, Swayze VW. Positive and negative symptoms: assessment and validity. In: Marneros A, Andreasen NC, Tsuang MT, eds. *Negative Versus Positive Schizophrenia.* Berlin, Germany: Springer-Verlag Berlin; 1991:28-51.
43. Carpenter WT Jr, Heinrichs DW, Wagman AMI. Deficit and nondeficit forms of schizophrenia: the concept. *Am J Psychiatry.* 1989;145:578-583.
44. Carpenter WT, Strauss JS, Bartko JJ. On the heterogeneity of schizophrenia. In: Alpert M, ed. *Controversies in Schizophrenia.* New York, NY: Guilford Press; 1985:25-37.
45. Lewine RR, Fogg L, Meltzer HY. Assessment of negative and positive symptoms in schizophrenia. *Schizophr Bull.* 1983;9:368-376.
46. Liddle PF. Schizophrenic syndromes, cognitive performance, and neurological dysfunction. *Psychol Med.* 1987;7:49-57.
47. Gibbons RD, Lewine RR, Davis JM, Schooler NR, Cole JD. An empirical test of a Kraepelinian vs a Bleulerian view of negative symptoms. *Schizophr Bull.* 1985;11:390-396.
48. Marneros A, Deister A, Rohde A. Long-term monomorphism of negative and positive schizophrenic episode. In: Marneros A, Andreasen NC, Tsuang MT, eds. *Negative Versus Positive Schizophrenia.* Berlin, Germany: Springer-Verlag Berlin; 1991:183-196.
49. Sommers AS. 'Negative symptoms': conceptual and methodological problems. *Schizophr Bull.* 1985;11:364-373.
50. Pogue-Geile MF, Harrow M. Negative symptoms in schizophrenia: their longitudinal course and prognostic importance. *Schizophr Bull.* 1985;11:427-439.
51. Goldberg SC. Negative and deficit symptoms in schizophrenia do respond to neuroleptics. *Schizophr Bull.* 1985;11:453-456.
52. Andreasen NC, ed. In: *Schizophrenia: Positive and Negative Symptoms and Syndromes. Modern Problems of Pharmacopsychiatry.* Basel, Switzerland: Karger; 1990.
53. Fish FJ. *Schizophrenia.* Bristol, England: John Wright & Sons Ltd; 1962.
54. Carpenter WT Jr, Strauss JS, Bartko JJ. Beyond diagnosis: the phenomenology of schizophrenia. *Am J Psychiatry.* 1981;138:948-953.
55. Andreasen NC. Brain imaging: applications in psychiatry. *Science.* 1988;239:1381-1388.
56. Andreasen NC. *Can Schizophrenia Be Localized in the Brain?* Washington, DC: American Psychiatric Press Inc; 1986.
57. Andreasen NC, Swayze VW II, Flaum M, O'Leary DS, Alliger R. The neural mechanisms of mental phenomena. In: Andreasen NC, ed. *Schizophrenia: From Mind to Molecule.* Washington, DC: American Psychiatric Press Inc; 1994:49-91.
58. Andreasen NC, Flaum M, Arndt S. The Comprehensive Assessment of Symptoms and History (CASH): an instrument for assessing psychopathology and diagnosis. *Arch Gen Psychiatry.* 1992;49:615-623.
59. Johnstone EC, Owens DGC, Frith CD, Crow TJ. The relative stability of positive and negative features in chronic schizophrenia. *Br J Psychiatry.* 1987;150:65-71.
60. Kirkpatrick B, Buchanan RW, McKenney PD, Alphs LD, Carpenter WT. The Schedule for the Deficit Syndrome: an instrument for research in schizophrenia. *Psychiatr Res.* 1989;30:119-124.
61. Lindenmayer JP, Kay SR, Friedman C. Negative and positive schizophrenic syndromes after the acute phase: a prospective follow-up. *Compr Psychiatry.* 1986;27:276-286.

62. Pogue-Geile MF, Harrow M. Negative and postive symptoms in schizophrenia and depression: a follow-up. *Schizophr Bull.* 1984;10:371-387.
63. Greden JF, Tandon R, eds. *Negative Schizophrenic Symptoms: Pathophysiology and Clinical Implications.* Washington, DC: American Psychiatric Press; 1990.
64. Meltzer HY. Dopamine and negative symptoms in schizophrenia: critique of the type I-type II hypothesis. In: Alpert M, ed. *Controversies in Schizophrenia: Changes and Constancies.* New York, NY: Guilford Press; 1985:110-136.
65. Meltzer HY, Sommers AA, Luchins DJ. The effect of neuroleptics and other psychotropic drugs on negative symptoms in schizophrenia. *J Clin Psychopharmacol.* 1986;6:329-338.
66. Trimble MR. Positive and negative symptoms in psychiatry. *Br J Psychiatry.* 1986;148:587-589.
67. Angrist B, Rotrosen J, Gershon S. Differential effects of amphetamine and neuroleptics on negative vs positive symptoms in schizophrenia. *Psychopharmacology (Berlin).* 1980;72:17-19.
68. Angrist B, Peselow E, Rubinstein M, Corwin J, Rotrosen J. Partial improvement in negative schizophrenic symptoms after amphetamine. *Psychopharmacology (Berlin).* 1982;78:128-130.
69. Buchanan RW, Kirkpatrick B, Tamminga CA. Differential patterns of glucose metabolism in deficit and non-deficit schizophrenia. *Biol Psychiatry.* 1989; 27(suppl):99A-100A.
70. Buchanan RW, Kirkpatrick B, Heinrichs DW, Carpenter WT. Clinical correlates of the deficit syndrome of schizophrenia. *Am J Psychiatry.* 1990;147: 290-294.
71. Kirkpatrick B, Buchanan RW. Anhedonia and the deficit syndrome of schizophrenia. *Psychiatry Res.* 1990;31:25-30.
72. Wagman AMI, Heinrichs DW, Carpenter WT. The deficit and non-deficit forms of schizophrenia: neuropsychological evaluation. *Psychiatry Res.* 1987;22: 319-330.
73. Gross G. The 'basic' symptoms of schizophrenia. *Br J Psychiatry.* 1989;155 (suppl 7):21-25.
74. Walker E, Lewine RJ. The positive/negative symptom distinction in schizophrenia: validity and etiological relevance. *Schizophr Res.* 1988;1:315-328.
75. Dworkin RH, Lenzenweger MF. Symptoms and the genetics of schizophrenia: implications for diagnosis. *Am J Psychiatry.* 1984;41:1541-1546.
76. Dworkin RH, Lenzenweger MF, Moldin SO, Skillings GF, Levick SE. A multidimensional approach to the genetics of schizophrenia. *Am J Psychiatry.* 1988; 145:1077-1083.
77. Johnstone EC, Owens DGC, Firth CD, Crow TJ. The relative stability of positive and negative features in chronic schizophrenia. *Br J Psychiatry.* 1986; 150:60-64.
78. Kemali D, Maj M, Galderisi S, Salvati A, Starace F, Valente A, Pirozzi R. Clinical, biological, and neuropsychological features associated with lateral ventricular enlargement in *DSM-III* schizophrenic disorder. *Psychiatry Res.* 1986; 21:137-149.
79. Mackay AVP. Positive and negative schizophrenic symptoms and the role of dopamine. *Br J Psychiatry.* 1980;137:379-383.
80. Tandon R, Greden JF. Cholinergic hyperactivity and negative schizophrenic symptoms: a model of cholinergic/dopaminergic interactions in schizophrenia. *Arch Gen Psychiatry.* 1989;46:745-753.
81. Tandon R, Goldman RS, Goodson JA, Greden JF. Mutability and relationship between positive and negative symptoms during neuroleptic treatment in schizophrenia. *Biol Psychiatry.* 1990;27:1323-1326.
82. van Kammen DP, Hommer DW, Malas KL. Effect of pimozide on positive and negative symptoms in schizophrenic patients: are negative symptoms dependent? *Neuropsychobiology.* 1987;18:113-117.
83. van Kammen DP, Peters JL, Rosen J, van Kammen WB, Neylan T, Shaw D, Linnoila M. Norepinephrine in acute exacerbations of chronic schizophrenia: negative symptoms revisited. *Arch Gen Psychiatry.* 1990;47:161-168.
84. Wing JK. The concept of negative symptoms. *Br J Psychiatry.* 1989;155 (suppl 7):10-14.
85. Liddle PF, Friston KJ, Frith CD, Frackowiak RSJ. Cerebral blood flow and mental processes in schizophrenia. *J R Soc Med.* 1992;85:224-226.
86. Liddle PF. The symptoms of chronic schizophrenia: a re-examination of the positive-negative dichotomy. *Br J Psychiatry.* 1987;151:145-151.
87. Liddle PF, Barnes TRE. Syndromes of chronic schizophrenia. *Br J Psychiatry.* 1990;157:558-561.
88. Liddle PF, Morris D. Schizophrenic syndromes and frontal lobe performance. *Br J Psychiatry.* 1991;158:340-345.
89. Frith CD, Done DJ. Towards a neuropsychology of schizophrenia. *Br J Psychiatry.* 1988;153:437-443.
90. Frith CR, Done DJ. Experiences of alien control in schizophrenia reflect a disorder in the central monitoring of action. *Psychol Med.* 1989;19:359-363.
91. McGlashan TH, Fenton WS. The positive-negative distinction in schizophrenia: review of natural history validators. *Arch Gen Psychiatry.* 1992;49:63-72.
92. Fenton WS, McGlashan TH. Natural history of schizophrenia subtypes: II, positive and negative symptoms and long-term course. *Arch Gen Psychiatry.* 1991; 48:978-986.
93. Bogerts B, Lieberman JA, Ashtari M, Bilder RM, Degreef G, Lerner G, Johns C, Masiar S. Hippocampus-amygdala volumes and psychopathology in chronic schizophrenia. *Biol Psychiatry.* 1993;33:236-246.
94. Ohta T, Okazaki Y, Anzai N. Reliability of the Japanese version of the Scale for the Assessment of Negative Symptoms (SANS). *Jpn J Clin Psychiatr.* 1984; 13:1123-1131.
95. Humbert M, Salvador L, Segui J, Obiols J, Obiols J. Estudio interfiabilidad version espanola evaluacion de sintomas positivos y negativos. *Rev Departmento Psiquiatria Facultad de Medicine, University of Barcelona.* 1986;13: 28-36.
96. Moscarelli M, Maffei C, Cesana BM. An international perspective on assessment of negative and positive symptoms in schizophrenia. *Am J Psychiatry.* 1987;144:1595-1598.
97. Arndt S, Alliger RJ, Andreasen NC. The distinction of positive and negative symptoms: the failure of a two-dimensional model. *Br J Psychiatry.* 1991; 158:317-322.
98. Miller DD, Arndt S, Andreasen NC. Alogia, attentional impairment, and inappropriate affect: their status in the dimensions of schizophrenia. *Compr Psychiatry.* 1993;34:221-226.
99. Bilder RM, Mukherjee S, Rieder RO, Pandurangi AK. Symptomatic and neuropsychological components of defect states. *Schizophr Bull.* 1985;11:409-491.
100. Kulhara P, Kota SK, Joseph S. Positive and negative subtypes of schizophrenia: a study from India. *Acta Psychiatr Scand.* 1986;74:353-359.
101. Lenzenweger MF, Dworkin RH, Wethington E. Models of positive and negative symptoms in schizophrenia: an empirical evaluation of latent structures. *J Abnorm Psychol.* 1989;98:62-70.
102. Schuldberg D, Quinlan DM, Morgenstern H, Glazer W. Positive and negative symptoms in chronic psychiatric outpatients: reliability, stability, and factor structure. *Psychological Assessment: J Consult Clin Psychol.* 1990;2:262-268.
103. Gur RE, Mozley D, Resnick SM, Levick S, Erwin R, Saykin AJ, Gur RC. Relations among clinical scales in schizophrenia. *Am J Psychiatry.* 1991;148: 472-478.
104. Minas IH, Stuart GW, Klimidis S, Jackson HJ, Singh BS, Copolov DL. Positive and negative symptoms in the psychoses: multidimensional scaling of SAPS and SANS items. *Schizophr Res.* 1992;8:143-156.
105. Brown KW, White T. Syndromes of chronic schizophrenia and some clinical correlates. *Br J Psychiatry.* 1992;161:317-322.
106. Peralta V, de Leon J, Cuesta MJ. Are there more than two syndromes in schizophrenia? a critique of the positive-negative dichotomy. *Br J Psychiatry.* 1992; 161:335-343.
107. Gorsuch RL. *Factor Analysis.* Philadelphia, Pa: WB Saunders Co; 1974.
108. Andreasen NC, Grove WM. Thought, language, and communication in schizophrenia: diagnosis and prognosis. *Schizophr Bull.* 1986;12:348-359.
109. Arndt S, Andreasen NC, Flaum M, Miller D, Nopoulos P. A longitudinal study of symptom dimensions in schizophrenia: prediction and patterns of change. *Arch Gen Psychiatry.* 1995;52:352-360.
110. Weinberger DR, Berman KF, Zec RF. Physiological dysfunction of dorsolateral prefrontal cortex in schizophrenia, I: regional cerebral blood flow (rCBF) evidence. *Arch Gen Psychiatry.* 1986;43:114-124.
111. Buchsbaum MS. The frontal lobes, basal ganglia, and temporal lobes as sites for schizophrenia. *Schizophr Bull.* 1990;16:379-384.
112. Andreasen NC, Flaum M, Arndt S, Alliger R, Miller D, O'Leary D. Positive and negative symptoms and syndromes: assessment and biological correlates. In: Ferrero F, Haynal AE, Sartorius N, eds. *Schizophrenia and Affective Psychoses: Nosology in Contemporary Psychiatry.* New York, NY: John Libbey; 1992.
113. Buchsbaum MS, Ingvar DH, Kessler R, Waters RN, Capelletti J, Kammen DP, King C, Johnson J, Manning RG, Flynn RW, Mann LS, Bunney WE, Sokoloff L. Cerebral glucography with positron tomography. *Arch Gen Psychiatry.* 1982; 39:251-259.
114. Robinson RG, Kubos KL, Starr LB, Rao K, Price TR. Mood disorders in stroke patients: importance of location of lesion. *Brain.* 1984;107:81-93.
115. Robinson RG, Starkstein SE. Current research in affective disorders following stroke. *J Neuropsychiatry Clin Neurosci.* 1990;2:1-4.
116. Walker EF, Harvey PD, Perlman D. The positive/negative symptom distinction in psychoses: a replication and extension of previous findings. *J Nerv Ment Dis.* 1988;176:359-363.
117. Klimidis S, Stuart GW, Minas IH, Copolov DL, Singh BS. Positive and negative symptoms in the psychoses: re-analysis of published SAPS and SANS global ratings. *Schizophr Res.* 1993;9:11-18.

A Longitudinal Study of Symptom Dimensions in Schizophrenia

Prediction and Patterns of Change

Stephan Arndt, PhD; Nancy C. Andreasen, MD, PhD; Michael Flaum, MD; Del Miller, PharmD, MD; Peg Nopoulos, MD

Background: Factor analytic studies have suggested that the symptoms of schizophrenia may be divided into three uncorrelated dimensions. This study examines the longitudinal course of the symptoms of schizophrenia using this three-dimensional perspective.

Methods: The sample was composed primarily of neuroleptic-naive patients suffering from schizophrenia. Subjects were studied in a prospective longitudinal design, with comprehensive structured assessments at index, discharge, and 6-month intervals after discharge over a 2-year period.

Results: Negative symptoms were already relatively prominent at the time of index evaluation; they tended to remain stable throughout the follow-up period. The two dimensions of positive symptoms, psychoticism and disorganization, although prominent at index evaluation, declined over the course of the follow-up period and tended to be less stable. A longitudinal factor analysis was conducted to determine whether the changes in symptoms followed any consistent pattern. We observed that all three groups of symptoms tended to change in unison and independently from one another.

Conclusions: These results suggest that these three dimensions of psychopathology show different patterns of exacerbation and remission during the course of schizophrenia. This independent pattern of evolution suggests that these three dimensions should be studied further with respect to response to treatment, cognitive mechanisms, psychosocial correlates, and neural substrates.

(Arch Gen Psychiatry. 1995;52:352-360)

From the Mental Health Clinical Research Center (Drs Arndt, Andreasen, Flaum, Miller, and Nopoulos) and the Departments of Preventive Medicine and Environmental Health (Dr Arndt) and Psychiatry (Drs Andreasen, Flaum, Miller, and Nopoulos), The University of Iowa Hospitals and Clinics, Iowa City.

THE STUDY of longitudinal course and outcome serves several purposes in the study of psychopathology. First, the observation of the evolution of symptoms may help us to identify homogeneous groups of patients, which may ultimately facilitate identification of the fundamental mechanisms that produce the disease. Second, the manner in which the symptoms change and evolve may in and of itself provide clues as to the fundamental mechanisms; for example, symptoms that are relatively persistent and stable are more likely to be caused by different neural mechanisms from symptoms that wax and wane. Third, the study of longitudinal course may assist in the identification of particular symptoms or patterns of symptoms that may have prognostic significance and can aid clinicians in the prediction of outcome. Fourth, the study of longitudinal course can provide important information about treatment efficacy, with the ultimate goal of developing improved medications or psychosocial treatment programs.

Studies of the course of schizophrenia fall into several different natural groups. One early group, typified by the work of Kraepelin et al[1] and Bleuler,[2] focused on the detailed description of symptoms accompanied by careful longitudinal observation whenever possible, with the goal of finding symptoms that were basic and fundamental to the disorder; the construct of fundamental, or basic, was usually taken to refer to symptoms that were more persistent and enduring, although Bleuler[2] and others[3,4] also emphasized the importance of specificity. Since neuroleptics were not available to affect course, patients were usually institutionalized for long periods of time, and definitions were relatively narrow and clear, observations from that era should be given careful attention.[1-13] Both

See Methods on next page

METHODS

SUBJECTS

Subjects underwent evaluation with the Iowa Prospective Longitudinal Study of recent-onset psychoses. Methods for selecting the overall population have been previously described in detail.[90] Briefly, subjects are recruited from consecutive admissions to the Psychiatry Inpatient Services at the University of Iowa Hospitals and Clinics, Iowa City. All patients who meet entry criteria and consent to participate are included. This longitudinal study emphasizes first-episode, recent-onset, and neuroleptic-naive patients; its goal is to acquire a cohort in whom symptoms, course, and outcome can be evaluated with a prospective design and minimal confounding of prior morbidity. Subjects are recruited into the study who are experiencing their first episode of psychosis or hospitalization or have experienced their first psychiatric hospitalization within the past 5 years and are less than 30 years of age. This report focuses on a subset of these patients who met *DSM-III-R* criteria for schizophrenia or schizophreniform disorder at index assessment.

The patients in this subset were typically young, acutely ill, and predominantly neuroleptic naive. The average age in the sample was 24.18 years (SD=5.2), and the median time since onset of the first psychotic symptom was 8.3 months. All but 11 of the subjects (85%) had never received neuroleptics before entering the study. Most subjects were male (77%) and never married (91%).

Sixty-five patients with a diagnosis of schizophrenia or schizophreniform disorder have been enrolled in this study and followed up for at least 6 months. These subjects have provided the sample for this report. This study is ongoing, and therefore the sample size for each of the follow-up periods varies. While 65 subjects have been followed up for 6 months, 53 have been followed up for 1 year, and 39 patients for 2 years. These decreasing sample sizes reflect study duration rather than subject attrition. Dropouts have been minimal. A total of four patients were unavailable for follow-up from this sample during the follow-up period: two patients committed suicide, one refused further participation, and one later received a diagnosis of another disorder that made her ineligible for the study. The available data for these four patients were maintained to reduce the bias of attrition. The 39 patients who have been followed up for 2 years are not different from the patients who were ascertained later, and therefore had shorter periods of observation, on any of the demographic or clinical variables (eg, age at onset, age at entrance into the study, gender, education, and severity of positive and negative symptoms at index evaluation). In over 40 comparisons, only one significant difference was found between the 39 subjects with 2-year follow-up data and those with shorter follow-up intervals. Consequently, the data for all 65 subjects were included in the statistical analyses.

INDEX ASSESSMENT

During the index hospitalization, all subjects underwent evaluation with the Comprehensive Assessment of Symptoms and History (CASH)[57,91] and the PSYCH-BASE.[92] Embedded within the CASH are expanded versions of the Scale for the Assessment of Negative Symptoms (SANS)[93] and the Scale for the Assessment of Positive Symptoms (SAPS),[94] rated at the subject's worst severity during the index period. All possible sources of information, including hospital records and interviews with informants, the patient, nurses, and social workers were used in completing the CASH, as elaborated in the companion article.[95] The *DSM-III-R* diagnosis was established by consensus of the clinical research team, using all available sources of information, as previously described. Treatment was not a controlled variable in this study. Consequently, during this index hospitalization, patients were treated using "clinician's choice" medications. Treatment typically consisted of neuroleptics (N=66), but also included antidepressants (N=7), lithium (N=4), antianxiety agents (N=3), and antiparkinsonians (N=35).

FOLLOW-UP EVALUATIONS

Every 6 months after discharge from the index hospitalization, the subject underwent reevaluation by an interviewer who made initial contact with the patient during the index hospitalization and participated in the completion of the consensus CASH at the time of discharge. Follow-up evaluations employed versions of the CASH and PSYCH-BASE that have been modified for longitudinal follow-up (the CASH-UP and PSYCH-UP). These instruments contain time lines that record global ratings of each positive and negative symptom at 1-week intervals covering the previous 6 months. The global ratings include: Hallucinations, Delusions, Positive Formal Thought Disorder, Bizarre (Disorganized) Behavior, Inappropriate Affect, Alogia, Anhedonia, Avolition, Affective Flattening, and Attention.

The data obtained using these instruments are both current (ie, describing the past week) and retrospective (ie, summarizing the past 6 months). These data were obtained at each of the 6-month follow-up periods by interviewing the subject concerning any changes in medication, hospitalizations, or exacerbations in symptoms that had occurred during the prior 6 months. Information was also obtained from an informant and medical records and used to establish a consensus rating, as described below. To reconstruct the retrospective weekly time line data, the PSYCH-UP is employed. Informants and patients are asked to identify any specific time period when a change occurred and describe the symptoms present, leading to a rating of level of severity at the peak time for each symptom, as well as the time and degree to which the symptom began to worsen or improve.

The CASH-UP covers symptoms during the past week, which provides a cross-sectional assessment of

Continued on next page

Kraepelin et al[1] and Bleuler[2] were especially impressed by the importance of fragmenting of thought, loss of volition, and loss of emotional responsiveness. A second group of studies, typified by the work of Vaillant[14] and Stephens et al,[15] emphasized the study of prognostic indicators and identified predictors of good vs poor outcome, such as premorbid adjustment or intact emotional responsiveness; these studies mark the beginning psychopathology in a series of 6-month "snapshots." Since the assessments are almost always obtained while the subject is an outpatient (rather than occurring at the time of hospital readmission during an exacerbation), they provide an unbiased estimate of the clinical status of the patient during the follow-up interval. That is, the time of assessment is not linked in any way to exacerbations or remissions. Because they describe current status at the time of assessment, they are very accurate; when analyzed over a 2-year time period, they provide the most valid repeated-measure data for longitudinal assessment.

The design of the follow-up evaluation has incorporated a systematic study of the effects of informant on the assessment of psychopathology; at the time of each 6-month follow-up, both the patient and an informant (most often the patient's mother, but potentially a sibling, spouse, or companion) underwent separate evaluation by two different interviewers. The same interviewer maintained contact with the patient or informant to ensure continuity, sustain rapport, and reduce dropout rate; these two different interviewers were, however, blind to one another's ratings. After these independent blind evaluations were completed, the two interviewers shared their information and established a consensus rating. In addition to the interviews, other sources of information (eg, medical records) also were used to establish consensus ratings. An analysis of the effects of informant on symptom reporting will be presented elsewhere. In this investigation, we have employed the "gold standard," or consensus ratings, in our analyses.

The reliability of the various symptom measures analyzed in this study has been carefully assessed; in general, reliability (determined by intraclass correlation coefficients) is good (.5 to .7) to excellent (.8 or greater), with higher estimates for interrater measures than for test-retest measures, as would be expected.[91] All interviewers participating in this follow-up study attend weekly calibration meetings coordinated by the Assessment and Training Core of the Iowa Mental Health Clinical Research Center, Iowa City. The assessment and training program developed by this core has extensive methods in place to ensure continuing reliability to and prevent "rater drift," including regular calibration checks on all instruments and raters. This program ensures that the high levels of reliability are maintained during the follow-up period. In addition, since this study also involves retrospective reporting of symptoms, the validity of such reporting is also being evaluated as a separate arm of the investigation and will be reported elsewhere. In general, the results indicate acceptable accuracy of assessment when all sources of information are used, as in the present report.

During the follow-up period, the majority of patients received some type of treatment that was prescribed by their primary physician. Thus, treatment in this study is naturalistic rather than controlled. The mainstay of treatment was neuroleptics, which the majority of the patients received throughout the follow-up period.

STATISTICAL ANALYSIS

One set of analyses addressed the questions of frequency of symptom categories at onset or early in the illness (ie, the extent to which negative symptoms may be primary) and the extent to which symptoms improve or worsen and to which some types of symptoms are persistent or enduring. Data from four evaluation periods (index, discharge, 1-year, and 2-year) were used to examine the change in symptoms over the 2-year time period. Means, intersubject SDs, and paired *t* tests were used for many of the descriptive analyses comparing index hospitalization or discharge ratings with the 1- and 2-year follow-up ratings.

To evaluate the issue of stability and predictability, we also conducted a "longitudinal factor analysis," in which the unit of analysis was the individual patient and time of measurement was the sample. The major purpose of this analysis was to determine whether groups of symptoms can be identified that show similar patterns of change over time. Correlations between symptoms over time were calculated by determining the intrasubject variance and covariances. These correlations (covariances) were generated for each subject separately, reflecting the intrasubject associations among the symptoms. The summary measures of association (covariances) were averaged across individuals according to the number of observation times and analyzed, using principal components analysis. The effective sample size for this analysis is very large (N=7098), since the correlations were based on the total number of observations for all subjects; statistically, it is therefore of a very optimal size for factor analysis. To determine the number of factors, we used an eigenvalue criterion for covariances analogous to the eigenvalue-greater-than-one rule for factoring correlations. A factor was included if the eigenvalue (variance accounted for) was greater than the average symptom variance (mean diagonal entry in the pooled intrasubject variance-covariance matrix). The extracted factors were analyzed with varimax rotation.

To examine the utility of the study of individual symptoms vs the three-dimensional model, we used two different approaches to exploring interrelationships between symptoms: global ratings for specific SANS/SAPS symptoms (eg, Delusions, Affective Flattening), and sums of global ratings that reflect the three dimensions of psychopathology suggested by our own cross-sectional factor analyses and those of others. In these analyses, global ratings of Delusions and Hallucinations were summed to characterize the dimension of psychoticism; Positive Formal Thought Disorder (disorganized speech), Bizarre (Disorganized) Behavior, and Inappropriate Affect were summed to measure disorganization; and Alogia, Affective Flattening, Avolition, Anhedonia, and Attention were summed to measure negative symptoms. The position of Attention with respect to other negative and positive symptoms is controversial, showing a relationship with some aspects of both in our own work and that of others. It was grouped with the negative symptoms here primarily for the sake of continuity and simplicity, anticipating that the longitudinal analyses might shed further light on its relationship.

of the early neuroleptic era and are characterized by a relatively broad conceptualization of schizophrenia. Other studies have sought to measure treatment efficacy, comparing various medications, psychotherapy, and psychosocial rehabilitation techniques.[16-24] Other studies from the postneuroleptic era have examined the capacity of various specific symptom groups, such as thought disorder or Schneiderian symptoms, to predict outcome.[25-30] Still others,[31-54] represented by the Iowa 500,[41] the International Pilot Study of Schizophrenia,[51] or the work of Ciompi,[39] have emphasized descriptive psychopathology or epidemiological techniques and attempted to provide a clear and accurate description of the pattern of symptoms and their relationship to psychosocial disability and outcome. During the past decade, interests have returned to the early formulations of Kraepelin et al[1] and Bleuler[2] and emphasized the study of fundamental symptoms, now usually referred to as negative or deficit symptoms.[29,55-70] One variant of this has been the study of the positive vs negative dichotomy, particularly the model of Crow,[71-73] which was an attempt to offer a heuristic simplification to facilitate studies of nosology, pathophysiology, outcome, and treatment.

While much has been learned from these studies, many issues are still debated. There is still no consensus as to whether schizophrenia leads to deterioration, whether particular symptoms respond to treatment, or whether any symptoms can be considered enduring or fundamental. Longitudinal studies are difficult to do well, since prospective studies require a long-term commitment with a slow return on the investment, whereas retrospective studies have obvious inherent limitations, because they are not based on direct observation of patients and may be handicapped by reporting biases. Studies done in the postneuroleptic era can no longer observe the natural history of untreated schizophrenia. Definitions of schizophrenia have also changed over time; the patient samples studied in the early work of Vaillant[14] or Stephens et al[15] are almost certainly quite different from those based on the recent narrow *DSM-III-R*[74] and *DSM-IV*[75] definitions. Although astute observers have worried since the time of Bleuler[2] that some symptoms may be secondary to others, very few investigators have attempted to develop designs that will disentangle actual primary from secondary symptoms. Finally, although many investigators pay lip service to the possibility that schizophrenia may be heterogeneous, the practicalities of assembling homogeneous samples are daunting. However, conclusions can vary widely if symptoms are assessed either cross-sectionally or longitudinally in patient samples that differ in terms of acuity, chronicity, hospitalization status, or phase of illness; conclusions about characteristic course or pattern will inevitably vary widely if samples of chronically institutionalized patients are compared with younger patients treated primarily in outpatient settings.

See also pages 341 and 361

In the present investigation, we report on a study of the longitudinal course of the symptoms of schizophrenia using a design and sample chosen to correct at least some of these problems. To reduce the confounding effects of chronicity, we have recruited a sample of patients who have been ill for less than 5 years and who are less than 30 years of age, with an emphasis on identifying patients at the time of first admission. To reduce the confounding effects of neuroleptic treatment, we have emphasized the recruitment of patients who have never received prior treatment with neuroleptics. To have maximally accurate documentation of symptoms, we assess the patients with a comprehensive interview at intake and follow up at regular intervals thereafter, using instruments with established reliability and validity. To keep the sample relatively homogeneous, this report is limited to those patients with a *DSM-III-R* diagnosis of schizophrenia or schizophreniform disorder at intake.

The primary purpose of this report is to extend our previous investigation of the interrelationships between positive and negative symptoms and obtain a longitudinal perspective. Research investigating the factor structure of the symptoms of schizophrenia has been remarkably consistent in showing that more than two factors are needed to account for the interrelationships among the symptoms.[58,76-86] Most of these studies have reported a three-factor solution. One is composed primarily of negative symptoms, whereas positive symptoms appear to split into two independent dimensions, "psychotic" and "disorganized." Hallucinations and delusions make up the former, while the latter typically include measures of disorganized speech, disorganized behavior, and inappropriate affect. These three factor solutions also appear consistently when different analytic methods are used.[87] Current research is actively exploring the pathophysiological and neuropsychological correlates of these three dimensions.[88,89]

The factor analytic studies published to date describe symptom interrelationships as they occur in a sample at a cross-sectional point in time. The course of schizophrenia, however, is typically characterized by chronicity and periods of relative exacerbations and remissions. Thus, cross-sectional analyses are limited in their predictive power or utility. Indeed, many of the most important questions about the symptoms of schizophrenia require a longitudinal research strategy, preferably one that can take a multivariate approach and will address patterns of change within individuals over time. For example, strong support for the three-dimensional model would be provided if individual symptoms that constitute a dimension covary or change together over time, but independently of symptoms within other dimensions.

The study of first-episode or recent-onset patients is the ideal laboratory in which to determine the course of these symptoms and their relationship to one another over time. We have investigated the change, stability, and patterns of change in psychotic, disorganized, and negative symptoms in such a sample. Specifically, we asked: Which symptoms are present at onset or early in the course of schizophrenia? How much do these symptoms change over time? How predictive (ie, stable) are the various symptoms or patterns of symptoms? How do changes in psychotic, disorganized, and negative symptoms correlate with one another (ie, do symptoms that cluster together cross-sectionally covary together over time and independently of other symptom dimensions)?

Table 1. Mean Symptom Ratings at Index Hospitalization, Discharge, and 1- and 2-Year Follow-up Evaluations*

	Symptom Ratings, Mean (SD)			
	Index Hospitalization (N=65)	Discharge (N=65)	1-Year Evaluation (N=53)	2-Year Evaluation (N=39)
Global rating measures				
Delusions	3.54 (1.19)	2.20 (1.15)†	1.81 (1.47)†‡	1.92 (1.46)†
Hallucinations	2.77 (1.59)	1.31 (1.25)†	1.40 (1.46)†	1.21 (1.40)†
Bizarre (Disorganized) Behavior	2.49 (1.24)	1.05 (1.08)†	1.17 (1.07)†	1.23 (1.04)†
Positive Thought Disorder	2.08 (1.33)	1.23 (1.16)†	0.89 (1.09)†‡	1.00 (1.15)†
Inappropriate Affect	1.58 (1.64)	0.66 (1.19)†	0.62 (1.08)†	0.69 (1.20)†
Alogia	2.89 (1.00)	2.38 (1.09)†	2.34 (1.04)†	2.05 (1.12)†‡
Anhedonia	3.78 (0.857)	3.34 (0.923)†	3.38 (0.985)†	3.41 (0.91)
Avolition	3.48 (1.24)	3.15 (1.16)†	2.89 (1.45)†	3.13 (1.17)
Affective Flattening	2.77 (1.07)	2.28 (1.19)†	2.17 (0.995)†	1.85 (1.09)†‡
Attention	2.49 (1.36)	1.86 (1.21)†	1.74 (1.24)†	1.69 (1.13)†‡
Psychotic symptoms§	3.15 (1.14)	1.75 (1.08)†	1.60 (1.35)†	1.56 (1.29)†
Disorganized symptoms‖	2.05 (0.945)	0.98 (0.860)†	0.89 (0.811)†	0.97 (0.962)†
Negative symptoms¶	3.08 (0.794)	2.60 (0.844)†	2.50 (0.891)†	2.43 (0.867)†‡

*Paired t tests were done for significance testing on complete pairs and not necessarily on the tabled means, which are based on all data. Global rating measures are from the Comprehensive Assessment of Symptoms and History, administered to each patient.
†For differences between index and follow-up ratings, $P<.05$ and $P<.01$, respectively.
‡For differences between discharge and follow-up ratings, $P<.05$ and $P<.01$, respectively.
§Psychotic symptoms are the mean of Delusions and Hallucinations ratings.
‖Disorganized symptoms are the mean of Bizarre (Disorganized) Behavior, Positive Thought Disorder, and Inappropriate Affect ratings.
¶Negative symptoms are the mean of the Alogia, Anhedonia, Avolition, Affective Flattening, and Attention ratings.

RESULTS

CHANGES IN SYMPTOM SEVERITY BASED ON ANALYSIS OF GROUP MEANS

The first step in the data analysis was to compare symptom severity across the four time periods to determine whether significant changes had occurred in any of the specific symptoms or the three dimensions. **Table 1** presents patients' symptom ratings at index hospitalization, discharge, and 1- and 2-year follow-ups. These results provide an index of the average degree of improvement or change in the various symptoms.

All symptoms showed an improvement from index hospitalization to discharge based on paired *t* tests ($P<.01$). Improvement, as assessed by comparison against index hospitalization, continued throughout the follow-up period, with the exception of two negative symptoms, anhedonia and avolition. These became nonsignificant at year 2, indicating that mean improvement in these two specific negative symptoms did not persist throughout the follow-up period and these symptoms may have begun to worsen or to progress by the time 2 years had elapsed.

The data are shown graphically in the **Figure**, which indicates that, while all symptoms improved significantly, both positive symptom dimensions (ie, psychoticism and disorganization) improved considerably more than negative symptoms. The average severity score of positive symptoms at discharge was almost halved compared with those at index hospitalization (from 3.15 to 1.75 for psychotic symptoms and from 2.05 to 0.98 for disorganization symptoms), while the average severity of negative symptoms showed only a modest improvement (from 3.08 to 2.6). Not only do these data indicate that negative symptoms are prominent in untreated first-episode and recent-onset patients, but they suggest that they tend to be more treatment resistant. Although positive and negative symptoms showed significant differences between follow-up and index ratings, there was no significant ongoing change in positive symptoms compared with discharge ratings; negative symptoms showed some improvement between discharge and follow-up at year 2, but the effect size is small. Similar results were obtained when a repeated-measures analysis of variance was applied to the 39 patients who were measured at index hospitalization, discharge, and 1- and 2-year follow-up.

PREDICTION OF CHANGES IN SYMPTOM SEVERITY BASED ON CORRELATIONAL ANALYSES

While changes in means provide one type of indicator of the extent to which positive and negative symptoms evolve over the course of time in a group of schizophrenic patients, it is also important to determine whether patterns of change occur at the level of the individual patient. Consequently, we also used correlational analysis to determine the extent to which the pattern of symptoms at index evaluation were predictive of the pattern at a later point in time. These results are shown in **Table 2**. Almost all individual positive and negative symptoms and all three dimensions are closely correlated between index and discharge evaluations, suggesting that patients tend to maintain their relative pattern of symptoms even when the severity decreases. After discharge, however, a different picture emerges. Correlations between index and 1- and 2-year follow-up evaluations tend to become nonsignificant, suggesting that the index presentation is not predictive of long-

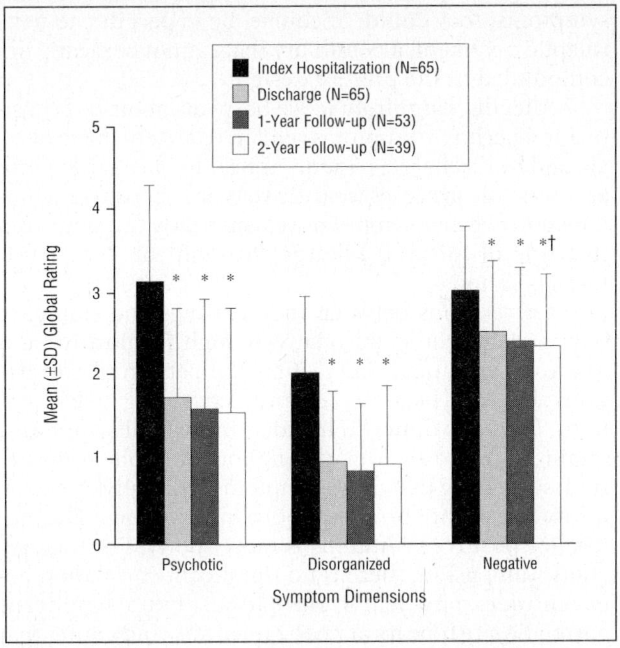

Symptom severity at index hospitalization, hospital discharge, and 1- and 2-year follow-up evaluations. Asterisk indicates P<.01 compared with symptoms at index hospitalization; dagger; compared with symptoms at discharge. Symptom dimensions are defined in the "Statistical Analysis" subsection of the "Methods" section of the text.

Table 2. Correlations of Index Hospitalization Ratings With Discharge, 1- and 2-Year Follow-up Ratings*

	Rating Correlations of Index Hospitalization		
	With Discharge (N=65)	With 1-Year (N=53)	With 2-Year (N=39)
Global rating measures			
Delusions	.564†	.085	.292‡
Hallucinations	.401†	.226	.353‡
Bizarre (Disorganized) Behavior	.193	.261‡	.130
Positive Thought Disorder	.651†	−.09	.209
Inappropriate Affect	.648†	.282‡	.417†
Affective Flattening	.685†	.524†	.408†
Alogia	.607†	.553†	.539†
Anhedonia	.762†	.234‡	.346‡
Avolition	.699†	.343†	.330‡
Attention	.697†	.516†	.425†
Psychotic symptoms	.502†	.097	.312‡
Disorganized symptoms	.401†	.105	.094
Negative symptoms	.774†	.542†	.467†

*Global rating measures and symptoms are described in Table 1.
†P<.01, one-tailed.
‡P<.05, one-tailed.

term outcome. The correlations between index and follow-up evaluations tend to remain significant for negative symptoms throughout the 2-year follow-up period, however, suggesting that negative symptoms tend to be more stable and traitlike. Since the negative symptoms tend to persist in the presence of diminishing positive symptoms, they are also less likely to be secondary, although the effects of akinesia cannot be excluded as an explanation.

PATTERNS OF INTRAINDIVIDUAL COURSE USING LONGITUDINAL RATINGS

Our final analysis explored the patterns of symptoms during the follow-up period available for each subject. This analysis used the weekly ratings to determine whether the changes in symptom pattern observed using the cross-sectional measures reflected a systematic and independent variation in the various individual symptoms. In this analysis, we examined the intercorrelations of the symptoms over time to determine whether any underlying factor structure was present.

The variance-covariance matrix for each patient over the weekly periods reflects how symptoms covary over time. Factor analysis of an individual's covariation over time has been referred to in the literature as the P-technique.[96] These individual matrices were pooled across individuals, and the results were used in a principal components analysis. Three factors met our criteria for inclusion, an analog of the eigenvalue-greater-than-one rule for covariance matrices. Factor loadings after varimax rotation are shown in **Table 3**.

The first factor correlates highly with the negative symptoms, although attentional impairment also loads on the second factor. This suggests that the negative symptoms tend to exacerbate and remit in unison. The second factor appears as a disorganized dimension, with high loadings for Bizarre (Disorganized) Behavior, Positive Thought Disorder, and Inappropriate Affect. Hallucinations and Delusions almost equally define the third factor. The loadings presented in Table 3 are based on an orthogonal rotation (varimax), so that these factors are statistically independent (uncorrelated). While symptoms within a factor tend to change together, changes occurring in one set of symptoms are not correlated with other symptoms. When we allowed the factors to become correlated using a promax rotation, the only change was a minor positive correlation between the negative and psychotic factors (r=.31), showing less than a 10% overlap of the factor's variance.

There is still the possibility that symptoms may not co-occur simultaneously, but the relationships are lagged in time. Some symptoms could precede others. For example, positive symptoms might be antecedents of negative symptoms or vice versa. An increase in positive symptoms during 1 week might correlate with negative symptoms increasing the following week. As a consequence, correlations between symptoms that were lagged an appropriate amount of time would be larger than the simultaneous correlations. We generated lagged correlations to investigate this possibility, lagging by 1-week intervals up to 4 weeks and then monthly intervals up to 4 months. There was no evidence of any time-lag structure to these data; all correlations tended to lower with more distal time points. This suggests that symptom clusters tended not to antecede other symptom clusters and provides further evidence that the clusters were independent.

Table 3. Patterns of Intrasubject Change in Symptom Severity Over the Weekly Periods: Loadings for Three Factors of Intraindividual (Variance-Covariance) Variation*

Factor	Factor Loading Correlations		
	Negative	Disorganized	Psychotic
Psychotic symptoms			
Delusions	.199	.203	.793
Hallucinations	.101	.143	.745
Disorganized symptoms			
Bizarre (Disorganized) Behavior	.103	.482	.317
Positive Thought Disorder	−.069	.859	.041
Inappropriate Affect	.073	.639	.080
Negative symptoms			
Alogia	.496	−.109	.182
Anhedonia	.646	.246	.056
Avolition	.902	.139	−.027
Affective Flattening	.599	−.071	.386
Attention	.334	.345	.183

**Global rating measures and symptoms are described in Table 1.*

COMMENT

This study provides support for conceptualizing the symptoms of schizophrenia as composed of three dimensions rather than two. The independence of the psychotic, disorganized, and negative dimensions previously demonstrated by a series of cross-sectional studies using factor analysis[77-79,81-86] has now been confirmed by our study using longitudinal factor analysis. The availability of detailed fine-grained ratings in a prospective longitudinal study of schizophrenic patients early in the course of illness has permitted us to observe that the evolution of the symptoms of schizophrenia over time occurs in three separate clusters. Positive symptoms break down into two dimensions that are uncorrelated with one another in their longitudinal progression, while negative symptoms form a third uncorrelated dimension. These three dimensions show different patterns in the way they exacerbate and remit during the course of schizophrenia.

Since patients in this study were all assessed during an acute hospitalization and 55 prior to receiving any neuroleptics, this sample provides us with an opportunity to observe the course of the symptoms of schizophrenia and the three dimensions independently of the effects of chronicity. The study demonstrates clearly that negative symptoms are present early in the illness. Further, when these patients are treated during a course of hospitalization, both negative symptoms and the two types of positive symptoms improve significantly. The improvement in positive symptoms is substantially greater than the improvement in negative symptoms, however, with a much larger effect size (more than 1 SD, compared with 0.5 or less). These findings suggest that negative symptoms tend to be less responsive to treatment, although they do not suggest that negative symptoms are necessarily treatment refractory. Since negative symptoms do not improve to the same degree as positive symptoms, these findings decrease the likelihood that the persistent negative symptoms are secondary to the positive symptoms; they could, of course, be in part due to neuroleptic treatment, a possibility that cannot be clearly deconfounded in the present design.

After discharge from index hospitalization, both positive and negative symptoms remain relatively stable overall, and by discharge, patients appear to have settled into a pattern. Mean scores for the two types of positive symptoms and negative symptoms remain nearly the same from the time of initial discharge through the 2-year follow-up period.

Correlations between index ratings and summary scores at discharge are relatively high for positive and negative symptoms. Thereafter, the pattern of correlations shifts and becomes less predictive. Negative symptoms, both as a dimension and as individual symptoms, retain high correlations throughout the follow-up period, suggesting that these symptoms are relatively stable; nevertheless, the correlations decline over time. The pattern for positive symptoms is more spotty. For the psychotic dimension, there is no significant correlation between index and year 1 evaluations, but a significant correlation reappears at year 2, probably indicating that a subset of patients has relapsed during this time period, with a reemergence of the symptoms that they originally manifested at index evaluation. Among the disorganized symptoms, only inappropriate affect remains consistently correlated throughout the follow-up period, indicating that this particular symptom is also relatively stable. The disorganized dimension as a whole remains poorly correlated with the index measure throughout the 2-year follow-up period; these results suggest that this particular dimension may be the most variable and unstable among the three. Reasons for this instability will require further study.

Interpretation of the results of this study is subject to limitations. First, all patients within the study were treated after the initial index assessment. Thus, the study does not provide us with information about the natural history of schizophrenia per se, but rather its course in the context of contemporary treatment approaches. This study design is naturalistic with respect to treatment, and all of the subjects were treated in a noncontrolled manner.

A second limitation of this study was that the weekly ratings used for the longitudinal factor analysis were determined retrospectively at the time of each 6-month follow-up evaluation. This method of acquiring data may have dampened changes in symptom variability over time. However, multiple sources, ie, informants, subjects, hospitals, and social workers, were used to construct the ratings, thereby increasing the diversity of information available and reducing the likelihood of dampening.

Rater effects also may have dampened the variability of changes during the period, since the same interviewer evaluated the patient's condition during the 2-year follow-up period whenever possible. This could produce a "halo effect" that could enhance the likelihood of finding longitudinal correlations. However, we believe that the advantages of interviewer continuity outweigh those of independent blind assessments. That is, as raters get to know the patient over time, building rapport with the patient and informants, they are more likely to pick up real, meaningful changes in the symptom profile and ability to function. Also, variability stemming from interrater differences in ratings is lowered. The use of informants (ie, family members) and other sources of information (eg, records from the referring psychiatrist following up the patient after discharge) also reduces the likelihood of halo effect.

In summary, these findings provide strong support for three separate dimensions of psychopathology in schizophrenia. The fact that the various positive and negative symptoms display a pattern of evolution that is independent suggests that they could reflect separate processes or even different neurobiological substrates. This study provides impetus for additional investigations using various types of neurobiological measures, as well as the exploration of the effects of treatments on these three dimensions of psychopathology.

Accepted for publication August 8, 1994.

Supported in part by grants MH31593, MH40856, MH46011, and MHCRC 43271 from the National Institute of Mental Health (NIMH), Rockville, Md, The Nellie Ball Trust Fund, Iowa State Bank and Trust Company (trustee), Iowa City (Dr Andreasen); and Research Scientist Award MH00625 from the NIMH (Dr Andreasen).

Reprint requests to 2911 JPP MHCRC, University of Iowa Hospitals and Clinics, 200 Hawkins Dr, Iowa City, IA 52242-1057 (Dr Arndt).

REFERENCES

1. Kraepelin E, Barclay RM, Robertson GM. *Dementia Praecox and Paraphrenia.* Edinburgh, Scotland: E & S Livingstone; 1919.
2. Bleuler E; Zinkin J, trans. *Dementia Praecox of the Group of Schizophrenias 1911.* New York, NY: International Universities Press; 1950.
3. Schneider K; Hamilton MW, trans. *Clinical Psychopathology.* New York, NY: Grune & Stratton; 1959.
4. Schneider K. Primary and secondary symptoms in schizophrenia. In: Hirsch SR, Shepherds M, eds. *Themes and Variations in European Psychiatry.* Littleton, Mass: John Wright–PSG Inc; 1974:40-46.
5. Huber G, Gross G, Schuttler R. A long-term follow-up study of schizophrenia: psychiatric course of illness and prognosis. *Acta Psychiatr Scand.* 1975;52:49-57.
6. Kleist K. Schizophrenic symptoms and cerebrapathology. *J Ment Sci.* 1960;106:246-255.
7. Langfeldt G. Schizophrenia: diagnosis and prognosis. *Behav Sci.* 1969;14:173-182.
8. Leonhard K. The question of prognosis in schizophrenia. *Int J Psychiatry.* 1966;2:633-635.
9. Fish FJ. *Schizophrenia.* Littleton, Mass: John Wright–PSG Inc; 1962.
10. Astrup C, Noreik K. *Functional Psychoses: Diagnostic and Prognostic Models.* Springfield, Ill: Charles C Thomas Publishers; 1966.
11. Babigian HM, Gardner EH, Miles HC, Romano J. Diagnostic consistency and change in a follow-up study of 1215 patients. *Am J Psychiatry.* 1965;121:895-901.
12. Fish FJ. The classification of schizophrenia: the views of Kleist and his coworkers. *J Ment Sci.* 1957;103:443-463.
13. Fish FJ. Leonhard's classification of schizohrenia. *J Ment Sci.* 1958;104:943-971.
14. Vaillant GE. Prospective prediction of schizophrenic remission. *Arch Gen Psychiatry.* 1964;11:509-518.
15. Stephens JH, Astrup C, Mangrum JC. Prognostic factors in recovered and deteriorated schizophrenics. *Am J Psychiatry.* 1966;122:1116-1121.
16. Klein DF, Rosen B. Premorbid asocial adjustment and response to phenothiazine treatment among schizophrenic inpatients. *Arch Gen Psychiatry.* 1973;29:480-485.
17. Pritchard M. Prognosis of schizophrenia before and after pharmacotherapy, I: short term outcome. *Br J Psychiatry.* 1967;113:1345-1352.
18. Pritchard M. Prognosis of schizophrenia before and after pharmacotherapy, II: three-year follow-up. *Br J Psychiatry.* 1967;113:1353-1359.
19. McGlashan TH. Intensive individual psychotherapy of schizophrenia: a review of techniques. *Arch Gen Psychiatry.* 1983;40:909-920.
20. Johnstone EC, Frith CD, Gold A, Stevens M. The outcome of severe acute schizophrenia illnesses after one year. *Br J Psychiatry.* 1979;134:28-33.
21. Goldberg SC, Frosch WA, Drossman AK, Schooler NR, Johnson GF. Prediction of response to phenothiazines in schizophrenia: a cross-validation study. *Arch Gen Psychiatry.* 1972;26:367-373.
22. Herz MI, Szymanski HV, Simon JC. Intermittent medication for stable schizophrenic outpatients: an alternative to maintenance medication. *Am J Psychiatry.* 1982;139:918-922.
23. Kane JM, Rifkin A, Quitkin F, Nayak D, Saraf K, Ramos-Lorenzi JR, Klein DF, Sachar EJ. Low dose fluphenazine decanoate and maintenance treatment in schizophrenia. *Psychiatry Res.* 1979;1:341-348.
24. Falloon IRH, Liberman RP. Interactions between drug and psychosocial therapy in schizophrenia. *Schizophr Bull.* 1983;9:543-554.
25. Silverstein ML, Harrow M. First-rank symptoms in the postacute schizophrenic: a follow-up study. *Am J Psychiatry.* 1978;135:1481-1484.
26. Harrow M, Bromet E, Quinlan D. Predictors of posthospital adjustment in schizophrenia. *J Nerv Ment Dis.* 1974;158:25-36.
27. McGlashan TH, Carpenter WT. An investigation of the postpsychotic depressive syndrome. *Am J Psychiatry.* 1976;133:14-19.
28. Strauss JS, Carpenter WT. Characteristic symptoms and outcome in schizophrenia. *Arch Gen Psychiatry.* 1974;30:429-434.
29. Strauss JS, Carpenter WT, Bartko JJ. The diagnosis and understanding of schizophrenia, III: speculations on the processes that underlie schizophrenia symptoms and signs. *Schizophr Bull.* 1974;1:61-69.
30. Chandrasena R, Rodrigo A. Schneider's first rank symptoms: their prevalence and diagnostic implications in an Asian population. *Br J Psychiatry.* 1979;135:348-351.
31. Pfohl B, Winokur G. The evolution of symptoms in institutionalized hebephrenic/catatonic schizophrenics. *Br J Psychiatry.* 1982;141:567-572.
32. Pfohl B, Winokur G. The micropsychopathology of hebephrenic/catatonic schizophrenia. *J Nerv Ment Dis.* 1983;171:296-300.
33. Carr VJ. Recovery from schizophrenia: a review of patterns of psychosis. *Schizophr Bull.* 1983;9:95-121.
34. Gittelman-Klein R, Klein DF. Premorbid asocial adjustment and prognosis in schizophrenia. *J Psychiatr Res.* 1969;7:35-53.
35. Zigler E, Glick M, Marsh A. Premorbid social competence and outcome among schizophrenic and nonschizophrenic patients. *J Nerv Ment Dis.* 1979;167:478-483.
36. Bland RC, Parker JH, Orn H. Prognosis in schizophrenia: prognostic predictions and outcome. *Arch Gen Psychiatry.* 1978;35:72-77.
37. Bland RC, Orn H. 14-year outcome in early schizophrenia. *Acta Psychiatr Scand.* 1978;58:328-338.
38. Bridge TP, Cannon E, Wyatt RJ. Burned-out schizophrenia: evidence for age effects on schizophrenic symptomatology. *J Gerontol.* 1978;33:835-839.
39. Ciompi L. Three lectures on schizophrenia. *Br J Psychiatry.* 1980;136:413-420.
40. Tsuang MT, Woolson RF. Excess mortality in schizophrenia and affective disorders: do suicides and accidental deaths solely account for this excess? *Arch Gen Psychiatry.* 1978;35:1181-1185.
41. Winokur G, Morrison J, Clancy J, Crowe R. Iowa 500: the clinical and genetic distinction of hebephrenic and paranoid schizophrenia. *J Nerv Ment Dis.* 1974;159:12-19.
42. Tsuang MT, Woolson RF, Fleming JA. Long-term outcome of major psychoses, I: schizophrenia and affective disorders compared wtih psychiatrically symptom-free surgical conditions. *Arch Gen Psychiatry.* 1979;36:1295-1301.
43. Waxler NE. Is outcome for schizohrenia better in nonindustrial societies? *J Nerv Ment Dis.* 1979;167:144-158.
44. Watt DC, Szulecka TK. The effect of sex, marriage and age at first admission on the hospitalization of schizophrenics during 2 years following discharge. *Psychol Med.* 1979;9:529-539.
45. Parnas J, Schulsinger F, Teasdale TW, Schulsinger H, Feldman PM, Mednick SA. Perinatal complications and clinical outcome within the schizophrenia spectrum. *Br J Psychiatry.* 1982;140:416-420.
46. Summers F, Hersh S. Psychiatric chronicity and diagnosis. *Schizophr Bull.* 1983;9:122-133.
47. McGlashan TH. The Chestnut Lodge Follow-Up Study, I: follow-up methodology and study sample. *Arch Gen Psychiatry.* 1984;41:573-585.
48. McGlashan TH. The Chestnut Lodge Follow-Up Study, II: long-term outcome of schizophrenia and the affective disorders. *Arch Gen Psychiatry.* 1984;41:586-601.
49. McGlashan TH. The prediction of outcome in chronic schizophrenia, IV: the

Chestnut Lodge Follow-Up Study. *Arch Gen Psychiatry.* 1986;43:167-176.
50. McGlashan TH. Schizotypal personality disorder: Chestnut Lodge Follow-Up Study, VI: long-term follow-up perspectives. *Arch Gen Psychiatry.* 1986;43: 329-334.
51. Wing JK, Cooper JE, Sartorius N. *The Measurement and Classification of Psychiatric Symptoms.* New York, NY: Cambridge University Press; 1974.
52. Fenton WS, McGlashan TH. Natural history of schizophrenia subtypes, I: longitudinal study of paranoid, hebephrenic, and undifferentiated schizophrenia. *Arch Gen Psychiatry.* 1991;48:969-977.
53. Harding CM, Strauss JS. The course of schizophrenia: an evolving concept. In: Alpert M, ed. *Controversies in Schizophrenia: Changes and Constancies.* New York, NY: Guilford Press; 1985.
54. Harding CM, Zubin J, Strauss JS. Chronicity in schizophrenia: fact, partial fact, or artifact? *Hosp Community Psychiatry.* 1987;38:477-486.
55. Andreasen NC. Negative symptoms in schizophrenia: definition and reliability. *Arch Gen Psychiatry.* 1982;39:784-788.
56. Andreasen NC, Olsen S. Negative *v* positive schizophrenia: definition and validation. *Arch Gen Psychiatry.* 1982;39:789-794.
57. Andreasen NC. *Comprehensive Assessment of Symptoms and History (CASH).* Iowa City, Iowa: The University of Iowa; 1985.
58. Andreasen NC. *Can Schizophrenia Be Localized in the Brain?* Washington, DC: American Psychiatric Press, Inc; 1986.
59. Andreasen NC. Method for assessing positive and negative symptoms. In: Andreasen NC, ed. *Positive and Negative Symptoms and Syndromes: Modern Problems in Pharmacopsychiatry.* New York, NY: S Karger AG; 1990:73-88.
60. Andreasen NC, Flaum M. Schizophrenia: the characteristic symptoms. *Schizophr Bull.* 1990;17:27-49.
61. Andreasen NC, Flaum M, Arndt S, Alliger R, Swayze VW. Positive and negative symptoms: assessment and validity. In: Marneros A, Andreasen NC, Tsuang MD, eds. *Negative Versus Positive Schizophrenia.* Heidelberg, Germany: Springer-Verlag Berlin; 1991:28-51.
62. Andreasen NC. Thought, language, and communication disorders, I: clinical assessment, definition of terms, and evaluation of their reliability. *Arch Gen Psychiatry.* 1979;36:1315-1321.
63. Andreasen NC. Thought, language, and communication disorders, II: diagnostic significance. *Arch Gen Psychiatry.* 1979;36:1325-1330.
64. Johnstone EC, Owens DGC, Firth CD, Crow TJ. The relative stability of positive and negative features in chronic schizophrenia. *Br J Psychiatry.* 1986;150:60-64.
65. Carpenter WT, Kirkpatrick B. The heterogeneity of the long-term course of schizophrenia. *Schizophr Bull.* 1988;14:645-659.
66. Buchanan RW, Kirkpatrick B, Heinrichs DW, Carpenter WT. Clinical correlates of the deficit syndrome of schizophrenia. *Am J Psychiatry.* 1990;147:290-294.
67. Carpenter WT Jr, Heinrichs DW, Alphs LD. Treatment of negative symptoms. *Schizophr Bull.* 1985;11:440-452.
68. McGlashan TH, Fenton WT. The positive-negative distinction in schizophrenia: review of natural history validators. *Arch Gen Psychiatry.* 1992;49:63-72.
69. Pogue-Geile MF, Harrow M. Negative symptoms in schizophrenia: their longitudinal course and prognostic importance. *Schizophr Bull.* 1985;11:427-439.
70. Sommers AS. 'Negative symptoms': conceptual and methodological problems. *Schizophr Bull.* 1985;11:364-373.
71. Crow TJ. Molecular pathology of schizophrenia: more than one disease process? *BMJ.* 1980;280:66-68.
72. Crow TJ. Positive and negative schizophrenic symptoms and the role of dopamine. *Br J Psychiatry.* 1980;137:383-386.
73. Crow TJ. The two syndrome concept: origins and current status. *Schizophr Bull.* 1985;11:471-486.
74. American Psychiatric Association. *Diagnostic and Statistical Manual of Mental Disorders, Revised Third Edition.* Washington, DC: American Psychiatric Association; 1987.
75. American Psychiatric Association. *Diagnostic and Statistical Manual of Mental Disorders, Fourth Edition.* Washington, DC: American Psychiatric Association; 1994.
76. Moscarelli M, Maffei C, Cesana BM. An international perspective on assessment of negative and positive symptoms in schizophrenia. *Am J Psychiatry.* 1987;144:1595-1598.
77. Arndt S, Alliger RJ, Andreasen NC. The distinction of positive and negative symptoms: the failure of a two-dimensional model. *Br J Psychiatry.* 1991;158: 317-322.
78. Miller DD, Arndt S, Andreasen NC. Alogia, attentional impairment, and inappropriate affect: their status in the dimensions of schizophrenia. *Comp Psychiatry.* 1993;34:221-226.
79. Bilder RM, Mukherjee S, Rieder RO, Pandurangi AK. Symptomatic and neuropsychological components of defect states. *Schizophr Bull.* 1985;11: 409-491.
80. Kulhara P, Kota SK, Joseph S. Positive and negative subtypes of schizophrenia: a study from India. *Acta Psychiatr Scand.* 1986;74:353-359.
81. Lenzenweger MF, Dworkin RH, Wethington E. Models of positive and negative symptoms in schizophrenia: an empirical evaluation of latent structures. *J Abnorm Psychol.* 1989;98:62-70.
82. Schuldberg D, Quinlan DM, Morgenstern H, Glazer W. Positive and negative symptoms in chronic psychiatric outpatients: reliability, stability, and factor structure: psychological assessment. *J Consult Clin Psychol.* 1990;2:262-268.
83. Gur RE, Mozley D, Resnick SM, Levick S, Erwin R, Saykin AJ, Gur RC. Relations amoung clinical scales in schizophrenia. *Am J Psychiatry.* 1991;148:472-478.
84. Minas IH, Stuart GW, Klimidis S, Jackson HJ, Singh BS, Copolov DL. Positive and negtive symptoms in the psychoses: multidimensional scaling of SAPS and SANS items. *Schizophr Res.* 1992;8:143-156.
85. Brown KW, White T. Syndromes of chronic schizophrenia and some clinical correlates. *Br J Psychiatry.* 1992;161:317-322.
86. Peralta V, de Leon J, Cuesta MJ. Are there more than two syndromes in schizophrenia? a critique of the positive-negative dichotomy. *Br J Psychiatry.* 1992; 161:335-343.
87. Gorsuch RL. *Factor Analysis.* Philadelphia, Pa: WB Saunders Co; 1974.
88. Liddle PF, Friston KJ, Frith CD, Frackowiak RSJ. Cerebral blood flow and mental processes in schizophrenia. *J R Soc Med.* 1992;85:224-226.
89. Andreasen NC, Rezai K, Alliger R, Swayze VW, Flaum M, Kirchner P, Cohen G, O'Leary DS. Hypofrontality in neuroleptic-naive and chronic schizophrenic patients: assessment with xenon 133 single-photon emission computed tomography and the Tower of London. *Arch Gen Psychiatry.* 1992;49:943-958.
90. Flaum M, Andreasen NC, Arndt S. The Iowa Prospective Longitudinal Study of recent onset psychoses: methodological and statistical strategies. *Schizophr Bull.* 1992;18:481-490.
91. Andreasen NC, Flaum M, Arndt S. The Comprehensive Assessment of Symptoms and History (CASH): an instrument for assessing diagnosis and psychopathology. *Arch Gen Psychiatry.* 1992;49:615-623.
92. Andreasen NC. *PSYCH-BASE.* Iowa City, Iowa: The University of Iowa; 1989.
93. Andreasen NC. *The Scale for the Assessment of Negative Symptoms (SANS).* Iowa City, Iowa: The University of Iowa; 1983.
94. Andreasen NC. *The Scale for the Assessment of Positive Symptoms (SAPS).* Iowa City, Iowa: The University of Iowa; 1984.
95. Andreasen NC, Arndt S, Alliger A, Miller D, Flaum M. Symptoms of schizophrenia: methods, meanings, and mechanisms. *Arch Gen Psychiatry.* 1995; 52:341-351.
96. Cattell RB. The structuring of change by P-technique and incremental R-technique. In: Harris CW, ed. *Problems of Measuring Change.* Madison, Wis: The University of Wisconsin Press; 1963.

COMMENTARY

Signs and Symptoms

What Can They Tell Us About the Clinical Course and Pathophysiologic Processes of Schizophrenia?

HISTORICALLY, psychiatry has emphasized phenomenologic description in its conceptualization and characterization of schizophrenia. Although Kraepelin[1] and Langfeldt[2] included longitudinal course as a diagnostic criterion, most students of schizophrenia focused on qualitative descriptions of the psychopathologic processes. Initial efforts to define the disorder by its neurobiologic characteristics were frustrated by the inability of classical neuropathologists to identify histopathologically distinct and replicable lesions.[3,4] Given the variable nature of the disorder, clinicians attempted to reduce its heterogeneity by delineating meaningful subtypes. The traditional subtypes of paranoid, undifferentiated, hebephrenic (disorganized), and catatonic schizophrenia were defined by qualitative differences in psychopathologic features and have endured despite the absence of validating evidence from investigations of treatment response, long-term outcome, pathophysiologic processes, or genetics. However, reductio ad absurdum, some skeptics suggest that phenomenological distinctions in schizophrenia may be meaningless in our efforts to understand the underlying nature and cause of the disease.

The efforts of Andreasen and Olsen[5] in the early 1980s to revive the Jacksonian model in our thinking of schizophrenia along with the two-syndrome disease typology proposed by Crow[6] provided a needed impetus at a time when the dominant models consisted of the traditional qualitative symptom subtypes[7,8] (ie, paranoid, undifferentiated, hebephrenic, and catatonic) and the dopamine hypothesis of schizophrenia.[9] Delineation of positive and negative symptom subtypes proved heuristic, giving rise to new ways to conceptualize schizophrenia. Carpenter et al's[10] definition of the "deficit state" provided an important elaboration and formalization of the negative symptom subtype. Subsequently, the positive/negative symptom model was reified to include a third symptom constellation (thought disorganization). This model has been replicated convincingly.[11-15] These lines of investigation have dovetailed with the burgeoning knowledge of the neurobiologic features of schizophrenia[16-20] and lead to comprehensive and detailed etiopathophysiologic models.[21-30]

At the same time, much remains to be reconciled and clarified in our understanding of schizophrenia. Articles by Andreasen and colleagues[31] and Arndt et al[32] in this issue of the ARCHIVES describe some of their efforts to extend our conceptual understanding of schizophrenia. Among the salient contributions of the first article[31] is the replication of the finding of the three symptom factors in a new large patient cohort. They point out that the symptom factors, although independent, are also overlapping and, therefore, do not constitute subtypes. They argue that the three symptom constellations, rather than reflecting subtypes or syndromes (symptoms that run together), represent symptom dimensions that may coexist and that derive from separate discrete loci of neurobiologic dysfunction. They further caution that the three symptom clusters must be considered purely descriptive (as are the traditional qualitative subtypes) until their relationships to other lines of evidence, eg, treatment response, illness course, family history, and neurobiologic measures, can be demonstrated. Although caution is warranted, it should

See also pages 341 and 352

be acknowledged that significant evidence linking the symptoms of these factors and treatment outcome, genetics, and neurobiology has already been reported.[33-42]

A limiting factor in our ability to identify relationships between symptoms and other factors is the ability to characterize accurately the relevant phenomenologic characteristics in a reliable manner. The Iowa group[5,14,32] has made important contributions to this effort. However, even the most sensitive and reliable instruments may be affected by factors that influence the expression of symptoms, such as clinical state (eg, acute, remitted, chronic, and residual state); medication status and side effects; and comorbid conditions such as depression and substance abuse. Cross-sectional and longitudinal studies of phenomenologic characteristics are both vulnerable to these methodologic pitfalls.

The second article[32] describes the longitudinal course of symptoms in recent-onset, predominantly first-episode patients who had no prior treatment exposure. This study is important for two reasons. First, patterns of symptom change can indicate the validity of symptom clusters such as in the three-factor model and can also reflect pathophysiologic changes occurring in the course of the illness. Second, previous long-term studies of schizophrenia indicate that most of the deterioration occurs in the early stage of the illness. Thus, in examining symptom change over the course of the illness, it is important to study patients during the period in which change might be expected to occur. Arndt et al[32] conclude from their findings, first, that negative symptoms are present early in the illness, are less responsive to treatment, and are stable over time and second, that the positive, negative, and disorganization symptoms are independent dimensions and remain so over the longitudinal course of schizophrenia. They interpret this as supporting the notion of certain symptoms being fundamental and enduring traitlike elements of the illness.

However, several considerations urge caution in the interpretation of these important results. First, negative symptom ratings during the index episode were made in a drug-free condition but when positive symptoms were active. Second, although high levels of negative symptoms were present, these were comparable to the severity levels of positive symptoms and could have been secondary to them. The fact that negative symptoms changed less than did positive symptoms over the follow-up period could indicate, as the authors suggest, that negative symptoms were not secondary to positive symptoms and are less responsive to treatment and more stable over time. However, the negative symptoms that initially were secondary to positive symptoms in the acute-phase pretreatment could have been secondary to extrapyramidal side effects of medication or depression, both of which are highly prevalent in first-episode patients[43-45] during the follow-up phase. Thus, secondary negative symptoms could have been present at all rating occasions. Consistent with this explanation are the results of earlier studies that reported that negative symptoms, although present in the early stage of schizophrenia, were predominantly secondary in nature and lower in prevalence and severity in first-episode patients than in multiepisode patients with chronic schizophrenia.[35,40,46] Moreover, negative symptoms have been shown to increase in frequency and severity over the course of the disorder.[40,47]

Changes seen in positive and disorganized symptoms over the index and follow-up periods parallel changes that would be expected when patients go from acute to remitted, partially remitted, or stable states. Beyond this, any potential for subsequent change in the pattern or severity of symptoms that may have occurred during the follow-up periods would be dependent on what happened to the patients during these intervals. Did the patients experience relapses and subsequent episodes? Did the patients continue to receive pharmacotherapy, and if so, what side effects did they incur? Based on prior studies of illness course, one would would expect that psychopathological change would be most likely to occur as a consequence of exacerbations of illness[48-51] and the development of neurologic side effects.[52-56]

Long-term outcome studies have described two various patterns of symptom evolution.[1,2,6,7,36,37,40,47,57] One is the previously described increase in negative symptoms over the illness course.[6,40,47] The second is the tendency in some patients who initially had paranoid or undifferentiated symptoms for symptoms of the disorganization and catatonic subtypes to develop in the latter stages of their illness.[36,57] Thus, the potential for psychopathologic change in the course of schizophrenia does appear to exist. However, acknowledging the potential for psychopathological change may be considerably easier than demonstrating it. Although the majority of patients with schizophrenia potentially may experience some degree of deterioration in the course of their illness, the deterioration is of a limited nature and may develop in a narrow and unpredictable time interval. Given this, the ability to demonstrate psychopathological change will be dependent on at what point in the trajectory of their illness patients are ascertained and over what period they are examined. The Arndt et al study[32] examined 65 patients with schizophrenia who had a median illness duration of 8 months and followed them up for 1 (82%) to 2 (60%) years. This time frame may have been too narrow a window to capture the potential change of the patient cohort.

Phenomenology has been the historical bootstrap that investigators have used in their efforts to understand the enigma of schizophrenia. Despite important advances in clinical neurobiology, it appears that phenomenology will remain the cornerstone of the diagnosis and research methods of schizophrenia for the foreseeable future.

Jeffrey A. Lieberman, MD
Department of Psychiatry
Hillside Hospital
75-59 263rd St
Glen Oaks, NY 11004

Reprint requests to Dr Lieberman.

REFERENCES

1. Kraepelin E; Barclay RM, trans. *Dementia Praecox.* Edinburgh, Scotland: E & S Livingstone Ltd; 1919.
2. Langfeldt G. *The Prognosis in Schizophrenia and the Factors Influencing the Course of the Disease.* Copenhagen, Denmark: Munksgaard International Publishers Ltd; 1937.
3. Bogerts B. The neuropathology of schizophrenia: pathophysiological and neurodevelopmental implications. In: Mednick SA, Cannon TD, Barr CE, eds. *Fetal Neural Development and Adult Schizophrenia.* New York, NY: Cambridge University Press; 1991:153-173.
4. Bogerts B, Lieberman J. Neuropathology in the study of psychiatric disease. In: Costa e Silva JA, Nadelson CC, eds. *International Review of Psychiatry.* Washington, DC: American Psychiatric Press; 1993:515-545.
5. Andreasen NC, Olsen S. Negative vs positive schizophrenia. *Arch Gen Psychiatry.* 1982;39: 789-794.
6. Crow JT. Molecular pathology of schizophrenia: more than one disease process? *BMJ.* 1980; 280:66-68.
7. Bleuler E; Zinkin J, trans. *Dementia Praecox or the Group of Schizophrenia.* New York, NY: International Universities Press; 1950.
8. McGlashan TH, Fenton WS. Classical subtypes for schizophrenia: literature review for *DSM-IV. Schizophr Bull.* 1991;17:609-632.
9. Snyder SH, Banarjee SP, Yamamura HT. Drugs, neurotransmitters and schizophrenia. *Science.* 1974;184:1243-1543.

10. Carpenter WT Jr, Heinrichs DW, Wagman AMI. Deficit and nondeficit forms of schizophrenia: the concept. *Am J Psychiatry.* 1988;145:578-583.
11. Bilder RM, Mukherjee S, Rieder RO, Pandurangi AK. Symptomatic and neuropsychological components of defect states. *Schizophr Bull.* 1985; 11:409-419.
12. Liddle PF, Barnes TRE. Syndromes of chronic schizophrenia. *Br J Psychiatry.* 1990;157:558-561.
13. Andreasen NC, Grove WM. Evaluation of positive and negative symptoms in schizophrenia. *Psychiatr Psychobiol.* 1986;2:108-121.
14. Andreasen NC, Flaum M, Swayze WV, Tyrrell G, Arndt S. Positive and negative symptoms in schizophrenia: a critical reappraisal. *Arch Gen Psychiatry.* 1990;47:615-621.
15. Arndt S, Alliger RJ, Andreasen NC. The distinction of positive and negative symptoms: the failure of a two-dimensional model. *Br J Psychiatry.* 1991;158:317-322.
16. Kendler KS, Diehl SR. The genetics of schizophrenia: a current, genetic-epidemiologic perspective. *Schizophr Bull.* 1993;19:261-285.
17. Gur RE, Pearlson GD. Neuroimaging in schizophrenia research. *Schizophr Bull.* 1993;19:337-353.
18. Kirch DG. Infection and autoimmunity as etiologic factors in schizophrenia: a review and reappraisal. *Schizophr Bull.* 1993;19:355-370.
19. Lieberman JA, Koreen AR. Neurochemistry and neuroendocrinology of schizophrenia: a selective review. *Schizophr Bull.* 1993;19:371-429.
20. Bogerts B. Recent advances in the neuropathology of schizophrenia. *Schizophr Bull.* 1993;19: 431-445.
21. Weinberger DR. Implications of normal brain development for the pathogenesis of schizophrenia. *Arch Gen Psychiatry.* 1987;44:660-669.
22. Carlsson M, Carlsson A. Schizophrenia: a subcortical neurotransmitter imbalance syndrome. *Schizophr Bull.* 1990;16:425-432.
23. Davis KL, Kahn RS, Ko G, Davidson M. Dopamine in schizophrenia: a review and reconceptualization. *Am J Psychiatry.* 1991;148:1474-1486.
24. Javitt DC, Zukin SR. Recent advances in the phencyclidine model of schizophrenia. *Am J Psychiatry.* 1991;148:1301-1308.
25. Lipska BK, Jaskiw GE, Weinberger DR. Postpubertal emergence of hyperresponsiveness to stress and to amphetamine after neonatal excitotoxic hippocampal damage: a potential animal model of schizophrenia. *Neuropsychopharmacology.* 1993;9:67-75.
26. Murray RM, Lewis SW. Is schizophrenia a neurodevelopmental disorder? *BMJ.* 1987;295:681-682.
27. Robbins TW. The case for frontostriatal dysfunction in schizophrenia. *Schizophr Bull.* 1990; 16:391-402.
28. Swerdlow NR, Koob GF. Dopamine, schizophrenia, mania, and depression: toward a unified hypothesis of cortico-striato-pallido-thalamic function. *Behav Brain Sci.* 1987;10:197-245.
29. Crow TJ. Sexual selection, Machiavellian intelligence, and the origins of psychosis. *Lancet.* 1993; 342:594-598.
30. Feinberg I. Schizophrenia: caused by a fault in programmed synaptic elimination during adolescence? *J Psychiatr Res.* 1983;17:319-334.
31. Andreasen NC, Arndt S, Alliger R, Miller D, Flaum M. Symptoms of schizophrenia: methods, meanings, and mechanisms. *Arch Gen Psychiatry.* 1995; 52:341-351.
32. Arndt S, Andreasen NC, Flaum M, Miller D, Nopoulos P. A longitudinal study of symptom dimensions in schizophrenia: prediction and patterns of change. *Arch Gen Psychiatry.* 1995;52:352-360.
33. Carpenter WT, Buchanan RW. Domains of psychopathology relevant to the study of etiology and treatment of schizophrenia. In: Schultz SC, Tamminga CT, eds. *Schizophrenia: Scientific Progress.* New York, NY: Oxford Press; 1989.
34. Buchanan RW, Breier A, Kirkpatrick B, Elkashef A, Munson RC, Gellad F, Carpenter WT. Structural abnormalities in deficit vs non-deficit schizophrenia. *Am J Psychiatry.* 1993;150:59-65.
35. Mayerhoff DI, Loebel AD, Borenstein M, Szymanski SR, Geisler SH, Alvir JMJ, Lieberman JA. The deficit state in first-episode schizophrenia. *Am J Psychiatry.* 1994;151:1417-1422.
36. Fenton WS, McGlashan TH. Natural history of schizophrenia subtypes, I: longitudinal study of paranoid, hebephrenic, and undifferentiated schizophrenia. *Arch Gen Psychiatry.* 1991;48: 969-977.
37. McGlashan TH, Fenton WS. Subtype progression and pathophysiologic deterioration in early schizophrenia. *Schizophr Bull.* 1993;19:71-84.
38. Waddington JL, Youssef HA. An unusual cluster of tardive dyskinesia in schizophrenia: association with cognitive dysfunction and negative symptoms. *Am J Psychiatry.* 1986;143:1162-1165.
39. Farmer A, McGuffin P, Gottesman II. Problems and pitfalls of the family history positive and negative dichotomy. *Schizophr Bull.* 1990; 16:367-370.
40. Fenton WS, McGlashan TH. Antecedents, symptom progression, and long-term outcome of the deficit syndrome in schizophrenia. *Am J Psychiatry.* 1994;151:351-356.
41. Catts SV, Shelley AM, Ward PB, Liebert B, McConaghy N, Andrews S, Michie PT. Brain potential evidence for an auditory sensory memory deficit in schizophrenia. *Am J Psychiatry.* 1995;152: 213-219.
42. Wolkin A, Sanfilipo M, Wolf AP, Angrist B, Brodie JD, Rotrosen J. Negative symptoms and hypofrontality in chronic schizophrenia. *Arch Gen Psychiatry.* 1992;49:959-965.
43. Lieberman JA, Jody D, Alvir JMJ, Ashtari M, Levy D, Bogerts B, Degreef G, Mayerhoff D, Cooper T. Brain morphology, dopamine, and eye tracking abnormalities in first episode schizophrenia: prevalence and clinical correlates. *Arch Gen Psychiatry.* 1993;50:357-368.
44. Chakos MH, Mayerhoff DI, Loebel AD, Alvir JM, Lieberman JA. Incidence and correlates of acute extrapyramidal symptoms in first episode schizophrenia. *Psychopharmacol Bull.* 1992;28:81-86.
45. Koreen AR, Siris SG, Chakos M, Alvir J, Mayerhoff D, Lieberman J. Depression in first episode schizophrenia. *Am J Psychiatry.* 1993;150: 1643-1648.
46. Kirkpatrick B, Buchanan RW, Breier A, Carpenter WT Jr. Case identification and stability of the deficit syndrome of schizophrenia. *Psychiatry Res.* 1993;47:47-56.
47. Pogue-Guile MF, Harrow M. Negative symptoms in schizophrenia: their longitudinal course and prognostic importance. *Schizophr Bull.* 1985; 11:427-439.
48. May RP, Tuma AH, Yale C, Potepan P, Dixon WJ. Schizophrenia—a follow up study of results of treatment, II: hospital stay over two to five years. *Arch Gen Psychiatry.* 1976;33:481-486.
49. Crow TJ, Macmillan JF, Johnson AL, Johnstone EC. A randomised controlled trial of prophylactic neuroleptic treatment. *Br J Psychiatry.* 1986; 148:120-127.
50. Loebel AD, Lieberman JA, Alvir JAJ, Mayerhoff DI, Geisler SH, Szymanski SR. Duration of psychosis and outcome in first episode schizophrenia. *Am J Psychiatry.* 1992;149:1183-1188.
51. Wyatt RJ. Neuroleptics and the natural course of schizophrenia. *Schizophr Bull.* 1991;17:325-351.
52. Lieberman JA, Alvir J, Geisler S, Ramos-Lorenzi J, Woerner M, Novacenko H, Cooper T, Kane JM. Methylphenidate response, psychopathology and tardive dyskinesia as predictors of relapse in schizophrenia. *Neuropsychopharmacology.* 1994;11:107-118.
53. Chakos MH, Lieberman JA, Bilder RM, Lerner G, Bogerts B, Degreef G, Wu H, Ashtari M. Increase in caudate nuclei volumes of first episode schizophrenic patients taking antipsychotic drugs. *Am J Psychiatry.* 1994;151: 1430-1436.
54. Paulsen JS, Heaton RK, Jeste DV. Neuropsychological impairment in tardive dyskinesia. *Neuropsychology.* 1994;8:227-241.
55. Waddington JL, Youssef HA, Dolphin C, Kinsella A. Cognitive dysfunction, negative symptoms, and tardive dyskinesia in schizophrenia. *Arch Gen Psychiatry.* 1987;44:907-912.
56. Buchanan RW, Kirkpatrick B, Heinrichs DW, Carpenter WT. Clinical correlates of the deficit syndrome of schizophrenia. *Am J Psychiatry.* 1990;147:290-294.
57. Pfohl B, Winokur G. The evolution of symptoms in institutionalized hebephrenic/catatonic schizophrenics. *Br J Psychiatry.* 1982;141: 5767-5772.

Introducing a selective
serotonin reuptake inhibitor for OCD

New LUVOX™

fluvoxamine maleate 50 mg & 100 mg SCORED TABLETS

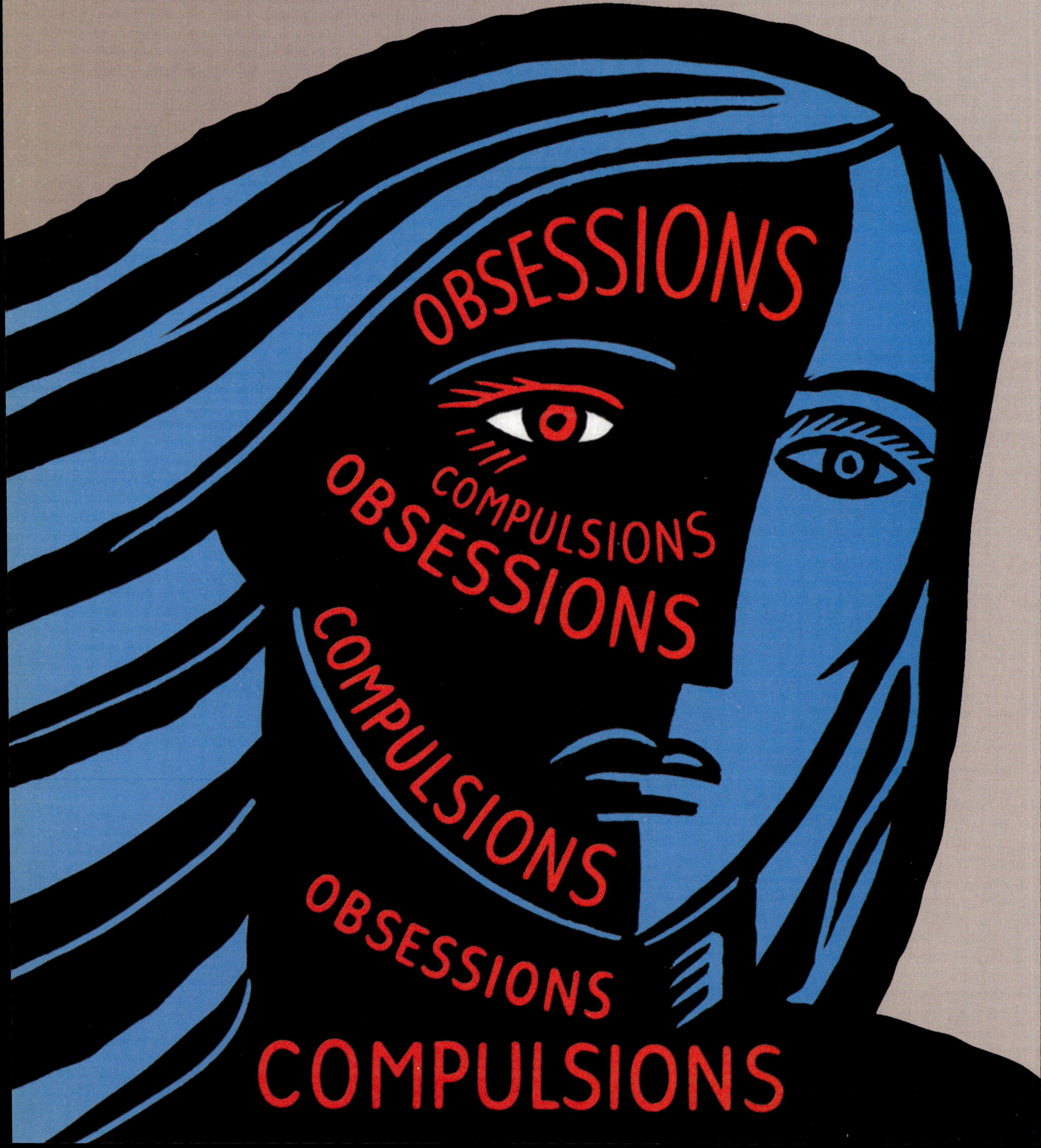

ORIGINAL ARTICLE

A Family Study of Manic-Depressive (Bipolar I) Disease

Is It a Distinct Illness Separable From Primary Unipolar Depression?

George Winokur, MD; William Coryell, MD; Martin Keller, MD; Jean Endicott, PhD; Andrew Leon, PhD

Objective: To determine whether bipolar I illness is autonomous or part of a multifactorial continuum with unipolar depression. In this study, we compare familial bipolar I illness and depression among three groups: probands with bipolar I disorder; probands with primary unipolar disorder; and controls. We also examine a continuum of severity between psychotic and nonpsychotic patients with bipolar I disorder. Considerable data suggest that bipolar I illness is distinct from unipolar illness as regards epidemiology, familial psychiatric illness, course, response to treatment, and biologic findings.

Method: Probands were separated into bipolar I and primary unipolar depressive groups. Personally interviewed family members of these patients were compared on variables of bipolar illness or schizoaffective mania and unipolar or schizoaffective depression. A personally examined control group was compared with the relatives of the two proband groups. Similar analyses were performed using data obtained by a systematic family history method. For the same familial variables, psychotic and nonpsychotic manic probands were compared.

Results: Familial mania is more frequent in families of patients with bipolar disease than in controls or in families of patients with primary unipolar disorder. The latter two groups did not differ in amount of mania. Unipolar depressive illness or schizoaffective depression was higher in families of probands with bipolar and unipolar disorder than in controls. Probands with bipolar disease separated into those who had psychotic symptoms (including schizoaffective mania) and no psychotic symptoms did not differ from each other in risk for familial mania or depression.

Conclusions: Bipolar I illness is a separate illness from primary unipolar illness because of an increase in familial mania. Patients with primary unipolar disease and controls show the same amount of familial mania. Lack of an increase in familial illness according to the severity of bipolar disease is against an affective continuum.

(Arch Gen Psychiatry. 1995;52:367-373)

A PERSISTENT debate continues over whether manic-depressive or bipolar illness should be considered a specific diagnostic entity, separable from other affective illnesses. Certainly, when compared with unipolar depression, manic-depressive disease differs in a variety of ways. It is less common in the population; it is associated with more premorbid hyperactivity; clinically, it is different because it shows manias whereas other affective disorders do not; it is more likely to show an acute onset and multiple episodes; cerebral metabolism during the depressive phase may be different from that in patients with unipolar depression.[1-4]

A major difference between bipolar and unipolar illness is that mania is found in the families of patients with bipolar disease but is not highly represented in the families of patients with unipolar disease.[5] To our knowledge, no studies contradict this last finding. Based on this plus the differences described above, a conservative conclusion would be to consider bipolar illness as a separate disease. However, some studies have been interpreted to suggest that bipolar illness is simply a part of an affective continuum. The problem has been approached in two ways.

Gershon et al[6] studied 1254 adult relatives of patients and controls and found that lifetime prevalences of major affective disorder (including schizoaffective) for relatives of probands with schizoaffective disorder, bipolar I illness, bipolar II illness, unipolar depression, and normal controls were 37%, 24%, 25%, 20%, and 7%, respectively. These data suggested that the different affective dis-

From the National Institute of Mental Health Collaborative Program on the Psychobiology of Depression—Clinical Studies, Bethesda, Md. For a complete list of participants, see p 373.

See Subjects and Methods on next page

SUBJECTS AND METHODS

The subjects in this study are affectively ill probands and their personally examined first-degree relatives. The probands were interviewed using the Schedule for Affective Disorders, and the RDC was used for diagnosis.[7,8] The probands were divided into those with bipolar I or schizoaffective manic disorder and those with primary unipolar depressive disorder or schizoaffective depression at intake or in a 10-year follow-up. Those patients who switched from unipolar to bipolar depression in the follow-up were included in the study as having bipolar disease. At intake, there were 231 patients with bipolar disease and 359 patients with primary unipolar disease. The patients with primary unipolar disease had their conditions diagnosed at intake by virtue of having had a major depressive disorder that was not preceded by another psychiatric diagnosis specifically noted in the RDC. A depression preceded by another psychiatric illness would be considered a "secondary" depression. Patients with secondary depression were excluded as probands. By the time of the 10-year follow-up, 20 patients had switched from unipolar to bipolar I depression, thus making the total number studied 251. Of course, by definition, having once shown a mania, a depressed patient with unipolar disease is permanently considered to have bipolar disease. As this change to mania is recorded by a personal follow-up at the time it occurs, it is more reliable than any change in diagnosis by a test-retest method. In addition to the loss of 20 patients with unipolar disease who became patients with bipolar I disease, 26 became patients with bipolar II disease and these were dropped from the study. This left 313 patients with primary unipolar disease in the study. Patients with bipolar II illness were excluded as probands as their relationship to bipolar and unipolar illness is open to question as to where they fit in the diagnostic scheme, ie, are they patients with bipolar disease, are they patients with unipolar disease, or do they constitute an independent group?[10] Furthermore, in a test-retest study of diagnostic reliability for 6 months, such reliability for the diagnosis of bipolar II disorder is very low (intraclass R=.06). For 5 years it remains low (κ=0.09). The reliability for a diagnosis of mania for 6 months is much higher (κ=0.88). For 5 years κ was 0.48, which, with a base rate of 2%, provides a specificity and sensitivity of 0.98.[11,12] Familial aggregation of affective disorders (bipolar I or schizoaffective manic and unipolar or schizoaffective depressed) in the two groups was compared.

All of the familial data in this article that were used for the survival curves (**Figure 1** through **Figure 5**) were derived from personally examined relatives. These relatives were evaluated with the SADS-L and their conditions were diagnosed using the RDC in the same way as the probands. In addition to the probands and first-degree relatives, a group of paired control subjects was matched to a subset of the first-degree relatives interviewed as part of the family study. Each relative provided the names of six acquaintances of similar age, sex, and socioeconomic status. These people were contacted at random order until a willing subject was identified. There were no exclusion criteria. The control subjects were evaluated with an SADS-L and diagnosed according to the RDC in the same fashion as the probands and the interviewed first-degree family members. The diagnoses in relatives and controls also took into account a 5- to 6-year follow-up. Thus, an illness occurred before intake, at intake, during the interval, or at the follow-up, when the subjects were again interviewed in a systematic fashion with the SADS-L.

Great care was taken to ensure that the relative raters were blind to the diagnostic status of the proband. The study coordinator at each site assigned raters to interview family members in such a way that no rater would interview a relative of a proband they had taken into the study or would be following in the longitudinal follow-up. Maintenance of this blinding was quite successful. Of 1682 first-degree relatives in the CDS, only 16 (0.9%) of the relatives (from 10 families) were interviewed by the same rater who interviewed the proband.

In addition to using the personally interviewed relatives, we also evaluated information that was gathered about the family history. In this case, as all relatives could not be interviewed directly, we obtained information about them by asking the proband and other family informants about the presence of psychiatric illness in the relatives. In the interview with the probands and other relatives, we used a systematic set of criteria (the Family History RDC) for the diagnosis of the noninterviewed relatives. The in-depth method of the family history and family study components have been presented thoroughly in a previous article.[13]

In a second part of this study, the patients with bipolar disorder were separated into three groups: those who had mood-incongruent psychotic features (including patients with schizoaffective mania, mainly affective); those with mood-congruent psychotic features; and those with no psychotic features. This was an effort made to separate the group with bipolar illness into severe (psychotic) and less severe (nonpsychotic) clinical groups. Family psychopathologic conditions in these groups were evaluated according to whether there was any difference in major depression or schizoaffective depression and separately in bipolar I or schizoaffective manic disorder. The probands used in this analysis were the patients with bipolar I or schizoaffective manic illness identified at index. Those with unipolar disease who switched to bipolar I in the 10-year follow-up were not rated as to whether they had mood-congruent or mood-incongruent psychotic symptoms.

The comparisons were accomplished using survival analysis to obtain Kaplan-Meier estimates of timed onset of affective disorder and mania. This is a nonparametric survival curve estimation method and presents the proportion of the group that developed illness, taking into account the differential follow-up times of the relatives (different ages at the time of diagnostic assessment). "Survival time" is defined as the time until first onset of the respective disorder. Technically, it is either the age at onset of illness for those who became ill or the age at the time of interview for those who did not develop the disorder. Subjects are considered "censored" if they did not develop the respective illness by the time of assessment. These analyses include all relatives and controls through the time that they became depressed or manic or left the study. The Wilcoxon χ^2 statistics were used as a nonparametric test for the differences in rates of illness.[14-16] The sampling unit in these survival curves is the individual, not the family. The individuals are differentiated by the type of ascertainment, either from a family with illness or from a control population.

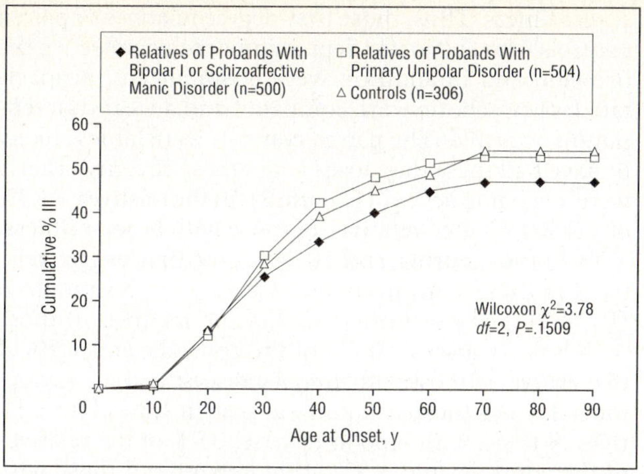

Figure 1. *Rates of first depressive episode by age (major depression or schizoaffective depression in relatives).*

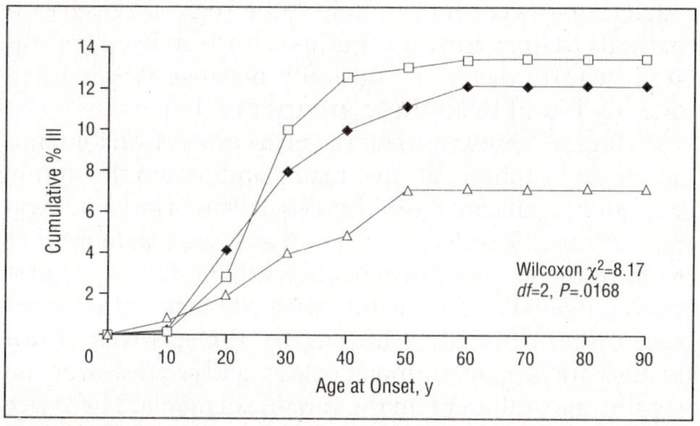

Figure 2. *Rates of severe depressive episode by age (major depression or schizoaffective depressed relatives who were hospitalized, incapacitated, or psychotic during a depressed period). See Figure 1 for key.*

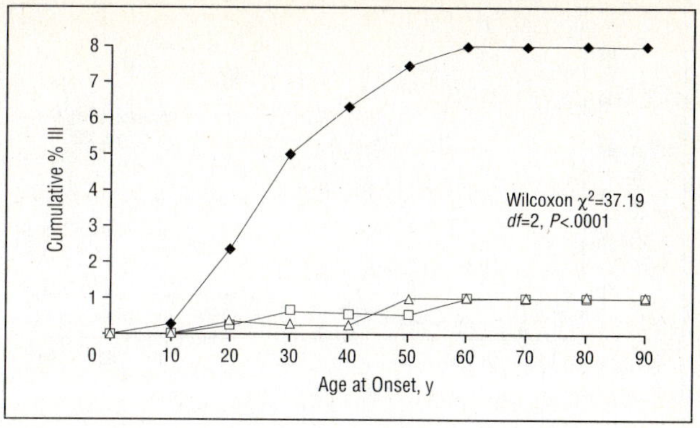

Figure 3. *Rates of mania or schizoaffective mania by age. See Figure 1 for key.*

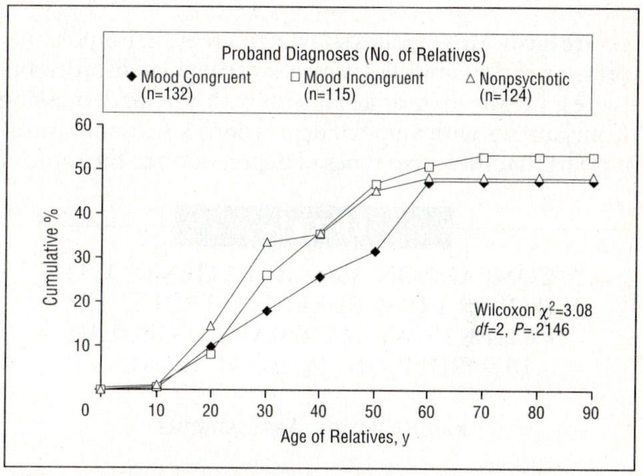

Figure 4. *Familial depression (major depression or schizoaffective depression) in the bipolar continuum.*

orders represented "thresholds on a continuum of underlying multifactorial vulnerability." The greatest vulnerability was for that of schizoaffective disorder and there was a systematic decrease as noted above. The patients were interviewed using the Schedule for Affective Disorders and Schizophrenia—Lifetime Version (SADS-L).[7,8] A diagnosis was made using a modified form of the Research Diagnostic Criteria (RDC) with an increased diagnostic threshold that required severe impairment in the major role. Familial bipolar illness was more frequent in probands with bipolar disease than in probands with unipolar disease and most frequent in family members of schizoaffective probands.

A second relevant study is that of Kendler et al,[9] who evaluated proband-wise concordance rates for affective illness in monozygotic and dizygotic twin pairs. They concluded that the results were not consistent with an independent transmission model of bipolar illness and unipolar illness because "the nonbipolar monozygotic co-twins of bipolar I probands are at an increased risk for unipolar illness." The risk for bipolar illness, however, was considerably increased in the co-twins of probands with bipolar illness. The increased risk for unipolar illness in the monozygotic co-twins with nonbipolar illness of the probands with bipolar illness was the major point suggesting that the two illnesses, bipolar and unipolar, are not independent as regards transmission.

The Collaborative Depression Study (CDS) is a large study of more than 900 patients who were examined at five participating clinical centers: University of Iowa, Iowa City; Rush Medical College, Chicago, Ill; Harvard Medical School, Cambridge, Mass; Washington University School of Medicine, St Louis, Mo; and Columbia University, New York, NY. In addition to diagnosing conditions in the probands, a family study was also accomplished, enabling an evaluation of independence of bipolar illness in a very large sample that was systematically assessed proband-wise and familially.

We will determine the presence of affective disorder, bipolar and primary unipolar, in the family members of probands with bipolar and primary unipolar illness. Also, we will evaluate a possible severity continuum by looking at patients with bipolar disorder who have mood-incongruent psychotic features, mood-congruent psychotic features, and no psychotic symptoms by determining amount of familial depression and mania in these proband groups.

If the familial risk for mania is equal between the controls and the relatives of probands with primary unipolar disease, it would lend support for separate diagnostic entities. If familial mania is significantly more frequent in relatives of those with unipolar disease than in the controls, it would lend support for an affective continuum. If probands with psychotic (more severe) and nonpsychotic (less severe) bipolar disease show familial risks for mania and depression that are equal, it would argue against the idea of a multifactorial hypothesis that includes unipolar nonpsychotic illness as the least severe form and schizoaffective mania as the most

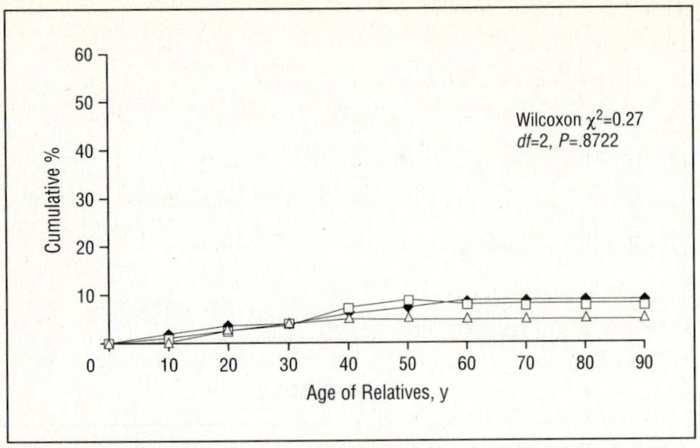

Figure 5. *Familial mania or schizoaffective mania in the bipolar continuum. See Figure 4 for key.*

severe form. Most studies show an increase in unipolar depression in the families of subjects with bipolar disorder, but there is no way to separate patients with bipolar depression from patients with unipolar depression; we cannot assume a priori that these two types of depression are the same.

RESULTS

A COMPARISON AMONG PATIENTS WITH BIPOLAR I DISORDER, CONTROLS, AND PATIENTS WITH PRIMARY UNIPOLAR DISORDER ON FAMILIAL ILLNESS

Family Study Assessments

For the 251 patients with bipolar I disorder, the mean (±SD) age was 36.6±13.2 years and for the 313 probands with primary unipolar disorder, the mean age was 41.3±16.0 years. The probands with bipolar I disease were significantly younger than the probands with primary unipolar disease (*P*=.0002). As regards the sex breakdown, for those with unipolar disease, 63% were female, and for those with bipolar disease, 53% were female (χ^2=6.06; *df*=1; *P*=.01). The older ages and the excess of female subjects in the probands with primary unipolar disorder are quite similar to numerous prior findings in the separation of bipolar and unipolar illnesses.

We compared the sex and age of the first-degree relatives with the controls. For the relatives of probands with unipolar and bipolar disorder and controls, the percent of female subjects, respectively, was 60.3%, 58.4%, and 66.8%. There is then a slight excess of female subjects in the control group (χ^2=5.65; *df*=2; *P*=.06). The mean (±SD) ages, respectively, were 46.9±16.0, 45.8±16.2, and 44.2±15.3 years (F=2.69; *df*=2, 1307; *P*=.07). The controls then are slightly younger than the relatives.

We compare rates of affective illness in relatives of probands with bipolar I or schizoaffective manic disease with relatives of probands with primary unipolar disorder and controls. On the RDC diagnoses of major depression or schizoaffective disorder depressed type taken together there was no difference between groups (Figure 1). In this figure as in all of the following figures, age at onset is defined as the time until the first onset of the respective disorder. As severity of depression may be a factor in the family history, we performed the same kind of comparison but used only criteria that indicated a more severe illness. Thus, those first-degree relatives or paired controls who had major depression or schizoaffective depression and in addition were hospitalized, incapacitated, or psychotic were compared and a clear differentiation occurred. The paired controls were far less likely to have had these diagnoses when these severity criteria were taken into account (Figure 2). In the relatives, 11.3% of the first-degree relatives of those with bipolar illness, 4.9% of the controls, and 10.4% of the first-degree relatives of those with unipolar disease were hospitalized (*P*=.005). For psychosis, 1.2% of the relatives of those with bipolar disease, 0.6% of the controls, and 1.9% of the relatives of those with unipolar disease had such symptoms (*P*=.34). Incapacitation was seen in 4.8% of the relatives of those with bipolar disease, 0.9% of the relatives of the controls, and 4.5% of the relatives of those with unipolar disease (*P*=.008). Thus, all of the criteria that made for severity—hospitalization, psychosis, and incapacitation—were more likely to be seen in relatives of patients than in controls, but psychosis in itself was not significantly different, possibly because it was infrequently found in all those groups of relatives.

Figure 3 presents material on a comparison for familial mania or schizoaffective mania and herein the finding was quite significant. First-degree relatives of probands with bipolar I or schizoaffective manic disease were far more likely to have mania or schizoaffective mania than were first-degree relatives of probands with primary unipolar disease or controls. Most important, the relatives of probands with primary unipolar disease and controls were not significantly different on the variable of mania. There were sufficient numbers of family members in Figures 1 through 3 to obtain stable estimates of the later portions of the survival curves for subjects with bipolar and unipolar disease and controls: 24%, 21%, and 26% were older than 60 years, respectively. The 2×2 comparisons are presented in **Table 1** for Figures 1 through 3.

Family History Assessments

We have also evaluated the proband groups and controls using the family as the unit of analysis. To accomplish this, we have used the information that was obtained by the family history method in which the proband and other available relatives were interviewed about all members of the family. First, there were no significant differences in the number of family members on whom we obtained information among any of the groups. For the subjects with bipolar disease, the family members numbered 6.4; for the subjects with unipolar disease, family members numbered 6.6; and for the controls, the family members numbered 6.3. We then assessed the number of families that contained mania or schizoaffective mania in first-degree relatives in the three proband groups and also the number of families that contained major depression and schizoaffective depression in the same groups (**Table 2**). As may be noted, mania and schizoaffective mania are highly increased in the families of patients with bipolar illness, but between the families of the controls and the patients with unipolar illness, there is no significant difference (χ^2=2.86; *df*=1; *P*=.09). Depression is increased in the family members of both patients with bipolar and unipolar disease, but these are not significantly different from

Table 1. Survival Analysis*

	MDD or SAD		Severe MDD or SAD		Mania or SAM	
	χ^2	*P*	χ^2	*P*	χ^2	*P*
Overall test (*df*=2)	3.8	.15	8.2	.02	36.7	<.0001
Pairwise tests (*df*=1)						
Relatives of probands with bipolar I disorder vs controls	2.0	.16	5.4	.02	15.8	<.0001
Relatives of probands with unipolar disorder vs controls	0.03	.86	8.3	.004	0.1	.76
Relatives of probands with bipolar I disorder vs relatives of probands with unipolar disorder	3.4	.07	0.4	.55	23.9	<.0001

**MDD indicates major depression; SAD, schizoaffective depression; and SAM, schizoaffective mania.*

each other (χ^2=1.15; *df*=1; *P*=.28). Notably, Table 2 is similar to Figure 2 in that the proband groups are more likely to contain major depression or schizoaffective depression than the families of the controls. This similarity suggests that in obtaining a family history, it is more likely that the family members will only know about people who have had more severe illnesses. Alternatively, the material obtained from the personal examination of the relatives picks up milder depressions that cause no social problem but do meet diagnostic criteria.

CONTINUUM FOR FAMILY HISTORY

Gershon et al[6] showed a severity continuum for family history among patients with schizoaffective disease, bipolar disease, unipolar disease, and controls. To explore this possibility, we separated the patients with bipolar disease into three groups according to the RDC: those who had mood-incongruent psychotic features or schizoaffective mania; those who had mood-congruent psychotic features; and those who had nonpsychotic mania. We termed this the bipolar psychosis continuum. In the mood-incongruent or schizoaffective manic group, 38 had mood-incongruent psychotic features; 14 of those 38 met the diagnosis of schizoaffective disorder manic type mainly affective. Forty-six probands had mood-congruent mania and 41 had nonpsychotic mania. The probands were all diagnosed as having mania or schizoaffective mania at intake and all had personally examined family members; the diagnosis of the family members took into account those who had been ill at intake or before and those who developed an affective illness in the 6-year follow-up. For neither major depression or schizoaffective depression nor for bipolar I disorder or schizoaffective mania was there any significant difference (Figures 4 and 5). Thus, in the data presented in this article, there is no support for a continuum of severity that manifests itself with a direct increase in familial affective disorder. This is consistent with a previous analysis of the CDS data that used other ways of assessing severity.[17]

COMMENT

Although there have been other studies comparing bipolar and unipolar illness, there are some advantages to this one. The number of probands and first-degree relatives who were personally evaluated is very large. It is possible to get rid of some of the heterogeneity within the diagnosis of depression by dealing only with probands with primary depressive disorder. This is a matter of consequence in that it excludes patients who start out with alcoholism or anxiety disorder and develop depressions in the course of these or some other illnesses that are frequently associated with depressions that follow the onset of another psychiatric problem (secondary depressions). By following up probands for 10 years and moving those with unipolar disease who over time switched to bipolarity, we have fewer subjects with primary unipolar disease who were inappropriately diagnosed as having unipolar disease. By following up the family members for 6 years, it is possible to increase the number of ill family members as some developed an affective illness in the 6 years. Finally, there is a large paired control group that was reasonably well matched to the relatives for age and sex, who themselves were personally evaluated with the use of systematic instruments, and who like the family members were followed up for a period of 6 years.

The findings are as follows. The variable of familial bipolar I or schizoaffective mania is significantly higher in the first-degree relatives of probands with bipolar I or schizoaffective mania than in either the first-degree relatives of subjects with primary unipolar disease or in paired controls. In fact, the last two are not significantly different from each other as regards familial bipolar or schizoaffective bipolar illness. These findings support the concept of bipolar illness as a separate and independent disease.

The findings as regards major depression and schizoaffective depression are more complex. In Table 1 and Figure 1, a comparison of these variables between relatives of probands with bipolar I illness and relatives of probands with primary unipolar illness reveals that these depressions may be more frequent in the latter (*P*=.07). However, this finding, which would suggest that unipolar depression breeds true in families, disappears when we evaluate the relatives with more severe forms of depression (Figure 2) where *P*=.55. In light of this inconsistency, we cannot say with confidence that unipolar depression or schizoaffective depression is more frequent in relatives of probands with primary unipolar illness than in relatives of probands with bipolar I illness. One possible explanation for the higher rate of milder depressions in the relatives of probands with primary unipolar disease is the heterogeneity in the group with primary unipolar disease. Relatives of patients with primary unipolar disease in families where alcoholism exists are more likely than other families with primary unipolar disease to show a high rate of mild depressions.[5]

Table 2. Presence of Mania or Schizoaffective Mania and Major Depression in Families of Probands and Controls*

	Family		
	Bipolar	Unipolar	Control
No. of families	251	311	305
Mania/schizoaffective mania, No. (%)	55 (21.9)	15 (4.82)	7 (2.30)
Depression, schizoaffective depression, No. (%)	162 (64.5)	187 (60.1)	119 (39.0)

*For mania or schizoaffective mania: χ^2=75.35; df=2; $P<.001$. For depression or schizoaffective depression: χ^2=43.50; df=2; $P<.001$.

There is ambiguity in the data. If one adds severity to the diagnosis of depression by including only those subjects with depression who have been incapacitated or hospitalized or psychotic, a clear difference emerges, with the family members of probands with both primary unipolar and bipolar I disorder being significantly more likely to show affective disorder than the controls. The problem of severity in diagnosis has been addressed before and it was for this reason that we analyzed the data using severity as a control. Leckman et al[18] added criteria for incapacitation and social functioning to the RDC.[18] Complete disruption of the principal social role or a noticeable impairment of function in this role for 4 weeks was a criterion for a diagnosis of depression. The importance of this now becomes clear. The expected difference between relatives of probands with bipolar and unipolar disease and controls on the variable of total affective disorder in the family appears in our data only when severity is taken into account. These data validate the need for more specific criteria for depression. Unless severity is taken into account, we find that the difference between relatives of subjects with bipolar and unipolar illness is specific only on the variable of mania or schizoaffective mania, not on the variable of depressive disorder. In itself, however, this is a major difference. Severity may not be a lifetime trait. We used the most severe episodes that were known for the relative or control. Thus, the same criteria for probands were used for relatives and controls. Reich et al,[19] in a preliminary analysis of segregation distribution of primary depressive disorder in the CDS, suggested that the mode of transmission of primary unipolar disorder in this sample was not compatible with a genetic explanation and they thought that this might be because the RDC for depression were so broad that "both genetic and nongenetic types of depression" are included in a single diagnostic entity. We have taken that finding one step further and noted that by adding severity to the diagnosis, a positive difference does emerge, with the relatives of patients having more depression than the controls.

In a blind assessment study, Tsuang et al[20] reported that total affective illness (bipolar and primary unipolar) in a personally interviewed control group was about 7%, but in family members of patients with bipolar and unipolar illness, it was double that, 14%. In that study, unipolar depression had to be present for an entire month; thus, it is possible that the patients with unipolar disease had more severe disease than those in the CDS. The RDC demands that the patient be ill only 1 to 2 weeks to qualify for a diagnosis. Thus, the finding in the present study supports the difference found in other studies, but only when another criterion, that of severity and psychosis, is added. Alternatively, no severity measure is needed to note the difference on the variable of bipolar disorder and schizoaffective mania. Herein the data are clear. The fact that the bipolar I or schizoaffective mania in the families of patients with bipolar I disease is high suggests that we are dealing with a specific illness. If unipolar disorder as a broad concept were related to bipolar disorder, in the families with unipolar disease, bipolar or schizoaffective mania in the relatives should be somewhere between the amount seen in the families with bipolar I disease and controls.

Rice et al[21] assessed the validity of the bipolar vs unipolar dichotomy from familial data in the CDS. They found an excess of bipolar I illness in relatives of patients with schizoaffective mania and probands with bipolar I illness, but not in the relatives of probands with schizoaffective depression. They concluded that schizoaffective mania lay on a continuum with bipolar illness. They also concluded that the hypothesis of a single multifactorial continuum between bipolar and unipolar affective disorder was not supported by the data. Rice et al,[22] in a subsequent article, evaluated the familial transmission of bipolar illness and concluded that a model that allowed for a single major locus with a multifactorial background was a possible type of transmission. In a controlled family study reported from Germany, Maier et al[23] selected their control sample from the general population. They showed equal amounts of unipolar depression in the relatives of probands with bipolar disorder and unipolar depression but an increase in bipolar disorder in the relatives of the probands with bipolar illness. Their general population figures for unipolar depression were lower by half than the figures for the relatives of the affectively ill probands. Diagnoses were made according to RDC and final diagnoses were based on a best-estimate procedure in which two experienced psychiatrists blind to subject status and relationship between subjects independently diagnosed the conditions of each subject. It is possible that there was an implicit criterion of severity in the judgments of the psychiatrists.

In the study by Gershon et al,[6] probands with schizoaffective illness showed more affected relatives than did probands with other kinds of affective disorders and there was a systematic decrease in proportion of affected relatives as one went from schizoaffective to bipolar I to bipolar II to unipolar to controls. We have tested this finding in a somewhat different fashion. We have separated the probands with bipolar I or schizoaffective mania into a severe group (those with psychotic bipolar illness, mood-incongruent psychotic features, and mood-congruent psychotic features) and a less severe group (those with nonpsychotic bipolar illness). There is no difference in amount of total affective disorder or mania between these groups in the family members. This suggests that within the bipolar diagnosis, there is no severity continuum.

Maier et al[24] compared schizoaffective disorder with affective disorders with mood-incongruent psychotic features. They noted that the unipolar vs bipolar distinction was reflected by distinct patterns of bipolarity in the relatives, with bipolar disorder being more frequently seen in the relatives of probands with schizoaffective bipolar disorder than in the relatives of subjects with schizoaffective unipolar depression. This was also true for the affective disorders with mood-

Study Participants

FROM THE NATIONAL INSTITUTE OF MENTAL HEALTH COLLABORATIVE PROGRAM ON THE PSYCHOBIOLOGY OF DEPRESSION—CLINICAL STUDIES

This study was conducted with the participation of the following investigators: **Brown University, Providence, RI:** Martin B. Keller, MD (*Chairperson*); Philip W. Lavori, PhD; Timothy I. Mueller, MD; M. Tracie Shea, PhD. **University of Iowa, Iowa City:** William Coryell, MD (*Cochairperson*); George Winokur, MD; James Haley. **University of California–San Diego:** Hagop S. Akiskal, MD. **National Institute of Mental Health, Washington, DC:** J. D. Maser, PhD. **Rush-Presbyterian-St Luke's Medical Center, Chicago, Ill:** Jan Fawcett, MD, William A. Scheftner, MD. **New York (NY) State Psychiatric Institute:** Jean Endicott, PhD; Andrew Leon, PhD; Jo Ellen Loth, MSW. **Washington University, St Louis, Mo:** John Rice, PhD, Theodore Reich, MD. Other contributors include the following: Nancy C. Andreasen, MD, PhD; P. J. Clayton, MD; J. Croughan, MD; G. L. Klerman, MD (deceased); R. M. A. Hirschfeld, MD; M. M. Katz, PhD; E. Robins, MD; R. W. Shapiro, MD (deceased); R. L. Spitzer, MD; and M. A. Young, PhD

incongruent psychotic features, the subjects with bipolar disease having more mania in their families. These authors noted only modest differences between patients with bipolar schizoaffective illness and patients with bipolar illness with mood-incongruent psychotic features. The CDS data suggest that the patients with bipolar disease with mood-incongruent illness and the patients with schizoaffective bipolar disease are essentially part of the same group.

We conclude on the basis of these data that the evidence supports the idea that bipolar I disorder is an independent illness. The fact that many characteristics are different from characteristics of patients with primary unipolar disease, ie, the epidemiology, the course, the premorbid characteristics, and the possible changes in brain function, support this viewpoint. Nevertheless, it is clear that there are certain subjects with depression who are related to subjects with bipolar illness. Patients with unipolar illness in a follow-up may become patients with bipolar disease, another way that patients with bipolar illness differ from patients with unipolar depression. We do not have any way of identifying these subjects with depression. They do not appear markedly different from the subjects with depression who are seen in the families of patients with unipolar illness or for that matter in controls. The subjects with unipolar depression in families with bipolar disease also pose a problem because of the relatively high frequency of affective illness in the general population.[25] It seems quite likely that in any family study of patients with bipolar illness, there will be a large amount of "contamination" from the patients with depression who would get into the study through normal expectation. In a genetic linkage study, there would be no way to discriminate between the patient with unipolar depression who is related to the patient with bipolar disorder through illness and those who are present in the family through chance. Until a method is devised to separate these two kinds of relatives with depression, there will be difficulty in using such subjects with depression as affected family members in linkage studies.

Accepted for publication January 20, 1995.

This article has been reviewed by the Publication Committee of the CDS and has its endorsement.

Correspondence to Department of Psychiatry, College of Medicine, University of Iowa, 1-457 Medical Education Bldg, Iowa City, IA 52242 (Dr Winokur).

REFERENCES

1. Tsuang M, Winokur G, Crowe R. Psychiatric disorders among relatives of surgical controls. *J Clin Psychiatry.* 1984;45:420-422.
2. Winokur G, Coryell W, Endicott J, Aksikal H. Further distinctions between manic-depressive illness (bipolar disorder) and primary depressive disorder (unipolar depression). *Am J Psychiatry.* 1993;150:1176-1181.
3. Winokur G, Coryell W, Keller M, Endicott J, Aksikal H. A prospective follow-up of patients with bipolar and primary unipolar affective disorder. *Arch Gen Psychiatry.* 1993;50:457-456.
4. Schwartz J, Baxter L, Mazziotta J, Gerner R, Phelps M. The differentiated diagnosis of depression, relevance of positron emission tomography studies of cerebral glucose metabolism to the bipolar-unipolar dichotomy. *JAMA.* 1987; 258:1368-1374.
5. Winokur G. *Mania and Depression: A Classification of Syndrome and Disease.* Baltimore, Md: The Johns Hopkins University Press; 1991.
6. Gershon E, Hamovit J, Guroff J, Dibble E, Leckman J, Sceery W, Targum S, Nurnberger J, Goldin L, Bunney W. A family study of schizoaffective, bipolar I, bipolar II, unipolar and normal control probands. *Arch Gen Psychiatry.* 1982; 39:1156-1167.
7. Spitzer R, Endicott J. *Schedule for Affective Disorders and Schizophrenia: Lifetime Version.* New York, NY: Biomatrics Research Division, New York State Psychiatric Institute; 1976.
8. Spitzer R, Endicott J, Robins E. Research Diagnostic Criteria: rationale and reliability. *Arch Gen Psychiatry.* 1978;35:773-782.
9. Kendler K, Pedersen N, Johnson L, Neale M, Mathe A. A pilot Swedish twin study of affective illness, including hospital and population-ascertained subsamples. *Arch Gen Psychiatry.* 1993;50:669-706.
10. Coryell W, Endicott J, Reich T, Andreason N, Keller M. A family study of bipolar II disorder. *Br J Psychiatry.* 1984;145:49-54.
11. Andreasen N, Grove W, Shapiro R, Keller M, Hirschfeld R, McDonald-Scott P. Reliability of lifetime diagnosis, a multicenter collaborative perspective. *Arch General Psychiatry.* 1981;38:400-405.
12. Rice J, McDonald-Scott P, Endicott J, Coryell W, Grove W, Keller M, Altis D. The stability of diagnoses with an application to bipolar II disorder. *Psychiatry Res.* 1986;19:285-296.
13. Andreasen N, Rice J, Endicott J, Coryell W, Grove W, Reich T. Familial rates of affective disorder. *Arch Gen Psychiatry.* 1987;44:462-469; correction 1988;45:776.
14. Kalbfleisch J, Prentice R. *The Statistical Analysis of Failure Time Data.* New York, NY: John Wiley & Sons Inc; 1980.
15. *SAS User's Guide: Statistics, Version 5.* Cary, NC: SAS Institute; 1985.
16. Kaplan E, Meier P. Nonparametric estimation from incomplete observations. *J Am Stat Assoc.* 1958;53:457-481.
17. Endicott J, Nee J, Coryell W, Keller M, Andreason N, Croughan J. Schizoaffective, psychotic and nonpsychotic depression. *Compr Psychiatry.* 1986;27:1-13.
18. Leckman J, Gershon E, McGinniss M, Targum S, Dibble E. New data do not suggest linkage between the Xg blood group and bipolar illness. *Arch Gen Psychiatry.* 1979;36:1435-1441.
19. Reich T, Rice J, Andreasen N, Clayton P. A preliminary analysis of the segregation distribution of primary major depressive disorder. *Psychopharmacol Bull.* 1980;16:34-36.
20. Tsuang M, Winokur G, Crowe R. Morbidity risks of schizophrenia and affective disorder among first degree relatives of patients with schizophrenia, mania, depression and surgical conditions. *Br J Psychiatry.* 1980;137:497-504.
21. Rice J, Reich T, Andreasen N, Coryell W, Endicott J. Validity of the bipolar/unipolar dichotomy: familial evidence. In: Shagass C, Josiassen R, Bridger W, Weiss K, Stoff D, Simpson G, eds. *Biological Psychiatry.* New York, NY: Elsevier Science Publishing Co Inc; 1986:850-852.
22. Rice J, Reich T, Andreasen N, Endicott J, Van Eerdewegh M, Fishman R, Hirschfeld R, Klerman G. The familial transmission of bipolar illness. *Arch Gen Psychiatry.* 1987;44:441-447.
23. Maier W, Lichtermann D, Minges J, Hallmayer J, Heun R, Benkert O, Levinson D. Continuity and discontinuity of affective disorders and schizophrenia. *Arch Gen Psychiatry.* 1993;50:871-883.
24. Maier W, Lichtermann D, Minges J, Hallmayer J, Heun R, Benkert O. Schizoaffective disorder and affective disorders with mood incongruent psychotic features. *Am J Psychiatry.* 1992;149:1666-1673.
25. Winokur G, Tsuang M, Crowe R. The Iowa 500: affective disorder in relatives of manic and depressed patients. *Am J Psychiatry.* 1982;139:209-212.

The Structure of the Genetic and Environmental Risk Factors for Six Major Psychiatric Disorders in Women

Phobia, Generalized Anxiety Disorder, Panic Disorder, Bulimia, Major Depression, and Alcoholism

Kenneth S. Kendler, MD; Ellen E. Walters, MS; Michael C. Neale, PhD; Ronald C. Kessler, PhD; Andrew C. Heath, DPhil; Lindon J. Eaves, PhD, DSc

Background: Although prior family and twin studies have examined the relationship between the genetic and environmental risk factors for pairs of psychiatric disorders, the interrelationship between these classes of risk factors for a broad range of psychiatric disorders remains largely unknown.

Methods: An epidemiologic sample of 1030 female-female twin pairs with known zygosity, ascertained from the Virginia Twin Registry, were evaluated by a personal interview conducted by mental health professionals, assessing lifetime history of phobia, generalized anxiety disorder, panic disorder, bulimia nervosa, major depression, and alcoholism.

Results: A multivariate twin analysis suggested the following: First, genetic, familial-environmental, and individual-specific environmental risk factors each cause a unique pattern of comorbidity among the six disorders. Second, genetic influences on these disorders are best explained by two factors, the first of which loads heavily on phobia, panic disorder, and bulimia nervosa and the second, on major depression and generalized anxiety disorder. Third, unlike other disorders, genetic influences on alcoholism are largely disorder specific. Fourth, familial-environmental influences on these disorders are best explained by a single factor that substantially influenced liability to bulimia nervosa only. Fifth, individual-specific environmental influences on the risk for these psychiatric disorders are best explained by a single factor, with highest loadings on generalized anxiety disorder and major depression and with large-disorder–specific loadings, especially on phobias, panic disorder, and alcoholism.

Conclusions: These results support the following hypotheses: First, each major risk factor domain (genes, family environment, and individual-specific environment) influences comorbidity between these disorders in a distinct manner. Second, genetic influences on these six disorders are neither highly specific nor highly nonspecific. Neither a model that contains a discrete set of genetic factors for each disorder nor a model in which all six disorders results from a single set of genes is well supported. Third, the anxiety disorders are not, from a genetic perspective, etiologically homogeneous. Fourth, most of the genetic factors that influence vulnerability to alcoholism in women do not alter the risk for development of other common psychiatric disorders. These results should be interpreted in the context of both the strengths and limitations of multivariate twin analysis.

(Arch Gen Psychiatry. 1995;52:374-383)

From the Department of Psychiatry (Drs Kendler, Neale, and Eaves and Ms Walters) and the Department of Human Genetics (Drs Kendler and Eaves), the Medical College of Virginia/Virginia Commonwealth University, Richmond; the Institute for Social Research, the University of Michigan, Ann Arbor (Dr Kessler); and the Department of Psychiatry, Washington University School of Medicine, St Louis, Mo (Dr Heath).

HISTORICALLY, psychiatric diagnostic systems have developed from clinical experience and intuition, which have only recently been guided by rigorously collected empirical evidence.[1] Although most nosologists agree that diagnoses should ultimately be based on etiologic characteristics, this has, with minor exceptions, been an unattainable goal in psychiatry. Genetic epidemiology has, however, begun to address systematically the relationship between the risk factors for the major psychiatric disorders, all of which have been shown to run in families.[2,3] The conceptual and analytic approach to these studies has, however, been largely limited to the consideration of two disorders at a time. For example, family studies have addressed the familial relationship between alcoholism and major depression (MD),[4,5] panic disorder and phobia,[6] and bulimia and MD.[7,8]

However, multivariate methods that permit a more definitive resolution of the structure of the genetic and environmental risk factors for a range of psychiatric disorders are now available.[9] In particular, such methods can be powerfully applied in twin

See Methods on next page

METHODS

As part of a longitudinal study of the genetic and environmental risk factors for common psychiatric disorders in women, we personally interviewed 2163 white female twins from the population-based Virginia Twin Registry who were born in the years 1934 to 1971.[16] This sample contained both members of 1033 pairs and had, at interview, a mean±SD age of 30.1±7.6 years. No male twins were studied. The refusal rate during the personal interview phase of this project, which was conducted by interviewers with master's degrees in social work or psychology or bachelor's degrees and 2 or more years' clinical experience, was 8%. Each twin was assessed by an interviewer who was blind to the psychopathologic status of her cotwin. Zygosity was determined by an algorithm based on questionnaire responses, photographs, and, when these sources were ambiguous, DNA polymorphisms,[22] and the algorithm yielded 590 monozygotic (MZ) pairs, 440 dizygotic (DZ) pairs, and three pairs of unknown zygosity. This zygosity distribution (57% MZ and 43% DZ) differs only slightly from that predicted for same-sex twins from records of white twin births in the Commonwealth of Virginia over the years 1940 to 1971 using Weinberg's rule[23] (53.5% MZ and 46.5% DZ). Our epidemiologically derived twin cohort did not suffer from the large excess of MZ twins usually seen in volunteer twin samples.[24] Our analyses herein will focus on the 1030 pairs with known zygosity.

The interview included, in modified form, sections of the Structured Clinical Interview for *DSM-III-R*[25] for MD, GAD, panic disorder, bulimia nervosa, and alcohol dependence. Phobias were assessed by an adaptation of the "Phobic Disorders" section of the Diagnostic Interview Schedule Version III-A,[26] which was based on the *DSM-III* criteria.[27] Phobia was defined as the presence of one of 17 specific fears that the respondent considered to be irrational and that in the interviewer's judgment, produced objective behavioral interference with the respondent's life.[18] Interviewers were trained to record symptoms as not present if they were due to the effects of medical illness or medication.

The diagnoses of MD, bulimia, panic disorder, and GAD were based on a blind review of the interview protocols by one of us (K.S.K.), using *DSM-III-R* criteria.[21] Thus, MD was not diagnosed when depressive symptoms resulted from uncomplicated bereavement. However, for GAD, we followed *DSM-III* convention, requiring only a 1-month minimum duration of illness, rather than *DSM-III-R* convention. Furthermore, the GAD section of the version of the Structured Clinical Interview for *DSM-III-R* from which we worked did not contain questions addressing whether the anxiety or worry affected two or more life circumstances. Thus, we considered twins to meet *DSM-III-R* criterion A for GAD if they responded positively to having had a time when they were "anxious, nervous, or worried more days than not." All diagnoses were made without regard to diagnostic hierarchies. The lifetime prevalence rates for MD, GAD, and any phobia in this sample were 31.4%,[16] 23.6%,[17] and 30.5%,[18] respectively.

Three of the six disorders examined in this sample had relatively low lifetime prevalence rates: bulimia (2.8%),[15] panic disorder (5.9%),[20] and alcohol dependence (9.0%).[19] Both power analyses[9,28] and previous experience in this sample[15,20] indicate that model fitting that is applied to disorders of this rarity usually yields results that are neither definitive nor stable. Therefore, to increase statistical power, the major analyses reported herein were based on broad definitions for these three disorders. For bulimia and panic disorder, cases diagnosed at the possible level were included because a multiple threshold model indicated that the possible cases were on the same continuum of liability as those diagnosed with greater certainty.[15,20] In addition, for bulimia, it was shown that a range of epidemiologic risk factors and patterns of comorbidity were similar for the narrowly and broadly diagnosed cases.[15] To maximize our statistical power for alcoholism, we chose the broad criteria of alcohol dependence, as defined by *DSM-III-R*,[21] or problem drinking, in which the respondent admits to having had or having been considered by others as having a significant drinking problem that is not limited to single isolated incidents. A multiple threshold model indicates that in these data, problem drinking reflects a milder disturbance on the same liability dimension that influences alcohol dependence.[19] For all three disorders, the results from univariate twin analysis were similar for the narrow and the broad definitions of illness. With the broader definitions of illness, the lifetime prevalence of bulimia, panic disorder, and alcoholism in this sample was 5.7%, 11.0%, and 17.3%, respectively.

Our approach to the analysis of twin data has been outlined in detail elsewhere,[9,16] as have the basic principles and goals of genetic multivariate analysis.[18] The models described herein are based on a liability-threshold model, the strengths and limitations of which have been discussed previously.[9,16] Whereas the goal of univariate genetic analysis is to decompose the variance of the liability to a disorder into genetic and environmental components, in multivariate genetic analysis, the focus expands to examine both the variance in liability of individual disorders and the

Continued on next page

studies, which, unlike family studies, can separate the etiologic roles of genetic and familial-environmental factors.

Based on personal interviews with both members of a large number of female-female pairs from a population-based twin registry, we examined the interrelationship between the genetic and the environmental risk factors for MD and several other disorders, examined one at a time.[10-13] In this article, using a multivariate twin analysis, we examined the interrelationship between the genetic and the environmental risk factors for the lifetime prevalence of all of the major psychiatric disorders assessed in this study to date: MD, generalized anxiety disorder (GAD), panic disorder, phobias, bulimia nervosa, and alcoholism. We sought to answer six questions:

1. Is the pattern of comorbidity that is due to genetic factors the same as that due to environmental factors? It is possible that one set of genetic risk factors may be common to several disorders, whereas environmental risk factors are disorder specific.[14] Or, a reverse pattern may be seen. To evaluate this hypothesis, we can formally test whether genetic and environmental risk factors influence these psychiatric disorders by a common pathway.[14]

2. How specific are the genetic risk factors for the common psychiatric disorders in women? Are they very

covariance of liability between disorders. Furthermore, when three or more disorders are simultaneously considered, general and disorder-specific genetic and environmental factors can be estimated. In traditional factor analysis, latent factors are assumed with the goal of explaining the covariation between a large number of variables by a small number of factors. Multivariate genetic analysis is similar to traditional factor analysis in that it seeks to explain covariation between multiple variables with a few factors. However, it differs from traditional factor analysis in that it provides separate estimates of the structure of genetic and environmental sources of covariation. Whereas traditional exploratory factor analysis is a descriptive statistical method, multivariate genetic analysis provides insight into the causes of resemblance.

In univariate analysis, information regarding the variation of liability to illness is obtained by comparing the tetrachoric correlations for that disorder in MZ and DZ twin pairs. In the multivariate case, entire matrices of tetrachoric correlations are used. By comparing the cross-twin, cross-variable correlations in MZ and DZ twins and contrasting them to the cross-twin, within-variable and the within-twin, cross-variable correlations, the covariation of two or more variables can be partitioned into its genetic and environmental components.

For example, if genetic factors are responsible for the comorbidity between two disorders, then the correlation in liability between the two disorders will be similar within individuals (eg, disorder 1 and disorder 2 in twin 1) and across MZ twins (ie, disorder 1 in twin 1 and disorder 2 in twin 2), who share all their genes in common, and both will be about twice as large as that seen in DZ twins, who share on average half their genes in common. If familial-environmental factors (eg, parental rearing style) cause the comorbidity, then the correlation between the two disorders will be similar in individuals and across MZ and DZ twins because MZ and DZ twins reared together share all their familial environment. If individual-specific environmental factors (eg, marital discord) are responsible for the comorbidity, then the liability to the two disorders should be correlated in individuals but not across MZ or DZ twins.

Genetic and environmental factors might influence the covariation between disorders in two different ways. First, genetic and environmental factors might influence the covariation of liability to two disorders by a common pathway through an intermediate phenotype.[14] For example, both genetic and environmental risk factors might influence the psychobiologic state of chronic dysphoria, which can manifest itself in MD and/or GAD. If the common pathway model fits best, this implies that the pattern of comorbidity produced by genetic and environmental factors is the same. Second, in the independent pathway model, genes and the environment contribute to covariation through separate genetic and environmental factors. For example, whereas genes might influence the liability to chronic dysphoria, environmental effects are specifically anxiogenic or depressogenic. If the independent pathway model fits best, this implies that genetic and environmental factors would, if separable, produce different patterns of comorbidity. The common pathway model can be parameterized as a series of constraints imposed on an independent pathway model. Therefore, the fit of the common pathway model can be formally compared with that of the more general independent pathway model.

Two 12×12 tetrachoric correlation matrices and their asymptotic covariance matrices (available on request) were calculated (separately for MZ and DZ twins) by PRELIS II,[29] giving the tetrachoric correlations within and across twins for the six disorders considered. To best describe how genes and environment influence the resemblance among the six disorders, a series of multivariate models were fitted to these matrices using Mx[30] by the method of asymptotic weighted least squares. The fit of the various models were compared by Akaike's information criterion (AIC),[31] with the goal of selecting the model that best combines the principles of both parsimony and goodness-of-fit. For selected comparisons, we also report the χ^2 difference test. Because no stable solution was found in this data for a full three-factor independent pathway model (containing three genetic, three familial-environmental, and three individual-specific environmental factors), we began by fitting two-factor independent and common pathway models.

Previous univariate and bivariate analyses of these disorders have uncovered no consistent evidence for dominance genetic variance. Therefore, in these analyses, we examine only additive genetic factors, which are, for the sake of simplicity, termed genetic. When multiple factors were present in a model, factor loadings were estimated by Mx and then rotated using VARIMAX criterion.[32]

As with univariate analyses, multivariate twin analyses are predicated on the validity of the equal environment assumption that MZ and DZ twins are approximately equally correlated in their exposure to environmental factors of etiologic relevance to the trait under study. This hypothesis has been empirically evaluated in several different ways for the psychiatric disorders assessed in this study,[15-20,33,34] with the results consistently supporting its validity.

nonspecific (ie, one common set of genes influences the liability to all disorders) or highly specific (ie, a different set of genes influences the liability to each disorder)?

3. Previous analyses in this sample suggest that familial-environmental factors are of little etiologic importance in common psychiatric disorders in women.[15-20] Would the greater power of the multivariate method uncover evidence that nongenetic familial factors were etiologically important in these disorders?

4. How specific is the effect of the environmental risk factors that are unique to the individual in these common psychiatric disorders? Are there environmental risk factors that are highly disorder specific in their impact, or is the action of most environmental stressors relatively nonspecific, thus increasing the risk for development of a variety of disorders?

5. The current grouping of GAD, panic disorder, and phobias in the anxiety disorders category[21] suggests that these three disorders might be etiologically related. Are the genetic and environmental risk factors for these three disorders sufficiently related to warrant their inclusion in this overarching nosologic category?

6. Alcoholism, a substance use disorder, is often conceptualized as differing from more typical psychiatric dis-

Table 1. The Comorbidity Between Six Major Psychiatric Disorders as Assessed by the Odds Ratio and the Tetrachoric Correlation*

	Phobia	GAD	Panic Disorder	Bulimia	Major Depression	Alcoholism
Phobia	...	3.00 (2.43-3.71)	5.62 (4.19-7.55)	1.87 (1.28-2.72)	2.24 (1.84-2.72)	2.02 (1.59-2.55)
GAD	.382	...	4.91 (3.69-6.53)	2.28 (1.55-3.35)	8.93 (7.11-11.22)	2.35 (1.84-3.00)
Panic disorder	.520	.484	...	2.32 (1.46-3.70)	3.98 (2.99-5.29)	2.47 (1.82-3.36)
Bulimia	.181	.234	.221	...	2.24 (1.54-3.25)	3.12 (2.10-4.61)
Major depression	.293	.677	.427	.232	...	2.67 (2.12-3.38)
Alcoholism	.237	.281	.275	.316	.329	...

**Tetrachoric correlations are below ellipses and are all positive; odds ratios with 95% confidence intervals are above ellipses. All tetrachorics are significant at P<<.000. GAD indicates generalized anxiety disorder.*

orders. Does alcoholism result from genetic and environmental risk factors that are very similar to or distinct from those that influence typical psychiatric disorders such as MD and panic disorder?

RESULTS

COMORBIDITY BETWEEN DISORDERS

Table 1 depicts the comorbidity between the six disorders assessed in this study, in terms of both odds ratios and tetrachoric correlations. The strongest associations using both measures were found between MD and GAD and between panic disorder and phobia.

MODEL FITTING

The two-factor common pathway model fit poorly (χ^2=180.2, *df*=104) compared with the two-factor independent pathway model (χ^2=138.8, *df*=87) and could be rejected against the more general model using both AIC (−23.8 vs −35.2, respectively) and the χ^2 difference test (χ^2=41.4, *df*=17, *P*<.001).

We then attempted to obtain the best-fitting independent pathway model, first by seeking the optimal number of genetic, familial-environmental, and individual-specific environmental factors, assuming the presence of disorder-specific loadings. Then, when the best factor model was found, we examined evidence for disorder-specific genetic, familial-environmental, and individual-specific environmental loadings. The details of the model fitting are given in **Table 2**.

Model 1 is the full two-factor independent pathway model, which we will now term the 2-2-2 model, with the digits indicating, respectively, the number of genetic, familial-environmental, and individual-specific environmental factors. In models 2 through 4, we attempted to simplify this model by reducing the number of factors from two to one for the individual-specific environment (model 2, a 2-2-1 model), the familial environment (model 3, a 2-1-2 model), and genes (model 4, a 1-2-2 model). Both models 2 and 3 produced a better (or more negative) AIC value than did model 1, indicating a better overall balance of fit and parsimony, with model 3 producing the best result. By contrast, model 4 produced a deterioration (or increase) in the AIC values compared with model 1. It should also be noted that model 4 can be rejected against model 1 by a χ^2 difference test (χ^2=11.8, *df*=5, *P*=.04).

Working from model 3, a 2-1-2 model, we attempted a further simplification by assuming either one individual-specific environmental factor (model 5, a 2-1-1 model) or one genetic factor (model 6, a 1-1-2 model). While model 5 produced an improvement in AIC value over that of model 3, model 6 produced a deterioration that was also highly significant by a χ^2 difference test (χ^2=18.3, *df*=5, *P*=.003).

We then tried to simplify model 5 in three ways: by eliminating the one individual-specific environmental factor (model 7, a 2-1-0 model), by eliminating the one familial-environmental factor (model 8, a 2-0-1 model), or by reducing the number of genetic factors to one (model 9, a 1-1-1 model). However, compared with model 5, models 7 through 9 all produced a worsening of the AIC value, indicating an overall poorer fit. Our results therefore suggest that the most parsimonious description of the covariation of these six common psychiatric disorders in women requires two genetic, one familial-environmental, and one individual-specific environmental factor.

Working from the 2-1-1 model (model 5), we then attempted to eliminate all disorder-specific unique-environmental, familial-environmental, and genetic factors, in models 10, 11, and 12, respectively. Model 10 produced a very large deterioration in the fit of the model. The AIC values for both models 11 and 12 were superior to that of model 5, but model 11 was the better of the two.

We then tried to further simplify model 11 (a 2-1-1 model with no familial-environmental–specific loadings), by eliminating the disorder-specific unique-environmental and genetic loadings in models 13 and 14. Both of these models, however, produced a considerably worse AIC value than did model 11, which was therefore the best-fit model. Of note, model 14 could also be strongly rejected against model 11 by a χ^2 difference test (χ^2=31.3, *df*=6, *P*<.0005).

PARAMETER ESTIMATES

Genetic Factors

The genetic parameter estimates of the best-fitting model 11 are seen in the **Figure**, top. The first genetic factor is dominated by high loadings (eg, >0.50) on phobia, panic disorder, and bulimia. Generalized anxiety disorder and alcoholism have more modest load-

Table 2. Results of a Model Fitting of a Multivariate Twin Analysis of Six Major Psychiatric Disorders*

Model	Additive Genetic Factor: Common Factors, No.	Additive Genetic Factor: Disorder-Specific Loadings	Familial-Environmental Factor: Common Factors, No.	Familial-Environmental Factor: Disorder-Specific Loadings	Unique Environmental Factor: Common Factors, No.	Unique Environmental Factor: Disorder-Specific Loadings	Fit of the Model: χ^2	Fit of the Model: *df*	Fit of the Model: AIC
1†	2	P	2	P	2	P	138.8	87	−35.2
2	2	P	2	P	1	P	143.4	92	−40.6
3†	2	P	1	P	2	P	141.8	92	−42.4
4	1	P	2	P	2	P	150.6	92	−33.4
5†	2	P	1	P	1	P	149.7	97	−44.3
6	1	P	1	P	2	P	160.1	97	−33.9
7	2	P	1	P	0	P	231.4	103	−25.4
8	2	P	0	P	1	P	164.9	103	−41.1
9	1	P	1	P	1	P	171.2	102	−32.8
10	2	P	1	P	1	A	306.6	103	100.6
11†	2	P	1	A	1	P	149.7	103	−56.3‡
12	2	A	1	P	1	P	156.9	103	−49.1
13	2	P	1	A	1	A	306.6	109	100.6
14	2	A	1	A	1	P	181.0	109	−37.0

**AIC indicates Akaike's Information Criterion[31]; P, disorder-specific loadings present; and A, disorder-specific loadings absent.*
†Models against which subsequent models are tested.
‡Best-fitting model by AIC.

ings and MD has almost no loading at all on this first genetic factor.

The second genetic factor is dominated by high loadings on MD and GAD. Panic disorder and alcoholism both have modest loadings, whereas the loadings of phobia and bulimia are small.

Disorder-specific genetic factors are nonzero only for GAD, where they are of only modest impact, and for alcoholism, where they constitute the single strongest loading. The liability to alcoholism is substantially influenced by genetic factors that do not contribute to the genetic vulnerability to the other psychiatric disorders considered.

Environmental Factors

As seen in the Figure, bottom, the single familial-environmental factor has a substantial loading only for bulimia, whereas the other loadings are small, with none exceeding 0.20. The single individual-specific environmental factor has high loadings (≈0.60) on GAD and MD, moderate loadings for phobia and panic disorder (≈0.40), and low loadings for alcoholism and bulimia. Although all of the disorders have substantial disorder-specific unique-environmental loadings, this loading is highest for phobia and lowest for MD.

ESTIMATED PROPORTION OF VARIANCE IN LIABILITY DUE TO GENETIC AND ENVIRONMENTAL RISK FACTORS

The Figure presents the path estimates from the best-fitting model. Another useful way to view these results is to divide the sources of variance in liability in each disorder into its component parts. This is displayed in **Table 3**, in which five results are worthy of note. First, with respect to the etiologic importance of genetic factors, the six disorders were divisible into three groups. For bulimia, GAD, and phobia, the estimated total heritability, 30% to 35%, was modest. For MD and panic disorder, total heritability was moderate and estimated at 41% to 44%. By contrast, the total heritability for alcoholism, estimated at 59%, was substantially higher than that for any other disorder.

Second, for both phobia and bulimia, nearly all of the genetic variation was from the first genetic factor. By contrast, for MD, nearly all of the genetic variation was from the second genetic factor.

Third, for alcoholism, over three fourths of the genetic variance was unique to that disorder and was not shared with any other disorders under consideration.

Fourth, using the increased power of multivariate analysis, the role of the familial environment still proved to be of little substantial importance for phobia, GAD, panic disorder, MD, or alcoholism, accounting at most for 4% of the variance in liability. However, for bulimia, our estimates suggest a substantial role for familial-environmental factors.

Fifth, the single individual-specific environmental factor accounted for a substantial proportion of variance only for GAD and MD. Disorder-specific unique environment was important for all disorders but was most important for phobia.

COMMENT

We applied multivariate twin analysis to the lifetime history of six major psychiatric disorders in a personally interviewed, population-based sample of twins from female-female pairs to clarify the structure of the genetic and environmental risk factors underlying these disorders. We examined, in turn, the answers obtained to the six questions outlined above.

GENES AND ENVIRONMENT: COMMON OR INDEPENDENT PATHWAYS?

We began our analysis by considering whether genetic and environmental risk factors for these six common psychiatric disorders acted via common or independent pathways. As previously outlined in the ARCHIVES[14] (see Figure therein), the common pathway model predicts that genetic and environmental risk factors should produce the same pattern of comorbidity between disorders, whereas the independent pathway model allows for the various risk factor domains to cause different patterns of comorbidity.

In our analyses, the common pathway model was rejected, suggesting that the genetic and environmental risk factors for these disorders are not influencing comorbidity in the same manner. This result is significant because it suggests that multivariate analyses of these disorders conducted on a phenotypic level may yield incomplete results. The implicit assumption of traditional multivariate analysis in the behavioral sciences, the assumption that the pattern of comorbidity (or covariance for quantitative traits) due to genetic and environmental risk factors is the same, is probably incorrect for the common psychiatric disorders in women.

THE SPECIFICITY OF GENETIC RISK FACTORS

A major goal of this analysis was to clarify the degree of specificity of the genetic risk factors for common psychiatric disorders in women. Consideration of two extreme hypotheses is heuristically useful. First, genetic influences on common psychiatric disorders could be entirely nonspecific. As predicted by unitary models for psychiatric disorders in general[35] or neuroses in particular,[36] genes might code for high or low levels of general liability to illness. Whether one disorder vs another develops in an individual with high liability would result solely from environmental experiences. Second, each of the individual disorders could be genetically distinct. For the six disorders under consideration, there might be six discrete sets of genetic factors that are unrelated to each other.

Previous work in this and other samples suggests that neither extreme hypothesis is likely to be true. For example, contrary to the prediction of the second extreme hypothesis (that of genetically distinct disorders), we and others have found evidence for common genetic and/or familial factors influencing MD and alcoholism,[4,5,13] panic disorder and phobia,[6] bulimia and MD,[7,8,11] and MD and GAD.[10] However, it was previously seen in this data that the genetic risk factors for MD and alcoholism[13] and MD and phobias[12] are partially distinct. Therefore, the first extreme hypothesis (that of one set of nonspecific genetic risk factors) is also unlikely to be true.

The results of our multivariate genetic analysis indeed support neither extreme hypothesis. The genetic risk factors for common psychiatric disorders in women are neither extremely nonspecific nor extremely specific. We found substantial statistical evidence for two genetic factors. The second genetic factor, which loaded most strongly on MD and GAD, was anticipated by a previous analysis[10] that suggested that the genes influencing liability to these two disorders were very closely related. This second genetic factor appears to influence the liability to intermittent and often recurrent episodes of dysphoria.

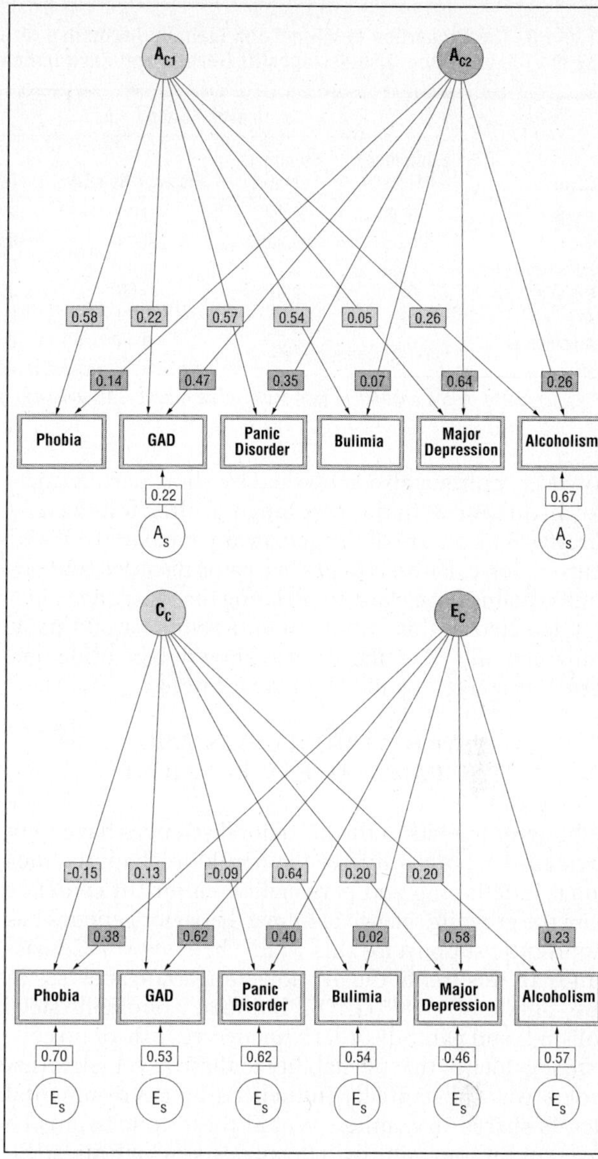

Top, Parameter estimates from the best-fitting multivariate twin model (model 11 [Table 2]) for the genetic common and disorder-specific factors. The model contains two additive genetic common factors (A_{C1} and A_{C2}), which load most strongly on phobia and panic disorder and on generalized anxiety disorder (GAD) and major depression, respectively. Disorder specific additive genes (A_S) are present for only two disorders, GAD and alcoholism. Bottom, Parameter estimates from the best-fitting multivariate twin model (model 11 [Table 2]) for the environmental common and disorder-specific factors. The model contains one familial-environmental common factor (C_C) and one individual-specific or unique-environmental common factor (E_C). No disorder-specific familial environmental loadings were obtained, whereas every disorder had disorder-specific unique-environmental loadings (E_S).

The validity of a genetically mediated, shared neurobiologic diathesis to GAD and MD is supported by results from both biological and pharmacologic treatment studies of depression and anxiety.[37-40]

The first genetic factor, which loads most heavily on phobia, panic disorder, and bulimia, appears conceptually more problematic. Unlike the second factor, the most prominent clinical manifestations of the disorders that load most heavily on this first factor are acute, short-lived, or even paroxysmal. Both phobia and panic disorder are characterized by a vulnerability to panic attacks.

Table 3. The Proportion of Variance in Liability Accounted for in Six Major Psychiatric Disorders by the Common and Disorder-Specific Genetic and Environmental Risk Factors*

	Genetic Factor					Individual-Specific Environmental Factor		
Disorder	Common Factor 1	Common Factor 2	Disorder-Specific	Total	Familial/Environmental Common Factor	Common Factor	Disorder-Specific	Total
Phobia	0.33	0.02	0.00	**0.35**	0.02	0.14	0.49	**0.63**
GAD	0.05	0.22	0.05	**0.32**	0.02	0.38	0.28	**0.66**
Panic disorder	0.32	0.12	0.00	**0.44**	0.01	0.16	0.39	**0.55**
Bulimia	0.29	0.01	0.00	**0.30**	0.41	0.00	0.29	**0.29**
MD	0.00	0.41	0.00	**0.41**	0.04	0.34	0.21	**0.55**
Alcoholism	0.07	0.07	0.45	**0.59**	0.04	0.05	0.32	**0.37**

**As estimated by the best-fitting twin multivariate model. GAD indicates generalized anxiety disorder; MD, major depression.*

However, bulimia also is marked by short paroxysmal-like disturbances, in this case binging, often followed by purging. The nature of the genetically mediated, shared neurobiologic diathesis to phobia, panic disorder, and bulimia remains to be clarified. Relating the two genetic factors detected in this sample to underlying variations in temperament,[41,42] which are also known to be under genetic influence,[43] would be of great interest.

PSYCHIATRIC ILLNESS AND THE FAMILIAL ENVIRONMENT

Although theorists in the behavioral sciences have long stressed the central role of the family in shaping emotional functioning and personality, empirical evidence from the growing science of human behavior genetics has found little support for this widely held view.[44] Consistent with this trend, the previous univariate analyses in this sample of MD,[16] GAD,[17] bulimia,[15] phobia,[18] alcoholism,[19] and panic disorder[20] uncovered little or no consistent evidence that the liability to these psychiatric disorders was substantially influenced by environmental factors shared in families. Would these conclusions be sustained in our multivariate analysis, which uses important data (eg, the cross-twin cross-disorder correlations) that was excluded from the previous analyses?

The multivariate analyses suggested that with one exception, familial environment played little or no etiologic role. This exception was bulimia nervosa. Previous univariate analysis of this disorder[15] had suggested a moderate familial environment component, but in part because of low rates of the disorder, evidence for this was not significant. Although still limited by the relatively small number of affected twins, our results do suggest that for bulimia, along with genetic factors, familial environmental factors play a significant etiologic role.[45]

PSYCHIATRIC ILLNESS AND THE INDIVIDUAL-SPECIFIC ENVIRONMENT

In accord with earlier analyses, the individual-specific environment appears to be a major risk factor for all of the six disorders considered. Furthermore, our results suggested that like the genetic risk factors, the impact of these environmental risk factors is neither highly disorder-specific nor highly nonspecific. We found evidence for one general environmental factor that was nonspecific in its impact. That is, there appears to be a set of environmental risk factors that increase the liability to a broad range of common psychiatric disorders. Of interest, these nonspecific environmental risk factors played a stronger etiologic role in MD and GAD than in phobia, panic disorder, bulimia, or alcoholism.

In addition, for each disorder, there was evidence for disorder-specific environmental risk factors. That is, our results suggest that a substantial proportion of individual-specific environmental risk factors for psychiatric disorders have an impact on the liability to only one disorder. It was intuitively reasonable that phobias had the highest such loading because many twins recounted idiosyncratic experiences (eg, being locked in a trunk by an older brother or diving into the water onto a corpse) that precipitated phobias but were probably unrelated to the risk for other psychiatric disorders. Our results suggest that environmental experiences that are not shared by a twin with her cotwin constitute a large proportion of the risk factors that are unique to individual psychiatric disorders. However, as detailed below, a certain proportion of what is herein interpreted as individual-specific environment may be error of measurement.

THE UNITY OF ANXIETY DISORDERS

In the *DSM-III*,[27] the old concept of anxiety neurosis was split into two new disorders, one reflecting chronic, free-floating anxiety (GAD) and the other characterized by acute, paroxysmal anxiety attacks (panic disorder). These two diagnoses were combined with phobias, obsessive-compulsive disorder, and posttraumatic stress disorder into the new diagnostic category of anxiety disorders.

Three of these diagnoses were among the six disorders examined in this study. Another goal of this analysis was to determine from the perspective of genetic and environmental risk factors whether the anxiety disorders constituted a cohesive nosologic category. Our results suggested otherwise. Although panic disorder and phobia appeared to share important etiologic factors, GAD was more closely related etiologically to MD than to either anxiety disorder. These results are broadly consistent with previous evidence from family,[46] developmental,[47,48] and biologic[49] studies that suggest important etiologic differences between GAD and panic disorder.

Our results validate the division in the *DSM-III*[27] of the broad category of anxiety neurosis into panic disorder and GAD.

ALCOHOLISM

Alcoholism can be conceptualized as either a psychiatric or a substance use disorder. Genetic factors may exist that influence the absorption, metabolism, or interaction of ethanol with the brain, which have little impact on the liability to psychiatric illness.[50,51] In Asian populations, for example, a variation at the aldehyde dehydrogenase locus (which metabolizes acetaldehyde to acetic acid) influences the risk for alcoholism.[52,53]

One of the most striking results of this analysis was the pattern of genetic risk factors for broadly defined alcoholism. Alcoholism was substantially more heritable than any other disorder. More importantly, although 12% of the genetic variation for alcoholism resulted from each of the two major genetic factors, the remaining 76% was due to genetic factors that are unique to alcoholism. That is, most of the genetic variation that influences vulnerability to broadly defined alcoholism in a general population of women is unrelated to the genetic factors that alter liability to the common mood, anxiety, and eating disorders. Our findings are consistent with the recent findings of Schuckit[54] that a reduced response to a standard dose of ethanol distinguishes offspring of alcoholic parents from those of controls and predicts future risk for alcohol abuse but does not predict future risk for MD or anxiety disorders.

Consistent with an earlier study,[13] the best-fitting multivariate model found that of the remaining disorders, alcoholism was, from a genetic perspective, most closely related to MD. The predicted genetic correlation between broadly defined alcoholism and MD from our multivariate model (.37) was reassuringly similar to that obtained from the previous analysis, which was limited to only these two disorders (.42).[13]

Our results also provided further insight into the environmental risk factors for alcoholism. In accord with previous findings, the family environment appeared to play little etiologic role in alcoholism in women.[19] Furthermore, consistent with earlier work that examined only alcoholism and MD,[13] the individual-specific environmental risk factors for alcoholism appeared to have little relationship to the common set of events that broadly influence vulnerability to most of the psychiatric disorders examined.

LIMITATIONS

The results of this analysis should be interpreted in the context of eight potentially significant methodologic limitations. First, the sample was entirely female. Because of gender differences in prevalence rates and risk factors for common psychiatric disorders,[55] the results obtained herein may not extrapolate to males.

Second, we presented only one of several plausible pathways through possibly appropriate models. We tried a number of different pathways and the results consistently led to the same best-fit model (model 11). In addition, although a full three-factor independent pathway model was not identified, models containing three genetic, familial-environmental, or individual-specific environmental factors were identified and fitted. In these cases as well, the pathway of model fitting led back to the same best-fit model explored above.

THIRD, DIFFERENCES of opinion exist in the field of structural equation modeling about the proper criteria with which to pick a best model.[56] We have herein relied on the AIC,[31] which, in our experience with genetic applications, provides a good balance between the demands of parsimony on the one hand and explanatory power on the other. Furthermore, in a recent detailed comparison of seven fit indexes in covariance structure analysis, AIC performed the best.[57] At the three key decision points in our model fitting (rejecting the common pathway model, rejecting a single genetic factor, and rejecting the elimination of all genetic-specific loadings), our decision was also supported by the χ^2 difference test. To explore this question further, we calculated three additional fit indexes: the Tucker-Lewis Index,[58] the Comparative Fit Index,[58] and the Consistent AIC.[59] Two of these indexes (the Tucker-Lewis Index and the Comparative Fit Index) agreed with the AIC both in preferring the independent over the common pathway model and in selecting model 11 from the 14 models described in Table 2. By contrast, the Consistent AIC differed substantially, choosing a common pathway model with a single genetic factor. Although the preponderance of the evidence supports our choice of model 11 as the best model for this data, a different interpretation of these results is possible.

Fourth, for maximal conceptual clarity, as well as to aid potential future models for gene action and for assortative mating, we used an orthogonal factor rotation to obtain loadings on the two genetic factors. However, an argument can be made that an oblique rotation might also be informative. Using the PROMAX routine in SAS,[32] an oblique rotation of the two genetic factors produced an overall pattern very similar to that seen in the Figure, top. As expected, most of the higher factor loadings were a bit higher, and the lower loadings, somewhat lower. The two factors were moderately correlated (.45).

Fifth, the lifetime prevalence rates for several of the disorders examined were higher than those obtained in women from the Epidemiologic Catchment Area study.[55] Our rates might be higher for several reasons, including the use of clinician interviewers and specific probes to encourage careful respondent recall and the youthfulness of our cohort. Our results are not outside the range reported by other investigators[18,60-64] and are, for all disorders except GAD, relatively close to those obtained in the National Comorbidity Survey.[65]

Sixth, because of concerns about the power and stability of estimates, we a priori used broad diagnostic criteria for the three rarest disorders in this sample: panic disorder, bulimia, and alcoholism. Previous analyses had indicated that for each of these three disorders, the broad and narrow definitions reflected the same underlying liability dimension.[15,19,20] Model fitting was repeated with all of the disorders narrowly defined, and broadly similar results were obtained with two exceptions. Evidence was found for two individual-specific environmental factors instead of one. This was unexpected because less statistical power usually results in the identification of fewer rather than more factors. Similar to the single individual-specific environmental factor seen in Table 2, the first factor loaded most strongly on GAD and MD. The second factor was dominated by a single high loading on phobia (0.83) and a more modest loading on panic disorder (0.35). There remains some uncertainty whether there is, in these data, evidence for one or two sets of environmental risk factors that influence vulnerability to more than one psychiatric disorder. A second set of common environmental risk factors that are largely specific to phobia and panic disorder may exist.

As in the analysis presented above, the analysis with narrow definitions of the rare disorders produced robust evidence for a large component of disorder-specific familial risk for alcoholism that was not shared with other disorders. However, with the narrower definition of alcoholism, the model could not clearly identify this component as genetic vs familial-environmental. None of the results in the twins[13,19] or in the twins and their parents[66] provided substantial evidence for familial-environmental risk factors for alcoholism. Therefore, we would argue that the conclusion reached above—that the disorder-specific familial risk factors for alcoholism are genetic—is probably correct.

Seventh, the lifetime prevalence for the six psychiatric disorders assessed in this sample was obtained at a single point in time. Although the interrater reliabilities of our assessments were high,[15-20] considerable evidence in this[67] and other data sets[68,69] indicates that the test-retest reliability would likely be lower. We have test-retest data on lifetime history for only MD and panic disorder in this data set,[67] so it was not possible to fit a full multivariate model to all disorders incorporating error of measurement. With single disorders, unreliability of measurement, if uncorrelated in twin pairs, leads to an overestimation of the individual-specific environment and an underestimation of heritability. This was precisely the effect seen when MD was analyzed based on two times of measurement.[67] Although it will also have that effect in multivariate models, measurement error can in addition produce other more subtle problems. For example, individuals in the interview may demonstrate a consistent self-report or recall bias, so that they are more or less likely to recall and report any disorders they have experienced. If not substantially correlated in twin pairs, such a bias would emerge as a general individual-specific environmental factor. By contrast, if errors of recall or reporting are largely random in nature and might easily affect reporting of one disorder but not another, then they will appear as disorder-specific unique-environmental factors. In our best-fit model, a substantial proportion of what we term individual-specific environmental effects are probably errors of measurement.

Finally, our model has not considered genotype-environment interaction[70] (eg, stressful life events predisposing to MD only individuals with a high genetic liability) or causal models[71] (eg, alcoholism developing as a form of self-medication for social phobia). Although both of the processes may be important in psychiatric disorders and are worthy of further inquiry, they were not included in this report because of the limitations of both our data set and our analytic models.

Accepted for publication August 1, 1994.

This work was supported by grants MH-40828 and AA-09095 from the US Alcohol, Drug Abuse and Mental Health Administration, Rockville, Md. The Virginia Twin Registry, established and maintained by Walter Nance, MD, PhD, and Linda Corey, PhD, is supported by grants HD-26746 and NS-25630 from the National Institutes of Health, Bethesda, Md.

Reprint requests to Box 980710, MCV Station, Richmond, VA 23298-0710 (Dr Kendler).

REFERENCES

1. Kendler KS. Toward a scientific psychiatric nosology: strengths and limitations. *Arch Gen Psychiatry.* 1990;47:969-973.
2. Slater E. *The Genetics of Mental Disorders.* London, England: Oxford University Press; 1971.
3. Vandenburg SG, Singer SM, Pauls DL. *The Heredity of Behavior Disorders in Adults and Children.* New York, NY: Plenum Medical Books; 1986.
4. Cloninger CR, Reich T, Wetzel R. Alcoholism and affective disorders: familial associations and genetic models. In: Goodwin DW, Erickson CK, eds. *Alcoholism and Affective Disorders: Clinical, Genetic, and Biochemical Studies.* New York, NY: Spectrum Publications Inc; 1979:57-86.
5. Merikangas KR, Gelernter CS. Comorbidity for alcoholism and depression. *Psychiatr Clin North Am.* 1990;13:613-632.
6. Noyes R, Crowe RR, Harris EL, Hamra BJ, McChesney CM, Chaudhry DR. Relationship between panic disorder and agoraphobia. *Arch Gen Psychiatry.* 1986;43:227-232.
7. Logue CM, Crowe RR, Bean JA. A family study of anorexia nervosa and bulimia. *Compr Psychiatry.* 1989;30:179-188.
8. Kassett JA, Gershon ES, Maxwell ME, Guroff JJ, Kazuba DM, Smith AL, Brandt HA, Jimerson DC. Psychiatric disorders in the first-degree relatives of probands with bulimia nervosa. *Am J Psychiatry.* 1989;146:1468-1471.
9. Neale MC, Cardon LR. *Methodology for Genetic Studies of Twins and Families.* Dordrecht, the Netherlands: Kluwer Academic Publishers Group; 1992.
10. Kendler KS, Neale MC, Kessler RC, Heath AC, Eaves LJ. Major depression and generalized anxiety disorder: same genes, (partly) different environments? *Arch Gen Psychiatry.* 1992;49:716-722.
11. Walters EE, Neale MC, Eaves LJ, Heath AC, Kessler RC, Kendler KS. Bulimia nervosa and major depression: a study of common genetic and environmental factors. *Psychol Med.* 1992;22:617-622.
12. Kendler KS, Neale MC, Kessler RC, Heath AC, Eaves LJ. Major depression and phobias: the genetic and environmental sources of comorbidity. *Psychol Med.* 1993;23:361-371.
13. Kendler KS, Heath AC, Neale MC, Kessler RC, Eaves LJ. Alcoholism and major depression in women: a twin study of the causes of comorbidity. *Arch Gen Psychiatry.* 1993;50:690-698.
14. Kendler KS, Heath AC, Martin NG, Eaves LJ. Symptoms of anxiety and symptoms of depression: same genes, different environments? *Arch Gen Psychiatry.* 1987;44:451-457.
15. Kendler KS, MacLean CJ, Neale MC, Kessler RC, Heath AC, Eaves LJ. The genetic epidemiology of bulimia nervosa. *Am J Psychiatry.* 1991;148:1627-1637.
16. Kendler KS, Neale MC, Kessler RC, Heath AC, Eaves LJ. A population-based twin study of major depression in women: the impact of varying definitions of illness. *Arch Gen Psychiatry.* 1992;49:257-266.
17. Kendler KS, Neale MC, Kessler RC, Heath AC, Eaves LJ. Generalized anxiety disorder in women: a population based twin study. *Arch Gen Psychiatry.* 1992;49:267-272.
18. Kendler KS, Neale MC, Kessler RC, Heath AC, Eaves LJ. The genetic epidemiology of phobias in women: the interrelationship of agoraphobia, social phobia, situational phobia, and simple phobia. *Arch Gen Psychiatry.* 1992;49:273-281.

19. Kendler KS, Heath AC, Neale MC, Kessler RC, Eaves LJ. A population-based twin study of alcoholism in women. *JAMA.* 1992;268:1877-1882.
20. Kendler KS, Neale MC, Kessler RC, Heath AC, Eaves LJ. Panic disorder in women: a population-based twin study. *Psychol Med.* 1993;23:397-406.
21. American Psychiatric Association. *Diagnostic and Statistical Manual of Mental Disorders, Revised Third Edition.* Washington, DC: American Psychiatric Association; 1987.
22. Spence JE, Corey LA, Nance WE, Marazita ML, Kendler KS, Schieken RM. Molecular analysis of twin zygosity using VNTR DNA probes. *Am J Hum Genet.* 1988;43:A159. Abstract.
23. Cavalli-Sforza LL, Bodmer WF. *The Genetics of Human Populations.* San Francisco, Calif: WH Freeman & Co; 1971.
24. Lykken DT, Tellegen A, DeRubies R. Volunteer bias in twin research: the rule of two thirds. *Soc Biol.* 1978;25:1-9.
25. Spitzer RL, Williams JB, Gibbon M. *Structured Clinical Interview for DSM-III-R.* New York, NY: Biometrics Research Dept, New York State Psychiatric Institute; 1987.
26. Robins LN, Helzer JE. *Diagnostic Interview Schedule (DIS): Version III-A.* St Louis, Mo: Washington University School of Medicine; 1985.
27. American Psychiatric Association. *Diagnostic and Statistical Manual of Mental Disorders, Third Edition.* Washington, DC: American Psychiatric Association; 1980.
28. Martin NG, Eaves LJ, Kearsey MJ, Davies P. The power of the classical twin study. *Heredity.* 1978;40:97-116.
29. Joreskog KG, Sorbom D. *PRELIS: A Preprocessor for LISREL.* Mooresville, Ind: Scientific Software; 1988.
30. Neale MC. *Statistical Modelling With Mx.* Richmond, Va: Dept of Psychiatry of the Medical College of Virginia/Virginia Commonwealth University; 1991.
31. Akaike H. Factor analysis and AIC. *Psychometrika.* 1987;52:317-332.
32. SAS Institute Inc. *SAS/STAT User's Guide, Version 6.* 4th ed. Cary, NC: SAS Institute Inc; 1990.
33. Kendler KS, Neale MC, Kessler RC, Heath AC, Eaves LJ. A test of the equal environment assumption in twin studies of psychiatric illness. *Behav Genet.* 1993;23:21-27.
34. Catania J, Gibson D, Chitwood D, Coates T. Methodological problems in AIDS behavioral research: influences on measurement error and participation bias in studies of sexual behavior. *Psychol Bull.* 1990;108:339-362.
35. Menninger K, Ellenberger H, Pruyser P, Mayman M. The unitary concept of mental illness. *Bull Menninger Clin.* 1958;22:4-12.
36. Tyrer P. Neurosis divisible? *Lancet.* 1985;1:685-688.
37. Breier A, Charney DS, Heninger GR. The diagnostic validity of anxiety disorders and their relationship to depressive illness. *Am J Psychiatry.* 1985;142: 787-797.
38. Lipman RS, Covi L, Rickels K, McNair DM, Downing R, Kahn RJ, Lasseter VK, Faden V. Imipramine and chlordiazepoxide in depressive and anxiety disorders, I: efficacy in outpatients. *Arch Gen Psychiatry.* 1986;43:68-77.
39. Kahn RJ, McNair DM, Lipman RS, Covi L, Rickels K, Downing R, Fisher S, Frankenthaler LM. Imipramine and chlordiazepoxide in depressive and anxiety disorders, II: efficacy in anxious outpatients. *Arch Gen Psychiatry.* 1986;43: 79-85.
40. Abelson JL, Glitz D, Cameron OG, Lee MA, Bronzo M, Curtis GC. Blunted growth hormone response to clonidine in patients with generalized anxiety disorder. *Arch Gen Psychiatry.* 1991;48:157-162.
41. Cloninger CR. A systematic method for clinical description and classification of personality variants: a proposal. *Arch Gen Psychiatry.* 1987;44:573-588.
42. Eysenck HJ, Eysenck SBG. *Manual of the Eysenck Personality Questionnaire.* London, England: Hodder & Stoughton Ltd; 1975.
43. Loehlin JC. *Genes and Environment in Personality Development.* Newbury Park, Calif: Sage Publications; 1992.
44. Plomin R, Daniels D. Why are children in the same family so different from each other? *Behav Brain Sci.* 1987;10:44-54.
45. Strober M, Humphrey LL. Familial contributions to the etiology and course of anorexia nervosa and bulimia. *J Consult Clin Psychol.* 1987;55:654-659.
46. Breslau N, Davis GC, Prabucki K. Searching for evidence on the validity of generalized anxiety disorder: psychopathology in children of anxious mothers. *Psychiatry Res.* 1987;20:285-297.
47. Silove D, Parker G, Hadzi-Pavlovic D, Manicavasagar V, Blaszczynski A. Parental representations of patients with panic disorder and generalised anxiety disorder. *Br J Psychiatry.* 1991;159:835-841.
48. Torgersen S. Childhood and family characteristics in panic and generalized anxiety disorders. *Am J Psychiatry.* 1986;143:630-632.
49. Cowley DS, Arana GW. The diagnostic utility of lactate sensitivity in panic disorder. *Arch Gen Psychiatry.* 1990;47:277-284.
50. Merikangas KR. The genetic epidemiology of alcoholism. *Psychol Med.* 1990; 20:11-22.
51. McGue M. Genes, environment and the etiology of alcoholism. In: Zucker R, Howard J, Boyd G, eds. *The Development of Alcohol Problems: Exploring the Biopsychosocial Matrix of Risk.* Washington, DC: National Institute on Alcohol Abuse and Alcoholism; 1994:1-40.
52. Harada S, Agarwal DP, Goedde HW, Tagaki S, Ishikawa B. Possible protective role against alcoholism for aldehyde dehydrogenase isozyme deficiency in Japan. *Lancet.* 1982;2:827.
53. Thomasson HR, Edenberg HJ, Crabb DW, Mai X-L, Jerome RE, Li T-K, Wang S-P, Lin Y-T, Lu R-B, Yin S-J. Alcohol and aldehyde dehydrogenase genotypes and alcoholism in Chinese men. *Am J Hum Genet.* 1991;48:677-681.
54. Schuckit MA. Low level of response to alcohol as a predictor of future alcoholism. *Am J Psychiatry.* 1994;151:184-189.
55. Robins LN, Regier DA, eds. *Psychiatric Disorders in America.* New York, NY: The Free Press; 1991.
56. Bollen KS. *Structural Equations with Latent Variables.* New York, NY: John Wiley & Sons Inc; 1989.
57. Williams LJ, Holahan PJ. Parsimony-based fit indices for multiple-indicator models: do they work? *Structural Equation Modeling.* 1994;1:161-189.
58. Tucker LR, Lewis C. A reliability coefficient for maximum likelihood factor analysis. *Psychometrika.* 1973;38:1-10.
59. Bandalos DL. Factors influencing cross-validation of confirmatory factor analysis models. *Multivariate Behav Res.* 1993;28:351-374.
60. Weissman MM, Myers JK. Affective disorders in a US urban community: the use of Research Diagnostic Criteria in an epidemiological survey. *Arch Gen Psychiatry.* 1978;35:1304-1311.
61. Rorsman B, Grasbeck A, Hagnell O, Lanke J, Ohman R, Ojesjo L, Otterbeck L. A prospective study of first-incidence depression: the Lundby Study, 1957-1972. *Br J Psychiatry.* 1990;156:336-342.
62. Andreasen NC, Endicott J, Spitzer RL, Winokur G. The family history method using diagnostic criteria: reliability and validity. *Arch Gen Psychiatry.* 1977; 34:1229-1235.
63. Pollock VE, Schneider LS, Gabrielli WF Jr, Goodwin DW. Sex of parent and offspring in the transmission of alcoholism: a meta-analysis. *J Nerv Ment Dis.* 1987;175:668-673.
64. Fairburn CG, Beglin SJ. Studies of the epidemiology of bulimia nervosa. *Am J Psychiatry.* 1990;147:401-408.
65. Kessler RC, McGonagle KA, Zhao S, Nelson CB, Hughes M, Eshleman S, Wittchen H-U, Kendler KS. Lifetime and 12-month prevalence of *DSM-III-R* psychiatric disorders in the United States: results from the National Comorbidity Survey. *Arch Gen Psychiatry.* 1994;51:8-10.
66. Kendler KS, Neale MC, Heath AC, Kessler RC, Eaves LJ. A twin-family study of alcoholism in women. *Am J Psychiatry.* 1994;151:707-715.
67. Kendler KS, Neale MC, Kessler RC, Heath AC, Eaves LJ. The lifetime history of major depression in women: reliability of diagnosis and heritability. *Arch Gen Psychiatry.* 1993;50:863-870.
68. Bromet EJ, Dunn LO, Connell MM, Dew MA, Schulberg HC. Long-term reliability of diagnosing lifetime major depression in a community sample. *Arch Gen Psychiatry.* 1986;43:435-440.
69. Mannuzza S, Fyer AJ, Martin LY, Gallops MS, Endicott J, Gorman J, Liebowitz MR, Klein DF. Reliability of anxiety assessment, I: diagnostic agreement. *Arch Gen Psychiatry.* 1989;46:1093-1101.
70. Kendler KS, Eaves LJ. Models for the joint effect of genotype and environment on liability to psychiatric illness. *Am J Psychiatry.* 1986;143:279-289.
71. Heath AC, Kessler RC, Neale MC, Hewitt JK, Eaves LJ, Kendler KS. Testing hypotheses about direction of causation using cross-sectional family data. *Behav Genet.* 1993;23:29-50.

ORIGINAL ARTICLE

Cingulotomy for Intractable Obsessive-compulsive Disorder

Prospective Long-term Follow-up of 18 Patients

Lee Baer, PhD; Scott L. Rauch, MD; H. Thomas Ballantine, Jr, MD; Robert Martuza, MD; Rees Cosgrove, MD; Edwin Cassem, MD; Ida Giriunas, RN; Peter A. Manzo; Charles Dimino, MD; Michael A. Jenike, MD

Background: The purpose of this study was to assess prospectively long-term change in obsessive-compulsive disorder (OCD) symptoms in patients with an OCD diagnosis that was confirmed by structured interview and with documented unsuccessful trials of multiple medications and attempts at behavior therapy.

Methods: We conducted an unblinded preoperative and follow-up assessment of comorbid diagnosis; OCD, depressive, and anxiety symptoms; and functional status in 18 patients who underwent cingulotomy.

Results: At a mean follow-up of 26.8 months, five patients (28%) met conservative criteria for treatment responders, and three others (17%) were partial responders. The group improved significantly in mean functional status, and few serious adverse events were found. Improvement in OCD symptoms was strongly correlated with improvement in depressive and anxiety symptoms.

Conclusions: The rate of clinical improvement was consistent with a previous retrospective study in the same setting, indicating that 25% to 30% of the patients who previously were unresponsive to medication and behavioral treatments are significantly improved after cingulotomy. Cingulotomy remains a last resort treatment for severely incapacitated patients who have not responded to all other state-of-the-art pharmacological and behavioral treatments for OCD and is not to be taken lightly.

(Arch Gen Psychiatry. 1995;52:384-392)

JENIKE ET al[1] recently reported the results of a retrospective follow-up of 33 patients who had undergone cingulotomy for refractory obsessive-compulsive disorder (OCD) at the Massachusetts General Hospital (MGH), Charlestown, between 1965 and 1986. With the use of conservative criteria, it was estimated that 25% to 30% of these patients benefited substantially from this procedure. However, Jenike et al also found that only six patients (18%) had received trials of clomipramine hydrochloride prior to cingulotomy, and only three patients (9%) had received a trial of behavior therapy before surgery (none of the current selective serotonin reuptake inhibitors were available during this time, and clomipramine only became widely available in the United States in the 1980s). Therefore, it was not possible to determine whether these patients' conditions would have been refractory to modern nonsurgical treatments. In addition, the retrospective nature of that study limited its conclusions.

After this retrospective study, we began a prospective evaluation of all patients with OCD referred to MGH for cingulotomy for two purposes: (1) to attempt to ensure that all patients, prior to undergoing cingulotomy, had undergone adequate trials of both medication and behavioral treatments with unsuccessful outcomes and (2) to assess these patients prospectively to determine their long-term outcome. In the earlier article,[1] in addition to data on 33 retrospectively studied patients, Jenike et al also reported preliminary data on the first four patients who were followed up prospectively; at 6- to 16-month follow-up, only one patient (25%) was classified as a responder, using strict criteria for improvement of OCD symptoms.

Recently, Hay et al[2] presented data on 26 patients with intractable OCD who were treated over two decades with psychosurgical procedures at the Prince Henry Hospital in Sydney, Australia. These procedures included six (23%) with cingulate lesions

From the Departments of Psychiatry (Drs Baer, Rauch, Cassem, and Jenike and Mr Manzo) and Neurosurgery (Drs Ballantine and Cosgrove and Ms Giriunas), Massachusetts General Hospital, Charlestown, Harvard Medical School (Drs Baer, Rauch, Ballantine, Cosgrove, Cassem, Dimino, and Jenike), and McLean Hospital (Dr Dimino), Boston, Mass; and Georgetown University Medical Center, Washington, DC (Dr Martuza).

See Subjects and Methods on next page

SUBJECTS AND METHODS

SUBJECTS

Patients were eligible for cingulotomy if they met *DSM-III-R*[4] criteria for OCD, they had severe OCD symptoms and functional impairment, and a rigorous regimen of medication and behavioral trials was unsuccessful. Eighteen consecutive patients were referred by their local psychiatrists to the MGH Neurosurgical Service for cingulotomy for severe OCD. Their mean age was 31.5 years; 11 were men and seven were women. Patients were reviewed by the MGH Cingulotomy Assessment Committee (three psychiatrists, two neurosurgeons, a neurologist, a nurse, and a secretary) via an extensive record review leading to preliminary approval. Next, to determine the appropriateness of their candidacy for neurosurgical treatment, patients were directly interviewed by a psychiatrist, a neurologist, and both neurosurgeons, and additional on-site tests and evaluations were performed as indicated. They were then assessed at the MGH OCD Clinic and Research Unit, where the Structured Clinical Interview for *DSM-III-R*[4] for diagnosis of Axis I disorders and the Structured Interview for Diagnosis of Personality Disorders–Revised[5] for Axis II disorders were administered by a single rater (to eliminate interrater variability). This rater was a research associate (P.A.M.) who was trained in the administration of these interviews as part of a large multicenter trial and who had experience administering more than 200 Structured Clinical Interviews for *DSM-III-R* to patients with OCD. They were also assessed by a behavior therapist (L.B.) who was familiar with OCD using a semistructured interview that included administration of the Yale-Brown Obsessive Compulsive Scale (YBOCS)[6]; the YBOCS Symptom Checklist[6]; the Beck Depression Inventory (BDI)[7]; and Clinical Global Improvement (CGI) scales[1] for obsessions and compulsions, depression, and anxiety.

Medication compliance history was obtained in conjunction with the referring psychiatrist and via a review of past records in addition to the history provided by the patient. In this regard, the Cingulotomy Assessment Committee was, in part, dependent on the assessment of the referring psychiatrist. Practically, the maximum dose tolerated was a subjective measure, in large part influenced by the patient's ability and/or willingness to tolerate adverse effects. The team sought, through its communication with the patient and referring physician, to ensure that the trials were not abandoned prematurely solely because of mild or nuisance side effects. In a more general sense, patients who were characterized as poorly compliant (eg, missing appointments, not taking their medications as prescribed, or not being genuine in terms of their effort to participate with behavior therapy) were not deemed appropriate candidates for surgery. If patients were accepted for cingulotomy, they provided informed consent for surgery and clinical follow-up. **Table 1** contains the criteria for required previous treatments.

Preoperatively, six of the 18 patients had not undergone an adequate trial of behavior therapy. Four (patients 1, 9, 14, and 18) were too anxious or depressed to comply adequately with exposure and response prevention; one (patient 3) was not referred for formal behavior therapy because she had almost constant obsessions that occurred during all waking hours, had no compulsions, and had made several attempts at self-administered behavior therapy techniques with no success; and one (patient 13) was referred for intensive behavior therapy but was unable to receive this because of financial problems. Patients who had not had a trial of behavior therapy previously and who agreed to a trial prior to surgery while in the Boston area were treated by experts in behavior therapy at the inpatient Behavior Therapy Unit of McLean Hospital, Belmont, Mass. Although we reviewed patient records of behavior therapy in the patients' local area and attempted to contact their behavior therapists, the reliability of local behavior therapy could not be fully ascertained in this open trial. **Table 2** lists the postoperative behavioral and pharmacologic treatments that each patient received and that had not been administered preoperatively.

Table 2 illustrates that none of the five patients who were categorized as responders were reported by their local psychiatrists to have had marked improvement in OCD symptoms as a result of any of these postoperative medication or behavior therapy changes. Among the three partial responders, one (patient 6) underwent a trial of intravenous administration of clomipramine, and she attributes her improvement in OCD symptoms to this medication trial rather than to the cingulotomy. Because the patients listed in Table 2 almost always continued to receive serotonin reuptake inhibitors after their first cingulotomy, it is impossible to determine whether improvement in responders may have been due to an interaction between these medications and the cingulotomy procedure.

OPERATIVE TECHNIQUE

Through bilateral bur holes that were 1.2 cm in diameter, 9.5 cm posterior to the nasion, and 1.5 cm to either side of the midline, electrically insulated thermistor electrodes were positioned in each cingulate bundle with either ventriculography or magnetic resonance imaging stereotactic guidance. The initial targets were located 0.7 cm lateral to the midline bilaterally, 2 cm posterior to the most anterior portions of the frontal horns, and 1.0 mm above the roof of the ventricles, as seen radiologically.

Lesions were created by heating the uninsulated 1.0-cm tip of the electrode to between 80°C and 85°C for 100 seconds by radio frequency current. The electrode was then withdrawn 1.0 cm, and the lesion was enlarged superiorly using the same lesion measurements. These steps were repeated for the opposite hemisphere. This produced symmetrical lesions in the anterior cingulate cortex bilaterally, approximately 1.0 cm in diameter and 2.0 cm in vertical height. Cingulotomies were performed by board-certified neurosurgeons who had extensive experience with this and similar surgical procedures.

FOLLOW-UP ASSESSMENTS

Magnetic resonance imaging scans were obtained from all patients to confirm lesion placement. An attempt was made to follow up all patients at 6-month intervals after their first

Continued on next page

cingulotomy. The initial 6-month follow-up point was chosen because it corresponded to the clinical practices of the MGH Cingulotomy Assessment Committee; specifically, the committee will not consider a patient for a second cingulotomy until 6 postoperative months have passed. Consequently, patients who are referred by their local physician for a second cingulotomy will typically initiate contact at the 6-month time point, thereby facilitating their follow-up assessment. At this reevaluation point, the MGH Cingulotomy Assessment Committee reviews the patient's progress since the first evaluation, along with the local physician's report, and decides whether a second cingulotomy is indicated. Because almost all of the patients lived a good distance from MGH, only those patients who were scheduled to return to the neurosurgery service for evaluation prior to a second cingulotomy procedure were followed up in person. All other patients were followed up via telephone (L.B. or P.A.M.) at or as near to 6-month intervals as possible.

The rating scales given at these follow-up visits or telephone calls were as follows:

- The YBOCS.[6] The YBOCS has been used as the main dependent variable in multicenter trials of clomipramine, fluvoxamine hydrochloride, fluoxetine hydrochloride, and sertraline hydrochloride and has demonstrated reliability and validity.[6]
- The MGH Visual Analog Assessment Scales.[1] To assess outcome in a variety of areas, we used a series of CGI scales that were developed for a previous study.[1] Patients were asked the following: "Compared with how you felt before your first neurosurgical operation, circle a number to describe how you are feeling now in each of the following areas." Three different areas that were assessed included OCD symptoms, depression, and anxiety. Each area was rated on the following scale: 1 indicates much better; 2, moderately better; 3, slightly better; 4, no change; 5, slightly worse; 6, moderately worse; and 7, much worse.
- The BDI.[7] The BDI is a widely used 20-item self-report scale to assess the severity of depression. This scale has demonstrated good reliability and validity for this purpose.
- The Sickness Impact Profile[8] (SIP). The SIP is a 136-item self-administered checklist that is one of the most widely used scales for functional status assessment. The SIP yields an overall score, 12 category scores, and three dimension scores: physical, psychosocial, and other (work, rest, recreational pastimes, and sleep), all of which have demonstrated excellent reliability, discriminant validity, and sensitivity to change.
- The SAFTEE Event List and Interview.[9] The SAFTEE Event List and Interview is a 62-item structured interview for the identification of side effects and adverse events that has been used widely in psychopharmacologic studies. Events are grouped by type (sleep-wake, mood, cognitive, psychological, sensory, neurological, musculoskeletal, thorax, gastrointestinal, genitourinary, skin and/or extremities, miscellaneous, and alcohol intake) and each event is assessed for severity (none, mild, moderate, or severe); any action taken is noted. The SAFTEE has good reliability and validity.[9]

Because we instituted administration of the SIP and SAFTEE after the beginning of this open trial, we asked patients to rate their functional status and adverse effects at the present time and then to also retrospectively rate themselves as they were just prior to the first cingulotomy.

The major clinical criterion pertaining to the severity of illness was functional impairment, with all patients' level of functioning being comparable to a *DSM-III-R* Global Assessment of Functioning (GAF)[4] score of less than 60, and for most patients, scores were less than 50. Although the YBOCS score is a general guide to symptom severity, there are cases in which the YBOCS score is an underestimate of severity, as it is for patients with obsessions only (and therefore with a score that is approximately one half of the true severity); in general, however, most patients must have had a YBOCS score of greater than 25.

DATA ANALYSIS

For clinical ratings of OCD and depression symptoms, we analyzed data at three times: (1) at baseline, before the first cingulotomy; (2) at the first postsurgical follow-up (a mean of 7.0 months after the first cingulotomy), at which point no patient had yet undergone a second cingulotomy; and (3) at the most recent follow-up (a mean of 26.8 months after the first cingulotomy), at which time seven patients (39%) had undergone two cingulotomies and one patient (6%) had undergone three cingulotomies. Functional status and adverse experiences were rated only at the most recent follow-up point and retrospectively at baseline. Information about the number of cingulotomies undergone by each patient, demographics, and the timing of follow-up assessments is contained in **Table 3**.

To classify patients as responders at the most recent follow-up, we employed conservative criteria that were used previously in medication trials for OCD[10]: an improvement of 35% or greater on the YBOCS and a CGI score of 1 (very much improved) or 2 (much improved). In addition, as in the previous study,[1] we also required that a patient must not have attributed improvement to a treatment other than cingulotomy.

We also classified patients as partial responders by employing less conservative criteria: (1) either an improvement of 35% or greater on the YBOCS or a CGI score of 1 or 2 or (2) adequate improvement on both the YBOCS and the CGI scales, but the patient attributed improvement to another treatment.

Patient 16 was unwilling to complete the YBOCS, SIP, or SAFTEE at her most recent telephone follow-up (42 months after surgery), although she did describe herself as much improved on the CGI for OCD symptoms. For the purposes of this study, we used her last YBOCS score available (at the 16-month follow-up), and classified her as a nonresponder.

Patient 18 had very severe contamination fears, and although he lived near the hospital, he refused to return to the clinic, to answer the telephone, or to have a home visit for the purposes of completing the rating instruments. Therefore, for this patient, we used the ratings provided by his parents, and classified him as a nonresponder.

only, three (12%) with bilateral orbitomedial lesions, and 17 (65%) with combined cingulate and orbitomedial lesions. They reported that at a mean follow-up of 10 years, 10 (38%) of their patients had clinically significant improvement, but another three patients (12%) had committed suicide. Hay et al rated clinical improvement on a global scale that assessed occupational and social functioning as well as OCD symptoms. They also reported that two patients had "personality change of the frontal lobe type" and that treated patients with only cingulate lesions did less well than those with orbitomedial or combined lesions.

We report herein the results of our prospective longitudinal follow-up of all 18 patients who underwent cingulotomy for OCD at MGH since 1989. In the absence of a sham surgical control condition (which is considered unethical in open neurosurgical procedures[3]), this method is our best assessment of the long-term outcome for OCD symptoms and functional status of these patients in whom we carefully documented that extensive trials of both medication and behavior therapy had been unsuccessful.

To our knowledge, this is the first report of a prospective study of cingulotomy in patients with a diagnosis of OCD that was confirmed by structured interview and with documented unsuccessful trials of multiple medications and behavior therapy. Our specific research questions were as follows:

1. How many patients undergoing cingulotomy for OCD will be classified as responders approximately 6 months after a single procedure?

2. How many patients will be responders at long-term follow-up?

3. Will patients undergoing cingulotomy show significant improvements or decrements in general or specific areas of functional status or quality of life at long-term follow-up?

4. Will patients undergoing cingulotomy show significant adverse effects at long-term follow-up?

5. Are there any significant predictors of outcome after cingulotomy?

Table 1. Previous Unsuccessful Treatment Trials Required of Patients Prior to Cingulotomy*

Medication Trials	
Minimum required trials (doses and duration as shown below)	
Three serotonin reuptake inhibitors, one of which must be clomipramine hydrochloride, and	
Two trials with different augmenting agents† added to a serotonin reuptake inhibitor, and	
One trial of an MAOI	
Medication dosage, mg/d‡ (duration, 10-12 wk)	
Clomipramine hydrochloride, 250	
Fluoxetine hydrochloride, 80	
Fluvoxamine hydrochloride, 300	
Sertraline hydrochloride, 200	
Paroxetine hydrochloride, 80	
MAOI	
Phenelzine sulfate, 90	
Tranylcypromine sulfate, 60	
Behavior Therapy Trials	
Minimum required trials	
Minimum of 20 hours of documented exposure and response prevention, or	
Demonstrated inability to tolerate the associated anxiety.	

**MAOI indicates monoamine oxidase inhibitor.*
†Augmenting agents include clonazepam, lithium carbonate, and buspirone hydrochloride.
‡Or maximum dosage tolerated.

RESULTS

HOW MANY PATIENTS WILL BE CLASSIFIED AS RESPONDERS APPROXIMATELY 6 MONTHS AFTER A SINGLE CINGULOTOMY?

Table 4 contains the OCD clinical rating scales for all patients at baseline and at first follow-up after one cingulotomy (mean, 7.0 months). This table illustrates that four patients (22%) met our criteria for responders at the first follow-up point. Another three patients (17%) were classified as partial responders at the first follow-up point.

In addition, the 18 patients improved significantly from baseline to latest follow-up on both the YBOCS (dependent $t[17]=4.1$, $P=.001$) and BDI (dependent $t[12]=3.8$, $P=.002$).

At first follow-up, the mean improvement in OCD measured by YBOCS was 26.2%, and the mean OCD CGI score was 3.1. Correlations between CGI ratings of OCD and depression improvement ($r=.50$, n=11, $P=.12$) and anxiety improvement ($r=.55$, n=9, $P=.12$) did not reach statistical significance.

HOW MANY PATIENTS WILL BE RESPONDERS AT LONG-TERM FOLLOW-UP?

Table 3 illustrates that five patients (28%) met our conservative criteria for being classified as responders at mean follow-up of 26.8 months. Three additional patients (patients 6, 7, and 8) met our more liberal criteria as partial responders.

One patient (patient 3) who met the criteria for being classified as a responder at the first follow-up continued to do well at a second follow-up at 32 months. However, at her most recent follow-up at 60 months, she reported a relapse of both OCD and depressive symptoms, and although she continued to meet our criteria for a responder, she was referred for a second cingulotomy procedure.

One patient (patient 18) was rated as 20% worse on YBOCS and slightly worse on the CGI scales. As a group, the 18 patients improved significantly from baseline to the most recent follow-up on both the YBOCS ($P<.001$) and BDI ($P<.002$). The CGI ratings of improvement of OCD symptoms and depression were correlated ($r=.72$, n=15, $P=.003$). The CGI ratings of improvement of OCD symptoms and anxiety were also significantly correlated ($r=.63$, n=15, $P=.01$).

At the most recent follow-up, the mean OCD improvement for the group was 27% by YBOCS, and the mean OCD CGI score was 2.8.

WILL PATIENTS IMPROVE OR DECLINE IN FUNCTIONAL STATUS OR QUALITY OF LIFE AT LONG-TERM FOLLOW-UP?

Table 5 contains the scores on the SIP at baseline (some obtained retrospectively) and at last follow-up for each

Table 2. Changes in Pharmacologic and Behavioral Treatments Following First Cingulotomy Based on the Local Psychiatrist's Report*

Patient No.	Pharmacologic Treatment	Behavioral Treatment
	Responders	
1	No medication changes	No behavior therapy changes
2	Repeated fluoxetine hydrochloride administration† at higher dose; discontinued at 3 wk because of side effects Added isocarboxazid (Marplan); no improvement Added pergolide mesylate; questionable OCD improvement	Inpatient trial; no OCD improvement
3	Added bupropion hydrochloride (Wellbutrin); no OCD improvement Added fluoxetine†; no OCD improvement Added diazepam (Valium); some OCD improvement when added to fluoxetine	No behavior therapy changes
4	No medication changes	No behavior therapy changes
5	No medication changes	No behavior therapy changes
	Partial Responders	
6	Intravenous administration of clomipramine hydrochloride†; attributes OCD improvement to this trial	No behavior therapy changes
7	Added sertraline hydrochloride†; no OCD improvement Added phenelzine sulfate; no OCD improvement	No behavior therapy changes‡
8	No medication changes	No behavior therapy changes
	Nonresponders	
9	No medication changes	No behavior therapy changes
10	Added pergolide mesylate; no OCD improvement	No behavior therapy changes
11	No medication changes	Outpatient trial; significant OCD improvement
12	Added paroxetine†; discontinued administration because of side effects	Day treatment trial; minimal OCD improvement
13	Added sertraline†; no OCD improvement Added paroxetine†; no OCD improvement	No behavior therapy changes
14	Added fluvoxamine†; no OCD improvement	No behavior therapy changes
15	Added phenelzine; no OCD improvement	Outpatient trial for 6 mo; mild OCD improvement
16	NA	
17	No medication changes	Inpatient trial; no OCD improvement
18	No medication changes	No behavior therapy changes

**OCD indicates obsessive-compulsive disorder; NA, not available (unable to collect data).*
†Serotonin uptake inhibitor.
‡Patient report.

of the specific areas of functional status and for overall status. The percentage impairment score was calculated as the obtained impairment score in a given area of functioning divided by the maximum obtainable impairment score in that area.

Table 5 illustrates that for the group as a whole, there were improvements in each subscale of the SIP, as well as in the total score. These improvements were significant (P=.03) for overall functional status. In addition, no individual area of functioning showed mean worsening. Among the five responders, the mean±SD score at baseline was 24.3±21.0 compared with 3.3±2.7 at follow-up. For the three partial responders, scores were 14.0±9.6 at baseline and 15.7±3.5 at follow-up.

WILL PATIENTS SHOW SIGNIFICANT ADVERSE EFFECTS AT LONG-TERM FOLLOW-UP?

We looked for either emergent symptoms or significant exacerbation of preexisting symptoms for each patient. The SAFTEE was administered to all patients, except for patients 16 and 18 who refused to complete this checklist. Patients were asked to report the adverse effects present at latest follow-up and to also report retrospectively which of these had also been present preoperatively. Of the 16 patients who were administered the SAFTEE, seven (44%) reported no emergent or significantly worsened symptoms at the most recent follow-up, and examination of the charts of the two patients who refused to take the SAFTEE found no reports of emergent or worsened symptoms following cingulotomy. Emergent adverse events and the patients who reported them were as follows: nightmares or night terrors (patient 3), hallucinations and flatulence (patient 6), muscle cramps (patient 9), inner tremulousness and/or shakiness (patient 10), urination problem (patient 14), weight increase (patient 15), and weight decrease (patient 16). The hallucinations experienced by patient 6 were nocturnal visual hallucinations that lasted 6 weeks and that began soon after starting a trial of intravenously administered clomipramine 20 months after cingulotomy. The urination problem of patient 14 consisted of nocturnal bed-wetting that began as a mild problem while in Florida immediately before coming to MGH for cingulotomy. It reportedly worsened after cingulotomy while at McLean Hospital; since discontinuing administration of lithium carbonate and starting carbamazepine administration in July 1993, bed-wetting is now again a mild problem. The 17-kg weight increase of patient 15 occurred after the operation, mostly during a 2-month trial of phenelzine sulfate that was begun 9 months after the second cingulotomy. This patient has now returned to his normal weight. Adverse

Table 3. Preoperative Characteristics of Subjects, Grouped by Response to Cingulotomy at Most Recent Follow-up*

Patient No./ Sex/Age,† y	Onset Age,‡ y	Disorders Comorbid With OCD: Axis I	Disorders Comorbid With OCD: Axis II
Responders			
1/M/27	17	MDD and panic disorder	None
2/M/40	13	MDD and panic disorder	NOS (avoidant, schizoid, and schizotypal)
3/F/28	14	MDD and dysthymia	None
4/M/37	5	MDD, Gilles de la Tourette's syndrome, and dysthymia	NOS (histrionic and borderline)
5/M/28	17	MDD and simple phobia	NOS (dependent and schizotypal)
Partial Responders			
6/F/60	8	MDD	Avoidant
7/M/22	15	MDD and dysthymia	Avoidant, paranoid, and schizotypal
8/F/50	37	MDD and agoraphobia without panic disorder	None
Nonresponders			
9/F/24	11	MDD (in the past)	NOS (avoidant)
10/F/35	19	MDD	NOS (paranoid and schizotypal)
11/M/36	15	MDD	None
12/M/70	13	Dysthymia and social phobia	Avoidant
13/M/30	7	MDD (in the past)	None
14/F/24	15	MDD and social phobia	Avoidant
15/M/22	10	MDD and social phobia	Avoidant and paranoid
16/F/41	20	MDD and GAD	Avoidant and dependent
17/M/29	19	MDD, tics, and simple phobia	None
18/M/25	10	MDD	None

**OCD indicates obsessive-compulsive disorder; MDD, major depressive disorder; NOS, not otherwise specified (significant traits listed in parentheses); and GAD, generalized anxiety disorder.*
†At time of cingulotomy. Mean age, 34.9 years.
‡Of OCD. Mean onset age, 14.7 years.

effects that were reported to have been mildly present preoperatively and severely present postoperatively were decreased libido (patient 4) and middle insomnia (patient 7). Because some patients underwent postoperative medication trials, which may have their own side-effects, except for the severe adverse effects that were explained above, it was impossible to be certain which adverse effects were attributable to surgery alone.

In addition, we searched the patients' medical records for reports of adverse experiences by their local physician. We found that in a left-handed 29-year-old man who was born prematurely with a weak, clumsy right hand (patient 13), a high-pitched, nasal voice with some protrusion and twitching of the tongue developed at 10 months after cingulotomy while the patient was receiving clomipramine and lithium. This effect disappeared after administration of both medications was stopped. The presumptive diagnosis was palatal dystonia. In addition, patient 8 suffered from daily, sometimes incapacitating, headaches for the first few months after cingulotomy, which then resolved. There were no suicides among the 18 patients.

ARE THERE ANY SIGNIFICANT PREDICTORS OF OUTCOME FOLLOWING CINGULOTOMY?

Using multiple regression, we found that neither the number of cingulotomies (entered either as a continuous measure or as a binary variable representing one vs more than one cingulotomy), baseline BDI score, nor improvement in either depression or anxiety (ie, CGI scores) were predictive of the final YBOCS score (over and above the baseline YBOCS score). When we entered the symptoms from the YBOCS Symptom Checklist, however, we found that the presence of preoperative symmetry obsessions (partial correlation, −.55; P=.03), ordering compulsions (partial correlation, −.55; P=.03), and hoarding compulsions (partial correlation, −.49; P=.06) were all predictive of lower YBOCS scores at final follow-up (ie, better outcome).

We also examined onset age and gender among patients in the responder or partial responder vs nonresponder groups in Table 3 and found no significant difference for either gender (corrected χ^2=0, df=1, P=.94) or onset age (t=0.8, df=14, P=.43).

COMMENT

Our finding that 28% of patients met conservative criteria for clinical improvement is consistent with a previous retrospective study.[1] Our patients showed overall improvement in functional status (with a return to near normal functional status in patients who were classified as responders) and few serious adverse events. Unlike the previous report,[1] there have been no suicides in this group of patients.

The only predictors of operative outcome were the presence of preoperative symmetry obsessions, ordering compulsions, and hoarding compulsions. These symptoms are of interest because, in varying combinations, they have been identified previously as being more common in patients with comorbid OCD and Tourette's syndrome.[11-13] Interestingly, one (patient 4) of two patients with comorbid tic or Tourette's syndrome (patients 4 and 17) in the present study was a responder. This patient's OCD

Table 4. YBOCS and CGI Measures Preoperatively and at Follow-up, Grouped According to Response to Cingulotomy at Most Recent Follow-up*

			First Follow-up				Most Recent Follow-up			
Patient No.	No. of Operations	Preoperative YBOCS Score	Months After Surgery	YBOCS Score	Decrease,†%	CGI Score	Months After Surgery	YBOCS Score	Decrease,† %	CGI Score
					Responders					
1	1	32	12	7	78	1	12‡	7‡	78‡	1‡
2	1	27	12	11	59	2	24	6	78	2
3	1	16	9	0	100	1	60	10	37	2
4	2	26	4	12	53	3	44	13	50	1
5	2	28	5	16	42	2	21	16	42	2
					Partial Responders					
6	1	27	5	21	22	2	25	15	44	1§
7	1	16	2	16	0	4	15	12	25	2
8	1	38	9	25	34	4	44	24	36	4
					Nonresponders					
9	1	26	5	12	54	3	20	20	23	5
10	2	37	16	36	2	4	47	27	27	3
11	2	34	8	27	20	4	30	25	26	3
12	1	29	5	24	17	3	8	24	17	3
13	2	28	5	29	−3	4	29	24	14	3
14	2	26	5	33	−27	5	32	24	7	3
15	2	16	4	13	18	3	17	15	6	3
16	3	31	6	27	13	3	16	33	−6	4
17	1	29	8	29	0	3	19	28	3	4
18	1	30	6	33‖	−10	4‖	19	36‖	−20	5‖
Overall mean	1.5	27.5	7.0	20.6	26.2	3.1	26.8	19.9	27.0	2.8

**YBOCS indicates the Yale-Brown Obsessive Compulsive Scale; CGI, Clinical Global Improvement.*
†From preoperative baseline (negative sign indicates worsened symptoms).
‡Only one follow-up.
§Patient responded after trial of intravenously administered clomipramine hydrochloride.
‖Rating from informant.

symptoms showed marked improvement at follow-up, but his Tourette's syndrome symptoms showed no improvement.[14]

Improvements in OCD clinical severity at the most recent follow-up were strongly and significantly related to self-ratings of improvements in both depression and anxiety. This raises the question as to whether OCD improvement was primary or secondary to changes in either depression or anxiety. It is not possible to resolve this question statistically based on the cross-sectional data collected in this study. However, all patients had a period of OCD that was not accompanied by depression at some point in the course of their illness. Also, because most patients received medication trials after surgery, it was not possible to determine whether clinical improvements were due to cingulotomy per se or rather to an interaction with medication that had not been effective preoperatively. This caveat in interpreting our results also holds true for patients who had undergone behavior therapy postoperatively when the follow-up evaluations were conducted.

Although we agree with Sachdev et al[15] that face-to-face assessments are preferable,[16] this was not possible for patients who did not return to MGH after being referred from throughout North America. For this reason, we were not able to assess these patients neuropsychologically at follow-up. However, previous careful neuropsychological assessment of patients undergoing cingulotomy at MGH found no evidence of lasting neurological, intellectual, personality, or behavioral deficits after surgery.[1,17] In addition, according to anecdotal evidence, negative personality changes following contemporary psychosurgical procedures are rare, and in fact, most of the changes have been in the direction of normalizing personality.[18-22] A widely used personality instrument, the Eysenck Personality Inventory,[23] was administered prospectively to 15 patients who underwent capsulotomy, another neurosurgical procedure used to treat patients with OCD[24,25]; in no case were negative personality changes observed after capsulotomy.

The pathophysiologic processes of OCD and the mechanisms by which antiobsessional treatments have their beneficial effects remain incompletely understood. Over the past decade, however, convergent data from pharmacologic, neuroimaging, neuropsychologic, and neurosurgical literature have been synthesized to produce integrated neurobiological models of OCD.[26-29] A circuit involving orbitofrontal cortex, caudate nucleus, pallidum, and thalamus as well as anterior cingulate cortex has been implicated in the pathophysiologic processes of OCD.[26-29] Indeed, functional neuroimaging findings suggest that aberrant activity within this system may distinguish the obsessional state from the resting state in subjects with OCD[30] and may distinguish cohorts with OCD from controls.[27,28,31] Moreover, the abnormal activity within this system may be attenuated with successful treatment.[27,28,30]

The rationale for the efficacy of anterior cingulate lesions follows from its role as the conduit for frontal cortical input to the Papez circuit and limbic system.[32,33] A variety of different neurosurgical procedures aimed at these regions have been used for the treatment of patients with intractable OCD, with purported efficacy. For example, Tan et al,[34] in the only study, to our knowledge, to employ an untreated control group, matched 13 inpatients who received intensive nonsurgical treatment for OCD with 24 patients who underwent modified, bimedial leucotomy (a procedure that is no longer in use[19]) and followed up both groups prospectively. At the 5-year follow-up, 50% of neurosurgical patients were rated as much improved in OCD symptoms compared with 23% of controls ($P<.05$), and maximum improvement was noted within the first 3 months. Herner[35] reviewed nine studies that included a total of 116 patients who underwent stereotactic interventions (limbic leucotomy, subcaudate tractotomy, and capsulotomy) and found 89 (77%) of 116 patients were markedly improved compared with seven patients (6%) who were rated as worse postoperatively. Waziri[36] recently reviewed 12 studies of stereotactic interventions in 253 cases of OCD and found that 3% of patients were reported to be worse or dead at follow-up, 10% were rated as unchanged, 29% were markedly improved, and 38% were free of symptoms.

Each of these operations entails making lesions that interrupt the neural systems described above. Specifically, anterior cingulotomy targets the anterior cingulate. Anterior capsulotomy and subcaudate tractotomy interrupt the frontothalamic fibers of passage at different sites. Limbic leucotomy is a multisite operation that combines the lesions of the anterior cingulate with those of the frontothalamic projections. The ability to draw meaningful comparisons between the various procedures with respect to efficacy and adverse effects is limited because no well-controlled head-to-head studies have been performed. Comparing results across studies and across the institutions where the procedures are performed is fraught with difficulties. Generally, however, the existing data support the notion that the different procedures have roughly comparable efficacy, whereas the issue of relative safety and side effect profile remains even less clear.[37] The multidisciplinary team at MGH has continued to offer cingulotomies, as opposed to other neurosurgical options, because of the large experience supporting its relative safety.

Despite the lack of adverse effects among our present group of patients, cingulotomy is not to be taken lightly and should be viewed as a treatment of last resort. To reflect the severity of impairment of our patients, one female patient had dropped out of college and, for several years, had remained in her home virtually every waking hour, frequently in darkness or with eyes closed in an attempt to shut out the ego-dystonic violent and sexual obsessions and images that she "saw" continuously in front of her. A male patient had remained in bed throughout the day (often not leaving to use the bathroom), communicating with no one but his parents for several years, because of severe fear of contamination.

We have sought to interpret our data conservatively and cautiously. Still, it is important to explicitly

Table 5. Sickness Impact Profile Scores at Last Follow-up*

Sickness Impact Profile	Baseline† Mean±SD Score	Follow-up, Mean±SD Score	t‡	P
Total score	21.7±13.2	12.9±8.3	2.3	.03
Subscales				
Emotional behavior	45.3±24.0	25.1±23.9	2.8	.01
Sleep and rest	51.0±31.4	23.0±20.1	2.4	.03
Home management	32.7±34.4	12.0±12.7	2.0	.05
Communication	10.0±10.4	4.6±6.0	2.1	.05
Social interaction	32.9±28.8	19.6±20.0	1.7	.10
Recreational activities	45.5±29.4	32.4±26.9	1.6	.11
Alertness	1.4±3.3	2.2±5.0	1.0	.33
Mobility	13.8±20.2	9.1±10.5	0.8	.41
Work	47.0±32.3	48.5±32.8	0.1	.88

*Scores represent percentage of interference in each area of functioning, calculated as total impairment score divided by total possible impairment score.

†Retrospective assessment of preoperative status.

‡Dependent t statistics; df=13.

acknowledge certain additional caveats. The data generated from this open study reflect results from anterior cingulotomies performed according to the specific conditions noted above. Therefore, these findings may not be generalizable to other neurosurgical treatments for OCD, including cingulotomies performed according to other methods or with different lesion measurements. For example, it is not known how changing lesion size or placement would impact the risk-benefit profile of this type of treatment. As an extreme example, there is at least one reported case of catastrophic adverse effects as a consequence of combining anterior cingulotomy with a subthalamic lesion site.[38] Furthermore, the candidacy of every patient receiving cingulotomy in this study was thoroughly scrutinized by a multidisciplinary team of experienced clinicians. Careful patient assessment and selection is a crucial factor in the outcome profile of this treatment modality. The process of multidisciplinary case review and clinical assessment aims to ensure that otherwise appropriate candidates will not receive neurosurgical treatment prematurely (ie, prior to undergoing an exhaustive array of other conventional therapies) and that inappropriate candidates will not be subjected to the risks of ill-advised neurosurgical treatment at all.

The strengths of this study include the careful diagnostic workup at baseline, documentation of adequate previous trials of medication and behavior therapy, and the prospective assessment of OCD and depressive symptoms.

A weakness is the fact that all patients had not undergone intensive trials of behavior therapy prior to cingulotomy; we did, however, examine the number of patients who underwent behavior therapy trials in the response categories and found no indication that patients who underwent behavior therapy had better outcomes: six (75%) of eight responders or partial responders vs six (60%) of 10 nonresponders underwent trials of behavior therapy (corrected χ^2=0.02, df=1, P=.86). In addition, because nonresponders were likely to return to our hospital for reevaluation, they, on average, were followed up sooner than responders. Although it is possible that this introduced systematic bias into our findings, our anecdotal experience was that most patients reported that clinical gains were present within approximately 2 months after cingulotomy.

Another weakness of our study was the absence of a sham control group. However, operations (ie, actual lesions) for which there is no likelihood or evidence of efficacy are considered to be unethical.[39] The Canadian Psychiatric Association has taken a strong stand on these matters: "It is difficult to see how experimental procedures involving the use of 'placebo operations' could be ethically and acceptably undertaken; we therefore have to rely on a more traditional method of evaluation by objectively reviewing the responses of patients who have already received these treatments."[3] Thus, although such procedures might well help us answer questions of efficacy, a sham operation (ie, bur holes only) has generally been considered to be unethical. However, with the development of modern technology, holes no longer need to be made in the cranium, and a controlled trial is now feasible and ethical. Because γ-capsulotomy lesions are made by cobalt radiation that comes from approximately 200 ports in an apparatus that surrounds the patient's head, the ports can be blocked by lead inserts prior to the operation by a technician. Using this mechanism, even the surgeon (as well as all raters) can be blind to the operative state (ie, capsulotomy vs sham). Because no actual lesion will be made in the brain itself or in the cranium (ie, bur holes) during this sham procedure, it now is feasible to do a sham operation,[19] and we have begun such a trial. Given that we have no such conclusive trials with cingulotomy, it appears that over a quarter of the patients who previously were unresponsive to optimal medication and behavioral treatments who underwent cingulotomy for OCD were much improved at follow-up using very conservative criteria, and if less stringent criteria are applied, over 40% of patients were improved.

Accepted for publication February 14, 1995.

This research was supported in part by the David Judah Research Fund, Boston, Mass (Dr Jenike).

Reprint requests to Massachusetts General Hospital–East, Bldg 149, Charlestown, MA 02129 (Dr Baer).

REFERENCES

1. Jenike MA, Baer L, Ballantine HT, Martuza RL, Tynes S, Giriunas I, Buttolph ML, Cassem NH. Cingulotomy for refractory obsessive-compulsive disorder: a long-term follow-up of 33 patients. *Arch Gen Psychiatry.* 1991;48:548-555.
2. Hay P, Sachdev P, Cumming S, Smith JS, Lee T, Kitchener P, Matheson J. Treatment of obsessive-compulsive disorder by psychosurgery. *Acta Psychiatr Scand.* 1993;87:197-207.
3. Earp JD. Psychosurgery: the position of the Canadian Psychiatric Association. *Can J Psychiatry.* 1979;24:353-365.
4. American Psychiatric Association. *Diagnostic and Statistical Manual of Mental Disorders, Revised Third Edition.* Washington, DC: American Psychiatric Association; 1987.
5. Stangl D, Pfohl B, Zimmerman M, Bowers W, Corenthal C. A structured interview for the *DSM-III* personality disorders. *Arch Gen Psychiatry.* 1985;42:591-596.
6. Goodman WK, Price LH, Rasmussen SA, Mazure C, Fleischmann R, Hill C, Heninger GR, Charney DS. The Yale-Brown Obsessive Compulsive Scale (YBOCS), I: development, use, and reliability. *Arch Gen Psychiatry.* 1989;46:1006-1011.
7. Beck AT, Ward CH, Mendelson M. An inventory for measuring depression. *Arch Gen Psychiatry.* 1961;41:561-571.
8. Bergner M, Bobbitt RA, Carter WB, Gilson BS. The Sickness Impact Profile: development and final revision of a health status measure. *Med Care.* 1981;19:787-805.
9. Guy W, Wilson WH, Brooking B, Manov G, Fjetland O. Reliability and validity of SAFTEE: preliminary analyses. *Psychopharmacol Bull.* 1986;22:397-401.
10. Clomipramine Collaborative Study Group. Clomipramine in the treatment of patients with obsessive-compulsive disorder. *Arch Gen Psychiatry.* 1991;48:730-738.
11. George MS, Trimble MR, Ring HA, Sallee FR, Robertson MM. Obsessions in obsessive-compulsive disorder with and without Gilles de la Tourette's syndrome. *Am J Psychiatry.* 1992;150:93-97.
12. Holzer JC, Goodman WK, McDougle CJ, Baer L, Boyarsky BK, Leckman JF, Price LH. Obsessive compulsive disorder with and without a chronic tic disorder: a comparison of symptoms in 70 patients. *Br J Psychiatry.* In press.
13. Baer L, Breiter HC, Goodman WK, Rasmussen SA, Eisen JL, Barr L, Shera D, Jenike MA. Identifying symptom subtypes in obsessive-compulsive disorder and their relationship to tourette and tic disorder: a factor analytic study. *J Abnorm Psychol.* In press.
14. Baer L, Rauch SL, Jenike MA, Cassem EH, Ballantine HT, Manzo PA, Martuza R. Cingulotomy in a case of concomitant obsessive-compulsive disorder and Tourette's syndrome. *Arch Gen Psychiatry.* 1994;51:73-74.
15. Sachdev P, Hay P, Cumming S. Psychosurgical treatment of obsessive-compulsive disorder. *Arch Gen Psychiatry.* 1992;49:582-583.
16. Jenike MA, Baer L. In reply. *Arch Gen Psychiatry.* 1992;49:583-584.
17. Corkin S, Twitchell TE, Sullivan EV. Safety and efficacy of cingulotomy for pain and psychiatric disorder. In: Hitchcock ER, Ballantine HT, Myerson BA, eds. *Modern Concepts in Psychiatric Surgery.* Amsterdam, the Netherlands: Elsevier Science Publishers; 1979:253-272.
18. Mindus P. *Capsulotomy in Anxiety Disorders: A Multidisciplinary Study.* Stockholm, Sweden: Karolinska Institute; 1991. Thesis.
19. Mindus P, Jenike MA. Neurosurgical treatments of malignant obsessive-compulsive disorder. *Psychiatr Clin North Am.* 1992;15:921-938.
20. Corkin S. A prospective study of cingulotomy. In: Valenstein ES, ed. *The Psychosurgery Debate.* New York, NY: WH Freeman & Co; 1980:264.
21. Göktepe EO, Young LB, Bridges PK. A further review of the results of stereotactic subcaudate tractotomy. *Br J Psychiatry.* 1975;126:270.
22. Kelly D. *Anxiety and Emotions: Physiological Basis and Treatment.* Springfield, Ill: Charles C Thomas Publisher; 1980.
23. Eysenck HJ, Eysenck SBG. *Manual of the Eysenck Personality Questionnaire (EPQ).* London, England: University of London Press; 1969.
24. Bingley T, Leksell L, Meyerson BA, Rylander G. Long-term results of stereotactic capsulotomy in chronic obsessive-compulsive neurosis. In: Sweet WH, Obrador S, Martin-Rodriguez JG, eds. *Neurosurgical Treatment in Psychiatry.* Baltimore, Md: University Park Press; 1977:287-299.
25. Rylander G. Stereotactic radiosurgery in anxiety and obsessive-compulsive states: psychiatric aspects. In: Hitchcock ER, Ballantine HT Jr, Meyerson BA, eds. *Modern Concepts in Psychiatric Surgery.* Amsterdam, the Netherlands: Elsevier Science Publishers; 1979:235.
26. Modell J, Mountz J, Curtis G, Greden J. Neurophysiologic dysfunction in basal ganglia/limbic striatal and thalamocortical circuits as a pathogenetic mechanism of obsessive-compulsive disorder. *J Neuropsychiatry Clin Neurosci.* 1989;1:27-36.
27. Baxter LR Jr, Schwartz JM, Bergman KS, Szuba MP, Guze BH, Mazziotta JC, Alazraki A, Selin CE, Ferng H-K, Munford P, Phelps ME. Caudate glucose metabolic rate changes with both drug and behavior therapy for obsessive-compulsive disorder. *Arch Gen Psychiatry.* 1992;49:681-689.
28. Insel TR. Toward a neuroanatomy of obsessive-compulsive disorder. *Arch Gen Psychiatry.* 1992;49:739-744.
29. Rauch SL, Jenike MA. Neurobiological models of obsessive compulsive disorder. *Psychosomatics.* 1993;34:20-32.
30. Rauch SL, Jenike MA, Alpert NM, Baer L, Breiter HC, Savage CR, Fischman AJ. Regional cerebral blood flow measured during symptom provocation in obsessive-compulsive disorder using oxygen 15–labeled carbon dioxide and positron emission tomography. *Arch Gen Psychiatry.* 1994;51:62-70.
31. Swedo SE, Pietrini P, Leonard HL, Schapiro MB, Rettew DC, Goldberger EL, Rapoport SI, Rapoport JL, Grady CL. Cerebral glucose metabolism in childhood-onset obsessive-compulsive disorder: revisualization during pharmacotherapy. *Arch Gen Psychiatry.* 1992;49:690-694.
32. Papez JW. Proposed mechanism of emotion. *Arch Neurol Psychiatry.* 1937;38:725-743.
33. Mesulam M-M. Patterns in behavioral neuroanatomy: association areas, the limbic system, and hemispheric specialization. In: Mesulam M-M, ed. *Principles of Behavioral Neurology.* Philadelphia, Pa: FA Davis Co; 1985:1-70.
34. Tan E, Marks IM, Marset P. Bi-medial leucotomy in obsessive-compulsive neurosis: a controlled serial inquiry. *Br J Psychiatry.* 1971;118:155-164.
35. Herner T. Treatment of mental disorders with frontal stereotactic thermolesions: a follow-up of 116 cases. *Acta Psychiatr Scand.* 1961;58(suppl):36.
36. Waziri R. Psychosurgery for anxiety and obsessive-compulsive disorders. In: Noyes R Jr, Roth M, Burrows GD, eds. *Handbook of Anxiety: Treatment of Anxiety.* Amsterdam, the Netherlands: Elsevier Science Publishers; 1990.
37. Chiocca EA, Martuza RL. Neurosurgical therapy of obsessive-compulsive disorder. In: Jenike MA, Baer L, Minichiello WE, eds. *Obsessive-Compulsive Disorders: Theory and Management.* St Louis, Mo: Mosby–Year Book; 1990:283-294.
38. Leckman JF, de Lotbiniere AJ, Marek K, Gracco C, Scahill L, Cohen DJ. Severe disturbances in speech, swallowing, and gait following stereotactic infrathalamic lesions in Gilles de la Tourette's syndrome. *Neurology.* 1993;43:890-894.
39. Levine RJ. *Ethics and Regulation of Clinical Research.* 2nd ed. New Haven, Conn: Yale Press; 1988.

Reduced Caudate Nucleus Volume in Obsessive-compulsive Disorder

Delbert Robinson, MD; Houwei Wu, MD; Rafael A. Munne, MD; Manzar Ashtari, PhD; Jose Ma. J. Alvir, DrPH; Gail Lerner, MS; Amy Koreen, MD; Karyl Cole, MD; Bernhard Bogerts, MD

Background: Current hypotheses about the neuroanatomical structures involved in obsessive-compulsive disorder (OCD) suggest abnormalities in cortical-striatal-thalamic-cortical circuits. This study examined selected brain regions within or adjacent to these circuits.

Methods: Magnetic resonance imaging scans from 26 patients with OCD and 26 healthy controls were analyzed to determine the volumes of the following structures: prefrontal cortex (cortex anterior to the genu of the corpus callosum), caudate nucleus, lateral and third ventricles, and whole brain.

Results: Patients with OCD had significantly smaller caudate nucleus volumes than controls ($F[1,48]=9.4$, $P=.004$) but did not differ in prefrontal cortex size or in volumes of the lateral or third ventricles. Structural volumes were not significantly correlated with the duration or severity of OCD symptoms.

Conclusion: Our findings provide additional evidence for pathological involvement of the caudate in OCD.

(Arch Gen Psychiatry. 1995;52:393-398)

NEUROLOGICAL diseases with obsessive-compulsive symptoms, neurosurgical procedures to treat obsessive-compulsive disorder (OCD), and functional brain imaging with single-photon emission computed tomography and positron emission tomography have been the primary bases for current hypotheses about abnormalities in cortical-striatal-thalamic-cortical loop circuits in OCD.[1-5] Structural brain imaging techniques can provide information about whether there are macroscopic anatomical differences in patients with OCD in structures within these circuits. Despite the importance of such information to developing theories of the pathophysiology of OCD, few structural brain imaging studies in OCD have been performed and their results have been contradictory. In two early studies using computed tomographic (CT) scans to measure ventricular brain ratio, Insel and coworkers[6] found no differences in ventricular brain ratio in adult OCD subjects compared with control subjects, while Behar and coworkers[7] found significantly greater ventricular brain ratios in adolescents with OCD. Using quantitative CT measures, Luxenberg and coworkers[8] found significantly smaller caudate nucleus volumes in OCD subjects compared with control subjects but no differences in lateral or third ventricular size; in contrast, Stein and coworkers[9] found increased ventricular volumes but no difference in caudate volumes using quantitative CT measures in OCD patients with neurological soft signs compared with healthy controls.

Magnetic resonance imaging (MRI) combined with current image assessment techniques could potentially allay some of the methodological limitations that may have contributed to the divergent findings in the CT literature. So far, however, the results of structural MRI studies in OCD have also been contradictory. Garber et al[10] obtained MRI scans on 32 patients with OCD and 14 healthy control subjects. No quantitative morphometric evaluations were done on the scans; radiological evaluations reported abnormalities in six of 14 healthy controls and 14 of 32 patients. Three MRI studies have reported on caudate measures; two[11,12] had direct assessments of caudate volume and one[13] used the bicaudate ratio as a mea-

From the Hillside Hospital, Psychiatry Research, Glen Oaks, NY (Drs Robinson, Wu, Munne, Alvir, Koreen, and Cole); Department of Psychiatry, Albert Einstein College of Medicine, New York, NY (Drs Robinson, Alvir, Koreen, and Cole); Department of Radiology, Long Island Jewish Medical Center, New Hyde Park, NY (Dr Ashtari); Department of Preventive Cardiology, St Francis Hospital, Roslyn, NY (Ms Lerner); and Department of Psychiatry, University of Magdeburg (Germany) (Dr Bogerts).

See Subjects and Methods on next page

SUBJECTS AND METHODS

SAMPLE SELECTION

Patients with OCD were obtained from the Hillside Hospital Research OCD Clinic, Glen Oaks, NY. Subject consent for the study was obtained using the guidelines of the Long Island Jewish Human Subjects Review Committee. The OCD patients were aged 18 years or older and had a *DSM-III-R* diagnosis of OCD by the Structured Clinical Interview for *DSM-III-R*: Patient Version (SCID-P) (4/1/88 revision, part 1).[14] Exclusion criteria included the following: (1) patients with cardiac pacemakers, metallic clips, or other metallic implants or artifacts in their bodies; (2) patients with significant medical illness—neurologic (including Gilles de la Tourette's syndrome, Huntington's disease, Parkinson's disease, and others), pulmonary, cardiac, renal, hepatic, endocrine, or metabolic (including dehydration) disorders; (3) patients with tardive dyskinesia; (4) patients who have had psychosurgery; (5) patients with current or past *DSM-III-R*–defined alcohol or psychoactive substance abuse or dependence; (6) patients with *DSM-III-R*–defined dementia, delirium, schizophrenia, schizoaffective disorder, delusional disorder, brief reactive psychosis, or psychotic disorder not otherwise specified; (7) *DSM-III-R*–defined mental retardation; and (8) pregnancy.

Control subjects were recruited from advertisements and medical center personnel, had no history of psychiatric disorders or psychotropic medication use, and were medically healthy. History of psychiatric disorders was assessed in the first 10 control subjects by use of a screening questionnaire followed by a clinical interview; all subsequent control subjects were assessed by an SCID-P interview.

MRI PROCEDURES

Magnetic resonance imaging scans were obtained using a 1.0-T whole-body MRI system (Magnetom, Siemens, Erlangen, Germany). For morphometric assessment of the brain, a three-dimensional gradient echo sequence named fast low angle shot (FLASH) was used, which provides excellent gray-white matter contrast and thin contiguous sections. Coronal slices through the head were collected using a 50° flip angle with a repetition time of 0.04 second, an echo time of 15 milliseconds, an effective slice thickness of 3.1 mm, one acquisition, a matrix of 256×256, and a field of view of 300 mm. This sequence produced 63 contiguous slices through the whole head. In addition, for standard morphological assessment of the brain, a standard T_2-weighted sequence was used that contained 16 to 20 parallel sections, 7 mm thick with a 3-mm gap in the axial plane.

ASSESSMENT OF SCANS

For morphometric analysis, images were input from a VAX11/750 onto a workstation (SUN Sparc 10, SUN Microsystems, Mountain View, Calif) via a 1.25-cm magnetic tape. Volumetric assessments were done using a semiautomated computer-operated mensuration system that provides valid and reliable volume measurements of specific structures (these methods have previously been described in detail[15,16]). Ratings were made under blinded conditions with patient and control cases randomly distributed. The images were also randomly flipped in the x-y axis prior to evaluation to eliminate any bias involving left-right evaluations.

All structures except whole brain and the third ventricle were divided into left and right subsections. Regions of interest included (1) whole brain: this was measured by two trained operators (H.W. and R.M.), whose interrater

sure of caudate volume. Of these studies, two[11,13] found no difference between patients and healthy controls, while one[12] found increased caudate volume in the right but not the left side in OCD patients compared with healthy control subjects.

Given these conflicting results, we performed a volumetric MRI study in patients with OCD, focusing on structures specified in the cortical-striatal-thalamic-cortical loop hypothesis of OCD.

RESULTS

SUBJECTS

The demographic characteristics of the 26 patients and 26 control subjects are presented in **Table 1**. Both the OCD and control samples were relatively young and overall were well educated. Twenty-two of the OCD patients and 21 of the control subjects were right-handed as assessed using a modified 20-item Edinburgh Inventory.[17] The OCD patients had been ill for an extended period of time (mean [±SD] onset of illness prior to the scans, 13.6±6.2 years; range, 3 to 28 years) and their symptoms were of moderate severity (mean [±SD] total of obsession and compulsion 10 items on the Yale-Brown Obsessive Compulsive Scale[18] was 22.3±6.4; range, 8 to 37). Twenty OCD patients had received prior medication treatment for their disorder. All OCD patients who had received prior medication treatment had taken selective serotonin reuptake inhibitors or clomipramine hydrochloride for 4 or more weeks; other classes of medications had been taken much less frequently (benzodiazepines, taken by six patients, was the next most frequently prescribed drug class). By SCID-P interview, seven OCD patients had a past episode of major depressive disorder and one had a current episode of major depression at assessment; two additional patients had dysthymic disorder. Other comorbid diagnoses included trichotillomania in two of the patients with past major depression; a history of panic disorder in the patient with current major depression; both trichotillomania and simple phobia in one patient; and past episodes of panic disorder, anorexia, and bulimia in one patient. Consistent with the infrequent occurrence of current mood disorders in the OCD sample, the mean (±SD) Hamilton Depression Rating Scale score (17 items minus the obsessive-compulsive item) was only 7.3±4.9.

reliability for this measure was .86 (*P*=.001, n=10); (2) prefrontal cortex: this consisted of the cortex anterior to the genu of the corpus callosum and extending to the frontal pole of the brain and was measured by the same two operators (H.W. and R.M.); (3) caudate nucleus: because the posterior parts of the caudate nucleus cannot be seen clearly on MRI scans, measurement of the caudate nucleus began at the first appearance of the cisterna pontis and continued anteriorly until the caudate head was no longer visible. At the slice anterior to the section where the anterior commissure crosses the midline, the nucleus accumbens was separated from the caudate by a line combining the most basal extents of the lateral ventricle and the internal capsule. All measurements were made by one of us (H.W.), whose interrater reliability with another rater on our system for this measure was .80 for the left caudate (*P*=.0001, n=20) and .83 for the right caudate (*P*=.0001 n=20); (4) ventricular volumes: the anatomic landmarks employed and typical reliability obtained for the third and lateral ventricular measurements (the fourth ventricle was excluded) on our system have been presented in detail previously.[16] The lateral ventricles were subdivided into occipital, frontal and temporal horns, and body. The occipital horn was measured from its most posterior extension to the slice posterior to the pulvinar section. It included the transition part to the inferior horn. Measurement of the body began at the first slice through the pulvinar and ended at the last slice caudal to the foramen Monro. Measurement of the frontal horn began at the slice where the entire foramen Monro was visualized and continued anteriorly until it ended in the prefrontal region. Temporal horn measurements began at the section through the pulvinar and extended to the last slice in the anterior pole of the amygdala. The third ventricle was measured on all slices anterior to the cerebral aqueduct up to and including the suprachiasmatic recess. All ventricular measurements were done by one of us (R.M.), whose interrater reliability with another operator for these measures ranged from .82 to .99 with a mean *r* of .90.

STATISTICAL PROCEDURES

The set of regional morphometric volumes (caudate, prefrontal cortex, lateral ventricle, and third ventricle) was analyzed using multivariate analysis of variance (MANOVA) to test for overall differences between OCD patients and control subjects. The overall MANOVA test was followed by *t* tests to specify which regions differed between groups. To demonstrate the precision with which between-group differences were estimated, 95% confidence intervals (CIs) were calculated for the differences (controls minus OCD subjects) in the regions of interest. Total brain volume was not used as a covariate because prior analysis showed no differences between groups. The major analyses were between-group comparisons, which were performed on total regional volumes (left+right hemispheres) because repeated-measures analyses of variance (ANOVA) done on each region separately showed no interaction between group and hemisphere. Subsequent analyses tested whether controlling for age and sex affected any between-group differences. Controlling for differences in educational attainment between groups was accomplished by limiting the analyses to subjects who had no more than 4 years of college. The analyses that controlled for education were done by limiting the sample because of differential patterns of correlation between brain volume and years of education that violated the assumptions of analysis of covariance. Further analyses subdivided the OCD group by history of depression and prior OCD medication use to test whether these factors affected brain volume.

MORPHOMETRY MEASURES

The results of the volumetric ratings are presented in **Table 2**. Ninety-five percent CIs are given for the differences between group means (control mean minus OCD mean).

Total brain volume did not differ between the OCD and control groups. The analyses we report therefore do not adjust for total brain volume. We examined interhemispheric differences in structural volumes by entering both left and right volumes in repeated-measures ANOVA in which the main effects of laterality (left vs right) and the interaction of laterality with group were tested. These analyses were done separately for each structure. There were no statistically significant interactions between hemisphere and group, which means that the effect of laterality, if present, did not differ between OCD patients and controls. There was a significant main effect for laterality in caudate volume (F[1,50]=8.33, *P*=.006), with larger caudate volumes on the right side in both patients and controls. Because of the absence of interaction effects between group and hemisphere, the major comparisons between groups were made on total volumes (right+left).

A MANOVA was performed wherein the OCD and control groups were compared on volumes of the caudate, prefrontal cortex, lateral ventricle, and third ventricle. The multivariate hypothesis of no overall group effect was rejected, indicating differential volumes between groups (F[4,47]=3.28, *P*=.02). Because of differences between groups in mean age and the slight imbalance in their sex distributions, a similar MANOVA was done controlling for age and sex. Neither age (F[4,45]=1.62, *P*=.19) nor sex (F[4,45]=1.13, *P*=.36) had significant effects on structural volumes, while the group effect remained significant (F[4,45]=2.92, *P*=.03). Post hoc univariate tests showed that the mean caudate volume in controls was 750 mm^3 (95% CI=164 to 1336) larger than in OCD patients (*t*=2.57, *df*=50, *P*=.01). Caudate volumes for each subject are presented in the **Figure**. The difference in caudate volume between groups remained significant after controlling for age and sex (F[1,48]=5.14, *P*=.03). Prefrontal cortex size did not differ between groups (*t*=0.15, *df*=50, *P*=.86). The OCD patients had substantially larger lateral ventricular size (4390 mm^3) but this difference was not statistically significant ($t_{\text{unequal variance}}$=1.68, *df*=32.9, *P*=.10).

Further analyses of caudate volume revealed significant differences between groups for both left (t=2.64, df=50, P=.01) and right (t=2.36, df=50, P=.02) caudate. The results for left and right caudate volume remained significant after controlling for age and sex. The differences in left and right caudate volume were similar within male and female subsamples; there were no significant interaction effects between group and sex.

Because the control group was more educated than the OCD group, we ran analyses that compared caudate volume controlling for years of education. The correlation between caudate volume and years of education differed between the control group (r=−.28; 95% CI=−0.60 to 0.11) and the OCD group (r=.31; 95% CI=−0.09 to 0.61). Therefore, the assumption in analysis of covariance of no interaction between group and years of education did not hold. We examined the distributions of years of education for the OCD and control groups; the main difference between the groups was for subjects who had postgraduate education. We therefore performed an analysis limited to subjects who were at most college graduates (12 controls and 23 OCD patients). The difference in caudate volumes between OCD and control groups was more pronounced in this subsample than in the entire sample because of the tendency toward smaller caudate volumes among the more educated control subjects. In the subsample, the control group had a mean caudate volume that was 1255 mm^3 larger than that of the OCD group (95% CI=548 to 1962). Similar results were seen for the left (difference in volume=622 mm^3; 95% CI=235 to 1008) and right (difference in volume=634 mm^3; 95% CI=296 to 971) caudate volumes.

Twenty OCD patients had ever taken any psychotropic medications; the history of ever having taken psychotropic drugs within the patient sample had no effect in multivariate analysis of caudate, prefrontal cortex, lateral ventricle and third ventricle size ($F_{[4,21]}$=0.56, P=.69). Since reduced caudate volumes have been reported in patients with current major depressive disorder,[19] we divided our OCD sample into those with a history of major depression (eight subjects) and those without a history of major depression (18 subjects). A history of major depression had no effect on our four regions of interest in multivariate analysis ($F_{[4,21]}$=0.87, P=.50). To assess the possible effects of duration of illness, we correlated duration of illness with our variables of interest; all correlations ranged from −.01 to −.10 and none were significant.

Table 1. Demographic Characteristics of Subjects*

	OCD Patients	Normal Controls
Gender		
M	14	16
F	12	10
Race		
W	22	21
B	1	2
Asian	3	0
Hispanic	0	2
Other	0	1
Age, y (range)	32.2±8.3 (19-44)	29.8±6.3 (20-45)
Education, y	14.7±2.3	17.1±2.8
Age at onset of illness, y	18.4±7.4	. . .
Duration of illness prior to scan, y	13.6±6.2	. . .

**Number of years are given as mean±SD. OCD indicates obsessive-compulsive disorder.*

COMMENT

To our knowledge, our findings are the first demonstration by MRI scanning of reduced caudate volume in OCD patients vs healthy control subjects; this is consistent with the CT study of Luxenberg et al[8] of reduced caudate volume in 10 OCD patients vs healthy control subjects. In contrast, other structural imaging studies by Kellner et al,[11] Aylward et al,[13] and Stein et al[9] found no differences in caudate measures, while Scarone et al[12] found increased right caudate volumes in OCD patients vs healthy controls. Different study methods and small sample sizes may account in part for these discrepant findings. Kellner et al[11] studied only 12 OCD patients, which limited their power to detect differences between groups. Aylward et al[13] did not report caudate volumes directly but reported percent caudate-to-brain ratio on a single MRI slice. This indirect measure of caudate volume may have decreased their ability to detect differences between groups. Their other measure of caudate size, the bicaudate ratio, did not differ between OCD patients, normal control subjects, and subjects with autism; however, this measure may not have been sensitive enough to detect differences of the magnitude found in our study. Stein et al[9] used CT images for their evaluations; the limited contrast resolution of their CT scans compared with MRI may have decreased their ability to detect differences in caudate volumes. Further, Stein and his coauthors themselves noted that their small sample size, 16 OCD cases and eight controls, and low test-retest reliability correlations for their caudate measures may have contributed to a type II error. Scarone et al[12] found increases in right but not left caudate size in 20 OCD patients compared with 16 control subjects. Measurements were made using 5-mm axial MRI scans with a 0.5-mm interslice gap; eight slices were obtained, three of which were chosen for the analyses. Their scans may therefore have not covered the entire caudate nucleus unlike our imaging protocol that produced a mean of 13 contiguous slices for each caudate evaluation. Scarone et al[12] did not directly report their patient or normal control caudate volumes but instead reported mean rank scores; this limits the ability to compare their results with ours.

We examined possible causes for the caudate volume reduction found in our OCD subjects. Among the factors not directly related to OCD, we considered the possibility of an effect of medication treatment and also the presence of a history of major depression in some of our patients with OCD; however, we found no evidence for either effect. If the decreases in caudate volume that we detected are directly related to the pathophysiology of OCD, our findings are not consistent with a progressive degenerative process occurring

Table 2. Morphometry Results for All Subjects

Region	Mean (±SD) Volume, mm³ OCD Patients	Mean (±SD) Volume, mm³ Normal Controls	95% Confidence Interval of Difference Between Groups
Total brain	1 320 864±122 372	1 324 130±122 749	−65 009 to 71 541
Prefrontal cortex	147 659±23 468	148 634±24 987	−12 528 to 14 478
Caudate total	5880±1092	6630±1012	164 to 1336*
Caudate left	2875±568	3284±547	98 to 720*
Caudate right	3005±549	3346±492	51 to 631†
Lateral ventricles	20 332±12 374	15 942±4993	−9714 to 934
Ventricle left	10 823±8192	8030±2712	−6247 to 661
Ventricle right	9509±5448	7912±2579	−3995 to 801
Body (lateral)	6375±4270	4744±1672	−3462 to 200
Left	3342±2465	2352±911	−2040 to 60
Right	3032±2042	2392±877	−1526 to 246
Frontal horns	5044±2760	4058±1490	−2231 to 259
Frontal horn left	2606±1558	2087±869	−1227 to 189
Frontal horn right	2438±1316	1971±739	−1066 to 132
Occipital horns	7781±5869	6138±2188	−4146 to 859
Occipital horn left	4342±4309	3121±1149	−3011 to 569
Occipital horn right	3439±2866	3017±1154	−1655 to 810
Third ventricle	1641±367	1509±354	−333 to 69

*P=.01.
†P=.02.

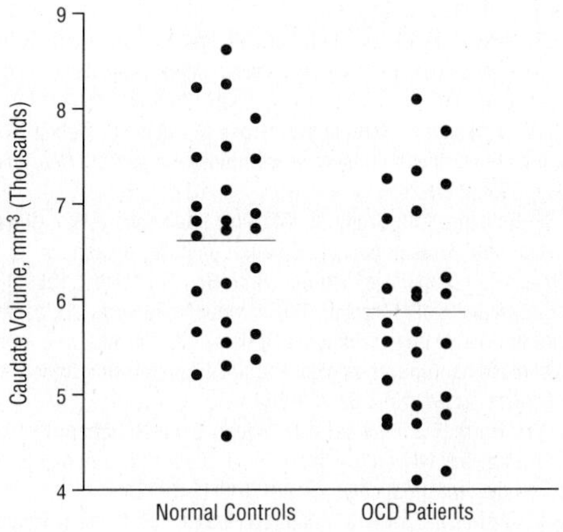

Caudate volume by group. Horizontal lines represent mean values.

in OCD since our caudate volumes were not correlated with illness duration. However, consonant with the long duration of symptoms most patients with OCD experience before seeking treatment, the patient with the shortest duration of symptoms in our study was 3 years. Thus, a degenerative process occurring during the first years of symptoms or prior to the onset of OCD symptoms would be consistent with our findings. Longitudinal follow-up studies would be needed to definitively address whether caudate volume changes in OCD are progressive; our data and those of Luxenberg et al[8] that show significant caudate reductions already in young men 17 to 24 years old with OCD suggest that younger OCD patients might be particularly appropriate for such longitudinal studies. Our caudate volumes were not correlated with the severity of symptoms on the Yale-Brown Obsessive Compulsive Scale; however, this lack of association must be interpreted cautiously since the majority of our patients had prior treatment that may have confounded assessment of the underlying severity of their illness.

Among the other structures we examined, our results are suggestive of possible lateral ventricular enlargement in OCD, which would be compatible with decreases in size of surrounding structures. Previous functional brain imaging studies have detected changes in frontal and orbital-frontal cortex metabolism in OCD subjects vs healthy controls.[20-26] Our failure to detect a difference in prefrontal cortex size between our patients and healthy controls may be because there are metabolic but not structural differences between OCD patients and healthy control subjects in the prefrontal cortex. However, functional imaging studies have implicated specific regions of the prefrontal cortex; thus, there may be morphological differences between patients with OCD and healthy controls in subregions of the prefrontal cortex that we were unable to detect with our prefrontal measure.

In summary, our findings provide additional evidence for the pathological involvement of basal ganglia structures in OCD. Given our results, future morphometric studies of the thalamus, cortical subdivisions, and other striatal structures besides the caudate would be of interest to assess further the macroscopic anatomy of structures within the cortical-striatal-thalamic-cortical loop hypothesis of OCD. Unfortunately, technical limitations prevented us from measuring the thalamus using the imaging protocol for this study. In addition to demonstrating the utility of MRI structural studies to examine structures specified in the cortical-striatal-thalamic-cortical loop hypothesis, our findings may have relevance for functional imaging studies in OCD. Our results suggest that volumetric differences in regions of interest between patient and control groups may need to be incorporated in functional imaging models.

Accepted for publication February 6, 1995.

This work was supported by grant MH46663-01A2 from the National Institute of Mental Health (Dr Robinson). The study was performed in association with The Brain Morphometry and Image Analysis Center of the Long Island Jewish Medical Center, New Hyde Park, NY, supported by a grant from the Helen and Irving Schneider Family.

We wish to acknowledge the contributions of Martin Redmond, MS, for computer system development and maintenance; JoAnn Weisbord, MSW, for subject recruitment; and Doris Galic, Mary Herling, Joni Schenkler, and Richard Goldstein for data management.

Reprint requests to Research Department, Hillside Hospital, Glen Oaks, NY 11004 (Dr Robinson).

REFERENCES

1. Rapoport JL, Wise SP. Obsessive-compulsive disorder: evidence for basal ganglia dysfunction. *Psychopharmacol Bull.* 1988;24:380-384.
2. Modell JG, Mountz JM, Curtis GC, Greden JF. Neurophysiologic dysfunction in basal ganglia/limbic striatal and thalamocortical circuits as a pathogenetic mechanism of obsessive-compulsive disorder. *J Neuropsychiatry Clin Neurosci.* 1989; 1:27-36.
3. Rapoport J. Recent advances in obsessive-compulsive disorder. *Neuropsychopharmacology.* 1991;5:1-10.
4. Insel TR. Toward a neuroanatomy of obsessive-compulsive disorder. *Arch Gen Psychiatry.* 1992;49:739-744.
5. Cummings JL. Frontal-subcortical circuits and human behavior. *Arch Neurol.* 1993;50:873-880.
6. Insel TR, Donnelly EF, Lalakea ML, Alterman IS, Murphy DL. Neurological and neuropsychological studies of patients with obsessive-compulsive disorder. *Biol Psychiatry.* 1983;18:741-751.
7. Behar D, Rapoport JL, Berg CJ, Denckla MB, Mann L, Cox C, Fedio P, Zahn T, Wolfman MG. Computerized tomography and neuropsychological test measures in adolescents with obsessive-compulsive disorder. *Am J Psychiatry.* 1984;141:363-369.
8. Luxenberg JS, Swedo SE, Flament MF, Friedland RP, Rapoport J, Rapoport SI. Neuroanatomical abnormalities in obsessive-compulsive disorder detected with quantitative x-ray computed tomography. *Am J Psychiatry.* 1988;145: 1089-1093.
9. Stein DJ, Hollander E, Chan S, DeCaria CM, Hilal S, Liebowitz MR, Klein D. Computed tomography and neurological soft signs in obsessive-compulsive disorder. *Psychiatry Res Neuroimaging.* 1993;50:143-150.
10. Garber HJ, Ananth JV, Chiu LC, Griswold VJ, Oldendorf WH. Nuclear magnetic resonance study of obsessive-compulsive disorder. *Am J Psychiatry.* 1989; 146:1001-1005.
11. Kellner CH, Jolley RR, Holgate RC, Austin L, Lydiard RB, Laraia M, Ballenger JC. Brain MRI in obsessive-compulsive disorder. *Psychiatry Res.* 1991;36:45-49.
12. Scarone S, Colombo C, Livian S, Ambruzzese M, Ronchi P, Locatelli M, Scotti G, Smeraldi E. Increased right caudate nucleus size in obsessive-compulsive disorder: detection with magnetic resonance imaging. *Psychiatry Res Neuroimaging.* 1992;45:115-121.
13. Aylward EH, Schwartz J, Machlin S, Pearlson G. Bicaudate ratio as a measure of caudate volume on MR images. *AJNR Am J Neuroradiol.* 1991;12:1217-1222.
14. Spitzer RL, Williams JBW, Gibbon M. *Structured Clinical Interview for* DSM-III-R*: Patient Version: SCID-P 4/1/88.* New York, NY: Biometrics Research Dept, New York State Psychiatric Institute; 1988.
15. Ashtari M, Zito JL, Gold BI, Lieberman JA, Borenstein MT, Herman PG. Computerized volume measurement of brain structure. *Invest Radiol.* 1990;25:798-805.
16. Degreef G, Ashtari M, Bogerts B, Bilder B, Jody DN, Alvir JMJ, Lieberman JA. Volumes of ventricular subdivisions measured from magnetic resonance images in first-episode schizophrenic patients. *Arch Gen Psychiatry.* 1992;49: 531-537.
17. Oldfield RC. The assessment and analysis of handedness: The Edinburgh Inventory. *Neuropsychologia.* 1971;9:97-114.
18. Goodman WK, Rasmussen SA, Price LH, Mazure C, Heninger GR, Charney DS. *Yale-Brown Obsessive Compulsive Scale (Y-BOCS).* New Haven, Conn: Clinical Neuroscience Research Unit, Connecticut Mental Health Center; 1988.
19. Krishnan KRR, McDonald WM, Escalona PR, Doraiswamy PM, Na C, Husain MM, Figiel GS, Boyko OB, Ellinwood EH, Nemeroff CB. Magnetic resonance imaging of the caudate nuclei in depression: preliminary observations. *Arch Gen Psychiatry.* 1992;49:553-557.
20. Baxter LR Jr, Phelps ME, Mazziotta JC, Guze BH, Schwartz JM, Selin CE. Local cerebral glucose metabolic rates in obsessive-compulsive disorder: a comparison with rates in unipolar depression and in normal controls. *Arch Gen Psychiatry.* 1987;44:211-218.
21. Baxter LR, Schwartz JM, Mazziotta JC, Phelps ME, Pahl JJ, Guze BH, Fairbanks L. Cerebral glucose metabolic rates in nondepressed patients with obsessive-compulsive disorder. *Am J Psychiatry.* 1988;145:1560-1563.
22. Nordahl TE, Benkelfat C, Semple WE, Gross M, King AC, Cohen RM. Cerebral glucose metabolic rates in obsessive-compulsive disorder. *Neuropsychopharmacology.* 1989;2:23-28.
23. Swedo SE, Schapiro MB, Grady CL, Cheslow DL, Leonard HL, Kumar A, Friedland R, Rapoport SI, Rapoport JL. Cerebral glucose metabolism in childhood-onset obsessive-compulsive disorder. *Arch Gen Psychiatry.* 1989;46:518-523.
24. Martinot JL, Allilaire JF, Mazoyer BM, Hantouche E, Huret JD, Legaut-Demare F, Deslauriers AG, Hardy P, Pappata S, Baron JC. Obsessive-compulsive disorder: a clinical, neuropsychological and positron emission tomography study. *Acta Psychiatr Scand.* 1990;82:233-242.
25. Machlin SR, Harris GJ, Pearlson GD, Hoehn-Saric R, Jeffery P, Camargo EE. Elevated medial-frontal cerebral blood flow in obsessive-compulsive patients: a SPECT study. *Am J Psychiatry.* 1991;148:1240-1242.
26. Rubin RT, Villanueva-Meyer J, Ananth J, Trajmar P, Mena I. Regional xenon 133 cerebral blood flow and cerebral technetium 99m HMPAO uptake in unmedicated patients with obsessive-compulsive disorder and matched normal control subjects. *Arch Gen Psychiatry.* 1992;49:695-702.

An In Vivo Study of the Prefrontal Cortex of Schizophrenic Patients at Different Stages of Illness via Phosphorus Magnetic Resonance Spectroscopy

Jeff A. Stanley, PhD; Peter C. Williamson, MD; Dick J. Drost, PhD; Tom J. Carr, MD; R. Jane Rylett, PhD; Ashok Malla, MD; R. Terry Thompson, PhD

Background: In this study, phospholipid metabolism of cell membranes, high-energy phosphate metabolism, and intracellular free magnesium concentration in the prefrontal cortex of first-episode drug-naive schizophrenic patients and medicated schizophrenic patients at different stages of illness were compared with those of controls.

Methods: Localized in vivo phosphorus 31 magnetic resonance spectra of the left dorsolateral prefrontal cortex of 11 drug-naive, eight newly diagnosed medicated, and 10 chronic medicated patients with schizophrenia were compared with controls of similar gender, education, parental education, and handedness.

Results: Significantly decreased levels of phosphomonoesters in drug-naive, newly diagnosed medicated, and chronic medicated patients and significantly increased levels of phosphodiesters in drug-naive patients were observed when compared with controls. There were no significant differences in the levels of high-energy phosphate metabolites between the groups except for a significant decrease in the inorganic orthophosphate levels of newly diagnosed medicated patients. A significant increase in the intracellular free magnesium concentration was observed in drug-naive, newly diagnosed medicated, and chronic medicated patients compared with controls. There were no correlations between the patients' negative and positive symptoms and the observed phosphorus-containing metabolites.

Conclusions: A reduction in precursors of membrane phospholipid are observed during the early and chronic stages of the schizophrenia illness, and breakdown products of membrane phospholipids are increased at the early stage of illness before medication treatment.

(Arch Gen Psychiatry. 1995;52:399-406)

One of the most consistent findings in schizophrenia has been a functional abnormality in the frontal lobes. Activation deficits have been demonstrated with quantitative electroencephalographic measures,[1,2] cerebral blood flow,[3-6] and positron emission tomography.[7-12] There is some evidence that this lack of activation is specific to schizophrenia.[13]

Reports of structural changes in the frontal lobes have been inconsistent. Most magnetic resonance (MR) imaging studies have failed to find volumetric differences in schizophrenics compared with controls.[14-17] However, more recent studies using thinner imaging slices to calculate volumes have suggested that there may be prefrontal volume deficits in at least some schizophrenic patients.[18,19] Both reduced gray matter[20] and white matter volumes[18,19] have been found in prefrontal regions in schizophrenic patients compared with controls. The spin-spin relaxation decay constant (T_2), an in vivo MR imaging measure reflecting the water environment in tissue, has also been reported to be longer in left prefrontal white matter of patients with schizophrenia compared with controls.[21]

While many studies of schizophrenia have shown functional and/or structural deficits in prefrontal regions, the nature of these deficits has remained elusive. One technique that offers some potential to understand these differences is phosphorus 31 MR spectroscopy.[22,23] This noninvasive technique provides quantitative information on the metabolism of high-energy phosphates, including adenosine triphosphate (ATP), phosphocreatine (PCr), and inorganic orthophosphate (Pi), and on membrane phospholipid metabo-

From the Magnetic Resonance Spectroscopy Unit (Dr Stanley), Montreal (Quebec) Neurological Institute; Department of Nuclear Medicine and Magnetic Resonance, St Joseph's Health Centre (Drs Drost, Carr, and Thompson); and the Departments of Psychiatry (Drs Williamson and Malla) and Physiology (Dr Rylett), University of Western Ontario, London.

See Subjects and Methods on next page

SUBJECTS AND METHODS

SUBJECTS

The schizophrenic patients participating in this study included 11 first-episode drug-naive patients, eight newly diagnosed patients taking medication, and 10 chronic patients taking medication. Two newly diagnosed medicated patients were also examined prior to receiving medication and, therefore, their previous measures were included in the drug-naive group. Patient characteristics are shown in **Table 1**. Of the 11 drug-naive patients (aged 18 to 39 years), nine were classified as having paranoid schizophrenia and two were classified as having as undifferentiated schizophrenia. The length of illness, the time between the onset of positive symptoms and the MR spectroscopy examination, ranged from 1 month to 6 years. None had been exposed to antipsychotic medication; however, six had received 1 to 3 mg of lorazepam in the 24 hours before assessment. Of the 18 patients taking medication (aged 17 to 59 years), eight were considered newly diagnosed, with a mean (±SD) length of illness of 4±2 years and 10 were considered chronic with a length of illness of 18±6 years (Table 1). All medicated patients were receiving antipsychotic medication (mean±SD equivalent dose of chlorpromazine, 560±410 mg). The mean (±SD) length of time on treatment with medication was 1.8±2.8 years for the newly diagnosed patients and 17.7±8.0 years for the chronic patients (Table 1). Fourteen patients reported that they were also taking an anticholinergic medication for side effects. Ten patients were diagnosed as having paranoid illness; two, undifferentiated; and six, residual.

The *DSM-III-R* diagnosis of schizophrenia was established with the Structured Clinical Interview for *DSM-III-R* (SCID)[27] administered by a psychiatrist (P.C.W.). The diagnoses of the drug-naive patients were reconfirmed by the treating psychiatrist 6 months after the MR experiments. Both the Scale for the Assessment of Negative Symptoms (SANS)[28] and the Scale for the Assessment of Positive Symptoms (SAPS)[29] were administered by a psychiatrist (P.C.W.) without any knowledge of the ^{31}P MR spectroscopy results. The mean total SANS and SAPS scores and handedness in terms of writing and throwing a ball for the three patient groups are reported in Table 1. Education level was rated on a four-point scale (1, ≤grade 10; 2, grades 11 to 13; 3, 1 to 3 years of college; and 4, >3 years of college). Parental education level for the most educated parent, or adoptive parent in three cases, was also rated (Table 1).

Twenty-one controls, ranging in age from 18 to 53 years, were recruited by advertisement. The absence of a psychiatric diagnosis was confirmed by a psychiatrist (P.C.W.) with the SCID.[27] The controls were comparably matched for gender, education level, parental education level, and handedness. Subject characteristics of the control group are shown in Table 1.

Patients and controls had no history of head injury, alcohol or other drug abuse, or serious medical illness based on information provided during the SCID interview. No gross abnormalities were detected on routine clinical MR images that were acquired for each subject. None of the drug-naive patients, all of the medicated patients, and eight of the 21 controls had undergone at least one previous MR imaging scan.

^{31}P MR SPECTROSCOPY

All the experiments were conducted using a whole-body MR spectrometer (Helicon SP System, Siemens AG, Erlangen, Germany) operating at a static magnetic field of 2 T with a 5-cm diameter transmit/receive surface coil tunable to both proton (^{1}H) and ^{31}P frequencies. The surface coil limited the depth of reception of the MR signal to cortical structures. In addition, the ^{31}P MR signal from the surface, which includes the scalp, skull, and frontalis muscle, was minimized with the use of the localized MR spectroscopy pulse sequence, fast rotating gradient spectroscopy (FROGS).[30] The FROGS sequence contains slice-selective pulses that saturate the ^{31}P MR signal within a specified slice. This saturation slice was oriented parallel with the surface coil and positioned between the surface coil and the cortex area.[26] Depending on the subject, the thickness of the saturation slice ranged from 2.0 to 3.0 cm. Correct positioning of the surface coil over the area of the left dorsolateral prefrontal cortex and the saturation slice was confirmed by ^{1}H MR sagittal images acquired with the surface coil. Immediately following the execution of the saturation slice, a nonselective excitation pulse, 300 microseconds, was applied. With a pulse repetition time of 2000 milliseconds, the amplitude of the excitation pulse was adjusted to maximize the ^{31}P MR signal. Therefore, the surface coil

lism through phosphomonoesters (PMEs) and phosphodiesters (PDEs). The intracellular pH and the intracellular free magnesium concentration ($[Mg^{2+}]_{intra}$) can also be calculated from the positions of spectral peaks.

Pettegrew and coworkers[24] observed decreased levels of PMEs, which are precursors to the synthesis of membrane phospholipids, and higher levels of PDEs, which are the breakdown products of membrane phospholipids, in the prefrontal region (left and right side combined) of first-episode drug-naive schizophrenic patients compared with controls. Increased levels of ATP and decreased levels of Pi were also observed. Williamson and coworkers[25] reported lower PME levels and higher PCr levels but no differences in PDE, Pi, or ATP levels from the left dorsolateral prefrontal region in 10 chronic medicated schizophrenic patients compared with seven controls. In addition, the $[Mg^{2+}]_{intra}$ was higher in these patients. In a preliminary follow-up unblinded study of schizophrenic patients taking medication, Stanley et al[26] observed lower PME levels in schizophrenics compared with controls, but PDE levels were increased only in patients early on in their illness. These findings suggest that the phospholipids of cell membranes may be involved in the prefrontal functional and/or structural deficits seen in schizophrenia. They also suggest that there may be differences in metabolic levels according to the stage of illness.

Our objectives were to examine the effects of stage of illness on the ^{31}P MR metabolites with blindly analyzed data and to examine the correlations between clinical symptom measures and ^{31}P MR spectroscopy and the FROGS sequence with its saturation slice enabled appropriate sampling of approximately 15 to 20 cm^3 of brain tissue in the left dorsolateral prefrontal cortex. The free induction decay signal, 300 milliseconds, was digitized with 4096 complex data points and 600 acquisitions were averaged. The preacquisition delay time was 1 millisecond. Furthermore, the static magnetic field homogeneity was maximized before data acquisition such that the full width at half maximum (FWHM) of the water resonance was approximately equal to 12 Hz.

POSTSPECTRAL PROCESSING

All the data files were coded to completely blind the operator to the status of the subjects. A noninteractive modeling technique based on linear prediction and singular value decomposition[31] was then applied to reconstruct the missing data points in the preacquisition delay time. The use of a 1-millisecond delay time minimized the contribution of any short T_2 species (ie, after a millisecond of relaxation, the time domain signal from bone and membrane phospholipids has predominantly decayed, whereas the attenuation of the PDE and PME signal is minimal) in the reconstruction, as demonstrated in the study by Stanley et al.[26] The free induction decay was exponentially filtered with 6-Hz line broadening, zero-filled from 4096 to 8192 data points, and then Fourier transformed. Reconstructing the initial data points on the free induction decay guaranteed a preacquisition delay time of zero; therefore, the adjustment of first-order phasing was within $\pm 1/2$ a dwell period. The operator then only adjusted the zero-order phase.

The area under each spectral peak is directly proportional to the concentration of that metabolite. Peak areas (amplitude multiplied by the FWHM) were obtained by modeling spectral peaks with Lorentzian line shapes. By varying the amplitude, line width, and position of each peak, the "best fit" between the sum of the modeled line shapes and the acquired spectrum was achieved with a nonlinear least squares fitting algorithm of Marquardt-Levenberg[32] (**Figure 1**). The triplet β-ATP was fitted with three Lorentzian line shapes of equal line widths; the doublets γ-ATP and α-ATP were fitted with two Lorentzian line shapes of equal line widths. All metabolite levels were expressed as a percentage of the total area of the observed ^{31}P MR signal. Quoted values of the peak's FWHM and chemical shift were taken from the modeled spectra. The intracellular pH was calculated from the chemical shift difference between Pi and PCr.[33] Each spectrum was modeled a second time using single Lorentzian line shapes for the fitting of the γ-, α- and β-ATP peaks to calculate the $[Mg^{2+}]_{intra}$ from the chemical shift difference between α-ATP and β-ATP.[34] The data were processed using a personal computer and the NMR-286 software package (SoftPulse Software, Guelph, Ontario).

To test the reliability of the methods and biological variations, ^{31}P MR spectroscopy measures were repeated in five chronic medicated schizophrenic patients and five controls. There were no statistically significant differences in metabolite levels between the first and second measures except for PCr, which was lower on the second measure.[35] κ Coefficients were calculated using an appropriate cutoff level for PME and $[Mg^{2+}]_{intra}$ to assign patient or control status on the first or second measure. The κ coefficients were 0.8 ($P<.01$) and 1.0 ($P<.001$) for PME levels and $[Mg^{2+}]_{intra}$, respectively.[35]

STATISTICAL ANALYSIS

A two-tailed *t* test was used to determine any significant differences in age, education level, and parental education level when comparing the drug-naive and the combined medicated group patients with the control group. If normality of the data failed (ie, $P<.05$), a Mann-Whitney rank-sum test was performed. Quantified ^{31}P MR parameters were modeled in a stepwise multiple regression analysis with subject group (ie, patient and control), age, gender, education level, and parental education level as independent parameters. This method enabled us to compare differences in the ^{31}P MR parameters between patient and control groups while adjusting for the covariables of age, gender, education level, and parental education level. *P* values of less than .05 were considered statistically significant and a threshold value of $P=.15$ was used to enter or remove independent variables from the multiple regression analysis. Pearson product moment correlations of age, length of illness, length of time taking medication, equivalent dose of chlorpromazine, SANS scores, SAPS scores, and total SANS and SAPS scores with levels of PME, Pi, PDE, PCr, ATP, and $[Mg^{2+}]_{intra}$ were evaluated for the control group and combined patient groups.

parameters. Additionally, we wished to investigate if our results on first-episode drug-naive schizophrenic patients compare with the findings of the pilot study of Pettegrew et al.[24] Therefore, ^{31}P MR spectra from the left dorsolateral prefrontal cortex of first-episode drug-naive, newly diagnosed medicated, and chronic medicated schizophrenic patients were acquired and compared with those of appropriately matched controls.

RESULTS

There were no significant differences in age, education level, and parental education level when comparing the drug-naive and the combined medicated patient groups with the control group. (The parental education levels of the controls and the medicated patient group failed the normality test.)

A typical in vivo ^{31}P MR spectrum from the left dorsolateral prefrontal cortex of a control is shown in Figure 1. In the spectrum, PME, Pi, PDE, PCr, and the three phosphate peaks from the ATP molecule are resolved (Figure 1). The signal-to-noise ratio of 100 for the PCr peak and 40 for the β-ATP peak is sufficient to reliably quantify the ^{31}P MR spectra. The mean ^{31}P metabolite levels of the patient groups and the control group are shown in **Figure 2**. Significantly decreased levels of PMEs were observed in the first-episode drug-naive group ($P<.001$), the newly diagnosed medicated group ($P<.001$), and the chronic medicated group ($P<.001$) compared with the control group. All 29 PME values from the patients failed to overlap within 1 SD of the PME values when com-

Table 1. Subject Characteristics*

Characteristic	Control Group	Schizophrenic Patients: First Episode Drug Naive	Newly Diagnosed Medicated	Chronic Medicated
Gender				
M	17	8	8	9
F	4	3	0	1
Age, y	31±9	26±7	23±6	43±7
Right-handedness	17	11	8	9
Education level†	2.7±1.0	2.4±0.8	2.3±0.7	2.8±0.6
Parental education level†	2.4±0.7	2.4±0.7	2.4±0.8	1.9±0.9
Length of illness, y	...	2±2	4±2	18±6
Length of time receiving medication, y	...	...	1.8±2.8	17.7±8.0
SANS score	...	41±11	35±14	19±10
SAPS score	...	31±10	9±10	5±7

Except for gender and handedness, data are given as mean±SD. SANS indicates Scale for the Assessment of Negative Symptoms; SAPS, Scale for the Assessment of Positive Symptoms.

†Education level was rated as follows: 1, ≤grade 10; 2, grades 11 to 13; 3, 1 to 3 years of college, and 4, >3 years of college.

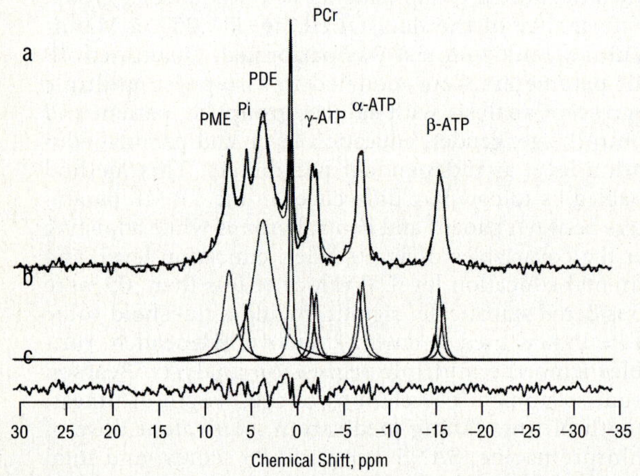

Figure 1. *a, A typical in vivo phosphorus 31 magnetic resonance (³¹P MR) spectrum (thick line) from the left dorsolateral prefrontal cortex of a control superimposed on the modeled spectrum (thin line). The spectral peaks are phosphomonoester (PME), inorganic orthophosphate (Pi), phosphodiester (PDE), phosphocreatine (PCr), and γ-, α- and β-adenosine triphosphate (ATP). b, The individual Lorentzian line shapes of the modeled spectrum. c, The difference between the acquired spectrum and the modeled spectrum.*

pared with those of the controls. When the three patient groups were combined, there was a significant decrease in the FWHM of the PME peak ($P<.001$) compared with the control group (**Table 2**). A significant increase in the PDE level of first-episode drug-naive schizophrenic patients was observed compared with the control group (Figure 2). However, no significant differences in PDE levels were observed between the newly diagnosed medicated and chronic medicated schizophrenic patients and the control group. When comparing the FWHM values and chemical shift of the PDE peak between the drug-naive patient group and the control group, significant differences were observed (Table 2). Except for a significant decrease in the Pi level in the newly diagnosed medicated group, no other significant differences in the high-energy phosphate metabolites were observed between any of the patient groups compared with the control group (Figure 2). The $[Mg^{2+}]_{intra}$ was significantly increased in first-episode drug-naive, newly diagnosed medicated, and chronic medicated patients ($P<.001$) compared with the controls (Table 2). No significant differences in the intracellular pH were observed.

In the combined patient group, ^{31}P metabolite levels and $[Mg^{2+}]_{intra}$ were not significantly correlated with the length of time taking medication, equivalent dose of chlorpromazine, or SANS or SAPS scores. In addition, the total SANS and SAPS scores of the combined patient groups, which reflect the severity of the illness, did not correlate with any of the ^{31}P metabolites. However, in this same group, the correlation between the PDE level and length of illness was −0.43 (P=.02), which is not significant with a Bonferroni correction for multiple comparisons. The PDE and age correlation was −0.28 (P=.2) in the combined patient group and 0.37 (P=.1) in the control group. In the first-episode drug-naive patients, there were no significant correlations between the dose of lorazepam and the ^{31}P metabolites and the $[Mg^{2+}]_{intra}$. Using a Mann-Whitney rank-sum test, there was no significant difference in the ^{31}P metabolites between the medicated patients who were (n=14) and were not (n=4) receiving anticholinergic medication.

COMMENT

A significant reduction in PME level in the left dorsolateral prefrontal cortex was observed in first-episode drug-naive, newly diagnosed medicated, and chronic medicated schizophrenic patients compared with the control group. The PME reduction of roughly 20% was striking as none of the 29 patients had PME values within 1 SD of the control group. In addition, the PME line width was significantly narrower and the PME chemical shift tended to be less than that of the chemical shift of the controls (Table 2). The PME line shape consists of a distribution of different PMEs, which cannot be resolved under these experimental conditions.[36] Phosphocholine, phosphoethanolamine, and L-phosphoserine are the predominant metabolites contributing to the observed PME line shape with their own distinct resonant frequencies.[37] Therefore, the evidence of a reduction in area and line width of the PME line shape and a trend in a shift in frequency away from the phosphoethanolamine resonant frequency of 6.78 ppm[36] suggest that the reduced levels of PME observed throughout the illness of schizophrenia could be due to a reduction in the phosphoethanolamine level. There are many processes that could result in a PME reduction: decreased kinase activity, decreased phospholipase-C activity, decreased phosphodiesterase activity, or increased phosphatase activity.[24,38]

Significantly increased levels of PDE were observed only in first-episode drug-naive patients compared with the control group. Similar to the line shape of PME, the PDE line shape is composed of a distribution of different PDEs. Metabolites dominating the PDE line shape include glycerol 3-phosphoethanolamine at 3.51 ppm[36] and glycerol 3-phosphocholine at 2.99 ppm.[35] The PDE line width was significantly broader and there was a significant shift in the PDE resonant frequency closer to the glycerol 3-phosphocholine resonant frequency in the drug-naive patients compared with the controls. Therefore, glycerol 3-phosphocholine could be implicated for the significant PDE increase in patients early in their illness. Processes that can increase the PDE level include a reduction of phosphodiesterase activity or increased phospholipase A_1 and A_2 activity.[24,38] Gattaz et al[39,40] have observed increased platelet phospholipase A_2 activity in schizophrenia. However, Bennett et al[41] reported no differences in the phospholipase A_2 activity in lymphoblast cell lines of schizophrenic patients compared with controls.

The differences observed in the PME and PDE levels are consistent with those of previous ^{31}P MR spectroscopy studies.[24-26] However, the reported increase in PDE level of newly diagnosed medicated patients[26] was not reproduced in this blind study. Phosphomonoesters are predominantly involved in the phospholipid synthesis of cell membranes and PDEs are predominantly found in the catabolic pathway of membrane phospholipids.[38] Therefore, only early in the illness of schizophrenia before medication treatment, membrane phospholipid breakdown products from phosphatidylcholine are increased and precursors to the synthesis of phosphatidylethanolamine, a phospholipid that is localized mainly on the cytoplasmic side of the membrane bilayer, are decreased. As the illness progresses to the chronic stage, the levels of breakdown products are normalized but precursors of membrane phospholipids are still reduced. It is possible that the process that causes the increase in breakdown products occurs much earlier in the illness and we are only observing the tail end of this process. A synaptic pruning process of excess axonal terminals occurs during normal development in late adolescence and in young adulthood.[42-46] Coinciding with this normal neurodevelopmental process, a pattern of decreased PMEs and increased PDEs are observed between the ages of 10 and 20 years.[47] Our ^{31}P MR spectroscopy findings and those of Pettegrew et al[24] show similar but enhanced patterns of decreased PMEs and increased PDEs in first-episode drug-naive schizophrenic patients. Pettegrew et al[24,47] suggested that this enhanced pattern observed in these patients is due to overexaggerated synaptic pruning of prefrontal axonal terminals, a hypothesis that was first introduced by Feinberg.[48] It may be argued that the medication has altered the level of PDEs since these levels are increased in the drug-naive patients and not in the medicated patients. However, PDE levels did not correlate with the medication dose or the length of time on medication treatment. The PDE–length of illness correlation observed in the schizophrenic patients is not a strong finding since the correlation was not significant after a Bonferroni correction. But, it does indicate that the PDE levels are more dependent on the length of illness than on the medication status.

It is of interest that numerous studies have observed differences in the composition of membrane phospholipids in erythrocytes and platelets of schizophrenic patients compared with controls.[49] Several authors have reported conflicting results, observing either a decrease in the phosphatidylethanolamine concentration[50-53] or no difference[54-56] in schizophrenic patients compared with controls. Significantly decreased concentrations of phosphatidylcholine in patients compared with controls have been observed in several studies[50,52,55,57] and no differences[53,54,56] and an increase[51] in concentrations have also been observed. Furthermore, the reduction in synthesis of phosphatidylethanolamine has the potential to reduce the synthesis of phosphatidylcholine via the phospholipid methylation pathway or the base-exchange process.[58] Several studies have observed a reduction in methylation activity in erythrocytes of schizophrenic patients relative to controls.[55,57,59,60]

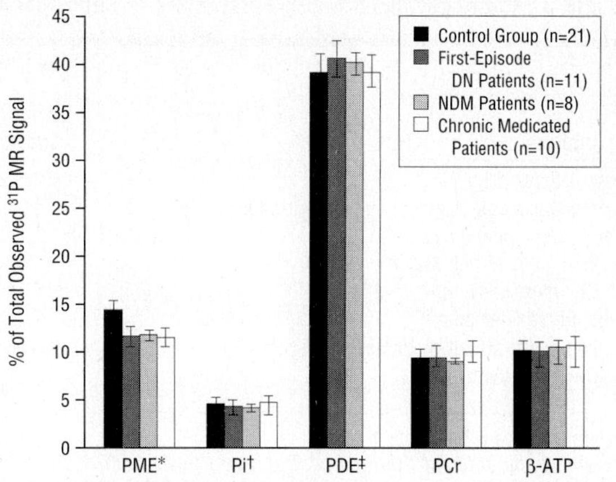

Figure 2. *The mean metabolite levels, expressed as a percentage of total observed phosphorus 31 magnetic resonance (^{31}P MR) signal, of the control group, drug-naive (DN), newly diagnosed medicated (NDM), and chronic medicated schizophrenic patients. The error bars represent 1 SD. PME indicates phosphomonoester; Pi, inorganic orthophosphate; PDE, phosphodiester; PCr, phosphocreatine; ATP, adenosine triphosphate; asterisk, significantly different between DN patients and controls (F=52.8; df=3,28; P<.001), significantly different between NDM patients and controls (F=48.4; df=3,25; P<.001), and significantly different between chronic medicated patients and controls (F=33.5; df=3,27; P<.001); dagger, significantly different between NDM patients and controls (F=4.03; df=1,27; P=.05); and double dagger, significantly different between DN patients and controls (F=4.27; df=2,29; P=.048) and nonsignificant between NDM patients and controls (F=2.58; df=2,26; P=.12).*

Under normal conditions, membrane phospholipids are constantly turning over at different metabolic rates with different metabolizing enzymes. Maintaining the proper structural integrity and functional activity of neuronal membrane phospholipids is crucial for neurotransmitter release, ion transport, calcium homeostasis, receptor binding, and membrane fusion.[58] Consequently, it is unclear how to interpret the reduced PME level observed throughout the illness of schizophrenia. The effect of the antipsychotic medication influencing the PME levels must be discounted since the PME levels were lower in the drug-naive and medicated patients. The PME levels also did not correlate with the clinical symptoms. If an altered neurodevelopmental process is present early in the illness of schizophrenia, then the reduction in membrane phospholipid precursors may reflect structural abnormalities as a result of this process. These abnormalities may include a deficit in gray matter volume, which

Table 2. Additional Quantifiable Parameters of Schizophrenic Patients and Controls*

		Schizophrenic Patients		
Parameter	**Control Group**	**First Episode Drug Naive**	**Newly Diagnosed Medicated**	**Chronic Medicated**
Intracellular pH	7.057±0.020	7.053±0.021	7.068±0.017	7.068±0.021
Intracellular free magnesium concentration, μmol	321±27	418±89†	352±36‡	375±32§
Phosphomonoester peak				
Full width at half maximum, Hz	51±6		44±4‖	
Chemical shift, ppm	6.71±0.04		6.69±0.03¶	
Phosphodiester peak				
Full width at half maximum, Hz	86±6	92±7#	88±6	
Chemical shift, ppm	2.96±0.04	2.91±0.04**	2.95±0.04	

*Data are given as mean±1 SD.
†Significantly different from the control group (F=21.5; df=1,30; P<.001).
‡Significantly different from the control group (F=6.94; df=2,26; P=.014).
§Significantly different from the control group (F=23.9; df=1,29; P<.001).
‖Significantly different between the combined patients and the control group (F=20.1; df=2,45; P<.001).
¶When comparing the combined patients with the control group, F=3.43; df=2,45; P=.07.
#Significantly different from the control group (F=7.74; df=2,29; P=.009).
**Significantly different from the control group (F=9.75; df=1,30; P=.004).

would be consistent with the volumetric MR imaging study by Zipursky et al.[20] However, Breier et al[18] and Buchanan et al[19] have observed a deficit only in white matter volume in the prefrontal region of schizophrenic patients compared with controls. Recently, Hinsberger and colleagues[61] have examined both gray and white matter volumes in the frontal lobes of schizophrenic patients compared with controls. That study included some of the patients in the study herein (ie, 10 drug-naive and nine chronic medicated patients). While PME levels were decreased and $[Mg^{2+}]_{intra}$ was increased in patients compared with controls, there were no differences in left gray or white matter volumes. With this result, the lower PME levels of approximately 20% observed throughout the illness would not be due to any gray or white matter deficit. This would suggest that reduced precursors of membrane phospholipids may reflect metabolic abnormalities rather than structural changes. Ultimately, direct in vitro or in vivo ^{31}P MR spectroscopy evidence is needed to determine if there is a relationship between the concentration of PMEs and the gray matter volume.

Inconsistencies have been observed in assessing the in vivo high-energy phosphate metabolism in the prefrontal region. Pettegrew and colleagues[24] first reported increased ATP levels and decreased Pi levels in drug-naive patients compared with controls, which suggests hypofrontality. However, subsequent ^{31}P MR spectroscopy studies have failed to reproduce these alterations in the high-energy phosphate metabolism. In this study, there were no differences in the levels of the high-energy phosphate metabolites between any of the patient groups and the controls except for the decreased Pi levels in the newly diagnosed medicated patients. This change in Pi level may be due to the initial administration of the medication. In a preliminary study, Williamson et al[25] reported an increase in the PCr level in chronic medicated patients compared with controls. Moreover, differences in the PCr level were observed between first and second measures in a reproducibility study.[35] Consequently, these observations do not provide evidence supporting a reduction in the utilization of ATP in the left dorsolateral prefrontal cortex of schizophrenic patients as previously reported.[24] Overall, the high-energy phosphate metabolites seem to behave as state-dependent variables. One would then expect factors such as SANS or SAPS scores to correlate with these high-energy phosphate metabolites, which was not the case in this study. In a preliminary study, Kato et al[62] did, however, report increased PCr levels in schizophrenic patients with a higher number of negative symptoms compared with patients with a lower number of negative symptoms.

The $[Mg^{2+}]_{intra}$ was increased in all three patient groups compared with controls. Mg^{2+} is an abundant intracellular and extracellular cation that is a necessary cofactor for many enzymes, including those involved in the transfer of phosphate groups.[63] In addition, abnormal regulation of the $[Mg^{2+}]_{intra}$ has the potential to block the signal transduction of glutamate subtype receptor channels (*N*-methyl-D-aspartate) and ion receptor channels in a voltage-dependent manner.[64] As a result, a reciprocal relationship exists between the $[Mg^{2+}]_{intra}$ and the binding of inositol-(1,4,5)-triphosphate to its receptor and subsequent release of calcium from intracellular stores.[65] Therefore, abnormal levels of $Mg^{2+}{}_{intra}$ could suggest that cellular metabolic activity is reduced, which could lead to further suppression of neuronal function(s). This would be consistent with the functional abnormalities observed in the frontal lobes of schizophrenic patients by other techniques, as noted in the introduction.

A number of limitations must be acknowledged. First, it is possible that lorazepam and the anticholinergic medication may have affected the ^{31}P MR spectroscopy results. However, there were no significant correlations between the dose of lorazepam and the ^{31}P metabolites and the $[Mg^{2+}]_{intra}$. There were no significant differences in the levels of the ^{31}P metabolites and $[Mg^{2+}]_{intra}$ between the patients who were and were not receiving the anticholinergic medication. Additionally, the decreased PME and increased $[Mg^{2+}]_{intra}$ were observed in the first-episode drug-naive patients and also in the patients taking medication, which would discount any effects due to the different medication status. Second, the sampled tissue volumes variy between subjects, and gray matter volume contribution varies within those tissue volumes. Cerebral spinal fluid has no contribution to the observed ^{31}P MR signal.[66] Normalizing the peak areas of the metabolites to the total observed peak areas corrects for the variation in volume of excitation from subject to subject but assumes there is a constant proportion of gray to white matter. The recent volumetric MR imaging study by Hinsberger et al[61] does, however, provide evidence to support the assumption of similar gray/white matter in patients and controls. Third, it is possible that the spin-lattice relaxation time constant (T_1) saturation effects may explain the observed differences in the PME area. The ^{31}P MR signal, which constitutes long T_1 species, does not fully recover its equilibrium magnetization because of the short repetition time used between acquisitions (ie, the observed ^{31}P MR signal is less than the ^{31}P MR signal at equilibrium). Consequently, an increase in the T_1 of the PMEs could account for the decrease in the PME level observed in the patients. However, to observe a change in T_1 would require an alteration in the physical and/or chemical environment of the PMEs (ie, to change the characteristics of the molecular motion of the PMEs), which could still affect the normal function of the precursors of membrane phospholipids. Fourth, in terms of T_2 relaxation effects, the ^{31}P MR signal was acquired immediately following the excitation pulse. Therefore, a change in T_2 of a metabolite does not reflect a change in spectral peak area (assuming that the attenuation difference due to the change in T_2 within the preacquisition delay time is negligible since the T_2 of the observed metabolites is much greater than 1 millisecond).[36] And fifth, although Mg^{2+} is an important cofactor in many enzymatic reactions in which ATP is a substrate, it must be noted that the observed differences in chemical shift from which $[Mg^{2+}]_{intra}$ is calculated could also be explained by an abnormal level of another cation binding to the β- and γ-phosphate sites of ATP rather than Mg^{2+}.

In summary, abnormalities were observed in the membrane phospholipid metabolism of schizophrenic patients relative to matched controls. First-episode drug-naive patients demonstrated decreased levels of PMEs and increased levels of PDEs. Newly diagnosed medicated patients and chronic medicated patients had decreased levels of only PMEs, suggesting that the stage of illness may be an important variable related to these changes. No differences in high-energy phosphate metabolism were observed between subject groups, except for lower Pi levels in newly diagnosed medicated patients. The measured $[Mg^{2+}]_{intra}$ was significantly higher in all the patient groups, which has the potential of influencing the signal transduction of N-methyl-D-aspartate receptors. Consequently, these in vivo findings suggest that the alterations in the membrane phospholipids metabolism are, in part, involved in the pathophysiology of schizophrenia.

Accepted for publication January 23, 1995.

This study was supported by the Ontario Mental Health Foundation, Medical Research Council of Canada (grant MT-12078) and The National Institute of Mental Health (grant 1 R01 MH50768-01).

The authors acknowledge the assistance of Harold Merskey, DM, Rahul Manchanda, MD, and Larry Stitt, MSc.

Reprint requests to Department of Psychiatry, University Hospital, 339 Windermere Rd, London, Ontario, Canada N6A 5A5 (Dr Williamson).

REFERENCES

1. Hoffman RE, Buchsbaum MS, Escobar MD, Makuch RWI, Nuechterlein KH, Guich SM. EEG coherence of prefrontal areas in normal and schizophrenic males during perceptual activation. *J Neuropsychiatry Clin Neurosci.* 1991;3:169-175.
2. Morrison-Stewart SL, Williamson PC, Corning WC, Kutcher SP, Merskey H. Coherence on electroencephalography and aberrant functional organisation of the brain in schizophrenic patients during activation tasks. *Br J Psychiatry.* 1991;159:636-644.
3. Berman K, Zec R, Weinberger D. Physiological dysfunction of dorsolateral prefrontal cortex in schizophrenia, II: role of neuroleptic treatment, attention, and mental effort. *Arch Gen Psychiatry.* 1986;43:126-135.
4. Berman K, Illowsky B, Weinberger D. Physiological dysfunction of the dorsolateral prefrontal cortex in schizophrenia, IV: further evidence for regional and behavioral specificity. *Arch Gen Psychiatry.* 1988;45:616-622.
5. Weinberger D, Berman K, Zec R. Physiological dysfunction of dorsolateral and prefrontal cortex in schizophrenia, I: regional cerebral blood flow evidence. *Arch Gen Psychiatry.* 1986;43:114-124.
6. Weinberger D, Berman K, Illowsky B. Physiological dysfunction of the dorsolateral prefrontal cortex in schizophrenia, III: a new cohort and evidence for a monoaminergic mechanism. *Arch Gen Psychiatry.* 1988;45:609-615.
7. Cohen SM, Semple W, Gross M, Nordahl TE, DeLisi LE, Holcomb HH, Morihisa JM, Pikar D. Dysfunction in a prefrontal substate of sustained attention in schizophrenia. *Life Sci.* 1987;40:2031-2039.
8. Volkow N, Wolfe S, van Gelder P, Brodie JD, Overall JE, Cancero R, Gomez-Mont F. Phenomenological correlates of metabolism activity in 18 patients with chronic schizophrenia. *Am J Psychiatry.* 1987;144:151-158.
9. Buchsbaum MS. The frontal lobes, basal ganglia, and temporal lobes as sites for schizophrenia. *Schizophr Bull.* 1990;16:379-389.
10. Buchsbaum MS, Neuchterlein KH, Haier RJ, Wu J, Sicotte N, Hazlett E, Asarnow R, Potkin S, Guich S. Glucose metabolic rate in normals and schizophrenics during the continuous performance test assessed by positron emission tomography. *Br J Psychiatry.* 1990;156:216-227.
11. Buchsbaum MS, Haier RJ, Potkin SG, Nuechterlein K, Bracha HS, Katz M, Lohr J, Wu J, Lottenberg S, Jerabek PA, Trenary M, Tafalla R, Reynolds C, Bunney WE Jr. Frontostriatal disorder of cerebral metabolism in never-medicated schizophrenics. *Arch Gen Psychiatry.* 1992;49:935-942.
12. Andreasen NC, Rezai K, Alliger R, Swayze VW, Flaum M, Kirchner P, Cohen G, O'Leary DS. Hypofrontality in neuroleptic-naive patients and in patients with chronic schizophrenia. *Arch Gen Psychiatry.* 1992;49:943-953.
13. Berman KF, Doran AR, Pickar O, Weinberger DR. Is the mechanism of prefrontal hypofunction in depression the same as in schizophrenia? regional cerebral blood flow during cognitive activation. *Br J Psychiatry.* 1993;162:183-192.
14. Kelsoe JR, Cadet JL, Pickar D, Weinberger DR. Quantitative neuroanatomy in schizophrenia: a controlled magnetic resonance imaging study. *Arch Gen Psychiatry.* 1988;45:533-541.
15. Suddath RL, Casanova MF, Goldberg TE, Daniel DG, Kelsoe J, Weinberger DR. Temporal lobe pathology in schizophrenia: a quantitative magnetic resonance imaging study. *Am J Psychiatry.* 1989;146:464-472.
16. Suddath RL, Christisan GW, Torrey EF, Casanova MF, Weinberger DR. Anatomic abnormalities in the brains of monozygotic twins discordant for schizophrenia. *N Engl J Med.* 1990;332:62-67.
17. Andreasen NC, Ehrhardt JC, Swayze VW, Alliger RJ, Yuh WTC, Cohen G, Ziebell S. Magnetic resonance imaging of the brain in schizophrenia. *Arch Gen Psychiatry.* 1990;47:35-44.
18. Breier A, Buchanan RW, Elkashef A, Munson RC, Kirkpatrick B, Gellad F. Brain morphology and schizophrenia: a magnetic resonance imaging study of limbic, prefrontal cortex, and caudate structures. *Arch Gen Psychiatry.* 1992;49:921-926.

19. Buchanan RW, Breier A, Kirkpatrick B, Elkashef A, Munson RC, Gellad F, Carpenter WT Jr. Structural abnormalities in deficit and nondeficit schizophrenia. *Am J Psychiatry.* 1993;150:59-66.
20. Zipursky RB, Lim KO, Sullivan EV, Brown BW, Pfefferbaum A. Widespread cerebral gray matter volume deficits in schizophrenia. *Arch Gen Psychiatry.* 1992; 49:195-205.
21. Williamson PC, Pelz D, Merskey H, Morrison S, Karlik S, Drost D, Carr T, Conlon P. Frontal, temporal, and striatal proton relaxation times in schizophrenic patients and normal comparison subjects. *Am J Psychiatry.* 1992;149:549-551.
22. Bottomley PA. Human in vivo NMR spectroscopy in diagnostic medicine: clinical tool or research probe? *Radiology.* 1989;170:1-15.
23. Keshavan MS, Shitij K, Pettegrew JW. Magnetic resonance spectroscopy in psychiatry: potential, pitfalls, and promise. *Am J Psychiatry.* 1991;148:976-985.
24. Pettegrew JW, Keshavan MS, Panchalingam K, Strychor S, Kaplan DB, Tretta MG, Allen M. Alterations in brain high-energy phosphate and membrane phospholipid metabolism in first-episode, drug-naive schizophrenics: a pilot study of the dorsolateral prefrontal cortex by in vivo phosphorus 31 nuclear magnetic resonance spectroscopy. *Arch Gen Psychiatry.* 1991;48:563-568.
25. Williamson PC, Drost D, Stanley J, Carr T, Morrison S, Merskey H. Localized phosphorus 31 magnetic resonance spectroscopy in chronic schizophrenic patients and normal controls. *Arch Gen Psychiatry.* 1991;48:578.
26. Stanley JA, Williamson PC, Drost DJ, Carr TJ, Morrison S, Merskey H. Membrane phospholipid metabolism and schizophrenia: an in vivo ^{31}P MR spectroscopy study. *Schizophr Res.* 1994;13:209-215.
27. Spitzer R, Williams J. *Structured Clinical Interview for* DSM-III-R. New York, NY: New York Psychiatric Institute; 1985.
28. Andreasen N. *Scale for the Assessment of Negative Symptoms (SANS).* Iowa City: The University of Iowa; 1984.
29. Andreasen N. *Scale for the Assessment of Positive Symptoms (SAPS).* Iowa City: The University of Iowa; 1984.
30. Sauter R, Mueller S, Weber H. Localization in vivo 31 P NMR spectroscopy by combining surface coils and slice-selective saturation. *J Magn Reson Imaging.* 1987;75:167-173.
31. Barkhuijsen H, de Beer R, Bovee WMMJ, van Ormondt D. Retrieval of frequencies, amplitudes, damping factors, and phases from time-domain signals using a linear least-squares procedure. *J Magn Reson Imaging.* 1985;61:465-481.
32. Marquardt DW. An algorithm for least-squares estimation of non-linear parameters. *J Soc Industrial Appl Math.* 1963;11:431-441.
33. Petroff OAC, Prichard JW, Behar KL, Alger JR, den Hollander JA, Shulman RG. Cerebral intracellular pH by ^{31}P nuclear magnetic resonance spectroscopy. *Neurology.* 1985;35:781-788.
34. Gupta RK, Gupta P, Moore RD. MRI studies of intracellular metal ions in intact cells and tissues. *Ann Rev Biophys Bioeng.* 1984;13:221-246.
35. Stanley JA, Williamson PC, Drost DJ, Carr T, Stitt L, Merskey H. In vivo ^{31}P MRS of schizophrenia: a reliability study. *Schizophr Res.* 1993;9:209. Abstract.
36. Merboldt KD, Chien D, Hänicke W, Gyngell ML, Bruhn H, Frahm J. Localized ^{31}P NMR spectroscopy of the adult human brain in vivo using stimulated-echo (STEAM) sequences. *J Magn Reson Imaging.* 1990;89:343-361.
37. Pettegrew JR, Kopp SJ, Minshew NJ, Glonek T, Feliksik JM, Tow JP, Cohen MM. ^{31}P nuclear magnetic resonance studies of phosphoglyceride metabolism in developing and degenerating brain: preliminary observations. *J Neuropathol Exp Neurol.* 1987;46:419-430.
38. Dawson RMC. Enzymatic pathways of phospholipid metabolism in the nervous system. In: Eichberg J, ed. *Phospholipids in Nervous Tissues.* New York, NY: John Wiley & Sons Ltd; 1985:45-78.
39. Gattaz WF, Köllisch M, Thuren T, Virtanen JA, Kinnunen PKJ. Increased plasma phospholipase-A2 activity in schizophrenic patients: reduction after neuroleptic therapy. *Biol Psychiatry.* 1987;22:421-426.
40. Gattaz WF, Hübner CVK, Nevalaineri TJ, Thursen T, Kinnunen PKJ. Increased serum phospholipase A2 activity in schizophrenia: a replication study. *Biol Psychiatry.* 1990;28:495-501.
41. Bennett ER, Yedgar S, Lerer B, Ebstein RP. Phospholipase A_2 activity in Epstein-Barr virus-transformed lymphoblast cells from schizophrenia patients. *Biol Psychiatry.* 1991;29:1058-1062.
42. Höttenlocher PR. Synaptic density in human frontal cortex: developmental changes and effects of aging. *Brain Res.* 1979;163:195-205.
43. Purves D, Lichtman JW. Elimination of synapses in the developing nervous system. *Science.* 1980;210:153-157.
44. Hüttenlocher PR, deCourten C, Garey LJ, Van Der Loos H. Synaptogenesis in human visual cortex: evidence for synapse elimination during normal development. *Neurosci Lett.* 1982;33:247-252.
45. Rakic P, Riley KP. Over-production and elimination of retinal axons in the fetal rhesus monkey. *Science.* 1983;219:1441-1444.
46. Cowan WM. Regressive events in neurogenesis. *Science.* 1984;225:1258-1265.
47. Pettegrew JW, Keshavan MS, Minshew NJ. ^{31}P Nuclear magnetic resonance spectroscopy: neurodevelopment and schizophrenia. *Schizophr Bull.* 1993;19: 35-53.
48. Feinberg I. Schizophrenia: caused by a fault in programmed synaptic elimination during adolescence? *J Psychiatr Res.* 1982;17:319-334.
49. Ryer H, Rotrosen J. Phospholipids and schizophrenia. In: Bazan NG, Horrocks LA, Toffiano G, eds. *Phospholipids in the Nervous System: Biochemical and Molecular Pathology.* Padova, Italy: Liviana Press; 1989;17:177-182.
50. Stevens JD. The distribution of phospholipid fractions in the red cell membrane of schizophrenics. *Schizophr Bull.* 1972;6:60-61.
51. Sengupta N, Datta SC, Sengupta D. Platelet and erythrocyte membrane lipid and phospholipid patterns in different types of mental patients. *Biochem Med.* 1981;25:267-275.
52. Tolbert LC, Monti JA, O'Shields H, Walter-Ryan W, Meadows D, Smythies JR. Defects in transmethylation and membrane lipids in schizophrenia. *Psychopharmacol Bull.* 1983;19:594-599.
53. Keshavan MS, Mallinger AG, Pettegrew JW, Dippold C. Erythrocyte membrane phospholipids in psychotic patients. *J Psychiatry Res.* 1993;49:89-95.
54. Lautin A, Mandio Cordasco D, Segarnick DJ, Wod L, Mason MF, Rotrosen J. Red cell phospholipids in schizophrenia. *Life Sci.* 1982;31:3051-3056.
55. Hitzemann R, Hirschowitz J, Garver D. Membrane abnormalities in the psychoses and affective disorders. *J Psychiatr Res.* 1984;18:319-326.
56. Pangerl AM, Steudle A, Jaroni HW, Rufer R, Gattaz WF. Increased platelet membrane lysophosphatidylcholine in schizophrenia. *Biol Psychiatry.* 1991; 30:837-840.
57. Hitzemann RJ, Mark C, Hirschowitz J, Garver DL. Characteristics of phospholipid methylation in human erythrocyte ghosts: relationship(s) to the psychoses and affective disorders. *Biol Psychiatry.* 1985;20:297-407.
58. Farooqui AA, Horrocks LA. Metabolic and functional aspects of neural membrane phospholipids. In: Horrocks LA, et al, eds. *Phospholipids in the Nervous System: Physiological Roles.* New York, NY: Raven Press Ltd; 1985;2:341-348.
59. Andreoli WM, Maffei T. Blood levels of S-adenosylmethionine in schizophrenia. *Lancet.* 1979;2:922.
60. Kelsoe JR Jr, Tolbert LC, Crews EL, Smythies JR. Kinetic evidence for decreased methionine adenosyltransferase activity in erythrocytes from schizophrenics. *J Neurosci Res.* 1982;8:99-103.
61. Hinsberger A, Williamson PC, Carr T, Stanley JA, Drost DJ, Densmore M, MacFabe G, Montemurro D. MRI volumetric measures and 31P MRS in schizophrenia. International Congress on Schizophrenia Research; April 1995; Warm Springs, Va. Abstract.
62. Kato T, Shioiri T, Murashita J, Hamakawa H, Inubushi T, Takahashi S. Phase-encoded ^{31}P-MRS of the frontal lobes in patients with schizophrenia. *Proc Soc Magn Reson.* 1994;2:602. Abstract.
63. Flatman PW. Mechanisms of magnesium transport. *Ann Rev Physiol.* 1991; 53:259-271.
64. Johnson JW, Ascher P. Voltage-dependent blocks by intracellular Mg^{2+} of *N*-methyl-D-aspartate-active channels. *Biophys J.* 1990;57(5):1085-1090.
65. White AM, Varney MA, Watson SP, Rigby S, Liu CS, Ward JG, Reese CB, Graham HC, Williams RJ. Influence of Mg^{2+} and pH on NMR spectra and radiological binding of inositol 1,4,5-triphosphate. *Biochem J.* 1991;278:759-764.
66. Hugg JW, Matson GB, Twieg DB, Maudsley AA, Sappey-Marinier D, Weiner MW. Phosphorous-31 MR spectroscopic imaging (MRSI) of normal and pathological brains. *Magn Reson Imaging.* 1992;10:227-243.

follows enumerates adverse events that occurred at an incidence of 1% or more, and were more frequent than in the placebo group, among SERZONE-treated patients who participated in short-term (6- to 8-week) placebo-controlled trials in which patients were dosed with SERZONE to ranges of 300 to 600 mg/day. This table shows the percentage of patients in each group who had at least one episode of an event at some time during their treatment. Reported adverse events were classified using a standard COSTART-based Dictionary terminology.

The prescriber should be aware that these figures cannot be used to predict the incidence of side effects in the course of usual medical practice where patient characteristics and other factors differ from those which prevailed in the clinical trials. Similarly, the cited frequencies cannot be compared with figures obtained from other clinical investigations involving different treatments, uses, and investigators. The cited figures, however, do provide the prescribing physician with some basis for estimating the relative contribution of drug and nondrug factors to the side-effect incidence rate in the population studied.

Treatment-Emergent Adverse Experience Incidence in 6- to 8-Week Placebo-Controlled Clinical Trials[1] SERZONE 300 to 600 mg/day Dose Range

Body System	Preferred Term	SERZONE (n=393)	Placebo (n=394)
Body as a Whole	Headache	36%	33%
	Asthenia	11%	5%
	Infection	8%	6%
	Flu syndrome	3%	2%
	Chills	2%	1%
	Fever	2%	1%
	Neck rigidity	1%	0%
Cardiovascular	Postural hypotension	4%	1%
	Hypotension	2%	1%
Dermatological	Pruritus	2%	1%
	Rash	2%	1%
Gastrointestinal	Dry mouth	25%	13%
	Nausea	22%	12%
	Constipation	14%	8%
	Dyspepsia	9%	7%
	Diarrhea	8%	7%
	Increased appetite	5%	3%
	Nausea & Vomiting	2%	1%
Metabolic	Peripheral edema	3%	2%
	Thirst	1%	<1%
Musculoskeletal	Arthralgia	1%	<1%
Nervous	Somnolence	25%	14%
	Dizziness	17%	5%
	Insomnia	11%	9%
	Lightheadedness	10%	3%
	Confusion	7%	2%
	Memory impairment	4%	2%
	Paresthesia	4%	2%
	Vasodilatation[2]	4%	2%
	Abnormal dreams	3%	2%
	Concentration decreased	3%	1%
	Ataxia	2%	0%
	Incoordination	2%	1%
	Psychomotor retardation	2%	1%
	Tremor	2%	1%
	Hypertonia	1%	0%
	Libido decreased	1%	<1%
Respiratory	Pharyngitis	6%	5%
	Cough increased	3%	1%
Special Senses	Blurred vision	9%	3%
	Abnormal vision[3]	7%	1%
	Tinnitus	2%	1%
	Taste perversion	2%	1%
	Visual field defect	2%	0%
Urogenital	Urinary frequency	2%	1%
	Urinary tract infection	2%	1%
	Urinary retention	2%	1%
	Vaginitis[4]	2%	1%
	Breast pain[4]	1%	<1%

[1] Events reported by at least 1% of patients treated with SERZONE and more frequent than the placebo group are included; incidence is rounded to the nearest 1% (<1% indicates an incidence less than 0.5%). Events for which the SERZONE incidence was equal to or less than placebo are not listed in the table, but included the following: abdominal pain, pain, back pain, accidental injury, chest pain, neck pain, palpitation, migraine, sweating, flatulence, vomiting, anorexia, tooth disorder, weight gain, edema, myalgia, cramp, agitation, anxiety, depression, hypesthesia, CNS stimulation, dysphoria, emotional lability, sinusitis, rhinitis, dysmenorrhea,[4] dysuria.

[2] Vasodilatation—flushing, feeling warm.

[3] Abnormal vision—scotoma, visual trails.

[4] Incidence adjusted for gender.

Dose Dependency of Adverse Events: The table that follows enumerates adverse events that were more frequent in the SERZONE (nefazodone hydrochloride) dose range of 300 to 600 mg/day than in the SERZONE dose range of up to 300 mg/day. This table shows only those adverse events for which there was a statistically significant difference (p≤0.05) in incidence between the SERZONE dose ranges as well as a difference between the high dose range and placebo.

Dose Dependency of Adverse Events in Placebo-Controlled Trials[1]

Body System	Preferred Term	SERZONE 300-600 mg/day (n = 209)	SERZONE ≤300 mg/day (n = 211)	Placebo (n = 212)
Gastrointestinal	Nausea	23%	14%	12%
	Constipation	17%	10%	9%
Nervous	Somnolence	28%	16%	13%
	Dizziness	22%	11%	4%
	Confusion	8%	2%	1%
Special Senses	Abnormal vision	10%	0%	2%
	Blurred vision	9%	3%	2%
	Tinnitus	3%	0%	1%

[1] Events for which there was a statistically significant difference (p≤0.05) between the nefazodone dose groups.

Vital Sign Changes: (See PRECAUTIONS Section, Postural Hypotension Subsection.)

Weight Changes: In a pooled analysis of placebo-controlled premarketing studies, there were no differences between nefazodone and placebo groups in the proportions of patients meeting criteria for potentially important increases or decreases in body weight (a change of ≥7%).

Laboratory Changes: Of the serum chemistry, serum hematology, and urinalysis parameters monitored during placebo-controlled premarketing studies with nefazodone, a pooled analysis revealed a statistical trend between nefazodone and placebo for hematocrit, i.e., 2.8% of nefazodone patients met criteria for a potentially important decrease in hematocrit (≤37% male or ≤32% female) compared to 1.5% of placebo patients (0.05<p≤0.10). Decreases in hematocrit, presumably dilutional, have been reported with many other drugs that block alpha$_1$-adrenergic receptors. There was no apparent clinical significance of the observed changes in the few patients meeting these criteria.

ECG Changes: Of the ECG parameters monitored during placebo-controlled premarketing studies with nefazodone, a pooled analysis revealed a statistically significant difference between nefazodone and placebo for sinus bradycardia, i.e., 1.5% of nefazodone patients met criteria for a potentially important decrease in heart rate (≤50 bpm and a decrease of ≥15 bpm) compared to 0.4% of placebo patients (p<0.05). There was no obvious clinical significance of the observed changes in the few patients meeting these criteria.

Other Events Observed During the Premarketing Evaluation of SERZONE

During its premarketing assessment, multiple doses of SERZONE were administered to 3496 patients in clinical studies, including more than 250 patients treated for at least one year. The conditions and duration of exposure to SERZONE varied greatly, and included (in overlapping categories) open and double-blind studies, uncontrolled and controlled studies, inpatient and outpatient studies, fixed-dose and titration studies. Untoward events associated with this exposure were recorded by clinical investigators using terminology of their own choosing. Consequently, it is not possible to provide a meaningful estimate of the proportion of individuals experiencing adverse events without first grouping similar types of untoward events into a smaller number of standardized event categories.

In the tabulations that follow, reported adverse events were classified using a standard COSTART-based Dictionary terminology. The frequencies presented, therefore, represent the proportion of the 3496 patients exposed to multiple doses of SERZONE who experienced an event of the type cited on at least one occasion while receiving SERZONE. All reported events are included except those already listed in the Treatment-Emergent Adverse Experience Incidence table, those events listed in other safety-related sections of this insert, those adverse experiences subsumed under COSTART terms that are either overly general or excessively specific so as to be uninformative, those events for which a drug cause was very remote, and those events which were not serious and occurred in fewer than two patients.

It is important to emphasize that, although the events reported occurred during treatment with SERZONE (nefazodone hydrochloride), they were not necessarily caused by it.

Events are further categorized by body system and listed in order of decreasing frequency according to the following definitions: frequent adverse events are those occurring on one or more occasions in at least 1/100 patients (only those not already listed in the tabulated results from placebo-controlled trials appear in this listing); infrequent adverse events are those occurring in 1/100 to 1/1000 patients; rare events are those occurring in fewer than 1/1000 patients.

Body as a Whole—*Infrequent:* allergic reaction, malaise, photosensitivity reaction, face edema, hangover effect, abdomen enlarged, hernia, pelvic pain, and halitosis. *Rare:* cellulitis.

Cardiovascular System—*Infrequent:* tachycardia, hypertension, syncope, ventricular extrasystoles, and angina pectoris. *Rare:* AV block, congestive heart failure, hemorrhage, pallor, and varicose vein.

Dermatological System—*Infrequent:* dry skin, acne, alopecia, urticaria, maculopapular rash, vesiculobullous rash, and eczema.

Gastrointestinal System—*Frequent:* gastroenteritis. *Infrequent:* eructation, periodontal abscess, abnormal liver function tests, gingivitis, colitis, gastritis, mouth ulceration, stomatitis, esophagitis, peptic ulcer, and rectal hemorrhage. *Rare:* glossitis, hepatitis, dysphagia, gastrointestinal hemorrhage, oral moniliasis, and ulcerative colitis.

Hemic and Lymphatic System—*Infrequent:* ecchymosis, anemia, leukopenia, and lymphadenopathy.

Metabolic and Nutritional System—*Infrequent:* weight loss, gout, dehydration, lactic dehydrogenase increased, SGOT increased, and SGPT increased. *Rare:* hypercholesteremia and hypoglycemia.

Musculoskeletal System—*Infrequent:* arthritis, tenosynovitis, muscle stiffness, and bursitis. *Rare:* tendinous contracture.

Nervous System—*Infrequent:* vertigo, twitching, depersonalization, hallucinations, suicide attempt, apathy, euphoria, hostility, suicidal thoughts, abnormal gait, thinking abnormal, attention decreased, derealization, neuralgia, paranoid reaction, dysarthria, increased libido, suicide, and myoclonus. *Rare:* hyperkinesia, increased salivation, cerebrovascular accident, hyperesthesia, hypotonia, ptosis, and neuroleptic malignant syndrome.

Respiratory System—*Frequent:* dyspnea and bronchitis. *Infrequent:* asthma, pneumonia, laryngitis, voice alteration, epistaxis, hiccup. *Rare:* hyperventilation and yawn.

Special Senses—*Frequent:* eye pain. *Infrequent:* dry eye, ear pain, abnormality of accommodation, diplopia, conjunctivitis, mydriasis, keratoconjunctivitis, hyperacusis, and photophobia. *Rare:* deafness, glaucoma, night blindness, and taste loss.

Urogenital System—*Frequent:* impotence[a] *Infrequent:* cystitis, urinary urgency, metrorrhagia,[a] amenorrhea,[a] polyuria, vaginal hemorrhage,[a] breast enlargement,[a] menorrhagia,[a] urinary incontinence, abnormal ejaculation,[a] hematuria, nocturia, and kidney calculus. *Rare:* uterine fibroids enlarged,[a] uterine hemorrhage,[a] anorgasmia, and oliguria.

[a]Adjusted for gender.

DRUG ABUSE AND DEPENDENCE

Controlled Substance Class

SERZONE (nefazodone hydrochloride) is not a controlled substance.

Physical and Psychological Dependence

In animal studies, nefazodone did not act as a reinforcer for intravenous self-administration in monkeys trained to self-administer cocaine, suggesting no abuse liability. In a controlled study of abuse liability in human subjects, nefazodone showed no potential for abuse.

Nefazodone has not been systematically studied in humans for its potential for tolerance, physical dependence, or withdrawal. While the premarketing clinical experience with nefazodone did not reveal any tendency for a withdrawal syndrome or any drug-seeking behavior, it is not possible to predict on the basis of this limited experience the extent to which a CNS-active drug will be misused, diverted, and/or abused once marketed. Consequently, physicians should carefully evaluate patients for a history of drug abuse and follow such patients closely, observing them for signs of misuse or abuse of SERZONE (e.g., development of tolerance, dose escalation, drug-seeking behavior).

OVERDOSAGE

Human Experience

There is very limited experience with nefazodone overdose. In premarketing clinical studies, there were seven reports of nefazodone overdose alone or in combination with other pharmacological agents. The amount of nefazodone ingested ranged from 1000 mg to 11,200 mg. Commonly reported symptoms from overdose of nefazodone included nausea, vomiting, and somnolence. One nonstudy participant took 2000–3000 mg of nefazodone with methocarbamol and alcohol; this person reportedly experienced a convulsion (type not documented). None of the patients died.

Overdose Management

Overdosage may cause an increase in incidence or severity of any of the reported adverse reactions (see ADVERSE REACTIONS Section).

There is no specific antidote for SERZONE (nefazodone hydrochloride). Treatment should be symptomatic and supportive in the case of hypotension or excessive sedation. Any patient suspected of having taken an overdose should have the stomach emptied by gastric lavage.

In managing overdosage, consider the possibility of multiple drug involvement. The physician should consider contacting a poison control center on the treatment of any overdose.

DOSAGE AND ADMINISTRATION

Initial Treatment

The recommended starting dose for SERZONE (nefazodone hydrochloride) is 200 mg/day, administered in two divided doses (BID). In the controlled clinical trials establishing the antidepressant efficacy of SERZONE, the effective dose range was generally 300 to 600 mg/day. Consequently, most patients, depending on tolerability and the need for further clinical effect, should have dose increased. Dose increases should occur in increments of 100 mg/day to 200 mg/day, again on a BID schedule, at intervals of no less than 1 week. As with all antidepressants, several weeks on treatment may be required to obtain a full antidepressant response.

Dosage for Elderly or Debilitated Patients

The recommended initial dose for elderly or debilitated patients is 100 mg/day on a BID schedule. These patients often have reduced nefazodone clearance and/or increased sensitivity to the side effects of CNS-active drugs. It may also be appropriate to modify the rate of subsequent dose titration. As steady-state plasma levels do not change with age, the final target dose based on a careful assessment of the patient's clinical response may be similar in healthy younger and older patients.

Maintenance/Continuation/Extended Treatment

There is no body of evidence available from controlled trials to indicate how long the depressed patient should be treated with SERZONE. It is generally agreed, however, that pharmacological treatment for acute episodes of depression should continue for up to six months or longer. Whether the dose of antidepressant needed to induce remission is identical to the dose needed to maintain euthymia is unknown. Although there are no efficacy data that specifically address maintenance antidepressant treatment with SERZONE, the safety of nefazodone in long-term use is supported by data from both double-blind and open-label trials involving more than 250 patients treated for at least one year.

Switching Patients to or from a Monoamine Oxidase Inhibitor

At least 14 days should elapse between discontinuation of an MAOI and initiation of therapy with SERZONE. In addition, at least 7 days should be allowed after stopping SERZONE before starting an MAOI.

HOW SUPPLIED

SERZONE® (nefazodone hydrochloride) tablets are hexagonal tablets imprinted with BMS and the strength (i.e., 100 mg) on one side and the identification code number on the other. The 100 mg (white) and 150 mg (peach) tablets are bisect scored on both tablet faces. The 200 mg (light yellow) and 250 mg (white) tablets are unscored.

Store at room temperature, below 40° C (104° F) and dispense in a tight container.

References: **1.** Data on file, Medical Affairs Department, Bristol-Myers Squibb Company. **2.** Fontaine R, Ontiveros A, Elie R, et al. A double-blind comparison of nefazodone, imipramine, and placebo in major depression. *J Clin Psychiatry.* 1994;55:234-241. **3.** Rickels K, Schweizer E, Clary C, Fox I, Weise C. Nefazodone and imipramine in major depression: a placebo-controlled trial. *Br J Psychiatry.* 1994;164:802-805. **4.** Mendels J, Reimherr F, Roberts D, et al. A double-blind comparison of high-dose nefazodone, low-dose nefazodone, and placebo in the treatment of depressed outpatients. Presented at the annual meeting of the ECNP: October 6-9, 1991. **5.** Armitage R, Rush AJ, Trivedi M, Cain J, Roffwarg HP. The effects of nefazodone on sleep architecture in depression. *Neuropsychopharmacology.* 1994;10:123-127. **6.** Ware JC, Rose FV, McBrayer RH. The acute effects of nefazodone, trazodone and buspirone on sleep and sleep-related penile tumescence in normal subjects. *Sleep.* 1994;17:544-550.

P8375-00 Issued: December 1994 Printed in U.S.A.

In a rare controlled study of methylphenidate (MPH) in adults with attention-deficit hyperactivity disorder (ADHD), **Spencer et al** (page 434) report a marked therapeutic response for the MPH treatment of ADHD symptoms that exceeded the placebo response. Response to MPH was independent of gender, psychiatric comorbidity with anxiety or moderate depression, or family history of psychiatric disorders. The study concludes that robust doses of MPH are effective in the treatment of adult ADHD.

One of the most controversial issues in pediatric psychopharmacology is the appropriateness of MPH for the treatment of ADHD in children with chronic tic disorder. In the largest double-blind, placebo-controlled study to date, **Gadow et al** (page 444) report that 0.1-, 0.3-, and 0.5-mg/kg dosages of MPH were each significantly more effective than placebo in suppressing ADHD, oppositional, and aggressive behavior. Although there was some indication that methylphenidate may modestly increase motor and decrease vocal tics, the drug had no adverse effects on the perceived severity of the tic disorder. Methylphenidate appears to be a safe and effective treatment for many children with ADHD and chronic tic disorder.

Cocaine, one of the most reinforcing and addictive of the abused drugs, has pharmacological actions very similar to those of MPH, one of the most commonly prescribed psychotropic medications for children in the United States. **Volkow et al** (page 456) used positron emission tomography (PET) to compare the regional distribution and the pharmacokinetics of these two drugs in the living human brain. While the percentage of uptake and regional distribution of these two drugs in the brain was almost identical, their pharmacokinetics were not. Both drugs entered the brain very rapidly, but the rate of clearance was significantly slower for MPH than for cocaine. Because it was the rate of uptake that was found to be associated with the subjective perception of the "high" and not the presence of the drug in brain, this study suggests that the slow clearance of MPH may not lead to its frequent repeated administration as occurs with cocaine.

A Commentary by Drs Rachael G. Klein and Paul Wender on the role of methylphenidate in psychiatry is included in this issue (page 429).

Compelling work by Sir Michael Rutter and colleagues suggests that family-environment adversity factors can lead to psychopathology and dysfunction in children and adolescents. **Biederman et al** (page 464) report on the impact of family adversity factors in ADHD. As predicted from Rutter's work, severe marital discord, low social class, large family size, paternal criminality, and maternal mental disorder had an increased prevalence in families of children with ADHD. Adversity factors also increased the risk for ADHD-associated psychopathology, impaired cognition, and dysfunction. These findings support Rutter's work and highlight the importance of adverse family-environment variables as risk factors for ADHD in children.

Clinical symptoms of schizophrenia may be related to dysfunctional activity of central dopaminergic systems, but disturbances in these systems are associated with symptoms of affective illness. **Pearlson et al** (page 471) used PET scanning to study the density of D_2 dopamine–related receptors in the basal ganglia of predominantly neuroleptic-naive patients who had bipolar disorder with or without psychotic symptoms and compared these subjects with matched schizophrenic patients and normal controls. Dopamine receptor density values were elevated in psychotic patients with bipolar disorder and in schizophrenic patients compared with both normal controls and patients with bipolar disorder without psychotic symptoms. Among the patients with bipolar disorder, dopamine receptor density values correlated significantly with the severity of psychotic symptoms but not with the severity of nonpsychotic (ie, mood-related) symptoms.

The elderly are at higher risk than younger patients for the development of tardive dyskinesia, a syndrome of abnormal involuntary movements, after treatment with neuroleptic medications. However, risk factors for the development of tardive dyskinesia in the elderly have not yet been well defined. **Sweet et al** (page 478) examined 386 elderly psychiatric patients and found that total lifetime duration of neuroleptic treatment was the strongest predictor of the risk for tardive dyskinesia, with the risk period beginning within the first months of neuroleptic use. Thus, there may be no absolutely safe duration of neuroleptic treatment for these patients. This study further underscores the need for research efforts to sharpen the indications for neuroleptic treatment in late life and to explore alternatives to neuroleptic medications in this population.

The questions of whether dysthymia should be classified as a mood or personality disorder and, if it is a mood disorder, whether it is sufficiently distinct from major depression to warrant a separate category have generated considerable controversy. In a family study of early-onset dysthymia, **Klein et al** (page 487) found that the rate of dysthymia in the relatives of outpatients with early-onset dysthymia was significantly greater than in the relatives of outpatients with episodic major depression and of normal controls. The relatives of dysthymic probands also exhibited significantly higher rates of major depression and most personality disorders than the relatives of normal controls. This suggests that despite the strong relationship between dysthymia and major depression, dysthymia is also somewhat distinct. In addition, there may be familial links between a variety of forms of mood and personality disorders.

The international disparities reported in the prevalence rates of both dementia and depression in the elderly are provocative but require further investigation. In the first psychiatric study of this kind in a Spanish-speaking country and in Southern Europe, **Lobo et al** (page 497) found that dementing disorders but not depression increase steeply after age 65 years. The prevalence rate of dementia was 5.5% (more than three fourths of the cases were of the Alzheimer's type), the rate of depression was 4.8%, and an intriguing overlap of cognitive and depressive disturbances was documented in a proportion of cases. With the exception of dementia, this investigation again challenges the once prevailing view that old age is inevitably accompanied by higher rates of psychiatric disturbance.

Notice to Authors

Length of Text. Ideally, the text of manuscripts (not including abstract, tables, figures, and references) should be under 5000 words. Include a word count on the title page.

Title. The title should be short, specific, and descriptive, emphasizing the main point of the article. Avoid two-part titles, if at all possible. Do not number titles, eg, "I" or "Part I." Title length, including punctuation and spaces, ideally should be under 100 characters and must not exceed 200 characters.

Abstract. The abstract should be structured into four parts and be no longer than 250 words.

Tables and Figures. Material should provide substantive data and not merely illustrate the text. While the main finding of a table or figure may be discussed in the narrative, the table or figure should not duplicate the text. Although no specific guideline applies to all articles, the number and length of tables and figures should be considered carefully and kept to a minimum.

References. All references should be selected carefully to acknowledge previous work or to document a specific point. They should not be exhaustive.

Please consult the "Instructions for Authors" on page 427 of this issue for other details regarding manuscript preparation.

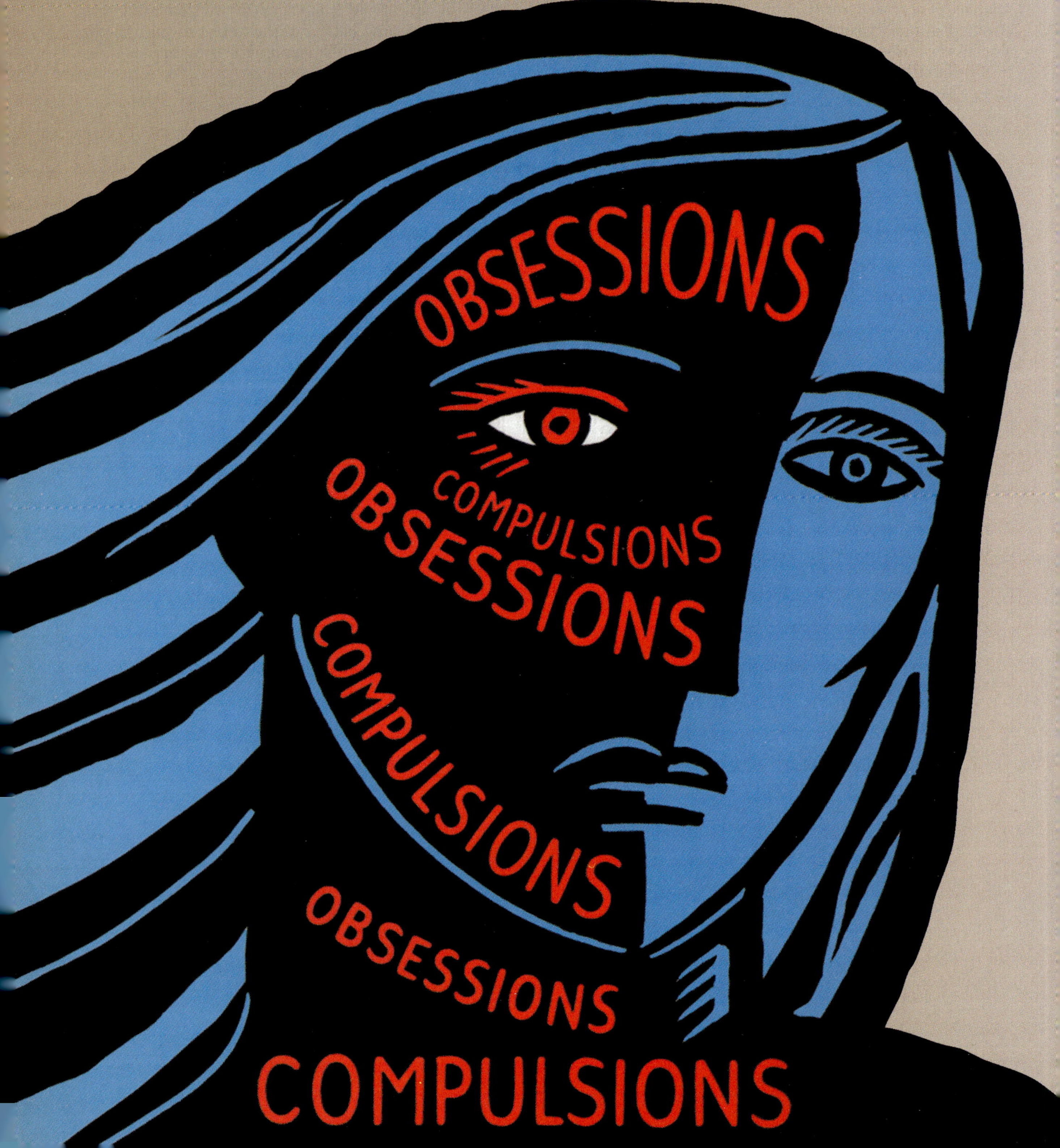
OBSESSIONS
COMPULSIONS
OBSESSIONS
COMPULSIONS
OBSESSIONS
COMPULSIONS

COMMENTARY

The Role of Methylphenidate in Psychiatry

SOME OF the articles appearing in this issue of the ARCHIVES document the current interest in the varied applications of methylphenidate hydrochloride in psychiatry. Together, the articles address questions that have been of concern to clinicians and scientists alike. The scope of the clinical use of methylphenidate in adult psychiatry is addressed in the study by Spencer and associates[1]; a potentially serious side effect (ie, tics) is examined carefully by Gadow et al[2]; and Volkow and colleagues[3] report on some mechanisms of methylphenidate activity and their contribution to our understanding of the drug's effects.

In an excellent review that appeared in the ARCHIVES in 1987, Chiarello and Cole[4] summarize the manifold uses of methylphenidate, as well as those of other psychostimulants. Although the literature consisted mostly of less than

See also pages 434, 444, 456, and 464

well-controlled studies conducted in imprecisely identified patient groups, the conclusions pointed to the likely usefulness of psychostimulants for a variety of clinical conditions and to their neglect in clinical as well as academic psychiatry. Based on an examination of the rates of methylphenidate prescriptions made over time, the message appears to have caught on. Sales of methylphenidate have mushroomed in the past decade (this escalating trend seems to have been reversed temporarily by negative media publicity).[5] However, the increase in methylphenidate prescriptions appears to be due mostly to an expansion of the diagnosis of childhood attention-deficit hyperactivity disorder (ADHD). It is not apparent that prescriptive practice in adult psychiatry has changed appreciably in the past decade.

ATTENTION-DEFICIT HYPERACTIVITY DISORDER

The efficacy of methylphenidate in ADHD of childhood needs no retelling. In spite of the periodic alarm expressed in the media, it is an unqualified success story for the following reasons, all amply documented: At appropriately high doses of methylphenidate, a large proportion of children with ADHD experience remission of symptoms of ADHD[6-8]; these children are not only better, many are well. In addition to having the cardinal features of their disorder eliminated, appropriately medicated children experience improvement in other important functional domains, such as in social interactions with parents, teachers, and peers, in academic performance, and in self-esteem.[9] Therefore, medication can be counted on to have a positive and broad effect in a large proportion of children with ADHD.

The first report of methylphenidate efficacy in adults with ADHD, which appeared almost 20 years ago,[10] and two subsequent placebo controlled studies with positive results had relatively little influence on clinical practice. Focus on ADHD in adults lagged until a flurry of popular books and national television programs appeared on the topic.[11,12] The resultant extensive public interest emphasizes the need for the establishment of rational bases for treatment.

The study by Spencer et al[1] is welcome as the first replication of the Utah group's findings of a substantial response of adults with ADHD to stimulant treatment, including treatment with methylphenidate[13] and pemoline,[14] and as the replication of clinical reports of the utility of monoamine oxidase inhibitors and pargyline hydrochloride,[15] selegiline hydrochloride,[16] and bupropion hydrochloride.[17] The relative greater proportion of responses in the study by Spencer et al may well be due to diagnostic differences because somewhat different standards were used. At the same time, it seems unwise to overinterpret the differences in response rates between studies that obtain significant drug-placebo differences unless these are replicated. Among effective interventions, variation in rates of treatment outcomes tends to be the rule rather than the exception—an observation that holds true for response rates in placebo as well as in actively treated groups. However, if methylphenidate effects superior to those reported by the Utah group[13] are obtained in other studies that apply the diagnostic standards of Spencer et al, implications for the diagnosis of ADHD in adults will become relevant.

Yet, the differences in diagnostic standards are not obvious. For example, Spencer et al note that the Utah criteria may identify a more heterogeneous group because, in addition to inattentiveness and impulsivity (hyperactivity was also required), they included affective lability, temper outbursts, and stress intolerance. It is not evident that these features were absent in the patients treated by Spencer et al. Mood and anxiety disorders, often associated with irritability, were not infrequent in the Boston sample.[1] The clinical criteria reported by each center do not provide clear differentiation of diagnostic features. It appears that both centers treated patients with high degrees of comor bidity. If diagnostic precision is desired, as appears to be the case, further delineation of the patients' clinical presentation will be necessary. This might be accomplished by the publication of a compendium of patients' autobiographical material. At present, it is not possible to pinpoint what aspects of the diagnostic standards are specific for predicting response to methylphenidate treatment in adult patients with ADHD.

ALTHOUGH both centers studied patients who all were white, they differed on socioeconomic status, an important demographic characteristic. The patients in the study by Spencer et al had an unusually high socioeconomic status (mean, 1.7, which indicates upper middle-class standing). This socioeconomic status level is all the more remarkable because the study was conducted in a clinic situated in a large urban medical center. Typically, the social class of samples drawn from such facilities is lower middle to lower class. Herein may lie the apparent superiority of methylphenidate in the trial by Spencer et al. It is conceivable that better educated individuals communicate subtleties in their clinical status more effectively than less educated individuals. In addition, because individuals from high socioeconomic strata hold positions that make relatively greater attentional demands, they may provide an ideal opportunity for the detection of positive effects of methylphenidate. If so, the results obtained in a group that represents a relatively small proportion of the general population may not be generalizable to patients from a broad socioeconomic spectrum.

The presence of childhood ADHD symptoms is not always confirmed by adults who present with current symptoms of ADHD. In such instances, it is difficult to know whether early history is negative for ADHD or forgotten. The probability of forgetting is not remote because, in a group of children who had been referred for treatment and who received diagnoses of ADHD, recall of childhood ADHD in young adulthood (between 23 and 30 years of age) occurred in only 60%.[18] At the same time, there are adults who give a clear negative, asymptomatic picture for ADHD until later in life. An interesting question concerns the therapeutic response of individuals who manifest adult ADHD symptoms but in whom there is no evidence for childhood ADHD symptoms. The Utah group[13] and Spencer et al[1] confined their studies to adults with a childhood history of ADHD. The only placebo-controlled study that included patients without a childhood history[19] did not detect any superiority of methylphenidate. Yet, we do not know that the case is closed. The symptoms of ADHD may be mimicked by other disorders. The ADHD symptoms that occur only in adulthood may be due to other chronic psychiatric disorders. Prominent among these are chronic depressive disorders, obsessive-compulsive disorders, narcolepsy, and long-standing language disorders. It is still undocumented whether individuals with a cluster of ADHD symptoms and no childhood history experience a therapeutic response to methylphenidate.

Another question to be resolved is the discrepancy in the rate of female patients among children and adults with ADHD. The sample of Spencer et al had an excess of women (57%). Yet, every clinical study of childhood ADHD to our knowledge, and there are literally hundreds, reports a markedly disproportionate number of male patients. Were such findings limited to clinical samples, one would suspect that gender-related referral biases accounted for the sex ratio of children in whom ADHD was identified. The possibility of such a bias is dispelled by the fact that every epidemiological study to our knowledge has documented a preponderance of boys among children with ADHD.[20-23] Furthermore, a difference in the relative prevalence of male and female patients in child and adult clinical samples does not appear attributable to gender differences in the course of ADHD (although data on this point are limited).[24] The marked contrast in gender representation in child and adult patients with ADHD is truly puzzling.

CONTROVERSY REGARDING METHYLPHENIDATE TREATMENT OF CHILDREN WITH TIC DISORDERS

Transient tics of a severity that does not reach diagnostic threshold are very common in children. Until recently, a history of tics, no matter how benign, was considered by some to contraindicate treatment with methylphenidate. The proscription went so far as to exclude from treatment consideration those with a family history of tics. This clinical caution was prompted by the observation that methylphenidate could aggravate tics or was associated with their emergence.[25] As a result, Tourette's syndrome was suspected of being a complication of exposure to methylphenidate in susceptible individuals.

By systematically examining the occurrence of tics in children with chronic tic disorder or Tourette's syndrome who were receiving methylphenidate, the study by Gadow and colleagues[2] addresses one of the contentious issues concerning the use of methylphenidate in children with ADHD who have tics and tic disorders. The work of investigators such as Gadow and his colleagues, as well as that of others cited in the article, has been influential in clarifying the risks associated with methylphenidate treatment with regard to worsening of tics. The message is somewhat mixed: on most measures, tics remained unchanged during treatment; on a couple of measures, they were significantly worse but to a degree that was not judged to be clinically meaningful. From their results, Gadow et al reach the reasonable conclusion that the presence of tics does not preclude treatment with methylphenidate when indicated by the presence of ADHD. The finding has substantial clinical importance and goes a long way toward providing a rational basis for treating children who pose major therapeutic dilemmas, while enabling clinicians to communicate in a knowledgeable fashion with understandably concerned parents.

The study was not designed to address the issue of whether methylphenidate administration causes Tourette's syndrome, one that has had a major influence on the use of the drug in children with a history of tics. Several naturalistic surveys have examined the theory by studying whether age at onset is earlier in individuals with Tourette's syndrome who were exposed to methylphenidate in childhood compared with those who were not.[25] The negative findings obtained in these surveys, together with those of Gadow et al,[2] provide a compelling case for the safe use of methylphenidate for the treatment of ADHD in children with tics or tic disorders. As noted by Gadow and colleagues, the experimental data are based on a very short exposure to methylphenidate hydrochloride: only 2 weeks at a typical clinical dosage. In fact, the highest dosage they used (single daily dosage of 5 mg/kg, with an upper limit of 20 mg) is less than is required for many children who may have to receive a total daily dosage of 60 mg or more. Therefore, the results are encouraging but not altogether reassuring for clinical practice. To rule out the risk of tics with methylphenidate treatment, it will be important to conduct studies with designs that reflect as closely as possible optimal clinical management.

Gadow et al[2] report that all children derived marked clinical benefit from methylphenidate treatment. This observation is important because a third of the children had concomitant anxiety disorders. The presence of the latter has been reported to have a deleterious influence on the efficacy of methylphenidate in children with anxiety symptoms.[26,27] As far as we know, this is the only study that used diagnoses of anxiety disorders rather than ratings of anxiety. The fact that these disorders were not a limiting factor to treatment efficacy should encourage clinicians to proceed with a trial of methylphenidate in ADHD even if it is comorbid with an anxiety disorder.

IS METHYLPHENIDATE LIKE COCAINE?

We find the title of the article by Volkow et al[3] potentially misleading because it implies relevance to psychiatric practice. As Volkow et al note, clinical administration of methylphenidate is always oral; therefore, comparisons of intravenous methylphenidate administration with intravenous administration of cocaine are not relevant to the clinical situation. This issue may seem to be beside the point because there is merit in examining brain distribution of various compounds in contexts that differ from clinical standards. However, in this instance, the criticism must stand because Volkow et al aver that the rationale for their study stems partly from concerns about methylphenidate abuse based on widespread use in children with ADHD. There is no basis for such concerns. There is a nearly total absence of methylphenidate abuse reported in methylphenidate-treated children and adolescents in spite of its very widespread application.[28] Furthermore, Volkow et al note that concerns about methylphenidate abuse stem from its pharmacological similarity to cocaine. Historically, such is not the case. The first drugs used to treat hyperactive children, the amphetamines, were known to be drugs of abuse. Therefore, questions about abuse potential followed whenever competing psychostimulants were introduced (eg, methylphenidate and pemoline).

The study by Volkow et al indicates that cocaine and methylphenidate may be acting on the same receptor systems, specifically in the striatum, and that methylphenidate has a longer clearance than cocaine. Of particular interest is that the data support a nonpharmacokinetic origin for the waning of the methylphenidate "high" (as other data do for cocaine). The speculations of Volkow et al that the rapid clearance of cocaine interferes with the development of this adaptive process and, thus, promotes readministration is not addressed by their data.

Unfortunately, we cannot assume that the same mechanisms account for a drug's reinforcing properties as for its other clinical activity. Therefore, the relevance of the data in furthering our understanding of the methylphenidate effect in patients with ADHD is unclear. At the same time, it is relevant to note that studies have implicated the striatum in ADHD[29] but not consistently.[30]

METHYLPHENIDATE IN GENERAL PSYCHIATRY

Since the 1987 review by Chiarello and Cole,[4] a sizable clinical literature has appeared on the use of methylphenidate in patients with a variety of clinical conditions. The use of methylphenidate in adults with major depression who derive only partial benefit from standard antidepressants (tricyclic antidepressants, monoamine oxidase inhibitors, and serotonin reuptake inhibitors) has continued to be reported.[31] In some of these individuals, methylphenidate may increase the therapeutic response to a clinically meaningful degree. Although appropriately controlled studies are lacking, these clinical reports must be taken seriously because stimulants are often the last drugs administered to patients who have not responded to trials with multiple antidepressant drugs. (It is important to note that the augmentation therapy is not limited to methylphenidate but pertains to psychostimulants in general.)

Clinical efficacy has been reported as well in elderly patients who are apathetic and withdrawn but who may not report hopelessness.[32] Another use of methylphenidate is in the treatment of medically ill depressed patients,[33-40] specifically those with acquired immunodeficiency syndrome.[41,42] The relevance of methylphenidate treatment in depressed medically ill patients to general psychiatry is highlighted by the publication of two articles on the psychiatric treatment of patients with cancer.[43,44] Clinical reports also have supported the safe use of methylphenidate in children with autism who are hyperactive.[45,46]

Methylphenidate (and dextroamphetamine) have been used experimentally to produce paranoid, schizophrenialike symptoms,[47] to determine the probability of relapse in patients with schizophrenia treated with neuroleptic medication, and in the treatment of the schizophrenias. With regard to the first, it has also been observed clinically that, in individuals with schizotypal personality disorder, low doses of stimulants may induce paranoid and other schizophrenic symptoms. To measure the probability of relapse, patients with schizophrenia treated with neuroleptic medication are given an intravenous bolus of methylphenidate.[48] Individuals who show an exacerbation of their symptoms are more likely to relapse when antipsychotic medication is diminished and then discontinued. Clinically, methylphenidate has been reported to be effective in patients with schizophrenia whose positive symptoms have been ameliorated by neuroleptic medications but who continue to have negative symptoms such as abulia, anhedonia, and withdrawal. No placebo-controlled or long-term trials have been conducted. Both would be useful.

IS METHYLPHENIDATE A SPECIAL CASE?

This Commentary has focused on methylphenidate. It would be unfortunate if the consequences of this focus led to the assumption that it holds a special place in clinical psychiatry compared with other psychostimulants. There is little reason to believe that this is the case, although it is possible, even likely, that other compounds may have even less abuse potential (eg, pemoline), whereas others may have more (eg, dextroamphetamine and methamphetamine). Yet, under proper supervision, the use of all psychostimulants has been found to be safe in patients without histories of substance abuse.[4] Interestingly, in children as well as adults, the failure to respond to one stimulant does not preclude response to another.[6,49,50] The clear implication is that a fair stimulant trial has not been conducted if it is limited to one compound.

RISKS ASSOCIATED WITH METHYLPHENIDATE USE

The spectrum of clinical application for methylphenidate use is broad. Therefore, an appreciation of the risks and problems associated with them is important. The cost-benefit ratio of methylphenidate is very favorable. As noted, tics do not constitute a uniform contraindication. Although the drug is believed by some to lower the seizure threshold, doses appropriate to the clinical management of AHDH in children and adults with seizures have not been found to increase seizure frequency.[51,52]

Another concern has been the potential for a reduction in growth velocity in methylphenidate-treated children. A significant relationship between methylphenidate exposure and growth was obtained in the only controlled study on the topic. The growth of a subgroup of children is significantly affected by long-term exposure to methylphenidate, but compensatory growth during adolescence reverses earlier decrements if treatment is interrupted.[25,53] No data are available concerning methylphenidate effects on growth when treatment is extended through adolescence.

As safe and at times effective as methylphenidate is, its use is not always straightforward. A major limitation is its short clinical activity, leading to multiple daily dosing in many cases. The slow-release preparation does not always provide a solution to this problem. Except when it is used as an augmentation therapy in depression, the clinical use of methylphenidate is seriously impeded by this clinical constraint.

Rachel G. Klein, PhD
Columbia University College of Physicians and Surgeons
722 W 168th St
New York, NY 10032
Paul Wender, MD
Salt Lake City, Utah

REFERENCES

1. Spencer T, Wilens T, Biederman J, Faraone SV, Ablon JS, Lapey K. A double-blind, crossover comparison of methylphenidate and placebo in adults with childhood-onset attention-deficit hyperactivity disorder. *Arch Gen Psychiatry.* 1995;52: 434-443.
2. Gadow KD, Sverd J, Sprafkin J, Nolan EE, Ezor SN. Efficacy of methylphenidate for attention-deficit hyperactivity disorder in children with tic disorder. *Arch Gen Psychiatry.* 1995;52:444-455.
3. Volkow ND, Ding Y-S, Fowler JS, Wang G-J, Logan J, Gatley JS, Dewey S, Ashby C, Liebermann J, Hitzemann R, Wolf AP. Is methylphenidate like cocaine? studies on their pharmacokinetics and distribution in the human brain. *Arch Gen Psychiatry.* 1995;52:456-463.
4. Chiarello RJ, Cole JO. The use of psychostimulants in general psychiatry. *Arch Gen Psychiatry* 1987;44:286-295.
5. Safer DJ, Krager JM. Effect of a media blitz and a threatened lawsuit on stimulant treatment. *JAMA.* 1992;268:1004-1007.
6. Elia J, Borcherding BG, Rapoport JL, Keysor CS. Methylphenidate and dextroamphetamine treatments of hyperactivity: are there true nonresponders? *Psychiatry Res.* 1991;36:141-155.
7. Abikoff H, Gittelman R. Does behavior therapy normalize the behavior of hyperactive children. *Arch Gen Psychiatry.* 1984;41:449-454.
8. Rapport MD, Denney C, DuPaul GJ, Gardner MJ. Attention deficit disorder and methylphenidate: normalization rates, clinical effectiveness, and response prediction in 76 children. *J Am Acad Child Adolesc Psychiatry.* 1994;33:882-893.
9. Klein RG. Pharmacotherapy of childhood hyperactivity: an update. In: Meltzer HY, Bunney W, Coyle J, Davis K, Kopin I, Shuster CR, Shader RI, Simpson G, eds. *Psychopharmacology: The Third Generation of Progress.* New York, NY: Raven Press; 1987:1215-1224.
10. Wood DR, Reimherr FW, Wender PH, Johnson GE. Diagnosis and treatment of minimal brain dysfunction in adults. *Arch Gen Psychiatry.* 1976; 33:1453-1460.
11. Hallowell EM, Ratey JJ. *Driven to Distraction.* New York, NY: Pantheon Books; 1994.
12. Weiss L. *Attention Deficit Disorder in Adults: Practical Help for Sufferers and Their Spouses.* Dallas, Tex: Taylor Publishing Co; 1992.
13. Wender PH, Reimherr FW, Wood D, Ward M. A controlled study of methylphenidate in the treatment of attention deficit disorder, residual type. *Am J Psychiatry.* 1985;142:547-552.
14. Wender PH, Reimherr FW, Wood DR. Attention deficit disorder ('minimal brain dysfunction') in adults: a replication study of diagnosis and drug treatment. *Arch Gen Psychiatry.* 1981;38:449-456.
15. Wender PH, Wood DR, Reimherr FW, Ward M. An open trial of pargyline in the treatment of attention deficit disorder, residual type. *Psychiatry Res.* 1983;9:329-336.
16. Wood DR, Reimherr FW, Wender PH. The use of L-deprenyl in the treatment of attention deficit disorder, residual type (ADD, RT). *Psychopharmacol Bull.* 1983;19:627-629.
17. Wender PH, Reimherr FW. Bupropion treatment of attention-deficit hyperactivity disorder in adults. *Am J Psychiatry.* 1990;147:1018-1020.
18. Klein RG, Mannuzza S. ADHD children in adulthood. Presented at the 146th Annual Meeting of the American Psychiatric Association; May 25, 1993; San Francisco, Calif.
19. Mattes JA, Boswell L, Oliver H. Methylphenidate effects on symptoms of attention deficit disorder in adults. *Arch Gen Psychiatry.* 1984;41: 1059-1063.
20. Anderson JC, Williams S, McGee R, Silva PA. *DSM-III* disorders in preadolescent children. *Arch Gen Psychiatry.* 1987;44:69-76.
21. Bird HR, Canino G, Rubio-Stipec M, Gould MS, Ribera J, Sesman M, Woodbury M, Huertas-Goldman S, Pagan A, Sanchez-Lacay A, Moscoso M. Estimates of the prevalence of childhood maladjustment in a community survey in Puerto Rico. *Arch Gen Psychiatry.* 1988;45:1120-1126.
22. McGee R, Feehan M, Williams S, Anderson J. *DSM-III* disorders from age 11 to age 15 years. *J Am Acad Child Adolesc Psychiatry.* 1992;31: 50-59.
23. Offord DR, Boyle MH, Szatmari P, Rae-Grant N, Links PS, Cadman DT, Byles JA, Crawford JW, Munroe Blum H, Byrne C, Thomas H, Woodward C. Ontario child health study: six month prevalence of disorder and rates of service uti-

lization. *Arch Gen Psychiatry.* 1987;44:832-836.
24. Mannuzza S, Gittelman R. The adolescent outcome of hyperactive girls. *Psychiatry Res.* 1984;13:19-29.
25. Klein RG, Bessler AW. Stimulant side effects in children. In: Kane JM, Lieberman JA, eds. *Adverse Effects of Psychotropic Drugs.* New York, NY: Guilford Press; 1992:470-496.
26. DuPaul GJ, Barkley RA, McMurray MB. Response of children with ADHD to methylphenidate: interaction with internalizing symptoms. *J Am Acad Child Adolesc Psychiatry.* 1994;33:894-903.
27. Pliszka SR. Effect of anxiety on cognition, behavior, and stimulant response in ADHD. *J Am Acad Child Adolesc Psychiatry.* 1989;28:882-887.
28. Jaffe SL. Intranasal abuse of prescribed methylphenidate by an alcohol- and drug-abusing adolescent with ADHD. *J Am Acad Child Adolesc Psychiatry.* 1991;30:773-775.
29. Castellanos FX, Giedd JN, Eckburg BS, Marsh WL, Vaituzis DK, Hamburger SD, Rapoport JL. Quantitative morphology of the caudate nucleus in attention deficit hyperactivity disorder. *Am J Psychiatry.* 1994;151:1791-1796.
30. Zametkin AJ, Liebenauer LL, Fitzgerald GA, King AC, Minkunas DV, Herscovitch P, Yamada EM, Cohen RM. Brain metabolism in teenagers with attention-deficit hyperactivity disorder. *Arch Gen Psychiatry.* 1993;50:333-340.
31. Thase ME, Rush AJ. Treatment-resistant depression. In: Bloom FE, Kupfer DJ, eds. *Psychopharmacology: Fourth Generation of Progress.* New York, NY: Raven Press; 1995:1081-1097.
32. Salzman C. Update on selected topics pertaining to geriatric psychopharmacology. *Curr Affective Illness.* 1995;14:5-13.
33. Breitbart W, Mermelstein H. An alternative psychostimulant for the management of depressive disorders in cancer patients. *Psychosomatics.* 1992;33:352-356.
34. Evans RW, Gualtieri CT, Patterson D. Treatment of chronic closed head injury with psychostimulant drugs: a controlled case study and an appropriate evaluation procedure. *J Nerv Ment Dis.* 1987;175:106-110.
35. Fernandez F, Adams F, Holmes VF, Levy JK, Neidhart M. Methylphenidate for depressive disorders in cancer patients. *Psychosomatics.* 1987;28:455-461.
36. Lazarus LW, Winemiller DR, Lingam VR, Neyman I, Hartman C, Abassian M, Kartan U, Groves L, Fawcett J. Efficacy and side effects of methylphenidate for poststroke depression. *J Clin Psychiatry.* 1992;53:447-449.
37. Masand P, Pickett P, Murray GB. Psychostimulants for secondary depression in medical illness. *Psychosomatics.* 1991;32:203-208.
38. Rosenberg PB, Ahmed I, Hurwitz S. Methylphenidate in depressed medically ill patients. *J Clin Psychiatry.* 1991;52:263-267.
39. Walling VR, Pfefferbaum B. The use of methylphenidate in a depressed adolescent with AIDS. *J Dev Behav Pediatr.* 1990;11:195-197.
40. White JC, Christensen JF, Singer CM. Methylphenidate as a treatment for depression in acquired immunodeficiency syndrome: an n-of-1 trial. *J Clin Psychiatry.* 1992;53:153-156.
41. Holmes VF, Fernandez F, Levy J. Psychostimulant response in AIDS-related complex patients. *J Clin Psychiatry.* 1989;50:5-8.
42. Rabkin JG. Psychostimulant medication for depression and lethargy in HIV illness: a pilot study. *Prog Notes Am Soc Clin Psychopharmacol.* 1993;4:1.
43. Fawzy FI, Fawzy NW, Arndt LA, Pasnau RO. Critical review of psychosocial interventions in cancer care. *Arch Gen Psychiatry.* 1995;52:100-113.
44. McDaniel JS, Musselman DL, Porter MR, Reed DA, Nemeroff CB. Depression in patients with cancer: diagnosis, biology, and treatment. *Arch Gen Psychiatry.* 1995;52:89-99.
45. Birmaher B, Quintana H, Greenhill LL. Methylphenidate treatment of hyperactive autistic children. *J Am Acad Child Adolesc Psychiatry.* 1988;27:248-251.
46. Strayhorn JM, Rapp N, Donina W, Strain PS. Randomized trial of methylphenidate for an autistic child. *J Am Acad Child Adolesc Psychiatry.* 1988;27:244-247.
47. Angrist B, Gershon S. The phenomenology of experimentally induced amphetamine psychosis: preliminary observations. *Biol Psychiatry.* 1970;2:95-107.
48. Robinson D, Jody D, Lieberman JA. Provocative tests with methylphenidate in schizophrenia and schizophrenia spectrum disorders. In: Greenhill LL, Osman BB, eds. *Ritalin: Theory and Patient Management.* New York, NY: Mary Ann Liebert; 1991:309-320.
49. Arnold LE, Christopher J, Huestis R, Smeltzer DJ. Methylphenidate vs dextroamphetamine vs caffeine in minimal brain dysfunction. *Arch Gen Psychiatry.* 1978;35:463-473.
50. Little KY. *d*-Amphetamine versus methylphenidate effects in depressed inpatients. *J Clin Psychiatry.* 1993;54:349-355.
51. Feldman H, Crumrine P, Handen BL, Alvin R, Teodori J. Methylphenidate in children with seizures and attention-deficit disorder. *AJDC.* 1989;143:1081-1086.
52. Wroblewski BA, Leary JM, Phelan AM, Whyte J, Manning K. Methylphenidate and seizure frequency in brain injured patients with seizure disorders. *J Clin Psychiatry.* 1992;53:86-89.
53. Klein RG, Landa B, Mattes J, Klein DF. Methylphenidate and growth in hyperactive children: a controlled withdrawal study. *Arch Gen Psychiatry.* 1988;45:1127-1130.

ORIGINAL ARTICLE

A Double-blind, Crossover Comparison of Methylphenidate and Placebo in Adults With Childhood-Onset Attention-Deficit Hyperactivity Disorder

Thomas Spencer, MD; Timothy Wilens, MD; Joseph Biederman, MD; Stephen V. Faraone, PhD; J. Stuart Ablon; Kathleen Lapey

Background: There are few controlled studies of methylphenidate hydrochloride in adults with attention-deficit hyperactivity disorder (ADHD), and their results have been equivocal. The discrepancies among these studies may be related to low doses, diagnostic uncertainties, and lack of attention to comorbid disorders.

Methods: We conducted a randomized, 7-week, placebo-controlled, crossover study of methylphenidate in 23 adult patients with *DSM-III-R* ADHD using standardized instruments for diagnosis, separate assessments of ADHD and depressive and anxiety symptoms, and a robust daily dose of methylphenidate hydrochloride, 1.0 mg/kg per day.

Results: We found a marked therapeutic response for methylphenidate treatment of ADHD symptoms that exceeded the placebo response (78% vs 4%, $P<.0001$). Response to methylphenidate was independent of gender, psychiatric comorbidity with anxiety or moderate depression, or family history of psychiatric disorders.

Conclusion: Robust doses of methylphenidate are effective in the treatment of adult ADHD.

(Arch Gen Psychiatry. 1995;52:434-443)

In recent years, an accumulating body of data suggest that the syndrome of attention-deficit hyperactivity disorder (ADHD) persists into adulthood in 30% to 60% of childhood-onset cases.[1-3] Considering current prevalence estimates that at least 5% of children may be affected with ADHD,[4,5] many adults also may have the disorder. In addition, studies have consistently reported that the persistence of ADHD into adulthood is associated with high rates of academic and work failure as well as high rates of psychiatric comorbidity, including substance use and antisocial disorders.[6,7]

While there is a growing appreciation that ADHD may be a common disorder in adults and it is associated with considerable disability and distress, it remains an underdiagnosed and undertreated adult psychiatric disorder. Despite increasing media attention (*The Wall Street Journal*. January 11, 1993:1), adult ADHD is an orphan diagnosis in both adult and child clinics. Child clinicians do not usually follow up patients into adulthood, and adult ADHD often is not considered in adult psychiatric settings. In addition, increasing recognition of the legitimacy of its diagnosis in adulthood has not been matched by similar advances in knowledge about its treatment. Therapeutic paralysis has resulted from concerns about the safety and efficacy of stimulants in adults with ADHD, along with medicolegal and ethical issues associated with the use of controlled substances in this population.

While there has been some debate about the validity of assessing the disorder retrospectively in adults, the weight of the available literature reveals adult ADHD to be a legitimate diagnosis that can be dependably made from historical self-reports of childhood symptoms.[1-3,6,8-12] For example, Biederman et al[12] recently reported findings from a large study of clinically referred adults with childhood-onset ADHD whose diagnoses were confirmed by structured interviews. The authors reported that the pattern of psychopathology, cognition, and functioning among the adults with ADHD closely approximated findings among children with ADHD. In addition, further support

See Methods on next page

From the Pediatric Psychopharmacology Unit of the Massachusetts General Hospital (Drs Spencer, Wilens, Biederman, and Faraone) and the Harvard Medical School (Mr Ablon and Ms Lapey), Boston, Mass.

METHODS

SUBJECTS

Subjects were 25 outpatient adults of both sexes with ADHD, between 18 and 60 years of age. They had been ascertained from clinical referrals to an adult psychopharmacology center at the Massachusetts General Hospital, Boston. Adults were either self-referred or referred by other clinicians for lifelong histories of inattention and underachievement. The *DSM-III-R* diagnosis of childhood-onset and current ADHD was determined by a psychiatrist's clinical evaluation and confirmed by a structured diagnostic interview. Subjects were not excluded for the presence of other psychiatric disorders unless treatment with methylphenidate was contraindicated or compliance with a double-blind protocol was judged to be jeopardized. We excluded prospective subjects if they had any clinically significant chronic medical conditions or abnormal baseline laboratory values or a history of tic disorders, mental retardation (IQ, <75), organic brain disorders, clinically unstable psychiatric conditions (ie, suicidal behaviors, psychosis, delinquency, criminality, or violence), or substance or alcohol abuse or dependence within the 6 months preceding the study or currently used psychotropics. We also excluded pregnant or nursing women.

ASSESSMENT MEASURES

Prior to inclusion in the study, patients underwent a standard clinical assessment consisting of a psychiatric evaluation by one of us who was a board-certified child and adult psychiatrist (J.B., T.S., or T.W.), a structured diagnostic interview, a medical history, and laboratory assessments (complete blood cell count, liver function tests, and electrocardiogram). The structured diagnostic interview used the Structured Clinical Interview for *DSM-III-R*[34] for adult diagnoses, supplemented by unmodified modules from the Kiddie Schedule for Affective Disorder and Schizophrenia–Epidemiologic Version (Kiddie SADS-E)[35] to assess ADHD and other childhood disorders. The structured interviews generate diagnostic information about both past and current (within the past month) disturbances. The rates of past illness are reported herein as lifetime prevalences. In addition, the level of associated impairment was recorded for each diagnosis (1 indicates mild; 2, moderate; and 3, severe). We assessed ADHD, mood disorders, adult and childhood anxiety disorders, antisocial disorders, substance and alcohol use disorders, obsessive-compulsive disorders, language disorders, and psychotic disorders.

To be given a full diagnosis of adult ADHD, the subject must have (1) met full *DSM-III-R* criteria (at least eight of 14 symptoms) for a diagnosis of ADHD by the age of 7 years and currently, (2) described a chronic course of ADHD symptoms from childhood to adulthood, and (3) endorsed a moderate or severe level of impairment attributed to the ADHD symptoms. To elicit ADHD symptoms, we used the ADHD module from the Kiddie SADS-E, wording questions in the past tense. If the subject endorsed a symptom to a clinically meaningful degree, we asked whether similar problems were currently present. For example, the childhood symptom of "difficulty playing quietly" would be consistent with an adult's inability to remain productively occupied in an unstructured setting. By using this method, we ensured that the syndrome observed in adulthood has some continuity with the syndrome reported in childhood. While major depression was diagnosed when full criteria were associated with at least moderate impairment, we also analyzed major depression associated with severe impairment, consistent with our previous work.[12,13] Also, we used two or more anxiety disorders to index the presence of a clinically meaningful anxiety syndrome.[36] Diagnostic reliability of the structured interviews was well established in a previous sample of 35 interviews of adults with ADHD, using the same diagnostic procedures as those used in this study. Diagnostic reliability between raters and board-certified child and adolescent psychiatrists was excellent. All κ values were higher than 0.81, with the exception of antisocial personality, for which κ was 0.71. The mean κ was 0.91. A κ of 1.0 was obtained for ADHD, with a 95% confidence interval of 0.8 to 1.0.

To assess intellectual functioning, we administered subtests of the Wechsler Adult Intelligence Scale–Revised (WAIS-R)[37] and the Wide Range Achievement Test–Revised (WRAT-R).[38] Academic underachievement was defined as a discrepancy of 20 points between intelligence (as measured by the WAIS-R) and achievement (as measured by the WRAT-R). The Vocabulary and Block Design subtests of the WAIS-R were used to estimate full-scale IQ. In addition, we assessed a family history of psychiatric disorder using the family history method.[39,40] A positive family history was defined as the presence of the disorder in at least one first-degree relative. Socioeconomic status was measured by the Hollingshead Four Factor Index of Social Status, with low values indicating high socioeconomic status.[41]

Continued on next page

for the validity of an ADHD diagnosis in adult subjects derives from evidence for genetic transmission[13-21] and abnormalities in brain structure and function.[22,23]

Despite the accumulating evidence for the validity of adult ADHD, little is known about its treatment.

See also pages 429, 444, 456, and 464

Although studies of methylphenidate hydrochloride in children and adolescents consistently report robust improvement of ADHD symptoms, equivocal results have been reported in the few trials of methylphenidate in adults with this disorder.[24-27] Among the four controlled studies of methylphenidate in adults with ADHD, the average rate of response is only 50%, much lower than the 70% rate among children and adolescents.[28] Plausible reasons for the lower response rate in adults include insufficient dosing and uncertain diagnostic criteria. For example, the estimated mean daily weight-corrected dose of methylphenidate hydrochloride in the available studies of adult patients with ADHD was 0.6 mg/kg per day. This dose is much lower than the 1.0 mg/kg per day commonly used in the treatment of children with this disorder.[28] Thus, it is possible that more aggressive pharma-

To assess change during treatment, we examined three main domains of symptoms: ADHD, depression, and anxiety. Overall severity in each of these domains was assessed with the Clinical Global Impression Scale (CGI) (CGI-ADHD, CGI-Depression, and CGI-Anxiety). The CGI has been extensively used in psychopharmacology research on adults and children and has been shown to be drug sensitive.[42] The CGI includes Global Severity (1 indicates not ill; 7, extremely ill) and Global Improvement (1 indicates very much improved; 7, very much worse) subscales. In addition, the following domain-specific rating scales were used. The ADHD Rating Scale[43] assesses each of the 14 individual criteria symptoms of ADHD in *DSM-III-R* on a severity grid (0 indicates not present; 3, severe; minimum score is 0; maximum score, 42). The psychometric properties of this scale have been established in children, and the scale has been shown to be sensitive to stimulant effects.[43] For depression, we used the physician-based 21-item Hamilton Depression Scale (HAM-D) (minimum score is 0; maximum, 64) and the paper-and-pencil 21-item Beck Depression Inventory (BDI) (minimum score is 0; maximum, 63). These are widely used scales with established psychometric properties. The physician-based 14-item Hamilton Anxiety Scale (HAM-A) (minimum score is 0; maximum, 56) assessed anxiety symptoms. While the structured interviews generate diagnostic information about disturbances within the past month, the rating scales reflect level of symptoms at the time of assessment. In addition, the physician recorded adverse experiences at each visit. For each such experience, the physician recorded its duration, severity, association with the treatment, action taken, and outcome. We administered the HAM-D, HAM-A, and BDI before and after each arm of the study. All other symptom rating scales were administered weekly.

PROCEDURES

Figure 1 provides an overview of our design: a double-blind, placebo-controlled, randomized, crossover trial comparing methylphenidate with placebo. There were two 3-week treatment periods with 1 week of washout between to avoid a carryover effect of medication. The order of treatment (methylphenidate followed by placebo or placebo followed by methylphenidate) was randomized. Weekly supplies of methylphenidate or placebo were dispensed by the pharmacy in identically appearing 5- and 10-mg capsules. Two of us (T.S and T.W.) prescribed medication under double-blind conditions in three times a day dosing. Compliance was monitored by pill counts at each physician visit. Study medication was titrated up to 0.5 mg/kg per day by week 1, 0.75 mg/kg per day by week 2, and up to 1.0 mg/kg per day by week 3, unless adverse effects emerged. Although drug or placebo status was randomized, the dose within each phase was not. Study treatment was always titrated from low to high doses to avoid exposure to high initial doses of active medication and to minimize side effects.

Serum samples were drawn for methylphenidate levels at the end of week 3. Since methylphenidate has a variable peak plasma concentration in 1 to 2 hours post ingestion, serum samples were obtained by venipuncture 1 hour after the last dose of drug. Samples were collected in 10-mL red-top tubes, allowed to coagulate, immediately centrifuged, and stored at −70°C until analysis. All samples were analyzed in one batch by gas chromatography with mass spectrometry by Met Path Laboratories (Teterboro, NJ).

STATISTICAL ANALYSIS

Sample size was based on power calculations. We estimated the main effect size to be moderate to large, based on our clinical experience and the past literature. Hence, we set the expected standardized difference to be 0.65 SDs in a paired design, with a two-tailed statistical significance set at the 1% level. Our final sample size of 23 had an 80% power to detect such a difference.

Improvement in ADHD and comorbid disorders was defined as a score on the disorder-specific CGI of 1 or 2 (very much or much improved) and a reduction in the corresponding rating scale of 30% or better. To compare the proportion of subjects improved while receiving methylphenidate vs placebo, we used the McNemar Test for correlated proportions. To compare individual symptom scores between two time points, we used the Wilcoxon Signed Rank Test for paired data. These individual scores can have only four ordinal values (0, 1, 2, and 3). For continuous outcome variables, we used the multivariate analysis of variance (MANOVA) to model the dependence of repeated measurements.[44,45] These analyses incorporated both treatment (methylphenidate vs placebo) and time (weeks) as within-subject factors. Since the distribution of the ADHD Rating Scale scores was skewed, we considered transformations from Tukey's ladder of powers[46] and found that squaring the values reduced skewness. Thus, for the MANOVA, values were squared prior to the analysis. All analyses were two tailed. We set statistical significance at the 1% level to account for multiple comparisons and to avoid type I errors. Unless otherwise indicated, data are presented as mean±SEM.

cotherapy in adult patients could result in a more positive outcome than that reported in the literature.

In addition, although the pioneering studies of methylphenidate treatment of adult ADHD provide valuable data, diagnostic issues hinder a straightforward generalization to *DSM-III-R* ADHD.[29] One of these studies did not require a clear history of childhood onset,[24] and others employed adult diagnostic criteria that diverge from those later established in *DSM-III* and *DSM-III-R*.[24-26] Moreover, there has been increasing concern that patients with ADHD and comorbid psychiatric disorders may have a differential response to stimulant therapy.[28,30] Both clinical and epidemiological studies show comorbidity to be a key feature of juvenile ADHD. This comorbidity goes beyond conduct disorder to include depressive and anxiety disorders.[31,32] Recently, Biederman et al[12] reported that adults with ADHD also have high rates of comorbid antisocial, depressive, and anxiety disorders. Despite these findings, little attention has been given to issues of comorbidity in the interpretation of drug trials for ADHD at any age.

The few controlled studies that address the impact of comorbidity on treatment response in children with ADHD report conflicting findings. There are no controlled studies that address the impact of comorbidity on treatment response in adults with ADHD. Pliszka[30] re-

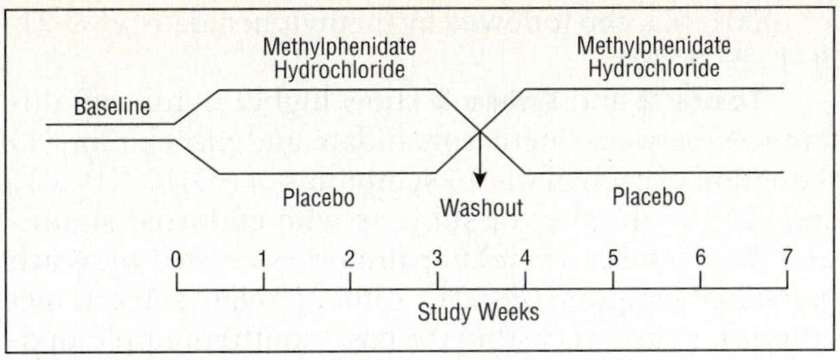

Figure 1. *Study design.*

ported that children with ADHD and comorbid overanxious disorder had a significantly poorer response to stimulant treatment than children with ADHD without overanxious disorder. Biederman et al[33] reported that the response to treatment of childhood ADHD with desipramine hydrochloride was independent of comorbidity. Thus, a comprehensive understanding of drug treatment for adults with ADHD requires careful attention to patterns of comorbidity.

In this study, we report results of a double-blind, placebo-controlled, crossover study of methylphenidate in well-characterized adults with ADHD, attending to issues of psychiatric comorbidity. We hypothesized that methylphenidate, in clinically meaningful doses, would be superior to placebo in the treatment of adults with ADHD.

RESULTS

Of 85 subjects who underwent screening for participation, 70% (n=60) were either ineligible or unable to meet the expectations of a controlled study. Major medical reasons for ineligibility included not meeting criteria for current ADHD (n=13), current use of other medication (n=31), current alcohol or substance abuse (n=4), medical conditions (n=4), and tic disorders (n=1).

Subjects were 25 white, non-Hispanic outpatient adults of both sexes between 18 and 60 years of age satisfying diagnostic criteria for ADHD. Of the 25 subjects enrolled in the study, 23 (92%) completed it. The two subjects who were dropped—one man and one woman—were both receiving methylphenidate. One had an episode of chest pain in the third week of the trial while receiving a dose of 1.0 mg/kg per day of methylphenidate hydrochloride. Although dropped from the study, he elected to have further treatment with methylphenidate after consultation with his internist. The second patient dropped out in the first week because of agitation, irritability, and general unease. Because these two patients did not complete the treatment protocol, they are not included in the data analysis.

Thus, the final sample consisted of 13 women and 10 men who ranged in age from 19 to 56 years (mean±SEM, 40±2 years). All met full criteria for a current *DSM-III-R* diagnosis of ADHD with at least eight of 14 *DSM-III-R* symptoms and an onset of the clinical picture in childhood by the age of 7 years. In all cases, the disorder was continuous until the time of assessment and associated with significant distress and disability. Only one subject had received a diagnosis in childhood of ADHD; none had been previously treated.

As depicted in **Table 1**, 74% (17 of 23) of subjects with ADHD had at least one past comorbid psychiatric disorder, and for 56% (13 of 23), the comorbid disorder was current. The average number of comorbid diagnoses was 2.6±0.3 per subject (Table 1). Baseline ratings of depressive (mean HAM-D score, 5.6±1.1; mean BDI score, 8.6±1.6) and anxiety (mean HAM-A score, 5.7±1.0) symptoms were relatively low. Using standard cutoff points for moderate severity on ratings of depression (HAM-D score, >16; BDI score, >19) and anxiety (HAM-A score, >21), only two subjects (9%) had scores of depression or anxiety above those cutoff points.

OUTCOME ASSESSMENT

Average daily doses of methylphenidate hydrochloride and placebo by the end of each week were 0.51±0.01 and 0.51±0.01 mg/kg, respectively, for week 1; 0.75±0.03 and 0.81±0.02 mg/kg, respectively, for week 2; and 0.92±0.04 and 1.00±0.04 mg/kg, respectively, for week 3. Methylphenidate treatment was more effective than placebo after the first week of treatment, and improvement was increasingly robust in subsequent weeks with increases in daily doses (**Figure 2**). Because data from the ADHD Rating Scale were skewed, we squared each value to achieve a normal distribution. Analysis of the transformed data by MANOVA showed highly significant effects for ADHD symptoms for the effects of drug (methylphenidate or placebo) ($F[1,21]=36$; $P=.0001$), time (weeks 0, 1, 2, or 3) ($F[3,19]=11$; $P=.0002$) and the drug by time interaction ($F[3,19]=12$; $P=.0001$). In addition, the MANOVA for ADHD symptoms found no significant order effect (methylphenidate first vs placebo first), no significant two-way interaction between drug and order, and no significant three-way interaction between drug, week, and order. Our analyses of the CGI-ADHD Global Severity score produced a similar pattern of results.

The effect of methylphenidate was robust enough to be detectable in a parallel group comparison of patients receiving methylphenidate vs placebo during the first 4 weeks of the protocol. This analysis showed highly significant effects for ADHD symptoms as measured by total score on the ADHD Rating Scale for the effects of drug (methylphenidate or placebo) ($F[1,21]=32$; $P=.0001$). There was also a significant effect of time (weeks 0, 1, 2, or 3) ($F[3,19]=11$; $P=.0001$) and a significant drug by time interaction ($F[3,19]=12$; $P=.0008$).

To further evaluate the absolute rate of improvement, we analyzed end-of-treatment results using a preestablished definition of improvement (CGI score, <2, and a reduction of at least 30% in individual rating scale scores). Using this definition, 78% (18 of 23) of patients showed meaningful improvement of ADHD symptoms while receiving methylphenidate, compared with only 4% (1 of 23) while receiving placebo ($\chi^2=25.91$; $df=1$; $P<.0001$). These results did not change when data were analyzed after stratification by order of randomization (methylphenidate followed by placebo, $\chi^2=17.14$, $df=1$,

Table 1. Clinical and Demographic Characteristics of Sample With Attention-Deficit Hyperactivity Disorder (ADHD) (N=23)

Characteristic	Value
Male, No. (%)	10 (43)
Mean (±SEM) age, y	40 (2.1)
Mean (±SEM) socioeconomic status*	1.7 (0.2)
Psychiatric disorders, No. (%)	
Major depression with severe impairment	
Past	6 (26)
Current	0 (0)
Major depression with at least moderate impairment	
Past	12 (52)
Current	3 (13)
Multiple anxiety disorders (≥2)	
Past	9 (39)
Current	8 (35)
At least one anxiety disorder	
Past	13 (56)
Current	11 (48)
Substance dependence	
Past	2 (9)
Current	...
Alcohol dependence	
Past	4 (17)
Current	...
Antisocial personality disorder	
Past	1 (4)
Current	0 (0)
Conduct disorder	
Past	3 (13)
Current	0 (0)
Any comorbid disorder	
Past	17 (74)
Current	13 (56)
Past Global Assessment of Functioning Scale score, mean (±SEM)	50 (1.4)
Current Global Assessment of Functioning Scale score, mean (±SEM)	55 (1.3)
Family history of disorders, No. (%)†	
ADHD	15 (71)
Depression	13 (65)
Anxiety	10 (50)
Antisocial personality disorder	5 (25)
Substance abuse and/or dependence	12 (60)
Cognitive testing, mean (±SEM) score‡	
Freedom From Distractibility IQ	106 (2.4)
Full-scale IQ	114 (2.1)
Achievement testing percentiles, mean (±SEM)§	
Arithmetic	52 (6.2)
Reading	66 (5.8)
Academic underachievement, No. (%)‖	
Arithmetic	7 (32)
Reading	2 (9)
School failure, No. (%)	
Repeated grade	4 (17)
Placement in special class	0 (0)
Tutoring	6 (26)

*Socioeconomic status was measured by the Hollingshead Four Factor Index of Social Status, with low values indicating high socioeconomic status.[41]

†Family history of ADHD was available in 21 subjects; of other disorders, 20 subjects.

‡Cognitive scores were derived from subscales of the Wechsler Adult Intelligence Scales–Revised.

§Achievement testing pecentiles are derived from subscales of the Wide Range Achievement Test–Revised.

‖Results of testing were available in 22 subjects.

$P<.0001$; placebo followed by methylphenidate, $\chi^2=9.21$, $df=1$, $P=.0039$).

Table 2 and **Table 3** show highly significant differences between methylphenidate and placebo for (1) reduction of each of the 14 symptoms of ADHD ($P<.01$) and (2) the number of subjects who endorsed significant (moderate or severe) impairment associated with each individual symptom ($P<.01$). Although eight subjects met criteria for current (within the past month) multiple anxiety disorders and three for current major depressive disorder with at least moderate impairment, only two subjects had severe HAM-A, HAM-D, or BDI symptoms of anxiety or depression at the baseline assessment. Thus, we could not evaluate the impact of treatment on these rating scale scores.

Results were also evaluated after stratification by sociodemographic characteristics, lifetime histories of comorbidity, and family histories of psychopathology to examine the role of these factors as potential confounders in accounting for the study findings. We analyzed end-of-treatment results using the preestablished definition of improvement (a CGI score of less than 2 and a reduction of at least 30% in the ADHD Rating Scale score). We compared the proportion of subjects who achieved this level of improvement of ADHD symptoms in subgroups with and without the individual factors. These analyses showed that similarly robust responses to methylphenidate could be established after stratification of subjects by gender; lifetime history of single and multiple anxiety disorders, moderate major depression, or academic underachievement; and family history of anxiety or ADHD (**Table 4**). Although similarly robust responses to methylphenidate were observed in subjects with and without severe major depression, conduct disorder, or substance use disorders, we lacked adequate statistical power to fully evaluate the impact of treatment on these subgroups.

Correlation analysis revealed no meaningful associations between improvement of symptoms of ADHD and age, number of ADHD symptoms, severity scores, and ratings of depression or anxiety ($r\leq.30$; $P>.05$).

Serum levels of methylphenidate in samples drawn 1 hour after dosing averaged 4.6±0.8 ng/mL (range, 1.0 to 16 ng/mL) at an average daily dose of 0.92±0.04 mg/kg. Methylphenidate levels did not correlate with dose or adverse effects or change the scores of psychiatric symptoms in the any of the domains (ADHD, depression, and anxiety) assessed.

ADVERSE EFFECTS

All but three subjects (13%, not including the two dropouts) were able to tolerate the target dose of 1.0 mg/kg. Although the rates of subjective adverse effects did not differ with methylphenidate and placebo, they were more pronounced with active medication. The most common adverse effects were loss of appetite (6/23 [26%]), insomnia (5/23 [22%]), and anxiety (5/23 [22%]). Five subjects receiving methylphenidate but no subject receiving placebo had the dose lowered because of side effects. Reasons for dose reduction included anxiety (n=3), insomnia (n=2), and euphoria (n=1).

While no meaningful changes in blood pressure were observed between methylphenidate or placebo conditions (systolic blood pressure, 123±2.6 vs 117±1.7 mm Hg, respectively; diastolic blood pressure, 77±2.0 vs 75±1.5 mm Hg, respectively), a small but statistically significant increase in heart rate (80±2.4 vs 76±1.5 beats/min) and decrease in weight (73.2±3.4 vs 74.3±3.6 kg) were observed in methylphenidate but not placebo conditions. However, none of these findings were clinically significant, and no subject required alteration of the dose of medication as a consequence.

COMMENT

In a double-blind, placebo-controlled, crossover trial in adults with ADHD, treatment with methylphenidate hydrochloride at an average oral daily dose of 0.92 mg/kg per day was consistently more effective than placebo. The overall response rate for ADHD symptoms was clinically and statistically higher during methylphenidate treatment than during placebo treatment (78% vs 4%, respectively; $P<.0001$). Improvement in ADHD symptoms was independent of gender, psychiatric comorbidity of anxiety or moderate depression, or family history of psychiatric disorders.

Our findings of a robust response to methylphenidate in adults with ADHD are somewhat discrepant, compared with the more equivocal findings reported in earlier studies. For example, of the four previous controlled studies evaluating the efficacy of methylphenidate in adults with ADHD, only one[24] reported a robust response to methylphenidate (73%) consistent with our results. In contrast, the other three studies reported levels of response ranging from 25%[26] to 57%.[25] This discrepancy could be due to various methodological differences between the studies such as ascertainment, diagnostic methods, sample characteristics, psychiatric comorbidity, and differences in daily doses.

Of note is that subjects in our study were referred for inattention or academic underachievement. This method of ascertainment may account for discrepant findings with one of the other reports of the subject. Mattes et al[26] studied patients who were referred to a general psychiatric clinic for a variety of symptoms and who also had symptoms of ADHD. More work needs to be done to determine the differential response to methylphenidate of subjects ascertained from a general psychiatric clinic or from a specialized ADHD clinic.

Diagnostically, two of the four previous studies of methylphenidate in adults with ADHD used the Utah criteria[24,25] for diagnosis. The Utah criteria contributed greatly to the recognition of ADHD in adulthood and operationalization of diagnostic criteria. However, in addition to the symptoms of inattentiveness and impulsivity that characterize ADHD, these criteria include symptoms of anxiety, mood, and personality disorders (eg, affective lability, hot or explosive temper, and stress intolerance). Thus, it is possible that, compared with the *DSM-III-R* diagnosis of ADHD, the Utah criteria may have identified a more heterogeneous syndrome with a more variable response to stimulants.

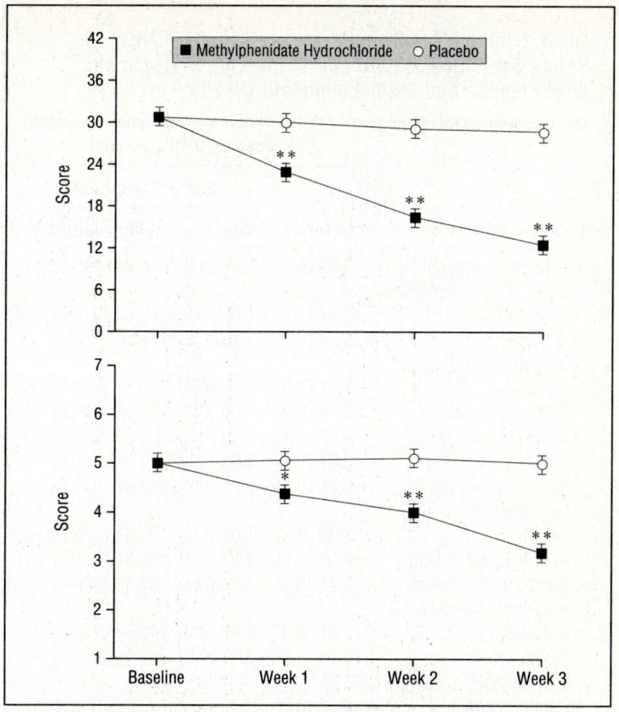

Figure 2. *Scores on the ADHD (attention-deficit hyperactivity disorder) Rating Scale (top) (maximum score, 42; minimum score, 0) and Global Severity subscale of the Clinical Global Impression Scale (bottom) (maximum score, 7; minimum score, 1), by week and dose. Single asterisk indicates* $P<.001$*; double asterisk,* $P<.0001$.

A third salient methodological difference between our work and previous studies was the difference in total daily dose. The target daily dose of 1.0 mg/kg used in our study was much higher than the average dose of 0.6 mg/kg used in previous reports. It is possible that the more equivocal findings previously reported were due to insufficient dosing. For example, we also observed only modest improvement in ADHD symptoms with methylphenidate hydrochloride at the daily dose of 0.5 mg/kg attained after the first week of treatment. In contrast, improvement of ADHD symptoms was far more robust at the end of treatment when higher doses of about 1.0 mg/kg were attained (Figure 2). This finding suggests that the response to methylphenidate in adults with ADHD may be dose dependent. These findings are consistent with pediatric studies in which cognitive, behavioral, and academic improvements occur in a stepwise fashion with increasing doses of methylphenidate.[28,46-48] Our data strongly suggest that adults, like younger patients, require robust dosing to attain an adequate clinical response.

Our analyses examined the effects of psychiatric comorbidity in light of emerging evidence that comorbidity is common in both pediatric[32] and adult[12] samples of subjects with ADHD. This comorbidity goes beyond antisocial and substance use disorders to include depressive and anxiety disorders. Our results suggest that methylphenidate response is independent of psychiatric comorbidity when comorbidity is defined in terms of lifetime diagnosis. However, we could not examine the effects of active, comorbid symptoms because few of our subjects had active comorbid symptoms when they started the protocol.

Table 2. Individual Symptom Scores on the ADHD Rating Scale at Baseline and at the End of Treatment With Placebo and Methylphenidate (N=23)*

	Mean (±SEM) Scores		
		End of Treatment	
Symptom Cluster	Baseline	Placebo	Methylphenidate
Hyperactivity (overall)	2.04 (0.2)	1.88 (0.2)	0.84 (0.2)†‡
Has difficulty remaining seated	1.87 (0.2)	1.61 (0.2)	0.78 (0.2)§‖
Is fidgety	2.13 (0.2)	2.13 (0.2)	0.83 (0.1)†¶
Has difficulty playing quietly	1.74 (0.3)	1.78 (0.2)	0.70 (0.2)§#
Talks excessively	2.44 (0.2)	2.00 (0.2)	1.04 (0.2)§‖
Impulsivity (overall)	2.55 (0.1)	1.99 (0.2)	0.91 (0.1)†‡
Interrupts or intrudes	2.57 (0.1)	2.00 (0.2)	0.96 (0.2)†§
Blurts out answers	2.44 (0.2)	2.05 (0.2)	0.87 (0.2)†§
Has difficulty waiting turn	2.39 (0.2)	1.96 (0.2)	0.83 (0.2)†§
Acts before thinking	2.39 (0.2)	1.91 (0.2)	0.87 (0.2)§‖
Inattentiveness (overall)	2.51 (0.1)	2.28 (0.1)	1.89 (0.1)†‡
Has difficulty sustaining attention	2.87 (0.07)	2.48 (0.2)	1.13 (0.2)†§
Shifts activities	2.96 (0.04)	2.17 (0.2)	1.04 (0.2)†§
Has difficulty following instructions	2.26 (0.2)	2.30 (0.2)	0.87 (0.2)‖¶
Is easily distracted	2.83 (0.08)	2.57 (0.2)	1.17 (0.2)†§
Loses things	2.22 (0.2)	2.22 (0.2)	0.70 (0.2)‖¶
Does not listen	2.39 (0.2)	1.83 (0.1)	0.70 (0.1)‖¶

**ADHD Rating Scale symptom scores range from 0 to 3. 1 indicates not a problem; 3, severe problem.*

†P≤.0001, compared with baseline, by Wilcoxon Signed Rank Test (z<3.2; P<.01).

‡P≤.0001, compared with end point of placebo treatment, by Wilcoxon Signed Rank Test (z>2.8; P<.01).

§P≤.01, compared with end point of placebo treatment, by Wilcoxon Signed Rank Test (z>2.8; P<.01).

‖P≤.001, compared with baseline, by Wilcoxon Signed Rank Test (z<3.2; P<.01).

¶P≤.001, compared with end point of placebo treatment, by Wilcoxon Signed Rank Test (z>2.8; P<.01).

#P≤.01, compared with baseline, by Wilcoxon Signed Rank Test (z<3.2; P<.01).

Table 3. Subjects With Moderately or Severely Impairing Symptom Scores on ADHD Rating Scale at Baseline and at the End of Treatment With Placebo and Methylphenidate (N=23)

	No. (%) of Subjects		
		End of Treatment	
Symptom	Baseline	Placebo	Methylphenidate
Has difficulty remaining seated	17 (74)	14 (61)	3 (13)*†
Is fidgety	19 (83)	19 (83)	3 (13)‡§
Has difficulty playing quietly	16 (70)	16 (70)	5 (22)†‡
Talks excessively	21 (91)	18 (78)	6 (26)*§
Interrupts or intrudes	22 (96)	17 (74)	6 (26)*§
Blurts out answers	21 (91)	17 (74)	5 (22)‡§
Has difficulty waiting turn	21 (91)	18 (78)	5 (22)*§
Acts before thinking	21 (91)	17 (74)	4 (17)*§
Has difficulty sustaining attention	23 (100)	21 (91)	8 (35)*§
Shifts activities	23 (100)	20 (87)	4 (17)‡§
Has difficulty following instructions	21 (91)	20 (87)	7 (30)*†
Is easily distracted	23 (100)	22 (96)	6 (26)‡§
Loses things	18 (78)	19 (83)	2 (9)§‖
Does not listen	20 (87)	17 (74)	3 (13)‡§

**P≤.01, compared with end point of placebo treatment, by χ^2 analysis (df, 1; $\chi^2 \geq 8.1$).*

†P≤.001, compared with baseline, by χ^2 analysis (df, 1; $\chi^2 \geq 11.0$).

‡P≤.001, compared with end point of placebo treatment, by χ^2 analysis (df, 1; $\chi^2 \geq 8.1$).

§P≤.0001, compared with baseline, by χ^2 analysis (df, 1; $\chi^2 \geq 11.0$).

‖P≤.0001, compared with end point of placebo treatment, by χ^2 analysis (df, 1; $\chi^2 \geq 8.1$).

The average 1-hour serum methylphenidate levels (4.6±0.8 ng/mL) in our study were lower than those reported in pediatric samples both in our laboratory and the literature[49] (approximately 10 ng/mL) for similar, single weight-corrected doses (0.3 mg/kg). While the reasons for this discrepancy remain unclear, it suggests that the dosage used in this study was not excessive. Our results failed to identify meaningful associations between methylphenidate serum levels and clinical response. These results are consistent with findings reported in pediatric samples of weak associations between methylphenidate serum levels and clinical response.[50] This absence of association, together with the wide interpatient variability in methylphenidate serum level and lack of association between methylphenidate serum level and daily dose (total or weight-corrected), does not suggest that the measurement of methylphenidate serum levels would be a useful indicator of response or development of adverse effects in subjects with ADHD. However, it is possible that a between-subjects, fixed-dose design would be a more powerful approach for detecting associations between serum levels and clinical response.[51]

Similar numbers of male and female subjects participated in this study. Although this balanced gender distribution is discrepant with the male preponderance in pediatric samples of subjects with ADHD,[2,10,14] similar gender distributions have been reported in previous studies of methylphenidate in adults with ADHD.[24-27] While the reasons for the discrepancy in gender representation between adult and pediatric samples of subjects with ADHD are unclear, one possibility can be proposed. Previous studies suggest that, compared with male subjects with ADHD, female subjects with ADHD are less likely to be severely conduct disordered.[31,52,53] Thus, lower levels of serious behavioral disturbance in girls could have led to gender referral biases and explain the underrepresentation of girls in pediatric samples of subjects with ADHD.[54,55]

Although the diagnosis of ADHD in adults remains controversial, current work provides converging evidence for its validity in adults. Biederman et al[12,56] reported that the retrospective diagnosis of ADHD among adults with ADHD resulted in a pattern of observations consistent with the literature on ADHD in children and adolescents. Compared with normal controls, adults with ADHD had significantly impaired cognitive performance (despite normal IQs), frequent school failures, poorer functioning on the Global Assessment of Functioning Scale, and high rates of antisocial, mood, and anxi-

Table 4. Proportion of Subjects With Improvement of Attention-Deficit Hyperactivity Disorder (ADHD) Symptoms Stratified by Sociodemographic Characteristics, Family History, and Comorbidity (N=23)

Stratification	No. of Subjects	% of Subjects Improved: Following Methylphenidate Treatment	% of Subjects Improved: Following Placebo Treatment
Sociodemographics			
Male	10	80*	10
Female	13	77†	0
Socioeconomic status I to II‡	17	82†	6
Socioeconomic status III to V‡	6	67	0
Family history§			
ADHD			
Yes	15	67‖	7
No	6	100*	0
Major depression			
Yes	14	71†	0
No	6	83	17
Anxiety			
Yes	11	73‖	0
No	9	78*	11
Comorbid disorders (lifetime history)			
Major depression with severe impairment			
Yes	6	67	0
No	17	82†	6
Major depression with at least moderate impairment			
Yes	12	67‖	0
No	11	91‖	9
Multiple (≥2) anxiety disorders			
Yes	9	67*	0
No	14	86†	7
At least one anxiety disorder			
Yes	13	69*	8
No	10	90†	0
Conduct disorder			
Yes	3	67	33
No	20	80†	0
Substance abuse			
Yes	5	60	0
No	18	83†	6
Academic underachievement¶			
Yes	8	100†	0
No	14	71†	0

*$P \leq .01$, by Fisher's Exact Test.
†$P \leq .0001$, by Fisher's Exact Test.
‡*Socioeconomic status was measured by the Hollingshead Four Factor Index of Social Status, with low values indicating high socioeconomic status.*[41]
§*Family history of ADHD was available in 21 subjects; of other disorders, 20 subjects.*
‖$P \leq .001$, by Fisher's Exact Test.
¶*Results of testing were available in 22 subjects.*

ety disorders. In addition, recent evidence of genetic transmission[13-21] and abnormalities in brain structure and function[22,23] further support the legitimacy of the adult diagnosis. These data, together with the robust treatment response to stimulants reported herein, further support the validity of the diagnosis of ADHD in adults using standardized instruments and operational criteria.

Our findings must be seen in light of methodological limitations. In our study, only 29% of subjects undergoing screening were enrolled. As presented herein, the reasons for exclusion consisted of (1) not meeting criteria for ADHD (22%), (2) current use of another medication (52%), (3) current substance use disorder, tic disorder, or medical condition (15%), or (4) inability to meet the expectations of a controlled study (11%), rather than refusal to participate. Thus, most subjects meeting eligibility participated. Nevertheless, more work needs to be done to characterize methylphenidate response in individuals who have subsyndromal ADHD or who are receiving other medications.

While our sample size was more than adequate to demonstrate a large main effect on ADHD symptoms, it was not large enough to fully evaluate all individual subtypes after stratification. Nevertheless, robust responses to methylphenidate treatment were observed after stratification of subjects by gender, lifetime history of single or multiple anxiety disorders or major depression with moderate impairment, academic underachievement, and family history of anxiety disorder or ADHD (Table 4).

Our results for major depression with severe impairment, conduct disorder, and substance use disorder may reflect low statistical power. Future studies will require larger sample sizes to better evaluate response to treatment in individual ADHD subtypes. Since we did not assess the Utah criteria, we cannot comment on their suitability for identifying stimulant-responsive adults with ADHD. This issue requires further investigation. In addition, because 74% of the subjects were from the two highest socioeconomic strata, these results may not be generalizable to lower socioeconomic strata. Further work also needs to be done to examine the response to methylphenidate in adults with ADHD from the lower socioeconomic strata.

The scarcity of subjects with severe depressive or anxiety symptoms did not permit evaluation of the impact of methylphenidate treatment on these non-ADHD domains. However, the low scores on symptoms of depression and anxiety in this sample further strengthen the evidence that the improvement observed is unlikely to be owing to the treatment of non-ADHD symptoms.

While our results are based on reports from affected individuals, it has been suggested that subjects with ADHD may not be ideal reporters of their disorder. Instead, family members may be more informative.[42,57] However, in contrast with the availability of teacher reports in pediatric samples, external evidence is not always available in adult samples. For instance, not all subjects are married, parents may not be available, and subjects may have concerns about asking employers to rate their impaired behaviors. Although this places some limits on the interpretation of our results, the highly significant effects on ADHD symptoms observed in this study under double-blind, placebo-controlled conditions suggest that adult subjects with ADHD are meaningful reporters of their own condition.

Finally, because subjects were not randomly assigned to low- or high-dose treatment, the design of our study does not permit complete separation of dose and time effects. Further investigation of the dose-response relationship may be important to assess in future studies of methylphenidate in adults with ADHD.

Despite these limitations, our double-blind, placebo-controlled trial using robust daily doses of methylphenidate in adults with ADHD shows methylphenidate to be well tolerated and associated with marked improvement in ADHD symptoms.

Accepted for publication October 12, 1994.

The authors thank Harold Demonaco, MS, and the pharmacy at the Massachusetts General Hospital for their assistance with this project.

Reprint requests to Pediatric Psychopharmacology Unit (ACC-725), Massachusetts General Hospital, Fruit Street, Boston, MA 02114 (Dr Spencer).

REFERENCES

1. Mannuzza S, Klein RG, Bonagura N, Malloy P, Giampino TL, Addalli KA. Hyperactive boys almost grown up, V: replication of psychiatric status. *Arch Gen Psychiatry.* 1991;48:77-83.
2. Gittelman R, Mannuzza S, Shenker R, Bonagura N. Hyperactive boys almost grown up, I: psychiatric status. *Arch Gen Psychiatry.* 1985;42:937-947.
3. Weiss G, Hechtman L, Milroy T, Perlman T. Psychiatric status of hyperactives as adults: a controlled prospective 15-year follow-up of 63 hyperactive children. *J Am Acad Child Adolesc Psychiatry.* 1985;24:211-220.
4. Bird HR, Canino G, Rubio-Stipec M, Gould MS, Ribera J, Sesman M, Woodbury M, Huertas-Goldman S, Pagan A, Sanchez-Lacay A, Moscoso M. Estimates of the prevalence of childhood maladjustment in a community survey in Puerto Rico: the use of combined measures. *Arch Gen Psychiatry.* 1988;45: 1120-1126.
5. Anderson JC, Williams S, McGee R, Silva PA. *DSM-III* disorders in preadolescent children: prevalence in a large sample from the general population. *Arch Gen Psychiatry.* 1987;44:69-76.
6. Klein RG, Mannuzza S. The long-term outcome of the attention deficit disorder/ hyperkinetic syndrome. In: Sagvolden T, Archer T, eds. *Attention Deficit Disorder: Clinical and Basic Research.* Hillside, NJ: Erlbaum Associates; 1989:71-89.
7. Weiss G, Hechtman L, Perlman T, Hopkins J, Wener A. Hyperactives as young adults: a controlled prospective 10-year follow-up of 75 children. *Arch Gen Psychiatry.* 1979;36:675-681.
8. Spencer T, Biederman J, Wilens T, Faraone S. Is attention deficit hyperactivity disorder in adults a valid disorder? *Harvard Rev Psychiatry.* 1994;1:326-335.
9. Klein RG, Mannuzza S. Long-term outcome of hyperactive children: a review. *J Am Acad Child Adolesc Psychiatry.* 1991;30:383-387.
10. Weiss G, Hechtman LT. *Hyperactive Children Grown Up.* New York, NY: The Guilford Press; 1986.
11. Thorley G. Review of follow-up and follow-back studies of childhood hyperactivity. *Psychol Bull.* 1984;96:116-132.
12. Biederman J, Faraone SV, Spencer T, Wilens T, Norman D, Lapey K, Mick E, Krifcher-Lehman B, Doyle A. Patterns of psychiatric comorbidity, cognition and psychosocial functioning in adults with attention deficit hyperactivity disorder. *Am J Psychiatry.* 1993;150:1792-1798.
13. Biederman J, Faraone SV, Keenan K, Benjamin J, Krifcher B, Moore C, Sprich-Buckminster S, Ugaglia K, Jellinek MS, Steingard R, Spencer T, Norman D, Kolodny R, Kraus I, Perrin J, Keller MB, Tsuang MT. Further evidence for family-genetic risk factors in attention deficit hyperactivity disorder: patterns of comorbidity in probands and relatives in psychiatrically and pediatrically referred samples. *Arch Gen Psychiatry.* 1992;49:728-738.
14. Biederman J, Faraone SV, Keenan K, Knee D, Tsuang MT. Family-genetic and psychosocial risk factors in *DSM-III* attention deficit disorder. *J Am Acad Child Adolesc Psychiatry.* 1990;29:526-533.
15. Goodman R. Genetic factors in hyperactivity account for about half of the explainable variance. *BMJ.* 1989;298:1407-1408.
16. Goodman R, Stevenson J. A twin study of hyperactivity, I: an examination of hyperactivity scores and categories derived from Rutter teacher and parent questionnaires. *J Child Psychol Psychiatry.* 1989;30:671-689.
17. Goodman R, Stevenson J. A twin study of hyperactivity, II: the aetiological role of genes, family relationships and perinatal adversity. *J Child Psychol Psychiatry.* 1989;30:691-709.
18. Faraone S, Biederman J, Chen WJ, Krifcher B, Keenan K, Moore C, Sprich-Buckminster S, Tsuang M. Segregation analysis of attention deficit hyperactivity disorder: evidence for single gene transmission. *Psychiatry Genet.* 1992; 2:257-275.
19. Faraone S, Biederman J. Is attention deficit hyperactivity disorder familial? *Harvard Rev Psychiatry.* 1994;1:271-287.
20. Deutsch CK, Matthysse S, Swanson JM, Farkas LG. Genetic latent structure analysis of dysmorphology in attention deficit disorder. *J Am Acad Child Adolesc Psychiatry.* 1990;29:189-194.
21. Manshadi M, Lippmann S, O'Daniel RG, Blackman A. Alcohol abuse and attention deficit disorder. *J Clin Psychiatry.* 1983;44:379-380.
22. Zametkin AJ, Nordahl TE, Gross M, King C, Semple WE, Rumsey J, Hamburger S, Cohen RM. Cerebral glucose metabolism in adults with hyperactivity of childhood onset. *N Engl J Med.* 1990;323:1361-1366.
23. Zametkin AJ, Liebenauer LL, Fitzgerald GA, King AC, Minkunas DV, Herscovitch P, Yamada EM, Cohen RM. Brain metabolism in teenagers with attention-deficit hyperactivity disorder. *Arch Gen Psychiatry.* 1993;50:333-340.
24. Wood DR, Reimherr FW, Wender PH, Johnson GE. Diagnosis and treatment of minimal brain dysfunction in adults: a preliminary report. *Arch Gen Psychiatry.* 1976;33:1453-1460.
25. Wender PH, Reimherr FW, Wood D, Ward M. A controlled study of methylphenidate in the treatment of attention deficit disorder, residual type, in adults. *Am J Psychiatry.* 1985;142:547-552.
26. Mattes JA, Boswell L, Oliver H. Methylphenidate effects on symptoms of attention deficit disorder in adults. *Arch Gen Psychiatry.* 1984;41:1059-1063.
27. Gualtieri CT, Ondrusek MG, Finley C. Attention deficit disorders in adults. *Clin Neuropharmacol.* 1985;8:343-356.

28. Wilens T, Biederman J. The stimulants. In: Schaffer D, ed. *Psychiatric Clinics of North America.* Philadelphia, Pa: WB Saunders Co; 1992:191-222.
29. American Psychiatric Association. *Diagnostic and Statistical Manual of Mental Disorders, Revised Third Edition.* Washington, DC: American Psychiatric Association; 1987.
30. Pliszka SR. Effect of anxiety on cognition, behavior, and stimulant response in ADHD. *J Am Acad Child Adolesc Psychiatry.* 1989;28:882-887.
31. Biederman J, Newcorn J, Sprich-Buckminster S. Comorbidity of attention deficit hyperactivity disorder with conduct, depressive, anxiety, and other disorders. *Am J Psychiatry.* 1991;148:564-577.
32. Biederman J, Newcorn J. Comorbidity in attention deficit hyperactivity disorder. In: Task Force on *DSM-IV*, ed. *Source Book for DSM-IV.* Washington, DC: American Psychiatric Association. In press.
33. Biederman J, Baldessarini RJ, Wright V, Keenan K, Faraone S. A double-blind placebo controlled study of desipramine in the treatment of attention deficit disorder, III: lack of impact of comorbidity and family history factors on clinical response. *J Am Acad Child Adolesc Psychiatry.* 1993;32:199-204.
34. Spitzer RL, Williams JB, Gibbon M, First MB. *Structured Clinical Interview for DSM-III-R–Non-Patient Edition (SCID-NP, Version 1.0).* Washington, DC: American Psychiatric Association; 1990.
35. Orvaschel H. Psychiatric interviews suitable for use in research with children and adolescents. *Psychopharmacol Bull.* 1985;21:737-745.
36. Biederman J, Rosenbaum JF, Hirshfeld DR, Faraone SV, Bolduc EA, Gersten M, Meminger SR, Kagan J, Snidman N, Reznick JS. Psychiatric correlates of behavioral inhibition in young children of parents with and without psychiatric disorders. *Arch Gen Psychiatry.* 1990;47:21-26.
37. Wechsler D. *Manual for the Wechsler Adult Intelligence Scale—Revised.* San Antonio, Tex: The Psychological Corp; 1981.
38. Jastak JF, Jastak S. *The Wide Range Achievement Test—Revised.* Wilmington, Del: Jastak Associates; 1985.
39. Faraone S, Biederman J. Genetics of attention-deficit hyperactivity disorder. *Child Adolesc Psychiatr Clin North Am.* 1994;3:285-302.
40. Faraone SV, Santangelo S. Methods in genetic epidemiology. In: Fava M, Rosenbaum JF, eds. *Research Designs and Methods in Psychiatry.* New York, NY: Elsevier Science Publishing Co Inc; 1992:93-118.
41. Hollingshead AB. *Four Factor Index of Social Status.* New Haven, Conn: Yale University Department of Sociology; 1975.
42. CGI (Clinical Global Impression) Scale—NIMH. *Psychopharmacol Bull.* 1985; 21:839-844.
43. Barkley RA. *Attention Deficit Hyperactivity Disorder: A Handbook for Diagnosis and Treatment.* New York, NY: The Guilford Press; 1990.
44. Ekstrom D, Quade D, Golden RN. Statistical analysis of repeated measures in psychiatric research. *Arch Gen Psychiatry.* 1990;47:770-772.
45. Lavori P. ANOVA, MANOVA, my black hen: comments on repeated measures. *Arch Gen Psychiatry.* 1990;47:775-778.
46. Tukey JW. *Exploratory Data Analysis.* Reading, Mass: Addison-Wesley Publishing Co; 1977.
47. Rapport MD, Jones JT, DuPaul GJ, Kelly KL, Gardner MJ, Tucker SB, Shea MS. Attention deficit disorder and methylphenidate: group and single-subject analyses of dose effects on attention in clinic and classroom settings. *J Clin Child Psychol.* 1987;16:329-338.
48. Barkley RA, DuPaul GJ, McMurray MB. Attention deficit disorder with and without hyperactivity: clinical response to three dose levels of methylphenidate. *Pediatrics.* 1991;87:519-531.
49. Gualtieri CT, Hicks RE, Patrick K, Schroeder SR, Breese GR. Clinical correlates of methylphenidate blood levels. *Ther Drug Monit.* 1984;6:379-392.
50. Patrick K, Mueller R, Gualtieri C, Breese GR. Pharmacokinetics and actions of methylphenidate. In: Meltzer H, ed. *Psychopharmacology: The Third Generation of Progress.* New York, NY: Raven Press; 1987:1387-1395.
51. Faraone SV, Simpson JC, Brown WA. Mathematical models of complex dose-response relationships: implications for experimental design in psychopharmacologic research. *Stat Med.* 1992;11:685-702.
52. Faraone SV, Biederman J, Keenan K, Tsuang MT. A family-genetic study of girls with *DSM-III* attention deficit disorder. *Am J Psychiatry.* 1991;148:112-117.
53. Wender PH, Reimherr FW, Wood DR. Attention deficit disorder ('minimal brain dysfunction') in adults: a replication study of diagnosis and drug treatment. *Arch Gen Psychiatry.* 1981;38:449-456.
54. Safer DJ, Krager JM. A survey of medication treatment for hyperactive/inattentive students. *JAMA.* 1988;260:2256-2258.
55. Shaywitz SE, Shaywitz BA. Attention deficit disorder: current perspectives. *Pediatr Neurol.* 1987;3:129-135.
56. Biederman J, Faraone SV, Knee D, Munir K. Retrospective assessment of *DSM-III* attention deficit disorder in non-referred individuals. *J Clin Psychiatry.* 1990; 51:102-107.
57. Wender P, Wood DR, Reimherr FW. Pharmacological treatment of attention deficit disorder, residual type (ADDRT, 'minimal brain dysfunction,' 'hyperactivity') in adults. *Psychopharmacol Bull.* 1985;21:222-232.

ORIGINAL ARTICLE

Efficacy of Methylphenidate for Attention-Deficit Hyperactivity Disorder in Children With Tic Disorder

Kenneth D. Gadow, PhD; Jeffrey Sverd, MD; Joyce Sprafkin, PhD; Edith E. Nolan, PhD; Stacy N. Ezor, MA

Background: The findings from case reports and patient questionnaire surveys have been interpreted as indicating that administration of stimulants is ill-advised for the treatment of attention-deficit hyperactivity disorder in children with tic disorder.

Methods: Thirty-four prepubertal children with attention-deficit hyperactivity disorder and tic disorder received placebo and three dosages of methylphenidate hydrochloride (0.1, 0.3, and 0.5 mg/kg) twice daily for 2 weeks each, under double-blind conditions. Treatment effects were assessed using direct observations of child behavior in a simulated (clinic-based) classroom and using rating scales completed by the parents, teachers, and physician.

Results: Methylphenidate effectively suppressed hyperactive, disruptive, and aggressive behavior. There was no evidence that methylphenidate altered the severity of tic disorder, but it may have a weak effect on the frequency of motor (increase) and vocal (decrease) tics.

Conclusion: Methylphenidate appears to be a safe and effective treatment for attention-deficit hyperactivity disorder in the majority of children with comorbid tic disorder.

(Arch Gen Psychiatry. 1995;52:444-455)

IN SPITE OF a relatively long and productive history of research on stimulant drug therapy for childhood behavior disorders, controversies remain, and none is more divisive than its appropriateness for the treatment of attention-deficit hyperactivity disorder (ADHD) in children with comorbid tic disorder. Historically, Bradley[1] was one of the first investigators to note that some children with behavior disorders who were receiving clinical doses of amphetamine "gave evidence of increased emotional tension by . . . accentuation of tic-like motor activities" (eg, nail biting, hair pulling, and nose picking). Later, Mattson and Calverly[2] described a case of drug-induced involuntary movements (lip smacking, grimacing, and eyelid twitching) in an 8-year-old boy who was treated with 5 mg of dextroamphetamine sulfate. Early studies of children treated with methylphenidate hydrochloride, which is currently the most widely prescribed drug for hyperactivity and/or ADHD,[3] also found that this stimulant significantly increased fingernail biting[4] and induced tics in a small percentage of subjects.[5] Golden[6] reported the first case of apparent methylphenidate-induced Tourette syndrome (TS) in a 9-year-old hyperactive boy. After 8 weeks of treatment, a variety of motor and vocal tics suddenly developed in the child and did not abate after administration of medication (10 mg, twice a day) was terminated. Additional cases have been described.[7,8]

Early case reports of stimulant drug therapy specifically for the treatment of tic disorder indicated limited efficacy and tic exacerbation in some individuals.[9-12] As an aside, it is noteworthy that these early reports also note that tic exacerbation is associated with almost all psychotherapeutic drugs,[9] which is an accurate description of currently popular medications as well.[13] The past two decades have witnessed a flurry of case reports, some of which were controlled drug evaluations,[11,14,15] questionnaire surveys, and chart reviews, that question the safety of

From the Department of Psychiatry and Behavioral Science, State University of New York–Stony Brook (Drs Gadow, Sverd, Sprafkin, and Nolan and Ms Ezor) and Sagamore Children's Psychiatric Center, Office of Mental Health, State of New York, Dix Hills (Dr Sverd).

See Subjects and Methods on next page

SUBJECTS AND METHODS

SUBJECTS

The subjects were 34 children (31 boys and three girls) between the ages of 6 years 1 month and 11 years 11 months, who were referred for evaluation to the Tic Disorders Clinic, Stony Brook, NY, by a clinician who specialized in the treatment of patients with tic disorders (J. Sverd) or to a child psychiatry outpatient service (**Table 1**). The diagnostic procedure included child and parent clinical interviews and a battery of psychometric instruments for assessing ADHD symptoms and tics. The study sample included 11 children who were described in preliminary reports.[37,39]

Prior to the children's enrollment in the study, parents were warned repeatedly of the possible risk of irreversible tic exacerbation as a result of stimulant treatment and were required to sign a written statement consenting to their child's participation. Once enrolled in the study, each child was monitored very closely. Parents had telephone access to clinicians (home and office) day and night for the duration of the drug evaluation, and the school was alerted to the possibility of tic exacerbation and the importance of immediate notification of changes in clinical status.

Acceptance Criteria

Potential subjects had to meet *DSM-III-R*[40] diagnostic criteria for ADHD and either chronic motor tic disorder or Tourette disorder (established on the basis of a clinical interview with the parent) and, in general, be above the cutoff on two of three parent- and teacher-completed hyperactivity and/or ADHD behavior rating scales. The ADHD measures that were part of the diagnostic evaluation included the Abbreviated Teacher Rating Scale (ATRS)/Abbreviated Parent Rating Scale (APRS),[41] the Inattention-Overactivity With Aggression (IOWA) Conners Teacher's Rating Scale,[42] the Conners (48-item) Parent Rating Scale,[43] the Mothers' Objective Method for Subgrouping (MOMS) checklist,[44] and the parent and teacher versions of the Stony Brook Child Psychiatric Checklist-3R.[45] All but two participating children were above the cutoff on at least two of three parent measures of hyperactivity and/or ADHD, and 26 were above the cutoff on at least two of three teacher measures.

The tic measures completed by one of us (J. Sverd) at the diagnostic evaluation included the Yale Global Tic Severity Scale,[46] the Tourette Syndrome–Clinical Global Impression Scale,[23(pp55-78)] the Shapiro Tourette Syndrome Severity Scale,[17] and the Tourette Syndrome Unified Rating Scale.[47] Each child also was videotaped during a 15-minute simulated classroom observation session during which the number of motor and vocal tics emitted was recorded. Briefly, our subjects' tic symptoms ranged from mild to severe (Table 1). All children met research diagnostic criteria[48,49] for either TS (definite or by history) or chronic multiple motor tic disorder (definite). The terms "definite" and "by history" were defined as follows: definite meant that motor and/or phonic tics must be witnessed by a reliable examiner directly at some point in the illness or be recorded by videotape or cinematography, and by history meant that tics were witnessed by a reliable family member or close friend and the description of tics as demonstrated are accepted by a reliable examiner. At least two reliable examiners in different settings witnessed motor tics in all of our subjects. A subsample of parents (n=22) were asked to evaluate the current status of their children's motor and vocal tics, respectively: less severe than usual (10%, 20%), average severity (76%, 70%), or more severe than usual (14%, 10%).

Comorbidities

The Diagnostic Interview for Children and Adolescents–Revised[50,51] was administered to the mothers (parent version) and children (child version) (n=21; 18 boys and three girls) and confirmed the diagnosis of ADHD in all cases. Most (81%) of the interviewed patients were comorbid for either oppositional defiant disorder (n=15) or conduct disorder (n=2). The number of children above the clinical cutoff on the aggression subscale of the IOWA Conners Teacher's Rating Scale and the MOMS aggression subscale was 23 and 20, respectively (Table 1). More than one third (n=8) also met diagnostic criteria (best estimate diagnosis based on the child and parent Diagnostic Interview for Children and Adolescents–Revised and child self-report) for an anxiety disorder (overanxious disorder, separation anxiety disorder, or simple phobia) and/or a depressive or dysthymic disorder. Three children met diagnostic criteria for obsessive-compulsive disorder.

Medication History

Children were not excluded from participation in the study if they had prior experience with stimulant drug therapy or if such therapy purportedly had exacerbated their tics. Thirteen of the children had a prior history of drug therapy for either ADHD (n=8) or ADHD and TS (n=5): 10 received stimulants; four, antipsychotic drugs; two, clonidine; and two, alprazolam. Seven children were receiving medication at the time of referral. In the case of stimulants (n=5), the minimum washout period was 1 week. The washout period for the children who were receiving an antipsychotic drug (pimozide) or clonidine was 3 and 2 weeks, respectively. Of the 10 children who were treated previously with stimulants, undocumented tic exacerbation was reported by parents in four children, and tic onset after drug exposure was reported in two children.

Rejection Criteria

Children who met one or more of the following criteria were excluded from consideration for the study: were believed to be too severely ill (dangerous to self or others); tics were the major clinical management concern; were psychotic or mentally retarded (IQ<70); or had a seizure disorder, major organic brain dysfunction, major medical illness, medical or other contraindication to medication (other than tics), or pervasive developmental disorder.

MEDICATION

Subjects received placebo and three dosages of methylphenidate hydrochloride (0.1 mg/kg [mean±SD, 4.4±1.5 mg], 0.3 mg/kg [mean, 9.0±3.3 mg], and 0.5 mg/kg [mean±SD,

Continued on next page

14.0±3.9 mg]) for 2 weeks each. For ease of administration, individual doses in milligrams were rounded off to the nearest 2.5 mg (0.1-mg/kg dosage) or 5 mg (0.3- and 0.5-mg/kg dosages). The upper limit for the 0.5-mg/kg dosage was 20 mg. Dose schedules were counterbalanced and assigned on a random basis. When the 0.5-mg/kg dosage was not preceded by a low-dose condition, the child was gradually built up to the moderate dose. Medication was administered twice daily, approximately 3.5 hours apart, 7 days a week. In most cases, the morning dose was given by parents before the child left for school, and the noon dose was administered by the school nurse. Medication and identically matching placebos were dispensed to the parents and school nurses in dated, sealed envelopes at 2-week intervals. Parents and nurses were asked to return unused medication envelopes, which allowed us to assess compliance. Medication was administered under double-blind conditions (ie, no one involved in the clinical management of the patient, data collection, or interaction with the school knew the identity of the treatment conditions). Given the possibility of a medical emergency, one investigator (K.D.G.) had access to the dosage code.

PROCEDURE

Once the medication evaluation began, each child with ADHD and at least one parent (typically the mother, who was designated as the respondent for all of the clinical assessments) were required to come to the clinic at 2-week intervals for clinical evaluation and to receive the next 2-week allotment of medication. During the clinical evaluation, the parent was interviewed by the clinician (J. Sverd), and the child's clinical status was determined. The parent was asked to complete separate rating scales for the child's ADHD and tic symptoms. The clinician also briefly interviewed the child, observed tics, and assessed weight, heart rate, and blood pressure.

Following the physician's evaluation, children were required to complete work activities in a simulated classroom, during which time they were videotaped for 15 minutes through a one-way window. Clinic observations were conducted approximately 1.25 hours after drug ingestion.

A subsample of children (n=28) completed a computerized version of the Continuous Performance Task (CPT) approximately 1.75 hours after drug ingestion. The CPT was first administered as part of the diagnostic evaluation. Prior to testing, the examiner demonstrated the task, gave the child a practice trial, and reminded him or her what the target was. The examiner remained in the room during testing, sat approximately 1.2 m behind the child, and engaged in a task while the child completed the CPT.

In addition to the rating scales that the parent completed as part of the clinic interview, parents were asked to provide behavioral, side effect, and tic ratings for each weekend. The parent completed one set of ratings for their child's behavior during the morning and early afternoon on Saturday and Sunday.

Teachers completed behavioral, side effect, and tic ratings for each subject's behavior 2 days per week for the duration of the drug evaluation.

MEASURES

Physician Evaluations

The tic measures (completed by J. Sverd) included the Yale Global Tic Severity Scale and the Tourette Syndrome Unified Rating Scale, which were completed for the entire sample, and the Global Tic Rating Scale (GTRS),[52,53] the Tourette Syndrome–Clinical Global Impression Scale, and the Shapiro Tourette Syndrome Severity Scale, which were added to the assessment battery for the last 22 subjects. Four subscales from the Yale Global Tic Severity Scale were used: the total motor tic score, the total phonic tic score, the overall impairment rating, and the global severity score. Three tic scales from the Tourette Syndrome Unified Rating Scale were administered: the Shapiro Symptom Checklist (total number of tics), the tic count (number of tics observed in 2 minutes during quiet conversation with the patient), and the LeWitt Disability Scale. The latter is a global symptom severity–impairment scale that assesses tics and tic-related features (eg, compulsive actions, obsessive thoughts, ritualistic behaviors, anxiety spells, disruptive behavior disorders, and attention deficits).

Obsessive-compulsive symptoms were evaluated using two scales from the Tourette Syndrome Unified Rating Scale. Parents were first asked five screening questions about the presence of obsessions and compulsions using the Obsessive-compulsive Disorder Screen, and then they evaluated the severity of these symptoms with the Clinical Global Impression Scale–Obsessive-compulsive Disorder.[23(pp55-78)] Because neither of these scales pertain to specific symptoms, they must be considered global assessment instruments.

Simulated Classroom

The playroom procedure developed by Routh and Schroeder[54] and modified by Roberts et al[55] and Milich and colleagues[56] was used to assess the effect of medication on tics. In this study, we used only the 15-minute restricted academic period. In the restricted academic setting, the child is instructed to complete worksheets and not to play with toys on an adjacent table. Worksheet items are similar to those on the coding subtest of the Wechsler Intelligence Scale for Children–Revised. Clinic sessions were videotaped to facilitate ease of scoring. For this study, videotapes were coded for the presence of motor and vocal tics. However, the latter were so infrequent that they precluded meaningful data analysis. The 15-minute observation sessions were divided into 180 five-second intervals, and tics were coded as either present or not present in each interval. Prior to coding the medication conditions, two experienced raters (J. Sprafkin and S.N.E.) reviewed a list of the child's known tics and coded the baseline (diagnostic) session. The two coders plus a third judge (K.D.G.) then met and reached a consensus on the identity of each tic (tic inventory). If interrater reliability for the baseline session was below criterion ($\kappa<0.60$), the baseline tape was recoded until the minimum reliability criterion was met. The four drug trials were then evaluated by the primary coder,

stimulants for the treatment of ADHD in children with tic disorder.[16,17] Briefly, the findings from questionnaire surveys and chart reviews suggest increased tics associated with stimulant medication in 40% to 50% and 10% to 30% of patients, respectively. Controlled studies that employed multiple challenge doses provided the most compelling evidence of tic exacerbation in specific individuals.[11] Perhaps the most influential proscription against stimulant drug therapy was a case review study by Lowe et al[18] of patients who and two randomly selected trials were scored by the secondary coder to assess reliability. Although the coders used the tic inventory as a guide, any new tics that emerged during the drug evaluation were also coded. The overall κ for the drug trials was 0.70 (range, 0.41 to 0.77).

Continuous Performance Task

The CPT used in this study was a computerized version developed by Halperin et al,[57] in which the child is instructed to press the space bar whenever the letter *A* follows the letter *X* on the screen. The CPT generates three measures (inattention, impulsivity, and dyscontrol) that are uncorrelated with each other and IQ. This version of the CPT has been shown to have good test-retest reliability, to correlate with teacher ratings of inattention, to be sensitive to stimulant drug effects, and to distinguish children with ADHD from controls.[58,59]

Parent and Teacher Ratings

The Conners[41] ATRS contains 10 items rated on a four-point scale (0 indicates not at all; 3, very much) that are summed to generate a total score. A factor analysis of the ATRS revealed two factors[60]: factor 1 refers to behaviors generally considered to be symptoms of hyperactivity, and factor 2 assesses emotional lability. The addition of five items to the ATRS permitted the determination of the inattention-overactivity and aggression subscale scores of the IOWA Conners Teacher's Rating Scale.[42] The IOWA Conners Teacher's Rating Scale has been shown to differentiate between the behavioral dimensions of hyperactivity and aggression and demonstrates adequate reliability and sensitivity to stimulant drug effects.[42,61-65] The ATRS was completed by the teacher 2 days per week for the child's behavior during school for each week of the dose-response evaluation.

Parents used the Conners APRS[41] to evaluate their child's behavior during morning and early afternoon on Saturday and Sunday. During their biweekly clinic evaluations, they also completed the MOMS for their child's behavior during the previous week. The MOMS contains 10 (hyperactivity and/or ADHD) symptoms arranged in a checklist format. The mother simply checks whether or not each item characterizes her child (1 indicates checked; 0, unchecked). The MOMS generates a hyperactivity scale score and an aggression scale score, both of which demonstrate convergent and divergent validity.[44]

The Peer Conflict Scale[65-67] was used by parents and teachers to assess aggressive interactions with other children. The Peer Conflict Scale shows adequate test-retest reliability and convergent validity with direct observations of negativistic behaviors.[65]

Parents and teachers recorded their perceptions of changes in tic status on the GTRS according to the same schedule as the behavior rating scales. Both parents and teachers were made aware of the behaviors and vocalizations that were considered tics during the diagnostic phase of the patient evaluation. Our own research shows the GTRS to be reliable.[53]

Parents and teachers evaluated adverse drug reactions using the Stimulant Side Effects Checklist (SSEC).[66,68] The SSEC contains 13 side effect items rated on a four-point scale (0 indicates not at all; 3, very much). Individual items are grouped to form three indexes of drug effects: the mood index, the attention-arousal index, and the somatic complaints index. One item pertains to abnormal movements.

STATISTICAL ANALYSES

The teacher- and parent-completed rating scale scores were first analyzed using a two-way (behavior by scale) repeated measures analysis of variance (ANOVA). Measures were grouped according to respondent (parent or teacher) and domain (ADHD behaviors or side effects). Both type of scale and dosage (placebo, 0.1 mg/kg, 0.3 mg/kg, or 0.5 mg/kg) were within-subjects factors. The data sets for a few children were incomplete because care providers did not complete the ratings. (Unless noted otherwise, all reported significant main effects are also significant using the Greenhouse-Geisser correction.) Tests for trend were also conducted to provide information about the form of the relation between doses of methylphenidate and the dependent variable. To localize the source of statistically significant dose effects, post hoc Newman-Keuls tests were performed to assess differences between doses in the rate of occurrence of specific behaviors.

Tics

The tic data were first analyzed using two-way (tic measure by dose) repeated measures ANOVAs; separate analyses were conducted for each respondent (observer, parent, or teacher). Given our concern about the possibility of making a type II error (ie, erroneously concluding that methylphenidate did not have an adverse effect on tics), follow-up repeated measures ANOVAs were performed on each respondent category even when the main effect of dose was not significant.

A power analysis (using published estimates of r=.5 to .8 for the 3-week stability [autocorrelation] of direct observations and ratings of tic frequency and severity)[69] indicated that a sample of 34 subjects provided 80% power to detect treatment effects of 0.33 SDs or larger assuming the stability equals .8. If the stability is as low as .5, an effect of at least 0.50 SDs could be detected with 80% power.

Multivariate Analyses of Variance

Separate two-way multivariate ANOVAs were conducted for the behavior rating scales for each of the three sets of raters (teachers, parents, and physician). Unless indicated otherwise, univariate ANOVAs were conducted only when the results of these analyses indicated that there was a significant main effect of dose (P<.01, using the Wilks' λ criterion).

were treated in university and community-based clinics that concluded "motor tics or diagnosed TS in a child should be a contraindication to the use of stimulant medication for alleviation of hyperactive symptoms." Much less attention was given to a literature review by Shapiro and Shapiro[16] that appeared about the same time and that noted the methodological problems and logical inconsistencies in the existing literature that is interpreted as supporting stimulant tic induction and/or exacerbation hypotheses. The

Table 1. Patient Characteristics at Diagnosis*

Characteristics	No. of Patients	Mean (SD)
Age	34	8 y 10 mo (1 y 11 mo)
IQ	28	105.9 (13.7)
Age at onset of tics	23	5 y 7 mo (2 y 7 mo)
Race/ethnicity, No. (%)	34 (100)	NA
White	29 (85)	NA
Hispanic	3 (9)	NA
Asian	1 (3)	NA
Black	1 (3)	NA
Research Diagnostic Criteria, No. (%)	34 (100)	NA
Tourette syndrome, definite	22 (65)	NA
Tourette syndrome by history	11 (32)	NA
Chronic multiple motor tics	1 (3)	NA
Hyperactivity/ADHD measures (cutoff score)		
Parent ADHD measures		
Stony Brook ADHD index (>7)	32	9.9 (2.4)
Conners hyperactivity index (>15)	33	18.1 (4.6)
MOMS hyperactivity subscale (>2)	34	4.1 (1.2)
Teacher ADHD measures		
Stony Brook ADHD index (>7)	30	9.8 (3.6)
ATRS (>15)	31	20.0 (6.0)
IOWA Conners I-O subscale (>6)	33	11.4 (3.0)
Tic measures		
Physician tic scale		
YGTSS	34	
Total motor tic score		13.8 (3.3)
Total phonic tic score		10.6 (3.8)
Overall impairment rating		18.0 (12.5)
Global severity score		42.3 (17.0)
TS-CGI	22	3.6 (0.7)
STSSS	22	2.9 (1.3)
Videotape tic counts	33	
Motor tics		18.9 (12.6)
Vocal tics		0.3 (0.7)
Comorbidities, agression (cutoff score)		
IOWA Conners aggression scale (>3)	33	7.4 (4.9)
MOMS aggression subscale (>2)	34	2.7 (1.9)
Special education, No. (%)	34 (100)	NA
Full time (self contained)	9 (26)	NA
Part time (resource room)	14 (41)	NA
None	11 (32)	NA
Family history tics/motor habits, No. (%)	32 (100)	NA
A first-degree relative	30 (94)	NA
Both biological parents	16 (50)	NA

**ADHD indicates attention-deficit hyperactivity disorder; MOMS, Mothers' Objective Method for Subgrouping; ATRS, Abbreviated Teacher Rating Scale; IOWA, Inattention-Overactivity With Aggression; I-O, inattention-overacting; YGTSS, Yale Global Tic Severity Scale; TS-CGI, Tourette Syndrome–Clinical Global Impression Scale; STSSS, Shapiro Tourette Syndrome Severity Scale; and NA, not applicable.*

relatively common co-occurrence of hyperactivity and tic disorder in children who are referred for psychiatric evaluation of behavioral disturbance[19-22] makes this controversy a significant issue in child psychiatry.

The debate over the safety and efficacy of stimulants for inattentive and/or disruptive behaviors in children with tic disorder has been further complicated by a major controversy over the pleiotropic manifestations of the TS diathesis. Children with TS experience a variety of behavioral, affective, and cognitive disabilities, and there is much disagreement as to which are intrinsic to the tic disorder (ie, phenocopies of other childhood disorders) and which are comorbidities.[17,23-26] For example, it was once argued that the attention deficits and disruptive behaviors seen in children with tic disorder are phenocopies of true ADHD and oppositional defiant disorder and/or conduct disorder, respectively, and that stimulants were ineffective for their clinical management.[27]

Response to stimulant medication also has played an important role in theory formulation concerning the neuropathologic characteristics of tic disorder. Most notable was the observation that stimulants exacerbated tics in some individuals,[11,14,15] which supported hyperdopaminergic dysfunction as a probable cause of tic expression.[24,28] Alternatively, evidence suggesting that the effect of stimulants on tics is heterogeneous and that some patients even experience tic amelioration[29-32] has led to more complex theories of dopaminergic involvement in the pathogenesis of tic disorder. For example, Comings[29] and Comings and Comings[30] suggested that early exposure to stimulant medications in children at risk for the development of TS might delay the onset of tics by preventing secondary hypersensitization of subcortical dopamine pathways, which results from genetically caused hypofunction of mesocortical dopamine pathways. Friedhoff[33] hypothesized that following transient worsening of tics on initial exposure to methylphenidate, the drug may induce a reduction in dopamine receptor sensitivity, resulting in tic amelioration, whereas others[34,35] suggested the corollary theory that stimulants might reduce the long-term severity of TS symptoms by desensitizing catecholamine receptors.

See also pages 429, 434, 456, and 464

Although the findings from controlled studies of stimulants in children with ADHD and tics or compulsive behaviors are encouraging,[32,36-39] this existing research is limited both in scope (relatively small patient samples) and in diagnostic clarity. The following is a report of the safety and efficacy of methylphenidate in a relatively large sample of children with ADHD and a diagnosed tic disorder. Participants were assigned at random to various sequences of placebo and three dosages of methylphenidate under double-blind conditions. To be eligible for the study, ADHD had to be a primary reason for seeking clinical services.

RESULTS

ADHD SYMPTOMS

Teacher Ratings

Analyses of the teacher behavior rating scale data revealed a significant main effect of behavior ($F[5,140]=54.76$, $P<.0001$) and dose ($F[3,90]=34.74$,

Table 2. Untransformed Means (SDs), Analyses of Variance, and Tests for Trend for Behavior Rating Scales and CPT and for Dosage of Methylphenidate*

	Placebo	Methylphenidate Hydrochloride 0.1 mg/kg	0.3 mg/kg	0.5 mg/kg	F Ratio	P	Trend Tests
Teacher ratings							
ATRS	14.2 (4.6)	10.0 (7.0)	9.3 (6.4)	7.1 (5.4)	18.91	.0001	L
Factor 1	11.4 (3.8)	7.9 (5.3)	7.1 (4.5)	5.7 (4.1)	20.59	.0001	L
Factor 2	2.9 (2.1)	2.2 (2.4)	2.2 (2.6)	1.4 (1.8)	5.94	.001	L
IOWA Conners							
I-O scale	8.7 (3.1)	6.2 (3.9)	5.8 (3.7)	4.6 (3.3)	18.7	.0001	L, C
Aggression scale	4.3 (3.7)	2.6 (3.4)	2.3 (3.5)	1.4 (2.0)	13.49	.0001	L
Peer Conflict Scale	5.2 (4.9)	3.6 (5.3)	2.7 (5.0)	1.7 (2.5)	8.94	.0001	L
Parent Ratings							
APRS	11.8 (7.3)	8.6 (5.0)	10.2 (5.4)	7.8 (4.6)	4.45	.006	L, C
MOMS							
Hyperactivity scale	2.8 (1.6)	2.7 (1.6)	2.6 (1.3)	2.0 (1.5)	4.17	.008	L
Aggression scale	2.4 (2.0)	1.9 (1.7)	1.9 (1.7)	1.5 (1.7)	3.90	.002	L
Peer Conflict Scale	5.6 (4.9)	4.3 (4.5)	4.5 (4.1)	3.0 (3.3)	3.50	.02	L
CPT							
Inattention	7.5 (5.7)	6.0 (5.2)	5.6 (6.0)	5.2 (6.1)	2.80	.045	L
Impulsivity	2.1 (3.1)	2.8 (4.5)	1.2 (1.6)	1.8 (4.8)	1.83	.15	NA
Dyscontrol	7.0 (9.4)	4.2 (5.9)	2.5 (2.8)	2.2 (5.4)	5.89	.001	L, Q

**CPT indicates Continuous Performance Task; ATRS, Abbreviated Teacher Rating Scale; IOWA, Inattention-Overactivity With Aggression; I-O, inattention-overactivity; APRS, Abbreviated Parent Rating Scale; L, significant linear trend; C, significant cubic trend; NA, not applicable; and Q, significant quadratic trend.*

$P<.0001$). The behavior-by-dose interaction was also significant ($F[15,450]=20.57$, $P<.0001$). Follow-up repeated measures ANOVAs were performed on each of the teacher rating scales (**Table 2**). Dose effects were significant for all of the teacher rating scales of hyperactivity, oppositionality, and aggressivity. Symptom severity decreased with each increment in dose, with the corresponding tests for linear trend being significant for each scale. For the inattention-overactivity subscale, the cubic trend was also significant ($F[1,30]=4.87$, $P=.04$). In general, there was a dramatic diminution of symptom severity with the 0.1-mg/kg dosage, little change in ratings of symptom severity (plateau) with the 0.3-mg/kg dosage, and continued but more modest additional improvement with the 0.5-mg/kg dosage. Post hoc analyses revealed that, with the exception of factor 2 of the ATRS, there were statistically significant differences between placebo and all three drug dosages and between dosages of 0.1 mg/kg and 0.5 mg/kg (**Table 3**) but no significant differences between dosages of 0.1 mg/kg and 0.3 mg/kg. It is noteworthy that comparisons between placebo and the 0.1-mg/kg dosage indicate a diminution in symptom severity of at least 30% on most measures of ADHD symptoms.

Parent Ratings

Analyses of these data revealed a significant main effect of dose ($F[3,72]=4.66$, $P=.005$). Follow-up repeated measures ANOVAs were performed, and dose effects were significant for all scales (Table 2). Post hoc analyses revealed significant differences between the 0.5-mg/kg dosage and placebo for all scales (Table 3). Even the placebo and the 0.1-mg/kg dosage comparison was significant for the APRS. Trend analyses indicated a significant linear function for the hyperactivity ($F[1,29]=7.15$, $P=.012$) and aggression ($F[1,29]=21.17$, $P<.0001$) subscales of the MOMS, the Peer Conflict Scale ($F[1,27]=4.59$, $P=.04$), and the APRS ($F[1,31]=6.90$, $P=.01$). The cubic function was also significant for the APRS ($F[1,31]=5.84$, $P=.02$) and was marginally significant for the Peer Conflict Scale ($F[1,27]=3.73$, $P=.06$).

Continuous Performance Task

Repeated measures ANOVAs were conducted for each of the three CPT scores (n=28) and the four treatment conditions (Table 2). There were significant dose effects for both the inattention and the dyscontrol measures. Tests for trend indicated significant linear functions: inattention ($F[1,27]=7.54$, $P=.01$) and dyscontrol ($F[1,27]=8.59$, $P=.007$). Performance improved with increasing dose. The quadratic function was also significant for the dyscontrol measure ($F[1,27]=5.16$, $P=.03$). Post hoc comparisons between placebo and the 0.5-mg/kg dosage were significant for both measures, as was the comparison between placebo and the 0.3-mg/kg dosage for the dyscontrol score (Table 3).

Severity of Tic Symptoms and Behavioral Drug Response

To examine the possibility that the response to medication may have been affected by the severity, frequency, or number of tics (as determined at diagnosis), subjects were separated into two groups on the basis of median splits for each tic variable: severity (Yale Global Tic Se-

Table 3. Mean Group Differences Between Treatment Conditions for Observations, Rating Scales, and CPT*

Behavior Category	Placebo vs 0.1 mg/kg	Placebo vs 0.3 mg/kg	Placebo vs 0.5 mg/kg	0.1 mg/kg vs 0.5 mg/kg
Teacher rating scales				
ATRS	4.18†	4.94†	7.14†	2.96‡
Factor 1	3.48†	4.31†	5.73†	2.25‡
Factor 2	0.64	0.67	1.43‡	0.79
IOWA Conners I-O subscale	2.59‡	2.93‡	4.19†	1.60‡
IOWA Conners aggression subscale	1.71‡	2.05†	2.92†	1.21‡
Peer Conflict Scale	1.58‡	2.49†	3.51†	1.93‡
Parent rating scales				
APRS	3.16‡	1.62	4.01†	0.85
MOMS hyperactivity subscale	0.11	0.23	0.84‡	0.73‡
MOMS aggression subscale	0.47	0.53	0.93‡	0.46
Peer Conflict Scale	1.27	1.08	2.58†	1.31
CPT				
Inattention	1.56	1.93	2.35‡	0.79
Dyscontrol	2.79	4.49†	4.76†	1.97
Physician tic ratings observations				
Shapiro Symptom Checklist, vocal tics	1.07‡	0.14	0.55	0.52
2-Minute tic count, motor tics	1.99	3.63	5.70‡	3.71
Teacher GTRS tic ratings				
Frequency of motor tic index	0.31	0.59	0.90‡	0.59
Frequency of vocal tics index	0.54†	0.54†	0.56†	0.02
Tic severity index	0.25	0.52	0.76‡	0.51

**Dosages are for methylphenidate hydrochloride. CPT indicates Continuous Performance Task; ATRS, Abbreviated Teacher Rating Scale; IOWA, Inattention-Overactivity With Aggression; I-O, inattention-overactivity; APRS, Abbreviated Parent Rating Scale; MOMs, Mothers' Objective Method for Subgrouping; and GTRS, Global Tic Rating Scale.*

†$P<.01$ using Newman-Keuls test.

‡$P<.05$ using Newman-Keuls test.

verity Score), frequency (number of tics observed during the 15-minute videotaping session in the clinic), and the total number of different tics (Shapiro Symptom Checklist from the Unified Tourette Syndrome Rating Scale). Separate three-way repeated measures ANOVAs with two within-subject factors (behavior and dose) and one between-subjects factor (group) were conducted for the behavior ratings scales for each of the three sets of raters (teachers, parents, and physician). The results of these analyses did not reveal a single statistically significant dose-by-group interaction.

FREQUENCY AND SEVERITY OF TICS

Physician Evaluations

A 9×4 (scale-by-dose) repeated measures ANOVA conducted on the tic scale scores revealed a significant main effect of scale ($F[8,224]=302.97$, $P<.0001$), a marginally significant main effect of dose ($F[3,84]=2.69$, $P=.06$), and a significant scale-by-dose interaction ($F[24,672]=1.85$, $P=.009$). (A multivariate ANOVA of the physician measures was not significant.) The means, SDs, and repeated measures ANOVAs for each tic scale are presented in **Table 4**. (With the exception of the LeWitt Disability Scale, increasing mean values indicate a worsening in tic status.) There was little evidence that methylphenidate exacerbated tics. This was also the case using the three physician scales (the Shapiro Tourette Syndrome Severity Scale, the Tourette Syndrome–Clinical Global Impression Scale, and the GTRS) that were added to the assessment battery. The only indication of tic worsening was the physician's 2-minute motor tic count. A linear trend provided a good fit to the data ($F[1,32]=5.98$, $P<.02$). The frequency of motor tics was significantly higher when the children received the 0.5-mg/kg dosage than when they received placebo (Table 3). The number of different vocal tics (Shapiro Symptom Checklist) exhibited during the previous week as reported by the parent to the physician was also dose-dependent, with the rate when the children received the 0.1-mg/kg dosage being significantly lower than that when they received placebo or the 0.3-mg/kg dosage. There was no main effect of dose or scale-by-dose interaction when the latter two scales were excluded from the analyses.

Exploratory analyses that were conducted on the component scales of the Yale Global Tic Severity Scale revealed a marginally significant phonic tics score ($F[3,90]=2.70$, $P=.05$), with lower levels of vocal tics when the children received medication: placebo (mean score, 1.68), 0.1-mg/kg dosage (mean score, 1.25), 0.3-mg/kg dosage (mean score, 1.58), and 0.5-mg/kg dosage (mean score, 1.64).

The physician's global assessment of obsessive-compulsive symptoms (Clinical Global Impression Scale–Obsessive-compulsive Disorder) also did not show drug effects ($F[3,84]=0.86$, $P=.46$).

Simulated Classroom

Although the frequency of motor tics was slightly higher in each of the three dose conditions compared with the placebo condition (Table 4), there was no significant effect of dose.

Table 4. Means (SDs) and Analyses of Variance for Observations and Ratings of Motor and Vocal Tics*

Measure	Placebo	Methylphenidate Hydrochloride 0.1 mg/kg	0.3 mg/kg	0.5 mg/kg	F Ratio	P	Trend Tests
Physician ratings							
YGTSS							
Total motor tics	11.6 (4.0)	12.3 (3.8)	11.9 (4.5)	12.0 (4.2)	0.57	.64	NA
Total phonic tics	7.9 (4.7)	6.7 (5.8)	7.5 (3.9)	8.6 (6.7)	2.04	.11	NA
Overall impairment rating	9.1 (9.5)	10.3 (8.8)	12.4 (10.9)	10.3 (10.6)	0.86	.46	NA
Global severity score	28.3 (15.9)	29.3 (15.6)	31.9 (17.4)	29.1 (16.5)	0.43	.73	NA
Tourette Syndrome Unified Rating Scale							
Shapiro Symptom Checklist							
No. of motor tics	11.6 (6.5)	11.5 (5.3)	11.6 (5.7)	11.7 (6.2)	0.02	.997	NA
No. of vocal tics	3.2 (2.7)	2.1 (2.8)	3.3 (3.4)	2.6 (3.3)	3.22	.03	NS
Motor tic count	9.4 (7.1)	11.3 (10.4)	13.0 (12.0)	15.0 (14.8)	2.96	.04	L
Vocal tic count	0.4 (0.8)	0.5 (1.6)	0.7 (2.0)	0.60 (0.9)	0.60	.60	NA
LeWitt Disability Scale	67.6 (11.5)	69.4 (9.7)	70.6 (11.4)	72.4 (9.7)	2.19	.09	NA
STSSS	1.7 (0.9)	1.9 (0.9)	1.9 (1.2)	1.9 (1.2)	0.48	.69	NA
Teacher ratings, GTRS							
Motor tic index	2.8 (2.6)	2.5 (2.6)	2.2 (2.1)	1.9 (2.0)	2.68	.05	L, C
Vocal tic index	1.3 (1.2)	0.7 (0.8)	0.7 (1.0)	0.7 (1.0)	5.66	.001	L
Tic severity index	2.0 (2.0)	1.8 (2.2)	1.5 (2.0)	1.3 (1.7)	2.68	.05	L
Parent ratings, GTRS							
Motor tic index	2.4 (1.7)	2.5 (1.8)	2.4 (1.7)	3.3 (2.5)	2.24	.09	NA
Vocal tic index	1.2 (1.1)	1.1 (1.1)	1.1 (1.3)	1.2 (1.1)	0.19	.90	NA
Tic severity index	1.6 (1.7)	1.9 (2.0)	1.9 (2.5)	2.2 (2.6)	0.70	.55	NA
Clinic observations							
Motor tic frequency	18.1 (13.3)	22.2 (17.8)	20.7 (18.0)	21.3 (18.0)	0.69	.56	NA

**YGTSS indicates Yale Global Tic Severity Score; STSSS, Shapiro Tourette Syndrome Severity Score; GTRS, Global Tic Rating Scale; NA, not applicable; NS, no significant trend; L, significant linear trend; and C, significant cubic trend.*

Teacher Ratings

Analyses of teacher ratings of tic frequency and severity on the GTRS indicated a main effect of dose ($F[3,87]=4.52$, $P=.006$). Follow-up ANOVAs indicated a significant dose effect for the frequency of vocal tic index (Table 4). Vocal tics were rated as less frequent for the three medication conditions compared with the placebo condition (Table 3), and a linear function provided a good fit to the data ($F[1,29]=8.20$, $P=.008$). Post hoc comparisons between placebo and all three doses of methylphenidate were significant.

There were marginally significant dose effects for the frequency of motor tics index and the tic severity index (Table 4). Ratings of motor tic frequency and tic severity improved with methylphenidate treatment. Post hoc comparisons between placebo and the 0.5-mg/kg dosage were significant for both indexes (Table 3). Linear trend functions were significant for both indexes, but the cubic function was also significant for the frequency of motor tics index ($F[1,29]=5.40$, $P=.03$).

Parent Ratings

Analyses of the parent ratings of tic frequency and severity as measured on the GTRS did not reveal a main effect of dose (Table 4). Descriptively, mean ratings of motor tic frequency ($P=.09$) and tic severity were higher for the 0.5-mg/kg dosage compared with the other treatment conditions.

In an effort to examine the possibility that tic exacerbation may be manifest as a rebound effect, a subsample of parents (n=21) also were asked during their children's biweekly clinic evaluation to compare their children's tics during the evening (on the weekend) with tic status during the day (1 indicates more severe; 2, about the same; and 3, less severe). The mean ratings for all four treatment conditions were virtually identical for both motor ($F[3,60]=0.41$, $P=.75$) and vocal ($F[3,60]=1.76$, $P=.17$) tics. Descriptively, for the placebo condition, six children were rated as having motor tics that are more severe in the evening, and two, as having less severe tics in the evening. With the 0.5-mg/kg dosage, six children were rated as having more-severe tics in the evening, but of these, only one was not so rated when receiving placebo.

Severity of Tic Symptoms and Drug Response

To examine the possibility that response to medication may have been affected by the severity, frequency, or number of tics (as determined at diagnosis), subjects were separated into two groups on the basis of median splits for each tic variable on the aforementioned tic measures. Separate three-way repeated measures ANOVAs with two within-subject factors (behavior and dose) and one between-subjects factor (diagnostic tic status) were conducted for the behavior rating scales for each of the three sets of raters (teachers, parents, and physician). The results of these analyses did not reveal a single statistically significant ($P<.05$) interaction between dose and diagnostic tic status.

ADVERSE DRUG REACTIONS

Teacher Ratings

There was a statistically significant effect of dose ($F[3,90]=3.56$, $P=.02$), behavior ($F[2,60]=8.00$, $P<.001$), and behavior-by-dose interaction ($F[6,180]=2.94$, $P=.009$) for the teacher-completed SSEC ratings. In general, SSEC ratings were more favorable for methylphenidate conditions than for the placebo condition, but only the ANOVA for the mood index was significant ($F[3,93]=6.01$, $P<.001$). Post hoc comparisons indicated that 0.5 mg/kg ratings were significantly ($P<.01$) lower than placebo and 0.1 mg/kg ratings, and a linear function provided a good fit to the data ($F[1,30]=9.92$, $P=.004$).

Parent Ratings

The analysis of the main effect of dose for the parent-completed SSEC ratings was not significant, but the main effect of behavior ($F[3,87]=12.56$, $P<.0001$) and the behavior-by-dose interaction ($F[9,261]=2.28$, $P=.02$) were. Similar to the teacher ratings, the mean parent SSEC ratings were generally lower for the drug conditions compared with the placebo condition, but only the ANOVA for the somatic complaints index was significant ($F[3,87]=4.88$, $P=.004$). Somatic complaints were significantly ($P<.01$) more severe with the 0.5-mg/kg dosage compared with placebo. A linear function provided a good fit to the data ($F[1,29]=10\text{-}66$, $P=.003$).

Physician Evaluations

Repeated measures ANOVAs were conducted for heart rate, blood pressure, and weight measurements for the four treatment conditions. Dose effects were evident only for heart rate ($F[4,84]=3.68$, $P=.008$). The rate for the 0.5-mg/kg dosage (mean±SD, 93.5±13.9) was significantly ($P<.05$) higher than that for placebo (mean±SD, 85.5±10.0).

COMMENT

All of the children in the study showed dramatic clinical improvement consequent to methylphenidate treatment; there were no nonresponders. Administration of methylphenidate was highly effective in the amelioration of inattentive, disruptive, and aggressive behaviors in children with ADHD and comorbid tic disorder as assessed by teacher- and parent-completed behavior rating scales and a computer-presented CPT evaluation in the clinic. These findings are consistent with the results of numerous studies of hyperactive children and/or children with ADHD.[70,71] It is noteworthy that treatment with the 0.1-mg/kg dosage resulted in significant improvement in teacher ratings of symptom severity. Credit for documenting the efficacy of relatively low dosages of methylphenidate (0.1 mg/kg) in short-term clinical trials goes to Werry and Sprague,[72] who showed that treatment effects even could be measured with teacher-completed behavior rating scales. Others also have reported significant treatment effects for the 0.1-mg/kg dosage on activity level.[73] Trend analyses of most dependent measures indicated dose effects to be linear, which lends additional support to previous investigations.[74,75] However, the magnitude of clinical improvement associated with the 0.3-mg/kg dosage compared with the 0.5-mg/kg dosage was generally trivial for many children. The 0.5-mg/kg dosage was associated with more side effects, but fortunately they were generally of limited clinical significance.

Even more gratifying than the finding that methylphenidate was effective for the management of ADHD behaviors in this clinical population is the compelling evidence that supports its relatively benign impact on the severity of tics. During the course of this short-term drug evaluation, physician, teacher, and parent ratings were in uniform agreement that methylphenidate did not lead to a worsening in the severity of the children's tic disorder. In fact, teacher ratings actually suggest improvement in the severity (and frequency) of motor and vocal tics when children were receiving methylphenidate compared with placebo. Although it may be tempting simply to dismiss this finding as a positive halo effect, at this juncture, such an interpretation is definitely premature.

The data pertaining to methylphenidate's effect on the frequency of motor tics are mixed. Detailed examination of videotapes of children performing an academic task for 15 minutes in a simulated classroom did not reveal any drug-related changes in tic frequency, which is consistent with caregiver ratings. However, the findings from the physician's 2-minute tic count of motor tics did indicate a statistically significant tic exacerbation with the 0.5-mg/kg dosage, which is consistent with our report on the initial sample of subjects.[39] Given the number of tic measures and the negative findings from the simulated classroom observations, this could be a spurious finding. However, it is also possible that stimulant medication interacts with specific somatic (eg, level of arousal) and environmental variables to produce tic exacerbations in certain situations, a hypothesis that warrants further study. For example, the children were present in the room as the physician interviewed the parent about changes in tic status, and occasionally, some even performed mock tics in response to specific questions when the physician was interviewing the parent. Most children were aware that the physician was observing them for tics during the tic-count procedure. Curiously, direct observations of these same children in public school settings did reveal a statistically significant increase in the frequency of occurrence of motor tics in the classroom with the 0.1-mg/kg dosage, but the magnitude of tic exacerbation was relatively small.[76] Furthermore, tic worsening was not observed in the lunchroom or on the playground and, according to teacher and parent reports, was evidently beyond the detection of care providers.

It is extremely difficult to determine whether changes in the observed frequency of tics in the physician's office or the simulated classroom represent true drug-induced tic exacerbation in specific individuals or simply natural fluctuations in tic frequency over time. (Unfortunately, the mean duration of cycles of waxing and waning is not known.) The fact that the frequency of motor tics emitted during the simulated classroom sessions conducted at diagnosis and when the children were receiving placebo differed by at least 0.5 SD (diagnostic) in 61% of the children does not bode well for the former interpretation. In other words, given the moderately high reliability of this type of assessment,[77] this finding indicates a great deal of instability over time (several weeks) and provides strong support for the natural waxing and waning in the frequency of tic symptoms during the course of a short-term drug study.

THE TENDENCY for methylphenidate to have a beneficial effect on vocal tics is inconsistent with our findings for motor tics. It is possible that parents inadvertently considered impulsive ADHD vocalizations when they reported vocal tics to the physician. Research on stimulant drugs and vocal behavior is contradictory, indicating both increased[78] and decreased[79-81] verbal productivity. However, as with other drug-induced changes in the behavior of hyperactive children and/or children with ADHD, these seemingly discrepant findings probably can be explained in terms of differences in task demands and setting characteristics. Although direct observations of the frequency of tic occurrence in the school setting also support a modest treatment-related suppression of vocal tics,[76] at this point, it is premature to draw any firm conclusions about the effect of methylphenidate on vocal tics.

The possibility that methylphenidate treatment may be associated with changes in the frequency but not the perceived severity of motor tics (at least in terms of behavior exhibited in the physician's office) has important assessment implications. In the clinical setting, it may be prudent to overlook insignificant changes in tic frequency, especially when alternative interventions carry a greater risk of behavioral or somatic toxic effects. Alternatively, the failure of clinician-completed tic rating scales to detect changes in the frequency of tic occurrence could obfuscate attempts to determine the cause of tic disorders, as in the case of a differential response to drugs.[33]

The generalizability of the findings from this study are subject to several qualifications. First, our data pertain to observed treatment effects over an 8-week period and therefore cannot address the issue of tic exacerbation as a function of long-term drug exposure. Although we have not had to terminate methylphenidate treatment for any of the children in this study for this reason, until the follow-up study in progress is completed, we are unable to comment with certainty about the potential risks of maintenance therapy. Second, our study was not designed specifically to address the issue of stimulant-induced tic exacerbation in individual children but rather to examine critically the notion that these drugs are contraindicated for the study population as a whole. To address adequately the individual drug reactions, we believe that specific treatment conditions should be repeated during the course of the evaluation.[82] Third, our findings pertain only to children with ADHD and with tics that are of mild to moderate severity and that occur frequently enough to be observed during 15-minute intervals. We specifically avoided children whose tics could only change in one direction on our dependent measures (ie, very mild cases could only get worse; severe cases could only get better). Fourth, although this study was not designed to address the possible exacerbation of comorbid anxiety and mood disorders, neither the global obsessive-compulsive disorder measure nor the LeWitt Disability scale showed a worsening of symptoms. The teacher-completed SSEC mood index actually indicated improvement in affect with methylphenidate administration, which is consistent with the findings of studies using caregiver and child self-report measures.[83] Finally, the use of a crossover design may have resulted in contamination of the placebo condition by prior exposure to medication (protracted carryover effects). However, comparison of the frequency of tic occurrence (simulated classroom) between baseline and placebo conditions for children who received placebo first (n=8) and last (n=9) indicated a small decrease in tics for both groups. This finding, combined with the absence of statistically significant rebound effects (daytime vs evening parent ratings) or tolerance (2 vs 6 weeks of drug exposure),[76] strongly suggests that this is not an issue.

Our findings also touch on theories pertaining to the neuropathologic causes of tic disorders. For example, dopamine receptor sensitivity modification theory[33] suggests that on initial exposure to methylphenidate, hyperdopaminergic receptors may be stimulated further to produce tic exacerbation in some patients. On continued exposure to this dopamine agonist, a reduction in dopamine sensitivity results. This, in turn, leads to the amelioration of tic symptoms. If this is true, tic exacerbation should occur at a higher rate during the early part of the dose evaluation than during the latter part. Our data indicate that this is not the case.[76] Another theory suggests that tic disorder and ADHD are both a result of a genetic deficit that causes an imbalance in mesencephalic-mesolimbic dopamine pathways, which leads to hypofunction of mesocortical dopamine pathways and disinhibition and hypersensitivity of subcortical dopamine pathways.[29] This theory predicts that psychostimulant treatment should ameliorate hyperactivity without adversely affecting tic status,[24] and our findings with regard to the severity of tic symptoms are consistent with this theory. Additional considerations that might explain the absence of tic exacerbation consequent to exposure to clinical doses of methylphenidate are the following: first, differential effects of dopamine on striatal outputs may be involved in differential clinical effects of exogenously administered drugs,[84] and second, evidence exists for a complex interaction of a number of neurotransmitter systems in the pathogenesis of hyperkinetic movement disorder and TS.[24,28,84-87]

In summary, the findings from this investigation indicate that methylphenidate is an effective treatment for ADHD and negativistic behaviors in children with ADHD and tic disorder. In spite of an intense effort using a lengthy battery of tic assessment measures, numerous evaluators, and a variety of settings, we were unable to document statistically or clinically significant adverse effects on the severity of tics pursuant to methylphenidate drug therapy. Nevertheless, the frequency of observed motor tic occurrence in the public school classroom was shown to be higher when patients received a low dose (0.1 mg/kg) of methylphenidate hydrochloride than when they received placebo.[76] Methylphenidate appears to have a differential effect on ADHD and motor and vocal tics, which suggests structural polymorphism in the neurochemical mechanisms and anatomical substrates involved in the genesis of tics and other pleiotropic manifestations of the TS diathesis. The findings from this study should not be interpreted as indicating that methylphenidate is universally benign with regard to tic exacerbation. Evidence from a multiple challenge study suggests that it can have an adverse effect on tics in specific children,[14] albeit, even with reliable and valid assessment procedures, it is often extremely difficult to determine whether methylphenidate is the cause of observed changes in tic frequency or severity.[13,32,54,82] Furthermore, it bears repeating that all psychotherapeutic drugs are capable of inducing or exacerbating comorbid conditions. Finally, this study does not address the possibility that tic exacerbations might result from longer-term drug exposure, but preliminary findings from our ongoing maintenance therapy study indicate that this is not a clinical issue in most cases.

Accepted for publication October 24, 1994.

This study was supported in part by a research grant from the Tourette Syndrome Association Inc, Bayside, NY, and US Public Health Service grant MH 45358 from the National Institute of Mental Health, Bethesda, Md.

Methylphenidate placebos were supplied by Ciba-Geigy Pharmaceutical Co, Summit, NJ.

We thank Joseph Schwartz, PhD, for assisting us with the data analyses, Linda Volkersz for conducting clinic evaluations, and Michele J. De Angelis and Michael V. De Angelis for providing pharmacy services. We are particularly indebted to the courageous families who made this study possible.

Reprint requests to Department of Psychiatry and Behavioral Science, Putnam Hall, South Campus, State University of New York–Stony Brook, Stony Brook, NY 11794-8790 (Dr Gadow).

REFERENCES

1. Bradley C. Benzedrine and Dexedrine in the treatment of children's behavior disorders. *Pediatrics.* 1950;5:24-36.
2. Mattson RH, Calverly JR. Dextroamphetamine sulfate–induced dyskinesias. *JAMA.* 1968;204:400-402.
3. Gadow KD. Prevalence of drug therapy. In: Werry JS, Aman M, eds. *Practitioner's Guide to Psychoactive Drugs for Children and Adolescents.* New York, NY: Plenum Publishing Corp; 1993:57-74.
4. Conners CK, Eisenberg L. The effects of methylphenidate on symptomatology and learning in disturbed children. *Am J Psychiatry.* 1963;120:458-464.
5. Weiss G, Minde K, Douglas V, Werry J, Sykes D. Comparison of the effects of chlorpromazine, dextroamphetamine, and methylphenidate on the behavior and intellectual functioning of hyperactive children. *Can Med Assoc J.* 1971;104:20-25.
6. Golden GS. Gilles de la Tourette's syndrome following methylphenidate administration. *Dev Med Child Neurol.* 1974;16:76-78.
7. Golden GS. The effect of central nervous system stimulants on Tourette syndrome. *Ann Neurol.* 1977;2:69-70.
8. Pollack MA, Cohen NL, Friedhoff AJ. Gilles de la Tourette's syndrome: familial occurrence and precipitation by methylphenidate therapy. *Arch Neurol.* 1977;34:630-632.
9. Abuzzahab FS, Anderson FO. Gilles de la Tourette's syndrome: cross-cultural analysis and treatment outcome. In: Abuzzahab FS, Anderson FO, eds. *Gilles de la Tourette's Syndrome.* St Paul, Minn, Mason Publishing Co; 1976;1:71-79.
10. Kelman DH. Gilles de la Tourette's disease in children: a review of the literature. *J Child Psychol Psychiatry.* 1965;6:219-226.
11. Meyerhoff JL, Snyder SH. Gilles de la Tourette's disease and minimal brain dysfunction: amphetamine isomers reveal catecholamine correlates in an affected patient. *Psychopharmacologia.* 1973;29:211-220.
12. Singer K. Gilles de la Tourette's disease. *Am J Psychiatry.* 1963;120:80-81.
13. Gadow KD, Sverd J. Stimulants for ADHD in child patients with Tourette's syndrome: the issue of relative risk. *J Dev Behav Pediatr.* 1990;11:269-271.
14. Caine ED, Ludlow CL, Polinsky RJ, Ebert MH. Provocative drug testing in Tourette's syndrome: *d*- and *l*-amphetamine and haloperidol. *J Am Acad Child Psychiatry.* 1984;23:147-152.
15. Feinberg M, Carroll BJ. Effects of dopamine agonists and antagonists in Tourette's disease. *Arch Gen Psychiatry.* 1979;36:979-985.
16. Shapiro AK, Shapiro E. Do stimulants provoke, cause or exacerbate tics and Tourette's syndrome? *Compr Psychiatry.* 1981;22:265-273.
17. Shapiro AK, Shapiro ES, Young JG, Feinberg TE. *Gilles de la Tourette Syndrome.* 2nd ed. New York, NY: Raven Press; 1988.
18. Lowe TL, Cohen DJ, Detlor J, Kremenitzer MW, Shaywitz BA. Stimulant medications precipitate Tourette's syndrome. *JAMA.* 1982;247:1729-1731.
19. Comings DE, Comings BG. A controlled study of Tourette syndrome, I: attention-deficit disorder, learning disorders, and school problems. *Am J Hum Genet.* 1987;41:701-741.
20. Conners CK. Symptom patterns in hyperkinetic, neurotic, and normal children. *Child Dev.* 1970;41:667-682.
21. Munir K, Biederman J, Knere D. Psychiatric comorbidity in patients with attention deficit disorder: a controlled study. *J Am Acad Child Adolesc Psychiatry.* 1987;26:844-848.
22. Sverd J, Curley AD, Jandorf L, Volkersz L. Behavior disorder and attention deficits in boys with Tourette syndrome. *J Am Acad Child Adolesc Psychiatry.* 1988;27:413-417.
23. Cohen DJ, Bruun RD, Leckman JF, eds. *Tourette's Syndrome and Tic Disorders.* New York, NY: John Wiley & Sons Inc; 1988.
24. Comings DE. *Tourette Syndrome and Human Behavior.* Duarte, Calif: Hope Press; 1990.
25. Kurlan R, ed. *Handbook of Tourette's Syndrome and Related Tic and Behavioral Disorders.* New York, NY: Marcel Dekker Inc; 1993.
26. Sverd J. Clinical presentations of the Tourette syndrome diatheses. *J Multihandicapped Pers.* 1989;2:311-326.
27. Golden GS. Tics and Tourette syndrome. *Hosp Pract (Off Ed).* 1979;14:91-93, 96-97, 100.
28. Anderson GM, Pollak ES, Chatterjee D, Leckman JF, Riddle MA, Cohen DJ. Postmortem analysis of subcortical monoamines and amino acids in Tourette syndrome. In: Chase TN, Friedhoff AJ, Cohen DJ, eds. *Tourette Syndrome: Genetics, Neurobiology, and Treatment.* New York, NY: Raven Press; 1992;58:123-133.
29. Comings DE. A controlled study of Tourette syndrome, VII: summary: a common genetic disorder causing disinhibition of the limbic system. *Am J Hum Genet.* 1987;41:839-866.
30. Comings DE, Comings BG. Tourette's syndrome and attention deficit disorder with hyperactivity: are they genetically related? *J Am Acad Child Psychiatry.* 1984;23:138-146.
31. Erenberg G, Cruse RP, Rothner AD. Gilles de la Tourette's syndrome: effects of stimulant drugs. *Neurology.* 1985;35:1346-1348.
32. Sverd J, Gadow KD, Paolicelli LM. Methylphenidate treatment of attention-deficit hyperactivity disorder in boys with Tourette's syndrome. *J Am Acad Child Adolesc Psychiatry.* 1989;28:574-579.
33. Friedhoff AJ. Receptor maturation in pathogenesis and treatment of Tourette syndrome. In: Friedhoff JA, Chase TN, eds. *Gilles de la Tourette Syndrome.* New York, NY: Raven Press; 1982;35:133-140.
34. Price RA, Leckman JF, Pauls DL, Cohen DJ, Kidd KK. Gilles de la Tourette's syndrome: tics and central nervous system stimulants in twins and nontwins. *Neurology.* 1986;36:232-237.
35. Waserman J, Lal S, Gauthier S. Gilles de la Tourette's syndrome in monozygotic twins. *J Neurol Neurosurg Psychiatry.* 1983;46:75-77.
36. Borcherding BG, Keysor CS, Rapoport JL, Elia J, Amass J. Motor/vocal tics and compulsive behaviors on stimulant drugs: is there a common vulnerability. *Psychiatry Res.* 1990;33:83-94.
37. Gadow KD, Nolan EE, Sverd J. Methylphenidate in hyperactive boys with comorbid tic disorder, II: short-term behavioral effects on school settings. *J Am Acad Child Adolesc Psychiatry.* 1992;31:462-471.
38. Konkol RJ, Fischer M, Newby RF. Double-blind, placebo-controlled stimulant

trial in children with Tourette's syndrome and attention-deficit hyperactivity disorder. *Ann Neurol.* 1990;28:424. Abstract.
39. Sverd J, Gadow KD, Nolan EE, Sprafkin J, Ezor SN. Methylphenidate in hyperactive boys with comorbid tic disorder, I: clinic evaluations. In: Chase TN, Friedhoff AJ, Cohen DJ, eds. *Tourette Syndrome: Genetics, Neurobiology, and Treatment.* New York, NY: Raven Press; 1992;58:271-281.
40. American Psychiatric Association. *Diagnostic and Statistical Manual of Mental Disorders, Revised Third Edition.* Washington, DC: American Psychiatric Association; 1987.
41. Conners CK. Rating scales for use in drug studies with children. *Psychopharmacol Bull.* 1973;9(special issue):24-84.
42. Loney J, Milich R. Hyperactivity, inattention, and aggression in clinical practice. In: Wolraich M, Routh DK, eds. *Advances in Developmental and Behavioral Pediatrics.* Greenwich, Conn: JAI Press Inc; 1982;3:113-147.
43. Goyette CH, Conners CK, Ulrich RF. Normative data on revised Conners Parent and Teacher Rating Scales. *J Abnorm Child Psychol.* 1978;6:221-236.
44. Loney J. A short parent scale for subgrouping childhood hyperactivity and aggression. Presented at the Annual Meeting of the American Psychological Association; August 1984; Toronto, Ontario.
45. Gadow KD, Sprafkin J. *Stony Brook Child Psychiatric Checklist-3R.* Stony Brook: Dept of Psychiatry, State University of New York–Stony Brook; 1987.
46. Leckman JF, Riddle MA, Hardin MT, Ort SI, Swartz KL, Stevenson J, Cohen DJ. The Yale Global Tic Severity Scale: initial testing of a clinic-rated scale of tic severity. *J Am Acad Child Adolesc Psychiatry.* 1989;28:566-573.
47. Kurlan R, Riddle M, Como P. *Tourette Syndrome Unified Rating Scale.* Bayside, NY: Tourette Syndrome Association Inc; 1988.
48. Tourette Syndrome Workshop Committee on Classification and Rating Scales. *Report of the Tourette Syndrome Workshop on Definitions of Tic Disorders.* Bayside, NY; Tourette Syndrome Association Inc; 1988.
49. Kurlan R. Tourette's syndrome: current concepts. *Neurology.* 1989;39:1625-1630.
50. Reich W, Welner Z. *Diagnostic Interview for Children and Adolescents: Revised Version for Children Ages 6-12 (DSM-III-R Version).* Saint Louis, Mo: Division of Child Psychiatry, Washington University; 1988.
51. Reich W, Welner Z. *Diagnostic Interview for Children and Adolescents: Revised Parent Version for Children Ages 6-17 (DSM-III-R Version).* Saint Louis, Mo: Division of Child Psychiatry, Washington University; 1988.
52. Gadow KD, Paolicelli LM. *Global Tic Rating Scale.* Stony Brook: Dept of Psychiatry, State University of New York–Stony Brook; 1986.
53. Nolan EE, Gadow KD, Sverd J. Observations and ratings of tics in school settings. *J Abnorm Child Psychol.* 1994;22:579-593.
54. Routh DK, Schroeder CS. Standardized playroom measures as indices of hyperactivity. *J Abnorm Child Psychol.* 1976;4:199-207.
55. Roberts MA, Ray RS, Roberts RJ. A playroom observational procedure for assessing hyperactive boys. *J Pediatr Psychol.* 1984;9:177-191.
56. Milich R, Loney J, Landau S. Independent dimensions of hyperactivity and aggression: a validation with playroom observational data. *J Abnorm Psychol.* 1982;91:183-198.
57. Halperin JM, Wolf LE, Pascualvaca DM, Newcorn JH, Healey JM, O'Brien JD, Morganstein A, Young JG. Differential assessment of attention and impulsivity in children. *J Am Acad Child Adolesc Psychiatry.* 1988;27:326-329.
58. Halperin JM, Matier K, Bedi G, Sharma V, Newcorn JH. Specificity of inattention, impulsivity, and hyperactivity to the diagnosis of attention-deficit hyperactivity disorder. *J Am Acad Child Adolesc Psychiatry.* 1992;31:190-196.
59. Matier K, Halperin JM, Sharma V, Newcorn JH, Sathaye N. Methylphenidate response in aggressive and non-aggressive ADHD children: distinctions on laboratory measures of symptoms. *J Am Acad Child Adolesc Psychiatry.* 1992;31:219-225.
60. Epstein MH, Cullinan D, Gadow KD. Teacher ratings of hyperactivity in learning disabled, emotionally disturbed, and mentally retarded children. *J Special Educ.* 1986;20:219-229.
61. Atkins MS, Pelham WE, Licht MH. The differential validity of teacher ratings of inattention/overactivity and aggression. *J Abnorm Child Psychol.* 1989;17:423-435.
62. Halperin JM, O'Brien JD, Newcorn JH, Healey JM, Pascualvaca DM, Wolf LE, Young JG. Validation of hyperactive, aggressive, and mixed hyperactive/aggressive childhood disorders: a research note. *J Child Psychol Psychiatry.* 1990;31:455-459.
63. Milich R, Fitzgerald G. Validation of inattention/overactivity and aggression ratings with classroom observations. *J Consult Clin Psychol.* 1985;53:139-140.
64. Milich R, Landau S. Teacher ratings of inattention/overactivity and aggression: cross validation with classroom observations. *J Clin Child Psychol.* 1988;17:92-97.
65. Nolan EE, Gadow KD. Relation between ratings and observations of stimulant drug response in hyperactive children. *J Clin Child Psychol.* 1994;23:78-90.
66. Gadow KD. A school-based medication evaluation program. In: Matson JL, ed. *Handbook of Hyperactivity in Children.* Needham Heights, Mass: Allyn & Bacon; 1993:186-219.
67. Gadow KD. *Peer Conflict Scale.* Stony Brook: Dept of Psychiatry, State University of New York–Stony Brook; 1986.
68. Gadow KD. *Stimulant Side Effects Checklist.* Stony Brook: Dept of Psychiatry, State University of New York–Stony Brook; 1986.
69. Goetz CG, Tanner CM, Wilson RS, Carroll VS, Como PG, Shannon KM. Clonidine and Gilles de la Tourette's syndrome: double-blind study using objective rating methods. *Ann Neurol.* 1987;21:307-310.
70. Barkley RA. *Attention Deficit Hyperactivity Disorder: A Handbook for Diagnosis and Treatment.* New York, NY: Guilford Press; 1990.
71. Gadow KD. *Hyperactivity, Learning Disabilities, and Mental Retardation.* Austin, Tex: PRO-ED; 1986;1.
72. Werry JS, Sprague RL. Methylphenidate in children: effects of dosage. *Aust N Z J Psychiatry.* 1974;8:9-19.
73. Solanto MV. Behavioral effects of low-dose methylphenidate in childhood attention deficit disorder: implications for a mechanism of stimulant drug action. *J Am Acad Child Psychiatry.* 1986;25:96-101.
74. Douglas VI, Barr RG, Amin K, O'Neill ME, Britton BG. Dosage effects and individual responsivity to methylphenidate in attention deficit disorder. *J Child Psychol Psychiatry.* 1988;29:453-475.
75. Rapport MD, Stoner G, DuPaul GJ, Kelly K, Tucker SB, Schoeler T. Attention deficit disorder and methylphenidate: multilevel analysis of dose-response effects on children's impulsivity across settings. *J Am Acad Child Adolesc Psychiatry.* 1988;27:60-69.
76. Gadow KD, Nolan EE, Sverd J, Sprafkin J. School observations of ADHD children with tic disorder: effects of methylphenidate treatment. *J Dev Behav Pediatr.* In press.
77. Chappell PB, McSwiggan-Hardin MT, Scahill L, Rubenstein M, Walker DE, Cohen DJ, Leckman JF. Videotape tic counts in the assessment of Tourette's syndrome: stability, reliability, and validity. *J Am Acad Child Adolesc Psychiatry.* 1994;33:386-393.
78. Creager RO, Van Riper C. The effect of methylphenidate on the verbal productivity of children with cerebral dysfunction. *J Speech Hear Res.* 1967;10:623-628.
79. Ludlow CL, Rapoport JL, Bassich CJ, Mikkelson EG. Differential effects of dextroamphetamine on language performance of hyperactive and normal boys. In: Knights RM, Bakker DJ, eds. *Treatment of Hyperactive and Learning Disordered Children.* Baltimore, Md: University Park Press; 1980:185-205.
80. Barkley RA, Cunningham CE, Karlsson J. The speech of hyperactive children and their mothers: comparison with normal children and stimulant drug effects. *J Learning Disabilities.* 1983;16:105-110.
81. Whalen CK, Collins BE, Henker B, Alkus SR, Adams D, Stapp J. Behavior observations of hyperactive children and methylphenidate (Ritalin) effects in systematically structured classroom environments: now you see them, now you don't. *J Pediatr Psychol.* 1978;3:177-187.
82. Sprafkin J, Gadow KD. Four purported cases of methylphenidate-induced tic exacerbation: methodological and clinical doubts. *J Child Adolesc Psychopharmacol.* 1993;3:231-244.
83. Gadow KD. Pediatric psychopharmacotherapy: a review of recent research. *J Child Psychol Psychiatry.* 1992;33:153-195.
84. Albin RL, Young AB, Penney JB. The functional anatomy of basal ganglia disorders. *Trends Neurosci.* 1989;12:366-375.
85. Young AB, Penney JB. Biochemical and functional organization of the basal ganglia. In: Jankovic J, Tolosa E, eds. *Parkinson's Disease and Movement Disorders.* Baltimore, Md: Urban & Schwarzenberg; 1988:1-11.
86. Haber SN, Wolfer D. Basal ganglia peptidergic staining in Tourette syndrome: a follow-up study. In: Chase TN, Friedhoff AJ, Cohen DJ, eds. *Tourette Syndrome: Genetics, Neurobiology, and Treatment.* New York, NY: Raven Press; 1992;58:145-150.
87. McConville BJ, Norman AB, Vogelson MH, Erenberg G. Sequential use of opioid antagonists and agonists in Tourette's syndrome. *Lancet.* 1994;343:601.

ORIGINAL ARTICLE

Is Methylphenidate Like Cocaine?

Studies on Their Pharmacokinetics and Distribution in the Human Brain

Nora D. Volkow, MD; Yu-Shin Ding, PhD; Joanna S. Fowler, PhD; Gene-Jack Wang, MD; Jean Logan, PhD; John S. Gatley, PhD; Stephen Dewey, PhD; Charles Ashby, PhD; Jeffrey Liebermann, MD; Robert Hitzemann, PhD; Alfred P. Wolf, PhD

Background: The purposes of this study were to investigate the pharmacokinetics of methylphenidate hydrochloride (Ritalin) in the human brain, to compare them with those of cocaine, and to evaluate whether cocaine and methylphenidate compete for the same binding sites.

Methods: We used positron emission tomography to measure the temporal and spatial distribution of carbon 11 (^{11}C)–labeled methylphenidate. These results were compared with those obtained previously for [^{11}C]cocaine. Eight healthy male subjects, 20 to 51 years of age, were scanned with [^{11}C]methylphenidate. Three were tested twice to assess test-retest variability, four were tested at baseline and after administration of methylphenidate, and one was tested with [^{11}C]methylphenidate and [^{11}C]cocaine. Two baboons were scanned to evaluate whether there was competition between cocaine and methylphenidate for the same binding sites in the brain.

Results: The uptake of [^{11}C]methylphenidate in the brain was high (mean±SD, 7.5%±1.5%), and the maximal concentration occurred in striatum. Pretreatment with methylphenidate decreased binding only in striatum (40%). Although the regional distribution of [^{11}C]methylphenidate was identical to that of [^{11}C]cocaine and they competed with each other for the same binding sites, these two drugs differed markedly in their pharmacokinetics. Clearance of [^{11}C]methylphenidate from striatum (90 minutes) was significantly slower than that of [^{11}C]cocaine (20 minutes). For both drugs, their fast uptake in striatum paralleled the experience of the "high." For methylphenidate, the high decreased very rapidly despite significant binding of the drug in the brain. In contrast, for cocaine, the decline in the high paralleled its fast rate of clearance from the brain.

Conclusion: We speculate that because the experience of the high is associated with the fast uptake of cocaine and methylphenidate in the brain, the slow clearance of methylphenidate from the brain may serve as a limiting factor in promoting its frequent self-administration.

(Arch Gen Psychiatry. 1995;52:456-463)

COCAINE, WHICH is one of the most reinforcing and addictive of the abused drugs,[1-3] has pharmacological actions that are very similar to those of methylphenidate hydrochloride, which is the most commonly prescribed psychotropic medication for children in the United States.[4] Methylphenidate is the drug of choice for the treatment of attention-deficit disorder,[5,6] which is estimated to affect 2% to 5% of school-age children.[5] Methylphenidate also is used for the treatment of narcolepsy,[7] and it has been used experimentally as an antidepressant[8] in the treatment of cocaine abusers,[9,10] for chronic fatigue, and in the treatment of medically ill, withdrawn, elderly patients.[11] Because of the pharmacological similarities between cocaine and methylphenidate, concerns have been raised about the abuse liability of methylphenidate, and methylphenidate is currently classified as a schedule 2 drug of the Controlled Substance Act.[12] Despite these concerns, little is known about the variables that influence the reinforcing and addictive properties of methylphenidate or other psychostimulant drugs.

The reinforcing effects of cocaine and cocaine analogues have been related to their ability to inhibit the dopamine transporter.[13,14] Because cocaine and methylphenidate have similar affinities for the dopamine transporter (K_i, the constant for drug concentration that would inhibit 50% of dopamine uptake, corresponds to 640 nmol/L for cocaine and 390 nmol/L for

From the Medical Department (Drs Volkow, Wang, and Ashby), the Chemistry Department (Drs Ding, Fowler, Logan, Gatley, Dewey, and Wolf), Brookhaven National Laboratory, Upton, NY; the Department of Psychiatry, State University of New York–Stony Brook (Drs Volkow and Hitzemann); and Hillside Hospital, Glen Oaks, NY (Dr Liebermann).

See Subjects and Methods on next page

SUBJECTS AND METHODS

SUBJECTS

Human Studies

Eight normal healthy male volunteers 20 to 51 years of age were included in this study. The age range for normal controls included in the [^{11}C]cocaine study was 26 to 45. Procedure selection for both studies was similar and has been published for the [^{11}C]cocaine study.[21] In summary, subjects were healthy male volunteers who were screened for absence of medical, neurological, or psychiatric disease. Care was taken to exclude subjects with a past or present history of alcohol or other drug use (except for caffeine). Urine toxicology tests were performed to ensure the absence of psychoactive drug use. Informed consent was obtained from the subjects, following the guidelines of the Human Studies Review Committee at Brookhaven National Laboratory, Upton, NY.

Each subject underwent scanning with [^{11}C]methylphenidate twice.[22] The scans were done 2 hours apart. Three subjects underwent two repeated scans to assess test-retest reproducibility, and four underwent one scan at baseline and the second scan 10 minutes after intravenous administration of 0.5 mg of methylphenidate hydrochloride per kilogram to assess specific to nonspecific binding. One subject underwent scanning with both [^{11}C]methylphenidate and [^{11}C]cocaine to compare the distribution and kinetics of these two compounds in the same individual.

Baboon Studies

To evaluate whether there was competition between cocaine and methylphenidate for the same binding sites in the brain, we evaluated the effects of pretreatment with pharmacological doses of cocaine on [^{11}C]methylphenidate binding and the effects of pretreatment with pharmacological doses of methylphenidate in [^{11}C]cocaine binding in the baboon brain. The PET studies were carried out in two anesthetized adult baboons (*Papio anubis*). One animal underwent scanning twice with [^{11}C]cocaine: at baseline and 5 minutes after administration of methylphenidate hydrochloride (0.5 mg/kg, intravenously). The other animal underwent scanning twice with [^{11}C]methylphenidate: at baseline and 5 minutes after administration of cocaine (0.2 mg/kg, intravenously). Protocols followed the guidelines of the Brookhaven National Laboratory Institutional Animal Care and Use Committee.

BEHAVIORAL EVALUATION

The mental state of the subject after injection of methylphenidate was evaluated using analog scales that assessed the subjective perception of high (defined as drug-induced euphoria). The interviewer (G.J.W.) asked the subject to rate the subjective experience of the high from 0 (felt nothing) to 10 (felt it extremely). The scales were completed 5 minutes prior to and every minute for 20 minutes after methylphenidate administration and thereafter at 5-minute intervals (total, 70 minutes). Electrocardiographic recordings, blood pressure, and pulse rate were obtained every 15 minutes for 30 minutes prior to and at 2, 4, 6, 8, 10, 15, 20, 30, 40, and 60 minutes after methylphenidate administration.

SCANNING

The PET studies were carried out with a whole-body, high-resolution positron emission tomograph (6.5×6.5×6.5 mm, full-width half maximum, 15 slices) (CTI 931, Computer Technologies Inc, Siemens, Knoxville, Tenn).

In the human studies, to ensure the accurate repositioning of subjects in the PET camera during the repeated scans, an individually molded head holder was made for each subject. The head of the subject was then positioned in the gantry with the aid of two orthogonal laser lines, one of which was placed parallel to the canthomeatal line and the other, parallel to the sagittal plane. Subjects underwent scanning twice, 2 hours apart, using 18.5×10^{10} to 37.0×10^{10} mBq of [^{11}C]methylphenidate (mass of methylphenidate hydrochloride injected, 9±2 μg). Prior to [^{11}C]methylphenidate injection, transmission scans were obtained to correct for attenuation. After injection of [^{11}C]methylphenidate, a series of 20 emission scans were obtained from the time of injection to 84 minutes after injection (four scans of 15 seconds, two scans of 30 seconds, four scans of 1 minute, four scans of 2 minutes, 5 scans of 10 minutes, and one scan of 20 minutes). Scanning with [^{11}C]cocaine was started after the injection of 22.2×10^{10} to 37.0×10^{10} mBq (mass of unlabeled cocaine injected, 17.8±12.2 μg) for a series of 14 sequential scans obtained from the time of injection to 45 minutes after injection (two scans of 30 seconds, nine scans of 1 minute, two scans of 10 minutes, and one scan of 15 minutes).[21] In preparation for the study, subjects had two catheters im-

Continued on next page

methylphenidate),[13] one might predict similar reinforcing properties for cocaine and methylphenidate if the only variables contributing to reinforcement are affinity for the dopamine transporter and bioavailability. Although methylphenidate is self-administered by animals[14-16] and abused by humans,[12,17,18] its abuse in humans appears to be much more limited[12] than that of cocaine and amphetamines. Although socioeconomic factors (eg, drug availability in the streets and fashions in the drug culture) could account for the higher rate of cocaine abuse than methylphenidate abuse, it is possible that pharmacological differences between the drugs are responsible. Although these two drugs differ in their affinities for the serotonin transporter as well as in their local anesthetic properties, neither of these properties has been related to the reinforcing properties of cocaine and/or methylphenidate.[13] It is more likely that differences in pharmacokinetics between these two drugs may account for differences in their reinforcing and addictive properties. Although cocaine and methylphenidate substitute for each other on discriminative experiments, no study, to our knowledge, has compared the reinforcing properties of these two drugs under conditions of free drug availability.

The importance of drug pharmacokinetics on the reinforcing properties of drugs of abuse has been recognized for a long time.[19,20] Specifically, the rapidity of drug delivery to the brain has been shown to affect the reinforcing properties of drugs. The shorter the interval beplanted, one in an antecubital vein for tracer injection and the other in the radial artery for blood sampling. Arterial sampling was used to quantitate levels of total ^{11}C and unchanged [^{11}C]methylphenidate or unchanged [^{11}C]cocaine in plasma. Arterial samples were obtained using an automated blood sampling device (Ole Dick, Hvidovre, Denmark) every 2.5 seconds for the first 2 minutes, every minute during the next 2 to 5 minutes, and then at 10, 15, 20, 30, 45, and 90 minutes after the injection.

In the baboon studies, the animals were initially anesthetized with ketamine hydrochloride and were maintained on gas anesthesia (nitrous oxide and isoflurane). Catheters were placed in an antecubital vein for tracer injection and in a femoral artery for blood sampling. Animals were positioned in the scanner using an individual head holder with the aid of two orthogonal laser beams. Transmission scans were obtained prior to the tracer injection to correct for attenuation. Emission scans were obtained immediately after injection of the tracer. Dynamic scans were obtained after the administration of 22.2×10^{10} to 37.0×10^{10} mBq of [^{11}C]cocaine (four scans of 30 seconds, four scans of 1 minute, four scans of 2 minutes, and four scans of 10 minutes). For [^{11}C]methylphenidate, dynamic scans were obtained after administration of 18.5×10^{10} to 37.0×10^{10} mBq of [^{11}C]methylphenidate (four scans of 15 seconds, two scans of 30 seconds, four scans of 1 minute, four scans of 2 minutes, five scans of 10 minutes, and one scan of 20 minutes). Arterial blood samples were obtained throughout the study, and selected plasma samples were analyzed for the presence of unchanged radiotracer. Blood sampling was performed in the same manner as that for the human studies. Vital signs were monitored throughout the length of the study (90303B monitor, SpaceLabs Medical, Redmond, Wash). Details about the procedures have been published.[23]

DATA ANALYSES

Regions of interest were drawn directly on the emission images. For this purpose, an averaged image was obtained that corresponded to the images obtained between 15 and 90 minutes after the injection. For the images obtained in the human subjects, regions for striatum, cerebellum, thalamus, occipital cortex, and whole brain were drawn in this averaged image as previously described.[21] Briefly, a template of geometric regions for five different planes was used. The templates were manually adjusted to each individual scan, and the weighted average for each anatomical region was computed. Regions in striatum and occipital cortex were obtained in three planes, and those in the thalamus and cerebellum were obtained in two planes. This multiplanar-method of analysis increases the reliability and reproducibility of the measures.[24] A similar procedure was used for the selection of regions of interest in the images obtained in the baboons. Regions of interest were obtained for the striatum and cerebellum as detailed previously.[23] Briefly, regions of interest for striatum were obtained in three sequential planes, and they were obtained for cerebellum in one plane, as previously described.[23] These regions were then projected to the dynamic images to compute time-activity curves.

The data from the time-activity curves in the brain and the data from the time-activity curves in the plasma were used to calculate the distribution volume (DV), using graphical analysis for reversible systems.[25] The ratio of the DV in striatum to that in cerebellum, expressed as DV(ST)/DV(CB), was used as the model measurement to calculate dopamine transporter availability at baseline and after pretreatment with methylphenidate. The analysis of tracer binding in terms of the DV provides a measure of binding that is a linear function of transporter availability, given by

$$(1) \qquad DV = K_1/k_2\ (1 + Bmax'/K_{d'})$$

for regions containing transporter sites that are characterized by an equilibrium dissociation constant, $K_{d'}$ ($K_{d'} = K_d/fNS$, where fNS is the free fraction of tracer in tissue and K_d is the equilibrium dissociation constant for ligand binding-site complex), and transporter concentration, Bmax′.[26] K_1 and k_2 are the plasma-to-tissue and the tissue-to-plasma transport constants, respectively. For regions with no transporter, the DV is given by

$$(2) \qquad DV = K_1/k_2.$$

A measurement that is proportional to free transporter concentration can be obtained from equations 1 and 2, giving

$$(3) \qquad Bmax'/K_{d'} = [DV(ST)/DV(CB)] - 1$$

where $K_{d'}$ and k_2 include the free fraction of tracer in tissue. Equations 1 and 2 are based on a classical compartmental analysis in which the effects of cerebral blood flow and capillary permeability are implicitly included in the kinetic constants K_1 and k_2.

Differences between the kinetic constants for [^{11}C]methylphenidate and those for [^{11}C]cocaine were tested with unpaired Student's *t* tests (two-tailed). Differences in the ratio of the DV in striatum to that in cerebellum at baseline and after methylphenidate administration were tested with paired *t* tests.

tween intake and the perceived effects of the drug, the greater the addictive potential of the drug.[20] Because classical human pharmacokinetic data for cocaine and methylphenidate are limited to that found in blood and urine, we used positron emission tomography (PET) to compare the pharmacokinetics of these two drugs in the human brain after intravenous administration.

Positron emission tomography is an imaging method that can be used to monitor noninvasively the temporal changes of the concentration of positron-labeled compounds in the living body. Because there are positron-emitting isotopes for some of the natural elements of life such as carbon 11 (^{11}C) (half-life, 20.4 minutes), drugs such as cocaine and methylphenidate can be labeled without changing their pharmacological properties. Thus, PET is ideally suited for investigating the distribution and pharmacokinetics of drugs in the human brain. Until recently, the determination of drug pharmacokinetics required the investigation of samples of tissue and fluids that were taken at particular times after drug administration, which precluded the investigation of the relation between the behavioral effects of drugs and their pharmacokinetics in the brain. With the availability of PET and appropriate labeled compounds, it is now feasible to assess the pharmacokinetics of drugs directly in the brain while, at the same time, monitoring behavioral effects and the relation with plasma bioavailability in a single individual. Furthermore, because the experiments are nonterminal, the same

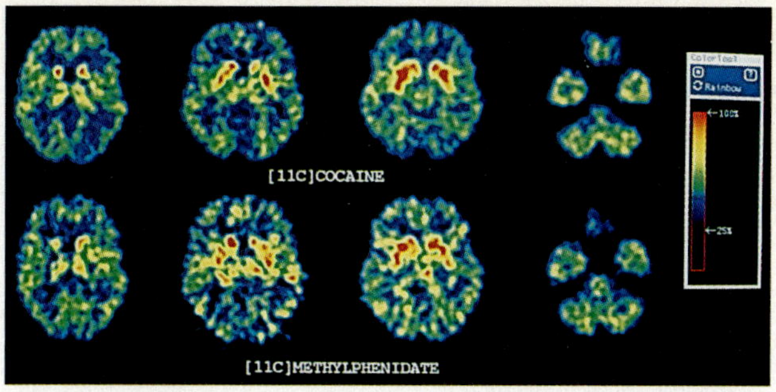

Figure 1. *Brain images obtained with carbon 11 (^{11}C)–labeled cocaine and with [^{11}C]methylphenidate hydrochloride for the normal control scanned with both tracers.*

subject can be used to investigate the effects of the drug on various neurochemical systems or the effects of drugs at different times after their administration. Position emission tomography and [^{11}C]cocaine were used to investigate the pharmacokinetics of cocaine in the human brain, and the striking similarity between the uptake and clearance of cocaine from striatum and the subjective experience of the "high" after its administration was pointed out.[21] It was postulated that the fast kinetics of cocaine in the brain contribute to its highly reinforcing properties.

This study compares the results that were obtained previously with PET for the pharmacokinetics of [^{11}C]cocaine in the human brain[21] with the pharmacokinetics of *d,l-threo*-[^{11}C]methylphenidate ([^{11}C]methylphenidate), the labeled form of the prescribed drug (Ritalin).[22] In parallel to the human studies, we performed studies in baboons to determine the degree of competition for binding between [^{11}C]cocaine and [^{11}C]methylphenidate.

RESULTS

The peak uptake of [^{11}C]methylphenidate in whole brain corresponded to a mean±SD of 7.5%±1.5% of the injected dose and was equivalent to that for the uptake of [^{11}C]cocaine (7.5%±3.0%). Binding of methylphenidate was heterogeneous; the highest concentration was in striatum, and relatively low levels were detected in cortex and cerebellum. The regional distribution of [^{11}C]methylphenidate in the human brain was almost identical to that of [^{11}C]cocaine. **Figure 1** shows the images from the subject scanned with [^{11}C]methylphenidate and [^{11}C]cocaine. The distribution and pharmacokinetics of [^{11}C]cocaine in this subject were comparable to the ones observed in our previous study.[21] **Table 1** provides the values for peak uptake of methylphenidate for the various regions and compares them with those of [^{11}C]cocaine.[21] Pretreatment with methylphenidate decreased binding in the striatum only. Values for the DV in striatum and cerebellum before and after methylphenidate administration, as well as the ratios for the DV in striatum to that in cerebellum are shown in **Table 2**, along with the values obtained for the test-retest measures. Pretreatment with methylphenidate significantly decreased the mean±SD ratio of the DV in striatum to that in cerebellum from 2.12±0.10 to 1.33±0.04 ($P<.05$).

In the baboon experiments, pretreatment with methylphenidate 5 minutes prior to the administration of [^{11}C]cocaine and pretreatment with cocaine 5 minutes prior to the administration of [^{11}C]methylphenidate significantly reduced binding of the corresponding tracer in striatum but not in cerebellum (**Figure 2**).

An analysis of the pharmacokinetic profiles in the brain revealed significant differences between [^{11}C]cocaine and [^{11}C]methylphenidate (**Figure 3**). The time to reach peak uptake in the brain was comparable for both drugs and corresponded to 4 to 10 minutes for [^{11}C]methylphenidate and 2 to 8 minutes for [^{11}C]cocaine. The peak concentration of [^{11}C]methylphenidate in the brain was maintained for 15 to 20 minutes, whereas for [^{11}C]cocaine, it was maintained for only 2 to 4 minutes. Also, [^{11}C]methylphenidate cleared from the brain much more slowly than did [^{11}C]cocaine. In the striatum, the half peak clearance of [^{11}C]cocaine corresponded to 20 minutes, whereas for [^{11}C]methylphenidate, it corresponded to 90 minutes. Times to reach peak uptake and halftimes for clearance of [^{11}C]methylphenidate and [^{11}C]cocaine are shown in Table 1.

The maximal high for methylphenidate was experienced 4 to 6 minutes after its administration, and the high had returned to baseline 30 to 40 minutes later. To investigate the relation between the drug-induced high and the kinetics of the drug in the brain, we plotted the time-activity curves for [^{11}C]methylphenidate in striatum and the curve for the high for the four subjects who received methylphenidate (**Figure 4**[21,27]). The sharp rise in the uptake of [^{11}C]methylphenidate in striatum almost paralleled the rapidly increasing high after methylphenidate administration (peak high preceded the peak for [^{11}C]methylphenidate uptake by 6 to 10 minutes). Interestingly, the high from methylphenidate decreased much faster than the rate of clearance of [^{11}C]methylphenidate. A similar comparison for [^{11}C]cocaine[21] showed that the high after cocaine administration[27] paralleled the kinetics of [^{11}C]cocaine in striatum for the uptake as well as for the clearance (Figure 4).

COMMENT

The regional distribution of [^{11}C]methylphenidate in the human brain was almost identical to that of [^{11}C]cocaine and corresponded to that previously described in autoradiographic studies.[28] The uptake of [^{11}C]methylphenidate was highest in striatum, which was also the only region for which pretreatment with methylphenidate decreased binding. Because pretreatment with methylphenidate decreased [^{11}C]methylphenidate binding in the baboon brain to the same extent as did pretreatment with drugs that inhibit dopamine transporters,[22] the accumulation of [^{11}C]methylphenidate in striatum is consistent with binding to the dopamine transporter.[22] These results are similar to those previously obtained when characterizing the binding of [^{11}C]cocaine in the baboon brain.[21] Furthermore, the fact that methylphenidate prevented binding of [^{11}C]cocaine and cocaine prevented binding of [^{11}C]methylphenidate indicates that both drugs bind to the same binding site in the dopamine transporter. Although this might be predicted based on the similar affinities of the two drugs for the dopamine transporter,[29] it cannot be assumed that drugs that inhibit up-

Table 1. Regional Uptake and Kinetics for [^{11}C]Cocaine (n=8) and [^{11}C]Methylphenidate*

	[^{11}C]Cocaine			[^{11}C]Methylphenidate Hydrochloride		
Regions	Peak Uptake, % of Dose/cm³	Time to Peak Uptake, min	Half Peak Clearance, min	Peak Uptake, % of Dose/cm³	Time to Peak Uptake, min	Half Peak Clearance, min
Global	0.005±0.002	2-8	15	0.005±0.001	4-10	75
Striatum	0.008±0.002	2-9	25	0.008±0.001	4-10	90
Cerebellum	0.007±0.002	2-6	15	0.006±0.001	4-8	50
Cortex	0.007±0.002	2-5	15	0.006±0001	4-10	55
Thalamus	0.008±0.002	2-6	15	0.007±0.001	3-10	60

**Data for carbon 11 (^{11}C)–labeled cocaine from Fowler et al.[21] Peak uptake is expressed as the mean±SD percentage of injected dose per cubic centimeter of tissue, and kinetics correspond to the time required to reach peak uptake and the time required for half peak clearance for the various brain regions.*

Table 2. Distribution Volumes (DVs) for Striatum (ST) and Cerebellum (CB) and the DV(ST)/DV(CB) Ratios for [^{11}C]Cocaine and [^{11}C]Methylphenidate

	DV(ST)	DV(CB)	DV(ST)/DV(CB)	Percentage Change
Test-Retest				
[^{11}C]cocaine*				
First test	5.1±1.3	3.08±0.70	1.70±0.22	−5.1±6.0
Second test	4.8±1.3	3.03±0.70	1.60±0.21	
[^{11}C]methylphenidate†				
First test	19.9±1.6	10.20±1.00	2.00±0.08	1.8±5.0
Second test	19.7±1.3	9.93±0.70	2.00±0.02	
[^{11}C]Methylphenidate Pretreatment				
[^{11}C]methylphenidate‡				
Without pretreatment	16.9±1.6	8.0±0.5	2.12±0.10	−37.0±1.0
With preteatment	11.7±1.2	8.7±0.7	1.33±0.04	

**Values represent mean±SD for four normal controls tested twice to assess test-retest reproducibility. Data from Fowler et al.[21]*
†Values represent mean±SD for three normal controls tested twice to assess test-retest reproducibility.
‡Values represent mean±SD for four normal controls tested twice, once with and once without pretreatment with carbon 11 (^{11}C)–labeled methylphenidate hydrochloride (0.5 mg/kg, intravenously).

take of a common neurotransmitter will necessarily inhibit each other.[30,31]

Despite the similarities between cocaine and methylphenidate in their affinity to the dopamine transporter, their absolute rate of brain uptake, and the rapidity with which they entered the brain, these two drugs differed markedly in their rate of clearance. [^{11}C]Methylphenidate cleared significantly more slowly from the brain than did [^{11}C]cocaine. These differences are in agreement with the pharmacokinetics of these two drugs in plasma. A review of these studies (**Table 3**)[4,32-42] reveals that although the time to reach peak drug concentration in plasma is similar for cocaine and methylphenidate, the rate of clearance is slower for methylphenidate than for cocaine.

Also, these studies[4,32-42] document marked differences in plasma pharmacokinetics as a function of the route of administration. The difference between the pharmacokinetics of cocaine and methylphenidate is interesting in light of the temporal pattern of the high induced by these two drugs. The high experienced after intravenous administration of methylphenidate was of a short duration, and the time pattern was similar to that reported for intravenous administration of cocaine.[27] For both drugs, the rate of drug uptake in striatum paralleled the rising portion of the high (because of the limited spatial resolution of the PET, we were unable to measure the nucleus accumbens). The association between the high and the rate of uptake of the drug in striatum and the lack of an association between the high and the rate of clearance of the drug suggests that the high induced by cocaine and methylphenidate is temporally related to the initial but not to the continuous binding to the dopamine transporters. This suggests that the experience of the high is related to the change in the concentration of dopamine (rate of change from baseline), which is secondary to the inhibition of dopamine transporters.

For cocaine, the time-response pattern for the increase in dopamine concentration has been shown to correspond to the time-response pattern of the actual presence of cocaine in striatum.[43,44] Although such studies, to our knowledge, have not been done for methylphenidate, one could predict that the increase in dopamine concentration after methylphenidate administration would last longer than that for cocaine. If the rate of change in dopamine is the predominant factor mediating the high, then rapid changes in synaptic dopamine concentration induced by cocaine could facilitate the frequent repeated administration of this drug as occurs during a binge. If this is the case, we could speculate that the persistence of methylphenidate in the brain may interfere with repeated administration and may explain the relatively low rate of abuse of methylphenidate when compared with that of cocaine.

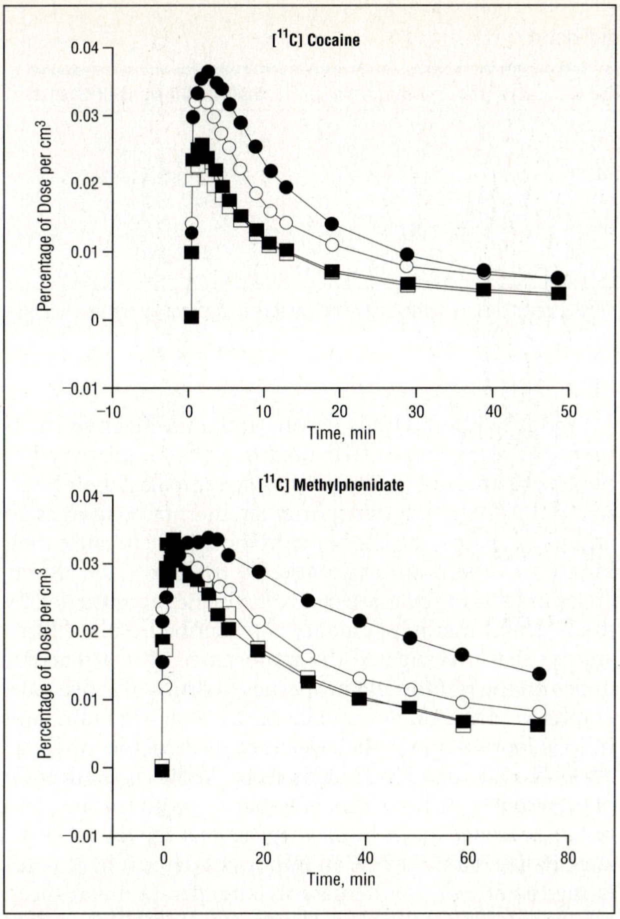

Figure 2. *Top, Time-activity curves for carbon 11 (^{11}C)–labeled cocaine in striatum and cerebellum on an animal tested at baseline (control) and after preadministration of methylphenidate hydrochloride. Solid circles indicate striatum at baseline; open circles, striatum after methylphenidate administration; solid squares, cerebellum at baseline; and open squares, cerebellum after methylphenidate administration. Bottom, Time-activity curves for [^{11}C]methylphenidate in striatum and cerebellum on an animal tested at baseline (control) and after preadministration of cocaine. Solid circles indicate striatum at baseline; open circles, striatum after cocaine administration; solid squares, cerebellum at baseline; and open squares, cerebellum after cocaine administration. Notice the decrease in striatum binding for both tracers with preadministration of methylphenidate and cocaine, while cerebellar uptake was not changed.*

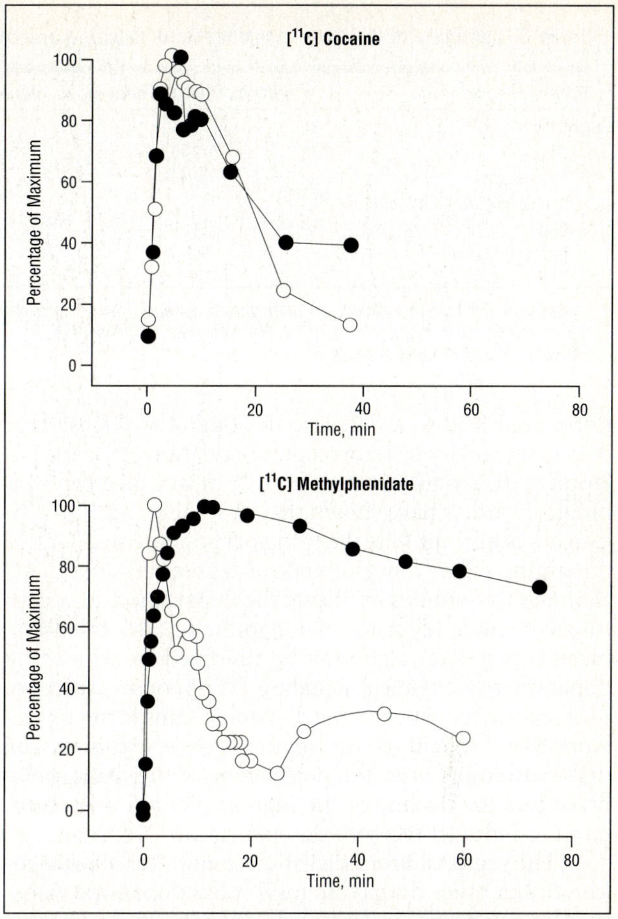

Figure 4. *Top, Time-activity curves for carbon 11 (^{11}C)–labeled cocaine in striatum (n=10) and the subjective experience of "high" after cocaine administration.[27] Notice the parallelism between the high after cocaine administration and the kinetics of [^{11}C]cocaine in striatum. The comparison between the high and the pharmacokinetics of [^{11}C]cocaine has been previously published.[21] Solid circles indicate uptake; open circles, subjective experience of high. Bottom, Time-activity curves (n=4) for [^{11}C]methylphenidate hydrochloride in striatum and the subjective experience of high after methylphenidate administration. The time-activity curve is measured at tracer doses, and the euphoria is measured after intravenous administration of 0.5 mg/kg of methylphenidate hydrochloride. Notice the dissociation between the high, which decreases rapidly after peaking, and the slow clearance of [^{11}C]methylphenidate from striatum.*

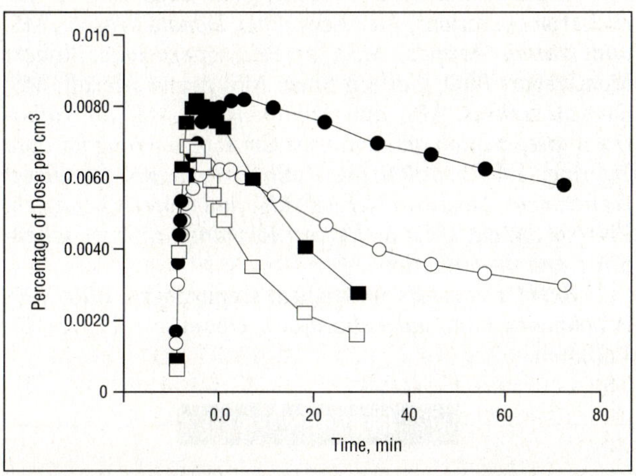

Figure 3. *Average time-activity curves for carbon 11 (^{11}C)–labeled methylphenidate hydrochloride in striatum (solid circles) and cerebellum (open circles) (n=8) and for [^{11}C]cocaine (n=10) in striatum (solid squares) and cerebellum (open squares).*

Documentation of a dissociation between the rate of decline of the high induced by methylphenidate and its rate of clearance from the brain is important because it might be expected that drugs that clear slowly from the dopamine transporter induce longer periods of the high than do drugs that have fast clearance rates, as does cocaine. Instead, it documents that it is only the initial inhibition of the dopamine transporter that is associated with the high. This dissociation suggests the occurrence of a fast adaptation process that occurs with methylphenidate. One could hypothesize that because cocaine clears from the brain very rapidly, the adaptation process is minimized. In support of this hypothesis are studies that document that when cocaine concentration in the brain is maintained constant by administering it in a continuous infusion, a similar dissociation occurs and the high declines despite constant levels of the drug in plasma.[45] The increase in dopamine concentration induced by either cocaine or methylphenidate administra-

Table 3. Summary of the Pharmacokinetics for Cocaine and Methylphenidate*

Drug	Brain: Plasma Ratio	Bioavailability, %	Peak (Plasma), min	Half-life Clearance (Plasma)
Cocaine				
Oral	5-7[32]†	20-30[34]	55-110 [34,38]	30-120 min[32,34,42]
Intravenous	NA	100[35,36]	<5 [39,40]	15-87 min[35,36]
Methylphenidate hydrochloride				
Oral	6-8[4,33]†	22-31[37]	60-170 [4,37,41]	3-4 h[4,37]
Intravenous	NA	NA	<5 [41]†	1.8-2.4 h[41]

**Values are for humans, except for brain measurements, which correspond to animal studies. Values vary for the different investigators so we provide the range of values most frequently reported. NA indicates not available.*

†Measurements done in animals.

tion could lead to a decrease in dopamine release that occurs secondary to autoreceptor regulation or via modulation of the striatonigral pathway.[46] In fact, electrophysiological studies have shown that short-term administration of cocaine inhibits the firing of spontaneously active dopamine cells from the ventral tegmental area.[47] Although most studies implicate the dopamine autoreceptor as the main regulator of dopamine release, the dopamine transporter also may be involved in regulating dopaminergic chemical signaling.[48] The consequences of prolonged occupation of the dopamine transporter on dopaminergic signaling require further investigation. The dissociation between the persistence of the drug in the brain and the decline of the high also could reflect dopamine-induced receptor desensitization.[49,50]

The regional brain distribution and the pharmacokinetics of other drugs that inhibit the dopamine transporters, such as nomifensine,[51] WIN 35428,[52] (1*R*)-2β-carbomethoxy-3β-(4-iodophenyl)tropane (β-CIT),[53] and GBR 12909 (M. Kilbourn, PhD, oral communication, 1994), have been investigated in the human brain. All of these drugs show a similar distribution, in the brain, with the highest uptake in striatum, but their pharmacokinetics differ markedly from each other. For [^{11}C]nomifensine and fluorine 18–labeled GBR 12909, peak uptake in striatum was reached within 15 minutes of injection; for iodine 123–labeled β-CIT, it was reached 1200 to 1500 minutes after injection; and for [^{11}C]WIN 35428, it was not reached at the end of the scanning period (100 minutes). Clearance of nomifensine from striatum was faster than that of methylphenidate and slower than that of cocaine (60%, 75%, and <5% of peak activity remained at 60 minutes, respectively), and clearance of GBR 12909 was similar to that of methylphenidate. Striatal clearance for the other drugs was not reported. Although all of these drugs appear to have reinforcing properties,[13,14,54] the extent to which they could induce frequent self-administration in humans, as is observed for cocaine during a binge, is unknown. For cocaine, we postulate that its unique pharmacokinetics in the brain (fast uptake and clearance) play a major role in its highly reinforcing properties and its ability to promote repeated administration. Studies on the rate of drug self-administration under conditions of free availability may enable investigators to evaluate the influence of the rate of clearance of these drugs from the dopamine transporters on their propensity to induce repeated administration.

Methylphenidate is a common and effective treatment for attention-deficit disorder. The similarity between cocaine and methylphenidate regarding their binding to the dopamine transporter should not be used as an argument against the use of methylphenidate because their kinetics in the brain are markedly different, and differences in their kinetics are probably further accentuated by the fact that methylphenidate is prescribed orally.[4] Most studies that investigated the importance of pharmacokinetics on the reinforcing properties of drugs of abuse have emphasized the rate of uptake of drugs in the brain, and little is known about the relevance of their rate of clearance. The fact that it is the initial rise in the concentration of the drug in the brain that is associated with the high and not its presence in the brain suggests that the rate of clearance in the brain may be an important determinant regulating the rate of repeated administration. In this respect, we speculate that the slow clearance of methylphenidate from the brain may serve as a limiting factor in promoting its frequent self-administration.

Accepted for publication October 10, 1994.

This study was supported by the US Department of Energy, Washington, DC, under contract DE-ACO2-76CH00016 and by grants 5RO1-DA06891 from the National Institute on Drug Abuse and NS15638 from the National Institute of Neurological Disorders and Stroke, Bethesda, Md.

We thank Robert Carciello and Babe Barrett for cyclotron operations; Alex Levy, PhD; Donald Warner, MS; and Naomi Pappas, MS, for PET operations; Robert MacGregor, PhD; Colleen Shea, MS; David Alexoff, MS; Darrin Jenkins, MS; and Payton King, MS, for radiotracer preparation and analysis; Cristopher Wong for data entering; Gale Burr, RN, and Kathy Pascani, RN, for subject recruitment; Noelwah Netusil, RN, and Noreen Pendzick, RN, for patient care; and Carol Redvanly, MS, for scheduling and organization.

Reprint requests to Medical Department, Bldg 490, Brookhaven National Laboratory, Upton, NY 11973 (Dr Volkow).

REFERENCES

1. Fischman MW, Schuster CR. Cocaine self administration in humans. *Fed Proc.* 1988;41:241-246.
2. Johanson CE, Fischman MW. The pharmacology of cocaine related to its abuse. *Pharmacol Rev.* 1989;41:3-52.

3. Koob GF, Bloom FE. Cellular and molecular mechanisms of drug dependence. *Science.* 1988;242:715-723.
4. Wilens TE, Biederman J. The stimulants. *Pediatr Psychopharmacol.* 1992;15: 191-222.
5. Barkley RA. A review of stimulant drug research with hyperactive children. *J Child Psychol Psychiatry.* 1977;8:137-165.
6. Safer DJ, Krager JM. Effect of a media blitz and a threatened lawsuit on stimulant treatment. *JAMA.* 1992;268:1004-1007.
7. Meyer JS, Sakai F, Karacan I, Derman S, Yamamoto M. Sleep apnea, narcolepsy, and dreaming: regional cerebral hemodynamics. *Ann Neurol.* 1980;7: 479-485.
8. Kaufman MW, Cassem NH, Murray GB, Jenike M. Use of psychostimulants in medically ill patients with neurological disease and major depression. *Can J Psychiatry.* 1984;29:46-49.
9. Pollack MH, Brotman AW, Rosenbaum JF. Cocaine abuse and treatment. *Compr Psychiatry.* 1989;30:31-44.
10. Khantzian EJ, Gawin FH, Riordan C, Kleber HD. Methylphenidate treatment of cocaine dependence: a preliminary report. *J Subst Abuse Treat.* 1984;1:107-112.
11. Chiarello RJ, Cole JO. The use of psychostimulant in general psychiatry. *Arch Gen Psychiatry.* 1987;44:266-295.
12. Parran TV, Jasinski DR. Intravenous methylphenidate abuse: prototype for prescription drug abuse. *Arch Intern Med.* 1991;151:781-783.
13. Ritz MC, Lamb RJ, Goldberg SR, Kuhar MJ. Cocaine receptors on dopamine transporters are related to self-administration of cocaine. *Science.* 1987;237: 1219-1223.
14. Bergman J, Madras B, Johnson SE, Spealman RD. Effects of cocaine and related drugs in nonhuman primates, III: self administration by squirrel monkeys. *J Pharmacol Exp Ther.* 1989;251:150-155.
15. Johanson CE, Shuster CR. A choice procedure for drug reinforcers: cocaine and methylphenidate in the rhesus monkey. *J Pharmacol Exper Ther.* 1975; 193:676-688.
16. Wilson MC, Hitomi M, Schuster CR. Psychomotor self administration as a function of dosage per injection in the rhesus monkey. *Psychopharmacology.* 1971; 22:271-281.
17. Jeffe RB, Koschmann EB. Intravenous drug abuse, pulmonary cardiac and vascular complications. *AJR Am J Roentgenol.* 1970;109:107-120.
18. Lewman LV. Fatal pulmonary hypertension from intravenous injection of methylphenidate (Ritalin) tablets. *Hum Pathol.* 1972;3:67-70.
19. Oldendorf WH. Some relationships between addiction and drug delivery to the brain. In: Frankenheim J, Brown RM, eds. *Bioavailability of Drugs to the Brain and the Blood Brain Barrier.* Rockville, MD: National Institute on Drug Abuse; 1992:13-25. Research Monograph 120.
20. Balster RL, Schuster CR. Fixed-interval schedule of cocaine reinforcement: effects of dose and infusion duration. *J Exp Anal Behav.* 1973;20:119-129.
21. Fowler JS, Volkow ND, Wolf AP, Dewey SL, Schlyer DJ, MacGregor RR, Hitzemann R, Logan J, Bendriem B, Gatley SJ, Christman D. Mapping cocaine binding sites in human and baboon brain in vivo. *Synapse.* 1989;4:371-377.
22. Ding Y-S, Fowler JS, Volkow ND, Gatley SJ, Dewey SL, Martin T, Jenkins D, Alexoff D, Salata C, Wolf AP. Synthesis of [^{11}C]*dl-threo*-methylphenidate: drug pharmacokinetics and binding to the presynaptic dopaminergic neuron. *Synapse.* 1994;18:152-160.
23. Dewey SL, MacGregor RR, Brodie JD, Bendriem B, King PT, Volkow ND, Schlyer DJ, Fowler JS, Wolf AP, Gately SJ, Hitzemann R. Mapping muscarinic receptors in human and baboon brain using [*N*-^{11}C-methyl]-benztropine. *Synapse.* 1990;5:213-223.
24. Bendriem B, Dewey SL, Schlyer DJ, Wolf AP, Volkow ND. Quantitation of the human basal ganglia with positron emission tomography: a phantom study of the effect of contrast and axial positioning. *IEEE Trans Med Imaging.* 1991; 10:216-222.
25. Logan J, Fowler JS, Volkow ND, Wolf AP, Dewer SL, Schlyer DJ, MacGregor RR, Hitzemann R, Bendriem B, Gatley SJ, Christman DR. Graphical analysis of reversible radioligand binding time-activity measurements applied to [*N*-^{11}C-methyl]-(−)-cocaine PET studies in human subjects. *J Cereb Blood Flow Metab.* 1990;10:740-747.
26. Logan J, Volkow ND, Fowler JS, Wang G-J, Dewey SL, MacGregor R, Schlyer D, Gatley S-J, Pappas N, King P, Hitzmann R, Vitkun S. Effects of blood flow on [^{11}C]raclopride binding in the brain: model simulations and kinetic analysis of PET data. *J Cereb Blood Flow Metab.* 1994;14:995-1010.
27. Cook CE, Jeffcoat AR, Perez-Reyes M. Pharmacokinetic studies of cocaine and phenylciclidine in man. In: Barnett G, Chiang CN, eds. *Pharmacokinetics and Pharmacodynamics of Psychoactive Drugs.* Foster City, Calif: Biomedical Publication; 1985:48-74.
28. Unis AS, Dawson TM, Gehlert DR, Wamsley JK. Autoradiographic localization of [3H]-methylphenidate binding sites in rat brain. *Eur J Pharmacol.* 1985; 113:155-157.
29. Seeman P. *Receptor Tables: Drug Dissociation for Neuroreceptors and Transporters.* Toronto, Ontario: Sz Research; 1993;2.
30. Laduron PM. Criteria for receptor sites in binding studies. *Biochem Pharmacol.* 1984;33:833-839.
31. Pristupa ZB, Wilson J, Hoffman B, Kish SJ, Niznik HB. Pharmacological heterogeneity of the cloned and native human dopamine transporter: dissociation of [^{3}H]WIN 35,428 and [^{3}H]GBR 12,935 binding. *Mol Pharmacol.* 1993;45: 125-135.
32. Benuck M, Lajtha A, Reith MEA. Pharmacokinetics of systemically administered cocaine and locomotor stimulation in mice. *J Pharmacol Exp Ther.* 1987; 243:144-149.
33. Kennerly PS, Ellington KR, Breese GR. *J Pharmacol Exp Ther.* 1984;231:61-67.
34. Van Dyke C, Jatlow P, Barash PG, Byck R. Oral cocaine: plasma concentrations and central effects. *Science.* 1978;100:211-213.
35. Javaid JI, Musa MN, Fischman M, Schuster CR, Davis JM. Kinetics of cocaine in humans after intravenous and intranasal administration. *Biopharm Drug Dispos.* 1983;4:9-18.
36. Jeffcoat AR, Perez Reyes M, Hill JM, Sadler BM, Cook CE. Cocaine disposition in humans after intravenous injection, nasal insufflation (snorting) or smoking. *Drug Metab Dispos Biol Fate Chem.* 1989;17:153-159.
37. Srinivas NR, Hubbard JW, Quinn D, Korchinski ED, Midha K. Extensive and enantioselective presystemic metabolism of dl-threo-methylphenidate in humans. *Prog Neuropsychopharmacol Biol Psychiatry.* 1991;15:213-220.
38. Holmstedt B, Lindgren JE, River L. Cocaine in blood of coca chewers. *J Ethnopharmacol.* 1979;1:69-78.
39. Javaid J, Fischman MW, Schuster CR, Dekirmenjian H, Davis JM. Cocaine plasma concentration: relation to physiological and subjective effects in humans. *Science.* 1978;201:227-228.
40. Foltin RW, Fischman M. Smoked and intravenous cocaine in humans: acute tolerance, cardiovascular and subjective effects. *J Pharmacol Exp Ther.* 1991; 257:247-261.
41. Wargin W, Kilts PC, Gualtieri CT, Ellington K, Mueller RA, Kraemer G, Breese GR. Pharmacokinetics of methylphenidate in man, rat and monkey. *J Pharmacol Exp Ther.* 1983;226:382-386.
42. Inaba T. Cocaine: pharmacokinetics and biotransformation in man. *Can J Physiol Pharmacol.* 1988;67:1154-1157.
43. Hurd YL, Kehr J, Ungerstedt U. In vivo microdialysis as a technique to monitor drug transport: correlation of extracellular cocaine levels and dopamine overflow in the rat brain. *J Neurochem.* 1988;51:1314-1316.
44. Nicolaysen LC, Pan HT, Justice JB. Extracellular cocaine and dopamine concentrations are linearly related in rat striatum. *Brain Res.* 1988;456:317-323.
45. Ambre JJ. Cocaine kinetics in humans. In: Redda KK, Walker CA, Barnett G, eds. *Cocaine, Marijuana, Designer Drugs, Chemistry, Pharmacology and Behavior.* Boca Raton, Fla: CRC Press Inc; 1989:53-69.
46. Chiodo LA. Dopamine-containing neurons in the mammalian central nervous system: electrophysiology and pharmacology. *Neurosci Biobehav Rev.* 1988; 12:49-91.
47. Einhorn LC, Johansen PA, White FJ. Electrophysiological effects of cocaine in the mesoaccumbens system: studies in the ventral tegmental area. *J Neurosci.* 1988;8:100-112.
48. Meiergerd SM, Patterson TA, Schenk JO. D2 receptors may modulate the function of the striatal transporter for dopamine: kinetic evidence from studies in vitro and in vivo. *J Neurochem.* 1993;61:764-767.
49. Parsons LH, Schad CA, Justice JB Jr. Co-administration of the D2 antagonist pimozide inhibits up-regulation of dopamine release and uptake induced by repeated cocaine. *J Neurochem.* 1993;60:376-379.
50. Memo M, Lovenberg W, Hanbauer I. Agonist-induced subsensitivity of adenylate cyclase coupled with a dopamine receptor in slices from rat corpus striatum. *Proc Natl Acad Sci U S A.* 1982;79:4456-4460.
51. Salmon E, Brooks DJ, Leenders KL, Turton DR, Hume SP, Cremer JE, Jones T, Frackowiak RSJ. A two-compartment description and kinetic procedure for measuring regional cerebral [^{11}C]nomifensine uptake using positron emission tomography. *J Cereb Blood Flow Metab.* 1990;10:307-316.
52. Wong RDF, Yung B, Dannals RF, Shaya EK, Ravert HT, Chen CA, Chan B, Folio T, Scheffel U, Ricaurte GA, Neumeyer JL, Wagner H, Kuhar MJ. In vivo imaging of baboon and human dopamine transporters by positron emission tomography using [^{11}C]WIN 35428. *Synapse.* 1993;15:130-142.
53. Innis RB, Seybel JP, Scanley BE, Laruelle M, Abi-Dargham A, Wallace E, Baldwin RM, Zea-Ponce Y, Zoghbi S, Wang S, Gao Y, Neumeyer JL, Charney DS, Hoffer PB, Marek KL. Single-photon emission–computed tomography imaging demonstrates loss of striatal dopamine transporters in Parkinson disease. *Proc Natl Acad Sci U S A.* 1993;90:11965-11969.
54. Spyraki C, Fibiger HC. Intravenous self-administration of nomifensine in rats: implications for abuse potential in humans. *Science.* 1981;212:1167-1168.

ORIGINAL ARTICLE

Family-Environment Risk Factors for Attention-Deficit Hyperactivity Disorder

A Test of Rutter's Indicators of Adversity

Joseph Biederman, MD; Sharon Milberger, ScD; Stephen V. Faraone, PhD; Kathleen Kiely; Jessica Guite; Eric Mick; Stuart Ablon; Rebecca Warburton; Ellen Reed

Background: This study investigated whether family-environment risk factors are associated with attention-deficit hyperactivity disorder (ADHD). Compelling work by Rutter and coworkers revealed that it was the aggregate of adversity factors (severe marital discord, low social class, large family size, paternal criminality, maternal mental disorder, and foster care placement) rather than the presence of any single factor that led to impaired development. Based on the work of Rutter, we hypothesized a positive association between indicators of adversity and the diagnosis of ADHD and ADHD-associated impairments.

Methods: We studied 140 ADHD and 120 normal control probands. Subjects were non-Hispanic white boys between the ages of 6 and 17 years. Rutter's indicators of adversity were used to predict ADHD-related psychopathology as well as impaired cognitive and psychosocial functioning.

Results: The odds ratio for the diagnosis of ADHD increased as the number of Rutter's adversity indicators increased. Higher scores on Rutter's adversity index predicted ADHD-related psychopathology (depression, anxiety, and conduct disorder), learning disabilities, cognitive impairment, and psychosocial dysfunction.

Conclusions: A positive association appears to exist between adversity indicators and the risk for ADHD as well as for its associated psychiatric, cognitive, and psychosocial impairments. These findings support the work of Rutter and stress the importance of adverse family-environment variables as risk factors for children with ADHD.

(Arch Gen Psychiatry. 1995;52:464-470)

IN RECENT YEARS, evidence has accumulated indicating that attention-deficit hyperactivity disorder (ADHD) is a familial disorder.[1] In two independent double-blind, controlled studies of *DSM-III*–defined attention-deficit disorder [2] and *DSM-III-R*–defined ADHD,[3] we documented the familiality of this disorder. However, many disorders run in families because of environmental—not genetic—factors.[4,5] Although twin, adoption, and segregation analysis studies implicate a genetic component in the cause of ADHD,[6] children with ADHD often come from families that are disorganized and have a parent who exhibits psychopathologic disorders. These families may create pathogenic environments.

The delineation of characteristics in the child's environment associated with more impaired outcome in children with ADHD has potentially important clinical, scientific, and public health implications. Such efforts can help identify the etiologic risk factors associated with more impaired outcome in ADHD and can characterize early predictors of persistence and morbidity of this disorder.[7] Moreover, finding environmental risk factors for ADHD could help design improved preventive and therapeutic intervention programs.

Perhaps the most compelling example of the delineation of psychosocial risk factors for childhood mental disorders comes from the now classic studies of Rutter and coworkers[8,9] (hereafter, Rutter) of the Isle of Wight and the inner borough of London, England. These studies examined the prevalence of mental disorders in children living in two very different geographic areas. That research revealed six risk factors within the family environment that correlated significantly with childhood mental disturbances: (1) severe marital discord, (2) low social class, (3) large family size, (4) paternal crimi-

From the Pediatric Psychopharmacology Unit of the Psychiatry Service, Massachusetts General Hospital and Harvard Medical School, Boston.

See Subjects and Methods on next page

SUBJECTS AND METHODS

SUBJECTS

We analyzed data from a family-genetic study of ADHD that we have presented previously.[3,14,16-18] We studied two groups of index children: 140 ADHD probands and 120 normal control probands. These groups had 174 and 129 biologic siblings, respectively. We obtained informed consent for all subjects prior to their enrollment in the protocol. All probands were white, non-Hispanic boys between the ages of 6 and 17 years. Potential probands were excluded if they had been adopted or if their nuclear family was not available for study. We excluded children if they had major sensorimotor handicaps (eg, paralysis, deafness, blindness), psychosis, autism, or an estimated full-scale IQ of less than 80. To minimize the potential confounds of social chaos, we excluded subjects from the lowest class of socioeconomic status (SES VI).[19] Each of the ADHD probands met diagnostic criteria for current ADHD at the time of the clinical referral; at the time of recruitment, each had active symptoms of the disorder.

ADHD PROBANDS

We selected psychiatrically referred ADHD probands from consecutive referrals to the Pediatric Psychopharmacology Unit, an outpatient clinic at the Massachusetts General Hospital (MGH) in Boston. The Pediatric Psychopharmacology Unit provides comprehensive diagnostic and treatment services for children with psychiatric disorders. It is not a tertiary care clinic; approximately 50% of referrals have never before been diagnosed or treated. The Harvard Community Health Plan (HCHP), one of the largest health maintenance organizations in the Boston area, provided the pediatrically referred ADHD probands.

A three-stage ascertainment procedure selected the ADHD probands. The first stage was the patient's referral to a psychiatric or pediatric clinic resulting in a clinical diagnosis of ADHD by a child psychiatrist (N=154) or a pediatrician (N=238) as recorded in the clinic record. The second stage confirmed the diagnosis of ADHD by screening all children who had a positive diagnosis for ADHD at the first stage using a telephone questionnaire with their mother that asked about the 14 *DSM-III-R*[20] symptoms of ADHD.

Among the referred pool of patients, 48% (n=74) at MGH and 66% (n=156) at HCHP were ineligible, unreachable, or refused to participate in the telephone interview. The most common reason for nonparticipation was refusal. Of those remaining and meeting study entry criteria, 4% (n=3) at MGH and 15% (n=12) at HCHP refused to participate further. In the third stage, subjects received the assessments described below. Only the patients who received a positive diagnosis of ADHD at all three stages were included in the final analysis. Among patients who received the comprehensive assessment, 1% (n=1) at MGH and 9% (n=6) at HCHP were not diagnosed as having ADHD and were not included in the final sample. The final ADHD sample consisted of 76 subjects at MGH and 64 at HCHP.

NORMAL CONTROL PROBANDS

We screened potential normal controls in three stages. First, we selected referrals to medical clinics for routine physical examinations (MGH, N=282; HCHP, N=261). Second, we administered the *DSM-III-R* ADHD telephone questionnaire to the mothers of the referred controls. Of the referred pool of normal controls, 83% (n=233) at MGH and 60% (n=157) at HCHP were ineligible, unreachable, or refused to participate. The most common reason for nonparticipation was refusal. Of those remaining and meeting study criteria, 20% (n=10) at MGH and 19% (n=20) at HCHP refused participation. In the third stage, subjects received the assessments described below. Among those who reached the third stage, 3% (n=1) at MGH and 2% (n=2) at HCHP were diagnosed as having ADHD; they were not included in the final control sample that comprised 38 MGH patients and 82 HCHP patients. We screened controls only for the purpose of ruling out ADHD. Screening for other conditions could spuriously produce evidence for familial coaggregation between the screened conditions and ADHD.[21]

DIAGNOSTIC AND SAMPLE SELECTION CONSIDERATIONS

We used three-stage ascertainment to maximize the probabilities of ADHD probands being "true cases" and of normal controls not having ADHD. The positive predictive power of a diagnosis (the proportion of those with the disorder among all patients receiving the diagnosis) increases as the base rate of the disorder being diagnosed increases.[22] Thus, our stepwise ascertainment procedure increases the positive predictive power by using both clinic and telephone interview diagnoses of ADHD to increase the proportion of true cases in the sample that is assessed through the structured psychiatric interview. Unavoidably, this method excludes subjects who have a disorder but are not referred to a clinic or referred but do not receive a clinical diagnosis. Thus, the generalizability of our results will be limited to the degree that these false negatives differ from the probands enrolled in our study.

Likewise, our three-stage screening of controls decreases the probability of misclassifying a child with ADHD as a control. Because our screened controls were selected for the absence of ADHD, they cannot be considered representative of the general population. However, unscreened controls frequently have rates of psychopathologic disorders that are above that expected in the general population.[23-25] We emphasize that controls were screened for ADHD only, not for other psychiatric disorders or conditions related to cognitive functioning.

ASSESSMENT PROCEDURES

The Kiddie Schedule for Affective Disorder and Schizophrenia for School-age Children (epidemiologic version)[26] was used for the psychiatric assessments of probands and siblings. Diagnoses were based on independent interviews with the mothers and direct interviews with probands and siblings, except for children younger than 12 years who were not directly interviewed. Diagnostic assessments of parents were based on direct interviews with each parent using the Structured Clinical Interview for *DSM-III-R*.[27] All assessments were made by raters who were blind to the proband diagnosis (ADHD or control) and ascertainment site (MGH or health maintenance organization). The raters had been trained to a high degree of clinician-to-rater reliability. κ Coefficients

Continued on next page

of agreement were computed between raters and experienced, board-certified child and adult psychiatrists who listened to audiotaped interviews made by the raters. Based on 75 interviews, all κ values were higher than 0.82 with the exception of alcohol abuse, which was 0.75. The mean κ was 0.90. A κ of 1.0 was obtained for ADHD (95% confidence interval [CI], 0.8 to 1.0), substance abuse (95% CI, 0.7 to 1.0), and substance dependence (95% CI, 0.7 to 1.0).

Diagnoses were considered positive if, based on the interview results, *DSM-III-R* criteria were unequivocally met. All diagnostic uncertainties were resolved by a committee of four board-certified child and adult psychiatrists who were blind to the subject's ascertainment group, ascertainment site, all data collected from other family members, and all nondiagnostic data (eg, cognitive functioning). Diagnoses presented for review were considered positive only if a consensus was achieved that criteria were met to a degree that would be considered clinically meaningful. As suggested by others,[28] the diagnosis of major depression was made only if the depressive episode was associated with marked impairment. Since the anxiety disorders comprise many syndromes with a wide range of severity, we also report results for two or more anxiety disorders to index the presence of a clinically meaningful anxiety syndrome.[29] For children older than 12 years, data from direct and indirect interviews were combined by considering a diagnostic criterion as positive if it was endorsed in either interview. The rates of illness reported here are lifetime prevalences.

Our interviewers assessed academic achievement with the arithmetic subtest of the Wide Range Achievement Test—Revised[30] and the Gilmore Oral Reading Test.[31] For subjects younger than 17 years, the interviewers assessed intellectual functioning with the vocabulary, block design, arithmetic, digit span, and coding subtests of the Wechsler Intelligence Scale for Children–Revised.[32] For subjects 17 years and older, the interviewers assessed intellectual functioning with the vocabulary, block design, arithmetic, digit span, and digit symbol subtests of the Wechsler Adult Intelligence Scale–Revised.[33] Using the methods of Sattler[34] we estimated full-scale IQ from the vocabulary and block design subtests and computed the Freedom From Distractibility IQ from the other subtests. All of our analyses of the Wechsler subtests use age-corrected scaled scores.

OPERATIONAL DEFINITIONS OF ADVERSITY AND OUTCOME

We performed analyses based on those adversity indicators identified by Rutter as being associated with childhood mental disturbances: severe marital discord, low social class, large family size, paternal criminality, maternal mental disorder, and foster care placement. Because none of our subjects had been placed in foster homes, the variable of foster care placement could not be used.

Low social class was defined as the lowest two socioeconomic classes in our sample (SES III and SES IV). Large family size was defined as three or more children. A history of antisocial personality in the father indexed paternal criminality. Maternal mental disorder was measured as the mother having at least two psychiatric disorders during the child's lifetime.

A summary measure of family conflict derived from the Moos Family Environment Scale (FES)[35] was used as a proxy for severe marital discord. This scale assessed the quality of interpersonal relationships among family members along three dimensions: (1) *cohesion* assessed the degree of commitment, help, and support family members provided for one another; (2) *expressiveness* measured the extent to which family members were encouraged to act openly and to express their feelings directly; and (3) *conflict* evaluated the amount of openly expressed anger, aggression, and conflict. We obtained FES ratings separately from mothers and fathers who rated family functioning twice: once to refer to the last month and once to summarize the entire past. For each rating, we used the worse of the mother and father reports as the final score. We defined persistent adversity as present if both the entire past and last month ratings exceeded the 1.5 SD of the controls. We defined our summary measure as a linear combination of the three FES persistence ratings and the six FES scale scores (conflict, expressiveness, and cohesiveness were rated twice; one rating described current functioning [the past month], the other described lifetime functioning). This variable was dichotomized by using the median in the normal control population as the cut point.

Because some of the adversity variables may be correlated with one another, we entered the individual adversity variables into a principal components analysis with varimax rotation. Two factors emerged: factor 1 (maternal psychopathology, paternal criminality, and SES) and factor 2 (family size and family conflict).

The psychopathologic outcomes were ADHD, conduct disorder, major depression, and multiple anxiety disorders. We indexed the severity of ADHD as the total number of ADHD symptoms. We measured psychosocial functioning with the Global Assessment of Functioning scale of *DSM-III-R*. Cognitive and school related outcomes were full-scale IQ, learning disability, and any school failure (ie, placement in special classes, in-school academic tutoring, or repeated grades). The definition of learning disabilities under Public Law 94-142 requires a significant discrepancy between a child's potential and achievement.[36] We used the procedure recommended by Reynolds[37] as we have elsewhere.[13,14] Although there is some overlap between our measures of learning disability and school failure, they differ in one important respect: the presence of a learning disability indicates a deficit in either reading or arithmetic achievement that cannot be accounted for by overall intelligence. In contrast, school failure indicates difficulties in learning regardless of intelligence.

To provide protection against type I errors, we used two-tailed statistical tests with .01 as the threshold probability level for asserting statistical significance.

nality, (5) maternal mental disorder, and (6) foster placement.

However, the work of Rutter also indicated that it was the aggregate of adversity factors, rather than the presence of any single factor, that impaired development. The studies[8,9] of Rutter showed that no single environmental risk factor significantly increased the risk for mental disorders in children, but the presence of two risk factors resulted in a fourfold increase in the likelihood of mental disorders and the presence of four risk factors yielded a 10-fold increase in risk.[8,9] Other studies also have found that as the number of adverse conditions accumulates, the risk for impaired outcome in the child increases proportionally.[10]

Association Between Rutter's Indicators and ADHD*

No. of Rutter's Indicators	Risk for ADHD, OR (99% CI)	No. of ADHD Probands (N=140)	No. of Control Probands (N=120)
0	...	38	94
1	7.4 (3.2-17.3)	57	19
2	9.5 (2.6-34.2)	23	6
3	34.6 (2.3-523.8)	14	1
4	41.7 (0.9-181.0)	8	0

**ADHD indicates attention-deficit hyperactivity disorder; OR, odds ratio; and CI, confidence interval. See Rutter et al[8,9] for further detail of indicators.*

In recent years, our group and others have reported on the heterogeneity of outcome in children with ADHD. These children manifest a wide range of psychiatric,[11,12] cognitive,[13,14] and functional[15] impairments. Although the reasons for these widely variable clinical manifestations are unclear, it is plausible that some of these complex outcomes are mediated by environmental factors.

The purpose of this study was to use Rutter's indicators of adversity to evaluate the impact of family-environment risk factors on ADHD. Based on Rutter's work, we hypothesized a positive association between Rutter's indicators of family adversity and the expression of ADHD and its associated dysfunction and impairment.

RESULTS

When compared with normal control children, ADHD probands were found to be from families with higher conflict (mean [±SD] FES score, 0.3±1.1 vs −0.3±0.8; χ^2=27.2, *df*=1, *P*=.0001; range, −9.19 to 21.1, with higher scores indicating more conflict) and lower SES (1.2±1.6 vs 0.45±0.84; χ^2=9.0, *df*=1, *P*=.003; range, 1 [high SES] to 4 [low SES] on the Hollingshead Scale[19]). The mothers of ADHD probands had a greater number of psychiatric diagnoses (1.2±1.6 vs 0.4±0.8; χ^2=16.9, *df*=1, *P*=.0001; range, 0 to 9). No significant differences were observed between ADHD and control children in rates of paternal antisocial personality disorder or in family size.

See also pages 429, 434, 444, and 456

The **Table** shows that the odds ratio for ADHD increased significantly with each increase in the number of Rutter's adversity indicators (χ^2=70.9, *df*=4, *P*<.0001). More specifically, the odds of having ADHD were 7.4 times greater in children having one indicator compared with children having none of Rutter's indicators, and the odds of having ADHD were 9.5, 34.6, and 41.7 times greater in children having 2, 3, and 4 indicators, respectively, compared with children having no adversity indicators.

The **Figure** shows a positive association between the number of Rutter's adversity indicators and impaired outcomes in both ADHD and normal control children as manifested by an increased risk for ADHD-related psychopathology (depression, anxiety, or conduct disorder) and impaired psychosocial functioning as measured by the Global Assessment of Functioning. In addition, there was a positive association between Rutter's index of adversity and the number of ADHD symptoms endorsed (Spearman correlation coefficient=.34, *P*=.0001).

Rutter's indicators of adversity were somewhat predictive of learning disability and cognitive functioning in ADHD and normal control probands. However, statistical significance could be established only for learning disability in control probands. An opposite finding occurred for impaired cognitive functioning in which statistical significance was attained in ADHD probands but not in control probands. No positive association was seen between the number of Rutter's indicators and school failure in either ADHD (χ^2=3.4, *df*=4, *P*=.5) or control probands (χ^2=4.3, *df*=3, *P*=.2).

Both factor 1 and factor 2 had positive associations with ADHD (χ^2=14.6, *df*=1, *P*=.0001 and χ^2=18.0, *df*=1, *P*=.0001, respectively). Factor 1 also was predictive of ADHD-related psychopathology (χ^2=14.6, *df*=1, *P*=.0001) and impaired psychosocial functioning (*t*=−4.6, *P*=.0001). We observed a trend for factor 2 to be associated with these variables (χ^2=4.2, *df*=1, *P*=.04, and *t*=−2.4, *P*=.02, respectively). Neither factor 1 nor factor 2 was associated with school failure.

A different pattern was observed between the adversity factors and learning disability and cognitive impairment. Factor 1 (maternal psychopathology, paternal antisocial personality disorder, and SES) was significantly associated with learning disability (χ^2=11.6, *df*=1, *P*=.0007) and impaired cognitive functioning (*t*=−4.7, *P*=.0001), while factor 2 was not associated with these outcomes.

When we controlled for family history, the significant positive associations between Rutter's index of adversity and ADHD and its associated impairment were still present. Statistical interaction between family history of ADHD and Rutter's index of adversity was seen only for learning disability: Rutter's index of adversity was a significant predictor of learning disability when there was no family history of ADHD (χ^2=12.5, *df*=1, *P*=.0004) but was not a significant predictor when family history was present (χ^2=0.11, *df*=1, *P*=.73).

COMMENT

We found a positive association between Rutter's index of adversity and ADHD, measures of ADHD-associated psychopathology, impaired cognition, and psychosocial dysfunction. These findings support the work of Rutter and stress the importance of adverse family-environment variables as risk factors in ADHD.

Our results deviate slightly from those reported by Rutter. We found positive associations between ADHD and some of the individual risk factors that are components of the adversity index. In contrast, Rutter found that the individual variables were not related to developing psychiatric disorder. Instead, a nonspecific environmental risk was conferred when variables were combined. This difference may be due to the samples studied.

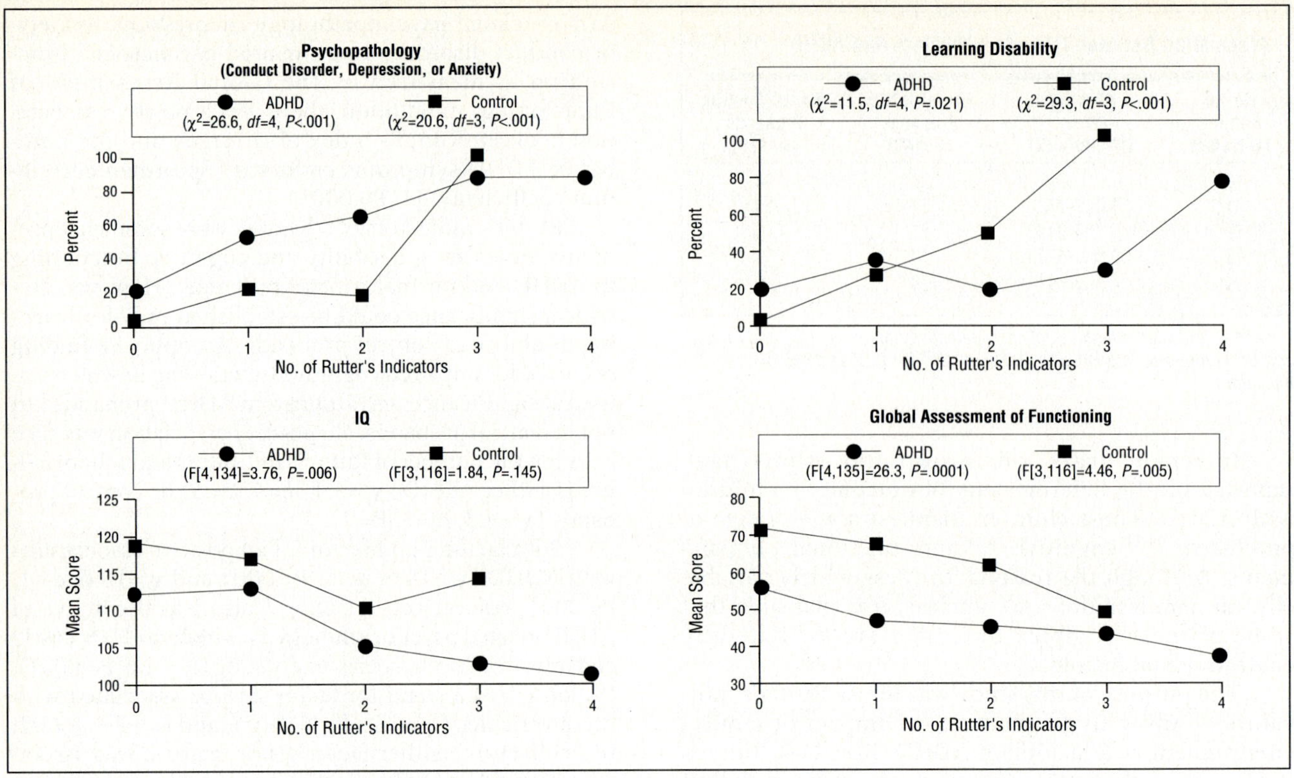

Association between Rutter's indicators of adversity[8,9] and psychopathology (conduct disorder, depression, or anxiety) and school, cognitive, and psychosocial functioning. ADHD indicates attention-deficit hyperactivity disorder.

Rutter used an epidemiologic sample and did not limit his psychopathologic outcome to ADHD. In contrast, we studied children who had been pediatrically or psychiatrically referred for ADHD. In addition, the variables we studied are only proxies for his adversity measures.

Although our results provide strong evidence for the importance of adversity factors on children's adaptive functioning and emotional health, they also show that this impact appears to be independent of ADHD; both children with ADHD and those without ADHD showed a similar positive association between the number of adversity indicators and measures of psychopathology and impaired psychosocial functioning. These results stress the universal importance of adversity for the adaptive functioning of children with and without psychopathologic disorders.

More intriguing results were seen in analyses that examined the impact of adversity factors on cognitive dysfunction. These analyses showed that with each increase in the number of adversity indicators, intellectual ability (as measured by IQ) decreased in children with ADHD but not in controls. In contrast, adversity significantly increased the risk for learning disability in controls, but only marginally in children with ADHD. Moreover, the absence of a significant association between the number of indicators of adversity and measures of school failure such as repeated grades, school-based tutoring, or placement in special classes in either ADHD or control probands is inconsistent with the commonly held psychosocial explanation for children's school dysfunction. These results raise clinically and educationally important questions about the complex interrelationships of ADHD, adversity, and psychoeducational functioning.

Our data suggest that, among ADHD children, adversity has differential effects on measures of intellectual ability (which was most sensitive to adversity), learning disability (which showed a moderate association with adversity), and school failure (which showed no association with adversity). Thus, adversity factors may worsen the already impaired intellectual functioning of children with ADHD, but these factors result only in modest exacerbations of learning disabilities beyond what is already associated with ADHD itself. In contrast, among controls, adversity had little impact on intellectual ability, but strongly predicted learning disability.

The differential effect of adversity on IQ in ADHD and normal controls together with the finding of lower IQs among children with ADHD[14] requires further comment. At a descriptive level, it suggests that the measured IQ of a child with ADHD is more malleable than that of a child without ADHD. This suggests that improvements in the psychosocial milieu of the child with ADHD could translate into increased intellectual abilities with its attendant psychoeducational relevance. Since IQ scores are frequently used for serious clinical and educational decisions, their interpretation should reflect the psychosocial context of the child.

Clearly, these results stress the complexity of the interactions between adversity factors and cognitive and academic functioning in children and emphasize the need for further longitudinal study. Moreover, the finding of a positive association between Rutter's index of adversity and learning disability only in those children without a family history of ADHD is intriguing. This indicates that when family history is present, psychosocial adversity does not have much influence on this deleterious outcome. In contrast, when family history is absent, the presence of psychosocial adversity has a significant impact on learning disability.

Both cross-sectional and longitudinal studies have identified variables such as marital distress, family dysfunction, and low social class as risk factors for psychopathologic disorders and dysfunction in children.[7,38-45] The Ontario Child Health Study showed that family dysfunction and low income predicted persistence and onset of one or more psychiatric disorders over a 4-year follow-up period.[46] Barkley[47] identified parental psychopathology, low maternal education, low social class, and single parenthood as important adversity factors in ADHD.[48,49] He also reported that the mothers of adolescents with ADHD had more negative communication patterns, more conflict with their child, and a greater intensity of anger than did control mothers.[50]

Compared with prior work, the nature of our sample provides a different perspective on the impact of adversity on children. First, by stratifying the sample into ADHD and non-ADHD groups, we could assess the impact of adversity above and beyond what could be accounted for by ADHD. Second, none of the children in our study were living in frank poverty or other extremes of social disadvantage. Thus, our work shows that more modest levels of adversity have important implications for psychiatric and psychosocial outcome.

Our results must be interpreted in the context of methodologic limitations. The cross-sectional nature of our study limits our ability to infer causality from statistical associations. However, a cross-sectional design can provide useful initial information and generate hypotheses to be tested longitudinally. Also, we used the FES as a proxy for Rutter's indicator of "marital discord." Although there is likely to be much overlap between the FES and marital discord, the FES also taps into other aspects of family functioning involving nonspousal family members.

We also do not know if our findings will generalize to nonreferred children with ADHD in the community. Previous studies of the family environment have mostly studied either population or clinic samples *not* selected for specific disorders. Moreover, since subjects in the lowest SES group were excluded from the study, our findings may have resulted in an underestimation of the impact of SES.

A potential source of bias stems from the lack of direct interviews with children younger than 12 years, which may have underestimated psychopathologic conditions, especially for "internalizing" disorders such as anxiety and depression. However, we found high rates of both these disorders. Moreover, children younger than 12 years have limited expressive and receptive language abilities, the inability to map events in time, limited powers of abstraction, and limited vocabulary. Thus, there is a real question about whether the young child's self-perceptions, memories, feelings, and reported behavior can be assessed reliably through self-report, especially for lifetime history of psychopathologic disorders.[51,52] Although limited, studies on the use of interview techniques among children younger than 12 years show that their replies are unreliable.[53]

Despite these limitations, we identified important associations between adversity and ADHD, suggesting that Rutter's factors may index important environmental features for ADHD families. Since adversity factors had a positive association with impaired outcome in children, intervention efforts aimed at reducing adversity may be useful.

Accepted for publication March 13, 1995.

This work was supported in part by grants from the US Public Health Service and by National Institute of Mental Health Health grant RO1 MH-41314-01A2 (Dr Biederman).

Reprint requests to Pediatric Psychopharmacology Unit (ACC 725), Massachusetts General Hospital, Fruit Street, Boston, MA 02114 (Dr Biederman).

REFERENCES

1. Faraone S, Biederman J. Is attention deficit hyperactivity disorder familial? *Harvard Rev Psychiatry.* 1994;1:271-287.
2. Biederman J, Faraone SV, Keenan K, Knee D, Tsuang MT. Family-genetic and psychosocial risk factors in *DSM-III* attention deficit disorder. *J Am Acad Child Adolesc Psychiatry.* 1990;29:526-533.
3. Biederman J, Faraone SV, Keenan K, Benjamin J, Krifcher B, Moore C, Sprich S, Ugaglia K, Jellinek MS, Steingard R, Spencer T, Norman D, Kolodny R, Kraus I, Perrin J, Keller MB, Tsuang MT. Further evidence for family-genetic risk factors in attention deficit hyperactivity disorder: patterns of comorbidity in probands and relatives in psychiatrically and pediatrically referred samples. *Arch Gen Psychiatry.* 1992;49:728-738.
4. Faraone SV, Tsuang MT. Methods in psychiatric genetics. In: Tohen M, Tsuang MT, Zahner GEP, eds. *Textbook in Psychiatric Epidemiology.* New York, NY: John Wiley & Sons. In press.
5. Faraone SV, Santangelo S. Methods in genetic epidemiology. In: Fava M, Rosenbaum JF, eds. *Research Designs and Methods in Psychiatry.* Amsterdam, the Netherlands: Elsevier Publishers; 1992:93-118.
6. Faraone S, Biederman J. Genetics of attention-deficit hyperactivity disorder. *Child Adolesc Psychiatr Clin North Am.* 1994;3:285-302.
7. Mrazek P, Haggerty R. *Reducing Risks for Mental Disorders: Committee on Prevention of Mental Disorders.* Washington, DC: National Academy Press; 1994.
8. Rutter M, Cox A, Tupling C, Berger M, Yule W. Attainment and adjustment in two geographical areas, 1: the prevalence of psychiatric disorders. *Br J Psychiatry.* 1975;126:493-509.
9. Rutter M, Quinton D. Psychiatric disorder: ecological factors and concepts of causation. In: McGurk H, ed. *Ecological Factors in Human Development.* Amsterdam, the Netherlands: North-Holland Publishing Co; 1977:173-187.
10. Blantz B, Schmidt MH, Esser G. Familial adversities and child psychiatric disorders. *J Child Psychol Psychiatr Disord.* 1991;32:939-950.
11. Biederman J, Faraone SV, Lapey K. Comorbidity of diagnosis in attention deficit hyperactivity disorder (ADHD). *Child Adolesc Psychiatr Clin North Am.* 1992; 1:335-360.
12. Biederman J, Faraone SV, Spencer T, Wilens T, Norman D, Lapey K, Mick E, Krifcher Lehman B, Doyle A. Patterns of psychiatric comorbidity, cognition and psychosocial functioning in adults with attention deficit hyperactivity disorder. *Am J Psychiatry.* 1993;150:1792-1798.
13. Faraone S, Biederman J, Krifcher Lehman B, Keenan K, Norman D, Seidman L, Kolodny R, Kraus I, Perrin J, Chen W. Evidence for the independent familial transmission of attention deficit hyperactivity disorder and learning disabilities: results from a family genetic study. *Am J Psychiatry.* 1993;150:891-895.
14. Faraone SV, Biederman J, Krifcher Lehman B, Spencer T, Norman D, Seidman L, Kraus I, Perrin J, Chen W, Tsuang MT. Intellectual performance and school failure in children with attention deficit hyperactivity disorder and in their siblings. *J Abnorm Psychol.* 1993;102:616-623.
15. Biederman J, Faraone S, Chen W. Social adjustment inventory for children and adolescents: concurrent validity in ADHD children. *J Am Acad Child Adolesc Psychiatry.* 1993;32:1059-1064.
16. Faraone S, Biederman J, Chen WJ, Krifcher B, Keenan K, Moore C, Sprich S,

Tsuang M. Segregation analysis of attention deficit hyperactivity disorder: evidence for single gene transmission. *Psychiatr Genet.* 1992;2:257-275.

17. Faraone SV, Biederman J, Krifcher B, Keenan K, Moore C, Sprich S, Ugaglia K, Jellinek MS, Spencer T, Norman D, Seidman L, Kolodny R, Benjamin J, Kraus I, Perrin J, Chen W, Tsuang MT. Evidence for independent transmission in families for attention deficit hyperactivity disorder (ADHD) and learning disability: results from a family-genetic study of ADHD. *Am J Psychiatry.* 1992; 150:891-895.
18. Biederman J, Faraone SV, Doyle A, Krifcher Lehman B, Kraus I, Perrin J, Tsuang MT. Convergence of the Child Behavior Checklist with structured interview-based psychiatric diagnoses of ADHD children with and without hyperactivity. *J Child Psychol Psychiatry.* 1993;34:1241-1251.
19. Hollingshead A. *Four Factor Index of Social Status.* New Haven, Conn: Yale University Press; 1975.
20. American Psychiatric Association. *Diagnostic and Statistical Manual of Mental Disorders, Revised Third Edition.* Washington, DC: American Psychiatric Association; 1987.
21. Kendler KS. The super-normal control group in psychiatric genetics: possible artifactual evidence for coaggregation. *Psychiatr Genet.* 1990;1:45-53.
22. Meehl P, Rosen A. Antecedent probability and the efficiency of psychometric signs, patterns or cutting scores. *Psychol Bull.* 1955;52:194-216.
23. Gibbons RD, Davis JM, Hedeker DR. A comment on the selection of 'healthy controls' for psychiatric experiments. *Arch Gen Psychiatry.* 1990;47:785-786.
24. Kruesi MJP, Lenane MC, Hibbs ED, Major J. Normal controls and biological reference values in child psychiatry: defining normal. *J Am Acad Child Adolesc Psychiatry.* 1990;29:449-452.
25. Shtasel DL, Gur RE, Mozley D, Richards J, Taleff MM, Heimberg C, Gallacher F, Gur RC. Volunteers for biomedical research: recruitment and screening of normal controls. *Arch Gen Psychiatry.* 1991;48:1022-1025.
26. Orvaschel H, Puig-Antich J. *Schedule for Affective Disorder and Schizophrenia for School-age Children–Epidemiologic.* 4th Version. Fort Lauderdale, Fla: Nova University, Center for Psychological Study; 1987.
27. Spitzer RL, Williams JB, Gibbon M, First MB. *Structured Clinical Interview for* DSM-III-R, *Non-Patient Edition* (SCID-NP, Version 1.0). Washington, DC: American Psychiatric Press; 1990.
28. Gershon ES, Hamovit J, Guroff JJ, Dibble E, Leckman JF, Sceery W, Targum SD, Nurnberg JI Jr, Goldin LR, Bunney WE Jr. A family study of schizoaffective, bipolar I, bipolar II, unipolar, and normal control probands. *Arch Gen Psychiatry.* 1982;39:1157-1167.
29. Biederman J, Rosenbaum JF, Hirshfeld DR, Faraone SV, Bolduc EA, Gersten M, Meminger SR, Kagan J, Snidman N, Reznick JS. Psychiatric correlates of behavioral inhibition in young children of parents with and without psychiatric disorders. *Arch Gen Psychiatry.* 1990;47:21-26.
30. Jastak JF, Jastak S. *The Wide Range Achievement Test-Revised.* Wilmington, Del: Jastak Associates; 1985.
31. Gilmore JV, Gilmore EC. *Gilmore Oral Reading Test.* New York, NY: Harcourt Brace & World Inc; 1968.
32. Wechsler D. *Manual for the Wechsler Intelligence Scale for Children–Revised.* New York, NY: Psychological Corporation; 1974.
33. Wechsler D. *Manual for the Wechsler Adult Intelligence Scale–Revised.* San Antonio, Tex: Psychological Corporation; 1981.
34. Sattler JM. *Assessment of Children's Intelligence.* San Diego, Calif: Jerome M Sattler; 1988.
35. Moos RH, Moos BS. *Manual for the Family Environment Scale.* Palo Alto, Calif: Consulting Psychologists Press; 1974.
36. Office of Education. *Assistance to States for Education for Handicapped Children: Procedures for Evaluating Specific Learning Disabilities.* Bethesda, Md: US Dept of Health Education and Welfare; 1977.
37. Reynolds CR. Critical measurement issues in learning disabilities. *J Special Educ.* 1984;18:451-476.
38. Graham P, Rutter M. Psychiatric disorder in the young adolescent: a follow-up study. *Proc R Soc Med.* 1973;66:1226-1228.
39. Hetherington EM, Cox M, Cox R. Effects of divorce on parents and children. In: Lamb M, ed. *Non-Traditional Families.* Hillsdale, NJ: Lawrence Erlbaum Associates; 1982:223-285.
40. Rutter M, Giller H. *Juvenile Delinquency: Trends and Perspectives.* New York, NY: Penguin Books; 1983.
41. Achenbach TM, Howell CT, Quay HC, Conners CK. National survey of competencies and problems reported by parents for normative and clinical samples of 4- to 16-year-olds. *Monogr Soc Res Child Dev.* 1991;56:1-131.
42. Bird HR, Gould MS, Yager T, Staghezza B, Canino G. Risk factors for maladjustment in Puerto Rican children. *J Am Acad Child Adolesc Psychiatry.* 1989; 28:847-850.
43. Costello EJ. Child psychiatric disorders and their correlates: a primary care pediatric sample. *J Am Acad Child Adolesc Psychiatry.* 1989;28:851-855.
44. Offord DR, Boyle MH, Racine Y. Ontario Child Health Study: correlates of disorder. *J Am Acad Child Adolesc Psychiatry.* 1989;28:856-860.
45. Velez CN, Johnson J, Cohen P. A longitudinal analysis of selected risk factors for childhood psychopathology. *J Am Acad Child Adolesc Psychiatry.* 1989; 28:861-864.
46. Offord DR, Boyle MH, Racine YA, Fleming JE, Cadman DT, Blum HM, Byrne C, Links PS, Lipman EL, Macmillan HL. Outcome, prognosis and risk in a longitudinal follow-up study. *J Am Acad Child Adolesc Psychiatry.* 1992;31:916-923.
47. Barkley RA. *Attention Deficit Hyperactivity Disorder: A Handbook for Diagnosis and Treatment.* New York, NY: Guilford Press; 1990.
48. Palfrey JS, Levine MD, Walker DK, Sullivan M. The emergence of attention deficits in early childhood: a prospective study. *Dev Behav Pediatr.* 1985;6:339-348.
49. Nichols PL, Chen TC. *Minimal Brain Dysfunction: A Prospective Study.* Hillsdale, NJ: Lawrence Erlbaum Associates Inc; 1981.
50. Barkley RA, Anastopoulos AD, Guevremont DC, Fletcher KE. Adolescents with attention deficit hyperactivity disorder: mother-adolescent interactions, family beliefs and conflicts, and maternal psychopathology. *J Abnorm Child Psychol.* 1992;20:263-288.
51. Loeber R, Green SM, Lahey BB, Stouthamer-Loeber M. Differences and similarities between children, mothers, and teachers as informants on disruptive child behavior. *J Abnorm Child Psychol.* 1991;19:75-95.
52. Institute of Medicine. *Research on Children & Adolescents With Mental, Behavioral & Developmental Disorders.* Washington, DC: National Academy Press; 1989.
53. Achenbach TM, McConaughy SH, Howell CT. Child/adolescent behavioral and emotional problems: implications of cross-informant correlations for situational specificity. *Psychol Bull.* 1987;101:213-232.

ORIGINAL ARTICLE

In Vivo D_2 Dopamine Receptor Density in Psychotic and Nonpsychotic Patients With Bipolar Disorder

Godfrey D. Pearlson, MB,BS; Dean F. Wong, MD, PhD; Larry E. Tune, MD; Christopher A. Ross, MD, PhD; Gary A. Chase, PhD; Jonathan M. Links, PhD; Robert F. Dannals, PhD; Alan A. Wilson, PhD; Hayden T. Ravert, PhD; Henry N. Wagner, Jr, MD; J. Raymond DePaulo, MD

Background: A prior positron emission tomographic study from The Johns Hopkins University, Baltimore, Md, using *N*-methylspiperone labeled with carbon 11 reported elevated basal ganglia D_2 dopamine receptor density (B_{max}) values in neuroleptic-naive schizophrenic patients compared with controls. We have now extended these studies to include patients with bipolar disorder.

Methods: Patients with bipolar disorder (n=14) either had never received neuroleptic medication or had been neuroleptic-free for more than 6 months, and they met *DSM-III* criteria for currently symptomatic affective disorder. Patients with bipolar disorder were compared with matched schizophrenic patients and normal controls. All received two positron emission tomographic scans, the second of which was preceded by oral administration of haloperidol lactate, to permit the calculation of D_2 dopamine receptor B_{max}.

Results: Diagnostic groups differed in B_{max} by analysis of variance ($P<.0001$); post hoc tests showed higher B_{max} values for psychotic patients with bipolar disorder and schizophrenic patients compared with normal controls and for schizophrenic patients and psychotic patients with bipolar disorder compared with nonpsychotic patients with bipolar disorder. Among patients with bipolar disorder, B_{max} values correlated significantly with the severity of psychotic symptoms (r=.63) on the Present State Examination but not with the severity of nonpsychotic mood symptoms.

Conclusions: We conclude that, like schizoprenic patients, patients with psychotic bipolar disorder have elevations of D_2 dopamine receptor B_{max} values and that such elevations in affective disorder are more closely associated with the presence of psychosis than with mood abnormality. Elevations in dopamine receptor values thus may occur in psychiatric states that are characterized by psychotic symptoms rather than being specific to schizophrenia.

(Arch Gen Psychiatry. 1995;52:471-477)

From the Departments of Psychiatry and Behavioral Sciences (Drs Pearlson, Tune, Ross, Chase, and DePaulo), Mental Hygiene (Drs Pearlson and Chase), Psychiatric Neuro-Imaging (Dr Pearlson), Radiology (Drs Wong, Links, Dannals, Wilson, Ravert, and Wagner), and Neuroscience (Dr Ross), The Johns Hopkins University, Baltimore, Md. Dr Tune is currently affiliated with Wesley Woods Geriatric Hospital, Emory University, Atlanta, Ga.

THE PROPOSAL that the clinical symptoms of schizophrenia could be related to the dysfunctional activity of central dopaminergic systems has been termed the *dopamine hypothesis of schizophrenia*. Evidence for this view has been summarized elsewhere.[1] Despite some reasonable evidence for the hypothesis,[2,3] it is not immune from criticism,[4,5] and lacking conclusive confirmation or refutation, it remains controversial. However, the question of the specificity of such dopaminergic disturbances to schizophrenia has received less attention. Cardinal symptoms of schizophrenia are hallucinations, delusions, and thought disorder, but these, including schneiderian first-rank symptoms, are also not uncommon in mania and can occur in depression.[6,7]

There are several reasons for postulating that disturbances in the dopaminergic system might be associated with symptoms of affective illness as well. These are summarized in several reviews.[8-10] First is the effectiveness of neuroleptic medications (D_2 dopamine [DA] receptor competitive antagonists) in treating mania as well as schizophrenia.[11] Many of Delay and Deniker's[12] original chlorpromazine hydrochloride responders were manic. Neuroleptic drugs of equivalent potencies appear to provide similarly effective symptomatic relief in mania and schizophrenia and are related to DA antagonist activity.[13] In a brief report,[14] it was suggested that only the D_2 DA receptor–blocking isomer of the neuroleptic medication clopenthixol has an antimanic

See Subjects and Methods on next page

SUBJECTS AND METHODS

SUBJECTS

Index subjects with bipolar disorder (n=14) met *DSM-III*[28] criteria for bipolar affective disorder and were currently manic (n=11) or depressed (n=3). Mean±SD length of the current episode was 5.4±7.8 months (range, 0.5 to 24 months). Successive patients from The Johns Hopkins Hospital psychiatric emergency department or inpatient units who met the study criteria were approached for inclusion. The majority of subjects were neuroleptic naive (n=11). Three subjects who were neuroleptic free had received neuroleptic treatment 6 months or more before the study (mean latency, 16 months). Treatment (including a detailed drug) history was obtained from the patient, at least one family member, and the previous psychiatrist or other treating physicians if applicable. Index patients were excluded if they had a history of electroconvulsive therapy, head injury leading to unconsciousness for longer than 1 hour, weight loss greater than 25% of body weight in the past 6 months, amphetamine or cocaine use in the past year, seizure disorder, dementia or other central nervous system disease, mental retardation, current oral use of steroids, or current alcohol or other drug abuse. Plasma screening using a radioreceptor assay[29] that was sensitive to any D_2 DA receptor–blocking agent was used to detect the presence of neuroleptic medication in the plasma of index patients, and the results were negative. In addition, index patients who had ever met criteria for schizophrenia, schizoaffective disorder, paranoid disorder, or any major mental illness other than affective disorder were excluded. Patients with rapid cycling or mixed affective states were also excluded. All subjects gave written informed consent to the protocol, which was approved by The Johns Hopkins Joint Committee on Clinical Investigation.

Index subjects were interviewed by a research psychiatrist (G.D.P. or C.A.R.) within 24 hours of the first PET scan. Subsequent to the scans, patients received outpatient follow-up either directly (by C.A.R. or G.D.P.) or by our maintaining regular contact with the patient's treating physician; in no case has the original diagnosis been changed.

The rating scales that were administered included the Montgomery and Asberg Depression Rating Scale,[30] the Hamilton Depression Rating Scale,[31] the Ross-Peyser-DePaulo Affective Symptom Rating Scale (C.A.R., C. E. Peyser, MD, J.R.D., unpublished data, 1986), the Young Mania Rating Scale,[32] the Blackburn Mania Rating Scale,[33] the Present State Examination (PSE),[34] including all items assessing psychotic symptoms (described by Tune et al[29]), the Montgomery and Asberg Psychopathology Rating Scale,[35] which assesses psychotic symptoms, and the Mini-Mental Status Examination.[36]

Patient characteristics are shown in **Table 1**. Six of the 11 manic patients and one of the three depressed patients (total, n=7) had psychotic symptoms (hallucinations, delusions, or thought disorder) on the PSE (PSE psychotic items, 28) at the time of PET scanning. All delusions and/or hallucinations were mood congruent. Patients classified as nonpsychotic had none of these symptoms and, according to chart review, had not had them in any prior affective episode.

Two comparison groups were used. Because of the decline in striatum-to-cerebellum ratios with N-methylspiperone (NMSP) administration that is associated with normal aging,[37] both groups were group age matched to index patients. The first comparison group consisted of 10 neuroleptic-naive patients with schizophrenia who consecutively underwent PET scanning and were described in earlier reports from the JHU group.[1,26] The second comparison sample consisted of 12 screened normal controls who were recruited by advertisements and word-of-mouth from the staff of The Johns Hopkins Hospital and the surrounding community. None had psychotic symptoms as defined by the PSE. Many were included in the

action. Drugs that inhibit DA synthesis may also reduce the severity of manic symptoms.[15] The Northwick Park "functional" psychosis study[16] showed that in a sample composed of both schizophrenic and affectively ill patients, the neuroleptic medication pimozide reduced psychotic symptoms (hallucinations, delusions, thought disorder, and affective incongruity) regardless of whether mood was elevated, depressed, or unchanged. The study concluded that "dopamine blockade seems relevant to the resolution of psychotic symptoms in all types of 'functional' psychosis."[16]

Second, mania, or symptomatic states resembling it, can be provoked by stimulant drugs that increase the amount of available DA.[17,18] Amphetamine-induced psychosis can resemble mania as well as schizophrenia.[2,4] Characteristic symptoms produced by prolonged administration or high doses of psychostimulants may include sleeplessness, euphoria, psychomotor activation, irritability, grandiosity, overtalkativeness, and hypersexuality, all of which occur more commonly in mania than in schizophrenia. Such amphetamine-induced euphoria is reduced by treatment with the neuroleptic medication pimozide.[19]

Evidence for a role of DA in depression also exists. Depression frequently accompanies Parkinson's disease.[20] Levodopa has modest antidepressant effects.[9,21] Bromocriptine mesylate and other DA agonists have some antidepressant effects in patients with bipolar disorder.[22] Depressed patients with psychosis are much less likely than depressed individuals without psychosis to respond to tricyclic antidepressant treatment alone. Such patients usually require additional treatment with neuroleptic drugs.[23]

Whereas numerous postmortem studies have investigated the role of D_2 DA receptors in schizophrenia,[3-5,24] few or none has examined D_2 receptors in autopsy specimens from patients with bipolar disorder. In general, there is a dearth of neuropathologic studies of affective disorder.[25] More recently, positron emission tomography (PET) has allowed the study of the DA system in the living human brain, including assessment of the caudate and putamen densities (B_{max}) of the D_2 DA receptor in earlier article,[26] and the remainder were added to ensure age and gender comparability between groups.

PET PROCEDURES

Each subject underwent a PET scan procedure as previously described.[26] This basically consisted of a localizing computed tomographic scan, a molded face mask, and PET imaging planes designed to pass through the maximum area of the caudate nucleus, the cerebellar cortex, and the frontal cortical regions. Each subject underwent two PET scans at high specific activity (approximately 7.4×10^{13} Bq/mmol) at the time of injection, with one study being preceded by the oral administration of haloperidol lactate to allow a calculation of B_{max} as per the previously published model.[38,39] Except for the 7.5 mg of orally administered haloperidol lactate, the subjects received no neuroleptic medication. Multiple PET images and blood sampling were obtained using the previously published methods.[38,39] Several patients received intramuscular injections of 50 mg of diphenhydramine hydrochloride (Benadryl) for akathisia or other extrapyramidal symptoms caused by the single oral dose of haloperidol. The B_{max} values in patients who did not receive diphenhydramine were not different from those who did (see the "Results" section). Five blood samples per subject were drawn for the measurement of haloperidol levels using gas chromatography (National Psychopharmacology Laboratories, Nashville, Tenn).

PET MODELING

The PET analysis was performed by investigators who were blind to diagnosis. Regions of interest were drawn bilaterally around the head of the caudate and cerebellum (as described previously[39]). Binding of NMSP to caudate receptors was described by a four-compartment model with four rate constants.[38,39] This model assumed irreversible binding (k_4=0) during the period of the scan.

Procedures carried out in this study differed from previously published methods[26,38,39] only in that many of the subjects underwent additional measurements during the PET scan procedure, including high-pressure liquid chromatographic measurement of levels of NMSP metabolites labeled with carbon 11 and ^{11}C-NMSP plasma protein binding. The calculations for B_{max}, however, are consistent with those of Wong et al,[38] so that the measurements of B_{max} in those drug-naive and drug-free schizophrenic patients and controls are comparable to this data set. The details of validation experiments relating to assumptions in this model and a summary of the theoretical aspects of the technique are described elsewhere (D.F.W., G.D.P., L.E.T., T. Young, MD, D. Young, PhD, C. Cidis-Meltzer, MD, A.A.W., B. Chan, MS, R.F.D., H.T.R., M. J. Kuhar, PhD, A. Gjedde, MD, PhD, unpublished data, 1990).

The B_{max} calculation was determined from the forward rate binding constant (k_3) to the D_2 DA receptor in both the unblocked case and the blocked (prior administration of haloperidol) case using the above quantitative model, an assumed blood-brain partition coefficient for haloperidol, and the k_{off} for haloperidol. The underlying assumptions of this method are detailed elsewhere (D.F.W., G.D.P., L.E.T., T. Young, MD, D. Young, PhD, C. Cidis-Meltzer, MD, A.A.W., B. Chan, MS, R.F.D., H.T.R., M. J. Kuhar, PhD, A. Gjedde, MD, PhD, unpublished data, 1990).

STATISTICAL ANALYSIS

We hypothesized that the B_{max} of D_2 DA receptors would be elevated in psychotic patients with bipolar disorder and that the severity of their psychotic symptoms (measured using the appropriate PSE subscale) would correlate with the magnitude of B_{max}. Data were analyzed using the χ^2 test, analysis of variance, and Pearson product-moment correlation coefficients. Post hoc testing was carried out using Fisher's least-significant difference post hoc test. A Kruskal-Wallis analysis of variance was also employed.

Table 1. Descriptive Characteristics and B_{max} Values of Patients With Bipolar Disorder

Patient No./ Sex/Age, y	Race	Current Episode*	Psychotic†	Neuroleptic Free vs Naive‡	B_{max},§ pmol/g
1/M/50	B	M	+	N	48.2
2/M/20	B	M	+	N	45.0
3/M/44	W	M	+	F	27.0
4/F/52	B	M	+	N	23.5
5/F/31	B	D	+	N	25.0
6/F/25	B	M	+	N	38.0
7/M/54	W	M	+	N	12.0
8/M/52	W	M	−	F	11.0
9/F/44	W	M	−	N	5.0
10/M/29	W	M	−	F	23.8
11/F/39	W	M	−	N	24.0
12/M/22	B	M	−	N	11.8
13/M/39	W	D	−	N	13.6
14/M/62	W	D	−	N	14.4

*M indicates manic; D, depressed.
†Plus sign indicates psychotic; minus sign, nonpsychotic.
‡Neuroleptic-free (F) patients had been drug free for at least 6 months. N indicates neuroleptic naive.
§B_{max} refers to measured receptor density of D_2-like dopamine receptors as assessed using carbon 11–labeled N-methylspiperone.

Table 2. Psychiatric Symptom Ratings in Patients With Bipolar Disorder at the Time of Positron Emission Tomographic Scan*

Patient No.†	Mini-PSE	MAPRS	Young	Blackburn	MADRS	Ross	HDRS
1	22	13	25	53	11	57	12
2	30	3	16	30	0	96	0
3	10	6	11	41	0	56	2
4	11	6	14	26	13	40	5
5	24	17	13	18	29	56	15
6	19	6	37	66	9	77	8
7	7	4	59	120	8	103	7
8	0	0	26	51	13	75	11
9	0	2	19	34	19	28	14
10	0	0	14	18	0	38	0
11	0	0	9	12	1	20	3
12	0	0	5	8	0	19	0
13	0	1	0	0	11	18	8
14	0	6	0	4	30	46	16

**Mini-PSE*[29] *is a subscale of the Present State Examination*[34] *measuring psychotic symptoms; MAPRS, Montgomery and Asberg Psychopathology Rating Scale*[35]*; Young, Young Mania Rating Scale*[32]*; Blackburn, Blackburn Mania Rating Scale*[33]*; MADRS, Montgomery and Asberg Depression Rating Scale*[30]*; Ross, Ross-Peyser-DePaulo Affective Symptom Rating Scale; and HDRS, Hamilton Depression Rating Scale.*[31]

†*Patient numbers correspond to those of Table 1. Patients 1 through 7 were psychotic at the time of scanning; patients 8 through 14 were nonpsychotic.*

Table 3. Descriptive Data for the Bipolar Disorder and Comparison Groups*

Group	No. of Patients	Age†, y	Years of Education‡	Socioeconomic Status§	Male,‖ %
Schizophrenic patients	10	31.1±11.4	12.0±3.2	3.1±1.0	60.0
Psychotic patients with bipolar disorder	7	39.4±13.9	11.9±2.0	3.6±0.5	57.1
Nonpsychotic patients with bipolar disorder	7	41.0±13.4	13.2±2.0	2.4±1.1	71.4
Controls	12	28.0±12.6	14.5±3.1	2.3±1.0	75.0

**Values are means±SDs.*
†*Between-group analysis of variance (ANOVA): df=3, 32; F=2.2; P was not significant.*
‡*Between-group ANOVA: df=3, 32; F=3.2; P<.05. Scheffé post hoc test: no significant between-group differences.*
§*Using Hollingshead classification. Between-group ANOVA: df=3, 32; F=3.4; P<.05. Scheffé post hoc test: psychotic patients with bipolar disorder vs controls, P<.05.*
‖χ^2*=0.9; df=3; P was not significant.*

neuroleptic-naive schizophrenic patients, as previously reported by The Johns Hopkins University (JHU) (Baltimore, Md) group.[1,26] Other groups, using a different ligand, did not replicate these results.[27] It recently has been suggested that these differences may reflect differential affinity of these two ligands for D_4 receptors, which are pharmacologically similar to D_2 receptors.[24] The current study applied methods that were similar to those used in previous JHU studies of schizophrenic patients[1,26] to symptomatic patients with bipolar disorder. We studied whether currently symptomatic patients with bipolar disorder had increased densities of D_2 DA receptors and whether such receptor density increases correlated with the severity of mood symptoms or the presence or severity of psychotic symptoms.

RESULTS

Characteristics of individual patients with bipolar disorder are shown in Table 1, and their psychiatric symptom ratings, in **Table 2**. As noted elsewhere,[40] within the normal control group, a statistically significant inverse relationship was established between the B_{max} of D_2 DA receptors and age. Demographic characteristics of all subject groups are illustrated in **Table 3**. A between-group analysis of variance for age showed no significant effect of age.

As shown in **Table 4** and the **Figure**, B_{max} values for D_2 DA receptors were similar in the seven psychotic patients with bipolar disorder and in the 10 schizophrenic patients, both of which were significantly greater than in the nonpsychotic group with bipolar disorder and the normal control group, which in turn were similar to each other. A between-group analysis of variance for B_{max} is shown in Table 4. Using the Fisher's least-significant difference post hoc test, the following B_{max} comparisons were significant at a level of $P<.05$: schizophrenic patients vs controls, schizophrenic patients vs nonpsychotic patients with bipolar disorder, psychotic patients with bipolar disorder vs nonpsychotic patients with bipolar disorder, and psychotic patients with bipolar disorder vs controls. A Kruskal-Wallis analysis of variance was used to further examine B_{max} by both psychosis and age group; for the latter, a median split was used. As predicted, there was a main effect of psychosis (df=1, H=10.1, $P<.01$) but no main effect of age group (df=1, H=2.2, P

Table 4. Values for Between-Group Analyses of Variance for D_2 Dopamine Receptor B_{max} and Age in the Bipolar Disorder and Comparison Groups*

Group	No. of Patients	B_{max},† pmol/g	Age, y
Schizophrenic patients	10	41.6±14.5	31.1±11.4
Psychotic patients with bipolar disorder	7	31.2±12.9	39.4±13.9
Nonpsychotic patients with bipolar disorder	7	14.8±6.9	41.0±13.4
Controls	12	16.7±9.8	28.0±12.6

*Values are means±SDs.

†See Table 1 for explanation of B_{max}. Between-group analysis of variance for B_{max}: df=3, 34; F=11.4; P=.0001. Fisher's least significant difference post hoc test: schizophrenic patients vs controls, 10.1, P<.05; schizophrenic patients vs nonpsychotic patients with bipolar disorder, 11.6, P<.05; psychotic patients with bipolar disorder vs nonpsychotic patients with bipolar disorder, 12.6, P≤.05; and psychotic patients with bipolar disorder vs controls, 11.1, P<.05. Schizophrenic patients vs psychotic patients with bipolar disorder and nonpsychotic patients with bipolar disorder vs controls both were not significant.

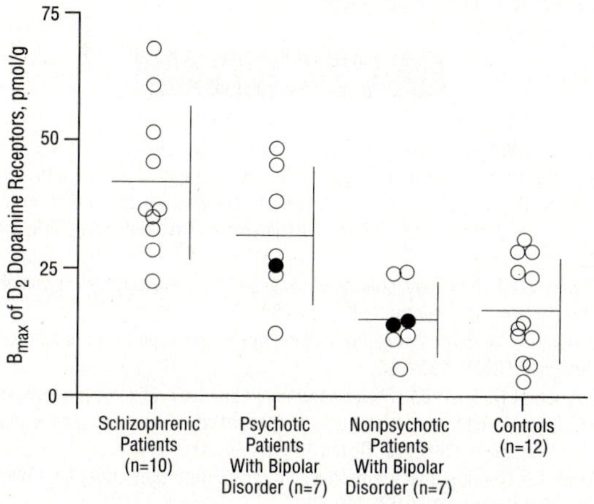

Scatterplot of caudate and putamen D_2 dopamine receptor density (B_{max}) values in schizophrenic patients, psychotic patients with bipolar disorder, nonpsychotic patients with bipolar disorder, and normal controls. For patients with bipolar disorder, open circles indicate manic patients and solid circles indicate depressed patients.

was not significant [NS]) and no interaction between diagnosis and age-group (*df*=1, H=0, *P* was NS). A correlation analysis examining the duration of illness (months since onset of current episode) in the patients with bipolar disorder revealed no relationship either to B_{max} (*r*=.20, *P* was NS) or to symptom severity on any clinical rating scale (*r*s, 0.04 to 0.23; all *P*s were NS).

Correlations between B_{max}, mood, and cognitive (Mini-Mental Status Examination) rating scales are shown in **Table 5**. Because 11 of the 14 patients with bipolar disorder were suffering from mania and thus were clinically homogeneous, values are shown for manic patients only. Significant correlations existed between B_{max} and the score for psychotic (but not nonpsychotic) items on the PSE. Correlation (*r*) between psychotic symptom severity and B_{max} was .78 (*P*<.05), with a similar trend (*r*=.65, *P*<.10) seen for the Montgomery and Asberg Psychopathology Rating Scale score. The same analysis was

Table 5. Correlations Between B_{max}, Mood, and Cognitive Rating Scales in the 11 Manic Patients*

Measure	*r*
PSE psychotic score[29]	.78†
PSE nonpsychotic score[34]	.20
Blackburn Mania Rating Scale score[33]	.03
Young Mania Rating Scale score[32]	.05
Ross-Peyser-DePaulo Affective Symptom Rating Scale score	.32
Montgomery and Asberg Psychopathology Rating Scale score[35]	.65
Mini-Mental Status Examination score[36]	−.28

*For the six psychotic patients with mania only, correlation between B_{max} and psychotic score on the Present State Examination (PSE) was r=.92; P<.001. See Table 1 for an explanation of B_{max}.

†P<.05.

repeated for the six psychotic patients with mania only, to avoid overly expanding the range of analysis because nonpsychotic patients scored 0's on the PSE psychotic subscale; the relationship remained significant (*r*=.92, *P*<.001).

With respect to the question of diphenhydramine administration, this drug was given to three subjects in the nonpsychotic group and three subjects in the psychotic group, all during the post–haloperidol administration PET scan. The mean±SD B_{max} values in the nonpsychotic group for those receiving and not receiving diphenhydramine were 16.7±6.3 (n=3) and 13.4±8.2 (n=4), respectively. For the psychotic patients with bipolar disorder, mean±SD B_{max} values for those receiving and not receiving diphenhydramine were 31.0±17.2 (n=3) and 31.5±11.2 (n=4), respectively.

COMMENT

The current study suggests an increased density (B_{max}) of D_2-like DA receptors in the caudate of patients who have bipolar disorder and psychotic symptoms compared with both normal controls and nonpsychotic patients who have bipolar disorder. Psychotic patients with bipolar disorder had elevations of D_2 DA B_{max} values that were comparable to those of similarly aged schizophrenic patients. Elevation of B_{max} in affective disorder correlated with the presence and the severity of psychosis but was unrelated to mood abnormality. Given the ongoing debate over quantitative PET measurements of DA receptors[26,27] and the emerging complexity of the D_2 DA receptor family,[24] we can conclude only that B_{max} measured by NMSP binding is a reflection of the density of D_2 or D_2-like DA receptor sites.

Although the number of subjects with affective disorder was not extensive, B_{max} findings were significant. Our report of increased receptor B_{max} in psychotic patients with bipolar disorder is not an artifact of prior neuroleptic treatment (which can elevate D_2 DA receptor B_{max}) because the majority of our patients were neuroleptic naive. Subjects were screened in such a way that we can be fairly confident in this assertion. Because most subjects are followed up clinically by the investigators, we are also confident about diagnoses. However, given the small sample size and subject heterogeneity of socioeconomic status and education, it will be important to study other patient populations to determine whether the results are generalizable. Analysis of PET data was done with the investigator blind to clinical symptomatic status (and vice versa). Although age matching was not ideal, no significant between-group differences on age existed.

We were concerned that diphenhydramine administration to subjects who experienced extrapyramidal side effects might have influenced B_{max} values. However, there was a balance in the number of patients who received short-term administration of diphenhydramine to counteract extrapyramidal side effects between the psychotic and the nonpsychotic group; furthermore, there was no significant difference in B_{max} between those subjects who received and those who did not receive diphenhydramine within both the nonpsychotic and the psychotic groups. It is our conclusion that administration of diphenhydramine had no obvious influence on our results. As expected, education and social class were not identical among the groups. Although it is conceivable that B_{max} measured via NMSP binding could be influenced by these variables, it is unlikely that such an effect would entirely explain our findings.

It is unlikely that primary changes in the DA system alone underlie the pathophysiologic processes of bipolar disorder. For instance, there exists convincing evidence for interactions between DA and other neurotransmitter systems whose involvement in the pathophysiologic processes of affective disorders has been hypothesized,[41,42] including serotonin-DA interactions in the nigrostriatal system and elsewhere.[43,44] It is possible that in affective disorders, primary abnormalities in the noradrenergic or serotonergic systems can lead to secondary changes in the DA system in some patients, which in turn are associated with psychotic symptoms.

The caudate nucleus and putamen are among the areas with the highest concentrations of D_2 DA receptors in the brain.[3] Autoradiographic studies with labeled 2-deoxy-D-glucose find a dose-related increase in the glucose metabolic rate of the caudate after administration of the DA agonists apomorphine hydrochloride and dextroamphetamine.[45,46] Both psychotic and affective symptoms are not uncommonly seen in diseases affecting the basal ganglia, such as Huntington's chorea.[47] Evidence exists from glucose metabolic PET studies for caudate involvement in affective and schizophrenic disorders.[48-50] A recently published single-photon emission computed tomographic study[51] offers partial support for the hypothesis of increased D_2 DA receptors in depression, although the issue of psychosis was not specifically addressed.

Abnormalities of brain DA systems may not be specific to schizophrenia but may be present in other forms of major mental illness with psychosis. In this sense, our findings are congruent with those of Johnstone et al[16] in being compatible with a DA theory of psychosis rather than a more narrow DA theory of schizophrenia. In our restatement of this hypothesis, a functional increase in levels of DA (either of the transmitter itself, the density of D_2 or the more recently described and pharmacologically D_2-like D_4 DA receptors,[24] or the sensitivity of those receptors) occurs in states characterized by hallucinations, delusions, or thought disorder across all types of functional psychosis.

Accepted for publication March 2, 1995.

This project was supported in part by grants MH40391 and MH43775 (Dr Pearlson) and MH42821 (Dr Wong) from the National Institute of Mental Health, grant DA05317 from the National Institute on Drug Abuse (Dr Pearlson), grant RR-00722 from the National Institutes of Health Division of Research Resources and The Johns Hopkins Outpatient Clinical Research Center (Dr Pearlson), National Institutes of Health Inpatient General Clinical Research Center Grant RR00035 (Dr Pearlson), grant P01 HD24061 from the Neuroimaging Core/Mental Retardation Research Center (Dr Wong), grant P01 HD23042 from the National Institute of Child Health and Development (Dr Wong), Bethesda, Md; and a Pew Scholarship in the Biomedical Sciences from Pew Charitable Trust, Los Angeles, Calif (Dr Ross).

Reprint requests to Division of Psychiatric Neuro-Imaging, Department of Psychiatry, The Johns Hopkins Hospital, 600 N Wolfe St, Meyer 3-166, Baltimore, MD 21287-7362 (Dr Pearlson).

REFERENCES

1. Tune LE, Wong DF, Pearlson GD, Strauss ME, Young T, Shaya EK, Dannals RF, Wilson AA, Ravert HT, Sapp J, Cooper T, Chase GA, Wagner HN Jr. Dopamine D_2 receptor density estimates in schizophrenia: a positron emission tomography study with ^{11}C-methylspiperone. *Psychiatry Res.* 1993;49:219-237.
2. McKenna PJ. Pathology, phenomenology and the dopamine hypothesis of schizophrenia. *Br J Psychiatry.* 1987;151:288-301.
3. Seeman P. Dopamine receptors in the dopamine hypothesis of schizophrenia. *Synapse.* 1987;1:133-152.
4. Pearlson GD, Coyle JT. The dopamine hypothesis and schizophrenia. In: Coyle JT, Enna S, eds. *Neuroleptics: Neurochemical, Behavioral and Clinical Perspectives.* New York, NY: Raven Press; 1983;3:297-324.
5. Crow TJ. The dopamine hypothesis survives, but there must be a way ahead. *Br J Psychiatry.* 1987;151:460-465.
6. Pope HG, Lipinski JF. Diagnosis and schizophrenia in manic-depressive illness: a reassessment of the specificity of 'schizophrenic' symptoms in the light of current research. *Arch Gen Psychiatry.* 1978;35:811-827.
7. Brockington IF, Wainwright S, Kendell RE. Manic patients with schizophrenic or paranoid symptoms. *Psychol Med.* 1980;10:73-83.
8. Silverstone T. Dopamine in manic depressive illness: a pharmacological synthesis. *J Affect Disord.* 1985;8:225-231.
9. Jimerson DC. Role of dopamine mechanisms in the affective disorders. In: Meltzer H, ed. *Psychopharmacology: The Third Generation of Progress.* New York, NY: Raven Press; 1987:505-511.
10. Miller R. Major psychosis and dopamine: controversial features and some suggestions. *Psychol Med.* 1984;14:779-789.
11. Cookson J, Silverstone T, Wells B. A double-blind comparative clinical trial of pimozide and chlorpromazine in mania: a test of the dopamine hypothesis. *Acta Psychiatr Scand.* 1981;64:381-397.
12. Delay J, Deniker P. Le traitement des psychoses par une méthode neurolytique derivee de l'hibernothérapie. In: Ossa PC, ed. Congrès de Mèdecins Aliénist et Neurologistes de France. Luxembourg et Paris, France: Maisson Editeurs Libraires et l'Académie de Mèdicine. 1952:497-502.
13. Wyatt RJ, Torgow JS. A comparison of equivalent clinical potencies of neuroleptics as used to treat schizophrenia and affective disorders. *J Psychiatr Res.* 1976;13:91-98.
14. Nolen WA. Dopamine and mania: the effects of trans- and cis-clopenthixol in a double-blind pilot study. *J Affect Disord.* 1983;5:91-96.
15. Sack RL, Goodwin FK. Inhibition of dopamine-hydroxylase in manic patients. *Arch Gen Psychiatry.* 1974;31:649-654.
16. Johnstone EC, Crow TJ, Frith CD, Owens DGC. The Northwick Park 'functional' psychosis study: diagnosis and treatment response. *Lancet.* 1988;2:119-125.

17. Carlsson A. Amphetamine and brain catecholamines. In: Costa E, Garattini S, eds. *Amphetamine and Related Compounds.* New York, NY: Raven Press; 1970: 389-400.
18. Van Kammen DP, Murphy DL. Attenuation of the euphoriant and activating effects of d-1-amphetamine by lithium carbonate treatment. *Psychopharmacology.* 1975;44:212-224.
19. Silverstone T, Fincham J, Wells B, Kryiakedes M. The effect of the dopamine receptor blocker pimozide on the stimulant and anorectic actions of dextroamphetamine. *Neuropharmacology.* 1980;19:1235-1237.
20. Swerdlow NR, Koob GF. Dopamine, schizophrenia, mania, and depression: toward a unified hypothesis of cortico-striato-pallido-thalamic function. *Behav Brain Sci.* 1987;10:197-245.
21. Butcher LL, Engel J. Behavioral and biochemical effects of L-dopa after peripheral decarboxylase inhibition. *Brain Res.* 1969;15:233-241.
22. Silverstone T. Response to bromocriptine distinguishes bipolar from unipolar depression. *Lancet.* 1984;1:903-904.
23. Chan CH, Janicak PG, Davis JM, Altman E, Andriukaitis S, Hedeker D. Response of psychotic and non-psychotic depressed patients to tricyclic antidepressants. *J Clin Psychiatry.* 1987;48:197-200.
24. Seeman P, Hong-Chang G, Van Tol HHM. Dopamine D_4 receptors elevated in schizophrenia. *Nature.* 1993;365:441-445.
25. Jeste DV, Lohr JB, Goodwin FK. Neuroanatomical studies of major affective disorders: a review and suggestions for further research. *Br J Psychiatry.* 1988; 153:444-459.
26. Wong DF, Wagner HN, Tune LE, Dannals RF, Pearlson GD, Links JM, Tamminga CA, Broussole EP, Ravert HT, Wilson AA, Tong TJK, Malat J, Williams JA, O'Tuama LA, Snyder SH, Kuhar MJ, Gjedde A. Positron emission tomography reveals elevated D_2 dopamine receptors in drug-naive schizophrenics. *Science.* 1986;234:1158-1563.
27. Farde L, Wiesel F-A, Hall H, Halldin C, Stone-Elander S, Sedvall G. No D_2 receptor increase in PET study of schizophrenia. *Arch Gen Psychiatry.* 1987;44: 671-672.
28. American Psychiatric Association. *Diagnostic and Statistical Manual of Mental Disorders, Third Edition.* Washington, DC: American Psychiatric Association; 1980.
29. Tune LE, Creese I, Coyle JT, Pearlson G, Snyder SH. Low neuroleptic serum levels in patients receiving fluphenazine decanoate. *Am J Psychiatry.* 1980; 137-1:80-82.
30. Montgomery SA, Asberg M. A new depression scale designed to be sensitive to change. *Br J Psychiatry.* 1979;134:382-389.
31. Hamilton M. A rating scale for depression. *J Neurol Neurosurg Psychiatry.* 1967;23:56-62.
32. Young RC, Biggs T, Ziegler VE, Meyer DA. A rating scale for mania: reliability, validity and sensitivity. *Br J Psychiatry.* 1978;133:429-435.
33. Blackburn IM, Loudon JB, Ashworth CM. A new scale for measuring mania. *Psychol Med.* 1977;7:453-458.
34. Wing JK, Cooper JE, Sartorius N. *The Measurement and Classification of Psychiatric Symptoms.* Cambridge, England: Cambridge University Press; 1974.
35. Montgomery SA, Taylor P, Montgomery D. Development of a schizophrenia scale sensitive to change. *Neuropharmacology.* 1978;17:1061-1063.
36. Folstein MF, Folstein SE, McHugh PR. Mini-Mental State: a practical method of grading the cognitive state of patients for the clinician. *J Psychiatry Res.* 1975;12:189-198.
37. Wong DF, Wagner HN Jr, Dannals RF, Links JM, Frost JJ, Ravert HT, Wilson AA, Rosenbaum AE, Folstein MF, Petronis JD, Douglas KH, Toung JKT, Kuhar MJ. Effects of age on dopamine and serotonin receptors measured by positron tomography in the living human brain. *Science.* 1984;226:1393-1396.
38. Wong DF, Gjedde A, Wagner HN Jr. Quantification of neuro-receptors in the living human brain, I: association rate of irreversibly bound ligands. *J Cereb Blood Flow Metab.* 1986;6:137-146.
39. Wong DF, Gjedde A, Wagner HN Jr, Dannals RF, Douglass KH, Links JM, Kuhar MJ. Quantification of neuroreceptors in the living human brain, II: assessment of receptor density and affinity using inhibition studies. *J Cereb Blood Flow Metab.* 1986;6:147-153.
40. Wong DF, Pearlson GD, Young LT, Singer H, Villemagne V, Tune L, Ross C, Dannals RF, Links JM, Chan B, Wilson AA, Ravert HT, Wagner HN Jr, Gjedde A. D_2 dopamine receptors are elevated in neuropsychiatric disorders other than schizophrenia. *J Cereb Blood Flow Metab.* 1989;9(suppl):S593.
41. Meltzer HY, Lowy MT. The serotonin hypothesis of depression. In: Meltzer H, ed. *Psychopharmacology: The Third Generation of Progress.* New York, NY: Raven Press; 1987:513-526.
42. Siever LJ. Role of noradrenergic mechanisms in the etiology of the affective disorders. In: Meltzer H, ed: *Psychopharmacology: The Third Generation of Progress.* New York, NY: Raven Press; 1987:493-504.
43. Waldmeier PC, Delini-Stula AA. Serotonin-dopamine interactions in the nigrostriatal system. *Eur J Pharmacol.* 1979;55:363-373.
44. Linnoila M, Oliver J, Adinoff B, Potter WZ. High correlations of norepinephrine, dopamine, and epinephrine and their major metabolite excretion rates. *Arch Gen Psychiatry.* 1988;45:710-714.
45. McCulloch J, Savaki HE, McCulloch MC, Jehle J, Sokoloff L. The distribution of alterations in energy metabolism in the rat brain produced by apomorphine. *Brain Res.* 1982:243:67-80.
46. Wechsler LR, Savaki HE, Sokoloff L. Effects of *d*-1-amphetamine on local cerebral glucose utilization in the conscious rat. *J Neurochem.* 1979;32:15-22.
47. Folstein MF, Robinson R, Folstein S, McHugh PR. Depression and neurological disorders: new treatment opportunities for elderly depressed patients. *J Affect Disord.* 1985;1(suppl):11-14.
48. Baxter LR, Phelps ME, Mazziotta JC, Schwartz JM, Gerner RH, Selin CE, Sumida RM. Cerebral metabolic rates for glucose in mood disorders: studies with positron emission tomography and flurodeoxyglucose F-18. *Arch Gen Psychiatry.* 1985;42:441-447.
49. Buchsbaum MS, Wu JC, DeLisi LE, Holcomb HH, Kessler R, Johnson J, King AC, Hazlett E, Langston K, Post RM. Frontal cortex and basal ganglia metabolic rates assessed by positron emission tomography with F-18 2-deoxyglucose in affective illness. *J Affect Disord.* 1986;10:137-152.
50. Buchsbaum MS, Wu JC, DeLisi LE, Holcomb HH, Hazlett E, Cooper-Langston K, Kessler R. Positron emission tomography studies of basal ganglia and somatosensory cortex neuroleptic drug effects: differences between normal controls and schizophrenic patients. *Biol Psychiatry.* 1987;22:479-494.
51. D'haenen HA, Bossuyt A. Dopamine D_2 receptors in depression measured with single photon emission computed tomography. *Biol Psychiatry.* 1994; 35:128-132.

ORIGINAL ARTICLE

Duration of Neuroleptic Treatment and Prevalence of Tardive Dyskinesia in Late Life

Robert A. Sweet, MD; Benoit H. Mulsant, MD; Babu Gupta, MD; Aicha H. Rifai, MD; Rona E. Pasternak, MD; Ann McEachran, MS; George S. Zubenko, MD, PhD

Background: Although increasing age is the most consistently cited risk factor for the development of tardive dyskinesia for patients in the second to sixth decades of life, this relationship may not hold within geriatric populations.

Methods: Consecutively admitted geropsychiatric inpatients were examined with the Abnormal Involuntary Movement Scale within 72 hours of admission; comprehensive demographic, diagnostic, and psychometric data were also obtained.

Results: Seventy-four (19.2%) of 386 patients received diagnoses of dyskinesia. Lifetime duration of neuroleptic use was strongly correlated with dyskinesia rates. After accounting for the effect of lifetime duration of neuroleptic use in a stepwise logistic regression, only associations with Global Assessment Scale score and presence of dental problems remained statistically significant. In comparison with the duration of neuroleptic use, however, the contribution of these factors was minor. Sixteen percent of patients with less than 3 months of neuroleptic use, 29% with 3 to 12 months of neuroleptic use, 30% with 1 to 10 years of neuroleptic use, and 41% with more than 10 years of neuroleptic use had dyskinesia. Compared with patients with no history of neuroleptic treatment, the relative risks for these durations of neuroleptic use were 1.62 (95% confidence limits [CL], 0.81, 3.24), 2.89 (95% CL, 1.50, 5.55), 3.08 (95% CL, 1.66, 5.70), and 4.11 (95% CL, 2.12, 7.96), respectively.

Conclusions: Within elderly populations, duration of exposure to neuroleptics is the strongest predictor of risk for tardive dyskinesia, and this risk increases rapidly within the first year of total lifetime neuroleptic use.

(Arch Gen Psychiatry. 1995;52:478-486)

NEUROLEPTICS remain the cornerstone of the pharmacotherapy for psychosis in late life. Elderly patients with schizophrenia of both early and late onset, major depression with psychotic features, or dementia complicated by delusions, hallucinations, or agitated behaviors may benefit from receiving neuroleptics.[1] As a consequence, neuroleptics are among the most widely prescribed psychotropic medications in elderly patients.[2] This places the elderly at substantial risk of developing the potential complications of neuroleptic treatment, among them tardive dyskinesia (TD).

Tardive dyskinesia is a syndrome of choreoid and athetoid involuntary movements that typically arise during sustained treatment with neuroleptics and persist after withdrawal of these medications. Following the recognition of the TD syndrome, numerous studies conducted from 1960 to 1980 and summarized by Smith and Baldessarini[3] and Kane and Smith[4] focused on identifying risk factors for the development of TD in neuroleptic-treated patients. Across studies, increasing age has been the most frequently cited risk factor for TD.[3,5] Reported TD prevalence rates in most elderly samples are quite high, typically ranging from 30% to 50%.[3,6,7] Most such studies, however, examined elderly patients institutionalized in state psychiatric hospitals or nursing homes. Prevalence rates reported in community-based samples have been lower, ranging from 16% to 21%.[5,8]

The discrepancy in TD prevalence between institutionalized and community-based elderly patients might be due to one of several factors. Long-term patients in psychiatric hospitals are likely to have re-

See Methods on next page

From the Department of Psychiatry, Western Psychiatric Institute and Clinic, University of Pittsburgh (Pa) School of Medicine.

METHODS

The Geriatric Clinical Research Unit at Western Psychiatric Institute and Clinic, Pittsburgh, Pa, is a 26-bed acute care unit for the assessment and treatment of elderly psychiatric patients. The current study was conducted over 23 months, from April 30, 1991, to March 31, 1993. All patients over the age of 60 years who were admitted to the Geriatric Clinical Research Unit for at least 72 hours during this period received a comprehensive multidisciplinary evaluation. This evaluation included a complete psychiatric history and mental status examination, medical history, physical and neurologic examinations, and laboratory testing and neuroimaging as previously described.[13] Axis I and Axis II diagnoses were determined for each patient according to *DSM-III-R* criteria,[14] using all available information from the patient, family or caregivers, outpatient physicians, and medical records, in addition to results of the evaluation performed on the unit. The diagnostic criteria of *DSM-III-R* were applied in weekly consensus diagnostic conferences attended by at least three faculty psychiatrists (including R.A.S., B.H.M., A.H.R., R.E.P., and G.S.Z.), including the patient's attending psychiatrist, all of whom have specialized expertise in geriatric psychiatry. The psychiatric diagnosis corresponding to the symptoms that led to admission was designated the "primary diagnosis." Axis III diagnoses were similarly determined at the weekly consensus diagnostic conference, using all available data to identify all active medical problems. A medical problem was classified as active if it was the focus of either diagnostic evaluation or treatment intervention (eg, an incidental finding of asymptomatic degenerative arthritis of the spine on chest radiograph would not be considered active, nor would a remote surgery for a resolved condition). Axis III diagnoses were coded according to the *International Classification of Diseases, Ninth Revision, Clinical Modification* system,[15] with the exception that mental disorders and diseases of the brain recorded on Axes I and II were not duplicated.

In addition to the above diagnostic assessment, all patients underwent evaluation and rating by a trained research clinician on a battery of psychometric scales within 72 hours of admission. This evaluation included ratings on the 17-item Hamilton Rating Scale for Depression (HRSD),[16] the Brief Psychiatric Rating Scale (BPRS),[17] the Global Assessment Scale (GAS),[18] and a standardized version of the Mini-Mental State Examination (MMSE).[19] During this 72-hour period, patients were also administered a comprehensive Geriatric Movement Disorders Assessment by a separate research clinician who was blind to the patient's clinical and neuroleptic history. The Geriatric Movement Disorders Assessment yields ratings on the Abnormal Involuntary Movement Scale (AIMS),[20] the Simpson Extrapyramidal Side Effect Scale (SEPSE),[21] and the Barnes Akathisia Scale.[22] Ratings on the AIMS included reports of current dental problems. For those patients admitted after July 1, 1992, this was extended to include additional information regarding edentulousness. Patients were categorized for the presence of dyskinesia according to the severity criteria of Schooler and Kane.[23] That is, patients receiving a rating of mild dyskinesia in two or more body areas on the AIMS or a rating of moderate or severe dyskinesia in any body area on the AIMS were rated as having dyskinesia on the AIMS Global Severity item.

The ability to train geriatric research clinicians to perform the Geriatric Movement Disorders Assessment reliably in comparison with an experienced geriatric psychiatrist has previously been demonstrated.[24] Throughout the study period, reliability was maintained by periodic retraining of the research clinicians. On repeated reliability testing conducted prior to, during, and near the conclusion of the study interval, intraclass correlation coefficients for the AIMS total score and the subtotal of scores for seven body areas ranged from .66 to .89 and .73 to .91, respectively. Simultaneously obtained intraclass correlation coefficients for the SEPSE and Barnes Akathisia Scale total scores ranged from .75 to .89 and .72 to .93, respectively. Intraclass correlation coefficients for the HDRS, BPRS, GAS, and MMSE ranged from .73 to less than .99.[25]

During the index hospitalization, histories of neuroleptic use for all patients were obtained by a research psychiatrist (including R.A.S., B.H.M., A.H.R., and R.E.P.) based

Continued on next page

ceived neuroleptic treatment over longer periods of time than their community counterparts. In addition, dyskinetic movements indistinguishable from TD can occur secondary to edentulousness or neurologic disorders in untreated schizophrenics and in patients without any identified causes.[9-11] It is possible that such factors may either lead to or result from institutionalization and therefore inflate rates of apparent TD in institutionalized elderly patients. This issue was recently addressed by Khot and Wyatt,[12] who performed a meta-analysis of nine studies of TD prevalence in which the rates of these "spontaneous" dyskinesias (ie, dyskinesias occurring in patients who have never been treated with neuroleptics) were also measured. They found that "true TD" rates, calculated by subtracting each age-specific rate of spontaneous dyskinesia from the corresponding age-specific rate of observed TD, were stable across all age groups, with prevalence rates in the 15% to 20% range.

To further determine the factors that contribute to the variability seen in TD rates in the elderly, we systematically studied all elderly patients admitted to an acute geropsychiatry inpatient unit. All patients underwent assessment for medical, psychiatric, and treatment factors that might contribute to the presence of TD. The independent contributions of these factors were evaluated using multivariate statistical approaches. Our main hypotheses were that the overall TD rate would be approximately 20%, with a low rate of spontaneous dyskinesia of approximately 1%,[8] that duration of neuroleptic treatment would be significantly associated with TD prevalence, and that there would be no independent effect of age on TD rate.

RESULTS

A sociodemographic and clinical description of the 386 subjects is presented in **Table 1**. Patients ranged in age from 60 to 100 years at the time of admission, with a mean age of 75 years. The group included twice as many women as men, and 16% of patients were African American. Almost one half of patients received a primary psychiatric on all available sources, including the patient, the patient's family, the treating physician, and old medical records. Whether the patient had ever received any neuroleptic, including amoxapine, metoclopramide hydrochloride, or prochlorperazine, was recorded. The lifetime duration of neuroleptic use, categorized as less than 3 months, 3 to 12 months, or more than 1 year, was determined. For those patients with more than 1 year of lifetime neuroleptic exposure, the number of years of total neuroleptic treatment was recorded. Finally, the interval since each patient last used neuroleptics, categorized as current, less than 3 months ago, 3 to 12 months ago, or more than 1 year ago, was noted.

Statistical analyses were conducted using the BMDP[26] and SPSS/PC[27] statistical software packages. A two-step approach was taken. First, all independent variables were examined in univariate analyses for their association with the presence of dyskinesia. The relationships of categorical variables to dyskinesia were examined using the χ^2 statistic. Ordinal and continuous variables (eg, age of onset, duration of neuroleptic use, MMSE, BPRS, HRSD, GAS, and SEPSE scores, and number of Axis III diagnoses), which assume an underlying linear association with the proportion of subjects having dyskinesia, were tested for this linear association using the linear trends test[28] for ordinal variables. The simpler *t* test, which would have tested for mean differences in the continuous variables in those with and without dyskinesia, fails to address the question of linearity, ie, does the proportion of subjects with dyskinesia increase with increasing age or with increasing duration of neuroleptic use? The grouping of each ordinal and interval variable was chosen both empirically and theoretically. Adjacent cells were collapsed where necessary to ensure that cell sizes were sufficiently large enough for the goodness-of-fit test, but the combination had to make theoretical sense. For example, HRSD ratings that would be considered indicative of depression (>15) would not be grouped with scores that would not indicate clinical depression for this group of patients (≤15). Observed proportions were also plotted in these cases to ensure that we had not missed some other possible relationship—a relationship that might be quadratic or one that might plateau, for example.

Those variables with significant associations were then entered into a stepwise logistic regression analysis with forward elimination. Variables were entered in order of the strength of their association with dyskinesia presence, with the variables with the strongest association entered first. This approach was taken to maximize the power of the analysis by minimizing the number of patients excluded from analysis owing to partially incomplete data sets. Receiver operating characteristic (ROC) methods were applied to those variables found to have significant effects in the stepwise logistic regression to determine the ability of the model to correctly predict the occurrence of dyskinesia.[29] Receiver operating characteristic curves evaluate the performance of a test, in terms of sensitivity and specificity, in such a way that the cutoff points used for the test do not alter the overall outcome (ie, estimating the probability of a correct classification given the equal probability of "present" vs "absent"). Further, the prevalence of the condition in question (in our case, dyskinesia) in the study population does not influence the prediction of its presence based on the equal probability of presence and absence. This latter circumstance can be seen as an endorsement of ROC methods or an objection, according to the expected application of the test in question. In a case such as this one, in which the goal is to determine if a variable is associated with outcome, not the prevalence of the outcome, ROC methods are certainly appropriate.

During the study period, there were 515 consecutive admissions of patients at least 60 years of age, with 101 (20%) repeated admissions (for patients admitted more than once during the study interval) that were not included in the data analysis. Fifteen patients (3%) were unable to complete the AIMS, and for eight patients (2%), a history of neuroleptic treatment could not be obtained. Finally, for five patients (1%), data were not available for logistic reasons, leaving a total study group of 386 patients. The data presented in this study were obtained as part of a clinical investigation of elderly patients admitted to the Geriatric Clinical Research Unit according to a protocol approved by the Biomedical Institutional Review Board of the University of Pittsburgh.

diagnosis of one of the organic mental disorders, with mood disorders diagnosed in close to 40% of patients. Patients with a diagnosis of schizophrenia, schizoaffective disorder, or delusional disorder constituted only 8% of the sample. Although the mean age at onset of the primary psychiatric diagnosis was 63.3 years, the range was broad (13 to 92 years).

At the time of admission, patients demonstrated clinically significant degrees of psychopathology and cognitive impairment that were reflected in their scores on a variety of psychometric measures. Mean BPRS score at admission was 43.8, with a mean HRSD score at admission of 18.7. Mean MMSE score at discharge, chosen over admission testing to better reflect the patients' persistent cognitive functioning, was 21.3. Patients also demonstrated a high degree of global impairment due to illness, with a mean GAS score at admission of 27.9. Finally, patients had substantial medical comorbidity, as indicated by a mean of 5.6 (range, 0 to 16) active medical problems diagnosed on Axis III.

Two hundred thirty-four (61%) of the patients had a history of neuroleptic use (**Table 2**). For 81 of these patients, total lifetime neuroleptic use had been less than 3 months. A similar number (86 patients) had more than 1 year of lifetime neuroleptic use, while the intermediate lifetime duration of neuroleptic use of 3 to 12 months was relatively less common, occurring in only 49 patients.

Slightly more than half (123/234 [53%]) of those patients with a history of neuroleptic treatment were receiving neuroleptics at the time of admission. Related in part to the current use of neuroleptics, patients on average demonstrated mild but clinically detectable parkinsonism, with a mean SEPSE score at admission of 5.7.

Seventy-four (19.2%) of the 386 subjects demonstrated dyskinesia on the AIMS. The 15 sociodemographic, clinical, and treatment variables included in Tables 1 and 2 were initially examined in univariate analyses for an association with the presence of dyskinesia. The following were associated with significantly higher dyskinesia rates: lower age (χ^2=5.61; *df*=1; *P*=.01), diagno-

Table 1. Association of Sociodemographic and Clinical Variables With Dyskinesia Presence*

Variables	Total	Subjects: With the Presence of Dyskinesia	Subjects: With the Absence of Dyskinesia	χ^2 Test Score	*df*	*P*
Sociodemographic						
No. of subjects	**386**	74	312			
Age at admission, y						
Mean (±SD)	75 (8)	73 (7)	75 (8)	5.61	1	.01**
Range	60-100	61-95	60-100			
Sex, No. (%) of subjects						
Female	266	54 (20)	212 (80)	0.70	1	.4
Male	120	20 (17)	100 (83)			
Race, No. (%) of subjects						
White	326	60 (18)	266 (82)	0.79	1	.4
African American	60	14 (23)	46 (77)			
Clinical						
Primary psychiatric diagnosis, No. (%) of subjects						
Organic mental disorder	181	36 (20)	145 (80)	15.3	3	.002
Mood disorder	146	23 (16)	123 (84)			
Schizophrenia or schizoaffective or delusional disorder	30	13 (43)	17 (57)			
Other disorder	29	2 (18)	27 (82)			
Mean (±SD) age at onset of primary diagnosis, y†	63.3 (18.6)	59.0 (18.3)	64.4 (18.5)	9.09	6	.2
Mean (±SD) MMSE score at discharge‡	21.3 (7.8)	20.0 (8.4)	21.6 (7.6)	1.92	3	.2
Mean (±SD) BPRS score at admission§	43.8 (10.0)	45.7 (8.8)	43.3 (10.2)	5.06	3	.2
Mean (±SD) HRSD score at admission‖	18.7 (5.5)	17.8 (5.3)	18.9 (5.6)	4.44	3	.2
Mean (±SD) GAS score at admission¶	27.9 (11.1)	24.0 (9.2)	28.9 (11.3)	17.3	3	.001
Mean (±SD) No. of Axis III diagnoses#	5.6 (2.9)	6.0 (3.6)	5.5 (2.8)	5.94	5	.3
Mean (±SD) SEPSE score at admission	5.7 (4.9)	7.0 (6.0)	5.4 (4.5)	5.05	3	.2
No. (%) of subjects with problem with mouth, teeth, or dentures						
Yes	80	24 (30)	56 (70)	9.72	1	.002
No	**266**	39 (15)	227 (85)			
Could not be determined	**40**	11 (28)	29 (72)			

**MMSE indicates Mini-Mental State Examination; BPRS, Brief Psychiatric Rating Scale; HRSD, Hamilton Rating Scale for Depression; GAS, Global Assessment Scale; and SEPSE, Simpson Extrapyramidal Side Effect Scale.*

†*N=384.*

‡*N=331.*

§*N=383.*

‖*N=384.*

¶*N=381.*

#*Indicates total number of consensus Axis III diagnoses, excluding mental disorders and diseases of the nervous system and sense organs in* International Classification of Diseases, Ninth Revision, Clinical Modification,[15] *which overlapped with the primary psychiatric diagnosis.*

***Derived from linear trends test.*

sis of a psychotic disorder (χ^2=15.3; *df*=3; *P*=.002), lower GAS score at admission (χ^2=17.3; *df*=3; *P*=.001), presence of dental problems (χ^2=9.72; *df*=1; *P*=.002), ever having received neuroleptic medication (χ^2=14.1; *df*=1; *P*=.0002), and duration of total lifetime use of neuroleptics (χ^2=23.2; *df*=4; *P*=.0001). In contrast, sex, race, age at onset of primary psychiatric illness, duration of psychiatric illness, MMSE score at discharge, BPRS score at admission, HRSD score at admission, number of medical diagnoses, the presence of extrapyramidal symptoms, and interval since last neuroleptic use were not associated with dyskinesia prevalence. In the subgroup of patients for whom the additional dental history regarding the presence of edentulousness (n=121) and use of dentures for the AIMS (n=123) was available, neither of these variables were associated with the presence of dyskinesia (*P*=.9 and *P*=.3, respectively).

Because of hypothesized links between diabetes, dopamine receptor function, and the development of dyskinesia,[30] we examined the association between TD and diabetes in our patients. Fifty-seven (14.8%) of our patients received an Axis III diagnosis of diabetes. Dyskinesia rates in diabetic and nondiabetic patients did not differ (21.0% vs 18.8%; χ^2=0.27; *df*=1; *P*=.7).

A stepwise multiple logistic regression was performed to determine the best-fitting model to predict the presence or absence of dyskinesia. Lifetime duration of neuroleptic use (β=0.41; χ^2=15.08; *df*=1; *P*=.0001), GAS score (β=−1.4; χ^2=13.13; *df*=1; *P*=.0003), and dental problems (β=0.87; χ^2=7.34; *df*=1; *P*=.007) all made significant independent contributions to the presence of dyskinesia. In contrast, neither age nor diagnosis remained significantly associated with dyskinesia (χ^2=2.22; *df*=1; *P*=.1; and χ^2=4.05; *df*=3; *P*=.3; respectively) after accounting for the effects of lifetime duration of neuroleptic use. Using ROC methods, duration of neuroleptic use was able to correctly predict the presence or absence of dyskinesia for 67.5% of the cases (**Figure**). When the dichotomous variable of dental problems was added to the model, the rate of correct prediction increased only slightly to

Table 2. Distribution of Neuroleptic Treatment Parameters and Their Association With Dyskinesia

Parameters	Total	No. (%) of Subjects: Dyskinesia Present	No. (%) of Subjects: Dyskinesia Absent	χ^2 Test Score	*df*	*P*
No. of subjects	**386**	74 (19)	312 (81)	...	...	...
Neuroleptics ever used						
No	**152**	15 (10)	137 (90)	14.1	1	.0002
Yes	**234**	59 (25)	175 (75)			
Total lifetime duration of neuroleptic treatment						
Never used	**152**	15 (10)	137 (90)	23.2	4	.0001
<3 mo	**81**	13 (16)	68 (84)			
3-12 mo	**49**	14 (29)	35 (71)			
1-10 y	**59**	18 (31)	41 (69)			
>10 y	**27**	11 (41)	16 (59)			
Could not be determined	**18**	3 (17)	15 (83)			
Last use of neuroleptics						
Never used	**152**	15 (10)	137 (90)	6.20	3	.1
>12 mo ago	**50**	9 (18)	41 (82)			
Within past 3-12 mo	**22**	8 (36)	14 (64)			
<3 mo ago	**34**	5 (15)	29 (85)			
Currently taking	**123**	37 (30)	86 (70)			
Could not be determined	**5**	0 (0)	5 (100)			

70.0%. Using all three predictive variables—duration of neuroleptic use, dental problems, and GAS score—increased the rate of correct prediction to 74.2%. **Table 3** presents the rate of observed dyskinesia and the rate of dyskinesia predicted by the logistic regression model for each of the combinations of the predictor variables.

The rate of dyskinesia in our patients increased for each category of increasing lifetime duration of neuroleptic use. Fifteen (9.9%) of 152 patients with no history of neuroleptic use demonstrated spontaneous dyskinesia. Thirteen (16.0%) of 81 patients with less than 3 months, 14 (28.6%) of 49 patients with 3 to 12 months, 18 (30.5%) of 59 patients with 1 to 10 years, and 11 (40.7%) of 27 patients with more than 10 years of lifetime neuroleptic use demonstrated evidence of neuroleptic-associated dyskinesia. In comparison with the rate of spontaneous dyskinesia in those patients with no history of neuroleptic treatment, the relative risks for neuroleptic-associated dyskinesia for each of these durations of lifetime neuroleptic use were 1.62 (95% confidence limits [CL], 0.81, 3.24), 2.89 (95% CL, 1.50, 5.55), 3.08 (95% CL, 1.66, 5.70), and 4.11 (95% CL, 2.12, 7.96), respectively.

When dyskinesia was present, it was generally mild or moderate. Thirty-nine (52.7%) of the 74 dyskinetic patients were rated as having mild dyskinesia, 30 (40.5%) were rated as having moderate dyskinesia, and five (6.8%) were rated as having severe dyskinesia. Similarly, only 10 patients (13.5%) reported their dyskinetic movements as mildly or moderately distressing. No patient reported being severely distressed by dyskinesia. Examiner ratings of disability due to dyskinesia revealed 56 dyskinetic patients (75.7%) with no or minimal disability, 15 patients (20.3%) with mild to moderate disability, and only one patient (1.4%) with severe disability (in two patients, disability due to dyskinesia could not be rated).

Although dyskinesia tended to be mild, severity was significantly correlated with the duration of lifetime neuroleptic use (r=.27; P=.03). While only three (20.0%) of 15 dyskinetic patients with no history of neuroleptic use had moderate or severe dyskinetic movements, three (23.1%) of 13 dyskinetic patients with less than 3 months of lifetime neuroleptic use, five (35.7%) of 14 dyskinetic patients with 3 to 12 months of lifetime neuroleptic use, and 22 (75.9%) of 29 dyskinetic patients with more than 1 year of lifetime neuroleptic use demonstrated moderate or severe dyskinetic movements.

COMMENT

Lifetime duration of neuroleptic use was the strongest predictor of TD risk in our sample of 386 well-characterized elderly inpatients. Untreated elderly patients were at low risk of developing spontaneous dyskinesias (9.9%). With neuroleptic treatment of increasing length, the risk for the development of TD progressively increased up to 40.7% for patients who had more than 10 years of treatment with neuroleptic medications. Although the presence of dental problems and evidence of increased global impairment were also associated with TD, the contribution of these factors was minor in comparison with the duration of neuroleptic use. Using duration of neuroleptic treatment alone to predict the presence of TD, 67.5% of patients could be correctly classified. When the presence of dental problems and global level of functioning were added to the model, an additional 6.7% of patients were correctly classified. Within our study group of elderly patients, increasing age did not make an independent contribution to the risk for TD.

While the mechanisms through which neuroleptic treatment and other factors lead to the development of TD remain undetermined, the relationship between neuroleptic treatment duration and TD prevalence resembles a

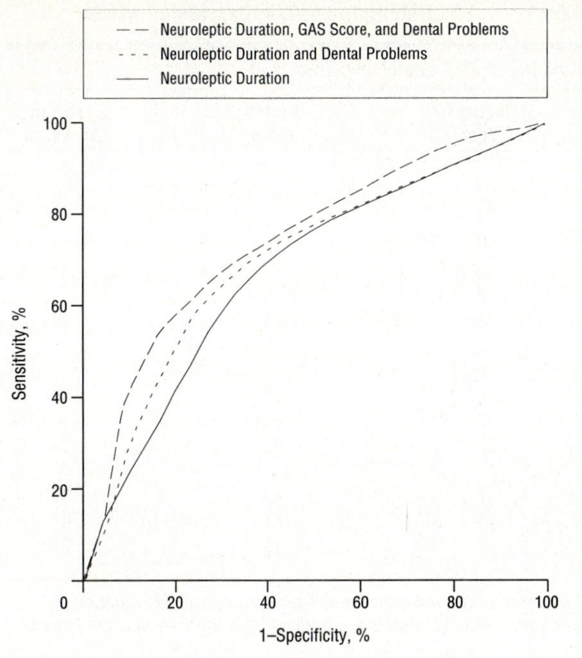

Receiver operating characteristic curves for multiple regression model in predicting the presence of dyskinesia. The area under each curve represents the likelihood of correct classification of random pairs of subjects, one with and one without dyskinesia. An area under the curve of 0.5 (line of no information) represents chance prediction of dyskinesia presence. The addition of the variables "dental problems" and "Global Assessment Scale (GAS) score" to the model based solely on lifetime cumulative duration of neuroleptic use can be seen to add only modestly to the overall predictive ability of the model.

"pack-years" model of dose-response relationship. Although we did not quantify average daily neuroleptic dose, our findings are consistent with those of two smaller prior studies that specifically addressed the relationship between neuroleptic treatment duration, total neuroleptic dose, and rates of TD in geriatric patients. Crane and Smeets[31] examined 39 patients ranging in age from 63 to 89 years and quantified total neuroleptic dose, maximum daily dose, and duration of neuroleptic treatment. Total dose was highly correlated with both maximum dose and duration of treatment (r=.78 and r=.79, respectively), and higher values of all three variables were associated with increased TD rates. Toenniessen et al[32] described 57 elderly inpatients with neuroleptic treatments of 1 to 301 months' duration. They also found that lifetime neuroleptic treatment duration correlated closely with lifetime neuroleptic dose (r=.94) and the AIMS score. Using multiple regression methods similar to those of the present study to control for the independent effects of age, sex, diagnosis, parkinsonism, and anticholinergic use, they found that only neuroleptic treatment duration (r=.30) and the presence of parkinsonism (r=−.39) were significantly correlated with the AIMS score. Together, these two variables were able to correctly classify 67% of TD cases, a percentage highly consistent with the results of the current study. Although in their study the risk for TD did not increase further when neuroleptic treatment histories extended beyond 2 years, we found that the risk for TD continues to rise in patients with longer neuroleptic treatment histories. Our finding is consistent with the recent work of Glazer et al[33] in patients ranging in age from 19 to 73 years. They found that even those patients who did not develop TD after up to 20 years of neuroleptic treatment were at risk of developing TD with further exposure to neuroleptics.

Our finding of a strong relationship between neuroleptic treatment duration and increasing TD prevalence may explain the discrepancy seen in TD rates when comparing studies of chronically institutionalized elderly patients with similar studies conducted in community-based populations. Long durations of neuroleptic use are common in institutionalized patients with chronic psychotic disorders in whom reported TD prevalence rates typically range from 30% to 50%.[3] These rates are consistent with those seen in our elderly patients with the longest durations of neuroleptic use. While institutionalization may also be associated with other factors contributing to higher TD rates, such as reduced level of global functioning or poor dental hygiene, our results suggest that the overall contribution of these factors to TD rates may be small.

The increase in TD risk in our elderly patients was not confined to those patients with a long lifetime duration of neuroleptic use. We noticed an increased risk for TD associated with lifetime neuroleptic treatment as brief as 3 to 12 months. This finding is consistent with those of two prospective studies of TD incidence in elderly patients.[34,35] In these two reports involving a total of 228 elderly patients, the investigators found cumulative TD incidence rates of 10% to 15% within the first 3 months of neuroleptic treatment. Although these studies did not control for the frequency of emergence of spontaneous dyskinesia, they suggest that the elderly may be prone to development of TD more rapidly than younger patients.[34,35] While the increased risk for TD among our patients with the shortest treatment durations (<3 months) did not reach significance, this may reflect limited power of our sample size. It is also possible that, as suggested by Ticehurst,[36] in highly impaired patients with cognitive comorbidity, a remote history of brief neuroleptic exposure may have been missed. These patients would then have been included in the group with no history of neuroleptic use, further decreasing the power to determine a significant difference in TD risk between truly neuroleptic-naive patients and those with brief past neuroleptic exposures. Our relatively high rate of spontaneous dyskinesia in comparison with findings of a prior report that used the same criteria for defining dyskinesia cases is consistent with this interpretation.[5] Accurate determination in elderly patients of the minimum duration of neuroleptic treatment associated with an increased risk for TD has important clinical, medicolegal, and health policy implications. For example, the Nursing Home Reform Amendments of the Omnibus Reconciliation Act of 1987[37] requires nursing homes to monitor for neuroleptic side effects, including TD, but provides no guidelines as to the frequency of such monitoring. Our findings suggest that with regard to TD, there may be no absolutely "safe" duration of neuroleptic treatment in the elderly. The increase in risk for the development of TD in elderly patients appears to begin within the first 3

Table 3. Observed and Predicted Rates of Dyskinesia Within Each Cell From the Final Multiple Logistic Regression Model*

GAS Scores	Never	Less than 3 Months	3 Months to 1 Year	1 to 10 Years	Greater than 10 Years
	Total Lifetime Duration of Neuroleptic Treatment				
>34 and no dental problems					
Observed rate, %	4	0	10	11	0
Predicted rate, %	3	5	7	10	14
No. of subjects	47	11	10	9	6
>34 with dental problems					
Observed rate, %	9	25	0	25	0
Predicted rate, %	7	10	15	21	28
No. of subjects	11	4	2	4	1
≤34 and no dental problems					
Observed rate, %	12	12	18	32	57
Predicted rate, %	11	16	22	30	40
No. of subjects	64	52	22	28	14
≤34 with dental problems					
Observed rate, %	19	50	57	43	40
Predicted rate, %	23	32	41	51	61
No. of subjects	5	14	7	10	22

**Values represent observed and predicted rates of presence of dyskinesia for each category of the following three variables: cumulative duration of neuroleptic exposure, Global Assessment Scale (GAS) score, and presence of dental problems. Predicted rates are derived from the final multiple logistic regression model.*

months of total lifetime neuroleptic treatment. Thus, the initiation of monitoring for TD in neuroleptic-treated elderly patients needs to occur within this interval.[38]

A noteworthy finding of our study is the lack of association between increases in age beyond 60 years and TD risk when controlling for the effect of duration of neuroleptic treatment. This finding is in contrast to the frequently reported relationship between age and TD rates in study populations drawn from across the life span.[3,5,33,39] There is a growing body of evidence that, within elderly groups, increasing age does not place patients at an increased risk of TD. Smith and Baldessarini[3] conducted a meta-analysis of nine studies of TD prevalence, totaling more than 4000 adult patients of all ages, predominantly with diagnoses of schizophrenia. The correlation between age and TD rate for age groups younger than 40 years, 40 to 49 years, 50 to 59 years, and 60 years or older was .99. When they confined the analysis to the six reports including elderly patients, there was no significant difference in TD rates between patients aged 60 to 69 years and 70 years and older. Khot and Wyatt[12] in a nonoverlapping sample of nine studies also found the prevalence of neuroleptic-associated dyskinesia to remain constant between ages 60 and 90 years, at a rate of approximately 35%. Three recent studies have examined the incidence of TD in neuroleptic-treated elderly.[34,35,40] None of these studies found a significant effect of increasing age on TD incidence.

Several other factors associated with increased risk for TD in other patient groups were not found to contribute to risk for TD in our patients. We found no association between TD and female gender,[5] a diagnosis of a mood disorder,[41-43] evidence of cognitive impairment,[44,45] or presence of an organic mental disorder.[46] We also found no association between a diagnosis of diabetes and increased risk for TD, despite a group including 57 diabetic and 329 nondiabetic patients. This stands in contrast to a prospective study conducted by Woerner et al[47] in 160 patients, 24 of whom had diagnoses of diabetes. In 54% of the diabetic patients in their sample, as opposed to 26% of nondiabetic patients, TD developed during 43 weeks of treatment. The authors did not, however, control for the emergence of spontaneous dyskinesia. Ganzini et al,[30] in a case-control study involving 38 patients with diabetes and an equal number of matched controls, also found that neuroleptic-treated diabetic patients had significantly higher rates of TD than nondiabetic neuroleptic-treated patients (79% vs 53%). In a concurrent sample of diabetic patients not treated with neuroleptics, however, the rate of spontaneous dyskinesia was 21%. This rate, roughly equivalent to the difference in TD rates between the two neuroleptic-treated groups, suggests that most of the increased risk for dyskinesia in diabetes may be secondary to spontaneous dyskinesia. Several important methodological differences between these studies should be noted. The three studies differ in sample size, inpatient vs outpatient setting, and cross-sectional vs prospective assessments. There may also be undefined differences in the populations studied with regard to severity of diabetes, extent of pharmacologic treatment of the diabetes, or timing of neuroleptic treatment relative to the onset of diabetes. Clearly the contrast in findings between our study and those of Ganzini et al[30] and Woerner et al[47] awaits clarification.

There are several possible limitations of the current study. Although our geropsychiatry inpatient unit serves as a primary admitting unit for an urban population of elderly patients, we also provide tertiary care to a large region of southwestern Pennsylvania and adjoining states. Thus, our population may not be truly representative of community geropsychiatry patient populations and therefore not generalizable to such settings. Our assessments of dyskinesia presence were performed cross-sectionally. While the use of the severity criteria of Schooler and Kane[23] to define dyskinesia cases in our sample should provide stability of diagnosis of TD,[48] it is possible that our rate of dyskinesia may have been inflated by factors such as mood or anxiety states associated with acute admission to a psychiatric unit.[43] The lack of association between dyskinesia and measures of depression and psychosis in the current study, however, would not support this contention. Alternatively, TD rates may have been suppressed by the high rate of current neuroleptic use at admission. While such an effect, if present, would work against our hypotheses and thus strengthen our findings, the lack of association between TD and the interval since last neuroleptic use or measures of parkinsonism suggests that this effect was not operative in our sample.

In conclusion, we found that TD remains a frequent complication of neuroleptic treatment in the elderly, with the risk for the development of TD increasing in direct relationship to the duration of neuroleptic treatment. This increased risk for the development of TD begins within the first months of neuroleptic treatment. Thus, for elderly patients, there may be no absolutely safe duration of neuroleptic treatment. While concern over neurologic side effects, including TD, has spurred the development of atypical neuroleptics, most effort has focused on the chronically ill or treatment-resistant younger patient with schizophrenia. Little attention has been paid to the development of atypical neuroleptics for use in the elderly, although this population may have the most to gain from a reduction in both extrapyramidal side effects and TD. Research efforts also need to better define the indications for neuroleptic treatment in late life, such as the separate roles for short-term and continuation neuroleptic treatment in elderly patients with major depression with psychotic features, and to explore alternatives to neuroleptics (for example, the use of selective serotonin agents in the treatment of behavioral syndromes associated with dementia).[49,50] Such efforts may ultimately reduce the prevalence of TD by providing clinical guidelines for the reduction of neuroleptic use in those elderly patients with transient psychoses.

Accepted for publication March 22, 1995.

Supported in part by grants MH 30915 and MH 49786 from the National Institute of Mental Health, Rockville, Md. Dr Sweet was the recipient of Scientist Development Award for Clinicians MH 01153 and Dr Zubenko was the recipient of Research Career Development Award MH 00540, both from the National Institute of Mental Health.

Presented in part at the Seventh Annual Meeting of the American Association for Geriatric Psychiatry, Tampa, Fla, February 19, 1994.

The authors acknowledge the contributions of the clinical and research staff of the Geriatric Clinical Research Unit at Western Psychiatric Institute and Clinic and thank Sharon Jenkins for her assistance in the preparation of the manuscript.

Correspondence to Western Psychiatric Institute and Clinic, 3811 O'Hara St, Pittsburgh, PA 15213 (Dr Sweet).

REFERENCES

1. Mulsant BH, Gershon S. Neuroleptics in the treatment of psychosis in late-life: a rational approach. *Int J Geriatr Psychiatry.* 1993;8:979-992.
2. Alvir JJ, Lieberman JA, Safferman AZ, Schwimmer JL, Schaaf JA. Clozapine-induced agranulocytosis: incidence and risk factors in the United States. *N Engl J Med.* 1993;329:162-167.
3. Smith JM, Baldessarini RJ. Changes in prevalence, severity, and recovery in tardive dyskinesia with age. *Arch Gen Psychiatry.* 1980;37:1368-1373.
4. Kane JM, Smith JM. Tardive dyskinesia: prevalence and risk factors, 1959 to 1979. *Arch Gen Psychiatry.* 1982;39:473-481.
5. Woerner MG, Kane JM, Lieberman JA, Alvir J, Bergmann KJ, Borenstein M, Schooler NR, Mukherjee S, Rotrosen J, Rubinstein M, Basavaraju N. The prevalence of tardive dyskinesia. *J Clin Psychopharmacol.* 1991;11:34-42.
6. Greenblatt DL, Dominick JR, Stotsky BA, DiMascio A. Phenothiazine-induced dyskinesia in nursing-home patients. *J Am Geriatr Soc.* 1968;16:27-34.
7. Bourgeois M, Bouilh P, Tignol J, Yesavage J. Spontaneous dyskinesias vs neuroleptic-induced dyskinesias in 270 elderly subjects. *J Nerv Ment Dis.* 1980; 168:177-178.
8. Sweet RA, Mulsant BH, Rifai AH, Zubenko GS. Dyskinesia and neuroleptic exposure in elderly psychiatric inpatients. *J Geriatr Psychiatry Neurol.* 1992;5: 156-161.
9. Koller WC. Edentulous orodyskinesia. *Ann Neurol.* 1982;13:97-99.
10. Owens DGC. Involuntary disorders of movement in chronic schizophrenia—the role of the illness and its treatment. In: Casey DE, Chase TN, Christensen AV, Gerlach J, eds. *Dyskinesia: Research and Treatment.* New York, NY: Springer-Verlag NY Inc; 1985:79-87.
11. Kane JM, Weinhold P, Kinon B, Wegner J, Leader M. Prevalence of abnormal involuntary movements ('spontaneous dyskinesias') in the normal elderly. *Psychopharmacology.* 1982;77:105-108.
12. Khot V, Wyatt J. Not all that moves is tardive dyskinesia. *Am J Psychiatry.* 1991;148:661-666.
13. Zubenko GS, Rosen J, Sweet RA, Mulsant BH, Rifai AH. Impact of psychiatric hospitalization on behavioral complications of Alzheimer's disease. *Am J Psychiatry.* 1992;149:1484-1491.
14. American Psychiatric Association. *Diagnostic and Statistical Manual of Mental Disorders, Revised Third Edition.* Washington, DC: American Psychiatric Association; 1987.
15. *International Classification of Diseases, Ninth Edition, Clinical Modification.* 3rd ed. Washington, DC: US Dept of Health and Human Services; 1989.
16. Hamilton M. Development of a rating scale for primary depressive illness. *Br J Soc Psychol.* 1967;6:278-296.
17. Overall JE, Gorham DR. The Brief Psychiatric Rating Scale. *Psychol Res.* 1962; 10:799-812.
18. Endicott J, Spitzer RL, Fleiss JL, Cohen J. The Global Assessment Scale: a procedure for measuring overall severity of psychiatric disturbance. *Arch Gen Psychiatry.* 1976;33:766-771.
19. Molloy DW, Alemayehu E, Roberts R. Reliability of a standardized Mini-Mental State Examination compared with the traditional Mini-Mental State Examination. *Am J Psychiatry.* 1991;148:102-105.
20. Guy W. Abnormal Involuntary Movement Scale. In: Guy W, ed. *ECDEU Assessment Manual for Psychopharmacology, Revised.* Rockville, Md: National Institute of Mental Health; 1976:534-537.
21. Simpson GM, Angus JWS. A rating scale for extrapyramidal side effects. *Acta Psychiatr Scand.* 1970;212:11-18.
22. Barnes TR. A rating scale for drug-induced akathisia. *Br J Psychiatry.* 1989; 154:672-676.
23. Schooler NR, Kane JM. Research diagnoses for tardive dyskinesia. *Arch Gen Psychiatry.* 1982;39:486-487.
24. Sweet RA, DeSensi EG, Zubenko GS. Reliability and applicability of movement disorder rating scales in the elderly. *J Neuropsychiatry Clin Neurosci.* 1993;5:56-60.
25. Mulsant BH, Sweet RA, Rifai AH, Pasternak RE, McEachran A, Zubenko GS. The use of the Hamilton Rating Scale for Depression in elderly patients with cognitive impairment and physical illness. *Am J Geriatr Psychiatry.* 1994;2: 220-229.
26. Brown MB, Engelman L, Jennrich RI. *BMDP Statistical Software Manual.* Los Angeles, Calif: University of California Press; 1990.

27. SPSS Inc. *SPSS for Windows Release 6.0.* Chicago, Ill: SPSS Inc; 1993.
28. Agresti A. *Categorical Data Analysis.* New York, NY: John Wiley & Sons Inc; 1990:100-101.
29. Houck PR, Reynolds CF, Mazumdar S, Kupfer DJ. Receiver operating characteristic analysis for validating EEG sleep discrimination of elderly depressed and demented patients. *J Geriatr Psychiatry Neurol.* 1991;4:30-33.
30. Ganzini L, Heintz RT, Hoffman WF, Casey DE. The prevalence of tardive dyskinesia in neuroleptic-treated diabetics: a controlled study. *Arch Gen Psychiatry.* 1991;48:259-263.
31. Crane GE, Smeets RA. Tardive dyskinesia and drug therapy in geriatric patients. *Arch Gen Psychiatry.* 1974;30:341-343.
32. Toenniessen LM, Casey DE, McFarland BH. Tardive dyskinesia in the aged: duration of treatment relationships. *Arch Gen Psychiatry.* 1985;42:278-284.
33. Glazer WM, Morgenstern H, Doucette JT. Predicting the long-term risk of tardive dyskinesia in outpatients maintained on neuroleptic medications. *J Clin Psychiatry.* 1993;54:133-139.
34. Harris MJ, Panton D, Caligiuri MP, Krull AJ, Tran-Johnson TK, Jeste DV. High incidence of tardive dyskinesia in older outpatients on low doses of neuroleptics. *Psychopharmacol Bull.* 1992;28:87-92.
35. Saltz BL, Woerner MG, Kane JM, Lieberman JA, Alvir JMJ, Bergmann KJ, Blank K, Koblenzer J, Kahaner K. Prospective study of tardive dyskinesia incidence in the elderly. *JAMA.* 1991;266:2402-2406.
36. Ticehurst SB. Is spontaneous orofacial dyskinesia an artefact due to incomplete drug history? *J Geriatr Psychiatry Neurol.* 1990;3:208-211.
37. Department of Health and Human Services. State operations manual: provider certification. In: *Health Care Financing Administration.* 7th ed. Dept of Health and Human Services; 1992. Transmittal 250.
38. Sweet RA, Pollock BG. Neuroleptics in the elderly: guidelines for monitoring. *Harvard Rev Psychiatry.* 1995;2:327-335.
39. Task Force on Tardive Dyskinesia. *Tardive Dyskinesia: A Task Force Report of the American Psychiatric Association.* Washington, DC: American Psychiatric Association; 1992.
40. Yassa R, Nastase C, Dupont D, Thibeau M. Tardive dyskinesia in elderly psychiatric patients: a 5-year study. *Am J Psychiatry.* 1992;149:1206-1211.
41. Davis KL, Berger PA, Hollister LE. Tardive dyskinesia and depressive illness. *Psychopharmacol Commun.* 1976;2:125-130.
42. Yassa R, Ghadirian AM, Schwartz G. Prevalence of tardive dyskinesia in affective disorder patients. *J Clin Psychiatry.* 1983;44:410-412.
43. Mukherjee S, Rosen AM, Caracci G, Shukla S. Persistent tardive dyskinesia in bipolar patients. *Arch Gen Psychiatry.* 1986;43:342-346.
44. Waddington JL, Youssef HA. Tardive dyskinesia in bipolar affective disorder: aging, cognitive dysfunction, course of illness, and exposure to neuroleptics and lithium. *Am J Psychiatry.* 1988;145:613-616.
45. Waddington JL, Youssef HA. An unusual cluster of tardive dyskinesia in schizophrenia: association with cognitive dysfunction and negative symptoms. *Am J Psychiatry.* 1986;143:1162-1165.
46. Richardson MA, Haugland G, Pass R, Craig TJ. The prevalence of tardive dyskinesia in a mentally retarded population. *Psychopharmacol Bull.* 1986;22:243-249.
47. Woerner MG, Saltz BL, Kane JM, Lieberman JA, Alvir JMJ. Diabetes and development of tardive dyskinesia. *Am J Psychiatry.* 1993;150:966-968.
48. Schooler NR. Evaluation of drug-related movement disorders in the aged. *Psychopharmacol Bull.* 1988;24:603-607.
49. Nyth AL, Gottfries CG. The clinical efficacy of citalopram in treatment of emotional disturbances in dementia disorders. *Br J Psychiatry.* 1990;157:894-901.
50. Houlihan DJ, Mulsant BH, Sweet RA, Rifai AH, Pasternak RE, Rosen J, Zubenko GS. A naturalistic study of trazodone in the treatment of behavioral complications of dementia. *Am J Geriatr Psychiatry.* 1994;2:78-85.

Family Study of Early-Onset Dysthymia

Mood and Personality Disorders in Relatives of Outpatients With Dysthymia and Episodic Major Depression and Normal Controls

Daniel N. Klein, PhD; Lawrence P. Riso, PhD; Shauna K. Donaldson, PhD; Joseph E. Schwartz, PhD; Rochelle L. Anderson, PhD; Paige Crosby Ouimette, PhD; Humberto Lizardi, MA; Thomas A. Aronson, MD

Background: The nosological status of dysthymia has generated considerable controversy. The major issues include whether dysthymia should be classified as a form of mood or personality disorder and, if dysthymia is classified as a mood disorder, whether it is sufficiently distinct from major depression to warrant a separate category.

Methods: We conducted a family study of 97 outpatients with early-onset dysthymia, 45 outpatients with episodic major depression, and 45 normal controls, and their 882 first-degree relatives. Axis I and II disorders were assessed in relatives using direct and informant interviews and all available medical records.

Results: The rate of major depression in the relatives of early-onset dysthymic probands was significantly greater than in the relatives of normal controls and nonsignificantly greater than in the relatives of episodic major depressive probands. The rate of dysthymia was significantly greater in the relatives of dysthymic probands than in relatives of both major depressive probands and normal controls. Rates of most personality disorders were increased in the relatives of the dysthymic and major depressive probands compared with relatives of normal controls. In addition, the relatives of dysthymic probands had significantly higher rates of any personality disorder and any cluster B disorder than those of episodic major depressive probands, although these differences disappeared after controlling for Axis II comorbidity in the probands. Finally, dysthymic probands with and without a lifetime history of major depression did not differ on rates of psychiatric disorders in relatives.

Conclusions: There is a strong familial relationship between dysthymia and major depression. However, dysthymia is also somewhat distinct in that it aggregates specifically in the families of patients with dysthymia. Finally, dysthymia and episodic major depression both appear to have a familial association with the personality disorders, although the link appears to be somewhat stronger for dysthymia.

(Arch Gen Psychiatry. 1995;52:487-496)

THE CATEGORY of dysthymic disorder was introduced in the *DSM-III* in 1980[1] as a rubric for chronic, mild depressive conditions. Epidemiological studies indicate that dysthymia is a common condition, with a 6- to 12-month prevalence of approximately 3%.[2,3] In addition, dysthymia is associated with high rates of health care utilization and significant psychosocial impairment.[3-6]

Despite its clinical and public health significance, the nosological status of dysthymia has been controversial.[7-10] On the one hand, a number of investigators have challenged whether dysthymia should be classified as a mood disorder, arguing that its chronic course and often early onset are more consistent with the personality disorders.[11-13] On the other hand, some investigators have questioned whether dysthymia is sufficiently distinct to warrant a separate category within the mood disorders, contending that it is simply a variant or phase of major depression.[14-17]

One of the most widely used approaches to validating nosological constructs is by examining patterns of familial aggregation.[18,19] Several studies have reported elevated rates of dysthymia in the relatives of probands with major depression.[20-22] However, few data on psychopathological disorders in the relatives of probands with dysthymia are available.[23] The four studies that have reported family history data on probands with dysthymia have yielded inconsistent findings.[14,24-26] Thus, the proportion of dysthymic probands with a family history of mood disorder has been reported to be lower,[24] similar,[14] higher,[25]

See Subjects and Methods on next page

From the Departments of Psychology (Drs Klein, Riso, Donaldson, Anderson, and Ouimette and Mr Lizardi) and Psychiatry and Behavioral Science (Drs Klein, Schwartz, and Aronson), State University of New York at Stony Brook.

and higher for antidepressant-responsive but lower for medication-nonresponsive dysthymic probands[26] than that of major depressive probands. Several studies have also suggested that a greater proportion of patients with dysthymia than with major depression have a family history of bipolar disorder[25,26] and antisocial personality.[25]

Unfortunately, these studies have significant limitations. First, all of them relied on the family history method instead of attempting to conduct personal interviews with relatives. Moreover, most employed a single data source, generally the proband. The family history method, particularly without the use of multiple informants, underestimates rates of psychopathological disorders in relatives,[27] and could produce biased results, as psychopathological disorders in informants may influence family history reports.[28,29] Second, most studies did not use reliable, systematic family history interviews such as the Family History Research Diagnostic Criteria.[30] Third, none of the studies used blind interviewers, raising the possibility of rater bias. Fourth, the samples in these studies were generally small, and only one[14] used normal or general population controls. Fifth, none of these studies distinguished between dysthymic subjects who did and did not have a history of major depression. Hence, it is unclear whether their findings are due to dysthymia per se or to comorbid major depression. Finally, none of these studies examined rates of dysthymia in relatives, and only one study[25] (which was limited to antisocial personality) examined any personality disorders in relatives. Hence, there are almost no data bearing on the specificity of transmission of dysthymia or its familial relationship to the personality disorders.

This article reports on what is, to our knowledge, the first family study of dysthymia. The study focused on the primary, early-onset subtype, as this is the prototypical form of dysthymia and has been the subject of most of the nosological controversy in this area.[7,10] Herein, we present the rates of mood and personality disorders in the relatives of outpatients with early-onset dysthymia and episodic major depression and normal controls. Data on non–mood Axis I disorders will be reported elsewhere. The article addresses five questions: (1) Is there familial aggregation of major mood disorders in dysthymia? (2) Do the rates of mood disorders in the relatives of dysthymic probands differ from those in the relatives of episodic major depressive probands? (3) Do the relatives of dysthymic probands exhibit an increased rate of dysthymia compared with the relatives of episodic major depressive probands and normal controls (ie, is there specificity of transmission)? (4) Is there an increased rate of personality disorders in relatives of dysthymic probands compared with relatives of episodic major depressive probands and normal controls? and

SUBJECTS AND METHODS

PROBANDS

The probands included 97 outpatients meeting *DSM-III-R*[31] criteria for primary early-onset dysthymia, 45 outpatients with *DSM-III-R* nonchronic major depression, and 45 subjects from the community with no lifetime history of Axis I disorder. Fifty-six (58%) of the dysthymic patients had concurrent major depression and 75 (77%) had a lifetime history of major depression. The patients with episodic major depression were required to have an onset prior to age 35 years to provide a better match with the dysthymic group on demographic variables and age of onset of major depression. In addition, their index major depressive episode could not have been attributable to a preexisting chronic Axis I or III disorder, and they could not have had a history of dysthymia. None of the early-onset dysthymic or episodic major depressive patients were currently psychotic or had ever been psychotic outside a major depressive episode. All the subjects were between the ages of 18 and 60 years, English speaking, and had knowledge of at least one first-degree relative. To obtain as representative a sample as possible, subjects were included even if they denied permission to contact their relatives.

Patients were recruited from consecutive admissions to the State University of New York at Stony Brook (SUSB) University Hospital Outpatient Psychiatric Clinic (50%) and the SUSB Psychological Center (41%). The sample was supplemented by a small number of referrals from the SUSB Student Counseling Center (7%) and a community mental health center outpatient clinic (2%). The proportions of dysthymic and episodic major depressive patients from each site were almost identical. Normal controls were recruited by randomly selecting households from the towns in which most of the patients lived using telephone directory listings. We attempted to match the normal and dysthymic groups for age and gender. Subjects were included in the normal group if there was no evidence of a lifetime history of Axis I disorder based on both an extensive telephone screening interview and a complete face-to-face structured diagnostic interview. Proband diagnoses were based on the Structured Clinical Interview for *DSM-III-R* (SCID),[32] the revised version of the Personality Disorder Examination (PDE),[33] and all available clinic records.

RELATIVES

All first-degree relatives older than 14 years were included in the study. The sample consisted of 446 relatives of patients with early-onset dysthymia, 207 relatives of patients with episodic major depression, and 229 relatives of normal controls. The relatives of the dysthymic group included 343 relatives of dysthymic patients with a history of major depression and 103 of dysthymic patients without such a history. We attempted to conduct personal interviews with all living relatives. Family history information was obtained from probands regarding all relatives. In addition, we attempted to obtain family history data from at least one other informant (generally the relative nominated by the proband as the person who knew the most about the other family members) for all relatives who did not receive personal interviews. Finally, treatment records were obtained whenever possible.

MEASURES

Direct interviews included the SCID (nonpatient version) and the PDE. Whenever possible, direct interviews were conducted in person; otherwise, they were conducted by telephone. Family history data were collected using an expanded version of the Family History Research Diagnostic Criteria interview guide[30] and the Family History Interview for Personality Disorders.[34] Direct and family history interviews were conducted blind to all information about the probands. Proband family histories and direct interviews with relatives were conducted by different interviewers, and all subjects were specifically instructed not to divulge any information about the proband to the interviewer.

Interviewers included a doctoral-level clinical psychologist, a master's-level psychiatric social worker, and graduate students in clinical psychology. All interviewers attended formal workshops on the use of the SCID and PDE that were conducted by the instruments' developers, completed an extensive training program that included corating interviews conducted by more experienced interviewers and being observed while conducting interviews, and participated in regular supervision sessions throughout the study. Data on the interrater reliability of our SCID, PDE, and family history interviews has been reported elsewhere.[34-36]

Blind lifetime best-estimate diagnoses[37] were derived for each relative using a team consensus method that has previously been described in detail.[35] The test-retest reliability of the best-estimate diagnoses was evaluated for 92 cases after a minimum 2-year interval. κ Values were 0.90 for major depression and 0.75 for dysthymia. The κ's for specific Axis II disorders ranged from 0.73 to 0.94, with a median of 0.87.[35]

DATA ANALYSIS

Diagnostic hierarchies were not employed, apart from those inherent in the *DSM-III-R* criteria. Categorical variables were analyzed using χ^2 (with Yates' correction for 2×2 tables) and Fisher's exact probability tests. Continuous variables were analyzed with *t* tests and one-way analyses of variance (using Tukey's Honestly Significant Difference Test for pairwise comparisons). The age-specific incidence of most forms of mood disorder in relatives was compared between groups using Cox's proportional hazards model, a semi-parametric multivariate regression model for survival data.[38] The proportionality assumption was examined using both graphical and statistical methods,[39,40] and generally appeared to be appropriate. In addition, similar results were obtained using χ^2 and multiple logistic regression[41] analyses. Rates of early-onset dysthymia and personality disorders were compared between groups using LR, as almost all subjects, by definition, were through the risk period for these conditions. Logistic regression was also used to compare the rates of bipolar disorder in relatives and for all the analyses stratifying the dysthymic probands by history of major depression because many of the proportional hazards models failed to converge owing to small Ns. Three covariates were included in all proportional hazards and logistic regression analyses: whether the relative received a direct interview, the sex of the relative, and the relative's birth cohort. Preliminary analyses indicated that proband gender, recruitment site, and relationship to the relative (offspring, sibling, or parent) were not associated with rates of psychopathological disorders in family members, hence, were not included in the models. The number of significant interactions between the covariates and proband group were no greater than would be expected by chance; therefore, only main effects were included in the models. To ensure that any differences in rates of personality disorders between groups of relatives were not simply due to differences in rates of comorbid Axis II disorders in probands,[42] we also conducted analyses including proband comorbidity as a covariate in the comparisons of personality disorders in relatives.

(5) Do these patterns of familial aggregation differ as a function of whether the dysthymic probands have a history of major depression?

RESULTS

COMPARISONS USING THE TOTAL DYSTHYMIC SAMPLE

Characteristics of Probands

The characteristics of the probands are described in detail elsewhere[36,43]; hence, only a brief summary is presented herein (**Table 1**). For demographic variables, the early-onset dysthymic, episodic major depressive, and normal control groups were similar on sex, age, race, and education. However, the groups differed significantly on marital status ($\chi^2[6]=31.7$, $P<.001$), reflecting the fact that a higher proportion of normal controls were married, and a lower proportion were single, separated, or divorced compared with the dysthymic and major depressive groups. The groups also differed on socioeconomic status[44] ($\chi^2[8]=23.7$, $P<.005$), with the normal controls exhibiting a significantly higher social class distribution than both the early-onset dysthymic and episodic major depressive groups.

In terms of clinical characteristics, the groups differed significantly on the 17-item Hamilton Rating Scale for Depression[45] ($F[2,146]=97.1$, $P<.001$), with the episodic major depressive group exhibiting a significantly higher level of depressive symptoms than the dysthymic group, who, in turn, exhibited a significantly higher level of symptoms than the normal controls.

The groups also differed on the Global Assessment of Functioning Scale[31] ($F[2,183]=178.9$, $P<.001$), with both groups of patients exhibiting a significantly lower level of functioning than the normal controls. With regard to comorbidity, the dysthymic group reported significantly higher rates of lifetime alcohol abuse or dependence ($\chi^2[1]=5.8$, $P<.02$), lifetime drug abuse or dependence ($\chi^2[1]=4.8$, $P<.03$), and personality disorders ($\chi^2[1]=20.21$ $P<.001$) than the episodic major depressive group. The groups did not differ on rates of lifetime anxiety, eating, and somatoform disorders.

Characteristics of Relatives

Of the 882 relatives in the sample, we were able to conduct personal interviews with 40%, a figure comparable to that

Table 1. Descriptive Characteristics of Probands*

Variable	Total DY (N=97)	DY−MD (n=22)	DY+MD (n=75)	EMD (N=45)	NC (N=45)
Sex, % female	75.3	54.5	81.3	66.7	82.2
Mean age, y	32.2 (9.8)	27.6 (7.2)	33.5 (10.1)	31.6 (9.2)	33.4 (10.1)
Race, % white	90.7	90.9	90.7	86.7	93.3
Mean education, y	13.2 (2.2)	13.6 (1.5)	13.1 (2.4)	14.0 (2.2)	13.6 (1.9)
Marital status, %					
Single	48.5	63.6	44.0	42.2	26.7
Married	29.9	22.7	32.0	31.1	73.3
Divorced/separated	19.6	13.6	21.3	26.7	0.0
Widowed	2.1	0.0	2.7	0.0	0.0
Social class, %					
I	9.1	21.1	5.8	17.1	9.3
II	28.4	15.8	31.9	29.3	51.2
III	25.0	42.1	20.3	24.4	32.6
IV	17.0	10.5	18.8	24.4	7.0
V	20.5	10.5	23.2	4.9	0.0
Mean GAF Scale	56.4 (9.6)	58.0 (9.5)	55.9 (9.6)	56.9 (12.6)	87.5 (3.8)
Mean HRSD score (17-item)	16.7 (8.1)	9.0 (4.9)	19.5 (7.2)	20.0 (6.5)	2.8 (2.6)
Recurrent MD, %	...	...	76.0	62.2	...
Mean age of onset of MD, y	...	...	20.6 (8.1)	23.9 (6.4)	...
Mean age of onset of dysthymia, y	10.2 (4.9)	11.5 (4.9)	9.9 (4.9)	...	...
Anxiety disorder, %†	43.3	18.2	50.7	28.9	...
Alcohol abuse/dependence, %†	37.1	50.0	33.3	15.6	...
Drug abuse/dependence, %†	35.1	45.5	32.0	15.6	...
Personality disorder, %	59.8	54.5	61.3	17.8	0.0

**Numbers in parentheses are SD. Total DY indicates all dysthymics; DY−MD, dysthymics with no history of major depression; DY+MD, dysthymics with a history of major depression; EMD, episodic major depressives; NC, normal controls; GAF, Global Assessment of Functioning; and HRSD, Hamilton Rating Scale for Depression.*

†Lifetime diagnoses.

of other recent family studies of depression in the United States.[22,46,47] Of the remaining relatives, the proband denied permission to contact 28%; 17% refused to participate; 9% were deceased; and 6% were otherwise inaccessible (eg, did not live in North America or did not speak English). Overall, we interviewed 70% of all living relatives who were accessible and whom we were permitted to contact.

In most cases, we were able to obtain data from multiple sources about each relative. Thus, we obtained either a direct interview and at least one family history interview or at least two family history interviews for 73% of the sample.

Overall, the mean age of the relatives was 42.2 (SD=16.9). Fifty percent were male and 41.8% were parents, 47.4% were siblings, and 10.4% were offspring of the probands. The relatives of the dysthymic, episodic major depressive, and normal control groups did not differ significantly on the type or number of data sources available, age, sex, or relationship to the proband.

Psychopathology in Relatives

Unadjusted rates of lifetime mood and personality disorders in the relatives of early-onset dysthymic, episodic major depressive, and normal control subjects are presented in **Table 2**. Because of space limitations, age-corrected rates are not presented. As would be expected, age correction produced higher rates overall, but the pattern of between-group differences was similar to that of the uncorrected rates.

The results of the multivariate analyses of mood disorders are shown in **Table 3**. The relatives of both the early-onset dysthymic and episodic major depressive probands exhibited significantly higher rates of any mood disorder, major mood disorder (bipolar disorder and major depression), and major depression than the relatives of normal controls. In addition, the relatives of dysthymic probands exhibited a significantly higher rate of any mood disorder, and a trend for a higher rate of major depression than the relatives of episodic major depressive probands. The rates of bipolar disorder were somewhat higher among the relatives of both the early-onset dysthymic and episodic major depressive probands than the relatives of normal controls, but neither difference approached statistical significance.

To explore whether the groups differed on type or severity of major depression, we also examined rates of recurrent major depression and major depression with treatment, medication, and incapacitation in major role functioning.[48] The relatives of dysthymic probands exhibited significantly higher rates of each of these conditions than the relatives of normal controls. In addition, there was a significantly higher rate of incapacitating major depression and a trend for a higher rate of recurrent major depression among the relatives of episodic major depressive probands than normal controls. Finally, the relatives of dysthymic probands exhibited a significantly higher rate of major depression with medication and a trend for a higher rate of recurrent major depression than the relatives of episodic major depressive probands.

Next, we compared the groups of relatives on rates of chronic depression overall, chronic major depression, dysthymia, and the early-onset dysthymia subtype. The number of subjects with late-onset dysthymia was too small to conduct proportional hazards or logistic regression analyses. The rate of chronic depression was significantly greater

Table 2. Unadjusted Rates of Lifetime Mood and Personality Disorders in Relatives of Patients With Dysthymia and Episodic Major Depression and Normal Controls*

Variable	Total DY (N=446)	DY−MD (n=103)	DY+MD (n=343)	EMD (N=207)	NC (N=229)
Mood disorders	37.4	34.0	38.5	27.1	16.6
Major mood disorders	31.2	24.3	33.2	26.1	15.7
Bipolar disorder	2.2	0.0	2.9	2.4	0.4
Major depression (MD)	28.9	24.3	30.3	23.7	15.3
Recurrent MD	14.3	12.6	14.9	9.7	5.2
MD with treatment	15.9	15.5	16.0	12.6	8.3
MD with medication	8.1	3.9	9.3	3.9	3.1
Incapacitating MD	10.6	6.8	11.7	7.7	4.4
Chronic depression	16.6	18.4	16.0	7.7	2.6
Chronic MD	6.7	5.8	7.0	5.3	1.7
Dysthymia	10.1	12.6	9.3	2.9	1.3
Early-onset dysthymia	6.7	9.7	5.8	1.4	1.3
Late-onset dysthymia	3.4	2.9	3.5	1.4	0.0
Personality disorders	47.2	48.5	46.8	38.6	14.8
Cluster A disorders	10.3	9.7	10.5	10.1	2.6
Paranoid	5.6	4.9	5.8	8.7	1.7
Schizoid	4.7	5.8	4.4	3.4	0.9
Schizotypal	2.2	1.0	2.6	0.0	0.0
Cluster B disorders	26.1	28.2	25.4	19.3	7.0
Antisocial	9.9	10.7	9.6	6.8	2.2
Borderline	11.7	9.7	12.3	7.7	1.7
Histrionic	12.6	11.7	12.9	9.7	1.7
Narcissistic	8.8	9.7	8.5	6.3	3.9
Cluster C disorders	21.8	18.4	22.8	17.4	8.3
Avoidant	8.8	8.7	8.8	5.8	5.2
Dependent	4.3	1.9	5.0	4.8	0.4
Obsessive-compulsive	9.2	6.8	9.9	9.7	2.6
Passive-aggressive	6.7	5.8	7.0	2.4	1.7

**Total DY indicates relatives of all dysthymics; DY−MD, relatives of dysthymics with no history of major depression; DY+MD, relatives of dysthymics with a history of major depression; EMD, relatives of episodic major depressives; and NC, relatives of normal controls.*

in the relatives of the early-onset dysthymic group than in the relatives of the episodic major depressive group, who, in turn, exhibited more chronic depression than the relatives of normal controls. However, the pattern differed as a function of the form of chronic depression. Thus, the relatives of both groups of depressed patients exhibited significantly higher rates of chronic major depression than the family members of normal controls, but did not differ from each other. In contrast, there appeared to be much more specificity in the familial aggregration of dysthymia, with the relatives of early-onset dysthymic probands exhibiting significantly higher rates of dysthymia in general, and of the early-onset subtype in particular, than the relatives of episodic major depressive probands and normal controls.

The results of comparisons of rates of personality disorders in relatives are shown in **Table 4**. The number of subjects with schizotypal personality disorder was too small to include in the analyses. Compared with relatives of normal controls, the relatives of early-onset dysthymic probands exhibited significantly higher rates of any personality disorder; any *DSM-III-R* cluster A, B, and C disorder; and all 10 of the specific personality disorders that were examined. The relatives of episodic major depressive probands exhibited significantly higher rates of any Axis II disorder; any cluster A, B, and C disorder; and paranoid, antisocial, borderline, histrionic, dependent, and obsessive-compulsive personality disorder, and a trend for a higher rate of schizoid personality disorder than the relatives of normal controls. Finally, the relatives of the early-onset dysthymic probands exhibited significantly higher rates of any personality disorder, any cluster B disorder, and passive-aggressive personality disorder, and a trend for a higher rate of borderline personality disorder than the relatives of the episodic major depressive probands.

When the comparisons of rates of personality disorders in relatives were conducted after controlling for Axis II comorbidity in the probands, all the differences between the relatives of the two groups of depressed probands and normal controls remained significant. However, the significant differences between the relatives of the early-onset dysthymic and episodic major depressive groups were eliminated.

Reporting Bias

Two recent studies[28,29] have suggested that informants' family history reports may be influenced by their own psychopathological condition. In particular, when family history and direct interview diagnoses were compared, informants with a disorder provided more sensitive but less specific reports of that disorder in relatives than subjects without the disorder.[28] To explore this issue, we examined the concordance between proband family history reports and SCID/PDE diagnoses based on direct interviews separately for each group for the diagnoses of major depression, dysthymia, any personality disorder, and the three Axis II clusters in rela-

Table 3. Relative Hazards for Onset of First Episode of Mood Disorders in First-Degree Relatives of Patients With Dysthymia and Episodic Major Depression and Normal Controls*

	Relative Hazard (95% Confidence Interval)		
Disorder	**Total DY vs NC**	**EMD vs NC**	**Total DY vs EMD**
Mood disorder	2.7 (1.9-3.9)†	1.7 (1.1-2.6)‡	1.6 (1.2-2.1)‡
Major mood disorder	2.3 (1.6-3.3)†	1.8 (1.2-2.7)‡	1.3 (0.9-1.8)
Bipolar disorder§	5.4 (0.7-42.8)	5.8 (0.7-50.1)	0.9 (0.4-2.8)
Major depression (MD)	2.1 (1.5-3.1)†	1.6 (1.0-2.5)‖	1.3 (0.9-1.8)¶
Recurrent MD	3.0 (1.6-5.6)†	2.0 (1.0-4.1)¶	1.5 (0.9-2.5)¶
MD with treatment	2.0 (1.2-3.3)‡	1.6 (0.9-2.8)	1.3 (0.8-2.0)
MD with medication	3.0 (1.3-6.8)‡	1.4 (0.5-3.9)	2.1 (1.0-4.6)‖
Incapacitating MD	3.7 (1.4-9.4)‡	3.1 (1.1-8.6)‖	1.2 (0.6-2.2)
Chronic depression	6.8 (3.0-15.7)†	3.1 (1.2-7.8)‡	2.2 (1.3-3.8)‡
Chronic MD	4.0 (1.4-11.4)‡	3.2 (1.0-10.0)‖	1.3 (0.6-2.5)
Dysthymia	8.0 (2.5-25.6)†	2.3 (0.6-9.2)	3.5 (1.5-8.1)†
Early-onset dysthymia§	5.4 (1.6-18.2)‡	1.1 (0.2-5.7)	4.8 (1.4-16.2)‡

Total DY indicates relatives of all dysthymics (N=446); EMD, relatives of episodic major depressives (N=207); and NC, relatives of normal controls (N=229). Interview status, sex, and birth cohort of relatives were controlled for in these analyses.

†$P \leq .001$.

‡$P \leq .01$.

§*A logistic regression rather than proportional hazards model was used for this variable; hence, the odds ratio rather than the relative hazard is reported in the table.*

‖$P \leq .05$.

¶$P < .10$.

tives. Sensitivity and specificity were generally comparable across groups for diagnoses of dysthymia and personality disorders in relatives. However, the dysthymic and major depressive probands exhibited somewhat greater sensitivity (35% to 39%) and lower specificity (77% to 81%) than the normal controls (28% and 97%, respectively) in reporting major depression in relatives.

Analyses Using Only Interviewed Relatives

In view of this potential bias in family history reports, we repeated the major proportional hazards and logistic regression analyses using only those relatives who had received direct interviews. The results of these analyses were similar to those reported for the total sample in terms of both statistical significance and the magnitude of the effects, with the following two exceptions: (1) there was a significantly higher rate of major depression among the relatives of early-onset dysthymic probands than among episodic major depressive probands (relative hazard=1.6, $P<.04$); and (2) the difference in rates of major depression between the relatives of episodic major depressive probands and normal controls was no longer significant.

Analyses Using Probands as the Unit of Analysis

As in most family studies, we treated relatives as independent observations in these analyses. Members of the same family are not independent, however. Hence, this may have caused a small reduction in the SEs and slightly inflated the estimates of statistical significance. In addition, a few very large families could have had a disproportionate influence on the results. Thus, we also ran a series of analyses using the proband as the unit of analysis. χ^2 Tests were used to compare the three proband groups on the proportion with a family history of each disorder. In addition, we compared the proband groups on the proportion of relatives in each family with the disorder using analysis of variance. The results were very similar to the analyses reported above, except that the differences between the episodic major depressive and normal control groups on family history of mood disorders did not achieve significance.

Effects of Covariates

Because of space limitations, the effects of the sex, birth cohort, and interview status of the relatives on rates of mood and personality disorders in family members will only be summarized here. For the most part, these associations were consistent with those reported in the literature. Thus, rates of major depression and dependent personality disorder were significantly higher among female subjects, while rates of antisocial, narcissistic, and obsessive-compulsive personality disorder were significantly higher among male subjects. A significant cohort effect[49] was observed for major depression, with a sharp escalation in rates being evident in relatives born after 1930 and remaining elevated in subsequent cohorts. Cohort effects were not significant for dysthymia or the personality disorders. Finally, among subjects with direct interviews, the rates of major depression and dysthymia were significantly higher, while the rate of antisocial personality disorder was significantly lower.

COMPARISONS STRATIFYING DYSTHYMIC PROBANDS ON HISTORY OF MAJOR DEPRESSION

Characteristics of Probands and Relatives

The demographic and clinical characteristics of dysthymic probands with and without a history of major de-

Table 4. Odds Ratios for Personality Disorders in First-Degree Relatives of Patients With Dysthymia and Episodic Major Depression and Normal Controls*

Disorder	Odds Ratio (95% Confidence Interval)		
	Total DY vs NC	EMD vs NC	Total DY vs EMD
Personality disorder	5.2 (3.4-7.8)†	3.6 (2.3-5.7)†	1.4 (1.0-2.0)‡
Cluster A disorder	4.4 (1.9-10.6)†	4.3 (1.7-11.0)§	1.0 (0.6-1.8)
Paranoid	3.4 (1.2-9.8)‡	5.3 (1.8-16.0)§	0.6 (0.3-1.2)
Schizoid	6.2 (1.4-26.7)‡	4.4 (0.9-21.9)‖	1.4 (0.6-3.4)
Cluster B disorder	4.6 (2.6-8.0)†	3.0 (1.6-5.6)†	1.5 (1.0-2.3)‡
Antisocial	4.9 (1.9-12.6)†	3.1 (1.1-8.9)‡	1.6 (0.8-3.0)
Borderline	7.1 (2.5-19.9)†	4.3 (1.4-13.1)§	1.6 (0.9-3.0)‖
Histrionic	8.0 (2.8-22.3)†	6.0 (2.0-18.0)†	1.3 (0.8-2.3)
Narcissistic	2.4 (1.1-5.0)‡	1.7 (0.7-4.1)	1.4 (0.7-2.7)
Cluster C disorder	3.1 (1.8-5.2)†	2.3 (1.3-4.2)§	1.3 (0.9-2.1)
Avoidant	1.8 (0.9-3.6)‖	1.2 (0.5-2.7)	1.6 (0.8-3.1)
Dependent	10.2 (1.4-76.8)‡	11.9 (1.5-94.4)‡	0.9 (0.4-1.9)
Obsessive-compulsive	3.9 (1.6-9.4)§	4.1 (1.6-10.6)§	0.9 (0.5-1.7)
Passive-aggressive	3.9 (1.3-11.2)§	1.3 (0.3-4.9)	3.0 (1.2-8.0)‡

**Total DY indicates relatives of all dysthymics (N=446); EMD, relatives of episodic major depressives (N=207); and NC, relatives of normal controls (N=229). Interview status, sex, and birth cohort of relatives were controlled for in these analyses.*

†*P*≤.001.

‡*P*≤.05.

§*P*≤.01.

‖*P*<.10.

pression are presented in Table 1. There was a significantly greater proportion of men in the dysthymic group without a history of major depression than in the dysthymic group with a history of major depression and the normal controls. Significantly smaller proportions of all three groups of patients than normals were married. The normal controls had a significantly higher social class distribution than the three groups of patients, and dysthymic subgroup without a history of major depression had a higher social class distribution than the dysthymic subgroup with a history of major depression. All three groups of patients exhibited significantly poorer functioning on the Global Assessment of Functioning Scale and greater symptomatology on the Hamilton Rating Scale for Depression than the normal controls, and the episodic major depressive group and the dysthymic subgroup with a history of major depression had higher Hamilton Rating Scale for Depression scores than the dysthymic subgroup without a history of major depression. The mean age of onset of major depression was slightly, but significantly, earlier in dysthymic patients with a history of major depression than in episodic major depressive patients. Finally, dysthymic patients with a history of major depression exhibited a significantly higher rate of lifetime anxiety disorders than those without a history of major depression and episodic major depressive probands; dysthymic patients without a history of major depression reported higher rates of lifetime alcohol and drug abuse and dependence than episodic major depressive patients; and both dysthymic subgroups exhibited a higher rate of personality disorders than the episodic major depressive group.

The relatives of dysthymic probands with and without a history of major depression, episodic major depressive probands, and normal controls did not differ significantly on sex, age, relationship to proband, or type and number of data sources available.

Psychopathology in Relatives

The results of comparisons between the relatives of the two groups of dysthymic probands, episodic major depressive probands, and normal controls on the major diagnostic categories are presented in **Table 5**. The results for the remaining mood and personality disorder diagnoses are not presented because of space limitations, but were similar to those included in the table.

The relatives of the dysthymic groups with and without a lifetime history of major depression did not differ on any of the mood or personality disorders. Similar to the findings for the dysthymic group as a whole, both the relatives of dysthymic probands with and those of dysthymic probands without a history of major depression exhibited significantly higher rates of mood disorders, major depression, dysthymia, and all three clusters of personality disorders than the relatives of normal controls. In addition, the relatives of both dysthymic subgroups exhibited significantly higher rates of dysthymia, and significantly, or trends for, higher rates of any personality disorder and cluster B personality disorders than the relatives of the episodic major depressive group. Finally, there was a trend for a higher rate of bipolar disorder among the relatives of dysthymic probands with a history of major depression than the relatives of normal controls.

COMMENT

To our knowledge, this is the first investigation of dysthymia using the family study method. The results indicate that there is a significantly higher rate of major depression in the first-degree relatives of outpatients with primary early-onset dysthymia than in those of normal controls. Moreover, the rate of major depression in the relatives of dysthymic outpatients was not significantly different from and, in fact, was somewhat greater than that in the relatives of outpatients

Table 5. Odds Ratios for Rates of Psychiatric Disorders in Relatives of Patients With Dysthymia With and Without a History of Major Depression, Patients With Episodic Major Depression, and Normal Controls*

	Odds Ratio (95% Confidence Interval)			
Disorder	DY−MD vs NC	DY+MD vs NC	DY−MD vs EMD	DY+MD vs EMD
Mood disorder	2.8 (1.6-4.9)†	3.5 (2.3-5.4)†	1.4 (0.8-2.3)	1.7 (1.2-2.6)‡
Bipolar disorder	§	7.1 (0.9-55.8)‖	§	1.2 (0.4-3.7)
Major depression (MD)	1.9 (1.0-3.4)¶	2.6 (1.7-4.1)†	0.9 (0.6-1.8)	1.4 (0.9-2.1)
Recurrent MD	2.8 (1.2-6.4)¶	3.5 (1.8-6.8)†	1.3 (0.6-2.7)	1.6 (0.9-2.8)
Chronic MD	3.8 (1.0-13.8)¶	4.4 (1.5-12.9)‡	1.1 (0.4-3.1)	1.3 (0.6-2.7)
Dysthymia	11.9 (3.3-43.5)†	8.2 (2.5-27.3)†	5.0 (1.8-13.7)‡	3.4 (1.4-8.4)‡
Early-onset dysthymia	8.2 (2.2-31.1)‡	4.6 (1.3-15.9)‡	7.3 (1.9-27.7)‡	4.1 (1.2-14.2)¶
Personality disorder	5.4 (3.2-9.3)†	5.1 (3.3-7.8)†	1.5 (0.9-2.5)‖	1.4 (1.0-2.0)¶
Cluster A disorder	4.3 (1.5-12.3)‡	4.5 (1.8-10.8)†	1.0 (0.5-2.2)	1.0 (0.6-1.8)
Cluster B disorder	4.9 (2.5-9.7)†	4.5 (2.6-7.9)†	1.6 (0.9-2.9)‖	1.5 (1.0-2.3)‖
Cluster C disorder	2.5 (1.3-5.1)‡	3.3 (1.9-5.6)†	1.1 (0.6-2.0)	1.4 (0.9-2.2)

**DY−MD indicates relatives of dysthymics with no history of major depression (n=103); DY+MD, relatives of dysthymics with a history of major depression (n=343); EMD, relatives of episodic major depressives (N=207); and NC, relatives of normal controls (N=229). Interview status, sex, and birth cohort of relatives were controlled for in these analyses.*

†$P \le .001$.

‡$P \le .01$.

§*Logistic regression was not used owing to the presence of an empty cell; however, the difference was not significant using a Fisher's exact probability test.*

‖$P < .10$.

¶$P \le .05$.

with episodic major depression. Importantly, these findings held even among the subgroup of dysthymic patients who reported never having experienced a major depressive episode. In addition, the major depressions in the relatives of dysthymic probands were no milder, and indeed appeared to be somewhat more severe, than those in the relatives of episodic major depressive probands. Thus, there was a significantly higher rate of major depression with medication and a trend for a higher rate of recurrent major depression in the relatives of dysthymic probands than in the relatives of episodic major depressive probands, and the relatives of both groups of depressed probands exhibited similar rates of chronic major depression, major depression with treatment, and incapacitating major depression. Taken together, these data provide compelling evidence for a familial link between dysthymia and major depression.

At the same time, dysthymia appears to aggregate specifically in the families of persons with dysthymia. Thus, the rate of dysthymia was significantly greater in the first-degree relatives of dysthymic probands than in the relatives of both episodic major depressive probands and normal controls. Interestingly, this was not the case for chronic major depression, which, like major depression in general, was elevated in the relatives of both dysthymic and episodic major depressive probands. This provides particularly striking evidence for the specificity of transmission of dysthymia in light of the difficulty of distinguishing between these two forms of chronic depression.[9] There also appeared to be some specificity in the aggregation of dysthymia subtypes. Most of the dysthymia in the relatives of early-onset dysthymic probands was of the early-onset type, and the rate of early-onset dysthymia was significantly greater among the relatives of early-onset dysthymic patients than among the relatives of episodic major depressive patients and normal controls. Taken together, the data on specificity of familial aggregation suggest that despite the close relationship between, and frequent co-occurrence of, dysthymia and major depression, these two conditions are also distinct and are not simply variants or different phases of the same disorder.

It has been argued that rather than conceptualizing dysthymia as a mood disorder, it should be more appropriately classified as a personality disorder. This position actually encompasses several distinct arguments.[9] One of these holds that dysthymia is the secondary consequence of a variety of preexisting chronic mental and physical disorders and life stressors, particularly personality disorders. The present findings on the familial relationship between dysthymia and the major mood disorders are inconsistent with this view. However, our data do support the possibility of some form of familial association between dysthymia and the personality disorders. Thus, the rates of most personality disorders were significantly greater among the relatives of early-onset dysthymic probands than among the relatives of normal controls. The rates of personality disorders in general, and cluster B disorders in particular, were also greater in the relatives of dysthymic probands than in the relatives of episodic major depressive probands, although these differences disappeared when Axis II comorbidity in the probands was controlled. However, the relatives of patients with episodic major depression also exhibited significantly higher rates of personality disorders than the relatives of normal controls, suggesting that the processes underlying the association between personality and mood disorders are not specific to dysthymia. Indeed, the fact that the rates of most Axis II disorders were elevated in the relatives of both groups with depression suggests that a common set of familial etiological factors may contribute to the development of a wide variety of forms of mood and personality disorder.

Two previous studies[50,51] have compared the rate of personality disorders in the relatives of inpatients with nonpsychotic major depression and normal controls. Although both studies found higher rates of personality disorders in the relatives of the patients with major depression, the differences were not significant in either study. However, differences were evident when subgroups of major depression that were probably more comparable to those in the study herein were examined. Thus, in both of those studies, the rate of personality disorders in the relatives of patients with nonmelancholic major depression was significantly or marginally significantly greater than that of the relatives of normal controls. In addition, one of the studies[50] also found a significantly higher rate of personality disorders in the relatives of major depressive patients with normal results on the dexamethasone suppression test compared with the relatives of normal controls.

It is noteworthy that the relatives of dysthymic probands with and without a lifetime history of superimposed major depression did not differ on rates of any disorder. Moreover, the pattern of differences between each of these subgroups and the episodic major depressive and normal control groups were generally quite similar. These data have important implications for the conceptualization of "double depression," as they support the view that dysthymia with a history of superimposed major depressive episodes may be much closer to dysthymia without a history of major depression than to episodic forms of major depression, and that the underlying pattern of mild, chronic depression may have greater significance than the superimposed episodes of florid symptoms.[8,52] We plan to explore this issue in greater detail in a future article in which we will specifically examine rates of "pure" dysthymia, double depression, and episodic major depression in our probands' relatives.

Several previous family history[25,26] and follow-up[53,54] studies have suggested that there may be a relationship between dysthymia and bipolar disorder. Our present findings are equivocal on this issue. Thus, the rates of bipolar disorder in the relatives of the dysthymic and episodic major depressive groups were similar and nonsignificantly higher than that in the relatives of normal controls. However, when the dysthmic probands were stratified by history of major depression, there was a trend for a higher rate of bipolar disorder among the relatives of dysthymic patients with a history of major depression than among the relatives of normal controls.

The rates of mood disorders in the relatives of both groups of depressed probands were well within the range reported in recent family studies of major depression and correspond particularly closely to the rates in relatives of patients with early-onset, recurrent major depression.[21,22,47] Our nonpatient controls were screened for Axis I disorders; hence, the rates of psychopathological disorders in their relatives should be slightly lower than those in the general population. In fact, the lifetime prevalence of mood disorders in the relatives of our normal controls was at the lower end of the range of a number of recent epidemiological studies in the United States.[2,55-57] The one major exception is the Epidemiological Catchment Area Study,[58] which reported a much lower rate of mood disorders in the general population. However, unlike our study and the others cited above, the Epidemiological Catchment Area project employed lay interviewers and a highly structured interview schedule that may have underestimated rates of mood disorders.[2,59] Although there are few data on the prevalence of most personality disorders in the general population, our rates among the relatives of normal controls are generally similar to those reported in previous studies.[50,60,61]

In evaluating the results of this study, several methodological factors should be considered. First, our dysthymic sample was limited to the primary, early-onset subtype. While this is the subgroup that has prompted the greatest controversy in the literature, and is the most common subgroup in clinical settings, our findings may not generalize to patients with late-onset dysthymia. Indeed, we have previously reported family history data indicating that patients with early-onset dysthymia have significantly higher rates of mood disorders in their relatives than those with late-onset dysthymia.[62]

Second, our normal controls were selected using telephone directory listings; hence, the sample was not entirely representative because subjects without telephones and with unlisted numbers were not included.

Third, recent studies have found that an earlier onset of major depression and recurrent major depressive episodes in probands are associated with higher rates of major depression in relatives.[63,64] In the present study, the dysthymic probands with a history of major depression were nonsignificantly more likely to have had recurrent episodes and they had a slightly but significantly earlier onset of major depression than the probands with episodic major depression. However, it is unlikely that these factors can account for our findings of similar, and in some cases higher, rates of mood disorders in the relatives of dysthymic probands than in the relatives of episodic major depressive probands, as similar results were obtained when comparisons were limited to the dysthymic subgroup with no lifetime history of major depression.

Finally, we conducted a large number of comparisons, raising the possibility of some type I errors. However, the pattern of findings was highly consistent, and most significant differences were well beyond the .05 level. Hence, this is unlikely to have had a substantial impact on our conclusions.

In summary, the results of the present study provide strong support for a familial link between early-onset dysthymia and major depression. At the same time, however, dysthymia appears to be somewhat distinctive in that it aggregates specifically in the families of persons with dysthymia. Finally, there also appears to be a familial association between dysthymia and the personality disorders, as the first-degree relatives of early-onset dysthymics exhibited elevated rates of most Axis II conditions. However, this relationship does not appear to be specific to dysthymia, as an increased rate of personality disorders was also evident in the relatives of patients with episodic major depression.

Accepted for publication March 13, 1995.

This work was supported by National Institute of Mental Health research grant RO1 MH45757 (Dr Klein).

The assistance of Aliza Cohn, Tova Ferro, MA, Rollin M. Gallagher, MD, Karen L. Kasch, Helen Salisbury Kelly, MA, Laura M. Klein, MSW, Kimberly A. Norden, MA, Carolyn M. Pepper, MA, and Charles L. Rich, MD, in the design of the study, data collection and processing, and the recruitment of subjects is gratefully acknowledged. Armand W. Loranger, PhD, and Robert M. A. Hirschfeld, MD, served as consultants on the diagnosis and assessment of personality disorders. James H. Kocsis, MD, Peter M. Lewinsohn, PhD, and Armand W. Loranger, PhD, provided helpful comments on an earlier draft of the manuscript.

Correspondence to Department of Psychology, SUNY at Stony Brook, Stony Brook, NY 11794-2500 (Dr Klein).

REFERENCES

1. American Psychiatric Association. *Diagnostic and Statistical Manual of Mental Disorders, Third Edition.* Washington, DC: American Psychiatric Association; 1980.
2. Kessler RC, McGonagle KA, Zhao S, Nelson CB, Hughes M, Eshleman S, Wittchen H-U, Kendler KS. Lifetime and 12-month prevalence of *DSM-III-R* psychiatric disorders in the United States. *Arch Gen Psychiatry.* 1994;51:8-19.
3. Weissman MM, Leaf PJ, Bruce ML, Florio L. Epidemiology of dysthymia in five communities. *Am J Psychiatry.* 1988;145:815-819.
4. Friedman RA. Social and vocational impairment in dysthymia. In: Kocsis JH, Klein DN, eds. *Diagnosis and Treatment of Chronic Depression.* New York, NY: Guilford Press. In press.
5. Howland RH. General health, health care utilization, and medical comorbidity in dysthymia. *Int J Psychiatry Med.* 1993;23:211-238.
6. Wells KB, Burnham MA, Rogers W, Hays M, Camp P. The course of depression in adult outpatients. *Arch Gen Psychiatry.* 1992;49:788-794.
7. Akiskal HS. Dysthymic disorder: psychopathology of proposed chronic depressive subtypes. *Am J Psychiatry.* 1983;140:11-20.
8. Akiskal HS. Towards a definition of dysthymia. In: Burton SW, Akiskal HS, eds. *Dysthymic Disorder.* London, England: Gaskell; 1990:1-12.
9. Klein DN. The diagnosis and classification of dysthymia. In: Kocsis JH, Klein DN, eds. *Diagnosis and Treatment of Chronic Depression.* New York, NY: Guilford Press. In press.
10. Kocsis JH, Frances AJ. A critical discussion of *DSM-III* dysthymic disorder. *Am J Psychiatry.* 1987;144:1534-1542.
11. Frances A, Cooper AM. Descriptive and dynamic psychiatry: a perspective on *DSM-III. Am J Psychiatry.* 1981;138:1198-1202.
12. Gunderson J. *DSM-III* diagnoses of personality disorders. In: Frosch JP, ed. *Current Perspectives on Personality Disorders.* Washington, DC: American Psychiatric Press; 1983:20-39.
13. Phillips KA, Gunderson JG, Hirschfeld RMA, Smith LE. A review of the depressive personality. *Am J Psychiatry.* 1990;147:830-837.
14. Angst J, Wicki W. The Zurich Study, XI: is dysthymia a separate form of depression? results of the Zurich Cohort Study. *Eur Arch Psychiatry Clin Neurosci.* 1990;240:349-354.
15. Keller MB, Lavori PW. Double depression, major depression, and dysthymia. *Psychopharmacol Bull.* 1984;20:399-402.
16. Murphy DGM. The classification and treatment of dysthymia. *Br J Psychiatry.* 1991;158:106-109.
17. Van Praag H. Diagnosing depression. *Psychiatr Dev.* 1989;4:375-394.
18. Leckman JF, Weissman MM, Pauls DL, Kidd KK. Family-genetic studies and identification of valid diagnostic categories in adult and child psychiatry. *Br J Psychiatry.* 1987;151:39-44.
19. Robins E, Guze SB. Establishment of diagnostic validity in psychiatric illness: its application to schizophrenia. *Am J Psychiatry.* 1970;126:983-987.
20. Klein DN, Clark DC, Dansky L, Margolis E. Dysthymia in the offspring of parents with primary unipolar affective disorder. *J Abnorm Psychol.* 1988;97:265-274.
21. Goldstein RB, Weissman MM, Adams PB, Horwath E, Lish JD, Charney D, Woods SW, Sobin C, Wickramaratne PJ. Psychiatric disorders in relatives of probands with panic disorder and/or major depression. *Arch Gen Psychiatry.* 1994;51:383-394.
22. Weissman MM, Gershon ES, Kidd KK, Prusoff BA, Leckman JF, Dibble E, Hamovit J, Thompson WD, Pauls DL, Guroff JJ. Psychiatric disorders in the relatives of probands with affective disorder. *Arch Gen Psychiatry.* 1984;41:13-21.
23. Goodman DW, Barnhill J. Family and genetic epidemiological studies. In: Kocsis JH, Klein DN, eds. *Diagnosis and Treatment of Chronic Depression.* New York, NY: Guilford Press. In press.
24. Murphy D, Checkley SA. Dysthymia presenting to the emergency clinic of the Maudsley Hospital. In: Burton SW, Akiskal HS, eds. *Dysthymic Disorder.* London, England: Gaskell; 1990:37-48.
25. Klein DN, Taylor ET, Dickstein S, Harding K. Primary early-onset dysthymia: comparison with primary nonbipolar nonchronic major depression on demographic, clinical, familial, personality, and socioenvironmental characteristics and short-term outcome. *J Abnorm Psychol.* 1988;97:387-398.
26. Rosenthal TL, Akiskal HS, Scott-Strauss A, Rosenthal RH, David M. Familial and developmental factors in characterological depressions. *J Affect Disord.* 1981;3:183-192.
27. Cohen PR. The effects of instruments and informants on ascertainment. In: Dunner DL, Gershon ES, Barrett JE, eds. *Relatives at Risk for Mental Disorders.* New York, NY: Raven Press; 1988:32-51.
28. Chapman TF, Mannuzza S, Klein DF, Fyer AJ. Effects of informant mental disorder on psychiatric family history data. *Am J Psychiatry.* 1994;151:574-579.
29. Kendler KS, Silberg JL, Neale MC, Kessler RC, Heath AC, Eaves LJ. The family history method: whose psychiatric history is measured? *Am J Psychiatry.* 1991;148:1501-1504.
30. Andreasen NC, Endicott J, Spitzer RL, Winokur G. The family history method using diagnostic criteria. *Arch Gen Psychiatry.* 1977;34:1229-1235.
31. American Psychiatric Association. *Diagnostic and Statistical Manual of Mental Disorders, Revised Third Edition.* Washington, DC: American Psychiatric Association; 1987.
32. Spitzer RL, Williams JBW, Gibbon M, First MB. *Structured Clinical Interview for* DSM-III-R. Washington, DC: American Psychiatric Press; 1990.
33. Loranger AW. *Personality Disorder Examination (PDE) Manual.* Yonkers, NY: DV Communications; 1988.
34. Ferro T, Klein DN, Norden K, Donaldson SK, Lizardi H. Development and reliability of the Family History Interview for Personality Disorders. *J Pers Disord.* In press.
35. Klein DN, Ouimette PC, Kelly HS, Ferro T, Riso LP. Test-retest reliability of team consensus best-estimate diagnoses of Axis I and II disorders in a family study. *Am J Psychiatry.* 1994;151:1043-1047.
36. Lizardi H, Klein DN, Ouimette PC, Riso LP, Anderson RL, Donaldson SK. Reports of the childhood home environment in early-onset dysthymia and episodic major depression. *J Abnorm Psychol.* 1995;104:132-139.
37. Leckman JF, Sholomskas D, Thompson WD, Belanger A, Weissman MM. Best estimate of lifetime psychiatric diagnoses. *Arch Gen Psychiatry.* 1982;39:879-883.
38. Kalbfleisch JD, Prentice RL. *The Statistical Analysis of Failure Time Data.* New York, NY: John Wiley & Sons; 1980.
39. Blossfeld H-P, Hamerle A, Mayer KU. *Event History Analysis.* Hillsdale, NJ: Lawrence Erlbaum Associates; 1989.
40. Friedman HS, Tucker JS, Tomlinson-Keasey C, Schwartz JE, Wingard DL, Criqui MH. Does childhood personality predict longevity? *J Pers Soc Psychol.* 1993;65:176-185.
41. Hosmer DW, Lemeshow S. *Applied Logistic Regression.* New York, NY: John Wiley & Sons; 1989.
42. Kendler KS. The super-normal control group in psychiatric genetics: possible artifactual evidence for coaggregation. *Psychiatr Genet.* 1992;1:45-53.
43. Pepper CM, Klein DN, Anderson RL, Riso LP, Ouimette PC, Lizardi H. Axis II comorbidity in dysthymia and major depression. *Am J Psychiatry.* 1995;152:239-247.
44. Hollingshead AB. *Four Factor Index of Social Position.* New Haven, Conn: Yale University, Department of Sociology; 1975.
45. Miller IW, Bishop S, Norman WH, Maddever H. The Modified Hamilton Rating Scale for Depression: reliability and validity. *Psychiatry Res.* 1985;14:131-142.
46. Andreasen NC, Rice J, Endicott J, Coryell W, Grove WM, Reich T. Familial rates of affective disorder: a report from the NIMH Collaborative Study. *Arch Gen Psychiatry.* 1987;44:461-469.
47. Weissman MM, Wickramaratne P, Adams PB, Lish JD, Horwath E, Charney D, Woods SW, Leeman E, Frosch E. The relationship between panic disorder and major depression: a new family study. *Arch Gen Psychiatry.* 1993;50:767-780.
48. Gershon ES, Weissman MM, Guroff JJ, Prusoff BA, Leckman JF. Validation of criteria for major depression through controlled family study. *J Affect Disord.* 1986;11:125-131.
49. Klerman GL, Weissman MM. Increasing rates of depression. *JAMA.* 1989;261:2229-2235.
50. Coryell WH, Zimmerman M. Personality disorder in the families of depressed, schizophrenic, and never-ill probands. *Am J Psychiatry.* 1989;146:496-502.
51. Maier W, Lichtermann D, Minges J, Heun R. The familial relation of personality disorders (*DSM-III-R*) to unipolar major depression. *J Affect Disord.* 1992;26:151-156.
52. Akiskal HS, Weise RE. The clinical spectrum of so-called 'minor' depressions. *Am J Psychother.* 1992;46:9-22.
53. Akiskal HS, Rosenthal TL, Haykal RF, Lemmi H, Rosenthal RH, Scott-Strauss A. Characterological depressions: clinical and sleep EEG findings separating 'subaffective dysthymias' from 'character spectrum disorders.' *Arch Gen Psychiatry.* 1980;37:777-783.
54. Kovacs M, Akiskal HS, Gatsonis C, Parrone PL. Childhood-onset dysthymic disorder: clinical features and prospective naturalistic outcome. *Arch Gen Psychiatry.* 1994;51:365-374.
55. Bromet E, Parkinson D, Curtis EC, Schulberg H, Blane H, Dunn L, Phelan J, Dew MA, Schwartz JE. The epidemiology of depression and alcoholism in a white-collar population. *J Occup Med.* 1990;32:989-995.
56. Kendler KS, Neale MC, Kessler RC, Heath AC, Eaves LJ. A population-based twin study of major depression in women: the impact of varying definitions of illness. *Arch Gen Psychiatry.* 1992;49:257-266.
57. Weissman MM, Myers JK. Affective disorders in a US urban community. *Arch Gen Psychiatry.* 1978;35:1304-1311.
58. Robins LN, Regier DA, eds. *Psychiatric Disorders in America: The Epidemiological Catchment Area Study.* New York, NY: The Free Press; 1991.
59. Parker G. Are the lifetime prevalence estimates in the ECA study accurate? *Psychol Med.* 1987;17:275-282.
60. Maier W, Lichtermann D, Klingler T, Heun R, Hallmayer J. Prevalences of personality disorders (*DSM-III-R*) in the community. *J Pers Disord.* 1992;6:187-196.
61. Samuels JF, Nestadt G, Romanoski AJ, Folstein MF, McHugh PR. *DSM-III* personality disorders in the community. *Am J Psychiatry.* 1994;151:1055-1062.
62. Klein DN, Taylor ET, Dickstein S, Harding K. The early-late onset distinction in *DSM-III-R* dysthymia. *J Affect Disord.* 1988;14:25-33.
63. Bland RC, Newman SC, Orn H. Recurrent and nonrecurrent depression: a family study. *Arch Gen Psychiatry.* 1986;43:1085-1089.
64. Weissman MM, Wickramaratne P, Merikangas KR, Leckman JF, Prusoff BA, Caruso KA, Kidd KK, Gammon GD. Onset of major depression in early adulthood: increased familial loading and specificity. *Arch Gen Psychiatry.* 1984;41:1136-1143.

ORIGINAL ARTICLE

The Prevalence of Dementia and Depression in the Elderly Community in a Southern European Population

The Zaragoza Study

Antonio Lobo, MD; Pedro Saz, MD; Guillermo Marcos, MD; José-Luis Día, MD; Concepción De-la-Cámara, MD

Background: Provocative international disparities reported in the prevalence rates of dementia and depression require further investigation. This is the first psychiatric study, to the best of our knowledge, about the prevalence of *DSM-III-R* dementing and depressive disorders and their relationships in a representative, stratified community sample of the elderly in both a Spanish-speaking country and southern Europe.

Methods: A two-stage screening was completed in 1080 elderly. Sampling with replacement was done, and the cumulative response rate was 88%. In phase 1, lay interviewers administered the Spanish versions of the Mini-Mental State examination and the Geriatric Mental State Schedule–Automated Geriatric Examination for Computer Assisted Taxonomy package. In phase 2, research psychiatrists administered the same instruments and the History and Aetiology Schedule to all the probable cases and a similar number of randomly selected, probably normal subjects.

Results: An estimated 5.5% of the elderly were considered to have a dementing disorder, the most prevalent types being primary degenerative dementia, Alzheimer's type (4.3%), and multi-infarct dementia (0.6%). Depressive disorders were found in 4.8% of the elderly. Psychiatric morbidity, specifically depression, was associated with lower educational levels. "Case levels" of depression were documented in 25.4% of the demented cases and case levels of "organic" disturbance were seen in 18.2% of cases of major depression.

Conclusions: Among the elderly, the prevalence of Alzheimer's disease and multi-infarct dementia, as opposed to depression, increases steeply with age. The overlap found between dementia and depression may have nosological implications. There could be an effect of lower education levels on psychiatric morbidity, particularly on depression.

(Arch Gen Psychiatry. 1995;52:497-506)

BECAUSE OF the rapid increase in the proportion of the aged in the world population,[1] more people are at risk of acquiring age-associated psychiatric and neurological disorders. Among these, dementia is probably the most devastating.[2] The prevalence rates of dementia derived from various studies differ markedly and invite epidemiological analysis, but authors such as Henderson and Jorm[3] have argued that methodological differences are so substantial that it is difficult to make any generalizations. Other authors have been less pessimistic about comparisons between studies,[4,5] but the reported international disparities require new epidemiological investigations. It is now clear that such studies should investigate representative community samples, which include institutionalized and noninstitutionalized elderly, and should use standardized structured methods of assessment specifically developed for the elderly and standardized diagnostic criteria and "case levels" of illness.[3]

Most studies report that Alzheimer's disease (AD) is the most frequent type of dementia in the elderly community,[6,7] but multi-infarct dementia (MID) has been found to be more common in other surveys.[8,9] While some authors have argued in favor of true regional differences in the relative prevalence of both,[10] the issue needs further investigation, since differences might be owing to sampling or methodological differences in surveys. The study of depression in a community investigation of dementia may also clarify the intricate relationships between both nosological entities.[11] Furthermore, recent epidemiological reports have suggested that depression is a risk factor for primary degenerative dementia.[12]

The principal aims of the Zaragoza

See Methods on next page

From the Psychosomatic Service and the Departments of Medicine and Psychiatry (Drs Lobo, Saz, and De-la-Cámara) and Preventive Medicine and Public Health (Dr Marcos), Faculty of Medicine, Universidad de Zaragoza and Hospital Clínico Universitario, Instituto Nacional de la Salud, and the Psychiatric Service, Hospital Miguel Servet (Dr Día), Zaragoza, Spain.

METHODS

STUDY CITY

The site of the study was Zaragoza, the capital of the historical kingdom of Aragon, situated in the northeastern part of Spain. This has been traditionally an agricultural area, but modern industrialization over the last 25 years has produced important migratory movements. Presently, more than half the total geriatric population of Aragon (68 954 [57.5%]) lives in Zaragoza, the fifth largest city in the country (close to 600 000 inhabitants).

DIAGNOSTIC AND SCREENING INSTRUMENTS

The following international instruments previously standardized in Spain by our research group were used:

- Mini-Examen Cognoscitivo (MEC),[13] the Spanish version of the Mini-Mental State examination, a reliable and valid indicator of cognitive disturbance[14] and probably the test of cognitive function in most widespread use.[15] The MEC has a maximum score of 35, and the best cutoff in the geriatric patient is considered to be 23 to 24.[16]
- Geriatric Mental State Schedule (GMS),[17] a semistructured, standardized clinical interview for assessing the mental state of elderly persons. Lay interviewers are able to administer this instrument. We used its shortened, community version, to which the computerized program Automated Geriatric Examination for Computer Assisted Taxonomy (AGECAT) can be applied.[18] This interview is also a syndrome case-finding instrument: the GMS threshold global score discriminates between subjects without mental disorder (noncases) (scores, 0 and 1) and subjects with mental disorder (cases). The latter are graded by severity as mild cases (score, 2) and moderate to severe cases (score, 3); cases also receive a probable diagnosis of dementia, depression, or others, which is recorded by the examiner in the final step of the GMS administration. The reliability and validity of the Spanish version of the GMS has been found to be adequate in hospital samples for both lay interviewers and psychiatrists.[19]
- AGECAT,[20,21] a set of computer programs that analyzes GMS data. The AGECAT groups the items of the GMS into components, which are gathered under eight diagnostic clusters (or syndromes), including organic (defined as cognitive disturbances) and depression syndromes. Each subject is awarded a level of confidence on a scale of 0 to 5 for most diagnostic clusters according to the certainty of diagnosis on that cluster. Therefore, a given subject may be shown to simultaneously have more than one diagnostic cluster or syndrome, for example, organic and depression syndromes. It has been found that levels of confidence of 3 and above correspond to what psychiatrists would usually recognize as a case. In the organic brain syndromes, it has been shown to correspond to diagnoses of dementia made according to the rules of *DSM-III*.[22] Experience with the GMS-AGECAT package includes community studies[18,23] and international comparisons.[5,24] Preliminary data about the validity of the Spanish version have also been reported.[25]
- History and Aetiology Schedule, a standardized method of collecting historical and etiological data from an informant to accompany the data obtained from the respondent with the GMS. It may also be directly administered to respondents when they are judged to be reliable. It is crucial to complete the GMS and facilitate a diagnostic process such as the one done in the present study with the *DSM-III-R* system.[18,26]
- Social Status Schedule,[26] a semistructured, standardized interview for assessing social characteristics and problems in the elderly. Lay interviewers are also able to administer this instrument. The validity of its Spanish version has been tested by the same researchers who standardized the GMS, with satisfactory results. Information provided by the Social Status Schedule is also helpful to document social difficulties required to diagnose dementia in systems such as that of the *DSM-III-R*.[27]

SAMPLING AND CASE-FINDING PROCEDURES

The study sample of the elderly (65 years or older) was proportionately stratified by sex and age (5-year age categories). Sampling size error was fixed at 2.5% and confidence levels at 95%, for a 25% probability of having a mental

(Spain) study were to assess the prevalence of mental illness (especially dementia) and the extent of the need for health and social services among the elderly living in the city and to develop hypotheses about the causation of illness. The main purpose of this article is to report (1) the final prevalence of psychiatric disorder (especially dementia) and the age- and sex-specific prevalence of dementia and depression, as well as the relative prevalence of types of dementia; (2) the validity of screening instruments used; and (3) data about relationships between cognitive and depressive syndromes in the elderly.

RESULTS

SAMPLE CHARACTERISTICS AND RESPONSE RATE

One thousand eighty individuals (95.2%) completed phase 1 of the study. The mean (±SD) age of the sample was 74.9±6.3 years, and the distribution by sex and 5-year age categories appears in **Table 1**. **Table 2** shows other demographic characteristics of the sample: most of the elderly had been born in rural areas and the majority had a limited, primary education. Only 48 individuals interviewed (4.4%) were institutionalized at the time of the study. Three hundred fifty-two elderly were selected for phase 2—198 (56.2%) were considered to be probable cases and 154 (43.7%) to be probable noncases in the first phase. Only 324 (92%) completed the interviewing procedure. Their mean (±SD) age was 75.7±6.5, and Tables 1 and 2 show their distribution by age, sex, and demographic characteristics.

At the end of phase 1 of the survey, 788 elderly responded (69.5% of the whole sample of 1134 individuals) to the first request for participation; another 193 (17%) were first substitutes and 99 (8.7%) were second substitutes. For 54 elderly selected (4.8%), no substitutes could be found. **Table 3** presents the distribution of the 553 nonresponders (346 among the elderly selected; 153

disturbance in some age groups. The sample was randomly selected from the municipal census list and included 1134 elderly (449 men and 685 women) living in the city. Difficulties in tracing the elderly were anticipated, but we had no previous estimates for nonresponse rate, and therefore two substitutes for each individual were also selected with identical procedures. Sampling with replacement has been advocated by other authors in this field.[28]

The elderly were initially informed about the study through an individually signed letter; then an appointment was made by telephone when possible, or the home address was visited. Up to three home visits were made before stopping attempts at contact. In accordance with Spanish laws, verbal informed consent was obtained from each participating individual (or a relative when the individual was unable to understand the terms of the agreement). Institutionalized elderly were interviewed in the institution.

A two-phase epidemiological screening design was used in this study. In phase 1, 10 lay interviewers who were medical students and had been previously taught the standardized methods[19,29] administered the Spanish versions of the GMS and MEC to the elderly. Individuals were nominated as being probable cases on the basis of their GMS threshold global score and/or MEC cutoff point (23-24), which we previously reported to have good validity coefficients.[13,19,25,29] For this particular study, the lay interviewers were instructed to be sensitive by accepting doubtful cases according to their GMS threshold global score as probable cases. They also recorded a probable diagnosis of dementia, depression, or others in all probable cases. Social work interviewers administered the Social Status Schedule in this stage.

All the probable cases and a similar number of randomly selected probable noncases were examined in phase 2, 2 months later, by three research psychiatrists taught the standardized methods and blind to the results of phase 1. They used the GMS and MEC as well as the History and Aetiology Schedule. The period of 2 months between phases was decided on to minimize the possibility of false-positive cases of dementia owing to acute brain syndromes. Outside informants were interviewed when the selected elderly responder was considered to be unreliable. In phase 2, a neurological examination was performed only when the psychiatrist considered it appropriate, specifically in cases of dementia. Medical reports, which are commonly kept at home by Spanish patients and may include laboratory data, were used in some cases to help in the diagnostic process.

At the end of phase 2, the psychiatrists diagnosed the identified cases according to *DSM-III-R* criteria.[27] The instruments used in this study generate enough information to diagnose according to these criteria the main nosological categories found in the elderly community. The psychiatrists were particularly careful to distinguish between AD and MID. In this respect, in all cases of dementia, the History and Aetiology Schedule data were collected from outside informants, a neurological examination was performed, and medical reports were examined when available. The last edition of the History and Aetiology Schedule includes sections covering onset and course of the present illness, psychiatric and neurological history, and the Hachinski Ischemic Score.[30] A hierarchical diagnostic classification was used. For example, if an individual had depression and another nonorganic disorder, he or she was assigned to a depression category. The research psychiatrists were previously considered to be reliable in the diagnoses of the main *DSM-III-R* categories in hospital samples.[19]

STATISTICAL ANALYSIS

Standard validity coefficients of the screening instruments were calculated. The prevalence rates (and confidence limits) of psychiatric disorders, dementia, dementia subtypes, and depression were estimated from the stratified sample of the elderly responders included in the clinical evaluation. Homogeneity of distribution by age and sex of responders and nonresponders was compared using χ^2 analyses during the screening procedure; these statistics were also used to test the independence of prevalence rates. Nass's correction factor[31] was applied when low frequencies appeared in some of the boxes. When sample size was small and/or the frequency of the characteristic being compared was low, Fisher's exact test[32] was used. Throughout, the $P=.05$ level was adopted as a reference point for considering results to be statistically significant.

among the first substitutes, and 54 among the second substitutes) in phase 1 by sex and reason for nonparticipation. Refusal rates did not differ by sex ($\chi^2=0.00003$; $df=1$; $P=.99$).

Table 3 also shows the distribution of the 28 nonresponders in phase 2 by sex, reason for nonparticipation, and psychiatric diagnosis by lay interviewers. More women than men refused the interview (Fisher's exact test, $P=.0116$). It is striking that all nonresponders but one were considered to be probable cases by the lay interviewers. Eleven of them had a probable diagnosis of dementia according to GMS criteria, and 14 had a probable diagnosis of depression.

VALIDITY OF INSTRUMENTS

Table 4 shows the validity coefficients of different screening instruments, calculated in the 324 individuals interviewed in phase 2, both cases and noncases. A psychiatrist's diagnosis of dementia was considered to be the gold standard for the lay interviewers' global score on the MEC, but also for their diagnostic impression of "organic case" (equivalent to dementia) after GMS administration and for the AGECAT organic score. A psychiatrist's diagnosis of depression (any of its *DSM-III-R* subtypes) was considered to be the gold standard for the lay interviewer's diagnostic impression of "case of depression" after GMS administration and for the AGECAT depression score. The efficiency of the screening instruments when using the standard cutoff points was satisfactory. The Spanish community version of the GMS, administered by the lay interviewers, was quite sensitive in detecting both dementia (93.2%) and depression (93.7%). The AGECAT for both dementia and depression (cutoff point 2 to 3, ie, level of confidence of 3 or above, was used to define syndrome cases) was less sensitive, but the specificity was satisfactory. As expected in a sample with a low prevalence of disorder, the positive predictive value of all of these screening instruments was also rather low, in contrast with very good negative predictive value coefficients.

Table 1. Distribution of the Samples by Age and Sex*

Age, y	No. (%) of Subjects Women†	Men†	Total
		Phase 1	
65-69	154 (14.2)	111 (10.3)	**265 (24.5)**
70-74	166 (15.4)	135 (12.5)	**301 (27.9)**
75-79	156 (14.4)	99 (9.2)	**255 (23.6)**
80-84	99 (9.2)	58 (5.4)	**157** (14.5)
85-89	56 (5.2)	26 (2.4)	**82 (7.6)**
≥90	14 (1.3)	6 (0.6)	**20** (1.8)
Total	**645** (59.7)	**435** (40.3)	**1080 (100)**
		Phase 2	
65-69	37 (11.4)	28 (8.6)	**65** (20.1)
70-74	49 (15.1)	37 (11.4)	**86 (26.5)**
75-79	44 (13.6)	39 (12.0)	**83 (25.6)**
80-84	36 (11.1)	20 (6.2)	**56 (17.3)**
85-89	16 (4.9)	9 (2.8)	**25 (7.7)**
≥90	8 (2.5)	1 (0.3)	**9 (2.8)**
Total	**190** (58.6)	**134** (41.4)	**324 (100)**

**Percentages have been rounded and may not sum totals.*
†Percentages are derived from total number of subjects.

PREVALENCE OF PSYCHIATRIC DISORDER

One hundred twenty-eight elderly (11.8%) were considered to be cases, all of them fulfilling *DSM-III-R* Axis 1 diagnostic criteria. As expected, dementia (59 cases) and depression (52 cases) were the most common psychiatric diagnoses. Taking the sampling into account, the final sampling error was 2.6%, and the prevalence rate for dementia was 5.5% (95% confidence limits, 2.9%, 8%). The prevalence rate for depression was 4.8% (95% confidence limits, 2.2%, 7.4%). The following tabulation shows the distribution of the specific *DSM-III-R* diagnoses:

Diagnoses	No.(%) of Subjects
Primary degenerative dementia	46 (4.2)
MID	7 (0.6)
Other dementias	6 (0.6)
Any dementia	**59 (5.5)**
Adjustment disorder with depressed mood	27 (2.5)
Dysthymic disorder	14 (1.3)
Major depression	11 (1.0)
Any depression	**52 (4.8)**
Adjustment disorder with anxious mood	7 (0.6)
Others	10 (0.9)
Any psychiatric disorder	**128 (11.8)**

Alzheimer's disease (46 cases [78%]) and MID (seven cases [11.9%]) were the most frequent types of dementia. Most cases of depression were considered to be adjustment disorders (27 cases [51.9%]). The category "others" includes two diagnoses of schizophrenia; one, delusional (paranoid) disorder; two, delirium; two, alcoholism; one, personality disorder; and two other diagnoses. Some cases diagnosed as dementia had depressive syndromes, and some cases diagnosed as depression had cognitive disturbances, but the overlap between dementia and depression is discussed further below.

AGE-SPECIFIC PREVALENCE OF DEMENTIA

Figure 1 shows the age-specific prevalence of dementing conditions for men, women, and both sexes combined. These results confirm the expected steep rise of prevalence with age. The overall rates for the groups aged 65 to 69 years, 70 to 74 years, 75 to 79 years, 80 to 84 years, 85 to 89 years, and 90 years and older were 0.7%, 3.0%, 4.7%, 11.5%, 14.6%, and 30.0%, respectively. Dementing conditions were more frequent in men (6.4%) than in women (4.8%), but the differences were not statistically significant (Fisher's exact test, $P=.9023$). The overall estimate is also larger for men than for women in all age groups until 89 years, when the trend becomes inverse from that age on, but there were only six demented individuals aged 90 years and older. However, no significant differences were found in the distribution by age and sex (χ^2 with Nass's correction, 5.1942; $df=5$; $P=.41$; [with age groups compacted due to low frequencies in some age groups, χ^2 with Nass's correction, 4.5663; $df=3$; $P=.22$]). The severity of dementia was documented with the GMS clinical criteria. Eleven cases (18.6% of total dementia) were considered to be mild, and 48 cases (81.4% of total dementia) were considered to be moderate to severe, the proportions being similar in men and women.

Figure 2 shows the age-specific prevalence of AD (senile and presenile types are pooled) for men, women, and both sexes combined. Taking the sampling into account, with a final sampling error of 2.6%, the prevalence rate for AD was 4.3% (95% confidence limits, 1.7% and 6.8%). The same trends observed in dementia in general are also observed here, with a rather steep rise of prevalence with age. The rates for the reported age groups were 0.7%, 2.3%, 2.7%, 11.5%, 8.5%, and 25.0%. Alzheimer's disease was more frequent in men (4.8%) than in women (3.9%), but the differences were not statistically significant (Fisher's exact test, $P=.8198$). Similarly, no significant differences were found in the distribution by age and sex (χ^2 with Nass's correction, 4.1982; $df=5$; $P=.52$ [with age groups collapsed due to low frequencies in some age groups, χ^2 with Nass's correction, 3.2961; $df=3$, $P=.37$]). Nine cases of AD (0.8%) were considered to be mild, and 37 cases (3.4%) were considered to be moderate to severe, the proportions being similar in men and women (for mild cases, Fisher's exact test, $P=.1015$; for moderate to severe cases, Fisher's exact test, $P=.5844$).

Seven cases (0.6%) were diagnosed as MID according to *DSM-III-R* criteria, and all were moderate to severe according to the GMS severity criteria. Four cases were diagnosed in men (0.9%) and three in women (0.5%), and the proportion of cases of MID tended to increase with age. Two cases (0.7%) were in the group aged 70 to 74 years; three cases (1.2%), in the group aged 75 to 79 years; one case (1.2%), in the group aged 85 to 89 years; and another case (5.0%), in the group aged 90 years and older.

AGE-SPECIFIC PREVALENCE OF DEPRESSION

Figure 3 shows the age-specific prevalence of depressive conditions (all *DSM-III-R* categories are pooled here)

Table 2. Demographic Characteristics of the Samples and Diagnostic Groups*

Characteristic	Phase 1, No. (%) of Subjects (n=1080)	Phase 2, No. (%) of Subjects: Total Subsample (n=324)	Diagnostic Group: Noncases (n=196)	Dementia (n=59)	Depression (n=52)	Others (n=17)	P†
Place of birth‡							
Urban	328 (30.4)	**100** (31.0)	65 (33.2)	12 (20.3)	19 (36.5)	4 (23.5)	.22
Rural	748 (69.5)	**223** (69.0)	131 (66.8)	46 (78.0)	33 (63.5)	13 (76.5)	
Marital status							
Single	101 (9.4)	**29** (9.0)	21 (10.7)	5 (8.5)	2 (3.8)	1 (5.9)	.43
Married or common law	551 (51.0)	**154** (47.5)	97 (49.5)	25 (42.4)	22 (42.3)	10 (58.8)	
Widowed	421 (39.0)	**140** (43.2)	77 (39.3)	29 (49.2)	28 (53.8)	6 (35.3)	
Separated or divorced	7 (0.6)	**1** (0.3)	1 (0.5)	0	0	0	
Education level							
Some primary	128 (11.8)	**43** (13.3)	19 (9.7)	14 (23.7)	9 (17.3)	1 (5.9)	.01
Primary	767 (71.0)	**242** (74.7)	146 (74.5)	39 (66.1)	41 (78.8)	16 (94.1)	
High school	95 (8.8)	**20** (6.2)	15 (7.6)	3 (5.1)	2 (3.8)	0	
Some college or higher	90 (8.3)	**19** (5.9)	16 (8.2)	3 (5.1)	0	0	

Diagnostic criteria are from DSM-III-R.[27] All dementia types are pooled. Major depression, dysthymic disorders, and adjustment disorders with depressed mood are pooled. Percentages are rounded and may not total 100.

†Determined by χ^2 with Nass's correction. Comparisons are between diagnostic groups.

‡The number of individuals listed for this characteristic does not always add up to the total number in the sample because the few individuals in whom information was uncertain were excluded.

for men, women, and both sexes combined. As hypothesized and opposite of dementing conditions, a rise of prevalence with age is not observed here. In fact, there is a trend for a decrease of frequency with increased age, with the following overall rates for the six age groups: 6.8%, 4.6%, 2.7%, 6.3%, 2.5%, and 5.0%. Depressive conditions were more frequent in women (5.7%) than in men (3.4%), and the differences almost reached statistical significance (Fisher's exact test, P=.0554). The age groups had to be collapsed for statistical comparison by age and sex, and the differences did not reach statistical significance (χ^2 with Nass's correction, 1.4322; df=3; P=.7). Twenty-nine cases of depression (2.7%) were considered to be mild according to the GMS clinical criteria, and a slightly lower number, 23 (2.1%) were considered to be of moderate to severe intensity. These proportions were similar in men and women (for mild cases, Fisher's exact test, P=.1096; for moderate to severe cases, Fisher's exact test, P=.2263).

ANALYSIS OF EFFECTS OF OTHER DEMOGRAPHIC CHARACTERISTICS ON PSYCHIATRIC MORBIDITY

Table 2 shows some sociodemographic characteristics by diagnostic group in the 324 elderly who underwent assessment by psychiatrists in phase 2. The elderly did not differ by place of birth (χ^2 with Nass's correction, 4.503; df=3; P=.29) or marital status (χ^2 with Nass's correction, 6.051; df=6; P=.43). The widowed and separated or divorced groups were collapsed for statistical analysis, since very few individuals were available in some diagnostic categories. Similarly, the group of high school graduates had to be collapsed for statistical analysis with the group of elderly having a college or university education. There were statistical differences by education (χ^2 with Nass's correction, 17.094; df=6; P=.01), the suggestion being that the prevalence of psychiatric morbidity decreases when the educational level increases. Further analyses were needed to explain this association.

Both AD and depression have been related to low educational levels in some reports.[6,33] Therefore, we tested this possible association. The prevalence of AD was higher in the elderly with primary education only, either complete or incomplete (41/285 [14.4%]) when compared with individuals with higher education levels (5/39 [12.8%]), but the differences were not statistically significant (Fisher's exact test, P=.51). Similarly, depression was more prevalent in the group with lower educational levels (50/285 [17.5%]) when compared with the individuals with higher educational levels (2/39 [5.1%]), and the differences were statistically significant (Fisher's exact test, P=.031).

RELATIONSHIPS BETWEEN DEMENTIA AND DEPRESSION

It had been hypothesized that depressive syndromes would be rather frequent in cases diagnosed as dementia, especially in the early or mild stages. Fifteen (25.4%) of 59 cases of dementia included syndrome case levels of depression in the AGECAT program output. Ten cases of dementia (16.9%) fulfilled GMS clinical criteria for a depressive condition, according to the psychiatrists who completed phase 2 evaluations. These cases with comorbidity were scattered across the age groups. There were more in women (seven cases) than in men (three cases), but the differences were not statistically significant (Fisher's exact test, P=.346).

It was also hypothesized that cognitive disturbances would be rather frequent in cases of depression, especially in the most severe. Only five (9.6%) of 52 cases of depression had syndrome case levels of organic disturbance (that is, of cognitive difficulties), according to

Table 3. Nonresponders by Sex and Lay Interviewers' Psychiatric Diagnosis*

Nonresponders	No. (%) of Nonresponders: Moved Away	Untraced	Dead	Refusals	Others†	Total
Phase 1‡						
Women	131 (23.7)	96 (17.4)	51 (9.2)	64 (11.6)	14 (2.5)	**356 (64.4)**
Men	52 (9.4)	63 (11.4)	35 (6.3)	42 (7.6)	5 (0.9)	**197 (35.6)**
Total	**183 (33.1)**	**159 (28.8)**	**86 (15.6)**	**106 (19.2)**	**19 (3.4)**	**553 (100)**
Phase 2§						
Women	7 (25.0)	...	4 (14.3)	8 (28.6)	3 (10.7)	**22 (78.6)**
Men	1 (3.6)	...	3 (10.7)	...	2 (7.1)	**6 (21.4)**
Total	**8 (28.6)**	...	**7 (25.0)**	**8 (28.6)**	**5 (17.9)**	**28 (100)**
Lay interviewers' diagnosis of nonresponders in phase 2						
Noncase						
Women	...	...	...	...	...	...
Men	...	...	1 (3.6)	...	...	**1 (3.6)**
Total	...	...	**1 (3.6)**	...	...	**1 (3.6)**
Dementia						
Women	4 (14.3)	...	1 (3.6)	4 (14.3)	1 (3.6)	**10** (35.7)
Men	...	...	...	...	1 (3.6)	**1 (3.6)**
Total	**4 (14.3)**	...	**1 (3.6)**	**4 (14.3)**	**2 (7.1)**	**11** (39.3)
Depression						
Women	3 (10.7)	...	3 (10.7)	4 (14.3)	2 (7.1)	**12** (42.9)
Men	...	...	2 (7.1)	...	...	**2 (7.1)**
Total	**3 (10.7)**	...	5 (17.9)	**4 (14.3)**	**2 (7.1)**	**14** (50.0)
Others						
Women	...	...	...	...	...	...
Men	1 (3.6)	...	...	...	1 (3.6)	2 (7.1)
Total	**1 (3.6)**	...	...	...	**1 (3.6)**	**2** (7.1)

**Percentages may not sum due to rounding.*
†*Includes census errors, subjects too ill to be interviewed, and monks secluded in monasteries.*
‡*Lay interviewers collected data.*
§*Psychiatrists collected data.*

Table 4. Validity Coefficients of Different Screening Instruments*

Instrument	Cutoff	Percentages: Sensitivity	Specificity	Positive Predictive Value	Negative Predictive Value	Overall Misclassification
MEC	23-24	89.8	83.9	51.2	97.8	15.1
GMS†						
Organic	1-2	93.2	89.4	66.3	98.3	9.8
Depression	1-2	93.7	89.2	68.2	98.3	9.8
AGECAT‡						
Organic	2-3	79.6	91.3	67.1	95.3	10.8
Depression	2-3	84.4	84.2	56.8	95.6	15.7

**Screening instruments were administered by lay interviewers. The gold standard is the psychiatrists' diagnosis. MEC indicates Mini-Examen Cognoscitivo; GMS, Geriatric Mental State Schedule; and AGECAT, Automated Geriatric Examination for Computer Assisted Taxomomy.*
†*Probable diagnoses are indicated as described in the "Diagnostic and Screening Instruments" subsection of the "Methods" section of the text.*
‡*Diagnostic clusters are indicated as described in the "Diagnostic Screening Instruments" subsection of the "Methods" section of the text.*

AGECAT results. The comorbidity cases were scattered across the age groups and all were found in women, the differences by sex being close to statistical significance (Fisher's exact test, $P=.067$). The cognitive problems were more frequent in *DSM-III-R* major depression (2/11 [18.2%]) than in dysthymic or adjustment disorders (3/41 [7.3%]).

In this article, we focus on the discrete entities approach. However, in view of the overlap between depression and dementia, we switched to a continuous approach to study the relationships between them. For this purpose, we looked at the psychopathological symptoms documented with the AGECAT program output and examined the results in all the elderly seen by the psychiatrists, that is, the 324 individuals who underwent screening in phase 2 of the study. The frequency of AGECAT depressive syndrome case levels for each of the AGECAT levels of organic syndromes was calculated. Depressive syndromes were rather frequent across all levels of organic psychopathological symptoms, but tended

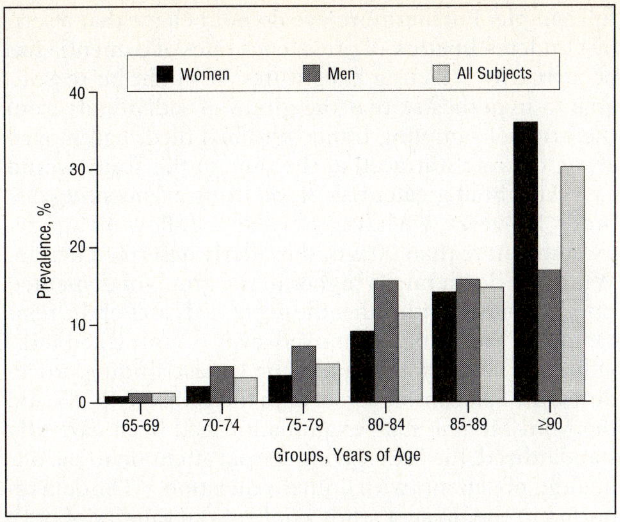

Figure 1. *Prevalence of dementia (*DSM-III-R *criteria*[27]*) in the elderly community by age and sex. All dementia types are pooled.*

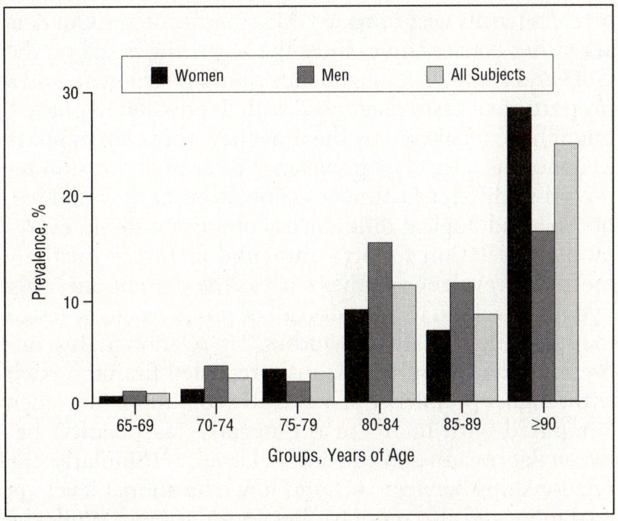

Figure 2. *Prevalence of primary degenerative dementia, Alzheimer's type (*DSM-III-R *criteria*[27]*), in the elderly community by age and sex.*

to be more frequent in the case levels (20/66 [30.3%]) than in the subcase levels (levels of confidence of less than 3) (55/258 [21.3%]), the differences not reaching statistical significance (χ^2=2.3851; *df*=1; *P*=.13). The highest prevalence (14/34 [41.2%]) was seen in AGECAT organic level 3 (equivalent to the mild GMS category of dementia).

From the opposite direction, the frequency of AGECAT organic syndrome case levels for each of the AGECAT levels of depressive syndromes was also calculated. Cognitive disturbances (called "organic" in the AGECAT terminology) also tended to be more frequent in the case levels of depression (20/75 [26.7%]) than in the noncase levels (46/249 [18.5%]), but the differences were not statistically significant (χ^2=2.3851; *df*=1; *P*=.13). However, contrary to the working hypothesis, the highest frequency of cognitive difficulties (42.8%) was seen in AGECAT subcase level 2 of depression, rather than in the most severe cases of depression. Comorbidity according to AGECAT criteria (syndrome case levels of both

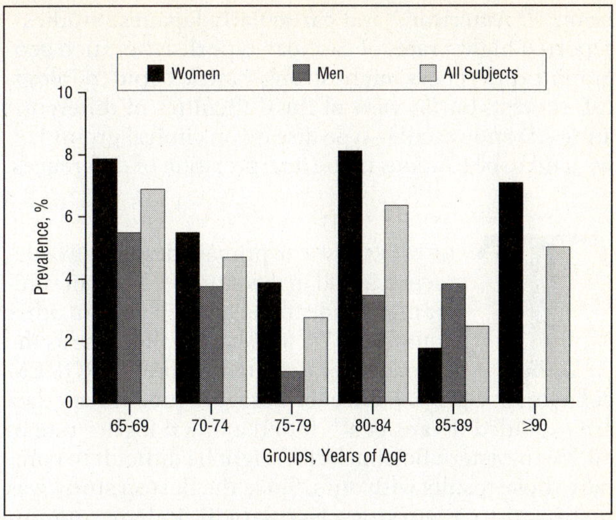

Figure 3. *Prevalence of depression (*DSM-III-R *criteria*[27]*) in the elderly community by age and sex. Major depression, dysthymic disorders, and adjustment disorders with depressed mood are pooled.*

organic and depressive disturbances) was documented in 20 individuals. They were scattered across the age groups; 14 were women and only six were men, but the differences by sex were not statistically significant (Fisher's exact test, *P*=.204).

COMMENT

To our knowledge, this is the first psychiatric report about the prevalence of dementia and other psychiatric conditions in either a Spanish-speaking country or in southern Europe in which a representative community sample of the elderly were investigated with standardized methods specifically developed for this age group. Comparable methods have been used in the Italian[34] and French[35] studies, as well as the present one, that were incorporated by the European Prevalence Research Group (EURODEM),[36] but both the Italian and French Studies were primarily neurological and have only addressed the issue of dementia. A substantial proportion (11.9%) of the elderly living in the city of Zaragoza was considered to have psychiatric morbidity, but some Spanish studies found a similar global prevalence in the adult, nongeriatric population.[37] Therefore, with the exception of dementia, our investigation in a similar sociocultural setting challenges the once prevailing view that old age is inevitably accompanied by higher rates of psychiatric disturbance. The prevalence of dementia documented in this study, 5.5%, and the finding that there is a steep rise of prevalence with advancing age tend to confirm our preliminary data included in two comparative, cross-cultural projects.[36,38] Similar estimates have been reported both in European[36] and non-European countries,[6,10,28,39] the overall similarity having implications for planners of health services.[10]

Seventy-eight percent of the cases of dementia in our study were considered to be AD, and 11.9% were considered to be vascular-type disease or MID. While AD has also been reported to be more common than vascular-type disease in a number of studies,[6,40] some European,[34,41] American,[9] and particularly Japanese studies[42] reported higher rates of vascular-type disease. Such geographic differences might strongly attract epidemiological interest, but in view of the difficulties of differentiating AD and vascular-type disease on clinical grounds,[43] we tend to be cautious in the interpretation of differences.

THE PREVALENCE of primary degenerative dementia found in this study, 4.3%, is of similar magnitude to the rate reported in other countries[28,44,45] and exactly the same as the one now recalculated by the EURODEM collaborative project[7] once the Zaragoza preliminary data are excluded. Evans et al[46] found a much higher rate of 10.3% in eastern Boston, but it might be difficult to compare those results with ours. Since the Boston study was restricted to a working-class, largely Italian community, sample attrition was rather high, and it appears that the functional impairment of a subject was inferred from the degree of cognitive impairment. Although the number of individuals in the group aged 90 years and older in our study is quite small and, therefore, the rates of dementia cannot be treated with the same degree of confidence as those generated from the younger groups, the Zaragoza study tends to confirm that the rates of AD (and similarly the rates of MID) increase steeply with advancing age in both men and women.[7,10]

This finding about the steep increase in the prevalence of AD with age is the most consistent one in the international literature. However, even if age is the most important risk factor for AD, it may conceal the effect of other, weaker risk factors in population studies.[47] In relation to distribution by sex, our study is discrepant, since most researchers documented higher rates of AD in women compared with men[7,10]: the Zaragoza rate of AD was 3.9% in women and 4.8% in men, although the differences did not reach statistical significance. The discrepant findings in our study might relate to greater geographic differences in the prevalence of AD in men than in women.[7] The differences reported in the rate and distribution of types of dementia in different countries generate epidemiological hypotheses, but prevalence studies may be influenced by factors related to duration and fatality rates. Therefore, it is generally agreed now that there is a need for follow-up studies on the incidence of dementia and studies of risk factors based on incident cases. This is the basis for the design of the new EURODEM protocol,[48] which includes the new Zaragoza incidence study.[49]

We do not believe that some methodological problems observed in epidemiological studies have seriously biased our results. The response rate was 95.2% in phase 1 and 92.0% in phase 2, with a cumulative response rate of 88% (0.95×0.92), which compares favorably with a number of previous reports.[18,28,46] The possibility that the inclusion of substitutes in phase 1 might bias the results has also been contemplated. However, the prevalence rate of disorders, as well as the distribution by sex and diagnostic group calculated in the 788 individuals randomly selected as the first choice (or 69.5% of the total sample) were quite similar to the ones reported for the full sample. Furthermore, we do not believe that a serious underestimation of prevalence rates of dementia has occurred by selecting substitutes. It might be reasonable to hypothesize that the group of individuals from the original sampling frame who had died, had moved away, or were untraced at the time of the study would especially be at greater risk of acquiring a dementing disorder. However, we have been able to follow up and reexamine more than 90% of the elderly described herein. While the death rate is higher in the group of demented cases compared with either the depressed cases or the noncases, the proportion of moved away or untracked individuals is not. Finally, in relation to case-finding procedures, the Spanish version of both the GMS-AGECAT and the Mini-Mental State examination had been carefully standardized, the MEC giving special attention to the difficulties of patients with limited education.[13] The data reported in the present study confirm the validity of both instruments in the general population.

The prevalence of depression found in this study was 4.8%, and close to one half the cases were of moderate to severe intensity according to GMS clinical criteria. Our data are rather conservative, since the screening based on the GMS and *DSM-III-R* diagnostic criteria is stringent, and a proportion of cases diagnosed with depression in phase 1 might have recovered by the time they were seen in phase 2, 2 months later. The prevalence rates of depression reported in different countries show important variations, but methodological differences complicate the interpretation in relation to environmental factors.[50] Furthermore, in prevalence studies such as the present one, only hypotheses about risk factors can be produced, to be tested in future, more analytical studies.[49] In relation to this, our present data support previously reported findings, such as the higher prevalence of depressive conditions in women compared with men[51] or the negative association between depression and educational level.[52,53] Similarly, the relationships between AD and low educational level are intriguing and also merit further consideration. While the relationships were not statistically significant in our study, they were in a previous report[34]; furthermore, significant relationships between low education level and cognitive deficits have been documented,[54] including a preliminary analysis in our data set.[55]

Our findings do not support the notion put forward by some authors[11] about the possibility that depression and dementia in the elderly might be common conditions due to dysfunction in an aging brain. First, the prevalence rate of depression documented herein is similar to the one found in studies in adult, nongeriatric individuals in Spain.[37] This coincides with the results of a recent review on community surveys in which a wide range of methods was used.[56] Second, in sharp contrast with the findings on dementia, a rise of prevalence of depression with age has not been observed in our investigation. Other studies have reported similar data in European countries[18] or in the United States.[2] Third, our data do not support an age effect on the comorbidity found. However, an overlap of dementia and depression had been hypothesized and is documented in this article by means of GMS clinical criteria and AGECAT criteria of syndrome clusters and case levels. This overlap complicates the diagnostic process[57,58] and has intriguing nosological implications, in view of the poor outcome of patients who receive diagnoses of depression.[26] Other implications relate to recent reports suggesting that depression is a risk factor for dementia.[12] While the depressive psychopathological symptoms documented primarily in the mildly severe cases of dementia might be interpreted as an emotional adjustment reaction, it is not possible at this stage to rule out the possibility that depression is an early manifestation of a diseased brain.[59] Among all disciplines involved in the epidemiological study of dementia, psychiatry is in a unique position to investigate this subject. The follow-up now under way of cases of both dementia and depression detected in the present study might clarify some of these issues.

Accepted for publication March 13, 1995.

Supported by grant 89-0524 from the Fondo de Investigación Sanitaria, Ministerio de Sanidad, Madrid, Spain, and by the Dirección General de Investigación Científica y Técnica, Secretaría General de Universidades, Madrid.

Presented in part at the 146th Annual Meeting of the American Psychiatric Association, San Francisco, Calif, May 24, 1993.

The authors acknowledge the contribution of the members of the team, psychiatrists and medical students, who participated in the field study as lay interviewers. We also thank Paul R. McHugh, MD, PhD, at the Department of Psychiatry and Behavioral Sciences, The Johns Hopkins Hospital and Medical School, Baltimore, Md, and Lenore J. Launer, PhD, at the Department of Epidemiology and Biostatistics, Erasmus University Medical School, Rotterdam, the Netherlands, for their encouragement and helpful criticisms of the final draft of this article.

Correspondence to Servicio de Psicosomática, Planta 11, Hospital Clínico Universitario, 50009 Zaragoza, Spain (Dr Lobo).

REFERENCES

1. Macfadyen D. International demographic trends. In: Kane RL, Evans JG, Macfadyen D, eds. *Improving the Health of Older People: A World View.* Oxford, England: Oxford University Press Inc and the World Health Organization; 1990: 19-29.
2. George LK, Blazer DG, Winfield-Laird I, Leaf PJ, Fischbach RL. Psychiatric disorders and mental health service use in later life: evidence from the Epidemiologic Catchment Area Program. In: Brody J, Maddox GL, eds. *Epidemiology and Aging.* New York, NY: Springer Publishing Co Inc; 1988:189-219.
3. Henderson AS, Jorm AF. Is case-ascertainment of Alzheimer's disease in field surveys practicable? *Psychol Med.* 1987;17:549-555.
4. World Health Organization. *Dementia in Later Life: Research and Action: Report of WHO Scientific Group on Senile Dementia.* Geneva, Switzerland: World Health Organization; 1985. Technical Reports Series.
5. Copeland JRM, Gurland BJ, Dewey ME, Kelleher MJ, Smith AMR, Davidson IA. Is there more dementia, depression and neurosis in New York? a comparative study of the elderly in New York and London using the computer diagnosis AGECAT. *Br J Psychiatry.* 1987;151:466-473.
6. Anthony JC, Aboraya A. The epidemiology of selected mental disorders in later life. In: Lebowitz BD, Niederehe G, eds. *Handbook of Mental Health and Aging.* 2nd ed. Orlando, Fla: Academic Press Inc; 1992:27-73.
7. Rocca WA, Hofman A, Brayne C, Breteler MMB, Clarke M, Copeland JRM, Dartigues JF, Engedal K, Hagnell O, Heeren T, Jonker C, Lindesay J, Lobo A, Mann AH, Mölsä PK, Morgan K, O'Connor DW, Da Silva Droux A, Sulkava R, Kay DWK, Amaducci L, for the European Prevalence Research Group. Frequency and distribution of Alzheimer's disease in Europe: a collaborative study of 1980-1990 prevalence findings. *Ann Neurol.* 1991;30:381-390.
8. Shibayama H, Kasahara Y, Kobayashi H. Prevalence of dementia in a Japanese elderly population. *Acta Psychiatr Scand.* 1986;74:144-151.
9. Folstein MF, Anthony JC, Parhad I, Duffy B, Gruenberg EM. The meaning of cognitive impairment in the elderly. *J Am Geriatr Soc.* 1985;33:228-235.
10. Jorm AF, Korten AE, Henderson AS. The prevalence of dementia: a quantitative integration of the literature. *Acta Psychiatr Scand.* 1987;76:465-479.
11. Mahendra B. Depression and dementia: the multi-faceted relationship. *Psychol Med.* 1985;15:227-236.
12. Jorm AF, van Duijn CM, Chandra V, Fratiglioni L, Graves AB, Heyman A, Kokmen E, Kondo K, Mortimer JA, Rocca WA, Shalat SL, Soininen H, Hofman A. Psychiatric history and related exposures as risk factors for Alzheimer's disease: a collaborative re-analysis of case-control studies. *Int J Epidemiol.* 1991; 20(suppl 2):43-47.
13. Lobo A, Ezquerra J, Gómez F, Sala JM, Seva A. El 'Mini-Examen Cognoscitivo:' un test sencillo, práctico, para detectar alteraciones intelectivas en pacientes médicos. *Actas Luso Esp Neurol Psiquiatr Cienc Afines.* 1979;3:189-202.
14. Folstein MF, Folstein SE, McHugh PR. 'Mini-Mental State:' a practical method for grading the cognitive state of patients for the clinician. *J Psychiatr Res.* 1975;12:189-198.
15. Oppenheimer C, Jacoby R. Assessment of the elderly patient: psychiatric examination. In: Jacoby R, Oppenheimer C, eds. *Psychiatry in the Elderly.* Oxford, England: Oxford Medical Publications; 1991:169-198.
16. Lobo A, Ventura T, Marco C. Psychiatric morbidity among residents in a home for the elderly in Spain: prevalence of disorder and validity of screening. *Int J Geriatr Psychiatry.* 1990;5:83-91.
17. Copeland JRM, Kelleher MJ, Kellett JM, Gourlay J, Gurland BJ, Fleiss JL, Sharpe L. A semi-structured clinical interview for the assessment of diagnosis and mental state in the elderly: the Geriatric Mental State Schedule, I: development and reliability. *Psychol Med.* 1976;6:439-449.
18. Copeland JRM, Dewey ME, Wood N, Searle R, Davidson IA, McWilliam C. Range of mental illness amongst the elderly in the community: prevalence in Liverpool using the GMS-AGECAT package. *Br J Psychiatry.* 1987;150:815-823.
19. Lobo A, Saz P, Día JL, González JL. El Geriatric Mental State en poblaciones españolas: estudio de validación de parámetros 'orgánicos' y 'afectivos.' *Actas XIII Reunión Nacional SE Psiquiatría Biológica.* Madrid, Spain; SE Psychiatría Biológica;1988;1:333-340.
20. Copeland JRM, Dewey ME, Henderson AS, Kay DWK, Neal CD, Harrison MAM, McWilliam C, Forshaw D, Schiwach R. The Geriatric Mental State (GMS) used in the community: replication studies of the computerised diagnosis AGECAT. *Psychol Med.* 1988;18:219-223.
21. Dewey ME, Copeland JRM. Computerised psychiatric diagnosis in the elderly: AGECAT. *J Microcomput Appl.* 1986;9:135-140.
22. Copeland JRM, Dewey ME, Griffiths-Jones HM. Dementia and depression in elderly persons: AGECAT compared with *DSM-III* and pervasive illness. *Int J Geriatr Psychiatry.* 1990;5:47-51.
23. Black SE, Blessed G, Edwarson JA, Kay DWK. Prevalence rates of dementia in an ageing population: are low rates due to the use of insensitive instruments? *Age Ageing.* 1990;19:84-90.
24. Magnússon H. Mental health of octogenarians in Iceland. *Acta Psychiatr Scand.* 1989;79(suppl 349):1-112.
25. Lobo A, Saz P, Día JL. The AGECAT 'organic' section as a screening instrument for minor cognitive deficits. *Psychiatr J Univ Ottawa.* 1990;15:212-215.
26. Copeland JRM, Davidson IA, Dewey ME, Gilmore C, Larkin BA, McWilliam C, Saunders PA, Scott A, Sharma V, Sullivan C. Alzheimer's disease, other dementias, depression and pseudodementia: prevalence, incidence and three-year outcome in Liverpool. *Br J Psychiatry.* 1992;161:230-239.
27. American Psychiatric Association. *Diagnostic and Statistical Manual of Mental Disorders, Revised Third Edition.* Washington, DC: American Psychiatric Association; 1987.
28. Folstein MF, Spear S, Anthony JC, Romanoski AJ, Nestadt GR. Dementia: case ascertainment in a community survey. *J Gerontol.* 1991;46:132-138.
29. Lobo A, Saz P, Día JL, Marcos G, Morales F, Pérez MJ, Pascual LF, Ventura T, Gracia E. The epidemiological study of dementia in Zaragoza, Spain. In: Stefanis CN, Soldatos CR, Rabavilas E, eds. *Psychiatry: A World Perspective.* New York, NY: Elsevier Science Publishing Co Inc; 1990;4:133-137.
30. Hachinski VC, Iliff LD, Zilhka E, Duboulay GH, McAllister VL, Marshall J, Russell RWR, Symon L. Cerebral blood flow in dementia. *Arch Neurol.* 1975;32: 632-637.
31. Nass CAG. The χ^2 test for small expectations in contingency tables with special reference to accidents and absenteeism. *Biometrika.* 1959;46:365-385.
32. Johnson EM. The Fisher-Yates exact test on unequal sample sizes. *Psychometrika.* 1971;37:103-106.
33. Zhang MY, Katzman R, Salmon D, Jin H, Cai GJ, Wang ZY, Qu GY, Grant I, Yu E, Levi P. The prevalence of dementia and Alzheimer's disease in Shangai,

China: impact of age, gender, and education. *Ann Neurol.* 1990;27:428-437.
34. Rocca WA, Bonaiuto S, Lippi A, Luciani P, Turtù F, Cavarzeran F, Amaducci L. Prevalence of clinically diagnosed Alzheimer's disease and other dementing disorders: a door-to-door survey in Appignano, Macerata Province, Italy. *Neurology.* 1990;40:626-631.
35. D'Artigues JF, Gagnon M, Barberger-Gateau P, Letenneur L, Commenges D, Sauvel C, Michel P, Salamon R. The PAQUID Epidemiological Program on Brain Ageing. *Neuroepidemiology.* 1992;11(suppl 1):14-18.
36. Hofman A, Rocca WA, Brayne C, Breteler MMB, Clarke M, Cooper B, Copeland JRM, Dartigues JF, Da Silva Droux A, Hagnell O, Heeren J, Engedal K, Jonker C, Lindesay J, Lobo A, Mann AH, Mölsä PK, Morgan K, O'Connor DW, Sulkava R, Kay DWK, Amaducci L, for the European Prevalence Research Group. The prevalence of dementia in Europe: a collaborative study of 1980-1990 prevalence findings. *Int J Epidemiol.* 1991;20:736-748.
37. Vázquez-Barquero JL, Díez-Manrique JF, Pena C, Aldama J, Samaniego-Rodríguez C, Menéndez-Arango J, Mirapeix C. A community mental health survey in Cantabria: a general description of morbidity. *Psychol Med.* 1987;17: 227-241.
38. Lobo A, Copeland JRM, Dewey M, Saz P, Día JL. The prevalence of dementia in the elderly people living in Zaragoza and Liverpool. *Psychol Med.* 1992;22: 239-243.
39. Hasegawa K, Honma A, Sato H, Aoba A, Iwai Y, Yamaguchi N, Itami A. The prevalence study of age-related dementia in the community. *Geriatr Psychiatry.* 1984;1:94-105.
40. Henderson AS. The epidemiology of Alzheimer's disease. *Br Med Bull.* 1986; 42:3-10.
41. Rorsman B, Hagnell O, Lanke J. Prevalence and incidence of senile and multi-infarct dementia in the Lundby Study: a comparison between the time periods 1947-1957 and 1957-1972. *Neuropsychobiology.* 1986;15:122-129.
42. Homma A, Niina R. International views: research on Alzheimer's disease in Japan. *Alzheimer Dis Assoc Disord.* 1988;2:366-374.
43. Henderson AS. Epidemiology of dementia disorders. In: Wurtman RJ, Corkin S, Growdon JH, Ritter-Walker E, eds. *Advances in Neurology: Alzheimer's Disease.* New York, NY: Raven Press; 1990;51:115-125.
44. Kokmen E, Beard M, Offord KP, Kurland LT. Prevalence of medically diagnosed dementia in a defined United States population: Rochester, Minnesota, January 1, 1975. *Neurology.* 1989;39:773-776.
45. Hasegawa K, Homma A, Imai Y. An epidemiological study of age-related dementia in the community. *Int J Geriatr Psychiatry.* 1986;15:122-129.
46. Evans DA, Funkenstein HH, Albert MS, Scherr PA, Cook NR, Chown MJ, Hebert LE, Hennekens CH, Taylor JO. Prevalence of Alzheimer's disease in a community population of older persons: higher than previously reported. *JAMA.* 1989;262:2551-2556.
47. Mortimer JA. Do psychosocial risk factors contribute to Alzheimer's disease? In: Henderson AS, Henderson JH, eds. *Etiology of Dementia of Alzheimer's Type.* New York, NY: John Wiley & Sons Inc; 1988:39-52.
48. Launer LJ, Brayne C, Breteler MMB. Epidemiologic approach to the study of dementing diseases: a nested case-control study in European incidence studies of dementia. *Neuroepidemiology.* 1992;11(suppl 1):114-118.
49. Lobo A, Saz P, Marcos G, Morales F. Incidence of dementia and other psychiatric conditions in the elderly: Zaragoza study. *Neuroepidemiology.* 1992; 11(suppl 1):52-56.
50. Kay DWK, Henderson AS, Scott R, Wilson J, Rickwood D, Grayson DA. Dementia and depression among the elderly living in the Hobart community: the effect of the diagnostic criteria on the prevalence rates. *Psychol Med.* 1985; 15:771-788.
51. Weissman MM, Klerman GL. Gender and depression. *Trends Neurosci.* 1985; 8:416-420.
52. Weissman MM, Bruce ML, Leaf PJ, Florio LP, Holzer CE. Affective disorders. In: Robins LN, Regier DA, eds. *Psychiatric Disorders in America.* New York, NY: The Free Press; 1991:53-80.
53. Kivela SL, Pahkala K. Dysthymic disorder in the aged in the community. *Soc Psychiatry Psychiatr Epidemiol.* 1989;24:77-83.
54. Bachman DL, Linn RT, Wolf PA, Knoefel JE, White LR, D'Agostino RB. Influence of education on cognitive decline with advancing age: preliminary results of the Framingham Study. *Neurology.* 1989;39(suppl 1):285.
55. Día JL. *Psicopatología Cognitiva en una Muestra Representativa de Ancianos de la Población General.* Zaragoza, Spain: Universidad de Zaragoza; 1992. Doctoral thesis.
56. Feinson MC. Are psychological disorders most prevalent among older adults? examining the evidence. *Soc Sci Med.* 1989;29:1175-1181.
57. Ames D, Dolan R, Mann A. The distinction between depression and dementia in the very old. *Int J Geriatr Psychiatry.* 1990;5:193-198.
58. Rabins PV, Merchant A, Nestadt G. Criteria for diagnosing reversible dementia caused by depression: validation by 2-year follow-up. *Br J Psychiatry.* 1984; 144:488-492.
59. Kral VA. The relationship between senile dementia (Alzheimer type) and depression. *Can J Psychiatry.* 1983;28:304-306.

Clozapine-Associated Postoperative Ileus: Case Report and Review of the Literature

It has long been known that long-term phenothiazine therapy can produce paralytic ileus, obstruction, obstipation, and constipation. It is hypothesized that this is mediated by phenothiazines' parasympatholytic action on the gastrointestinal tract. However, in animal models, potent anticholinergic action alone is not sufficient to account for the tissue damage (inflammation, edema, and hemorrhage) produced by phenothiazines.[1]

Clozapine, an atypical neuroleptic medication with potent anticholinergic properties, is known to produce constipation in approximately 14% of patients. As of September 1, 1992, there have been at least 19 cases of severe complications of constipation associated with clozapine therapy (M. B. Krassner, MD, written communication, 1993). These included eight cases of bowel obstruction, seven cases of fecal impaction, three cases of paralytic ileus, and one case of obstipation. Several of these patients required hospitalization, four required surgical intervention, and in four cases, the outcome was fatal. Of the four patients who required surgical intervention, data on the postoperative course are unavailable.

To date, no studies have addressed the possible additive or synergistic effects of long-term treatment with neuroleptic drugs (phenothiazines or other classes) on postoperative gastrointestinal function. Postoperative ileus, which is not uncommon, is presumed to be secondary to intestinal sympathetic neuronal hyperactivity, but its pathophysiologic processes remain incompletely understood. After colon resection, a postoperative ileus may take up to 6 days to resolve, but peristalsis usually returns within 48 hours.[2]

The following case is, to the best of our knowledge, the first report of a prolonged postoperative paralytic ileus in a patient receiving long-term clozapine therapy. Additionally, the ileus occurred later postoperatively than is commonly seen (within the first 3 to 4 days[3]) in surgical patients not receiving a neuroleptic medication.

Report of a Case. A 42-year-old man with schizophrenia began clozapine therapy in January 1991. He has received 450 mg of clozapine daily since the fall of 1991. Preoperatively, he had no history of gastrointestinal tract symptoms. In January 1993, a right hemicolectomy was performed for a Dukes' class C_2 adenocarcinoma of the cecum. Hypoactive bowel sounds were noted on postoperative day 2. By day 4, the patient had normoactive bowel sounds and was passing flatus. Accordingly, on postoperative day 4, the patient began receiving a liquid diet, and he progressed to a regular diet on day 5. Discharge from the hospital was postponed on day 6 because of several orthostatic-induced syncopal episodes. On day 7, an adynamic ileus was diagnosed in the patient; oral intake was withheld. His ileus resolved on day 13, and he again began receiving a liquid diet. He progressed to a regular diet the next day and was discharged on postoperative day 15.

Clozapine treatment was interrupted for 2 days (the day prior to surgery and the day of surgery). Other medications included atenolol and ferrous sulfate, and their administration was discontinued prior to surgery.

Pain medication was limited to three 1-mg doses of morphine sulfate on days 1, 3, and 4. There were no other confounding variables; no electrolyte imbalances, inflammation, or severe pain was present. During his hospital stay, the patient experienced no change in mental status and was able to communicate his symptoms, primarily hunger and mild discomfort. Through 14 months of follow-up after surgery, he has experienced no subsequent gastrointestinal tract symptoms or evidence of carcinoma recurrence.

Comment. Because postoperative ileus is potentially life threatening, the physician should be aware that the use of clozapine has been associated with severe gastrointestinal tract complications. This case report suggests that administration of clozapine may potentiate adynamic ileus postoperatively. The character of the postoperative adynamic ileus may also differ from that occurring in non–clozapine-treated patients after abdominal surgery. The ileus may be prolonged and/or may occur later than expected. An ileus of any origin promotes fluid movement from the intravascular to the extravascular compartment. This, in turn, can lead to orthostatic hypotension, the above patient's first clinical sign of an ileus. We believed that the risk of discontinuing the administration of clozapine in this patient (including the clinical management of psychosis on a surgical ward) was greater than the increased risk of a prolonged paralytic ileus after bowel resection.

Brenda Erickson, MD
Department of Psychiatry
University of New Mexico
2400 Tucker Blvd NE
Albuquerque, NM 87108
Don M. Morris, MD
Alison Reeve, MD
Albuquerque, NM

1. Szanto P, Ehrenpreis E, Krakow M, Rubinstein O, Ehrenpreis S. Histologic changes in the guinea pig gastrointestinal tract following 1 weeks' administration of chlorpromazine, haloperidol, or atropine. *Psychopharmacology*. 1988; 95:351-355.
2. Way LW. *Current Surgical Diagnosis and Treatment*. 10th ed. Los Altos, Calif:

Lange Medical Publications. 1994;616-617.
3. Nadrowski L. Paralytic ileus: recent advances in pathophysiology and treatment. *Curr Surg*. 1983;40:260-273.

The Prevalence of Schizophrenia in Ireland: Readdressing the Enigma

Consequent to the recent report by Kendler and colleagues in the ARCHIVES,[1] Torrey[2] challenges their assertion that there is not a high rate of schizophrenia in the general population in Ireland, while Walsh and Kendler[3] defend their position; curiously, these antagonists fail to note data published previously in the ARCHIVES that is not only highly relevant to this important, long-standing, and apparently still unresolved controversy, but may also offer some resolution of the impasse.

The most recent systematic (*DSM-III-R*) catchment area epidemiological study of both the incidence and the prevalence of schizophrenia in rural Ireland[4] reports overall rates that are entirely unremarkable and fall well within the midrange of values recorded previously on a worldwide basis, eg, a lifetime morbid risk (±SE) of 0.7%±0.1% that is virtually identical to the value derived by Walsh and Kendler[3]; thus, there would appear to be little contemporary evidence for generally high rates of schizophrenia in Ireland, contrary to the position of Torrey. However, this overall, macroscopic estimate obscures significant geographical variations in the rate of occurrence that become evident on examining the spatial microstructure of the individual cases that constitute the total patient population within the study region.[4,5] That there appear to be significant geographically discrete pockets of high (eg, 2.6%±0.9%) and low (eg, 0.0%±0.0%) rates[4,6] would now appear to support aspects of Torrey's position[2] and contradict that of Walsh and Kendler.[3] As for many aspects of scientific inquiry, the answer depends on precisely what question one asks and how one asks it; Torrey and Walsh and Kendler may not actually be debating the same question.

Just as local geographical variations in the rate of occurrence of schizophrenia may be obscured by too macroscopic an analysis, so might secular variations be obscured similarly. Integrated over a 50-year period, the risk for schizophrenia in rural Ireland was again entirely unremarkable but this obscured a significant fall in risk for persons born since 1940,[7] as noted by Torrey.[2] These are complex issues for which substantial patient populations aggregated over large areas or long periods can superficially reassure as to the results derived, but may actually "flatter to deceive" by obscuring potentially important dimensional variations; as both geographical[6] and temporal[7] variations in rate of occurrence of schizophrenia appear more prominent among women than among men, it may also be unwise to pool the genders in such analyses.

Ireland presents rare opportunities for studying the epidemiology of schizophrenia, but the yield therefrom will not be maximized without eclectic consideration of all of the available data; Torrey and Walsh and Kendler may only *appear* to be antagonists, as the findings discussed above offer a route to reconciling several elements of their respective positions.

John L. Waddington, PhD, DSc
Department of Clinical Pharmacology
Royal College of Surgeons in Ireland
St Stephen's Green
Dublin 2, Ireland
Hanafy A. Youssef, DM, FRCPsych
Monaghan, Ireland
Anthony Kinsella, MSc
Dublin

1. Kendler KS, McGuire M, Gruenberg AM, O'Hare A, Spellman M, Walsh D. The Roscommon Family Study, I: methods, diagnosis of probands, and risk of schizophrenia in relatives. *Arch Gen Psychiatry*. 1993;50:527-540.
2. Torrey EF. The prevalence of schizophrenia in Ireland. *Arch Gen Psychiatry*. 1994;51:513.
3. Walsh D, Kendler KS. The prevalence of schizophrenia in Ireland. *Arch Gen Psychiatry*. 1994;51:513-515.
4. Youssef HA, Kinsella A, Waddington JL. Evidence for geographical variations in the prevalence of schizophrenia in rural Ireland. *Arch Gen Psychiatry*. 1991;48:254-258.
5. Waddington JL, Youssef HA, Kinsella A. Geographic variations in the prevalence of schizophrenia. *Arch Gen Psychiatry*. 1992;49:907-908.
6. Youssef HA, Kinsella A, Waddington JL. Gender specificity of geographical variation in morbid risk for schizophrenia in rural Ireland. *Acta Psychiatr Scand*. 1993;88:135-139.
7. Waddington JL, Youssef HA. Evidence for a gender-specific decline in the rate of schizophrenia in rural Ireland over a 50-year period. *Br J Psychiatry*. 1994; 164:171-176.

In reply

Waddington and his colleagues take us to task for omitting to refer to their recent work on the topic of the general population rate of schizophrenia in Ireland. We regret this omission, the more so as their findings are confirmatory of our own work on the same topic.

They rightly point out that overall general population rates may obscure pockets of high incidence and/or prevalence in localized areas and they note their own findings in an Irish county in this regard. However, observations of this kind on a microscale may throw up variations between contiguous regions of small population size simply by chance, as has been pointed out by Lin and Goodman[1] in this journal when commenting on the original presentation by Youssef and colleagues.[2] An additional difficulty arises with the diagnostic cross-reliability between studies, although this of course is not relevant to the interregional variation observed in the work by Youssef et al, which was carried out by one diagnostician only. In any case, observations of high rates in local geographic areas are not in any way in conflict with the lower national rates found by ourselves and by Waddington and colleagues. Finally, these comments are equally relevant to the findings of Torrey, which were also based on a geographic isolate.

Dermot Walsh, MB, FRCPI
The Health Research Board
73 Lower Baggot St
Dublin 2, Ireland
Kenneth S. Kendler, MD
Richmond, Va

1. Lin SP, Goodman AB. Geographic variations in the prevalence of schizophrenia. *Arch Gen Psychiatry*. 1992;49:906-907.
2. Youssef HA, Kinsella A, Waddington JL. Evidence for geographical variations in the prevalence of schizophrenia in rural Ireland. *Arch Gen Psychiatry*. 1991;48:254-258.

Professional Opportunities

Physician Recruitment

Psychiatry
Multiple Specialties/Group Practice
Locum Tenens Wanted
Graduate Training/Residencies/Fellowships
Chiefs/Department Heads/Directors
Academic/Faculty
CME Corner
Courses/Symposia/Seminars
Practices For Sale
Notices

1995 Professional Opportunity Rates

Regular	1x	1.10/wd	*3x	1.00/wd
Bold	1x	1.25/wd	*3x	1.15/wd

*In order to receive the 3 time frequency price, the request must be made upon initial placement. The minimum charge is 20 words. A word consists of one or more letters surrounded by space on each side.

For information on display advertising and our network buys contact an account representative.

Policy

Orders for classified advertising must be submitted in writing. Although the American Medical Association believes the classified advertisements in these pages to be from reputable sources, the Association does not investigate the offers made and assumes no liability concerning them. Acceptance of advertising is restricted to professional opportunities, practices for sale, and medical office space available. The Association reserves the right to decline, withdraw, or edit advertisements at its discretion. Every care is taken to avoid mistakes but responsibility cannot be accepted by the Association for clerical or printer's errors.

Blind Box Service

Confidential box numbers are available for an additional $20 per issue, plus the words - Box ____, c/o AGNP.

When responding to a box number, please send to Archives of General Psychiatry, Box ____, c/o AGNP, 515 N State St, Chicago, IL 60610.

Cancellations/Changes

Cancellations/changes must be received in writing at least 25 days prior to the date of the issue. In order to expedite, please fax to 312-464-5909 to the attention of your account representative.

General Information

To contact a Physician Recruitment Advertising account representative, call 312-464-2475/2490/2491/4485 or **800-AMA-2260.** Or fax your insertion order to **312-464-5909**. Mail your materials to **AMA Physician Recruitment Advertising, 12th Floor, 515 N State St, Chicago, IL 60610**.

Psychiatry

JACKSON: BE/BC GENERAL PSYCHIATRIST POSITION AND DEVELOPMENTAL NEUROPSYCHIATRIST position available at state-operated JCAHO accredited 300-bed inpatient facility. 40 hrs/week; salary negotiable via competitive pay plan based on training, experience, and certification. Deferred retirement membership and leave package. Private practice allowed after hours. Louisiana license required. Low-cost housing available on grounds. East Louisiana State Hospital is located in East Feliciana Parish and serves as a primary psychiatric facility for adults that serves all 64 parishes. Historic Jackson is primarily a residential community within 30 minutes from Baton Rouge, one hour and 20 minutes from New Orleans, and five miles from Audubon State Commemorative Park. The area emphasizes family life and has a large number of churches. Fishing, water sports, and hunting activities nearby. EO/AA Employer. Send vitae to Denise M. Graham, MD, Clinical Director, or Fred Calcote, CEO, ELSH, PO Box 498, Jackson, LA 70748. Telephone 504-634-2651, ext 200 or ext 216; fax 504-634-5827.

Nationwide
PSYCHIATRY
&
NEUROLOGY
Positions
We know how busy you are.
Let us do the mundane busy work.
1 (800) 428-4406
Physician Search Associates

ILLINOIS: Outstanding opportunity for a BC/BE psychiatrist to join two other psychiatrists in a newly developed Regional Mental Health Center in Peru, Illinois. Includes a 20-bed psychiatry unit, a 1:3 call schedule, competitive salary or income guarantee, and a comprehensive benefits package. Peru, with a draw of 120,000, is located in the beautiful Illinois Valley where recreational activities abound, including sailing and cross country skiing. Together with excellent schools, diverse cultural opportunities, and a low cost of living, Peru offers superb quality of life. Contact Steve Baker at 800-430-6587 or Marie Noeth at 800-438-3745 or fax your CV to 309-685-2574.

PSYCHIATRIST: General psychiatrist, BC/BE, needed to develop a practice in conjunction with local community 231-bed hospital with the largest mental health system in the region, one hour from Pittsburgh, PA. This Ohio opportunity has attractive compensation, medical directorships, private, group, and salaried opportunities, very attractive family lifestyle with the best of both a big city and a small town atmosphere. For more information, call 800-443-9346 or send CV to Richard L. Shrum, Vice President, Diamond Healthcare Corporation, 700 East Main Street, Suite 900, Richmond, VA 23219.

TEXAS, the SOUTHEAST, and the SUNBELT STATES- There are Excellent Private Practice Opportunities Available in Psychiatry. Major Cities and Rural Communities Are Available.

Call 1-800-284-4560/Houston 713-493-2797

Or send CV to:
P.O. Box 42314
Houston, TX 77242-2314
FAX 713-493-2234

Reuben Bronstein & Associates

Blind Box Service
is available for an
additional $20 per insertion.

PSYCHIATRISTS: The California Department of Corrections has immediate opportunities at the California Men's Colony at San Luis Obispo, located on the scenic central California coast, midway between San Francisco & Los Angeles. Our largest outpatient multidisciplinary mental health facility offers a spectacular environment with beaches, sailing, cultural activities, clean air, and excellent schools. BE/BC, CA licensed. For more information, contact Karl Weaver, MD, 805-547-7957 x 7297, or Anne Perez, 916-327-7081. EOE.

GEROPSYCHIATRY FACULTY
University of Michigan

Position available immediately for academic geropsychiatrist for tenure-track position (Assistant Professor) at the Ann Arbor VA Medical Center (VAMC) and University of Michigan in Ann Arbor, MI. Position involves participation in clinical care, education, and research in a growing Geriatric Psychiatry division with an active, ACGME-accredited fellowship training program. The Medical Center and University provide an extraordinarily rich academic environment, fostering collaborations among faculty both within Psychiatry and in other departments. University has NIA-funded Alzheimer's Disease Research Center and Geriatric Research and Training Center, as well as NIAAA-funded Alcohol Research Center, specializing in aging. VAMC has a Geriatric Research, Educational, and Clinical Center (GRECC). Successful candidate will have adequate protected time and should have demonstrated potential for developing an independent research program in a clinical or preclinical area related to geriatric psychiatry. MD or MD-PhD applicants with clinical and/or laboratory-based research interests are appropriate. Preference will be given to candidates with fellowship training in geriatric psychiatry and holding the ABPN Certificate of Added Qualifications in Geriatric Psychiatry. Successful applicant must be eligible for a full-time faculty appointment in University of Michigan Medical School. The Ann Arbor VAMC and The University of Michigan are equal opportunity employers. Please send CV to:

Alan M. Mellow, MD, PhD, Chief
Psychiatry Service (116A)
Ann Arbor VA Medical Center
2215 Fuller Road
Ann Arbor, MI 48105

Locum Tenens Wanted

HKA LOCUM TENENS is looking for quality general psychiatry physicians to do Locum Tenens. We have opportunities coast-to-coast. We furnish Occurence Malpractice Insurance (no tail necessary). Please call **HKA LOCUM TENENS at (800)226-6347, Extension AM7.1.**

For more
Professional Opportunities
please refer to
the Physician Recruitment
sections in ***JAMA***
and ***AMNews***.

THIS MONTH IN

ARCHIVES OF GENERAL PSYCHIATRY

Lithium is the most effective treatment for bipolar affective disorder. **Manji et al** (page 531) review and integrate the exciting recent progress in the identification of second-messenger generating systems as targets for lithium's actions. Lithium can thus regulate multiple neurotransmitter systems in critical regions of the brain, and Manji et al propose that these effects play a major role in the treatment of recurrent affective disorders. The identification of these targets may lead to the development of novel, improved therapeutics and may facilitate our understanding of the biological factors predisposing individuals to bipolar affective disorder.

Since Kraepelin's description of the course of schizophrenia (dementia praecox) at the beginning of this century, there has been controversy regarding whether some schizophrenic patients show a progressive neurodegenerative course after the onset of the illness. To examine this, **O'Donnell et al** (page 544) used a neurophysiological measure of mental processing speed, P300 latency, whose prolongation is usually associated with neural damage or degeneration. Evaluation of groups of adult male schizophrenic patients and age-matched normal control subjects showed that the rate of prolongation of P300 latency was greater among schizophrenic patients than control subjects. These findings provide neurophysiological evidence that male patients with chronic schizophrenia experience a neurodegenerative process that becomes evident in adulthood.

Functional brain imaging studies of memory dysfunction in schizophrenia have focused primarily on high-order association regions such as prefrontal cortex or hippocampus. Using electrophysiological imaging, **Javitt et al** (page 550) now find that memory disturbances can be demonstrated even at the level of auditory sensory cortex. Auditory cortex normally maintains a short-duration representation of recent events and automatically detects events that differ from those in memory. Schizophrenic patients experience less automatic activation than do controls to novel events, indicating widespread memory dysfunction, which is consistent with the predictions of the phencyclidine/*N*-methyl-D-aspartate model of schizophrenia.

A Commentary by Adolf Pfefferbaum et al on event-related potentials in the study of psychiatric disorders is included in this issue.

The current classification of phobias departs from earlier systems in defining simple phobia, social phobia, and agoraphobia with panic disorder as separate disorders. Although these changes have stimulated research, their validity remains uncertain. In particular, the higher than expected comorbidity among these disorders suggests some causal overlap. Using the family study method, **Fyer et al** (page 564) found that when each of these disorders occurs without lifetime anxiety comorbidity, it is familial and "breeds true." These findings support a specific familial contribution to each phobic disorder and suggest that there may be causally discrete syndromes within the group of cases identified by each of these criteria sets.

Prior study has shown that relatives of persons with panic disorder have a higher risk for social phobia than relatives of persons without panic disorder. **Horwath et al** (page 574) report on a family study in which they found that social phobia frequently co-occurs with panic disorder in relatives of persons with panic disorder and/or major depression but the risk for comborbidity does not vary across different proband groups. They conclude that further family studies are needed to determine whether the co-occurrence of social phobia and panic disorder is caused by a shared familial diathesis.

The neurobiological abnormalities of posttraumatic stress disorder (PTSD) may be quite different from those observed in major depression or classic stress responses. **Yehuda et al** (page 583) evaluated the plasma cortisol and lymphocyte glucocorticoid responses to low doses of dexamethasone of combat veterans with PTSD, combat veterans without PTSD, and demographically similar normal men. Combat veterans with PTSD showed a significantly greater cortisol suppression and a significant decline in the number of cytosolic glucocorticoid receptors following dexamethasone administration. The data suggest that combat veterans with PTSD show an enhanced sensitivity of the hypothalamic-pituitary-adrenal axis that can be distinguished from general effects produced by the traumatic experience of combat.

The high prevalence of mental illness observed in Western societies among persons who commit suicide has never been examined in Eastern countries. **Cheng** (page 594) reports a biographical case-control study of consecutive suicides among two aboriginal groups and the Han Chinese in East Taiwan. In all three groups, a very high proportion of suicides had mental illness before committing suicide. This finding strongly indicates that suicide is universally linked with mental illness, in particular with comorbid depression and alcoholism.

Because

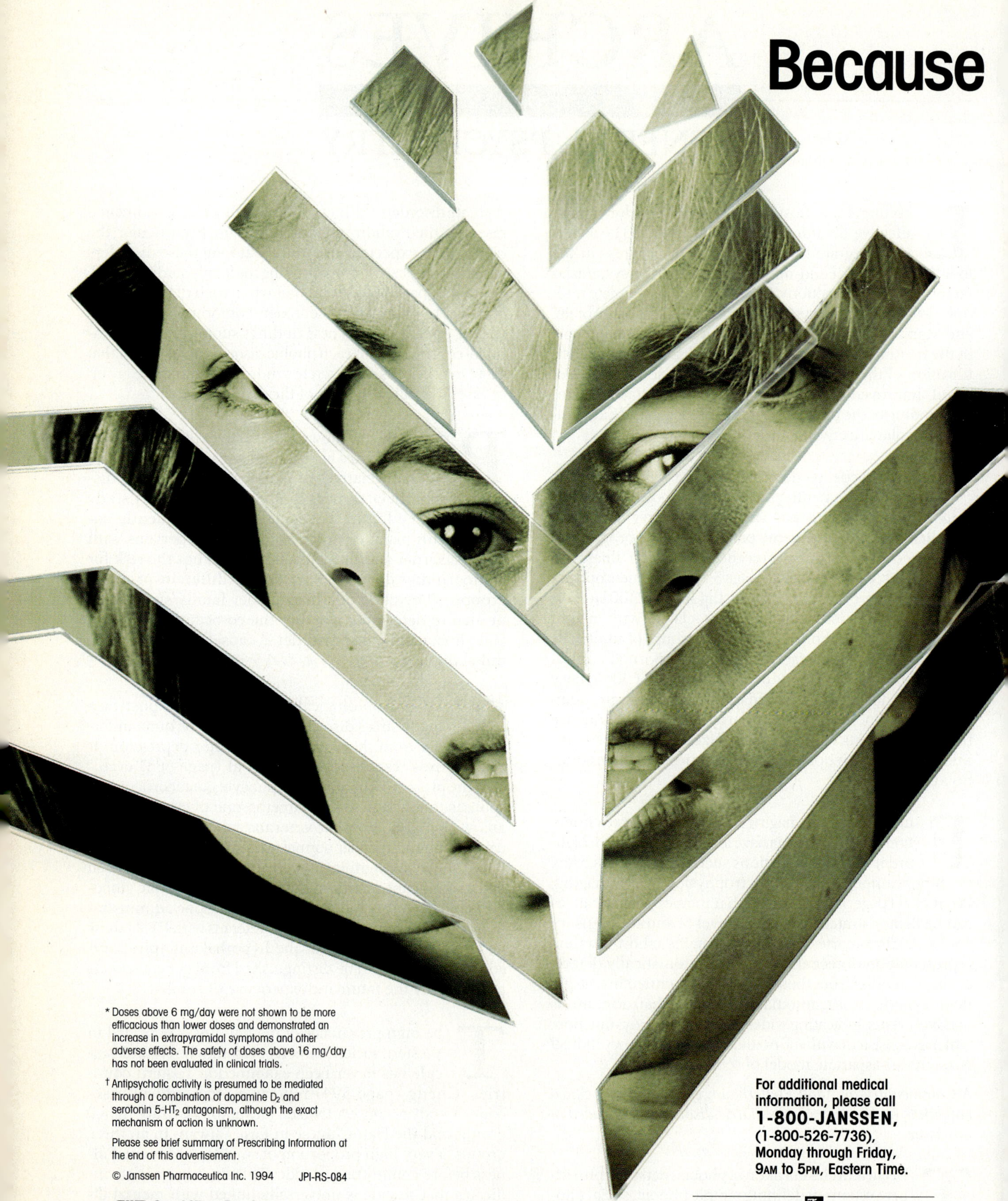

* Doses above 6 mg/day were not shown to be more efficacious than lower doses and demonstrated an increase in extrapyramidal symptoms and other adverse effects. The safety of doses above 16 mg/day has not been evaluated in clinical trials.

† Antipsychotic activity is presumed to be mediated through a combination of dopamine D_2 and serotonin 5-HT_2 antagonism, although the exact mechanism of action is unknown.

Please see brief summary of Prescribing Information at the end of this advertisement.

For additional medical information, please call 1-800-JANSSEN, (1-800-526-7736), Monday through Friday, 9AM to 5PM, Eastern Time.

Signal Transduction Pathways

Molecular Targets for Lithium's Actions

Husseini K. Manji, MD, FRCPC; William Z. Potter, MD, PhD; Robert H. Lenox, MD

Lithium remains the most widely used treatment for bipolar disorder, and this monovalent cation represents one of psychiatry's most important treatments. Despite its demonstrated efficacy in reducing both the frequency and severity of recurrent affective episodes and decades of clinical use, the molecular mechanisms underlying its therapeutic actions have not fully been elucidated. In this report, we review the exciting recent progress in the identification of key components of signal transduction pathways (in particular, guanine nucleotide–binding proteins [G proteins], adenylyl cyclases, and protein kinase C isozymes) as targets for lithium's actions and attempt to integrate these effects with the large body of data emphasizing alterations in various neurotransmitter (particularly monoaminergic) systems. Regulation of signal transduction within critical regions of the brain by lithium affects the function of multiple neurotransmitter systems and may thus explain lithium's efficacy in protecting susceptible individuals from spontaneous, stress-induced, and drug-induced cyclic affective episodes. Recent evidence has also demonstrated significant effects of lithium on the regulation of gene expression in the central nervous system, effects that may play a major role in the long-term stabilization of mood. The identification of these intracellular targets for lithium's actions offers the potential for the development of novel, improved therapeutic agents and, in conjunction with molecular genetic approaches, may facilitate our understanding of the biological factors predisposing individuals to manic-depressive illness.

(Arch Gen Psychiatry. 1995;52:531-543)

Lithium remains the most widely used treatment for bipolar affective disorder, and this monovalent cation represents one of psychiatry's most important treatments. Although it is far from the perfect drug, it has clearly revolutionized the treatment of this disorder.[1] Lithium not only treats the acute episode of mania, but also reduces the frequency and severity of recurrent episodes of mania and depression in patients with bipolar and unipolar disorders.[1] Numerous placebo-controlled studies have unequivocally documented the efficacy of lithium in the long-term prophylactic treatment of bipolar affective disorder, and the beneficial effects appear to involve both a reduction in the number of episodes, as well as in their intensity, with approximately 60% to 80% of all patients with bipolar affective disorder showing at least a partial response.[1] Adequate lithium treatment, particularly in the context of a lithium clinic, is also reported to reduce the excessive mortality observed in the illness,[2,3] and it has been estimated that in most industrialized countries, 0.1% of the population is undergoing lithium treatment.[4]

Despite lithium's remarkable efficacy and decades of use, the molecular mechanisms underlying its therapeutic actions have not been fully elucidated.[5-8] In recent

From the Section on Clinical Pharmacology, Experimental Therapeutics Branch, National Institute of Mental Health, Bethesda, Md (Drs Manji and Potter), and the Molecular Neuropsychopharmacology Program, Department of Psychiatry, Pharmacology, and Neuroscience, University of Florida College of Medicine, Gainesville (Dr Lenox). Dr Manji is currently with the Molecular Pathophysiology Program, Department of Psychiatry and Pharmacology, Wayne State University School of Medicine, Detroit, Mich.

years, it has become increasingly clear that rather than any single neurotransmitter system's being responsible for depression or mania, multiple interacting and overlapping systems are involved in regulating mood[9-12] and that most effective drugs do not work on any particular neurotransmitter system in isolation but rather affect the functional balance between interacting systems.[7,9-14] Advances in our understanding of the cellular basis of neuronal communication have also led to a reconceptualization of the mechanisms by which neuronal function is regulated, and it has become increasingly appreciated that neurotransmitter function can be indirectly regulated through alterations in intracellular signaling.[11,15-17] In this context, signal transduction pathways are in a pivotal position in the central nervous system (CNS) and represent attractive targets to explain lithium's efficacy in treating multiple aspects of bipolar affective disorder.[6,11,15,18,19] It is thus not surprising that, over the past several years, research aimed at the elucidation of the molecular mechanisms underlying lithium's therapeutic effects has focused on signal transduction pathways and that these studies have generally found that the function of second-messenger generating systems in the brain are affected by the chronic administration of "therapeutic" concentrations of lithium; however, the attribution of therapeutic relevance to any observed biochemical effect needs to account for certain key features of the drug when used clinically in the treatment of bipolar affective disorder. One of the major considerations is the time course of lithium's actions; thus, both the antimanic (generally days to weeks) and antidepressant (generally weeks when used as monotherapy) actions of lithium require a lag period for onset.[1] In addition, the long-term mood-stabilizing effect of lithium can continue indefinitely without tolerance and is generally not immediately reversed on discontinuation of therapy, although increasing evidence suggests that there may be a rebound increase in risk for recurrence of affective episodes (in particular, manic episodes) in the several months following discontinuation of lithium maintenance therapy.[20]

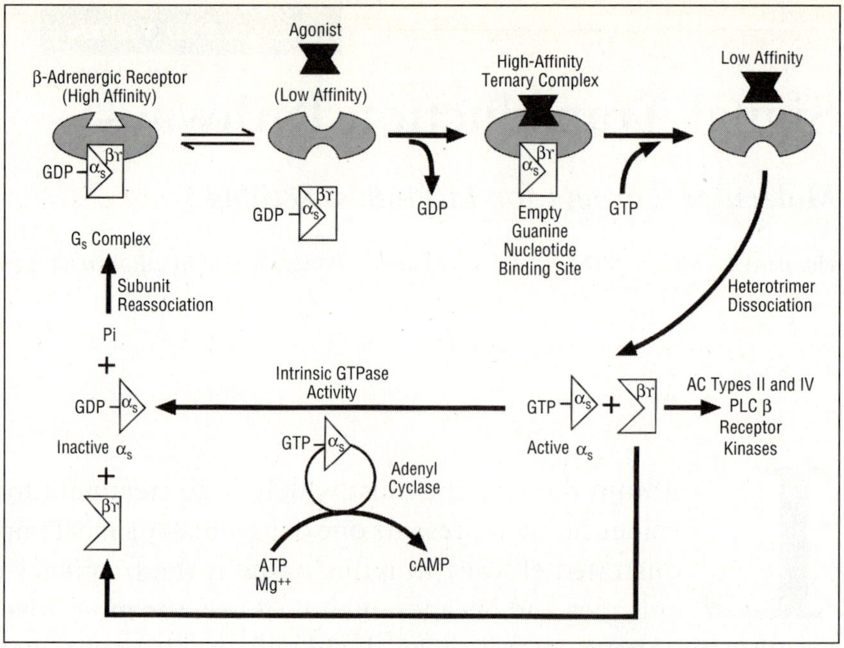

Figure 1. *Activation of the stimulatory G protein (G_s) by the β-adrenergic receptor. A similar activation-deactivation cycle is thought to occur with most (if not all) G proteins. The G protein α subunit cycles between an inactive guanosine diphosphate (GDP)–bound heterotrimeric (αβγ) and an active guanosine triphosphate (GTP)–bound monomeric form. At rest, an equilibrium exists between the receptor in the high-affinity (coupled to the G protein) and the low-affinity (uncoupled) states. Activation of receptors by an agonist induces a conformational change in the receptor, allowing it to interact with the G protein, leading to the release of GDP and the formation of a high-affinity ternary complex (agonist-receptor-G protein). This high-affinity state is short lived, and binding of GTP to the empty nucleotide site on the α subunit of the G protein leads to a destabilization of the high-affinity complex and a dissociation of the G protein into α-GTP and βγ subunits. It is now well established that both the α-GTP and βγ subunits are able to regulate the activity of various effectors. To date, the best-characterized effects of the G protein βγ subunits are the potentiation of the activity of adenylyl cyclases (AC) types II and IV and the activation of certain phospholipase C (PLC) isozymes and receptor kinases. The α-GTP is shown to activate ACs in this Figure, but there is also evidence demonstrating the direct activation of L-type Ca^{++} channels by α-GTP (at least in certain tissues). The continued activation of effectors by α-GTP is terminated by the action of a GTPase enzyme intrinsic to the α subunit. The formation of α-GDP causes its dissociation from AC; the reassociation of α-GDP with βγ is thermodynamically stable and completes the cycle with the formation of the inactive GDP–bound heterotrimeric (αβγ) G protein. ATP indicates adenosine triphosphate; cAMP, cyclic adenosine monophosphate; α_s, α subunit of stimulatory G protein; PLC β, PLC β isozyme; Mg^{++}, magnesium^{++}; Ca^{++}, calcium; and Pi, inorganic phosphate.*

Thus, any *relevant mechanism* postulated to explain the therapeutic actions of this drug must account for this pattern of treatment response, ie, changes induced during chronic administration that persist beyond abrupt discontinuation of treatment.[6,21,22]

In this report, we critically review and appraise the exciting recent progress in the identification of key components of signal transduction pathways as targets for lithium's therapeutic effects. In particular, we discuss the increasing body of data identifying protein kinase C (PKC) isozymes, guanine nucleotide–binding proteins (G proteins), and adenylyl cyclases (ACs) as targets for lithium's actions and attempt to integrate these effects with the large body of data emphasizing alterations in various neurotransmitter (particularly monoaminergic) systems. The identification of these targets offers hope not only for the development of novel, improved therapeutic agents but also for the identification of molecular sites underlying the pathophysiology and/or etiology of manic-depressive illness. We now provide a brief overview of transmembrane cellular signal transduction pathways before discussing the evidence for second-messenger generating systems as targets for lithium's actions.

TRANSMEMBRANE CELLULAR SIGNAL TRANSDUCTION

One of the most exciting recent advances in neuroscience has been the elucidation of the molecular mechanisms underlying neuronal communication, particularly with respect to

Table 1. Key Features of G Protein Subunits*

G Protein Class	Members	Toxin	Effectors	Examples of Receptors
α_s	$G\alpha_s$, $G\alpha_{olf}$	Cholera toxin	AC(+), L-type Ca^{++} channels (+)	β_1, D_1, A_2, olfactory signals
α_i	$G\alpha_{i1\text{-}3}$, $G\alpha_o$, $G\alpha_z$, $G\alpha_{t1\text{-}2}$	Pertussis toxin (except $G\alpha_z$)	AC(−), K^+ channels (+), Ca^{++} channels (−), cyclic GMP, phosphodiesterase (+) ($G\alpha_{t1\text{-}2}$)	α_2, D_2, A_1, μ, M_2, 5-HT_{1A}, $GABA_B$, retinal rods, cones, (rhopdopsins)
α_q	$G\alpha_q$, $G\alpha_{11}$ $G\alpha_{14}$, $G\alpha_{15}$, $G\alpha_{16}$	...	PLCβ (+)	TxA_2, 5-HT_{2c}, M_1, M_3, M_5, α_1
α_{12}	$G\alpha_{12}$, $G\alpha_{13}$	...	?Na^+/H^+ exchange, ?Ca^{++} channels (−)	TxA_2, thrombin
β	$\beta(\times 4)$	...	AC type I (−), AC types II and IV (potentiation), PLC (+), receptor kinases (+), inactivates α_s	...
γ	$\gamma(\times 7)$	...	β and γ required for interaction of α subunit with receptor	...

**AC indicates adenylyl cyclase; PLC, phospholipase C; $G\alpha_t$, transducins; β_1, α_1, and α_2, adrenergic receptor subtypes; D_1 and D_2, dopaminergic receptor subtypes; A_1 and A_2, adenosine receptor subtypes; M_1, M_2, M_3, and M_5, muscarinic receptor subtypes; 5-HT_{1A} and 5-HT_{2c}, serotonin receptor subtypes; $GABA_B$, γ-aminobutyric acid receptor; TxA_2, thromboxane A_2 receptor; K^+, potassium+; Na^+, sodium+; H^+, hydrogen+; Ca^{++}, calcium++; plus sign, stimulation; and minus sign, inhibition. ?Na^+/H^+ exchange and ?Ca^{++} channels (−) indicate that, although regulation of Na^+/H^+ exchange and Ca^{++} channels by $G\alpha_{12}$, and $G\alpha_{13}$ has been demonstrated in artificial systems in vitro, these findings await definitive confirmation.*

defining the obligatory role of G proteins in the transduction of a vast array of extracellular, receptor-detected signals across cell membranes to intracellular effectors. Most neurotransmitters and neuromodulators that initiate cellular signaling cannot penetrate the hydrophobic plasma membrane lipid bilayer but rather transmit their message via cell surface receptors. It has been estimated that about 80% of all known hormones, neurotransmitters, and neuromodulators (numbering over 100) elicit cellular responses through G proteins coupled to a variety of intracellular effectors.[23] The G proteins are a ubiquitous family of proteins that serve the critical role of transducers of information across the plasma membrane, coupling receptors to various effectors.[12,18,23-26] The G proteins are heterotrimers localized to the inner surface of the plasma membrane consisting of an α subunit that binds (and hydrolyzes) guanosine triphosphate (GTP) and β and γ subunits that form a tightly but noncovalently linked dimer. The α subunits have generally been assumed to confer receptor and effector specificity to the G protein, but recent evidence has also demonstrated critical roles for $\beta\gamma$ subunits in signal transduction pathways.[27-30] Information traverses catalytically across a G protein–coupled system in a GTP cycle (**Figure 1**), resulting in a several thousandfold amplification of the original signal. The G proteins that coordinate receptor-effector activity are derived from a large gene family,[31] and recent cloning and sequencing of complementary DNAs encoding the α subunits have defined four major *subfamilies* (G_s, G_i, G_q, and G_{12}) based on degree of amino acid sequence identity, with at least 16 isotypes (**Table 1**). Seminal work by Alfred Gilman (discussed in Katada et al[32]) and Martin Rodbell[33] initially identified the G proteins as distinct proteins that mediated either the stimulation (G_s) or inhibition (G_i) of AC. It is now clear, however, that the G protein α and $\beta\gamma$ subunits regulate a variety of effectors (Table 1). The G protein cycle at the center of receptor-effector communication represents the unique compromise of a carefully timed molecular switch, allowing the cell to respond both rapidly and to low-stimulus concentration.[26] Given the variety of functions subserved by G protein–coupled signal transduction, it is not surprising that abnormalities in G protein–coupled pathways have been implicated in the pathophysiological features of a variety of human diseases.[11,24]

The signal-transducing G proteins also play a critical integrative role in the CNS.[11,15-17] Since a single receptor subtype can be coupled to multiple G proteins and since multiple G proteins can converge to activate or inactivate a single effector,[12,16-18] the G protein–coupled interactions form complex networks. The high degree of complexity generated by the interactions of G protein–coupled receptors may be one mechanism by which neurons aquire the flexibility to generate the wide range of responses observed in the CNS. This finding has led to the proposal that G proteins may be involved in pathways regulating such diverse vegetative functions as mood, appetite, and wakefulness and, by extrapolation, in the molecular mechanisms of action of mood-stabilizing drugs like lithium.[11] We now discuss the evidence supporting second-messenger generating systems as targets for lithium's actions.

LITHIUM AND THE PHOSPHOINOSITIDE (PI) CYCLE

In recent years, research on the molecular mechanisms underlying lithium's therapeutic effects has focused on intracellular second-messenger generating systems and, in particular, receptor-coupled hydrolysis of phosphatidylinositol 4,5-bisphos-

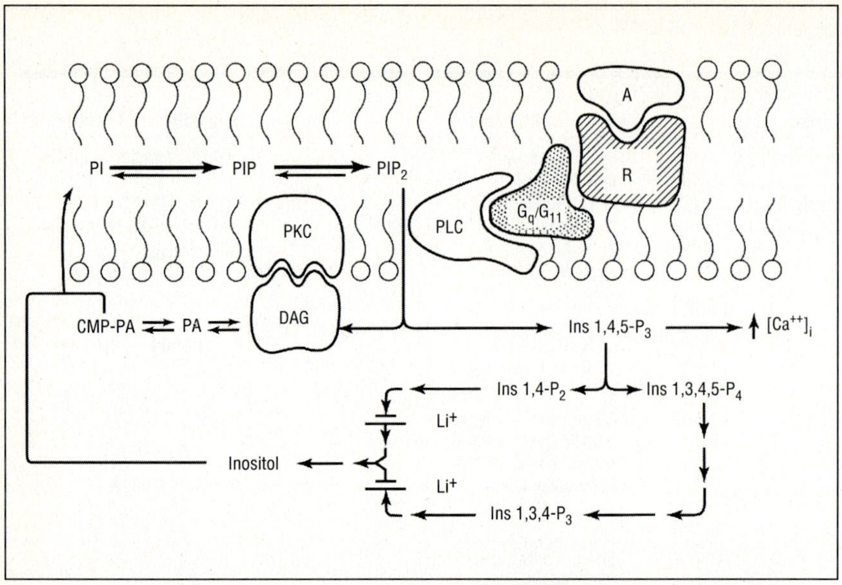

Figure 2. *Effects of lithium$^+$ (Li$^+$) on receptor-mediated phosphoinositide (PI) hydrolysis. Agonists such as acetylcholine, norepinephrine, or serotonin (5-HT) bind to specific cell surface receptors (including muscarinic [M_1, M_3, and M_5], α_1-noradrenergic, and 5-HT_{2c}), which interact with guanine nucleotide–binding proteins (G_q and/or G_{11}) and thereby stimulate certain isoforms of the enzyme phospholipase C (PLC) to produce the intracellular second messengers* sn*-1,2-diacylglycerol (DAG) (an endogenous activator of protein kinase C [PKC]) and inositol 1,4,5-trisphosphate (Ins 1,4,5-P_3), which facilitates the release of intracellular stored calcium^{++} (Ca^{++}). Lithium is an inhibitor of inositol monophosphatases, and this results in an accumulation of inositol 1-monophosphate as well as a reduction in levels of free inositol. Due to the limited ability of inositol to cross the blood-brain barrier, the conservation of inositol in the central nervous system CNS depends strongly on recycling via dephosphorylation of inositol phosphates. As a result of inositol depletion in the presence of lithium, levels of metabolites within the phospholipid portion of the hydrolytic pathway, which include DAG, phosphatidic acid (PA), and cytidine monophosphate-phosphatidate (CMP-PA), have been shown to be significantly elevated in a variety of cell types, including brain cells. This might be expected since the end metabolite in this pathway, CMP-PA, requires free* myo*-inositol to resynthesize inositol phosphates for the regeneration of phosphatidylinositol 4,5-bisphosphate (PIP_2). Thus, depletion of cellular* myo*-inositol interferes with the recycling of the system, resulting in the consequent accumulation of CMP-PA and its interconvertible metabolite, DAG. The DAG is an endogenous activator of PKC, and the lithium-induced elevations in DAG levels may therefore activate PKC; interestingly, PKC is known to activate phospholipase D, which liberates DAG from phosphatidylcholine (PC). It has been demonstrated that the DAG generated from PC hydrolysis remains elevated for a prolonged period, resulting in a more sustained activation of PKC. Since PKC activation is often followed by its rapid proteolytic degradation, a prolonged increase in DAG levels by lithium may lead to an increased membrane translocation and subsequent degradation of PKC isozymes. PIP indicates phosphatidylinositol 4-monophosphate; G_q/G_{11}, G proteins coupled to stimulation of PI turnover; A, agonist; and R, receptor.*

phate (PIP_2) (**Figure 2**). Although inositol phospholipids are relatively minor components of cell membranes, they play a major role in receptor-mediated signal transduction pathways and are involved in a diverse range of responses in the CNS. Activation of a variety of neurotransmitter receptor subtypes (including muscarinic [M_1, M_3, M_5], α_1-noradrenergic, and serotonergic [5-HT]$_{2c}$ subtypes) induces the hydrolysis of membrane phospholipids. Agonist-stimulated PIP_2 hydrolysis has been extensively reviewed elsewhere, and interested readers are referred to these reports for details.[18,34-36] In brief, agonists such as acetylcholine, norepinephrine, or 5-HT bind to specific cell surface receptors, which interact with G proteins (both pertussis toxin–insensitive [G_q and/or G_{11}] and pertussis toxin–sensitive [G_o and/or G_i]) and thereby stimulate certain isoforms of the enzyme phospholipase C to produce the two intracellular second messengers *sn*-1,2-diacylgycerol (DAG) (an endogenous activator of PKC) and inositol 1,4,5-trisphosphate (which facilitates the release of intracellular stored calcium^{++}). Lithium, at therapeutically relevant concentrations (0.6 to 1.2 mmol/L in plasma), is an inhibitor of the intracellular enzyme inositol monophosphatase (concentration of lithium needed to inhibit the enzyme activity by 50%, 0.8 mmol/L), which plays a major role in the recycling of inositol phosphates.[37,38] Since the brain has limited access to inositol other than what it derives from recycling of inositol phosphates, the ability of a neuron to maintain sufficient supplies of *myo*-inositol (the isoform that is the physiological substrate for the generation of PIP_2) can be crucial to the resynthesis of the PIs and the maintenance and efficiency of signaling.[39] Furthermore, since the mode of enzyme inhibition is *uncompetitive*, lithium's effects have been postulated to be most pronounced in systems undergoing the highest rate of PIP_2 hydrolysis.[40,41] Thus, Berridge and associates[42,43] first proposed that the physiological consequence of lithium's action is derived through a depletion of free inositol and that its selectivity could be attributed to its preferential action (due to the uncompetitive nature of the inhibition) on the most active receptor-mediated neuronal pathways. Since several subtypes of adrenergic, cholinergic, and 5-HT receptors are coupled to PIP_2 hydrolysis in the CNS,[34-36] such a hypothesis offers a plausible explanation for lithium's therapeutic efficacy in treating multiple aspects of bipolar affective disorder.

Numerous studies have examined the effects of lithium on receptor-mediated PI responses, and although some report a reduction in agonist-stimulated PIP_2 hydrolysis in rat brain slices following acute or chronic lithium treatment, these findings have often been small, inconsistent, and subject to numerous methodological differences.[6,44-50] It should be noted, however, that various species (and subtypes of cells) differ markedly in the regulation of inositol levels,[51,52] perhaps contributing to some of the differences in the outcomes of various studies. In addition, several lines of evidence suggest that the action of chronic lithium administration may not simply be directly manifest in receptor-mediated PI turnover. Whereas investigators have observed that levels of inositol in the brain remain reduced in rats receiving chronic lithium treatment,[39,53] it has been difficult to demonstrate that this results in a reduction in the resynthesis of PIP_2, which is the substrate for agonist-induced PI turnover. This, however, may be due to the methodological difficulties in accurately mea-

Table 2. Effects of Lithium on Adenylyl Cyclase*

Tissue (Reference)	Lithium Administration Paradigm	Lithium Effects	Comments
Rat cortex (Risby et al,[7] Mork et al[69])†	In vitro incubation with "therapeutic" dose	Attenuation of AC activity in response to isoproterenol, GTP analogues, and forskolin	Effects appear to be due to competition with Mg^{++} for a site on AC
Rat and human kidney (Dousa,[72] Goldberg et al[73])	In vitro incubation with >2 mmol/L	Attenuation of AC activity in response to vasopressin	Contributes to nephrogenic diabetes insipidus?
Dog thyroid tissue (Tseng et al[74])	In vitro incubation with >2 mmol/L	Attenuation of AC activity in response to thyrotropin	May contribute to lithium-induced subclinical hypothyroidism
Human platelets (Ebstein et al[65])	In vitro incubation with therapeutic dose	Attenuation of AC activity in response to forskolin	Effects may be due to competition with Mg^{++} for a site on AC
SD rats (Ebstein et al,[63] Mork and Geisler,[66-68] Mork et al[69])	Therapeutic levels for >2 weeks	Attenuated norepinephrine-, GTP analogue-, and forskolin-stimulated AC in cortex	Lithium's effects on G_s may also contribute
SD Rats (Colin et al[75])	Therapeutic levels for 4 weeks	Increased AC types I and II protein levels in cortex	Lithium treatment also increased types I and II AC mRNA levels in cortex
Human subjects (Belmaker,[64] Friedman et al,[76] Belmaker et al[77])	Chronic therapeutic levels	Attenuation of plasma cAMP response to epinephrine	Effects on receptor-G protein coupling may also contribute
Human platelets (Ebstein et al[65])	3-week treatment of manic patients	Decreased AC affinity for lithium	Adaptive changes in AC may occur over time
Human subjects (Ebstein et al[70])	Chronic therapeutic levels	Attenuation of platelet receptor-, fluoride-, and forskolin-stimulated AC activity	Effects may be due to competition with Mg^{++} for a site on AC

**AC indicates adenylyl cyclase; GTP, guanosine triphosphate; Mg^{++}, magnesium^{++}; G_s, subunit of G protein mediating the stimulation of AC; mRNA, messenger RNA; cAMP, cyclic adenosine monophosphate; and SD, Sprague-Dawley.*

†Findings by Mork and Geisler[66-68] and Newman and Belmaker[71] are reviewed in these references.

suring alterations in a rapidly turning over, small, signal-related pool of PIP_2 and/or recent evidence that resynthesis of inositol phospholipids may also occur through base exchange reactions from other larger pools of phospholipids such as phosphatidylcholine.[21,54] Interestingly, some[55,56] (but not all[47]) studies have demonstrated that the addition of high concentrations of exogenous inositol can attenuate some of lithium's effects on the PI cycle. However, although pharmacological concentrations of extracellular inositol appear to attenuate some of lithium's effects in recent animal studies, the addition of inositol *prevented* but did not *reverse* the effects of lithium on the PI system,[56-59] suggesting that lithium may induce long-term changes beyond simple inositol depletion.

Investigators have also examined lithium's effects on the PI system distal to the receptor since, as noted above, experimental evidence has shown that lithium may alter receptor coupling to PI turnover. Since the fluoride ion will directly activate G protein–coupled second-messenger responses, efforts have been made to examine the effect of lithium on sodium fluoride–stimulated PI responses in the brain. Although Godfrey et al[46] reported a reduction of fluoride-stimulated PI response in cortical membranes of rats treated with lithium for 3 days, no change in response was observed in cortical slices from rats administered lithium for 30 days. More recently, Song and Jope[60] have attempted to elucidate the mechanisms underlying the effects of chronic lithium administration on receptor-mediated PI turnover; using ^3H (hydrogen 3–labeled)-PI as a substrate (which should bypass any putative inositol depletion), these investigators found that cortical membranes prepared from rats receiving chronic lithium treatment showed diminished PI turnover in response to GTP analogues. Taken together, these results suggest that although chronic lithium administration may affect receptor-mediated PI signaling, these effects are unlikely to be simply due to an inositol depletion in the CNS.[6,21,22] Most importantly, the therapeutic actions of lithium occur only after chronic treatment and generally remain in evidence long after discontinuation; these actions cannot be attributed only to inositol reductions evident in the presence of lithium. Thus, although the preponderance of the data suggests that the initial actions of lithium may occur with a relative depletion of inositol and thereby alterations in receptor-coupled PI response, the effects of chronic lithium administration (and likely those representing the most relevant ones in the treatment of bipolar affective disorder) are more likely to be mediated by changes distal to the receptor such as at the G protein level or modification of PKC isozymes (discussed below).

LITHIUM AND AC

The other major receptor-coupled second-messenger system on which lithium exerts significant effects is the cyclic adenosine monophosphate (cAMP) generating system. Forn and Valdecasas[61] were the first to report that lithium in vitro attenuated norepinephrine-stimulated cAMP accumulation; since then, numerous studies[7,62-77] have clearly demonstrated that cAMP accumulation by various neurotransmitters and hormones is inhibited by lithium at therapeutic concentrations both in vivo and in vitro (**Table 2**). Norepinephrine- and adenosine-stimulated cAMP accumulations in rat cortical slices are inhibited significantly by 1- to 2-mmol/L lithium, although the generalizability of this finding to human brain tissue has not yet been fully determined.[78]

Table 3. Effects of Lithium on G Proteins*

Tissue (Reference)	Lithium Administration Paradigm	Lithium Effects	Comments
SD rats (Risby et al,[7] Mork et al[69])†	"Therapeutic" levels for >10 days	Attenuation of receptor-mediated AC activity	Effects may also be due in part to direct inhibition of ACs by lithium
SD rats (Mork and Geisler[66,68])	Chronic at therapeutic levels	Attenuation of βAR-mediated AC activity in washed membranes	Effects of lithium on AC were overcome by GTP but not Mg^{++}
SD rats (Song and Jope[60])	Chronic at therapeutic levels	Attenuation of G protein–mediated PI turnover in membranes	Used ^{3}H–PI, which should bypass any putative inositol depletion
SD rats (Masana et al[86,88])	Chronic at therapeutic levels	Increase in pertussis toxin–catalyzed ^{32}P-ADP ribosylation in cortical membranes	No effects on levels of G protein α subunits; increases in basal cAMP levels suggest reduced G_1 function
SD rats (Colin et at[75])	Therapeutic levels for 21 days	Reduced $G\alpha_{i1}$ and $G\alpha_{i2}$ protein levels in cortex	Also observed reduced $G\alpha_{i1}$ and $G\alpha_{i2}$ mRNA levels
Wistar rats (Li et al[89,90])	Therapeutic levels for 21 days	Reduced $G\alpha_s$, $G\alpha_{i1}$, and $G\alpha_{i2}$ mRNA levels in cortex	Did not observe any effects on G protein α subunit protein levels
Healthy humans (Risby et al,[7] Hsiao et al[91])	2 weeks at therapeutic levels	Increase in pertussis toxin–catalyzed ^{32}P-ADP ribosylation in platelet membranes	No effects on G protein α subunit levels; increases in basal cAMP levels suggests reduced G_i function

**AC indicates adenylyl cyclase; βAR, β-adrenergic receptor; GTP, guanosine triphosphate; Mg^{++}, magnesium^{++}; PI, phosphoinositide; ADP, adenosine diphosphate; cAMP, cyclic adenosine monophosphate; mRNA, messenger RNA; and SD, Sprague-Dawley.*

†Findings by Mork and Geisler[66-68] and Newman and Belmaker[71] are reviewed in these references.

Studies in humans have demonstrated that lithium treatment at therapeutic levels results in an attenuation of the plasma cAMP level increase in response to epinephrine,[76,77,79] and there is also evidence for an attenuation of receptor coupling to AC in peripheral cells.[7,64,80,81] In fact, lithium inhibition of vasopressin-[82] or thyrotropin-sensitive AC is generally believed to underlie two of lithium's more common side effects in humans, namely, nephrogenic diabetes insipidus and subclinical hypothyroidism.[72-74]

Lithium attenuation of β-adrenoceptor–stimulated AC activity has been shown in membrane, slice, and synaptosomal preparations from rat cerebral cortices.[7,66,69] Lithium in vitro inhibits the stimulation of AC by the poorly hydrolyzable analogue of GTP, guanyl imidodiphosphate, and also by calcium^{++}-calmodulin, suggesting that lithium in vitro is directly able to inhibit the catalytic unit of AC. Since these inhibitory effects of lithium in vitro can be overcome by magnesium^{++},[66,69,71,83-85] they appear to be mediated (at least in part) by a direct competition with magnesium (whose hydrated ionic radius is similar to that of lithium) for a binding site on the catalytic unit of AC.[66,69,71,83] However, the inhibitory effects of *chronic* lithium treatment on rat brain β-adrenoceptor–stimulated AC are not reversed by magnesium^{++} and still persist after washing of the membranes but are reversed by increasing concentrations of GTP.[66,69] These results suggest that the inhibitory effects of chronic lithium administration on the cAMP generating system may also be mediated at the level of signal-transducing G proteins.

Most recently, Colin and associates[75] have demonstrated that chronic lithium administration results in an increase in the levels of AC types I and II and in their messenger RNA (mRNA) levels. The mechanism(s) underlying the alterations in AC subtypes following chronic lithium administration is presently unknown; however, these elevations in the levels of the AC subtypes may have physiological significance, since several studies have demonstrated tissue- and region-selective *increases* in basal cAMP levels after chronic lithium administration.[63,71,86] These increases in basal cAMP levels may also represent the manifestations (at least in part) of a lithium-induced attenuation of the tonic inhibitory input of G_i.[71,86] It is thus clear that the net effect of chronic lithium administration on the cAMP generating system depends on the subtypes of ACs present and on the relative abundance and activity of various G protein subtypes.

Do these complex effects of lithium on the cAMP generating system have any clinical relevance? The commonly observed side effects of polyuria and subclinical hypothyroidism[72-74] suggest that lithium's effects on the cAMP generating system do indeed have physiological effects in humans, but an important issue to address is whether they have any demonstrable CNS manifestations. Considerable caution is obviously required when attempting to correlate biochemical changes in rodents with the complex symptoms observed in bipolar affective disorder; nevertheless, the increases in the levels of AC types I and II following chronic lithium administration may result in a long-term sensitization of the cAMP generating system, which only becomes fully manifest following discontinuation of lithium therapy. This may represent one factor contributing to the significantly increased risk for manic episodes following rapid lithium therapy discontinuation and is worthy of further study.

LITHIUM AND G PROTEINS

As noted above, experimental evidence has shown that lithium attenuates receptor-mediated AC activity and PI turnover in rodents and in humans in the absence of consistent changes in the density of the receptors themselves. The first direct evidence that G proteins may be the targets of lithium's actions was provided by Avissar and colleagues,[87] who reported that lithium

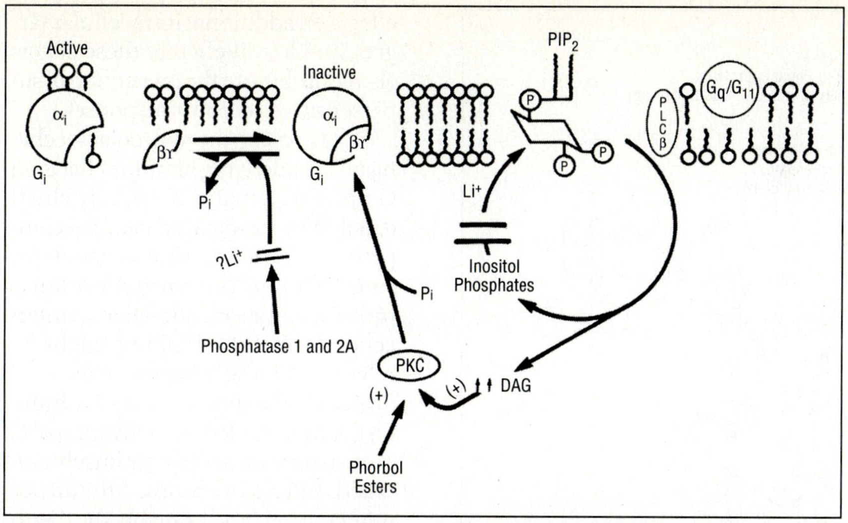

Figure 3. *Mechanisms by which chronic lithium (Li) administration may produce an inactivation of the inhibitory G protein (G_i). Activation of G_i (by receptors or by guanosine triphosphate [GTP] or its nonhydrolysable analogues) shifts the equilibrium to the left, toward the dissociated, active form of G_i. Chronic lithium treatment has been demonstrated to attenuate G_i function, while increasing pertussis toxin (PT)–catalyzed ^{32}P-adenosine diphosphate (ADP) ribosylation. Since PT selectively ADP ribosylates the undissociated, inactive form of G_i, these results suggest that the effects of chronic lithium administration involve a stabilization of the inactive $\alpha\beta\gamma$ conformation of G_i. Activation of protein kinase C (PKC) by phorbol esters also inactivates G_i, and in several tissues also leads to an increase in PT-catalyzed ^{32}P-ADP ribosylation. Thus, one possible mechanism for lithium's effects on G_i may be the modulation of the phosphorylation state of G_i. Lithium via its inhibition of inositol 1-phosphatase produces an elevation of diacylglycerol (DAG) levels, which may regulate the activity of PKC. In addition to the potential enhancement of the phosphorylation state of G_i by activation of PKC, it is also possible that lithium interferes with the* dephosphorylation *of G_i. Protein phosphatases 1 and 2A have been demonstrated to dephosphorylate G_i, and inhibiting their activity (for example by the use of okadaic acid) increases the phosphorylation state of G_i. It should be noted that there are at present no data regarding lithium's effects on the activity of protein phosphatases 1 or 2A, but this represents a testable hypothesis worthy of study. PIP_2 indicates phosphatidylinositol 4,5-bisphosphate; G_q/G_{11}, G proteins coupled to stimulation of phosphoinositide turnover; PLC β, phospholipase C β isozyme; Pi, inorganic phosphate; and plus sign, stimulatory.*

dramatically *eliminated* isoproterenol- and carbachol-induced increases in ^{3}H-GTP binding to various G proteins in rat cerebral cortical membranes. These effects were reported to occur both in vitro in the presence of 0.6-mmol/L lithium and in washed cortical membranes from rats treated with lithium carbonate for 2 to 3 weeks, suggesting that the function of several G proteins (eg, G_s, G_i, and G_o) might be modified by this mood-stabilizing drug. In animals withdrawn from lithium treatment for 2 days, the agonist-stimulated response (^{3}H-GTP binding) returned. Whereas these studies[75,86,88-91] have been of considerable heuristic interest and the preponderence of data *does* suggest an action of *chronic* lithium administration at the level of G proteins (**Table 3**), such a *direct* action of lithium on G protein function has been difficult to replicate in light of a number of methodological problems[22,50]; moreover, the fact that routine assays of agonist-stimulated PI hydrolysis in brain slices are conducted in the presence of 10 mmol/L lithium suggests that the lithium ion does not directly exert any major effects on G protein function.

There is, however, considerable evidence that chronic lithium administration affects G protein function, and numerous investigations have addressed the role of G proteins in the attenuated receptor-mediated AC activity and PI responses observed after chronic lithium administration in rodents and in humans.[6,7,45,60,64,66,71,92,93] Using in vivo microdialysis measurements of cAMP levels, Masana and associates[86,88] found that chronic lithium treatment produced a significant increase in basal- and post–receptor-stimulated (cholera toxin or forskolin) AC activity while attenuating the β-adrenergic–mediated effect in rat frontal cortex. Moreover, chronic lithium treatment resulted in an almost absent cAMP response to pertussis toxin[86,88]; taken together, these results suggest a lithium-induced attenuation of G_i function and of the β-adrenergic receptor–G_s interaction. These investigators did not observe alterations in the amounts of $G\alpha_s$, $G\alpha_{i1\text{-}3}$, or $G\alpha_o$, but observed a significant increase in pertussis toxin–catalyzed ^{32}P (phosphorus 32-labeled) adenosine diphosphate ribosylation in frontal cortex. Since pertussis toxin selectively adenosine diphosphate ribosylates the undissociated, inactive $\alpha\beta\gamma$ heterotrimeric forms of G_i and G_o,[25,94] it has been postulated that lithium inactivates G_i via a stabilization of the inactive conformation (**Figure 3**).[7,86,91]

At present, the possible effects of chronic lithium administration on the absolute *levels* of $G\alpha_s$ and $G\alpha_i$ remain unclear—two laboratories have not observed any alterations,[89,91] whereas another one has observed small but significant decreases in the levels of $G\alpha_{i1}$ and $G\alpha_{i2}$ in rat frontal cortex.[75] However, chronic lithium administration has been reported to reduce the mRNA levels of several G protein α subunits in rat brain, including $G\alpha_{i1}$,[75,89,90] $G\alpha_{i2}$,[75,89,90] and $G\alpha_s$,[89,90] suggesting that lithium produces complex transcriptional and posttranscriptional effects after chronic administration (discussed below).

Recent studies have also examined the effects of chronic lithium administration on G protein function in humans and have generally observed reduced receptor–G protein coupling.[7,64,65,81,82,91,95-97] The effects of 2 weeks of lithium administration on G protein measures have also recently been examined in healthy volunteers (which overcomes the potentially confounding, significant effects of alterations in mood-state–dependent biochemical and neuroendocrine parameters).[7,98] Chronic lithium administration resulted in an increase in both basal and postreceptor-stimulated AC activity in platelets, most compatible with an attenuation of G_i function.[7,98] Similar to the findings in rat brain, lithium did not affect the levels of platelet G protein α subunits but produced a significant 40% increase in pertussis toxin–catalyzed ^{32}P-ADP ribosylation, once again compatible with a stabilization of the inactive undissociated $\alpha\beta\gamma$ heterotrimeric forms of G_i.[91,94]

Overall, considerable evidence argues for an effect of chronic lithium administration on the G protein function in both humans and rodents

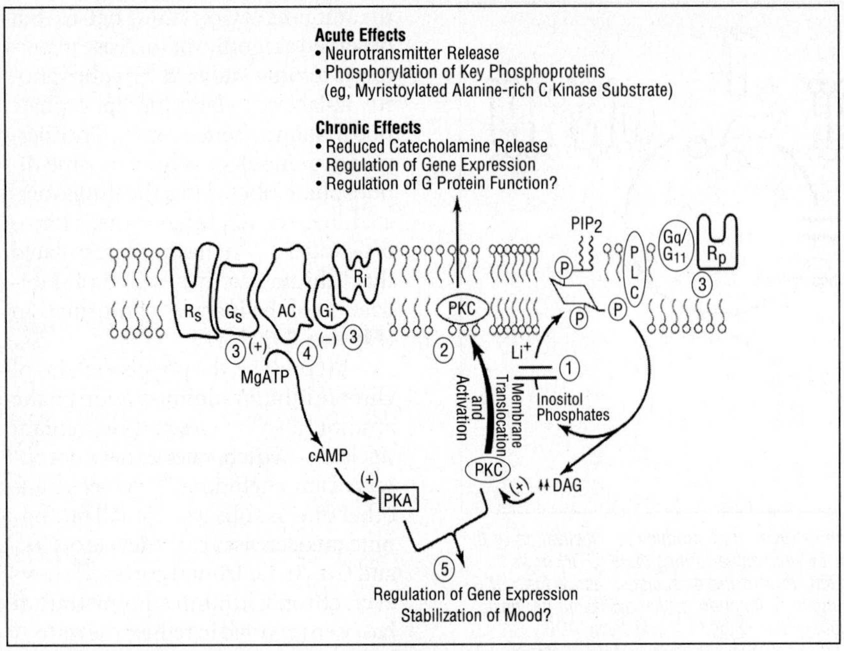

Figure 4. *Major intracellular cellular signaling pathways affected by lithium (Li). 1, Lithium, at therapeutically relevant concentrations, inhibits the activity of inositol monophosphatases, resulting in a depletion of cellular* myo*-inositol. The interference with the recycling of the phosphoinositide (PI) system by lithium results in an accumulation of* sn*-1,2-diacylglycerol (DAG) (an endogenous activator of protein kinase C [PKC]). 2, Acute lithium administration activates PKC, resulting in the phosphorylation of key proteins and facilitating neurotransmitter (eg, serotonin) release; since PKC activation is often followed by its rapid proteolytic degradation, a prolonged increase in DAG levels by lithium may lead to subsequent degradation of PKC isozymes. 3, Chronic administration of lithium affects the function of several G proteins, including those coupled both to adenylyl cyclases (ACs) (G_s and G_i) and phospholipase C (PLC) isozymes (G_q and/or G_{11}). The allosteric modulation of G proteins might serve to explain lithium's long-term prophylactic efficacy in protecting susceptible individuals from spontaneous, stress-induced, and drug-induced cyclic affective episodes. 4, Lithium exerts complex effects on AC in vitro and in vivo. Lithium in vitro inhibits the stimulation of AC, likely by a direct competition with magnesium (Mg) (whose hydrated ionic radius is similar to that of lithium) for a binding site on the catalytic unit of AC. This direct inhibitory effect of lithium on AC may persist with chronic in vivo administration of lithium; however, chronic lithium administration also increases the expression of AC types I and II protein and messenger RNA. 5, Drugs such as lithium that require prolonged administration (days to weeks) for therapeutic efficacy may exert significant effects at the genomic level. A growing body of evidence has shown that lithium affects gene expression, likely via second- and third-messenger–induced alterations in nuclear transcription regulatory factors responsible for modulating the expression of specific genes. Thus, via its transcriptional and posttranscriptional effects, lithium brings about long-term changes in the regulation of processes such as neurotransmitter release and receptor coupling and responses; these effects may play a major role in lithium's mood-stabilizing effects. ATP indicates adenosine triphosphate; R_s and R_i, receptors coupled to stimulation and inhibition, respectively, of AC; P, PI turnover; R_p, receptor coupled to PI turnover; PIP_2, phosphatidylinositol 4,5-bisphosphate; PKA, protein kinase A; plus sign, stimulation; and minus sign, inhibition.*

(Table 3). The allosteric modulation of G proteins might serve to explain lithium's long-term prophylactic efficacy in protecting susceptible individuals from spontaneous, stress-induced, and drug-induced (eg, antidepressant or stimulant) cyclic affective episodes. In addition, although speculative, it might be postulated that these effects on G proteins represent the mechanistic basis by which chronic lithium administration blocks the development of supersensitive dopaminergic, adrenergic, and cholinergic receptors. Thus, many (but not all) previous studies have demonstrated that chronic lithium administration is able to block the development of lesion- or drug-induced supersensitive receptor responses.[5,22] These supersensitive responses have been assayed by biochemical, electrophysiological, and behavioral studies; interestingly, most receptor-binding studies have not generally demonstrated lithium-induced alterations in the density of the receptors themselves, suggesting that lithium exerts its effects at postreceptor sites, in particular at the level of the signal-transducing G proteins. Such a contention also receives support from the observation that lithium's effects appear to involve different classes of receptors coupled both to AC and phospholipase C isozymes (**Figure 4**); however, it is clear that lithium exerts effects on additional intracellular targets, and it is likely that these effects also contribute to the prevention of supersensitive receptor responses.

At present, the molecular mechanism(s) underlying lithium's effects on G proteins remains to be fully elucidated. Whereas data indicate that competition with magnesium accounts for some of lithium's in vitro effects on G proteins and speculation that an interaction with GTP binding might be relevant to the chronic effects of lithium,[66,75] a direct effect of lithium on guanine nucleotide activation of G protein remains at this time unsubstantiated. Effects of chronic lithium administration (and arguably the therapeutically relevant effects) may more likely be attributable to an indirect posttranslational modification of the G proteins. Since receptor and G protein function is known to be regulated by phosphorylation,[99-103] one *potential* mechanistic explanation for lithium's effects on G protein subunit dissociation is phosphorylation by PKC, an enzyme responsible for considerable convergence and "crosstalk" between multiple second messenger systems (Figure 3).[11,54,101] It is also possible that the effects of lithium on G protein α subunit mRNA levels are mediated via PKC, since recent studies have demonstrated that PKC activation produces a similar decrease in $G\alpha_s$ and $G\alpha_{i2}$ mRNA levels in cells in vitro.[104] We now discuss the evidence for an effect of lithium on PKC isozymes.

LITHIUM AND PKC

Calcium-activated phospholipid-dependent PKC is a ubiquitous enzyme, highly enriched in the brain, where it plays a major role in regulating presynaptic and postsynaptic aspects of neurotransmission.[54,105,106] Protein kinase C is one of the major intracellular mediators of signals generated on external stimulation of cells via a variety of neurotransmitter receptor subtypes that induce the hydrolysis of membrane phospholipids. Protein kinase C is now known to exist as a family of closely related subspecies, has a heterogenous distribution in the brain (with particularly high levels in presynaptic nerve terminals), and together with other kinases plays a crucial role in the regulation of synaptic plasticity. Molecu-

Table 4. Effects of Lithium on PKC and PKC-Mediated Responses*

Tissue (Reference)	Lithium Administration Paradigm	Duration (Dose)	Lithium Effects	Comments
SD rats (Evans et al[107])	Electrophysiological characterization of pilocarpine's effects	Acute (1-5 mmol/L)	Attenuation of pilocarpine's presynaptic inhibitory effects	PKC inhibitor (H7) or phorbol ester pretreatment blocks lithium's effects
AtT 20 cells (Reisine and Katz[108])	ACTH secretion and desensitization of ACTH secretion	Acute and prolonged (2 mmol/L)	Facilitates ACTH secretion	Cross-desensitization with lithium's secretory effects
SD rats (Anderson et al,[109] Wang and Friedman[110])	Phorbol ester–induced ^{3}H–5-HT release	3 days and chronic (therapeutic)	3-day dose facilitates, but decreases ^{3}H–5-HT release	Decreased translocation of PKC also reported
SD rats (Lenox et al[111])	In vitro PKC-mediated ^{32}P phosphorylation	3 weeks (therapeutic)	Decreased in vitro PKC-mediated phosphorylation of 83- and 45-kd substrates	Decreased levels of MARCKS protein also
SD rats (Manji et al[112])	^{3}H-PDBU binding and immunoblotting of PKC isozymes	4-5 weeks (therapeutic)	Reduced ^{3}H-PDBU binding and reduced membrane PKC α levels	No significant effects on PKC β or PKC γ levels in subcortical areas
SD rats (Casebolt and Jope[113])	In vitro PKC-mediated ^{32}P phosphorylation	4 weeks (therapeutic)	Reduced PKC-mediated phosphorylation of 87-, 18-, and 19-kd membrane proteins	No effect on relative cytosol-membrane PKC activity

**PKC indicates protein kinase C; ACTH, corticotropin; 5-HT, serotonin; MARCKS, myristoylated alanine-rich C kinase substrate; PDBU, phorbol 12, 13-dibutyrate; and SD, Sprague-Dawley.*

lar cloning has recently revealed the presence of multiple, closely related PKC isoforms; the differential tissue distribution of PKC isozymes as well as the fact that several isoforms are expressed within a single cell type suggest that each isozyme may exert distinct cellular functions.[54,105,106] At rest, the PKC isozymes exist in both cytosolic and membrane-bound forms, but with partitioning predominantly in the cytosolic form. Activation of receptors coupled to phospholipase C (which results in the production of DAG) facilitates the translocation of cytosolic PKC to the membrane and its activation.

Recent evidence accumulating from various laboratories[107-113] has demonstrated that lithium exerts significant effects on PKC in a number of cell systems, including the brain (**Table 4**).[21] Currently available data suggest that acute lithium exposure facilitates a number of PKC-mediated responses, whereas longer-term exposure results in an attenuation of phorbol ester–mediated responses that may be accompanied by a down-regulation of PKC isozymes.[21,105-115] Interestingly, this pattern of effects is seen both in cultured cells in vitro and in brain in vivo. Biochemical studies have revealed biphasic effects of lithium on PKC-mediated events in rat hippocampus; 3-day lithium administration augments 5-HT release, whereas chronic (3-week) lithium administration at therapeutic levels attenuates both the phorbol ester–induced cytosol to membrane PKC translocation and ^{3}H–5-HT release in hippocampus.[109,110,113] Activation of PKC is now known to facilitate the release of a number of neurotransmitters, although the precise mechanisms remain to be fully elucidated; it has been postulated, however, that the phosphorylation of myristoylated alanine-rich C kinase substrate (MARCKS) and growth-associated protein (GAP-43) by PKC plays a key role in facilitating neurotransmitter release.[115,116] In this context, it is noteworthy that Lenox and associates[111] have recently demonstrated reduced in vitro phosphorylation of two major protein substrates for PKC in rat hippocampus, following chronic in vivo exposure to lithium at therapeutic levels. Using immunoblot analysis, they also demonstrated that the levels of MARCKS, a protein implicated in synaptic transmission, was significantly reduced after chronic lithium exposure.[111] Using quantitative autoradiographic techniques, Manji and associates[112] have recently demonstrated that chronic (5-week) lithium administration results in a significant decrease in membrane-associated PKC levels in several hippocampal structures, most notably the subiculum and CA1 regions, in the absence of any significant changes in the various other cortical and subcortical structures examined. Furthermore, immunoblotting using monoclonal anti-PKC antibodies revealed an isozyme-specific decrease in PKC α (which has been particularly implicated in facilitating neurotransmitter release)[117,118] in the absence of significant alterations in PKC β or PKC γ.[112] It is noteworthy that, presumably as a result of inositol depletion in the presence of lithium, metabolite levels within the phospholipid portion of the hydrolytic pathway that include DAG, phosphatidic acid, and cytidine monophosphate-phosphatidate levels have been shown to be significantly elevated in a variety of cell types, including brain cells (Figure 1).[119-123] Since PKC activation is often followed by its rapid proteolytic degradation,[54,105,106,124] a prolonged increase in DAG levels by lithium may lead to an increased membrane translocation and subsequent degradation of PKC isozymes. Such a mechanism would also be consistent with the accumulating evidence that lithium acutely activates PKC, whereas prolonged treatment is associated with decreased PKC-mediated responses, including neurotransmitter release (Figure 4).[21]

Do these effects of lithium on PKC have any clinical relevance? Interestingly, both the short-term activation of PKC and the decrease in the

Table 5. Effects of Lithium on Gene Expression in Rodent Brain*

Tissue (Reference)	Lithium Administration Paradigm	Lithium Effects	Comments
SD rats (Pfeiffer et al[127])	6 mmol/L per kilogram per day for 10 days	Increased glucocorticoid type II mRNA levels in selected areas of rat brain	Sex differences in lithium's regional effects
SD rats (Colin et al[75])	"Therapeutic" levels for 4 weeks	Increased AC types I and II mRNA levels in cortex	Lithium treatment also increased AC type I and II protein levels
SD rats (Colin et al[75])	Therapeutic levels for 4 weeks	Reduced $G\alpha_{i1}$ and $G\alpha_{i2}$ mRNA levels in cortex	Also observed reduced $G\alpha_{i1}$ and $G\alpha_{i2}$ protein levels
Wistar rats (Li et al[89,90])	Therapeutic levels for 3 weeks	Reduced $G\alpha_{s1}$, $G\alpha_{i1}$, and $G\alpha_{i2}$ mRNA levels in cortex	PKC regulates $G\alpha_s$ and $G\alpha_i$ mRNA levels in a similar manner in isolated systems
Fisher rats (Sivam et al[128])	4 mmol/kg per day for 6 days	Increased prodynorphis mRNA levels in basal ganglia	PKC regulates prodynorphin expression
SD rats (Weiner et al[129])	Acute injection	Marked augmentation of pilocarpine-induced *fos* mRNA levels in cortex	Acute lithium potentiation of M_1-PKC–mediated *fos* gene expression
SD rats (Weiner et al[129])	6 days	Augmentation of pilocarpine-induced *fos* mRNA in cortex, but less than after 1 day of lithium administration	Suggests an attenuation of previously enhanced M_1-PKC responses (due to reduced PKC levels?)
Fisher 344 rats (Sivam et al[130])	4 mmol/kg per day for 1-4 days	Increased expression of striatal preprotachykinin gene expresson	Activation of PKC also increases preprotachykinin gene expression

**mRNA indicates messenger RNA; AC, adenylyl cyclase; $G\alpha_i$, α subunit of G protein mediating the inhibition of AC; PKC, protein kinase C; $G\alpha_s$, α subunit of G protein mediating the stimulation of AC; M_1, muscarinic receptor subtype; and SD, Sprague-Dawley.*

levels of PKC α and MARCKS following chronic lithium administration *may* underlie (at least in part) certain well-documented effects of lithium on monoaminergic systems. With respect to the short-term effects, de Montigny and associates[125] (using electrophysiological recordings) have demonstrated that lithium enhances the release of 5-HT in the hippocampus, an effect that would be entirely consistent with an activation of PKC by subacute lithium administration. These observations led to the proposal that lithium might increase the efficacy of other antidepressants[125]; this postulate has, of course, been borne out in several open and double-blind clinical investigations.[126] By contrast, the decrease in the levels of PKC α and MARCKS observed after chronic lithium administration may represent one mechanism by which chronic lithium administration attenuates the release of catecholamines and, along with its effects on receptor-G protein coupling, may be relevant to lithium's protective effects against spontaneous, stress-induced, and drug-induced (eg, stimulant) manic episodes. Since PKC is known to regulate the induction of a variety of genes and since lithium's therapeutic effects generally require chronic administration, it is also noteworthy that increasingly, recent research has demonstrated that lithium affects gene expression in the CNS.

LITHIUM AND GENE EXPRESSION

As noted already, there has been a growing appreciation that any relevant biochemical model of lithium's actions must account for the observation that both its antimanic and antidepressant effects generally require days to weeks to develop[1,6,21]; biochemical changes requiring such prolonged administration of a drug suggest the potential for alterations at the genomic level. In this context, it is noteworthy that increasing evidence[77,91,92,127-130] suggests that lithium affects gene expression (**Table 5**), possibly via PKC-induced alterations in nuclear transcription regulatory factors responsible for modulating the expression of specific genes.[131] Several recent studies have demonstrated that lithium alters the expression of the early response gene, c-*fos*, in different cell systems, including the brain, through a PKC-mediated mechanism.[21] For example, preincubation of cultured PC12 cells (a rat pheochromocytoma cell line) with lithium for 16 hours markedly potentiates *fos* expression in response to the muscarinic agonist, carbachol. Lithium pretreatment in these cells also potentiates *fos* expression in response to phorbol esters, which directly activate PKC and thus bypass PI turnover.[132] Moreover, lithium's effects show a selectivity for the PKC signal transduction pathway and do not appear to be due to a nonspecific alteration in mRNA stability, since the *fos* expression in response to AC activation is unaffected under identical conditions.[132] Perhaps adding more relevance to the results observed in cell culture, a single intraperitoneal injection of lithium results in an augmentation of pilocarpine-induced *fos* gene expression in rat brain, which can be antagonized by the M_1 antagonist, pirenzepine.[129] These lithium-induced effects on the expression of *fos* mRNA, generally thought to represent a "master switch" to turn on a "second wave" of specific neuronal genes of functional importance, offer a mechanism for affecting long-term events in the brain.[131] In this regard, incubation of cerebellar granule cells with 1.5 mmol/L lithium has recently been shown to result in biphasic effects on the levels of both *fos* mRNA and M_3 receptor mRNA, consistent with the previously noted acute vs chronic effects of lithium on PKC-mediated responses.[133]

Chronic administration of lithium at therapeutic levels also significantly changes the expression of a number of genes in rat brain[21]; these include the gene expression of a number of neuromodulatory peptide hormones (prodynorphin, preprotachykinin, and neuropeptide Y) and hormone receptors (glucocorticoid type II).[127,128,130,134,135] In view of lithium's proposed actions on synaptic function and signal-transducing systems, it is also noteworthy that chronic lithium administration (3 to 4 weeks) has been reported to alter the expression of various components of second-messenger generating systems, including $G\alpha_{i1}$,[75,89,90] $G\alpha_{i2}$,[75,89,90] and $G\alpha_s$[89,90] mRNA and AC types I and II mRNA in rat brain.[75] It must be acknowledged that, at present, the therapeutic relevance of these lithium-induced alterations in gene expression remains to be established; nevertheless, the demonstration of the long-term modulation of the genetic expression of critical proteins involved in the regulation of synaptic function in the brain is of considerable heuristic importance and allows for the design of future studies to delineate their potential roles in the therapeutic actions of lithium.

CONCLUDING REMARKS

Lithium remains our most effective treatment for reducing the frequency and severity of recurrent affective episodes but, despite extensive research, the underlying biological basis for the therapeutic efficacy of this drug remains unknown. In recent years, however, there has been considerable progress in the identification of signal transduction pathways as targets for lithium's actions. Regulation of signal transduction within critical regions of the brain by lithium affects the intracellular signal generated by multiple neurotransmitter systems; these effects represent attractive targets for its therapeutic efficacy, since the behavioral and physiological manifestations of the illness are complex and are likely mediated by a network of interconnected neurotransmitter pathways. The biological processes in the brain responsible for the episodic clinical manifestation of mania and depression may be due to an inability to mount the appropriate compensatory responses necessary to maintain homeostatic regulation, with the resultant clinical picture being reflected in disruption of behavior, circadian rhythms, neurophysiological features of sleep, and neuroendocrine and biochemical regulation within the brain.[1,22,136,137] The molecular targets underlying lithium's ability to stabilize an underlying dysregulation of limbic and limbic-associated function is thus critical to our understanding of its mechanism of action.

There have been significant advances in our understanding of the long-term action of lithium on PKC-mediated events, particularly the posttranslational modification of key synaptic proteins. Biochemical changes requiring prolonged administration of a drug such as lithium also suggest alterations at the genomic level, which may be mediated in large part by the activation and inactivation of subsets of genes with temporal specificity. In this context, the complex effect of lithium on PKC isozymes represents both an attractive and heuristic mechanism by which the expression of various proteins involved in long-term neuronal plasticity and cellular response is modulated, thereby compensating for as yet genetically undefined physiological abnormalities in critical regions of the brain.

Many questions still remained to be answered. For example, do the observed effects of chronic lithium administration on signal transduction pathways and gene expression stem exclusively from lithium's demonstrated efficacy as an inhibitor of inositol monophosphatase and resultant changes in the DAG pathway, or does lithium under therapeutic conditions have other, more direct effects? Studies currently under way examining the effects of other inositol monophosphatase inhibitors (with no structural similarity to lithium) should soon yield important clues and offer insights into new drug development. Nevertheless, it is clear that our understanding of the mechanisms of action of lithium has gained much from the rapid technological advances in both biochemistry and molecular biology. Studies designed to examine a potential action of lithium on the genetically defined defect underlying the dysregulation inherent in bipolar affective disorder must await the ultimate identification of the aberrant protein(s) through advanced genetic strategies and the use of new experimental approaches, including the development of transgenic animals. In the meantime, since lithium is so effective in the treatment of this illness, using cellular and molecular pharmacological studies to identify molecular targets for the long-term action of chronic lithium administration in the brain holds the potential for the development of newer, more potent therapeutics. In conjunction with molecular genetic approaches, this will facilitate our understanding of the biological factors predisposing individuals to cyclic affective disorders such as bipolar affective disorder.

Accepted for publication April 13, 1995.

Reprint requests to Molecular Pathophysiology Program, Department of Psychiatry and Pharmacology, Wayne State University School of Medicine, UHC-9B, 4201 St Antoine, Detroit, MI 48201 (Dr Manji).

REFERENCES

1. Goodwin FK, Jamison KR. *Manic-Depressive Illness.* New York, NY: Oxford University Press; 1990.
2. Muller-Oerlinghausen B, Ahrens B, Grof E, Grof P, Lenz G, Schou M, Simhandl C, Thau K, Volk J, Wolf R. The effect of long-term lithium treatment on the mortality of patients with manic-depressive and schizoaffective illness. *Acta Psychiatr Scand.* 1992;86:218-222.
3. Vestergaard P, Aagaard J. Five-year mortality in lithium-treated manic-depressive patients. *J Affect Disord.* 1991;21:33-38.
4. Schou M. Clinical aspects of lithium in psychiatry. In: Birch NJ, ed. *Lithium and the Cell.* Orlando, Fla: Academic Press Inc; 1991:1-6.
5. Bunney WE, Garland-Bunney BL. Mechanisms of action of lithium in affective illness: basic and clinical implications. In: Hy M, ed. *Psychopharmacology: The Third Generation of Progress.* New York, NY: Raven Press; 1987: 553-565.
6. Jope RS, Williams MB. Lithium and brain signal transduction systems. *Biochem Pharmacol.* 1994;47:429-441.
7. Risby ED, Hsiao JK, Manji HK, Bitran J, Moses F, Zhou DF, Potter WZ. The mechanisms of action of lithium, II: effects on adenylate cyclase activity and β-adrenergic receptor binding in normal subjects. *Arch Gen Psychiatry.* 1991; 48:513-524.
8. Wood AJ, Goodwin GM. A review of the biochemical and neuropharmacological actions of lithium. *Psychol Med.* 1987;17:579-600.
9. Hsiao JK, Agren H, Bartko JJ, Rudorfer MV, Linnoila M, Potter WZ. Monoamine neurotransmitter interactions and the prediction of antidepressant response. *Arch Gen Psychiatry.* 1987; 44:1078-1083.
10. Janowsky DS, El-Yousef MK, Davis JM, Sekerke HJ. A cholinergic-adrenergic hypothesis of mania and depression. *Lancet.* 1972;2:632-635.
11. Manji HK. G proteins: implications for psychiatry. *Am J Psychiatry.* 1992;149:746-760.
12. Prange AJ, Wilson IC, Lynn CL, Alltop LB, Stikeleather RA. L-tryptophan in mania: contributions to a permissive hypothesis of affective disorders. *Arch Gen Psychiatry.* 1974;30: 56-62.
13. Meltzer HY. The importance of serotonin-dopamine interactions in the action of clozapine. *Br J Psychiatry.* 1992;17(suppl):22-29.
14. Hsiao JK, Colison J, Bartko JJ, Doran AR, Konicki PE, Potter WZ, Pickar D. Monoamine neurotransmitter interactions in drug-free and neuroleptic-treated schizophrenics. *Arch Gen Psychiatry.* 1993;50:606-614.
15. Bourne HR, Nicoll R. Molecular machines in-

tegrate coincident synaptic signals. *Cell.* 1993; 72(suppl):65-75.
16. Ross EM. Signal sorting and amplification through G protein-coupled receptors. *Neuron.* 1989;3:141-152.
17. Taylor CW. The role of G proteins in transmembrane signalling. *Biochem J.* 1990;272:1-13.
18. Baraban JM, Worley PF, Snyder SH. Second messenger and psychoactive drug action: focus on the phosphoinositide system and lithium. *Am J Psychiatry.* 1989;146:1251-1260.
19. Lachman HM, Papolos DF. Abnormal signal transduction: a hypothetical model for bipolar affective disorder. *Life Sci.* 1991;45:1413-1426.
20. Suppes T, Baldessarini RJ, Faedda GL, Tohen M. Risk of recurrence following discontinuation of lithium treatment in bipolar disorder. *Arch Gen Psychiatry.* 1991;48:1082-1088.
21. Manji HK, Lenox RH. Long-term action of lithium: a role for transcriptional and posttranscriptional factors regulated by protein kinase C. *Synapse.* 1994;16:11-28.
22. Lenox RH, Manji HK. Lithium. In: Nemeroff CB, Schatzberg AF, ed. *American Psychiatric Press Textbook of Psychopharmacology.* Washington, DC: American Psychiatric Press Inc; 1995: 303-350.
23. Birnbaumer L. G proteins in signal transduction. *Annu Rev Pharmacol Toxicol.* 1990;30: 675-705.
24. Spiegel AM, Shenker A, Weinstein LS. Receptor-effector coupling by G proteins: implications for normal and abnormal signal transduction. *Endocr Rev.* 1992;13:536-565.
25. Iyengar R, Birnbaumer L. *G Proteins.* Orlando, Fla: Academic Press Inc; 1990.
26. Gilman AG. G proteins and regulation of adenylyl cyclase. *JAMA.* 1989;262:1819-1825.
27. Iniguez-Lluhi J, Kleuss C, Gilman AG. The importance of G protein βγ subunits. *Trends Cell Biol.* 1993;3:230-236.
28. Pitcher JA, Inglese J, Higgins JB, Arriza JL, Casey RJ, Kim C, Benovic JL, Kwatra MM, Caron MG, Lefkowitz RJ. Role of beta gamma subunits of G proteins in targeting the beta-adrenergic receptor kinase to membrane-bound receptors. *Science.* 1992;257:1264-1267.
29. Birnbaumer L. Receptor-to-effector signaling through G proteins: roles for beta gamma dimers as well as alpha subunits. *Cell.* 1993;71:1069-1072.
30. Simonds WF, Manji HK, Lupas A, Garritsen A. G proteins and βARK: a new twist for the coiled-coil. *Trends Biochem Sci.* 1993;18:315-317.
31. Simon MI, Strathmann MP, Gautam N. Diversity of G proteins in signal transduction. *Science.* 1991;252:802-808.
32. Katada T, Bokoch GM, Northup JK, Ui M, Gilman AG. The inhibitory guanine nucleotide-binding regulatory component of adenylate cyclase: properties and function of the purified protein. *J Biol Chem.* 1984;259:3568-3577.
33. Rodbell M. The role of hormone receptors and GTP-regulatory proteins in membrane transduction. *Nature.* 1980;284:17-22.
34. Rana RS, Hokin LE. Role of phosphoinositides in transmembrane signaling. *Physiol Rev.* 1990; 70:115-164.
35. Chuang DM. Neurotransmitter receptors and phosphoinositide turnover. *Annu Rev Pharmacol Toxicol.* 1989;29:71-110.
36. Fisher SK, Heacock AM, Agranoff BW. Inositol lipids and signal transduction in the nervous system: an update. *J Neurochem.* 1992;58:18-38.
37. Allison JH, Stewart MA. Reduced brain inositol in lithium-treated rats. *Nat New Biol.* 1971; 233:267-268.
38. Hallcher LM, Sherman WR. The effects of lithium ion and other agents on the activity of *myo*-inositol-1-phosphatase from bovine brain. *J Biol Chem.* 1980;255:10896-10901.
39. Sherman WR. Inositol homeostasis, lithium and diabetes. In: Michell RH, Drummond AH, Downes CP, eds. *Inositol Lipids in Cell Signalling.* Orlando, Fla: Academic Press Inc; 1989:39-80.
40. Nahorski SR, Jenkinson S, Challiss RA. Disruption of phosphoinositide signalling by lithium. *Biochem Soc Trans.* 1992;20:430-434.
41. Nahorski SR, Ragan CI, Challiss RAJ. Lithium and the phosphoinositide cycle: an example of uncompetitive inhibition and its pharmacological consequences. *Trends Pharmacol Sci.* 1991; 12:297-303.
42. Berridge MJ, Downes CP, Hanley MR. Lithium amplifies agonist-dependent phosphatidylinositol responses in brain and salivary glands. *Biochem J.* 1982;206:587-595.
43. Berridge MJ, Downes CP, Hanley MR. Neural and developmental actions of lithium: a unifying hypothesis. *Cell.* 1989;59:411-419.
44. Casebolt T, Jope RS. Chronic lithium reduces norepinephrine-stimulated inositol phospholipid hydrolysis in rat cortex. *Eur J Pharmacol.* 1987;140:245-246.
45. Casebolt T, Jope RS. Long-term lithium treatment selectively reduces receptor coupled inositol phospholipid hydrolysis in rat brain. *Biol Psychiatry.* 1989;25:329-340.
46. Godfrey PP, McClue SJ, White AM, Wood AJ, Grahame SD. Subacute and chronic in vivo lithium treatment inhibits agonist- and sodium fluoride-stimulated inositol phosphate production in rat cortex. *J Neurochem.* 1989;52:498-506.
47. Kendall DA, Nahorski SR. Acute and chronic lithium treatments influence agonist and depolarization-stimulated inositol phospholipid hydrolysis in rat cerebral cortex. *J Pharmacol Exp Ther.* 1987;241:1023-1027.
48. Whitworth P, Kendall DA. Lithium selectively inhibits muscarinic receptor-stimulated inositol tetrakisphosphate accumulation in mouse cerebral cortex slices. *J Neurochem.* 1988;51: 258-265.
49. Whitworth P, Kendall DA. Effects of lithium on inositol phospholipid hydrolysis and inhibition of dopamine D1 receptor-mediated cyclic AMP formation by carbachol in rat brain slices. *J Neurochem.* 1989;53:536-541.
50. Ellis J, Lenox RH. Receptor coupling to G proteins: interactions not affected by lithium. *Lithium.* 1991;2:141-147.
51. Lee CH, Dixon JF, Reichman M, Moummi C, Los G, Hokin LE. Li^+ increases accumulation of inositol 1,4,5-trisphosphate and inositol 1,3,4,5-tetrakisphosphate in cholinergically stimulated brain cortex slices in guinea pig, mouse and rat: the increases require inositol supplementation in mouse and rat but not in guinea pig. *Biochem J.* 1992;282:377-385.
52. Gray DW, Challiss RA, Nahorski SR. Differential effects of lithium on muscarinic cholinoceptor-stimulated CMP-phosphatidate accumulation in cerebellar granule cells, CHO-M3 cells, and SH-SY5Y neuroblastoma cells. *J Neurochem.* 1994;63:1354-1360.
53. Sherman WR. Lithium and the phosphoinositide signaling system. In, Birch NJ, ed. *Lithium and the Cell.* Orlando, Fla: Academic Press Inc; 1991:121-157.
54. Nishizuka Y. Intracellular signaling by hydrolysis of phospholipids and activation of protein kinase C. *Science.* 1992;258:607-614.
55. Varney MA, Godfrey PP, Drummond AH, Watson SP. Chronic lithium treatment inhibits basal and agonist-stimulated responses in rat cerebral cortex and GH_3 pituitary cells. *Mol Pharmacol.* 1992;4:671-678.
56. Kennedy ED, Challiss RAJ, Ragan CI, Nahorski SR. Reduced inositol polyphosphate accumulation and inositol supply induced by lithium in stimulated cerebral cortex slices. *Biochem J.* 1990;267:781-786.
57. Kofman O, Belmaker RH. Biochemical, behavioral, and clinical studies of the role of inositol in lithium treatment and depression. *Biol Psychiatry.* 1993;34:839-852.
58. Maslanski JA, Leshko L, Busa WB. Lithium-sensitive production of inositol phosphates during amphibian embryonic mesoderm induction. *Science.* 1992;256:243-245.
59. Tricklebank MD, Singh L, Jackson A, Oles RJ. Evidence that a proconvulsant action of lithium is mediated by inhibition of *myo*-inositol phosphatase in mouse brain. *Brain Res.* 1991;558: 145-148.
60. Song L, Jope RS. Chronic lithium treatment impairs phosphatidylinositol hydrolysis in membranes from rat brain regions. *J Neurochem.* 1992;58:2200-2206.
61. Forn J, Valdecasas FG. Effects of lithium on brain adenyl cyclase activity. *Biochem Pharmacol.* 1971;20:2773-2999.
62. Dousa T, Hechter O. Lithium and brain adenyl cyclase. *Lancet.* 1970;1:834-835.
63. Ebstein RP, Hermoni M, Belmaker RH. The effect of lithium on noradrenaline-induced cyclic AMP accumulation in rat brain: inhibition after chronic treatment and absence of supersensitivity. *J Pharmacol Exp Ther.* 1980;213:161-167.
64. Belmaker RH. Receptors, adenylate cyclase, depression, and lithium. *Biol Psychiatry.* 1981; 16:333-350.
65. Ebstein RP, Moscovich D, Zeevi S, Amiri Z, Lerer B. Effect of lithium in vitro and after chronic treatment on human platelet adenylate cyclase activity: postreceptor modification of second messenger signal amplification. *Psychiatry Res.* 1987; 21:221-228.
66. Mork A, Geisler A. The effects of lithium in vitro and ex vivo on adenylate cyclase in brain are exerted by distinct mechanisms. *Neuropharmacology.* 1989;28:307-311.
67. Mork A, Geisler A. Effects of GTP on hormone-stimulated adenylate cyclase activity in cerebral cortex, striatum, and hippocampus from rats treated chronically with lithium. *Biol Psychiatry.* 1989;26:279-288.
68. Mork A, Geisler A. Effects of lithium ex vivo on the GTP-mediated inhibition of calcium-stimulated adenylate cyclase activity in rat brain. *Eur J Pharmacol.* 1989;168:347-354.
69. Mork A, Geisler A, Hollund P. Effects of lithium on second messenger systems in the brain. *Pharmacol Toxicol.* 1992;71(suppl 1):4-17.
70. Ebstein RP, Lerer B, Bennett ER, Shapira B, Kindler S, Shemesh Z, Gerstenhaber N. Lithium modulation of second messenger signal amplification in man: inhibition of phosphatidylinositol-specifec phospholipase C and denylate cyclase activity. *Psychiatry Res.* 1988;24:45-52.
71. Newman ME, Belmaker RH. Effects of lithium in vitro and ex vivo on components of the adenylate cyclase system in membranes from the cerebral cortex of the rat. *Neuropharmacology.* 1987;26:211-217.
72. Dousa TP. Interaction of lithium with vasopressin-sensitive cyclic AMP system of human renal medulla. *Endocrinology.* 1974;95:1359-1366.
73. Goldberg H, Clayman P, Skorecki K. Mechanism of Li inhibition of vasopressin-sensitive adenylate cyclase in cultured renal epithelial cells. *Am J Physiol.* 1988;24:F995-F1002.
74. Tseng FY, Pasquali D, Field JB. Effects of lithium on stimulated metabolic parameters in dog thyroid slices. *Acta Endocrinol (Copenh).* 1989; 121:615-620.
75. Colin SF, Chang HC, Mollner S, et al. Chronic lithium regulates the expression of adenylate cyclase and G_i-protein alpha subunit in rat cerebral cortex. *Proc Natl Acad Sci U S A.* 1991; 88:10634-10637.
76. Friedman E, Oleshansky MA, Moy P, Gershon S. Lithium and catecholamine-induced plasma cyclic AMP elevation. In: Cooper TB, Gershon S, Kline NS, Schou MA, eds. *Lithium Controversies and Unresolved Issues.* Princeton, NJ: Excerpta Medica; 1979:730-736.
77. Belmaker RH, Kon M, Ebstein RP, Dasberg H. Partial inhibition by lithium of the epinephrine-stimulated rise in plasma cyclic GMP in humans. *Biol Psychiatry.* 1980;15:3-8.
78. Newman M, Klein E, Birmaher B, Feinsod M, Belmaker RH. Lithium at therapeutic concentrations inhibits human brain noradrenaline-sensitive cyclic AMP accumulation. *Brain Res.* 1983;278:380-381.

79. Ebstein RP, Lerer B, Shlaufman M, Belmaker RH. The effect of repeated electroconvulsive shock treatment and chronic lithium feeding on the release of norepinephrine from rat cortical vesicular preparations. *Cell Mol Neurobiol.* 1983; 3:191-201.
80. Newman ME, Lerer B, Lichtenberg P, Shapira B. Platelet adenylate cyclase activity in depression and after clomipramine and lithium treatment. *Psychopharmacology.* 1992;109:231-234.
81. Lonati GM, Emrich HM, Raptis C, Pirke KM. Effect of in vivo lithium treatment on (−) isoproterenol-stimulated cAMP accumulation in lymphocytes of healthy subjects and patients with affective psychoses. *Pharmacopsychiatry.* 1989;22:241-245.
82. Singer I, Rotenberg D, Puschett JB. Lithium-induced nephrogenic diabetes insipidus: in vivo and in vitro studies. *J Clin Invest.* 1972;51: 1081-1091.
83. Andersen PH, Geisler A. Lithium inhibition of forskolin-stimulated adenylate cyclase. *Neuropsychobiology.* 1984;12:1-3.
84. Geisler A, Klysner R, Andersen PH. Influence of lithium in vitro and in vivo on the catecholamine-sensitive cerebral adenylate cyclase systems. *Acta Pharmacol Toxicol.* 1985;56:80-97.
85. Mork A, Geisler A. Effects of lithium on calmodulin-stimulated adenylate cyclase activity in cortical membranes from rat brain. *Pharmacol Toxicol.* 1987;60:17-23.
86. Masana MI, Bitran JA, Hsiao JK, Mefford IN, Potter WZ. Lithium effects on noradrenergic-linked adenylate cyclase activity in intact rat brain: an in vivo microdialysis study. *Brain Res.* 1991; 538:333-336.
87. Avissar S, Schreiber G, Danon A, Belmaker RH. Lithium inhibits adrenergic and cholinergic increases in GTP binding in rat cortex. *Nature.* 1988;331:440-442.
88. Masana MI, Bitran JA, Hsiao JK, Potter WZ. In-vivo evidence that lithium inactivates G_i modulation of adenylate cyclase activity in brain. *J Neurochem.* 1992;59:200-205.
89. Li PP, Young LT, Tam YK, Sibony D, Warsh JJ. Effects of chronic lithium and carbamazepine treatment on G-protein subunit expression in rat cerebral cortex. *Biol Psychiatry.* 1993; 34:162-170.
90. Li PP, Tam YK, Young LT, Warsh JJ. Lithium decreases G_s, G_{i-1} and G_{i-2} alpha-subunit mRNA levels in rat cortex. *Eur J Pharmacol.* 1991; 206:165-166.
91. Hsiao JK, Manji HK, Chen GA, Bitran JA, Risby ED, Potter WZ. Lithium administration modulates platelet G_i in humans. *Life Sci.* 1992;50: 227-233.
92. Newman ME, Shapira B, Lerer B. Effects of lithium and desimipramine on second messenger responses in rat hippocampus: relation to G protein effects. *Neuropharmacology.* 1991; 30:1297-1301.
93. Manji HK, Bitran JA, Masana MI, Chen G, Hsiao JK, Risby ED, Rudorfer MV, Potter WZ. Signal transduction modulation by lithium: cell culture, cerebral microdialysis and human studies. *Psychopharmacol Bull.* 1991;27:199-208.
94. Ui M. Pertussis toxin as a valuable probe for G protein involvement in signal transduction. In: Moss J, Vaughn M, eds. *ADP-Ribosylation Toxins and G Proteins.* Washington, DC: American Society for Microbiology; 1990:45-79.
95. Wang YC, Pandey GN, Mendels J, Frazer A. Effect of lithium on prostaglandin F1-stimulated adenylate cyclase activity of human platelets. *Biochem Pharmacol.* 1974;23:845-855.
96. Garcia-Sevilla JA, Guimón J, García-Vallejo P, Fuster MJ. Biochemical and functional evidence of supersensitive platelet α_2-adrenoceptors in major affective disorder: effect of long-term lithium carbonate treatment. *Arch Gen Psychiatry.* 1986;43:51-57.
97. Smith CB, Hollingsworth PJ, Garcia-Sevilla JA, Zis AP. Platelet alpha$_2$ adrenoreceptors are decreased in number after antidepressant therapy. *Prog Neuropsychopharmacol Biol Psychiatry.* 1983;7:241-247.
98. Manji HK, Hsiao JK, Risby ED, Oliver J, Rudorfer MV, Potter WZ. The mechanisms of action of lithium, I: effects on serotoninergic and noradrenergic systems in normal subjects. *Arch Gen Psychiatry.* 1991;48:505-512.
99. Garcia-Sainz JA, Gutierrez VG. Activation of protein kinase C alters the interaction of alpha$_2$-adrenoceptors and the inhibitory GTP-binding protein (G_i) in human platelets. *FEBS Lett.* 1989; 257:427-430.
100. Halenda SP, Volpi M, Zavoico GB, Shaafi RI, Feinstein MB. Effects of thrombin, phorbol myristate acetate, and prostaglandin D_2 on 40-41 kDa protein that is ADP ribosylated by pertussis toxin in platelets. *FEBS Lett.* 1986;204:341-346.
101. Houslay MD. 'Crosstalka': pivotal role for protein kinase C in modulating relationships between signal transduction pathways. *Eur J Biochem.* 1991;195:9-27.
102. Sagi-Eisenberg R. GTP-binding proteins as possible targets for protein kinase C action. *Trends Biochem Sci.* 1989;14:355-357.
103. Huganir RL, Greengard P. Regulation of neurotransmitter receptor desensitization by protein phosphorylation. *Neuron.* 1990;5:555-567.
104. Thiele EA, Eipper BA. Effect of secretagogues on components of the secretory system in AtT-20 cells. *Endocrinology.* 1990;126:809-817.
105. Stabel S, Parker PJ. Protein kinase C. *Pharmacol Ther.* 1991;51:71-95.
106. Huang KP. The mechanism of protein kinase C activation. *Trends Neurosci.* 1989;12:425-432.
107. Evans MS, Zorumski CF, Clifford DB. Lithium enhances neuronal muscarinic excitation by presynaptic facilitation. *Neuroscience.* 1990;38:457-468.
108. Reisine T, Zatz M. Interactions between lithium, calcium, diacylglycerides and phorbol esters in the regulation of ACTH release from AtT-20 cells. *J Neurochem.* 1987;49:884-889.
109. Anderson SMP, Godfrey PP, Grahame-Smith DG. The effects of phorbol esters and lithium on 5-HT release in rat hippocampal slices. *Br J Pharmacol.* 1988;93(suppl):96P.
110. Wang HY, Friedman E. Lithium inhibition of protein kinase C activation-induced serotonin release. *Psychopharmacology.* 1989;99:213-218.
111. Lenox RH, Watson DG, Patel J, Ellis J. Chronic lithium administration alters a prominent PKC substrate in rat hippocampus. *Brain Res.* 1992; 570:333-340.
112. Manji HK, Etcheberrigaray R, Chen G, Olds JL. Lithium decreases membrane-associated Protein kinase C in hippocampus: selectivity for the α isozyme. *J Neurochem.* 1993;61:2303-2310.
113. Casebolt TL, Jope RS. Effects of chronic lithium treatment on protein kinase C and cyclic AMP-dependent protein phosphorylation. *Biol Psychiatry.* 1991;25:329-340.
114. Bitran JA, Potter WZ, Manji HK, Gusovsky F. Chronic Li^+ attenuates agonist- and phorbol ester–mediated Na^+/Ha^+ antiporter activity in HL-60 cells. *Eur J Pharmacol.* 1990;188:193-202.
115. Robinson PJ. The role of protein kinase C and its neuronal substrates dephosphin, B-50, and MARCKS in neurotransmitter release. *Mol Neurobiol.* 1991;5:87-130.
116. De Graan PN, Schrama LH, Heemskerk FM, Dekker LV, Gispen WH. The role of protein kinase C substrate B-50 (GAP-43) in neurotransmitter release and long-term potentiation. *Adv Exp Med Biol.* 1990;268:347-358.
117. Ben-Shlomo H, Sigmund O, Stabel S, Reiss N, Naor Z. Preferential release of catecholamine from permeabilized PC12 cells by alpha- and beta-type protein kinase C subspecies. *Biochem J.* 1991;280:65-69.
118. Oda T, Shearman MS, Nishizuka Y. Synaptosomal protein kinase C subspecies, B: down-regulation promoted by phorbol ester and its effect on evoked norepinephrine release. *J Neurochem.* 1991;56:1263-1269.
119. Brami BA, Leli U, Hauser G. Influence of lithium on second messenger accumulation in NG108-15 cells. *Biochem Biophys Res Commun.* 1991; 174:606-612.
120. Brami BA, Leli U, Hauser G. Elevated phosphatidyl-CMP is not the source of diacylglycerol accumulation induced by lithium in NG108-15 cells. *J Neurochem.* 1993;60:1137-1142.
121. Downes CP, Stone MA. Lithium-induced reduction in intracellular inositol supply in cholinergically stimulated parotid gland. *Biochem J.* 1986;234:199-204.
122. Drummond AH, Raeburn CA. The interaction of lithium with thyrotropin releasing hormone-stimulated lipid metabolism in GH3 pituitary tumor cells. *Biochem J.* 1984;224:129-136.
123. Watson SP, Shipman L, Godfrey PP. Lithium potentiates agonist formation of [^{3}H]CDP-diacylglycerol in human platelets. *Eur J Pharmacol.* 1990;188:273-276.
124. Young S, Parker PJ, Ullrich A, Stabel S. Down-regulation of protein kinase C is due to an increased rate of degradation. *Biochem J.* 1987; 24:775-779.
125. de Montigny C, Cournoyer G, Morissett R, Langlois R, Caillé G. Lithium carbonate addition in tricyclic antidepressant-resistant unipolar depression: correlations with the neurobiologic actions of tricyclic antidepressant drugs and lithium ion on the serotonin system. *Arch Gen Psychiatry.* 1983;40:1327-1334.
126. Price LH. Lithium augmentation in tricyclic-resistant depression. In: Extein IL, ed. *Treatment of Tricyclic-Resistant Depression.* Washington, DC: American Psychiatric Press; 1989:49-79.
127. Pfeiffer A, Veilleux S, Barden N. Antidepressant and other centrally acting drugs regulate glucorticoid receptor messenger RNA levels in rat brain. *Psychoneuroendocrinology.* 1991;16:505-515.
128. Sivam SP, Takeuchi K, Li S, Douglass J, Civelli O, Calvetta L, Herbert E, McGinty JF, Hong JS. Lithium increases dynorphin A(1-8) and prodynorphin mRNA levels in the basal ganglia of rats. *Brain Res.* 1988;427:155-163.
129. Weiner ED, Kalasapudi VD, Papolos DF, Lachman HM. Lithium augments pilocarpine-induced *fos* gene expression in rat brain. *Brain Res.* 1991;553:117-122.
130. Sivam SP, Krause JE, Takeuchi K, Li S, McGinty JF, Hong JS. Lithium increases rat striatal beta- and gamma-preprotachykinin messenger RNAs. *J Pharmacol Exp Ther.* 1989;248: 1297-1301.
131. Hunter T, Karin M. The regulation of transcription by phosphorylation. *Cell.* 1992;70:375-387.
132. Divish MM, Sheftel G, Boyle A, Kalasapudi VD, Papolos DF, Lachman HM. Differential effect of lithium on *fos* protooncogene expression mediated by receptor and postreceptor activators of protein kinase C and cyclic adenosine monophosphate: model for its antimanic action. *J Neurosci Res.* 1991;28:40-48.
133. Gao XM, Fukamauchi F, Chuang DM. Long-term biphasic effects of lithium treatment on phospholipase C-coupled M3-muscarinic acetylcholine receptors in cultured cerebellar granule cells. *Neurochem Int.* 1993;22:395-403.
134. Weiner ED, Mallat AM, Papolos DF, Lachman HM. Acute lithium treatment enhances neuropeptide Y gene expression. *Mol Brain Res.* 1992; 12:209-214.
135. Kislauskis E, Dobner P. Mutually dependent response elements in the *cis*-regulatory region of the neurotensin/neuromedin N gene integrate environmental stimuli in PC12 cells. *Neuron.* 1990;4:783-795.
136. Depue R, Karuss S, Spoont M. A two-dimensional threshold model of seasonal bipolar affective disorder. In: Magnusson D, Ohman A, eds. *Psychopathology: An Interactional Perspective.* Orlando, Fla: Academic Press Inc; 1987:95-123.
137. Mandell A, Knapp S, Ehlers C, Russo PV. The stability of constrained randomness: lithium prophylaxis at several neurobiological levels. In: Post R, Ballenger J, eds. *Neurobiology of Mood Disorders.* Baltimore, Md: Williams and Wilkins; 1984:744-776.

ORIGINAL ARTICLE

Increased Rate of P300 Latency Prolongation With Age in Schizophrenia

Electrophysiological Evidence for a Neurodegenerative Process

Brian F. O'Donnell, PhD; Steven F. Faux, PhD; Robert W. McCarley, MD; Matthew O. Kimble; Dean F. Salisbury, PhD; Paul G. Nestor, PhD; Ron Kikinis MD; Ferenc A. Jolesz, MD; Martha E. Shenton, PhD

Background: The latency of the P300 event-related potential is prolonged in disorders associated with neural damage and degeneration and also becomes prolonged in the course of neural changes that accompany aging. We tested whether the rate of P300 latency increase with age was greater in male schizophrenic patients than in normal subjects because a steeper slope in schizophrenia would suggest a progressive neurodegenerative process. We also evaluated a subset of these subjects for changes in brain volumes as determined by magnetic resonance imaging.

Method: The P300 component was elicited during an auditory "oddball" paradigm and was recorded from 47 male patients with chronic schizophrenia whose mean age at onset was 22.4 years and from 47 age-, handedness-, and gender-matched control subjects. The relation of P300 latency and amplitude to age within each group was evaluated using correlation and regression analyses. Brain volumes determined via magnetic resonance imaging were evaluated by quantitative volumetric analyses of images acquired with three-dimensional Fourier transform and double echo-spin echo-pulse sequences.

Results: The slope of P300 latency on age was steeper for schizophrenic patients than for normal control subjects at midline frontal and central electrode sites. The slope of N100 latency did not differ, implying that the P300 differences were not likely to be due to peripheral hearing loss or damage affecting the initial stages of neural processing. Posterior superior temporal gyrus gray matter volume determined via magnetic resonance imaging significantly diminished with age on the left side in patients with schizophrenia but not on the right side or in controls; these slopes were not, however, statistically significantly different from each other.

Conclusions: These findings provide preliminary evidence that male patients with chronic schizophrenia experience a neurodegenerative process that becomes evident in adulthood and is reflected by the rate of change of P300 latency with age. Whether this process is due to the primary effects of schizophrenia or is secondary to factors associated with schizophrenia's chronic course and treatment remains a question for future investigation.

(Arch Gen Psychiatry. 1995;52:544-549)

From the Departments of Psychiatry (Drs O'Donnell, McCarley, Salisbury, Nestor, and Shenton and Mr Kimble) and Radiology (Drs Kikinis and Jolesz), Harvard Medical School, Boston, Mass; the Brockton (Mass) Veterans Affairs Medical Center (Drs O'Donnell, McCarley, Salisbury, Nestor, and Shenton and Mr Kimble); the Department of Radiology, Magnetic Resonance Imaging Division, Surgical Planning Center, Brigham and Women's Hospital, Boston (Drs Kikinis and Jolesz); and the Department of Psychology, Drake University, Des Moines, Iowa (Dr Faux).

SINCE KRAEPELIN'S description of the course of schizophrenia (dementia praecox) at the beginning of the century,[1] the question of whether schizophrenia is a neurodegenerative disorder has elicited sustained interest and controversy. Although the long-term course of schizophrenia shows great heterogeneity among patients,[2-9] a significant number of patients, sometimes termed *kraepelinian*, experience very poor outcomes.[10,11] In particular, a subset of elderly patients institutionalized on a long-term basis shows severe cognitive impairment that is suggestive of a progressive neurodegenerative disorder and that is not associated with any known dementing illness.[5,12-20]

A major problem in evaluating the course of schizophrenia has been the lack of a noninvasive physiological marker for neurodegenerative changes in humans. One candidate marker is the P300 component of the event-related potential (ERP). This component is a large positive peak in the electroencephalogram about 300 to 500 milliseconds following the onset of task-relevant stimuli. In clinical studies, the P300 component is most commonly elicited using an "oddball" paradigm. In this paradigm, a subject is asked to count or respond to infrequent target stimuli that are randomly interspersed among frequent nontarget stimuli; the target stimuli produce a large P300 response in normal subjects. Because P300 latency can be measured without requiring a behavioral

See Subjects and Methods on next page

SUBJECTS AND METHODS

SUBJECTS

Forty-seven right-handed male schizophrenic patients between the ages of 20 and 60 years were recruited from the Brockton, Mass, and the Bronx, NY, Veterans Affairs Medical Centers. They were drawn from previously reported samples[34-37] and from a new series of evaluations. Seventeen were outpatients and 30 were inpatients at the time of testing. Twelve were not receiving medication at the time of testing; the remainder were receiving neuroleptic medication, with a mean±SD daily dose equivalent to 576±668 mg of chlorpromazine.[38] The *DSM-III-R*[39] diagnosis was ascertained on the basis of a structured psychiatric interview and the Schedule for Affective Disorders and Schizophrenia[40] and by a review of patients' medical charts. Mean±SD age at onset was 22.4±4.0 years (range, 16 to 33 years), mean±SD illness duration was 17.2±7.4 years, and mean±SD percentage of time hospitalized since first episode was 31.4%±25.0%. None of the subjects had a history of electroconvulsive shock treatment, alcohol or other drug abuse (*DSM-III-R* criteria) within the last 5 years, addiction, or a neurologic illness affecting the central nervous system.

The normal control group (NL group) included 47 age-, handedness-, and gender-matched subjects who were recruited from newspaper advertisements. Information obtained from structured interviews were used to exclude control subjects if they had a history of alcohol or other drug abuse, psychiatric or neurologic illness, or psychiatric illness in a first-degree relative.

The NL group did not differ from patients with schizophrenia (SZ group) in mean±SD age (NL group, 39.6±9.1 years; SZ group, 39.5±8.0 years). Although none of the schizophrenic patients was demented at the time of testing, patients had slightly worse (*P*=.009) mean±SD Mini-Mental State scores (NL group, 28.9±1.5; SZ group, 27.6±3.0)[41] and Wechsler Adult Intelligence Scale–Revised (WAIS-R) information subscale scores (NL group, 11.4±2.5; SZ group, 9.8±2.7).[42]

ERP EVALUATION

Recording Procedures

The ERPs were recorded using an auditory oddball paradigm. Infrequent (*P*=.15) target tones (1500 Hz, 97-dB sound pressure level) were presented among frequent nontarget tones of a lower pitch (1000 Hz, 97-dB sound pressure level). Tone pips were of 40 milliseconds' duration and presented with a 1.2-second interstimulus interval through insert earphones (Neuroscan, Herndon, Va) against a background of continuous 70-dB binaural white noise. Three blocks of 200 tones were presented. Subjects silently counted the tones (NL group, 36 patients; SZ group, 35 patients) or responded to target tones with a button press (NL group, 11 patients; SZ group, 12 patients). While listening to the tones, subjects stared at a central fixation point to reduce eye movements. The ERPs were recorded from 28 tin plate scalp electrodes using an electrode cap (Electro-Cap International Inc, Dallas, Tex) referenced to linked ear electrodes. Scalp electrode placements included 20 electrodes in the International 10-20 system[43] with eight additional interpolated electrodes. A vertical electro-oculogram (EOG) was recorded using right eye supraorbital and infraorbital electrodes. A horizontal EOG was recorded from electrodes at the right and left external canthi. Electrode impedance was maintained at less than 4 kΩ. Right and left ear impedances were matched within 1 kΩ. The electroencephalogram was filtered using a bandpass of 0.15 to 40 Hz, with 36 dB per octave roll-off for low pass and 6 dB per octave roll-off for high pass. Single trial epochs were digitized and stored on hard disk for later off-line processing. Each ERP consisted of 256 electroencephalogram samples over a 700-millisecond epoch, including a 100-millisecond prestimulus baseline interval.

Thirteen control subjects and 10 patients from the sample described in Faux et al[34] received an ERP protocol that differed from that described above in the following ways: the interstimulus interval was 1.0 second, the baseline interval was 16 milliseconds, the high-pass filter cutoff was 0.3, and on-line vertical EOG artifact rejection was used.

Data Processing

All single-trial epochs were baseline corrected prior to subsequent processing. The ERP responses with vertical EOG artifact were corrected using individually computed weighting coefficients at each electrode site using the procedure of Semlitsch et al.[44] After correction for vertical EOG artifact, all epochs with voltages in excess of ±50 μV at any site were rejected. Epochs were then sorted into infrequent target ERP and frequent nontarget ERP averages. Each averaged ERP was then digitally low-pass filtered at 16 Hz to attenuate high-frequency electromyographic artifact.

P300 latency and amplitude were measured at F_z, C_z, and P_z as the most positive voltage sampled in the latency range of 300 to 500 milliseconds. P300 most commonly has been evaluated at these sites in ERP studies of aging, and the component is largest at midline sites. Because P300 latency might be delayed by peripheral factors such as conductive hearing loss or alterations in subcortical neurotransmission, we also measured the N100 component, which precedes the P300 component in the waveform. Unlike P300, N100 latency is usually unaffected by age or dementia.[45,46]

STATISTICAL ANALYSIS

Mixed-model analyses of variance were used to compare latency and amplitude values of the P300 component between groups among midline sites (F_z, C_z, and P_z). Linear regression coefficients were computed to determine the slope of component latency on age. The percentage of variance explained was not increased using logarithmic or quadratic regression, and linear regression was thus selected as the simplest model. In the SZ group, the relation between measures of clinical status and ERP component values were evaluated using Pearson correlation coefficients or independent *t* tests. All *P* values reported are two tailed. Data are presented as mean±SD.

response, it provides an index of information processing that is not affected by slowed or abnormal response production, as is the case with behavioral measures of function.

P300 latency is prolonged in adult-onset neurodegenerative disorders, including heterogeneous dementias,[21,22] Alzheimer's dementia,[23] multiple sclerosis,[24] Huntington's chorea,[25] Parkinson's disease,[26,27] hydrogen sulfide intoxication,[28] and progressive supranuclear palsy.[29] P300 latency also becomes prolonged in the course of neural changes accompanying aging at a rate of 1 to 2 ms/y.[30-33] Consequently, if a sample of schizophrenic patients experienced a neurodegenerative process in adulthood, P300 latency would be likely to show an increased rate of prolongation (increased slope) with age. To test this hypothesis, we investigated the relation of auditory P300 latency to age in patients with chronic schizophrenia and in normal control subjects between 20 and 60 years of age.

RESULTS

GROUP DIFFERENCES

An analysis of variance on P300 latency at F_z, C_z, and P_z revealed a main effect of electrode site ($F[2,184]=14.1$, $P<.001$), with earlier P300 latencies recorded at F_z than P_z in both groups, and no group or interaction effects. At C_z, control latency was 379±32 milliseconds, and patient latency was 393±52 milliseconds. An analysis of variance on P300 amplitude across electrode sites revealed a main effect for group ($F[1,92]=36$, $P<.001$) and electrode site ($F[2,184]=55.6$, $P<.001$). The SZ group had lower P300 amplitudes at all three sites, and P300 amplitude was largest at P_z and smallest at F_z. At C_z, control amplitude was 10.8±4.7 μV, and patient amplitude was 6.1±4.0 μV.

AGE AND P300

The slope of P300 latency on age was steeper in schizophrenic subjects, particularly at F_z and C_z. The slope of P300 latency on age at F_z was 0.65 ms/y ($P=.16$) for control subjects and 2.98 ms/y ($P=.001$) for schizophrenic subjects. At C_z, the slope was 1.21 ms/y ($P=.02$) for control subjects and 3.18 ms/y ($P<.001$) for schizophrenic subjects. The difference between slopes in the SZ and the NL groups was significant at both F_z ($P=.03$) and C_z ($P=.04$), using the *t* test for comparison of regression coefficients.[47] While the slope (b) of P300 latency on age at P_z was steeper in patients (b=2.11 ms/y, $P=.03$) than in control subjects (b=1.54 ms/y, $P=.002$), the difference between slopes was not statistically significant. The **Figure** shows scatterplots, linear regression coefficients, and least square regression lines for P300 latency on age at F_z and C_z. P300 amplitude did not correlate with age at any site in either group.

It is possible that variations in experimental protocols across studies might affect the slope of P3 on aging. We compared slopes at F_z separately for two samples evaluated before 1990 at this site[34,35] and for subjects evaluated since 1990 (NL group, 23 subjects; SZ group, 26 subjects). In the 1990 Faux et al study,[34] the interstimulus and baseline interval, high-pass setting, and artifact correction procedure differed slightly from more recent studies, as described in the "Subjects and Methods" section. In the 1993 Faux et al study,[35] patients were tested after they had stopped receiving medication and responded with a key press rather than a silent count. In each study, the slope of P300 on age was three to four times steeper in schizophrenic patients than in control subjects. For schizophrenic patients, the average slope of P300 latency on age was 3.2 ms/y ($P=.01$ in Faux et al,[34] $P=.07$ in Faux et al,[35] and $P=.02$ in the new sample) in contrast to the mean control slope of 0.76 ms/y ($P=.25$ in Faux et al,[34] $P=.32$ in Faux et al,[35] and $P=.29$ in the new sample).

We next tested whether the N100 component increased with age in schizophrenia. N100 latency is sensitive to conductive hearing loss or disturbances of neurotransmission within the peripheral auditory pathways but not to aging or dementia. The regression of N100 latency on age was not significant in either group at any of the three electrode sites.

P300 AND CLINICAL STATUS

One specific issue raised by the finding of an increased rate of P300 latency change in schizophrenic subjects is whether this could be attributed to differences in institutionalization, clinical status, or other patient characteristics. We thus evaluated the relation of P300 latency at F_z and C_z to the following variables: percentage of time hospitalized since onset, current chlorpromazine-equivalent dosage of neuroleptic medication, an estimate of lifetime dosage (current dosage multiplied by duration of illness), illness duration, age at illness onset, Mini-Mental State score, information subscale score from the WAIS-R and educational attainment.

See also pages 550 and 559

P300 latency in outpatients did not differ from P300 latency recorded in inpatients. There was no correlation between an estimate of lifetime neuroleptic medication exposure and P300 latency. Current dosage and P300 latency were not correlated in medicated patients, but patients who were no longer receiving medication showed prolonged P300 latency compared with patients receiving medication at all three recording sites (F_z: $P=.002$; C_z: $P=.004$; P_z: $P=.03$). P300 amplitude, in contrast to latency, did appear to be related to clinical status. P300 amplitude decreased with increased percentage of time hospitalized at P_z ($r=-.42$, $P=.01$) and was also reduced in inpatients compared with outpatients at C_z and P_z ($P<.01$ on *t* tests). Mini-Mental State score, the information subscale score from the WAIS-R, and educational attainment did not correlate with P300 latency or with amplitude.

Because current (testing) age equals age at illness onset plus illness duration, the latter two variables are, by definition, highly interrelated with age. In stepwise multiple regression analyses with P300 latency at F_z and C_z, with all three variables entered, current age was the only retained variable (P's$<.01$), with the contributions of onset age and duration being redundant (not significant). The colinearity (both duration and onset were significantly correlated with age, univariate P's $<.005$) and the limited range of the onset variable (all onsets at ages younger than 33 years) made valid multiple regression measurements of the relative strength of the contribution of these two variables not possible. For comparative purposes, we did perform stepwise multiple re-

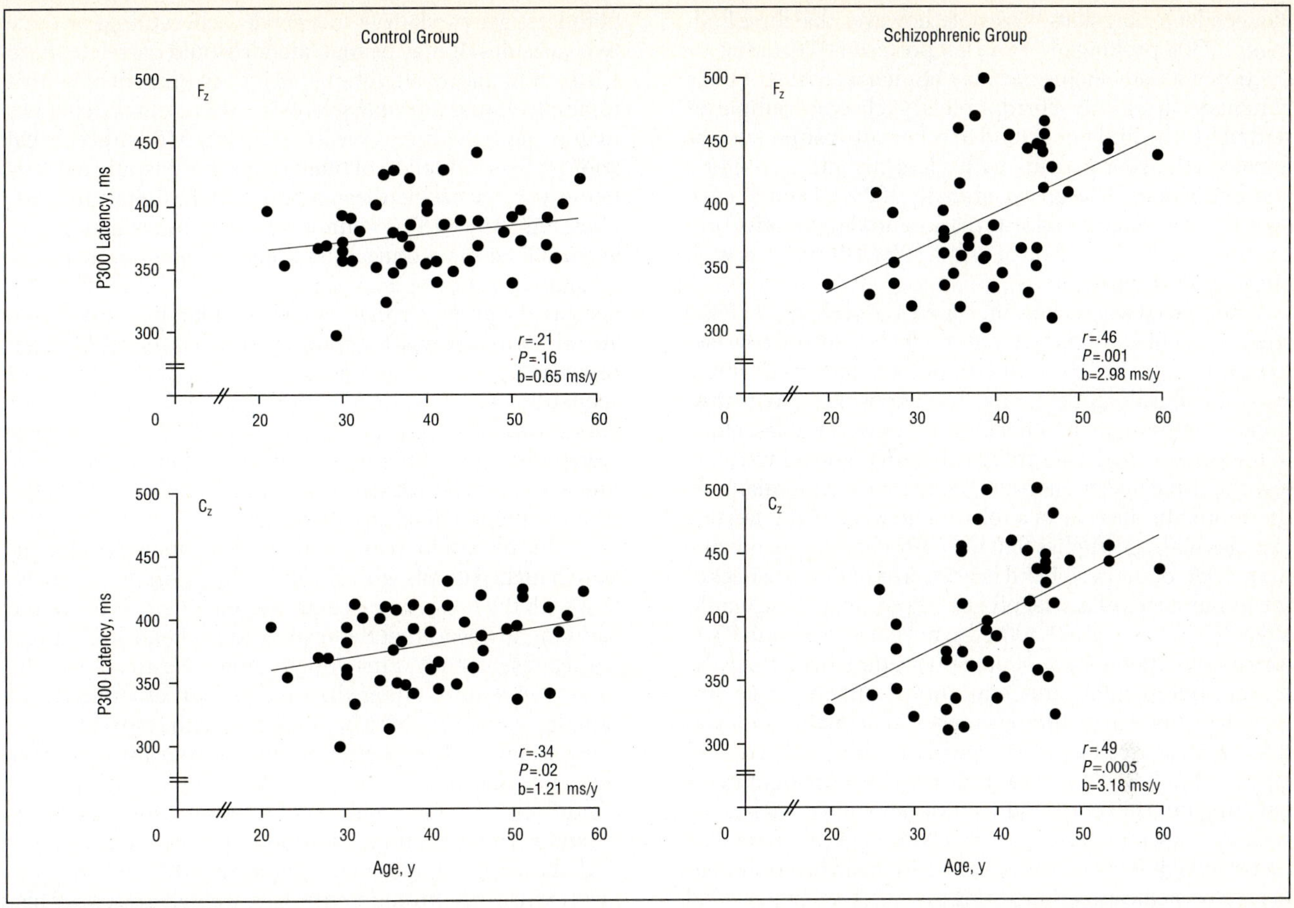

Scatterlots and linear regression lines showing the relationship of P3 latency to age in both groups at F_z and C_z. b indicates the slope.

gression analyses that compared the effects of forced entry as the first variable, of duration of illness, and of age of onset. The mean percentages of variance explained (R^2) were similar (duration, 11.5%; onset, 11%); also, the mean absolute magnitudes of the univariate correlation coefficients were similar ($|r|\approx.28$) for duration and onset.

AGING AND GRAY MATTER VOLUMES DETERMINED BY MRI

In a subset of 15 schizophrenic patients who received MRI evaluations, we previously reported that reductions in gray matter volume of the left posterior superior temporal gyrus (STG) were correlated with P300 amplitude, particularly at electrode sites over the left temporal region.[37,48] In the original MRI study,[49] group differences had been tested using age as a covariate, with no change in the results, but the univariate relation of age to gray matter volumes was not explicitly evaluated. However, in view of these P300 findings, we examined whether aging had a differential impact on the absolute gray matter volume (in milliliters) of the left and right posterior STG in these 15 schizophrenic patients compared with 15 control subjects in the same study.

Posterior STG gray matter volume significantly diminished with age in the schizophrenic patients on the left side ($r=-.61$, b=−0.07 mL/y, $P=.02$) but not on the right side ($r=-.39$, b=−0.05 mL/y, $P=.15$). The difference between these correlation coefficients and slopes in the SZ group was not significant. P300 latency in the SZ group did not correlate with left posterior STG volume in these patients. Control subjects showed no statistically significant decrease in posterior STG gray matter volume with age, either on the left side ($r=-.20$, b=−.02 mL/y, $P=.48$) or on the right side ($r=-.37$, b=−0.05 mL/y, $P=.17$); these correlation coefficients and slopes were not significantly different from zero. In the SZ group, there was a trend for total brain gray matter volume to diminish with age ($r=-.46$, b=−4.7 mL/y, $P=.08$), but the NL group showed no such trend level significance ($r=-.26$, b=−3.0 mL/y, $P=.35$) in this relatively small sample; control-schizophrenic differences between slopes and correlation coefficients were not statistically significant.

COMMENT

The rate of increase of P300 latency with age in schizophrenic patients was greater than that in control subjects. These findings support the hypothesis that schizophrenia has a progressive course, at least in the subgroup of male patients with chronic schizophrenia who we studied. The slope of P300 latency on age in schizophrenic patients ranged from 2.1 to 3.2 ms/y across midline electrode sites, whereas in control subjects the range was 0.7 to 1.5 ms/y. This difference in slope was significant at F_z ($P=.03$) and C_z ($P=.04$). Because prolonged P300 latency has been demonstrated to be a reliable sign of a neurodegenerative process, this increased prolongation may be the first sign of a pathophysiological process that will later become manifest as a severe cognitive impairment[17,18] or as more severe negative symptoms and lack of independent living skills.[11] We note, however, that these findings of P300 prolongation and left posterior STG tissue reduction with advancing age may be characteristic of male patients with chronic schizophrenia, such as the sample reported herein, and not extend to other subgroups, such as female patients or patients with a less chronic course or a later age of onset. The great variability of P300 latency, even among older patients, suggests that a neurodegenerative process may be characteristic of only a subset of patients with chronic schizophrenia.

We tested whether the increased rate of change of P300 latency in schizophrenic patients might be explained by factors other than the schizophrenic process, such as the presence of a neurologic dementia, long exposure to an institutional environment, or other clinical status variables. None of the patients had a neurologic disorder, and all were below the usual age of onset for Alzheimer's dementia. Furthermore, the absence of a relation between N100 latency changes with age implies that the P300 changes are not due to such factors as peripheral hearing loss or disturbances of the initial stages of neural processing because these would affect N100[50] as well as P300. Also not correlated with P300 latency were percentage of time institutionalized since the first episode, mental status, educational attainment, and inpatient status. These findings suggest that institutionalization (as measured by percentage of time hospitalized) and current functional status (as indicated by outpatient vs inpatient status) did not account for variations in P300 latency with age. Patients who stopped receiving medication showed increased P300 latency relative to patients who continued to receive medication, suggesting that medication may tend to normalize P300 latency.[35] An estimate of lifetime neuroleptic medication exposure did not correlate with latency. Although subjects were screened to rule out addiction and recent substance abuse, the extent of any lifetime subaddictive use could not be ascertained from patient records. Although the current literature[51-54] does not indicate that nonaddictive lifetime use of alcohol or other substances influences P300 latency, we cannot exclude the possibility that nonaddictive use was greater in the patient than in the NL group and may have had an unknown degree of influence on P300 latency. We note also that the absence of correlation with the Mini-Mental State score and the information subscale score of the WAIS-R could reflect the constricted range of scores in the group, which excluded patients with signs of dementia or other severe cognitive impairment.

We note that in the present cross-sectional sample, it was not possible to reliably disentangle the relative contributions of duration of illness and age of illness onset to the strong age-related correlations of P300 latency. Such a differentiation may be possible in the population of first-episode schizophrenic and age-matched control subjects[55] we are currently studying in the same P300 paradigm because we plan to do long-term, repeated follow-up measurements.

Gray matter volume of the left posterior STG, one probable determinant of the amplitude of the scalp-recorded auditory P300 component, showed an age-related decline that was significant in the SZ but not in the NL group. These MRI structural data are thus supportive of (although they do not prove) a neurodegenerative process and complement the functional P300 measures. That P300 latency in the SZ group did not correlate with left posterior STG volume (as did amplitude) suggests relatively independent effects of age on these two variables. It may be that latency would correlate more with white matter alterations, as it does in cases of neurotoxic effects and multiple sclerosis,[24] than with the changes in gray matter volumes measured in our MRI study. Focal and/or gross reduction of brain tissue in schizophrenic patients with age has also been reported in the literature. Test-retest reduction of STG volume was noted by DeLisi and colleagues.[56] Less anatomically specific evidence of a neurodegenerative process, including decreased brain volume, decreased gray matter, increased ventricular size, or increased atrophy with age in schizophrenic subjects, have also been reported by some[57-60] but not all investigators.[61-63] It is consequently of interest that left posterior STG volume in our data showed a greater decline with age than did total gray matter. Although this difference did not attain statistical significance in this small sample, it is compatible with the possibility of regional brain differences.

Our data of increased rate of P300 latency prolongation in male patients with chronic schizophrenia is consistent with the presence of a neurodegenerative process. We caution, however, that there are methodologic limitations to the present study. First, longitudinal investigation of the same population, rather than the present cross-sectional sample, would provide a better design with respect to sampling and would also better be able to determine whether these findings reflect a primary effect of schizophrenia or conditions associated with this disorder, including administration of neuroleptic medication and other treatment. Second, the slope of P300 latency should also be studied in patients with a less chronic course, with well-characterized histories of alcohol or other substance use, and with detailed histories of lifetime neuroleptic medication use and in women because the presentation and course of schizophrenia differs between men and women.[64] Although our data do not provide firm proof of a neurodegenerative process, they should motivate further functional and structural studies of the neural consequences of aging in schizophrenia, particularly given the paucity of empirical data bearing on the question of the pathophysiological evolution of schizophrenia across the life span.

Accepted for publication January 20, 1995.

Supported by grants 40799 (Dr McCarley) and IR29 MH50747-01 (Dr Shenton) from the National Institute of Mental Health, Bethesda, Md, the Department of Veterans Affairs Medical Research Service and Schizophrenia Center, Brockton, Mass (Dr McCarley), the Commonwealth of Massachusetts Research Center, Boston (Dr McCarley), the National Alliance for Research on Schizophrenia and Depression (Chicago, Ill) Young Investigator Award (Dr O'Donnell), the National Institute of Mental Health Research Scientist Development Award K02-MH0110-01 (Dr Shenton), and the Stanley Foundation, Arlington, Va (Drs Kikinis and Shenton).

Presented in part at the 1993 Annual Meeting of the American Psychiatric Association, San Francisco, Calif, May 25, 1993, and the 1993 Annual Meeting of the Society of Biological Psychiatry, San Francisco, May 21, 1993.

REFERENCES

1. Kraepelin E; Barclay E, Barclay S, trans. *Dementia Praecox*. New York, NY: Churchill Livingstone Inc; 1971.

2. Bland RC, Orn H. Fourteen-year outcome in early schizophrenia. *Acta Psychiatr Scand.* 1979;58:327-338.
3. Bleuler M. *The Schizophrenic Disorders: Long-term Patient and Family Studies.* New Haven, Conn: Yale University Press; 1978.
4. Breier A, Schreiber JL, Dyer J, Pickar D. National Institute of Mental Health longitudinal study of chronic schizophrenia: prognosis and predictors of outcome. *Arch Gen Psychiatry.* 1991;48:239-246.
5. Ciompi L. Catamnestic long-term study on the course of life and aging of schizophrenics. *Schizophr Bull.* 1980;6:606-618.
6. Engelhardt DM, Rosen B, Feldman J, Engelhardt JAZ. A 15-year follow-up of 646 schizophrenic outpatients. *Schizophr Bull.* 1982;8:493-503.
7. Harding CM, Brooks WW, Ashikaga T, Strauss JS, Breier A. The Vermont longitudinal study of persons with severe mental illness, II. *Am J Psychiatry.* 1987; 144:727-735.
8. Huber G, Gross G, Schuttler R, Linz M. Longitudinal studies of schizophrenic patients. *Schizophr Bull.* 1980;6:592-605.
9. McGlashan TH. The Chestnut Lodge follow-up study, II: long-term outcome of schizophrenia and the affective disorders. *Arch Gen Psychiatry.* 1984;41:585-601.
10. Keefe RSE, Mohs RC, Losonczy MF, Davidson M, Silverman JM, Kendler KS, Horvath TB, Nora R, Davis KL. Characteristics of very poor outcome in schizophrenia. *Am J Psychiatry.* 1987;144:889-895.
11. Keefe RSE, Lobel DS, Mohs RC, Silverman JM, Harvey PD, Davidson M, Losonczy M, Davis KL. Diagnostic issues in chronic schizophrenia. *Schizophr Res.* 1991;4:71-79.
12. Angst J. European long-term follow-up studies of schizophrenia. *Schizophr Bull.* 1988;14:501-513.
13. Casanova MF, Carosella NW, Gold JM, Kleinman JE, Weinberger DR, Powers RE. A topographical study of senile plaques and neurofibrillary tangles in the hippocampi of patients with Alzheimer's disease and cognitively impaired patients with schizophrenia. *Psychiatry Res.* 1993;49:41-62.
14. Davidson M, Powchik P, Losonczy MF, Katz S, McCrystal J, Parella M, Frecska E, Haroutunian V, Bierer L, Perl D, Goldstein M, Davis KL. Dementia in elderly schizophrenic patients. *Biol Psychiatry.* 1991;29:91A. Abstract.
15. Heaton RK, Drexler M. Clinical neuropsychological findings in schizophrenia and aging. In: Miller NE, Cohen GD, eds. *Schizophrenia and Aging.* New York, NY: Guilford Press; 1987:145-161.
16. Johnstone EC, Cunningham DG, Gold A, Crow TJ, Macmillan JF. Institutionalization and the defects of schizophrenia. *Br J Psychiatry.* 1981;139:195-203.
17. Liddle PF, Crow TJ. Age disorientation in chronic schizophrenia is associated with global intellectual impairment. *Br J Psychiatry.* 1984;144:193-195.
18. Purohit DP, Davidson M, Perl DP, Powchik P, Haroutunian VH, Bierer LM, McCrystal J, Losonczy M, Davis K. Severe cognitive impairment in elderly schizophrenic patients: a clinico-pathological study. *Biol Psychiatry.* 1993;33:255-260.
19. Bruton CJ, Crow TJ, Frith CD, Johnstone EC, Owens DGC, Roberts GW. Schizophrenia and the brain. *Psychol Med.* 1990;20:285-309.
20. El-Mallakh RS, Kirch DG, Shelton R, Fan KJ, Pezeshkpour G, Kanhouwa S, Wyatt RJ, Kleinman JE. The nucleus basalis of Meynert, senile plaques and intellectual impairment in schizophrenia. *J Neuropsychiatry Clin Neurosci.* 1991; 3:383-386.
21. O'Donnell BF, Friedman S, Squires NK, Maloon A, Drachman DA, Swearer JM. Active and passive P3 latency in dementia. *Neuropsychiatry Neuropsychol Behav Neurol.* 1990;3:164-179.
22. Pfefferbaum A, Wenegrat BG, Ford JM, Roth WT, Kopell BS. Clinical application of the P3 component of the event-related potentials, II: dementia, depression and schizophrenia. *Electroencephalogr Clin Neurophysiol.* 1984;59:104-124.
23. Patterson JV, Michalewski HJ, Starr A. Latency variability of the components of auditory event-related potentials to infrequent stimuli in aging, Alzheimer-type dementia, and depression. *Electroencephalogr Clin Neurophysiol.* 1988; 71:450-460.
24. Polich J, Romine JS, Sipe JC, Aung M, Dalessio DJ. P300 in multiple sclerosis: a preliminary report. *Int J Psychophysiol.* 1992;12:155-163.
25. Homberg V, Hefter H, Granseyer G, Strauss J, Lange P, Hennerici R. Event-related potentials in patients with Huntington's disease and relatives at risk in relation to detailed psychometry. *Electroencephalogr Clin Neurophysiol.* 1986; 63:552-569.
26. Hansch EC, Syndulko K, Cohen SN, Goldberg ZI, Potvin AR, Tourtellotte WW. Cognition in Parkinson's disease. *Ann Neurol.* 1982;11:599-607.
27. O'Donnell BF, Squires NK, Martz MJ, Chen JR, Phay AJ. Evoked potential and neuropsychological performance in Parkinson's disease. *Biol Psychol.* 1987; 24:23-37.
28. Wasch H, Estrin W, Yip P, Bowler R, Cone J. Prolongation of the P300 latency associated with hydrogen sulfide exposure. *Arch Neurol.* 1989;46:902-904.
29. Pierrot-Deseilligny C, Turell E, Penet C, Lebrigand D, Pillon B, Chain F, Agid Y. Increased wave P300 latency in progressive supranuclear palsy. *J Neurol Neurosurg Psychiatry.* 1989;52:656-658.
30. Goodin DS, Squires KC, Henderson BH, Starr A. Age-related variations in evoked potentials to auditory stimuli in normal subjects. *Electroencephalogr Clin Neurophysiol.* 1978;44:447-458.
31. O'Donnell BF, Friedman S, Maloon A, Drachman DA. P3 latency and neuropsychological performance. *Int J Psychophysiol.* 1992;12:187-195.
32. Pfefferbaum A, Ford JM, Wenegrat BG, Walton WT, Kopell BS. Clinical application of the P3 component of event-related potentials, I: normal aging. *Electroencephalogr Clin Neurophysiol.* 1984;59:85-103.
33. Polich J. P300 in the evaluation of aging and dementia. In: Brunia CHM, Mulder G, Verbaten MN, eds. *Event-Related Brain Potential Research.* Amsterdam, the Netherlands: Elsevier Science Publishers; 1991:304-323.
34. Faux SF, Shenton ME, McCarley RW, Nestor PG, Marcy B, Ludwig A. Preservation of P300 event-related potential topographic asymmetries in schizophrenia with use of either linked-ear or nose reference sites. *Electroencephalogr Clin Neurophysiol.* 1990;75:378-391.
35. Faux SF, McCarley RW, Nestor PG, Shenton ME, Pollak SD, Penhune V, Mondrow E, Marcy B, Peterson A, Horvath T, Davis KL. P300 topographic asymmetries are present in unmedicated schizophrenics. *Electroencephalogr Clin Neurophysiol.* 1993;88:32-41.
36. Shenton ME, Faux SF, McCarley RW, Ballinger R, Coleman M, Torello M, Duffy FH. Correlations between abnormal auditory P300 topography and positive symptoms in schizophrenia: a preliminary report. *Biol Psychiatry.* 1989;25:710-716.
37. McCarley RW, Shenton ME, O'Donnell BF, Faux SF, Kikinis R, Nestor PG, Jolesz FA. Auditory P300 abnormalities and left posterior superior temporal gyrus volume reduction in schizophrenia. *Arch Gen Psychiatry.* 1993;50:190-197.
38. Bernstein JG. *Handbook of Drug Therapy in Psychiatry.* 2nd ed. St Louis, Mo: Mosby–Year Book; 1988.
39. American Psychiatric Association. *Diagnostic and Statistical Manual of Mental Disorders, Revised Third Edition.* Washington, DC: American Psychiatric Association; 1987.
40. Spitzer RL, Endicott J. *Schedule for Affective Disorders and Schizophrenia: Lifetime Version.* New York, NY: Biometric Research, New York State Psychiatric Institute; 1978.
41. Folstein MF, Folstein SE, McHugh PR. Mini-Mental State. *J Psychiatr Res.* 1975; 12:189-198.
42. Wechsler D. *The Wechsler Adult Intelligence Scale–Revised Manual.* New York, NY: Psychological Corp; 1982.
43. Duffy FH, Iyer VG, Surwillo WW. *Clinical Electroencephalography and Topographic Brain Mapping.* New York, NY: Springer-Verlag NY Inc; 1989.
44. Semlitsch HV, Anderer P, Schuster P, Presslich O. A solution for reliable and valid reduction of ocular artifacts applied to the P300 ERP. *Psychophysiology.* 1986;23:695-703.
45. Iragui VJ, Kutas M, Mitchiner MR, Hillyard SA. Effects of aging on event-related potentials and reaction times in an auditory oddball task. *Psychophysiology.* 1993;30:10-22.
46. O'Donnell BF, Friedman S, Squires NK, Maloon A, Drachman DA, Swearer JM. Active and passive P3 latency in dementia: relationship to psychometric, EEG, and CT measures. *Neuropsychiatry Neuropsychol Behav Neurol.* 1990;3:164-179.
47. Howell DC. *Statistical Methods for Psychology.* Boston, Mass: Duxbury Press; 1982.
48. O'Donnell BF, Shenton ME, McCarley RW, Faux SF, Smith RS, Salisbury DF, Nestor PG, Pollak SD, Kikinis R, Jolesz FA. The auditory N2 component in schizophrenia. *Biol Psychiatry.* 1993;34:26-40.
49. Shenton ME, Kikinis R, Jolesz FA, Pollak SD, LeMay M, Martin J, Metcalf D, Coleman M, McCarley RW. Left temporal lobe abnormalities in schizophrenia. *N Engl J Med.* 1992;327:604-612.
50. Regan D. *Human Brain Electrophysiology.* New York, NY: Elsevier Science Publishing Co Inc; 1989.
51. Patterson WP, Williams HL, McLean GA, Smith LT, Schaeffer KW. Alcoholism and family history of alcoholism. *Alcohol.* 1987;4:265-274.
52. Pfefferbaum A, Ford JM, White P, Mathalon D. Event-related potentials in alcoholic men. *Alcohol Clin Exp Res.* 1991;15:839-850.
53. Polich J, Bloom FE. P300 from normals and adult children of alcoholics. *Alcohol.* 1987;4:301-305.
54. Steinhauer SR, Hill SY. Auditory event-related potentials in children at high risk for alcoholism. *J Stud Alcohol.* 1993;54:408-421.
55. Salisbury DF, Shenton ME, McCarley RW, Tohen M, Matthusse SW, Yurgelin-Todd DA, Chang W. Does P3 topography discriminate schizophrenic psychosis from affective psychosis? *Society for Neuroscience 24th Annual Meeting Abstracts.* Washington, DC: Society for Neuroscience; 1994;20(part 1):25. Abstract.
56. Delisi LE, Grimson R, Kushner M, Lee G, Sakuma M, Gao T, Kantawala K. Is there progressive brain change following a first hospitalization for schizophrenia? a 4-year follow-up. *Schizophr Res.* 1994;11:135-136.
57. Keshavan MS, Pettegrew K, Beckwith K, Bagwell W, Haas GL, Sweeney J, Schooler NR. Gray matter abnormalities in first-episode schizophrenia. *Schizophr Res.* 1994;11:136.
58. Nasrallah HA. Progressive and static ventriculomegaly in schizophrenia: clinical and methodological variables. *Schizophr Res.* 1991;5:191-192.
59. Waddington JL, O'Callaghan E, Buckley P, Larkin C, Redmond O, Stack J, Ennis JT. The age dependencies of MRI abnormalities in schizophrenia suggest early ventricular enlargement but later prominence of cortical atrophy. *Schizophr Res.* 1991;5:188-189.
60. Woods BT, Yurgelin-Todd D. Brain volume loss in schizophrenia: when does it occur and is it progressive? *Schizophr Res.* 1991;5:202-203.
61. Goldberg TE, Hyde TM, Kleinman JE, Weinberger DR. Course of schizophrenia. *Schizophr Bull.* 1993;19:797-804.
62. Vita A. Cerebral ventricular abnormalities in schizophrenia: evidence of their early origin and stability over time. *Schizophr Res.* 1991;5:189-190.
63. Andreasen NC, Swayze VW, Flaum M, Yates WR, Arndt S, McChesney C. Ventricular enlargement in schizophrenia evaluated with computed tomographic scanning. *Arch Gen Psychiatry.* 1990;47:1008-1015.
64. Goldstein JM, Tsuang MT. Gender and schizophrenia: an introduction and synthesis of findings. *Schizophr Bull.* 1990;16:179-183.

ORIGINAL ARTICLE

Impaired Mismatch Negativity Generation Reflects Widespread Dysfunction of Working Memory in Schizophrenia

Daniel C. Javitt, MD, PhD; Paolina Doneshka, MD, PhD; Sandra Grochowski; Walter Ritter, PhD

Background: Impaired P300 (P3) generation is one of the most robust indices of brain dysfunction in schizophrenia. This study investigates the integrity of cognitive event-related potentials that precede P3 in an "oddball" paradigm to determine the earliest stages at which auditory information processing is impaired in schizophrenia.

Methods: Cognitive event-related potential components including mismatch negativity (MMN), N2, and P3 were recorded from subjects with chronic schizophrenia who were receiving medication (n=20), from those who were withdrawn from drug treatment (n=11), and from healthy volunteers (n=11) during an auditory oddball paradigm. Recordings were made in both passive and active response conditions. The MMN, N2, and P3 amplitudes were compared across groups and the degree of MMN deficit was correlated with the degree of P3 reduction as a function of diagnostic group.

Results: Schizophrenic subjects showed severe impairments in the generation of MMN and N2 as well as P3. Across groups, the decrement in MMN amplitude correlated significantly with the decrement in P3 amplitude. There were no significant between-group differences in MMN topography.

Conclusions: The present study demonstrates that the neurophysiological deficits associated with schizophrenia, as reflected in cognitive event-related potential generation, are pervasive, extending even to the level of the sensory cortex. Mismatch negativity indexes the functioning of an automatic alerting mechanism designed to stimulate individuals to explore unexpected environmental events. Dysfunction of this mechanism may contribute to the deficit state associated with schizophrenia.

(Arch Gen Psychiatry. 1995;52:550-558)

PERSISTENT neurocognitive dysfunction represents one of the major predictors of chronic disability and impaired long-term outcome in schizophrenia.[1-3] Event-related (evoked) potentials (ERPs) provide an objective index of cognition-related brain activity and a mechanism for investigating underlying neurophysiological mechanisms. Much research in schizophrenia has focused on P300 (P3), a long-latency ERP component that is elicited by unexpected, novel, and/or behaviorally significant events.[4] P3 is so named because it is positive (P) in polarity over the surface of the scalp and occurs approximately 300 milliseconds following the presentation of a significant, novel event. Over the past 20 years, it has been established that decreased P3 amplitude is one of the most consistent and robust biological abnormalities associated with schizophrenia.[4] At the time when the P3 deficit in schizophrenia was first described, little was known about the cognitive processing operations that occurred during the 300 milliseconds preceding P3 generation. Subsequent studies have demonstrated that P3 is preceded by several components that reflect earlier stages of information processing.[5] Mismatch negativity (MMN) is a short-latency cognitive auditory ERP component that represents the earliest cortical response to stimulus novelty. The present study investigates MMN generation, relative to that of P3, to determine the earliest stages at which cortical information processing is impaired in schizophrenia.

Decreased P3 amplitude in schizophrenia was first demonstrated over two decades ago[6] and has been confirmed since that time in at least 30 independent investigations.[4,7] In schizophrenic subjects, the deficits persist despite neuroleptic treatment or overall clinical improvement.[8-12] In one study of more than 300 patients and

From the Departments of Psychiatry and Neuroscience, Albert Einstein College of Medicine, and Bronx Psychiatric Center, Bronx, NY.

See Methods on next page

METHODS

SUBJECTS

Subjects consisted of 20 medicated and 11 unmedicated patients with schizophrenia (mean [±SD] age, 36.2±8.8 years) diagnosed according to *DSM-III-R*[40] criteria and 11 age-matched controls (mean age, 38.3±9.73 years). Schizophrenic and control subjects did not differ in terms of dextrality (control, 10 right-handed and one left-handed; schizophrenic, 29 right-handed and two left-handed). The Quick Test[41] IQ, however, was significantly higher ($P<.02$) among the controls (110.8±8.9) than among the schizophrenic subjects (98.1±12.9). The control group also had a significantly higher proportion of women than the schizophrenic group (control, six men and five women; schizophrenic, 27 men and four women). Medicated subjects consisted entirely of inpatients. The mean neuroleptic dose among the medicated schizophrenic group was 885.0 chlorpromazine-equivalent milligrams per day (range, 150 to 4000). Eleven of the medicated schizophrenic subjects were also receiving anticholinergic medication (benztropine mesylate) at the time of testing. Eight of the unmedicated patients were inpatients, while three were outpatients. The mean (±SD) duration of withdrawal from drug treatment for inpatient subjects was 13.5±7.3 days (minimum, 7 days; maximum, 30 days); outpatient subjects were drug free for at least 6 months prior to testing. The mean (±SD) Brief Psychiatric Rating Scale scores for the medicated and unmedicated subjects were 52.3±11.0 and 37.0±12.8, respectively ($t=3.50$, $P<.002$). There were no significant correlations between Brief Psychiatric Rating Scale scores and any of the ERP components measured. Four subjects were studied both prior to and following drug treatment withdrawal. Medicated and unmedicated schizophrenic subjects did not differ in terms of age, sex, dextrality, or IQ.

DATA ACQUISITION

The ERPs were collected under "passive" and "active" conditions. In the passive condition, the subjects were instructed to ignore presented stimuli. In the active discrimination condition, the subjects were requested to press a button within 750 milliseconds following the presentation of deviant, target stimuli. For both paradigms, the auditory stimuli consisted of 1000-Hz standard and 1024-Hz deviant stimuli presented in pseudorandom order with a fixed interstimulus interval of 1.3 seconds; deviant stimuli occurred on average every 9 seconds (15% sequential probability). All tones were 50 milliseconds in duration with 5-millisecond rise/fall time presented binaurally with intensity of 75-dB sound pressure level through intra-aural stimulators. Tones were presented in two blocks of 667 stimuli each. All of the subjects were tested first in the passive, and second in the active discrimination conditions. Because of technical difficulties, ERPs were not obtained from one schizophrenic subject and one control subject during the active condition.

The ERPs were recorded using the montage of Naatanen.[5] Gold cup electrodes were applied to four midline sites (F_{pz}, F_z, C_z, and P_z) and the left (LM) and right (RM) mastoids. Coronal electrodes were placed one third (R_1, L_1) and two thirds (R_2, L_2) of the distance between F_z and the mastoids. The R_1 and L_1 corresponded to parasagittal locations between F_3 and C_3 or F_4 and C_4, respectively, of the international 10-20 System. The R_2 and L_2 corresponded to temporal locations between T_3 and T_5 or T_4 and T_6, respectively. Eye movements were monitored using an electrode located 1 cm below the left outer canthus. Electrical activity from all contacts was amplified relative to a nose reference with a bandpass (2 dB down) of 0.3 to 35 Hz using an electroencephalograph (Grass model 8-10E, Quincy, Mass). Activity was digitized continuously at a sampling rate of 256 Hz using the "SCAN" digital acquisition system (Neuroscan, Herndon, Va) implemented on an IBM compatible 80386 computer. Digitized waveforms along with 0.01-millisecond duration timing pulses and digital stimulus identification tags were stored on a hard disk for subsequent analysis. Analysis epochs were constructed off-line from the stored, digitized waveforms. Epochs incorporated a 75-millisecond prestimulus period and a 750-millisecond analysis period. Following rejection of sweeps containing amplitudes exceeding ±100 μV at any electrode including the eye moni-

Continued on next page

controls, over 70% could be differentiated from controls based on P3 measures alone.[13] In that study, as well as other studies, P3 deficits were observed not only in schizophrenic subjects but in first-degree relatives as well. In schizophrenic subjects receiving medication (hereafter, medicated subjects), the degree of P3 deficit correlates with the severity of thought disturbance[14,15] and negative symptoms.[12,16] P3 and other cognitive ERP components may serve, therefore, as markers for the neurophysiological abnormalities underlying persistent negative and cognitive symptoms in schizophrenia.

See also pages 544 and 559

A major current controversy is whether neurocognitive dysfunction in schizophrenia reflects cortical disturbances within specific, circumscribed cortical regions, such as the left temporal lobe[17-21] or prefrontal cortex,[17,18,20,22-24] or whether it results from more generalized cortical dysfunction.[25-27] Deficits that are primarily focal in nature would support suggestions that localized, structural damage to specific brain regions might be etiologic in schizophrenia.[28] By contrast, a more generalized pattern of deficit would suggest that schizophrenia might be associated with widespread neurochemical and/or microcellular disturbances distributed throughout the cortex. Generators for P3 have been localized to frontotemporal and temporoparietal association regions.[29-32] The deficit in P3 generation thus supports other lines of research indicating that information processing is impaired by the time information reaches association cortex in schizophrenia. The question of whether information processing deficits are limited to association cortex can be addressed by analyzing ERP components that precede P3.

tor lead, epochs were averaged off-line for each subject. The number (mean±SD) of sweeps included per average per subject did not differ significantly between schizophrenic and control subjects for either deviant (schizophrenic, 72.4±45.0; control, 79.2±32.8) or standard (schizophrenic, 403.5±225.1; control, 453.7±166) waveforms.

DATA ANALYSIS

Responses to the standard and deviant stimuli were averaged separately for each subject on each of the two behavioral conditions. The primary analysis was performed by averaging the peak amplitude and latency values for each component across subjects within each group. Sensory components were determined from waveforms to standard stimuli. N1 was defined as the peak negativity at F_z during the 50- to 150-millisecond latency range; P2 was defined as the peak positivity at C_z during the 150- to 250-millisecond latency range. Cognitive components were determined from deviant minus standard difference waveforms. The MMN amplitude was defined as the peak negativity at F_z during the 50- to 200-millisecond latency range in the passive condition difference waveform. N2 was defined as the peak negativity at F_z during the 150- to 250-millisecond latency range in the active condition difference waveform; P3 was defined as the peak positivity during the 300- to 450-millisecond range at P_z. N1 and MMN are known to invert in polarity between F_z and LM and RM. For those components, waveforms were rereferenced to a mathematically computed average mastoid derivation prior to peak detection.

Between-group amplitude and latency comparisons were performed using one-way across-group analysis of variance (ANOVA) for each of the seven defined components, of which four were sensory in nature and three were cognitive in nature. When significant across-group results were detected, preplanned contrast analyses were performed using one-way ANOVAs collapsed across medication status. Post hoc comparisons were performed using the Least Significant Difference statistic with a significance threshold of $P<.05$ unless otherwise specified. Topographical analyses were performed using repeated-measures (electrode) multivariate analysis of variance (MANOVA) according to the method of Faux and McCarley.[42] In addition, parasagittal and temporal laterality indices were defined as $(L_1-R_1)/(L_1+R_1)$ and $(L_2-R_2)/(L_2+R_2)$, respectively. Statistical comparisons were performed using the *SPSS/PC+* statistical program (SPSS Inc, Chicago, Ill). Power computations for tests that did not find significant between-group differences were performed using the Statistical Power Analysis software program (Erlbaum Associates, Hillsdale, NJ). Power computations are based on comparisons of within-group and between-group variance and indicate the smallest magnitude of effect that could have been detected given the observed data distributions, as measured by the effect-size index f. Effect-size values were interpreted using the convention that a small effect size corresponds to 0.10, a medium effect size corresponds to 0.25, and a large effect size corresponds to 0.40.[27]

A secondary analysis was performed by constructing across-subjects average (grand mean) waveforms for each group. Across-subjects average waveforms were compared between the control and schizophrenic groups using running *t* tests, which compare group mean values independently at each of the 256 sampling points. Running *t* tests are less likely to be affected by single, outlier points than are peak measurements, and indicate whether between-group differences are confined to a latency range of interest. However, because running *t* tests entail multiple comparisons, differences were considered significant only if they exceeded the $P<.05$ level of significance for at least 15 milliseconds of the specified latency ranges.[43] Values represent mean±SD unless otherwise specified.

P3 and other cognitive ERP components are elicited most commonly in an auditory "oddball" paradigm in which a sequence of repetitive standard stimuli is interrupted infrequently or unexpectedly by physically deviant "oddballs." In such a paradigm, both standard and deviant stimuli elicit sensory potentials that reflect processing of the physical properties of each individual stimulus. Deviants, however, elicit additional components that reflect cortical processing of the relationships among stimuli. In an oddball paradigm, P3 is preceded by several components that reflect discrete stages of information processing including two well-characterized early cognitive components: MMN, a frontocentral negativity with a latency as short as 50 milliseconds following stimulus delivery,[5] and N2, a central negativity with a latency of approximately 200 milliseconds.[33] Like P3, MMN and N2 are elicited by deviant, but not standard, stimuli. Like P3, therefore, MMN and N2 reflect cognitive information processing rather than simple sensory registration within the cortex. Mismatch negativity amplitude is unaffected by task demands and may be elicited even by deviant stimuli that are not consciously detected; therefore, MMN appears to index an automatic, preattentive stage of auditory information processing.[5] Nevertheless, when the difficulty of deviance detection is increased, eg, when the pitch separation between standard and deviant stimuli is made less extreme, the latencies of MMN and N2 increase in parallel with that of P3. Thus, MMN, N2, and P3 index sequentially organized events in the processing of unexpected stimulus change.[34]

The MMN, N2, P3 sequence of cognitive ERP components is superimposed on a sequence of obligatory sensory components that includes N1, a frontal negativity with a peak latency of approximately 100 milliseconds, and P2, a frontocentral positivity with a peak latency of approximately 200 milliseconds. Obligatory sensory components differ from cognitive components in that they are elicited by standard and deviant stimuli. Moreover, the amplitude of obligatory components depends primarily on the physical characteristics of individual stimuli such as pitch or intensity. By contrast, the amplitude of cognitive components depends primarily on the relationship between stimuli as defined by the stimulus sequence and behavioral paradigm. Although MMN and N1 may overlap temporally and spatially, electroencephalographic[35] and magnetoencephalographic[36] dipole mapping studies have confirmed that MMN and N1 are generated from distinct regions of the supratemporal auditory cortex.

The temporal overlap of cognitive and obligatory components necessitates the use of subtraction procedures in which responses to standard stimuli are subtracted from those to deviant stimuli. Two studies[8,37] have investi-

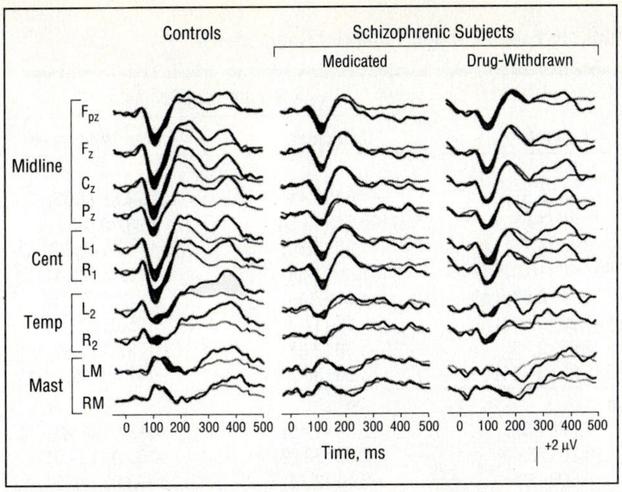

Figure 1. *Event-related potentials obtained during the passive condition in response to standard (thin lines) and deviant (thick lines) stimuli from schizophrenic subjects and normal controls at midline, paracentral (Cent), temporal (Temp), and mastoid (Mast) electrodes. Waveforms are shown relative to a nose reference. Shaded regions indicate latency range of mismatch negativity. Positive polarity corresponds to an upward deflection. LM indicates left mastoid; RM, right mastoid.*

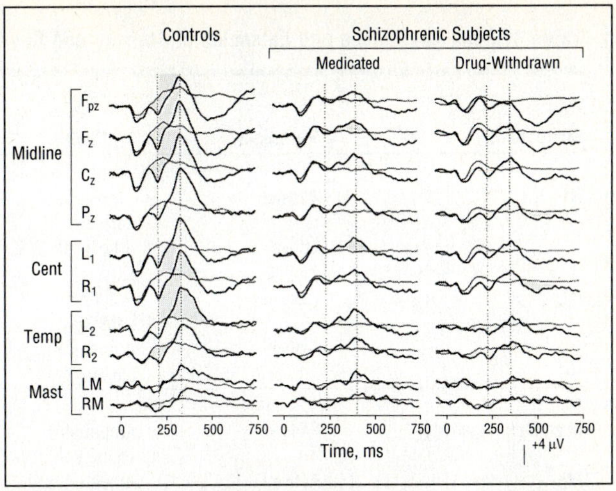

Figure 2. *Event-related potential waveforms obtained during the active discrimination condition in response to standard (thin lines) and deviant (thick lines) stimuli from schizophrenic subjects receiving medication and those withdrawn from drug treatment and from normal controls at midline, paracentral (Cent), temporal (Temp), and mastoid (Mast) electrodes. Waveforms are shown relative to a nose reference. Dotted lines indicate latencies of N2 and P3. Note that epoch length and calibration size differ from those in Figure 1. LM indicates left mastoid; RM, right mastoid.*

gated N2 generation in schizophrenia using subtraction methods. Both studies demonstrated decreased N2 amplitude, suggesting that the cortical information processing deficits in schizophrenia are not limited to specific P3 generator regions. Mismatch negativity has been the subject of only two brief preliminary studies,[38,39] both of which observed decreased MMN amplitude in medicated schizophrenic subjects relative to age-matched controls. However, neither investigated MMN relative to the generation of temporally overlapping sensory components or P3. The present study confirms the deficits in MMN and N2 generation in subjects withdrawn from drug treatment (hereafter, drug-withdrawn subjects), as well as medicated schizophrenic subjects, and, additionally, suggests that the deficits in the early stages of cortical information processing might contribute to impaired P3 generation.

RESULTS

N1 AND P2

In response to standard stimuli, peak N1 amplitude occurred approximately 100 milliseconds after stimulus onset in schizophrenic subjects and controls in both the passive (**Figure 1**) and active behavioral (**Figure 2**) conditions. There was no significant between-group difference in peak N1 latency (**Table 1**). Peak N1 amplitude to standard stimuli did not differ significantly among schizophrenic and control groups in either the passive ($F[2,39]=0.20$, $P=.82$) or active ($F[2,37]=0.42$, $P=.66$) behavioral conditions (Table 1). For both controls and schizophrenic subjects, N1 amplitude was unaffected by the behavioral condition. The between-group ANOVAs had sufficient power (>0.8) to detect small (f=0.03) effect-size changes in the passive condition and small to medium (f=0.15) effect-size changes in the active condition, were such differences present.

N1 was followed by a frontocentral positivity, P2. There was no across-group difference in P2 amplitude in either the passive ($F[2,39]=1.62$, $P=.45$) or active ($F[2,37]=0.77$, $P=.55$) conditions. In the passive condition, P2 latency did not differ between schizophrenic subjects and controls. However, in the active condition, the P2 latency was significantly longer in controls than schizophrenic subjects (Table 1).

MISMATCH NEGATIVITY

Mismatch negativity amplitude was determined by analysis of peak amplitude at the frontal midline (F_z) electrode for both the control and schizophrenic groups. There was a significant across-group amplitude difference ($F[2,39]=5.78$, $P=.006$) in MMN amplitude reflecting a significant decrease in medicated and drug-withdrawn subjects compared with controls ($F[1,40]=11.4$, $P=.002$). The MMN amplitude at F_z was decreased by 46% in drug-withdrawn subjects and by 37% in medicated subjects compared with controls (Table 1). There was no significant difference in MMN amplitude between medicated and drug-withdrawn schizophrenic subjects. The MMN latency did not differ significantly across groups. Optimal between-group separation was obtained with an MMN amplitude cutoff of -5.0 μV, which correctly identified 29 of 30 schizophrenic subjects and five of 10 controls (Fisher's Exact Test, $P=.002$).

Separate analyses were conducted to assess the potential contribution of medication, gender, and IQ. Within the medicated group, there was no correlation between neuroleptic or anticholinergic dosage and MMN amplitude. Within the drug-withdrawn group, there was no correlation between prior neuroleptic dosage or length of drug-free period and MMN amplitude. A diagnostic group-by-gender ANOVA showed a significant effect of diagnostic group ($F[1,39]=12.49$, $P=.001$) but not of gender on MMN amplitude. There was no significant effect

Table 1. Peak Amplitudes and Latencies of Sensory and Cognitive Auditory Event-Related Potential Components

Component	Paradigm	Peak	Controls	Schizophrenic Subjects: Medicated	Schizophrenic Subjects: Drug-Withdrawn
Sensory					
N1	Passive	Amplitude	−4.34 (2.55)	−4.53 (2.41)	−4.95 (2.55)
		Latency	103.80 (14.91)	100.50 (13.24)	93.20 (26.10)
	Active	Amplitude	−4.85 (1.75)	−4.65 (3.16)	−5.41 (2.32)
		Latency	103.90 (10.02)	101.40 (17.97)	102.75 (20.41)
P2	Passive	Amplitude	4.11 (2.63)	4.51 (2.39)	2.09 (3.56)
		Latency	196.20 (32.52)	183.60 (17.72)	195.81 (23.50)
	Active	Amplitude	4.60 (2.28)	3.58 (2.28)	3.51 (2.39)
		Latency*	235.20 (34.44)	196.90 (30.22)	192.39 (22.77)
Cognitive					
Mismatch negativity	Passive	Amplitude†	−4.76 (2.52)	−2.38 (1.40)	−2.96 (1.28)
		Latency	126.20 (27.63)	113.80 (33.97)	108.90 (39.64)
N2	Active	Amplitude‡	−7.66 (4.88)	−3.15 (2.75)	−3.99 (4.05)
		Latency	216.40 (18.13)	207.20 (33.07)	208.98 (34.96)
P300	Active	Amplitude‡	12.15 (4.36)	5.66 (3.63)	4.38 (4.15)
		Latency	354.72 (29.62)	359.22 (64.62)	353.15 (38.80)

*$P<.05$, schizophrenic group vs control group.
†$P<.01$, schizophrenic group vs control group.
‡$P<.005$, schizophrenic group vs control group.

of either gender or IQ on MMN amplitude within either the control or schizophrenic groups. Moreover, there was no significant difference (F[1,20]=0.19, *P*=.95) in MMN amplitude among schizophrenic subjects in the lower (mean IQ, 90.3±4.2) compared with the upper (mean IQ, 108.8±10.9) half of scores. Finally, the difference in MMN amplitude between the control and schizophrenic groups remained significant even if comparisons were restricted to schizophrenic subjects in the top half of IQ scores (F[1,19]=5.48, *P*=.03).

Across-group topographical comparisons were performed by repeated-measures MANOVA with factors of electrode and diagnosis. There was a significant across-group amplitude difference (F[2,39]=4.11, *P*=.02) but no significant electrode-by-group interaction. The parasagittal and temporal laterality indices did not differ significantly from zero for any of the experimental groups, and there were no across-group differences in laterality scores. The laterality comparisons had sufficient power to detect small effect-size between-group differences in MMN topography at parasaggital (f=0.03) and temporal (f=0.02) electrodes, were such differences present.

To exclude the possibility that MMN in schizophrenic subjects might occur outside the predetermined latency window, running *t* tests were performed on grand-mean difference waveforms derived from controls and medicated and drug-withdrawn schizophrenic subjects (**Figure 3**). For controls, the difference waveform showed a significant negativity during the 125- to 160-millisecond latency range, peaking at 140 milliseconds. For schizophrenic subjects, difference waveforms did not show significant negative deflections either during the predefined latency range of control MMN or at any other time during the recording epoch. Running between-group *t* tests revealed a significant difference in MMN between controls and medicated schizophrenic subjects, and a trend toward reduction between controls and drug-withdrawn subjects.

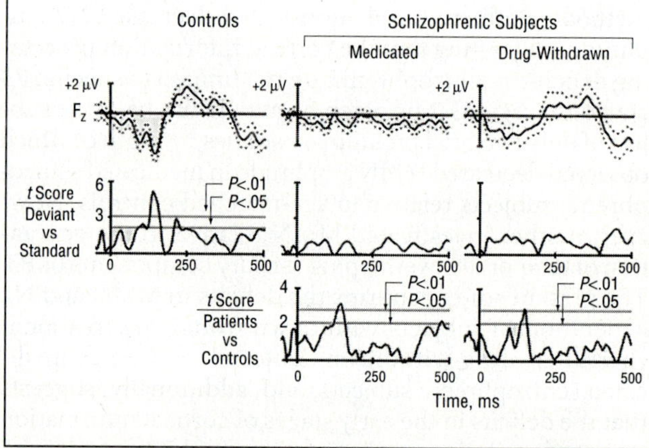

Figure 3. *Deviant minus standard difference waveforms at F_z during the passive condition for schizophrenic subjects receiving medication and those withdrawn from drug treatment and for normal controls. Solid and dotted lines in top panels represent across-subjects average (grand mean±SEM) waveforms. Deviant vs standard* t *scores represent absolute paired* t *values comparing waveforms elicited by deviant and standard stimuli across subjects within indicated groups. The* t *score for schizophrenic vs control group represents absolute* t *values resulting from between-group comparison of the across-subjects average difference waveforms. Waveforms are shown relative to a derived average mastoid reference.*

N2

N2 amplitude was determined by analysis of the deviant minus standard difference waveform at F_z (Table 1). There was a significant across-group difference in N2 amplitude (F[2,37]=5.14, *P*=.01), reflecting a significant difference between medicated and drug-withdrawn subjects compared with controls (F[1,38=10.02, *P*=.003). Compared with controls, N2 amplitude was decreased

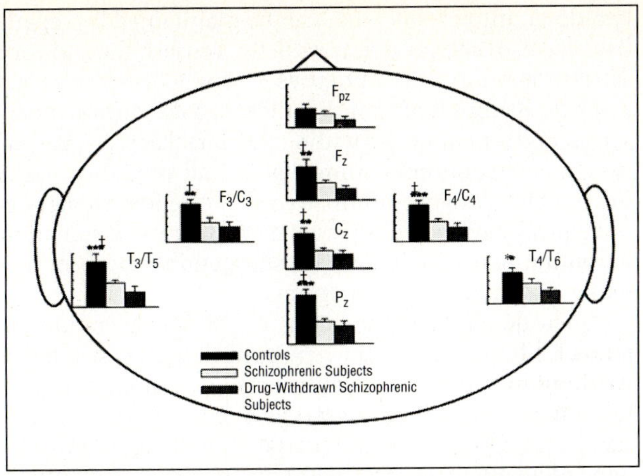

Figure 4. *Peak amplitude of P3 for schizophrenic subjects receiving medication and those withdrawn from drug treatment and normal controls at indicated electrodes during the active discrimination condition. Vertical calibration is 12 mV. Asterisk indicates $P<.05$; dagger, $P<.01$; and double dagger, $P<.005$.*

by 59% in medicated subjects and by 48% in drug-withdrawn subjects. There was no significant across-group difference in N2 latency. Studies of N2 topography showed a significant across-group amplitude difference ($F[2,37]=4.24$, $P=.02$) with no significant group-by-electrode interaction ($F[14,60]=1.65$, $P=.18$). Laterality scores were not significantly different from zero for any group and did not differ significantly across groups.

P3

P3 elicited during the active discrimination condition was maximal at P_z (Table 1). There was a significant across-group difference in P3 amplitude ($F[2,37]=12.29$, $P<.001$), with significant reduction in both medicated and drug-withdrawn subjects ($P<.001$). Compared with controls, P3 amplitude was decreased by 55% in medicated subjects and by 57% in drug-withdrawn subjects. P3 latency was greater in schizophrenic subjects than in control subjects, although the difference did not reach statistical significance (Table 1). Optimal between-group separation was obtained using a P3 cutoff of 10.0 μV, which correctly identified 27 of 30 schizophrenic subjects and seven of 10 controls (85%; Fisher's Exact Test, $P=.001$).

There was a highly significant group-by-electrode interaction (Hotelling's T^2-equivalent $F[14,60]=3.10$, $P=.001$). The across-group differences reached significance at all scalp locations other than the prefrontal and right temporal electrodes (**Figure 4**), suggesting a possible differential deficit in schizophrenic subjects over the left compared with the right temporal regions. Profile analysis of parallelism using normalized data[42] did not show a significant laterality effect (Hotelling's T^2-equivalent $F[8,66]=0.41$, $P=.95$). Moreover, laterality indices were not significantly different across groups for parasagittal ($F[2,38]=1.40$, $P=.50$) or temporal ($F[2,38]=0.46$, $P=.65$) electrodes. Finally, when topographical analyses were restricted alternately to the midline (F_{pz}, F_z, C_z, P_z) or coronal (L_2, L_1, F_z, R_1, R_2) chains, a significant group-by-electrode interaction was detected along the midline chain (Hotelling's T^2-equivalent $F[6,68]=5.67$, $P<.001$]) but not the coronal chain (Hotelling's T^2-equivalent $F[8,66]=0.79$, $P=.91$). Power computations suggest that the study would have had sufficient power (>0.8) to detect a small to medium effect-size between-group difference in P3 topography at parasagittal electrodes (f=0.18) were such an abnormality present but would have been able to detect only a large effect-size between-group difference in P3 topography at temporal electrodes (f=0.4).

Table 2. Performance of Schizophrenic and Control Subjects on Auditory Continuous Performance Task During the Active Discrimination Task

Performance Measure	Controls, Mean (SD)	Schizophrenic Subjects, Mean (SD)
Correct detections, %	99.9 (2.0)*	69.6 (26.7)
Correct rejections, %	93.2 (1.9)	83.9 (16.1)
Reaction time, ms	430 (8.0)*	556 (14.0)

*$P<.02$, schizophrenic group vs control group.

RELATIONSHIPS AMONG ERP MEASURES, DIAGNOSIS, AND BEHAVIORAL PERFORMANCE

To determine the potential interrelationship among ERP measures, a principal components analysis was performed using the seven ERP component variables. Following varimax rotation, three factors emerged with eigenvalues greater than 1. The first factor consisted of MMN amplitude and P3 amplitude (factor loadings greater than 0.7 in all cases), supporting the interpretation that these variables reflect the operation of a common underlying dimension. N2 amplitude loaded with moderate power into the first factor as well (loading score=0.36). Factor loadings for MMN and P3 were less than 0.3 for the other two factors. The second factor consisted of N2 amplitude, P2 amplitude in the passive condition, and P2 amplitude in the active condition, all of which had factor loadings greater than 0.7. The third factor consisted on N1 amplitude in the active and passive conditions, which had factor loading of 0.9 or greater. Together, the three factors accounted for 70.0% of the total variance. When diagnosis was added as a factor in the principal components analysis, it loaded significantly (loading score, >0.7) with the first factor (MMN and P3) but not with either of the two subsequent factors (loading scores less than 0.3).

The relationship among cognitive and sensory ERP component amplitudes and diagnosis was further investigated using linear regression analysis both across and between groups. There was a significant across-group correlation in the expected direction between MMN and P3 amplitudes ($r=-.38$, $P<.02$). There were also across-group trends in the expected direction between MMN and N2 amplitude ($r=+.29$, $P=.075$) and between N2 and P3 amplitude ($r=-.27$, $P=.09$). Correlations among cognitive components did not reach statistical significance in either the control or schizophrenic group considered individually. There were no significant correlations between the sensory components, N1 and P2, and MMN or P3, either across or within groups ($P>.25$).

Compared with controls, schizophrenic subjects showed a significantly lower percentage of correct detections of targets and prolonged reaction time (**Table 2**). Behavioral performance was a significant predictor of P3 amplitude across groups. Thus, there were significant correlations between P3 amplitude and the percentage of correct detections ($r=+.44$, $P<.005$), the percentage of correct rejections ($r=.37$, $P<.02$), and reaction time ($r=-.39$, $P<.02$). Within the schizophrenic group, but not the control group, there was also a nearly significant correlation ($r=.33$, $P=.09$) between the percentage of correct detections and P3 amplitude. The lower accuracy of schizophrenic subjects, compared with controls, raises the possibility that the between-group difference in P3 amplitude might reflect differential performance. However, the between-group difference in P3 amplitude remained strongly significant even following covariation for between-group difference in behavioral performance ($F[1,33]=11.4$, $P=.002$). There were no significant correlations between MMN amplitude and indices of behavioral performance either across or within groups.

COMMENT

Because of their millisecond-level temporal resolution, ERPs are ideally suited to analyzing the brain activity related to information processing activity.[28] The major finding of the present study is that the amplitude of MMN, an index of early cortical processing, is decreased in schizophrenia, along with that of N2 and P3. Mismatched negativity reflects activation of neural structures within primary auditory cortex (Heschl's gyrus) or adjacent supratemporal auditory regions,[35,36] as opposed to N2, which reflects activity primarily within auditory association cortex[37] and P3, which reflects activity in prefrontal, temporoparietal, and, potentially, other polysensory association regions of cortex.[29-32] The present findings, therefore, indicate that the neurophysiological dysfunction associated with schizophrenia is widespread and extends even to the level of the sensory cortex.

Generation of MMN depends on the ability of the auditory cortex to maintain a modality-specific short-duration representation of recent auditory events in the form of a "mnemonic template"[5] or short-duration sensory memory. Mismatch negativity is elicited when an individually presented stimulus differs from the working stimulus representation that has developed over the preceding several seconds. The demonstration of impaired MMN generation in schizophrenia thus supports the concept that impairments of short-duration, working-type memories may be a crucial role in the psychophysiology of schizophrenia.[44] The sensory memory on which MMN is based integrates auditory information over a period of approximately 10 seconds and corresponds to the neuropsychologically defined "echoic" or auditory sensory memory.[45,46] The deficit in MMN generation suggests that schizophrenia is associated with a deficit in the formation or maintenance of the sensory memory underlying MMN generation. It should be noted that the type of auditory working memory implicated in MMN generation differs from immediate recall-type short-term memory that is evaluated during mental status examination using digit span.[47] In immediate recall-type short-term memory, also termed *phonological loop memory*,[48] information is broken down into chunks that can be maintained by repetitive, vocal, or subvocal rehearsal. By contrast, the auditory sensory memory that underlies MMN generation stores acoustic attributes of stimuli rather than the stimuli themselves, and is maintained without rehearsal or subvocalization. In schizophrenia, immediate recall-type short-term memory is relatively unimpaired.[17,49,50] Echoic memory is not typically evaluated as part of mental status examination or routine neuropsychological testing, and has not been formally evaluated in schizophrenia.

The demonstration of impaired MMN generation extends findings from other neurophysiological studies of working memory in schizophrenia. Schizophrenic subjects show impaired generation of processing negativity,[51,52] an index of selective, working memory–dependent attention, and N400,[53,54] an index of attention-dependent semantic processing and decreased accuracy of memory-guided saccades.[50] Processing negativity, like MMN, is elicited only by stimuli that are presented with interstimulus intervals below approximately 10 seconds,[5] suggesting that the processing negativity deficits, like those of MMN, may reflect impaired short-duration memory in schizophrenia. Moreover, like MMN, the processing negativity deficits are present in drug-withdrawn,[16] as well as medicated subjects, and are more evident at long rather than short interstimulus intervals.[52]

An advantage of MMN over other neurophysiological indices of cortical dysfunction in schizophrenia is that MMN generation is largely independent of sustained attention or conscious motivation. Mechanisms underlying MMN generation can also be studied in lower animals using stimulation conditions identical to those used for clinical studies. Both cats[55] and monkeys[56] generate MMN-like activity that is highly similar to human MMN. Based on animal studies, one receptor type that appears to be specifically involved in the generation of MMN is the *N*-methyl-D-aspartate (NMDA) type glutamate receptor.[57] The NMDA channels show unique, dual-voltage and ligand sensitivity, allowing them to generate "conditional" neuronal depolarizations. Intracortical injection of NMDA antagonists into auditory cortex results in a selective disruption of MMN generation without affecting simultaneously generated obligatory components.[57] A widespread cortical deficit in NMDA receptor-mediated neurotransmssion, therefore, might account for the severe abnormalities in working and long-term memory formation that are associated with schizophrenia, as well as the pervasive deficits in cognitive ERP generation observed in the present study (reviewed in Javitt and Zukin[58]).

For the present study, stimulation and recording parameters were optimized for analysis of MMN generation in schizophrenic subjects relative to normal controls. In normal controls, MMN amplitude increases sharply as the pitch separation between standard and deviant stimuli is increased to just above the discrimination threshold, but begins to plateau once the degree of separation exceeds the easy discrimination threshold for all subjects.[5] The degree of pitch separation chosen for the present study, 1000 vs 1024 Hz, produces an approximately half-maximal MMN amplitude in normal controls, minimizing the degree to which floor or ceiling effects would interfere with between-group statistical comparisons. Mismatch negativity inverts in polarity between F_z and mastoid electrodes consistent with a predominant generator within the Heschl's gyrus region of the superior temporal plane.[5] The montage used for this study interpolates electrodes between F_z and the mastoids to analyze the left-right symmetry of the MMN polarity reversal. The absence of a between-group topographical difference in MMN amplitude suggests that the neurophysiological deficit associated with schizophrenia is not lateralized at the level of the primary sensory cortex. There was a significant across-group correlation between MMN and P3 amplitude and a nearly significant correlation between MMN and N2 amplitude, suggesting that deficits in the early stages of auditory information processing in schizophrenia might contribute to subsequent neurophysiological dysfunction. However, the correlation accounted for only a modest percentage of the variance in P3 amplitude (approximately 14%), indicating that other factors might affect P3 amplitude to an equal or greater extent.

In the present study, the reduction in P3 amplitude was greatest over the left temporal region, as has been reported previously.[15,42,59] While the left-right asymmetry tests did not reach statistical significance, a power analysis suggests that a large effect would have had to be present for a significant between-group difference to have been detected. Several factors may have contributed to the relatively low power of the present study for detecting lateralization of the P3 deficit. First, because electrode placements were optimized for the detection of MMN, no electrodes were placed in the regions at which deficits were most strongly lateralized in prior studies. Second, because the behavioral task was relatively difficult, schizophrenic subjects performed far worse than controls. Finally, the control group for the present study was relatively small and not fully matched for gender. However, the relatively small group size cannot fully account for the lack of power since this study had sufficient statistical power to detect even a small to moderate between-group difference in MMN topography, were such an abnormality present.

The decreased P2 latency for standard stimuli observed in the present study has been found by others in both schizophrenic subjects[12-14] and nonschizophrenic college students with high levels of allusive thinking.[60] Several previous studies have found abnormalities of N1 generation in schizophrenia, including both increased[61] and decreased[8,12-14,28,62,63] amplitude, while others have not.[6,11,51,52] In the study herein, there was no significant decrease in N1 amplitude in schizophrenic subjects relative to controls and no significant effect of medication status on N1 amplitude. Differences in findings regarding obligatory ERP components may relate to differences in stimulus type (tone vs click), intensity, duration, or interstimulus interval.[61] Further, schizophrenic subtype may be an important consideration, with decreased N1 amplitude being characteristic of paranoid but not residual-type schizophrenic subjects.[64]

The finding of decreased MMN generation in schizophrenia has significant relevance to schizophrenia at both the research and clinical levels. On a research level, this study demonstrates that cortical information processing is impaired even at the level of the sensory cortex, and that impairments in the early stages of information processing may contribute to subsequent "high-order" deficits such as impaired P3 generation. The finding that NMDA antagonists, injected into auditory cortex, induce a pattern of auditory dysfunction similar to that observed in schizophrenia[57] supports the hypothesis that dysfunction or dysregulation of NMDA receptor-mediated neurotransmission may play a crucial role in the pathophysiology of schizophrenia.[58]

On a clinical level, the demonstration of deficient MMN generation indicates that a basic system designed to draw an individual's attention to significant environmental events is severely impaired in schizophrenia. Under normal conditions, auditory cortex maintains a transient representation of environmental background sounds even when such sounds are outside the focus of attention or are consciously ignored. When a significant change in background stimulation occurs, specific neuronal ensembles within the auditory cortex are automatically activated. These neurons, in turn, activate ensembles within secondary and higher cortical centers, leading to a shift in attention toward the source of the novel events. Because unexpected events occur continually in real-world settings, the MMN generation system normally provides individuals with a constant impetus to explore their environment. The lack of MMN generation in schizophrenia indicates that persons with schizophrenia do not experience the same level of automatic cortical activation in response to new or unexpected events and so do not have the same constant impetus for environmental exploration. The lack of this basic alerting mechanism, and the corresponding lack of a constant pull to explore new environmental stimuli, may contribute significantly to the isolation, passive withdrawal, and lack of interest in the environment that are characteristic of the deficit syndrome of schizophrenia. As demonstrated in the present study, the deficit in automatic activation persists despite treatment with conventional antipsychotic agents. The development of new treatment approaches aimed at reversing this deficit in automatic activation might yield significant benefit in the management of persistent deficit symptoms of schizophrenia.

Accepted for publication December 27, 1994.

Funding for this study was provided by grant R29 MH49334 from the US Public Health Service, a National Alliance for Research on Schizophrenia and Affective Disorders Young Investigator Award (Dr Javitt), and the Zara and Bernad Jakubovitz Fund for Schizophrenia Research (Dr Javitt).

The authors acknowledge the valuable contributions of Herbert G. Vaughan, Jr, MD, to study design, data interpretation, and manuscript preparation.

Reprint requests to Department of Psychiatry, Room K322, Albert Einstein College of Medicine, 1300 Morris Park Ave, Bronx, NY 10461 (Dr Javitt).

REFERENCES

1. Harvey PD, Doherty NM, Serper MR, Rasmussen M. Cognitive deficits and thought disorder, II: an 8-month followup study. *Schizophr Bull.* 1990;16:147-156.
2. Kay SR, Murrill LM. Predicting outcome of schizophrenia: significance of symptom profiles and outcome dimensions. *Compr Psychiatry.* 1990;31:91-102.
3. Carpenter WT, Heinrichs DW, Wagman AM. Deficit and non-deficit forms of schizophrenia: the concept. *Am J Psychiatry.* 1988;145:578-583.
4. Pritchard WS. Cognitive event-related potential correlates of schizophrenia. *Psychol Bull.* 1986;100:43-66.

5. Naatanen R. The role of attention in auditory information processing as revealed by event-related potentials and other measures of cognitive function. *Behav Brain Sci.* 1990;13:201-288.
6. Roth WT, Cannon EH. Some features of the auditory evoked response in schizophrenics. *Arch Gen Psychiatry.* 1972;27:466-471.
7. Blackwood DHR, Muir WJ. Cognitive brain potentials and their application. *Br J Psychiatry.* 1990;157(suppl 9):96-101.
8. Ogura C, Nageishi Y, Matsubayashi M, Omura F, Kishimoto A, Shimokochi M. Abnormalities in event-related potentials, N100, P200, P300 and slow wave in schizophrenia. *Jpn J Psychiatry Neurol.* 1991;45:57-65.
9. St Clair D, Blackwood D, Muir W. P300 abnormality in schizophrenic subtypes. *J Psychiatr Res.* 1989;23:49-55.
10. Duncan CC. Event-related brain potentials: a window on information processing in schizophrenia. *Schizophr Bull.* 1988;14:199-203.
11. Blackwood DH, Whalley LJ, Christie JE, Blackburn IM, St Clair DM, McInnes A. Changes in auditory P3 event-related potential in schizophrenia and depression. *Br J Psychiatry.* 1987;150:154-160.
12. Pfefferbaum A, Ford JM, White PM, Roth WT. P_3 in schizophrenia is affected by stimulus modality, response requirements, medication status, and negative symptoms. *Arch Gen Psychiatry.* 1989;46:1035-1044.
13. Blackwood DH, St Clair DM, Muir WJ, Duffy JC. Auditory P300 and eye tracking dysfunction in schizophrenic pedigrees. *Arch Gen Psychiatry.* 1991;48:899-909.
14. Roth WT, Horvath TB, Pfefferbaum A, Kopell BS. Event-related potentials in schizophrenics. *Electroencephalogr Clin Neurophysiol.* 1980;48:127-139.
15. McCarley RW, Shenton ME, O'Donnell BF, Faux SF, Kikinis R, Nestor PG, Jolesz FA. Auditory P300 abnormalities and left posterior superior temporal gyrus volume reduction in schizophrenia. *Arch Gen Psychiatry.* 1993;50:190-198.
16. Ward PB, Catts SV, Fox AM, Michie PT, McConaghy N. Auditory selective attention and event-related potentials in schizophrenia. *Br J Psychiatry.* 1991; 158:534-539.
17. Gruzelier J, Seymour K, Wilson L, Jolley A, Hirsch S. Impairments on neuropsychological tests of temporohippocampal and frontohippocampal functions and word fluency in remitting schizophrenia and affective disorders. *Arch Gen Psychiatry.* 1988;45:623-629.
18. Kolb B, Whishaw IQ. Performance of schizophrenic patients on tests sensitive to left or right frontal, temporal or parietal functions in neurological patients. *J Nerv Ment Dis.* 1983;171:435-443.
19. Saykin AJ, Gur RC, Gur RE, Mozley D, Mozley LH, Resnick SM, Kester B, Stafiniak P. Neuropsychological function in schizophrenia. Selective impairment in memory and learning. *Arch Gen Psychiatry.* 1991;48:618-624.
20. Buchsbaum MS. The frontal lobes, basal ganglia, and temporal lobes as sites for schizophrenia. *Schizophr Bull.* 1990;16:379-389.
21. Crow TJ. Temporal lobe asymmetries as the key to the etiology of schizophrenia. *Schizophr Bull.* 1990;16:433-443.
22. Beatty WW, Jocic Z, Monson N, Staton RD. Memory and frontal lobe dysfunction in schizophrenia and schizoaffective disorder. *J Nerv Ment Dis.* 1993;181:448-453.
23. Levin S. Frontal lobe dysfunction in schizophrenia, II: impairments of psychological and brain functions. *J Psychiatr Res.* 1984;18:57-72.
24. Weinberger DR, Berman KF, Zec RF. Physiologic dysfunction of dorsolateral prefrontal cortex in schizophrenia, I: regional cerebral blood flow evidence. *Arch Gen Psychiatry.* 1986;43:114-124.
25. Braff DL, Heaton R, Kuck J, Cullum M, Moranville J, Grant I, Ziszook S. The generalized pattern of neuropsychological deficits in outpatients with chronic schizophrenia with heterogeneous Wisconsin Card Sorting Test results. *Arch Gen Psychiatry.* 1991;48:891-898.
26. Chelune GJ, Heaton RK, Lehman RA, Robinson A. Level versus pattern of neuropsychological performance among schizophrenic and diffusely brain-damaged patients. *J Consult Clin Psychol.* 1979;47:155-163.
27. Blanchard JJ, Neale JM. The neuropsychological signature of schizophrenia: generalized or differential deficit? *Am J Psychiatry.* 1994;151:40-48.
28. McCarley RW, Faux SF, Shenton ME, Nestor PG, Adams J. Event-related potentials in schizophrenia: their biological and clinical correlates and a new model of schizophrenic pathophysiology. *Schizophr Res.* 1991;4:209-231.
29. Knight RT, Scabini D, Woods DL, Clayworth CC. Contributions of temporal-parietal junction to the human auditory P3. *Brain Res.* 1989;502:109-116.
30. Smith ME, Halgren E, Sokolik M, Baudena P, Musolino A, Liegeois-Chauvel C, Chauvel P. The intracranial topography of the P3 event-related potential elicited during auditory oddball. *Electroencephalogr Clin Neurophysiol.* 1990;76:235-248.
31. Neshige R, Luders H. Recording of event-related potentials (P300) from human cortex. *J Clin Neurophysiol.* 1992;9:294-298.
32. Simson R, Vaughan HG, Ritter W. The scalp topography of potentials associated with missing visual or auditory stimuli. *Electroencephalogr Clin Neurophysiol.* 1976;40:33-42.
33. Naatanen R, Picton TW. N2 and automatic versus controlled processes. *Electroencephalogr Clin Neurophysiol Suppl.* 1986;38:169-186.
34. Novak G, Ritter W, Vaughan HG Jr. The chronometry of attention-modulated processing and automatic mismatch detection. *Psychophysiology.* 1992;29:412-430.
35. Scherg M, Vajsar J, Picton TW. A source analysis of the late human auditory evoked potentials. *J Cog Neurosci.* 1989;1:336-355.
36. Sams M, Kaukoranta E, Hamalainen M, Naatanen R. Cortical activity elicited by changes in auditory stimuli: different sources for the magnetic N100m and mismatch responses. *Psychophysiology.* 1991;28:21-29.
37. O'Donnell BF, Shenton ME, McCarley RW, Faux SF, Smith RS, Salisbury DF, Nestor PG, Pollak SD, Kikinis R, Jolesz FA. The auditory N2 component in schizophrenia: relationship to MRI temporal lobe gray matter and to other ERP abnormalities. *Biol Psychiatry.* 1993;34:26-40.
38. Javitt DC, Doneshka P, Zylberman I, Ritter W, Vaughan HG Jr. Impairment of early cortical processing in schizophrenia: an event-related potential replication study. *Biol Psychiatry.* 1993;33:513-519.
39. Shelley AM, Ward PB, Catts SV, Michie PT, Andrews S, McConaghy N. Mismatch negativity: an index of a preattentive processing deficit in schizophrenia. *Biol Psychiatry.* 1991;30:1059-1062.
40. American Psychiatric Association. *Diagnostic and Statistical Manual of Mental Disorders, Revised Third Edition.* Washington, DC: American Psychiatric Association; 1987.
41. Ammons RB, Ammons CH. The Quick Test (QT): provisional manual. *Psychol Rep.* 1962;11:111-162.
42. Faux SF, McCarley RW. Analysis of scalp voltage asymmetries using Hotelling's T^2 methodology. *Brain Topography.* 1990;2:237-245.
43. Guthrie D, Buchwald JS. Significance testing of difference potentials. *Psychophysiology.* 1991;28:241-244.
44. Goldman-Rakic PS. Prefrontal cortical dysfunction in schizophrenia: the relevance of working memory. In: Carroll BJ, Barrett JE, eds. *Psychopathology and the Brain.* New York, NY: Raven Press; 1991:1-24.
45. Cowan N, Winkler I, Teder W, Naatanen R. Memory prerequisites of the mismatch negativity in the auditory event-related potential. *J Exp Psychol Learn Mem Cogn.* 1993;19:909-921.
46. Naatanen R, Paavilainen P, Reinikainen K. Do event-related potentials to infrequent decrements in duration of auditory stimuli demonstrate a memory trace in man? *Neurosci Lett.* 1989;107(1-3):347-352.
47. Strub RL, Black FW. *The Mental Status Examination in Neurology.* Philadelphia, Pa: FA Davis; 1981.
48. Baddeley A. Working memory. *Science.* 1992;255:556-559.
49. Tamlyn D, McKenna PJ, Mortimer AM, Lund CE, Hammond S, Baddeley AD. Memory impairment in schizophrenia: its extent, affiliations and neuropsychological character. *Psychol Med.* 1992;22:101-115.
50. Park S, Holzman PS. Schizophrenics show spatial working memory deficits. *Arch Gen Psychiatry.* 1992;49:975-982.
51. Michie PT, Fox AM, Ward PB, Catts SV, McConaghy N. Event-related potential indices of selective attention and cortical lateralization in schizophrenia. *Psychophysiology.* 1990;27:209-227.
52. Baribeau-Braun J, Picton TW, Gosselin J-Y. Schizophrenia: a neurophysiological evaluation of abnormal information processing. *Science.* 1983;219:874-876.
53. Gaillard AW, Naatanen R. Some baseline effects on the CNV. *Biol Psychol.* 1980;10:31-39.
54. Mitchell PF, Andrews S, Fox AM, Catts SV, Ward PB, McConaghy N. Active and passive attention in schizophrenia: an ERP study of information processing in a linguistic task. *Biol Psychol.* 1991;32(2-3):101-124.
55. Csépe V, Karmos G, Molnár M. Evoked potential correlates of stimulus deviance during wakefulness and sleep in cat—animal model of mismatch negativity. *Electroencephalogr Clin Neurophysiol.* 1987;66:571-578.
56. Javitt DC, Schroeder CE, Steinschneider M, Arezzo JC, Vaughan HG Jr. Demonstration of mismatch negativity in the monkey. *Electroencephalogr Clin Neurophysiol.* 1992;83:87-90.
57. Javitt DC, Schroeder CE, Steinschneider M, Arezzo JC, Ritter W, Vaughan HG Jr. Cognitive event-related potentials in human and non-human primates: implications for the PCP/NMDA model of schizophrenia. In: Karmos G, Molnar M, Csepe V, Czigler Z, Desmedt JE, eds. *Perspectives of Event-Related Potentials Research.* Amsterdam, the Netherlands: Elsevier Science Publishers; 1994. (EEG suppl 44).
58. Javitt DC, Zukin SR. Recent advances in the phencyclidine model of schizophrenia. *Am J Psychiatry.* 1991;148:1301-1308.
59. Faux SF, McCarley RW, Nestor PG, Shenton ME, Pollak SD, Penhune V, Mondrow E, Marcy B, Peterson A, Horvath T. P300 topographic asymmetries are present in unmedicated schizophrenics. *Electroencephalogr Clin Neurophysiol.* 1993;88:32-41.
60. Catts SV, Armstrong MS, Ward PB, McConaghy N. Reduced P200 latency and allusive thinking: an auditory evoked potential index of a cognitive predisposition to schizophrenia. *Int J Neurosci.* 1986;30:173-179.
61. Adler G, Adler J, Schneck M, Armbruster B. Influence of stimulation parameters on auditory stimulus processing in schizophrenia and major depression: an auditory evoked potential study. *Acta Psychiatr Scand.* 1990;81:453-458.
62. Shagass C, Roemer RA, Straumanis JJ, Amadeo M. Evoked potential correlates of psychosis. *Biol Psychiatry.* 1978;13:163-184.
63. Barrett K, McCallum WC, Pocock PV. Brain indicators of altered attention and information processing in schizophrenic patients. *Br J Psychiatry.* 1986;148:414-420.
64. Kessler C, Steinberg A. Evoked potential variation in schizophrenic subgroups. *Biol Psychiatry.* 1989;26:372-380.

COMMENTARY

Event-Related Potentials in the Study of Psychiatric Disorders

TWO ARTICLES in this issue of the ARCHIVES[1,2] use a common method for studying neurophysiological processes in the intact brains of human subjects. This method is based on the fact that slowly changing membrane potentials of dendrites and nerve cell bodies generate extracellular current flow. Excitatory and inhibitory postsynaptic potentials cause outflows of ionic charges into extracellular fluid, which are then pumped back into the cell. The movement of charges constitutes current flow and in a summated form results in volume-conducted potentials recorded at the scalp as the electroencephalogram (EEG).

WHAT ARE EVENT-RELATED POTENTIALS?

Event-related potentials (ERPs) are EEG changes that are time-locked to sensory, motor, or cognitive events and provide a neurophysiological reflection of the processing of these events. At the scalp, ERPs are relatively small compared with the background EEG. Therefore, signal averaging is used to enhance the signal-to-noise ratio (SNR). This process assumes that the ERP (signal) is invariant and the EEG (noise) is random, that EEG amplitude will approximate zero, and that the ERP amplitude will emerge unaffected by the EEG after sufficient ERP trials are averaged. The smaller the signal, the more trials are needed. The repeated trials are synchronized to the stimulus event, and an ensemble average, time-locked to the synchronizing event, is calculated across stimulus repetitions (trials) for each time point in the trial. If X_{jt} is the electrical potential (voltage) at some electrode location at time t and trial j, the signal average over J trials is defined as follows:

$$\bar{X}_t = \frac{1}{J}\sum_{j=1}^{J} X_{jt}$$

For example, if a tone is repeated 30 times, the averages of all 30 trials (j=1, 30) could be calculated at 1-millisecond intervals (t=1, 500) following tone onset, yielding a 500-millisecond epoch. If X_{jt} is considered the sum of true signal plus random noise (background EEG and measurement error), signal averaging improves the SNR ratio. The validity of the method rests on the assumptions that the signal is invariant across trials and that the background EEG is random noise with respect to the stimulus.

In addition to the EEG, electrodes on the scalp will also record nonbrain activity, especially from eye movement (the electro-oculogram) and muscle activity (the electromyogram). These electrical signals are often generated in response to external stimuli; eg, a subject might blink when a tone is sounded. This can be especially problematic when studying psychiatric patients who are often less able than controls to cooperate and refrain from blinking and moving when stimuli are presented. Thus, care must be taken to either exclude trials with electro-oculogram or electromyogram activity or to compensate for them. In recent years several mathematical techniques have been developed to correct ERPs for the influence of electro-oculogram activity.[3,4]

Signal averaging of the EEG allows one to examine small electrical potentials in response to a variety of sensory stimuli. Auditory, visual, and somatosensory stimuli are most commonly used, although any sensory stimulation with a fairly abrupt onset that can be administered repeatedly can be used. The averaged EEG response from simple sensory stimulation is often referred to as an evoked potential (EP) or evoked response (ER), especially in the neurology literature and early psychiatry literature. More recently, the term *event-related potential* has been used to convey the importance of the psychological meaning of the stimulus; an event can actually be the absence of a stimulus when one is expected.[5]

Simple sensory evoked potential components usually occur earlier in time than cognitive ERP components. For instance, auditory brain-stem responses occur between 1 and 8 milliseconds after stimulation and are little affected by attention. In contrast, cognitive ERPs usually do not develop until 50 or 100 milliseconds after stimulation and can last for several seconds. While the sensory vs cognitive distinction represents a continuum rather than a true dichotomy, the latency of evoked potentials is in the temporal range of perception and the latency of ERPs is in the temporal range of attention and cognition.

HOW HAVE ERPs BEEN APPLIED TO THE STUDY OF INFORMATION PROCESSING?

Event-related potentials have been used to study many aspects of information processing that are relatively inaccessible using self-report or traditional behavioral techniques. Different components of the ERP reflect different aspects of information processing. A component is usually defined as a reliably observed positive- or negative-going deflection in the ERP waveform. One of the most prominent components is the N100 that is elicited by simple auditory stimuli (eg, tones or clicks); it is negative (N) and occurs at about 100 milliseconds after tone onset, hence, the name "N100." Although it is affected in a

See also pages 544 and 550

predictable manner by stimulus intensity (amplitude increases and latency decreases with increasing intensity[6]) the amplitude of the N100 component also reflects the direction of attention to stimuli even when no behavioral response is made.[7]

The mismatch negativity (MMN) response occurs in the same latency range as the N100 component and represents an early response to stimulus novelty. It is generated when an auditory stimulus is deviant in frequency, intensity, or duration from the preceding stimuli in a sequence.[8] It is small in amplitude and usually is presented as a difference waveform created by the subtraction of the deviant stimulus ERP from the frequent stimulus ERP. Unlike P300, it does not require that the deviant stimulus be unexpected, and it is used as a reflection of early sensory memory that is often beyond awareness.

P300 is a positive ERP component that occurs between 300 and 500 milliseconds after stimulus onset. It is elicited when a stimulus is relevant to a task or is surprising, ie, unexpected.[9] Its latency has been used to supplement reaction-time measurements in studies of mental chronometry, ie, how long it takes a subject to make a decision about a particular stimulus.[10] Like other ERP components, it can be elicited in the absence of a behavioral response. When an overt response such as a button press is required, P300 latency is coupled to reaction time in some situations and uncoupled in others.[11,12] When tightly coupled, it provides little extra information beyond reaction time, although it can be used as a substitute for an overt response when a response is not possible or practical. When uncoupled from an overt response, the latency of P300 provides additional information, namely, an estimate of the time required to evaluate the stimulus. Further, when one wants information about the mental chronometry of withholding a response, ERPs may be the only metric available.[13]

In addition to its polarity, latency, and lawful relationship to its eliciting events, an ERP component is defined by its amplitude distribution across the scalp. The scalp distribution of the various components (sometimes referred to as its "topography") can help localize brain function and distinguish one cognitive process from another. The P300 associated with a simple button press is maximal over midline parietal scalp, whereas the P300 associated with withholding a response is more centrally distributed. This suggests subtle neurophysiological differences in the decision to produce or withhold a response to a task-relevant stimulus.[13]

HOW HAVE ERPs BEEN APPLIED TO PSYCHIATRY?

Since the mid-1960s, cognitive psychologists have made considerable progress toward understanding the psychological correlates of these physiological phenomena (ie, ERPs). For just as long, clinically oriented investigators have attempted to use these tools to investigate psychopathological disorders. In 1976, Shagass[14] proposed that clinical electrophysiological investigations could proceed under two distinct conceptual approaches, "psychophysiological" or "pathophysiological." The psychophysiological approach applies the knowledge about lawful relationships between electrophysiological and psychological events to understand some of the manifestations of mental illness. The pathophysiological approach assumes that biological abnormalities in mental illness may have neurophysiological expressions that do not lie on a continuum with normal psychophysiology, eg, the EEG signs of an epileptic focus. To date, no "signature" ERP for a psychiatric disorder has been discovered, and ERP research in psychiatry has mainly taken the psychophysiological approach. However, with the advent of localization studies using many scalp electrodes, the pathophysiological approach may yet yield distinct pathological electrophysiological signatures for specific psychiatric diseases.

The psychophysiological-pathophysiological dichotomy is similar to the contrast between quantitative vs qualitative alterations in disease states. In the absence of qualitatively abnormal ERPs in any psychiatric disorder, ERP research has focused on quantitative differences, assessing the amplitude or latency of ERP components during the presentation of stimuli or performance of some mental task. Results have been easiest to interpret in diseases with known pathological characteristics such as multiple sclerosis, where delay of P100 latency to visual checkerboard reversal is considered a "hard sign" of the disease, presumably due to delayed neuronal transit time, and related to demyelination. Similarly, as mentioned above, P300 is delayed with normal aging with yet more delay in certain dementing disorders. These are quantitative deviations of normal physiological functions recorded from the scalp electrodes.

In this issue, O'Donnell et al[1] and Javitt et al[2] have both used variations of Shagass' psychophysiological approach. O'Donnell et al use P300 latency as a physiological index of the speed of stimulus evaluation and compare its delay with age in patients with schizophrenia and controls. Thus, they have used an ERP variable in a quantitative fashion to test a hypothesis about a "normal" physiological function in abnormal people. In their paradigm, the subjects were asked to keep a mental count of the number of rare events in a sequence. Since the subjects did not press a reaction time button, P300 latency was the only measure of cognitive speed. In patients with schizophrenia, P300 latency may be the better measure because motor responses are more likely to be affected by motivation, cooperation, and attention.

The observation that, in normals, P300 latency decreases from childhood to the teenage years and then increases throughout adulthood was first noted by Goodin et al[15] and has been replicated by many others since.[16,17] In dementing disorders, there can be P300 latency prolongation over and above that expected with normal aging.[18-21] O'Donnell et al report that the rate of P300 latency prolongation with age is exaggerated in male patients with chronic schizophrenia compared with normal controls. Although this excessive prolongation did not correlate with clinical severity, they interpreted it as consistent with a progressive neurodegenerative process in schizophrenia.

If neurons do degenerate progressively in schizophrenia, one might also expect to see morphological age-related changes with brain magnetic resonance imaging (MRI) or x-ray computed tomography (CT) studies. However, relevant data from structural imaging are inconclusive in that some studies show progression of dysmorphology with age or duration of illness while others do not. The data of O'Donnell et al imply that ERPs are more sensitive than structural imaging to age-related changes associated with schizophrenia. This would not be at all surprising, given the current sensitivity of morphological studies and the fact that physiological changes would be expected to precede loss of structural volume. As O'Donnell and colleagues point out, caution is in order given the limitations of this and most clinical studies. Their observations were cross-sectional, the range of age of illness onset and age at testing were restricted, and knowledge about subjects' medication and substance abuse history was limited. Only longitudinal study with adequate controls can address these concerns.

One might take issue with the use of the term "neurodegenerative" since the underlying physiology giving rise to the observations is unknown. This is not unlike the problem of tissue volume reduction seen with CT and MRI in schizophrenia. In the early literature, it was common to refer to enlarged ventricles, for example, as a sign of "atrophy." However, without knowing the underlying pathology or the previous morphological features of the brain, it is uncertain whether true atrophy (ie, cell loss) has taken place or whether the observed tissue volume decrement was due to agenesis or other processes such as changes in intracellular hydration.

In the past, the O'Donnell research group found a relationship between P300 *amplitude* and gray matter volume in the left posterior superior temporal gyrus in patients with schizophrenia.[22] In the current report,[1] P300 *latency* was not related to the amount of gray matter volume in the left posterior superior temporal gyrus in the same subjects (a subset of the larger group on which the current report is based). They speculate that white rather than gray matter changes are more likely to be reflected in P300 latency. The lack of relationships between P300 latency and gray matter has been noted by others.[23] Another possibility is that complex neural systems are responsible for generating P300 and abnormalities in several elements of these systems will alter P300 latency and amplitude.[23] These are testable hypotheses being investigated in several laboratories.[23,24]

In summary, the report of O'Donnell et al is interesting, provocative, and challenging. It gives support to the contention that at least a subset of patients with schizophrenia have a progressive disorder with electrophysiological evidence of excessive cognitive decline associated with advancing age.

Javitt et al[2] also use ERPs to assess a psychophysiological function and conclude that it is deficient in schizophrenia by virtue of reduced amplitude of certain ERP components. They build on the observations in normals that the P300 is temporally preceded by other components, some of which are obligatory sensory responses and others of which are reflections of earlier cognitive processing stages, including N100, P200, MMN, and N200. Mismatch negativity (MMN) is sensitive to auditory sensory memory and is augmented when a stimulus mismatches a template residing in memory. Using a paradigm similar to that of O'Donnell et al, but with a passive and active response condition and different analysis techniques, Javitt et al demonstrate decreased amplitude in MMN and N200, as well as P300, in a group of schizophrenic patients. The reduction in amplitude of MMN and N200 is offered as evidence that the cognitive deficit associated with schizophrenia and manifested by decreased P300 amplitude is present early in the chain of cognitive events and is not unique to P300. The deficit is in a sense "pervasive" and extends to several brain regions. There is some evidence, primarily from magnetoencephalogram (MEG) and ERP dipole localization studies, that points to separate neural sources for P300, MMN, and the sensory N100. Thus, Javitt et al conclude that the neurophysiological deficit of schizophrenia extends to the level of sensory cortex. This assertion would be consistent with the MRI and CT findings of diffuse rather than circumscribed brain dysmorphology in schizophrenia.[25]

The most intriguing aspect of the report by Javitt et al is that there appears to be a fairly robust animal model for MMN. Further, the amplitude of this component can be selectively disrupted by the injection of *N*-methyl-D-aspartate (NMDA) antagonists. Thus, Javitt and colleagues speculate that a widespread cortical deficit in *N*-methyl-D-aspartate receptor–mediated neurotransmission might account for some memory impairment in schizophrenia. If these observations are confirmed, their paradigm might lead to a model for investigation of certain types of auditory memory deficits in a variety of disorders in which drug manipulation and parallel animal investigations can be carried out.

NEW DIRECTIONS: IMAGES OF BRAIN ACTIVITY

The two articles[1,2] in this issue of the ARCHIVES relied on the traditional measures of ERP component amplitudes and latencies to answer specific questions about mental chronometry and memory function. Nerve cells also generate intracellular current flow from dendrites to cell body, resulting in a magnetic field that can be detected at the scalp as a MEG. Magnetoencephalogram recording has been made practical by the development of superconducting quantum interference devices (SQUIDs) that are sensitive to minute magnetic fields. Like ERPs constructed from the EEG, MEG activity can be averaged to enhance the SNR ratio to produce event-related magnetic fields (ERFs).

With modern technological advances, ERPs and ERFs can be used to create temporally meaningful images of brain activity that can be coordinated with images of brain structure and images of blood flow or chemical concentrations. For localization studies relating ERP or ERF data to brain structures visualized by MRI, electrodes must be aligned according to skull landmarks, with fiducial markers visible in MRI scans. Event-related potentials and ERFs from multiple EEG leads or MEG sensors can be subjected to mathematical analysis to reduce these data to images, eg, current source density maps, or to model dipole sources. While the conventional 10-20 system of Jasper[26] used 19 electrodes with a typical distance of 6 cm between them, recent investigators have expanded the electrode arrays to 124, or even 256, electrodes, which yield interelectrode distances of 2.25 and 1.6 cm. Magnetoencephalogram systems also began with a few channels, but this number has increased quickly as the technology has been perfected; a 122-channel MEG system is online in Finland.[27]

Images from multiple electrodes are usually constructed in one of three ways: simple voltage amplitude maps, current source density maps, and dipole modeling. *Current source density maps* (also called surface Laplacian or radial current estimate maps) act as spatial filters emphasizing localized components with a high spatial frequency. For this to work well, of course, electrodes must be placed with a high spatial frequency. Maps can be made of unaveraged activity such as epileptic spikes or of signal averages. Using current source density maps, sensory ERP components show a more localized distribution than that achieved with simple voltage maps. Further, the current source density map has a physical interpretation—local radial current flow from the brain into the scalp and vice versa—but it is different from dipole modeling (described below) and free of dipole modeling's ambiguities.

Dipole modeling is a method for reducing data from multilead ERP or multisensor ERF by deducing the dipole sources that may have produced them. Although the "forward problem," calculating scalp distribution from known dipoles, has a unique solution whose accuracy is limited only by the approximations of skull geometry and conductivities, the "inverse problem," has multiple mathematically valid solutions as was pointed out by Helmholz[28] more than a century ago. The reason is that a single scalp distribution can be produced by different numbers of dipoles in different combinations of locations and orientations. Thus, various constraints must be applied as to the number of sources allowed and their approximate location to reach a solution. Sometimes these constraints are so severe as to specify that the source be a single dipole located somewhere in the brain. For MEG, it is not necessary to consider the conductivities of various layers of tissues between the brain and the scalp because magnetic permeability is unaffected by variations in conductivity. In practice only, the radial component of the field is measured because it is convenient to place pickup coils parallel to the scalp (reviewed in Kaufman et al[29]).

The power of dipole modeling has been demonstrated by using it to map the sensory projections to the human cortex of different pitched tones. Using MEG ERFs coordinated with MRI scan data, Pantev et al[30] located dipoles ordered in depth according to pitch (ie, tonotopic) just below the surface of the transverse temporal gyrus (Heschl's gyrus), the assumed location of the primary auditory cortex. Verkindt et al[31] were able to show similar tone pitch results for dipoles derived from ERPs.

WHAT IS THE PLACE OF ERPs AMONG OTHER METHODS OF ASSESSING BRAIN FUNCTION?

Other functional imaging methods include positron emission tomography (PET) and functional MRI (fMRI). Together with ERPs, ERFs and structural MRI, these methods provide different advantages and disadvantages that ensure a place for each in the next decade of human brain research. Magnetic resonance imaging has the best spatial resolution, but it provides only structural information and will most likely only reflect relatively enduring cognitive and psychological abnormalities. Event-related potential and ERF spatial localization is comparable to oxygen 15–labeled PET resolution (6 to 100 mm), but both ERPs and ERFs have advantages over PET in terms of temporal resolution: the sample time of ^{15}O PET is 45 to 60 seconds in contrast to the millisecond resolution of the EEG and MEG. Functional MRI reflects transient changes in blood flow or blood oxygen saturation with a resolution on the order of seconds rather than milliseconds. However, important neural events that can be picked up electrically or magnetically may not be concentrated enough to increase blood flow regionally.[32]

Thus, ERPs have a dual role in psychophysiological research of psychiatric disorders. They can be used to examine mental chronometry and cognitive resource allocation and they can be used to specify where in the brain psychophysiologically relevant activity occurs. Structural brain images with MRI become the first-order observation and functional brain images with PET, fMRI, ERP, and ERF are the second, offering information about neurochemical, blood flow or oxygen saturation, electrical physiology, and magnetic physiology, respectively. Each approach has a different sensitivity as well as temporal and spatial resolution. The primary advantage of ERPs and ERFs is their fine temporal resolution, which is fast enough to capture multiple, sequential stages of human sensory and cognitive phenomena. The future use of combinations of the functional methods (each with its special attributes) superimposed on high-resolution structural brain images will serve to validate and extend the information gained by each singly.

Adolf Pfefferbaum, MD
Walton T. Roth, MD
Judith M. Ford, PhD
Psychiatry Service (116A)
Department of Veterans Affairs Medical Center
3801 Miranda Ave
Palo Alto, CA 94304

Supported by the National Institutes of Health (grants MH30854, MH40052, and AA05965), Bethesda, Md, and the Department of Veterans Affairs.

Reprint requests to Dr Pfefferbaum.

REFERENCES

1. O'Donnell BF, Faux SF, McCarley RW, Kimble MO, Salisbury DF, Nestor PG, Kikinis R, Jolesz FA, Shenton ME. Increased rate of P300 latency prolongation with age in schizophrenia: electrophysiological evidence for a neurodegenerative process. *Arch Gen Psychiatry.* 1995;52:544-549.
2. Javitt DC, Doneshka P, Grochowski S, Ritter W. Impaired mismatch negativity generation reflects widespread dysfunction of working memory in schizophrenia. *Arch Gen Psychiatry.* 1995;52:550-558.
3. Gratton G, Coles MGH, Donchin E. A new method for off-line removal of ocular artifact. *Electroencephalogr Clin Neurophysiol.* 1983;55:468-484.
4. Miller GA, Gratton G, Yee CM. Generalized implementation of an eye movement correction procedure. *Psychophysiology.* 1988;25:241-243.
5. Ford JM, Roth WT, Kopell BS. Attention effects on auditory evoked potentials to infrequent events. *Biol Psychol.* 1976;4:65-77.
6. Butler RA. Effect of changes in stimulus frequency and intensity on habituation of the human vertex potential. *J Acoust Soc Am.* 1968;44:945-950.
7. Hillyard SA, Hink R, Schwent VL, Picton TW. Electrical signs of selective attention in the human brain. *Science.* 1973;182:177-180.
8. Näatanen R, Paavilainen P, Tiitinen H, Jiang D, Alho K. Attention and mismatch negativity. *Psychophysiology.* 1993;30:436-450.
9. Johnson R. The amplitude of the P300 component of the event-related potential: review and synthesis. In: Ackles PK, Jennings JR, Coles MGH, eds. *Advances in Psychophysiology.* Greenwich, Conn: JAI Press; 1987;3.
10. Kutas M, McCarthy G, Donchin E. Augmenting mental chronometry: the P300 as a measure of stimulus evaluation time. *Science.* 1977;197:792-795.
11. Pfefferbaum A, Ford J, Johnson R, Wenegrat B, Kopell BS. Manipulation of P3 latency: speed vs accuracy instructions. *Electroencephalogr Clin Neurophysiol.* 1983;55:188-197.
12. Pfefferbaum A, Christensen C, Ford JM, Kopell BS. Apparent response incompatibility effects on P3 latency depend on the task. *Electroencephalogr Clin Neurophysiol.* 1986;64:424-437.
13. Pfefferbaum A, Ford JM, Weller BJ, Kopell BS. ERPs to response production and inhibition. *Electroencephalogr Clin Neurophysiol.* 1985;60:423-434.
14. Shagass C. An electrophysiological view of schizophrenia. *Biol Psychiatry.* 1976;11:3-30.
15. Goodin D, Squires K, Henderson B, Starr A. Age-related variations in evoked potentials to auditory stimuli in normal human subjects. *Electroencephalogr Clin Neurophysiol.* 1978;44:447-458.
16. Pfefferbaum A, Ford J, Wenegrat B, Roth WT, Kopell BS. Clinical application of the P3 component of event-related potentials, I: normal aging. *Electroencephalogr Clin Neurophysiol.* 1984;59:85-103.
17. Picton TW, Stuss DT, Champagne SC, Nelson RF. The effects of age on human event-related potentials. *Psychophysiology.* 1984;21:312-325.
18. Polich J. P3 in the evaluation of aging and dementia. In: Brunia CHM, Mulder G, Verbaten MN, eds. *Event-Related Brain Research.* Amsterdam, the Netherlands: Elsevier Science Publishers; 1991:304-323.
19. Pfefferbaum A, Wenegrat B, Ford J, Roth WT, Kopell BS. Clinical application of the P3 component of event-related potentials, II: dementia, depression and schizophrenia. *Electroencephalogr Clin Neurophysiol.* 1984;59:104-124.
20. Goodin D, Squires K, Starr A. Long latency event-related components of the auditory evoked potential in dementia. *Brain.* 1978;101:635-648.
21. Pfefferbaum A, Ford JM, Kraemer HC. Clinical utility of long latency 'cognitive' event-related potentials (P3): the cons. *Electroencephalogr Clin Neurophysiol.* 1990;76:6-12.
22. Shenton ME, Kikinis R, Jolesz FA, Pollak SD, LeMay M, Wible CG, Hokama H, Martin J, Metcalf D, Coleman M, McCarley RW. Abnormalities of the left temporal lobe and thought disorder in schizophrenia: a quantitative magnetic resonance imaging study. *N Engl J Med.* 1992;327:604-612.
23. Ford JM, Sullivan EV, Marsh L, White PK, Lim KO, Pfefferbaum A. The relationship between P300 amplitude and regional gray matter volumes depends upon the attentional system engaged. *Electroencephalogr Clin Neurophysiol.* 1994;90:214-228.
24. McCarley RW, Shenton ME, O'Donnell BF, Faux SF, Kikinis R, Nestor PG, Jolesz FA. Auditory P300 abnormalities and left posterior superior temporal gyrus volume reduction in schizophrenia. *Arch Gen Psychiatry.* 1993;50:190-197.
25. Zipursky RB, Lim KO, Sullivan EV, Brown BW, Pfefferbaum A. Widespread cerebral gray matter volume deficits in schizophrenia. *Arch Gen Psychiatry.* 1992;49:195-205.
26. Jasper HH. The ten-twenty electrode system of the International Federation. *Electroencephalogr Clin Neurophysiol.* 1957;10:371-375.
27. Wikswo JP, Gevins A, Williamson SJ. The future of the EEG and MEG. *Electroencephalogr Clin Neurophysiol.* 1993;87:1-9.
28. Helmholz H. Über einigen Gesetze der Verteilung elektrischer Ströme in körperlichen Leitern mit Anwendung auf die tierelektrische Versuche. *Ann Phys Chem.* 1853;29:211-233.
29. Kaufman L, Kaufman JH, Wang JZ. On cortical folds and neuromagnetic fields. *Electroencephalogr Clin Neurophysiol.* 1991;79:211-226.
30. Pantev C, Hoke M, Lehnertz K, Lutkenhoner B, Fahrendorf G, Stober U. Identification of sources of brain neuronal activity with high spatiotemporal resolution through combination of neuromagnetic source localization (NMSL) and magnetic resonance imaging (MRI). *Electroencephalogr Clin Neurophysiol.* 1990;75:173-184.
31. Verkindt C, Bertrand O, Perrin F, Echallier J-F, Pernier J. Tonotopic organization of the human auditory cortex: N100 topography and multiple dipole model analysis. *Electroencephalogr Clin Neurophysiol.* 1995;96:143-156.
32. Eulitz C, Elbert T, Bartenstein P, Weiller C, Muller SP, Pantev C. Comparison of magnetic and metabolic brain activity during a verb generation task. *Neuroreport.* 1994;6:97-100.

ORIGINAL ARTICLE

Specificity in Familial Aggregation of Phobic Disorders

Abby J. Fyer, MD; Salvatore Mannuzza, PhD; Tim F. Chapman, PhD; Lynn Y. Martin, RNCS; Donald F. Klein, MD

Background: To investigate whether each of three *DSM-III-R* phobic disorders (simple phobia, social phobia, and agoraphobia with panic attacks) is familial and "breeds true."

Design: Rates of each phobic disorder were contrasted in first-degree relatives of four proband groups: simple phobia, social phobia, agoraphobia with panic attacks, and not ill controls. Phobia probands were patients who had one of the phobia diagnoses but no other lifetime anxiety comorbidity.

Results: We found moderate (two- to fourfold increased risk) but specific familial aggregation of each of the three *DSM-III-R* phobic disorders.

Conclusions: These results support a specific familial contribution to each of the three phobia types. However, conclusions are limited to cases occurring without lifetime anxiety comorbidity and do not imply homogeneity within categories.

(Arch Gen Psychiatry. 1995;52:564-573)

From the Department of Psychiatry, Columbia University College of Physicians and Surgeons (Drs Fyer, Mannuzza, and Klein), and the Department of Therapeutics at New York State Psychiatric Institute (Drs Fyer, Mannuzza, Chapman, and Klein and Ms Martin), New York, NY.

THE *DSM-III* (1980)[1] and *DSM-III-R* (1987)[2] classification of phobic disorders departs from earlier systems (*ICD-9*,[3] *DSM-II*[4]) by subdividing the unitary phobic neurosis category into four disorders: agoraphobia with and without panic attacks, simple phobia, and social phobia. Although these changes stimulated empirical research, their etiologic validity remains uncertain.

Despite common features of irrational fear and avoidance, simple, social, and agoraphobia differ with regard to age at onset, sex, range and type of phobic stimuli, association with spontaneous panic attacks, and response to treatment.[5,6] However, recent studies also indicate both considerable heterogeneity within categories and a significant number of cases that exhibit symptoms of more than one phobic disorder but fit neatly into none. More importantly, there is far greater than expected comorbidity among anxiety disorders in both clinical and epidemiologic populations.[7-11] Taken together these observations suggest a more complex relationship between clinical presentation and etiology than is implied by either discrete categorical or unitary (ie, one common underlying process despite differing manifest symptomatic and developmental pictures) theories of anxiety.

Family studies can address this question. A first step is to determine if each of the phobia types "breeds true." If simple phobia, social phobia, and agoraphobia were the same familial illness in different manifestations, then one would not expect true breeding but simply an enhanced familial propensity for any phobia. To test for true breeding, that is, distinct separable syndromes, we would have to show that proband diagnosis A is associated with increased familial risk for A but not for B or C. Further, proband diagnosis of B would be associated with increased familial risk for B but not for A or C, and so on.

Family studies can challenge categorical distinctions when a particular proband diagnosis increases familial risk for another category. For example, if proband diagnosis A is associated with increased familial risk for A, B, and C, it would imply either a shared etiologic diathesis (eg, general phobia proneness or neurotic syndrome) or the existence of "phenocopies" (ie, disorders that are clinically similar but causally distinct).

As previously noted,[12-14] this type of interpretation of family study data depends on

See Subjects and Methods on next page

SUBJECTS AND METHODS

SUBJECTS

Subjects came from a family study of anxiety disorders conducted at the Anxiety Disorders Clinic of the Columbia College of Physicians and Surgeons/New York State Psychiatric Institute, New York.

Social phobia and panic disorder with agoraphobia (panic-agoraphobia) probands were recruited from the treatment and biological research programs of this clinic. All patients entering these studies between 1983 and 1988 and the last 6 months of 1989 who met *DSM-III-R* (1985)[18] criteria for social phobia, agoraphobia, or panic disorder with or without agoraphobia; were of European descent; English speaking; and had at least one living first-degree relative were asked to participate in the family study.

Simple phobia probands were recruited from among participants in treatment studies at the Phobia Clinic at the Long Island Jewish Medical Center (LIJMC) between 1973 and 1978.[19,20] A detailed description of this sample is given elsewhere.[15] Briefly, a letter requesting participation in the family study was sent by one of us (D.F.K.) to all located LIJMC treatment study subjects who had originally met criteria for specific phobias. Consenting subjects who on reinterview met both 1985 *DSM-III-R* simple phobia and family study entry criteria (European descent, one living first-degree relative) were asked to participate.

Not ill control probands were individuals with neither past nor current history of any *DSM-III-R* or Research Diagnostic Criteria[21] diagnoses who were recruited using a modification of the National Institute of Mental Health Collaborative Study of Psychobiology of Depression Acquaintance method.[22,23] A randomly chosen acquaintance from the list given by each participating relative was blindly interviewed using the Schedule for Affective Disorders and Schizophrenia–Lifetime Anxiety Version (SADS-LA).[24,25] Those acquaintances with no lifetime psychiatric diagnosis, who were also of European descent and had one living first-degree relative, were asked to participate as NIC probands in the family study. Informed consent was obtained from all participating subjects following an explanation of study procedures.

INTERVIEW AND BEST-ESTIMATE PROCEDURES

Interview Procedures

Proband data are from direct interview of subjects using the semistructured SADS-LA interview schedule. Proband interviews were conducted by one of three specially trained senior clinicians who were not blind to the proband's participation in the clinic program. Narrative case histories and interview forms were reviewed (blind to relative diagnosis) for diagnostic consistency and completeness by the principal investigator (phobia probands) (A.J.F.) or a co-investigator (control probands) (S.M.).

Diagnoses of relatives were derived from a best-estimate procedure that combines both direct interview and family informant reports on each subject. Only relatives for whom direct interview data were available were included in this report.

Direct interviews of acquaintances and relatives of both patients and controls were conducted using the SADS-LA by trained clinician raters who were blind to proband diagnosis status (see "Assessment of Blind vs Blind-Broken Interview Status" below).

Family informant data were collected using the Family Informant Schedule and Criteria.[26] Probands were asked to provide data about all first-degree relatives. Relatives were requested to provide information about all first-degree relatives except the proband.

Best-Estimate Procedure

Best-estimate ratings were made for all major *DSM-III-R* anxiety, mood, substance use, and psychotic disorders as well as a variety of subthreshold anxiety symptoms (irrational fears, isolated panic attacks, compulsions, etc) at definite, probable, and possible levels. The cases reported here met either probable or definite best-estimate criteria.

The best-estimate diagnoses are consensus ratings derived as follows. All case materials (direct interview narrative, SADS-LA, and family informant) on each directly interviewed relative were independently reviewed by two specially trained senior clinician "best-estimate" raters who were blind to both patient vs control status and anxiety diagnosis status of the proband through whom the relative was connected to the study. Each rater completed a "best-estimate diagnosis" form. After this, the two met to arrive at a consensus best-estimate rating for each 1987 *DSM-III-R* and subthreshold diagnosis. If consensus could not be reached, the case was submitted to a senior investigator (D.F.K.) for final assessment.

A review conducted after completion of these first two thirds of the subjects indicated that there were no between-rater disagreements on best-estimate diagnoses of those subjects for whom the case materials contained no evidence of psychiatric symptomatology. Therefore, for the remaining subjects, if there was no direct interview SADS-LA symptom or diagnosis rating, packets were first sent to a single best-estimate rater. If this first rater considered the subject to have a best-estimate diagnosis of any symptomatology (disorder or subthreshold), the case was sent to a second rater for independent review, followed by the usual consensus procedure. If, however, the first rater arrived at a best-estimate diagnosis of no disorder or symptoms, the case was considered complete at that point.

DIAGNOSTIC CRITERIA

Direct interview diagnoses were based on the 1985 *DSM-III-R* in progress.[18] Best-estimate diagnoses were made using the 1987 *DSM-III-R*.[2] For the disorders discussed in this report, the only diagnostically significant difference between the 1985 and 1987 criteria sets concerns the classification of avoidance in panic disorder. The 1985 *DSM-III-R* delineates three types of panic disorder with respect to avoidance: uncomplicated (with no avoidance), with extensive avoidance (with agoraphobia), and limited avoidance (with some avoidance but does not meet criteria for extensive type). In contrast, the 1987 *DSM-III-R* defines two categories: panic disorder with (any degree of avoidance) and without (no avoidance) agoraphobia. To facilitate comparison with other studies, we reclassified our subjects using the 1987 categories as follows: subjects classified as having uncomplicated panic disorder by the 1985 system are considered to have panic disorder without agoraphobia and

Continued on next page

those with limited avoidance panic disorder or extensive avoidance panic disorder are grouped under panic disorder with agoraphobia.

ASSESSMENT OF BLIND VS BLIND-BROKEN INTERVIEW STATUS

The current study was designed so that raters who conducted the diagnostic interviews of the relatives and controls were initially blind to group status (ie, whether an interviewee was a relative of an anxiety proband vs a relative of an NIC proband vs an acquaintance).

However, previous experience indicated that despite considerable rater efforts to the contrary, subjects did on occasion "break the blind" during interviews.[27] To evaluate the possible effects of this on observed patterns of familial psychopathology, two items that ask the rater to indicate whether or not the blind was broken during the interview were included in the SADS-LA: (1) Did the subject indicate that he or she had a relative in treatment at the Anxiety Clinic? (2) Did the subject say anything to indicate the diagnosis of the relative who is in treatment?

On the basis of the response to the first question, each relative interview was subsequently classified as "blind" or "blind broken."

Interviews of relatives of NIC acquaintance probands could not be classified since the complementary question (ie, Did the subject indicate that he or she was recruited into the study through an acquaintance?) was not included in the schedule.

DATA ANALYSIS

Demographic Variables

Chi-square tests were used to assess possible differences in dichotomous variables among the four groups of relatives (eg, gender, interview compliance). A 2×4 χ^2 test was used initially. If this test indicated significant differences ($P<.10$, two tailed), individual pairwise tests (comparing each group with all of the other three groups) were undertaken. Differences among the four groups in continuous variables (eg, age at interview) were analyzed with pairwise Student's *t* tests. To minimize the likelihood of type II error in all planned comparisons, two-tailed *P* values to the $P<.10$ level are reported. In cases of small cell size (less than five), we report statistics for Fisher's exact test.

Familial Prevalence

Familial contrasts implying specificity of transmission involve a priori directional hypotheses of increased aggregation. However, the remaining familial contrasts are null rather than directional. To facilitate exposition, two-tailed *P* values to $P\leq.10$ are reported for all familial contrasts, rather than a mix of one- and two-tailed tests.

Proportional hazards analyses[28] were used to test the hypotheses of familiality and distinctness. To test if each phobic disorder is familial, we calculated the relative risk (RR) for the proband's phobia in relatives of each phobia proband group vs relatives of NIC (Table 1, question A).

The contrasts needed to test the hypothesis of specificity of transmission are listed in Table 1, questions B and C. The proportional hazards model was used to calculate RRs for each of these contrasts.

In each of the proportional hazards analyses, survival time for each relative was defined as age at onset of disorder (ie, the specific disorder whose prevalence was being compared) or age at interview for individuals who do not have the specific disorder (ie, censored cases). Proband disorder status was treated as a dichotomous covariate (risk factor) in all the models. Age and sex of relatives were controlled for by using each as a covariate in each of the proportional hazards analyses.

To assess the effect of the blind having been broken during the direct interview on familial prevalence, two dummy variables describing potential blind-broken status were included in all the proportional hazards analyses. The first variable was scored as positive only if the subject revealed to the interviewer that a relative (ie, the proband) was in treatment at the anxiety clinic, but did not indicate the relative's specific diagnosis; the second was scored as positive only if the subject also revealed the proband's diagnosis.

Another way in which we approached the question of specificity was to investigate how concordant proband and relative diagnoses were with regard to each of the three phobias considered. Concordance between proband phobia and single anxiety cases of the same phobia in relatives was assessed using the κ coefficient. The κ statistic is a chance-corrected measure of agreement that is used in measuring interrater reliability and that can readily be generalized to multicategory nominally scaled data.[29,30] In a 3×3 array (relating proband to relative diagnosis), the hypothesis of specific familial transmission is tested by an unweighted κ for agreement, across all three phobic diagnoses. Because of the as yet unexplored possibility of syndromal complexity,[31] comorbid cases (eg, an individual with a lifetime diagnosis of both social and simple phobia) were classified as disagreements.

For completeness, familial aggregation was examined in two additional ways. Unadjusted rates of each phobic disorder in relatives of each proband group were contrasted with rates in relatives of controls using a 2×2 χ^2 test (or Fisher's exact test for contrasts with cell sizes of less than five). The same set of contrasts was done using the family as the unit of analysis, ie, contrasting the proportion of families with at least one member affected by the diagnosis under study. This latter method is an approximate adjustment for family size. In both analyses, two-tailed *P* values to the $P<.10$ level are reported.

An additional more rigorous test of specificity was used in one case in which there was a trend suggesting the possibility of shared familial vulnerability between simple and social phobia (ie, relatives of probands with one phobia showed a trend toward increased risk for another).[32] In this test, the relatives of each of the two phobia proband groups and the NIC probands were considered to be three independent multinomial samples. Members of each sample were classified as simple phobic only, social phobic only, doubly phobic, or doubly negative. Two null hypotheses were tested: (1) the proportion of simple phobics (whether doubly phobic or not) is the same among the relatives of social phobics and controls and (2) the proportion of social phobics (whether doubly phobic or not) is the same among the relatives of simple phobic controls. The covariance matrix of these two differences was estimated assuming the null hypotheses and assuming the proportion of doubly phobic relatives is the same in all three groups. Where d is the column vector of observed differences in proportions and S is the estimates covariance matrix of d, $d'S^{-1}d$ is distributed as χ^2.

Table 1. Predictions of Hypothesis of Specific Familial Aggregation: Prevalence of Phobic Disorders in Relatives of Simple, Social, and Panic Disorder With Agoraphobia Probands

	Diagnosis Assessed in Relatives		
Questions	Simple Phobia	Social Phobia	Panic With Agoraphobia
A. Is there familial aggregation?	SIP>NIC	SOCP>NIC	PDA>NIC
B. Is familial loading specific to proband diagnosis?	SOCP=NIC PDA=NIC (SOCP+PDA)=NIC	SIP=NIC PDA=NIC (SIP+PDA)=NIC	SOCP=NIC SIP=NIC (SOCP+SIP)=NIC
C. Does familial loading for proband's phobic disorder distinguish relatives of each phobia proband group from relatives of the other two?	SIP>SOCP SIP>PDA	SOCP>PDA SOCP>SIP	PDA>SOCP PDA>SIP

**SIP indicates simple phobia; SOCP, social phobia; PDA, panic disorder with agoraphobia; and NIC, not ill controls.*

appropriate diagnostic restrictions in proband groups. For example, to examine whether proband diagnosis A increases familial risk for B or C, we must use *only* probands who have A but not B or C. Therefore, in this study we have restricted our probands to individuals who have one of the three phobic disorders (simple, social, or agoraphobia) but no other lifetime phobic or anxiety diagnosis. For ease of exposition we will refer to these as "single anxiety cases" of each disorder. The effects of proband comorbidity on familial transmission will be reported later.

Our previous data from direct interview of relatives of single anxiety case simple and social phobia probands indicate moderate, yet specific familial aggregation.[15,16] The current report extends this earlier work by adding a third phobic disorder (panic disorder with agoraphobia), enlarging our social phobia sample, and using best-estimate (all sources of information) rather than direct interview diagnoses.

Best-estimate diagnosis and the blinding of relative interviewers to proband diagnosis are two widely used strategies developed to minimize bias and halo effect in family study data. However, each may introduce its own difficulties, which are also examined.

There are no major differences between the *DSM-IV*[17] specific (simple) and social phobia criteria and the *DSM-III-R* criteria for these disorders that were used in this study. The *DSM-IV* criteria for panic disorder with agoraphobia require recurrent unexpected panic attacks as well as 1 month of panic-related worry or behavioral change. The *DSM-III-R* required either four attacks in 4 weeks *or* one attack followed by 1 month of worry about the next attack.

HYPOTHESES

If each of the three phobic disorders (simple, social, and panic with agoraphobia) is familial and breeds true, then familial loading will be specific to proband diagnosis. That is, a proband diagnosis of one type of phobia will be associated with increased familial risk for the proband's phobia but *not* for either of the other types of phobia.

This hypothesis can be tested by comparing familial loading for each disorder in relatives of each of the phobia proband groups and controls. These comparisons and predicted outcomes (consistent with our hypothesis) are presented in equation form in **Table 1**. Our hypothesis of specificity of familial aggregation can be broken down into three component questions (or predictions). For ease of exposition, Table 1 and the "Results" section below are organized in terms of these three questions.

For example, if simple phobia is familial and distinct from social phobia and agoraphobia, then relatives of simple phobia probands will have significantly increased rates of simple phobia but not social phobia or agoraphobia as compared to both relatives of not ill controls (NIC) and social phobia and agoraphobia probands. Relatives of simple phobia probands will also have a significantly increased rate of simple phobia as compared to the combined relatives of both the social and agoraphobia probands.

This last strategy (combining relatives of the two "other" patient proband groups) is useful since the increased power acquired through the larger combined sample size may reveal relationships missed by smaller separate group contrasts. The separate group contrasts do allow for the possibility that a particular diagnosis may occur in the relatives of one but not the other of the two phobia contrast groups. Using only combined groups might obscure such specific findings. Therefore, we do both analyses. The same hypotheses follow in parallel, respectively, for social phobia and panic disorder with agoraphobia.

RESULTS

PROBANDS

One hundred thirteen probands who entered the Anxiety Family Study through the Anxiety Disorders Clinic of the Columbia College of Physicians and Surgeons/New York State Psychiatric Institute met criteria for panic-agoraphobia. Of these, 49 (43%) had panic-agaoraphobia but no additional lifetime anxiety disorder diagnosis (ie, single anxiety case panic-agoraphobia probands) and 64 (57%) had at least one additional anxiety disorder.

Table 2. Demographic Characteristics of Probands and First-Degree Relatives and Compliance of Relatives by Proband Diagnosis

	Proband Diagnosis*			
	Simple Phobia	Social Phobia	Panic With Agoraphobia	Not Ill Controls
Probands, No.	15	39	49	77
Mean age, y (±SD)	48 (8)[ab]	33 (8)[b]	35 (10)[a]	42 (17)[ab]
Sex, % female	87[ce]	38[ef]	76[df]	55[cd]
Total Relatives, No.	**79**	**178**	**195**	**380**
All living relatives, No.	62	160	164	309
Interviewed, No.	49	105	131	231
Mean age, y (±SD)	41 (21)	43 (16)	46 (18)	46 (17)
Sex, % female	53	60[g]	59[h]	54
Uninterviewed,† No.	13	55	33	78
Mean age, y (±SD)	47 (22)	44 (20)	45 (18)	49 (19)
Sex, % female	46	42[g]	39[h]	44
Compliance of Relatives, %				
Interviewed/total	62	59	67	61
Interviewed/living	79	66	80	75

*Proband groups are mutually exclusive. Phobia probands had no additional lifetime anxiety diagnoses. Age and sex items with same superscript (a, b, c, etc) differ from each other in two-way χ^2 at P<.10 level. The 2×4 χ^2 contrasting proband age and sex across diagnostic groups were significant at P<.05. All P values are two tailed.

†Includes only living uninterviewed relatives.

Social phobia as a lifetime diagnosis was found in 90 of the entering probands. Thirty-nine (43%) of these probands were single anxiety cases of social phobia, 50 (56%) had comorbid anxiety diagnoses, and one (1%) had social phobia and recurrent spontaneous panic attacks.

Thirty-four of 70 patients with specific phobia who participated in the LIJMC treatment studies during the 1970s were located and consented to participate in the family study. Of these 34, 30 met *DSM-III-R* (1985) simple phobia criteria and were eligible. Fifteen (50%) of the 30 were single anxiety cases of simple phobia.

Of 133 not ill acquaintances evaluated to date, 52 (39%) refused to participate, four (3%) were ineligible, and 77 (58%) entered the study as NIC probands.

Several significant age and sex differences were found among the phobia and NIC proband groups (**Table 2**). The panic-agoraphobia and social phobia probands, who were enrolled from the clinic treatment-seeking population, were both significantly younger than the simple phobia probands who had been recruited through 10-year follow-up of previously treated LIJMC subjects. The NIC group, derived from an acquaintance sample that was originally age matched to relatives of patient probands was midway between, ie, they were significantly older than the social phobia and agoraphobia probands and younger than the simple phobia probands. In addition, paralleling previous experience in treated samples,[5,19,20,33] agoraphobia and simple phobia probands were more likely and social phobia probands less likely to be female than the NIC group (Table 2).

RELATIVES

Direct interview data were obtained from 62% (516/832) of the total (living and dead) or 74% (516/695) of living first-degree relatives of the combined proband group (Table 2). There were no significant age or sex differences between the interviewed relatives of the four proband diagnostic groups.

For each proband diagnostic group, a higher proportion of potential female interviewees (ie, living female relatives) were actually interviewed than potential male interviewees. However, this difference reached significance only in relatives of the social phobia and agoraphobia probands (Table 2). No significant age differences were found between interviewed and uninterviewed living relatives.

Raters indicated that the blind was broken in 18% (50/285) of the interviews of relatives of phobia probands. In 18 (6%) cases the interviewee revealed the proband's specific anxiety diagnosis. In the remaining 32 cases (11%), the proband's patient status but not the type of anxiety disorder was revealed. Only the 18 blind-broken cases in which the specific anxiety diagnosis was revealed would be expected to systematically affect our hypothesis of specificity in familial aggregation. However, to be conservative, the effect of each type of blind breaking was separately assessed in the proportional hazards analyses described below (see "Effects of Blind Breaking on Outcome").

Statistically significant differences were not found in contrasts of age and sex for blind vs blind-broken relatives of each proband diagnostic group.

PHOBIC DISORDER IN RELATIVES

The unadjusted lifetime rates (percent) of each of the three phobic disorders in interviewed relatives of phobia and NIC proband groups are presented in **Table 3**.

Table 4, A through C, presents the proportional hazards analyses testing the hypothesis of specific familial aggregation of each of the three phobic disorders. Table

Table 3. Unadjusted Rates of Phobic Disorders Among Directly Interviewed First-Degree Relatives of Phobic Disorder Probands

	Proband Groups			
	Simple Phobia	Social Phobia	Panic With Agoraphobia	Not Ill Controls
Diagnosis in Relatives,* %				
Simple phobia	31†	13	10	9
Social phobia	10	15‡	8	6
Panic with agoraphobia§	0	2	10‡	3
Agoraphobia without panic	0	1	2	1
Not ill‖	39¶	34†	40†	58
(No. of probands)	(15)	(39)	(49)	(77)
(No. of relatives)	(49)	(105)	(131)	(231)

**Best-estimate diagnoses,* DSM-III-R *criteria, includes both definite and probable cases.*
†*P*≤*.001; two tailed for 2×2* χ^2 *contrast to rates in relatives of not ill controls.*
‡*P*≤*.01; two tailed for 2×2* χ^2 *contrast to rates in relatives of not ill controls.*
§DSM-III-R *panic disorder with agoraphobia.*
‖*No lifetime diagnosis of psychosis, alcohol or drug abuse, major depression, bipolar disorder, bulimia, anorexia, somatization disorder, or any* DSM-III-R *anxiety disorder.*
¶*P*≤*.05; two tailed for 2×2* χ^2 *contrast to rates in relatives of not ill controls.*

4 is organized in terms of our three predictions or questions (see the "Hypotheses" section) necessary to test the study hypothesis. The first column on the left in Table 4 lists the diagnosis in relatives for which risk is being assessed (eg, simple phobia in the first row). The headings indicate the three questions. For each question, the "Predicted Outcome" column indicates the results predicted by the hypothesis of specific familial aggregation when the risk for the "assessed diagnosis" is compared between the relatives of the listed proband groups. The actual results of these contrasts in this sample are given in the right-hand column ("Observed Outcome").

Table 5 presents the proportion of families of each phobia proband group in which at least one member was affected with each of the phobic disorders.

IS THERE FAMILIAL AGGREGATION OF PHOBIC DISORDERS?

Moderate but statistically significant familial aggregation was found for all three phobic disorders (Table 4, A). Relatives of each phobia proband group had a significantly increased risk for the proband's particular phobia as compared to relatives of NIC probands. The magnitude of the increased risk varied somewhat by disorder: fourfold in the case of simple phobia, threefold in the case of panic-agoraphobia, and only twofold for social phobia.

A similar pattern is seen for simple phobia and panic with agoraphobia using the family as the unit of analysis (Table 5). However, in the case of social phobia, although there is a higher rate of affected families among social phobia probands, the difference (Fisher's exact test, *P*=.244) does not reach significance.

IS FAMILIAL LOADING SPECIFIC TO PROBAND PHOBIA DIAGNOSIS?

Familial aggregation of panic-agoraphobia occurred only in relatives of panic-agoraphobia probands (Table 4, B). The rates of panic-agoraphobia in relatives of the social and simple phobia probands groups did not differ from those in the relatives of NIC probands. A similar pattern was seen for social phobia. The rates of social phobia in relatives of simple phobia and panic-agoraphobia probands taken separately or combined did not differ significantly from those in relatives of NIC probands (Table 4, B).

The rate of simple phobia in the relatives of panic-agoraphobia probands did not differ significantly from that in the relatives of NIC probands. Combining the relatives of the panic-agoraphobia and social phobia probands did not change the results. However, a weak trend (RR=1.8, *P*=.109 (Table 4) toward an increased rate of simple phobia was found in the relatives of social phobia probands when this group was considered separately compared with relatives of NIC probands. Given this trend and the slight (though nonsignificant *P*=.4) elevation in the rate of social phobia in relatives of simple phobics (Table 4, B), a second analysis was conducted to more rigorously test the possibility of shared familial vulnerability between these disorders (simple and social phobia). When this method (see "Familial Prevalence" in the "Subjects and Methods" section) is applied to our data, the univariate χ^2 values were 0.81 and 1.73 in relatives of social phobia and simple phobia probands, respectively. The joint test led to a χ^2 of 2.54. None of these tests reached statistical significance.

Also consistent with specificity of aggregation was the significant 3×3 unweighted κ (0.34, *P*=.01) for exact concordance between single-case phobia diagnoses in probands and relatives.

DOES FAMILIAL LOADING FOR THE PROBAND'S PHOBIA DISTINGUISH RELATIVES OF EACH PHOBIC DISORDER PROBAND GROUP FROM THE OTHER TWO?

Relatives of each of the three phobic disorder proband groups had higher rates of the proband's phobic disorder than did relatives of the other phobia probands (Table 4, C). In all but one of these contrasts this dif-

Table 4. Prevalence of Phobic Disorders in Relatives of Simple Phobia, Social Phobia, and Panic With Agoraphobia Probands: Comparison of Observed Outcome to Predictions of Hypothesis of Specific Familial Aggregation*

	A. Familial Aggregation?			B. Is Familial Loading Specific to Proband Diagnosis?		
		Observed Outcome			Observed Outcome	
Diagnosis in Relatives	Predicted Outcome	Relative Risk	95% Confidence Interval	Predicted Outcome	Relative Risk	95% Confidence Interval
Simple phobia	SIP>NIC	3.9†	1.8-8.1	SOCP=NIC	1.8	0.9-3.6
				PDA=NIC	1.1	0.5-2.3
				(SOCP+PDA)=NIC	1.4	0.8-2.5
Social phobia	SOCP>NIC	2.4‡	1.2-5.0	SIP=NIC	1.6	0.6-4.4
				PDA=NIC	0.7	0.2-1.8
				(SIP+PDA)=NIC	0.9	0.4-2.1
Panic with agoraphobia	PDA>NIC	3.0‡	1.0-8.7	SOCP=NIC	0.9	0.2-4.3
				SIP=NIC	§	
				(SOCP+SIP)=NIC	0.6	0.1-2.8

(continued)

Table 4. Prevalence of Phobic Disorders in Relatives of Simple Phobia, Social Phobia, and Panic With Agoraphobia Probands: Comparison of Observed Outcome to Predictions of Hypothesis of Specific Familial Aggregation* (cont)

	C. Does Familial Loading for the Proband's Phobic Disorder Distinguish Relatives of Each Phobia Proband Group From Relatives of the Other Two?		
		Observed Outcome	
Diagnosis in Relatives	Predicted Outcome	Relative Risk	95% Confidence Interval
Simple phobia	SIP>SOCP	2.8‖	1.3-5.7
	SIP>PDA	4.2†	2.0-9.1
Social phobia	SOCP>PDA	2.3‡	1.0-5.1
	SOCP>SIP	2.1	0.7-5.8
Panic with agoraphobia	PDA>SOCP	5.3‡	1.2-23.8
	PDA>SIP	¶	

**SIP indicates simple phobia; SOCP, social phobia; PDA, panic disorder with agoraphobia; and NIC, not ill controls. Each row gives the predicted and observed relative frequencies of the "diagnosis assessed in relatives" in the two listed proband groups; eg, in the first row the equation SIP>NIC indicates that the rate of SIP is expected to be greater in relatives of SIP probands vs relatives of NIC and 3.9 is the observed relative risk for simple phobia in relatives of simple phobia probands compared with relatives of NIC in this sample. The relative risks are derived from proportional hazards analyses controlling for age, sex, and blind-vs-"blind broken" status of relatives.*

†$P \leq .001$, two tailed.

‡$P \leq .05$, two tailed.

§*There were no cases of PDA in relatives of SIP probands; Fisher's exact test, 0% vs 3%,* $P=.60$, *two tailed.*

‖$P \leq .01$, two tailed.

¶*There were no cases of PDA in relatives of SIP probands; Fisher's exact test, 10% vs 0%,* $P=.03$, *two tailed.*

ference reached at least the .05 level of significance. The exception was the comparison of rates of social phobia in relatives of social vs simple phobia probands (*P*=.17).

There were no cases of panic-agoraphobia in relatives of simple phobia probands. Therefore, an RR contrasting the rate of this disorder in relatives of panic-agoraphobia vs simple phobia probands could not be calculated. However, a Fisher's exact test indicated a significantly higher rate of panic-agoraphobia among relatives of the panic-agoraphobia proband group (10% vs 0%; *P*<.03, two tailed).

AGORAPHOBIA WITHOUT PANIC ATTACKS

Only four cases of agoraphobia without panic attacks were found among the 516 interviewed relatives. Two occurred in relatives of panic-agoraphobia probands, one in a relative of a social phobia proband, and the fourth in an NIC relative (Table 3).

Table 5. Familial Prevalence of Phobic Disorders Using the Family as the Unit of Analysis

	Proband Groups			
	Simple Phobia	Social Phobia	Panic With Agoraphobia	Not Ill Controls
Affected families,* %				
Simple phobia	73†	26	20	22
Social phobia	20	31	20	19
Panic with agoraphobia	0	5	23‡	6
(No. of families)	(15)	(39)	(49)	(77)

*Percentage of families with at least one relative with the diagnosis.
†$P \leq .001$, two tailed from χ^2 (2×2) comparing rates in families of simple phobia probands to rates in not ill control families.
‡$P \leq .005$, two tailed from χ^2 (2×2) comparing rates in families of panic-agoraphobia probands to rates in not ill control families.

COMORBIDITY OF PHOBIC DISORDERS AMONG RELATIVES

For each of the three types of phobic disorder, the majority of "familial" cases occurred without lifetime comorbidity for other phobias or anxiety disorders. Thirteen of the 15 cases of simple phobia in relatives of simple phobia probands were without anxiety comorbidity. For social phobia and panic-agoraphobia, these figures were 14 of 16 and 10 of 13, respectively.

These rates of anxiety comorbidity in familial cases are not inconsistent with those expected from chance co-occurrence calculated from base rates of each of the phobic disorders in this population. However, the number of cases is too small for meaningful statistical estimates.

To further investigate this issue, the proportional hazards analyses presented in Table 4 were redone to assess the familial prevalence of single anxiety cases of phobic disorders in relatives. For example, in this reanalysis a relative with simple phobia and no other lifetime phobia diagnosis would be counted as a case of simple phobia; a relative with both simple and social phobia would not. As expected, given the small number of comorbid phobia cases in relatives, the results of this reanalysis did not differ from those in Table 4, thus reaffirming specificity of familiality.

EFFECTS OF BLIND BREAKING ON OUTCOME

The more restrictive blind-broken covariate (ie, whether the interviewee revealed his or her relative's specific diagnosis) had no significant effect on diagnostic status in any of the proportional hazards analyses shown in Table 4, A through C. A significant effect for the broader blind-broken covariate (ie, the interviewee revealed the relative's clinic treatment status, but did not indicate diagnosis) was found in three of the proportional hazards models. One of these reflected the fact that relatives of panic-agoraphobia probands with whom the blind was broken were more likely to receive a social phobia diagnosis than those with whom the blind was maintained. The other two reflected that simple phobia was more likely to be diagnosed in "blind-broken" relatives of both panic-agoraphobia and simple phobia probands.

These differences indicate some potential associations between proband diagnosis and magnitude of familial aggregation, but did not alter our basic findings or lead to any substantive change in our conclusions. A more detailed discussion will be presented in a future article.

CONTRAST OF DIRECT INTERVIEW AND BEST-ESTIMATE OUTCOMES

The major substantive findings in the direct interview and best-estimate data sets were also similar, both indicating moderate but specific familial aggregation of each phobia. However, two differences may merit further investigation.

The magnitude of familial aggregation of panic-agoraphobia was higher in the best-estimate (Table 4, A) than in direct interview data (RR=2.6; P=.05, two tailed). There was also some variation between the data sets in the rates of simple phobia in relatives of "nonsimple phobia" phobia probands. In the direct interview data, there was a trend for simple phobia to aggregate in the relatives of panic-agoraphobia (16% vs 9%, RR=1.9, P<.08) but not social phobia probands (as in the best-estimate data, Table 4, B). However, in both data sets the rates of simple phobia in relatives of simple phobia probands were significantly higher than those in the other three relative groups.

COMMENT

These data indicate specific but moderate (two- to fourfold increased risk) familial aggregation of each of three *DSM-III-R* phobic disorders (simple phobia, social phobia, and panic disorder with agoraphobia) in families of probands who have each of these disorders but no other lifetime anxiety disorder comorbidity (ie, single anxiety cases). Also supporting specificity is the finding that the majority of familial cases of simple phobia, social phobia, and panic-agoraphobia occurred without anxiety comorbidity.

For simple phobia, an insignificant trend was found for aggregation in the relatives of social phobia probands (best-estimate data only) and a weaker trend in relatives of panic-agoraphobia probands (direct interview data only). Attempting to maximize the chances to show nonspecific aggregation by combining the tendency for simple phobics to aggregate in the families of social phobics with the tendency for social phobics to aggregate in the families of simple phobics did not prove significant even at a trend level. Further, the rates of simple phobia in the families of simple phobia probands were consistently and significantly higher than those in the relatives of the other two phobia proband groups. However, as will be discussed below, our finding of specificity in familial aggregation does not necessarily imply transmissional homogeneity within each of the phobia proband groups. We cannot rule out the possibility that a small subset of our simple and social phobia probands have some degree of familial overlap.

IMPLICATIONS FOR CLASSIFICATION OF PHOBIAS

The main objective of this study was to use the family study method to investigate the validity of three *DSM-III-R* phobic disorder categories by seeing if they bred true. Our findings suggest the existence of separable, etiologically discrete syndromes within the group of cases identified by each of the three *DSM-III-R* criteria sets. However, at present, this conclusion must be limited to the subset of clinically identified phobias, which occur without lifetime anxiety disorder comorbidity (ie, single anxiety cases). The extent to which these findings will be applicable to phobias that co-occur with other anxiety disorders requires further study in samples which include both prospectively stratified anxiety comorbid and single anxiety case phobia proband groups.

These data should *not* be interpreted as demonstrating etiologic homogeneity within each phobia group. For example, if two subtypes of simple phobia (blood injury and animal) are both familial but etiologically discrete, then relatives of blood injury phobia probands would be expected to have an increased risk for blood injury but not animal phobias and vice versa. However, this separation would not be evident if analyses were limited to the assessment of rates of "all simple phobias." Unfortunately, our sample size is inadequate for this type of fine-grained exploration of subgroups within the *DSM-III-R* categories.

Family studies do not distinguish between genetic vs environmental contributions. The moderate elevations of familial risk reported here are consistent with any of several "models" of transmission (eg, multifactorial complex, combined common and specific environmental effects, heterogeneous mix of the latter two plus a rare single-locus type).[34-37] However, distinguishing among these will require twin, adoption, epidemiologic, and molecular genetic techniques.

COMPARISON WITH RESULTS OF PREVIOUS FAMILY/TWIN STUDIES OF PHOBIAS

Several family history[38,39] and direct interview[40-42] family studies have compared the risk for phobic disorders among relatives of a single phobia proband group with that among relatives of controls. These data are consistent with ours in that they indicate an increased familial risk for the proband's phobia, but not other phobia types.

We are aware of only one previous report, an epidemiologically based twin study of phobias by Kendler and colleagues,[37] which has used patterns of heritability to address the distinctness and/or interrelationships of these three disorders. Results of the two studies (Kendler et al[37] and ours) are consistent in indicating a heritable contribution to each of the three disorders that does not depend on inclusion of nonimpairing irrational fears. However, in contrast to our study, Kendler et al found evidence of both partial distinctness *and* overlap with respect to the genetic contribution to the etiology of these three disorders. Both "common" (ie, increased liability for *any* phobia) and "specific" genetic factors made substantial contributions to three (agoraphobia, social and situational phobias) of the four studied phobia types. The fourth (animal phobias) evidenced only a common genetic contribution.

Translated into a family study context, this outcome would predict, in contrast to our results, that relatives of each phobia proband group would have an increased risk for all phobia types. However, the magnitude of the increased risk for phobias other than the proband's would vary. The weak and inconsistent trend for increased risk for simple phobia observed in relatives of our social phobia (best-estimate data only) and panic-agoraphobia (direct interview data only) probands do not clearly address the findings of Kendler et al. However, the absence of a significant elevation of social phobia or panic-agoraphobia in relatives of simple phobia probands directly contradicts one of the stronger predictions of the Kendler model.

One possible explanation for these differences is the handling of proband anxiety comorbidity. We excluded comorbid cases; Kendler et al did not. Comorbid simple phobia may be associated with different patterns of familial transmission than single simple phobia. Also, undetected confounding variables may arise from differences in clinical vs epidemiologic samples.

Andrews et al[43] reported a second epidemiologically based twin study that included two (panic-agoraphobia and social phobia) of the three phobia groups. They found no genetic contribution that was specific to either phobia. Differences between this study and ours are difficult to interpret. As in the Kendler et al report,[37] single and comorbid cases are not separately reported and the source of subjects is different (epidemiologic vs clinic). In addition, Andrews et al excluded simple phobias and used a diagnostic procedure (modules from the Diagnostic Interview Schedule),[44] which may have been less sensitive to social phobia diagnosis than the SADS-LA.

LIMITATIONS

Several limitations affect the interpretation of these data. One important concern is the possible impact of proband comorbidity. Our control probands were selected to have no psychiatric disorder (ie, "supernormals"). Since our central questions concerned interrelationships between anxiety disorders, our phobia probands were chosen for the presence of phobias and the absence of any other anxiety disorder. It was not feasible (in terms of sample size) to also exclude phobia probands who had other psychiatric disorders and still conduct meaningful statistical tests. Therefore, proband comorbidity for these other disorders (nonanxiety) might be responsible for some of the observed differences in familial psychopathology. The most common types of comorbidity were affective and substance abuse disorders. Previous studies have suggested that affective disorder comorbidity may be associated with differences in course[45] and familiality[46-48] of certain anxiety disorders. To clarify this issue with respect to the different phobia types will require larger samples and inclusion of proband groups with affective or substance use disorders but no phobia diagnosis.

Additional limitations are the restriction of phobia probands to clinically rather than epidemiologically sampled subjects[7] and the difficulties of retrospective lifetime diagnosis.[49,50] Epidemiologic studies indicate that the majority of individuals with phobias do not seek treatment. Therefore, generalizing to untreated subjects requires empirical testing. Phobias may also be particularly susceptible to retrospective errors. Often untreated and circumscribed in impact, they are more likely to be forgotten by the interviewer and unknown to relatives. However, this would probably attenuate real findings rather than produce artifactual ones. Prospective studies are necessary.

Despite these reservations, the data support the existence of a specific familial contribution to particular phobia types.

Accepted for publication April 7, 1995.

This work was supported in part by grants MH-30906 and MH-37592 from the National Institute of Mental Health, Bethesda, Md.

The authors thank Donald Ross, PhD, for statistical consultation and Jean Endicott, PhD, and Theodore Reich, MD, for their ongoing assistance.

Reprint requests to New York State Psychiatric Institute, 722 W 168th St New York, NY 10032 (Dr Fyer).

REFERENCES

1. American Psychiatric Association. *Diagnostic and Statistical Manual of Mental Disorders, Third Edition.* Washington, DC: American Psychiatric Association; 1980.
2. American Psychiatric Association. *Diagnostic and Statistical Manual of Mental Disorders, Revised Third Edition.* Washington, DC: American Psychiatric Association; 1987.
3. World Health Organization. *Manual of the International Statistical Classification of Diseases, Injuries, and Causes of Death, Based on the Recommendations of the Ninth Revision Conference, 1975.* Geneva, Switzerland: World Health Organization; 1977.
4. American Psychiatric Association. *Diagnostic and Statistical Manual of Mental Disorders, Second Edition.* Washington, DC: American Psychiatric Association; 1968.
5. Marks IM. *Fears and Phobias.* Orlando, Fla: Academic Press Inc; 1969.
6. Klein DF, Rabkin JG, eds. *Anxiety: New Research and Changing Concepts.* New York, NY: Raven Press; 1981.
7. Boyd JH, Burke JD, Gruenberg E, Holzer CE, Rae DS, George LK, Karno M, Stoltzman R, McEvoy L, Nestadt G. Exclusion criteria of *DSM-III*: a study of co-occurrence of hierarchy-free syndromes. *Arch Gen Psychiatry.* 1984;41:983-989.
8. Mannuzza S, Fyer AJ, Liebowitz MR, Klein DF. Delineating the boundaries of social phobia: its relationship to panic disorder and agoraphobia. *J Anxiety Disord.* 1990;4:1-59.
9. Barlow DH. *Anxiety and Its Disorders: The Nature and Treatment of Anxiety and Panic.* New York, NY: Guilford Press; 1988.
10. Weissman MM. Evidence for comorbidity of anxiety and depression: family and genetic studies of children. In: Maser JD, Cloninger CR, eds. *Comorbidity of Mood and Anxiety Disorders.* Washington, DC: American Psychiatric Press Inc; 1990.
11. Klerman GL, Weissman MM, Ouellette R, Johnson J, Greenwald MA. Panic attacks in the community: social morbidity and health care utilization. *JAMA.* 1991;265:742-746.
12. Kendler KS. The super-normal control group in psychiatric genetics: possible artifactual evidence for coaggregation. *Psychiatr Genet.* 1990;1:45-53.
13. Klein DF. The utility of the super-normal control group in psychiatric genetics. *Psychiatr Genet.* 1993;3(1):17-19.
14. Wickramaratne PJ. Selecting control groups for studies of familial aggregation of disease. *J Clin Epidemiol.* In press.
15. Fyer AJ, Mannuzza S, Gallops SM, Martin LY, Aaronson C, Gorman JM, Liebowitz MR, Klein DF. Familial transmission of simple phobias and fears. *Arch Gen Psychiatry* 1990;47:252-256.
16. Fyer AJ, Mannuzza S, Chapman TF, Liebowitz MR, Klein DF. A direct interview family study of social phobia. *Arch Gen Psychiatry.* 1993;50:286-293.
17. American Psychiatric Association. *Diagnostic and Statistical Manual of Mental Disorders, Fourth Edition.* Washington, DC: American Psychiatric Association; 1994.
18. American Psychiatric Association, Work Group to Revise *DSM-III.* DSM-III-R *in Development.* 2nd draft. Washington, DC: American Psychiatric Association; 1985.
19. Klein DF, Zitrin CM, Woerner MG, Ross DC. Treatment of phobias, II: behavior therapy and supportive psychotherapy: are there any specific ingredients? *Arch Gen Psychiatry.* 1983;40:139-145.
20. Zitrin CM, Klein DF, Woerner MG, Ross DC. Treatment of phobias, I: comparison of imipramine hydrochloride and placebo. *Arch Gen Psychiatry.* 1983;40:125-138.
21. Spitzer RL, Endicott J. *Schedule of Schizophrenic and Affective Disorders-Lifetime Version.* 3rd ed. New York, NY: Research Assessment and Training Unit, New York State Psychiatric Institute; 1979.
22. Katz MM, Klerman GL. Introduction: overview of the clinical studies program. *Am J Psychiatry.* 1979;136:49-51.
23. Mannuzza S, Fyer AJ, Endicott J, Gallops MS, Martin LY, Reich T, Klein DF. An extension of the acquaintanceship procedure in family studies of mental disorder. *J Psychiatr Res.* 1992;26:45-57.
24. Fyer AJ, Endicott J, Mannuzza S, Klein DF. *Schedule for Affective Disorders and Schizophrenia-Lifetime Version (Modified for the Study of Anxiety Disorders).* New York, NY: Anxiety Disorders Clinic, New York State Psychiatric Institute; 1985.
25. Mannuzza S, Fyer AJ, Endicott J, Klein DF. Schedule for Affective Disorders and Schizophrenia-lifetime version (modified for the study of anxiety disorders) (SADS-LA): rationale and conceptual development. *J Psychiatr Res.* 1986; 20:317-325.
26. Mannuzza S, Fyer AJ, Endicott J, Klein DF. *Family Informant Schedule and Criteria (FISC).* New York, NY: Anxiety Disorders Clinic, New York State Psychiatric Institute; 1985.
27. McDonald-Scott P. Informed versus blind: the reliability of cross-sectional ratings of psychopathology. *Psychiatry Res.* 1984;12:207-217.
28. Kalbfleish JD, Prentice RL. *The Statistical Analysis of Failure Time Data.* New York, NY: John Wiley & Sons Inc; 1980.
29. Fleiss JL. *Statistical Methods for Rates and Proportions.* 2nd ed. New York, NY: John Wiley & Sons Inc; 1981.
30. Siegel S, Castellan NJ Jr. *Nonparametric Statistics for the Behavioral Sciences.* 2nd ed. New York, NY: McGraw-Hill International Book Co; 1988.
31. Fyer AJ, Liebowitz MR, Klein DF. Treatment trials, comorbidity, and syndromal complexity. In: Maser JD, Cloninger CR, eds. *Comorbidity of Mood and Anxiety Disorders.* Washington, DC: American Psychiatric Press Inc; 1990.
32. Rao CR. *Advanced Statistical Methods in Biometric Research.* New York, NY: John Wiley & Sons Inc; 1952.
33. Ost LG. Age at onset in different phobias. *J Abnorm Psychol.* 1987;96:223-229.
34. Kendler KS, Neale MC, Kessler RC, Heath AC, Eaves LJ. Panic disorder in women: a population-based twin study. *Psychol Med.* 1993;23:397-406.
35. Hall JM, Lee MK, Newman B, Morrow JE, Anderson LA, Huey B, King MC. Linkage of early-onset familial breast cancer to chromosome 17q21. *Science.* 1990;250:1684-1689.
36. King RA, Rotter JI, Motulsky AG. The approach to genetic bases of common diseases. In: King RA, Rotter JI, Motulsky AG, eds. *The Genetic Basis of Common Diseases.* New York, NY: Oxford University Press; 1992.
37. Kendler KS, Neale MC, Kessler RC, Heath AC, Eaves LJ. The genetic epidemiology of phobias in women: the interrelationship of agoraphobia, social phobia, situational phobia, and simple phobia. *Arch Gen Psychiatry.* 1992;49:273-281.
38. Reich J, Yates W. Family history of psychiatric disorders in social phobia. *Comp Psychiatry.* 1988;29:72-75.
39. Munjack DJ, Moss HB. Affective disorder and alcoholism in families of agoraphobics. *Arch Gen Psychiatry.* 1981;38:869-871.
40. Noyes R Jr, Crowe RR, Harris EL, Hamra BJ, McChesney CM, Chaudhry DR. Relationship between panic disorder and agoraphobia: a family study. *Arch Gen Psychiatry.* 1986;42:227-232.
41. Carey G, Gottesman II. Twin and family study of anxiety, phobic, and obsessive disorders. In: Klein DF, Rabkin JG, eds. *Anxiety: New Research and Changing Concepts.* New York, NY: Raven Press; 1981:117-136.
42. Wheeler EO, White PD, Reed E, Cohen ME. Familial incidence of neurocirculatory asthenia 'anxiety neurosis,' 'effort syndrome.' *J Clin Invest.* 1948;27:262.
43. Andrews G, Stewart G, Allen R, Henderson AS. The genetics of six neurotic disorder: a twin study. *J Affect Disord.* 1990;19:23-29.
44. Robins LN, Helzer JE, Weissman MM, Orvaschel H, Gruenberg E, Burke JD, Regier DA. Prevalence of specific psychiatric disorders in three sites. *Arch Gen Psychiatry.* 1984;41:949-958.
45. Angst J, Vollrath M, Merikangas KR, Ernst C. Comorbidity of anxiety and depression in the Zurich cohort study of young adults. In: Maser JD, Cloninger CR, eds. *Comorbidity in Anxiety and Mood Disorders.* Washington, DC: American Psychiatric Press Inc; 1989.
46. Weissman MM, Merikangas KR, John K, Wickramarante P, Prusoff B, Kidd KK. Family-genetic studies of psychiatric disorders: developing technologies. *Arch Gen Psychiatry.* 1986;43:1104-1116.
47. Weissman MM, Wickramaratne P, Adams PB, Lish JD, Horwath E, Charney D, Woods SW, Lehman E, Frosch E. The relationship between panic disorder and major depression: a new family study. *Arch Gen Psychiatry.* 1993;50:767-780.
48. Maier W, Lichtermann D, Meyer A, Oehrlein A, Klinger T. A controlled family study in panic disorder. *J Psychiatr Res.* 1993;27:79-87.
49. Rubin DC, ed. *Autobiographical Memory.* New York, NY: Cambridge University Press; 1986.
50. Fyer AJ, Mannuzza S, Martin LY, Gallops MS, Endicott J, Schleyer B, Gorman JM, Liebowitz MR, Klein DF. Reliability of anxiety, II: symptom agreement. *Arch Gen Psychiatry.* 1988;46:1102-1110.

Is the Comorbidity Between Social Phobia and Panic Disorder Due to Familial Cotransmission or Other Factors?

Ewald Horwath, MD, MSc; Susan I. Wolk, MD; Risë B. Goldstein, PhD, MPH; Priya Wickramaratne, PhD; Christina Sobin, PhD; Phillip Adams, PhD; Jennifer D. Lish, PhD; Myrna M. Weissman, PhD

Background: We previously reported significantly elevated rates of social phobia in relatives of probands with panic disorder compared with relatives of other proband groups. This study further investigates the relationship between social phobia and panic disorder.

Method: This sample is from a family study that included 193 probands from four mutually exclusive groups (patients with panic disorder, patients with panic disorder and major depression, patients with early-onset major depression, and normal controls) and 1047 of their adult first-degree relatives. Best-estimate diagnoses were completed using *DSM-III-R* criteria.

Results: Social phobia and agoraphobia aggregate in the families of probands with panic disorder without major depression. Social phobia frequently co-occurs with panic disorder in relatives, but the risk for comorbidity does not vary across proband groups.

Conclusions: The familial aggregation of social phobia with panic disorder may be explained by the aggregation of panic disorder in relatives of probands with panic disorder combined with the tendency for panic disorder to occur comorbidly with social phobia in individuals.

(Arch Gen Psychiatry. 1995;52:574-582)

SEVERAL STUDIES have demonstrated substantial comorbidity between social phobia and panic disorder. Schneier and colleagues,[1] in an analysis of the Epidemiologic Catchment Area (ECA) data, found that subjects with social phobia had a greater than threefold increased risk for lifetime panic disorder when compared with those without social phobia. In a clinical sample of 57 patients with social phobia, Van Ameringen and associates[2] found that 49% had a lifetime diagnosis of panic disorder. Other investigators[3-7] have reported rates of social phobia ranging from 6% to 53% in subjects with panic disorder.

Clinical, epidemiologic, and biologic data support a diagnostic boundary between social phobia and panic disorder, suggesting that these two disorders are distinct even though they frequently co-occur.[8-11] There is evidence that social phobia and panic disorder have different ages at onset, prevalence rates, gender ratios, sensitivities to sodium lactate infusion and carbon dioxide inhalation, patterns of help-seeking behavior, and pharmacologic-response profiles.[8,12]

The consensus seems to be that social phobia and panic disorder are two distinct syndromes with substantial comorbidity. It is not clear, however, whether social phobia and panic disorder co-occur because they share common risk factors, whether one disorder causes the other, or whether social phobia comorbid with panic disorder is a distinct syndrome that is different from either disorder alone.

Family studies can help differentiate the cause for co-occurrence from among these alternative explanations of comorbidity by providing data on familial cotransmission of the two disorders. To date, family studies have not established a familial relationship between social phobia and panic disorder.

There is considerable evidence that panic disorder is highly familial.[13-19] However, the familiality of social phobia has been less well studied. Fyer and colleagues,[20] in the only published direct interview family study of social phobia, found that relatives of probands with social phobia had a threefold increased risk

See Methods on next page

From the Department of Psychiatry, the College of Physicians and Surgeons of Columbia University (Drs Horwath, Wolk, Wickramaratne, Sobin, Adams, and Weissman), and the Division of Clinical and Genetic Epidemiology, New York State Psychiatric Institute (Drs Goldstein, Wickramaratne, Sobin, Adams, and Weissman), New York, NY; and the Department of Psychiatry, the Medical College of Pennsylvania, Philadelphia (Dr Lish).

METHODS

PROBAND SELECTION

The study methods have been described in detail elsewhere.[13,14] Probands were selected from research clinics at Yale University, New Haven, Conn, and the New Haven site of the ECA study. Probands selected were white, were between 18 and 70 years of age, and met the criteria for one of the four groups.

Persons who initially met the demographic and diagnostic inclusion criteria were reinterviewed blindly using the Schedule for Affective Disorders and Schizophrenia–Lifetime Version for Anxiety Disorders (SADS-LA).[26] The SADS-LA generated RDC and was modified to incorporate *DSM-III* and *DSM-III-R* criteria as well.

DIAGNOSTIC CRITERIA FOR PROBANDS

Probands were excluded from all groups if they met criteria for schizophrenia, mania, Briquet's syndrome, antisocial personality disorder, or anorexia. Substance abuse was not considered exclusionary if it was secondary to the primary diagnosis, primary but mild, or followed by a significant period of recovery prior to the onset of the inclusion diagnosis. The diagnostic criteria for each specific group were as follows.

Early-Onset MDD

A history of MDD by modified RDC with the first episode having occurred at or before the age of 30 years was required.[27] The modification to the RDC included duration of illness of at least 4 weeks and impairment of social functioning in the major social role. Probands were excluded from this group if they had panic attacks or panic disorder during their lifetime by any diagnostic criteria at any level of certainty.

Panic Disorder With or Without MDD

Probands were required to meet *DSM-III* criteria for panic disorder. For the comorbid group, probands were additionally required to meet RDC for MDD, modified as described above. Probands in the panic disorder without MDD group were excluded if they reported any evidence of MDD during their lifetime by any diagnostic system at any level of certainty.

Never Mentally Ill Controls

Probands were included if they had received no lifetime psychiatric diagnosis during any of the three waves of the ECA interviews based on the Diagnostic Interview Schedule[28] and on reinterview with the SADS-LA. Some controls who were classified as never mentally ill may have had phobia symptoms, but these symptoms were insufficient to meet *DSM-III* criteria for a phobic disorder.

RELATIVES

After acceptance of the proband into the study, all first-degree relatives (FDRs), living or deceased, aged 6 years and older were enumerated systematically using the Pedigree Collection Form.[29] Permission to contact relatives was obtained from the proband, and all consenting relatives were directly interviewed by SADS-LA. This resulted in direct SADS-LA interviews in 52% of all living FDRs, a percentage that did not vary across proband groups. In addition to the SADS-LA, family history on all probands and FDRs was collected from all probands and interviewed relatives using a modified Family History Method for RDC.[30-32] The interviewers were clinicians with master's degrees in social work or doctor of philosophy degrees in clinical psychology or were advanced doctoral students in clinical programs. Interviewers were blind to the diagnostic group of the proband.

BEST-ESTIMATE DIAGNOSES

Best-estimate diagnoses were made by a psychiatrist or a clinical psychologist with a doctor of philosophy degree on each proband or relative based on all available information from the interview, the family history, and medical records.[33] The best estimator was blind to the diagnostic group and to the status of the individual as proband or relative. Thirty-six of the 229 probands were dropped from the study because they did not meet criteria for any of the four groups when the best-estimate diagnoses were completed. Thus, the final sample consisted of 193 probands and 1047 adult FDRs.

DATA ANALYSIS

Crude lifetime rates of disorders were compared using χ^2 tests. Age-corrected lifetime rates were derived from Kaplan-Meier analyses. Adjusted hazard ratios were derived from proportional hazards regression models that controlled for gender, age, and interview status of relatives and proband ascertainment source. This method applies multiple regression to a survival distribution to yield the age-specific incidences of disorders in relatives while controlling for potentially confounding variables. We controlled for proband ascertainment source because of a previous finding that ascertainment source confounded the effect of proband group, although it did not independently influence the rates of social phobia in relatives.[34] The strength of the association between panic disorder and social phobia in relatives was measured by odds ratios calculated from 2×2 tables stratified by proband group. The homogeneity of the odds ratio across proband groups was evaluated with the Breslow-Day statistic.

for social phobia compared with relatives of the never mentally ill subjects. Another study,[21] which used a less sensitive family history method, found rates of social phobia in the relatives of probands with social phobia that were higher than those in the relatives of probands with panic disorder but not different from the rates in the relatives of normal controls.

The few studies on the cotransmission of phobias and other anxiety disorders have produced findings that are difficult to interpret. Family studies that used

Research Diagnostic Criteria (RDC),[22] which do not distinguish one phobic subtype from another, have found aggregation of phobias in the relatives of probands with panic disorder or generalized anxiety disorder (GAD).[10,11,15] However, these studies did not control for the effect of comorbid phobic disorders or major depression (MDD) among probands. Family studies that have differentiated between phobic subtypes using *DSM-III*[23] or *DSM-III-R*[24] criteria have not found elevated rates of social phobia in the relatives of probands with panic disorder or agoraphobia.[7,16,21,25] Similarly, Fyer et al[20] did not find aggregation of panic disorder in the relatives of probands with social phobia.

Weissman et al[13] recently reported results from a family study indicating that the rates of social phobia were significantly higher in the relatives of probands with panic disorder than in the relatives of normal controls, and this finding was not explained by the presence of comorbid social phobia in the probands with panic disorder.[14] To the best of our knowledge, this is the first specific report of a familial association between social phobia and panic disorder.

The purpose of this article is to explore the possible explanations for this association. We propose several alternative hypotheses that could explain our finding of familial coaggregation of social phobia and panic disorder:

Hypothesis 1. The coaggregation of social phobia with panic disorder reflects a general tendency for phobic disorders to coaggregate with panic disorder. This hypothesis predicts that rates of social phobia, panic disorder with agoraphobia, agoraphobia without panic disorder, and simple phobia would be higher in relatives of probands with panic disorder than in relatives of normal controls.

Hypothesis 2. The co-occurrence of social phobia and panic disorder in families is not due to familial cotransmission. In this case, social phobia and panic disorder would co-occur in relatives of each proband group at rates greater than that which would be expected by chance alone, but the strength of the association between social phobia and panic disorder would not vary across the relatives of the four proband groups.

Hypothesis 3. The reported association between social phobia and panic disorder is spurious. One potential cause of a spurious association would be the misdiagnosis of agoraphobia, which is known to co-occur with panic disorder, as social phobia.

Herein, we further analyze data from our family study to test these alternative hypotheses.

RESULTS

DEMOGRAPHIC AND CLINICAL CHARACTERISTICS OF PROBANDS AND RELATIVES

The demographic and clinical characteristics of the probands and relatives have been described in detail elsewhere.[13,14] **Table 1** presents the demographic and clinical characteristics pertinent to this set of analyses. In brief, there were no differences among proband groups in age, marital status, number of marriages, social class, education, or religion. Proband groups were initially matched for gender and age; however, gender differences emerged when best estimators' diagnoses required reclassification or elimination of some probands. Significantly more female probands were left in the two proband groups with MDD. **Table 2** shows the demographic and clinical characteristics of the FDRs by proband group. The mean current age, age at onset of panic disorder, and social class differed in the relatives of the different proband groups.

Table 1. Demographic and Clinical Characteristics of Probands by Group*

	Proband Group				
	Panic Disorder Without MDD (n=30)	Panic Disorder With MDD (n=77)	Early-Onset MDD (n=41)	Never Mentally Ill (n=45)	*P*
Gender, No. (%)					
M	10 (33)	13 (17)	5 (12)	25 (56)	<.001
F	20 (67)	64 (83)	36 (88)	20 (44)	
Mean (SD) age, y	43.3 (12.5)	42.6 (8.8)	43.9 (12.5)	48.0 (10.5)	.06
Marital status, No. (%)					
Single	5 (17)	7 (9)	7 (17)	6 (13)	.40
Married, remarried, or common-law marriage	23 (77)	55 (71)	28 (68)	34 (76)	
Separated or divorced	1 (3)	13 (17)	5 (12)	2 (4)	
Widowed	1 (3)	2 (3)	1 (2)	3 (7)	
Social class, No. (%)†					
1 and 2	7 (24)	24 (31)	15 (36)	23 (51)	.28
3	12 (41)	29 (38)	14 (34)	10 (22)	
4 and 5	10 (35)	24 (31)	12 (29)	12 (27)	
Mean (SD) age at onset of panic disorder, y	27.2 (8.9)	28.1 (10.4)	NA	NA	.83

**MDD indicates major depression; NA, not applicable.*
†Defined by the five-level Hollingshead Index.

TEST OF HYPOTHESIS 1

Rates of Disorders in FDRs

Table 3 shows the age-corrected lifetime rates of social phobia, panic disorder with and without agoraphobia, agoraphobia without panic disorder, and simple phobia in FDRs of each proband group. The lifetime rate of social phobia in the adult FDRs of probands with panic disorder without MDD is 5.9%, which is significantly higher than the rates in the adult FDRs of the other three proband groups.

In Table 3, row 2, we excluded probands with comorbid social phobia from the analysis to eliminate the possibility that the higher rate of social phobia in relatives of probands with only panic disorder was due to the presence of social phobia in the probands. The lifetime rate of social phobia in the adult FDRs of probands with panic disorder remained significantly higher than in the adult FDRs of the other three proband groups.

As expected, the rates of panic disorder with and without agoraphobia are both significantly greater in the adult FDRs of the probands with panic disorder alone or panic disorder with MDD. Although the rates of agoraphobia without panic disorder and simple phobia were highest in relatives of the probands with panic disorder without MDD, the differences among the four proband groups did not reach statistical significance for these disorders.

Adjusted Hazard Ratios in FDRs

Table 4 presents the results of proportional hazards regression models, from which hazard ratios with 95% confidence intervals were derived. These analyses test whether the relatives of each ill proband group have a higher risk for social phobia, panic disorder with and without agoraphobia, agoraphobia without panic disorder, or simple phobia than the relatives of normal controls. The regression models in Table 4 control for source from which the proband was recruited and for age, gender, and interview status of the relatives.

Table 4 shows that relatives of probands with panic disorder without depression are more than five times as likely to have social phobia than relatives of the never mentally ill probands. This risk remains significantly elevated when the probands with comorbid social phobia and their relatives are excluded from the analysis. Relatives of the other two ill proband groups do not differ significantly from relatives of the never mentally ill probands with regard to risk for social phobia.

Table 4 also shows that relatives of probands with panic disorder with or without depression have an increased risk for panic disorder when compared with relatives of normal controls. When the FDRs with panic disorder are subdivided into those with or without agoraphobia, the proportional hazards remain elevated in the relatives of the two proband groups with panic disorder, although the smaller number of subjects in each group limits the statistical power of these comparisons. The risk for agoraphobia without panic disorder is also increased in relatives of probands with panic disorder without MDD when compared with relatives of normal controls. The risk for simple phobia is not significantly different in relatives of probands with panic disorder without depression from that in relatives of normal controls.

TEST OF HYPOTHESIS 2

The adjusted hazard ratios in Table 4 show that relatives of probands with panic disorder (without MDD) have

Table 2. Demographic and Clinical Characteristics of Adult First-degree Relatives by Proband Group*

	Proband Group				
	Panic Disorder Without MDD	Panic Disorder With MDD	Early-Onset MDD	Never Mentally Ill	*P*
All relatives (N=1047)					
Gender, No. (%)					
M	74 (52)	224 (51)	97 (46)	133 (52)	.59
F	67 (48)	218 (49)	112 (54)	122 (48)	
Mean (SD) age, y	50.0 (18.4)	48.1 (18.4)	49.1 (18.5)	52.5 (19.5)	.03
Diagnosis of panic disorder					
Number	20	33	5	3	
Mean (SD) age at onset, y	23.3 (9.7)	27.1 (9.6)	22.2 (7.7)	39.7 (16.7)	.003
Interviewed relatives (n=435)					
Marital status, No. (%)					
Single	11 (15)	47 (26)	21 (24)	28 (30)	.36
Married, remarried, or common-law marriage	51 (69)	106 (59)	54 (61)	47 (50)	
Separated or divorced	9 (12)	15 (8)	8 (9)	14 (15)	
Widowed	3 (4)	11 (6)	5 (6)	5 (5)	
Social class, No. (%)†					
1 and 2	20 (27)	38 (21)	30 (34)	35 (37)	.054
3	32 (43)	73 (41)	37 (42)	34 (36)	
4 and 5	22 (30)	68 (38)	21 (24)	25 (27)	

**Information on age, gender, and age at onset of panic disorder is available for all relatives. Information on other demographics is available only for interviewed relatives. MDD indicates major depression; NS, not significant.*

†Defined by the five-level Hollingshead Index.

Table 3. Age-Corrected Lifetime Rates of *DSM-III-R* Phobias and Panic Disorder in Interviewed and Uninterviewed Relatives (N=1047) by Proband Group*

	Proband Group				
	Panic Disorder Without MDD	Panic Disorder With MDD	Early-Onset MDD	Never Mentally Ill	P
Subjects					
No. of probands	30	77	41	45	
No. of relatives	141	442	209	255	
Disorder in relatives, %					
Social phobia (n=23)	5.93	1.62	2.00	1.59	.02
Social phobia (probands with comorbid social phobia and their FDRs excluded) (n=22)†	6.58	1.93	2.27	1.59	.04
Panic disorder with or without agoraphobia (n=61)	16.14	9.28	2.61	1.82	<.001
Panic disorder with agoraphobia (n=31)	8.97	4.12	2.06	1.40	<.001
Panic disorder without agoraphobia (n=30)	7.70	5.28	5.49	4.17	<.001
Agoraphobia without panic disorder (n=16)‡	5.45	1.27	1.03	0.39	.07
Simple phobia (n=64)	10.73	7.15	8.14	4.14	.08

**MDD indicates major depression; FDR, first-degree relative.*

†Six probands with comorbid social phobia and panic disorder (without MDD) and their FDRs excluded.

‡Includes cases with any evidence of limited-symptom, near, spontaneous, or situational panic attacks in persons with agoraphobia who do not meet the full criteria for panic disorder.

an increased risk for both social phobia and panic disorder when compared with relatives of normal controls. From the ECA study, we know that social phobia is often comorbid with panic disorder in the community.[1] We hypothesized that the higher rates of social phobia in relatives of probands with panic disorder without MDD might be explained by shared nonfamilial risk factors or by one disorder causing the other in individuals. **Table 5** presents a test of this hypothesis.

The analyses shown in Table 5 test whether social phobia and panic disorder co-occurred with greater probability than that due to chance alone in relatives of the different proband groups. Furthermore, these analyses examine whether the strength of the association between the two disorders in relatives varied across proband groups. Table 5 presents a series of 2×2 contingency tables arrayed by proband group. Each table shows the social phobia status of relatives cross-classified by whether they had panic disorder. A measure of the extent to which comorbidity greater than that due to chance alone exists is given by the odds ratio (odds of a relative having social phobia given that he or she has panic disorder compared with the odds of the relative having social phobia given that he or she does not have panic disorder). If the value of the odds ratio is significantly greater than 1, it can be concluded that the comorbidity is greater than that due to chance alone. Furthermore, the greater the value of the odds ratio, the stronger the association between social phobia and panic disorder in the relatives.

As Table 5 shows, the odds ratios for the relatives of the three ill proband groups are all significantly greater than 1. The odds ratio for the relatives of the never mentally ill probands cannot be calculated because there were no relatives with comorbid panic disorder and social phobia. At the bottom of Table 5, the Breslow-Day test for the homogeneity of the odds ratios shows no significant differences in the odds ratios in the relatives across the different proband cells. These results suggest that, although there is a strong association between social phobia and panic disorder, as reflected by the common odds ratio of 9.99 (ie, almost a tenfold increased risk for social phobia if the relative also has panic disorder), the strength of this association does not differ significantly by proband group.

TEST OF HYPOTHESIS 3

To test whether diagnostic misclassification of agoraphobia as social phobia contributed to finding higher rates of social phobia in relatives of probands with panic disorder, we reviewed all of the available diagnostic information on the 23 relatives in whom social phobia was diagnosed. Twenty-two of the 23 relatives with social phobia had been directly interviewed. Eleven of the 23 relatives with social phobia met the criteria for panic disorder (n=9) or experienced subsyndromal panic attacks (n=2). In eight relatives, both agoraphobia and social phobia were diagnosed. Eleven relatives with social phobia did not have comorbid diagnoses of either panic disorder or agoraphobia.

We compared the demographic and clinical characteristics of the FDRs with social phobia, panic disorder, or agoraphobia. Several differences increased our confidence in the diagnostic distinctions: (1) the mean age at onset of social phobia was earlier than the mean ages at onset of panic disorder or agoraphobia; (2) the female-male ratio for social phobia was closer to unity than the gender ratios for panic disorder or agoraphobia; and (3) the percentage of relatives with social phobia who had never married was higher than that of the relatives with panic disorder or agoraphobia. These demographic and clinical differences between the subjects with social phobia, panic disorder, or agoraphobia suggest that the cases of social phobia were clinically distinct from agoraphobia.

Early drafts of the *DSM-IV* proposed discrete and generalized subtypes of social phobia,[35] and the *DSM-IV* in-

Table 4. Adjusted Hazard Ratios With 95% CIs Comparing Rates of *DSM-III-R* Phobias and Panic Disorder in Relatives of Ill and Relatives of Normal Control Probands (N=1047) by Proband Group*

Disorder in Relatives	Proband Group, Hazard Ratio† (95% CI): Panic Disorder Without MDD	Panic Disorder With MDD	Early-Onset MDD
Social phobia (n=23)	5.44 (1.38-21.54)‖	1.52 (0.37-6.27)	0.98 (0.21-4.52)
Social phobia (probands with comorbid social phobia and their FDRs excluded) (n=22)‡	6.70 (1.64-27.35)¶	2.04 (0.49-8.51)	1.20 (0.27-5.37)
Panic disorder with or without agoraphobia (n=61)	8.77 (2.28-33.78)	5.66 (1.51-21.16)‖	2.14 (0.49-9.34)
Panic disorder with agoraphobia (n=31)	8.28 (1.53-44.72)‖	4.25 (0.80-22.42)#	2.88 (0.51-16.35)
Panic disorder without agoraphobia (n=30)	9.48 (0.97-92.43)#	7.51 (0.81-69.97)#	1.06 (0.06-18.47)
Agoraphobia without panic disorder (n=16)§	13.73 (1.38-136.97)‖	5.39 (0.55-53.29)	3.01 (0.26-35.30)
Simple phobia (n=64)	1.95 (0.70-5.40)#	1.57 (0.62-3.97)	1.06 (0.42-2.70)

*CI indicates confidence interval; MDD, major depression; and FDR, first-degree relatives.
†Adjusted for source from which proband was recruited and gender, age, and interview status of relative.
‡Six probands with comorbid social phobia and panic disorder (without MDD) and their FDRs were excluded.
§Includes cases with any evidence of limited-symptom, near, spontaneous, and situational panic attacks in persons with agoraphobia who do not meet the full criteria for panic disorder. Because of the small number of cases, only gender and interview status of the relative could be controlled for.
‖$P<.05$.
¶$P<.01$.
#$.05<P<.10$.

cludes a specification for a generalized type.[36] The discrete subtype involves one or two specific fears, whereas the generalized subtype includes most social situations and may be more difficult to distinguish from agoraphobia. Data from the ECA study support the validity of the discrete and generalized subtypes of social phobia.[37] In our sample of relatives, 17 of the 23 cases of social phobia were of the discrete subtype, which involved fear and avoidance of public speaking, eating in public, the use of public lavatories, performing, speaking on the telephone, or asking directions. This preponderance of cases with discrete social phobias further supports the validity of our diagnostic distinction between social phobia and agoraphobia.

COMMENT

In this study, we tested several alternative hypotheses in an attempt to explain our previously reported finding of familial coaggregation of social phobia and panic disorder.

HYPOTHESIS 1

We found that there is a fivefold increased risk for social phobia in relatives of probands with panic disorder without MDD compared with relatives of never mentally ill probands. The increased risk for social phobia in relatives of probands with panic disorder is not accounted for by the occurrence of comorbid social phobia in probands. As previously reported, relatives of probands with panic disorder had a higher risk for panic disorder than relatives of the never mentally ill probands. Relatives of probands with panic disorder had an increased risk for agoraphobia without panic disorder when compared with relatives of the never mentally ill probands. There was no significant difference in the risk for simple phobia when comparing relatives of probands who have panic disorder with relatives of controls. These results suggest that social phobia and agoraphobia aggregate in relatives of probands with panic disorder without MDD but that simple phobia does not.

HYPOTHESIS 2

We found that social phobia and panic disorder co-occurred in relatives of all three ill proband groups at a higher-than-chance level. Relatives with panic disorder had an almost tenfold increased risk for social phobia compared with relatives without panic disorder. However, the strength of the association between social phobia and panic disorder in relatives did not vary across different proband cells.

The uniformly strong association between social phobia and panic disorder in relatives regardless of proband group suggests that nonfamilial factors may account for the high comorbidity of these two disorders. Therefore, the increased rate of social phobia in relatives of probands with only panic disorder compared with relatives of normal controls may be accounted for by the high rates of panic disorder in the relatives of probands with only panic disorder combined with a tendency for these two disorders to co-occur. In other words, panic disorder in the relatives may be a risk factor for social phobia.

HYPOTHESIS 3

We found that cases of social phobia in relatives were clearly differentiable from agoraphobia based on clinical factors such as the fear and avoidance of specific social situations as opposed to the more general avoidance behaviors usually seen in agoraphobia. Furthermore, the gender ratio, mean ages at onset, and marital status of the relatives with social phobia are consistent with the demographic characteristics that have been reported by other investigators and are distinct from those of the relatives with panic disorder or agoraphobia.

Our finding that relatives of probands with panic dis-

Table 5. Association Between Panic Disorder and Social Phobia in Relatives by Proband Group*

Proband Group	Relatives†		Social phobia: Yes	Social phobia: No	Total	Odds Ratio (95% Confidence Interval)	χ^2 Test for Association	*P*
Panic disorder without MDD	Panic disorder	Yes	4	16	**20**	7.31 (1.98-26.95)	8.938	.003
		No	4	117	**121**			
			8	**133**	**141**			
Panic disorder with MDD	Panic disorder	Yes	3	30	**33**	10.13 (2.86-35.85)	12.895	<.001
		No	4	405	**409**			
			7	**435**	**442**			
Early-onset MDD	Panic disorder	Yes	2	3	**5**	67.33 (18.14-245.04)	39.582	<.001
		No	2	202	**204**			
			4	**205**	**209**			
Never mentally ill	Panic disorder	Yes	0	3	**3**	NA	0.048	.826
		No	4	248	**252**			
			4	**251**	**255**			

**Breslow-Day test for homogeneity of the odds ratio:* χ^2*=3.940,* df=3, P=*.268. Estimate of the common odds ratio: odds ratio (95% confidence interval): 9.99 (4.59, 21.73),* P<*.001. MDD indicates major depression; NA, not applicable.*

†Values are numbers of relatives. Boldfaced numbers outside the box are totals.

order have an increased risk for social phobia is consistent with previously published studies in children by Weissman et al[10] and in adults by Coryell et al[11] and Leckman et al.[15] These studies found increased risks for RDC phobias in relatives of probands with panic disorder. However, these studies did not differentiate social phobia from other phobic disorders and, therefore, are not directly comparable. Furthermore, all of the probands in these studies had comorbid MDD. We did not find elevated rates of social phobia in the relatives of probands with comorbid panic disorder and MDD.

In contrast to our finding of an increased rate of social phobia in relatives of probands with panic disorder without MDD, Mendlewicz et al[25] did not find increased rates of social or simple phobias in relatives of probands with panic disorder. However, their report did not distinguish social from simple phobias so that distinct risks for social phobia could not be determined from their study. This is important because of our finding that the risk for simple phobia was not significantly higher in relatives of probands with panic disorder when compared with relatives of the never mentally ill probands.

Other studies that used *DSM-III* or *DSM-III-R* criteria did not find an increased risk for social phobia in relatives of probands with panic disorder.[7,16,21] This conflicts with our finding that social phobia aggregated in the relatives of probands with panic disorder without comorbid MDD, but the discrepancy may be explained by methodological differences. Bellodi and colleagues[7] and Reich and Yates[21] did not find a familial aggregation of social phobia with panic disorder, but their results were based on the family history method. Relatives were not directly interviewed as was done in our study, probably resulting in underestimation of the prevalence of social phobia and other disorders compared with our direct interview study.[38,39]

Noyes et al[16] determined diagnoses of anxiety disorders according to the hierarchy outlined in the *DSM-III*, with a single primary anxiety diagnosis assigned according to the predominant anxiety symptoms. De Ruiter and colleagues[4] found that in patients with comorbid panic disorder, agoraphobia, and social phobia, social phobia more frequently was considered the primary illness when primacy was determined temporally than when primacy was assigned according to the greatest interference with functioning. Noyes and colleagues may have underestimated the rates of social phobia in the relatives of probands with panic disorder by defining social phobia as the secondary anxiety diagnosis. Social phobia is frequently assigned as an additional diagnosis in patients in whom another anxiety disorder is judged as principal.[40]

Fyer and associates[20] found an increased risk for social phobia in relatives of probands with social phobia. Recognizing the evidence for the familiality of social phobia, we controlled for comorbid social phobia in the probands in our study, but this did not account for our finding of an increased risk for social phobia in relatives of probands with panic disorder.

LIMITATIONS

In this study, we tested three alternative hypotheses regarding the familial coaggregation of social phobia and panic disorder. A fourth hypothesis suggests that social phobia comorbid with panic disorder is a distinct syndrome that aggregates in families independently of either disorder alone. We could not fully test this hypothesis for lack of a social phobia proband group.

However, we were able to partially test this hypothesis by comparing rates of panic disorder without social phobia, panic disorder with social phobia, and social phobia without panic disorder in relatives of probands with panic disorder with and without social phobia. The rates of these three syndromes were not significantly different when comparing relatives of probands with panic disorder with and without social phobia.

This limited test suggests that social phobia comorbid with panic disorder is not a single, distinct syndrome with independent familial aggregation. A study with a social phobia proband group without panic disorder would be necessary to test this hypothesis fully. This study was not designed originally with a social phobia proband group because the finding of coaggregation of social phobia with panic disorder was unexpected.

Several authors[8,12] have commented on the difficulties in differentiating between social phobia and panic disorder with agoraphobia. Although we had concerns that misdiagnosis might have contributed to our finding, we found that differences in ages at onset, gender ratio, marital status, and discreteness of social fears supported the diagnostic distinctions we made between social phobia and agoraphobia.

It is not clear why social phobia did not aggregate in the relatives of probands with panic disorder and MDD. One possible explanation is heterogeneity in the proband group with panic disorder and MDD, which may have included subtypes of panic disorder with differing associations with social phobia.

Rosenbaum and colleagues[41] have suggested that behavioral inhibition in children may be a precursor to the development of panic disorder and social phobia in adults. Several family studies have shown an association between panic disorder and social phobia in parents and behavioral inhibition in children.[42,43] Behavioral inhibition in children of parents with social phobia or panic disorder may be a marker for the familial transmission of a shared diathesis for these disorders.

Although familial transmission of a shared diathesis for panic disorder and social phobia is a possible explanation for the findings of our study, we could not test this hypothesis because of the lack of a social phobia proband group without panic disorder. However, Fyer and colleagues[20] did not find an increased risk for panic disorder in the relatives of patients with social phobia, which would be expected if the two disorders are alternate expressions of an underlying trait that is transmitted familially.

Comorbidity may be due to common nonfamilial risk factors or one disorder causing the other. Early nonfamilial environmental stressors may predispose individuals to both social phobia and panic disorder. Social phobia may be a risk factor for development of panic disorder or vice versa. Our study could not differentiate among these possible explanations for comorbidity. Longitudinal follow-up studies would be required to explore these possibilities more fully.

Given the small number of cases of social phobia on which we report, these results should be regarded cautiously and require replication. Family studies with the full range of mutually exclusive proband groups (panic disorder with no social phobia, panic disorder with social phobia, social phobia without panic disorder, and normal controls) are needed to clarify the relationship between social phobia and panic disorder.

Accepted for publication April 11, 1995.

This work was supported by grants MH-438781, MH-28274, and MH-30906 from the National Institute of Mental Health, Bethesda, Md, and National Institute of Mental Health Research Training grant 5T32MH16434 (Dr Wolk), administered through Columbia University, New York, NY.

Reprint requests to New York State Psychiatric Institute, Unit 14, 722 W 168th St, New York, NY 10032 (Dr Horwath).

REFERENCES

1. Schneier FR, Johnson J, Hornig CD, Liebowitz MR, Weissman MM. Social phobia: comorbidity and morbidity in an epidemiologic sample. *Arch Gen Psychiatry.* 1992;49:282-288.
2. Van Ameringen M, Mancini C, Styan G, Donison D. Relationship of social phobia with other psychiatric illness. *J Affect Disord.* 1991;21:93-99.
3. Barlow DH, DiNardo PA, Vermilyea BB, Vermilyea J, Blanchard EB. Comorbidity and depression among the anxiety disorders. *J Nerv Ment Dis.* 1986; 174:63-72.
4. de Ruiter C, Rijken H, Garssen B, van Schaik A, Kraaimaat F. Comorbidity among the anxiety disorders. *J Anxiety Disord.* 1989;3:57-68.
5. Stein MB, Shea CA, Uhde TW. Social phobic symptoms in patients with panic disorder: practical and theoretical implications. *Am J Psychiatry.* 1989;146: 235-238.
6. Reiter SR, Otto MW, Pollack MH, Rosenbaum JF. Major depression in panic disorder patients with comorbid social phobia. *J Affect Disord.* 1991;22:171-177.
7. Bellodi L, Battaglia M, Diaferia G, Draisci A, Sciuto G. Lifetime prevalence of depression and family history of patients with panic disorder and social phobia. *Eur Psychiatry.* 1993;8:147-152.
8. Uhde TW, Tancer ME, Black B, Brown TM. Phenomenology and neurobiology of social phobia: comparison with panic disorder. *J Clin Psychiatry.* 1991;52 (suppl):31-40.
9. Fyer AJ, Mannuzza S, Gallops MS, Martin LY, Aaronson C, Gorman JM, Leibowitz MR, Klein DF. Familial transmission of simple phobias and fears: a preliminary report. *Arch Gen Psychiatry.* 1990;47:252-256.
10. Weissman MM, Leckman JF, Merikangas KR, Gammon GD, Prusoff BA. Depression and anxiety disorders in parents and children: results from the Yale family study. *Arch Gen Psychiatry.* 1984;41:845-852.
11. Coryell WH, Endicott J, Andreassen NC, Keller MB, Clayton PJ, Hirschfeld RMA, Scheftner WA, Winokur G. Depression and panic attacks: the significance of overlap as reflected in follow-up and family study data. *Am J Psychiatry.* 1988; 145:293-300.
12. Mannuzza S, Fyer AJ, Liebowitz MR, Klein DF. Delineating the boundaries of social phobia: its relationship to panic disorder and agoraphobia. *J Anxiety Disord.* 1990;4:41-59.
13. Weissman MM, Wickramaratne P, Adams P, Lish J, Horwath E, Charney D, Woods SW, Leeman E, Frosch E. The relationship between panic disorder and major depression: a new family study. *Arch Gen Psychiatry.* 1993;50:767-780.
14. Goldstein RB, Weissman MM, Adams PB, Horwath E, Lish JD, Charney D, Woods SW, Sobin C, Wickramaratne PJ. Psychiatric disorders in relatives of probands with panic disorder and/or major depression. *Arch Gen Psychiatry.* 1994;51:383-394.
15. Leckman JF, Weissman MM, Merikangas KR, Pauls DL, Prusoff BA. Panic dis-

order and major depression: increased risk of depression, alcoholism, panic, and phobic disorders in families of depressed probands with panic disorder. *Arch Gen Psychiatry.* 1983;40:1055-1060.

16. Noyes R, Crowe RR, Harris EL, Hamra BJ, McChesney CM, Chaudhry DR. Relationship between panic disorder and agoraphobia: a family study. *Arch Gen Psychiatry.* 1986;43:227-232.
17. Crowe RR, Noyes R, Pauls DL, Slymen D. A family study of panic disorder. *Arch Gen Psychiatry.* 1983;40:1065-1069.
18. Hopper JL, Judd FK, Derrick PL, Burrows GD. A family study of panic disorder. *Genet Epidemiol.* 1987;4:33-41.
19. Moran C, Andrews G. The familial occurrence of agoraphobia. *Br J Psychiatry.* 1985;146:262-267.
20. Fyer AJ, Mannuzza S, Chapman TF, Liebowitz MR, Klein DF. A direct interview family study of social phobia. *Arch Gen Psychiatry.* 1993;50:286-293.
21. Reich J, Yates W. Family history of psychiatric disorders in social phobia. *Compr Psychiatry.* 1988;29:72-75.
22. Spitzer RL, Endicott J, Robins E. *Research Diagnostic Criteria for a Selected Group of Functional Disorders.* 3rd ed. New York, NY: Biometrics Research Division, New York State Psychiatric Institute; 1977.
23. American Psychiatric Association. *Diagnostic and Statistical Manual of Mental Disorders, Third Edition.* Washington, DC: American Psychiatric Association; 1980.
24. American Psychiatric Association. *Diagnostic and Statistical Manual of Mental Disorders, Revised Third Edition.* Washington, DC: American Psychiatric Association; 1987.
25. Mendlewicz J, Papadimitriou G, Wilmotte J. Family study of panic disorder: comparison with generalized anxiety disorders, major depression, and normal subjects. *Psychiatr Genet.* In press.
26. Mannuzza S, Fyer AJ, Klein DF, Endicott J. Schedule for affective disorders and schizophrenia-lifetime version (modified for the study of anxiety disorders): rationale and conceptual development. *J Psychiatr Res.* 1986;20:317-325.
27. Weissman MM, Wickramaratne P, Merikangas KR, Prusoff BA, Caruso KA, Kidd KK, Gammon GD. Onset of major depression in early adulthood: increased familial loading and specificity. *Arch Gen Psychiatry.* 1984;41:1136-1143.
28. Robins LN, Helzer JE, Croughan J, Ratcliff KS. National Institute of Mental Health Diagnostic Interview Schedule: its history, characteristics, and validity. *Arch Gen Psychiatry.* 1981;38:381-389.
29. Thompson DG, Kidd JR, Weissman MM. A procedure for the efficient collection and processing of pedigree data suitable for genetic analysis. *J Psychiatr Res.* 1980;15:291-303.
30. Andreasen NC, Endicott J, Spitzer RL, Winokur G. The family history method using diagnostic criteria: reliability and validity. *Arch Gen Psychiatry.* 1977; 34:1229-1235.
31. Weissman MM, Gershon ES, Kidd KK, Prusoff BA, Leckman JF, Dibble E, Hamovit J, Thompson WD, Pauls DL, Guroff JJ. Psychiatric disorders in the relatives of probands with affective disorders. *Arch Gen Psychiatry.* 1984;41:13-21.
32. Mannuzza S, Fyer AJ, Endicott J, Klein DF. *Family Informant Schedule and Criteria (FISC).* New York, NY: Anxiety Disorders Clinic, New York State Psychiatric Institute; 1985.
33 Leckman JF, Sholomskas D, Thompson WD, Belanger A, Weissman MM. Best estimates of lifetime psychiatric diagnosis: a methodological study. *Arch Gen Psychiatry.* 1982;39:879-883.
34. Wickramaratne PJ, Weissman MM, Horwath E, Adams P. The familial aggregation of panic disorder by source of proband ascertainment. *Psychiatr Genet.* 1994;4:125-133.
35. American Psychiatric Association Task Force on *DSM-IV. DSM-IV Options Book: Work in Progress.* Washington, DC: American Psychiatric Association; 1991.
36. American Psychiatric Association. *Diagnostic and Statistical Manual of Mental Disorders, Fourth Edition.* Washington, DC: American Psychiatric Association; 1994.
37. Horwath E, Johnson J, Hornig CD, Weissman MM. Social phobia diagnostic subtypes and the relationship between social phobia and panic disorder/agoraphobia. In: Frances A, Pincus H, Widiger TA, eds. *DSM-IV Sourcebook.* Washington, DC: American Psychiatric Press Inc. In press.
38. Mendlewicz J, Fleiss JL, Cataldo M, Rainer JD. Accuracy of the family history method in affective illness. *Arch Gen Psychiatry.* 1975;32:309-314.
39. Lavori PW, Keller MB, Endicott J. Improving the validity of FH-RDC diagnosis of major affective disorder in uninterviewed relatives in family studies: a model-based approach. *J Psychiatr Res.* 1988;22:249-259.
40. DiNardo PA, Moras K, Barlow DH, Rapee RM, Brown TA. Reliability of *DSM-III-R* anxiety disorder categories: using the Anxiety Disorders Interview Schedule-Revised (ADIS-R). *Arch Gen Psychiatry.* 1993;50:251-256.
41. Rosenbaum JF, Biederman J, Hirshfeld DR, Bolduc EA, Chaloff J. Behavioral inhibition in children: a possible precursor to panic disorder or social phobia. *J Clin Psychiatry.* 1991;52(suppl):5-9.
42. Rosenbaum JF, Biederman J, Gersten M, Hirshfeld DR, Meminger SR, Herman JB, Kagan J, Reznick JS, Snidman S. Behavioral inhibition in children of parents with panic disorder and agoraphobia. *Arch Gen Psychiatry.* 1988;45: 463-470.
43. Rosenbaum JF, Biederman J, Hirshfeld DR, Bolduc EA, Faraone SV, Kagan J, Snidman N, Reznick JS. Further evidence of an association between behavioral inhibition and anxiety disorders: results from a family study of children from a non-clinical sample. *J Psychiatr Res.* 1991;25:49-65.

ARCHIVES Circulation

The ARCHIVES is available by request to nonfederal physicians in the United States (50 states and Washington, DC) whose official American Medical Association masterfile record shows a primary specialty of psychiatry or child psychiatry in an office- or hospital-based practice as a staff physician, resident in training beyond the first year, or clinical fellow.

If you meet the above qualification criteria and are not currently receiving the ARCHIVES and would like to receive it each month, you must complete a free subscription request card. To receive a request card, please write to Kathryn Osten, American Medical Association, Circulation Processing Department, 515 N State St, Chicago, IL 60610 (fax 312-464-2580). A subscription request card will be sent to you in response. If you are a resident or fellow, please include verification of your training program and a complete mailing address.

Dose-Response Changes in Plasma Cortisol and Lymphocyte Glucocorticoid Receptors Following Dexamethasone Administration in Combat Veterans With and Without Posttraumatic Stress Disorder

Rachel Yehuda, PhD; David Boisoneau; Martin T. Lowy, PhD; Earl L. Giller, Jr, MD, PhD

Background: Our previous studies have suggested that combat veterans with posttraumatic stress disorder (PTSD) have alterations in hypothalamic-pituitary-adrenal axis functioning that are different from the well-documented biological changes observed in major depressive disorder and following exposure to stress.

Methods: In the present study, we examined cortisol and lymphocyte glucocorticoid receptor number before and after the administration of 0.50 and 0.25 mg of dexamethasone in 14 combat veterans with PTSD, 12 combat veterans without PTSD, and 14 nonpsychiatric healthy men. All subjects were medication free at the time of testing and none met diagnostic criteria for major depression or substance dependence.

Results: Combat veterans with PTSD suppressed cortisol to a greater extent than did combat veterans without PTSD and normal controls in response to both doses of dexamethasone. Differences in cortisol suppression could not be attributed to substance dependence history or differences in dexamethasone bioavailability. Combat veterans with PTSD showed a larger number of baseline glucocorticoid receptors compared with normal men. Combat veterans without PTSD also had a larger number of baseline glucocorticoid receptors compared with normal men and in fact were comparable to combat veterans with PTSD on this measure. However, only veterans with PTSD showed a decrease in lymphocyte glucocorticoid receptor number following dexamethasone administration.

Conclusion: The data support the hypothesis of an enhanced negative feedback sensitivity of the hypothalamic-pituitary-adrenal axis in PTSD.

(Arch Gen Psychiatry. 1995;52:583-593)

From the Departments of Psychiatry, Mount Sinai School of Medicine and Bronx Veterans Affairs Medical Center, New York, NY (Dr Yehuda), and University of Connecticut Health Center, Farmington (Mr Boisoneau); the Burroughs Wellcome Co, Research Triangle Park, NC (Dr Lowy), and CNS Research, Pfizer Inc, Groton, Conn (Dr Giller).

STUDIES OF the hypothalamic-pituitary-adrenal (HPA) axis in posttraumatic stress disorder (PTSD) have demonstrated a series of alterations that are distinct from those reported in major depressive disorder (MDD). Compared with normal subjects and other psychiatric patients, individuals with chronic PTSD show lower mean 24-hour urinary cortisol excretion,[1,2] lower baseline plasma cortisol levels,[3] increased numbers of cytosolic lymphocyte glucocorticoid receptors (GRs),[4,5] and an increased suppression of cortisol in response to the administration of dexamethasone.[6] These changes are different from the higher cortisol levels,[7-9] decreased lymphocyte GR number,[10-12] and dexamethasone nonsuppression[13,14] observed in MDD. On the other hand, some of the HPA alterations observed in PTSD are similar to those seen in depressive and anxiety disorders. For example, a blunted corticotropin response to corticotropin-releasing factor (CRF) was observed in combat veterans with PTSD compared with that of normal subjects.[15] More recently, an increased concentration of cerebrospinal fluid CRF has been reported in combat veterans with PTSD.[16]

We have hypothesized that HPA alterations in chronic PTSD may represent an enhanced negative feedback at one or more sites along the axis.[17-19] According to the model of enhanced negative feedback,[17] chronic increases in the release of hypothalamic CRF, resulting from differences in neuropeptide modulation, lead to an altered responsiveness of the pituitary, as evidenced by the blunted response of corticotropin to CRF challenge. However, because of a primary alteration in GR responsivity, there is a

See Methods on next page

METHODS

SUBJECTS

Twenty-six nonmedicated, nonhospitalized Vietnam combat veterans (age range, 40 to 50 years; mean±SD age, 44.1±0.56 years) and 14 nonpsychiatric, age-comparable men (age range, 30 to 49 years; mean±SD age, 37.6±1.4 years) participated in the study. Veterans were recruited from the Vietnam Veterans Outreach Center in Hartford, Conn (a facility that offers counseling and social services for veterans), and the Middletown (Conn) Vietnam Veterans group housed at the local armory (which meets for social and recreational purposes). Normal volunteers were recruited via advertisements in local newspapers and by word of mouth within the University of Connecticut Health Center in Farmington. All subjects provided written informed consent prior to undergoing a medical and psychiatric evaluation that included history taking, physical examination, and routine clinical laboratory tests (including urine toxicological studies). All the subjects were free from major medical illness, endocrinological disorder, psychotic or organic psychiatric illness, and psychoactive substance dependence (including alcohol) for at least 12 months. None were being treated with psychoactive medications for at least 4 weeks prior to their participation in the study.

The subjects were interviewed using the Structured Clinical Interview for *DSM-III-R*[41] and combat veterans were subdivided into groups of those meeting and those not meeting current *DSM-III-R* criteria for PTSD. Interrater reliability (κ statistic) for PTSD for the two raters (R.Y. and E.L.G.) using this instrument was 0.85. Nine of the 12 non-PTSD subjects had sought treatment for readjustment problems in the past, but none had been hospitalized for psychiatric-related problems in the 5 years prior to the study. No veteran met current *DSM-III-R* criteria for a primary current major comorbid mood (major depressive disorder or bipolar mania) or anxiety disorder as determined by the Structured Clinical Interview for *DSM-III-R*.

The severity of PTSD symptoms was determined using the Impact of Event Scale (IES)[42] and the Figley PTSD Scale.[43] Exposure to combat during the Vietnam War was quantified on a scale of 1 to 56 using the Combat Exposure Scale (CES).[44] Each veteran reported exposure to at least one specific traumatic event while in Vietnam.

THE DEXAMETHASONE SUPPRESSION TEST (DST)

The testing took place at the John Dempsey Hospital of the University of Connecticut Health Center. Two doses of dexamethasone (0.50 and 0.25 mg) were administered in randomized order, usually within 1 to 2 weeks of each other. State symptoms were determined on the following day of each of the two DSTs.

Fifty milliliters of whole blood was obtained by venipuncture at 8 AM and mononuclear cells were isolated using a cell separation medium (Ficoll-Hypaque, Pharmacia, Piscataway, NJ) within 1 hour following the drawing of blood. White blood cells were centrifuged at 300*g* at 4°C, washed four times in ice-cold Hanks' buffer solution, and pelleted. An aliquot of the lymphocyte suspension was counted using a hemocytometer, and the final pellet was stored at −70°C for subsequent determination of GR number. Plasma samples for cortisol determination were collected on ice, spun, aliquoted, and stored at −70°C for subsequent assay. At 11 PM, blood was drawn for cortisol determinations, and subjects received oral doses of 0.50 mg or 0.25 mg of dexamethasone. Blood samples for cortisol and dexamethasone levels were obtained at 8 AM and 4 PM the following morning. Lymphocytes were again isolated from post-dexamethasone 8 AM blood samples for the subsequent determination of cytosolic GR.

BIOCHEMICAL ASSAYS

Plasma cortisol levels were determined by radioimmunoassay using a commercially available kit (IncStar Inc, Minneapolis, Minn). The interassay and intra-assay coefficients of variation in our laboratory for this procedure were 6.8% and 4.0%, respectively. The dexamethasone levels were determined by radioimmunoassay using a commercially available antibody (IgG Corporation, Nashville, Tenn) as

stronger negative feedback resulting in attenuated baseline corticotropin and cortisol levels. Under conditions of enhanced negative feedback inhibition, the pituitary gland would be expected to show an augmented responsiveness to dexamethasone.

An enhanced sensitization of the HPA axis as reflected by a stronger negative feedback inhibition is compatible with some preclinical models of stress. Although stress is generally associated with an overactivation of the HPA axis and a resultant resistance of the HPA axis to glucocorticoid feedback signals,[20-24] the HPA axis may become sensitized under certain conditions of stress. For example, chronic stress in both adult[25-30] and developing[31-34] rats has been shown to result in exaggerated plasma corticosterone responses to subsequent, primarily acute and novel stressors.[25-30] Thus, depending on the type and timing of the stressor, either adaptation or sensitization of the HPA axis can occur.[35,36] Furthermore, some components of the HPA axis may become desensitized in response to stress, whereas others become more sensitized.[37] For example, a desensitization of the pituitary corticotroph following long-term CRF infusion has been demonstrated in in vivo and in vitro studies of the rat.[37] However, superimposition of a novel acute stressor can increase the attenuated corticotropin levels following chronic stress.[38,39]

The present study evaluated the cortisol and GR response to low doses of dexamethasone in combat veterans and normal volunteers. We previously reported an enhanced suppression of cortisol in severely symptomatic inpatients with PTSD (with and without comorbid MDD) following administration of 0.50 mg of dexamethasone.[6] However, a limitation of that study was that subjects had chronic and severe substance dependence histories. Because liver damage secondary to chronic alcohol abuse may lead to a decreased metabolism of dexamethasone and a resultant hypersuppression of cortisol,[40] it was not possible to evaluate the extent to which cortisol previously described.[6] The sensitivity of the dexamethasone assay as defined by the concentration of dexamethasone to decrease reference binding by 10% is approximately 5 to 10 pg per tube. The cross-reactivity of the antibody with cortisol is 0.04%, and with other endogeneous steroids (ie, progesterone, estradiol, aldosterone, and testosterone), less than 0.01%. The interassay and intraassay coefficients of variation in our laboratory were 8.2% and 6.0%, respectively.

Binding of lymphocyte GR was measured using a cytosolic radioligand binding assay as previously described.[4] Briefly, the frozen lymphocyte pellets (containing 50 to 100 million cells) were suspended in the assay buffer (consisting of TRIS, 10 mmol/L; ethylenediaminetetraacetic acid, 1 mmol/L; 1,4-dithiothreitol, 2.5 mmol/L; 10% glycerol; and sodium molybdate, 20 mmol/L; ph 7.4 [TEDGM]), mixed vigorously in the cold for 30 minutes, then spun at 250 000g for 30 minutes. Total binding of the ligand was measured in 0.25-mL aliquots of cytosol that were incubated overnight at 4°C with ligand, 10 nmol/L. Specific binding was defined as that inhibited by a 500-fold excess of unlabeled RU 28362. Following overnight incubation, bound steroid was separated from free-using columns packed with Sephadex LH-20 (Pharmacia), and washed with TEDGM buffer at 4°C. Most of the samples were assayed using tritiated RU 28362 as the ligand; however, owing to a shortage of this product from the only manufacturer and distributor of this ligand (Roussel Uclaf, Romanville, France), three of the 14 assays were run using tritiated dexamethasone. Prior to running samples with tritiated dexamethasone, our laboratory conducted the necessary quality-control study in which several concentrations of both ligands were evaluated in the same assay on pooled rat thymus and human lymphocytes. The results showed comparable specific-bound disintegrations per minute from pooled lymphocyte preparations when tritiated RU 28362, 10 nmol/L, and tritiated dexamethasone, 20 nmol/L, were used (ie, for the thymus sample, GR/cell=192.1 using 10-nmol/L tritiated RU 28362 and GR/cell=196.4 using 20-nmol/L tritiated dexamethasone; for the lymphocyte sample, GR/cell=5327 using 10-nmol/L tritiated RU 28362 and GR/cell=6387 using tritiated dexamethasone). Other laboratories have also shown comparable estimates of Type II receptors on lymphocytes with these two ligands (M.T.L. et al, oral communication, June 1992), reflecting the commonly held view that only a few Type I receptors are present in lymphoid tissue.[45-48] Samples from all three groups were always represented in each of the assays. The interassay and intraassay coefficients of variation for the GR assay were 22.0% and 14.0% using tritiated RU 28362, and 25.0% and 14.6% using tritiated dexamethasone.

DATA ANALYSIS

Cortisol data were subjected to three-way repeated-measures analysis of covariance (ANCOVA) (group×time×dose) with baseline cortisol values and dexamethasone levels as covariates. Dexamethasone and GR data were analyzed using a three-way repeated-measures analysis of variance (ANOVA) (group×time×dose). The percent cortisol suppression and percent glucocorticoid suppression were determined by dividing the 8 AM postdexamethasone values by the baseline values. Post hoc testing was performed using Tukey's test (two tailed), alpha $P<.05$. The impact of past substance dependence on the biological and clinical variables was also assessed by two-way ANOVAs using diagnoses and presence of past substance dependence.

Correlational analyses were performed to evaluate relationships among pairs of biological variables and between pairs of biological and clinical measures. For analyses of postdexamethasone variables, partial correlation controlled for dexamethasone level. There were four tests, one for each of the three individual subject groups and one for the total sample, for each pair of biological variables. To determine correlations between biological variables and clinical measures, each of four biological variables (percent cortisol suppression or percent GR suppression) were correlated with four symptom rating scale scores. Scores on the CES were correlated with cortisol and GR at each dosage level, and then with the four biological measures describing suppression to dexamethasone (ie, percent cortisol suppression and percent GR suppression at each dosage). After applying Bonferroni corrections, the results were considered significant only at the .0125 level.

suppression may have been related to changes associated with substance abuse.

In the present study we examined dose-dependent changes in cortisol levels and lymphocyte GR number following the administration of 0.50 and 0.25 mg of dexamethasone in nonhospitalized combat Vietnam veterans who were free from alcohol and other drug dependence for at least 1 year and in age-comparable nonpsychiatric men. We hypothesized that veterans with PTSD would show a hypersuppression of cortisol following dexamethasone administration compared with both veterans without PTSD and normal men, and that this response would be related to baseline lymphocyte GR number. Based on studies that show a positive association between cortisol suppression and percentage decline of GR following dexamethasone administration (hereafter also termed postdexamethasone),[10,12] we further predicted that cytosolic GR number would be decreased following dexamethasone administration (ie, reflecting the translocation of the bound steroid-complex into cell nucleus), particularly in subjects showing cortisol hypersuppression.

RESULTS

CLINICAL DATA

Clinical information is summarized in **Table 1**. Fourteen of the 26 veterans met *DSM-III-R* criteria for current PTSD. Veterans with PTSD showed significantly greater scores (mean±SD) on both the Figley PTSD Scale (33.7±10.6 PTSD vs 18.54±10.2 non-PTSD; $t=3.53$, $df=22$, $P=.002$) and the IES compared with veterans without PTSD (44.5±11.7 PTSD vs 25.9±13.8 non-PTSD; $t=3.57$, $df=22$, $P=.002$). Analysis of the IES subscales showed that the larger score in the PTSD groups was primarily owing to a higher severity of "intrusive" symptoms (20.9±8.0 PTSD vs 9.5±5.8 non-PTSD; $t=3.8$, $df=22$,

Table 1. Clinical and Descriptive Data for Combat Veterans

Subject No./ Age, y	Current PTSD*	Past PTSD	Past Substance Dependence	Figley Scale†	Impact of Event Scale‡ Intrusive	Impact of Event Scale‡ Avoidance	Combat Exposure Scale§
With PTSD							
1/41	Y	Y	N	20	13	18	14
2/42	Y	Y	Y	47	31	34	33
3/42	Y	Y	N	39	19	24	22
4/40	Y	Y	Y	31	16	25	47
5/42	Y	Y	Y	35	18	22	39
6/45	Y	Y	Y	51	35	22	45
7/46	Y	Y	N	31	14	21	42
8/44	Y	Y	Y	12	11	18	42
9/44	Y	Y	N	24	14	19	28
10/46	Y	Y	Y	...	30	29	37
11/50	Y	Y	Y	38	32	18	52
12/45	Y	Y	N	42	24	36	36
13/44	Y	Y	N	35	21	14	49
14/43	Y	Y	N	33	15	28	40
Without PTSD							
15/44	N	N	N	4	0	0	32
16/44	N	Y	N	15	4	6	21
17/43	N	N	Y	25	17	30	10
18/44	N	Y	Y	...	...	...	11
19/44	N	N	Y	38	12	20	11
20/46	N	N	N	11	19	5	33
21/45	N	Y	N	27	9	23	46
22/41	N	Y	Y	28	...	...	22
23/48	N	Y	Y	19	13	22	9
24/48	N	N	N	8	7	10	20
25/42	N	Y	Y	10	5	33	44
26/44	N	N	N	19	9	16	25

*PTSD indicates posttraumatic stress disorder.
†Figley PTSD Scale: range, 0-51.
‡Impact of Event Scale: range, 0-75 (intrusive subscale: range, 0-35; avoidance subscale: range, 0-40).
§Combat Exposure Scale: range, 0-56 (light combat, 0-6; moderate combat, 7-25; heavy combat, 26-56).

P=.001). The subjects with PTSD scored higher on the CES than those without PTSD (37.6±10.57 PTSD vs 23.67±12.8 non-PTSD; t=3.03, df=24, P=.006), but both group means reflected moderate to high combat exposure.

Although *DSM-III-R* criteria were not met by the 12 veterans in the non-PTSD group, half of these veterans met diagnostic criteria for past PTSD (Table 1). Table 1 also shows that half of the 26 veterans had a prior history of substance dependence (seven of 14 in the PTSD group and six of 12 in the non-PTSD group).

BIOLOGICAL DATA

Figure 1 and **Figure 2** show individual cortisol levels before and after dexamethasone administration at the 0.50- and 0.25-mg doses for subjects in all three groups. **Table 2** summarizes group means, SDs, and post hoc comparisons for all biological variables measured in this study. An initial ANOVA determined significant group differences in baseline cortisol levels; therefore, these values were used as covariates in analyzing the cortisol response to 0.50 and 0.25 mg of dexamethasone. Dexamethasone levels at 8 AM and 4 PM were also used as covariates to control for potential individual differences in dexamethasone bioavailability, although ANOVA failed to reveal significant group differences in dexamethasone levels in the present study. The final three-way ANCOVA of the cortisol data revealed significant effects for both the baseline cortisol covariate (T=2.381, P=.02) and the dexamethasone covariate (T=3.25, P=.002). Nonetheless, after correcting for these contributions to the cortisol response to dexamethasone, ANCOVA revealed significant main effects for group (F=10.57; df=2,36; P=.002) and time of day (F=28.51, df=1,36; P=.000). There were also significant group-by-dose (F=8.5; df=2,36; P=.001) and time-by-dose (F=20.94; df=1,36; P=.0001) interactions. Post hoc testing confirmed that the mean cortisol levels of the PTSD group were significantly lower than those of the two non-PTSD groups, and that the cortisol responses to dexamethasone in the veteran group without PTSD were comparable to those of the normal men following administration of both doses of dexamethasone. Significant main effects for group (F=4.62; df=2,37; P=.01) and dose (F=77; df=2,37; P=.0001) were also observed when the data were expressed as percent cortisol suppression at 8 AM. Again, post hoc testing confirmed that veterans with PTSD were significantly different from the two non-PTSD groups (Table 2). Thus, 0.25 mg of dexamethasone decreased plasma cortisol lev-

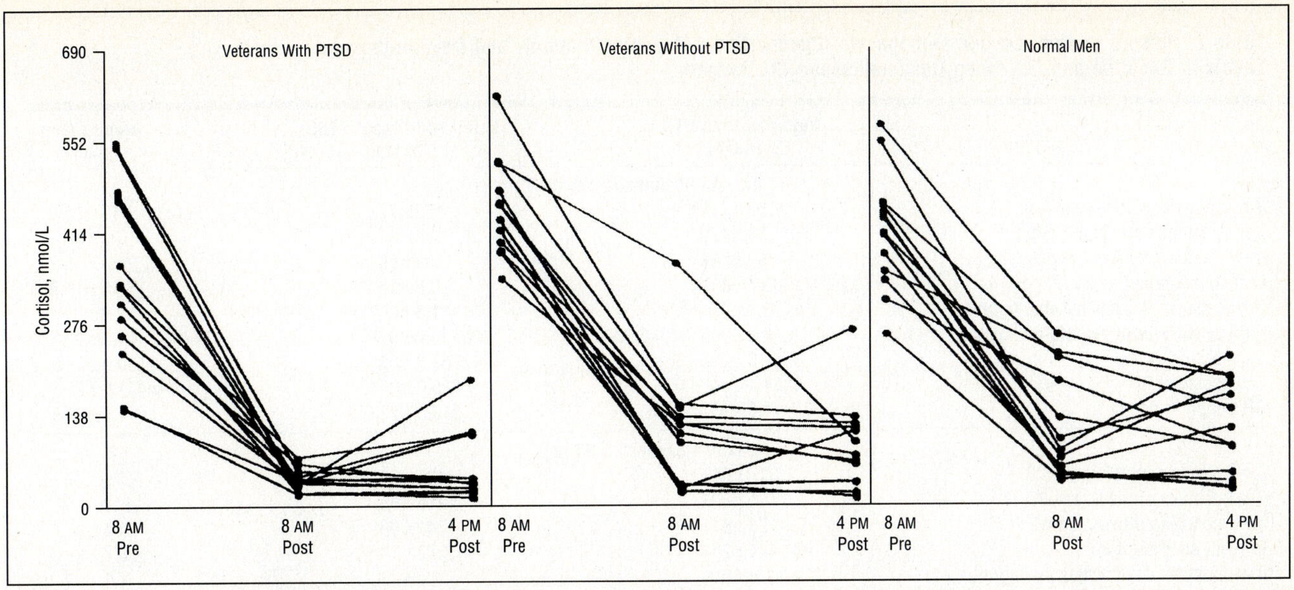

Figure 1. *Individual cortisol blood levels before (pre) and after (post) the administration of 0.50 mg of dexamethasone in male Vietnam veterans with and without posttraumatic stress disorder (PTSD) and age-comparable normal men.*

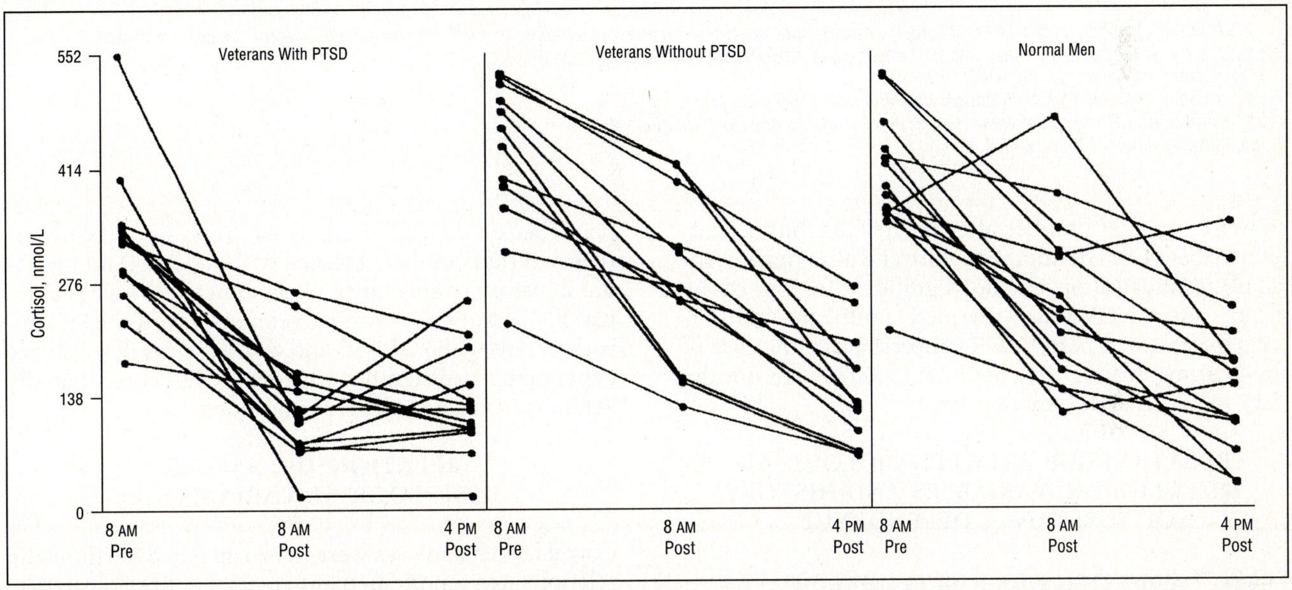

Figure 2. *Individual cortisol blood levels before (pre) and after (post) the administration of 0.25 mg of dexamethasone in male Vietnam veterans with and without posttraumatic stress disorder (PTSD) and age-comparable normal men.*

els at 8 AM in PTSD subjects, which is earlier than the time course for dexamethasone suppression in the non-PTSD veterans and normal controls.

Figure 3 and **Figure 4** show individual GR levels before and after dexamethasone administration at the 0.50-mg and 0.25-mg doses for subjects in all three groups. Because of missing observations, ANOVAs were conducted on data for each of the doses separately. Analysis of GR number before and after the administration of 0.50 mg of dexamethasone revealed a significant main effect of time (F=38.3; *df*=1,27; *P*=.0001) and a significant group-by-time interaction (F=16.7; *df*=2,27; *P*=.0001). Post hoc analysis showed that veterans with and without PTSD did not differ in mean baseline GR number; however, both groups had significantly higher GR numbers compared with the normal group (Table 2). All three groups showed a smaller number of cytosolic lymphocyte GRs following the administration of 0.50 mg of dexamethasone; however, only PTSD subjects had a significantly smaller number of post-dexamethasone GRs compared with baseline levels.

Analysis of lymphocyte GR number before and after the administration of 0.25 mg of dexamethasone showed significant main effects for group (F=3.5; *df*=2,32; *P*=.04) and time (F=6.1; *df*=1.32; *P*=.02). Post hoc analysis revealed that PTSD subjects showed a significantly greater number of receptors at baseline compared with normal subjects. The non-PTSD combat veteran group was not significantly different from either the PTSD group or the nonveteran normal group. Following the administration of 0.25 mg of dexamethasone, all the groups

Table 2. Plasma Cortisol Levels, Lymphocyte Glucocorticoid Receptor Number, and Dexamethasone Levels at Baseline and Following Dexamethasone Challenge*

	Veterans With PTSD (n=14)	Veterans Without PTSD (n=12)	Normal Men (n=14)
	Dexamethasone, 0.50 mg		
8 AM baseline cortisol, nmol/L	350±116†	452±77	413±88
8 AM postdex cortisol, nmol/L	30±17‡	108±97	108±80
4 PM postdex cortisol, nmol/L	52±52‡	88±69	108±74
Cortisol suppression, %	89.7±6.5‡	76.6±18.7	73.4±19.9
8 AM postdex dexamethasone, ng/mL	2.1±0.7	1.8±0.7	1.8±0.8
4 PM postdex dexamethasone, ng/mL	0.9±0.4	0.7±0.4	0.7±0.5
8 AM baseline GR§	8761.0±2987.0‖	7783.0±3048.0‖	4480.0±2326.0
8 AM postdex GR	5034.4±2462.0	6535.0±3019.0	4431.0±2804.0
GR suppression, %	44.0±15.2‡	11.33±22.0	14.0±25.5
	Dexamethasone, 0.25 mg		
8 AM baseline cortisol, nmol/L	317±86‡	425±94	395±77
8 AM postdex cortisol, nmol/L	124±69‡	276±99	248±102
4 PM postdex cortisol, nmol/L	124±61‡	141±69	154±94
Cortisol suppression, %	54.4±25.7‡	35.2±17.6	36.7±26.3
8 AM postdex dexamethasone, ng/mL	1.4±0.4	1.4±1.1	1.2±0.5
4 PM postdex dexamethasone, ng/mL	0.5±0.3	0.5±0.6	0.4±0.2
8 AM baseline GR	9440.9±4015.0‖	6797.0±2682.0	5027.0±3839.0
8 AM postdex GR	7487.0±6050.0	6126.0±2210.0	4131.0±2827.0
GR suppression, %	26.1±41.6	5.5±36.2	8.9±37.3

**PTSD indicates posttraumatic stress disorder; postdex, after dexamethasone administration; and GR, glucocorticoid receptor. Values are mean±SD. Post hoc testing for all biological variables was performed using Tukey's test (two tailed), alpha P<.05.*
†Significantly different from non-PTSD veterans.
‡Significantly different from both normal men and non-PTSD veterans.
§All lymphocyte GR values are expressed as number of receptors per lymphocyte.
‖Significantly different from normal men.

showed a smaller number of cytosolic GRs, but the difference between GR number before and after dexamethasone administration was not significant for any of the groups. An ANOVA also revealed significant main effects for group in percent GR suppression in the case of the 0.50-mg dose (F=6.0; *df*=2,27; *P*=.0075) but not the 0.25-mg dose of dexamethasone.

RELATIONSHIP BETWEEN BIOLOGICAL AND CLINICAL VARIABLES AND HISTORY OF SUBSTANCE DEPENDENCE

Table 3 shows the results of the two-way ANOVAs exploring the impact of past substance dependence on the biological and clinical variables. There were no significant main effects of past substance dependence behavior on any of the biological variables measured. There was one significant interaction (*P*=.05), which was GR number following the administration of 0.25 mg of dexamethasone. However, at least one significant result among 36 tests of significance (18 main effects and 18 interactions) would be expected by chance.

An ANOVA revealed a significant main effect of past substance dependence on the avoidant subscale of the IES. A significant interaction on this measure further indicated that high scores on this subscale were only observed in the non-PTSD combat veterans with a history of substance dependence. Combat veterans without PTSD and without a substance dependence history were significantly different from the other veterans. There was a significant interaction of diagnosis and past substance dependence on the CES. In this case, analysis of the means revealed that combat veterans without PTSD and without a history of substance dependence had scores comparable to those for combat veterans with PTSD. Combat veterans without PTSD and with a history of substance dependence had significantly lower CES scores than the veterans in the other three subgroups.

RELATIONSHIP AMONG BIOLOGICAL VARIABLES

Correlational analyses were performed to determine the relationships among percent cortisol suppression, percent GR suppression, baseline cortisol levels, baseline GR levels, postdexamethasone cortisol levels, and postdexamethasone GR levels in each of the subject groups separately and in the entire group as a whole. After adjusting the alpha level to correct for the number of comparisons, the only significant relationship observed was that between the percent suppression of cortisol and percent suppression of GR following the administration of 0.50 mg of dexamethasone when the entire sample was considered as a whole (r=.47, P=.009).

RELATIONSHIP BETWEEN SUPPRESSION TO DEXAMETHASONE AND CLINICAL SYMPTOMS IN COMBAT VETERANS WITH AND WITHOUT PTSD

The relationship between percent cortisol suppression and percent GR suppression and clinical variables (ie,

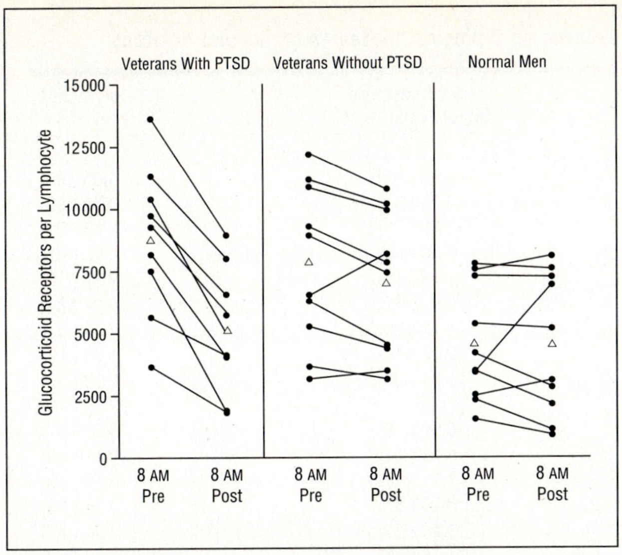

Figure 3. *Individual values of glucocorticoid receptors per lymphocyte before (pre) and after (post) the administration of 0.50 mg of dexamethasone in male Vietnam veterans with and without posttraumatic stress disorder (PTSD) and age-comparable normal men. Triangles represent group means.*

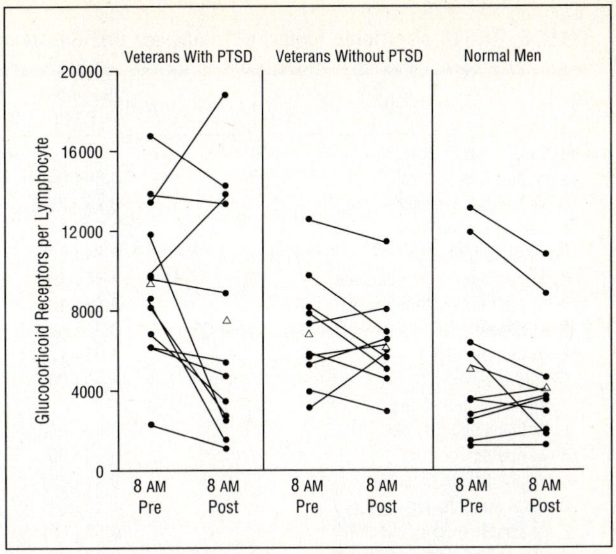

Figure 4. *Individual values of glucocorticoid receptors per lymphocyte before (pre) and after (post) the administration of 0.25 mg of dexamethasone in male Vietnam veterans with and without posttraumatic stress disorder (PTSD) and age-comparable normal men. Triangles represent group means.*

scores on the Figley PTSD Scale and the two subscales of the IES) was determined using correlational analysis controlling for dexamethasone levels as appropriate. After adjusting the criterion for significance to correct for multiple comparisons, there were no significant correlations between scores on any of the four symptom rating scales and the percent suppression of cortisol or GR following 0.50-mg dexamethasone administration.

There was a significant relationship between total IES scores and percent cortisol suppression following the administration of 0.25 mg of dexamethasone (r=.66, df=23, P=.0025). There was also a trend for a relationship between Figley PTSD Scale score and percent suppression to 0.25 mg of dexamethasone (r=.47, df=23, P=.04). Further analysis of the IES subscale scores revealed that the relationship between symptoms and cortisol suppression was owing to an association between "intrusive" symptoms and cortisol suppression (**Figure 5**). There were no significant relationships between clinical symptoms and percent GR suppression following the administration of 0.25 mg of dexamethasone.

RELATIONSHIP BETWEEN EXPOSURE TO TRAUMA AND BIOLOGICAL VARIABLES IN COMBAT VETERANS WITH AND WITHOUT PTSD

Scores on the CES were negatively correlated with baseline cortisol levels (r=.49, df=24, P=.01) and positively correlated with baseline GR number (r=.50, df=22, P=.01) at the 0.25-mg dose. After correcting for multiple comparisons, there were no significant relationships between CES scores and percent suppression of either cortisol or GR at either of the doses.

COMMENT

These results demonstrate that combat veterans with PTSD show a dose-related hypersuppression of cortisol in response to the administration of dexamethasone compared with both nonpsychiatric normal men and combat veterans without PTSD. These findings agree with previous data of cortisol hypersuppression following the administration of 0.50 mg of dexamethasone in inpatient combat veterans with PTSD,[6] and with the failure to observe a high rate of nonsuppression to the standard 1.0-mg dose in patients with PTSD.[49-53] The 0.25-mg dose allowed for the determination that cortisol hypersuppression following dexamethasone administration is significantly associated with the severity of PTSD symptoms. Baseline differences in plasma cortisol levels at 8 AM were also noted. The low cortisol levels observed in the PTSD group are consistent with prior observations of low urinary[1,2] cortisol excretion in PTSD. It is also possible, however, that the higher plasma cortisol levels at the 8 AM baseline in the two non-PTSD groups reflected a significant group difference in the stress of venipuncture.

Cortisol hypersuppression in PTSD appears to reflect the presence and severity of PTSD symptoms and is not likely an artifact of past substance dependence or individual differences in dexamethasone bioavailability. Although in the present study dexamethasone levels were found to be significantly associated with cortisol hypersuppression, reflecting the fact that individuals markedly differ in their ability to metabolize dexamethasone,[6,54] there were no significant *group* differences in dexamethasone levels that could account for the hypersuppression observed in subjects with PTSD. Furthermore, significant group differences in postdexamethasone cortisol levels were present after correcting for individual variation in dexamethasone levels.

Table 3. ANOVA Describing Impact of Diagnoses and Substance Dependence on Biological Measures on Combat Veterans*

	Diagnosis, F (*P*)	Past Substance Dependence, F (*P*)	Interaction, F (*P*)
Main effects (*df*=1,22)			
8 AM baseline cortisol	4.86 (.04)	0.01 (.92)	0.05 (.83)
8 AM postdex cortisol	8.28 (.009)	0.35 (.56)	0.69 (.69)
4 PM postdex cortisol	2.77 (.11)	3.28 (.08)	1.68 (.21)
Cortisol suppression	5.84 (.02)	0.56 (.46)	0.53 (.47)
8 AM postdex dexamethasone	1.81 (.19)	2.13 (.15)	2.87 (.10)
4 PM postdex dexamethasone	2.53 (.12)	0.05 (.82)	0.04 (.84)
8 AM baseline GR	0.35 (.55)	1.72 (.208)	2.00 (.17)
8 AM postdex GR	2.00 (.17)	2.39 (.14)	1.63 (.22)
GR suppression	11.48 (.004)	1.34 (.26)	0.29 (.59)
0.25-mg Dexamethasone			
8 AM baseline cortisol	8.46 (.008)	0.07 (.79)	0.03 (.87)
8 AM postdex cortisol	19.20 (.000)	0.13 (.72)	0.19 (.66)
4 PM postdex cortisol	0.51 (.48)	3.11 (.09)	0.50 (.49)
Cortisol suppression	4.42 (.04)	0.26 (.61)	0.00 (.99)
8 AM postdex dexamethasone	0.02 (.89)	1.60 (.21)	0.81 (.37)
4 PM postdex dexamethasone	0.00 (.94)	1.75 (.19)	0.29 (.59)
8 AM baseline GR	3.40 (.08)	0.04 (.84)	1.21 (.28)
8 AM postdex GR	0.66 (.43)	2.02 (.17)	4.55 (.04)
GR suppression	1.87 (.18)	3.05 (.10)	1.73 (.20)
Clinical symptoms			
Figley PTSD Scale	12.43 (.002)	2.64 (.11)	0.57 (.46)
IES intrusive subscale	15.11 (.0009)	3.93 (.06)	0.51 (.51)
IES avoidant subscale	3.24 (.09)	8.70 (.008)	6.56 (.01)
Combat Exposure Scale	10.74 (.003)	0.08 (.76)	6.01 (.02)

**Values represent the F values generated by two-way analysis of variance (ANOVA) with diagnosis (with and without posttraumatic stress disorder [PTSD]) and past substance dependence as independent variables. Postdex indicates after dexamethasone administration; GR, glucocorticoid receptor; and IES, Impact of Event Scale.*

The lack of difference between combat veterans without PTSD and nontraumatized normal men and the lack of correlation between suppression of cortisol and severity of combat exposure suggest that the response of cortisol to dexamethasone is unrelated to trauma exposure per se. An important question arising in all biological studies of PTSD is the extent to which the alterations being observed are related to the severity of trauma exposure, or rather to the subsequent development of a prolonged and debilitating disorder following such an experience. Epidemiological studies have now clearly demonstrated that PTSD, as currently described by *DSM-III-R*, develops in only a proportion of individuals exposed to trauma.[55-57] Approximately 15% of Vietnam combat veterans currently meet diagnostic criteria for PTSD.[57] The present findings suggest that cortisol suppression following dexamethasone administration is associated with the characteristics of PTSD, rather than the severity of the stressor that precipitated this condition.

On the other hand, cytsolic lymphocyte GR number at baseline does appear to be related to severity of trauma, rather than state symptoms of PTSD.[4] In contrast to the marked difference between veterans with and without PTSD in the response of cortisol to dexamethasone, the two combat veteran groups were not significantly different from each other in regard to the number of baseline lymphocyte GRs. To the extent that changes in lymphocyte and brain GR are similar,[58,59] the present findings of a larger number of GRs in combat veterans without PTSD compared with normal subjects and the positive correlation between lymphocyte GR number and severity of combat exposure support the idea that the increased baseline GR number in combat veterans may reflect a relatively permanent change in HPA axis regulation in response to the traumatic event.

Indeed, there is precedence in the preclinical literature for a permanent up-regulation of hippocampal GR in adult rats exposed to chronic early neonatal handling.[60,61] The up-regulation of GR following early handling is considered an exception to the general finding that stress and glucocorticoids result in a down-regulation of GR in brain and peripheral tissue in adult rats.[62,63] Although there are no prima facie parallels between the early neonatal handling paradigm and chronic PTSD as it occurs in war veterans, a careful consideration of potential similarities between this animal model of stress and PTSD is warranted (as discussed in Yehuda et al[64]). For example, future studies of GR regulation might consider the impact of early childhood trauma or pretrauma factors in patients with PTSD. Recent evidence indicates that the development of PTSD following war may be associated with a greater frequency of early childhood physical and sexual abuse.[65] To the extent that the development of PTSD in adulthood depends on earlier experiences, animal studies showing that stress-induced HPA axis activation is facilitated by prior chronic stress may be relevant to an understanding of PTSD.[18,19,25-30,66]

A substantial difference between the veteran groups with and without PTSD was that the increased number of GRs in the latter group was not accompanied by a decrease in basal cortisol secretion as it was in the combat veterans with PTSD. One of the major confounds in in-

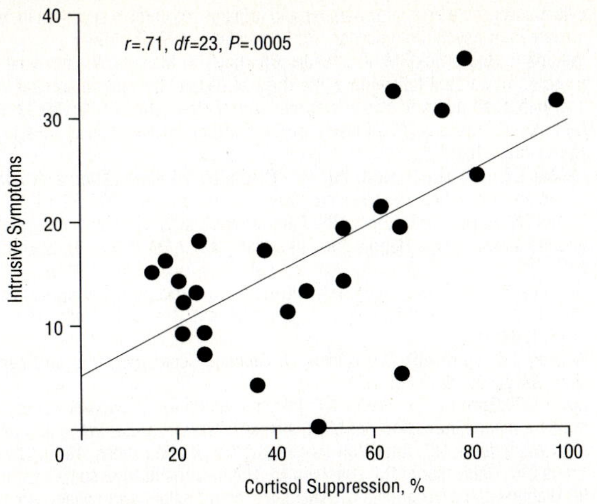

Figure 5. *Relationship between percent cortisol suppression following the administration of 0.25 mg of dexamethasone and the severity of intrusive symptoms (intrusive subscale of the Impact of Event Scale[42]) in Vietnam veterans with and without posttraumatic stress disorder.*

terpreting GR measurements in humans is that circulating steroids may be occupying the cytosolic receptor and translocating into the nucleus where GR can no longer bind to steroid.[67] In the present study, non-PTSD and normal subjects had comparable plasma cortisol levels, suggesting that ambient cortisol concentrations within a modest range do not likely have a major effect on the steady-state levels of cytosolic GR and, therefore, that lymphocyte GR numbers measured are not simply a result of alterations in circulating cortisol levels at the time the lymphocytes are collected.

Cytosolic lymphocyte GR number was not related to the response of cortisol to dexamethasone, as initially predicted. Rather, the extent of cortisol suppression to dexamethasone was related to group differences in the *reduction* of GR following dexamethasone administration. Previous studies in normal DST suppressors have also demonstrated a decrease in lymphocyte cytosolic GR following a 1-mg dose of dexamethasone, whereas DST nonsuppressors failed to show such a decrease.[10,12] The normal decrease in cytosolic GR following dexamethasone administration apparently occurs with no change in binding affinity.[68] Studies using cultured cells have also demonstrated a decrease in GR messenger RNA (mRNA) and total GR protein within 24 hours of glucocorticoid exposure, suggesting that homologously induced regulation occurs within a short time.[69,70] In the present study, the 0.50-mg dose of dexamethasone only produced a significant decrease in lymphocyte GR in veterans with PTSD. It will be important in future studies to determine if the increased number of GRs in subjects with PTSD is associated with a functional increase in GR sensitivity. Previous studies have used mitogen-induced lymphocyte proliferation as a functional test of in vitro GR sensitivity as it relates to DST status.[71]

The exact mechanism for the apparent heightened sensitivity of GR following dexamethasone administration in the PTSD group is not clear, but several possibilities can be explored in future studies. First, differences in receptor affinity (Kd) could account for these findings. Second, the observed decrease in cytosolic GR in the subjects with PTSD may be related to the relative proportion of receptors that are activated. One interpretation of the data is that the decrease in cytosolic GR observed following the administration of dexamethasone reflects dexamethasone-induced translocation of the cytosolic receptor to the nucleus, where it is incapable of binding radioligand.[67] Future studies that use in vitro translocation experiments in living cells or DNA-cellulose binding assays are needed to more firmly test the hypothesis that there is a greater degree of GR activation and nuclear translocation in response to glucocorticoids in patients with PTSD.

The larger decrease in cytosolic GR in the PTSD group may also represent a true down-regulation of the total GR content in the cells (ie, both cytosolic and nuclear GRs are decreased subjects with PTSD following dexamethasone administration). Examination of the total cellular amount of GR protein levels or GR mRNA expression will provide additional information concerning the dynamic regulation of GR gene expression in lymphocytes in veterans with and without PTSD. Finally, increased receptor down-regulation in patients with PTSD may be related to differences in subpopulations of lymphocytes and monocytes that are preferentially influenced by dexamethasone in the PTSD group.[72]

Future studies should also address the mechanisms that might contribute to enhanced negative feedback sensitivity of the HPA axis and, in particular, consider the role of neuromodulators and neuropeptides, in addition to CRF, which regulate the anterior pituitary gland. For example, basic research has shown that the coregulation of parvocellular CRF and vasopressin in the hypothalamus is important in adaptation to chronic stress.[73,74] Because the expression and release of CRF and vasopressin in hypothalamic parvocellular neurons appear to be differentially regulated by glucocorticoids,[75] it is possible that at least some of the negative feedback effects observed result from differences in the release of vasopressin. For example, increases in vasopressin expression in parvocellular CRF neurons may increase corticotroph responsiveness in postsynaptic CRF receptor sites.

The current findings have several important implications. First, there may be permanent changes in the regulation of the HPA axis following exposure to trauma that are qualitatively different from those associated with stressors of lower magnitude. Although some of the changes observed (ie, in GR number) may not necessarily be associated with the subsequent development of PTSD, they may contribute to the regulation of biological systems that are more directly associated with manifest symptoms of PTSD. For example, there is now substantial evidence for state-related catecholamine alterations in PTSD.[76-79] Furthermore, GR immunoreactivity has been demonstrated in the locus caeruleus and other brain areas known to contain catecholamines.[80] The state-related changes observed in HPA axis regulation may involve the interaction of multiple neurotransmitter-neuromodulatory systems that contribute to the induction of PTSD symptoms.

Second, some aspects of HPA axis functioning following exposure to extreme trauma (ie, the cortisol and GR responses to dexamethasone) are specifically related to the presence and severity of PTSD. The presence of state-related changes in HPA axis functioning in this disorder raises a question regarding the reversibility of this effect following successful pharmacological or other treatments. In this regard, the low-dose DST may be potentially useful as a measurement of treatment outcome.

Third, individuals with a history of trauma and/or PTSD can be clearly differentiated from patients with MDD. Thus, the low-dose DST may be useful in the differential diagnosis of PTSD vs MDD. The findings further suggest that assessment for trauma and PTSD symptoms is clearly warranted in biological studies of MDD. It has been striking that only a proportion of depressed patients studied to date show the classic features of hypercortisolemia and nonsuppression of cortisol following dexamethasone administration. It may be, therefore, that depressed patients with a history of trauma and/or PTSD symptoms would not show HPA axis changes that are consistent with a blunted negative feedback or hypercortisolemia.

Finally, the results suggest that the response to dexamethasone challenge appears to be bidirectional and that using moderate to very low doses of dexamethasone may allow for the discrimination of enhanced negative feedback from normal feedback. Although factors influencing this bidirectionality are still largely unknown, it would be important in future studies to determine if other traumatic stress response disorders, such as multiple personality disorder or borderline personality disorder, are similar to PTSD in regard to HPA axis regulation. It may be that nonsuppression vs hypersuppression to exogenous steroids may be dependent on baseline characteristics of the HPA axis that, in turn, are substantially influenced by prior history of stress and adaptation.

Accepted for publication April 11, 1995.

This work was performed at the University of Connecticut Health Center and was supported by a Health Center Faculty Research Award (Dr Yehuda), grant MH 49536 from the National Institute of Mental Health (Dr Yehuda), and Veterans Affairs Merit Review (Dr Yehuda).

We gratefully acknowledge Jane Thompson, MSW, of the Hartford Outreach Center for her assistance in patient recruitment. We also thank James Schmeidler, PhD, of Mount Sinai School of Medicine, New York, NY, for his expert statistical consultation.

Reprint requests to Psychiatry Department 116/A, Bronx VAMC, 130 W Kingsbridge Rd, Bronx, NY 10468 (Dr Yehuda).

REFERENCES

1. Mason JW, Giller EL, Kosten TR, Ostroff RB, Podd L. Urinary free-cortisol levels in post-traumatic stress disorder patients. *J Nerv Ment Dis.* 1986;174:145-159.
2. Yehuda R, Southwick SM, Nussbaum G, Giller EL, Mason JW. Low urinary cortisol excretion in PTSD. *J Nerv Ment Dis.* 1991;178:366-369.
3. Yehuda R, Teicher M, Trestman RL, Levengood RA, Siever LJ. Cortisol regulation in post-traumatic stress disorder: a chronobiological analysis. *Ann N Y Acad Sci.* 1994;746:378-380.
4. Yehuda R, Lowy MT, Southwick SM, Shaffer S, Giller EL. Increased number of glucocorticoid receptor number in post-traumatic stress disorder. *Am J Psychiatry.* 1991;149:499-504.
5. Yehuda R, Boisoneau D, Mason JW, Giller EL. Relationship between lymphocyte glucocorticoid receptor number and urinary-free cortisol excretion in mood, anxiety, and psychotic disorder. *Biol Psychiatry.* 1993;34:18-25.
6. Yehuda R, Southwick SM, Krystal JH, Charney DS, Mason JW. Enhanced suppression of cortisol following a low dose of dexamethasone in combat veterans with posttraumatic stress disorder. *Am J Psychiatry.* 1993;150:83-96.
7. Gibbons JL, McHugh PR. Plasma cortisol in depressive illness. *J Psychiatry Res.* 1962;1:162-171.
8. Sachar EJ, Hellman L, Roffwarg HP. Disrupted 24-hour patterns of cortisol secretion in psychotic depression. *Arch Gen Psychiatry.* 1973;28:19-24.
9. Kathol RG, Jaeckle RS, Lopez WF. Pathophysiology of HPA axis abnormalities in patients with major depression: an update. *Am J Psychiatry.* 1989;146:311-317.
10. Gormley GJ, Lowy MT, Reder AT. Glucocorticoid receptors in depression: relationship to the dexamethasone suppression test. *Am J Psychiatry.* 1985;142:1278-1284.
11. Whalley LJ, Borthwick N, Copolov D. Glucocorticoid receptors and depression. *BMJ.* 1986;292:859-861.
12. Lowy MT, Gormley GJ, Reder AT. Immune function, glucocorticoid receptor regulation and depression. In: Miller AH, ed. *Depressive Disorders and Immunity.* Washington DC: American Psychiatric Association Press; 1989:105-134.
13. Arana GW, Baldessarini RJ, Ornsteen M. The dexamethasone suppression test for diagnosis and prognosis in psychiatry: commentary and review. *Arch Gen Psychiatry.* 1985;42:1193-1204.
14. Carroll BJ. The dexamethasone suppression test for melancholia. *Br J Psychiatry.* 1982;140:292-304.
15. Smith MA, Davidson J, Ritchie JC, Kudler H, Lipper S, Chappell P, Nemeroff CB. The corticotropin releasing hormone test in patients with post-traumatic stress disorder. *Biol Psychiatry.* 1989;26:349-355.
16. Darnell A, Bremner JD, Licinio J, Krystal J, Nemeroff CB, Owens M, Erdos J, Charney DS. CSF levels of corticotropin releasing factor in chronic post-traumatic stress disorder. *Neurosci Abs.* 1994;20:15.4.
17. Yehuda R, Giller EL, Levengood RA, Southwick SM, Siever LJ. Hypothalamic-pituitary-adrenal functioning in PTSD: expanding the concept of the stress response spectrum. In: Friedman MH, Charney DS, Deutch AY, eds. *Neurobiological and Clinical Consequences of Stress: From Normal Adaptation to PTSD.* New York, NY: Raven Press. In press.
18. Yehuda R, Giller EL, Southwick SM, Lowy MT, Mason JW. Hypothalamic-pituitary-adrenal dysfunction in posttraumatic stress disorder. *Biol Psychiatry.* 1991;30:1031-1048.
19. Yehuda R, Resnick H, Kahana, B, Giller EL. Long-lasting hormonal alterations to extreme stress in humans: normative or maladaptive? *Psychosom Med.* 1993;55:287-297.
20. Young EA, Akana S, Dallman MF. Decreased sensitivity to glucocorticoid fast feedback in chronically stressed rats. *Neuroendocrinology.* 1990;51:536-542.
21. Vernikos J, Dallman MF, Bonner C, Katzen A, Shinsako J. Pituitary-adrenal function in rats chronically exposed to cold. *Endocrinology.* 1982;110:413-420.
22. Armario A, Restrepo C, Castellanos JM, Balasch J. Dissociation between adrenocorticotropin and corticosterone responses to restrain after previous chronic exposure to stress. *Life Sci.* 1985;36:2085-2092.
23. Natelson BH, Ottenweller JW, Cook J, Pirm SL, McCarty R, Tapp WNL. Effect of stressor intensity on habituation of the adrenocortical stress response. *Physiol Behav.* 1988;43:41-46.
24. Pitman DL, Ottenweller JE, Natelson BH. Plasma corticosterone levels during repeated presentation of two intensities of restraint stress: chronic stress and habituation. *Physiol Behav.* 1988;43:47-56.
25. Daniels-Severs A, Goodwin A, Keil LC, Vernikos-Danellis J. Effect of chronic crowding and cold on the pituitary-adrenal system: responsiveness to an acute stimulus during chronic stress. *Pharmacology.* 1973;9:348-356.
26. Sakellaris PC, Vernikos-Danellis J. Increased rate of response of the pituitary-adrenal system in rats adapted to chronic stress. *Endocrinology.* 1975;97:597-602.
27. Caggiula AR, Antelman SM, Aul E. Prior stress attenuates the analgesic response but sensitizes the corticosterone and cortical dopamine responses to stress 10 days later. *Psychopharmacology (Berl).* 1989;99:233-237.
28. Dallman MF, Jones MT. Corticosteroid feedback control of ACTH secretion: effect of stress-induced corticosterone secretion on subsequent stress responses in the rat. *Endocrinology.* 1973;92:1367-1375.
29. Katz RJ, Roth A, Carrol BJ. Acute and chronic stress effects on open field activity in the rat: implications for a model of depression. *Neurosci Biobehav Rev.* 1981;5:247-251.
30. Armario A, Hidalgo J, Giralt M. Evidence that the pituitary-adrenal axis does not cross-adapt to stressors: comparison to other psychological variables. *Neuroendocrinology.* 1988;47:263-267.
31. Levine S, Haltmeyer CG, Karas GG, Denenberg VH. Physiological and behavioral effects of infantile stimulation. *Physiol Behav.* 1976;2:55-59.
32. Haltmeyer GC, Denenberg VH, Zarrow MX. Modification of the plasma corticosterone response as a function of infantile stimulation and electric shock parameters. *Physiol Behav.* 1967;2:61-63.
33. Hess JL, Denenberg VH, Zarrow X, Pfeifer WD. Modification of the corticosterone response curve as a function of handling in infancy. *Physiol Behav.* 1969;4:109-111.
34. Ader R. The effects of early experience on the adrenocortical response to dif-

ferent magnitudes of stimulation. *Physiol Behav.* 1970;5:837-839.
35. Kant GJ, Eggleston T, Landman-Roberts L. Habituation to repeated stress is stressor specific. *Pharmacol Biochem Behav.* 1985;22:631-634.
36. Mason JW. Psychoendocrine approaches in stress reseach. *Symposium of Medical Aspects of Stress in the Military Climate.* Washington, DC: Walter Reed Army Institute of Research, US Government Printing Office; 1965:375-417.
37. Wynn PC, Harwood JP, Catt KJ, Aguilera G. Corticotropin-releasing factor (CRF) induces sensitization of the rat pituitary CRF-receptor adenylate cyclase complex. *Endocrinology.* 1988;122:351-358.
38. LeMevel JC, Abitbol S, Veraud G, Maneity J. Temporal changes in plasma adrenocorticotropin concentration after repeated neurotropic stress in male and female rats. *Endocrinology.* 1979;105:812.
39. Vernikos J, Dallman MF, Bonner C, Katzen A, Shinsako J. Pituitary-adrenal function in rats chronically exposed to cold. *Endocrinology.* 1972;110:413-420.
40. Carson SW, Halbreich U, Yeh CM, Galanter M. Liver function, plasma dexamethasone, and DST results in detoxified alcoholics. *Psychiatry Res.* 1989; 30:217-221.
41. Spitzer RL, Williams JBW. *Structured Clinical Interview for* DSM-III-R. New York: New York State Psychiatric Institute, Biometrics Research; 1985.
42. Horowitz M, Wilner N, Alvarez W. Impact of Event Scale: a measure of subjective distress. *Psychosom Med.* 1979;41:209-218.
43. Figley CR, Stretch RH. *Vietnam Veterans Questionnaire.* West Lafayette, Ind: CR Figley, Family Research Institute, Purdue University; 1980.
44. *Long-term Stress Reactions: Some Causes, Consequences and Naturally Occurring Support Systems: Legacies of Vietnam: Comparative Adjustment of Veterans and Their Peers.* Washington, DC: US Government Printing Office; 1981;14.
45. Lowy MT, Meltzer HY. Dexamethasone bioavailability: implications for DST research. *Biol Psychiatry.* 1987;22:373-385.
46. Miller AH, Spencer RL, Stein M, McEwen BS. Adrenal steroid receptor binding in spleen and thymus after stress or dexamethasone. *Am J Physiol.* 1990;14: E405-E412.
47. Murakami T, Brandon D, Rodbard D, Loriauz DL, Lipsett MB. Glucocorticoid receptor in circulating mononuclear leukocytes. *Endocrinology.* 1979;104:500-505.
48. Armanini D, Strasser T, Weber PC. Characterization of aldosterone binding sites in circulating human mononuclear leukocytes. *Am J Physiol.* 1985;248:E388-E390.
49. Kudler H, Davidson J, Meador K, Lipper S, Ely T. The DST and posttraumatic stress disorder. *Am J Psychiatry.* 1987;144:1068-1071.
50. Halbreich U, Olympia J, Carson S, Glogowski J, Yeh CM, Axelrod S, Desu MM. Hypothalamo-pituitary-adrenal activity in endogenously depressed posttraumatic stress disorder patients. *Psychoneuroendocrinology.* 1989;14:365-370.
51. Kosten TR, Wahby V, Giller E Jr, Mason J. The dexamethasone suppression test and thyrotropin-releasing hormone stimulation test in posttraumatic stress disorder. *Biol Psychiatry.* 1990;28:657-664.
52. Olivera AA, Fero D. Affective disorders, DST, and treatment in PTSD patients: clinical observations. *J Traumatic Stress.* 1990;3:407-414.
53. Dinan TG, Barry S, Yatham LN, Mobayed M, Brown I. A pilot study of a neuroendocrine test battery in posttraumatic stress disorder. *Biol Psychiatry.* 1990; 28:665-672.
54. Meikle AW. Dexamethasone suppression tests: usefulness of simultaneous measurement of plasma cortisol and dexamethasone. *Clin Endocrinol.* 1982;16: 401-408.
55. Breslau N, David GC, Andreski P, Peterson E. Traumatic events and posttraumatic stress disorder in an urban population of young adults. *Arch Gen Psychiatry.* 1991;48:216-222.
56. Helzer JE, Robins LN, McEvoy L. Post-traumatic stress disorder in the general population: findings of the Epidemiological Catchment Area survey. *N Engl J Med.* 1987;317:1630-1634.
57. Kulka RA, Schlenger WE, Fairbank JA, Hough RL, Jordan BK, Marmor CR, Weiss DS. *Trauma and the Vietnam War Generation.* New York, NY: Brunner/ Mazel; 1990.
58. Lowy MT. Reserpine induced decrease in type I and II corticosteroid receptors in neuronal and lymphoid tissue of adrenalectomized rats. *Neuroendocrinology.* 1990;51:190-196.
59. Lowy MT. Quantification of type I and II adrenal steroid receptors in neuronal, lymphoid, and pituitary tissues. *Brain Res.* 1989;503:191-197.
60. Meany MJ, Aitken DH, Bodnoff SR, Iny LJ, Sapolsky RM. The effects of postnatal handling on the development of the glucocorticoid receptor systems and stress recovery in the rat. *Prog Neuropsychopharmacol Biol Psychiaty.* 1985; 9:731-734.
61. Meaney MJ, Aitken DH, Bodnoff SR, Iny LJ, Taterewicz JE, Sapolsky RM. Early postnatal handling alters glucocorticoid receptor concentrations in selected brain regions. *Behav Neurosci.* 1985;99:765-77.
62. Saplosky RM, Krey LC, McEwen BS. Stress down regulates corticosterone receptors in a site specific manner in the brain. *Endocrinology.* 1984;114:287-292.
63. Sapolsky RM, Krey LC, McEwen BS. Prolonged glucocorticoid exposure reduces hippocampal neuron number: implications for aging. *J Neurosci.* 1985; 5:1221-1226.
64. Yehuda R, Southwick SM, Perry BD, Mason JW, Giller EL. Interactions of the hypothalamic-pituitary-adrenal axis in the catecholaminergic system in posttraumatic stress disorder. In: Giller EL, ed. *Biological Assessment and Treatment of Posttraumatic Stress Disorder.* Washington DC: American Psychiatric Association; 1990.
65. Bremner JD, Southwick SM, Johnson DR, Yehuda R, Charney DS. Childhood physical abuse and combat-related posttraumatic stress disorder in Vietnam veterans. *Am J Psychiatry.* 1993;150:235-239.
66. Yehuda R, Antelman S. Criteria for rationally evaluating animal models of posttraumatic stress disorder. *Biol Psychiatry.* 1993;33:479-486.
67. Svec F. Minireview: glucocorticoid receptor regulation. *Life Sci.* 1985;36:2359-2366.
68. Schlecte JA, Ginsburg BH, Sherman BML. Regulation of the glucocorticoid receptor in human lymphocytes. *J Steroid Biochem.* 1982;16:69-74.
69. Burnstein KL, Jewell CM, Cidlowski JA. Human glucocorticoid receptor cDNA contains sequences sufficient for receptor downregulation. *J Biol Chem.* 1990; 266:7284-7291.
70. Bellingham DL, Sar M, Cidlowski JA. Ligand-dependent down-regulation of stably transfected human glucocorticoid receptors is associated with the loss of functional glucocorticoid responsiveness. *Mol Endocrinol.* 1992;6:2090-2102.
71. Lowy MT, Reder MT, Gormley GJ, Meltzer HY. Comparison of in vivo and in vitro glucocorticoid sensitivity in depression: relationship to the dexamethasone suppression test. *Biol Psychiatry.* 1988;24:619-630.
72. Distelhorst CW, Benutto BM. Glucocorticoid receptor content of T lymphocytes: evidence for heterogeneity. *J Immunol.* 1991;126:1630-1634.
73. Rivier C, Vale W. Modulation of stress-induced ACTH release by corticotropin-releasing factor, catecholamines and vasopressin. *Nature.* 1983;305:325-327.
74. Dimphena CE, de Goeij DJ, Tilders FJH. Repeated stress enhances vasopressin synthesis in corticotropin releasing factor neurons in the paraventricular nucleus. *Brain Res.* 1992;577:165-168.
75. Sawchenko PE. Evidence for a local site of action for glucocorticoids in inhibiting CRF and vasopressin expression in the paraventricular nucleus. *Brain Res.* 1987;403:213-224.
76. Yehuda R, Southwick SM, Giller EL, Ma X, Mason JW. Urinary catecholamine excretion and severity of PTSD symptoms in Vietnam combat veterans. *J Nerv Ment Dis.* 1992;180:321-325.
77. Yehuda R. Neuroendocrinology of post-traumatic stress disorder. *Curr Opin Psychiatry.* 1992;5:109-112.
78. Murburgh MM. *Catecholamine Function in Posttraumatic Stress Disorder: Emerging Concepts.* Washington, DC: American Psychiatric Association Press; 1993.
79. Southwick SM, Krystal JH, Morgan CA, Johnson D, Nagy LM, Nicolaou A, Heninger GR, Charney DS. Abnormal noradrenergic function in posttraumatic stress disorder. *Arch Gen Psychiatry.* 1993;50:266-274.
80. Harfstrand A, Fuxe K, Cintra A, Agnati LF, Zini AC, Wikstrom S, Okret ZY, Yu M, Goldstein W, Steinbus A, Verhofstad A, Gustafsson JA. Glucocorticoid receptor immunoreactivity in monoaminergic neurons of rat brain. *Proc Natl Acad Sci U S A.* 1986;83:9779-9783.

Conversions From Système International (SI) Units to Traditional Units (Modified From *The SI Manual in Health Care*)

System	Component	SI Reference Interval*	SI Unit	Conversion Factor (Divide by)	Traditional Reference Interval*	Traditional Unit
Serum	Cortisol					
	8 AM	110-520	nmol/L	27.59	4-19	μg/dL
	4 PM	50-410	nmol/L	27.59	2-15	μg/dL
	Midnight	<140	nmol/L	27.59	<5	μg/dL

**These reference values are not intended to be definitive since each laboratory determines its own values. They are provided for illustration only.*

ORIGINAL ARTICLE

Mental Illness and Suicide

A Case-Control Study in East Taiwan

Andrew T. A. Cheng, MD, PhD, MRCPsych

Background: As part of the Taiwan Aboriginal Study Project, a case-control study of suicide among two aboriginal groups and the Han Chinese was carried out in East Taiwan.

Methods: Biographical reconstructive interviews were conducted for consecutive suicides from each of the three ethnic groups (a total of 116 suicides), 113 of whom were matched with two controls for age, sex, and area of residence.

Results: In all three groups, a high proportion of suicides suffered from mental illness before committing suicide (97% to 100%). The two most prevalent psychiatric disorders were depression and alcoholism, and the most common comorbid pattern was depression with substance use disorders. The risk for suicide was significantly associated with all of these psychiatric conditions, previous suicide attempts, and a family history of suicide and depression. Fifty-one percent of all suicides had consulted medical professionals in the previous month.

Conclusion: Despite the widely different rates of depressive illness and alcoholism in different cultures previously reported, the psychiatric antecedents of suicide are the same in the West and the East.

(Arch Gen Psychiatry. 1995;52:594-603)

PREVIOUS STUDIES using biographical reconstructive methods among consecutive suicides in Western societies have reported that most persons who commit suicide suffer from mental illness before committing suicide.[1-10] The two most common mental disorders preceding suicide have consistently been found to be depressive illness and alcoholism, with most suicides seeking medical treatment before committing suicide.

The relationship between mental illness and suicide has not been well investigated in non-Western societies, in which biographical studies of consecutive suicides in the community have never been conducted, nor has the impact of depressive illness and alcoholism on suicide been examined. Previous epidemiological studies of mental disorders in Chinese communities have consistently reported much lower prevalences of alcoholism and depressive illness than their Western counterparts.[11-16] Furthermore, according to hospital records, the prevalence of mental illness among suicides is only 10% in Taiwan.[17] I therefore hypothesized that rates of mental disorders among suicides should be much lower in Chinese societies than in Western societies. This hypothesis is tested in this biographical study in East Taiwan.

From the Institute of Biomedical Sciences, Academia Sinica, Taipei, Taiwan.

RESULTS

Of all the suicides, 72 were men and 45 were women. More men committed suicide than women in all three groups, but the difference was mainly evident in the Chinese. The peak age for suicide was older than 65 years in the Chinese group, but between 25 and 44 years in the two aboriginal groups (**Table 1**). The age-standardized incidence rate of suicide in the Atayal (68.2 per 100 000) was significantly higher than in the Ami (15.6 per 100 000) and the Chinese (18.0 per 100 000).

SYMPTOM PROFILE AND DIAGNOSES

Wide-ranging psychiatric symptoms in suicides before death were reported by key informants. The most frequent moderate to

See Subjects and Methods on next page

SUBJECTS AND METHODS

THE SAMPLE

Two aboriginal groups (the Atayal and the Ami) and the Han Chinese in Taiwan were selected for the study on the basis of a preliminary inquiry into official vital statistics for 1981 to 1985, which had found a high suicide rate in Atayal (46.3 per 100 000) and a low rate in Ami (5.3 per 100 000).[18] The study took place in the adjacent counties of Hualien and Taitung in eastern Taiwan. Consecutive suicides were first identified in all three ethnic groups between July 1989 and June 1990 in Hualien County, including residents of that county who committed suicide elsewhere. Visitors and transients who committed suicide there were then excluded. Fifty-seven cases from the Chinese remained. To obtain totals of 30 cases for each aboriginal group, consecutive suicides of Atayal and Ami in Hualien County and Ami in Taitung County, between July 1990 and December 1991, were similarly collected. Each suicide was matched with two living controls for age (±5 years), sex, and area of residence during the year before committing suicide. Controls were randomly selected from the census record.

ASCERTAINMENT OF SUICIDE

In Taiwan, a death verdict of unnatural causes is jointly assigned by a prosecutor and coroner, whose main concern is the possibility of homicide. Since suicide has never been a crime in Taiwan, a suicide verdict helps only in excluding this possibility. Therefore, although prosecutors and coroners may identify suicide as the cause of unnatural death and may record this in confidential inquest notes, often this is not recorded on the official death certificate that is delivered to the health department.

As the first stage in ascertaining suicide, the research team reclassified all unnatural nonhomicidal deaths into suicide, accident, and undetermined groups. The inquest notes, which included postmortem reports, were jointly examined and prosecutors and coroners were interviewed within a few days of the suicide. The final classification was reached by joint discussion among research team members. The second stage of case identification included all potential suicides and undetermined deaths. All death records of each ethnic group at the Hualien and Taitung Health Office during the investigation period also were reviewed, and unnatural deaths (except for victims of traffic accidents) without a legal examination were also included in this stage of inquiry, conducted through fieldwork.

THE FIELDWORK

Key informants of potential cases, including close relatives and significant others, were contacted approximately 1 month after the death occurred. A direct home visit introduced by a public health nurse or local civil servant was conducted. A biographical reconstructive interview was conducted for those deaths that were judged to be either suicides or undetermined. Informed consent was obtained after the research team had expressed concern about the suicides' living family members and explained the purpose of the study. Confidentiality about interview records was assured. Key informants of the controls were also interviewed in the same month. A psychiatrist (A.T.A.C.) and two clinical psychologists (one of whom is an aborigine) conducted the interviews separately. All interviewers have had years of experience in field interviews related to mental illness.

The interview inventory was first thoroughly discussed, then a joint pretest was conducted using 10 suicides (from all three groups) that had occurred just before July 1989. Medical professionals who had seen the suicide victim before death were interviewed and their records were reviewed. Suicide notes were also reviewed. To further improve the reliability of the assessment, audiotape recordings of many of the interviews were made with informed consent.

The fieldwork was completed in December 1991, and the results were jointly discussed by the three interviewers to decide which cases were suicides. Only one case was classified as an undetermined death because of disagreement between the interviewers. Altogether, 117 suicides were identified during the survey period. One young man had committed suicide with a gun during his military service. His medical record was not available until recently,

Continued on next page

severe symptoms were those commonly observed in patients with major depression. Other common symptoms included anxiety, irritability, and somatic symptoms. Panic, excessive concern with physical health, aggressive behavior, and organic/psychotic symptoms were less frequent. None of the suicides had obsessional symptoms (excluding depressive rumination). Most symptoms were similarly prevalent in suicides from all groups. However, rates of irritability, agitation, and aggressive behavior were significantly higher in the aboriginal than in the Chinese suicides; the reverse was observed for somatic concern.

Nearly all the suicides had had one or more forms of mental disorder. **Table 2** lists percentages of individual *DSM-III-R* Axis I diagnoses among the suicides. In all groups, the most prevalent disorder was major depression, followed by alcohol use disorders, dysthymia, organic mental disorders, and schizophrenia. None of the suicides had anxiety or dissociative disorders. For comparison, the most prevalent mental disorder among the controls of all the groups was alcohol use disorders (25.2%), followed by major depression (22.1%), adjustment disorder (9.3%), dysthymia (8.0%), anxiety disorders (6.6%), and organic mental disorders (2.2%). None of the controls had functional psychoses. The major differences between the suicides and controls were the suicides' much higher rates of major depression and alcohol use disorders.

DEPRESSIVE DISORDERS

Major depression was the predominant diagnosis in all groups. If dysthymia is added, the percentages increased to more than 90% in each group. There was no significant difference in rates of single-episode and recurrent major depression between the groups. However, the prevalence of dysthymia was significantly higher in the aboriginal groups than in the Chinese group ($P<.01$). Conversely, and all his close relatives were dead. The other 116 suicide cases had satisfactory data and were therefore included in the clinical study. Three of the 116 suicides, long-institutionalized psychotic patients, were excluded from the case-control study because their controls could not be properly selected. Informants of controls for the 113 suicides were all successfully interviewed.

Several key informants were identified for most suicide cases. The mean number interviewed was six for the suicides and five for the controls. In 92.2% of the suicide cases and 92.5% of the controls, family members who had lived with them were interviewed. For a further 6.9% of suicides and 0.9% of controls, the people who visited the candidates daily were interviewed.

THE INTERVIEW

The interview used a semi-structured biographical inventory, initially constructed as a considerably modified version of that used by Barraclough et al[3] in their suicide study in England, to fulfill the requirements for *DSM-III-R*[19] diagnoses. A second revision was performed according to the pretest results. Revisions also incorporated psycholinguistic equivalents and native idioms for major emotional symptoms in Chinese and aborigines, gathered in previous epidemiological studies.[13,14,18,20]

Based on the pretest, psychiatric symptoms were rated as follows: severe, 3; moderate, 2; mild, 1; or absent, 0. A rating of 0 was given when the subject (suicide or control) did not complain of and did not manifest the symptom; 1 indicates that the subject mildly manifested or complained of the symptom and his or her social function remained intact or only slightly less effective; 2 denotes an observable and self-reported symptom frequently moderate or sometimes severe, with somewhat impaired social function; and 3 refers to an observable and self-reported symptom frequently severe, with marked impairment of social function. Although symptoms in suicides are likely to be underestimated if mild, the principle of "always rate down" was followed.

The inventory included 295 items covering suicidal behavior (27 items), medical and psychiatric history and clinical conditions at the time of death (122 items), and associated psychosocial factors (146 items). The interviewers allocated scores and also recorded relevant descriptive information (including audiotape transcription) for all the items.

RELIABILITY AND PSYCHIATRIC DIAGNOSIS

Using the results of the pretest, the interrater reliability was examined. The κ coefficients for the three raters ranged from 0.78 to 1.00. The main items with disagreement largely concerned suicidal behavior (such as assessment of preparatory actions before suicide, preventability of the suicidal act, and the suicide's knowledge about the fatality of the suicide method used). The interview records of all 116 suicides were jointly reviewed by the interviewers to reach a final agreement. Any residual disagreement was then clarified by audiotape records and/or further visits to the interviewees. The remaining slight disagreement mainly included assessment of symptoms in two suicides lacking psychiatric diagnosis.

Not blind to subjects' case or control status, I made the psychiatric diagnoses of suicides and controls according to *DSM-III-R*. However, the clinical data of 15 suicides and 15 controls randomly selected from the three groups were given to another senior psychiatrist who was blind to their case or control status for independent diagnoses. Interrater reliability between us was satisfactory, with 100% agreement for major depression, substance use disorder, adjustment disorder, schizophrenia, and organic mental disorder.[21]

DATA ANALYSIS

Descriptive statistics were used to investigate the incidence of suicide, the distribution of psychiatric symptoms and diagnoses, and other independent variables in suicides and controls. Conditional logistic regression was then applied to evaluate the relationship between different clinical variables and suicide.[22] Student's *t* test, which does not take into account the matching design, was performed on mean values of age at onset and duration of illness between suicides and controls with major depression and alcoholism.

prevalences of major depression among controls in the aboriginal groups were significantly higher than among controls in the Chinese group ($P<.01$). Rates of dysthymia did not differ between the three groups.

Among all 102 depressive suicides, one had dysthymia and 72 had major depression only; the other 29 had dysthymia superimposed with major depression. The prevalence of "double depression" in depressive suicides was significantly higher in the Atayal (37%) and the Ami (50%) than in the Chinese (12%) ($P<.002$). Among the suicides with double depression, three quarters had recurrent major depression and the rest had single-episode major depression in all three groups.

Major depression was diagnosed in 60 male and 41 female suicides, with a prevalence sex ratio (F/M) of 1.1. The female-male ratios in all groups were very similar. The mean age at death for all the suicides with major depression was 47.1 years (SD=18.7); for men it was 49.1 years (SD=18.3) and for women it was 44.1 years (SD=19.2). This mean age differed significantly among the groups only for men ($F=4.19$; $df=2,57$; $P=.02$), being higher in the Chinese group (54.8, SD=19.0) than in the Atayal group (39.2, SD=16.1) (Scheffé's test). There was no sex difference in mean age of the suicides with major depression in any group.

The age at onset of the first episode of major depression was higher in Chinese suicides than in the Ami and Atayal suicides. Such difference was only statistically significant for men ($F=4.01$; $df=2,57$; $P=.024$), with the onset in the Chinese (49.4, SD=19.1) being later than in the Atayal (34.0, SD=14.3) (Scheffé's test). The mean duration of current episode of major depression was 5.3 months (SD=5.7): 24% of the episodes in cases had lasted less than 1 month; 52%, less than 3 months; and 73%, less than 6 months. Only 7% of episodes had lasted more than 1 year. The mean duration of illness was similar in

Table 1. Age and Sex Distribution of Consecutive Suicides Among Three Ethnic Groups in East Taiwan (1989-1991)

Age Group, y	Atayal M	Atayal F	Ami M	Ami F	Han Chinese M	Han Chinese F	Total M	Total F
15-24	4	5	1	1	3	2	**8**	**8**
25-44	9	4	9	7	11	7	**29**	**18**
45-64	4	2	5	6	8	5	**17**	**13**
≥65	1	1	1	0	16	5	**18**	**6**
Total	**18**	**12**	**16**	**14**	**38**	**19**	**72**	**45**

Table 2. Percentage of *DSM-III-R* Diagnoses Among 116 Consecutive Suicides in East Taiwan

DSM-III-R Categories*	Atayal (n=30)	Ami (n=30)	Han Chinese (n=56)	Total (N=116)
Organic mental disorders	10.0	3.3	7.1	6.9
Dementia (290)	0.0	0.0	1.8	0.9
Alcoholic psychosis (291)	10.0	3.3	3.6	5.2
Drug psychosis (305.90)	0.0	0.0	1.8	0.9
Mental retardation (317)	0.0	0.0	1.8	0.9
Schizophrenia (295)	6.7	6.7	5.4	6.0
Schizophreniform disorder (295.40)	0.0	0.0	1.8	0.9
Major depression	83.3	86.7	89.3	87.1
Single episode (296.2)	36.7	40.0	50.0	44.0
Recurrent (296.3)	46.7	46.7	39.3	43.1
Dysthmia (300.4)	36.7	43.3	10.7	25.9†
Alcoholic use disorders	70.0	53.3	25.0	44.0‡
Abuse (305.00)	30.0	16.7	8.9	16.4
Dependence (303.00)	40.0	36.7	16.1	27.6
Drug abuse (305.70, 304.60, 304.90)	10.0	0.0	3.6	4.3
Adjustment disorder (309)	3.3	3.3	0.0	1.7
Pathological gambling (312.31)	0.0	0.0	3.6	1.7
No mental disorder	3.3	3.3	0.0	1.7

**Each case may have more than one diagnosis.*
†*P*<.001.
‡*P*<.002.

all groups, with no significant difference across all sex and ethnic groups.

The prevalence of dysthymia in all the suicides was 21.1% in men and 33.3% in women. Rates of dysthymia in men were significantly higher in the aboriginal groups than in the Chinese group (*P*<.02). There was no significant difference in current age, onset age, and duration of illness in the suicides with dysthymia either among the three groups or between the sexes.

According to univariate conditional logistic regression analysis, the risk for suicide for any type of depressive disorder was highly significant in each group, except for dysthymia in the Chinese group (**Table 3**). The odds ratio (OR) of suicide for major depression was 11 times that for dysthymia. The OR of suicide for any depressive illness was 13.4 times that for nondepressive illness.

A simple comparison between the suicides and controls with major depression found that the age at onset was not significantly different between cases and controls in the three groups (**Table 4**). However, the mean duration of current episode was significantly higher in controls, a difference mainly evident in the Atayal and Chinese groups. For dysthymia, the onset age and duration of illness were not significantly different between the suicides and controls.

ALCOHOL USE DISORDERS

The prevalence of alcohol use disorders in the suicides was significantly different between the groups (Table 2). For both abuse and dependence, the Atayal had the highest rate, the Chinese the lowest. The alcoholic suicides included 40 men and 11 women, with a prevalence sex ratio (M/F) of 2.3 (*P*<.001). The male-female ratios in the Atayal, Ami, and Chinese groups were 2.8, 1.9, and 3.1, respectively. The difference between the three groups in the prevalence of alcoholism was significant for men only, in both suicides (*P*<.0001) and controls (*P*<.001).

The mean age of the male alcoholic suicides was 38.5 years (SD=13.9). More than one third (38%) were younger than 20 years at onset, and only 18% had onset at older than 30 years. Two thirds (65%) of the male alcoholic suicides had been alcoholic for more than 10 years and 28% for more than 20 years. No significant difference was found between the groups in age at suicide, onset age, or duration of alcoholism.

The risk for suicide was significant for alcohol dependence but not for alcohol abuse (Table 3). This trend was consistent in all three groups. In fact, the prevalence of alcohol abuse was similar in the suicides and controls (17.7%), whereas the controls had a much lower prevalence of alcohol dependence than the suicides. The age at onset of alcoholism in the male alcoholics was significantly earlier in cases than in controls for all groups (Table 4). In the aboriginal groups, the duration of alcoholism was significantly longer in cases than in controls.

MISCELLANEOUS DIAGNOSES

Seven suicides had schizophrenia. According to the *International Classification of Diseases, 10th Edition (ICD-10), Diagnostic Criteria for Research,*[23] one of them had postschizophrenic depression (F20.4, a comorbid condition of 311.00 in *DSM-III-R*) and two had schizoaffective disorder, depressive type (F25.11). One suicide suffered from schizophreniform psychosis (the diagnosis is schizophrenia according to *ICD-10*). The prevalence of "functional psychoses" in the suicides was almost the same in all ethnic groups.

Four of the schizophrenic suicides were paranoid and the remaining three were of undifferentiated type. All seven committed suicide under the influence of auditory hallucinations and/or paranoid delusions. Five schizophrenic suicides also had depression, as did the case with schizophreniform psychosis. Altogether, 75% of the suicides with functional psychoses manifested vivid depressive syndrome preceding the suicide. Alcoholism was found in three (38%) schizophrenic suicides, all of whom were aborigines. Among the eight psychotic suicides, three had been institutionalized for more than 10 years, and

Table 3. Odds Ratio of Suicide for Mental Disorders in Three Ethnic Groups: Univariate Conditional Logistic Regression Analysis*

	Atayal			Ami			Han Chinese	
***DSM-III-R* Diagnosis**	**Suicides**	**Controls**	**OR (95% CI)**	**Suicides**	**Controls**	**OR (95% CI)**	**Suicides**	**Controls**
Major depression, single episode								
No	19	52	1.0	18	53	1.0	25	101
Yes	11	8	4.2 (1.3-13.4)†	12	7	3.8 (1.4-10.1)‡	28	5
Major depression, recurrent								
No	16	48	1.0	16	49	1.0	31	99
Yes	14	12	6.6 (1.8-23.8)‡	14	11	5.1 (1.6-16.1)‡	22	7
Dysthymia								
No	19	54	1.0	17	53	1.0	47	101
Yes	11	6	4.4 (1.5-12.7)‡	13	7	5.5 (1.8-17.0)‡	6	5
Alcoholism								
None	9	38	1.0	14	38	1.0	39	93
Abuse (305)	9	16	2.0 (0.7-6.1)	5	19	1.0 (0.3-3.7)	5	5
Dependence	12	6	6.5 (1.9-21.6)‖	11	3	7.2 (1.8-29.8)‡	9	8
Adjustment disorder								
No	29	54	1.0	29	52	1.0	53	99#
Yes	1	6	0.3 (0.0-2.7)	1	8	0.3 (0.03-2.0)	0	7
Organic and psychotic disorders								
No	25	60#		27	59	1.0	48	102
Yes	5	0	. . .	3	1	6.0 (0.6-57.7)	5	4
Single and comorbid disorders								
No morbidity	1	21	1.0	1	21	1.0	0	54#
Single morbidity	6	21	7.4 (0.8-65.4)	6	21	5.0 (0.6-41.7)	34	46
Comorbidity	23	18	25.3 (3.0-215.6)‡	23	18	12.6 (1.7-93.3)†	19	6
Total	**30**	**60**		**30**	**60**		**53**	**106**

**OR indicates odds ratio; CI, confidence interval.*
†*P*<.02.
‡*P*<.01.
§*P*<.001.
‖*P*<.002.
¶*P*<.05.
#There was no convergence.

the rest had been ill for 2 to 24 months (mean, 7.5 months).

Eight suicides, all men, had organic mental disorders. They included six who had chronic alcoholism with alcoholic psychoses, one with inhalant (glue) intoxication and dependence coexisting with alcohol dependence, and one who had dementia of senile onset with delusions (most probably 290.20). The six alcoholic suicides included two with alcoholic hallucinosis (290.30) and four with alcohol withdrawal delirium (291.00). They had been alcoholic long before the onset of depression and probably committed suicide under the influence of both psychotic symptoms and depression. Seven of these eight suicides also had depressive syndrome (three with double depression, three with major depression, and one with dysthymia). In contrast, all five controls with organic mental disorders had dementia of senile onset (one with depression and four were probably uncomplicated).

Contrary to the male predominance in alcoholic suicides, four of the five suicides with substance abuse were young women. The substances used included glue (two), amphetamines (two), and barbiturates (two). Four were also alcoholics and all five suicides with drug abuse were comorbid with depression. Other suicides with psychiatric diagnoses included two young men with adjustment disorder (one combined with alcoholic abuse), two men with pathological gambling (312.13), and one elderly man with mild mental retardation (the last three were also comorbid with major depression). The two cases with adjustment disorder manifested vivid agitation and aggressive behavior (one machine-gunned his military colleagues before shooting himself). Frequencies of adjustment disorder and anxiety disorders were conversely higher in the controls.

COMORBIDITY

Comorbidity (56%) was more common in the suicides than single morbidity (42%), whereas the reverse was true in the controls ($P<.001$). However, whereas there was more comorbidity in the aboriginal suicide groups, the Chinese suicide group had more single morbidity (Table 3). The most frequent single morbid condition in the suicides was major depression in all groups (67% to 100%), and other diagnoses were few (except for functional psychoses). For the suicides with a comorbid condition, major depression with substance use disorders was most common (43%), followed by double depression with substance use disorders (26%), and double depression (17%). The percentage of depressive

OR (95% CI)	Total: Suicides	Total: Controls	Total: OR (95% CI)
1.0	62	206	1.0
13.6 (4.8-38.9)§	51	20	6.6 (3.7-12.1)§
1.0	63	196	1.0
8.2 (3.1-21.8)§	50	30	6.8 (3.6-12.9)§
1.0	83	208	1.0
2.7 (0.7-9.7)	30	18	4.2 (2.2-8.1)§
1.0	62	169	1.0
3.1 (0.7-14.3)	19	39	1.6 (0.8-3.4)
3.2 (1.0-10.1)¶	32	18	5.5 (2.7-11.2)§
...	111	205	1.0
	2	21	0.2 (0.04-0.8)¶
1.0	100	221	1.0
2.5 (0.7-9.3)	13	5	5.2 (1.9-14.6)∥
	2	96	1.0
...	46	88	42.0 (5.7-309.3)§
	65	42	169.6 (21.8-1321)§
	113	**226**	

illness with substance use disorders comorbidity in the three groups ranged from 65% to 78%. Among the suicides with major depression, the rates of comorbidity with substance use disorders in the Atayal, Ami, and Chinese groups were consistently higher in men (100%, 71%, and 31%, respectively) than in women (36%, 42%, and 17%, respectively).

Clearly almost all (96%) the suicides who had substance use disorders also had other psychiatric conditions (mainly depressive disorders) in all groups. Their clinical history usually indicated that the onset of alcoholism preceded depression, which often appeared to be a complication of the former, as did marked deterioration in physical health and social functioning.

Overall, the most prevalent psychiatric morbid condition in the Chinese suicide group was a single morbid condition of major depression (55%), and that in the aboriginal suicide groups was depressive illness with substance use disorders comorbidity (56.7% in the Atayal and 50.0% in the Ami). These differences correspond to the much higher prevalence of alcoholism among the aborigines.[24]

The risk for suicide for comorbidity was four times that for single morbidity (Table 3). Comorbidity of depression and substance use disorders had the highest risk for suicide (OR=470.2, 95% confidence interval [CI]=44.7 to 4942), followed by major depression only (OR=168, 95% CI=17.0 to 1664), and all other comorbid conditions (OR=112.6, 95% CI=11.0 to 1156). The risk for suicide was not significant for any other single morbidity.

SUICIDES WITH NO PSYCHIATRIC DIAGNOSIS

Two aboriginal female suicides were not diagnosed as having mental illness. A 17-year-old Atayal woman committed suicide to force her grandmother to submit to her demands. No morbid symptoms were observed before the event, except a possibly subclinical dysphoric mood. A 42-year-old Ami housewife killed herself immediately after a severe quarrel with her husband during a celebration party with heavy drinking. Her mental condition was judged to be normal, except for a sensitive personality trait, and without drinking problems before the event. These two suicides both ingested pesticide. Previous studies have often found a small proportion of suicides with serious medical conditions but no mental illness, but these two suicides were physically healthy before committing suicide.

FAMILY HISTORY, PREVIOUS SUICIDE ATTEMPTS, AND WARNINGS

The percentages of suicides with a family history of suicide, depressive illness, and alcoholism in first-degree relatives were consistently highest in the Atayal group and lowest in Chinese group (**Table 5**). In case-control analysis, the risk for suicide was significant for a family history of suicide and depression, but not for alcoholism. Such risk was only significant for family history of suicide in the Atayal group, and not for history of depression or alcoholism in any group.

Twenty-one percent of the suicides had previous suicide attempt(s) verified by key informants; no significant interethnic difference existed. The risk for suicide was significant for previous suicide attempts in the Atayal and Chinese groups. More than half of the suicides gave warnings (direct or indirect) before the event. The Atayal were significantly more likely to give warning than the Ami or Chinese ($P<.05$), and the risk for suicide was highly significant for both direct and indirect warnings.

MEDICAL CONSULTATION

The frequencies of medical consultation among the suicides in the previous 1, 3, and 6 months of life were 43%, 43%, and 43% in the Atayal group; 47%, 53%, and 53% in the Ami group; and 55%, 66%, and 70% in the Chinese group, respectively. Hence, most consultation in each group was made within the last month of life. Compared with the controls, the consultation frequency in the suicides was significantly higher for the last 3 and 6 months among the Chinese group only. The suicides most commonly visited general practitioners and medical specialists in general hospitals (47%); only 13% had seen a psychiatrist. Chinese men but not women had significantly more consultations than the two aboriginal groups ($P<.05$). Altogether, 8% of the suicides sought help from nonmedical institutions (eg, the church or Lifeline International

Table 4. Age at Onset and Duration of Illness in Suicides and Controls With Major Depression and Alcoholism

	Atayal		Ami		Han Chinese		Total	
	Suicides	Controls	Suicides	Controls	Suicides	Controls	Suicides	Controls
Suicides With Major Depression								
Age at onset, y								
Mean (SD)	34.0 (14.3)	33.9 (13.3)	41.3 (13.5)	41.6 (17.6)	49.4 (19.1)	53.1 (18.5)	43.5 (17.7)	41.2 (17.6)
t Value	0.05		−0.05		−0.60		0.75	
Duration of current episode, mo								
Mean (SD)	5.0 (6.3)	12.5 (16.4)	5.1 (4.7)	7.1 (6.5)	5.6 (5.9)	15.1 (13.0)	5.3 (5.7)	11.2 (12.9)
t Value	−2.10*		−1.17		−3.81†		−3.84†	
Total No.	**25**	**20**	**26**	**18**	**50**	**12**	**101**	**50**
Male Alcoholic Suicides								
Age at onset, y								
Mean (SD)	20.9 (5.4)	29.5 (10.8)	24.4 (7.7)	32.5 (7.6)	24.8 (11.2)	38.2 (17.6)	23.0 (8.1)	32.9 (12.5)
t Value	−2.98‡		−2.68§		−2.25*		−4.28†	
Duration, y								
Mean (SD)	15.2 (9.3)	7.6 (8.0)	16.7 (7.8)	8.7 (6.5)	14.8 (11.7)	12.6 (10.7)	15.5 (9.5)	9.3 (8.5)
t Value	2.62§		2.84‡		0.48		3.17‖	
Total No.	**17**	**19**	**11**	**15**	**12**	**13**	**40**	**47**

*P<.05.
†P<.0001.
‡P<.01.
§P<.02.
‖P<.002.

in Hualien). Only one quarter of the suicides were taking any psychotropic drugs. More Chinese suicides (34%) were receiving drug treatment than those in the two aboriginal groups (13% and 17%). The percentage of the suicides receiving psychotropic medication was significantly higher than that of the controls in the Chinese and Ami groups.

Benzodiazepines (22%) were the most commonly prescribed drugs, followed by neuroleptics (12%). Tricyclic antidepressants were prescribed for only 4% of all the suicides. Of the different diagnostic groups, psychotic subjects were most commonly receiving medication (53%), followed by depressive subjects (20%). Among the 25 suicides receiving psychotropic medication, nonpsychiatric physicians had prescribed the drug for 64%, and psychiatrists for 52%. All had received benzodiazepines, and 64% received neuroleptics and/or tricyclic antidepressants from psychiatrists. The remaining 36% were prescribed only benzodiazepines by nonpsychiatric physicians. Among the 14 suicides receiving neuroleptic medication, 10 were psychotic and the rest were nonpsychotic depressive. None of the latter received tricyclic antidepressants, but three of them were given a low dose of chlorpromazine (50 mg) for insomnia and one received thioridazine (175 mg) for severe depression.

The mean chlorpromazine equivalent dose of neuroleptics for the 10 psychotic suicides was 205 mg (SD=109 mg), and the doses of tricyclic antidepressants for five suicides with severe depression ranged from 25 to 100 mg. These doses were insufficient for treatment. For many cases, the duration of medication treatment before committing suicide was too short: 60% of those receiving a tricyclic antidepressant had taken it for less than 1 week, and 50% of the 10 psychotic suicides had taken neuroleptics for less than 3 weeks. The drug compliance of these psychotic and depressive suicides was largely poor and without adequate supervision. Furthermore, 80% of the depressive suicides receiving tricyclic antidepressants and 50% of the psychotic suicides receiving neuroleptics had stopped taking the medication for over 1 week before committing suicide.

COMMENT

METHODOLOGICAL VALIDITY OF THE STUDY

The validity of this study mainly depends on the accuracy of reporting from coroners and key informants and the reliability of the interview and psychiatric diagnosis. Barraclough et al[3] argued that the effects of mental illness, life insurance companies, and social stigma on the misclassification of suicide by coroners were negligible. This study reaches the same conclusion in Taiwan, but for quite different reasons. Coroners in Taiwan rarely inquire about a suicide's psychological condition and there is no social stigma on suicide in Chinese and aboriginal societies nowadays. However, they do quite accurately inquire about suicide intentions to exclude the possibility of homicide. Only two elderly suicides were misclassified as accidental deaths. They committed suicide by drowning and the coroners failed to discover their depressive illness before the event. Coroners frequently do not document suicide unless the suicidal behavior is quite obvious (eg, hanging). Other causes of death (usually "accident") are often put on the death certificate for official uses to avoid any argument with insurance agencies and suicides' relatives. It is therefore highly likely that the underestimation of suicide in Taiwan reflects methods of suicide. This issue is currently under investigation.

In previous studies, relatives of suicides have been found to underestimate psychiatric symptoms and illness, owing partly to memory effects and their difficulty in recognizing nonobservable symptoms and abnormal behaviors and partly to reluctance to admit any mental problems of suicides.[3] Such biases might also exist in the study herein, particularly because mental illness bears a strong social stigma in Chinese society. Relatives usually attributed the suicide act to life events or misfortunes, and rarely spontaneously mentioned suicides' abnormal behavior. Explicit mention of mental illness was avoided in this study's interview, which always started by inquiring about physical health and somatic symptoms. The high rate of mental illness in the suicides described herein implies that false negatives are few, if any. However, I do not think mental illness was overdiagnosed.

Informants for the controls were interviewed to obtain the same level of recall information for controls and suicides. Even so, resistance to reporting psychiatric conditions by informants was comparatively minor for the controls. Moreover, because of the delay between the suicides' death and the interview, the recall of events by informants probably was less accurate for the suicides than for controls. These potential information biases would underestimate the strength of association between clinical variables and suicide.

The possibility of a systematic bias from the interviewer seems unlikely, since interrater reliability among the three interviewers in the pretest was satisfactory, and the reliability between independent diagnoses by me and another psychiatrist in this study was very satisfactory.[21] I made the psychiatric diagnoses, having carried out thousands of psychiatric interviews in Chinese[13] and aboriginal communities,[18,20] and am trained in the use of several well-known psychiatric interview schedules such as the Schedule for Affective Disorders and Schizophrenia,[25] the Schedules for Clinical Assessment in Neuropsychiatry,[26] and the Clinical Interview Schedule.[27] The interrater reliability between me and British psychiatrists was satisfactory.[28] Comparability between the findings herein and those in Western surveys can thus be reasonably ensured. Although Student's *t* test for mean age at onset and duration of illness might have underestimated the true association for subsets of suicides and controls with major depression and alcoholism, this would not materially affect the positive findings. Overall, therefore, the methodological validity of this study appears satisfactory.

COMPARISONS WITH OTHER STUDIES

Table 6 lists findings in 10 biographical studies of suicide.[1-10] The overall prevalences of mental disorders were similarly high (82% to 100%). In all the studies except one,[4] the most prevalent principal diagnosis was depressive illness, followed by substance use disorders. Differences in the frequencies of principal and individual diagnoses might be attributed in part to differences in the diagnostic criteria that were used and the demographic characteristics of the sample subjects. However, the rates of main principal diagnoses were similar between surveys in England[3] and East Taiwan. The prevalence of depressive illness was greater than 80% in England and East Taiwan, and prevalences of substance use disorders were greater than 40% in several places including East Taiwan.[2,4,6,8] The percentages of suicides with either of these diagnoses ranged from 65% in Sweden[4] (male suicides only) to 94% in East Taiwan. The rates of these two disorders in

Table 5. Attempted Suicides, Warnings, and Family History of Mental Disorders Among Suicides*

	Atayal (n=30)	Ami (n=30)	Han Chinese (n=56)	Total (N=116)
Family history†				
Suicide	12 (40)	3 (10)	1 (2)	16 (14)‡
Depression	14 (47)	5 (17)	4 (7)	23 (20)‡
Alcoholism	26 (87)	20 (67)	9 (16)	55 (47)‡
Previous suicide attempt	6 (20)	4 (13)	14 (25)	24 (21)
Threats and warnings	23 (77)	16 (53)	26 (46)	65 (56)§

*Data are given as number (percent).
†In parent, sibling, or child.
‡$P<.001$ for comparison between the three ethnic groups.
§$P<.05$ for comparison between the three ethnic groups.

the suicides presented herein, contrary to my initial speculation, were high in comparison with those reported in other studies. Such findings cannot be solely attributed to the much higher prevalence of depression and alcoholism among the aboriginal population[20,24] since the figures were also high among the Chinese suicides.

In several studies, most depressive disorders among suicides were severe. For instance, depressive suicides in the English survey[3] had much worse symptoms than their matched living "endogenous" depressive controls, and 63% of the former were of the recurrent type. All the depressive suicides in the St Louis, Mo, series[1] had a major depressive episode before committing suicide and 46% had previous episodes of mania or depression. All except one of the depressive suicides in the present study had had a major depressive episode before committing suicide and 49% of them had had recurrent depressions.

Some studies have emphasized a higher risk for suicide in older persons with depression (92% older than 40 years in the St Louis study,[1] 75% older than 45 years in the English study[3]), a notion supported by our findings for the Chinese suicides (70% over age 40 years), but not for the aboriginal suicides (32% and 46% over age 45 years in the Atayal and Ami groups, respectively). Just over 50% of depressive suicides in the Brisbane, Australia, study[5] were older than 45 years, and 43% were older than 59 years in the Swedish study of Asgard.[10] The evidence therefore suggests that the age-specific risk for suicide in depressive subjects varies in different ethnic groups and societies. This also might apply to duration of the last depressive episode preceding suicide, which was significantly longer in the English study[3] (50%, <6 months) and the St Louis study[1] (57%, <6 months) than in East Taiwan (73%, <6 months) ($P<.05$). However, the English analysis included all types of depressives, whereas only those with major depression were included in the other two studies.

Most alcoholic suicides in this study were men, and they had a significantly earlier onset age and longer duration of alcoholism than the alcoholic controls. Alcoholic suicides in the English[3] and St Louis[1] studies also had such trends. The mean durations of alcoholism in all three studies were between 16 and 25 years, and the proportions of alcoholic suicides aged less than 20 years or younger than 30 years at the onset of alcoholism are *similar* between the English study (33% and 80%) and the study herein (33% and 75%). These

Table 6. Psychiatric Disorders Among Consecutive Suicides*

Study	Years of Study	Site of Study	N†	Depressive Disorders	Substance Use Disorders	Schizophrenic Disorders‡	Other Disorders	No Disorders
Unselected cases								
Robins et al[1]	1956-1957	St Louis, Mo	134	45	25	2	22	6
Dorpat and Ripley[2]	1957-1958	Seattle, Wash	108	30	27 (42)	12	31	0
Barraclough et al[3]	1966-1968	England	100	70 (80)	16 (19)	4	3	7§
Chynoweth et al[5]	1973-1974	Brisbane, Australia	135	45 (55)	24 (34)	4	15	12
Rich et al[7]	1981-1983	San Diego, Calif	198	. . . (47)	. . . (51)	6	20	6‖
Arato et al[8]	1985	Budapest, Hungary	200	64	8 (20)	9	1	19¶
Current study	1989-1991	East Taiwan	116	65 (89)	24 (45)	7	3	2#
Age <30 y, both sexes								
Runeson[9]	1984-1987	Göteborg, Sweden	58	24 (64)	3 (47)	16	55	2#
Males, all ages								
Beskow[4]	1970-1971	Sweden	271	28 (45)	37 (49)	3	29	3§
Females, all ages								
Asgard[10]	1982	Stockholm, Sweden	104	57	12	5	22	5¶

**Values represent percentages of principal (primary) diagnosis and those in parentheses are based on individual diagnostic entities.*
†*Includes only suicides with sufficient clinical information.*
‡*Including schizoaffective and schizophreniform psychoses.*
§*Using* International Classification of Diseases, Eighth Revision *criteria.*
‖*Using* DSM-III *criteria, only multiple diagnoses were reported.*
¶*Using Research Diagnostic Criteria.*
#*Using* DSM-III-R *criteria.*

figures suggest that the risk for suicide for alcoholism is higher for early-onset alcoholics, and is mainly confined to later periods of the disease.[29]

Contrary to the usual pervasive female preponderance of depressive disorders, generally no significant sex difference in the rates of major depression is found among suicides.[1,3,7,8] The higher suicide rate in men might partly derive from men's greater rate of alcoholism.[7] Our findings further suggest that the similar rates of major depression in male and female suicides might reflect a male excess in comorbidity involving major depression with substance use disorders.

The frequency of functional psychoses among suicides is generally low. Similar to suicides in the St Louis,[1] San Diego, Calif,[6] and Budapest, Hungary,[8] studies, none of the suicide cases reported herein had anxiety or dissociative disorders. Three percent of the English suicides had a phobic disorder (one had comorbid drug dependence).[3] Therefore, while the risk for suicide has been attested in patients with panic disorder,[30,31] anxiety disorders probably neither protect against nor provoke suicide, but do have considerable comorbidity with risky disorders.[32]

Family history of suicide in first-degree relatives differs significantly among suicides in the East Taiwan (14%), England[3] (4%), and Budapest[8] (27%) ($P<.001$) studies. Corresponding figures for depression were identical between studies in England and East Taiwan. The proportion of suicides in this study with a history of suicide attempts resembled that reported in the St Louis study (22%) and was less than that reported in all other studies. The frequency of the suicides in the present study giving warnings was similar to that reported in the English study (55%).

Overall, despite some differences in case definition, diagnosis, and demographic distribution, *similarities* in clinical features of mental illness among suicides are much more common than differences among these studies. Therefore, to my knowledge, this is the first study that has obtained broadly similar findings in a non-Western society. The evidence strongly implies that suicide is almost exclusively associated with severe depressive illness and long-term substance use disorders (mainly alcoholism) worldwide.

Among these studies, only the present one investigated controls for clinical variables in detail. Despite possible underestimation on statistical power, the risk for suicide for mental disorders, previous suicide attempts and warnings, and family history of suicide and depression were generally highly significant in case-control analysis. These findings further suggest that the risk for suicide is much higher for comorbidity, especially for depression and alcoholism in all three groups. Since similar surveys have put less emphasis on psychiatric comorbidity in suicides, how far these findings can be generalized to other ethnic groups and societies needs further inquiry.

It is not easy to explain the much higher rate of suicide in the Atayal. There was no interethnic difference in the total prevalence of major depression and clinical severity, distribution of subtypes, and duration of illness among the suicides with such morbidity. There was also no such difference in current age, onset age, and duration of illness among the male alcoholic suicides. Previous epidemiological studies have suggested a role of genetics in suicide.[33-35] Herein, significantly higher rates of suicide and depression were found in the first-degree relatives of Atayal suicides. This, plus their higher rate of alcoholism comorbid with earlier onset of major depression, might substantially contribute to the Atayal's higher suicide rate. The implications of these results for the genetic and environmental bases of suicide in different ethnic groups await investigation.

IMPLICATIONS FOR SUICIDE PREVENTION

Although most suicides in this study had suffered from major mental disorders contributing to the suicide intention, only 13% of them received psychiatric treatment, fewer than in Western surveys. The proportion of suicides who made any medical contact during their last 3 months was, however, quite high (58% in East Taiwan, 83% in England,[2] and 44% in Brisbane[5]). In the present study, the proportion of the suicides receiving psychotropic medication was much lower than that reported in the England[3] (82%) and Brisbane[5] (61%) studies. These psychotropic prescriptions were judged to be generally inadequate in Taiwan and in England.

All these findings strongly imply that suicide prevention through the early detection and effective treatment of severe mental disorders is feasible.[36] This strategy has now been officially advocated in the United Kingdom.[37,38] I emphasize that this preventive measure cannot be realized without a comprehensive psychiatric service in primary care settings, since most suicides contact medical doctors other than psychiatrists. Improvement of postgraduate psychiatric education for general practitioners has recently been reported to have lowered the suicide rate in Gotland, Sweden.[39] Other approaches, such as restricting access to lethal suicide methods, should also have their place.[40]

CONCLUSIONS

Despite widely different rates of depressive illness and alcoholism previously reported in different cultures, these findings strongly indicate that the psychiatric antecedents of suicide are the same in the East and the West. This work reveals a more universal nature of suicide than could previously have been assumed.

Accepted for publication March 22, 1995.

This work was supported by a grant (NSC79-0301-H002-04/NSC80-0301-H002-07) from the National Science Council, Taiwan, Republic of China.

Presented in part at the Sixth Congress of the International Federation of Psychiatric Epidemiology, Lisbon, Portugal, April 17, 1993, and the Symposium of the World Psychiatric Association, Section of Epidemiology and Community Psychiatry, Groningen, the Netherlands, September 3, 1993.

I thank Brian Barraclough, MD, and his team for their permission to revise and use the questionnaire from their suicide study in England and for providing their invaluable fieldwork experience. Statistical advice was offered by K. Y. Liang, PhD, Department of Biostatistics, The Johns Hopkins University, and K. A. Chan, MD, Dsc, Institute of Public Health, National Taiwan University. I also acknowledge C. Fletcher, PhD, for editing the manuscript and the excellent performance of my assistants J. Y. Kao and H. M. Lin.

Reprint requests to Division of Epidemiology and Public Health, Institute of Biomedical Sciences, Academia Sinica, Taipei 11529, Taiwan, Republic of China (Dr Cheng).

REFERENCES

1. Robins E, Murphy GE, Wilkinson RH, Gassner S, Kayes J. Some clinical considerations in the prevention of suicide based on a study of 134 successful suicides. *Am J Public Health.* 1959;49:888-898.
2. Dorpat T, Ripley HS. A study of suicide in the Seattle area. *Compr Psychiatry.* 1960;1:349-359.
3. Barraclough B, Bunch J, Nelson B, Sainsbury P. A hundred cases of suicide: clinical aspects. *Br J Psychiatry.* 1974;125:355-373.
4. Beskow J. Suicide and mental disorder in Swedish men. *Acta Psychiatr Scand.* 1979:277(suppl):1-138.
5. Chynoweth R, Tonge JI, Armstrong J. Suicide in Brisbane: a retrospective psychosocial study. *Aust N Z J Psychiatry.* 1980;14:37-45.
6. Rich CL, Young D, Fowler RC. San Diego suicide study, I: young vs old subjects. *Arch Gen Psychiatry.* 1986;43:577-582.
7. Rich CL, Ricketts JE, Fowler RC, Young D. Some differences between men and women who commit suicide. *Am J Psychiatry.* 1988;145:718-722.
8. Arato M, Demeter E, Rihmer Z, Somogyi E. Retrospective psychiatric assessment of 200 suicides in Budapest. *Acta Psychiatr Scand.* 1988;77:454-456.
9. Runeson B. Mental disorder in youth suicide: *DSM-III-R* Axes I and II. *Acta Psychiatr Scand.* 1989;79:490-497.
10. Asgard U. A psychiatric study of suicide among urban Swedish women. *Acta Psychiatr Scand.* 1990;82:115-124.
11. Lin T, Rin H, Yeh EK, Hsu CC, Chen CC, Chu HM. Mental disorders in Taiwan, fifteen years later. In: Caudill W, Lin TY, eds. *Mental Health Research in Asia and the Pacific.* Honolulu, Hawaii: East-West Center Press; 1969:66-91.
12. Singer K. Drinking patterns and alcoholism in the Chinese. *Br J Addiction.* 1972; 67:3-14.
13. Cheng TA. A community study of minor psychiatric morbidity in Taiwan. *Psychol Med.* 1988;18:953-968.
14. Cheng TA. Symptomatology of minor psychiatric morbidity: a crosscultural comparison. *Psychol Med.* 1989;19:697-708.
15. Helzer JE, Cunino GJ, Yeh E-K, Bland RC, Lee CK, Hwu H-G, Newman S. Alcoholism—North America and Asia: a comparison of population surveys with the Diagnostic Interview Schedule. *Arch Gen Psychiatry.* 1990;47:313-319.
16. Chen C-N, Wong J, Lee N, Chan-Ho M-W, Lau J, Fung M. The Shatin community mental health survey in Hong Kong, II: major findings. *Arch Gen Psychiatry.* 1993;50:125-133.
17. Rin H. Suicide in Taiwan. In: Headley LA, ed. *Suicide in Asia and Near East.* Berkeley: University of California Press; 1983:60-86.
18. Cheng TA, Hsu M. A community study of mental disorders among four aboriginal groups in Taiwan. *Psychol Med.* 1992;22:255-263.
19. American Psychiatric Association. *Diagnostic and Statistical Manual of Mental Disorders, Revised Third Edition.* Washington, DC: American Psychiatric Association; 1987.
20. Cheng TA, Hsu M. Sex differences in minor psychiatric morbidity among three aboriginal groups in Taiwan: the effects of lineage. *Psychol Med.* 1993;23:449-457.
21. Cheng TA, Chong MY. Reliability of the Chinese biographical reconstructive inventory for use in Taiwan. *Chin J Mental Health.* In press.
22. Kleinbaum DG, Kupper LL, Morgenstern H. *Epidemiologic Research: Principles and Quantitative Methods.* New York, NY: Van Nostrand Reinhold; 1982.
23. World Health Organization. *The ICD-10 Classification of Mental and Behavioural Disorders: Diagnostic Criteria for Research.* Geneva, Switzerland: World Health Organization; 1993.
24. Cheng TA, Chen WJ. Alcoholism among four aboriginal groups in Taiwan: high prevalences and their implications. *Alcohol Clin Exp Res.* 1995;19:81-91.
25. Endicott J, Spitzer RL. A diagnostic interview: the Schedule for Affective Disorders and Schizophrenia. *Arch Gen Psychiatry.* 1978;35:837-844.
26. Wing JK, Babor T, Brugha T, Burke J, Cooper JE, Giel R, Jablenski A, Regier D, Sartorius N. SCAN: Schedules for Clinical Assessment in Neuropsychiatry. *Arch Gen Psychiatry.* 1990;47:589-593.
27. Goldberg DP, Cooper B, Eastwood MR, Kedward HB, Shepherd M. A standardized psychiatric interview for use in community surveys. *Br J Prev Soc Med.* 1970;24:18-23.
28. Cheng TA, Williams P, Clare AW. Reliability of the Clinical Interview Schedule (CIS) between British and Chinese psychiatrists. *Bull Chin Soc Neuro Psychiatry.* 1983;9:54-55.
29. Murphy GE. *Suicide in Alcoholism.* Oxford, England: Oxford University Press; 1992.
30. Coryell W. Panic disorder and mortality. *Psychiatr Clin North Am.* 1988;11: 433-440.
31. Allgulander C, Lavori PW. Excess mortality among 3302 patients with 'pure' anxiety neurosis. *Arch Gen Psychiatry.* 1991;48:599-602.
32. Appleby L. Panic and suicidal behaviour: risk of self-harm in patients who complain of panic. *Br J Psychiatry.* 1994;164:719-721.
33. Roy A. Family history of suicide. *Arch Gen Psychiatry.* 1983;40:971-974.
34. Tsuang MT. Risk of suicide in the relatives of schizophrenics, manics, depressives, and controls. *J Clin Psychiatry.* 1983;44:396-400.
35. Wender PH, Kety SS, Rosenthal D, Schulsinger F, Ortmann J, Lunde I. Psychiatric disorders in the biological and adoptive families of adopted individuals with affective disorders. *Arch Gen Psychiatry.* 1986;43:923-929.
36. World Health Organization. *Prevention of Mental, Neurological and Psychosocial Disorders.* Copenhagen, Denmark: World Health Organization; 1985.
37. Royal College of Psychiatrists. *Report on Prevention and Mental Health.* London, England: Royal College of Psychiatrists; 1993.
38. Department of Health. *Key Area Handbook: Mental Illness.* London, England: Her Majesty's Stationery Office; 1993.
39. Rutz W, von Knorring L, Malinder J. Frequency of suicide on Gotland after systematic postgraduate education of general practitioners. *Acta Psychiatr Scand.* 1989;81:151-154.
40. Lester D, Murrell ME. The influence of gun control laws on suicidal behavior. *Am J Psychiatry.* 1980;137:121-122.

Premenstrual Dysphoric Disorder and Response to Cholecystokinin-Tetrapeptide

We read with interest the article by Leibenluft and colleagues[1] in the October 1994 issue of the ARCHIVES, which summarized the clinical data on how menstrual cycles can influence biochemical responses to biological challenges. Although the review emphasized mood disorder studies, the authors' conclusions can be extended to biological research in panic disorder. An overlooked area in biological studies of panic disorder is the influence of menstrual cycles and premenstrual syndrome on behavioral sensitivity to panicogenic agents. In this regard, we conducted a study to compare the behavioral response of normal women with and without premenstural dysphoric disorder (PDD) to systemic administration of cholecystokinin-tetrapeptide (CCK-4), a well-validated panicogenic agent. We present herein preliminary data collected from 12 women with PDD and 13 women without PDD.

All of our subjects were screened with the Structured Clinical Interview for *DSM-III-R*, Non-Patient Edition[2] to exclude those with Axis I disorders. The diagnosis of PDD was made following the prospective monitoring of at least four completed menstrual cycles using the Prism Calendar, a validated tool employed in PDD research. A randomized placebo-controlled three-period design was used. All the subjects received placebo in the first study period, which coincided with the luteal phase of the menstrual cycle (2 to 5 days before the end of the cycle). In periods 2 and 3, the subjects received a 35-μg dose of CCK-4 under two conditions: during the luteal phase and during the follicular phase (7 to 10 days after the onset of menses) of the menstrual cycle. Subjects were blind to the order in which placebo and CCK-4 were administered, and the cycle in which the subjects received the CCK-4 injections was randomized. The accuracy of the timing of the placebo and CCK-4 injections was ensured by using a kit for detecting leutinizing hormone peak in urine.

Behavioral response to CCK-4 was evaluated with an 18-item *DSM-III-R*–derived Panic Symptom Scale.[3] The occurrence of a panic attack following CCK-4 administration was based on *DSM-III-R* criteria for a panic attack and a score of 2 or more on the fear/anxiety/apprehension rating of the Panic Symptom Scale. Preliminary analysis of sum intensity scores (ie, the sum of the intensity ratings) revealed that women with PDD were behaviorally hypersensitive to CCK-4, irrespective of menstrual cycle phase ($F[1,21]=10.49$, $P<.004$). The mean (±SEM) sum intensity scores during the follicular and luteal phases of the menstrual cycle were 20.4±2.8 and 22.9±4.0, respectively, for women with PDD and 14.1±2.2 and 15.5±2.0, respectively, for women without PDD. The frequency of CCK-4–induced panic attacks was also higher among women with PDD compared with those without PDD during both the follicular (50% vs 8%) and luteal (58% vs 15%) phases of the menstrual cycle.

These preliminary data provide evidence to suggest that the presence of PDD can account for a significant proportion of the variance in behavioral response to CCK-4 in female subjects. Conceivably, the enhanced behavioral responsivity to CCK-4 evident in women with PDD is attributable, at least in part, to supersensitivity of CCK_B receptors and/or alterations in neurotransmitter systems that interface with CCK. Such a proposal is consistent with the view that PDD might be associated with a dysfunction of central neurotransmitter activity and that pharmacological interventions correct the underlying dysfunction.[4] It would be of considerable interest to determine if the behavioral sensitivity of female patients with panic disorder exposed to CCK-4 varies as a function of menstrual cycles and comorbid PDD. In view of the observation that women with comorbid generalized anxiety disorder and PDD experience higher levels of anxiety, as measured by the Hamilton Anxiety Scale, relative to women with generalized anxiety disorder alone,[5] we would expect panic disordered patients with coexisting PDD to exhibit an augmented panicogenic response to CCK-4.

In conclusion, our data suggest that researchers must give greater consideraton to the possible influence of PDD in biological studies of psychiatric disorders, including panic disorder. It is our impression that current methods for screening female patient and control subjects for biological studies may not be sufficient, and methods that incorporate specific questions about PDD should be used. On a final note, our data appear to be relevant to clinical trials, in which the behavioral response to pharmacological interventions might be expected to vary with menstrual cycles and the presence of PDD may be associated with poor therapeutic effect. We recommend that pharmacological-based efficacy studies pay greater attention to the potential influence of menstrual cycles and PDD on behavioral outcome measures, particularly at a time when regulatory agencies legitimately demand the inclusion of a greater number of women of childbearing age in clinical trials to ensure a more equitable representation of women.

Jean-Michel Le Melledo, MD
St Mary's Hospital
McGill University
3830 Lacombe Ave
Montreal, Quebec, Canada H3T 1M5
Jacques Bradwejn, MD
Diana Koszycki, PhD
Toronto, Ontario
Daniel Bichet, MD
Montreal

1. Leibenluft E, Fiero PL, Rubinow DR. Effects of the menstrual cycle on dependent variables in mood disorder research. *Arch Gen Psychiatry*. 1994;51:761-781.
2. Spitzer RL, Williams JB, Gibbon M, First MB. *Structured Clinical Interview for* DSM-III-R, *Non-Patient Edition* (SCID-NP, Version 1.0). Washington, DC: American Psychiatric Press; 1990.
3. Bradwejn J, Koszycki D, Shriqui C. Enhanced sensitivity to cholecystokinin-tetrapeptide in panic disorder: clinical and behavioral findings. *Arch Gen Psychiatry*. 1991;48:603-607.
4. Halbreich U, Tworek H. Altered serotonergic activity in women with dysphoric premenstrual syndromes. *Int J Psychiatry Med*. 1993;23:1-27.
5. McLeod DR, Hoehn-Saric RF, Foster GV, Hipsley PA. The influence of premenstural syndrome on ratings of anxiety in women with generalized anxiety disorder. *Acta Psychiatr Scand*. 1993;88:248-251.

Premenstrual Dysphoric Disorders, Anxiety, and Depressions: Vulnerability Traits or Comorbidity

An association between premenstrual dysphoric disorder (PDD) (or premenstrual syndrome [PMS]) and major depressive disorder (MDD) has been demonstrated by several groups.[1] Various biological factors that have been shown to be abnormal in patients with MDD were also reported to be abnormal in women with dysphoric PMS,[2,3] and several antidepressants have been shown to be effective for the treatment of PMS. However, women with PMS also have been reported to be more sensitive to develop anxiety symptoms in response to lactate infusions[4] and carbon dioxide inhalation[5]—stimuli that were reported to distinguish patients with panic disorders. Now, increased sensitivity of women with PDD to the panicogenic compound cholecystokinin-tetrapeptide is reported by Le Melledo et al in their letter above.

Levels of some of the variables that are abnormal in patients with MDD fluctuate along the menstrual cycles,[6] but it is of importance that some variables are abnormal in women with dysphoric PMS also during the asymptomatic phases of their menstrual cycle (eg, the midfollicular phase). Therefore, they might indicate a vulnerability trait to dysphoria.[7,8] The case of a trait might be supported by the many reports of consistent distinct personality characteristics[9] and cognitive impairment[10] in women with PMS, even during the follicular phase. Interestingly, as Le Melledo and colleagues point out, so far the association between PDD and affective disorders has been emphasized, while a possible association between PDD and anxiety disorders seems to attract less attention. They interpret this association as comorbidity. Another, and, in my opinion a more plausible interpretation, might be that women with PDD represent a vulnerability trait to MDD or anxiety disorders. The difference between women who meet criteria for general anxiety disorders or panic disorders and those who meet criteria for PDD might be in the level of sensitivity to develop symptoms, but the underlying processes might be similar.

As is the case with MDD, abnormalities in systems that are putatively involved in the pathophysiology of affective disorders (and anxieties) have been found in a selective subgroup but not in all women with PDD. It is still unclear if women who present a specific biological abnormality also have some other abnormalities. For instance, it might be of heuristic and clinical interest to determine the overlap between the 50% of women with PDD who are sensitive to cholecystokinin-tetrapeptide stimuli and those who are sensitive to stimuli that are more characteristic of affective disorders. (Such studies might also contribute to the knowledge on the common underlying mechanisms of overlap between anxiety and affective disorders in general.) Instead of interpretation of these abnormal data in terms of "sensitivity" and "specificity" to the particular descriptive disorder, it might be suggested that diversified premenstrual symptoms (more than 200 have been reported) might be related to diversified biological abnormalities or vulnerabilities that might be expressed as symptoms in response to a common menstrually related trigger.[8] If this is the case, then some women might be vulnerable to develop mostly anxiety PMS and also panic or anxiety disorders, while others might be vulnerable to develop depressive PMS (or PDD) and eventually MDD. Regretfully, it is almost a cliché to conclude that the pathophysiology of PDD is still obscure and more studies are needed.

Uriel Halbreich, MD
Department of Psychiatry
Erie County Medical Center, K Annex
SUNY at Buffalo
4624 Griden St
Buffalo, NY 14215

1. Halbreich U, Endicott J. The relationship of dysphoric premenstrual changes to depressive disorders. *Acta Psychiatr Scand*. 1985;71:331-338.
2. Halbreich U, Alt T, Paul L. Premenstrual changes in impaired hormonal homeostasis. *Endocrinol Metab Clin North Am*. 1988;17:173-194.
3. Parry BL. Biological correlates of premenstrual complaints. In: Gold JH, Severino SK, eds. *Premenstrual Dysphorias: Myths and Realities*. Washington DC: American Psychiatric Press; 1994:47-66.
4. Sandberg D, Endicott J, Harrison W, Nee J, Gorman J. Sodium lactate infusion in late luteal phase dysphoric disorder. *Psychiatry Res*. 1993;46:79-88.
5. Harrison WM, Sandberg D, Gorman JM, Fyer M, Nee J, Uy J, Endicott J. Provocation of panic with carbon dioxide inhalation in patients with premenstrual dysphoria. *Psychiatry Res*. 1989;27:183-192.
6. Leibenluft E, Fiero PL, Rubinow DR. Effects of the menstrual cycle on dependent variables in mood disorder research. *Arch Gen Psychiatry*. 1994;51:761-781.
7. Halbreich U, Piletz J, Carson S, Halaris A, Rojansky N. Increased imidazoline and alpha$_2$ adrenergic binding in platelets of women with dysphoric premenstrual syndromes. *Biol Psychiatry*. 1993;34:676-686.
8. Halbreich U. Menstrually related changes and disorders: conceptualization and diagnostic considerations. *Neuropsychopharmacology*. 1993;9:25-29.
9. Coppen A, Kessel N. Menstruation and personality. *Br J Psychiatry*. 1963;109:711-721.
10. Keenan PA, Stern RA, Janowsky DS, Pedersen CA. Psychological aspects of premenstrual syndrome, I: cognition and memory. *Psychoneuroendocrinology*. 1992;17:179-187.

THIS MONTH IN

ARCHIVES

OF

GENERAL PSYCHIATRY

Clinicians find it difficult to formulate recurrent problems in interpersonal relationships. An obstacle to this has been individual case variation in how emotional transactions occur in different states of mind. **Horowitz et al** (page 625) use person schemas theory in an innovative approach that surmounts this obstacle. They provide a system for shaping clinical inferences into configurations of role-relationship models. These models can contain multiple self-other beliefs and explain the cycles of changing emotion commonly observed. The method has empirical findings that indicate reliability and validity and so offers a new useful approach. Commentaries about this article prepared by a number of investigators are included in this issue of the ARCHIVES.

Functional neuroimaging has suggested that persons with schizophrenia have abnormally low activity in frontal regions of the cerebral cortex. In a positron emission tomography study of glucose metabolism, **Gur et al** (page 657) report relative left hemispheric overactivity in temporal lobe of patients but no hypofrontality. This finding related to symptoms, suggesting that lateralized dysregulation of temporal lobe activity may underlie the neural substrate of schizophrenia. Both first-episode neuroleptic-naive patients and previously treated patients showed the abnormality, indicating brain dysfunction was evident at presentation of the illness. The results support a neurodevelopmental deficit in schizophrenia.

Autoimmunity may play a pathogenic role in some patients with schizophrenia. In the largest study yet of never-medicated first-episode schizophrenic patients, **Ganguli et al** (page 668) found that these patients had lower levels of interleukin-2 (IL-2) production when compared with matched controls. The level of IL-2 production in individual patients correlated with the age at onset of schizophrenia. There was also a negative correlation with the severity of negative symptoms. The results lend support to the autoimmune hypothesis of schizophrenia, at least in a subgroup of patients.

A major therapeutic challenge in the treatment of schizophrenia is prediction and prevention of psychotic relapses. Many patients discontinue administration of their antipsychotic medication on their own. **van Kammen et al** (page 673) compared both biochemical and behavioral measures obtained in medicated schizophrenic patients and produced a better prediction rate than either set of variables alone. This suggests that a biochemical assessment of schizophrenic patients obtained before discharge may aid the clinician in identifying those patients at increased risk for relapse due to medication noncompliance.

McFarlane et al (page 679) tested a multiple-family group version of psychoeducational treatment for patients with schizophrenia and determined that providing social support in the treatment process was feasible and cost-effective and would improve outcomes. This approach was more effective in preventing relapse than either the single-family version or standard treatment. In multiple-family groups, patients with poorer symptomatic response to medication relapsed at less than one-third the expected rate. Furthermore, that approach allowed lower drug doses, more effectively promoted medication compliance, and fostered better work outcomes. By 2 years, the cost-benefit ratio reached 1:34 (treatment costs–savings in hospitalizations).

It has been suggested that obsessive-compulsive disorder (OCD) involves abnormal levels of arousal. **Hoehn-Saric et al** (page 688) report that when patients with OCD were compared with matched controls while at rest, patients with OCD exhibited higher ratings of psychic and somatic anxiety but no elevated physiological measures (heart interbeat interval, skin conductance, respiration, blood pressure, and muscle tension). During psychologically stressful tasks, psychophysiological measures changed less in patients with OCD than in controls, indicating decreased physiological flexibility. The findings suggest that hyperarousal, measured peripherally, is not essential for the pathology of OCD.

Assessment of the quality of care delivered to patients with mental disorders has become increasingly important for both policy and research purposes. **Norquist et al** (page 695) studied the care delivered to several thousand elderly patients with depression in general medical beds and acute psychiatric units of general hospitals. They found the quality of psychological and general medical aspects of treatment differed between the two settings. This study demonstrates the ability to assess quality of care in mental health from a research perspective and emphasizes the need for such data to inform improvements in treatment.

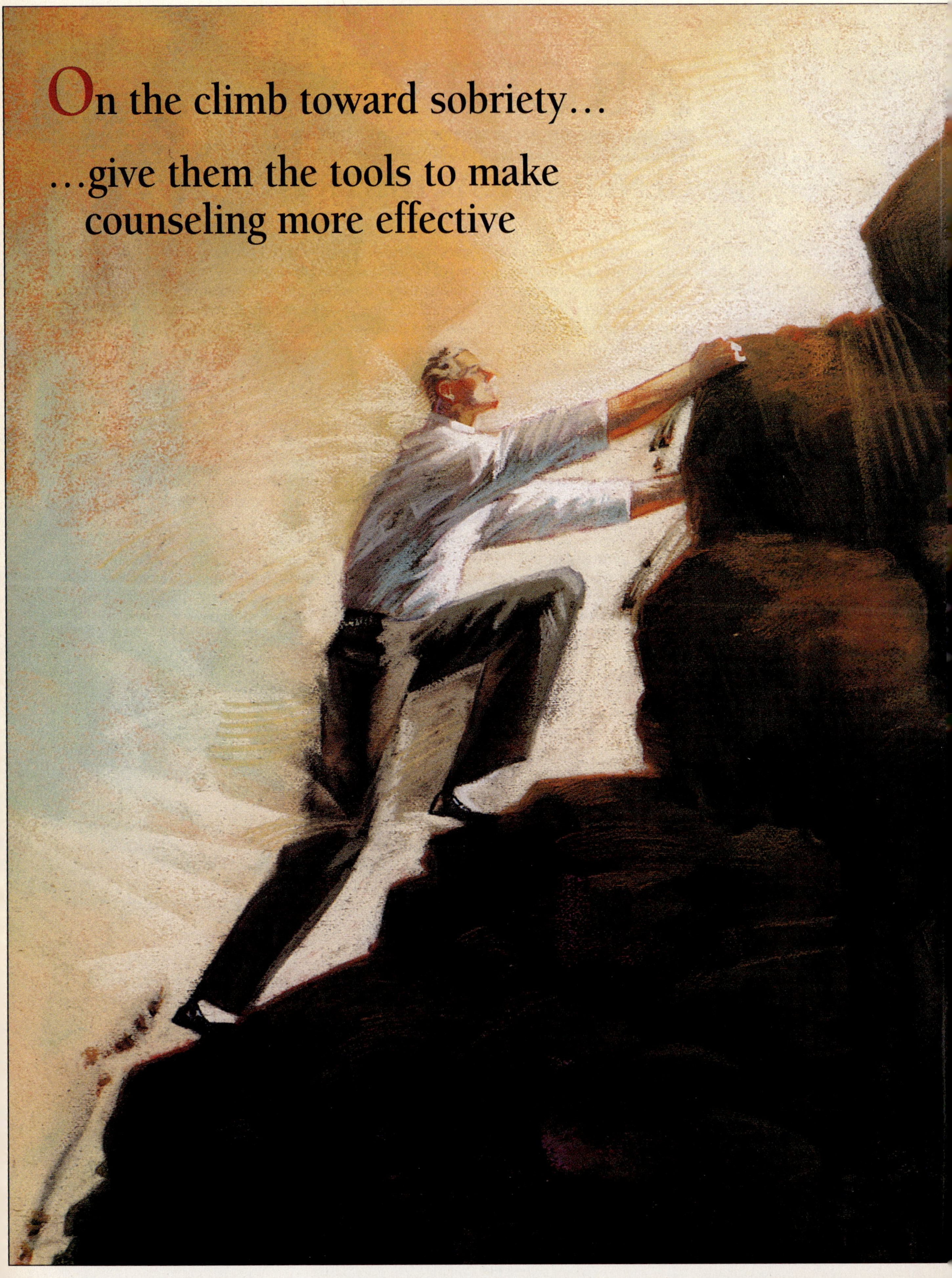
On the climb toward sobriety…
…give them the tools to make counseling more effective

ORIGINAL ARTICLE

Role-Relationship Models for Case Formulation

Mardi J. Horowitz, MD; Tracy Eells, PhD; Jerome Singer, PhD; Peter Salovey, PhD

Background: Personality disorders are important because they occur frequently and often complicate psychiatric symptom disorders. They are difficult to diagnose and formulate because unitary core traits and themes are hard to define for individual patients. A multiple-selves approach helps clinicians define core contradictions in belief that are frequently present.

Method: A configurational system for case formulation was used with an approach of states and person schemas. Transactions and stories involving self and others were observed for recurrent elements of identity, attribution, and action. These elements were systematically arranged as role relationship models for each important state of behavior. Cyclic repetitions of maladaptive interpersonal behavior patterns were then explained in terms of motivations and social events that activate enduring, but erroneous, beliefs.

Results: Reliable and valid individualized formulations were derived by means of configurations of role relationship models. Inferring several levels of diverse self and other beliefs clarified the complexity usually found in disorders of personality.

Conclusions: The role relationship models method of formulation is compatible with integrative approaches to treatment planning.

(Arch Gen Psychiatry. 1995;52:625-632)

Diagnosis of a personality disorder represents a first step toward treatment; however, it is not sufficient for the effective planning of therapy. An essential step toward effective therapy is proper formulation. While diagnoses are descriptive generalizations, formulations are efforts at partial explanatory models. They inform us about how and why an individual repeats a maladaptive pattern.

Most schools of practice recognize that personality disorders are prevalent and play a major role in the evocation and resolution of Axis I symptom disorders. The presence of a personality disorder influences treatment success or failure. Although personality disorders are difficult to diagnose and formulate, the task of doing so is extremely important. This article provides a method using role-relationship models (RRMs).

Role relationship models contain beliefs about self and others. Formulating several role relationship models allows specification of multiple self-concepts, roles for others, and transactional sequences. This multiplicity of person schemas solves some problems resulting from attempts to formulate a case in terms of only one dominant scheme. Inferring multiple role relationship models allows formulations that include characterologic contradictions and habitual avoidances of threat. Personal dilemmas of wish and fear are clarified as a partial explanation of recurrent cycles of maladaptive behaviors.

SALIENT OBSERVATIONS

Observation of phenomena of disturbances in identity and interpersonal relationships led to the classification of personality disorders in *DSM-III* and *DSM-IV*. This nosology is based on typologic clusters of disturbances—in love, caretaking, and work relationships. Psychoanalytic explanations of such patterns emphasized enduring, dynamically active, but unconscious fantasies, as summarized by Arlow[1] and Inderbitziw and Levy.[2] More recent efforts have in turn explained what is meant by "unconscious fantasy" in terms of internalized, mental representations or schemas based on residues of past and present social transactions.[3,4]

To make inferences about internal

From the Department of Psychiatry, University of California, San Francisco (Dr Horowitz); Department of Psychiatry, University of Louisville (Ky) (Dr Eells); and Department of Psychology, Yale University, New Haven, Conn (Drs Singer and Salovey).

mental models and the motives that infuse them, clinicians review a patient's interpersonal relationship patterns, emphasizing recurrent but maladaptive patterns. An obstacle to clear inference about meaning structures concerning identity and affiliation in the mind is that maladaptive interpersonal patterns often include contradictions in how the patient views self and others. The behavioral patterns of an individual, even within one relationship, may vary from one state to another. That is why multiple schemas are used in the RRM approach to formulation.

Recurrent but maladaptive interpersonal patterns are hard to observe when a cycle of changes occurs over a relatively long period, such as months or years. In *love relationships*, a person may begin with behavioral patterns that produce social and mental states in which they court, love, and happily live with a partner. Then there may be a patterned way in which this story sours, negative actions and states prevail, and coldness, anger, rejection, or provoked abandonment destroys the affiliation. In a story of just one relationship, this pattern may appear to have been caused by a single personal trait of the self, of the other, or in interaction with the social context. In ensuing relationships, the repetition of the pattern may clarify that there is something that is not a single, static trait that endures within the person or that is a characteristic of another; instead, there may be contradictory traits and complex motives of wish, fear, and avoidance of wish-fear dilemmas.

See also pages 633, 637, 639, 642, 645, 646, 649, 651, and 654

In a *parent* role, a person may display initially positive and responsible caregiving and derive pleasure from the reciprocal responses of a child. At a certain age or milestone of the child's development, the person may alter parental behavior. Again, the relationship may sour. The parent may repeat the cycle of positive-to-negative behavioral sequences with each successive child. Only after years with different children may it become clear that there is some motivated belief structure within the parent that causes the eventual deterioration of each relationship. That "something within" may involve multiple self and other concepts, contradictions among those representations, and discords between these internal schematizations and the actual relationship contexts.

Work relationships also may begin with adaptive patterns of both cooperation and controlled competition. People with character and temperament disturbances may then shift to states in which they systemically misinterpret others. A given person might manifest, in different jobs, the same pattern of being too aggressive, then too submissive, and then too hurt and outraged. The interpersonal symptomatic phenomena as seen in intimate, caretaking, and work relationships may also be repeated in evaluation and therapy sessions. It can be directly observed as psychiatric signs.[5-9] Repetition allows recognition and inference of the intrapersonal basis of the interpersonal pattern, with the person-schema theory aiding the inferential process.

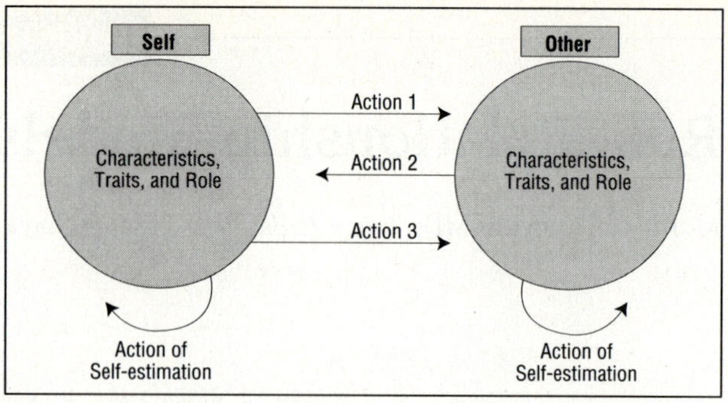

Figure 1. *A role-relationship model. The actions and traits depicted are a mental schema of what form real events* might *take. The patterned expected sequence of the events is labeled with the successive numbers. Actions include emotional expressions and conscious experiences. Self-estimation may include pride, guilt, bolstering of self, or attacks on self.*

PERSON-SCHEMA THEORY

Person-schema theory helps provide an integrative dynamic and cognitive basis for formulating intrapersonal repertoires of multiple views of self and other. The result uses and advances from psychoanalytic discoveries and explanations of transference phenomena.[10-13] Person schemas are belief structures about self and other; they are organized, feature-linking, enduring, slowly changing, and generalized knowledge structures about people.[4,14] According to empiric research, schemas are distillates of memory and fantasy processing that appear to be stored as nested hierarchies of meaning.[15] Simple subordinate forms combine systematically, through linkages, to form complex supraordinate packages. The information contained can be physical, as in body image, or mental, as in a sense of identity. The larger package can fill in information derived from perceptions in a social context. The internal and external sources of self and other information provide a coherent, but not necessarily correct, internalized model. The internalized working model of a relationship active in a state guides behavior, including felt and expressed emotion, in that state.

The person modeled in a person schema may be the self or another. There may also be person schemas of a "we" in a relationship.[16] Schemas include scripts for action sequences.[14,17] Schemas are a form of knowledge that coordinates features of perception, thought, emotion, and action. Schemas help form conscious experiences and actions, but they are a part of preconscious processing and implicit rather than explicit representations. Schemas themselves are slowly changed by processing new information. The mourning process is one example of reschematization by modifying affiliative behavioral patterns and learning by identification with another.

One may be fully conscious of secondary *symbolic derivatives* of person schemas. Examples are a sense of identity, a self-concept or a body image, and an attitude toward others. Labeling the meanings of inferred schemas may be an important component in gaining conscious control over mood and in altering otherwise automatized repetitions of maladaptive interpersonal patterns.

This article describes a method of formulating person schemas as RRMs that contain the roles of parties and

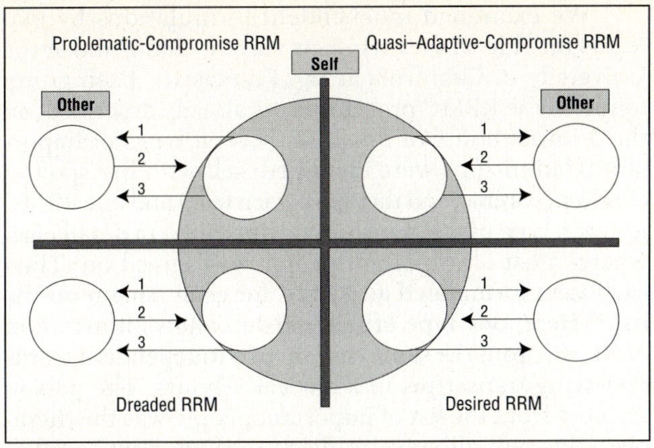

Figure 2. *A role-relationship model (RRM) configuration format. The desired and dreaded RRM may link as a wish-fear dilemma.*

their likely transactive scripts. The theoretical base is the concept that personality structure is, in part, a combination of such schemas and schemas used to organize processes of control of emotion over time.

The raw information used to formulate RRMs stems from observations of repeated patterns in narratives and from direct observation of transactional processes. **Figure 1** shows the RRM format. In any type of interpersonal relationship, there may be different states. Cycles may occur. Different RRMs may be inferred as different states of phenomena about identity and social interaction are observed, and as state cycles are described. Wish-fear dilemmas and defensive layerings may be identified. To arrive at motivational layering, RRMs are organized into a configuration of dreaded, desired, problematic-compromise, and quasi–adaptive-compromise RRMs (**Figure 2**).

BACKGROUND

Federn's ego states,[18] Berne's transactional analysis,[19] and Luborsky's Core Conflictual Relationship Theme (CCRT)[3,20] influenced the development of the RRM configurations method. The CCRT system contains five elements: an individual's core wish, positive and negative responses to the wish from the self, and positive and negative responses to the wish expected by the self from others. In addition to these elements of the CCRT, the use of configurations of RRMs added a systematic approach to inferring multiple selves and motivational layering of RRMs, including characterologic avoidance strategies.

The bottom of an RRM configuration (RRMC) is often a wish-fear dilemma composed of linking between desired and dreaded RRMs. In response to a similar motive for affiliation, the desired RRM could organize a state of satisfaction while the dreaded RRM organizes a state of suffering and loss of control. The link between wish and fear—the dilemma of wishes having dreaded consequences—leads to defensive avoidances. These are placed in the top or "surface" part of the figuration.

The avoidant RRMs in the top half of the RRMC are compromises divided into (1) the less adaptive and more problematic RRM that often relates to presenting complaints and (2) the quasi-adaptive RRM that reduces emotional problems at the expense of walling the self off from others or from fuller expressions of desire.[4,21,22] Thus, the desired RRM contains wishes and goals of satisfaction, the dreaded RRM contains the worst fears, and compromises avoid a wish-fear dilemma.

Wishes may occur early in the script schema of a dreaded RRM, and feared consequences may occur later in the script sequence.[23] Also, anticipated consequences of acting on a wish may lead from desired RRMs to dreaded RRMs in a script sequence that, when activated, leads to a cycle of behavioral states. The RRMs that serve as compromises avoid the threat of such scripts running to their dreaded conclusions.

METHOD OF CONSTRUCTING RRMS AND RRMCS

Finding elements for making RRMs begins with reducing observations to just those words and phrases that relate to the RRM elements. These categories include *traits of self, traits of other,* and *actions* stemming from either source. The semantics and metaphors of the subject and the nonverbal behaviors that fit these categories are paraphrased. The paraphrased elements are then assembled into a standard, repeated order by use of a mapping sentence.

In such a map, an "I" in the paraphrasing effort stands for the subject person, the patient. The sentence reads: "I, [self] who am [enter adjectives of trait and nouns of role] do and/or feel [enter adverbs of quality of expression and verbs of action] toward other [specify who], who is [enter adjectives of trait and nouns of role]." The sequence continues the response of other to the self: "Other, who is [enter roles, etc] does [enter expressions and actions] to self, who is [enter roles, etc]." The sequence can extend to reactions of self, to the responses of the other, and to critical appraisals about what was expressed or done. At each step in this sequence, the actual or imagined nature of acts may be designated.[21,22]

Elements that have significant repetitions in the stories and behaviors of a patient are used to form RRMs. The result, even for one relationship, will be several RRMs. These RRMs can then be designated as those that relate to desired, dreaded, or compromise aspects of a configuration. All RRMs for each important type of relationship can then be put together by means of the format in Figure 2.

EXAMPLE OF RRMC CONSTRUCTION

Subject

The patient was a young married woman with children. She had worked, but at the time of therapy she devoted herself to responsible caretaking within the home. She met criteria for both social phobia and avoidant personality disorder. She felt painfully shy in meeting people and had withdrawn from possible work opportunities. She sometimes explained her isolation as resulting from eccentricity; at other times she complained of it as a symptom. She gave written informed consent and was seen

Problematic Compromise	Quasi-Adaptive Compromise
• Shy, Sick Patient	• Eccentric Woman • Passive Girl
Dreaded	**Desired**
• Inferior Girl • Worthless Woman • Sexually or Aggressively Bad Girl or Out-of-Control Woman	• Capable Woman • Talented Girl • Sexual Woman • Strong, Assertive Woman

Figure 3. *Multiple self schemas in a case formulation.*

twice per week in individual long-term psychotherapy in a research context.

Procedure

Formulation proceeds first by selective observation, then by clustering of similar observations, and then by rearrangements that best link different clusters. In this illustrative case, self and other descriptions were selected from transcripts of the first 5 hours. This replicates what a clinician might selectively "listen for."

As is common in most disorders of personality,[24-27] there were systematic inconsistencies in the words the patient used to describe herself (and in her directly observable and shifting demeanors of expressing herself). Her first descriptions identified herself as too shy and in need of psychiatric help. At other times, however, she dismissed what she had referred to as symptoms, identifying herself as "eccentric rather than sick," or perhaps just on the passive side of a normal distribution of temperament. At still other times she described herself as strong and assertive, a capable, talented, and sexually vivid woman, more active than passive. In yet other states, she cast herself as a worthless woman, inferior and immature, or a person who might become bad and out of control.

The task of formulation is not to choose which identity is "right." All of the above attributions of self were important. The discrepancies of self-description were not mere defenses, not mere clouding of the clinical picture, but were at the heart of the clinical picture. These contradictions might be clarified through treatment and, eventually, better integrated. With the use of a system that accepts multiple self schemas, such descriptions can be put into a motivational arrangement. The result is shown in **Figure 3**.

Combining alternative identities with schemas for relationships can lead to formulations that identify recurrent dilemmas of patients with personality problems. A format, the RRMC, helps clarify the contradictions and conflicts and the motivational-defensive layerings involved. Having the same format allows one to check, empirically, how well different clinicians reviewing the same case may come up with similar RRM formulations.

We examined independent formulations by two teams (at Yale University, New Haven, Conn, and at the University of California at San Francisco). Each group followed the RRMC procedures, as already described, on the 5 initial hours of this case. Several types of important relationships were identified: self with her spouse, children, parents, and therapist. Each team and one RRMC for each type of relationship. As described in detail elsewhere, a list of important people was agreed on. Then each item formulated an RRMC for each person on the list.[28] Here, one type of relationship allows illustration of RRMC from the same case by two independent teams reviewing transcripts of a few early hours. The person selected from the list of important people was the therapist (this will allow us to discuss below how "predictive" early session formulations were for this patient's way of relating to the therapist in the later hours of treatment).

For her early expressed views of her actual or potential relationship with the therapist, one group of clinicians produced the RRMC in **Figure 4**. The other group produced the RRMC in **Figure 5**. We can begin this illustration by looking at the problematic role relationship in Figure 4, which contains the shy, sick identity of herself already shown in Figure 3. This is found in the upper-left quadrant, where a sick and shy patient seeks help from an ambiguous mentor. The response she expects from this ambiguous mentor is that he will pressure her. Her reaction is to feel suspicious of the intentions of the mentor and to resist or oppose pressure. The next response of the mentor, to that resistance, is to not appreciate or adequately support her. Because of this lack of support, she expects to repeat social failure. She will not counteract her problems and will remain too fearful.

In a richly complex approach to formulation, we cannot expect perfect independent agreement. Selection of elements is essential, and, working independently, clinicians will vary.

The other RRM (Figure 5) for the problematic compromise (upper-left quadrant) begins with herself as a patient who is "socially uncomfortable." This is similar to but not exactly the same words as the "shy, sick patient" used by the team that produced Figure 4. It is acceptably close. This "socially uncomfortable woman" in this RRM attempts to trust and seek the approval of a person (the therapist) who might not be entirely on her side, who might see her as psychopathologic and who might take the side of her husband against her. The therapist's apparent interest in her is expected to be at times insincere. Her reaction is to indicate her inability to make progress with this therapist. In return, the therapist might disdain her as abnormal, leading to her anxious response. As in the formulation in Figure 4, she expects failure and remains in a fearful or anxious state in the problematic RRM. In both RRMs the patient is avoidant and anxious because she appraises the therapist as unreliable and herself as vulnerable.

The approach-avoidance conflict in the problematic RRM is distressing but not as potentially distressing as a state of mind organized by a dreaded RRM. The dreaded RRM in Figure 4 contains an inferior identity. As in the problematic RRM, the initial wish is to gain help,

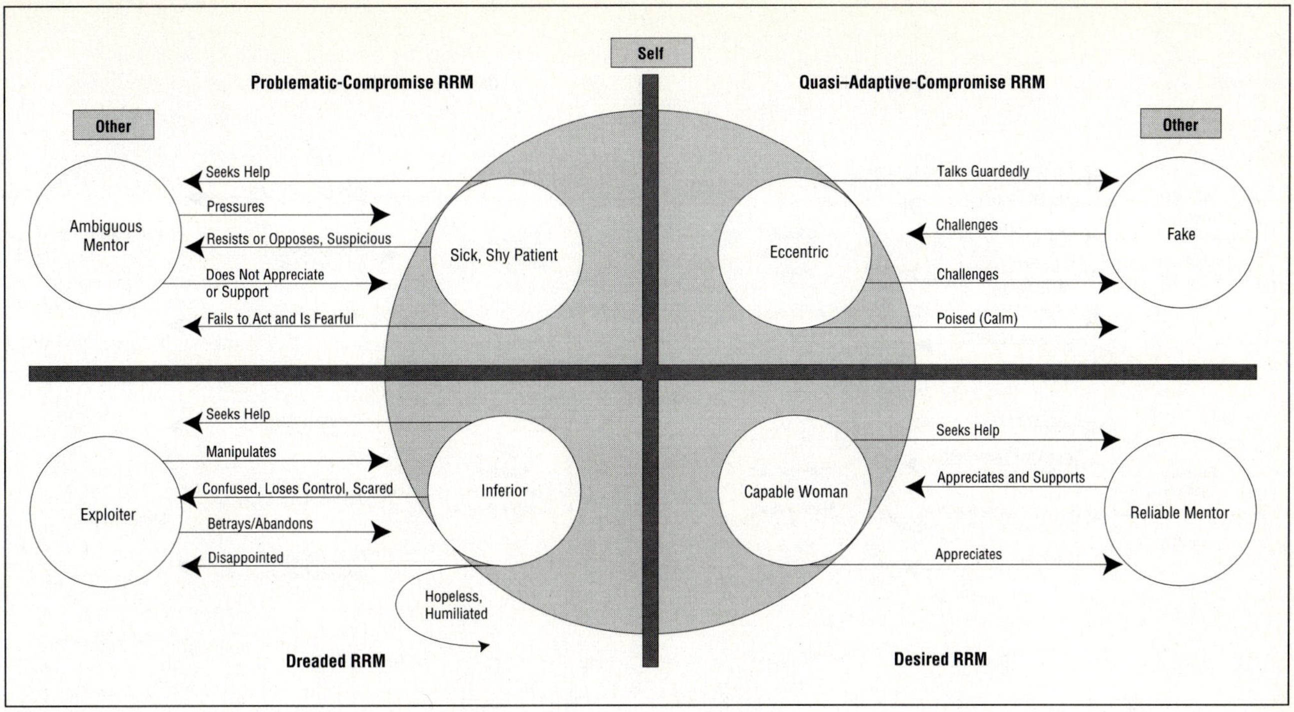

Figure 4. *Role-relationship model (RRM) configuration of a patient with social phobia, team 1.*

but the person from whom the help is sought is an exploiter who then manipulates this inferior woman to subordinate herself to his selfish purposes. She feels confused, loses control, and becomes frightened. He betrays and abandons her. She then experiences bitter disappointment and hopeless humiliation.

The dreaded RRM in Figure 5 also portrays the patient's sense of powerlessness in the face of manipulation. She is forced to comply with the intentions of a selfish lover who would betray her. She is forced by the therapist to change in ways she does not wish and so feels increasingly vulnerable.

In the independent formulations by both teams of clinicians, the problematic-compromise RRM prevents the even more dangerous closeness of the dreaded RRM. By being unable to make progress, by seeing the therapist as disdainful and judgmental, by opposing him, she wards off the dreaded consequence of submitting, being exploited and then abandoned.

In the quasi–adaptive-compromise RRM of Figure 4, the patient's identity is as an eccentric woman. This self-concept disavows the sick-shy "patient" self of the problematic compromise: she is not symptomatic, but rather the way she actively chooses to be. The other person was so ambiguous that no clear role could be attributed to him. She spoke guardedly to this figure, he challenged her, she challenged back, yet felt "calm."

In Figure 5, for this quadrant, she is adaptive and capable. She trusts and divulges things to a potential mentor, he provides guidance but challenges her, and she is able to get better. One team (Figure 4) emphasized the patient's resistive challenging; the other team (Figure 5) formulated her as expecting the therapist to challenge her.

The desired RRM of Figure 4 lists the patient as a capable woman seeking help from a reliable mentor. The therapist responds with appreciative support and the patient reacts with appreciation. The desired RRM of Figure 5 has her as a capable, admired woman who engages in treatment without fear. She views the therapist as an ally who provides protective reassurance. With his support she feels better and becomes productive.

The independent RRMCs of Figures 4 and 5 are not exactly the same. Each is richly complex. As whole gestalts, they have good accord and might lead to similar treatment plans of where to direct attention and what relationship patterns might emerge as problems in treatment.

SHIFT IN RRMS

Figure 3 illustrated various identity schemas, and Figure 4 placed these into an RRMC. Both are from one team of clinicians (Figure 5 provided a view of what a different team came up with using the same system). Now we can examine cycles of change in identity schemas and RRMs that might lead to the recurrent maladaptive interpersonal pattern. We use the ingredients shown in Figures 3 and 4 to do this. We added material reviewed from midtherapy to confirm repetitions of the cyclic pattern.

Figure 6 shows the results. We formulated a repeated cycle through wish, fear, defense, and back to wish. It integrates a psychodynamic attention to wish-fear-defense motivational configurations with cognitive-behavioral attention to dysfunctional beliefs, schemas, and acts.

Figure 6 begins with the patient conceptualizing herself as a talented youth. She shows herself to an idealized mentor in the hope of being taught. As that appears to happen, she becomes enthralled. This activates erotic

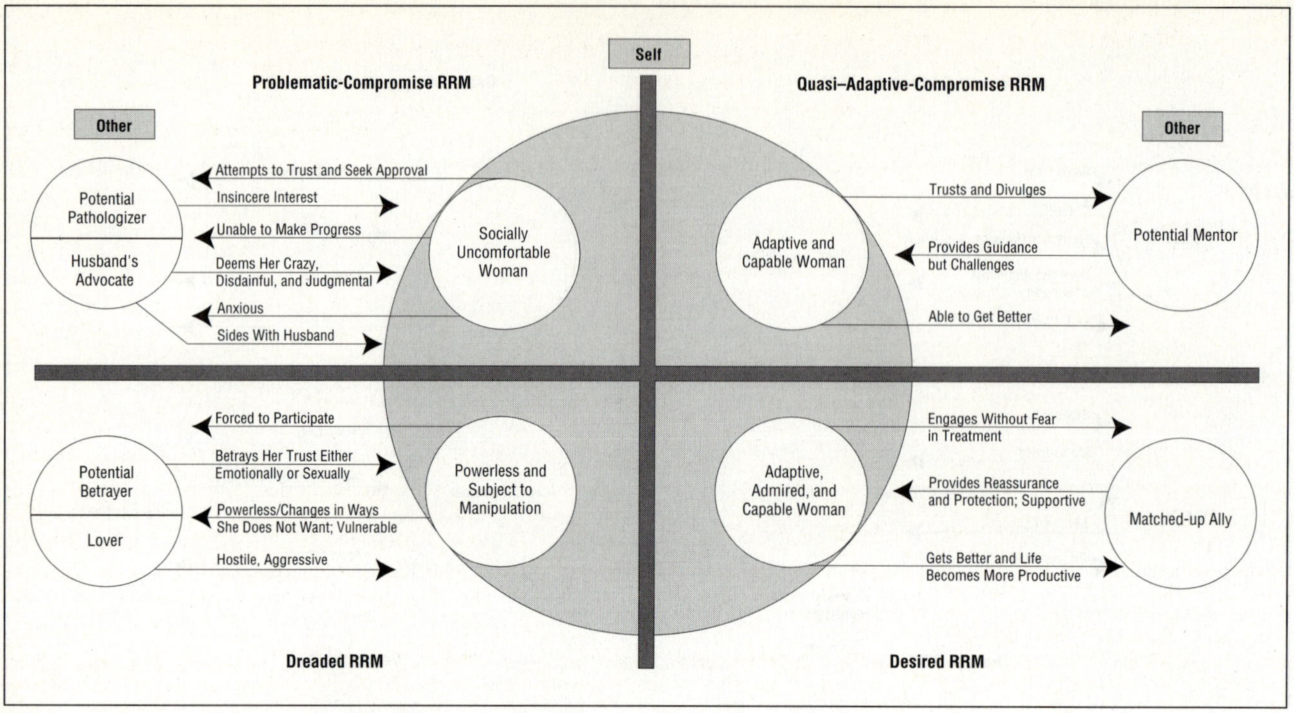

Figure 5. *Role-relationship model (RRM) configuration of a patient with social phobia, team 2.*

schemas and dreaded consequences. Emotions related to seeing, being seen, sexual excitement, pride, and admiration are associated with a fear of loss of control, being overpowered, and going too far too fast.

The fear of states in which she would experience a loss of control keeps her from feeling like an active sexual woman; rather, she has a self-concept as a passive, helpless youth in danger. Instead, to ward off sexual identity as a grown woman, she conceptualizes herself as an inferior girl who must ward off her tendency to romantic enthrallment by reducing closeness. She can do this either through a *weak* set of maneuvers (in which she acts vague and hopeless) or a *strong* set of maneuvers (in which she takes a challenging position, an eccentric who disparages the conventional roles).

As the cycle unfolds, she wards off the pining for the loss of the idealized relationship by devaluing the mentor into a fake. At the same time, that the self has succumbed to the initial advances of a devalued fake may lead to despair and self-loathing. To restore self-esteem, she seeks a new mentor and may repeat the script. The "mentor" may represent past figures, such as either parent.

RELIABILITY AND VALIDITY OF THIS METHOD

We compared RRMCs with other measures, such as the CCRT from which it is in part derived,[29,30] and found convergent validity. The RRMC contained important additional features, such as inference of multiple selves, and inference of some to ward off the emergence into experience and behavior of others.[31] In a separate study of four socially and diagnostically similar cases, Horowitz and Eells[32] had 20 judges relate correct and incorrect RRMCs to videotape records of the psychotherapy sessions from which the RRMC had been formulated. Judges were unaware of what was a correct match, were reliable in their goodness of fit ratings, and significantly rated correct RRMCs higher than RRMCs drawn from other cases.

In a second reliability study, teams took five transcripts of discourse from each of two subjects and followed RRMC derivation procedures.[32] Each team independently produced six to eight RRMCs for each case, one for each self-other relationship repeatedly described in the transcripts. One case was the source of the RRMCs for the relationship with the therapist shown in Figures 4 and 5. These RRMCs are not reported there, since that article[32] dealt with issues of reliability methods and statistics across the cases. To do that, the many RRMs and RRMCs produced by the two teams, each having multiple types of relationships, were arranged into 206 pairs for ratings of accord. New judges reliably (intraclass correlation=.89 for RRMs and .79 for RRMC judgments) agreed in rating these pairs. The 56 correct pairings were from the same relationship, same patients, and same RRMC quadrant and contrasted the two teams' formulations. The 153 incorrect pairings shuffled these criteria systematically. The judges rated the correct pairs as having a significantly higher accord than the indirect ones (P=.001).

Studies confirming convergence between RRMs and responses of subjects in tasks where they give and rate attributions about selves and significant others have also been reported (T.E., B. Fridhandler, PhD, M.J.H., unpublished data, 1993, and Hart et al,[33] Merluzzi,[34] and Tunis et al[35]). For example, a hierarchical-cluster analysis was conducted on a single subject's ratings of herself in nine different "stimulus" contexts. The four-cluster solution of her "response" ratings revealed separate clus-

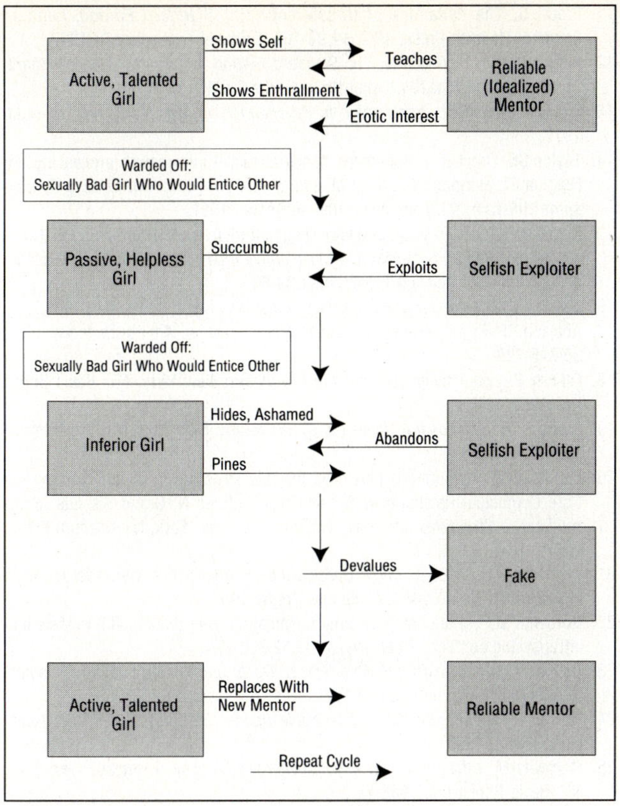

Figure 6. *Cycle through states of mind for a patient with social phobia.*

tering of different "selves" defined by attributes. There was a three-way convergence among (1) this result from a hierarchical-cluster analytic solution, (2) the subject's ratings separately on a modified version of the Structural Analysis of Social Behavior categories of Interpersonal Transaction, and (3) narrative-based formulations of her person schemas.[35]

RELATIONSHIPS WITH THE THERAPIST DURING TREATMENT SESSIONS

One reason that personality disorders are hard to treat is that the disorder itself may make it difficult to develop a trusting relationship. The patient may even seem to spoil, in a characteristic way, the opportunity for change through working with the clinician over time. A variety of transferences may occur and a variety of countertransferences may be evoked. Early formulations may be inexact but nonetheless may usefully predict problems to be expected in treating the patient. Plans for dealing with these problems can be formed early and followed as the need arises or as the expectable crises can be averted by preparations.

As an aspect of testing the validity of such assertions, we took the individualized formulations for the patient-therapist relationship of the illustration case as shown already in Figures 4 and 5. We added three formulations from other cases with the same Axis I diagnosis of social phobia and the same gender. We had judges rate these five formulations, in configurations on videotapes drawn from the middle of the patient's psychotherapy. We used two separated 5-hour sequences.

To recapitulate, the RRMCs in Figures 4 and 5 were formulated by observing records from the first five therapy sessions. Five-hour sets of sessions from the middle thirds of the same patient's therapy were then examined. We used two "case-correct" (Figures 4 and 5) and three "case-incorrect" RRMCs from different patients with social phobia diagnoses. Judges were four new clinicians operating as pairs in two teams rating each of five formulations against videotapes of therapy sessions. They were to rate the goodness of fit of each formulation to the transactional patterns observed in dialogue between patient and therapist. Interteam reliabilities were satisfactory (κ=.6). Judges watched each of 10 sessions in their entirety, rating each one for goodness of fit to each RRMC. The sessions were one third (sessions 67 through 71) and two thirds (sessions 138 through 142) of the way along the therapy. The case-correct formulations were rated as having a significantly greater goodness of fit. The average rating of goodness of fit of the correct RRMC was 3.8 in sessions 67 through 71 and 3.7 in sessions 138 through 142, two thirds into the therapy. This contrasted to the mean of the case-incorrect formulations, which was 1.6 for sessions 67 through 71 and 1.7 for sessions 138 through 142 (F=3.6, P<.0001). The RRMCs for formulating problems of the relationship with the therapist from transcripts of the first five sessions predicted style of interaction with the therapist in midtherapy.

COMMENT

This article presents a method of using RRMCs for case formulation. A person-schema theory that integrates dynamic and cognitive perspectives underlies this method. The assumptions of this theory and method can be summarized as follows.

1. Person schemas include traits and characteristics of self and others as well as scripts of likely transactions.

2. Any one person has multiple self schemas and RRMs.

3. Role relationship models, like other schemas, may operate outside of conscious awareness, but they can have symbolic derivatives in conscious awareness and expressive derivatives in social transactions.

4. A person may interpret any one situation in parallel channels of information processing according to his or her multiple RRMs. Contradictions in interpretation of the situation may occur. Appraisals of an affiliation and sense of identity will vary in different states.

5. One view usually dominates a state, but shimmering states may occur when contradictory schemas are active and produce expressive discords.

6. Persons can inhibit features that might instantiate a dreaded RRM and can facilitate features that might instantiate a protective alternative RRM.

7. Wishful motives may infuse a usually inhibited RRM. The result may be instability or shimmering states in which derivatives of desired, dreaded, and compromise RRMs appear as active, expressed contradictions and discords.

8. Personality is a plurality of possible states, possible selves, possible relationship patterns, and possible styles of defensive control of emotion.

Individualized case formulation can fill a gap between diagnoses and treatment planning. In personality disorders, psychotherapy will be a key modality. Planning that psychotherapy will be assisted by formulations that can capture individual complexity, including recurrent discords in self-organization. The RRM method can contain and characterize that complexity. It can be used to clarify systematically contradictions in views of self and others. Using systematic formulations, therapists can then help patients set aside defensive avoidances and gradually modify these contradictions.

Accepted for publication July 1, 1994.

This research was supported by the Program on Conscious and Unconscious Mental Processes of the John D. and Catherine T. MacArthur Foundation, sited at the Langley Porter Psychiatric Institute of University of California at San Francisco.

Nigel Field, PhD, Dianna Hartley, PhD, and Alan Skolnikoff, MD, made important contributions to the University of California at San Francisco formulations reported in this article. An anonymous reviewer provided important conceptualizations used toward revising the paper.

Reprint requests to University of California at San Francisco, Box F-LPPI, San Francisco, CA 94143 (Dr Horowitz).

REFERENCES

1. Arlow J. Unconscious fantasy and disturbances of conscious experience. *J Am Psychoanal Assoc.* 1969;38:1-27.
2. Inderbitziw LB, Levy ST. Unconscious fantasy: a reconsideration of the concept. *J Am Psychoanal Assoc.* 1990;15:113-130.
3. Luborsky L, Crits-Christoph P, eds. *Understanding Transference: The CCRT Method.* New York, NY: Basic Books Inc; 1990.
4. Horowitz MJ, ed. *Person Schemas and Maladaptive Interpersonal Patterns.* Chicago, Ill: University of Chicago Press; 1991.
5. Bird B. Notes on transference: universal phenomenon and hardest part of analysis. *J Am Psychoanal Assoc.* 1972;15:267-301.
6. Jacobs TJ. Transference relationships: the relationships between transferences, and reconstruction. In: *The Use of the Self: Constructions and Communications in the Analytic Situation.* New York, NY: International Universities Press; 1991;sect 2.
7. Brenner C. Transference and countertransference. In: *The Mind in Conflict.* New York, NY: International Universities Press; 1983.
8. Stone L. The psychoanalytic situation and transference. *J Am Psychoanal Assoc.* 1967;15:3-55.
9. Knapp P. Self and other schemas. In: Horowitz M, ed. *Person Schemas and Maladaptive Interpersonal Patterns.* Chicago, Ill: University of Chicago Press; 1991:81-104.
10. Abraham K. A short study of the develop of libido, viewed in light of mental disorders. In: Jones E, ed. *Selected Papers of Karl Abraham.* London, England: Hogarth Press; 1942. Originally published in 1924.
11. Freud S. The dynamics of transference. In: *Standard Edition.* London, England: Hogarth Press; 1962;12:97-108. Originally published in 1912.
12. Freud S. The unconscious. In: *Standard Edition.* London, England: Hogarth Press; 1962;14:161-204. Originally published in 1915.
13. Freud S. *A General Introduction to Psychoanalysis.* New York, NY: Liveright; 1917.
14. Taylor SE, Crocker J. Schematic bases of social information processing. In: Higgins ET, Herman CP, Zanna M, eds. *Social Cognition: The Ontario Symposium.* Hillsdale, NJ: Lawrence Erlbaum Assoc; 1981.
15. Singer J, Salovey P. Organized knowledge structures and personality. In: Horowitz M, ed. *Person Schemas and Maladaptive Interpersonal Patterns.* Chicago, Ill: University of Chicago Press; 1991:33-80.
16. Bowlby J. *Attachment and Loss.* New York, NY: Basic Books Inc; 1969;2.
17. Abelson RP. Psychological status of the script concept. *Am Psychologist.* 1981; 36:715-729.
18. Federn P. *Ego Psychology and the Psychoses.* New York, NY: Basic Books Inc; 1952.
19. Berne E. *Transactional Analysis in Psychotherapy.* New York, NY: Grove Press; 1961.
20. Luborsky L. Measuring a pervasive psychic structure in psychotherapy: the Core Conflictual Relationship Theme. In: Freedman N, Grand SS, eds. *Communicative Structures and Psychic Structures.* New York, NY: Plenum Press; 1977.
21. Horowitz MJ. *States of Mind: Configurational Analysis of Individual Psychology.* 2nd ed. New York, NY: Plenum Press; 1987.
22. Horowitz MJ. Relationship schema formulation: role-relationship models and intrapsychic conflict. *Psychiatry.* 1989;52:260-274.
23. Shank RC, Abelson RP. *Scripts, Plans, Goals and Understanding.* Hillsdale, NJ: Lawrence Erlbaum Assoc; 1977.
24. Rowan J. *Subpersonalities: The People Inside Us.* London, England: Routledge Press; 1990.
25. Horowitz M. *Introduction to Psychodynamics: A New Synthesis.* New York, NY: Basic Books Inc; 1988.
26. Kernberg OF. *Aggression in Personality Disorders and Perversions.* New Haven, Conn: Yale University Press; 1992.
27. Greenberg JR, Mitchell SA. *Object Relations in Psychoanalytic Theory.* Cambridge, Mass: Harvard University Press; 1983.
28. Eells T, Horowitz MJ, Singer JL, Salovey P. The Role-Relationship Model method: a comparison of independently derived case formulations. *Psychother Res.* In press.
29. Luborsky L, Crits-Christoph P, Friedman SH, Mark D, Schaffler P. Freud's concept of a transference template and vicissitudes of the Core Conflictual Relationship Theme (CCRT) for two specimen cases. In: Horowitz MJ, ed. *Person Schemas and Maladaptive Interpersonal Patterns.* Chicago, Ill: University of Chicago Press; 1991:167-196.
30. Crits-Christoph P, Demorest A. Qualitative assessment of relationship theme components. In: Horowitz MJ, ed. *Person Schemas and Maladaptive Interpersonal Patterns.* Chicago, Ill: University of Chicago Press; 1991:197-212.
31. Horowitz MJ, Luborsky L, Popp C. A comparison of the Role-Relationship Models Configuration and the Core Conflictual Relationship Theme. In: Horowitz MJ, ed. *Person Schemas and Maladaptive Interpersonal Patterns.* Chicago, Ill: University of Chicago Press; 1991:213-220.
32. Horowitz MJ, Eells TD. Case formulations using role-relationship model configurations: a reliability study. *Psychother Res.* 1993;3:57-68.
33. Hart D, Field N, Ewert M, Stinson CH, Horowitz MJ. A semantic space approach to representations of self and other in pathological grief. In press.
34. Merluzzi TV. Representation of information about self and other: a multidimensional scaling analysis. In: Horowitz MJ, ed. *Person Schemas and Maladaptive Interpersonal Patterns.* Chicago, Ill: University of Chicago Press; 1991: 155-166.
35. Tunis SL, Fridhandler B, Horowitz M. Identifying schematized views of self with significant others: convergence of qualitative and clinical methods. *J Pers Soc Psychol.* 1990;59:1279-1286.

COMMENTARY

Personality Theory

Clinical Practice, Social Development, and the Biology of Individual Differences

THE ARTICLE by Horowitz et al[1] in this issue of the ARCHIVES is intended to introduce a complex procedure of personality assessment, the role-relationship method, to a wide and varied readership. Horowitz et al give a glimpse of the scientific and theoretical background of this approach, present a single example of how this approach is used, and finally give a brief summary of a novel program to assess the reliability and validity of this procedure. Since all these sections are intended to be introductory, none is detailed enough to provide a basis for a systematic clinical or scientific critique. Rather, in the spirit of this contribution, it is more productive to consider the article itself as a configuration of carefully arranged parts and to examine this configuration of clinical ideas and procedures as a whole.

See also pages 625, 637, 639, 642, 645, 646, 649, 651, and 654

In this spirit, I phrase a general question: where does this work fit in current clinical efforts to understand and treat personality disorders? The current article is best understood as a contribution to the long-term individual psychotherapy of personality disorders. Its concepts and procedures are both derived from and support the assessment of this therapeutic approach. It strengths lie in its singular contributions to this field. However, when this approach is considered as an effort to develop a broader theory of personality and its disorders, its close association to dynamic psychotherapy can be seen as a constraint as well as a strength. To clarify the constraints, I will touch briefly on some trends of research in the origin of personality and its disorders in social relationships and the possible biological roots of individual differences in temperament and personality.

CLINICAL PRACTICE

Horowitz et al present their work as a theory-guided system of case formulation; that is, their work is not intended as an approach to the diagnosis of personality disorder. Indeed, the Horowitz team appears to accept that system of diagnosis as it stands; thus, the exemplar patient receives a diagnosis of avoidant personality disorder drawn directly from *DSM-IV*.[2] The role-relationship method is intended to take us three steps beyond *DSM-IV:* (1) to understand ("formulate") the patient's personality disorder in preparation for psychotherapy, (2) to monitor the ongoing progress of psychotherapy, including predicting some of its possible impasses, and, presumably, (3) to provide a more complete assessment of the ultimate impact of psychotherapy. The intimate relationship between the role-relationship method and long-term individual dynamic therapy is manifest in its emphasis on conflict, in its use of psychotherapy as the most important source of data for case formulation as well as for the assessment of the reliability and validity of the formulations, and in its centering on transference.

At the core of this approach is the fundamental precept of dynamic psychology: the origin of a psychiatric disorder and its cure lies in understanding intrapsychic conflict. The conflict process in the role-relationship model is between the *desired* and *dreaded* self; this conflict is an echo of the tension Freud posited 72 years ago between the wishes and impulses in the *id* and the fearful injunctions of the *superego*.[3] Horowitz and colleagues formulated their own ideas about intrapsychic conflict with less metapsychological baggage than the Freudian system.

Horowitz and colleagues have drawn on contemporary cognitive research, particularly its focus on how people organize and store their experiences of significant social relationships and on how children and adults come to understand and express their understanding of the likely sequences of interactions between themselves and others. Horowitz and colleagues thoughtfully integrate these two areas of research into a conception of personality as a net of schemata and narratives that are relatively stable over time and that predict perceptions, feelings, and actions of individuals in relationship to significant others.

The contribution of Horowitz and his team has been to use their own clinical research to hypothesize four types of personal schemata, each with its own narrative or expected sequence of interaction between self and others. As they point out, their theory has two levels of inferences. In their diagram of four schemata or role-relationship models (Figure 2 in the article by Horowitz et al), the bottom two "selves" represent each individual's core conflict between wishes—the "desired" self—and fears—the "dreaded" self. Although the current article does not make this clear, it seems likely that these more submerged selves are manifest in less direct ways: through fantasies, dreams, and behavior patterns. It also seems likely that these selves do not typically emerge in articulate, conscious self-descriptions and may often elude the well-developed standard interviews and questionnaires on which our field currently relies to characterize personality disorders.[4,5] The top two selves—the "problematic" self and the "adaptive" self—can be recognized as the defensive layer of personality and may generate much of the conventional picture of personality disorders.

The second link of this system to dynamic psychotherapy is its method of collecting data. The prime data, with some exceptions, do not come from research interviews or clinical diagnostic sessions. Rather, the prime data come from psychotherapy once it is initiated; that is, the patient and therapist have already decided to work with one another, and the patient's productions are intensely colored by an emotionally meaningful dyadic relationship with a "mentor" or "tormentor" or "healer" or "savior," depending on the patient and, within the patient, which self is emergent. Moreover, much of the psychometric evaluation of the role-relationship method is conducted with additional material from psychotherapy. It should be noted that this research team—quite appropriately—does not use conventional approaches to assess the reliability and validity of simpler instruments. Rather, they rely on expert judges to use sophisticated and complex pattern recognition skills to match role-relationship formulations with each other or with clinical observations. With some exceptions, this psychometric evaluation relies heavily on correct and incorrect matches, requiring complex judgments by expert clinicians.

Finally, the links between the role-relationship method and dynamic psychotherapy are manifest in the method's focus on transference phenomena. This approach seeks to understand how the patient conceives of the therapist as the "other" in the self-other models in different ways at different points in the therapy. Indeed, one suspects that a major motive for the research team is to aid themselves as therapists and their colleagues in understanding the complexity of clinical phenomena when more than one self is emergent. These are called *shimmering states*. It is equally important to understand the cycles in therapy, which regularly go from positive to "spoiled" transactions between patient and therapist. These cycles were identified as early as 40 years ago[6] and have been reaffirmed by careful empirical studies of psychoanalytic process.[7]

It is intriguing to contemplate that, through its contribution to the understanding and measurement of transference phenomena, the role-relationship model may enter into its most productive dialogue with general psychiatry. Currently, *DSM-IV* defines personalities disorders thus (emphasis added)[2]: "an *enduring* pattern of inner experience and behavior. . . . This enduring pattern is *inflexible and pervasive* across a broad range of personal and social situations . . . is *stable* and of long duration." Undoubtedly, transference phenomena are inherent in the diagnostic situation as well as the therapeutic situation. These transference phenomena may illuminate other clinical data and may help clinicians of all theoretical persuasions to recognize more clearly the multiple and cyclical disorders of personality inherent in many patients; this may untangle some of the problems of personality disorder that now masquerade as comorbidity and diagnostic unreliability. In other words, the surface manifestations of personality disorder may not be as enduring, inflexible, and stable as most of us believe, and diagnostic instruments that presume this to be the case may be inherently flawed.

However closely linked the role-relationship model is to case formulation in psychodynamic psychotherapy, it is difficult to avoid the impression that it is also being presented as a more general theory of personality and its disorders. The more complete development of the role-relationship model as a general theory requires its proponents to confront other lines of research on personality disorders and, hopefully, to recognize some of the constraints caused by the abiding intimacy of the role-relationship model with long-term individual dynamic psychotherapy. To illustrate, I draw briefly and schematically on two other important lines of investigation of personality and its disorders. An examination of the role-relationship model in the light of recent research on the social development of self-representations raises questions about the model's concepts of the self-other dyad. Comparison of the role-relationship model with biologically rooted efforts to understand individual differences in personality raises questions about stable attributes of individuals that may tie together each of the four selves.

SOCIAL DEVELOPMENT AND THE SELF

With respect to recent data on the social origins of self-representations, it seems clear that from a young age, children can represent themselves not just in relationship to a single important other, such as a parent, but also as part of a more ordered system of relationships. For example, by the age of 2 years, children recognize conflict between a parent and older sibling; they take sides in these disputes and often comfort the party they perceive as injured. They develop skills to draw positive attention to themselves and deflect negative attention by a parent to their siblings.[8-10] As children mature, they become able to represent clearly differences between themselves and their siblings in how they were treated by their mother and father. Moreover, these triadic representations (self-parent-sibling) are strongly associated with measures of depression, positive psychological adjustment, and personality functioning.[11-14] As an extension of this, children in large families represent themselves in position of birth order. While birth order does not have large and uniform effects across all families,[15] it does have a major impact in cultures that emphasize birth order privileges, such as primogeniture, or in families in which a parent suffers from a stigmatizing condition, such as alcoholism.[16] As children move into adolescence, they experience their own position in complex social systems outside the family, both in intimate cliques and in larger, impersonal crowds.[17]

As the authors of the role-relationship model reach for an understanding of the social or interpersonal origins of the individual differences in role configurations, the dyadic emphasis of their theory, itself an outgrowth of a focus on dyadic therapies, may bias their inquiries toward an exclusive focus on parent-child relationships or other important dyadic relationships in social development. The centrality in the theory of the self-other dyad may not only seal the theory off from a wide range of social experiences beyond the dyad that influence self-representations, but it may also be difficult to reconcile with empirical evidence that focuses on these multiperson representations in the development of personality. To be sure, the role-relationship dyad can be stretched to accommodate hints of triadic perceptions. Note, for example, that in Figure 5 in the article by Horowitz et al, one of the formulation teams depicts a problematic self-other model in which the other (in this case the therapist) may favor the self's husband. However, this is not an adequate effort to represent a triadic perception. We learn nothing in this role model of the patient's construction of her husband vis-à-vis her construction of her therapist. The husband does not emerge as a clearly conceived second other but is barely a pretext in this formulation for the patient's mistrust of the other in the dyad, the therapist.

BIOLOGY OF INDIVIDUAL DIFFERENCES

When we turn to biologically rooted theories of personality and personality disorders, another constraint of the role-relationship model becomes evident. Many biologically informed theories of personality are rooted in conceptions and measurement of temperament. It is instructive to turn to a line of investigation in this tradition that was summarized by a pair of articles in published in the ARCHIVES 2 years ago. Cloninger and his team[18,19] presented a summary of years of work on a temperament-based theory of personality that stylistically parallels the article by Horowitz et al.

Cloninger and his group build their model on typical or characteristic reaction patterns of individuals. In contrast to Horowitz et al, Cloninger et al appear to agree that the *DSM-IV* criteria of personality and its disorders are enduring, inflexible, pervasive, and stable. To some extent, Cloninger et al are the victims of their own methods. They use questionnaires that include such comments as (emphasis added), "I *often* feel that I am victim of circumstances" or "I *usually* accept other people as they are." By emphasizing the frequent or usual state, the questionnaire asks subjects to average their own responses and interactional behavior over time. When the Cloninger team reads about fluctuating or shimmering mental states in the data of Horowitz et al, one wonders whether they are tempted to explore momentary or long-term fluctuations.

Despite these limitations, the Cloninger group identified four temperaments: novelty seeking, harm avoidance, reward dependence, and persistence. All are substantially heritable but there are few or no overlapping genetic influences on these temperamental attributes, suggesting that each reflects a distinct biological system.[20] These temperaments predict different behavioral and response styles in normal and in pathological personalities. It would greatly spur the field of personality study to link findings such as these to psychodynamic formulations such as those of the role-relationship model. (Cloninger and colleagues recently added their own concepts of self to their theory.) However, as presented by Horowitz et al, the role-relationship model lacks a concept (and associated measures) to tie the four selves together. Is there some attribute of individuals—one that is enduring, inflexible, pervasive, and stable—that colors or inflects each of the selves or lowers the threshold for persons to slip from the adaptive to the problematic or even the dreaded self? In other words, can the role-relationship model be further specified to focus on dimensional differences among individuals, differences that may be biologically rooted, in addition to complex conflicts and changes within individuals?

All theories and, for that matter, all commentary have strengths and constraints. In summary, it seems fair to say that the Horowitz team has developed an imaginative, perceptive, and clinically rich approach to understanding personality and its disorders along with a commendable program of measurement development and testing. They have forged a link between the needs of general psychiatry to understand and treat some of the most intractable disorders on the one hand and the ongoing development of dynamic psychology on the other hand. This link is an enduring contribution. As an emerging general theory of personality and its disorders, the role-relationship model needs revision to accommodate scientific findings on the social development of the self and on the biological roots of individual differences in personality functioning and disorder.

David Reiss, MD
Division of Research
Department of Psychiatry
George Washington University
Ross Hall #613
2300 Eye St NW
Washington, DC 20037

REFERENCES

1. Horowitz MJ, Eells T, Singer J, Salovey P. Role-relationship models for case formulation. *Arch Gen Psychiatry.* 1995;52:625-632.
2. American Psychiatric Association. *Diagnostic and Statistical Manual of Mental Disorders, Fourth Edition.* Washington, DC: American Psychiatric Association; 1994.
3. Freud S. *The Ego and the Id.*
4. Stangle D, Pfohl B, Zimmerman M, Bowers W, Corenthal C. A structured interview for the *DSM-III* personality disorders: a preliminary report. *Arch Gen Psychiatry.* 1985;42:591-596.
5. Hyler SE, Rieder RO, Spitzer RL, Williams JB. *The Personality Disorder Questionnaire.* New York: New York State Psychiatric Institute; 1983.
6. French T. *The Reintegrative Process in a Psychoanalytic Treatment.* Chicago, Ill: University of Chicago Press; 1958.
7. Schlessinger N, Robbins FP. *A Developmental View of the Psychoanalytic Process: Follow-up Studies and Their Consequences.* New York, NY: International Universities Press; 1983.
8. Dunn J, Munn P. Becoming a family member: family conflict and the development of social understanding in the second year. *Child Dev.* 1985; 56:480-492.
9. Dunn J, Munn P. Development of justification in disputes with mother and sibling. *Dev Psy-*

chol. 1987;23:791-798.

10. Dunn J, McGuire S. Young children's nonshared experiences: a summary of studies in Cambridge and Colorado. In: Hetherington EM, Reiss D, Plomin R, eds. *Nonshared Environments.* Hillsdale, NJ: Lawrence Erlbaum Associates Inc Publishers; 1993:111-128.
11. Baker LA, Daniels D. Nonshared environmental influences and personality differences in adult twins. *J Pers Soc Psychol.* 1990;58:103-110.
12. Daniels D, Dunn J, Furstenberg F, Plomin R. Environmental differences within the family and adjustment differences within pairs of adolescent siblings. *Child Dev.* 1985;56:764-774.
13. Daniels D, Plomin R. Differential experiences of siblings in the same family. *Dev Psychol.* 1985; 21:747-760.
14. Daniels D. Differential experiences of children in the same family as predictors of adolescent sibling personality differences. *J Pers Soc Psychol.* 1987;51:339-346.
15. Schooler C. Birth order effects: not here, not now! *Psychol Bull.* 1972;78:161-175.
16. Bennett LA, Wolin SJ, Reiss D, Teitelbaum MA. Couples at risk for transmission of alcoholism: protective influences. *Fam Proc.* 1987;26:111-129.
17. Brown BB. Peer groups and peer cultures. In: Feldman SS, Elliott GR, eds. *At the Threshold: The Developing Adolescent.* Cambridge, Mass: Harvard University Press; 1991:171-196.
18. Svrakic DM, Whitehead C, Przybeck TR, Cloninger CR. Differential diagnosis of personality disorders by the seven-factor model of temperament and character. *Arch Gen Psychiatry.* 1993;50:991-999.
19. Cloninger CR, Svrakic DM, Przybeck TR. A psychobiological model of temperament and character. *Arch Gen Psychiatry.* 1993;50:975-990.
20. Heath AC, Cloninger CR, Martin NG. Testing a model for the genetic structure of personality: a comparison of the personality systems of Cloninger and Eysenck. *J Pers Soc Psychol.* 1993;66:762-75.

COMMENTARY

Diagnosis, Assessment, and Individual Complexity

THE CLINICIAN'S diagnostic process involves both the identification and classification of the disorder and the assessment of individual functioning. Both aspects are important for planning treatment and for evaluating outcomes. The multiaxial system of diagnosing mental disorders has arisen in recognition of the need for a standardized system of classification for communication among professionals. Hence, the classifications in *DSM-IV* (axes 1 through 3) are supplemented by the assessment of an individual's life stressors and functioning (axes 4 and 5).[1] Axes 4 and 5, however, are wanting. Criteria for judgments are less specific than for the first three axes, and axes 4 and 5 occupy little attention in our manuals and do not take account of individual complexity.

See also pages 625, 633, 639, 642, 645, 646, 649, 651, and 654

The article by Horowitz and colleagues[2] presents a method to bolster our systematic assessment of individual functioning. It is remarkably ambitious, for it aims to make use of both psychodynamic and cognitive-behavioral approaches to capture individual complexity in context, and all of this in a way that will be useful for clinicians. Not only is the conceptual background for the method far-reaching, but its empirical background is also extensive. The work of the authors and others they have collaborated with spans more than two decades of research and clinical experience. The authors make the point that their method is being designed for "case formulation" in personality disorders, but the implications are much broader. Clearly, it is meant to be used in individual assessment across a spectrum of disorders.

A major question remains. Can the proposed method be developed so that it can be used widely by clinicians? As I think about this question, two paradoxes come to mind.

The first paradox is that the authors' method is designed to take account of individual complexity, yet it must be simplified to make it more user friendly if it is to be applied widely in either research or clinical work. The method encompasses complexity in compelling ways. Role-relationship models (RRMs) and recurrent maladaptive interpersonal behavior patterns are inferred from observations of repeated patterns in patient narratives and also from direct observations of interactions in the course of evaluation or treatment. The RRMs vary from one state (ie, a mental or interpersonal context) to another and thus may be typified for a given individual according to love roles, parent roles, or work roles. Moreover, typical RRMs can then be categorized by an observer into a configuration according to sectors in which RRMs can be seen as (1) dreaded, (2) desired, (3) compromised adaptively, or (4) compromised in a problematic way. Research teams can communicate about a patient using this method, and the case illustration convinces us that some measure of agreement can be achieved using transcripts. Still, practical questions remain. Can the method be simplified even further so that it can be understood more easily? Can it be applied outside of a dedicated research setting in an efficient and reliable way? There are additional questions of validity. To what extent would a simplified method be appropriate given the goal of capturing complexity? Can a simplified method be shown to have validity in terms of individual meaning and outcome?

The second paradox is that the authors' method of assessment is relational, yet it is to be applied in a diagnostic tradition in which the focus has been on the individual. As noted above, RRMs vary according to social relationships; correspondingly, maladaptive interpersonal relationship patterns may in considerable part be interpersonally based, ie, located within particular relationships. During the diagnostic process and in planning treatment, it would be wise to take such assessment into account, and the authors' method holds promise in this area. However, this kind of broadening of the traditional diagnostic process will be difficult. Can we determine the boundaries between individually based and interpersonally based diagnostic understanding? Can we establish more detailed criteria for interpersonal assessment? Such considerations are not yet included in the RRM configuration method. A shift in our thinking to include a relational-based system of assessment in the diagnostic process is timely, however. Clinicians working with young children have recently published schemes for dealing with such an assessment, in which many common disorders of mental health and development are embedded in problematic relationships with caregivers.[3-5] Clinical trials in the next years will determine the adequacy and usefulness of early childhood criteria for such an assessment.

The proposed method, with its ambitious conceptual scheme, is likely to push mainstream clinicians into new territory. I have raised some awkward questions, but unless we deal with individual complexity and unless we attempt to evaluate social relationships, our diagnostic process will be impoverished. Can the scheme be simplified? Can relationship-based criteria be developed? Given the programmatic and dedicated work of these investigators, I believe that time will tell us how well these difficult questions can be addressed.

Robert N. Emde, MD
Health Sciences Center
University of Colorado
4200 E Ninth Ave
Denver, CO 80262

REFERENCES

1. American Psychiatric Association. *Diagnostic and Statistical Manual of Mental Disorders, Fourth Edition.* Washington, DC: American Psychiatric Association; 1994.
2. Horowitz MJ, Eells T, Singer J, Salovey P. Role-relationship models for case formulation. *Arch Gen Psychiatry.* 1995;52:625-632.
3. Sameroff AJ, Emde RN, eds. *Relationship Disturbances in Early Childhood: A Developmental Approach.* New York, NY: Basic Books; 1989.
4. National Center for Clinical Infant Programs. *Diagnostic Classification: 0-3: Diagnostic Classification of Mental Health and Developmental Disorders of Infancy and Early Childhood.* Arlington, Va: Zero to Three/National Center for Clinical Infant Programs; 1993.
5. Emde RN, Bingham RD, Harmon RJ. Classification and the diagnostic process in infancy. In: Zeanah C, ed. *The Handbook of Infant Mental Health.* New York, NY: The Guilford Press; 1993: 225-235.

Progress on Case Formulation

READERS of the ARCHIVES may be unfamiliar with some of the recent advances in methods for psychodynamic formulation. Horowitz and colleagues[1] continue to make important contributions to this developing field, and therefore we hope to highlight the strengths and weaknesses of their article.

BACKGROUND

Some background on the history of research on psychodynamic formulation may help to put the work by Horowitz and colleagues in context. Many earlier attempts[2] to assess the agreement of clinicians in arriving at a psychodynamic formulation resulted in poor interjudge reliability. This failure to achieve adequate agreement was likely a function of three major issues: (1) There is not one psychodynamic theory but many theories, often quite distinct and often only loosely articulated, thus leading to different clinicians formulating dynamic issues in discrepant ways based on their discrepant theories. (2) Even among clinicians of the same theoretical persuasion, an approach that allows judges to derive formulations without focusing their attention on specific clinical material and structuring the nature of the formulation is likely to result in substantial disagreements. (3) The phenomena of interest are inherently elusive, leading to marginal agreement between clinicians even under the best of circumstances. More recent attempts to create methods for psychodynamic formulation have used structured methods based on specified theories and have limited judges to inferences in specific domains of interest. This shift has resulted in a variety of methods with more acceptable levels of reliability.[3] The article by Horowitz and colleagues continues in this vein.

The purpose of the article by Horowitz et al is first to present the theory of "person schemas" on which their assessment method is based. The general elements of the role-relationship models configuration (RRMC) method, derived from person schemas theory, are presented next. The authors then give procedural details for formulating RRMCs, including an example of an RRMC construction. Reliability and validity studies performed to date with the instrument are reviewed, and some data are presented showing convergence between an RRMC and aspects of the patient-therapist relationship for a single case.

ADVANTAGES OF THE RRMC METHOD

There are a number of ways in which we believe the RRMC approach has the potential to be important. One notable way in which this method differs from other dynamic formulation methods is that rather than relying on the language and theories articulated by previous psychodynamic clinical writings, the RRMC method is tied to person schemas theory. Person schemas theory integrates dynamic and cognitive theories and generally avoids the language of psychoanalytic theories, relying instead on more clearly defined terms from social cognition, such as *scripts* and *schemas,* as well as terms specific to Horowitz and his colleagues (eg, *shimmering states*). While at times it hinders understanding of the RRMC approach for general readers, this new language serves the useful function of distinguishing the approach from more traditional psychoanalytic approaches. Furthermore, the integration of dynamic and cognitive constructs might help the field move beyond the "brand names" that dominate the clinical arena to focus more on the variables that are relevant for treatment planning and intervention.

See also pages 625, 633, 637, 642, 645, 646, 649, 651, and 654

A second major advantage of the RRMC method is that it is specifically oriented toward the assessment of multiple person schemas for an individual. By assuming the existence of multiple person schemas, the RRMC method has the potential to understand contradictory behaviors and conflicts between wishes. On the other hand, the complexity of the RRMC approach is an inherent disadvantage because it makes the method cumbersome and time-consuming and makes it difficult if not impossible to achieve high reliability for all aspects of the model.

LIMITATIONS OF THE RRMC METHOD

Several limitations of the RRMC theory, method, and data presented by Horowitz and colleagues are also apparent. These limitations, however, are primarily a function of the early stage of development of the RRMC method and of psychodynamic formulation methods in general. Thus, a discussion of these limitations may serve to inform future research on the RRMC method.

Horowitz and colleagues link the RRMC approach to personality disorders, although in previous writings Horowitz[4] has applied the RRMC approach to stress response syndromes. Although the connection to Axis II disorders seems intuitively appealing since Axis II disorders are defined in terms of enduring maladaptive patterns of relating to the environment and viewing oneself, Horowitz and colleagues do not specify in what ways the RRMC of a patient with an Axis II disorder would differ from the RRMC of a patient without an Axis II diagnosis. It is possible that the contents of RRMCs would map onto the different Axis II diagnoses in systematic ways or that Axis II disorders would be characterized by higher prevalence (within an individual over time) of one role-relationship model (RRM) (eg, problematic-compromise) across many interpersonal relationships in the patient's life.

Another issue is that Horowitz and colleagues suggest that the RRMC method of formulation is compatible with integrative approaches to treatment planning, but they do not discuss what treatment techniques would be integrated as a function of RRMC formulation. The RRMC terminology resembles the language of cognitive therapy,[5] with the use of terms such as *dysfunctional beliefs* and *schemas*. However, it is not clear whether Horowitz and colleagues are advocating the integration of cognitive therapy techniques with psychodynamic techniques and why such integration would follow from the formulation method.

Although the data on the reliability of the RRMC method seem promising, several limitations should be noted. The procedure used involves first having a team of judges work together to produce an RRMC for each case. In the second step, another set of judges working independently make similarity ratings between RRMCs (or their component RRMs) and the videotapes of psychotherapy sessions[6] or the RRMCs created by another team of judges.[7] Both correct (same case) and incorrect (different case) pairings are rated for similarity. Reliability is then reported in terms of the interjudge agreement on the similarity ratings and also in terms of the mean difference in similarity between correctly and incorrectly matched pairs.

IT IS USEFUL for research purposes that these elaborate procedures produce one type of reliability assessment, but such reliability results cannot be generalized to the use of the RRMC method by a clinician. First, the similarity ratings might be artificially inflated because of idiosyncrasies in the vocabularies used by different patients. If the RRMCs are developed based on patients' descriptions of their interpersonal interactions, judges may extract language that is unique to that patient, thus increasing the probability that future judges will match the RRMC to the patient session based merely on the uniqueness of the language. Both reliability studies obtained adequate interjudge agreement on the similarity scores by pooling the ratings of 20 judges. Reliability for a single judge matching an RRMC with the correct patient would be quite low. Furthermore, the mean differences between correctly matched and incorrectly matched cases might be a function of the sample of cases rated. Since only a small number of cases have been included in the reliability studies (four patients in the first reliability study, two patients in the second), it is uncertain to what extent judges can adequately match the RRMCs of relatively unselected patients presenting for treatment. In addition, the authors report $P<.0001$ for the comparison of case-correct similarity ratings with case-incorrect similarity ratings. It is unclear why this result is so highly significant when only two case-correct and three case-incorrect pairings were rated. Finally, the authors report that in both reliability studies, the complexity of the method prevents the judges from reliably constructing *independent* case formulations. However, it is unlikely that the method will have much clinical utility if clinicians cannot independently formulate the RRMC in a reliable way. At the moment, then, the RRMC is best seen as a research tool for the intensive analysis of a small number of cases, and the generalization of this technique to larger numbers of cases and to clinical practice remains a goal for future research.

Similarly, studies of the validity of the RRMC method are at an early stage of development. Two of the four validity studies cited by Horowitz and colleagues were currently published and available for our review; both were single case studies. One of these studies[8] did not actually assess RRMs, so it provides little if any validation of the RRMC method per se. The second study[9] showed that items derived from a clinical team's RRMC for a patient could be rated by that patient, resulting in clusters that correspond to the original RRMC formulation. Although this result appears promising, a stronger test of validity would examine whether patients independently describe themselves in ways similar to an RRMC formulation. It is not clear whether the similarity in clustering produced by the patient's ratings is an artifact of the stimuli rated. Would the items cluster differently if rated by other patients (ie, is the clustering of the items more a function of items that would go together for many patients rather than evidence of this patient's self-schema?)?

In addition, the similarity between the patient's ratings and the original RRMC does not validate the structure of the RRMC model. For example, it does not seem likely that all patients experience four states (ie, the four RRMC quadrants) in their relationships with others. Moreover, the authors suggest that the RRMC method can be used to understand the patient's motivational system, ie, that various RRMs serve a defensive function to ward off alternative RRMs. The authors have not presented data to validate this aspect of the model. In one validation study, Merluzzi[9] suggests that the absence of recognition on the patient's part of stimuli that would be contained in the "dreaded" RRM category validated the defensive function of the RRMC to ward off undesirable aspects of the self-schema. However, in the absence of external validation of the RRMC, this result could also be interpreted as a failure of the RRMC judges to correctly assess the patient's interpersonal patterns. Further work is needed to validate both the format of the RRMC and the content of reliably rated RRMCs with more objective external criteria.

In summary, we commend Horowitz and colleagues for making progress in an important yet difficult area of research. The results presented so far suggest areas for future efforts. The reliability of independent case formulations can be explored across larger patient samples to determine the usefulness of the RRMC method in both clinical and research settings. Furthermore, research on the construct validity of the RRMC can be useful in understanding the complexity of patients' schemas and in developing integrated treatment techniques.

Paul Crits-Christoph
Mary Beth Connolly
Center for Psychotherapy Research
Department of Psychiatry
University of Pennsylvania
3600 Market St
Philadelphia, PA 19104-2648

REFERENCES

1. Horowitz MJ, Eells T, Singer J, Salovey P. Role-relationship models for case formulation. *Arch Gen Psychiatry.* 1995;52:625-632.
2. Seitz PF. The consensus problem in psychoanalytic research. In: Gottschalk L, Auerbach L, eds. *Methods of Research and Psychotherapy.* East Norwalk, Conn: Appleton & Lange; 1966:209-225.
3. Barber J, Crits-Christoph P. Recent advances in the evaluation of psychodynamic formulations. *J Consult Clin Psychol.* 1993;61:574-585.
4. Horowitz MJ. *Stress Response Syndromes.* Northvale, NJ: Jason Aronson Inc; 1986.
5. Beck AT, Rush AJ, Shaw BF, Emery G. *Cognitive Therapy of Depression.* New York, NY: Guilford Press; 1979.
6. Horowitz MJ, Eells TD. case formulations using the role-relationship model configurations: a reliability study. *Psychother Res.* 1993;3:57-68.
7. Eells TD, Horowitz MJ, Singer J, Salovey P, Daigle D, Turvey C. The role-relationship models method: a comparison of independently derived case formulations. *Psychother Res.* In press.
8. Tunis SL, Fridhandler B, Horowitz M. Identifying schematized views of self with significant others: convergence of qualitative and clinical methods. *J Pers Soc Psychol.* 1990;59:1279-1286.
9. Merluzzi TV. Representation of information about self and other: a multidimensional scaling analysis. In: Horowitz MJ, ed. *Person Schemas and Maladaptive Interpersonal Patterns.* Chicago, Ill: University of Chicago Press; 1991:155-166.

Between the Past and the Future of Psychotherapy Research

THE overarching goal of psychotherapy research is to understand the mechanisms through which such treatment operates and to assess the impact of moderating influences on maladaptive and adaptive functioning. During the past two decades, there has been a dramatic increase in empirically based outcome- and process-oriented psychotherapy research. Outcome-oriented research[1-4] concerns itself with the scientific evaluation of the effectiveness of psychotherapy. Moving beyond this approach, process-oriented psychotherapy research[5-9] investigates the extent to which outcome is determined by the interaction of the patients' psychopathologic characteristics and personality on the one hand, and the therapists' skills, personality, and particularly their technique on the other.

See also pages 625, 633, 637, 639, 645, 646, 649, 651, and 654

Both approaches have contributed much to our understanding in this realm. At the same time, both have demonstrated the difficulties inherent in the systematic investigation of psychotherapy, an enterprise that subsumes over 400 techniques for adults and over 200 for children and adolescents.[10,11] Consider, too, that there are almost 300 different psychological syndromes or symptom patterns currently recognized to which psychotherapy may be applied. Regardless of all this, both paradigms do point to important research paths for the future. The kind of research advocated by either and exemplified in the article by Horowitz et al[12] will become increasingly crucial if we are to demonstrate the efficacy of psychotherapy to those who make important health care policies in our society.

Emerging from process-oriented psychotherapy research are a number of studies that focused on mapping out the topography of the patients' interpersonal relationships. The oldest reliably guided system for deriving central relationships and the early patterns from which they develop was the Core Conflictual Relationships Theme measure.[13-15] At least 15 similar measures have since evolved from the Core Conflictual Relationships Theme, including Horowitz's[16,17] Role-Relationship Model Configuration, a method that examines psychotherapy data from three points of view: psychic states, relationship patterns, and information processing. In discussing this current elucidation by Horowitz et al[12] of their Role-Relationship Model Configuration, we will proceed in a concentric fashion from broad issues to more specific points.

HISTORY AND LANGUAGE

The contribution by Horowitz et al is a sophisticated application of complex psychodynamic principles that are largely derived from psychoanalysis to the understanding of metaprocesses in psychotherapy. At the same time, their article is strikingly aloof from overlapping and prior psychoanalytic concepts. Although the psychoanalytic writings and psychotherapy research literature have indeed diverged and although no article can have an entirely complete literature review, the omissions in the article by Horowitz et al[12] are far from being marginal. The authors seem insistent on disavowing the psychoanalytic lineage of their concepts.

This disavowal is evident in their use of phrases like "self and other concepts," "multiple selves," and "multiple self schemas," instead of the widely accepted "self and object representations" and "multiple self-representations."[18,19] Their use of "self" instead of "self-representation" is, in addition, historically retrogressive because it blurs the important distinction between the self as it exists in the external world and as it is experienced, piecemeal, in the individual's psychic reality.[18] The same applies to using "others" rather than "object representations." Another example of avoiding established vocabulary is the use of "outside of conscious awareness" instead of "unconscious." The fact that the word transference appears only once in this article betrays a similar tendency.

A strategy that is parallel to creating new terms for existing constructs is the lack of appropriate citations. Noticeable in this regard is the omission of Slap and Saykin's[20] thorough delineation of internal schemas and of Piaget's[21] notions of accommodation and assimilation as effects of intrapsychic factors on perception and vice versa, in relevant sections of the article. Similarly striking is the fact that Horowitz et al talk of discrepancies in self-description due to underlying "multiple self schemas" without correlating this with Kernberg's[19] "borderline personality organization." Moreover, it is historically inaccurate to suggest that the notion of "unconscious fantasy"[22] preceded the elucidation of "internalized, mental representations or schemas based on residues of past and present social transactions."[12] This overlooks the fact that Fairbairn[23] had, as early as 1944, outlined that all internalizations involve dyadic units of ego and objects (self and object representations, in current terminology) engaged in an affective interaction with each other. Jacobson's[18] and Kernberg's[24] later related ideas also preceded the literature on unconscious fantasy cited by Horowitz et al.

By omitting important references, creating a new language, and presenting the history of psychoanalytic ideas in a questionable manner, the authors' ideas do achieve a sense of novelty, but they also lose an important theoretical and historical anchor.

CONCEPTS AND METHODS

The article by Horowitz et al[12] has a number of methodological strengths and limitations. A major strength of this model lies in the exciting promise of attempting to operationalize constructs that are central to psychodynamic psychotherapy. If successful, the model could greatly increase our understanding of the factors involved in the process of successful treatment. Another strength of the model is that it adheres to actual clinical data and thus has the potential to avoid theoretical prejudice. Analyzing psychotherapy in terms of factors that cause changes in "states of mind" (a term Horowitz et al took from Eric Berne's phrase "ego states"[25]) by means of configurational analysis can introduce a much higher level of objectivity into the field than the customary psychodynamic formulations. It reaches for objectivity through reducing the necessity for inference to a minimum.

Horowitz's model takes the clinician and patient close to the here-and-now clinical data. By extension, it helps the clinician develop a flexible, pragmatic map rather than a rigid, theoretical explanation. The model provides an organizational schema for collecting multiple relationship patterns (in contrast to Luborsky's single Core Conflictual Relationships Themes[13-15]), each of which may be studied and used to learn more about the patient.

Parallel to these strengths, there exist conceptual and methodological weaknesses in the article. Most striking is the fact that the conclusions of Horowitz et al are based on only the first 5 hours of psychotherapy with a single patient. Despite the long recognized heuristic value of single case studies (eg, Freud's renowned cases), this method, especially when limited to very short duration vignettes, is inadequate as a basis for valid scientific conclusions. Relationships between independent and dependent variables are often difficult to discern, and threats to internal validity are difficult to rule out. These data seem best understood, therefore, as a point of departure from which hypotheses and alternate explanations would emerge. Relatedly, a critical issue not addressed in the article is suggested in the statement regarding consensual agreement. Given that the constructs suggested are less abstract than many metapsychological premises, can observers independently concur as to their presence and intensity? If one were to have verbatim transcripts of the work of Horowitz et al, would we agree about the presence of warded-off states and their changes? It is this movement from the therapists' observations to those of independent raters that is crucial for the next state of development of this model.

In more general terms, it also remains unclear whether the model proposed in this article implies any change in the customary ways of doing psychotherapy or whether it provides a different way of analyzing the therapeutic procedure. From another perspective, would not the relationship model outlined by Horowitz et al inhibit or distort transference judgments made by clinicians? Relatedly, there is some concern regarding whether such a system includes truly unconscious aspects of the interactions described. Finally, to define conflict only in terms of wish-defense dynamic seems narrow because conflicts also exist between contradictory wishes and between wishes and needs.

CONCLUSION

The study by Horowitz et al seems promising insofar as it creates a theoretically lively point of departure from which additional research seems clearly warranted. Another strength of their work lies in its elaboration of and building on the more established Core Conflictual Relationships Theme model of Luborsky et al.[13-15] Furthermore, although there remain problems with a single case method, the strategy does draw attention to the frequently lamented hiatus between clinical practice and research. At the same time, one regrets the authors' insistence on new terminology in favor of the more established language in this realm. Moreover, the model proposed is highly complex and requires much further research to determine whether it is possible to catalog states and their accompanying features in such a way that they can be reliably identified, that is, so that a sufficiently high interrater reliability can be achieved.

Salman Akhtar, MD
Steven Samuel, PhD
Department of Psychiatry and Human Behavior
Jefferson Medical College
1201 Chestnut St, Suite 1503
Philadelphia, PA 19107

REFERENCES

1. Smith NL, Glass GV, Miller TT. *The Benefits of Psychotherapy.* Baltimore, Md: The Johns Hopkins University Press; 1988.
2. Persons JB. Psychotherapy outcome studies do not accurately represent current models of psychotherapy: a proposal remedy. *Am Psychol.* 1991; 46:99-106.
3. Jones EE, Hall SA, Parke LA. The process of change: the Berkeley Psychotherapy Research Group. In: Beutler L, Crago M, eds. *Psychotherapy Research: An International Review of Programmatic Studies.* Washington, DC: American Psychological Association; 1991:99-106.
4. Whitson S, Sexton T. An overview of psychotherapy outcome research: implications for practice. *Professional Psychol Res Pract.* 1993;24:43-51.
5. Grunzig H. Time series analysis of psychoanalytic treatment processes: sampling processes and first findings in a single case. In: Dahl H, Kachele H, Thoma M, eds. *Psychoanalytic Process Research Strategies.* New York, NY: Springer Publishing Co Inc; 1988.213-226.

6. Hill CE, Nutt EA, Jackson S. Trends in psychotherapy process research: samples, measures, researchers and classic publications. *J Counseling Psychol.* 1994;31:364-377.
7. Gruenberg L. Research on the process of change. *Psychother Res.* 1991;1:3-16.
8. Lambert M. The individual therapist's contribution to psychotherapy process and outcome. *Clin Psychol Rev.* 1989;9(special issue):469-485.
9. Rounsaville B, Chevron E, Prusoff B, Elkin I, et al. The relation between specific and general dimensions of the psychotherapy process in interpersonal psychotherapy of depression. *J Consult Clin Psychol.* 1987;55:379-384.
10. Karasu TB, ed. *Treatment of Psychiatric Disorders: A Task Force Report of the American Psychiatric Association.* Washington, DC: American Psychiatric Association; 1990;vol 1-4.
11. Kazdin AE. *Child Psychotherapy: Developing and Identifying Effective Treatments.* Elmsford, NY: Pergamon Press; 1988.
12. Horowitz MJ, Eells T, Singer J, Salovey P. Role-relationship models for case formulation. *Arch Gen Psychiatry.* 1995;52:625-632.
13. Luborsky L. Measuring a pervasive psychic structure in psychotherapy: the core conflictual relationship theme. In: Freedman N, Grand S, eds. *Communicative Structures and Psychic Structures.* New York, NY: Plenum Press; 1977:367-395.
14. Luborsky L, Crits-Cristoph P. *Understanding Transference: The CCRT Method.* New York, NY: Basic Books; 1990.
15. Luborsky L, Luborsky E. The era of measures of transference: the CCRT and other measures. *J Am Psychoanal Assoc.* 1993;41(suppl):329-352.
16. Horowitz MJ. Relationship schema formulation: role-relationship models and intrapsychic conflict. *Psychiatry.* 1989;52:260-274.
17. Horowitz MJ, ed. *Person Schemas and Maladaptive Interpersonal Patterns.* Chicago, Ill: University of Chicago Press; 1991.
18. Jacobson E. *The Self and the Object World.* New York, NY: International Universities Press; 1964.
19. Kernberg OF. *Borderline Conditions and Pathological Narcissism.* New York, NY: Jason Aronson; 1975.
20. Slap JW, Saykin A. The schema: basic concept in nonmetapsychological model of the mind. *Psychoanal Contemp Thought.* 1983;6:305-325.
21. Piaget J. *The Construction of Reality in the Child.* New York, NY: Basic Books; 1954.
22. Arlow J. Unconscious fantasy and disturbances of conscious experience. *J Am Psychoanal Assoc.* 1969;38:1-27.
23. Fairbairn WRD. Endopsychic structure considered in terms of object-relationships (1944). In: *Psychoanalytic Studies of the Personality.* London, England: Routledge and Kegan Paul Ltd; 1952:82-136.
24. Kernberg OF. Borderline personality organization. *J Am Psychoanal Assoc.* 1967;18:800-822.
25. Berne E. *Transactional Analysis in Psychotherapy.* New York, NY: Grove Press; 1961.

COMMENTARY

Are Case Formulations Useful for Outcomes Research?

THE ARTICLE by Horowitz and colleagues[1] is most helpful in defining and illustrating some of the difficulties facing clinical researchers who are investigating psychodynamic constructs and psychotherapy. Horowitz et al rightly point out the gap between symptoms and the in-therapy focus on psychotherapeutic intervention. Even when the final goal of treatment is symptom reduction, eg, reduction in depression, the various schools of psychotherapy approach this final goal with quite different mediating goals of treatment. How to measure these mediating goals is extremely important to the advancement of the field. Horowitz and colleagues attempt to bridge dynamic and cognitive-behavioral constructs and to measure these constructs in a reliable manner.

See also pages 625, 633, 637, 639, 642, 646, 649, 651, and 654

Horowitz and colleagues' own work highlights some of the difficulties they and others have faced. Is their method reliable? The data suggest that it is reliable, although one gets the impression that the raters were trained for many hours. The difficulties in dealing with complex constructs and the idiosyncratic verbalizations of patients provide obstacles to be overcome.

Is the method of Horowitz et al too time consuming for others to use? Only time will tell. A comparable method is Luborsky's core conflictual relationship theme (CCRT) method, which was briefly associated with a flurry of activity (see Miller et al[2] for a recent review). In contrast, self-report instruments, such as those described by Benjamin[3] and by Benjamin and Wonderlich,[4] seem to provide a more practical approach to assessment of the self-object paradigms of patients with personality disorders.

In the model of Horowitz et al, does the therapist contribute to the role-relationship verbalizations made by the patients? Data collection is focused solely on the patient's verbalizations. Perhaps different aspects of the patient's self are brought out and fostered by different therapists.

The most serious issue for me, however, is that the labor-intensive methods of describing in detail the various aspects of the self that are verbalized by the patient during therapy sessions may be seen as solipsistic musings of abstract psychodynamic thinkers. Unless the role-relationship model can be seen as useful in the context of assessing psychotherapy *outcome* rather than *process* alone, the method will probably be used only for a short time. However, there is every reason to believe that such a method, applied in the context of outcomes research, could be useful and informative. For example, in the multisite National Institute of Mental Health Treatment of Depression Collaborative Research Program (Elkin et al[5] and Elkin[6]), we know that depressed patients with comorbid Axis II disorders did not respond readily to treatment (Shea et al[7]). It would be interesting to examine the role-relationship themes between patient and therapist and to compare them in the patients with and without comorbid personality disorders. Furthermore, it is possible that the therapists using interpersonal psychotherapy addressed the role-relationship themes in a different way than those using cognitive behavior therapy. On the other hand, it is possible that the role-relationship themes were addressed in a way that depended more on therapist characteristics than on the specific treatment (interpersonal psychotherapy or cognitive behavior therapy) being used. The more general point is that efficacy research (ie, carefully defined, small samples of patients treated by highly selected therapists) must lead to effectiveness research (ie, large groups of patients treated by more typical therapists in the community). Detailed, labor-intensive process research has a place, but only when the efficacy of the treatment is firmly established.

John F. Clarkin, PhD
Department of Psychiatry
Westchester Division
Cornell Medical Center
21 Bloomingdale Rd
White Plains, NY 10605

REFERENCES

1. Horowitz MJ, Eells T, Singer J, Salovey P. Role-relationship models for case formulation. *Arch Gen Psychiatry.* 1995;52:625-632.
2. Miller NE, Luborsky L, Barber JP, Docherty JP. *Psychodynamic Treatment Research.* New York, NY: Basic Books; 1993.
3. Benjamin LS. *The Intrex User's Manual: Parts I and II.* Salt Lake City, Utah: Intrex Interpersonal Institute; 1983.
4. Benjamin LS, Wonderlich SA. Social perceptions and borderline personality disorder: the relation to mood disorders. *J Abnorm Psychol.* 1994;103:610-624.
5. Elkin I, Shea TM, Watkins JT, Imber SD, Sotsky SM, Collins JF, Glass DR, Pilkonis PA, Leber WR, Docherty JP, Fiester SJ, Parloff MB. National Institute of Mental Health Treatment of Depression Collaborative Research Program: general effectiveness of treatments. *Arch Gen Psychiatry.* 1989;46:971-982.
6. Elkin I. The NIMH treatment of depression collaborative research program: where we began and where we are. In: Bergin AE, Garfield SL, eds. *Handbook of Psychotherapy and Behavior Change.* 4th ed. New York, NY: John Wiley & Sons Inc; 1994:114-139.
7. Shea MT, Pilkonis PA, Beckham E, Collins JF, Elkin I, Sotsky SM, Docherty JP. Personality disorders and treatment outcome in the NIMH Treatment of Depression Collaborative Research Program. *Am J Psychiatry.* 1990;147:711-718.

COMMENTARY

Role-Relationship Models

Are They Useful for Research and Practice?

CLINICAL theories, psychological formulations of patients, and inferences about their mental processes, until recently, could be evaluated only informally. Such assessments necessarily relied largely on clinical understanding and experience. Important strides are now being made in the formidable task of testing, in scientifically acceptable ways, inferences and assumptions that are made routinely in clinical practice about patients' mental processes. The method of Horowitz and his colleagues[1] for generating psychological formulations that are reliable and replicable is an important exemplar of this development. Alternative approaches to this problem include, among others, the Core Conflictual Relationship Theme,[2] the Plan Formulation Method,[3] the Structural Analysis of Social Behavior,[4] and Fundamental Repetitive and Maladaptive Emotion Structures.[5] All of these approaches apply an organizing framework for specific constructs and capture repetitive structures of motivation, cognition, emotion, or interpersonal transactions.

See also pages 625, 633, 637, 639, 642, 645, 649, 651, and 654

The role-relationship model (RRM) configurational method derives from an extensive research program, and during the last 10 years, a series of publications has appeared presenting the model and its theoretical underpinnings. Significant effort clearly has been invested in the development of this approach to diagnosis and formulation, and it represents a step forward in the ongoing attempt to operationalize complex and subtle clinical constructs. Nevertheless, it continues to be characterized by conceptual and methodological ambiguities that raise questions about the model's usefulness for clinical work and research and that persist in giving the impression that the approach remains preliminary in a number of important respects: in its assumption that cognitive science and psychoanalytic theory have been sufficiently integrated to permit direct and pragmatic application; in its implications for the conduct of psychotherapy; and methodologically, in terms of the adequacy and replicability of its empirical strategies.

THEORETICAL CONUNDRUMS AT THE INTERFACE OF COGNITIVE SCIENCE AND PSYCHOANALYSIS

Underlying this new approach to case formulation is an ambitious attempt at creating a new theory of mind that borrows constructs, terminology, and metaphors from psychoanalytic theory, cognitive science, and information processing models. In this mix of often ambiguous and sometimes confusing theoretical paradigms and language, the reader is flung precipitously between widely varying levels of conceptualization. The many problems in achieving a useful amalgamation of some of our biggest and most important theories obviously have not yet been worked out successfully. Although there is little firm ground, the reader is expected to go along with the assumption that, at least in some key respects, such an integration has been accomplished.

The central construct in this approach to case formulation is that of *schemas*, which are defined as structures of meaning that affect thinking, planning, and action concerning the self and others. The difficulty with the concept is that it appears to be (and to do) too much: schemas are unconscious and are part of preconscious processing; they organize processes of control of emotions over time; they help form conscious experience; they are (conscious) belief structures; they are self and other in multiple combinations; they are scripts for action sequences; and they are forms of knowledge that coordinate features of perception, thought, emotion, and action. This key construct and its functions, processes, and motivational sources remain, in many important aspects, ambiguously conceptualized.

Role-relationship models are a method for identifying schemas, giving them an organizing framework, and presenting them diagrammatically. The RRMs capture attributes of the self (as seen by the self) and attributes of other persons. They also include a script for the expected interaction between oneself and the other. In short, how we behave or act toward others depends on how we view ourselves in relation to the other person. How we experience an event that occurs in reality depends on what latent person schema is activated by the event.

The problem of conceptual blurring and ambiguity can be seen in the definition of the various categories and constructs and in the relations among these entities. It is said that

> schemas are distillates of memory and fantasy processing that appear to be stored as nested hierarchies of meaning. Simple subordinate forms combine systematically, through linkages, to form complex supraordinate package.[1]

The language is difficult and strikes one as a forced attempt to graft some of the ideas of cognitive science and artificial intelligence onto psychodynamic theory, as is the invocation of pathway models and information processing flow charts. Terminology is used without specific referent, and conceptualizations are often disconcertingly vague.

The description of the symptoms of personality disorders and thinking about the underlying motivation of behavior seem oversimplified, possibly in an effort to accommodate such descriptions to the constraints necessarily inherent in RRM configurations (RRMCs). Still, it is as if all personality disorders are similar and only vary from one another in terms of the specific content of the individual's RRMC. Horowitz et al[2] assert that "observation of phenomena of disturbances in identity and interpersonal relationships led to the classification of personality disorders in *DSM-III* and *DSM-IV*." This is a serious overgeneralization. Although the majority of *DSM* criteria across personality disorders describe symptomatic behavior that affects an individual's ability to relate (or style of relating) to others, the only personality disorder that includes disturbances in identity as one of its criteria is borderline personality disorder. Most researchers who have studied the traits that are descriptive of the various personality disorders do not include identity disturbance or diffusion among their criteria.[6]

A central premise of the RRM method is that identity disturbance is identifiable in contradictory statements made about the self. Again, identity disturbances are not uniformly or essentially descriptive of all personality disorders. Second, the assumption that identity disturbances can be assessed from contradictory statements about oneself has thus far not been supported empirically, nor is it commonly accepted clinically. There is evidence that traits of individuals with personality disorder vary only in terms of degree (rather than categorically) from those of individuals with normal or adaptive personalities.[7,8] If a person can be considered to be located somewhere on a spectrum of traits, where on this continuum does an appreciation for inner contradictions or the complexity of one's identity become a cluster of contradictory multiple selves? Research on cognitive bias shows that individuals make more situational or state attributions for their varying behavior, whereas others observing their behavior make more trait attributions. This may be relevant to the RRM method, which requires that judgments be made about identity disturbances or intraindividual contradictions in patients who describe themselves as being different in different situations. Pragmatically speaking, it is not easy to judge inconsistency among a patient's self-descriptions, and moreover, it cannot be concluded that such inconsistencies indicate the presence of a personality disorder.

A great deal more clear thinking is needed about the specific relations that are likely between certain kinds of RRMs and Axis II diagnoses. A serious effort to link the two would require another kind of research program, one that generated data, systematically tying particular sets of characteristics, traits, roles, and transactions to certain categories of personality disorder. Indeed, it is difficult to assess how interested Horowitz et al[1] really are in creating meaningful links between their method and *DSM* personality disorder diagnoses. One is left wondering whether the RRM method is not actually intended to be a potential alternative to *DSM* Axis II diagnoses. Developing alternative models to *DSM* will, of course, help in continuing to advance the field. The problem is that the link between RRMs and *DSM* diagnoses is merely asserted and not actually demonstrated.

THE USEFULNESS OF RRMCs FOR CLINICAL PRACTICE IS UNCERTAIN

Horowitz et al[1] open their article with a statement to which all clinicians could give assent:

> Diagnosis of personality disorders represents a first step toward treatment; however, it is not sufficient for the effective planning of therapy. An essential step toward effective therapy is proper formulation.

Unfortunately, the treatment implications of RRMC-derived formulations are nowhere addressed. How might an RRMC inform a therapist's approach to a case? Would it, for example, aid in finding a more systematic way to judge when to make an intervention or how to frame an interpretation? The several figures, diagrams, and cycle charts illustrating the RRMC of a patient are of little help. It would be useful if the idiom of the RRM approach included more traditional clinical language, eg, how is the RRM similar to the familiar construct of mental representations? In view of the uneasy theoretical amalgamation RRMs represent, there is no obvious reason why the concept of transference could not be invoked to explain why particular RRMs emerge or predominate in certain interpersonal contexts and why they repeatedly reoccur. It would also help if the model spoke more directly to current clinical concerns. One could imagine, for example, RRMCs serving as a framework for contemporary intersubjective theories of psychotherapy.[9] It will be difficult for this approach to enter clinical thinking until it becomes further integrated into the more usual modes of clinical discourse, and clear links are made to other, more conventional methods of formulation.

LIMITATIONS IN METHOD

It is difficult to assess the adequacy or replicability of the methods used to establish RRMCs based on the description of research methods presented. Basic procedures are not described in sufficient detail. The first step in creating an RRM requires identifying "systematic inconsistencies in the words the patient used to describe herself."[1] The criteria and procedure for identifying inconsistencies is not spelled out here or elsewhere. Are all self-representations that are contained in the voluminous material made available in videotapes (or transcripts) of treatment hours identified and coded? How many occur in a typical hour? How many judges are needed? No mention is made whether this task, so basic to the RRM approach, can be accomplished reliably.

In the illustration of the procedure provided, two independent teams freely create their own RRMCs. One team arrives at an RRM of "shy sick patient"; the other team generates "socially uncomfortable." These formulations are then deemed "acceptably close."[1] This is a weak approach to establishing consensus; the strategy is defended by the rationalization that "in a richly complex approach to formulation, we cannot expect perfect independent agreement." Perhaps, however, methods could be devised to determine how close these formulations are, for example, by submitting them to another independent panel of judges who could assess their similarity in ways that would yield conventional reliability indexes.

In the one report cited that describes a reliability study in some detail,[10] the procedure entailed assessing the rate of agreement among a panel of clinical judges in pairing RRMCs with four patients whose videotaped therapy sessions were observed. Reliability for these four patients was described as "fair to poor"; reliability for some treatment hours was less than zero. In short, even when a less than stringent test of reliability (a matching task involving a small number of patients) is applied, reliability for the RRM method does not appear to be strong. Moreover, while such procedures assess agreement among clinicians as to which (previously constructed) RRMCs fit reasonably well with which patients, it does not address the more difficult problem of determining whether RRMCs can be reliably constructed in the first place using the RRM format to freely generate configurations for patients. Could independent groups using RRMC procedures achieve consensus? The question remains, then, whether the method is transportable and user friendly.

COMMENT

The RRM method attempts to address an important problem for clinical science. It is creative, complex, and intriguing. Identifying and articulating the method's problems is not always easy, given the sometimes loose conceptualization and often vague terminology. One is left with the uncomfortable feeling that grand theorizing obscures limitations in methods. A real disappointment is its failure to advance: problems in the theory, in the operationalization of its constructs, and in their quantification, which were evident in previous publications, persist unmitigated. The disappointment becomes even more pronounced with the realization that the RRM model, with all its promise for clinical research and practice, is, by virtue of its often obscure theory and language, inaccessible to most clinicians.

Enrico E. Jones, PhD
Jennifer Dyer-Friedman, MA
Department of Psychology
University of California–Berkeley
3210 Tolman Hall, No. 1650
Berkely, CA 94720-1650

Reprint requests to Dr Jones.

REFERENCES

1. Horowitz MJ, Eells T, Singer J, Salovey P. Role-relationship models for case formulation. *Arch Gen Psychiatry.* 1995;52:625-632.
2. Luborsky L, Crits-Christoph P. *Understanding Transference: The CCRT Method.* New York, NY: Basic Books Inc; 1990.
3. Weiss J, Sampson H, Mount Zion Psychotherapy Research Group. *The Psychoanalytic Process: Theory, Clinical Observation and Empirical Research.* New York, NY: Guilford Press; 1986.
4. Benjamin L. *Interpersonal Diagnosis and Treatment of Personality Disorders.* New York, NY: Guilford Press; 1993.
5. Dahl H, Teller V. The characteristics, identification, and application of FRAMES. *Psychother Res.* 1994;3-4:253-276.
6. Wiggins J, Pincus A. Conceptions of personality disorders and dimensions of personality. *Psychol Assess.* 1989;1:305-316.
7. Livesly W, Jackson D, Schroeder M. Factorial structure of traits delineating personality disorder in clinical and general population samples. *J Abnorm Psychol.* 1992;101:432-440.
8. Trull T, Widiger T, Guthrie P. Categorical vs dimensional status of borderline personality disorder. *J Abnorm Psychol.* 1990;99:40-48.
9. Stolorow R, Brandchaft B, Atwood G. *Psychoanalytic Treatment: An Intersubjective Approach.* Hillsdale, NJ: Analytic Press; 1987.
10. Horowitz M, Eels T. Case formulations using role-relationship model configurations: a reliability study. *Psychother Res.* 1993;3:57-68.

COMMENTARY

'Richly Complex' but Needs an Emotion Theory

At a time when health maintenance organizations of all kinds are paying little or nothing for psychotherapy of Axis I, much less Axis II, disorders, many, if not most, psychiatry departments seem to be cooperating by emphasizing *DSM-IV*[1] diagnoses and drug treatment. In my own department, 11 of 25 psychiatric grand rounds in the past academic year were sponsored by drug companies. Guess what diagnoses they are interested in?

Therefore, it is refreshing to read the focus by Horowitz et al[2] on avowed personality problems. For the last 10 years, with MacArthur Foundation support, Horowitz and colleagues have pursued "configurational analysis," by which they mean a case formulation method that is also, to some extent, an explanatory model of the patient's pathological, maladaptive interactions with other people. The role-relationship model (RRM) configurations, as they call them, are designed "to inform us about how and why an individual repeats a maladaptive pattern" of relationships with others.

They are not alone. The Fall 1994 issue of *Psychotherapy Research* contains seven different but enticingly similar approaches to systematically, reliably, and rigorously studying, measuring, and characterizing patients' recurring maladaptive behaviors.[3-5] Each of these seven different research groups (including two simpler methods by Dahl and Teller[3] and Luborsky et al[5]) applied their own research methods to the same patient's 10 000-word initial interview. It is also striking that the majority of these researchers have doctorates in psychology, not psychiatry. With National Institute of Mental Health funding for such work a near thing of the past, it is clear that clinical psychology departments hold whatever future there is for such research, not psychiatry departments.

One major implication of all this work is that, despite its best efforts to ignore and not support such work, psychiatry may in the long run benefit from others not letting the psyche die. It is less clear to me that the model of Horowitz et al[2] will be one of the survivors. It yields configurations that are, in their own words, "richly complex." To them, it is a virtue that their methods can capture multiple contradictory trends in the RRM's predetermined structure. One of the method's strengths lies in what they call the "mapping sentence." This is a way to systematically capture and organize "*traits of self, traits of others,* and *actions* stemming from either source." Also, it leads to a personality description that has the same structure for every patient, but different contents. Horowitz et al are correct; this method yields complex descriptions that do indeed seem to capture some of the apparent complexity of personality organization.

See also pages 625, 633, 637, 639, 642, 645, 646, 651, 654

However, in his article in *Psychotherapy Research*, Horowitz[4] throws doubt on the method's practical application to actual, real-life patients, as he proposes. First, there is the dubious prospect that any health organization in the near future will pay for the extra clinical work (recording and transcribing interviews, searching these transcripts for data to map into the RRM structures, etc) that this method entails. Second, it will take a large body of research to convincingly demonstrate, if it can be done, that these formulations will actually help clinicians and save money in the long run. Third, most of the judgments involved in the mapping are in effect clinical judgments, not much different from those that all psychotherapists tend to make automatically, if not so systematically. It is, in the end, a method that uses very familiar clinical categories. Finally, and this might be the last nail in the coffin, Horowitz[4] himself wrote that the 10 000-word interview used by all seven research groups did "not provide enough information for configurational analysis." He did his best, but in the detailed study by Luborsky et al[6] of the degree of similarity among the different groups' formulations of the patient's problems and personality, that of Horowitz[4] ranked six of seven. A 10 000-word interview is extensive, and, if this is not enough for his procedure, he will have a hard time selling it to clinicians.

There is, however, another, less obvious set of problems, which Horowitz shares with most researchers in this field. All psychiatrists and psychotherapists implicitly (and most of the time explicitly) use basic concepts like "wish," "emotions," "beliefs," and of course, "conflict." However, there are almost never real definitions of these terms, and they are rarely embodied in coherent theories. I am particularly troubled by the common (shared by Horowitz et al[2]) lack of a functional theory of emotions. The terms their judges use in Figures 4 and 5 are almost all emotion labels or descriptions of behaviors designed to satisfy wishes implicit in emotions. It is true that there is a rough division into positive, eg, "desired RRM," and negative, eg, "dreaded RRM," but otherwise they are not represented by their functions. Moreover, the authors[2] mention a "wish-fear dilemma composed of linking between desired and dreaded RRMs," as if wishes and fears were polar opposites. Of course we can guess that they simply mean the commonsense idea that a wish is something to be desired and a fear is something to be avoided. The problem is that this is a too simple (and probably false) formula. It does not account for the obvious fact that people often wish for very fearful experiences if they think they can escape the danger involved. Witness skydiving, bungee jumping, rock climbing, and driving 60 mph on the streets of Brooklyn.

I am particularly biased because 17 years ago, I first published an emotion classification scheme based on three empirically independent dimensions of mental life, yielding eight major categories of emotions.[7,8] I have also presented an information feedback theory of emotions that views one large class of emotions such as anger, love, surprise, and fear as *appetitive wishes* about objects, with many different consummatory acts to fulfill them.[9-12] The other large class of emotions such as anxiety, depression, contentment, or joy represent *beliefs about the state of fulfillment of the wishes*. The theory offers a rationale for noting the differing functions of each class of emotions. In addition to my own ongoing research on the expressions of emotions during psychotherapy, an increasing amount of research, particularly in Germany, is being done using this scheme. In addition, my own FRAMES (Fundamental Repetitive and Maladaptive Emotion Structures)[3] represent the enduring plots of the stories that people in psychotherapy tell about their encounters with others. A central reason these recurrent plots effectively capture a patient's maladaptive personality structure is that the great majority of events in each plot are in fact emotion events, just as Horowitz et al[2] have aptly demonstrated in Figures 4 and 5. It seems a pity to me that psychotherapy researchers, whose raw material deals so much in people's feelings, do not avail themselves of the power of a coherent functional model of emotions.

In their article, Horowitz et al[2] show that it does indeed make a difference how one formulates a case. By comparing "case-correct" and "case-incorrect" formulations, they show that judgments of correct formulations "fit" much better. This is surely a minimum requirement if this or a similar method were to be actually used to evaluate real-life patients. However, they also make clear that a lot of work is involved in these judgments, a lot of data are needed (five recorded and transcribed sessions in their examples), and the question is, for clinical purposes, who is going to pay for it all?

Hartvig Dahl, MD
Health Science Center
State University of New York
450 Clarkson Ave
Brooklyn, NY 11203-2098

REFERENCES

1. American Psychiatric Association. *Diagnostic and Statistical Manual of Mental Disorders, Fourth Edition.* Washington, DC: American Psychiatric Association; 1994.
2. Horowitz MJ, Eells T, Singer J, Salovey P. Role-relationship models for case formulation. *Arch Gen Psychiatry.* 1995;52:625-632.
3. Dahl H, Teller V. The characteristics, identification and applications of FRAMES. *Psychother Res.* 1994;3-4:252-274.
4. Horowitz M. Configurational analysis and the use of role-relationship models to understand transference. *Psychother Res.* 1994;3-4:184-196.
5. Luborsky L, Popp C, Luborsky E, Mark D. The core conflictual relationship theme. *Psychother Res.* 1994;3-4:172-183.
6. Luborsky L, Popp C, Barber J. Common and special factors in different transference-related measures. *Psychother Res.* 1994;3-4:277-286.
7. Dahl H. A new psychoanalytic model of motivation: emotions as appetites and messages. *Psychoanal Contemp Thought.* 1978;1:373-408.
8. Dahl H, Stengel B. A classification of emotion words: a modification and partial test of de Rivera's decision theory of emotions. *Psychoanal Contemp Thought.* 1978;1:269-312.
9. Dahl H. An information feedback theory of emotions and defenses. In: Conte H, Plutchik R, eds. *Ego Defenses: Theory and Measurement.* New York, NY: John Wiley and Sons Inc; 1995:98-119.
10. Dahl H. The appetite hypothesis of emotions: a new psychoanalytic model of motivation. In: Izard CE, ed. *Emotions in Personality and Psychopathology.* New York, NY: Plenum Press; 1979:201-225.
11. Dahl H. The key to understanding change: emotions as appetitive wishes and beliefs about their fulfillment. In: Safran J, Greenberg L, eds. *Emotions, Psychotherapy and Change.* New York, NY: Guilford; 1991:130-165.
12. Dahl H, Hölzer M, Berry JW. *How to Classify Emotions for Psychotherapy Research.* Ulm, Germany: Ulmer Textbank-Verlag; 1992:1-100.

Personality: Psychodynamic Perspectives

The personality disorder literature bulges with arguments concerning the aptness of the dimensional or the categorical view as a basis for classification.[1] Now Horowitz and his team[2] ask yet another question that goes beyond the issue of discriminant validity in personality taxonomy, raising the issue of the usefulness of our current classification for intervention. Other matters are also considered in their criticism, such as the idea that static personality profiles do not account for the multiple reaction patterns that may arise in any one person with a so-called personality disorder. They reintroduce the role-relationship model (RRM), about which Horowitz[3] has written so eloquently before, and acknowledge his debt to the core conflictual relationship theme (CCRT) of Luborsky et al.[4] This report is not a fully original contribution, but rather a summary of new and prior reliability and validity studies that recommend the scientific claim of the method, and further demonstrates the efficacy of the approach for therapeutic intervention. I will by and large leave any quibbling about the adequacy of the demonstration for other audiences. I instead will attempt to approach the RRM in terms of where it fits in modern psychoanalytic theory, also try to place it in the framework of current psychiatric personality theory, and finally inquire into its pragmatic value for psychiatric clinicians.

Currently, psychoanalysis can be said to operate among a number of related theories. They include classical ego psychology, with emphasis on conflict resolution and compromise formation as its foundation; self-psychology, with emphasis on deficit in early experience as the pathogenic agent and seeking self-cohesion as an aim; Kleinian theory, with emphasis on inner state and its projections as the distorting effect on relationships; and, finally, object-relations theory, with emphasis on the distorting effect of rigidly established tendencies for interaction, based on internalized patterns that are believed to have their origins in past relationships. All models share three common premises of unconscious contribution to overt behavior, the centrality of childhood experience, and the role of defensive operations that are called into play outside of awareness to protect the person from facing unacceptable thoughts and wishes. This should serve as a sufficient reminder of the major theories in current use. I should now like to turn to Horowitz's proposal about the usefulness of the RRM for personality theory and to determine where his attempt to render the clinical wisdom carried in these theories stands scientifically and which models seem to dominate his thinking as derived from systematic observation of the actual interchanges between patients and therapists.

Horowitz's view of personality differs from the standard *DSM* categorical approach and also from the dimensional trait approach espoused by others. In taking this stance, he highlights the Galtonian pitfall of averaging to cover blemishes and differences. Instead, he emphasizes the interpersonal configurations of personality expression in various interactions, rendering each personality as a conglomerate of action and reaction patterns. As the authors of the study[2] note, "Schemas include scripts for action," and "Person schemas are [enduring] belief structures about self and other." This approach avoids hypostasizing static structures. Instead, they offer a syntagmatic dynamic view that, like any standard sentence, contains a subject, verb, and object. It allows for a variety of interactional schemas to define the person. Horowitz and his team do not limit the number of patterns in this study. However, if there are more than three or four dispositions, we open the door to a most complex personality theory that is boundless in its dimensions. How can we reconcile this model with existing models, and how does the Horowitz model stand up to existing data?

See also pages 625, 633, 637, 639, 642, 645, 646, 649, and 654

First, I will consider a psychoanalytic frame to find his coordinates and follow with a consideration of a general psychiatric frame. In its infancy, psychoanalysis had a characterology that was based on libidinal-stage configurations. We are all acquainted with such rubrics as anal and oral personalities and recognize that their descriptive components certainly have some validity. However, analysts have not sought to verify the soundness of the relationship between developmental stages and the specific adult personality outcomes. Horowitz's schemas go much beyond static variables in an attempt to capture the patient in action, and here he seems to be strongly attached to the object-relationist vantage, coupled with a firm classical belief in wish-defense compromise.

When Freud discovered the transference tendencies of patients, he allowed for the inclusion of a firm focus within psychoanalysis of a set of restrictive patterns of interaction that were tainted by past experiences with early caretakers as remembered. Many then offered that these restrictive patterns discovered in interaction were the true stuff of patients as defined in their behavior with others. Among analysts, the discussion arose as to whether we were discovering the past in the present or whether the interpersonal field was determining. This is a central debate currently. Those who worked with difficult borderline patients, such as Kernberg,[5] focused on internalized self-object oscillations in which patients enacted either pole of the distorted constellations. Kleinians invented projective identification, best modified by Sandler,[6] as the tendency of the analyst to respond in a "role responsive" way if not aware of his or her own countertransference. All these ideas have a kinship to Horowitz's RRM, if we also include his strong plea for wish-defense configurations. In the foregoing, I hope that I have placed Horowitz in a psychoanalytic frame. Most importantly, he belongs also to too small a cadre of scientists who have diligently attempted to convert the clinical anecdote into firmer data for public scrutiny and scientific advance.[7]

I will now approach the RRM model from the vantage of modern psychiatry. The multiaxial format in *DSM-III*[8] and *DSM-IV*[9] did much to help clinicians get some descriptive soundness into diagnoses. Nonetheless, its categorical frame of reference leaves much to be desired in regard to discriminant validity and in capturing personality. As Cantwell[10] wrote about *DSM-III* concerning children, it describes disorders and not children. Indeed, too many persons must be squeezed into procrustean patient beds. Many dynamic psychiatrists argued for a dynamic or a defense axis to cover the larger field not considered in the five Axes, and then Perry et al[11] and Shapiro,[12] representing respectively adults and children, opted for a dynamic formulation to round out the inadequacies of static categorical description.

Horowitz, in his espousal of a set of schemas to define the personality, offers a dimensionlike description similar to those personality theorists who, though descriptive in their vantage, wish to capture more of the person. Most significantly, as noted above, this is a model based on observations over time and in interaction with a therapist. Thus, the diagnosis cannot be captured in a single interview. In this sense, the basic method is similar to those of Kernberg[5] and Kohut,[13] whose approaches to diagnoses are defined by a sequence of interactions with examiners. Can we say that these are more ecologically sound? Do they better describe personalities and/or offer better prognostic predictive valence for understanding future action patterns? Indeed, in large strokes, can a description derived from a single clinical interview match a novelist's description? Closer to our home ground, can a questionnaire or a diagnostic schedule capture the personality?

There is no doubt that such schedules achieve reliable concordance but, once done, what else do they predict? I think that most taxonomists of personality would answer, "What do we wish to include in the basic description, and what use shall we put it to?" Horowitz is clearly interested in the interaction potentials, the distorting influence of fixed response patterns to anticipated categories of wish and dread, etc. Parenthetically, Horowitz's model also is close to the cognitive behavioral school in this dimension insofar as distorted cognitive organizations are said to be the seat of emotional miscarriage.

His, as I noted earlier, is a syntagmatic dynamic model of personality. Nonetheless, there are other problems that arise in relation to the remainder of our personality network. For Horowitz, traits are the atoms that are not further defined, not the molecules of the system, whereas the descriptive personality theorists use traits in a reverse manner. Behavioral genetic studies[14] probably would falter if confronted with a rich array of RRMs that were state dependent as the only means of classification; developmental continuities could probably be followed up from early interaction patterns, but we still do not have the language of translation of trait to personality or the determinants of interaction patterns except in the broadest strokes. The early attempt by Brody[15] to define "baby" by patterns of mothering may have some kinship to this method.

Thus I am led to the conclusion that the RRM and its sister CCRT[4] are extremely innovative and useful research tools that will offer a means of understanding how persons act with each other and will alert the new wave of psychotherapists to a firmer ground on which to base their interpretations and descriptions. Such methodological advances should remove the mystery from the psychotherapeutic approaches and solidify the next wave of research in this area. This, however, is a pragmatic application of the method to a unique task. It does not cover all bases in our need to have a personality theory.

A final caution: even if research of this kind does not lead to widespread use by clinicians, it remains an impressive antidote to the naysayers who only offer criticism of psychoanalytically driven research. Similarly, Horowitz and his colleagues,[2] I am sure, are well aware that every investigative approach reduces data to an algorithm, or else the ideas could not be statistically manipulated to diminish bias or be considered to be generally applicable. The RRMs that define any human being are still coded statements within a specific frame of reference that is method bound and therefore selective in its general usefulness. Insofar as this proviso is specified, we can see both its prospects and its limits.

Theodore Shapiro, MD
Department of Psychiatry
Cornell University
Medical College
525 E 68th St, Box 147
New York, NY 10021

REFERENCES

1. Shapiro T. Psychoanalytic classification and empiricism with borderline personality disorder as a model. *J Consult Clin Psychol.* 1989;57:187-194.
2. Horowitz MJ, Eells T, Singer J, Salovey P. Role-relationship models for case formulation. *Arch Gen Psychiatry.* 1995;52:625-632.

3. Horowitz MJ, ed. *Person Schemas and Maladaptive Interpersonal Patterns.* Chicago, Ill: University of Chicago Press; 1991.
4. Luborsky L, Crits-Christoph P, Friedman SH, Mark D, Schaffler P. Freud's transference template compared with the core conflictual relationship theme (CCRT): illustrations by the two cases. In: Horowitz MJ, ed. *Person Schemas and Maladaptive Interpersonal Patterns.* Chicago, Ill: University of Chicago Press; 1991:167-196.
5. Kernberg OF. Psychic structure and structural change: an ego psychology-object relations theory viewpoint. *J Am Psychoanal Assoc.* 1988;36 (suppl):315-337.
6. Sandler J. Countertransference and role responsiveness. *Int Rev Psychoanal.* 1976;3:43-47.
7. Shapiro T, Emde R, eds. *Research in Psychoanalysis: Process, Development, Outcome.* Madison, Conn: International Universities Press; 1994.
8. American Psychiatric Association. *Diagnostic and Statistical Manual of Mental Disorders, Third Edition.* Washington, DC: American Psychiatric Association; 1980.
9. American Psychiatric Association. *Diagnostic and Statistical Manual of Mental Disorders, Fourth Edition.* Washington, DC: American Psychiatric Association; 1994.
10. Cantwell DP. The diagnostic process and diagnostic classification in child psychiatry: *DSM-III. J Am Acad Child Psychiatry.* 1980;19:345-355.
11. Perry S, Cooper A, Michels R. The psychodynamic formulation: its purpose, structure and clinical application. *Am J Psychiatry.* 1987;144:543-550.
12. Shapiro T. The psychodynamic formulation in child and adolescent psychiatry. *J Am Acad Child Adolesc Psychiatry.* 1989;28:675-680.
13. Kohut H. *How Does Analysis Cure?* Chicago, Ill: University of Chicago Press; 1984.
14. Lochlin JC, Nichols RC. *Heredity, Environment, and Personality.* Austin, Tex: University of Texas Press; 1976.
15. Brody S. *Patterns of Mothering.* New York, NY: International Universities Press; 1956.

Role-Relationship Model Configurations

A Summation

WE ARE most grateful for the opportunity provided by the ARCHIVES for this dialogue. The commentaries accord on the importance, future potential, and difficulty of research in this area. The difficulty is worth confronting because we need to understand the psychological core of psychiatric disorders as well as the biological and social cores. Emotions and personal meanings in conflict are a part of the psychological domain.

Some commentators said we moved too far from psychodynamics, others said we were too psychodynamic. That range of assessments seems about right to us. We are on the move toward an integration of theories and aim to preserve valid aspects of psychodynamic formulations. Consider the authors of our article[1]: Horowitz is trained as a psychoanalyst, Salovey is a cognitive-behaviorist, and Eells and Singer are interpersonal and cognitive clinicians. We worked together because we sought a sober and objective pursuit of truth, as do the commentators. This kind of debate in the journal is a good tool for forging an eventual consensus.

We will summarize the debate and respond to the commentaries by first touching on language and theory. Then we will address the issues of research methods and practical clinical utility.

LANGUAGE AND THEORY

In developing a shared terminology, some habitual usages must change. Our terms were agreed on, in workshops consisting of both psychodynamic and cognitive scientists, though never unanimously.[2] In those workshops, we learned that it is important to use separate terms for the conscious representation of self-concepts and personal identity and for nonconscious linkages between associated meaning elements that can constitute self-schemas. This differentiation of terminology is important in scientific domains that recognize the importance of constructive mental activities based on brain substrates as well as the social contexts of meanings. It acknowledges that relationship schemas may be implicit rather than explicit, procedural rather than declarative, and based on connections between meanings that do not necessarily have a primary semantic basis.

Several commentaries focused on our use of the word *schemas* instead of *representations*. This terminology is based on a willingness to articulate connectionism in neuroscience with psychological models based on associationism. The word representation is then used in the sense of a conscious awareness of meaning. There can be visual image representations, auditory image representations, lexical representations, and representations as bodily enactions. This array of conscious experiences is formed by constructive processes. Yet we still need words to refer to meanings that are not conscious and that are used in formation of conscious experiences. It is best not to call unconscious meaning structures by the same word, representations.

The modern term schemas was agreed on (rather than the latinized word *schemata*) to indicate enduring and slowly changing packages of generalized information that may be used in the construction of conscious representations. Thus, self-representations would refer to conscious self-concepts in any mode of representation (words, images, enactions) while self-schemas would refer to organized, nonconscious, generalized, and patterned associations that can combine and construct many bits of knowledge derived from several modular brain activities. We use the term *other* rather than *object* to facilitate interdisciplinary communication. Yet, we retain the essentials of both a dynamic and "object relations" psychoanalytic point of view, which are these: we look for configurations between wishes, fears, wish-fear dilemmas, and defensive compromises in which various enduring views of self and others in a relationship can be seen as key motivational components.

See also pages 625, 633, 637, 639, 642, 645, 646, 649, and 651

Some commentators raised issues of biological and social-contextual determinants. We agree that biological, temperamental, cultural, and other influences are important codeterminants of personality and psychopathological organization. Temperament may serve as a road map that bends individuals toward certain self-schemas and role-relationship models, all else being held constant. All else is never constant. Social practices specific to families, ethnic groups, gender, generational age cohorts, and cultures also shape internalized meanings about self and other, and in turn are shaped by what individuals do. With bio-psycho-social—each codetermines the other two.

But beyond saluting any particular terminological or theoretical flag whenever it is hoisted, we must get down to some content. What are the stars, bars, and colors of the flag?

Role-relationship models, and configurations of possibly contradictory beliefs, provide a system for inferring aspects of such content at the psychological level, including what may lie beyond immediate conscious representations.

So if it is difficult and not in a yet fully shared language, why bother? The reason is that formulation must occur somewhere between our current diagnoses and any case-specific treatment planning. We all know that *DSM-IV* diagnoses are almost all descriptive, not etiological. They are the product of debate and compromise in committees as well as field trials. Surely, we place psychiatry on weak footing if we teach our trainees that these compromise diagnostic categories are true disease entities. That is why, until the development of an etiological nosology, we need systems for formulation during this interim, as most commentators agreed. The question is, which systems?

The most salient area considered by the commentators is disorders of personality. *DSM-IV* Axis II categories are a transitory menu couched in a static language of convenience. They serve useful actuarial purposes. We need to use, revise, and go beyond them to plan individual treatments. That is where formulation comes in. We agree with the commentators that configurations of role-relationship models, when standing alone, are insufficiently narrow constructions to capture all that is important in an individual's maladaptive functioning. While the article[1] you have read focused on the role-relationship models configuration (RRMC), that method is just part of a five-step approach to formulation, called configurational analysis, summarized in the **Table** and reported elsewhere.[3-5] Configurational analysis is not restrictively psychological. Biological issues such as temperament or current brain toxicities and social issues such as stigmatization, stressors, and current three-party conflictual contexts can be integrated.

Configurational Analysis for Case Formulation

Step	Activity
Phenomena	Select and describe the symptoms and problems to be explained
States of mind	Describe states in which the selected phenomena do and do not occur as well as recurrent maladaptive cycles of states
Themes and defensive control processes	Describe themes of concern during problematic states; describe how actions and expressions of ideas and emotions are avoided or obscured; infer how states of compromise may function to ward off dreaded undermodulated states
Identity and relationship configurations	Describe the organizing roles, beliefs, and scripts of expression and action that occur in each state; describe wish-fear dilemmas in relation to desired and dreaded role-relationship models; infer how defensive control processes and compromise role-relationship models may ward off such dangers; construct a configuration of role-relationship models for important but conflicted relationships and themes; identify dysfunctional attitudes and how these are involved in maladaptive state cycles
Therapy technique planning	Consider the interactions of phenomena, states, controls, and role-relationship models; explain biological and social-contextual contributions; plan how to stabilize working states by support, how to counteract defensive avoidances by direction of attention, and how to alter dysfunctional attitudes by interpretation, trials of new behavior, and repetitions; integrate psychological plan with biological and social plans

RESEARCH METHODOLOGY

The RRMC method can be used by any investigator interested in mental representations of the self and others: members of psychodynamic, cognitive-behavioral, ethnographic, or family systems schools as well as those ready for integration. Many of the commentaries supported the method, since it can contain elements derived from simpler methods, enriching the formulation by allowing for multiple selves and defensive layers. Others opposed it as too time consuming. Personality disorders may be complex enough to demand more time devoted to formulation, certainly complex stress response syndromes that combine recent traumas with enduring personality features are hard enough to formulate that time should be given to inferences about causation. Therefore, time is necessary both in formulating what to treat and how to treat it. The argument that managed care now does not permit long evaluations or treatments is not relevant; good science can and should change how care is managed.

The two alternative relational formulation systems mentioned most by commentators were the Structural Analysis of Social Behavior (SASB) of Benjamin and the Core Conflictual Relationship Theme (CCRT) of Luborsky. Neither of these systems incorporates the attention to identity and possible contradictory views of self that the RRMC fosters. That means they are less able to deal with an important aspect of motivation, the attempt to develop in the future a more coherent sense of identity and set of integrated and clear personal intentionalities with regard to relationships. Not dealing with that kind of motivation may mean overlooking important causes of interpersonal anxiety and depressions influenced by loss.

The SASB is a polarities-based system for categorization of social actions and appraisals. Its categories can be used to form the transactional scripts in an RRMC, or in a CCRT, as illustrated elsewhere.[6,7] Such use in research would probably increase reliability. In clinical practice, however, it would inevitably restrict the individual specificity of formulations. Thus, reliability is only one issue to consider when evaluating a measure; clinical utility, practicality, and the comprehensiveness with which the measure captures important phenomena must also be weighed.

The CCRT includes several elements, among which are social actions. It begins with a wish and then systematizes inferences about the positive and negative responses of self and other. As outlined in the configurational analysis approach,[5] the CCRT is contained. What the RRMC adds is (1) multiplicity of beliefs about self in any specific attachment bond of a relationship and (2) the configuration of wishes, fears, and defenses that may include antithetical, contradictory, and discrepant beliefs about likely social actions and emotional responses.

We have always acknowledged that containing simpler elements (SASB, CCRT) in a larger and layered format makes for more complex methodological problems. Although good reliability is more difficult to achieve, clinical utility may be increased. The real test, as pointed out by several commentators, is going to be in outcomes research in the future.

In the commentaries, there are a couple of minor errors we should note here. Our article summarized two reliability studies, reported in full detail elsewhere. In the first of these,[8] the reliability of the judges was not "fair to poor" as erroneously stated by Jones and Dyer-Friedman. Rather, the mean intraclass correlation coefficient for groups of five judges was .63, which is considered good reliability. Furthermore, clinical judges were able to correctly match each of four RRMCs to psychotherapy tapes that provided material for the construction of the RRMCs. All four patients in the study were treated for pathological grief.

The second reliability study,[9] not mentioned by Jones and Dyer-Friedman, contained the kind of test of independent formulation they asked for.

Another error was inadvertently made by Crits-Christoph and Connolly because our summary was too pared down. These authors were correct in noting that reliability increases with the number of judges providing ratings. However, they are wrong in stating that we pooled 20 judges to obtain reliability levels in the first study. These judges were in five-member panels (a total of 20 judges were divided into four sets of five each). A five-judge group is similar to the size of outpatient teams who might pool inferences in case conferences about the aptness of a specific case formulation.

In addition, Crits-Christoph and Connolly spoke of idiosyncratic clues in the RRMC. We anticipated this in the first reliability study and removed such clues in the wordings of RRMC as stated in that article.[7] The design of the second reliability study was such that this concern was not relevant.[8]

CLINICAL PRACTICE

As several commentaries mentioned, while some role-relationship models and configurations might be sketched out in a single session that is focused on relationship histories, it is unlikely that a valid configuration can be completed without more information. The Internal Revenue Service cannot audit a person in a single session; a complex medical condition is not decisively diagnosed in a single session; and it is ridiculous to demand that complex psychiatric disorders may be formulated in a single session. When one is dealing with a personality disorder and with an Axis I symptom disorder complicated by a personality disorder, it will be necessary to take some time with a patient before having confidence in how to formulate the case.

The procedure requires listening and observing as a patient tells and perhaps enacts with the clinician patterned stories about identity, relationships, and action traits. That is not a fault of the procedure but an advantage. Formulations are gradually developed through a sequence of revisions. As interventions are made, patients respond and more information is gained.

You, dear reader, are a clinician. Please try the format on a case you know over several sessions, at least. Stay with it a bit in spite of early hesitation and cloudiness due to the unfamiliar procedure. Think in terms of a mapping sentence with a spatial, relational topography. Start with the patient having a role in relation to another person; does the patient feel or want something to happen; the other person gives some response; the self reacts; and the self evaluates the actions of self leading to a range from pride to guilt or shame. Struggle a bit with the format (Figure 2 in our article,[1] perhaps amplified to triadic rather than diadic models if that is required). If you do so, you may find that it can call forth recognitions. See for yourself if it has clinical utility.

Suppose you find that with the first struggle to do something a bit new, or at least different from what you were doing, that it "works." You may then find the result has immediate clinical use. You can identify cycles of states based on shifts in the RRMC that organize current views and emotions of your patient. You can clarify dilemmas. You can anticipate how you might help your patient develop new beliefs about self and other. You can consider whether to encourage trials of new behavior that can, by repetitions, alter the function and nature of person schemas. You may use the language of the inferences directly in discourse that helps patients to integrate previously isolated, dissociated, discrepant, ambivalent, and otherwise contradictory beliefs about identity and relationships.

Mardi J. Horowitz, MD
University of California, San Francisco
Center on Stress and Personality
Langley Porter Institute
401 Parnassus Ave, Box F-0984
San Francisco, CA 94143

Tracy Eells, PhD
Louisville, Ky

Jerome Singer, PhD
Peter Salovey, PhD
New Haven, Conn

REFERENCES

1. Horowitz MJ, Eells T, Singer J, Salovey P. Role-relationship models for case formulation. *Arch Gen Psychiatry.* 1995;52:625-632.
2. Horowitz MJ. *Psychodynamics and Cognition.* Chicago, Ill: University of Chicago Press; 1988:16-18.
3. Horowitz MJ, ed. *Person Schemas and Maladaptive Interpersonal Patterns.* Chicago, Ill: University of Chicago Press; 1991.
4. Horowitz MJ. *Case Formulation for Psychotherapy.* Washington, DC: American Psychiatric Press Inc. In press.
5. Horowitz MJ. *States of Mind.* 2nd ed. New York, NY: Plenum Press; 1987.
6. Hartley D. Assessing the interpersonal behavior patterns using structural analysis of social behavior (SASB). In: Horowitz MJ, ed. *Person Schemas and Maladaptive Interpersonal Patterns.* Chicago, Ill: University of Chicago Press; 1991:221-260.
7. Horowitz MJ. Converging several methods for inferring person schemas. In: Horowitz MJ, ed. *Person Schemas and Maladaptive Interpersonal Patterns.* Chicago, Ill: University of Chicago Press; 1991:303-311.
8. Horowitz MJ, Eells TD. Case formulations using role-relationship model configurations: a reliability study. *Psychother Res.* 1993;3:57-68.
9. Eells TD, Horowitz MJ, Singer J, Salovey P, Daigle D, Turvey C. The role-relationship models method: a comparison of independently derived case formulations. *Psychother Res.* 1995;5:161-175.

Resting Cerebral Glucose Metabolism in First-Episode and Previously Treated Patients With Schizophrenia Relates to Clinical Features

Raquel E. Gur, MD, PhD; P. David Mozley, MD; Susan M. Resnick, PhD; Lyn Harper Mozley, PhD; Derri L. Shtasel, MD; Fiona Gallacher, MS; Steven E. Arnold, MD; Joel S. Karp, PhD; Abass Alavi, MD; Martin Reivich, MD; Ruben C. Gur, PhD

Background: Functional neuroimaging can elucidate brain dysfunction in schizophrenia. The frontal, temporolimbic, and diencephalic regions have been implicated. There is a lack of prospective samples of first-episode and previously treated patients followed up longitudinally.

Methods: Patients and controls (42 per group) were studied. Positron emission tomography with fluorodeoxyglucose, cross-registered with magnetic resonance imaging, measured metabolism. Scales assessed clinical features, premorbid adjustment, and outcome.

Results: There were no differences between groups in whole-brain metabolism or regional ratios or in anterior-posterior gradients, but left midtemporal metabolism was relatively higher in patients. This was pronounced in the negative and Schneiderian and absent in the paranoid subtypes. Higher metabolism and lower relative left hemispheric values were associated with better premorbid adjustment and outcome. A higher subcortical-cortical gradient was noted in first-episode patients.

Conclusions: There are no resting metabolic abnormalities in any brain region, but abnormal gradients are evident. These vary in subtypes, and laterality is associated with functioning. The results support the hypothesis of temporolimbic disturbance in schizophrenia that is already present at the onset of illness.

(Arch Gen Psychiatry. 1995;52:657-667)

From the Department of Psychiatry, Neuropsychiatry Program, Mental Health Clinical Research Center (Drs R. E. Gur, P. Mozley, Resnick, Shtasel, Arnold, and R. C. Gur and Ms Gallacher), the Department of Neurology, Cerebrovascular Research Center (Dr Reivich), and the Department of Radiology, Center for Functional and Metabolic Imaging (Drs L. Mozley, Karp, and Alavi), University of Pennsylvania School of Medicine, Philadelphia. Dr Resnick is currently affiliated with the Gerontology Research Center, National Institute of Aging, Baltimore, Md.

POSITRON EMISSION tomography (PET) studies of cerebral glucose metabolism with fluorodeoxyglucose (FDG) in schizophrenia[1,2] have implicated cortical and subcortical regions, suggesting abnormalities in the frontal lobes,[3,4] temporolimbic structures,[5,6] and diencephalic regions.[7,8] Studies that have examined metabolic gradients indicated abnormalities in the anterior-posterior, subcortical-cortical, and laterality dimensions.[1-8]

The value of such studies has been questioned, given the inconsistent results and the advances in technology for studying neuroreceptors.[9] Furthermore, resting measures may not be meaningful without cognitive challenges.[10,11] However, such measures obtained in a standardized setting can contribute to an understanding of the pathophysiological features by providing reliable parameters of brain activity[8] related to clinical, neurobehavioral, and neuroanatomic features.[12,13]

The topography of resting glucose metabolism has been correlated with clinical variables, including illness duration,[14] symptoms,[5,6] and treatment response.[15,16] Most studies had small, chronic, cross-sectional samples and applied single assessment scales, while few report longitudinal data in prospective samples, including neuroleptic-naive patients. Given the heterogeneity of schizophrenia, its understanding as a brain disorder necessitates assessment along multiple dimensions.

In previous cerebral blood flow[10,17] and PET FDG studies,[8,18-20] abnormalities in the laterality and subcortical-

See Subjects and Methods on next page

SUBJECTS AND METHODS

SUBJECTS

Data are given as mean±SD.

The sample included 42 patients, 22 FE and 20 PT, and 42 healthy controls (29 men and 13 women per diagnostic group), balanced sociodemographically. Age was 30.5±8.1 years for patients and 28.5±7.2 years for controls. As expected, patients attained a lower educational level than controls (12.5±2.2 vs 14.6±2.0 years, respectively), but the groups did not differ in paternal (12.8±2.8 vs 12.7±3.2 years, respectively) or maternal (12.3±2.6 vs 12.7±2.5 years, respectively) education. There were 20 white and 22 African-American subjects in the patient group and 24 and 18, respectively, in the control group.

Patients were consecutively admitted to the Mental Health Clinical Research Center, Philadelphia, Pa, with a *DSM-III-R*[22] diagnosis of schizophrenia. They included 27 inpatients and 15 outpatients examined during exacerbation in symptoms. They received previously described medical, neurological, and psychiatric[23] evaluations.[24] Participants had no history of another disorder or event that may affect brain function, including substance abuse or head trauma with loss of consciousness. Age at onset was 24.3±7.6 years (men, 22.5±6.2 years; women, 28.3±9.2 years). For FE patients, enrollment in the study was during their first psychiatric presentation. The number of previous hospitalizations for the PT patients was 3.8±5.4. Duration of illness was 2 years or less for 12 patients (all FE) and 9.5±5.4 years (range, 2 to 19 years) for the remainder. The FE patients were studied while neuroleptic naive. The PT patients were studied while not receiving neuroleptics, with the following distribution of medication-free periods: 1 week for one patient; 2 weeks for three patients; 3 weeks for one patient; 4 weeks for two patients; and more than 4 weeks for 13 patients (range, 1 to 442 weeks, for a mean of 71.9±116.8 weeks). Patients were free of any movement disorder at admission to the protocol. Four other FE patients were excluded because follow-up indicated that they did not have schizophrenia.

The controls were consecutively admitted to the Mental Health Clinical Research Center in response to newspaper advertisements and underwent a comprehensive screening.[25,26] They were healthy, with no history of schizophrenia or affective illness in a first-degree relative. There were 37 right-handed and five left-handed patients, and 40 and two controls, respectively. Informed consent was obtained prior to participation in the study.

CLINICAL RATINGS AND TYPOLOGY

The following scales were completed on admission to the Mental Health Clinical Research Center: Brief Psychiatric Rating Scale,[27] Scale for the Assessment of Negative Symptoms,[28] Scale for the Assessment of Positive Symptoms,[29] Premorbid Adjustment Scale,[30] and Abnormal Involuntary Movements Scale.[31] **Table 1** presents clinical features. None of the differences between FE and PT patients were significant when Bonferroni corrected.

Patients were followed up with repeated structured assessment of symptoms and level of functioning at 6-month intervals for a minimum of 2 years. This ensured diagnostic accuracy, permitted the typology of deficit and nondeficit,[32] and provided data on the course of illness and outcome as assessed with the Level of Function Scale.[33]

Ratings of symptoms during intake were used to form a factor-referenced subtype classification previously detailed.[21] The procedure yielded four statistically independent categories with adequate reliabilities (negative symptoms, disorganization, Schneiderian delusions and hallucinations, and suspicion and/or hostility). Patients were divided into three subgroups based on their scores on these symptom dimensions. Scores in the moderate to severe range were judged to be clinically relevant. Seven patients were classified as having negative subtypes; 19, paranoid subtypes; 11, Schneiderian subtypes; and five were not classifiable. The three groups did not differ in age at onset (22.4±8.2, 25.5±8.7, and 22.7±6.0 years for negative, paranoid, and Schneiderian subgroups, respectively) ($F[2,36]<1$), number of previous hospitalizations (0.9±1.7, 1.0±1.5, 1.5±2.1, respectively) ($F[2,36]<1$), or illness duration (6.7±3.8, 5.2±5.3, 7.6±6.4 years, respectively) ($F[2,36]<1$). The number of FE patients in the three groups was 4, 11, and 5, respectively, and the number of weeks in which no medication was received by the PT subjects were 31.4±42.3, 39.3±42.6, and 98.8±124.9, respectively ($F[2,14]=1.16$; $P=.34$).

PET PROCEDURES

Subjects underwent scanning after an overnight fast. The radial artery was catheterized with a 20-gauge Teflon cannula under local anesthesia (2% lidocaine [Xylocaine]). A venous line was placed in the contralateral antebrachium. Lines were kept patent with a solution of physiological saline. Approximately 185 MBq (5 MCi) of fluorine 18–labeled 2-fluoro-2-deoxy-D-glucose (FDG) was administered intravenously while subjects lay recumbent in a quiet, dimly lit room with eyes open and ears unoccluded. Arterial samples were obtained initially every 15 seconds and then at progressively increasing time intervals over the next 90 minutes. Samples were aspirated through a three-way stopcock coupled to the arterial cannula. The activity of ^{18}F in 250-μL aliquots was measured in a well counter (Tennelec 707, Memphis, Tenn) after a 3- to 4-hour decay interval.

Image acquisition began 40 minutes later. Subjects were positioned in a custom-molded, rigid foam head holder, using for alignment two lasers focused on the head at right angles to each other. Images were acquired on the PENN-PET scanner (built at the University of Pennsylvania, Philadelphia).[34] Its fixed gantry had a 9-cm axial field of view, and the data were sorted into 45 transaxial slices 2 mm apart. The spatial full-width half-maximum resolution averaged

cortical gradients were associated with severity of symptoms. Interpretation of physiological data requires knowledge of the neuroanatomic substrate measurable by magnetic resonance imaging (MRI). Results of subtyping our patients on a dimensional approach have suggested distinct neuroanatomic abnormalities for three subtypes: negative, Schneiderian, and paranoid.[21] The present study relates these clinical dimensions to cerebral activity in a new prospective sample, using a scanner with improved resolution and cross-registration with MRI. First-episode (FE) neuroleptic-naive patients were compared with

5.5 mm in all directions near the center of the field.[35] An average of 30 million counts was collected over the next 50 minutes. The projection data were corrected for nonuniform sensitivity that resulted from the decreasing number of coincident angles toward the axial edges of the field. Background subtraction was performed on the sinogram to compensate for scatter. Metabolic rates were calculated[36] using experimentally determined values of lumped and rate constants.[37] A standardized correction for attenuation was placed around the head to account for skull density. An optimized Hanning filter was applied during back projection. Data were averaged in the axial direction, retaining sampling of 2 mm. The fine axial sampling minimizes quantitative errors due to partial volume effects[35] and interpolation errors in registering PET image to the region of interest (ROI) template. Count rates were calculated as a product of the mean counts per pixel divided by the duration of the scan. The calibration needed to transform the count rates into units of radioactivity and dead-time correction were done regularly by phantom studies. Normalization per unit of mass in each brain region was derived from the known volume of each voxel by assuming that the density of the brain was 1.0. The images were then exported electronically into a graphics workstation (Sun Microsystems, Mountain View, Calif) for processing, together with the corresponding MRI of each subject.

IMAGE PROCESSING

Magnetic Resonance Imaging

Proton and T_2-weighted scans were acquired on a 1.5-tesla instrument (GE Medical Systems, Milwaukee, Wis), with a repetition time of 3000 milliseconds and echo times of 30 and 80 milliseconds, and processed as previously detailed.[21] Each transaxial slice was constructed by adding six 0.78-mm thick pixels. The resliced images were subsequently overlapped by 1 pixel for a final distance between slice centers of 5 pixels, or 3.9 mm.

Registration

The MRI scans and PET images were rotated in three orthogonal directions, resliced in planes parallel to the line connecting the anterior and posterior commissures, and fixed in the same orientation relative to the interhemispheric fissure. A set of templates with 42 ROIs per hemisphere was custom fitted to each MRI slice by operators blind to diagnosis.[38] Of the original set of ROIs, three were excluded for questionable validity (considered possibly too small or not well defined). The operators were trained on a set of 10 scans to an interrater reliability criterion of more than .85 (intraclass correlation) for 36 of the remaining 39 ROIs studied. Reliability calculations were based on the counts per pixel for each region, volume averaged across all slices in which the region appeared. The ROIs in representative slices are illustrated in **Figure 1**.

The MRI-based ROIs were transposed onto the resliced PET images after they were displayed on a trichotomous color scale that used a cutoff for color of 50% of the counts in the pixel of maximum intensity. The fit between MRI and PET images was accomplished by overlaying the whole-brain boundaries. All the other ROIs were moved in synchrony with the whole-brain boundaries as a single unit. The counts per pixel in these regions were imported automatically into a relational database slice by slice, region by region. Regional rates were calculated by volume-weighted averaging across all slices in which the region was present. We consider this method to be more appropriate for quantitative PET data than the within-slice averaging method necessary in nonquantitative studies. The individual fitting of PET with MRI avoids errors associated with averaging across brains with realignment methods.

DATA ANALYSIS

Absolute metabolic rates and region–whole-brain (R-WB) ratios were calculated for the 36 ROIs. We will follow the convention of presenting quantitative data for whole-brain analyses, whereas for regional analyses we will report the results of the R-WB ratios. For the primary analysis testing the hypothesis of frontal, temporal, and subcortical abnormalities in schizophrenia, we selected four subcortical, four cortical, and one control region. We limited the number of ROIs to preserve a favorable subject-to-variable ratio. The subcortical regions included the basal ganglia (caudate nucleus), the medial lenticular region that consists predominantly of the globus pallidus, the lateral lenticular region that is predominantly putamen, and the hippocampus. Cortical regions included the medial and lateral dorsal prefrontal cortex and the superior temporal and midtemporal gyri. The occipital lobe served as a control region (Figure 1).

To test the hypothesis of differential topography of activity between FE and PT patients and controls, each set of regions (subcortical, cortical, and control) was entered as the dependent measure in a repeated-measures analysis of variance (ANOVA), with diagnosis as a grouping factor and hemisphere as a within-group (repeated measures) factor. This was followed by a contrast of the FE and PT groups with controls and each other, using the same design. For the subcortical and cortical ROIs, region (four levels) served as an additional within-group factor. To limit the number of comparisons for decomposing significant interactions, we used averages of left and right hemispheres for decomposing diagnosis-by-region interactions and the laterality score, defined as (left hemisphere minus right hemisphere)/mean of (left hemisphere and right hemisphere), to decompose diagnosis-by-region-by-hemisphere interactions. Greenhouse-Geisser adjusted *P* values were used.

Testing of the hypothesis of association between metabolic activity and clinical variables was done by calculating product moment correlations between the metabolic data and summary scores of the clinical scales. Correlations were computed separately for average regional values (mean of left and right hemispheres) and the laterality index. Regional specificity of correlations was tested using the method of Olkin and Finn[39] for contrasting "correlated correlations."

previously treated (PT) patients to examine the effects of chronicity and treatment. Patients were followed up to ensure diagnosis and examine outcome. We tested the hypothesis that clinical features relate to regional abnormalities, including basal ganglia, relative hypofrontality, and increased left temporal activity.

RESULTS

WHOLE-BRAIN METABOLISM

Metabolic rates did not differ between the combined sample of FE and PT patients (4.97±2.27 mg/100 g

Table 1. Clinical Characteristics of Patients

Scale	Mean (±SD) Ratings: First-Episode Patients	Mean (±SD) Ratings: Previously Treated Patients
Brief Psychiatric Rating Scale	47.5 (7.7)	50.3 (6.5)
Scale for the Assessment of Negative Symptoms		
Affective flattening or blunting	2.4 (1.3)	2.7 (1.1)
Alogia	2.0 (1.6)	2.2 (1.6)
Avolition-Apathy	2.5 (1.8)	2.5 (1.4)
Anhedonia-Asociality	3.3 (1.0)	3.4 (1.3)
Attention	2.1 (0.9)	1.9 (1.7)
Scale for the Assessment of Positive Symptoms		
Global hallucinations	3.0 (1.3)	2.3 (1.5)
Delusions	3.5 (1.0)	3.1 (1.1)
Bizarre behavior	1.6 (1.2)	1.5 (1.5)
Positive formal thought disorder	1.8 (1.3)	3.0 (1.2)
Premorbid Adjustment Scale		
Childhood	1.8 (1.0)	1.6 (1.1)
Early adolescence	2.2 (1.1)	2.8 (2.3)
Late adolescence	2.4 (1.3)	2.5 (1.7)
Adulthood	3.2 (1.5)	4.1 (1.2)
General	2.3 (0.9)	2.5 (1.2)
Level of Function Scale		
Short-term	3.1 (0.8)	2.8 (0.7)
Long-term	3.1 (0.8)	2.8 (0.7)
Abnormal Involuntary Movements Scale	1.1 (0.2)	1.2 (0.2)

per minute) and controls (4.51±1.05 mg/100 g per-minute) (t[46.6]=1.12; P=.27). Degrees of freedom were based on the inequality of the variances, with patients having a significantly higher variance (F'[40,40]=4.73; P<.001). This was produced by one patient with a low whole-brain metabolic rate of 1.9 mg/100 g per minute and one with a high rate of 15.0 mg/100 g per minute. However, when these subjects were removed, the variances were equal, but the difference between the groups was still not significant (t[80]<1). Therefore, the data analysis and presentation include the outliers.[40] Neither FE (4.98±1.52 mg/100 g per minute) nor PT patients (4.39±0.96 mg/100 g per minute) differed significantly from controls (t[62]=1.41 and t[60]<1, respectively), nor did FE differ from PT patients (t=1.20; df=40).

REGIONAL TOPOGRAPHY

The means of absolute metabolic rates for the hemispheric ROIs in the three groups are presented in **Table 2**.

Subcortical Regions

Results of ANOVA showed main effects for region (F[3,246]=277.33; P<.001), reflecting variability among the four regions in metabolism, and hemisphere (F[1,82]=43.09; P<.001), with relatively higher right hemispheric rates. The region-by-hemisphere interaction was also significant (F[3,246]=55.23; P<.001), as this asymmetry was more pronounced for the two lenticular regions (**Figure 2**). However, there were no interactions of these effects with diagnosis. Thus, patients and controls had a similar subcortical topography.

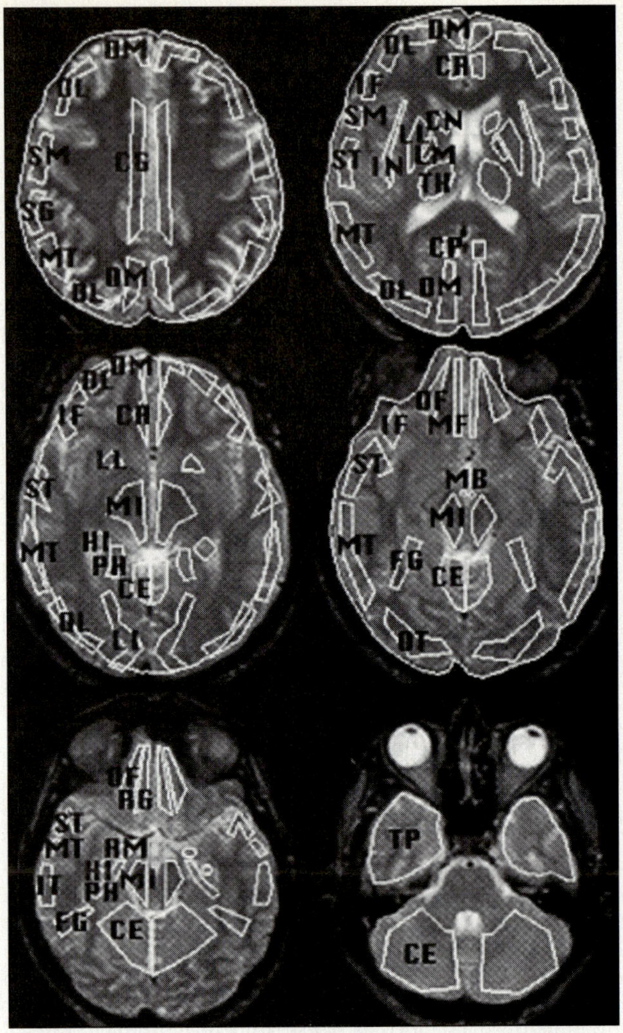

Figure 1. *Placement of regions of interest. AM indicates amygdala; CA, anterior cingulate gyrus; CE, cerebellum; CN, caudate nucleus; CG, cingulate gyrus; CP, posterior cingulate gyrus; DM, medial dorsal prefrontal cortex; DL, lateral dorsal prefrontal cortex; FG, fusiform gyrus; HI, hippocampus; IF, inferior frontal gyrus; IN, insula; IT, inferior temporal gyrus; LI, lingual gyrus; LL, lateral lenticular region (putamen); LM, medial lenticular region (globus pallidus); MB, mammillary body; MF, medial frontal region; MI, midbrain; MT, midtemporal gyrus; OF, orbital frontal region; OL, lateral occipital cortex; OM, medial occipital cortex; OT, occipital temporal cortex; PH, parahippocampal gyrus; RG, rectal gyrus; SG, supramarginal gyrus; SM, sensorimotor region; ST, superior temporal region; TH, thalmus; and TP, temporal lobe.*

Cortical Regions

There were main effects of region (F[3,216]=48.46; P<.001) and hemisphere (F[1,82]=3.98; P=.049), with relatively higher values in the left hemisphere. The region-by-diagnosis interaction was significant (F[3,246]=3.78; P=.03), although none of the individual regions showed a significant difference between patients and controls (Figure 2, top). In support of the hypothesis of *lateralized* abnormality in schizophrenia, the diagnosis-by-region-by-hemisphere interaction was significant (F[3,246]=5.23; P=.003). As seen in Figure 2 (bottom), this is attribut-

Table 2. Cerebral Metabolic Rates of Glucose in the Standard Set of Regions*

Region of Interest	Controls, Left, Mean (±SD)	Controls, Right, Mean (±SD)	First-Episode Patients, Left, Mean (±SD)	First-Episode Patients, Right, Mean (±SD)	Previously Treated Patients, Left, Mean (±SD)	Previously Treated Patients, Right, Mean (±SD)
Frontal lobe						
SF	4.08 (0.98)	4.17 (1.14)	4.64 (1.64)	4.73 (1.77)	4.51 (2.36)	4.46 (2.37)
DL	**4.78 (1.38)**	**4.75 (1.48)**	**5.39 (1.81)**	**5.43 (1.94)**	**5.16 (2.61)**	**5.19 (2.95)**
DM	**4.25 (1.18)**	**4.24 (1.27)**	**4.97 (1.87)**	**5.03 (2.06)**	**4.69 (2.58)**	**4.84 (2.73)**
MF	5.51 (1.58)	5.07 (1.61)	5.86 (1.72)	5.47 (1.87)	5.77 (3.16)	5.22 (2.72)
IF	5.15 (1.51)	5.05 (1.65)	5.86 (2.18)	5.61 (2.10)	5.72 (3.06)	5.39 (2.77)
Sensorimotor region	5.12 (1.29)	4.93 (1.40)	5.44 (1.64)	5.10 (1.58)	5.61 (3.11)	5.26 (3.18)
Parietal lobe						
SP	4.74 (1.36)	4.62 (1.42)	4.66 (1.51)	4.46 (1.14)	5.01 (3.32)	4.75 (3.54)
SG	4.60 (1.15)	4.46 (1.27)	4.54 (1.30)	4.28 (1.21)	4.65 (3.36)	4.56 (3.41)
Occipital lobe						
OL	**5.41 (1.32)**	**5.14 (1.25)**	**5.55 (1.77)**	**5.39 (1.61)**	**5.79 (3.94)**	**5.59 (3.76)**
OM	**3.95 (1.11)**	**4.19 (1.18)**	**4.11 (1.34)**	**4.24 (1.38)**	**4.36 (3.36)**	**4.56 (3.44)**
LI	5.22 (1.76)	5.11 (1.86)	5.46 (1.80)	5.35 (1.59)	5.73 (3.96)	5.81 (4.41)
FG	4.98 (1.66)	5.16 (1.75)	5.38 (2.29)	5.73 (2.57)	5.77 (5.09)	5.88 (5.29)
Corpus callosum						
C1	3.44 (1.03)	3.35 (1.03)	3.71 (1.16)	3.57 (1.23)	3.89 (2.26)	3.73 (2.41)
C2	3.78 (1.22)	3.31 (1.12)	3.91 (1.49)	3.39 (1.11)	4.48 (2.83)	3.84 (2.71)
Temporal lobe						
TP	4.72 (1.92)	4.90 (2.17)	5.55 (2.90)	5.84 (3.17)	4.54 (2.28)	4.74 (2.39)
ST	**5.14 (1.41)**	**5.05 (1.56)**	**5.53 (1.85)**	**5.29 (1.87)**	**5.80 (3.77)**	**5.60 (3.72)**
MT	**4.78 (1.25)**	**4.88 (1.50)**	**5.21 (1.77)**	**4.95 (1.65)**	**5.59 (4.05)**	**5.28 (3.61)**
IT	5.11 (1.88)	4.94 (1.99)	5.79 (2.56)	5.14 (2.18)	5.11 (2.15)	4.74 (2.27)
OT	4.41 (1.48)	4.48 (1.56)	4.53 (1.50)	4.77 (1.72)	5.01 (4.23)	5.05 (3.87)
Limbic						
PH	4.55 (1.35)	4.98 (1.54)	4.88 (1.65)	5.32 (1.90)	4.94 (3.02)	5.48 (4.37)
HI	**4.48 (1.32)**	**4.47 (1.34)**	**4.91 (1.69)**	**4.89 (1.81)**	**4.95 (3.43)**	**4.93 (3.90)**
AM	4.04 (1.33)	4.21 (1.48)	4.51 (1.99)	4.86 (2.12)	5.09 (3.92)	4.91 (3.45)
IN	5.20 (1.39)	5.90 (1.55)	5.89 (1.89)	6.53 (2.10)	5.78 (3.46)	6.24 (4.01)
OF	5.14 (1.75)	5.11 (1.84)	6.19 (3.11)	6.03 (3.25)	4.89 (2.09)	4.71 (2.03)
RG	5.48 (1.87)	5.34 (1.83)	7.26 (3.12)	7.03 (3.13)	5.28 (2.37)	5.06 (2.36)
CA	5.28 (1.55)	4.86 (1.48)	5.84 (1.91)	5.37 (1.84)	5.72 (3.19)	5.29 (2.98)
CG	5.25 (1.26)	4.05 (1.13)	5.34 (1.76)	4.44 (1.67)	5.63 (3.41)	4.59 (2.29)
CP	5.69 (1.57)	5.35 (1.44)	6.06 (2.06)	5.59 (1.64)	6.35 (3.98)	6.06 (4.27)
Basal ganglia						
CN	**5.39 (1.41)**	**5.42 (1.45)**	**6.06 (2.13)**	**6.15 (2.09)**	**5.89 (4.06)**	**5.89 (3.90)**
LM	**5.16 (1.40)**	**5.77 (1.55)**	**5.85 (1.84)**	**6.59 (1.84)**	**5.93 (3.70)**	**6.23 (3.97)**
LL	**5.74 (1.51)**	**6.11 (1.56)**	**6.54 (2.13)**	**6.86 (2.23)**	**6.38 (3.95)**	**6.53 (4.09)**
Diencephalon						
MB	3.73 (1.28)	3.73 (1.39)	4.05 (1.80)	4.13 (1.50)	4.23 (2.40)	4.33 (2.99)
TH	5.13 (1.35)	5.19 (1.33)	5.42 (1.39)	5.64 (1.51)	5.64 (3.86)	5.78 (3.85)
Brain stem						
MI	4.53 (1.49)	4.38 (1.38)	4.99 (1.99)	4.95 (2.01)	5.26 (4.04)	5.19 (3.91)
PO	4.07 (1.75)	3.75 (1.49)	4.57 (2.32)	4.24 (2.45)	3.97 (2.33)	3.79 (2.31)
Cerebellum	4.38 (1.30)	4.75 (1.47)	4.90 (2.04)	5.28 (2.26)	5.22 (3.79)	5.65 (4.37)

Rates, mg/100 g per Minute.

**The main regions of interest for hypothesis testing are given in boldface. Left indicates left hemisphere; right, right hemisphere; SF, superior frontal region; SP, superior parietal region; PO, pons; C1, anterior corpus callosum; and C2, posterior corpus callosum. Abbreviations for other regions of interest are described in Figure 1.*

able to the midtemporal region's having relatively higher left than right hemispheric activity in patients than controls (F[1,82]=7.60; *P*=.001). The occipital control region showed no main effects or interactions.

FE Patients

The ANOVA (FE patients vs controls) for subcortical regions showed no main effects or interactions. For cortical regions, there was no main effect of grouping, but there was a group-by-region interaction (F[3,186]=4.23; *P*=.006) and a group-by-region-by-hemisphere interaction (F[3,186]=3.17; *P*=.025). This interaction (Figure 2) emanates from a relatively higher left-right gradient in FE patients compared with controls, specifically in the midtemporal region. Indeed, the laterality index was significantly higher in FE patients than controls (*t*[62]=2.33; *P*=.023).

PT Patients

The ANOVA (PT patients vs controls) for subcortical regions likewise showed no main effects or interactions.

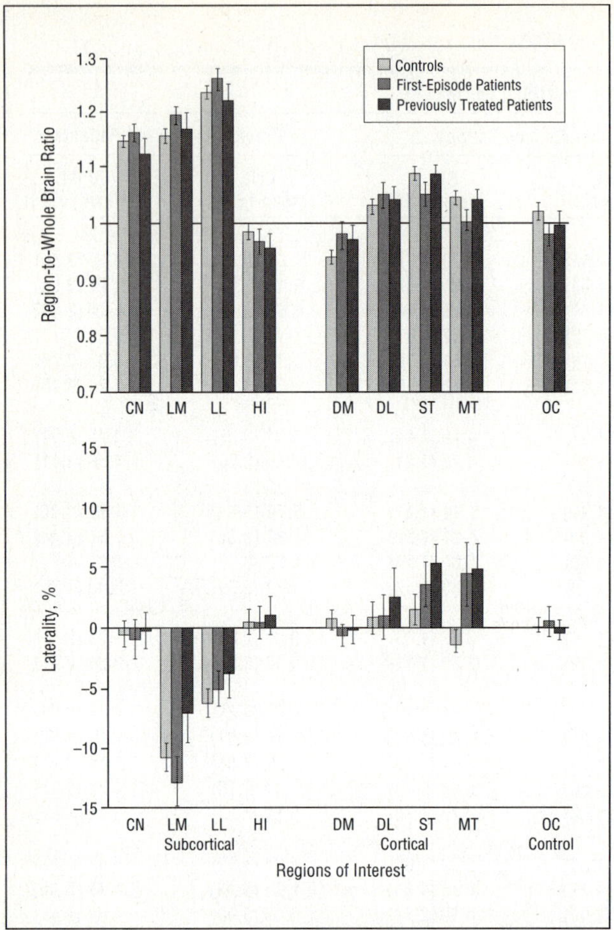

Figure 2. *Topography of metabolic activity for region–whole-brain ratio (mean±SEM) in controls and first-episode and previously treated patients with schizophrenia for the 10 main regions of interest, a subset of those presented in Table 2 and delineated in Figure 1. OC indicates occipital region (average of lateral and medial occipital cortex from Figure 1). Other abbreviations are described in Figure 1. Top graph shows region–whole-brain ratios averaged for the two hemispheres; bottom graph, laterality differences (left minus right), ie, 100 (left minus right)/mean of (left and right).*

For the cortical regions, there was no main effect of grouping, but a group-by-hemisphere interaction (F[1,60]=3.82; *P*=.05). This interaction (Figure 2) reflects a relatively higher left-right gradient in PT patients. This was again most pronounced in the midtemporal region, where the laterality index was significantly higher in PT patients than in controls (t[60]=2.73; *P*=.008). The ANOVA for FE vs PT patients showed no main effects or interactions with grouping.

Given the consistency of the laterality effect in the midtemporal region for both patient groups, we examined separately the two hemispheres in this region (**Figure 3**). Whereas for controls there was no significant difference in metabolism between the two hemispheres (*t*[40]=1.11; *P*=.27), the left hemisphere had relatively higher metabolism than the right for both FE patients (*t*[20]=1.75; *P*=.045) and PT patients (*t*[18]=2.31; *P*=.015). Examination of group differences for each hemisphere separately showed no difference between FE patients and controls for the left midtemporal values (*t*[62]<1) but reduced right midtemporal values in the patients compared with controls (t[62]=2.81; *P*=.007 [two-tailed]). Neither comparison of midtemporal values was significant for PT patients vs controls (left, *t*[60]=1.16; *P*=.25; and right, *t*[60]=1.62; *P*=.11).

Since the results suggested no evidence of hypofrontality, this hypothesis was further tested as in earlier studies reporting hypofrontality by calculating the ratio of the occipital region to each of the frontal regions, using *t* tests to compare FE and PT patients with controls for these ratios. None of the results of the *t* tests approached significance.

RELATIONSHIP WITH SUBTYPES

The ANOVA comparing deficit vs nondeficit groups showed no effects or interactions with grouping. However, the division into the factor-referenced subtypes showed a significant subtype-by-region-by-hemisphere interaction for the subcortical regions (F[6,102]=3.19; *P*=.007). As can be seen in **Figure 4**, the interaction reflects a difference between the paranoid subtype and the other two subtypes, with more negative laterality values (relatively higher right than left hemisphere metabolism) in both lenticular regions for the paranoid patients. Post hoc univariate contrasts between the paranoid subtype and the other two subtypes showed no significant differences for any region considered bilaterally (average of the two hemispheres), but the difference in laterality between the subtypes was significant for the medial lenticular region (globus pallidus) (F[1,35]=4.48; *P*=.04). For cortical regions, there was also a subtype-by-region-by-hemisphere interaction (F[6,102]=2.79; *P*=.015). This interaction reflected symmetrical metabolism in the paranoid patients compared with greater relative left hemispheric activity in the other patient subtypes. As can be seen in Figure 4 (bottom), relative overactivity in the left midtemporal region is most pronounced in the negative subtype, which also showed higher relative left hemispheric activity for the lateral dorsal prefrontal region. Post hoc contrasts between the paranoid patients and the other subtypes showed both bilateral and hemispheric differences. Paranoid patients had higher metabolism in the medial aspect of the dorsal prefrontal cortex (F[1,35]=5.94; *P*=.020). For the laterality scores, paranoid patients differed from the other patients in showing relatively lower left hemispheric metabolism both in the lateral aspect of the dorsal prefrontal cortex (F[1,35]=7.44; *P*=.009) and in the midtemporal region (F[1,35]=6.66; *P*=.009). Thus, the increased relative left midtemporal activity, which differentiated patients from controls, was not observed in the paranoid patients and is accounted for by only two of the subtypes. The paranoid patients did not differ from controls in the laterality of metabolism in any cortical region. No differences among the clusters were found for the occipital control region.

RELATIONSHIP WITH CLINICAL VARIABLES

In view of reports of correlations between temporal lobe measures, hallucinations, and thought disorder,[41,42] we computed this correlation between superior temporal metabolism (R-WB ratio) and the global hallucinations rating from the Scale for the Assessment of Positive Symptoms. The correlation was significant ($r[40]=-.29$; $P=.02$), suggesting that relatively lower superior temporal lobe metabolism is associated with more severe hallucinations. It is noteworthy that the correlation between metabolism in this region and thought disorder was positive ($r[40]=.32$; $P=.012$), higher metabolism being associated with more severe thought disorder. Furthermore, laterality of metabolism correlated with severity of hallucinations both for the lateral dorsal prefrontal and midtemporal regions ($r[40]=.30$ and $r[40]=.31$, respectively; $P=.02$), suggesting greater left hemispheric activity associated with more severe symptoms.

Premorbid Functioning

The correlations of the "general" Premorbid Adjustment Scale score with metabolism showed no regional specificity for the R-WB ratios, but it did for laterality ($\chi^2[8]=18.37$; $P=.02$), with a higher than average correlation for the midtemporal region ($r[40]=.40$; $z=2.51$; $P=.006$). Thus, relatively higher left midtemporal metabolism was associated with poorer premorbid adjustment.

Duration of Illness

We applied linear regression to remove the association between age and duration. The only significant correlations were between laterality and duration for both the medial and lateral lenticular regions ($r[40]=.44$ [$P=.002$] and $r[40]=.35$ {$P=.009$], respectively). This suggested that greater duration was associated with relatively higher left hemispheric activity.

Medication

Weeks during which no medication was received were correlated with metabolism in the PT patients. The correlations were significant for the caudate, superior temporal, and midtemporal regions ($r[18]=-.37$ [$P=.05$], $r[18]=-.47$ [$P=.04$], and $r[18]=-.45$ [$P=.04$], respectively [one-tailed]). Thus, a prolonged period during which neuroleptics were not received was associated with lower relative metabolism in these regions. For laterality, these correlations were significant for caudate and superior temporal regions ($r[18]=-.48$ [$P=.04$] and $r[18]=-.47$ [$P=.04$], respectively). However, examination of the scatterplots indicated that these correlations were attributable to three patients with prolonged illness who refused medication. These results should be interpreted with caution because of the variability in treatment.

Outcome

Several correlations between the R-WB ratios and outcome factors were significant both for short term (0.5 to 1 year) and long term (>1.5 year). Higher metabolism was generally associated with better outcome, with the highest correlation between lateral lenticular

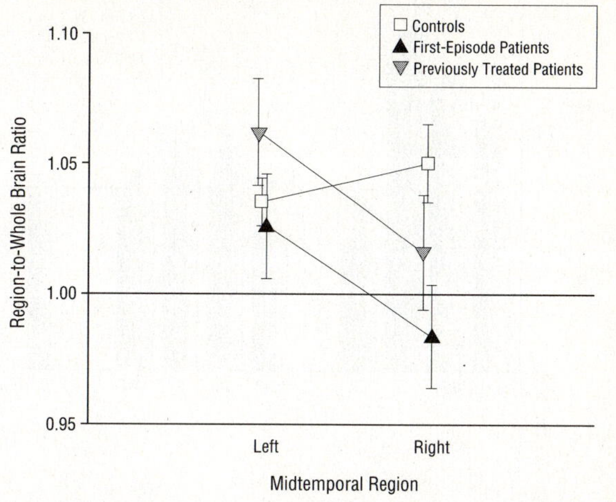

Figure 3. *Metabolic activity (mean±SEM) expressed as region–whole-brain ratio (mean±SEM) in the left and right midtemporal regions for controls and first-episode and previously treated patients.*

metabolism and freedom from hospitalizations ($r[40]=.41$; $P=.004$ [two-tailed]), but there was no significant regional specificity. Most comparable correlations with laterality were negative, indicating better outcome associated with relatively lower left than right hemispheric metabolism. Regional specificity of these correlations was significant only for long-term freedom from hospitalizations ($\chi^2[8]=29.76$; $P=.003$). This variability was attributable to the correlation for the lateral lenticular region ($r[40]=-.41$; $P=.004$ [one-tailed]), which was differentially negative ($z=3.49$; $P<.001$) compared with the other correlations.

COROLLARY AND EXPLORATORY ANALYSES

Corollary analyses were performed on age, education, and parental education in view of their potential effects on the relationship between brain and behavior. Negative correlations were found between age and whole-brain metabolism across groups ($r[82]=-.27$; $P<.01$), as well as within patients ($r[40]=-.32$; $P=.01$) and controls ($r[40]=-.27$; $P=.02$). There was significant regional variability in these correlations for controls ($\chi^2[8]=17.02$) and patients ($\chi^2[8]=16.64$) ($P=.03$), indicating highest negative correlation with age for the lateral dorsal prefrontal region in controls ($r[82]=-.31$; $z=2.15$; $P=.02$) and in patients ($z=3.14$; $P=.001$). Correlations of age with laterality showed significant variability for controls ($\chi^2[8]=17.10$; $P=.03$), with a higher than average correlation for the lateral dorsal prefrontal region only, suggesting that aging is accompanied by relatively greater reduction in right hemispheric metabolism in this region. Patients showed no significant regional variability.

Neither group showed significant correlations with education. For parental education, in both groups the correlations were significantly more positive in both dorsal prefrontal regions (medial and lateral) ($r[40]=.33$ and $r[40]=.32$, $z=2.76$ [$P=.003$] and $z=2.81$ [$P=.003$] [for con-

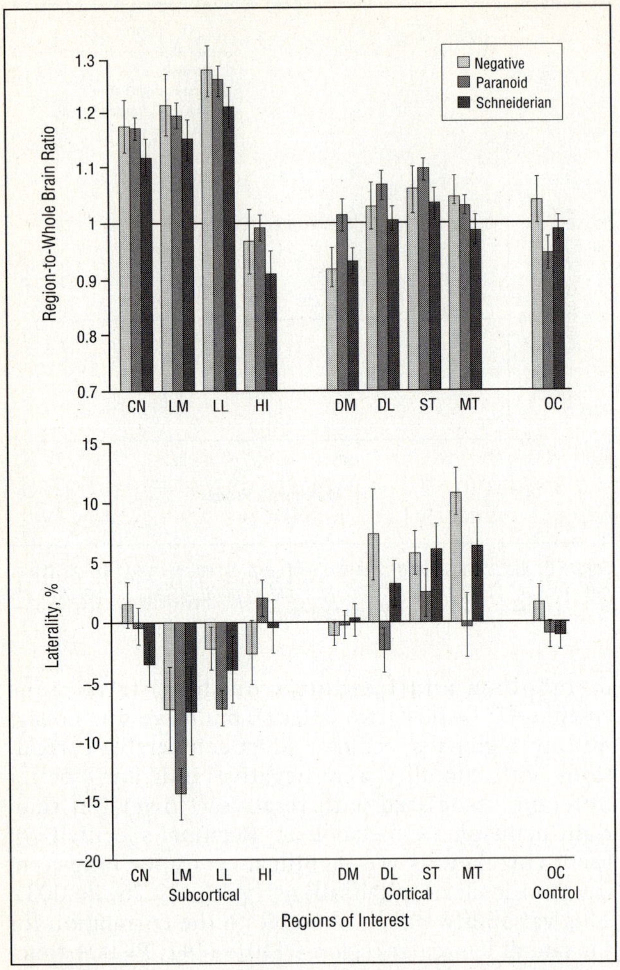

Figure 4. *Topography of metabolic activity (mean±SEM) in patients with the following three subtypes of schizophrenia: negative, paranoid, and Schneiderian. Abbreviations are described in Figure 1; parameters, in Figure 2.*

trols]; *r*=.35 and *r*=.44, *z*=2.13 [*P*=.017] and *z*=2.98 [*P*=.001] [for patients]). The laterality correlations with parental education showed no regional variability.

There were no significant sex differences and exclusion of the left-handed participants did not change the results. However, given the inadequate numbers of women and left-handed participants, this could be a type II error.

For exploratory analyses, diagnosis-by-hemisphere ANOVAs were performed on each of the regions not included in the hypothesis testing phase. Setting the *P* value at .01 to protect from type I error, no other region showed a significant effect of or interaction by diagnosis except the cingulate gyrus, which showed a significant hemisphere-by-diagnosis interaction (F[1,82]=8.03; *P*=.005), with patients having an attenuated left greater than right asymmetry relative to controls (Table 2).

COMMENT

Past PET studies of cerebral glucose metabolism have reported several abnormalities in schizophrenia, but the findings have been inconsistent. Discrepancies have been attributed to variability in samples and methods. The heterogeneity of relatively small samples, considering variables such as chronicity, treatment history, clinical status, and comorbidity, could explain differences in findings. In this respect, the present study contributes data from a relatively large sample of FE and PT patients without comorbidity who were followed up longitudinally and compared with sociodemographically balanced healthy controls. Method variability can be found in study conditions as well as scanner resolution, brain tissue sampled, quantitation, image processing, and analysis. This investigation used a standard resting condition, a high-resolution scanner that enabled evaluation of metabolism in the entire brain, and coregistration with anatomic measures. Thus, we believe that the results reflect the rate and topographic distribution of resting metabolism in schizophrenia.

We found no whole-brain differences in resting glucose metabolism between FE and PT patients and controls. This finding differs from some reports of abnormal metabolism but is consistent with others.[1,2] In our previous, smaller sample with an older scanner, we did not find group differences in whole-brain metabolism, but when subjects with the highest and lowest metabolic rates in each group were deleted (using the robust *t* test procedure), patients did have significantly lower values.[18] This perhaps underscores the undesirability of removing outliers in analyses of small samples.[40] The "gold standard" quantitation of whole-brain metabolism defined by Kety et al[43] did not find differences between patients and controls. The absence of metabolic differences in our study is unlikely to be explained by limited sensitivity of measures, since the corollary analyses showed the expected negative correlation with age. Furthermore, the means and ranges of values are comparable to those established by Kety and Schmidt.[44] Because our patients underwent screening for comorbidity with other conditions that may affect brain function, we conclude that schizophrenia in itself, as represented in this sample of both FE and PT patients, is not associated with global abnormalities in the rates of cerebral glucose utilization.

REGIONAL TOPOGRAPHY

The metabolic activity of any brain region averaged across hemispheres, either in raw absolute rates or when expressed as R-WB ratios, did not differ between patients and controls. This included the lateral dorsal prefrontal cortex. These negative findings fail to replicate studies reporting hypofrontality,[3,4] which have been considered to be a majority of studies,[45] and we cannot confirm reports of bilateral abnormalities in basal ganglia or other subcortical regions.[6-8] Thus, the results are consistent with those of studies of resting metabolism and blood flow that reported no regional differences.[1,2] Again, the corollary analyses suggest that our measures do show sensitivity to regional effects. For both patients and controls, age was associated with a reduction in frontal metabolism but not in temporal metabolism. This age effect, including its magnitude, is consistent with studies using anatomic[46] and physiological[47,48] measures of regional brain function. Unless normal aging, even within the truncated age range of this sample, has more devastating effects than schizophrenia on frontal metabolism, we can rule out bilateral hypofrontality as underlying schizophrenia in this sample.

The Anterior-Posterior Gradient

It is possible that while no single region differs between patients and controls, there are abnormalities in metabolic gradients. We examined the anterior-posterior gradient and found no evidence of abnormalities. These results would seem to contrast most directly with those of Siegel et al,[49] who reported "lower hypofrontality scores," which were measured as ratios of lateral frontal to occipital metabolism, in 70 men with schizophrenia who had received no medication. It is noteworthy that frontal metabolism of patients in their study did not differ from that of controls, while occipital metabolism was higher in patients. Our data did not show frontal or occipital differences or diagnosis effects on ratios. A difference between the study conditions may explain the discrepancy. During the FDG uptake, their subjects performed an attentional task while our subjects were resting. Since patients have impaired attentional performance, the task is more difficult and may require greater cerebral activation. It is also possible that while bilateral regional abnormalities do not characterize patients as a group, the severity of specific clinical features can correlate with metabolic activity. Both the negative and Schneiderian subtypes of patients had lower relative metabolism in the medial dorsal prefrontal region, while paranoid patients had normal values. Furthermore, the significant correlations between prefrontal measures and clinical features suggest that higher metabolism in frontal regions is associated with better premorbid adjustment during childhood and adolescence and less likelihood of hospitalization at short-term follow-up. Perhaps abnormal anterior-posterior gradients could characterize subgroups of patients with a chronic course.

The Laterality Gradient

The hypothesis of relative left hemispheric overactivation was supported both for the whole brain in the FE group and the midtemporal cortex in both patient groups. The hemispheric effect for the averaged cortical regions is consistent with the finding in our laboratory using the xenon 133 clearance method for measuring cerebral blood flow.[10] It also replicated the previous PET FDG study for the high-severity group.[8] The specificity of the effect for the midtemporal region was not examined in these studies but is consistent with another recent ^{133}Xe cerebral blood flow study that noted failure of this region to show task-appropriate activation for memory of words and faces.[50] It is also consistent with neurobehavioral deficits observed in these patients, including learning and memory, primarily in the verbal domain.[51] Neuroanatomic studies have also suggested lateralized temporal lobe abnormalities.[41,42] The relevance of this resting asymmetry in midtemporal lobe metabolism to schizophrenia is buttressed by its correlation with clinical features, including premorbid functioning and outcome.

We emphasize that at this stage we can support the *relative* asymmetry, but we cannot determine whether this reflects lower than normal right hemispheric activity or higher left hemispheric activity. Whereas for PT patients higher left and lower right hemispheric midtemporal metabolism was observed, FE patients showed bilateral reduction relative to controls, with right hemispheric values being significantly lower than in controls. It would be tempting to conclude that in this group, there is right hemispheric hypometabolism for this region, and hence that the hypothesis of relative left hemispheric overactivation needs to be modified as reflecting absolute right hemispheric underactivation. However, this would be premature, given evidence for lateralized reductions in temporal lobe volume,[41,42] which is more pronounced in the left hemisphere.[52] There is also a need to establish specificity for gray and white matter, which differ substantially in their metabolic rates.[36] Thus, conclusions on the absolute effects contributing to the differences between patients and controls in the laterality gradient must await the development of methods for making such corrections.

SUBTYPES AND CLINICAL VARIABLES

The metabolic topography, except for the subcortical-cortical ratio, did not differ for FE compared with PT patients. The groups likewise did not differ in symptom severity. This is consistent with the clinical profile,[24] neurobehavioral functioning,[53] and neuroanatomic measures[21] reported for FE patients. Lack of differences between FE and PT patients is also seen in functional studies evaluating response to cognitive challenges.[45,50] Brain dysfunction in schizophrenia seems to exist at first presentation and prior to treatment with neuroleptics. Consonant with this interpretation is the paucity of correlations between the length of time in which medications are not received and regional metabolism. The study did not examine the effect of specific pharmacologic interventions, but others have suggested the potential utility of metabolic measures for examining such effects.[15,16]

Categorization of patients as deficit or nondeficit types did not distinguish between the groups. This contrasts with a previous report with a smaller sample.[6] However, factor-referenced clusters yielded significant differences among three patient subtypes. Patients with severe negative symptoms, without marked positive symptoms, showed increased relative left hemispheric metabolism in both the midtemporal and medial frontal regions. Schneiderian patients showed only increased left temporal relative metabolism. Paranoid patients had normal cortical activity and were only distinguishable from controls by relatively higher right hemispheric metabolism in the medial lenticular region encompassing the globus pallidus. It is noteworthy that MRI volumetric measures also showed abnormal asymmetry in the temporal lobe, which included both reduced volume and increased cerebral spinal fluid levels for the patients with negative symptoms but only reduced volume without increased cerebral spinal fluid levels for paranoid patients.[52] The heterogeneity of schizophrenia may thus have neural substrates that merit further investigation. However, such studies require larger samples targeted prospectively at specific subtypes. This may be particularly important for correlating metabolism and clinical features within subtypes.

Lower overall metabolism, averaging the two hemispheres, and higher laterality scores, indicating more relative left hemispheric activity, were associated with poorer premorbid functioning and worse outcome. These correlations had some regional specificity. Worse premorbid functioning was differentially associated with relatively higher left hemispheric activity in the midtemporal region. Worse outcome was differentially associated with higher lateral lenticular and higher left lateral lenticular metabolism. Higher left lenticular metabolism was also associated with longer duration of illness. These findings have not been predicted and merit replication.

LIMITATIONS

The main limitation of the present study is sample size, even though it is second only to that of Siegel et al[49] in the published literature. The size still does not permit simultaneous investigation of gender-related differences that have been reported in clinical and neurobiologic studies of schizophrenia and has insufficient power to decompose all region-by-hemisphere interactions in the large number of regions that can be measured with PET. Larger samples would also be necessary to establish with some reliability the relation of metabolic measures to anatomic, neurobehavioral, and clinical features. Another limitation is the use of the template approach to placing the ROIs. A more precise method would be to outline the boundaries of each region on the MRI, with segmentation of cerebral spinal fluid and white matter. This, however, requires detailed definitions and guidelines to establish acceptable interoperator reliability.

CONCLUSIONS

Patients with schizophrenia have normal rates of whole-brain resting glucose metabolism and do not differ from controls in frontal activity or in anterior-posterior gradient. This is unlikely because the measures lack sensitivity to individual differences in variables related to behavior, since they were correlated with age in this study and showed sex differences.[13] Therefore, resting measures of metabolism are unlikely to elucidate the pathophysiological features of schizophrenia unless they are combined with other measures. The increased relative activity of the midtemporal left compared with right hemisphere, which is associated with clinical features, supports the hypothesis of lateralized brain dysfunction in schizophrenia.[54-57]

Accepted for publication March 2, 1995.

Supported by grants MH-42191, MH-43880, MH-00586, MH-48539, NS-14867, and MO1RR0040 from the National Institutes of Health, Bethesda, Md, and by the EJLB Foundation, Montreal, Quebec.

We thank Diane Sandefur for her contribution, Kimberly Hambrose Martin, MSN, RN, for assessment, Teony Thew for programming, and Helen Mitchell-Sears for assistance in manuscript preparation.

Reprint requests to Neuropsychiatry Program, University of Pennsylvania, 10th Floor, Gates Building, Philadelphia, PA 19104 (Dr R. E. Gur).

REFERENCES

1. Buchsbaum MS. The frontal lobes, basal ganglia, and temporal lobes as sites for schizophrenia. *Schizophr Bull.* 1990;16:377-387.
2. Gur RE, Pearlson GD. Neuroimaging in schizophrenia research. *Schizophr Bull.* 1993;19:337-353.
3. Buchsbaum MS, Haier RJ, Potkin SG, Nuechterlein K, Bracha HS, Katz M, Lohr J, Wu J, Lottenberg S, Kerabek PA, Trenary M, Tafalla R, Reynolds C, Bunney WE. Frontostriatal disorder of cerebral metabolism in never-medicated schizophrenics. *Arch Gen Psychiatry.* 1992;49:935-942.
4. Wolkin A, Angrist B, Wolf A, Brodie JD, Wolkin B, Jaeger J, Cancro R, Rotrosen J. Low frontal glucose utilization in chronic schizophrenia: a replication study. *Am J Psychiatry.* 1988;145:251-253.
5. DeLisi LE, Buchsbaum MS, Holcomb HH, Langston KC, King AC, Kessler R, Pickar D, Carpenter WT, Morihisa JM, Margolin R, Weinberger DR. Increased temporal lobe glucose use in chronic schizophrenic patients. *Biol Psychiatry.* 1989;25:835-851.
6. Tamminga CA, Thaker GK, Buchanan R, Kirkpatrick B, Alphs LD, Chase TN, Carpenter WT. Limbic system abnormalities identified in schizophrenia using positron emission tomography with fluorodeoxyglucose and neocortical alterations with deficit syndrome. *Arch Gen Psychiatry.* 1992;49:522-530.
7. Buchsbaum MS, Ingvar DH, Kessler R, Water RN, Cappeletti J, Van Kammen DP, King AC, Johnson JL, Manning RG, Flynn RN, Mann LS, Bunney WE, Sokoloff L. Cerebral glucography with positron tomography. *Arch Gen Psychiatry.* 1987;39:251-259.
8. Gur RE, Resnick SM, Gur RC, Alavi A, Caroff S, Kushner M, Reivich M. Regional brain function in schizophrenia, II: repeated evaluation with positron emission tomography. *Arch Gen Psychiatry.* 1987;44:126-129.
9. Sedvall GC. The current status of PET scanning with respect to schizophrenia. *Neuropsychopharmacology.* 1992;7:41-54.
10. Gur RE, Skolnick BE, Gur RC, Caroff S, Rieger W, Obrist WD, Younkin D, Reivich M. Brain function in psychiatric disorders, I: regional cerebral blood flow in medicated schizophrenics. *Arch Gen Psychiatry.* 1983;40:1250-1254.
11. Weinberger DR, Berman KF, Zec RF. Physiologic dysfunction of dorsolateral prefrontal cortex in schizophrenia, I: regional cerebral blood flow evidence. *Arch Gen Psychiatry.* 1986;43:11.
12. Gur RE, Gur RC. Neurotransmitters are important, but so is metabolism. *Neuropsychopharmacology.* 1992;7:63-65.
13. Gur RC, Mozley LH, Mozley PD, Resnick SM, Karp JS, Alavi A, Arnold SE, Gur RE. Sex differences in regional cerebral glucose metabolism during a resting state. *Science.* 1995;267:528-531.
14. Wiesel FA, Wik G, Sjrgren I, Blomqvist G, Greitz T, Stone-Elander S. Regional brain glucose metabolism in drug free schizophrenic patients and clinical correlates. *Acta Psychiatr Scand.* 1987;76:628-641.
15. Buchsbaum MS, Potkin SG, Siegel BV Jr, Lohr J, Katz M, Gottschalk LA, Gulasekaram B, Marshall JF, Lottenberg S, Teng Cy, Bunney WE, Abel L, Plon L. Striatal metabolic rate and clinical response to neuroleptics in schizophrenia. *Arch Gen Psychiatry.* 1992;49:966-974.
16. Wik G, Wiesel FA, Sjogren I, Blomqvist G, Greitz T, Stone-Elander S. Effects of sulpride and chlorpromazine on regional cerebral glucose metabolism in schizophrenic patients as determined by positron emission tomography. *Psychopharmacology.* 1989;97:309-318.
17. Gur RE, Gur RC, Skolnick BE, Caroff, S, Obrist WD, Resnick S, Reivich M. Brain function in psychiatric disorders, III: regional cerebral blood flow in unmedicated schizophrenics. *Arch Gen Psychiatry.* 1985;42:329-334.
18. Gur RE, Resnick SM, Alavi A, Gur RC, Caroff S, Dann R, Silver FL, Saykin AJ, Chawluk JB, Kushner M, Reivich M. Regional brain function in schizophrenia, I: a positron emission tomography study. *Arch Gen Psychiatry.* 1987;44:119-125.
19. Resnick SM, Gur RE, Alavi A, Gur RC, Reivich M. Positron emission tomography and subcortical glucose metabolism in schizophrenia. *Psychiatry Res.* 1988;24:1-11.
20. Gur RE, Resnick SM, Gur RC. Laterality and frontality of cerebral blood flow and metabolism in schizophrenia: relationship to symptom specificity. *Psychiatry Res.* 1989;27:325-334.

21. Gur RE, Mozley PD, Shtasel DL, Cannon TD, Gallacher F, Turetsky B, Grossman R, Gur RC. Clinical subtypes of schizophrenia differ in brain and cerebrospinal fluid volume. *Am J Psychiatry.* 1994;151:343-350.
22. American Psychiatric Association. *Diagnostic and Statistical Manual of Mental Disorders, Revised Third Edition.* Washington, DC: American Psychiatric Association; 1987.
23. Spitzer R, Williams J, Gibbon M. Structured clinical interview for *DSM-III-R.* New York, NY: New York Psychiatric Institute; 1986.
24. Shtasel DL, Gur RE, Gallacher F, Heimberg C, Cannon T, Gur RC. Phenomenology and functioning in first episode schizophrenia. *Schizophr Bull.* 1992; 18:449-462.
25. Spitzer RL, Williams JBW, Gibbon M. *Structured Clinical Interview for DSM-III-R–Nonpatient Version (SCID-NP).* New York, NY: Biometrics Research Department, New York State Psychiatric Institute; 1987.
26. Shtasel DL, Gur RE, Mozley PD, Richards J, Taleff MM, Heimberg C, Gallacher F, Gur RC. Volunteers for biomedical research: recruitment and screening of normal controls. *Arch Gen Psychiatry.* 1991;48:1022-1025.
27. Overall JR, Gorham DR. The Brief Psychiatric Rating Scale. *Psychol Rep.* 1962; 10:799-812.
28. Andreasen NC. *The Scale for the Assessment of Negative Symptoms (SANS).* Iowa City, Iowa: The University of Iowa; 1984.
29. Andreasen NC. *The Scale for the Assessment of Positive Symptoms (SAPS).* Iowa City, Iowa: The University of Iowa; 1984.
30. Harris JG. An abbreviated form of the Phillips Rating Scale of Premorbid Adjustment in schizophrenia. *J Abnorm Psychol.* 1975;84:129-137.
31. Simpson GM, Lee JH, Zoubek B, Gardos G. A rating scale for tardive dyskinesia. *Psychopharmacology.* 1979;64:171-179.
32. Carpenter WT, Heinrichs DW, Wagman AMI. Deficit and nondeficit forms of schizophrenia: the concept. *Am J Psychiatry.* 1988;145:578-583.
33. Strauss JS, Carpenter WT. Characteristic symptoms and outcome in schizophrenia. *Arch Gen Psychiatry.* 1974;30:429-434.
34. Karp JS, Muehllehner G, Mankoff DA, Ordonez CE, Ollinger JM, Daube-Witherspoon ME, Haigh AT, Beerbohm DJ. Continuous-slice PENN-PET: a positron tomograph with volume-imaging capability. *J Nucl Med.* 1990;31:617-627.
35. Karp JS, Daube-Witherspoon ME, Muehllehner G. Factors affecting accuracy and precision in PET volume imaging. *J Cereb Blood Flow Metab.* 1991;11 (suppl):A38-A44.
36. Reivich M, Kuhl D, Wolf AP, Greenberg J, Phelps M, Ido T, Casella V, Fowler J, Hoffman E, Alavi A, Som P, Sokoloff L. The ^{18}F-fluorodeoxyglucose method for the measurement of local cerebral glucose utilization in man. *Circ Res.* 1979;44:127-137.
37. Reivich M, Alavi A, Wolf AP, Fowler JS, Russell J, Arnett C, MacGregor RR, Shive CY, Atkins H, Anand A, Dann R, Greenberg JH. Glucose metabolic rate kinetic model parameter determination in man: the lumped constants and rate constants for ^{18}F-fluorodeoxyglucose and ^{11}C-deoxyglucose. *J Cereb Blood Flow Metab.* 1985;5:179-192.
38. Resnick SM, Karp JS, Turetsky B, Gur RE. Comparison of anatomically-defined versus physiologically-based regional localization: effects on PET-FDG quantitation. *J Nucl Med.* 1993;34:2201-2207.
39. Olkin I, Finn J. Testing correlated correlations. *Psychol Bull.* 1990;108:330-333.
40. Dalal SR, Fowlkes EB, Hoadley B. Risk analysis of the space shuttle: pre-Challenger prediction of failure. *J Am Stat Assoc.* 1989;84:945-957.
41. Shenton ME, Kikinis R, Jolesz FA, Pollack SD, LeMay M, Wible CG, Hokama H, Martin J, Metcalf D, Coleman M, McCarley RW. Left-lateralized temporal lobe abnormalities in schizophrenia and their relationship to thought disorder: a computerized, quantitative MRI study. *N Engl J Med.* 1992;327:604-612.
42. Barta PE, Pearlson GD, Richards SS, Powers RE, Tune LE. Reduced superior temporal gyrus volume in schizophrenia: relationship to hallucinations. *Am J Psychiatry.* 1990;147:1457-1462.
43. Kety SS, Woodford RB, Harmel MH. Cerebral blood flow and metabolism in schizophrenia. *Am J Psychiatry.* 1948;104:765-770.
44. Kety SS, Schmidt CF. The nitrous oxide method for the quantitative determination of cerebral blood flow in man: theory, procedure and normal values. *J Clin Invest.* 1948;27:476-483.
45. Andreasen NC, Rezai K, Alliger R, Swayze VW, Flaum M, Kirchner P, Cohen G, O'Leary DS. Hypofrontality in neuroleptic-naive patients and in patients with chronic schizophrenia. *Arch Gen Psychiatry.* 1992;49:943-958.
46. Cowell PE, Turetsky BI, Gur RC, Grossman RI, Shtasel DL, Gur RE. Sex differences in aging of the human frontal and temporal lobes. *J Neurosci.* 1994; 14:4748-4755.
47. Gur RC, Gur RE, Obrist WD, Skolnick BE, Reivich M. Age and regional cerebral blood flow at rest and during cognitive activity. *Arch Gen Psychiatry.* 1987; 44:617-621.
48. Kuhl DE, Metter EJ, Riege WH, Phelps ME. Effects of human aging on patterns of local cerebral glucose utilization determined by the [^{18}F]fluorodeoxyglucose method. *J Cereb Blood Flow Metab.* 1982;2:163-171.
49. Siegel BV Jr, Buchsbaum MS, Bunney WE Jr, Gottschalk LA, Haier RJ, Lohr JB, Lottenberg S, Najafi A, Nuechterlein KH, Potkin SG, Wu JC. Cortical-striatal-thalamic circuits and brain glucose metabolic activity in 70 unmedicated male schizophrenic patients. *Am J Psychiatry.* 1993;150:1325-1336.
50. Gur RE, Jaggi JL, Shtasel DL, Ragland JD, Gur RC. Cerebral blood flow in schizophrenia: effects of memory processing on regional activation. *Biol Psychiatry.* 1994;35:3-15.
51. Saykin AJ, Gur RC, Gur RE, Mozley D, Mozley LH, Resnick SM, Kester DB, Stafiniak P. Neuropsychological function in schizophrenia: selective impairment in memory and learning. *Arch Gen Psychiatry.* 1991;48:618-624.
52. Turetsky BI, Cowell PE, Gur RC, Grossman RI, Gur RE. Frontal and temporal lobe brain volumes in schizophrenia: relationship to symptomatology and clinical subtype. Presented at the 49th Annual Meeting for the Society for Biological Psychiatry; May 21, 1994; Philadelphia, Pa.
53. Saykin AJ, Shtasel DL, Gur RE, Kester DB, Mozley LH, Stafiniak P, Gur RC. Neuropsychological deficits in neuroleptic naive, first episode schizophrenic patients. *Arch Gen Psychiatry.* 1994;51:124-131.
54. Flor-Henry P. Lateralized temporal-limbic dysfunction and psychopathology. *Ann N Y Acad Sci.* 1976;280:777-797.
55. Gur RE. Left hemisphere dysfunction and left hemisphere overactivation in schizophrenia. *J Abnorm Psychol.* 1978;87:226-238.
56. Crow TJ. Temporal lobe asymmetries as the key to the etiology of schizophrenia. *Schizophr Bull.* 1990;16:433-443.
57. Friston KJ, Liddle PF, Frith CD, Hirsch SR, Frackowiak S. The left medial temporal region and schizophrenia: a PET study. *Brain.* 1992;115:367-382.

ORIGINAL ARTICLE

Mitogen-Stimulated Interleukin-2 Production in Never-Medicated, First-Episode Schizophrenic Patients

The Influence of Age at Onset and Negative Symptoms

Rohan Ganguli, MD; Jaspreet S. Brar, MD; K. N. R. Chengappa, MD; Marcia DeLeo, RN; Zan Wei Yang, PhD; Galina Shurin, PhD; Bruce S. Rabin, MD, PhD

Background: Decreased interleukin-2 (IL-2) production is characteristic of active autoimmune diseases and has previously been reported in patients with schizophrenia. We attempted to replicate this finding in never-medicated schizophrenic patients and examine the possible correlation between IL-2 production and clinical variables.

Methods: The production of IL-2 was measured in equal numbers (N=33) of *DSM-III-R*–diagnosed schizophrenic patients and controls who were matched for age, race, and gender. Patients were also assessed for positive, negative, and depressive symptoms.

Results: The production of IL-2 was significantly lower in patients than in controls. There was a significant positive correlation between IL-2 production and age at onset, and significant negative correlation between IL-2 production and negative symptom scores. In multivariate analyses, the predictive power was stronger for age at onset than for negative symptoms. Positive or depressive symptoms were unrelated to IL-2 production.

Conclusions: Our finding of low IL-2 production in neuroleptic-naive schizophrenic patients confirms that this finding is not confounded by medications. The correlation of low IL-2 production with younger age at onset suggests that this may be a marker for a subtype of the illness or for severity.

(Arch Gen Psychiatry. 1995;52:668-672)

From the Departments of Psychiatry (Drs Ganguli, Brar, Chengappa, Yang, Shurin, and Rabin and Ms DeLeo) and Pathology (Drs Ganguli and Rabin), University of Pittsburgh (Pa) School of Medicine, and the Brain, Behavior, and Immunity Center (Drs Ganguli, Brar, Chengappa, Yang, Shurin, and Rabin), Pittsburgh.

NEARLY 60 years ago, Lehman-Facius suggested that schizophrenia may have an autoimmune component to its pathophysiology.[1,2] Several clinical features, namely, an adolescent onset (sometimes referred to as the "juvenile grace gap"); remitting and relapsing course; season of birth; triggering by infections, drug abuse, and physical injury; and an association with other autoimmune disorders are common to both schizophrenia and known autoimmune diseases, such as Graves' disease and systemic lupus erythematosus.[3,4] Abnormalities in the results of laboratory tests of immune function have also frequently been reported to occur in a proportion of patients with schizophrenia.[4,5] However, the notion that these findings represent evidence for an autoimmune pathogenesis has not gained wide acceptance. This skepticism is probably the result of the inconsistent replication of most reported abnormalities; the fact that in most studies, immune abnormalities, if found, occur only in a small subgroup of patients with schizophrenia; and because no antigen-specific antibody has been found to be exclusively associated with schizophrenia. In reviewing this extensive literature, several methodologic shortcomings can easily be identified in a large proportion of studies with both negative and positive results, thus failing to either weaken or strengthen the purported association between autoimmune findings and schizophrenia.

Of all the immunologic findings reported in association with schizophrenia, abnormalities of lymphokine physiology have been the most consistently replicated. These findings include decreased lymphocyte production of interleukin-2 (IL-2) following mitogenic stimulation[6-9] and increased serum IL-2 receptor[10,11] and serum IL-6[12,13] concentrations. In fact, decreased IL-2 production has been reported by four different groups[6-9] in as many countries, and no negative studies have appeared as yet.

In this study, we examined the lymphocyte production of IL-2 in drug-naive

See Methods on next page

METHODS

RECRUITMENT

Patients

Drug-naive individuals experiencing their first psychotic episode were recruited from the Schizophrenia Treatment and Research Center (STRC) at the Western Psychiatric Institute and Clinic, Pittsburgh, Pa. The STRC is a comprehensive service located in an urban area that provides inpatient, outpatient, partial hospital, rehabilitation, drug and alcohol, and other services to individuals with a diagnosis of schizophrenia and related psychotic disorders. Because it is the community mental health center for a section of Pittsburgh that includes a wide range of ethnic and social classes, the STRC population is fairly representative of the population of the region. The study was described to the patients orally and in writing, and informed consent was documented by their signing a consent form approved by the University of Pittsburgh Institutional Review Board for Biomedical Research. The patients were administered a modified Schedule for Affective Disorders and Schizophrenia[16] interview designed to allow the application of both Research Diagnostic Criteria[17] and *DSM-III-R*[18] criteria. Final *DSM-III-R* diagnoses were assigned by consensus at a staff conference that reviewed the results of the structured interview along with all other available information about the patients. The majority of patients in this cohort received their outpatient care at the STRC, either as part of an ongoing first-break study or in the clinic. The initial diagnosis was reevaluated 6 to 12 months later, and only subjects who still met *DSM-III-R* criteria for schizophrenia were retained in the sample. Interleukin-2 production and autoantibodies were assayed in a resulting sample of 33 patients who met *DSM-III-R* criteria for schizophrenia at follow-up. Schizophrenic patients who had other forms of psychiatric and/or medical comorbid disorders including substance and alcohol abuse (and/or dependence) were excluded from this study. Refusal or inability to give informed consent, recent infectious illness, or serious debilitating diseases that might have affected the immune system, and recent treatment with immunomodulating drugs were also grounds for exclusion.

Controls

Healthy nonpsychiatric controls who matched the schizophrenic patients on three demographic characteristics (age, race, and gender) were specifically recruited for this study from the greater Pittsburgh metropolitan area. They were interviewed regarding psychiatric and medical symptoms by trained mental health workers. Each patient was matched with a healthy control of the same race and gender and within 2 years for age. Control subjects who had an existing autoimmune disorder, infections, or a history of substance and/or alcohol abuse (or dependence) were excluded, as were those who were currently receiving treatment with antibiotics or immunomodulatory drugs. Controls who met the above inclusion criteria reviewed and signed a consent form that had been approved by the University of Pittsburgh Institutional Review Board for Biomedical Research. Controls were paid for their participation.

CLINICAL ASSESSMENTS

Age at onset (of illness) was defined as the age at which psychotic symptoms first appeared, as reported by the patient or family. Positive symptoms and overall severity of illness were assessed using the Brief Psychiatric Rating Scale.[19] The severity of "psychosis" was operationally defined as the sum of the scores for six items: conceptual disorganization, suspiciousness, hallucinatory behavior, unusual thought content, mannerisms and posturing, and grandiosity. Negative symptoms were assessed using negative symptom items from the Manchester Scale,[20] and the summed score was used to rate severity. Depression was assessed using the Montgomery-Asberg Scale.[21]

GENERATION AND QUANTITATION OF IL-2 PRODUCTION

After an overnight fast, venous blood was collected from subjects between 7:30 and 9:30 AM in sterile heparinized tubes (Vacutainer). The procedure for generating IL-2 from whole blood has been described previously.[7,14,22] Briefly, aliquots of venous blood were mixed with RPMI 1640 media (GIBCO, Grand Island, NY) in a ratio of 1:9 (vol/vol). The media was supplemented with 10-mmol/L HEPES (GIBCO), 2-mmol/L glutamine (GIBCO), and 50-ng/mL gentamicin. To generate IL-2 production, 0.5 mL of diluted blood was stimulated with phytohemagglutinin in a final concentration of 5 μg/mL in 24-well plates for 48 hours at 37°C in 5% carbon dioxide. At the end of the incubation period, the well contents were placed into polypropylene tubes and immediately freeze-thawed twice in liquid nitrogen to obtain the supernatant, which was stored at −70°C until assayed. The IL-2 thus obtained was quantified in picograms per milliliter using a commercially available enzyme-linked immunosorbent assay kit (Research & Diagnostic Systems). This sandwich immunoassay employed a specific monoclonal antibody that bound the IL-2 (if any) in the aliquot, and a second enzyme-conjugated specific polyclonal antibody captured the bound IL-2. An enzyme substrate solution then detected colorimetrically the amount of IL-2 bound in the initial step after the reaction was terminated. The optical density was read at 405 nm using a microplate reader (Flow Labs, Mclean, Va). A standard calibration curve was calculated for each plate and the average of duplicate determinations for each aliquot was plotted against the curve to obtain the quantity of IL-2 in picograms per milliliter. The laboratory assays were conducted without knowledge of the subject's status. The interassay variation was less than 8% for the six-point calibration curve that was run in every plate.

STATISTICAL ANALYSIS

The distribution of IL-2 production was examined separately in the patient and control samples by using Tukey's box plot. In both samples, the mean values closely approximated the median (50th percentile) value, suggesting a normal distribution (**Figure**). Differences in group means (of IL-2 production) between the patients and controls were examined using matched-pairs *t* tests. Subsequently, the analysis carried out among each group (patients and controls separately) employed independent group *t* tests. Pearson's product-moment correlations as well as partial correlations were used to examine the relationship between IL-2 production and clinical variables within the patient sample. Finally, a multiple linear regression was used to examine the relative significance of each clinical variable in explaining IL-2 production in patients.

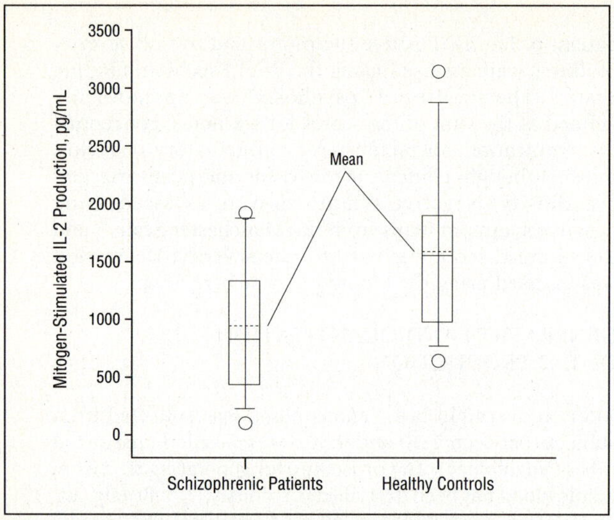

Tukey's box plots of mitogen-stimulated interleukin-2 (IL-2) production in never-medicated schizophrenic patients and healthy controls. Circles represent the fifth and 95th percentiles of the range.

first-episode patients and healthy, age-, gender-, and race-matched controls employing a widely used, commercially available, enzyme-linked immunosorbent assay kit (Research & Diagnostic Systems, Minneapolis, Minn). We undertook this study because previous studies of IL-2 production by Villemain et al[8] and our group[7,14] had only small numbers of drug-naive schizophrenic patients. We believed that a larger sample would help to establish the robustness of the findings. A definitive demonstration of low IL-2 production in drug-naive patients seemed especially needed since it has been reported, in animal studies, that high concentrations of antipsychotic drugs (10^{-6} mol) can inhibit IL-2 production.[15] Another difference between this study and previous investigations of phytohemagglutinin-stimulated IL-2 production is that the latter have employed the CTLL-2 bioassay to measure IL-2. The bioassay, which indirectly measures IL-2 concentration based on the proliferation of IL-2-dependent murine cytotoxic T cells (CTLL), does not provide a quantitative measure of IL-2, and thus accurate comparison of results across studies is difficult. The CTLL-2 cell lines used in these bioassays are also known to be not entirely specific to IL-2 and may proliferate in response to other cytokines (especially IL-4). Thus, an additional reason for conducting this investigation was to confirm that it is really IL-2, the production of which is deficient in patients with schizophrenia.

RESULTS

The mean (±SD) IL-2 production in the schizophrenic patients (935.8±646.9 pg/mL) was significantly lower than their matched controls (1566.5±832.1 pg/mL; matched-pairs *t* test; *t*=3.80; *P*=.0006) (Figure).

The effects of demographic characteristics on IL-2 production are presented in **Table 1**. There were no differences in the mean IL-2 production between black and white control subjects. There were trends for lower IL-2 production among men when compared with women. There was no association between current age and IL-2 production (Pearson's product-moment correlation; *r*=.03, *P*=.87). Since these variables were not found to have significant effects on IL-2 production, they were not used as covariates in the subsequent analyses.

Table 1. Effects of Demographic Characteristics on Interleukin-2 (IL-2) Production

Group Characteristic	Mean±SD IL-2 Production, pg/mL	*t*	*P*
Healthy controls (N=33)	1566.5±832.1*		
Black (n=12)	1779.7±1051.5	0.99	.34
White (n=21)	1444.6±675.9		
Male (n=19)	1317.7±713.7	2.04	.05
Female (n=14)	1904.0±886.6		
Schizophrenic patients (N=33)			
Black (n=12)	903.3±549.4	0.23	.82
White (n=21)	954.5±708.8		
Male (n=19)	931.9±700.3	0.04	.97
Female (n=14)	941.2±592.4		

**Matched-pairs* t *test,* t*=3.80;* P*=.006.*

We next examined the correlation between age at onset, duration of illness, positive symptoms, negative symptoms, depressive symptoms, and IL-2 production. The correlation matrix as seen in **Table 2** suggests that IL-2 production is related to both age at onset (positively) as well as to the severity of negative symptoms (negatively).

To examine the relative explanatory power of negative symptom score and age at onset on IL-2 production, a multiple linear regression analysis was carried out. The overall fit of the regression equation was significant. The results are presented in **Table 3**. As can be seen, the effect of age at onset was stronger than that of negative symptoms.

In view of the observed gender trends of IL-2 production among the control subjects, and the knowledge of the existing relationship between gender and age at onset in the patients with schizophrenia, a partial correlation between IL-2 production and age at onset (controlling for the effects of gender) was determined. The positive correlation (*r*=.55; *P*=.0009) observed was found to be slightly stronger than that found without correction for gender (Table 2).

COMMENT

To our knowledge, this is the largest study to date of IL-2 production in never-medicated patients with schizophrenia, and the first to use age-, race-, and gender-matched controls from the community. Our results confirm the association between acute schizophrenia and low IL-2 production and suggest that this finding is not explained by prior neuroleptic treatment. Our findings also indicate that low IL-2 production occurs at an early stage in the course of schizophrenia.

Originally called T-cell growth factor, IL-2 is produced by activated T cells (both CD4 and CD8, but especially CD4) and acts on T cells to stimulate proliferation. Interleukin-2 also promotes cell division of other

Table 2. Correlation Matrix of Mitogen-Stimulated Interleukin-2 (IL-2) Production and Clinical and Demographic Variables*

	Negative Symptoms	Positive Symptoms	Depression Score	Age at Onset	Duration of Illness
IL-2 production	−.38 (.03)	−.09 (.61)	.18 (.33)	.54 (.001)	.09 (.61)
Negative symptoms		.07 (.68)	.16 (.37)	−.28 (.11)	−.17 (.34)
Positive symptoms			.35 (.05)	−.19 (.29)	−.13 (.47)
Depression score				−.08 (.65)	.07 (.71)
Age at onset					.20 (.27)

Values are Pearson's product-moment correlation coefficients (two-tailed significance).

cells, including natural killer cells and B cells. Low IL-2 production in response to mitogenic stimulation is a characteristic finding in several autoimmune diseases, eg, insulin-dependent diabetes mellitus,[23] systemic lupus erythematosus,[24] rheumatoid arthritis,[25] and Graves' disease.[26] Furthermore, in NZB mice, which are genetically predisposed to develop autoimmune disease, the defect in IL-2 production is not present at birth but develops a few weeks in advance of the appearance clinical symptoms of the disease.[27] In humans, identical twins who are discordant for insulin-dependent diabetes mellitus show a similar discordance for low IL-2 production,[28] again suggesting that this defect is associated with the clinical expression of autoimmune disease rather than just the presence of a genetic predisposition. Based on this and other evidence, it has been suggested that defects in IL-2 synthesis and release may represent a core feature of the pathophysiology of systemic autoimmunity.[29] Thus, our findings, while not conclusive in this regard, do suggest the possibility of an autoimmune process active in the early stages of schizophrenia.

Only a few studies have examined the clinical correlations of immune dysfunction in schizophrenia. However, this may be important, as only a proportion of the patients have findings that fall outside the normal range and immunologic dysfunction may be associated with a subtype of schizophrenia. The reported association by Rapaport et al[30] between negative symptoms and increased IL-2 receptor concentration in schizophrenic subjects is intriguing, especially since Ganguli and Rabin[10] found a similar abnormality in subjects with brain damage. However, the confounding effects of neuroleptic medication and chronicity of illness in producing secondary negative symptoms cannot be ruled out in those studies.

The mechanism of lowered IL-2 production in autoimmune diseases remains unclear. One hypothesis is that, on stimulation in vitro, lowered IL-2 production may be a result of the inability of the T cells to produce IL-2. Another theory is that in autoimmune disease, low IL-2 production is a reflection of the "exhausted" state of T cells, which have been driven to overproduce IL-2 in vivo. In one experiment, preculture of cells from patients with systemic lupus erythematosus resulted in normal levels of IL-2 production on subsequent stimulation,[31] providing support for the "exhaustion" hypothesis. In another experiment, however, Warrington[32] used limited dilution analysis to see if cells from patients with systemic lupus erythematosus were normally responsive to IL-2 and found evidence for both the exhaustion hypothesis combined with an intrinsic defect in IL-2 production capacity. The underlying pathophysiology of low IL-2 production in schizophrenia remains to be investigated, but might be clarified by measurement of the signal for the messenger RNA (mRNA) for IL-2 in lymphocytes from these patients, a strategy that we intend to pursue.

Table 3. Regression Analysis of Interleukin-2 Production on Age at Onset and Negative Symptoms in Patients With Schizophrenia*

Variable	B	SE B	β	*t*	Sig† of *t*
Negative symptoms	−50.21	30.88	−0.25	−1.63	.11
Age at onset	47.27	15.74	0.47	3.00	.005
(Constant)	53.78	386.49	...	0.14	.89

*$F_{[2,29]}$=7.88; R^2=.35; P=.002.
†Sig indicates significance.

How is low IL-2 production involved in the pathogenesis of schizophrenia? Clearly the answer is not yet available. It has been proposed that IL-2 might function as a neuromodulator.[33] The finding of high concentrations of IL-2 receptors in the hippocampus[34] and other brain regions such as the striatum,[35] provides evidence for the possibility that IL-2 could affect central nervous system function. Infusion of IL-2 is associated with a variety of psychiatric and neuropsychologic abnormalities in the recepients.[36] However, caution must be exercised in any attempt to extrapolate from this to the pathophysiology of naturally occurring psychoses, as extremely high and unphysiologic concentrations of IL-2 were used in these clinical trials.

Lesions in the central nervous system of mice are known to impair IL-2 production by splenic lymphocytes.[37] In view of this, the association between negative symptoms, early age at onset, and decreased IL-2 production raises some additional interesting possibilities. Negative symptoms and early age at onset are often associated with a more deteriorating form of schizophrenia.[38] Negative symptoms have also been associated with structural brain abnormalities. We have also previously observed an inverse relationship between IL-2 production and titers of antihippocampal antibody (IgG) in schizophrenic patients, a phenomenon not seen in healthy controls.[39] Could the association between reduced IL-2 production and schizophrenia be incidental, with both resulting from a common underlying brain abnormality? Neuroimaging studies of brain structure and function could be combined with clinical and immunologic measures to address this question.

Could low IL-2 production be a nonspecific effect

of stress? We believe that this is unlikely, since, in human studies, stress has been found to be associated with an *increase* rather than a decrease in IL-2 production.[40] In this study, the subject's perception of stress was assessed at the time of the initial drawing of blood,[41] and no association was found between measures of stress and IL-2 production in either the patient or control population (data not shown). Scores on anxiety and tension from the Brief Psychiatric Rating Scale also did not correlate with IL-2 production in patients. Thus, low IL-2 production in this study was not explained by nonspecific stress.

In conclusion, low IL-2 production appears to be consistently associated with acute schizophrenia, independent of medication treatment or other treatment effects. It is also found early in the course of the disorder and appears to be associated with an earlier age at onset and with more severe negative symptoms. The pathophysiology of this abnormality in schizophrenia, and its possible role in the pathophysiology of the disorder, remains to be explored. Since low IL-2 production is associated with specific clinical features, it may prove to be useful as a marker for a distinct subtype of the disorder and may also help to explore the etiologic heterogeneity of the schizophrenic syndrome.

Accepted for publication April 11, 1995.

This study was partially supported by grants from the National Institute of Mental Health (MH-41883), a Research Scientist Development Award (MH-00710), and a National Alliance for Research in Scizophrenia and Affective Disorders Established Investigator Award to Dr Ganguli.

The authors wish to thank David J. Kupfer, MD, for scientific and editorial advice and Linda Koerbel and Erin Petrelle for secretarial assistance.

Reprint requests to Western Psychiatric Institute and Clinic, 3811 O'Hara St, Pittsburgh, PA 15213-2593 (Dr Ganguli).

REFERENCES

1. Lehman-Facius H. Liquaruntersuchumben bei Destructiven Erkrankurgen des Nerwensystems Besonders bei Schizophrenien. *Neurol Psychiatry.* 1937;157: 109-115.
2. Lehman-Facius H. Serologischanalytis che Versuche mit Liquoren und Seren von Schizophrenien. *Allq Z Psychiatry.* 1939;110:232-243.
3. Knight JG. Dopamine receptor stimulating autoantibody: a possible cause of schizophrenia. *Lancet.* 1982;2:1073-1075.
4. Ganguli R, Brar JS, Chengappa KNR, Yang ZW, Nimgaonkar VL, Rabin BS. Autoimmunity in schizophrenia. *Ann Med.* 1993;25:489-496.
5. Kirch DG. Infection and autoimmunity as etiologic factors in schizophrenia. *Schizopr Bull.* 1993;19:355-370.
6. Kolyaskina, GI, Morozov TP, Sekirina TP, Burbayeya GS. Immunological and virological studies in schizophrenia. Presented at the Second World Congress on Viruses, Immunity, and Mental Health; October 6, 1988; Quebec, Quebec.
7. Ganguli R, Rabin BS, Belle SH. Decreased interleukin-2 production in schizophrenic patients. *Biol Psychiatry.* 1989;26:427-430.
8. Villemain F, Chatenoud L, Galinowski A, Homo-Delarche F, Ginistet D, Loo H, Zarifian E, Bach JF. Aberrant T cell-mediated immunity in untreated schizophrenic patients: deficient interleukin-2 production. *Am J Psychiatry.* 1989; 146:609-616.
9. Sirota P, Fishman P, Elizur A, Djaldetty M. Lymphokine production in schizophrenic patients. *Biol Psychiatry.* 1990;27:173A. Abstract.
10. Ganguli R, Rabin BS. Increased serum interluekin-2 receptor concentration in schizophrenic and brain damaged subjects. *Arch Gen Psychiatry.* 1989;46: 292.
11. Rapaport MH, McAllistar C, Pickar D, Nelson DL, Paul SM. Elevated levels of interleukin-2 receptors in schizophrenia. *Arch Gen Psychiatry.* 1989;46:291-292.
12. Shintani F, Kanba S, Maruo N, Nakaki T, Nibuya M, Suzuki E, Kinoshita N, Yagi G. Serum interleukin-6 in schizophrenic patients. *Life Sci.* 1991;49:661-664.
13. Ganguli R, Yang ZW, Shurin G, Chengappa KNR, Brar JS, Gubbi AV, Rabin BS. Serum interleukin-6 concentration in schizophrenia. *Psychiatry Res.* 1994;51: 1-10.
14. Ganguli R, Brar JS, Solomon W, Chengappa KNR, Rabin BS. Altered interleukin-2 production in schizophrenia. *Psychiatry Res.* 1992;44:113-123.
15. Boukhris W, Kouassi E, Revillard JP. Differential effect of mixed D1/D2 and selective D2 dopaminergic antagonists on mouse T and B lymphocyte proliferation and interleukin production in vitro. *Immunopharmacol Immunotoxicol.* 1988;10:501-512.
16. Endicott J, Spitzer RL. A diagnostic interview: the Schedule for Affective Disorders and Schizophrenia. *Arch Gen Psychiatry.* 1978;35:837-844.
17. Spitzer RL, Endicott J, Robins E. *Research Diagnostic Criteria (RDC) for a Selected Group of Functional Disorders.* 3rd ed. New York: New York State Psychiatric Institute; 1978.
18. American Psychiatric Association. *Diagnostic and Statistical Manual of Mental Disorders, Third Edition.* Washington, DC: American Psychiatric Association; 1980.
19. Overall JE, Gorham DR. The Brief Psychiatric Rating Scale. *Psychol Rep.* 1962; 10:799-812.
20. Krawiecka M, Goldberg D, Vaughan M. A standardized psychiatric assessment scale for rating chronic psychotic patients. *Acta Psychiatr Scand.* 1977;55: 299-308.
21. Montgomery SA, Asberg M. A new depression scale designed to be sensitive to change. *Br J Psychiatry.* 1979;134:382-389.
22. Chengappa KNR, Ganguli R, Yang ZW, Shurin G, Cochran J, Brar JS, Rabin BS. Non-right sidedness: an association with lower IL-2 production. *Life Sci.* 1992;51:1843-1849.
23. Zier KS, Leo MM, Spielman RS, Baker L. Decreased synthesis of interleukin-2 (IL-2) in insulin-dependent diabetes mellitus. *Diabetes.* 1984;33:552-555.
24. Alcocer-Varela J, Alarcon-Segovia D. Decreased production of and response to interleukin-2 by cultured lymphocytes from patients with systemic lupus erythematosus. *J Clin Invest.* 1982;69:1388-1392.
25. Cathely GB, Amor B, Fournier C. Defective IL2 production in active rheumatoid arthritis: regulation by radiosensitive suppressor cells. *Clin Rheumatol.* 1986; 5:482-492.
26. Eisenstein Z, Engelsman E, Weiss M, Kalechman Y, Svedni B. Production of and response to interleukin-2 in Graves' disease. *J Clin Immunol.* 1988;8:349-355.
27. Dauphinee MJ, Kipper SB, Wofsy D. Interleukin-2 deficiency is a common feature of autoimmune mice. *J Immunol.* 1981;127:2483.
28. Kaye WA, Adri MN, Soeldner JS, Rabinowe SL, Kaldany A, Kahn CR, Bistrian B, Srikanta S, Ganda OP, Eisenbarth GS. Acquired defect in interleukin-2 production in patients with type I diabetes mellitus. *N Engl J Med.* 1986;315:920-924.
29. Kroemer G, Andreu JL, Gonzalo JA, Gutierrez RJ, Martinez C. Interleukin-2, autotolerance, and autoimmunity. *Adv Immunol.* 1991;50:147-235.
30. Rapaport MH, Torrey EF, McAllister C, Nelson DL, Pickar D, Paul SM. Increased serum soluble interleukin-2 receptors in schizophrenic monozygotic twins. *Eur Arch Psychiatry Clin Neurol.* 1993;243:7-10.
31. Huang YP, Miescher PA, Zubler RH. The interleukin 2 secretion defect in vitro in systemic lupus erythematosus is reversible in rested cultured T cells. *J Immunol.* 1986;137:3515-3520.
32. Warrington RJ. Interleukin-2 abnormalities in systemic lupus erythematosus and rheumatoid arthritis. *J Rheumatol.* 1988;15:616-620.
33. Nistico G, DeSarro G. Is interleukin-2 a neuromodulator in the brain? *Trends Neurosci.* 1991;14:146-150.
34. Araujo DM, Lapchak PA, Collier V, Quirrion R. Localization of interleukin-2 immunoreactivity and interleukin-2 receptors in the rat brain: interaction with the cholonergic system. *Brain Res.* 1989;498:257-266.
35. Lapchak PA. A role for IL-2 in the regulation of striatal dopaminergic function. *Neuroreport.* 1992;3:165-168.
36. Rosenberg SA, Lotze MT, Muul LM. A progress report on the treatment of 157 patients with advanced cancer using lymphokine-activated killer cells and IL-2 or IL-2 alone. *N Engl J Med.* 1987;316:889-897.
37. Neveu PJ, Barncoud P, Vitiello S, Kelley KW, LeMoal MA. Brain neocortex modulation of mitogen-induced interleukin 2, but not interleukin 1, production. *Immunol Lett.* 1989;21:307-310.
38. Crow TJ. A current view of the type II syndrome. *Br J Psychiatry.* 1989;7 (suppl):15-20.
39. Yang ZW, Chengappa KNR, Shurin G, Brar JS, Rabin BS, Gubbi AV, Ganguli R. An association between antihippocampal antibody level and lymphocyte production of IL-2 in patients with schizophrenia. *Psychol Med.* 1994;24:449-455.
40. Kiecolt-Glaser JK, Garner W, Speicher C, Penn GM, Holliday J, Glaser R. Psychosocial modifiers of immunocompetence in medical students. *Psychosom Med.* 1984;46:7-14.
41. Michaux MW. *The First Year Out: Mental Patients After Hospitalization.* Baltimore, Md: The Johns Hopkins Press; 1969.

ORIGINAL ARTICLE

Behavioral vs Biochemical Prediction of Clinical Stability Following Haloperidol Withdrawal in Schizophrenia

Daniel P. van Kammen, MD, PhD; Mary E. Kelley; John A. Gurklis, MD; Mark W. Gilbertson, PhD; Jeffrey K. Yao, PhD; Jeffrey L. Peters, MD

Background: We sought to identify haloperidol-treated subjects who relapsed within 6 weeks of placebo replacement and those who did not, using multivariate analysis.

Methods: In the week prior to discontinuation of haloperidol treatment, global behavioral ratings and a lumbar puncture for cerebrospinal fluid monoamine metabolites were obtained in 88 patients with chronic schizophrenia. Logistic regression analyses were used to evaluate two competing models of relapse prediction. The models were then compared using receiver operating characteristic analysis and a final combined model was derived.

Results: The behavioral model was less variable in its prediction than the cerebrospinal fluid monoamine model. The final model consisted of increased psychosis, decreased anxiety, higher cerebrospinal fluid homovanillic acid levels, and lower cerebrospinal fluid 5-hydroxyindoleacetic acid levels.

Conclusions: Several monoamine systems are involved in psychotic relapse within 6 weeks of haloperidol withdrawal. Future studies of relapse prediction should include both clinical and biological measures to fully assess relapse risk.

(Arch Gen Psychiatry. 1995;52:673-678)

THE COURSE of schizophrenia is marked by periods of clinical stability that are interrupted by psychotic exacerbations or relapses.[1-3] A major therapeutic challenge in schizophrenia is to prevent such relapses. The risk for relapse is affected by medication status, the dose of antipsychotic drug, increased stress or life events,[4] and changes in the internal biochemical milieu.[5] The present recommendations for the prevention of relapse suggest continued neuroleptic treatment for up to 1 year following the first episode, for up to 5 years after the second episode, and indefinitely after the third episode. Many patients, however, prefer not to take medication or are not consistently compliant. Still others who are compliant may relapse in spite of antipsychotic drug treatment. Relapses during antipsychotic drug treatment are more associated with increases in independent life events (ie, stress) than are relapses without medication treatment.[4]

For many years clinicians have noted that relapses are preceded by changes in behavior or prodromes.[6] Several groups have designed studies to evaluate the possibility of medicating patients only when the patient or the therapist believed that relapse was imminent.[7-10] While antipsychotic maintenance treatment clearly prevents psychotic relapses,[11] clinically identifying patients who relapse before the fact is nearly impossible[12]: too many patients relapsed before they could be returned to neuroleptic treatment, in spite of careful clinical supervision.[7-10,13] Others tried to predict relapse following drug withdrawal with behavioral prodromes,[14-17] with limited results. Unfortunately, many patients in the prodromal phase do not share emerging psychotic symptoms with therapists.

In our series of studies of relapse prediction, we have found that in 32 haloperidol-treated schizophrenic patients, cerebrospinal fluid (CSF) norepinephrine (NE) levels and paranoia subscale scores of the Brief Psychiatric Rating Scale (BPRS)[18] were higher but that BPRS anxiety ratings were lower in patients who relapsed after haloperidol withdrawal than those who did not relapse.[19] By adding CSF

From the Veterans Affairs Medical Center, Pittsburgh, Pa, and the Western Psychiatric Institute and Clinic, University of Pittsburgh, School of Medicine.

See Methods on next page

METHODS

SUBJECTS

Eighty-eight physically healthy male psychiatric patients with a diagnosis of chronic schizophrenia according to *DSM-III-R* criteria[23] receiving antipsychotic maintenance treatment participated in the study following admission to the Schizophrenia Research Unit at the Department of Veterans Affairs Medical Center, Highland Drive, in Pittsburgh, Pa. All lived in the community prior to the study and gave written informed consent. Clinical and demographic information on the sample is provided in **Table 1**. Seventy-nine of the subjects were white, seven were black, and two were Hispanic. All the subjects were screened with a complete physical, neurological, and psychiatric evaluation conducted by board-certified psychiatrists. Trained staff obtained the diagnostic data from a structured interview using the Schedule for Affective Disorders and Schizophrenia–Lifetime Version,[24] and a *DSM-III-R* checklist. Patients who met *DSM-III-R* criteria for alcohol or substance abuse/dependence were excluded at the time of the study unless they had been in remission for at least 6 months. All the subjects were put on a low-monoamine, caffeine- and alcohol-free diet on admission, and their medication was converted to haloperidol for at least 3 months if they were not already being treated with haloperidol. Following this, they were switched to treatment with haloperidol in unmarked capsules for 2 to 4 weeks. If benztropine mesylate (1 to 3 mg/d) was given, this was discontinued at least 2 weeks prior to the lumbar puncture. No other medications were given. Identical-looking placebo capsules replaced the haloperidol capsules overnight within days following the lumbar puncture.

RATINGS

Patients were rated daily by the nursing staff on the global psychosis scale of Bunney and Hamburg.[21] The 1- to 15-point psychosis item of this scale is subdivided into five consecutive levels of intensity, each consisting of three points. Relapse was considered to have taken place if there was a 3-day mean increase in 3 points in the global psychosis ratings compared with the mean of those psychosis ratings of the last 7 days of haloperidol treatment done by the nursing staff. A rating of 6 and higher was required, indicating a clear presence of psychotic symptoms, which ensured that an increase into the range of psychotic behavior had taken place.[25] These criteria have been previously validated.[20,26] Of the 88 subjects, 54 relapsed within 6 weeks. The 34 patients who did not meet the criteria for relapse by 6 weeks were considered to be clinically stable for the purpose of the study.

Therapists who were blinded to patients' status independently rated patients weekly on the Bunney-Hamburg Global Rating Scale[21] and the Scale for the Assessment of Negative Symptoms.[22] Weekly meetings were conducted to ensure interrater reliability, computed using intraclass correlation coefficients; the interrater reliability was greater than 85% for all behavioral measures. The ratings of the last week of haloperidol treatment were used in the analysis.

LUMBAR PUNCTURES

Lumbar punctures were obtained during the last week of haloperidol treatment, with the patient in the lateral decubitus position between 7:30 and 8:30 AM after overnight fasting and bed rest as previously described.[27] The CSF was collected on ice and stored at −80°C. The CSF measures included HVA, 5-HIAA, NE, and MHPG, assayed according to the modified assays by Scheinin et al[28] from aliquots of the first 12-mL pool.

STATISTICAL PROCEDURES

Logistic regression[29] (SPSS-PC, SPSS Inc, Chicago, Ill) was used to predict dichotomous relapse status using various biochemical and behavioral measures as independent predictors. Logistic regression models, using relapse as the dependent variable, were performed with the following groups of independent variables: (1) a biochemical model consisting of CSF HVA, 5-HIAA, MHPG, and NE and dosage of haloperidol in milligrams per kilograms per day; (2) a behavioral model consisting of the global items of the Bunney-Hamburg scale[21] (except for mania, which had insufficient variance), as well as the Scale for the Assessment of Negative Symptoms total score; and (3) a reduced combination of the variables from the behavioral and biochemical models. The probability of relapse was calculated as $1/[1+e^{-(exp)}]$, where the exponent of the logit function (exp) is a linear combination of the independent variables (see the "Results" section).

The Hosmer-Lemeshow goodness-of-fit χ^2 statistic[29] was used to determine whether any of the models presented had a global lack of fit, which would result if the error or residual deviance (analogous to the residual sum of squares in linear regression) was high. Likelihood ratio χ^2 statistics were used to evaluate each individual variable's contribution to the model as well as the significance of the model as a whole.

The evaluation of the success of classification produced by the logistic regression model is often presented as a 2×2 table, indicating the number of correctly predicted members in each group. However, the data in the 2×2 table are based on an arbitrary cutoff point for the probability of relapse computed by the model. The steps involved are depicted in **Figure 1**; the equation resulting from the logistic regression procedure gives a probability for relapse between 0 and 1 for each subject based on the levels of his covariates.

To assess the number of subjects correctly predicted, subjects must be assigned to a group based on their probability score. A reasonable cutoff point, and the cutoff used as the default in the majority of logistic regression output results (the SPSS, SAS, BMDP statistical software programs), can be made at the probability level of .5 (or 50%), with those receiving a probability lower than .5 being classified as nonrelapsers and those with a probability above .5 being classified as relapsers. However, other cutoffs are often not explored. Receiver operating characteristic (ROC) analysis[30] is a graphical representation of a series of 2×2 tables, each table being generated by using a different cutoff point. Thus, each point on the curve represents a sensitivity and (1−specificity) combination that defines the ability of the model to discriminate at the given cutoff point. In this assessment of the logistic regression model, there is no specific sensitivity or specificity associated with the model, but rather a set of values that can be tested against the null hypothesis of a random allocation. Comparison of the ROC curves allows us to compare the discriminating ability of the models at all cutoff points, and one can judge by the smoothness of the curve how sensitive each model is to the choice of the cutoff point, ie, the consistency of the model.

Table 1. Clinical and Biochemical Variables Prior to Haloperidol Withdrawal*

Variable	Relapsers (n=54)	Nonrelapsers (n=34)
Age, y	35.7±7.1	34.6±9.1
Age of onset, y	22.7±5.1	23.4±4.9
Duration of illness, y	13.1±6.3	11.2±7.6
Haloperidol dosage, mg/kg per day	0.15±0.09	0.13±0.14
CSF NE, nmol/L	0.64±0.51	0.52±0.38
CSF HVA, nmol/L	177.0±85.6	163.8±61.1
CSF 5-HIAA, nmol/L	87.4±39.0	97.5±39.8
CSF MHPG, nmol/L	40.7±14.0	42.7±17.0
Psychosis† (BH)	6.1±1.7	5.6±1.9
Depression† (BH)	4.8±1.9	4.6±1.7
Anxiety† (BH)	5.0±1.8	5.5±1.8
Negative symptoms score (SANS total)†	8.6±3.9	7.9±3.9

**Data are given as mean±SD. CSF indicates cerebrospinal fluid; NE, norepinephrine; HVA, homovanillic acid; 5-HIAA, 5-hydroxyindoleacetic acid; MHPG, 3-methoxy-4-hydroxyphenylglycol; BH, Bunney-Hamburg Global Rating Scale[21]; and SANS, Scale for the Assessment of Negative Symptoms.*

†Ratings made by blinded therapists, not nurses' ratings used for establishing relapse.

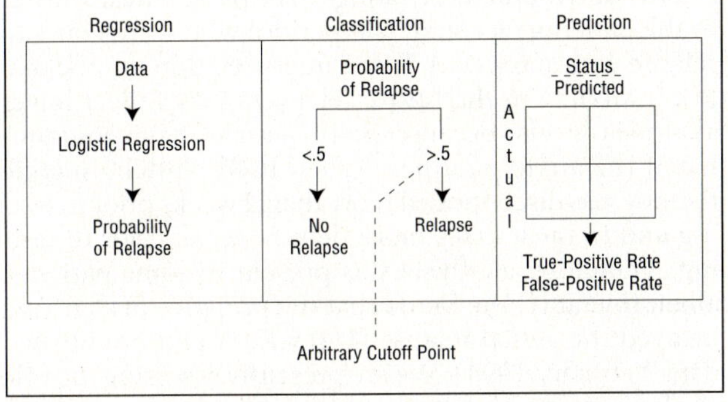

Figure 1. *The steps from regression to prediction of relapse in schizophrenia.*

3-methoxy-4-hydroxyphenylglycol (MHPG) and chromogranin A–like immunoreactivity and the dose of haloperidol to those items, we developed a logistic regression model in 50 schizophrenic patients that correctly identified relapsers and nonrelapsers with high specificity.[20] We decided to test both biochemical (CSF homovanillic acid [HVA], 5-hydroxyindoleacetic acid [5-HIAA], MHPG, and NE) and behavioral models of relapse prediction and compare their abilities to discriminate between those patients who would relapse and those who would not. We hypothesized that changes in serotonin (5-HT) and NE levels in addition to dopamine turnover would be involved based on the observations that 5-HT and NE affect dopamine activity and that indirect dopamine agonists and serotonin–dopamine antagonists affect psychosis more profoundly than more specific or direct dopaminergic agents. We report herein on a group of 88 well-diagnosed and carefully screened neuroleptic-treated schizophrenic patients. Fifty of these patients participated in a previous exploratory study.[20] For this study, we used the therapists' global ratings of psychosis, depression, and anxiety[21] and the total score of the Scale for the Assessment of Negative Symptoms[22] during antipsychotic treatment for the behavioral prediction model; it has been our experience that the BPRS clusters do not always reflect changes in global clinical behavior as well as do these items. We believe that these once-a-week ratings more resembled the clinical practice setting. These patients were stabilized on treatment with haloperidol and participated in a 6-week placebo replacement study of relapse prediction, using operationally defined psychotic relapse criteria.

RESULTS

LOGISTIC REGRESSION

The behavioral and CSF monoamine models are presented in **Table 2**. In the behavioral model, anxiety and psychosis were significant contributors, while CSF HVA, 5-HIAA, and NE contributed significantly to the biochemical model. The probability of relapse can be calculated for each subject; for example, for the biochemical model the probability of relapse=$1/[1+e^{-(exp)}]$, where the exponent of the logit function (exp) = 0.5466 + 0.0144 (CSF HVA) + 1.1773 (CSF NE) − 0.0282 (CSF MHPG) − 0.0274 (CSF 5HIAA) + 3.5109 (dose/weight). None of the models had a significant lack of fit.

ROC CURVES

The cutoff points used for classification were the quintiles (those values that separate the subjects into five equal-sized groups) of the distribution of predicted values for each model. The resulting quintiles were 0.502, 0.572, 0.644, 0.724, for the biochemical model and 0.454, 0.594, 0.681, 0.783 for the behavioral model. The curves are depicted in **Figure 2**; the gray diagonal line represents a 50-50 chance, or random curve. A random curve is expected if the variables have no predictive value; thus, the larger the area under the curve, the larger the significance. The area under the ROC curve is a measure of the model's predictive value; by testing this area vs the null hypothesis of the area=0.5 (no prediction), we arrive at the significance values presented in Table 2.[31]

The use of the ROC curves allows us to see that the biochemical model is more varied in its predictability, ie, it is more sensitive to the choice of cutoff point, while the behavioral model is not. In addition, one can choose the cutoff point that has the highest sensitivity and specificity combination (the highest value of the two added) to be considered the "best" cutoff point.

COMBINED MODEL

We used all the independent variables from the first two models as competing predictors in a backward stepwise procedure; the remaining variables were CSF HVA and 5-HIAA, anxiety, and psychosis (Table 2). The quintiles for the combined model were 0.472, 0.591, 0.689, 0.768, respectively. The area under the ROC curve was more

Table 2. Logistic Regression Models Significance of β Coefficient*

Variable	Biochemical Model			Behavioral Model			Reduced Combined Model		
	β	χ^2	*P*†	β	χ^2	*P*†	β	χ^2	*P*†
CSF HVA	0.014	8.248	**.004**	...	...	...	0.011	5.736	**.017**
CSF NE	1.177	3.668	.055	...	...	...	...	...	...
CSF MHPG	−0.028	2.273	.132	...	...	...	...	...	...
CSF 5-HIAA	−0.027	8.791	**.003**	...	...	...	−0.025	7.447	**.006**
Dose/weight	3.511	2.455	.117	...	...	...	...	...	...
Psychosis (BH)	...	...	...	0.272	2.974	.085	0.333	4.368	**.037**
Anxiety (BH)	...	...	...	−0.369	4.668	**.031**	−0.387	5.544	**.018**
Depression (BH)	...	...	...	0.108	0.374	.541	...	...	...
SANS total	...	...	...	0.029	0.155	.694	...	...	...
Intercept	0.547	...	...	0.080	...	...	0.979	...	...
Model χ^2	12.900	...	...	6.460	...	...	13.777	...	...
Significance	0.024	...	...	0.167	...	...	0.008	...	...
Area under the ROC curve	...	0.667	...	...	0.653	...	...	0.685	...
SE (area)	...	0.060	...	...	0.059	...	...	0.057	...
Significance level	...	**0.003**	...	...	**0.005**	...	...	**0.001**	...

**ROC indicates receiver operating characteristic. See Table 1 for expansion of other abbreviations.*
†P values are based on the significance of the likelihood ratio χ^2 statistic; boldface values indicate P≤.05.

significant for the combined model than either the biochemical or behavioral models (Figure 2).

BENEFIT OF ROC

It can be seen from the "best" cutoff values for the curves (0.502, 0.681, 0.591) that the default value of 0.5 is not always the best cutoff point, and thus examination of different cutoff points, using ROC, is beneficial in interpreting the logistic regression results.

COMMENT

BEHAVIORAL VS BIOCHEMICAL PREDICTION OF RELAPSE

A variety of behavioral measures have been found to predict relapse. Among others, Dencker et al[14] reported higher paranoia and Subotnik and Nuechterlein[12] reported higher levels of BPRS hostility and grandiosity prior to psychotic relapse following drug withdrawal. Buchanan et al[15] reported nonsignificantly higher BPRS thinking disturbance cluster values in the relapsers prior to drug withdrawal. In the logistic regression model, it is the combination of variables and the weights that each carry in the equation that determines the risk for relapse. The variables by themselves do not need to be significantly different between the two groups, which may lead to seemingly paradoxical observations; ie, there may be a complex relationship among predictors. This relationship may explain why clinical assessment of specific symptoms cannot reliably indicate relapse risk in drug-free patients.

The relapse rates reported in this sample seem higher than those usually reported.[11] This may be because the criteria for relapse reported in the literature varies considerably. Our criteria are based on specific behavioral criteria that are conservative in nature, thus, one would expect the relapse rate to be increased in our sample.

We have previously included (BPRS) anxiety because of its potential relationship with locus coeruleus activity and found these ratings to be paradoxically lower in the patients receiving haloperidol who were going to relapse within 6 weeks.[19] One interpretation may be that lower anxiety in the future relapsers may reflect lower akathisia levels, because akathisia may have contaminated the anxiety ratings. When used, anticholinergic therapy was discontinued more than 2 weeks prior to testing and in most cases more than 3 weeks prior to testing. Therefore, akathisia was present in some patients, albeit tolerably. We found that the presence of akathisia delayed the actual relapse (D.P.v.K. et al, unpublished data, February 1994). We are presently assessing the role of akathisia in the relapse process.

Negative symptoms were not included in the model, suggesting that negative symptoms associated with haloperidol treatment have no predictive value. This may be because the negative symptoms observed with neuroleptic treatment may be partially induced by the treatment itself, rather than by a primary phenomenon.

Higher neuroleptic doses have been associated with relapse following drug withdrawal,[15,20,32,33] but this phenomenon was observed within different dosage ranges.[32] Although the simplest explanation is that clinicians treat the most symptomatic patients with higher doses, the actual differences between the groups do not support this notion. In the current study, dose/weight was not a significant predictor of relapse, either by itself (mean±SD, 0.15±0.9 vs 0.13±0.14 mg/kg per day; t=0.79, P=.43) or in the models (Table 2). This may be because median doses for the relapsers and nonrelapsers were 10 and 7 mg/d, respectively, neither of which is a relatively high dose. Recent evidence indicates that most patients are effectively treated with haloperidol in doses between 5 and 15 mg/d. The generalizability of our results obtained in an all-chronic, male, veteran patient sample may be limited. Similar studies will have to be done in women, par-

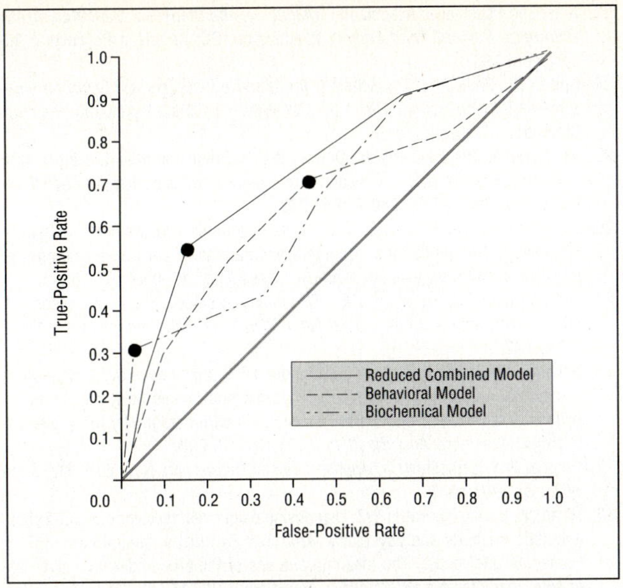

Figure 2. *Receiver operating characteristic curves. The larger the area under the curve, the more discriminating the model; the best discriminating points are those that are the farthest from the gray diagonal (random) curve and are marked with solid circles. The best discriminating points refer to cutoff points of 0.502 for the biochemical model, 0.681 for the behavioral model, and 0.591 for the combined model.*

ticularly because women in general require lower doses of antipsychotic drugs. However, gender-specific relapse rates are not available from the literature.

We have previously shown in 50 patients that a model consisting of CSF NE, MHPG, chromogranin A, dose of haloperidol, weight, and the BPRS paranoia subscale and anxiety item predicted relapse at 6 weeks with 86% accuracy using a cutoff value of 0.5.[20] The purpose of the present study was to examine the options of different cutoff values and their ability to predict relapse. It can be seen from Figure 2 that the traditionally used 0.5 value is not the best discriminating point of the distribution. Cerebrospinal fluid NE was almost significant at $P=.06$ in the biochemical model, but did not add significantly to the final model, suggesting that the noradrenergic contribution was the result of its relationship to other items that were significant in the model. Possibly, this is because HVA is derived in part from dopamine broken down in noradrenergic neurons.

The inclusion of a serotonergic measure (ie, CSF 5-HIAA) in the biochemical model is of particular interest, considering the pharmacological properties of the newer antipsychotic agents, such as clozapine, risperidone, sertindole, olanzapine, and others.[34] Because these atypical agents have strong 5-HT_2 receptor blockade as well as α_1 and α_2 receptor blockade and may be more effective antipsychotics, in addition to the fact that the NE, 5-HT, and dopamine systems interact, a role for 5-HT in psychotic decompensation is plausible. Further support for a role of 5-HT in psychotic relapse, if psychotic relapse represents a loss of impulse control, may come from the association of impulsive behaviors with decreased 5-HT turnover.[35] Furthermore, Hsiao et al[36] have shown that the relationships between these CSF monoamines decrease with psychotic deterioration, while Joyce[37] has reported that the 5-HT systems were altered in autopsy results of the brains of schizophrenics. Because haloperidol does not have discernible 5-HT_2 or α_2 receptor blockade, our data imply that patients with lower 5-HT turnover or higher 5-HT_2 receptor activity are more likely to relapse following haloperidol discontinuation. Dopamine receptor blockade may normalize the relationships between the 5-HT and dopamine systems.[36]

This multimonoamine involvement in the psychotic relapse process supports the notion that during relapse, relationships between these neurotransmitters are disturbed[38] and that the interactions among the monoaminergic systems are more important than each neurotransmitter by itself.[39] The more compromised these relationships are, the more likely the patient will relapse. Patients who are in a prerelapse state may have failing feedback systems that maintain behavioral and biochemical homeostasis.[40,41] Conceivably, dopamine involvement in schizophrenia reflects the failure of a homeostatic mechanism that allows for integration of different brain functional parts as needed.

CONCLUSIONS

If antipsychotic drugs raise the stress threshold and "normalize" relationships between monoamines, and if relapse risk is also a function of this stress sensitivity, then relapse is a failed attempt to contain stress. We have proposed that clinical instability, as exposed by the state-dependent response to stimulant challenges, is due to biochemical instability, reflecting increased stress sensitivity.[42,43] We hypothesize now that increased stress sensitivity and decreased impulse control (ie, relapse risk) causes relapse when the stress threshold is lowered with haloperidol withdrawal. If we can identify when patients change into a high-risk condition, appropriate stress and performance demand reduction can be implemented while receiving medication,[4] and drug-free patients can be returned to medication treatment in a timely fashion.

We are continuing our search for a measure or measures that will reflect stress sensitivity to identify those patients who will remain clinically stable without antipsychotic drug treatment, or inversely will relapse early following haloperidol withdrawal.

Accepted for publication March 29, 1995.

Funding for this project was provided to Dr van Kammen in part by the National Institute of Mental Health (RO1MH44-841), the Department of Veterans Affairs Research and Development Service (Merit Review), and the American Defenders of Bataan and Corregidor Medical Fund.

The authors thank the patients and nursing staff of the Schizophrenia Research Unit under the leadership of Doris McAdam, RN, for their participation and collaboration.

Reprint requests to Professor of Psychiatry, Chief of Staff, VAMC, 7180 Highland Drive, Pittsburgh, PA 15206 (Dr van Kammen).

REFERENCES

1. Meyer A. Constructive formulation of schizophrenia. *Am J Psychiatry.* 1922; 78:355-364.
2. Bleuler M. *The Schizophrenic Disorders: Long-term Patient and Family Studies.* New Haven, Conn: Yale University Press; 1978.
3. Strauss JS, Hafez H, Lieberman P, Harding CM. The course of psychiatric disorder, III: longitudinal principles. *Am J Psychiatry.* 1985;142:289-296.
4. Ventura J, Nuechterlein KH, Hardesty JP, Gitlin M. Life events and schizophrenic relapse after withdrawal of medication. *Br J Psychiatry.* 1992;161:615-620.
5. van Kammen DP. The biochemical basis of relapse and drug response in schizophrenia: review and hypothesis. *Psychol Med.* 1991;21:881-895.
6. Docherty JP, van Kammen DP, Siris SG, Marder SR. Stages of onset of schizophrenia psychosis. *Am J Psychiatry.* 1978;135:420-426.
7. Herz MI, Glazer WM, Mostert A, Sheard MA, Szymanski HV, Hafez H, Mirza M, Vana J. Intermittent vs maintenance medication in schizophrenia: two-year results. *Arch Gen Psychiatry.* 1991;48:333-339.
8. Heinrichs DW, Carpenter WT Jr. Prospective study of prodromal symptoms in schizophrenic relapse. *Am J Psychiatry.* 1985;142:371-373.
9. Hirsch SR, Jolley AG, Morrison E, McRink A, Wilson L. Trial of brief intermittent neuroleptic prophylaxis for selected schizophrenic outpatients: clinical and social outcome at 2 years. *Schizophr Res.* 1990;3:40.
10. Müller P, Bandelow B, Gaebel W, Köpcke W, Linden M, Müller-Spahn F, Pietzcker A, Schaefer E, Tegeler J. Intermittent medication, coping and psychotherapy: interactions in relapse prevention and course modification. *Br J Psychiatry.* 1992;161(suppl 18):140-144.
11. Davis JM. Overview: maintenance therapy in psychiatry: schizophrenia. *Am J Psychiatry.* 1975;132:1237-1245.
12. Subotnik KL, Nuechterlein KH. Prodromal signs and symptoms of schizophrenic relapse. *J Abnorm Psychol.* 1988;97:405-412.
13. Gaebel W, Frick W, Kopcke W, Linden M, Müller P, Müller-Spahn F, Pietzcker A, Tegeler J. Early neuroleptic intervention in schizophrenia: are prodromal symptoms valid predictors of relapse? *Br J Psychiatry.* 1993;163:8-12.
14. Dencker SJ, Malm U, Lepp M. Schizophrenic relapse after drug withdrawal is predictable. *Acta Psychiatr Scand.* 1986;73:181-185.
15. Buchanan RW, Kirkpatrick B, Summerfelt A, Hanlon TE, Levine J, Carpenter WT Jr. Clinical predictors of relapse following neuroleptic withdrawal. *Biol Psychiatry.* 1992;32:72-78.
16. Nuechterlein KH, Dawson ME. A heuristic vulnerability/stress model of schizophrenic episodes. *Schizophr Bull.* 1984;10:300-312.
17. Johnson DAW, Pasterski G, Ludlow JM, Street K, Taylor RDW. The discontinuance of maintenance neuroleptic therapy in chronic schizophrenic patients: drug and social consequences. *Acta Psychiatr Scand.* 1983;67:339-352.
18. Overall JE, Gorham DR. The Brief Psychiatric Rating Scale. *Psychol Rep.* 1962; 10:799-812.
19. van Kammen DP, Peters J, van Kammen WB, Nugent A, Goetz KL, Yao J, Linnoila M. CSF norepinephrine in schizophrenia is elevated prior to relapse after haloperidol withdrawal. *Biol Psychiatry.* 1989;26:176-188.
20. van Kammen DP, Ågren H, Yao JK, O'Connor DT, Gurklis JA, Peters JL. Noradrenergic activity and prediction of psychotic relapse following haloperidol withdrawal in schizophrenia. *Am J Psychiatry.* 1994;151:379-384.
21. Bunney Jr WE, Hamburg DA. Methods for reliable longitudinal observation of behavior. *Arch Gen Psychiatry.* 1963;9:280-294.
22. Andreasen NC. Negative symptoms in schizophrenia: definition and reliability. *Arch Gen Psychiatry.* 1982;39:784-794.
23. American Psychiatric Association. *Diagnostic and Statistical Manual of Mental Disorders, Revised Third Edition.* Washington, DC: American Psychiatric Association; 1987.
24. Spitzer RL, Endicott J. *The Schedule for Affective Disorders and Schizophrenia–Lifetime Version.* 3rd ed. New York, NY: New York State Psychiatric Institute, Biometrics Research; 1979.
25. van Kammen DP, Docherty JP, Bunney WE Jr. Prediction of early relapse after pimozide discontinuation by response to d-amphetamine during pimozide treatment. *Biol Psychiatry.* 1982;17:233-242.
26. van Kammen DP, Peters JL, Yao JK, van Kammen WB, Neylan T, Shaw D, Linnoila M. Norepinephrine in acute exacerbations of chronic schizophrenia: negative symptoms revisited. *Arch Gen Psychiatry.* 1990;47:161-168.
27. van Kammen DP, Sternberg DE. CSF studies in schizophrenia. In: Wood JH, ed. *Neurobiology of Cerbrospinal Fluid.* New York, NY: Plenum Press; 1980; 1:719-742.
28. Scheinin M, Chang W-H, Kirk JL, Linnoila M. Simultaneous determination of 3-methoxy-4-hydroxyphenylglycol, 5-hydroxyindoleacetic acid, and homovanillic acid in CSF with high performance liquid chromatography using electrochemical detection. *Anal Biochem.* 1983;131:246-253.
29. Hosmer DW, Lemeshow S. *Applied Logistic Regression.* New York, NY: John Wiley & Sons; 1989.
30. Hsiao JK, Bartko JJ, Potter WZ. Diagnosing diagnoses: receiver operating characteristic methods and psychiatry. *Arch Gen Psychiatry.* 1989;46:664-667.
31. Hanley JA, McNeil BJ. The meaning and use of the area under a receiver operating characteristic (ROC) curve. *Radiology.* 1982;143:29-36.
32. Prien RF, Cole JO, Belkin NF. Relapse in chronic schizophrenics following abrupt withdrawal of tranquillizing medication. *Br J Psychiatry.* 1968;115:679-686.
33. Andrews P, Hall JN, Snaith RP. A controlled trial of phenothiazine withdrawal in chronic schizophrenic patients. *Br J Psychiatry.* 1976;128:451-455.
34. Meltzer HY. The mechanism of action of novel antipsychotic drugs. *Schizophr Bull.* 1991;17:263-287.
35. Linnoila M, Dejong J, Virkkunen M. Monoamines, glucose metabolism, and impulse control. *Psychopharmacol Bull.* 1989;25:404-406.
36. Hsiao JK, Colison J, Bartko JJ, Doran AR, Konicki PE, Potter WZ, Pickar D. Monoamine neurotransmitter interactions in drug-free and neuroleptic-treated schizophrenics. *Arch Gen Psychiatry.* 1993;50:606-614.
37. Joyce J. The dopamine hypothesis of schizophrenia: limbic interactions with serotonin and norepinephrine. *Psychopharmacology.* 1993;112(suppl):S16-S34.
38. Potter WZ, Manji HK. Are monoamine metabolites in cerebrospinal fluid worth measuring? *Arch Gen Psychiatry.* 1993;50:653-656.
39. Joyce JN, Shane A, Lexow N, Winokur A, Casanova MF, Kleinman JE. Serotonin uptake sites and serotonin receptors are altered in the limbic system of schizophrenics. *Neuropsychopharmacology.* 1993;8:315-336.
40. Davidson M, Davis KL. A comparison of plasma homovanillic acid concentrations in schizophrenic patients and normal controls. *Arch Gen Psychiatry.* 1988; 45:561-563.
41. Davis KL, Kahn RS, Ko G, Davidson M. Dopamine in schizophrenia: a review and reconceptualization. *Am J Psychiatry.* 1991;148:1474-1486.
42. Angrist B, van Kammen DP. CNS stimulants as tools in the study of schizophrenia. *Trends Neurosci.* 1984;7:388-390.
43. van Kammen DP, van Kammen WB. The amphetamine challenge test in schizophrenia: a stress response? In: Usdin E, Kvetnansky R, Axelrod J, eds. *Stress: The Role of Catecholamines and Other Neurotransmitters.* New York, NY: Gordon & Breach Science Publishers; 1984:957-966.

ORIGINAL ARTICLE

Multiple-Family Groups and Psychoeducation in the Treatment of Schizophrenia

William R. McFarlane, MD; Ellen Lukens, PhD; Bruce Link, PhD; Robert Dushay, PhD; Susan A. Deakins, MD; Margaret Newmark, CSW; Edward J. Dunne, PhD; Bonnie Horen, MA; Joanne Toran, MPA

Objective: To compare outcomes in psychoeducational multiple-family group treatment vs psychoeducational single-family treatment.

Method: A total of 172 acutely psychotic patients, aged 18 to 45 years, with *DSM-III-R* schizophrenic disorders were randomly assigned to single- or multiple-family psychoeducational treatment at six public hospitals in the state of New York. Psychotic relapse, symptom status, medication compliance, rehospitalization, and employment were assessed independently during 2 years of supervised treatment.

Results: The multiple-family groups yielded significantly lower 2-year cumulative relapse rates than did the single-family modality (16% vs 27%) and achieved markedly lower rates in patients whose conditions had not remitted at index hospital discharge (13% vs 33%). The relapse hazard ratio between treatments was 1:3. The relapse rate for both modalities was less than half the expected rate (65% to 80% for 2 years) for patients receiving individual treatment and medication. Rehospitalization rates and psychotic symptoms decreased significantly, and medication compliance was high, to an equal degree in both modalities.

Conclusion: Psychoeducational multiple-family groups were more effective than single-family treatment in extending remission, especially in patients at higher risk for relapse, with a cost-benefit ratio of up to 1:34.

(Arch Gen Psychiatry. 1995;52:679-687)

MOUNTING evidence suggests that family psychoeducation is more effective in the prevention of relapse in schizophrenia than is individual treatment or medication alone.[1-10] The common elements in several cited approaches include social support, detailed education on clinical aspects, direct guidance, and training in coping skills. Building on these studies and earlier work by multiple-family group (MFG) clinicians,[11-17] we conducted a small-sample study that demonstrated that the psychoeducational MFG was more effective in the prevention of relapse than were the same techniques conducted in single-family treatment (SFT) or in traditional MFG therapy without psychoeducation.[10] In that study and in the one reported herein, treatment methods in the psychoeducational MFGs and SFT were the same, consisting primarily of training in coping skills and problem solving. The principal difference between MFGs and SFT was in the membership of the treatment groups. In SFT, single families met alone with a single clinician; MFGs comprised six families meeting together with two clinicians. Patients were strongly encouraged but not required to attend meetings in both approaches.

Our previous study[10] suggested that two components of psychoeducational MFGs—expansion of social networks and family psychoeducation as a clinical framework—had separate effects during different phases of a long-term treatment process. The social network of the MFGs had effects later and for more prolonged periods than did psychoeducation. We hypothesized that the effects of MFGs derive from the larger number of individuals involved in problem solving and from the development of a social support network.

However, Leff et al[7] found no difference in outcome between single-family behavioral management and psychoeducational relatives groups (in which patients were absent) and raised the question of

See Patients and Methods on next page

From the Biosocial Treatment Research Division of the Department of Epidemiology of Mental Disorders, Department of Psychiatry, College of Physicians and Surgeons, Columbia University and the New York State Psychiatric Institute, New York. Dr McFarlane is now affiliated with Maine Medical Center, Portland.

PATIENTS AND METHODS

INCLUSION CRITERIA, SAMPLE, AND RANDOM ASSIGNMENT

The criteria for inclusion in the study were (1) a diagnosis of schizophrenia, schizoaffective disorder, or schizophreniform disorder according to *DSM-III-R* criteria[20]; (2) age 18 to 45 years; (3) admission to an inpatient psychiatric unit for an acute psychotic episode; (4) patients living with their family of origin or in contact with a family member for at least 10 hours per week during the 2 months preceding the index admission; (5) patient and family consent to participate; and (6) attendance, at a minimum, by one member of the family, of five face-to-face contacts. Stabilization with medication after hospital discharge was not required. Patients with a history of substance abuse were excluded only if they were physically dependent, as judged by the inpatient psychiatrist, thus including a significant proportion who were not compliant with antipsychotic drug regimens and used alcohol and other illicit drugs in clinically significant quantities.[21] At four of the five state hospitals, treatment had already failed in all cases in brief-stay acute inpatient units in general hospitals.

The total eligible sample consisted of 191 patients and their families, comprising six subsamples drawn from serial admissions to one of the six clinical sites. The study sites were five New York state hospitals: Kings Park Psychiatric Center, Long Island; Hudson River Psychiatric Center, Poughkeepsie; South Beach Psychiatric Center, Staten Island; Creedmoor Psychiatric Center, Queens; and Rochester Psychiatric Center, Rochester; and one municipal hospital: Harlem Hospital, Manhattan. The sample represented a wide range of demographic characteristics found in the eastern United States. We placed no limit on the duration of the index hospital admission; 11 patients were not discharged within 2 years of the index admission date. In eight cases, the patient and family dropped out of treatment during the engagement phase; these 19 cases were excluded from the data sample, yielding a final at-risk sample of 172. A categorical description of the sample and the two experimental cohorts is included in **Table 1**.

Recruitment procedures were consistent across sites. With the patient's permission, families were contacted by a family clinician immediately after the index admission to obtain informed consent. The patient was then solicited by the study psychiatrist to obtain informed consent. Following the diagnostic interview and baseline assessments, patients and their families were randomly assigned to a psychoeducational MFG or to psychoeducational SFT.

TREATMENTS

Both SFT and MFG treatment were expected to reduce symptom levels and frequency of relapse, enhance psychosocial functioning, and lower expressed emotion.[22] To achieve these goals, the treatments were designed to help families and patients improve their coping and illness-management skills. This general strategy was derived largely from work previously reported by Goldstein et al,[1] Leff et al,[2] Falloon et al,[3] and Hogarty et al.[4]

Specific treatment interventions in MFGs and SFT were to (1) engage key members of the family within 7 days of an acute admission; (2) provide information about the biologic aspects of schizophrenia and the treatment process, via a standardized videotape, lectures, and written coping guidelines; (3) intervene early in incipient relapse[23]; (4) provide ongoing support and formal clinical problem solving[24] for at least 2 years; and (5) expand the family's social network. A "family clinician,"[25] a regularly employed member of the social work, psychology, or nursing staff at the site hospital, was assigned to each case and was expected to act as (1) the patient's primary case coordinator and therapist during inpatient and outpatient phases, (2) the family's educator and consultant, (3) a leader of SFT or MFG treatment sessions, and (4) the principal liaison to the treating psychiatrist and rehabilitation agencies. At each site, a full-time psychiatrist provided pharmacologic treatment for the entire subsample. These arrangements ensured continuity of care through the 2-year protocol and into the post-study period.

Both treatments initially concentrated on helping the patients reenter the community after discharge by promoting family interactions that supported recovery from the acute episode. In the second phase, corresponding roughly to the second year of treatment, the focus shifted to the patients' vocational and social functioning. At the earliest sign of decompensation, the clinical team instituted a combination of pharmacologic, family, and crisis interventions, including hospitalization, if indicated. Patients continued to undergo the assigned treatment during and after relapses. After the 2-year course of the research treatment, many patients were referred to rehabilitation programs while continuing in, or entering, MFGs. The clinical methods in both versions of psychoeducation were derived from the approaches of Anderson and Falloon and are more fully described elsewhere.[25,26]

PSYCHOEDUCATIONAL MFG TREATMENT

The MFG protocol began with two study-trained family clinicians, each meeting separately with three families, without patients present, for three weekly single-family sessions, commencing within 7 days of the index admission. On completion of these sessions, the clinicians presented an educational workshop to these six families, again without patients present, using the standard videotape and coping guidelines. This presentation was modeled on the Survival Skills Workshop developed by Anderson et al.[25] Two weeks later, the six-family MFG began to meet biweekly, co-led by the same two clinicians. Meetings were organized around a formal problem-solving procedure, designed to develop individualized coping methods that were derived from suggestions by most members of the MFG. (The MFG model has been described elsewhere[8]; a detailed treatment manual is available on request.)

PSYCHOEDUCATIONAL SFT

As in the MFG modality, SFT began with at least three engagement sessions, involving one clinician and the patient's family members. Then, the Survival Skills Workshop was presented by the family clinician to the members of an individual family, without the patient present, using the same content and informational videotape as in the MFGs. Two weeks later, the patient and his or her family began to meet biweekly with a single therapist. The overall treatment was similar to that in MFGs, except that education was more individualized and the therapist was somewhat more involved in working out and following up problem solutions. The clinicians did not arrange contact between their study families to allow a comparison of psychoeducation with and without clinician-aided interfamily social support. Whenever appropriate, clinicians in both modalities emphasized enlarging and reactivating the family's natural social network.

FAMILY CLINICIAN TRAINING AND SUPERVISION

To establish a common orientation, each family clinician read the relevant treatment manual(s) and was trained by the principal investigator, study clinical supervisors, and Carol Anderson, PhD, of the University of Pittsburgh (Pa). Thereafter, training and fidelity control consisted of systematic review of videotapes by the study supervisors of (1) all family-engagement sessions, (2) every MFG meeting, and (3) every other SFT session throughout the study period. Supervision occurred weekly via telephone consultation, augmented by live, on-site supervision every 3 months. Clinicians were not required to meet competency criteria before beginning treatment, although supervision was especially intense during the initial phases of each clinician's early cases. The 24 clinicians, four at each site, assigned themselves to the respective modalities on the basis of personal interest to minimize the effects of bias on motivation.

MEDICATION

The design called for a standard-dose strategy for antipsychotic medication. The study psychiatrist at each site adjusted maintenance dosages after index hospital discharge to the lowest dose that controlled psychotic symptoms and agitation; there was no major effort to reduce dosages below that level. The goal was to achieve as high a level of compliance as possible with a standard-dosage regimen. For that reason, injectable preparations were used extensively in instances of poor compliance. The study psychiatrists were masked to the treatment assignment of the patients.

ANCILLARY TREATMENTS

By protocol, patients in the study could not receive any intensive outpatient individual or family psychotherapy. Other treatments, including day hospital admissions and vocational or recreational therapies, were allowed. The clinicians routinely coordinated treatment plans with the staff of these programs. There were no differences between modalities in the number or type of these interventions; each type had relatively low frequencies.

MEASURES

The primary outcome variables were rates of relapse and rehospitalization, positive and negative symptoms, medication dosage and compliance, and patient employment. Scales were drawn from existing instruments; some were selected to foster comparison with other studies of this type, especially the National Institute of Mental Health Treatment Strategies in Schizophrenia Study.[9]

DIAGNOSIS

The Psychotic Disorders version of the Structured Clinical Interview for *DSM-III-R* (SCID-PD)[27] was completed during the index admission by the site psychiatrists, who were trained to administer the SCID-PD and tested for reliability by the staff of the Biometrics Division at New York State Psychiatric Institute. The SCID-PD was also used to measure substance abuse.

RELAPSE ASSESSMENT

Patients were considered at risk for relapse for 2 years after they were discharged from the index hospital admission. Our intent was to make the relapse assessment procedure as sensitive as possible to alterations in clinical status. Using a method developed by Kane et al[28] for assessing drug treatment effects, we defined relapse as the reemergence of frank psychotic symptoms, whether or not the episode required rehospitalization. Brief Psychiatric Rating Scale (BPRS)[29] criteria were used: a rating of 5 or higher for unusual thought content, or 6 or higher for conceptual disorganization or hallucinatory behavior, or 7 for suspiciousness. However, if a patient had ongoing symptoms that met these criteria when stabilized, relapse was defined as a two-point summed increase across any of these four items. Patients were deemed to have relapsed if they met either set of criteria for any duration, providing a conservative and sensitive assessment.

The members of the clinical team of each project site, regular clinical staff, families, patients themselves, and ancillary treating staff were charged with bringing a suspected relapse to the attention of the on-site project director. Independent field raters, masked to treatment condition, then performed an immediate assessment. This procedure was repeated every 3 or 4 days up to 2 weeks (ie, for a maximum of four ratings) or until the patient no longer met criteria.

HOSPITALIZATION

Hospitalization is a complex event, often occurring in response to medication noncompliance, family stress, and substance abuse, as well as psychosis. Nevertheless, we are reporting data on hospital admissions because hospitalization is of such great economic importance and because it is the only means in this study of comparing the effects of family psychoeducation to standard treatment. Rehospitalizations are reported as the mean per-patient rate of all admissions occurring in the sample during each of eight consecutive 6-month periods, 2 years before and after study entry. Those data create a mirror-image, quasi-experimental comparison spanning 4 years. Hospitalizations occurring before the index admission were compiled from the medical record and patient and family interviews. Previous admissions may be underestimated; the index admission is not included.

POSITIVE AND NEGATIVE SYMPTOMS

Positive and negative symptoms were measured at index hospital admission, at discharge from index hospital admission, and at 1 year and 2 years after initiation of treatment. The BPRS was used to assess positive symptoms of schizophrenia, while negative symptoms were assessed using the Schedule for the Assessment of Negative Symptoms.[30] Raters in pairs independently evaluated a minimum of five patients to determine interrater reliability,

Continued on next page

achieving .71 mean per item intraclass correlation across both scales.

MEDICATION COMPLIANCE

At 12 and 24 months after initiation of treatment, the treating psychiatrist assessed medication compliance during the previous 6 months based on all available sources of information. Compliance was reported on a six-point ordinal scale, with 1 indicating noncompliant; 2, 25% compliant; 3, 50% compliant; 4, 75% compliant; 5, 90% compliant; and 6, 100% compliant. Compliance was measured globally, as a percentage of the total prescribed drug dosage actually taken. Thus, a 50% rating could reflect any pattern of compliance that led to consumption of 50% of the total prescribed dosage. Blood levels were not measured routinely.

STATISTICAL ANALYSIS

We used a form of survival analysis, the Cox Proportional Hazards Model,[31] to test our major hypotheses. The main advantage of this technique is that it takes into account information concerning the time to relapse. Specifically, it compares the sequencing of relapses. Moreover, given that patients are often unavailable for follow-up before the end of a study, this approach can accommodate variable periods of observation for different patients. Patients who dropped out are only censored from the relapse survival analysis after the point of dropout. The procedure allowed us to examine the influence of SFT vs MFG treatment on relapse while controlling for other variables.[32] Moreover, a simple transformation of the regression coefficients (the antilog) from the Cox regression model defines the risk of relapse that can be attributed to a one-unit change in the independent variable. The assumption of proportional hazards was not violated. Standard statistical procedures, especially Student's t tests, χ^2 tests, and analysis of variance, were used to test other hypotheses and to check the similarity of the two cohorts following randomization.

Table 1. Sociodemographic Characteristics of Patients in FPSP by Therapy Mode*

Variable	MFG	SFT	Total
No. of cases	83	89	**172**
Mean (SD) age, y†	26.5 (5.8)	28.1 (6.0)	27.3 (6.0)
Sex			
F	26.5	27.0	26.7
M	73.5	73.0	73.3
Race			
White	51.8	53.9	52.9
African American	43.4	38.2	40.7
Hispanic American	3.6	5.6	4.7
Asian American	1.2	2.2	1.7
Marital status‡			
Never married	91.6	83.1	87.2
Separated, divorced, widowed	8.4	14.6	11.7
Married	0.0	2.2	1.2
Education			
Pre–high school dropout	13.2	10.1	11.6
Some high school	18.1	22.5	20.3
High school graduate	36.1	30.3	33.1
Some college	27.7	27.0	27.3
College graduate	4.8	7.8	6.4
Missing data	0.0	2.2	1.2
Employment‡			
Competitive employment	13.2	14.6	14.0
Sheltered employment	1.2	2.2	1.7
Unemployed	80.7	75.3	77.9
Other	3.6	3.4	3.5
Missing data	1.2	4.5	2.9
Residence‡			
With family	83.1	82.0	82.6
Without family, supervised§	4.8	10.1	7.6
Without family, unsupervised	12.0	7.8	9.9
Substance abuse‡			
No history of abuse	59.0	67.4	63.4
History of abuse	41.0	32.6	36.6
Diagnosis			
Schizophrenia	80.7	87.6	84.3
Schizoaffective disorder	14.5	9.0	11.6
Schizophreniform disorder	4.8	3.4	4.1
Mean (SD) age at onset of symptoms, y‖	18.7 (4.7)	20.2 (4.8)	19.5 (4.8)
Mean (SD) duration of index admission, d	68.0 (80.6)	66.4 (80.7)	67.2 (80.4)

**There are no significant differences between therapy modes for most variables. Values are percentages unless otherwise noted. FPSP indicates Family Psychoeducation in Schizophrenia Project; MFG, multiple-family group treatment; and SFT, single-family treatment.*

†$t(170)=1.73$, $P=.08$.

‡*Data reflect status during the 2 months before index admission.*

§*Refers to professional or paid supervision.*

‖$t(167)=2.00$, $P<.05$.

whether MFGs increase the effectiveness of psychoeducational intervention. In addition, it remained to be determined whether either approach is effective in ordinary clinical settings with regular staff[18,19] and whether MFGs are more cost-effective.

To address these questions, our present study—the New York State Family Psychoeducation in Schizophrenia Project—experimentally compared SFT and MFG psychoeducational treatment during a 2-year period at five state psychiatric hospitals and one city hospital. The study involved a large and representative sample. This design varied the key factors in MFG treatment, social network expansion and problem solving in a group format, allowing assessment of differences in relapse and other outcomes and delineation of interaction between treatment type and family and patient variables. The protocol included full specification of the test therapies in treatment manuals, extensive training, and close supervision of experienced clinicians at the field sites and multidimensional measurement of patient and family outcome. The main hypotheses were that (1) MFG treatment would yield lower relapse rates, levels of psychiatric symptoms, and functional disabilities than would SFT and (2) psychoeducational family intervention in either format would produce fewer rehospitalizations than previous standard treatment.

RESULTS

SYMPTOMATIC RELAPSE OUTCOME

Relapse outcome is reported in three forms: symptomatic, clinical, and total relapses. The symptomatic rates for

Table 2. Relapse Status by Treatment Modality*

	Total Sample		Medication-Compliant Patients Only		Treatment Completers Only	
	MFG	SFT	MFG	SFT	MFG	SFT
0-12 mo						
Full treatment, no relapse	59 (71)	57 (64)	50 (71)	51 (68)	51 (86)	46 (69)
Partial treatment, no relapse before dropout	11 (13)	7 (8)	10 (14)	5 (7)	...	...
Relapse	13 (16)	25 (28)	10 (14)	19 (25)	8 (14)	21 (31)
Total	**83 (100)**	**89 (100)**	**70 (99)**	**75 (100)**	**59 (100)**	**67 (100)**
0-24 mo						
Full treatment, no relapse	41 (49)	35 (39)	37 (53)	33 (44)	41 (70)	35 (52)
Partial treatment, no relapse before dropout	19 (23)	17 (19)	17 (24)	13 (17)	...	...
Relapse	23 (28)	37 (42)†	16 (23)	29 (39)‡	18 (30)	32 (48)§
Total	**83 (100)**	**89 (100)**	**70 (100)**	**75 (100)**	**59 (100)**	**67 (100)**

Values are number (percent). MFG indicates multiple-family group treatment; SFT, single-family treatment. All tests are two-tailed.
†*β=−.49, SE=.27,* P=.06.
‡*β=−.57, SE=.31,* P=.06.
§*β=−.57, SE=.27,* P=.05.

1 and 2 years, shown in **Table 2** and **Figure 1**, support our first hypothesis: of 172 eligible cases at risk, 23 patients (27.7%) of the MFG cohort experienced at least one relapse compared with 37 (41.6%) in SFT, ie, the MFG relapse rate was 67% of the SFT rate. Controlling for medication compliance (a significant predictor of relapse), SFT cases had a 60% higher risk of relapse than did MFG cases, but the result fell just short of statistical significance (model $\chi^2_{(1)}$=6.76; β=−.49, SE=.27, *P*=.06, two-tailed test). As expected, patients who did not comply with medication regimens were more than twice as likely to suffer relapse as were compliant patients (β=−.76, SE=.30, *P*<.01). Previous hospitalization frequency, substance abuse, diagnosis, and the patient's place of residence (with family vs other) did not predict relapse.

Positive symptoms at index discharge did not predict risk of relapse (β=.11, SE=.15, *P*=.46). However, as is evident in **Figure 2**, they markedly influenced relapse outcome in MFG treatment and SFT (interaction of treatment modality and positive symptoms: β=−.85, SE=.39, *P*<.05). For each one-point increase in the mean per-item score in the discharge BPRS, the risk of relapse increased by 39% in the SFT group, but, in stark contrast, *decreased* by 42% in MFGs. For those 96 patients discharged with essentially no positive symptoms (BPRS score ≤2), there was no difference in relapse rate (32.7% in MFGs vs 31.8% in SFT). However, for those 76 patients whose psychosis was only partially remitted during the index hospital admission (BPRS score, <2), the difference was marked: 19% in MFGs vs 51% in SFT; in MFGs, relapse was *less* likely in the more symptomatic subsample. In this subsample, assignment to an MFG conferred a relapse risk only 28% of that of SFT (β=−1.28, SE=.46, *P*<.01). This higher symptom subgroup substantially accounts for the difference in relapse outcomes between MFGs and SFT.

Relapse rates were significantly lower in MFGs when families and/or patients participated in the test treatment for 2 years ("treatment completers," Table 2): 31% in MFGs vs 48% in SFT (therapy modality: β=−.57, SE=.27, *P*<.05; medication compliance: β=−.87, SE=.30, *P*<.01). Differential outcomes were similar for fully medication-compliant cases (>50% compliance) but with lower absolute rates: 23% in MFGs vs 39% in SFT (β=−.57, SE=.31, *P*=.06) (medication compliant cases only, see Table 2). For the total sample, relapse rates were roughly the same in the first (24.6%) and second (22.5%) years. Relapse was less frequent in MFGs at five of the six sites. A nearly constant relapse rate for each modality meant that the difference in relapse rates between modalities increased over time.

CLINICAL RELAPSE

In other research studies of this type, patients were required to have met relapse criteria for a minimum length of time, often 1 or 2 weeks.[3,4] To allow comparisons between this study and others, we selected relapses that met our BPRS criterion for at least 7 consecutive days and, thereby, represented clinically significant episodes; 61.7% of all relapses met this higher severity criterion. The respective rates were 15.7% for MFGs and 26.8% for SFT, similar to the effect noted using the symptomatic criterion for relapse, although neither treatment modality nor medication compliance alone was statistically significant (therapy modality: β=−.58, SE=.35, *P*=.09; medication compliance: β=−.73, SE=.39, *P*=.06). The subsample whose psychosis did not fully remit during the index hospital admission (BPRS score, <2) had significantly fewer relapses if assigned to MFGs (13% vs 33% in SFT; therapy modality: β=−1.14, SE=.56, *P*<.05), yielding a risk of relapse 32% of that in SFT. A total of 70.5% of relapses required rehospitalization, with no significant differences between the two treatments.

TOTAL RELAPSES

We assessed all relapses occurring within the 2-year protocol to disclose late-arriving treatment effects in patients with early relapse as well as treatment failures. The MFG modality generated significantly fewer total relapse episodes (MFG vs SFT: 38 vs 60 episodes, or 0.46 vs 0.67 episode per sample patient) than SFT (therapy modality: β=−.42, SE=.22, *P*=.05; medication compliance: β=−.69, SE=.23, *P*<.01), by 31.3%. Once patients dropped out, we

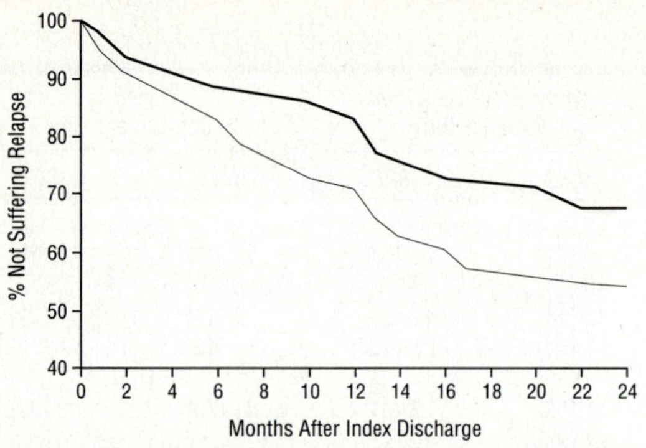

Figure 1. *Remission during a 2-year period in psychoeducational multiple-family groups and single-family treatment. Thin line indicates single-family treatment cohort (n=89); heavy line, multiple-family group cohort (n=83). For the multiple-family group cohort vs the single-family treatment cohort, β=−.49,* P<.06.

were no longer able to track them for relapse, so this analysis may underestimate the total number of relapses. Once relapse occurred, the risk of subsequent relapse in both modalities within the 2-year study interval was similar to, or higher than, the risk of having the first relapse. In the MFG modality, 10 (43.5%) of 23 patients who had one relapse had at least one other episode; in SFT, the comparable figures were 15 (40.5%) of 37, eliminating the modality difference. Of the total sample, 25 patients (14.5%) had more than one relapse and were considered treatment failures.

ATTRITION

In Table 2, the relapse rates of patients who did *not* suffer a relapse before dropping out are separated from those for treatment completers; patients who had a relapse before dropping out are included in the "relapse" section of the table. Twenty-four patients from the MFG cohort (29%) and 22 from the SFT cohort (25%) discontinued participation in the research protocol during the 2-year period. We were able to collect data on the reason for discontinuing treatment in 54% of the patients who dropped out. Only 11% of that subsample discontinued participation contrary to the recommendations of the clinicians. The relapse rate of the dropouts before discontinuing participation was similar to that of the completers ($\chi^2_{(1)}$=.34, *P*=.56).

HOSPITALIZATIONS

Before entering the protocol, patients who had at least one prior hospitalization (n=144) had experienced 4.2 admissions during a mean duration of illness of 5.4 years, or 1.3 mean admissions per year of illness, with a median of 0.83. This rate is higher than those reported in other family-intervention clinical studies of this type (eg, approximately 0.47 in the Hogarty et al[4] project). This constant rate suggested that the pretreatment condition was a valid control against which to compare family treatment effects.

Because there was no difference in hospitalization rates between therapy modalities, the hospitalization analysis compared pretreatment and in-treatment differences for all available study cases. **Figure 3** shows that the first-year in-treatment rate was essentially unchanged from the rate before admission into the study (F[1,114]=.15, *P*=.70). However, the second-year rate is significantly less than the pretreatment rate (F[1,114]=4.20, *P*<.05). Furthermore, the rate for the final 6 months of treatment was half that of the pretreatment rate and was significantly lower than that of the first 18 months of treatment (F[1,114]=6.00, *P*<.05). The proportion of patients who had at least one hospitalization was 36.0% for the first year, 24.4% for the second year (*t*[125]=1.26, *P*=.21), and 48.8% for the 2-year study period.

PSYCHIATRIC SYMPTOMS

The BPRS and the Schedule for the Assessment of Negative Symptoms ratings taken at index hospital admission and discharge and at the 2-year end point gave a more detailed picture of the course of illness than could relapse rates alone. We report mean per-item scores to facilitate interpretation of the results. (Scores range from 1.0 to 7.0, and an asymptomatic rating, ie, the normal range, is between 1.0 and 2.0.) Symptoms were analyzed with a series of multivariate analyses of variance, with therapy modality and site as the independent variables and the discharge BPRS rating as a covariate. Thirty-five patients who could not tolerate the initial rating procedure could not be included in the analysis.

Positive symptoms decreased 0.33 point during the 2-year study period (F[1,135]=25.74, *P*<.001). The MFG patients at the 2-year point had nearly significantly lower BPRS scores than did SFT patients (F[1,135]=2.98, *P*=.09). The relatively small decline in symptoms has much to do with the low levels measured at index discharge. However, the subsample of 22 patients who were discharged from the index admission while still noticeably symptomatic (BPRS score, <3.0; mean score, 3.59) showed significant improvement at 2 years, reaching a mean BPRS score of 1.83 (F[1,22]=136.73, *P*<.001), similar to the 1.74 score of the rest of the sample (*t*[166]=.77, *P*=.44).

Negative symptoms showed a similar pattern. Patients in the MFG cohort had fewer negative symptoms than did SFT patients at index discharge (F[1,171]=5.14, *P*<.05). During the 2-year period, negative symptoms in the SFT cohort improved, while the MFG cohort remained at the lower index discharge level throughout the study, with the result that the scores in the two modalities were identical at 2 years (2.12 for both modalities) and that negative symptoms for the total sample demonstrated a trend toward improvement (F[1,145]=2.88, *P*<.09).

MEDICATION DOSAGE AND COMPLIANCE

Dosage levels were followed up at 6-month intervals, with use of data recorded by the study psychiatrists and converted to mean chlorpromazine equivalents. At index discharge, the mean chlorpromazine equivalent was 850 mg (SD=902 mg) for the MFG cohort and 751 mg (SD=711 mg) for the SFT cohort (*t*[163]=.75, *P*=.46). Among treatment completers, mean MFG dosage during the 2-year period decreased by 194 to 656 mg, while the SFT dosage increased by 124 to 875 mg (MFG vs SFT, using mean dosages at 2 years: *t*[140]=1.54, *P*=.12). There were no significant changes in medication compliance over time (F[1,116]=0.56, *P*=.46) and no treatment modality effect (F[1,116]=2.05, *P*=.16). Compliance was maintained at a high level for 2 years: MFG

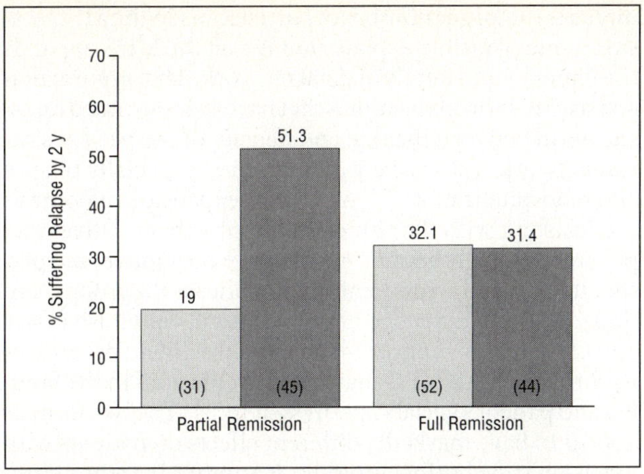

Figure 2. *Interactions of positive symptoms and treatment modality: effects on relapse. Light shaded bars indicate multiple-family group cohort; dark shaded bars, single-family treatment cohort (β=−.85,* P*<.05). Partial remission is indicated by a Brief Psychiatric Rating Scale score higher than 2 at discharge; full remission, a Brief Psychiatric Rating Scale score of 2 or lower at discharge. Numbers in parentheses indicate numbers in subsample.*

patients reached a compliance rate higher than 90%, and none of the patients who completed 2 years of treatment was totally noncompliant with medication. These levels of compliance compare favorably with those reported in the drug maintenance literature, in which there is a noncompliance range of 10% to 76%, with a median of about 46%.[33]

EMPLOYMENT OUTCOME

An important goal for patients in family psychoeducation is to be increasingly able to pursue normal activities, especially those related to employment, by experiencing long periods of remission and reduced family stress. Work became one of the prime targets of clinical effort during the second year of treatment, once clinical stability was achieved.

Employment data were collected with use of a dichotomous scale—either "unemployed" or "engaged in work-related activities"—for the 2 months preceding the index admission and at the 1- and 2-year follow-up visits. Data for 139 patients were available for analysis. Although the analyzed data were similar to the missing data on both negative and positive baseline symptom scales, the results must be interpreted cautiously.

There were no differences in level of work-related activity between therapy modalities for the 2 months before index admission (16% for the MFG cohort vs 21% for the SFT cohort; $F[1,127]=0.41$, $P=.52$) or at the 2-year point (34% for the MFG cohort vs 28% for the SFT cohort; $F[1,127]=1.82$, $P=.18$). However, there was significant improvement over time ($F[1,127]=12.23$, $P<.01$) in the total sample and a trend toward an interaction effect of therapy modality and time (18% increase in the MFG cohort vs 7% increase in the SFT cohort; $F[1,127]=3.08$, $P=.08$) favoring the MFG cohort.

COST-EFFECTIVENESS

The lower relapse rates in the MFG cohort are promising in view of the lower potential cost of that format. The MFG approach is designed to require exactly one half the staff time per patient compared with the SFT format: 1 hour per month per patient for MFG compared with 2 hours for SFT. In New York State, it costs about $240 per year per patient in direct staff salary (at $20/h) to conduct a psychoeducational MFG. Arbitrarily assuming a $350/d cost for inpatient hospitalization and comparing the rehospitalization rates during the prestudy to the 18- to 24-month study periods, we derived a 1:34 cost-benefit ratio for MFG and a 1:17 cost-benefit ratio for SFT ([0.34−0.17 hospitalization per patient per 6 months] × [68.5 mean days per admission × $350]/$120=34). Note that this represents only a rough estimate of costs because it does not include costs for ancillary treatments and costs to family and compares the most favorable period within the study interval.

COMMENT

The principal finding of our study was that psychoeducational MFG treatment extended remission and enhanced functioning more effectively than its SFT counterpart. The MFG advantage occurs most dramatically among patients with higher levels of psychiatric symptoms at the time of hospital discharge. Moreover, the benefit derived from the MFG appears to increase with time across three measures of relapse: symptomatic, clinically significant, and total relapses. This observation replicates an earlier study in which we found that relapse rates diverged in a similar pattern during a longer 4-year period.[10] The MFG cohort consistently demonstrated trends toward greater positive symptom reduction, medication compliance, dosage reduction, and employment. Because these trends are in different outcome domains, it seems unlikely that they are solely chance findings.[34]

The finding that MFGs induce a lower rate of relapse than does SFT psychoeducation is validated by comparison with aspects of the study reported by Hogarty et al.[5] First, our SFT modality yielded the same clinically significant 2-year relapse rate (27%) that was observed by Hogarty et al (29%) in a large, diverse, and clinically and demographically representative sample. That finding established a valid standard against which to compare MFG outcome. Second, the findings of Hogarty et al appear to be replicable by the permanent clinical staff of six different public outpatient clinics. That conclusion supports the feasibility of using these treatments in the settings where they are most likely to be needed and negates the assumption that these outcomes are the result of the skills of exceptional therapists. Third, unlike previous family intervention trials, this is a multisite study in which the lower relapse rate of the MFG cohort was replicated at five of the six sites. Fourth, the relapse findings are validated by the rehospitalization rates, which, when compared with the sample's high prior hospitalization rate, decreased dramatically in both modalities during the second year of the intervention. Fifth, at least 36% of the patients began the study with a documented history of moderate to heavy substance abuse. Finally, there was no sample selection based on medication compliance or stabilization, as required in comparable studies.[3,4,9] These characteristics describe a sample that entered the study with greater, and perhaps more typical, morbidity, which may explain the modest vocational outcomes.

We are able to describe subsamples that responded differentially to the two formats. The MFGs were markedly

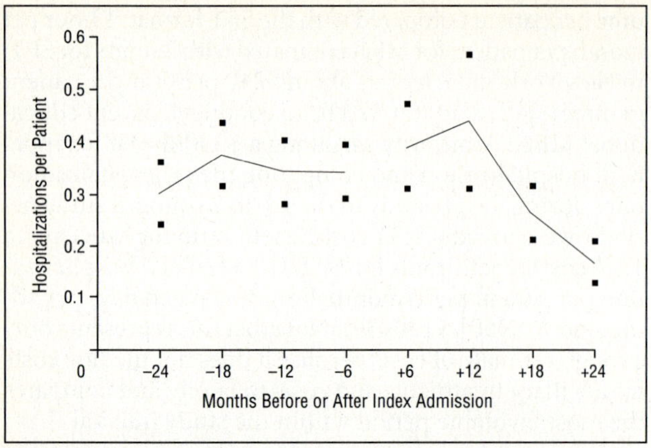

Figure 3. *Pretreatment and in-treatment rehospitalizations for the total sample. Differences between the multiple-family group cohort and the single-family treatment cohort were not statistically significant. Points represent hospitalizations per patient and SDs, in the previous 6 months, counting from the index admission. For the 2-year pretreatment period vs the second in-treatment year,* $P<.05$*; for the first 18 in-treatment months vs the last 6 in-treatment months,* $P<.05$.

more effective in the subsample with persistent psychotic symptoms. Also, MFGs performed significantly better under conditions of full compliance with either pharmacologic or family treatment. In the noncompliant group, there was no outcome differential between family treatment types. The condition of full compliance is the most appropriate test within a comparative design, eliminating the confounding effects of inadequate drug treatment and dropping out.

The fact that patients who were discharged with relatively high ratings of psychotic symptoms showed improvement during the course of the study suggests that there is a long-term symptom-stabilizing effect for family intervention. This finding is consistent with that in the study by Falloon et al[3]: in their study, symptoms in the family-management cohort remitted early and tended to decrease progressively, unlike outcome in the non–family-management comparison group. The finding that symptomatic patients responded to MFGs markedly better than to SFT suggests that the specific treatment effect of the MFGs will be especially valuable in managed settings where brief hospital stays and more severe discharge symptoms are the rule.

In any study involving so many clinicians, bias may be responsible for some of the main effects. In this study, the clinicians were aware of the comparative design. However, clinicians chose which modality they preferred to use and received the same amount of supervision. The supervisors' assessment was that the clinicians demonstrated equal skill and enthusiasm for their chosen treatment modality. There was no confounding of results by clinicians' or raters' awareness of interim outcome. A direct test of the independent raters' knowledge of cohort assignment at study completion confirmed that they had remained masked throughout the study. In short, the available indexes do not suggest that bias was a significant influence.

INTERVENING PROCESSES

What are the intervening processes that might account for the differences in outcome between MFG and SFT treatments? Because the fundamental difference between treatments is the larger number of participants in the MFG sessions, one plausible explanation is that the MFG expands the patient's and family's social network. That argument is consistent with other studies that have demonstrated an association between the size and density of the patient's social network and a variety of outcomes, especially relapse and rehospitalization.[35-40] A network expansion hypothesis is consistent with the clinicians' reports that relatives and patients gradually became more open, cooperative, and personally involved across family boundaries as the groups continued to meet. Extended networks usually diminish in size and capacity for support as the patient's illness progresses to chronicity. An MFG may fill a specific void in the family's and patient's social support system.[40,41] The two formats appear to have markedly different effects on patients with persistent psychotic symptoms. It appeared to many clinicians that the MFGs absorbed anxiety and stress generated by psychotic symptoms in a given family's midst. Conversely, the same level of symptoms in an SFT session tended to generate more family tension than the clinician and an already-stressed family could dissipate with available techniques.

Three other theories may explain the MFG therapeutic effect. They include expanded problem-solving capacity, effects on the emotional overinvolvement component of expressed emotion, and the positive emotional tone that characterizes most MFGs. For instance, MFGs generate a greater variety of alternatives during problem solving than occurs in SFT. Also, we have consistently observed that overinvolved families become more functional as they develop relationships with members of the other families in MFGs, which are usually characterized by more humor and warmth than SFT sessions. It is presently unclear how these network effects might operate, whether via the patient, family, or both. A parsimonious explanation for MFG efficacy will require sophisticated research because several of the explanations are consistent with one another and may operate simultaneously.[42]

DIFFERENCES OF OUTCOME WITH OTHER FAMILY INTERVENTION STUDIES

The most important comparisons with this study are to be made with those of Leff et al[7] and Hogarty et al.[5] Leff and his colleagues in London, England, did not observe a difference between a relatives group and home-based single-family behavioral management[7]; 2-year relapse rates were 33% and 36%, respectively. The relatives groups experienced a 50% nonengagement and dropout rate. However, the psychoeducational MFGs differed from the British relatives group approach in several ways: patients in MFGs attended meetings, there were at least three separate single-family and single-patient engagement sessions before the MFG commenced, and the group leaders were also the primary therapists for the patients. We believe that these clinical features account for the lower family dropout rate and lower patient relapse rates observed herein. Patients, in our experience, need to attend the MFG to benefit from its social rehabilitation effects and participation in constructing illness-management strategies.

In the SFT study by Hogarty et al,[5] relapse rates *increased* during the second year. This was attributed to the impending termination of the family clinician's involvement. In the study reported herein, we found *decreasing* rates. However, this protocol offered the same treatment in the same clinic with the same therapist after the data collection period ended. The difference in outcomes is best attributed to the promise and reality of continuity of care after the study.

CONCLUSION

In two studies with a total sample of more than 200 patients and at six of seven sites, the MFG has consistently yielded lower morbidity than SFT psychoeducation.[10] Indeed, patients with more severe and persistent positive symptoms and poor response to medication were specifically protected from relapse by MFGs, experiencing a 7% per year clinical relapse rate. Eighty-five percent of all cases experienced substantial reduction in the risk for relapse. This study, with its naturalistic sample, settings, and staff, demonstrates that family psychoeducational intervention is widely indicated and feasible and that there are substantial cost-effectiveness advantages for single-family[43] and, to a greater degree, multiple-family intervention. The unusually consistent evidence for the efficacy and feasibility of family intervention in schizophrenia[1-10] has now demonstrated an effect, in medicated patients, equivalent to antipsychotic medication itself. We propose that empiric experience confirms a biosocial treatment paradigm that obligates clinicians to train, support, and expand the patient's immediate social network.

Accepted for publication March 9, 1995.

The authors are grateful to the entire staff of the Family Psychoeducation in Schizophrenia Project for their unflagging assistance and support. Special recognition goes to the project directors at each site: Norman Ackerman, MD, Kathryn Alexander, MSW, Linda Breslin, MSW, Carolyn Crummey, PhD, Terry Holbrook, MSW, Stella Hughes, MSW, Gene Kaplan, MSW, Katharine Kelly, RN, Susan Kurtz, MSW, Henry McCurtis, MD, Joan Nachtman, RN, Janice Oursler, PhD, James Regan, PhD, and Susan Schiff, MSW. The authors extend special appreciation to Elmer Struening, PhD, for his scientific and organizational support and assistance in editing the manuscript. Finally, we are deeply indebted to the New York State Office of Mental Health and the New York State Alliance for the Mentally Ill for their vision, commitment, and generous funding support.

Reprint requests to Maine Medical Center, 22 Bramhall St, Portland, ME 04102 (Dr McFarlane).

REFERENCES

1. Goldstein MJ, Rodnick E, Evans J, May P, Steinberg M. Drug and family therapy in the aftercare of acute schizophrenics. *Arch Gen Psychiatry.* 1978;35:1169-1177.
2. Leff JP, Kuipers L, Berkowitz R, Sturgeon D. A controlled trial of social intervention in the families of schizophrenic patients: two year follow-up. *Br J Psychiatry.* 1984;146:594-600.
3. Falloon I, Boyd J, McGill C, Williamson M, Razani J, Moss HB, Gilderman AM, Simpson GM. Family management in the prevention of morbidity of schizophrenia. *Arch Gen Psychiatry.* 1985;42:887-896.
4. Hogarty GE, Anderson CM, Reiss DJ, Kornblith SJ, Greenwald DP, Javna CD, Madonia MJ. Family psychoeducation, social skills training and maintenance chemotherapy in the aftercare treatment of schizophrenia. *Arch Gen Psychiatry.* 1986;43:633-642.
5. Hogarty GE, Anderson CM, Reiss DJ, Kornblith SJ, Greenwald DP, Ulrich RF, Carter M, EPICS Research Group. Family psychoeducation, social skills training, and maintenance chemotherapy in the aftercare treatment of schizophrenia, II: two-year effects of a controlled study on relapse and adjustment. *Arch Gen Psychiatry.* 1991;48:340-347.
6. Tarrier N, Barrowclough C, Vaughn C, Bamrah JS, Porceddu K, Watts S, Freeman H. Community management of schizophrenia: a two-year follow-up of a behavioral intervention with families. *Br J Psychiatry.* 1989;154:625-628.
7. Leff J, Berkowitz R, Shavit N, Strachan A, Glass I, Vaughn C. A trial of family therapy v a relatives group for schizophrenia. *Br J Psychiatry.* 1989;154:58-66.
8. McFarlane WR. Multiple family groups in the treatment of schizophrenia. In: Nasrallah HA, ed. *Handbook of Schizophrenia.* Amsterdam, the Netherlands: Elsevier; 1990;4:167-189.
9. Schooler NR, Keith SJ, Severe JB, Matthews S. Acute treatment response and short-term outcome in schizophrenia: first results of the NIMH Treatment Strategies in Schizophrenia Study: Treatment Strategies in Schizophrenia Collaborative Study Group. *Psychopharmacol Bull.* 1989;25:331-335.
10. McFarlane WR, Link B, Dushay R, Marchal J, Crilly J. The multiple family group and psychoeducation in the treatment of schizophrenia: four year outcome in a small sample. *Fam Process.* 1995;34:127-144.
11. Laqueur HP. Mechanisms of change in multiple family therapy. In: Sager CJ, Kaplan HS, eds. *Progress in Group and Family Therapy.* New York, NY: Brunner/Mazel; 1972.
12. Detre T, Sayer J, Norton A, Lewis H. An experimental approach to the treatment of the acutely ill psychiatric patient in the general hospital. *Conn Med.* 1961;25:613-619.
13. Beels CC. Family and social management of schizophrenia. *Schizophr Bull.* 1975; 13:97-118.
14. Berman KK. Multiple family therapy: its possibilities in preventing readmission. *Ment Hygiene.* 1966;50:367-370.
15. Lansky MR, Bley CR, McVey GG, Botram B. Multiple family groups as aftercare. *Int J Group Psychother.* 1978;29:211-224.
16. Levin EC. Therapeutic multiple family groups. *Int J Group Psychother.* 1966; 19:203-208.
17. Lurie A, Ron H. Socialization program as part of after-care planning. *Gen Psychiatr Assoc J.* 1972;17:157-162.
18. Braun P. Deinstitutionalization of psychiatric patients: a critical review of outcome studies. *Am J Psychiatry.* 1981;138:736-749.
19. Bachrach LL. Assessment of outcomes in community support systems: results, problems and limitations. *Schizophr Bull.* 1982;8:41-60.
20. American Psychiatric Association. *Diagnostic and Statistical Manual of Mental Disorders, Revised Third Edition.* Washington, DC: American Psychiatric Association; 1987.
21. Regier DA, Farmer ME, Rae DS, Locke BZ, Keith SJ, Judd LL, Goodwin FK. Comorbidity of mental disorders with alcohol and other drug abuse: results from the Epidemiologic Catchment Area (ECA) Study. *JAMA.* 1990;264:2511-2518.
22. Leff J, Vaughn C. The interaction of life events and relatives' expressed emotion in schizophrenia and depressive neurosis. *Br J Psychiatry.* 1980;136:146-153.
23. Herz M. Recognizing and preventing relapse in patients with schizophrenia. *Hosp Community Psychiatry.* 1984;35:344-349.
24. Falloon IRH, Liberman R. Behavioral family interventions in the management of chronic schizophrenia. In: McFarlane WR, ed. *Family Therapy in Schizophrenia.* New York, NY: Guilford Press; 1983:141-172.
25. Anderson C, Hogarty G, Reiss D. *Schizophrenia and the Family.* New York, NY: Guilford Press; 1986.
26. Falloon I, Boyd J, McGill C. *Family Care of Schizophrenia.* New York, NY: Guilford Press; 1984.
27. Spitzer RL, Williams JBW, Gibbon M, Burke J, Keith SJ, Schooler N. *Structured Clinical Interview for* DSM-III, *Psychotic Disorders Version (SCID-PD, 3/1/85).* New York, NY: Biometric Research Dept, New York State Psychiatric Institute; 1985.
28. Kane J, Rifkin A, Woerner M. Low-dose neuroleptic treatment of outpatient schizophrenics. *Arch Gen Psychiatry.* 1983;40:893-900.
29. Overall J, Gorham D. The Brief Psychiatric Rating Scale. *Psychol Rep.* 1962; 10:799-812.
30. Andreasen N. *Scale for the Assessment of Negative Symptoms (SANS).* Iowa City: University of Iowa; 1981.
31. Cox DR. Regression models and life tables. *J R Stat Soc B.* 1972;34:187-202.
32. Allison P. *Event History Analysis: Regression for Longitudinal Event Data.* Beverly Hills, Calif: Sage Publications; 1984.
33. Young JL, Zonana HV, Shepler L. Medication noncompliance in schizophrenia: codification and update. *Bull Am Acad Psychiatry Law.* 1986;14:105-122.
34. Cohen J. Things I have learned (so far). *Am Psychol.* 1990;45:1304-1312.
35. Hammer M. Social supports, social networks, and schizophrenia. *Schizophr Bull.* 1981;7:45-57.
36. Garrison V. Support systems of schizophrenic and non-schizophrenic Puerto Rican women in New York City. *Schizophr Bull.* 1978;4:561-596.
37. Dozier M, Harris M, Bergman H. Social network and rehospitalization among young adult patients. *Hosp Community Psychiatry.* 1987;38:61-64.
38. Anderson C, Hogarty G, Bayer T. Expressed emotion and social networks of parents of schizophrenic patients. *Br J Psychiatry.* 1984;144:247-255.
39. Lipton F, Cohen C, Fischer E. Schizophrenia: a network crisis. *Schizophr Bull.* 1981;7:144-151.
40. Pattison E, Llama R, Hurd G. Social network mediation of anxiety. *Psychiatr Ann.* 1979;9:56-67.
41. Granovetter M. The strength of weak ties. *Am J Sociol.* 1973;78:1360-1380.
42. Reiss D, Costell R. The multiple family group as a small society: family regulation of interaction with nonmembers. *Am J Psychiatry.* 1977;134:21-32.
43. Falloon IRH. *Family Management of Mental Illness: A Study of Clinical Social and Family Benefits.* Baltimore, Md: The Johns Hopkins University Press; 1984.

ORIGINAL ARTICLE

Is Hyperarousal Essential to Obsessive-compulsive Disorder?

Diminished Physiologic Flexibility, but Not Hyperarousal, Characterizes Patients With Obsessive-compulsive Disorder

Rudolf Hoehn-Saric, MD; Daniel R. McLeod, PhD; Pamela Hipsley

Objective: To examine the hypothesis that the pathologic features of obsessive-compulsive disorder (OCD) are facilitated by abnormal levels of arousal, we compared patients with OCD with controls on self-reports and psychophysiologic measures.

Methods: Twenty-three patients with OCD were compared with 21 controls on rating scales and on psychophysiologic measures (ie, heart interbeat interval, skin conductance, respiration, blood pressure, and electromyographic activity) during rest and during two psychologically stressful tasks.

Results: Patients rated themselves higher on psychic and somatic anxiety scales. Mean physiologic activities were not elevated at rest. During tasks, changes in electrodermal, cardiovascular (except blood pressure), and muscle activities were smaller in patients with OCD, indicating decreased physiologic flexibility.

Conclusions: Hyperarousal, measured peripherally, is not an essential pathologic feature of OCD. Decreased physiologic flexibility indicates an anxiety-related, but not OCD-specific, impairment of psychophysiologic reactivity to one's environment.

(Arch Gen Psychiatry. 1995;52:688-693)

Despite arguments by many investigators that obsessive-compulsive disorder (OCD) is not an anxiety disorder,[1] it is classified as such in *DSM-III-R*.[2] These reservations are based on the fact that the psychopathologic features of OCD differ substantially from those of other anxiety disorders and that in some patients obsessions and compulsions cause irritation or disgust rather than anxiety. Nevertheless, OCD generally is associated with heightened anxiety, and most researchers agree that anxiety plays an important contributory role in OCD; however, the nature of this role remains controversial. Learning theorists see obsessions as conditioned responses to anxiety-provoking stimuli and compulsions as mechanisms that reduce anxiety, at least temporarily.[3] There is some support for this theory. Stimuli that evoke obsessive thoughts increase subjective anxiety in conjunction with an increase in skin conductance levels, skin conductance fluctuation, and heart rate.[4,5] A trend for increased heart rate variability after exposure to a feared stimulus[6] could not be replicated in a different patient population.[7] On the other hand, giving in to obsessive thoughts by engaging in compulsions leads to a reversal of these manifestations, while attempts by the patient to control the compulsions increase anxiety.[5] Successful behavior therapy also tends to reduce subjective and physiologic responses to stimuli that evoke obsessions.[7]

Other investigators[8] have suggested that patients with OCD are in a state of abnormal arousal that facilitates sensitization, which in turn results in failure to adapt to unwanted thoughts. For these theories to be correct, heightened autonomic arousal should be observed in these patients, at least in response to stressful stimuli. Experimental evidence, however, is contradictory. Clinical observations have shown that higher levels of anxiety increase the severity of OCD,[9] while relaxation leads to the reduction of symptoms.[10] Many patients with OCD have generalized anxiety and some experience panic attacks, but a small number of patients

See Subjects and Methods on next page

From the Department of Psychiatry and Behavioral Sciences, The Johns Hopkins Medical Institutions, Baltimore, Md.

SUBJECTS AND METHODS

SUBJECTS

Two groups of subjects were compared. All subjects were between the ages of 18 and 65 years and were free of all centrally acting drugs for at least 2 weeks before entry into the study. In addition, results of routine laboratory tests and electrocardiographic findings had to be within normal limits. Subjects were diagnosed as having OCD according to *DSM-III-R*,[2] and symptoms had to be present for more than 1 year. To be included, patients with OCD also had to score at least 7 on the National Institute of Mental Health Global Obsessive-compulsive Scale,[21] at least 16 on the Yale-Brown Obsessive-compulsive Scale,[22] below 21 on the Hamilton Scale of Depression,[23] and below 3 on the Depressive Mood subscale of the Hamilton Scale of Depression.

Twenty-three subjects with OCD and 21 subjects with no psychiatric disorders participated in the study. Each group included 10 men. The OCD group included 13 women, and the control group included 11 women. The mean (±SD) ages were 35.5±9.6 years and 35.6±10.8 years for the control and OCD groups, respectively. The average (±SD) level of education was 15.0±2.4 years and 14.6±2.2 years for the control and OCD groups, respectively. The control group consisted of 11 whites, eight blacks, and two Asian Americans; the OCD group consisted of 22 whites and one Asian American.

PROCEDURE

During the initial visit, all subjects underwent psychiatric and physical examinations, electrocardiography, and routine laboratory tests. Patients with OCD were also assessed with the Yale-Brown Obsessive-compulsive Scale, the National Institute of Mental Health Global Obsessive-compulsive Scale, and the Hamilton Scale of Depression at this time. Their mean (±SD) scores on these scales were 26.9±3.4, 9.4±1.5, and 12.0±4.1, respectively. All subjects were then assessed with the Somatic Symptoms Scale,[24] the Marks-Sheehan Phobia Scale,[25] the Childhood Disturbance Scale,[26] the Eysenck Personality Inventory,[27] the Mastery-Powerlessness Scale,[28] the State-Trait Anxiety Inventory–Trait Scale,[29] and the Tridimensional Personality Questionnaire.[30] All subjects signed a consent form approved by the Joint Committee on Clinical Investigation before entry into the study.

Within 1 week of the initial visit, subjects underwent a psychophysiologic examination. They reported to the laboratory at 8:30 AM. After a rest period of 15 minutes (baseline 1), subjects were exposed to two stress tasks, each lasting 5 minutes (Divided Attention Task and Risk-Taking Task), followed by a 5-minute rest period (baseline 2). Following baseline 2, the OCD group was exposed to two 3-minute visualization periods. Results of the visualization periods before and after treatment were presented by Hoehn-Saric et al.[13] Physiologic measures were taken during the last 5 minutes of baseline and during each of the subsequent session segments. The Divided Attention and Risk-Taking tasks are nonspecific stress tasks, presented by means of a microcomputer (Apple IIe, Apple Computer Inc, Cupertino, Calif), and are described below. The following physiologic measures were taken: heart interbeat interval (IBI), heart IBI range, skin conductance, skin conductance range, skin conductance fluctuations, frontalis and gastrocnemius electromyographic (EMG) activity, and respiratory frequency. For each subject, IBI and skin conductance ranges were computed as the difference between the largest and smallest values obtained during each session segment. These ranges were used because we have found them to be sensitive measures of physiologic flexibility.[18,20] Interbeat interval artifacts were detected and removed as follows: each IBI that was less than 75% of the preceding IBI or greater than 137% of the preceding IBI was set equal to the preceding IBI (for the reasoning behind this procedure, see Cheung[31]). Blood pressure was measured at the end of baseline 1, Divided Attention, Risk-Taking Task, baseline 2, and visualization 2 by means of a commercial blood pressure monitor (Infrasonde, Puritan Bennet Co, Baltimore, Md). This monitor was operated from an adjoining room. Blood pressure was measured after, rather than during, the session segments so as not to interfere with the recording of other physiologic measures. Recordings were obtained while the subjects sat in a comfortable reclining chair in a dimly lit room. Details of the recording procedures have been described by McLeod et al.[32] Following the physiologic recording session, subjects were assessed by the following psychomotor tasks: the automated Digit Symbol Substitution Task[33] and automated versions of Digits Forward and Choice Reaction Time.[32]

STRESS TASKS

The stress tasks were chosen to examine physiologic changes resulting from stress induced by cognitive activity and stress resulting from decisions whose consequences can be either positive or negative. In the Divided Attention Task, subjects were asked to press the 0 key on a numeric keypad as quickly as possible when they detected a 0 in a stream of numbers presented on a video screen. In addition, they had to keep track of how many times a number higher than 5 followed the occurrence of 5. In the Risk-Taking Task, subjects pressed the 1 (left key) to earn points and the 3 (right key) to save points that were earned by pressing the 1 key. With P=.05, ie, with a probability of one time in 20, the left key presses could produce a red line, which meant that twice the number of points accumulated on that trial were subtracted from the subject's saved total. Thus, the greater the number of times a subject pressed the left key before pressing the right key, the higher the potential gain but the greater the potential loss should a left key press produce the red line. To assess risk, the number of left key presses before switching over and saving the trial points was measured, as was the variability (SD) in risk responses from trial to trial. Further details of these tasks have been described by McLeod et al.[32]

DATA ANALYSIS

Two-way analyses of variance (ANOVAs) with repeated measures were used to compare physiologic measures of the two subject groups across tasks. Student's t tests were used to compare the two subject groups on clinical ratings and psychomotor performance. Student's t tests were also used to compare groups during tasks when indicated by significant interactions in the ANOVA. Differences were considered significant if the probability of their occurring by change was less than .05. Relationships between changes in blood pressure and changes in other physiologic measures were assessed by means of Pearson Product-Moment Correlation Coefficients.

manifest little or no anxiety.[9] Insel et al[1] found that 12 of 30 patients with OCD also had generalized anxiety disorder, but they did not report how many patients complained of increased but subclinical anxiety. Mellett[11] reported that all 20 of his patients complained of "generalized tension," but only four experienced somatic symptoms. In previous studies, we have found that patients with OCD score high on scales describing anxiety symptoms.[12,13]

Several laboratory studies have failed to find evidence of autonomic hyperarousal in untreated patients with OCD, despite high levels of anxiety.[6,14,15] Other studies have reported higher levels of skin conductance[1] or heart rate[1,14,16] at rest as well as heightened physiologic reactivity to stressors.[1,4,8] Three studies,[3,8,17] but not a fourth,[1] reported that patients with OCD habituated more slowly than did controls. Also contradictory were reports of the effects of stressful mental activity on patients' physiologic measures. In one study, stressful mental activity attenuated spontaneous skin conductance fluctuations.[8] In another study, it increased skin conductance levels but lowered the heart rate.[1] We[13] found that clinical improvement with clomipramine hydrochloride treatment was independent of the physiologic state of the patients and was not associated with autonomic down-regulation. Thus, while anxiety frequently accompanies OCD, exacerbates its manifestations, or becomes activated by obsessions or the inability to engage in compulsions, it remains unclear whether and to what degree the psychopathologic features of OCD are caused or at least induced by heightened arousal. An alternative interpretation of findings reported in the literature is that OCD symptoms trigger anxiety and that clinically observable anxiety in patients with OCD is a consequence rather than the cause of OCD. If this is the case, we should find no evidence of hyperarousal in patients with OCD at times when they do not experience obsessions or compulsions.

Our aim was to examine the presence of generalized anxiety and physiologic hyperarousal in a group of patients who exhibited OCD according to *DSM-III-R* but had no other Axis I diagnoses, except generalized anxiety disorder or simple phobias. Based on our previous studies of patients with OCD[12,13] and of patients with generalized anxiety disorder,[18] we predicted that patients with OCD, uncomplicated by comorbid disorders other than generalized anxiety disorder or simple phobias, would differ physiologically from controls during resting periods only in muscle tension. In addition, because patients with generalized anxiety disorder,[18,19] as well as those with panic disorder,[20] react to non–disorder-specific stressors, such as laboratory tasks with diminished rather than exaggerated physiologic responsivity, we predicted that patients with OCD also would, under such conditions, exhibit decreased physiologic flexibility. A disorder-specific stressor is one that triggers a disorder-related response, eg, dirt would evoke a response in a person with a contamination phobia.

RESULTS

Table 1 presents differences between OCD and control groups on a variety of rating scales. The OCD group rated themselves higher on the Neuroticism subscale but not on the Extroversion subscale of the Eysenck Personality Inventory. They were more externally oriented on locus of control, as measured by the Mastery-Powerlessness Scale. They rated themselves as more anxious on the State-Trait Anxiety Inventory–Trait Scale and Somatic Symptoms Scale and rated themselves higher on all three subscales of the Marks-Sheehan Phobia Scale. The groups did not differ on the Childhood Disturbance Scale, but the patients with OCD rated themselves higher on the Harm Avoidance and Reward Dependence subscales of the Tridimensional Personality Questionnaire. No group differences were found on the Novelty subscale.

Table 1. Comparison of Clinical Ratings in Subjects With and Without Obsessive-compulsive Disorder (OCD)*

	OCD Group	Control Group	*t*	*P*†
EPI (Neuroticism subscale)	11.5 (6.1)	4.9 (2.8)	4.08	<.001
EPI (Extroversion subscale)	13.4 (5.8)	11.1 (4.0)	1.44	.16
Mastery-Powerlessness Scale	13.9 (3.4)	17.7 (2.6)	3.82	.001
STAI Trait Scale	56.9 (11.6)	31.3 (5.8)	9.04	<.001
Childhood Disturbance Scale	8.6 (4.9)	6.6 (6.1)	1.23	.23
Phobia (Fear)	48.2 (24.6)	16.8 (17.2)	4.60	<.001
Phobia (Avoid)	15.9 (8.4)	7.6 (7.3)	3.33	.004
Phobia (State)	5.7 (2.7)	0.8 (1.2)	7.20	<.001
Somatic Symptoms Scale	18.7 (10.4)	5.1 (5.4)	5.34	<.001
TPQ (Novelty subscale)	13.2 (4.5)	15.6 (3.8)	1.22	.23
TPQ (Harm Avoidance subscale)	21.0 (6.5)	7.7 (4.2)	4.98	<.001
TPQ (Reward Dependence subscale)	21.2 (3.9)	15.4 (4.8)	3.16	.008

**EPI indicates Eysenck Personality Inventory; STAI, State-Trait Anxiety Inventory; Phobia, Marks-Sheehan Phobia Scale; and TPQ, Tridimensional Personality Questionnaire. Values are means (SDs).*

†Significance was defined as P<.05.

Two-way ANOVAs (subject group×task, with repeated measures on tasks) were used to assess between-group differences in subjective and physiologic measures. The Greenhouse-Geisser correction[34] was used for repeated measures. As seen in the degrees of freedom, not all measures could be obtained for all subjects at all times. No main effects representing an overall group difference were found.

Baseline physiologic measures are presented in **Table 2**. Although there is a tendency for patients with OCD to show higher frontalis EMG activity and more frequent spontaneous fluctuations in skin conductance, these differences did not reach statistical significance.

Main effects for tasks were found in mean IBI ($F[3,123]=14.43$, $P<.001$), mean skin conductance ($F[3,126]=83.88$, $P<.001$), skin conductance range ($F[3,126]=17.09$, $P<.001$), skin conductance fluctuations per minute ($F[3,126]=10.41$, $P<.001$), frontalis EMG ($F[3,126]=7.88$, $P<.001$), systolic blood pressure ($F[3,126]=24.10$, $P<.001$), and diastolic blood pressure ($F[3,126]=11.20$, $P<.001$). In general, **Figure 1** through **Figure 3** show that the tasks tended to produce increases in skin conductance and blood pressure, along with decreases in heart IBI (increases in heart rate).

Significant subject group×task interactions were found for mean IBI ($F[3,123]=2.69$, $P<.05$), skin con-

Table 2. Comparison of Physiologic Measures in Subjects With and Without Obsessive-compulsive Disorder (OCD) During Initial Baseline Conditions*

	OCD Group	Control Group	t	P†
Mean IBI, ms	875.4 (132.0)	893.6 (133.6)	0.26	.79
Mean SC, microsiemens	3.2 (2.9)	2.7 (1.3)	0.71	.48
SC range, microsiemens	0.9 (1.3)	0.6 (0.9)	0.88	.38
SC fluctuations/min	1.3 (2.5)	0.1 (0.3)	1.90	.06
Systolic BP, mm Hg	109.4 (14.8)	109.9 (10.4)	0.46	.65
Diastolic BP, mm Hg	67.2 (12.6)	71.0 (7.9)	1.50	.14
Frontalis EMG, μV	9.4 (3.1)	7.7 (3.2)	1.82	.08
Gastrocnemius EMG, μV	3.2 (3.0)	4.0 (6.3)	0.14	.09

**IBI indicates heart interbeat interval; SC, skin conductance; fluctuations, spontaneous fluctuations in SC; BP, blood pressure; and EMG, electromyographic. Values are means (SDs).*

†Significance was defined as P<.05.

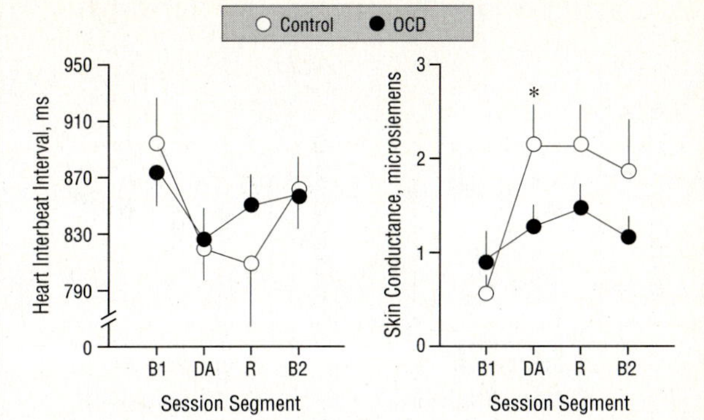

Figure 1. *Comparison of mean heart interbeat interval and skin conductance range in patients with obsessive-compulsive disorder and control subjects during initial baseline (B1), the Divided Attention Task (DA), the Risk-Taking Task (R), and second baseline (B2). Asterisk indicates that the obsessive-compulsive group differs from the control group at* P<.05.

ductance range (F[3,126]=5.63, *P*<.001), frontalis EMG (F[3,126]=5.88, *P*<.001), gastrocnemius EMG (F[3,111]=2.97, *P*<.04), systolic blood pressure (F[3,126]=3.63, *P*<.02), and diastolic blood pressure (F[3,126]=3.00, *P*<.03). Change scores reflecting differences between tasks and baseline were calculated, and group *t* tests were used to compare these change scores across subject groups.

As Figures 1 and 2 show, patients with OCD exhibited smaller changes in IBI, skin conductance range, frontalis EMG, and gastrocnemius EMG during the tasks. When performing the Divided Attention Task, patients with OCD showed smaller increases than did the healthy volunteers in skin conductance range (*t*=3.54, *P*<.001), frontalis EMG (*t*=2.09, *P*<.04), and gastrocnemius EMG (*t*=2.67, *P*<.01). When performing the Risk-Taking Task, patients with OCD showed smaller increases than did the healthy volunteers in heart rate (*t*=2.54, *P*<.02), skin conductance range (*t*=2.44, *P*<.02), frontalis EMG (*t*=2.09, *P*<.04), and gastrocnemius EMG (*t*=2.45, *P*<.02). On the other hand, blood pressure changes were greater in the patients with OCD immediately following the tasks (Figure 3). After performing the Risk-Taking Task, patients with OCD showed greater increases in both systolic (*t*=2.41, *P*<.02) and diastolic (*t*=3.47, *P*<.001) blood pressures. After performing the Divided Attention Task, no between-group differences in blood pressure were seen.

Blood pressure changes following the Risk-Taking Task were the only physiologic measure that was higher in patients with OCD compared with controls. To determine whether resting blood pressure was related to changes in other physiologic variables, correlations were calculated between absolute systolic and diastolic blood pressure values at baseline 1 and change scores for all physiologic measures from baseline 1 to each task and to baseline 2. Only the correlation between diastolic blood pressure at baseline 1 and the change scores of diastolic blood pressure from baseline 1 to the completion of the Divided Attention Task was significant (*r*=−.62, *P*>.001). Thus, the greater the diastolic blood pressure at rest, the smaller its change after completion of the task.

To determine whether changes in blood pressure were related to changes in other physiologic variables, correlations were calculated between changes from baseline 1 to each task and baseline 2 for all physiologic variables. Only changes in systolic blood pressure and IBI from baseline 1 to baseline 2 were significantly correlated (*r*=.43, *P*<.04). Thus, greater changes in blood pressure were associated with greater change in heart rate from the rest period before the tasks to the rest period after the tasks.

No between-group differences were noted in psychomotor performance.

COMMENT

Our study confirmed the presence of heightened anxiety in patients with OCD that had been noted in other studies.[1,11-13] In addition to higher ratings of psychic and somatic anxiety, patients with OCD also were more phobic. On personality scales, they rated themselves higher on neuroticism, harm avoidance, and reward dependency and had a more external locus of control than did the control subjects. However, they were not more introverted and did not differ from controls in novelty seeking or childhood disturbances. The ratings of the patients with OCD in our study resemble those previously obtained in nonimpulsive patients with OCD[12] and in patients with generalized anxiety disorder.[18,24] This finding may be attributed to the selection of patients with "pure" OCD who had no other Axis I disorders, except generalized anxiety disorder or simple phobias. The advantage of the strict selection criteria was that they permitted us to examine psychophysiologic variables of OCD without contamination by other disorders, such as major depression, panic attacks, or the presence of neurologic disorders, including tics and Tourette's syndrome.

Physiologically, patients with OCD did not differ from controls during resting conditions. As in other anxiety disorders,[35] stress tasks changed physiologic measures in the predicted direction by increasing blood pressure, heart rate, skin conductance, and muscle tension. The actual degree of changes, however, differed considerably not only between anxiety disorders but also between individuals and was poorly correlated between

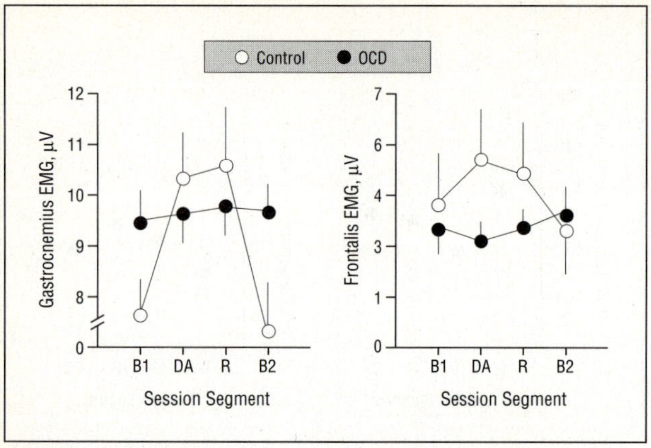

Figure 2. *Comparison of frontalis and gastrocnemius electromyographic (EMG) activity in patients with obsessive-compulsive disorder and control subjects during initial baseline (B1), the Divided Attention Task (DA), the Risk-Taking Task (R), and second baseline (B2). Values are given as means.*

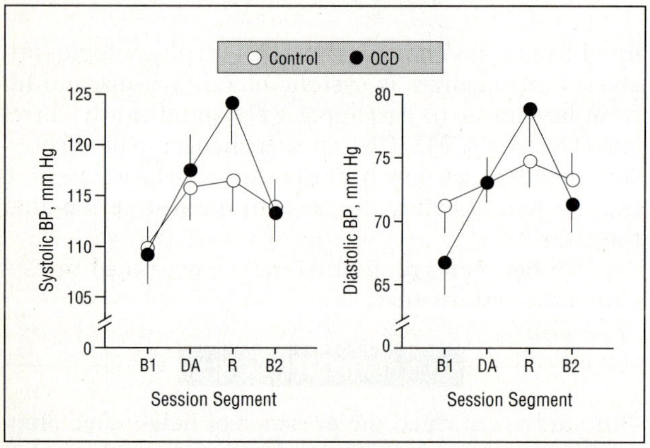

Figure 3. *Comparison of systolic and diastolic blood pressures (BPs) in patients with obsessive-compulsive disorder and control subjects during initial baseline (B1), the Divided Attention Task (DA), the Risk-Taking Task (R), and second baseline (B2).*

physiologic systems, such as between the cardiovascular and sudomotor systems. Unlike patients with generalized anxiety disorder,[18] patients with OCD did not differ from controls in EMG activity. However, like patients with generalized anxiety disorder and panic disorder, patients with OCD exhibited smaller changes in skin conductance range during both Divided Attention and Risk-Taking tasks. In addition, patients with OCD exhibited smaller changes in mean IBI, frontalis EMG, and gastrocnemius EMG during the tasks. Blood pressure changes following the tasks were greater in the patients with OCD. This was not the case for patients with generalized anxiety disorder[18] but was the case for patients with panic disorder.[20]

The psychophysiologic findings speak against the hyperarousal theory of OCD.[8] To the contrary, patients with OCD exhibited the same physiologic levels at rest and lower levels in response to stressors than did controls. Their response pattern to the laboratory-induced psychological stressors was similar to that observed in generalized anxiety disorder by us and other investigators[18,19] and by us in patients with panic disorder,[20] namely, a decreased physiologic flexibility. Decreased physiologic flexibility under stress has been demonstrated not only in autonomic measures but also in EMG[36] and electroencephalography[37] in patients with generalized anxiety disorder and in catecholamine excretion in persons with "poor" adjustment.[38] It is not disorder-specific but occurs in a variety of anxiety disorders and in conditions in which individuals feel stressed or worry excessively.[19,39] Diminished physiologic flexibility may be the consequence of diminished attention or the lack of emotional involvement in tasks that are unrelated to a person's disease. If this is the case, then the preoccupation of our patients with OCD with their inner world rather than with the tasks may be even more intense than that of patients with other anxiety disorders, as diminished physiologic flexibility was even more pronounced in our patients with OCD than in patients with other anxiety disorders. Decreased physiologic flexibility may also represent a constitutional bodily inadequacy in responding to stressors that predispose individuals to develop anxiety disorders.[40]

In the past, we have observed an increase in blood pressure at the end of task performance in patients with panic disorder. Increases in blood pressure following the Risk-Taking Task were also observed in these patients with OCD. While patients with panic disorder also exhibited higher heart rate and systolic blood pressure at rest, this was not the case in the patients with OCD. Moreover, correlations with other physiologic measures showed no relationship between higher initial blood pressure levels or greater blood pressure changes during tasks and changes in other physiologic measures. Thus, it is unlikely that a unitary sympathetic drive, occurring during the Risk-Taking Task, is responsible for the increase in blood pressure. Moreover, so as not to disturb other measures by the inflation of the cuff, blood pressure was measured at the end of and not during the tasks. Therefore, it may not accurately reflect the blood pressure levels during the tasks. Our findings may demonstrate a true increase in blood pressure during the task and a delayed habituation, a rebound effect after the task, or a chance finding. It also may demonstrate the independence of physiologic systems in their responses to stress. Therefore, studies examining blood pressure and other physiologic changes during a variety of laboratory stressors, including decision-making tasks, are indicated. We have only limited information on physiologic reactions of patients with OCD to obsessive thoughts and to attempts to control compulsions and how such reactions compare with reactions when patients face everyday stressors. Studies that involve the use of ambulatory monitors will help to clarify these questions.

In conclusion, patients with OCD do not exhibit hyperarousal on peripheral measures when at rest. Similar to patients with other anxiety disorders, patients with OCD react with less physiologic flexibility to non–disease-specific stressors. Thus, physiologic hyperarousal, as reflected by peripheral measures, may have little bearing on the psychopathologic features of OCD. Our findings do not diminish the importance of regional hyperactivity in the central nervous system that may not manifest itself in peripheral arousal. Using single photon emission computed tomography and positron emission tomography imaging techniques, we and other investigators (for reviews, see Hoehn-Saric and Benkelfat[41]) have demonstrated, in untreated patients with OCD, increased cerebral blood flow and glucose metabolism in prefrontal cerebral regions that diminished during successful treatment with fluoxetine hydrochloride or clomipramine hydrochloride. Thus, hyperactivity in patients with OCD may be limited largely to certain brain areas and extend to the peripheral autonomic system only during disorder-specific stress. Probably because of preoccupation with disorder-specific stressors, nonspecific stressors cause a decrease rather than an exaggeration of physiologic response.

Accepted for publication April 19, 1995.

This study was supported in part by grant MH42579-03 from the National Institute of Mental Health, Rockville, Md.

Reprint requests to the Department of Psychiatry and Behavioral Sciences, The Johns Hopkins Medical Institutions, 600 N Wolfe St/Meyer 144, Baltimore, MD 21287-7144 (Dr Hoehn-Saric).

REFERENCES

1. Insel TR, Zahn T, Murphy DL. Obsessive-compulsive disorder: an anxiety disorder? In: Tuma AT, Maser J, eds. *Anxiety and the Anxiety Disorders.* Hillsdale, NJ: Lawrence Erlbaum & Associates; 1985:577-589.
2. American Psychiatric Association. *Diagnostic and Statistical Manual of Mental Disorders, Revised Third Edition.* Washington, DC: American Psychiatric Association; 1987:245-247.
3. Carr A. Compulsive neurosis: a review of the literature. *Psychol Bull.* 1974; 81:311-318.
4. Boulougouris JC, Rabavilas AD, Stefanis C. Psychophysiological responses in obsessive-compulsive patients. *Behav Res Ther.* 1977;15:221-230.
5. Rabavilas A, Boulougouris J, Stefanis C. Synchrony and concordance on subjective and psychophysiological measures after beta-blockade and flooding in obsessive-compulsive patients. In: Boulougouris JC, Rabavilas AD, eds. *The Treatment of Phobic and Obsessive-compulsive Disorders.* Elmsford, NY: Pergamon Press Inc; 1977:115-125.
6. Hodgson RJ, Rachman S. The effects of contamination and washing in obsessional patients. *Behav Res Ther.* 1972;10:111-117.
7. Rachman SJ, Hodgson RJ. *Obsessions and Compulsions.* Englewood Cliffs, NJ: Prentice-Hall International Inc; 1980:235-249.
8. Beech HR, Liddell A. Decision-making, mood states and ritualistic behaviour among obsessional patients. In: Beech HR, ed. *Obsessional States.* London, England: Methuen & Co Ltd; 1974:143-160.
9. Marks I. *Fears, Phobias and Rituals.* New York, NY: Oxford University Press; 1987:281-322.
10. Leger LA. Spurious and actual improvement in the treatment of preoccupying thoughts by thought-stopping. *Br J Soc Psychol.* 1978;17:373-377.
11. Mellett PG. The clinical problem. In: Beech HR, ed. *Obsessional States.* London, England: Methuen & Co Ltd; 1974:55-94.
12. Hoehn-Saric R, Barksdale VC. Impulsiveness in obsessive-compulsive patients. *Br J Psychiatry.* 1983;143:177-182.
13. Hoehn-Saric R, McLeod DR, Zimmerli WD, Hipsley PA. Symptoms and physiologic manifestations in obsessive-compulsive patients before and after treatment with clomipramine. *J Clin Psychiatry.* 1993;54:272-276.
14. Benkelfat C, Mefford IN, Masters CF, Nordhal TE, King AC, Cohen RM, Murphy OL. Plasma catecholamines and their metabolites in obsessive-compulsive disorder. *Psychiatry Res.* 1991;37:321-331.
15. Hollander E, DeCaria C, Nitescu A, Cooper T, Stover B, Gully R, Klein DF, Liebowitz MR. Noradrenergic function in obsessive-compulsive disorder: behavioral and neuroendocrine responses to clonidine and comparison to healthy controls. *Psychiatry Res.* 1991;37:161-177.
16. Kelly D. *Anxiety and Emotions.* Springfield, Ill: Charles C Thomas Publisher; 1980:121-180.
17. Lelliott PT, Noshirvani HF, Marks IM, Monteiro WO, Basoglu M, Cohen SD. Relationship of skin conductance activity to clinical features in obsessive-compulsive ritualizers. *Psychol Med.* 1987;17:905-914.
18. Hoehn-Saric R, McLeod DR, Zimmerli WD. Somatic manifestations in women with generalized anxiety disorder. *Arch Gen Psychiatry.* 1989;46:1113-1119.
19. Roemer L, Borkovec TD. Worry: unwanted cognitive activity that controls unwanted somatic experience. In: Wegner DW, Pennebaker J, eds. *Handbook of Mental Control.* Englewood Cliffs, NJ: Prentice-Hall International Inc; 1993: 220-238.
20. Hoehn-Saric R, McLeod DR, Zimmerli WD. Psychophysiological response patterns in panic disorder. *Acta Psychiatr Scand.* 1991;83:4-11.
21. Zohar J, Insel TR, Zohar-Kadouch RC, Hill JL, Murphy DL. Serotonergic responsivity in obsessive-compulsive disorder: effects of chronic clomipramine treatment. *Arch Gen Psychiatry.* 1988;45:167-172.
22. Goodman WK, Price LH, Rasmussen SA, Mazure C, Fleischmann RL, Hill CL, Heninger GR, Charney DS. The Yale-Brown Obsessive-compulsive Scale. *Arch Gen Psychiatry.* 1989;46:1006-1016.
23. Hamilton M. A rating scale for depression. *J Neurol Neurosurg Psychiatry.* 1960;23:56-62.
24. Hoehn-Saric R. Characteristics of chronic anxiety patients. In: Klein DF, Rabkin J, eds. *Anxiety; New Research and Changing Concepts.* New York, NY: Raven Press; 1981:399-409.
25. Sheehan DV. *The Anxiety Disease and How to Overcome It.* New York, NY: Charles Scribner's Sons; 1984.
26. Tarter RE, McBride H, Buonpane N, Schneider DU. Differentiation of alcoholics. *Arch Gen Psychiatry.* 1977;34:761-768.
27. Eysenck SBG, Eysenck HJ. *Manual of the Eysenck Personality Questionnaire.* London, England: Hodder & Stoughton; 1975.
28. Hoehn-Saric R, McLeod DR. Locus of control in chronic anxiety disorders. *Acta Psychiatr Scand.* 1985;72:529-535.
29. Spielberger CD, Gorsuch RL, Lushene RE. *Manual for the State-Trait Anxiety Inventory.* Palo Alto, Calif: Consulting Psychologists Press; 1970.
30. Cloninger CR, Svrakic DM, Przybeck TR. The Tridimensional Personality Questionnaire: US normative data. *Psychol Rep.* 1991;69:1047-1057.
31. Cheung MN. Detection of and recovery from errors in cardiac interbeat intervals. *Psychophysiology.* 1981;18:341-346.
32. McLeod DR, Hoehn-Saric R, Labib AS, Greenblatt DJ. Six weeks of diazepam treatment in normal women: effects on psychomotor performance and psychophysiology. *J Clin Psychopharmacol.* 1988;8:83-99.
33. McLeod DR, Griffiths RR, Bigelow GE, Yingling J. An automated version of the Digit Symbol Substitution Test (DSST). *Behav Res Methods Instrum.* 1982; 14:463-466.
34. Greenhouse SW, Geisser S. On methods in the analysis of profile data. *Psychometrica.* 1959;24:95-112.
35. McLeod DR, Hoehn-Saric R. Perception of physiological changes in normal and pathological anxiety. In: Hoehn-Saric R, McLeod DR, ed. *Biology of Anxiety Disorders.* Washington, DC: American Psychiatric Press; 1993:223-243.
36. Hazlett R, McLeod DR, Hoehn-Saric R. Muscle tension in generalized anxiety disorder: elevated muscle tonus or agitated movement? *Psychophysiology.* 1994; 31:189-195.
37. Inz J. *EEG Activity in Generalized Anxiety Disorder.* University Park, Pa: Penn State University; 1990. Doctoral dissertation.
38. Frankenhaeuser M. Psychoneuroendocrine approaches to the study of emotion as related to stress and coping. In: Howe HEJ, ed. *Nebraska Symposium on Motivation.* Lincoln, Neb: University of Nebraska Press; 1979:123-161.
39. Shapiro D, Crider A. Psychophysiological approaches in social psychology. In: Lindzey G, Aronson E, eds. *The Handbook of Social Psychology.* 2nd ed. Reading, Pa: Addison-Wesley Publishing Co; 1969:1-49.
40. Hoehn-Saric R, McLeod DR. Somatic manifestations of normal and pathological anxiety. In: Hoehn-Saric R, McLeod DR, eds. *Biology of Anxiety Disorders.* Washington, DC: American Psychiatric Press; 1993:177-222.
41. Hoehn-Saric R, Benkelfat C. Structural and functional brain imaging in obsessive compulsive disorder. In: Hollander E, Zohar J, Marazzati D, Olivier B, eds. *Current Concepts in Obsessive-compulsive Disorder.* New York, NY: John Wiley & Sons Inc; 1994:183-211.

ORIGINAL ARTICLE

Quality of Care for Depressed Elderly Patients Hospitalized in the Specialty Psychiatric Units or General Medical Wards

Grayson Norquist, MD, MSPH; Kenneth B. Wells, MD, MPH; William H. Rogers, PhD; Lois M. Davis, PhD; Katherine Kahn, MD; Robert Brook, MD

Background: Studies to assess quality of care have become increasingly important for research and policy purposes.

Objective: To evaluate the difference in quality of care between elderly depressed patients hospitalized in specialty psychiatric units and those hospitalized in general medical wards.

Methods: We reviewed retrospectively the medical charts of 2746 patients with depression hospitalized in 297 general medical hospitals in five different states. Quality of care was assessed by clinical review of explicit and implicit information contained in the medical records of patients in specialty psychiatric units (n=1295) and general medical wards (n=1451). We also used other secondary data sources to determine postdischarge outcomes.

Results: We found that (1) a higher percentage of admissions on the psychiatric units were considered appropriate, (2) overall psychological assessment was better on the psychiatric unit, (3) patients were more likely to receive psychological services on the psychiatric wards but more likely to receive traditional general medical services on medical wards, (4) there were more inpatient general medical complications on the psychiatric wards, and (5) implicit measures of clinical status at discharge were better for those on the psychiatric unit.

Conclusions: Although limited by reliance on medical record abstraction and a retrospective study design, our data indicate that the quality of care for the psychological aspects of the treatment of depression may be better on psychiatric units, while the quality of general medical components of care may be better on general medical wards.

(Arch Gen Psychiatry. 1995;52:695-701)

STUDIES TO assess the quality of care in the treatment of mental disorders have become increasingly important for research and policy purposes. As clinical treatment and systems of care change, it is imperative to understand the factors that affect the quality of care provided. This has been emphasized by the request for quality-of-care data from such organizations as the Joint Commission on Accreditation of Healthcare Organizations and the recommendation for a national quality monitoring program as part of the president's original health care reform proposal.[1]

Components of quality of care are traditionally divided into structure, process, and outcome.[2,3] *Process* relates to clinical treatment approaches and transactions between providers and patients, while *outcome* indicates patient status during or after treatment. Previous work in the non-mental health care area has shown the feasibility and utility of explicit criteria and implicit review for measuring clinical processes of care and the ability to correlate variations in process to variations in outcomes.[4,5]

A critical quality issue that has policy and clinical implications is whether people with mental disorders receive better quality of care when treated on specialty mental health units than when treated on general medical wards. Previous studies conducted with inpatients have had a limited focus in attempting to address this issue, comparing the prescribing practices for psychotropic medications of specialists and generalists. In patients with depression, studies of inpatients and outpatients have shown that generalists may provide inadequate or inappropriate treatment.[6-18] Because some studies were conducted at single sites and different studies used different methods, it is difficult to generalize findings across studies. In addition, a more comprehensive evaluation of quality of care

From the National Institute of Mental Health, Rockville, Md (Dr Norquist); the Departments of Psychiatry (Dr Wells) and Medicine (Drs Kahn and Brook), University of California–Los Angeles; and RAND, Santa Monica, Calif (Drs Wells, Rogers, Davis, Kahn, and Brook).

See Patients and Methods on next page

PATIENTS AND METHODS

Data used herein are from the Prospective Payment Quality of Care Study.[22] We selected regions within five states (California, Florida, Indiana, Pennsylvania, and Texas) and within these regions selected hospitals so that their patients were as representative as possible of Medicare patients nationally with six study conditions. The study included 297 general medical hospitals. We oversampled hospitals with a large Medicaid caseload and those with large numbers of patients with depression, but we did not include free-standing psychiatric hospitals. We elected to focus on the acute-care general medical hospitals because approximately 80% of all psychiatric inpatient care reimbursed by Medicare is provided in this sector alone.[21]

The Prospective Payment Quality of Care Study was designed to evaluate the impact of the prospective payment system (PPS). Thus, we divided the sample into a pre-PPS period (January 1, 1981, to December 31, 1982) and a post-PPS period (July 1, 1985, to June 30, 1986). We obtained hospital-specific lists of Medicare patients who had a discharge diagnosis of unipolar or unspecified depression (*International Classification of Diseases, Ninth Revision,* codes 296.2, 296.3, 298.0, 300.04, 309.0, 309.1, and 311)[23] within the first five listed codes. Our sample consisted of 3626 Medicare patients with a discharge diagnosis of depression. We obtained their medical records and required that they contain evidence that depressive affect or suicidal ideation was present at the time of admission. We excluded patients if they had at least one current life-threatening general medical condition, such as cardiac arrest within 24 hours before admission or surgery during the admission, because these conditions make it difficult to evaluate the quality of care for depression. We required that patients be at least 65 years of age and hospitalized during the specified periods. These criteria caused exclusion of 880 (24%) patients, yielding a study sample of 2746 patients with depression. The most common reason for exclusion (n=405) was the absence of evidence that depression was active at the time of admission.

We developed explicit measures (ie, specific, objective indicators) of sickness at the time of admission, quality of care during the admission, and outcomes of care. We formulated these measures from review of the scientific literature, guidelines for peer review programs, findings of clinical consensus conferences, and recommendations of practicing clinicians familiar with the medical records of depressed elderly patients.[24] Clinicians included board-certified psychiatrists nominated by the Professional Standard Review Organizations of the participating states, a clinical psychologist, and an academic geropsychiatrist. We developed and pretested a medical record abstraction form to collect data for the study.[25] We also trained the five psychiatrists nominated by the Professional Standard Review Organizations to provide implicit judgments of sickness at the time of admission, quality of care during the admission, and outcomes of care. Their judgments (ie, implicit judgments) were based on review of photocopies of parts of the medical record (ie, admitting history and physical examination findings, discharge summary, first psychiatric consultation, and last 2 days of clinician notes) and the completed medical record abstraction form. We developed a set of detailed written guidelines to standardize these judgments. We abstracted 32 medical records twice to evaluate interrater reliability and used the κ statistic to evaluate agreement.

QUALITY OF CARE AND OTHER MEASURES

We divided our measures into three general categories (**Table 1**): (1) clinical assessment, (2) services provided, and (3) outcomes. The first two categories represent the traditional process component of quality. Although some measures under the "services provided" category are not considered traditional quality-of-care measures, we believed that the provision of these services in a population of depressed elderly inpatients did indicate process components of quality and so we include them herein.

To evaluate the completeness of the admission assessment of psychological status (item 5 under "Clinical assessments" in Table 1), we asked the psychiatric reviewers whether the admission history and mental status examination provided an acceptable general impression of the patient's depression at the time of admission. For the other measures, we used data from the medical record abstraction form and developed measures of whether specific components of the initial history and physical examination were recorded in the medical record. These included assessment of suicide status, psychosis, the psychiatric history, history of alcohol use, examination of the heart, neurologic examination, recording of vital signs, assessment of cognitive status, and prior medication history. Interrater reliabilities of these quality-of-care measures ranged from 0.35 to 1.00 (fair to excellent).[26]

is needed to identify a broader range of differences in the care provided to patients with serious mental disorders in these two different treatment sectors.

Consistent with the recommendations of McGlynn et al,[3] we used a clinically detailed approach to compare the quality of care between psychiatric units of general medical hospitals and general medical wards. We focused our study on a national sample of elderly inpatients with depression. The elderly are a critical population for study because they represent a growing segment of the US population and are often treated in the general medical sector for mental health problems.[19]

Given current concerns about the financing of inpatient mental health care within health care reform, it is important to know what kinds of settings should be promoted. If specialty care is more costly than care provided in the general medical sector, then the quality of care should be higher to warrant the added costs associated with treating patients in specialty settings.[20,21] Research such as that presented herein can help in understanding the strengths and weaknesses of these various provider settings and further inform providers and policymakers.

RESULTS

Elderly people with depression treated on medical wards were older and more likely to be white than those treated in psychiatric units of general hospitals (**Table 2**). The

We included measures of process that occurred during the hospitalization (see "Services provided" in Table 1). The measure of the quality of psychotropic medication management (item 2 under "Services provided" in Table 1) represented an average of the implicit ratings for the quality of administration of psychotropic medications during the admission and at the time of discharge.[27] Unacceptable care was defined as that likely to place the patient at risk owing to severe untreated depression, severe medication side effects, or complications of unusual or inappropriate forms of therapy. We also assessed the percentage of hospital days of the first 3 and last 2 (specified days) during which a variety of clinical services were provided. We used these particular hospital days because they are easy to find in the medical record and because we believed that recording of therapeutic services would be more complete at the beginning and end of the hospitalization.

We also assessed outcomes (Table 1). Mortality and readmission data were obtained from national secondary databases. Because inpatient complications were rare, we used a dichotomous indicator of whether any occurred. We also determined whether those admitted from home were discharged to another hospital or nursing home. Psychiatric reviewers provided two implicit ratings of the patient's clinical status at the time of discharge. One measure indicated whether the treating physician, psychologist, or nurse noted that clinical status was unimproved at the time of discharge, as interpreted by the study's implicit reviewers (item 1 under "Outcomes" in Table 1). The judgments were based on statements made at the time of discharge, such as "still very depressed" or "no change in status." The psychiatric reviewers also evaluated the acceptability of the patient's general clinical status at the time of discharge, implicitly assigning a code of "unacceptable" if the patient still had a depression that merited an acute-care hospitalization (item 2 under "Outcomes" in Table 1). For example, a patient with a first episode of severe depression who at the time of discharge was still suicidal or gravely disabled was rated as having an unacceptable outcome. Reliabilities of the outcome measures were good to excellent. The construct validity of the implicit ratings of outcome were supported by their significant associations with the more objective outcome measures.[24]

We also included in this study a measure of the appropriateness of the acute admission (data not shown). This particular measure combined implicit clinical judgments with data from the abstraction form on the presence of serious symptoms and comorbid disorders. Patients with a potentially life-threatening general medical illness or a depression that could not safely be treated on an outpatient basis were considered to have a clearly appropriate admission. Patients with a mild depression, no major psychiatric comorbidity, and no potentially life-threatening general medical illness were considered to have a clearly inappropriate admission.

TREATMENT LOCATION

We used data from the medical record to place patients into one of two exclusive categories: (1) ever treated in the specialty psychiatric ward of a general hospital or (2) treated on a general medical ward ("scatter bed"). Patients treated in free-standing psychiatric hospitals were not included in this study.

STATISTICAL METHODS

We performed multiple regression analyses (logistic or log linear) with assessment measures, services measures, and outcome measures as the dependent variables. We included as covariates patient demographic characteristics (age, sex, Medicaid status, and race) and state and hospital characteristics (percentage of total hospital admissions that are Medicare patients, percentage of Medicaid admissions, geographic region size, bed size, teaching status, and profit status). We controlled for level of sickness at the time of admission, using scales that have been described previously.[28] The explicit measures used to determine level of sickness included a single-item measure of suicide attempt at the time of admission, a general depression severity scale, a measure of substance abuse, and a physical illness scale. In addition, we included implicit clinical judgments of the presence at the time of admission of serious depression and/or acute general medical illness and judgments of moderate to severe dementia. For the analysis of appropriateness at the time of admission, we did not control for sickness at the time of admission because the two types of measures were based on the same items. To adjust inference statistics and SEs for the multistage clustered sampling design, we used the intraclass correlation model.[29,30] We tested the differences in all measures not only by ward placement but also for time period effects. Data were weighted to the national sample of elderly patients hospitalized in acute-care general medical hospitals, using data from the 1981 to 1982 and 1985 to 1986 Medicare Provider Analysis and Review files to derive the weights.

two groups did not differ in the proportion that was female or in the percentage receiving Medicaid.

CLINICAL ASSESSMENTS

Our analysis of clinical assessments conducted at the time of admission or during the first 2 days of admission are shown in **Table 3**. Results are predictions, based on parameters of the regression models. Except for three assessments (admission and discharge suicide assessment by physician or psychologist and assessment of the psychiatric history), differences between the wards did not vary by time period and are reported by ward combining time periods. We had a number of nursing assessment measures but due to their poor κ values, we report in this study only those with good κ values (assessment for suicide and cognitive status).[31]

Patients on the psychiatric units were more likely to receive what are traditionally considered psychological components of the clinical assessment (assessment of suicide status, assessment of psychosis, and assessment of psychiatric history) than patients on the medical wards. Yet, the differences in the assessment of psychiatric history and suicide assessment were only found in the pre-PPS period (psychiatric history: 85% on psychiatric ward vs 65% on medical ward, $P<.0001$; admission suicide status: 50% on psychiatric ward vs 25% on medical ward, $P<.001$; discharge suicide status: 6% on psychiatric ward vs 1% on medical ward, $P<.001$). Regardless of time period, a greater percentage of

Table 1. Measures of Quality of Care

Measure	Data Source	Definition	Interrater Reliability (κ)
Clinical assessments			
1. Suicide status†	1	Assessment of suicide attempt or ideation	0.78
2. Psychosis	1	Assessment of hallucinations, delusions, or bizarre behaviors	0.76
3. Psychiatric history	1	Assessment of psychiatric disorders, symptoms, or treatment before admission	0.44
4. Alcohol use	1	Documentation of whether patient used alcohol	0.64
5. Admission assessment of psychological status	2	Acceptability of the initial mental status examination, psychiatric history, and diagnosis	0.52
6. Heart examination	1	Auscultation of the heart	0.74
7. Neurologic examination	1	Count of assessment of pupils, limb deep tendon reflexes, and coordination or gait	0.50
8. Weight	1	Weight measured	1.00
9. Vital signs	1	Count of vital signs recorded	1.00
10. Cognitive status†	1	Assessment of orientation to time, person, or place; level of alertness; or acute neurologic change or coma status at admission	0.58
11. Prior medications	1	Documentation of whether patient was receiving any medication before or at time of admission	0.59
Services provided			
1. Rehabilitation services	1	Percentage of specified days that patient received rehabilitation, vocational, or recreation therapy	0.42
2. Psychotropic medication management	2	Acceptability of the inpatient psychotropic medication management	0.82
3. Hematological test	1	Ever had hematocrit and hemoglobin test	0.43
4. Other laboratory test	1	Ever had serum sodium, potassium, urea nitrogen, or creatinine determinations	0.60
5. Thyroid test	1	Ever had blood thyroid test	0.81
6. Intake/output	1	Intake and output measured at least once during hospitalization	0.60
7. Blood pressure/postural blood pressure	1/1	Percentage of specified days that blood pressure was measured/postural blood pressure measured at least once	0.5/0.35
8. MD/PhD visit	1	Percentage of specified days with visit by physician or psychologist	0.68
Outcomes			
1. Unimproved clinical status at discharge (as noted by treating providers)	2	Treating clinician or nurse states that depression, overall status, grooming, or nutrition status is unimproved or worse at discharge; rated only if a problem is present at admission and if discharged alive	0.78
2. Unacceptable or equivocal clinical status at discharge (rated by study psychiatrist)	2	Study psychiatrist's opinion of whether clinical status at discharge is unacceptable or equivocal vs acceptable; rated only if discharged alive	0.68
3. Any inpatient complication	1	A very serious adverse physical (eg, death or stroke) or psychological (eg, suicide attempt) problem occurring after day 2 and not present at admission	0.84
4. Discharge to hospital or nursing home	1	If admitted from home or board and care facility and discharged alive, then discharged to any acute, subacute, or long-term care hospital or nursing home	0.74
5. Mortality	3	Dead within 365 days of discharge if discharged alive	...
6. Any readmission	3	Any acute care admission (medical or psychiatric) within 365 days of discharge	...

**1 indicates medical record, explicit review; 2, medical record, implicit review; and 3, Health Care Financing Administration secondary data sources.*
†Nurse and MD/PhD assessment; admission and discharge assessment.

patients on the psychiatric unit received an implicit rating of acceptable overall assessment of their psychological status than did patients on the medical wards.

Traditional general medical components (ie, nonpsychological components) of the assessment (eg, heart examination, neurologic examination, and measuring weight and vital signs) were performed equally on the two types of wards, although the level of assessment for some items, such as auscultation of the heart, was lower on both types of wards than one might expect in this population. Assessment of cognitive status and prior medication history would not be considered a unique component of either the psychological or general medical part of the assessment. Yet, patients on the psychiatric unit were more likely to have their cognitive status assessed by physicians on admission, while those on the medical wards were more likely to have a history taken of their prior medication use.

Although not shown in Table 1, we also assessed the appropriateness of the acute admission. A higher percentage of admissions on the psychiatric units were considered appropriate than on the medical wards (ie, the patients were sicker) (93% vs 81%, $P<.01$). In addition, about 9% of patients on both wards were admitted with a history of a suicide attempt.

SERVICES PROVIDED

In terms of services provided during the admission, those treated on psychiatric wards were more likely to receive psychological services, such as rehabilitation or vocational or recreation therapy, and the management of their psychotropic medications was better. Although the absolute difference across ward types in the implicit rating of medication management is small, this measure has a high correlation with better outcomes ($P<.01$ for all outcome measures, except readmission [$P<.05$]; correlation with postdischarge mortality was not significant). In addition, we assessed other measures of medication management at the time of discharge (data not shown. We found that patients on the medical ward were significantly more likely to have antidepressant therapy started within the 48 hours before discharge than were those on psychiatric wards (20% on medical ward vs 2% on psychiatric ward, $P<.001$). Patients were visited with equal frequency by primary providers on both wards, but only 48% of patients with depression on the general medical wards ever had a consultation by a psychiatrist or psychologist.

Patients on medical wards were more likely to receive traditional general medical services (hematological test, intake and output measurement, and blood pressure measurement) than those on psychiatric wards (Table 3). Yet, we found that patients on the psychiatric unit were more likely to have postural blood pressure measurement (16% vs 7%, $P<.01$), but the κ value for this measure was low (κ=0.35).

OUTCOMES

The only explicit outcome measure that showed a statistically significant difference was the trend toward more serious inpatient complications (primarily general medical, eg, stroke and hypotensive syncopal episode) on the psychiatric units compared with general medical wards (item 3 in Table 3). Although the implicit measures show that the clinical status at the time of discharge was better for patients who were on psychiatric units (items 1 and 2 in Table 3), many patients in both types of settings were rated as having unacceptable or unimproved clinical status at the time of discharge. A rating of unacceptable on these implicit outcome measures was significantly associated with all explicit outcome measures, except postadmission mortality ($P<.01$ compared with inpatient complication and discharge to hospital or nursing home; $P<.05$ compared with any postdischarge readmission).

COMMENT

Data from our study indicate that elderly depressed inpatients on psychiatric units of general medical hospitals may receive better quality of care for the psychological aspects of the treatment of their depression than similar patients on general medical wards. On the other hand, quality of general medical components of care (ie, nonpsychological) may be better on medical wards, suggesting that each type of ward setting has a unique strength.

In this section, we first outline several important methodologic issues in assessing the quality of care received by inpatients with depression and then discuss the policy implications of our findings. One measures quality by assessing how well the care conforms to accepted standards for such care. We used an extensive literature review and a consensus panel to formulate explicit criteria that represent important components of treating elderly people with depression in the hospital setting. These included key clinical aspects of treatment, such as assessment of current psychiatric and physical status and antidepressant therapy. To make sure we captured broader concepts of treatment and outcome, we incorporated reviews by psychiatrists of major parts of the medical record to derive implicit judgments of process and outcome. Although psychiatric reviewers were not blinded to ward setting, they were not looking for ward differences but instead were focused on differences before and after the implementation of prospective payment.

Table 2. Characteristics of Depressed Patients by Ward Setting

Patient Characteristics	Psychiatric Unit (n=1295)	Medical Ward (n=1451)
Age ≥80 y, %	12	20*
% Female	75	76
% Nonwhite	10	6†
% Receiving Medicaid	11	8

*$P<.001$.
†$P<.01$.

Although the process measures had face validity as indicators of quality, we wanted to further ensure their construct validity by linking them to outcome measures. The implicit judgments of medication management had good predictive validity for most of the outcomes and were highly associated with more explicit indicators of such management (eg, whether antidepressant medication was started within 2 days before discharge). In addition, the implicit reviews of outcome were significantly associated with other explicit outcome measures.

An overall assessment of quality is based on more than a summary count. Thus, the ward with the greatest absolute number of high-quality measures is not necessarily rated as better. Some measures are more important than others. For example, when determining the ward on which patients received better quality of psychological treatment, if only clinical assessment measures were used, then the differences would be minimal and not clinically important. Yet, when we combined findings from implicit judgments of clinical assessment, appropriateness of admission, implicit judgment of medication management, explicit discharge medication management measures, and clinical status at the time of discharge, the data support the conclusion that patients on psychiatric wards received better quality of care for psychological aspects of treatment than did those on the medical wards. The data also support the conclusion that general medical components of treatment were better on the medical wards.

Our standards were set at a level to find major deficiencies in quality of care. For example, we expected there to be at least one assessment of a person's suicide status, but we did not expect daily accounting of such status. The retrospective study design and use of the medi-

Table 3. Comparison of Quality of Care Between Psychiatric and Medical Wards

	Psychiatric Unit, %	Medical Ward, %
Clinical assessments*		
1. Suicide status		
Admission (MD/PhD)	†	†
Discharge (MD/PhD)	†	†
(RN)	4	0.7‡
2. Psychosis	51	27§
3. Psychiatric history	†	†
4. Alcohol use	48	49
5. Admission assessment of psychiatric status	75	66‖
6. Heart examination	55	59
7. Neurologic examination (mean count)	1.4	1.4
8. Weight	78	78
9. Vital signs (mean count)	2.9	2.9
10. Cognitive status		
Admission (MD/PhD)	74	61§
(RN)	86	91‡
Discharge (MD/PhD)	15	11
(RN)	42	68§
11. Prior medications	69	76‖
Services provided		
1. Rehabilitation services	45	13§
2. Psychotropic medication management (mean score) (higher score=higher quality)	1.5	1.4‡
3. Hematological test	90	95‖
4. Other laboratory test	68	65
5. Thyroid test	52	46
6. Intake/output	14	21¶
7. Blood pressure	88	93¶
8. MD/PhD visit (% of days with visit)	86	86
Outcomes		
1. Clinical status at discharge (provider) (unimproved or worse)	33	43‖
2. Clinical status at discharge (rater) (unacceptable or equivocal)	47	52‡
3. Any inpatient complication	23	17‡
4. Discharged to hospital or nursing home	13	10
5. Mortality (1 year)	9	9
6. Any readmission (1 year)	58	55

All assessments at the time of admission or during the first 2 days, unless otherwise noted.

†*Comparisons differed by time period (see text).*

‡$P<.05$.

§$P<.0001$.

‖$P<.01$.

¶$P<.001$.

cal record did not permit us to evaluate a comprehensive range of treatment process and outcomes. To do so would have required the use of multiple data sources. In spite of this, we believe that our measures provide a useful multidimensional profile of quality of care.

There are methodologic issues related to reliance on medical record abstraction.[32] Psychiatric units that were not exempt from prospective payment in the later study period may have had greater incentive for better recording than units that were exempt, because payment to those units was tied to diagnosis and complications.[33] Also, a given component of treatment could be performed but not recorded in the chart. Most of the components of care that we measured are ones that one might expect to be recorded in the medical record. Some had to be recorded to be provided (eg, laboratory tests and medication). Although there are no data in the mental health area, previous studies in the physical health field show that the medical record is a good indicator of what actually happens during treatment, and good medical recording is associated with good medical performance.[34,35] Because length of stay tended to be longer on specialty wards, there is a possibility that more information was available for those with longer stays on these wards. More comprehensive assessments of the full spectrum of treatment and outcome require multiple data sources collected prospectively. Such assessments would be prohibitively expensive and impractical for large-scale studies of quality such as this one. In addition, quality measures that could be used to monitor care provided by health plans would require readily accessible sources of data. Medical records provide useful and somewhat inexpensive sources of such data. Yet, our finding that some data have poor reliability calls into question whether some data should be collected in routine accreditation reviews.

Our findings have important clinical and policy implications. From a clinical perspective, the care and outcomes of psychological aspects of treatment for depression (eg, management of psychotropic medications and clinical status at the time of discharge) on psychiatric units appear to be better than that provided on general medical wards, even when adjusting for severity of illness. However, patients on general medical wards have their physical health status assessed and are provided with general medical services (eg, certain laboratory tests) as well as or better than the patients on psychiatric units. In addition, inpatient complication rates (representing primarily new general medical illnesses or abnormal laboratory or vital sign values) are less frequent on the general medical wards. In essence, both wards do what providers on those wards are traditionally trained to do.

Although findings from this study indicate the need for improvement of care on the general medical wards in the treatment of depression and care on the psychiatric units for general medical complications, there is evidence that at least clinical assessment of depression on general medical wards is already improving. We found that the level of assessment of suicide status and psychiatric history improved with time to the point where it was equivalent on both types of wards by the later study period. In addition, there are indications that quality of care may not be the best possible in either setting. For example, 48% of people with depression on the psychiatric unit did not have an assessment of suicide status recorded on admission, and 33% of patients on these units were rated by the provider as unimproved at the time of discharge. Both settings clearly have room for improvement.

Because we did not separate clinical subtypes of depression, it is possible that only some elderly patients (eg, those with psychotic symptoms) receive better care on psychiatric units, while others receive comparable care in both types of settings. Future studies should focus on these clinically important subgroups. Also, specific interventions not studied herein (eg, consultation by mental health specialists) may improve the care received by elderly patients on general medical wards. We found that less than half of the patients on medical wards received consultation from mental health specialists. More studies are needed to determine whether our findings are characteristic for other populations treated in free-standing psychiatric hospitals (excluded from this study).

With the advent of health care reform at the state level and current private market trends, it is likely that more people with mental disorders will be treated in the general medical sector. Thus, data such as ours indicate the increasing importance of efforts to improve mental health care in this sector. In addition to improved postgraduate training for general medical providers, there is a need for the development and implementation of practice guidelines for treatment of depression. To date, these efforts have not focused specifically on the elderly, but our data suggest that such a focus would be clinically appropriate. Furthermore, our results suggest that development of guidelines should also address issues of the quality of management of general medical problems and complications in elderly people hospitalized with depression—an issue largely ignored in current versions of depression guidelines.[36,37]

Our study was designed to provide a descriptive analysis of the quality of care provided in different treatment settings. Ours was not a longitudinal, course-of-illness study, so we were unable to answer specific questions about why outcomes were poor in certain settings. Yet, studies such as ours show that the field has the technology to measure and compare the quality of care provided to people with mental disorders. Future research should seek to refine the technology, to test the methods in other settings, to determine whether processes can be linked to outcomes, and to attempt to ascertain the factors that account for differences in quality. Findings from such research can help to ensure that people with mental disorders receive the best care possible.

Accepted for publication March 31, 1995.

Reprint requests to Room 10-105, 5600 Fishers Ln, Rockville, MD 20857 (Dr Norquist).

REFERENCES

1. Health Security Act, Title 5, Subtitle A, October 1993.
2. Donabedian A. *Explorations in Quality Assessment and Monitoring: The Definition of Quality and Approaches to Its Assessment.* Ann Arbor, Mich: Health Administration Press; 1980.
3. McGlynn EA, Norquist GS, Wells KB, Sullivan G, Liberman RP. Quality-of-care research in mental health: responding to the challenge. *Inquiry.* 1988;25:157-170.
4. Kahn KL, Rogers WH, Rubenstein LV, Sherwood MJ, Reinisch EJ, Keeler EB, Draper D, Kosecoff J, Brook RH. Measuring quality of care with explicit process criteria before and after implementation of the DRG-based prospective payment system. *JAMA.* 1990;264:1969-1973.
5. Rubenstein LV, Kahn KL, Reinisch EJ, Sherwood MJ, Rogers WH, Kamberg C, Draper D, Brook RH. Changes in quality of care for five diseases measured by implicit review, 1981 to 1986. *JAMA.* 1990;264:1974-1979.
6. Johnson DAW. Treatment of depression in general practice. *BMJ.* 1973;2:18-20.
7. Johnson DAW. A study of the use of antidepressant medication in general practice. *Br J Psychiatry.* 1974;125:186-192.
8. Davidson JRT, Raft D, Lewis BF, Gelbhardt M. Psychotropic drugs on general medical and surgical wards of a teaching hospital. *Arch Gen Psychiatry.* 1975; 32:507-511.
9. Raft D, Davidson J, Toomey TC, Spencer RF, Lewis BF. Inpatient and outpatient patterns of psychotropic drug prescribing by non-psychiatrist physicians. *Am J Psychiatry.* 1975;132:1309-1312.
10. Weissman MM, Klerman GL. The chronic depressive in the community: unrecognized and poorly treated. *Compr Psychiatry.* 1977;13:523-532.
11. Gullick EL, King LJ. Appropriateness of drugs prescribed by primary care physicians for depressed outpatients. *J Affect Disord.* 1979;1:55-58.
12. Holt RJ, Gaskins JD. Neuroleptic drug use in a family-practice center. *Am J Hosp Pharm.* 1981;38:1716-1719.
13. Keller MB, Klerman GL, Lavori PW, Fawcett JA, Coryell W, Endicott J. Treatment received by depressed patients. *JAMA.* 1982;248:1848-1855.
14. Wells KB, Goldberg G, Brook RH, Leake B. Quality of care for psychotropic drug use in internal medicine group practices. *West J Med.* 1986;145:710-714.
15. Callies AL, Popkin MK. Antidepressant treatment of medical-surgical inpatients by nonpsychiatric physicians. *Arch Gen Psychiatry.* 1987;44:157-160.
16. Wells KB, Goldberg G, Brook R, Leake B. Management of patients on psychotropic drugs in primary care clinics. *Med Care.* 1988;26:645-656.
17. Broadhead WE, Clapp-Channing NE, Finch JN, Copeland JA. Effects of medical illness and somatic symptoms on treatment of depression in a family medicine residency practice. *Gen Hosp Psychiatry.* 1989;11:189-195.
18. Magruder-Habib K, Zung WWK, Feussner JR, Alling WC, Stevens S, Saunders WB. Management of general medical patients with symptoms of depression. *Gen Hosp Psychiatry.* 1989;11:196-202.
19. German PS, Shapiro S, Skinner EA. Mental health of the elderly: use of health and mental health services. *J Am Geriatr Soc.* 1985;33:246-252.
20. Sturm R, Wells KB. How can care for depression become more cost-effective? *JAMA.* 1995;273:51-58.
21. Goldman HH, Taube CA, Jencks SF. The organization of the psychiatric inpatient services system. *Med Care.* 1987;25(suppl 9):S6-S21.
22. Draper D, Kahn KL, Reinisch EJ, Sherwood MJ, Carney MF, Kosecoff J, Keeler EB, Rogers WH, Savitt H, Allen H, Wells KB, Reboussin D, Brook RH. Studying the effects of the DRG-based prospective payment system on quality of care: design, sampling, and fieldwork. *JAMA.* 1990;264:1956-1961.
23. World Health Organization. *Manual of the International Statistical Classification of Diseases, Injuries, and Causes of Death, Based on the Recommendations of the Ninth Revision Conference, 1975.* Geneva, Switzerland: World Health Organization; 1977.
24. Wells KB, Rogers WH, Davis LM, Kahn K, Norquist G, Keeler E, Kosecoff J, Brook RH. Quality of care for hospitalized depressed elderly before and after implementation of prospective payment system. *Am J Psychiatry.* 1993;150: 1799-1805.
25. Wells KB, Kosecoff J, Sherwood M, Roth CP, Chew CF, Essock-Vitale S, Brook RH, Kahn KL. *Medical Record Abstraction Form and Guidelines for Assessing Quality of Care for Hospitalized Patients With Depression.* Santa Monica, Calif: RAND; 1988. Publication N-2803-HCFA.
26. Landis JR, Koch GG. The measurement of observer agreement for categorical data. *Biometrics.* 1977;33:159-174.
27. Wells KB, Norquist GS, Benjamin B, Rogers W. Quality of antidepressant medications prescribed at discharge to depressed elderly patients in general medical hospitals before and after prospective payment system. *Gen Hosp Psychiatry.* 1994;16:4-15.
28. Davis LM, Wells KB, Rogers WH, Benjamin B, Norquist GS, Kahn K, Kosecoff J, Brook RH. Length of stay and intensity of clinical services for depressed elderly inpatients before and after implementation of Medicare PPS. *Psychiatr Serv.* In press.
29. Searle SR. *Linear Models.* New York, NY: John Wiley & Sons Inc; 1971.
30. Huber PJ. The behavior of maximum likelihood estimates under nonstandard conditions. In: *Fifth Berkeley Symposium on Mathematical Statistics and Probability.* Berkeley, Calif: University of California Press; 1967.
31. Parker LE, Wells KB, Buchanan JL, Benjamin B. Institutional and economic influences on quality of nursing documentation. *Health Care Manage Rev.* 1994; 19:9-19.
32. Romm FJ, Putnam SM. The validity of the medical record. *Med Care.* 1981; 19:310-315.
33. Wells KB, Rogers WH, Davis LM, Benjamin B. Quality of care for depressed elderly pre-post prospective payment system: differences in response across treatment settings. *Med Care.* 1994;32:257-276.
34. Lyons TF, Payne BC. The relationship of physicians' medical recording performance to their medical care performance. *Med Care.* 1974;12:463-469.
35. Kosecoff J, Fink A, Brook RH, Chassin MR. The appropriateness of using a medical procedure. *Med Care.* 1987;25:196-201.
36. Depression Guideline Panel. *Depression in Primary Care: Volume 2: Treatment of Major Depression. Clinical Practice Guideline, Number 5.* Rockville, Md: US Dept of Health and Human Services, Public Health Service, Agency for Health Care Policy and Research; 1993. AHCPR publication 93-0551.
37. Work Group on Major Depressive Disorder. Practice guideline for major depressive disorder in adults. *Am J Psychiatry.* 1993;150(suppl):1-26.

Professional Opportunities

Physician Recruitment

Psychiatry
Multiple Specialties/Group Practice
Locum Tenens Wanted
Graduate Training/Residencies/Fellowships
Chiefs/Department Heads/Directors
Academic/Faculty
CME Corner
Courses/Symposia/Seminars
Practices For Sale
Notices

1995 Professional Opportunity Rates

Regular	1x	1.10/wd	*3x	1.00/wd
Bold	1x	1.25/wd	*3x	1.15/wd

*In order to receive the 3 time frequency price, the request must be made upon initial placement. The minimum charge is 20 words. A word consists of one or more letters surrounded by space on each side.

For information on display advertising and our network buys contact an account representative.

Policy

Orders for classified advertising must be submitted in writing. Although the American Medical Association believes the classified advertisements in these pages to be from reputable sources, the Association does not investigate the offers made and assumes no liability concerning them. Acceptance of advertising is restricted to professional opportunities, practices for sale, and medical office space available. The Association reserves the right to decline, withdraw, or edit advertisements at its discretion. Every care is taken to avoid mistakes but responsibility cannot be accepted by the Association for clerical or printer's errors.

Blind Box Service

Confidential box numbers are available for an additional $20 per issue, plus the words - Box ____, c/o AGNP.

When responding to a box number, please send to Archives of General Psychiatry, Box ____, c/o AGNP, 515 N State St, Chicago, IL 60610.

Cancellations/Changes

Cancellations/changes must be received in writing at least 25 days prior to the date of the issue. In order to expedite, please fax to 312-464-5909 to the attention of your account representative.

General Information

To contact a Physician Recruitment Advertising account representative, call 312-464-2475/2490/2491/4485 or **800-AMA-2260.** Or fax your insertion order to **312-464-5909**. Mail your materials to **AMA Physician Recruitment Advertising, 12th Floor, 515 N State St, Chicago, IL 60610.**

Psychiatry

OCHSNER CLINIC OF BATON ROUGE: Seeks a BC/BE child psychiatrist to see children, adolescents, and adults. Ochsner Clinic is a physician directed, integrated health care system which includes its own health plan and is an established multispecialty group practice in the Gulf South. Competitive salary, excellent fringe benefits package, liberal paid vacation and CME time. Opportunity for partnership status. All malpractice insurance is provided. Abundant cultural and recreational activities. CVs should be sent to Ochsner Clinic, Physician Recruiting, Ref #A3PSYC, 16777 Medical Center Drive, Baton Rouge, LA 70816. 1-800-488-2240 or 504-755-5441 (fax). All inquiries are confidential.

SOUTH FLORIDA, EAST COAST: Well-established psychiatrist seeks an associate, full- or part-time, to join solo private practice (with coverage) in beautiful area of Fort Lauderdale, Florida. Practice focus is on medicine and involves primarily office work along with inpatient visits and consultations. Qualifications include BC/BE psychiatrist with concentration in biological medical treatments. Interested candidates may send CV to North Broward Hospital District, Physician Recruitment, 303 SE 17th Street, Suite 305, Fort Lauderdale, FL 33316.

PSYCHIATRIST: General psychiatrist, BC/BE, needed to develop a practice in conjunction with local community 231-bed hospital with the largest mental health system in the region, one hour from Pittsburgh, Pa. This Ohio opportunity has attractive compensation, medical directorships, private, group, and salaried opportunities, very attractive family lifestyle with the best of both a big city and a small town atmosphere. For more information, call 800-443-9346 or send CV to Richard L. Shrum, Vice President, Diamond Healthcare Corporation, 700 East Main Street, Suite 900, Richmond, VA 23219.

GENERAL/CHILD PSYCHIATRIST: Immediate opening in an expanding, fiscally sound, community hospital in the beautiful South West Virginia. Comprehensive diagnostic and treatment services provided in collaboration with local mental health agencies. Inpatient privileges at the local psychiatric facility possible, along with research opportunities. Salary range $100,000 plus, in addition to fringe benefits and incentives. For further information contact Sally Sturgill, 703-546-1815 or fax your CV 703-546-2048.

ILLINOIS: Outstanding opportunity for a BC/BE psychiatrist to join two other psychiatrists in a newly developed Regional Mental Health Center in Peru, Illinois. Includes a 20-bed psychiatry unit, a 1:3 call schedule, competitive salary or income guarantee, and a comprehensive benefits package. Peru, with a draw of 120,000, is located in the beautiful Illinois Valley where recreational activities abound, including sailing and cross country skiing. Together with excellent schools, diverse cultural opportunities, and a low cost of living, Peru offers superb quality of life. Contact Steve Baker at 800-430-6587 or Marie Noeth at 800-438-3745 or fax your CV to 309-685-2574.

TEXAS, the SOUTHEAST, and the SUNBELT STATES- There are Excellent Private Practice Opportunities Available in Psychiatry. Major Cities and Rural Communities Are Available.

Call 1-800-284-4560/Houston 713-493-2797

Or send CV to:
P.O. Box 42314
Houston, TX 77242-2314
FAX 713-493-2234

Reuben Bronstein & Associates

CHILD AND ADOLESCENT PSYCHIATRIST: Foote Hospital is a 488-bed, acute care facility in Jackson, Michigan. This financially strong, dynamic community hospital features a 210-member medical staff and a draw area of 285,000 people. Currently we are seeking a second Child/Adolescent Psychiatrist, either BE or BC, to join a hospital-employed group psychiatric practice which is part of The Center for Mental Health at Foote Hospital. This is a continuum-of-care program which includes a 50-bed inpatient psychiatric facility with a distinct adolescent unit. This position includes both inpatient and outpatient duties with at least 80% emphasis in child and adolescent psychiatry. The employment arrangement includes an excellent salary, bonus potential, comprehensive benefits package, and 1:7 on-call responsibility. You'll live and work in a safe, comfortable, and affordable community and enjoy an expanding recreation area filled with many lakes, golf courses, sports, and family facilities. For additional information, please call or send your CV to Kim Keller, Physician Recruiter, at 800-894-2694 or Elliot Wolf, MD, at 517-789-5910; WA Foote Memorial Hospital, 205 N East Avenue, Jackson, MI 49201; fax 517-789-5966. Equal Opportunity Employer.

Locum Tenens Wanted

HKA LOCUM TENENS is looking for quality general psychiatry physicians to do Locum Tenens. We have opportunities coast-to-coast. We furnish Occurence Malpractice Insurance (no tail necessary). Please call **HKA LOCUM TENENS at (800)226-6347, Extension AM7.1.**

© 1995 MAILSTAR

Chiefs/Department Heads/Directors

CHIEF OF PSYCHIATRY vacancy in 339-bed general medical-surgical VA facility with a tertiary psychiatric mission located at Fort Meade, SD, near Mount Rushmore in the Black Hills. Inpatient, outpatient, and outreach psychiatry services offered. Treatment programs include chemical dependency, PTSD, and ECT. Board certification and US citizenship required. JCAHO accredited. Affiliated with USD School of Medicine. Relocation assistance. No state income tax. Excellent secondary schools and colleges. Low crime rate, rural setting within 30 minutes of metro area. VA-maintained family quarters available. Contact Michael Davies, MD, Chief of Staff, 605-347-7172 or VA Medical Center (11), 113 Comanche Road, Fort Meade, SD 57741-1099. Equal Opportunity Employer.

THIS MONTH IN

ARCHIVES
OF
GENERAL PSYCHIATRY

In 1990, the National Institute of Mental Health embarked on the *National Plan for Research on Child and Adolescent Mental Disorders*, a widely heralded program to capitalize on opportunities to better understand the causes of these disorders and to enhance prevention and treatment efforts. **Leckman et al** (page 715), assessing the plan's impact at the midpoint of its implementation, found that the climate for child-related research has improved, but financial support for such research has fallen far short of that recommended in the plan. They conclude that both clinicians and the general public have much to gain from full implementation of the plan. Four commentaries discuss this update.

Patients with schizophrenia have been reported to have global, diffuse brain structure abnormalities. In a meta-analysis, **Elkis et al** (page 735) conclude that groups of patients with depression also have these brain abnormalities, but the size of the effect is smaller than that seen in patients with schizophrenia. These findings are relevant to the pathophysiology of depression and reinforce the suggestion that these abnormalities may be nonspecific.

For many years, psychiatrists have sought to understand the neurological basis of mood disorders. **Dupont et al** (page 747) found abnormalities in the white matter and thalamus of patients with bipolar mood disorder. In patients with unipolar disorder without accompanying medical illness, no abnormalities were found. The presence of structural abnormalities found in some reports of unipolar mood disorder may define a subgroup in which clinical depression reflects one outcome of brain injury.

Antipsychotic-induced tardive dyskinesia (TD) is a serious and potentially persistent movement disorder. In a study of middle-aged and elderly outpatients treated with typical or conventional antipsychotics, **Jeste et al** (page 756) found that in 26% of the patients, TD developed within 1 year; in 52%, within 2 years; and in 60%, within 3 years of treatment. This incidence was five to eight times greater than that reported in younger adults. Tardive dyskinesia was most likely to develop in patients treated with higher amounts of antipsychotics, especially high-potency ones, and in those with alcohol abuse or dependence or subtle movement disorder at baseline.

Self-injurious and autistic behavior are frequent problems in mentally retarded subjects who, according to pilot studies, might be treated with opioid antagonists such as naltrexone. In the largest double-blind, placebo-controlled, fixed-dose study to date, **Willemsen-Swinkels et al** (page 766) report that neither a single dose of 100 mg of naltrexone nor treatment with 50 mg or 150 mg for 4 weeks had therapeutic effects. Since treatment with 50 mg of naltrexone even appeared to aggravate behavior problems, the findings indicate that naltrexone cannot be recommended for the treatment of self-injurious or autistic behavior in mentally retarded subjects.

Despite substantial loss of noradrenergic locus ceruleus neurons in Alzheimer's disease, resting concentrations of norepinephrine in cerebrospinal fluid are normal or even increased. **Peskind et al** (page 774) measured cerebrospinal fluid norepinephrine concentrations following yohimbine, clonidine, and placebo administration in persons with Alzheimer's disease and in both young and older normal persons. Yohimbine increased cerebrospinal fluid norepinephrine levels more in Alzheimer's disease and normal older subjects than in young subjects and produced substantial agitation only in subjects with Alzheimer's disease. Central noradrenergic systems respond robustly to stimulation in Alzheimer's disease and may contribute to the agitated behaviors commonly present in this disorder.

Report Card on the *National Plan for Research on Child and Adolescent Mental Disorders*

The Midway Point

Members of the Committee for the Study of Research on Child and Adolescent Mental Disorders

A strong argument can be made that given the long-term impact of child and adolescent mental disorders, it is essential for the National Institutes of Health and other funding agencies in the public and private sectors to identify this as a priority in need of greater financial support. This document uses data provided by the National Institute of Mental Health and other sources to assess the impact of the National Plan for Research on Child and Adolescent Mental Disorders that was presented to Congress in 1990. Major gains are noted, particularly in the areas of services research and prevention. Investment in research training and career development has been modest and many deserving career development proposals have not been funded. A major shortcoming in the implementation of the national plan, thus far, has been that the National Institute of Mental Health has not yet taken steps to inform the public concerning the nature and impact of child and adolescent mental disorders. This report ends with an examination of the declining indicators of the status of children in the United States and the conclusion that concerted efforts are needed to educate all segments of society concerning the latest knowledge about these potentially devastating conditions and what can be done to prevent and treat them. Our most precious natural resource, our children and youth, is in jeopardy. It is time to build on advances in related fields of scientific inquiry and to continue to develop the knowledge-base needed to intervene effectively and lessen the enormous human and financial costs associated with these conditions.

(Arch Gen Psychiatry. 1995;52:715-723)

In response to requests from the US Senate and House of Representatives, the National Institute of Mental Health (NIMH), Rockville, Md, issued the *National Plan for Research on Child and Adolescent Mental Disorders* in 1990.[1] The impetus for this plan came from the growing recognition that

> Our Nation is needlessly wasting its most precious natural resource: our children and youth. We are permitting more than 12 percent of our children and adolescents—7.5 million young Americans—to suffer from mental disorders, often for life. And we are doing far too little to develop the scientific knowledge needed to treat or prevent their illness or lessen its enormous human and financial costs.

The plan was prepared by the National Advisory Mental Health Council of NIMH and was based on a report from the Institute of Medicine (IOM), *Research on Children and Adolescents With Mental, Behavioral, and Developmental Disorders,*[2] and on the recommendations of a National Advisory Mental Health Council ad hoc advisory group.

The 5-year national plan focused on three immediate goals: (1) develop and sustain a critical mass of basic and clinically oriented researchers focused on mental disorders that afflict children and adolescents, (2) stimulate a wide range of basic and clinical research at the frontiers of scientific inquiry, and (3) form an institute-wide consortium of NIMH program staff concerned with child and adolescent mental health research to implement the national plan.

A complete list of participants in the preparation of this report card are listed at the end of the article. This is not an "official" Institute of Medicine document, and it did not go through the National Research Council review process. The opinions expressed are those of the Institute of Medicine committee members.

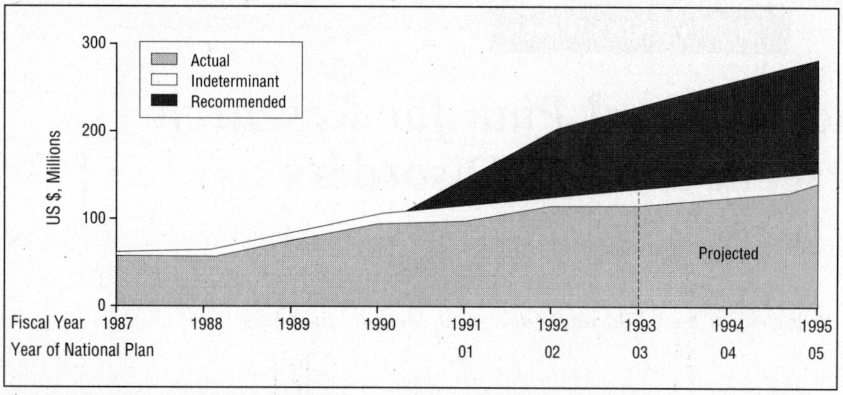

Figure 1. *Actual vs recommended funding for research on child and adolescent mental disorders by the National Institute of Mental Health (NIMH): FY 1987 to FY 1995 (projected). Based on figures made available by NIMH, the institute has fallen well short of its funding objectives as presented in the* National Plan for Research on Child and Adolescent Mental Disorders.[1] *The indeterminant zone refers to NIMH awards that in some way involve children or adolescent populations but whose major focus is on adult forms of mental disorder (see text).*

The recommended budget for the full implementation of the national plan called for a dramatic increase in monies directed toward research on child and adolescent mental disorders—from $57.7 million in fiscal year (FY) 1987 and $92.3 million in FY 1990 to $152.5 million in the first year (FY 1991) to $232.9 million in the third year (FY 1993) to $283.3 million in the final and fifth year (FY 1995) (**Figure 1**).

This "report card" and the invited commentaries are based on information provided by NIMH in the form of narrative summaries and financial data. Detailed information was provided for FY 1987 (before the national plan was envisioned) and FY 1993 (the midpoint of the national plan). It is hoped that this critique will serve to inform the field and assist NIMH in planning how best to achieve the remaining goals as outlined in the national plan.

OVERVIEW

Consonant with the aims of the national plan, there has been a 103% to a 120% overall increase in funding over FY 1987 levels for research on child and adolescent mental disorders (Figure 1). The greatest gain has been a nearly sevenfold increase in services research. Research on prevention and the acquired immunodeficiency syndrome also increased substantially. Basic behavioral and biomedical research has shown a slower rate of growth (79%). The Intramural Research Program has shown the slowest rate of growth (21%). Growth in research training and career development has also been modest, with many promising scientists failing to receive support because of a shortage of funds.

Given the targets established in the national plan, the funding levels for the first 3 years have consistently fallen short of those envisioned. In the third year of the national plan (FY 1993), at most 58% of the target level was achieved (Figure 1). This percentage (actual/target×100) steadily declined from 78% in the first year (FY 1991) to 63% in the second year (FY 1992) (Figure 1). These estimates, however, are almost certain to be overly generous given the difficulties associated with precisely dividing the amount of existing support for clinical research into child and adult categories. Indeed, these figures include the *entire* funding for any grant that has at least some component focused on children and/or adolescents.

For commentary see pages 724, 727, 729 and 732

To place these figures in perspective, it is important to consider the overall growth in the NIMH budget and the effects of inflation. From FY 1987 to FY 1993, the total research budget of NIMH increased 103%, from $288 million in FY 1987 to $583 million in FY 1993. Furthermore, when the effects of inflation are taken into account, the actual percentage increase in the total NIMH research budget approximates 52%. The comparable range for the inflation-adjusted increase in research funding for child and adolescent mental disorders is between 52% and 65%. Thus, it is reasonable to conclude that during this period of increased funding for research on mental disorders as a whole, funding for child and adolescent mental disorders research simply kept pace (or perhaps did slightly better) than the institute as a whole.

CAREER DEVELOPMENT

From FY 1987 to FY 1993, funding for research training and career development increased 88% (or a 41% increase after adjusting for the effects of inflation), with a 46% increase in the number of awards (summing across all relevant funding mechanisms). This level of funding is approximately 70% of what was called for in the national plan (**Figure 2**). Specific points include those discussed below.

In most areas, the proportion of funding devoted to research training and career development is approximately 20%. However, in the areas of services research and prevention, the proportions are markedly lower: 12% and 2%, respectively. Initiatives are needed to ensure that adequate numbers of new investigators enter these crucially important areas of research.

Since 1990, at least 20 worthy career development proposals ("K" Awards and R29 FIRST Awards) have not been funded, despite having received priority scores in the "outstanding" or the high end of the "excellent" range. While some of these grants have subsequently been funded on resubmission, many (10 to 15) have not. Additional support is needed to take full advantage of well-trained investigators who are just entering or who have made a commitment to this area of research.

Additional training initiatives are needed to foster interdisciplinary research. Specific gaps include the need to train developmental neuroscientists in the clinical features and natural history of the various child and adolescent mental disorders. In addition, patient-oriented researchers need to become more acquainted with the advances in the basic developmental neurosciences and in vivo neuroimaging techniques.

In sum, partly as a result of the national plan of the NIMH, there has been considerable growth in the area of career development of basic and clinical researchers interested in child and adolescent mental disorders. More efforts are needed to recruit, train, and sustain the careers of promising individuals early in their scientific careers. Good opportunities remain, particularly in the areas of services research and prevention. The more we can increase the number of investigators in these key areas, the greater will be the opportunities to develop and refine successful treatment and prevention programs.

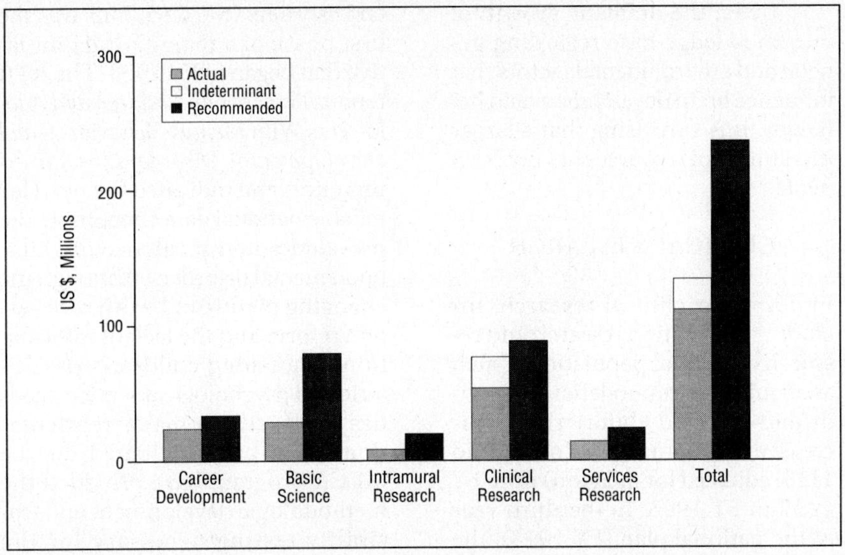

Figure 2. *Actual vs recommended funding for the third year of the* National Plan for Research on Child and Adolescent Mental Disorders[1] *of the National Institute of Mental Health (NIMH). Based on figures made available by NIMH, the institute has fallen well short of its funding objectives in the third year of the national plan. The categories are taken from Table 1 (p 47) of the publication describing the national plan.[1] The figures for clinical research include funds for prevention and acquired immunodeficiency syndrome research. The indeterminant zone (clinical research and total) refers to NIMH awards that in some way involve children or adolescent populations but whose major focus is on adult forms of mental disorder (see text). When these figures are adjusted for the effects of inflation, the actual amount of money spent on the intramural child and adolescent research programs of the NIMH has actually suffered a 9% decline.*

BASIC RESEARCH

Basic behavioral and biomedical research focused on issues of development increased 79% (or a 34% increase after adjusting for the effects of inflation) from FY 1987 to FY 1993. In the third year of the national plan (FY 1993), the projected level of support was $78 million, but the actual level of support was $26.1 million (not counting $8.2 million spent on research training and career development), or just 33% of the target (Figure 2). Most of the funded grants in this area are project grants (R01s), with only one center grant (P50) currently funded. Specific points include those discussed below.

The past several years have produced substantial gains in the basic understanding of the biologic (genetic, hormonal, and neurochemical) and environmental (family and social settings, as well as exposure to violence and trauma) factors that influence brain development. Advances in neurobiologic research have changed the way we view and understand the interactions between the brain and the environment. Much of this work is highly relevant to understanding the interactions between brain development, children's growth and development (normal and pathologic), and the larger environmental context. For example, while science has traditionally sought to discern the physiologic and hormonal influences that affect behavior, investigators are demonstrating the wide array of circumstances in which social structure and social behavior directly influence physiologic and hormonal processes. Understanding how children develop and how that process can lead to pathologic outcomes frequently includes broad multidisciplinary perspectives. To advance behavioral science in the child and adolescent area, there is a great need for the development of methods and measures that capture the complexities of multilevel (physiologic, behavioral, subjective, and contextual) approaches for studies of infants, children, adolescents, and their families. The NIMH needs to continue and expand efforts that address the persistent gap between research paradigms in developmental psychology and the other developmental neurosciences. Work performed in concert with other institutes, such as the National Institute of Neurological Disease and Stroke and the National Institute of Child Health and Human Development, and private foundations is needed to take advantage of this opportunity through mechanisms such as the Decade of the Brain and the Human Brain Project.

Funding for basic behavioral and social science research often involves longitudinal studies, which are inherently expensive and require stable funding. Recent accomplishments highlight the importance of early interpersonal relationships in shaping later behavioral outcomes. Specifically, an ongoing longitudinal study of low-income families has found that the strongest predictor of hostile behavior in childhood was the quality of the early mother-child relationship. Other studies of risk and protective factors have shown that neighborhood characteristics, such as the level of social disorganization and violence, in addition to family and individual characteristics, affect the pathways taken by urban adolescents in achieving academic success and personal competence. Child maltreatment is another understudied phenomenon. To move this area of science ahead, grant mechanisms may need to be modified or developed to encourage and support longitudinal research given the time constraints usually associated with traditional research awards.

Given the dramatic growth of our knowledge base regarding genetic and environmental factors that influence brain development and behavior, it is surprising that a larger investment of resources has not been made.

CLINICAL RESEARCH

Funding for clinical research, including prevention research and research on special populations (such as acquired immunodeficiency syndrome–infected children), has increased 150% to 180% (or 92% to 112% adjusted for inflation) from FY 1987 to FY 1993. In the third year of the national plan (FY 1993), the projected level of support was $85 million, and the actual support was between $50 million and $72 million. The precision of all of these estimates is limited by uncertainties about how much actual support for child and adolescent mental disorders research is contained in certain awarded grants coded by NIMH as falling in the child and adolescent mental disorders domain. In many instances, the principal focus of the grant is on adult mental disorders, but the grants have been included in the NIMH totals because, to a limited extent, they touch on developmental issues. Depending on how these figures are weighted, this level of funding is 59% to 85% of the target, with the 59% figure probably being more accurate (Figure 2). The program staff of NIMH have indicated that there are many project grants (R01s) rated in the "outstanding" or "excellent" range by study sections that are not being awarded because of a shortage of funds. Currently, only three program projects (P01s) and two center grants (P50s) focus on the clinical mental disorders of children and adolescents. These figures are well below the goals of the national plan. Specific points include those described below.

In the past several years, major programmatic efforts have been implemented in the area of epidemiology of child and adolescent mental disorders. In particular, a key study has been the Cooperative Agreement for Methodologic Research in Child and Adolescent Mental Disorders (MECA). This was the first phase of a major NIMH initiative that began in FY 1989. The IOM report, *Research on Children and Adolescents With Mental, Behavioral, and Developmental Disorders*, endorsed this effort and indicated the need for reliable national data concerning the prevalence and incidence of childhood mental disorders. Although the changing picture of health care system reform and the lack of information concerning children's psychiatric and psychological service needs has resulted in a major reorientation of this program, data from the MECA program have provided the methodologic development and feasibility testing necessary for the implementation of the Service Use, Need, Outcomes, and Costs for Child and Adolescent Populations (UNO-CAP) study, described below.

Substantial development is needed in the field of child and adolescent psychopharmacology. The number of funded psychopharmacologic studies has grown modestly from nine to 16 between 1987 and 1993, including a three-site multicenter study of lithium therapy for adolescent bipolar disorder. A number of substantial difficulties remain, however, in the development of pharmacologic research for children and adolescents. A major problem concerns the failure of pharmaceutical companies, NIMH, or others to fund research focused on the safety and efficacy of potentially useful psychotropic medications in the pediatric age range. This is an important public health concern because despite the lack of safety and efficacy data, millions of prescriptions are written each year for children and adolescents. While some of this use is for Food and Drug Administration–"approved" indications, most of these prescriptions are for "off-label" indications. The fact that many children appear to benefit from the use of psychoactive medications places parents and prescribing physicians in a dilemma as to the best course of action for specific children suffering from severe childhood mental or emotional disabilities. The NIMH is to be commended for its initiatives in bringing together representatives from the Food and Drug Administration, the Office of Protection From Research Risks, representatives from the pharmaceutical industry, child psychopharmacology researchers, and the lay community to enlist their help in addressing these issues. Partly as a result of consultative meetings, some encouraging signs of change have been observed. The Food and Drug Administration has begun to request pharmaceutical companies seeking new clinical indications for adult populations to examine the safety and efficacy of these medications in children and adolescents during "phase IV" trials. Continued efforts in this area are essential.

Somewhat greater growth has occurred in the area of psychosocial treatments, where the number of grants has increased from 10 to 20 in 1987 through 1993. This area shows real promise, as investigators are now beginning to adapt cognitive behavioral treatments developed initially for adult populations to adolescents. Findings are preliminary, but early evidence indicates that cognitive behavioral treatments are an effective treatment for adolescent major depressive disorder. Likewise, investigators have modified interpersonal therapy for use in adolescents, and clinical trials involving groups of depressed adolescents are under way.

Another important indicator of the growth of treatment research has been the increased number of research studies testing the efficacy of combined pharmacologic and psychosocial treatments. Currently, there are nine funded studies in this area, compared with zero in 1987. A major initiative in this area, the six-site multimodal treatment study of attention-deficit hyperactivity disorder, is the most complex and sophisticated treatment study undertaken to date by NIMH, incorporating recent advances in theory, method, and design to address major questions of relevance to national health care system reform and practitioners' "real-world" treatment concerns. This study is cofunded by the Department of Education. Similar studies are needed in adolescent depression and obsessive-compulsive disorder.

Advances in the area of in vivo neuroimaging hold promise for researchers focused on the neurobiologic origins of many childhood disorders, including schizophrenia, autism, attention-deficit hyperactivity disorder, Tourette's syndrome, obsessive-compulsive disorder, and specific mental retardation syndromes. At present, three-dimensional volumetric measurements of subcortical structures and ventricular spaces with the use of noninvasive magnetic resonance imaging have been the most extensively utilized. Ligand-based single photon emission computed tomography and positron emission tomography have gained some measure of acceptance in adolescent populations, despite their use of radioactive tracers. The most promising technologic developments have been in the area of functional magnetic resonance imaging and its remarkable temporal and spatial resolution. These noninvasive functional imaging techniques will be powerful tools to study aspects of normal development and psychopathologic states.

The NIMH has a broad program of theory-driven prevention research in children and adolescents that recognizes that multiple outcomes can arise from single risk factors and single outcomes can arise from multiple risk factors across multiple domains. Prevention research funded by NIMH is closely tied to advances in basic, clinical, and epidemiologic research. The 4 years since the issuance of the IOM report on child and adolescent mental disorders have seen a fourfold expansion in the area of prevention research. Currently, 83% of the funds and 57% of the grants in the prevention research branch portfolio are focused on children and adolescents.

In addition to the earlier IOM report, two subsequent reports have also given an account of the field of prevention research: the NIMH Prevention Steering Committee Report entitled *The Prevention of Mental Disorders: A National Research Agenda* and a congressionally mandated IOM report entitled *Reducing Risks for Mental Disorders: Frontiers for Preventive Intervention Research*.[3] These reports have major implications for the future directions of prevention research involving children, adolescents, and their families, and additional funds are needed to implement these initiatives.

INTRAMURAL RESEARCH

The NIMH Intramural Research Program has shown a 21% growth in funding from FY 1987 to FY 1993. In constant 1987 dollars, this actually represents a 9% decrease in funding. In the third year of the national plan (FY 1993), the projected level of support was $18 million, and the actual level of support was $5.1 million. This level of funding is just 28% of the target (Figure 2). Specific points include those discussed below.

The intramural program has a rich history of scientific accomplishment and a unique set of studies not easily duplicated elsewhere. These studies span clinical research (genetics, neurochemistry, neuroimmunology, neuroimaging, and treatment) with difficult-to-study populations, basic research, epidemiology, and prevention. Examples include studies of children with autism, childhood-onset schizophrenia, attention-deficit hyperactivity disorder, affective disorders, obsessive-compulsive disorder, and Tourette's syndrome.

Rather than expanding the number of child-focused intramural programs from two to three, as recommended in the national plan, it appears that NIMH is on the verge of decreasing the number from two to one (following the anticipated retirement of a senior laboratory director in the near future).

The NIMH intramural program is under enormous pressure to reduce its overall budget. Despite efforts to lessen the impact of these cuts on senior scientists (grades GS-14 and above), the resulting salary caps, hiring freeze, and actual layoffs have had a devastating impact on morale throughout the program. This austerity has affected virtually every laboratory at the NIMH, but the child and adolescent program has been particularly hard hit with the phasing out of an entire program of research.

In other respects, this crisis has been met with creativity and much-needed reforms. The creation of a consortium of investigators focused on child and adolescent disorders is sensible and long overdue. The formation of multidisciplinary groups is appropriate, and the inclusion of investigators with expertise in psychosocial and developmental perspectives can only strengthen this scientific effort. The anticipated reduction in support, however, of the intramural scientific program at NIMH with regard to child and adolescent mental disorders is shortsighted and wholly inconsistent with the spirit and letter of the national plan. These programs require a fair share of the available resources.

The intramural programs remain a premiere site for research training and career development, although their status in this regard has been jeopardized by below-par financial incentives and by the poor morale in the clinically oriented intramural research programs of NIMH generally.

SERVICES RESEARCH

Services research funding has increased 656% (467% increase, adjusting for the effects of inflation) from FY 1987 to FY 1993. In the third year of the national plan (FY 1993), the projected level of support was $20 million, and the actual level of support was $11 million. This level of funding is 54% of the target (Figure 2). As detailed below, three center grants (P50s) are currently funded, and a major national initiative is well under way. As in other research areas, funding for research training and career development has been tallied separately (see above). Specific points include those discussed below.

Service system integration models are being studied at the local county and state levels. These projects are investigating community-based service system models and linking these integrated programs with family and child outcomes. Private foundations working in conjunction with NIMH and the Substance Abuse and Mental Health Services Administration, such as the Robert Wood Johnson Foundation Mental Health Services for Youth program, have also taken the lead in this area.

Service utilization studies include examination of the types of services used by children and families across the major service sectors. For example, researchers in western North Carolina are examining service use by adolescents with mental and addictive disorders in a rural area of southern Appalachia. The goal of the study is to describe service use and to examine how the amount of service use (type of care, restrictiveness, intensity, and duration) is influenced over time by the interaction of disease comorbidity with individual, family, and community factors. Preliminary results indicate that the strongest predictor of service use among adolescents with severe mental disorders is the ability of family members to mobilize resources to care for their child.

Controlled studies of service effectiveness are still rare. Recent meta-analyses have found consistent evidence of the positive effects of psychotherapy from carefully controlled laboratory studies involving children and adolescents. However, similar analyses of the effect of therapy involving clinic samples in nonresearch settings have shown weaker or even negative effects. The reasons for these discrepant findings are unclear, but such findings suggest the need to bridge the gap between the laboratory and the clinic and to conduct research that is targeted for use in real-world practice settings.

DESPITE THESE advances, many research questions have not been studied. Such investigations could contribute to the formulation of public policies, such as the current debate on health care system reform. Areas in which knowledge is greatly needed include the effectiveness of services provided by the educational, foster care, and juvenile justice systems; comparative studies of community-based services vs residential treatment or hospital-based services; the effectiveness of services used by minority children and families; the impact of more direct parental involvement in treatment, service delivery planning, and service system design; and studies of alternative treatments and services, such as family preservation, therapeutic foster care, or wraparound services using flexible funding. There is also a need to examine the effects of cost-containment strategies on the provision of children's mental health services. The impact of alternative reimbursement and funding strategies within the public and private sectors also needs to be evaluated.

The recently funded UNO-CAP study should address some of these gaps in our knowledge. Specifically, this study involves a systematic study of children's mental health needs and services based on a representative national sample of children as well as a more in-depth examination of service needs and utilization in four regions across the country (Los Angeles, Calif; Baltimore, Md; St Louis, Mo; and Chapel Hill, NC). Results of this study will help delineate the extent of unmet need for mental health services in this country (including the prevalence and incidence of child and adolescent psychopathology at local and national levels), the patterns of service use provided across the major service sectors, and the barriers families face in accessing services. Furthermore, it will supply information on the socioeconomic, ethnic, family, community, and service system characteristics that influence entry into one or more service sectors; the clinical, developmental, functional, and service-related outcomes for children and adolescents who do and do not receive care; and the costs of care. The chance to follow up longitudinally a national sample of 7000 boys and girls, aged 4 to 17 years, provides unprecedented research opportunities to examine a range of putative risk and protective factors. Funding for the UNO-CAP study began in September 1994.

Given the continued interest in comprehensive, integrated services for children, joint activities are planned to coordinate the child and adolescent services research program with major initiatives emanating from the Center for Mental Health Services, a component of the Substance Abuse and Mental Health Services Administration. Through a joint program announcement, this combined effort by the Center for Mental Health Services and the NIMH will encourage investigators to refine the models of integrated service provision for children and adolescents, while incorporating effectiveness and outcome studies into the overall interventions.

DISSEMINATION AND ADVOCACY

The national plan called for the allocation of funds ($0.3 million to $1.3 million) to support the dissemination of scientific knowledge in the area of child and adolescent mental disorders. Although many programs and initiatives could be identified as responses to this mandate, NIMH has thus far missed the opportunity to engage Center for Mental Health Services and interested lay and professional organizations in a well-organized effort to inform the public concerning the magnitude and consequences of child and adolescent mental disorders and to convey in appropriate media settings the results of empiric research and the need to take advantage of advances in related scientific disciplines. Given the motivation and resources of such organizations as the National Alliance for the Mentally Ill and its Children and Adolescent Network, the National Mental Health Association and its Federation of Families for Child Mental Health, the National Alliance for Research on Schizophrenia and Affective Disorders, the National Depressive and Manic Depressive Association, the Tourette Syndrome Association, the Obsessive Compulsive Foundation, and others, much more can be done. The NIMH has failed to capitalize on its unique ability to convene these organizations and develop joint funding mechanisms to provide an impetus for concerned lay and professional organizations to work together to educate and inform both practitioners and the public. The initiative of the NIMH to increase the public's awareness of the signs and symptoms of depression and the availability of safe and efficacious treatments could serve as a useful model.[4-6]

LEADERSHIP

By 1990, the leadership of NIMH had developed a broad range of strategies to implement the national plan. As recommended in the original IOM report, an institute-wide Consortium for Research in Child and Adolescent Mental Disorders was established. A major goal of this consortium was to unify the field and provide national leadership for the many NIMH research activities related to children and adolescents. Specific strategies adopted by the consortium have included the following.

1. The development of new program announcements in specific, high-priority research areas. Many of these initiatives are reflected in the range of basic, epidemiologic, clinical, prevention, and services research documented above, including the MECA study, UNOCAP study, and the six-site multimodal treatment study of attention-deficit hyperactivity disorder described above.

2. Creation of a new initial research review committee. The Childhood Psychopathology and Treatment Committee convened for the first time in March 1992. It has had a substantial number of proposals to review (40 to 55) in each subsequent grant cycle.

3. Coordination of research initiatives in collaboration with other National Institutes of Health (NIH) institutes and government agencies. Specifically, contacts have begun with the National Institute of Child Health and Human Development, the National Institute of Neurological Disease and Stroke, Substance Abuse and Mental Health Services Administration, and the Department of Education to explore joint research approaches and funding strategies to address high-priority areas.

4. Developing funding partnerships with foundations. For example, the Child Consortium has begun collaborating with several major foundations (W. T. Grant and the John D. and Catherine T. MacArthur foundations) to consider mechanisms whereby private and public sources of funding can collaborate to develop the much-needed research in the areas of child and adolescent mental disorders. Preliminary work in this regard has led one foundation to sponsor and fund two Developmental Child Centers in early FY 1992.

A major challenge to the viability and effectiveness of the national plan is and will be the impact of leadership changes at NIMH (there have been two directors and two acting directors at NIMH since the inception of the national plan) and adjustments that will be necessary with the reintegration of NIMH within the NIH. The consortium and its chair, Peter Jensen, MD, have played an essential and vital role in moving ahead the recommendations of the IOM report. Its continued health will be essential for the success of the national plan and in formulating the next phase of development as this scientific field matures.

A PRIORITY AREA—FOR OUR CHILDREN, FAMILIES, AND OUR FUTURE

The scientific community has repeatedly identified research on child and adolescent mental disorders as a priority area for increased funding.[1,2] A strong argument can be made that, given the long-term impact of child and adolescent mental disorders, anything short of the level of funding called for the national plan would be unwise.[2] In some instances, such as in autistic disorder, the impact is obvious, devastating, and lifelong. Other conditions, such as prepubertal major depression, are associated with significant levels of morbidity and mortality. For many other conditions, including mood and anxiety disorders, affected children and adolescents are at increased risk to develop adult mental disorders, while a significant proportion of children and adolescents diagnosed as having conduct disorder will enter the criminal justice system. As a result, it is appropriate to include not only the direct costs to families and society associated with these disorders but also a portion of the costs associated with adult psychiatric morbidity and mortality (decreased productivity in the workplace and the need for social welfare supports) and criminal outcomes to measure the true cost to society of child and adolescent mental disorders.

This argument is further strengthened by an examination of the declining indicators of the status of children in this country: the high rate (>20%) of children living in poverty,[7] increasing rates of child maltreatment,[8] the high rates of dropping out of school[9] and teenage pregnancy,[10] the increasing violence of urban youth culture,[11] and the knowledge that these risk factors are and will be associated with increasing rates of child and adolescent mental disorders. These figures emphasize that it is time to *overinvest* in our children if we care about their future.

Alternatively, the promising advances in related fields of genetics and the developmental neurosciences suggest that this is an especially propitious time to invest in research on the biologic determinants of child and adolescent mental disorders. Indeed, there is compelling evidence that the mechanisms responsible for some adult-onset disorders, such as schizophrenia and Alzheimer's disease, involve abnormalities in early brain development.

The argument can also be made that this field of research has long been underfunded. Based on the demographic yardstick, in 1990, there were 65 million children and adolescents younger than 18 years, or 26% of the total US population of 253 million.[12] In contrast, the proportion of the total research budget of NIMH that has been allocated to child and adolescent mental disorders has been consistently less during the past 7 years (FY 1987, 19% to 22%; FY 1988, 17% to 20%; FY 1989, 19% to 22%; FY 1990, 19% to 24%; FY 1991, 19% to 23%; FY 1992, 19% to 23%; and FY 1993, 19% to 23%). Depending on the year, the shortfall between the actual funding vs what might be expected based on the demographic yardstick of 26% of the total research budget ranges between $15 million and $38 million per year for each of the past 7 years.

It is a critically important time for the federal government to invest in our families. Advances in clinical, prevention, and services research have had and will continue to have direct benefits for families. The provision of state-of-the-art services tailored to local and regional needs is an important priority that must be supported by basic and clinical research at the frontiers of scientific inquiry.

CONCLUSIONS

Overall, the report card for NIMH on the national plan is mixed, with some components nearly fully realized and others scarcely addressed.

1. The *National Plan for Research on Child and Adolescent Mental Disorders* announced in 1990 has had a discernable impact on the level of funding for this area. Greatest gains have occurred in services research and prevention programs. The NIMH is to be commended for moving ahead with the UNO-CAP study, which will provide for the first time national prevalence, service, and needs assessment data for child and adolescent mental disorders. Other bright spots include the multisite trial of combined cognitive-behavioral and pharmacologic treatment of attention-deficit hyperactivity disorder. On the whole, clinical research has fared better than basic research.

2. The formation of the institute-wide consortium has provided essential leadership for the implementation of the plan. The creation of an initial review committee devoted to assessing the scientific merit of grant proposals in this area has also had a major positive impact. Care is needed to preserve these gains, given leadership changes at NIMH and the reintegration of the institute into the larger NIH structure.

3. Gains in the funding of research for child and adolescent mental disorders have been commensurate with an overall increase in the total research budget for NIMH. The proportion of research funds (19% to 23%) directed toward child and adolescent mental disorders has not changed during the past 7 years. These figures fall short of what was called for as part of the national plan and do not reflect the priority that research in this area should receive and do not meet a more basic standard, given that 26% of the US population is younger than 18 years.

4. Investment in research training and career development has been modest, and many excellent career development proposals have not been funded. This is a critical issue if the capacity-building aspects of the national plan are to be realized.

5. The intramural NIMH programs focused on child and adolescent mental disorders are in crisis and are absorbing a disproportionate share of the cuts in funding. One of the two existing programs is being phased out. Innovative efforts are under way to diminish the adverse impact and improve morale, but valuable national resources that have been premier sites for scientific progress and research training are at risk.

6. A major shortcoming in the implementation of the national plan has been the failure of NIMH to facilitate dissemination of knowledge concerning child and adolescent mental disorders and their treatment. Concerted efforts of many public and private organizations are needed to educate all segments of society—both lay and professional—concerning the latest knowledge about these devastating conditions and what can be done to prevent and treat them. A national program such as that undertaken to educate and disseminate knowledge concerning depression and other major affective disorders is needed.

7. Research on child and adolescent mental disorders remains a priority area in need of greater funding. Our nation continues to waste needlessly its most precious natural resource: our children and youth. For the millions of young Americans suffering from mental disorders, we are doing far too little to develop the scientific knowledge needed to treat or prevent their illness or lessen its enormous human and financial costs. In the mid-1990s, in a time of increasingly scarce resources for research, what is the appropriate yardstick to measure how much support is needed? A strong argument can be made that, given the long-term impact of child and adolescent mental disorders, it is essential for NIH and other funding agencies in the public and private sectors to identify this as a priority area in need of greater funding. It is time to invest *fully* in our children if we care about their future and the future of our society.

Accepted for publication January 23, 1995.

This report card was commissioned by the American Academy of Child and Adolescent Psychiatry in the spring of 1994. The authors thank Peter Jensen, MD, and other members of the NIMH Consortium for Research on Children and Adolescent Mental Disorders for their hard work on behalf of children and adolescents with mental, behavioral, and developmental disorders. We are also grateful for their assistance in preparing the materials used to compile this report card. Thanks to Rex Cowdry, MD, the acting director of NIMH, and Michael Brownstein, MD, PhD, the former acting intramural chief of NIMH, for their candor, advice, and support of this effort. We are also grateful for the encouragement and support of Virginia Q. Anthony, executive director, American Academy of Child and Adolescent Psychiatry, and her critique of an earlier version of the report.

Members of the original IOM committee who assisted in the preparation of this report card include James F. Leckman, MD (chair)*; Glen R. Elliott, MD* (vice-chair)*; Evelyn J. Bromet, PhD; Magda Campbell, MD; Dante Cicchetti, PhD; Donald J. Cohen, MD; John J. Conger, PhD; Joseph T. Coyle, MD; Felton J. Earls, MD; Ronald Feldman, PhD; Morris Green, MD; Beatrix Hamburg, MD; Alan E. Kazdin, PhD; David R. Offord, MD; Dominick Purpura, MD; Albert J. Solnit, MD; and Frederic Solomon, MD. Robert M. Cook-Deegan, MD, former director of the Division of Biobehavioral Sciences and Mental Disorders at the IOM, also assisted in the preparation of this report card.*

The full text of this report card has been formally endorsed by the following organizations: the American Academy of Child and Adolescent Psychiatry, the American Academy of Pediatrics, the American Family Foundation, the American Medical Association, the American Psychiatric Association, the American Psy-

chological Association, the American Society for Adolescent Psychiatry, the Association of Child and Adolescent Psychiatric Nurses, Bazelon Center for Mental Health Law, Children and Adults With Attention-Deficit Disorder, the Federation of Families for Children's Mental Health, the International Association of Child and Adolescent Psychiatry and Allied Professions, the Leon Lowenstein Foundation, the National Alliance for the Mentally Ill, the National Alliance for Research on Schizophrenia and Depression, the National Association of School Psychologists, the National Association of Psychiatric Treatment Centers for Children, the National Mental Health Association, the National Depressive and Manic Depressive Association, the Obsessive Compulsive Foundation, the Society for Neuroscience, the Society for Research on Child and Adolescent Psychopathology, the Society for Research in Child Development, the Tourette Syndrome Association, and the W. T. Grant Foundation.

Reprint requests to Sterling Hall of Medicine, Child Study Center, Room I-269, Yale University School of Medicine, New Haven, CT 06520-7900 (James F. Leckman, MD).

REFERENCES

1. National Institute of Mental Health. *National Plan for Research on Child and Adolescent Mental Disorders: A Report Requested by the US Congress Submitted by the National Advisory Mental Health Council.* Rockville, Md: US Dept of Health and Human Services, Alcohol, Drug Abuse, and Mental Health Administration; 1990. US Dept of Health and Human Services publication 90-1683.
2. Institute of Medicine. *Research on Children and Adolescents With Mental, Behavioral, and Developmental Disorders.* Washington, DC: National Academy Press; 1989.
3. Institute of Medicine. *Reducing Risks for Mental Disorders: Frontiers for Preventive Intervention Research.* Washington, DC: National Academy Press; 1994.
4. Depression Guideline Panel. *Clinical Practice Guideline: Depression in Primary Care: Detection and Diagnosis.* Rockville, Md: US Dept of Health and Human Services, Agency for Health Care Policy and Research; 1993:1. Agency for Health Care Policy and Research publication 93-0550. Depression Guideline Panel. *Clinical Practice Guide*
5. line: Depression in Primary Care: Treatment of Major Depression. Rockville, Md: US Dept of Health and Human Services, Agency for Health Care Policy and Research; 1993:1. Agency for Health Care Policy and Research publication 93-0550.
6. Depression Guideline Panel. *Clinical Practice Guideline: Depression Is a Treatable Illness: A Patient's Guide.* Rockville, Md: US Dept of Health and Human Services, Agency for Health Care Policy and Research; 1993. Agency for Health Care Policy and Research publication 93-0553.
7. US Department of Commerce, Bureau of the Census. *Current Population Reports, Ser P-60, Number 168, Money Income and Poverty Status in the United States.* Washington, DC: US Printing Office; 1989.
8. US Department of Health and Human Services. *Child Abuse and Neglect: Critical First Steps in Response to a National Emergency.* Washington, DC: US Printing Office; 1990.
9. Kaufman P, Frase MJ. *Dropout Rates in the United States: 1989.* Washington, DC: US Printing Office; 1990.
10. Hayes CD, ed. *Risking the Future: Adolescent Sexuality, Pregnancy, and Childbearing.* Washington, DC: National Academy Press; 1987.
11. US Department of Health and Human Services, National Center for Health Statistics. *Firearm Mortality Among Children, Youth, and Young Adults 1-34 Years of Age, Trends and Current Status: United States, 1979-1988.* Washington, DC: US Printing Office. Monthly Vital Statistics Report 39, No. 11.
12. US Department of Commerce, Bureau of the Census. *Census 1990.* Washington, DC: US Printing Office; 1993.

The Report Card

Progress Report or Final Grade?

IT IS NO coincidence that the appraisal[1] of the *National Plan for Research on Child and Adolescent Mental Disorders*[2] should be referred to as "a report card." As all of us recall, report cards are what we got in school to let us know how our performance stacked up against teacher and curriculum expectations. In this case, the curriculum designers were the Institute of Medicine (IOM) Committee (IOM) for the Study of Research on Child and Adolescent Mental Disorders, chaired by James Leckman, MD, and Glen R. Elliot, MD, in consort with eminent committee members and task forces. The National Institute of Mental Health (NIMH), Bethesda, Md, which developed the national plan, is presumably getting the report card.

See also pages 715, 727, 729, and 732

By way of history, the NIMH had asked the IOM to study the current status of research on child and adolescent mental disorders. The committee was convened in July 1988, and its report[3] was published 1 year later. The report was submitted to the House Committee on Appropriations, which directed the NIMH's National Advisory Mental Health Council to prepare a 5-year plan implementing the IOM's recommendations, which was to be acted on prior to the 1991 budget. It was published in 1990,[2] and a program announcement from the NIMH implementing the national plan was released in April 1991.

Unfortunately, the report card, although written at the "midway point," is being disseminated not only at the end of the term but possibly at the end of the course. Given that this was a 5-year plan, it would appear that there is little time left for the grade to be improved. It is unclear whether we have the option of repeating the course or asking for an extension before the final grade is submitted or whether the interim report card is, in fact, the final grade. I would hope that it is not the latter.

It is difficult to argue with the conclusions of the IOM report. The bottom line was that it is imperative to boost the knowledge base by which serious child mental health problems could be prevented and treated. The national plan goals that were designed to execute this, as summarized in the report card, were to form an "institute-wide consortium of NIMH program staff concerned with child and adolescent mental health research to implement the national plan" (the Child/Adolescent Disorders Research Branch is an outgrowth of this), stimulate a wide range of basic and clinical research, and develop and maintain a critical mass of interdisciplinary researchers focused on child and adolescent mental health problems.[1] Of these, the last has failed most miserably, partly because of funding problems and partly because it takes much longer than 5 years to grow and sustain dedicated scientists. To implement the national plan, the NIMH was empowered to put its budget where its mouth was and vastly increase the funding and initiatives to best utilize the increased funding.

The report card basically catalogs the budgetary shortfall that has occurred, in some areas more than others, over the past 4 years. If one looks at the cup as half full, one sees that as a result of the 5-year plan, spending definitely has increased. The half-empty version says that the increase was not as much as was promised or needed. The lowest grades go to the inadequate funding given to research career development and to the lack of NIMH support for intramural research in child psychiatry. It is not clear whether this state of affairs is solely the result of budgetary allocations within the NIMH, indicating a less-than-wholehearted response to the national plan, or of the emergence of new, competing priorities elsewhere. It is unfortunate that the need to expand resources for such research and training has come at a time when Congress has been focused on budget cutting and the NIMH has been without permanent leadership. Discretion being the better part of valor, one assumes that the report card drafters chose not to place blame but merely to indicate where the deficiencies were.

The demise of the intramural child development research program appears to represent a reality (retirement of the "senior laboratory director"). However, although the program could have been reoriented under new leadership, it is likely that the opportunity the "retirement" presented in terms of funding reallocation was too good to miss.

Another criticism leveled at the NIMH by the report card is that "a major shortcoming in the implementation of the national plan has been the failure of NIMH to facilitate dissemination of knowledge concerning child and adolescent mental disorders and their treatment."[1] Interestingly, the same could be said for the report card. What is missing is what kind of bang we have gotten so far for the buck that has been spent. As a taxpayer, clinical researcher, and practicing child psychiatrist, I would like to know what kinds of information I am likely to have that would not have been forthcoming without this initiative. Communication of the findings emanating from this presumably crème de la crème of proposals is likely to be long in coming because grant writers spend an ever-increasing amount of time submitting and resubmitting grants and not writing the peer-reviewed, scientific papers needed to disseminate results. Worse yet is the fact that specialty journals are multiplying like rabbits. Although these provide an outlet for more papers to be published, they are unlikely to be very widely read. Finally, and most troubling, is the fact that we have not developed a mechanism to communicate to the general public what we are doing.

To return to positive accomplishments, if the NIMH has been somewhat hampered by lack of permanent leadership, leadership in the Child/Adolescent Disorders Research Branch has been capable, energetic, and creative. Actually, most of the NIMH branches have solicited an interesting distribution of child-related grants. According to the 1994 Active Grants Listing (Peter Jensen, MD, written communication [available on request from Dr Jensen's office, NIMH]), of all the proposals devoted exclusively or in part to the younger-than-18-year-old population, about 45% are in basic behavioral science and child/adolescent disorders; 11%, in basic prevention or prevention research; approximately 4% to 6% each, in basic sciences and epidemiology and basic sciences; and 7.5%, in violence and traumatic stress research (**Table**). However, this represents only the numbers of grants in each branch, not the amount of dollars allocated to them. For instance, I do not know what percentage of child research moneys are being devoted to the massive epidemiologic services survey UNO-CAP (Service Use, Need, Outcomes, and Costs for Child and Adolescent Populations) project.

Child-Related Grants*

NIMH, No. (%)	
Affective disorders	52 (9.2)
Behavioral neuroscience	22 (3.9)
Basic behavioral science	115 (20.2)
Child and adolescent disorders	141 (24.8)
Epidemiology	34 (6.2)
Health services research	53 (9.3)
Molecular cell biology	15 (2.6)
Minority training	9 (1.5)
Basic prevention	29 (5.1)
Prevention Research Branch	33 (5.8)
Instrumentation and small business	11 (1.9)
Schizophrenia	10 (1.8)
Violence and trauma	43 (7.6)
Child/Adolescent Disorders Research Branch, %	
Attention-deficit hyperactivity disorder	14
Psychopharmacology	8.5
Anxiety disorders	7
Autism, fragile X syndrome, and developmental disabilities	14.9
Suicidal behavior	6.3
Training and research	10
Depression	8.5
Aggression and conduct disorder	14
Other	17

**Data are from the National Institute of Mental Health (NIMH), Bethesda, Md (Peter Jensen, MD, written communication, 1994), and include grants devoted exclusively or in part to the younger-than-18-year-old population.*

As a child and adolescent psychiatrist, I find even more fascinating the types of projects that have been funded by the Child/Adolescent Disorders Research Branch. Although many proposals cut across numerous categories in my classification system, it appears that about 14% of grants each addressed attention-deficit hyperactivity disorder, conduct disorder and aggression, and autism and fragile X syndrome. Approximately another 6% to 8% each addressed suicidal behavior, depression, anxiety disorders, and psychopharmacology. About 10% of the studies funded in this branch were dedicated to training programs, and the remaining 17% covered a multitude of areas (Table). As indicated earlier, the proportion of funding devoted to each of these areas is not necessarily correlated with the number of grants. The fact that many more exciting proposals have gone unfunded is indeed unfortunate.

Will there be another 5-year plan? Just as a few doses of methylphenidate are not going to reverse years of attention-deficit hyperactivity disorder, it would be woefully shortsighted to think that a relatively brief, somewhat tempered bit of attention could reverse the long-term problems associated with inattention to child mental health. Moreover, besides the need to continue to advocate for the items that were originally proposed, there are at least two new questions that our NIMH leadership (and perhaps the leadership of private foundations as well) should be asking: (1) In the land of the shrinking research dollar, where should we be putting our focus? and (2) In charting a course for the next 5 years, of what land mines should we be mindful? Certainly, the shifting priorities of health care are shaping the kinds of research we are doing, and there are a plethora of serious problems that need to be addressed.

When I see a child with the usual combination of behavior problems, mood problems, learning difficulties, and family disruption, I frequently ask him or her, "If a fairy godmother could remove one problem, which would it be?" In a similar vein, if the "fairy godmother" could eliminate one symptom or behavior, which would have the greatest consequences for child mental health? Irritable, impulsive aggression would be highest on my list. In cooperation with the various mental health leaders of Suffolk County, New York, I conducted a 1-month (March 1991) survey of reasons children and adolescents (n=1263) were being treated by emergency psychiatric services, county and state mental health clinics, and state and private psychiatric hospitals. Aggression—in particular, irritable, explosive aggression—was the No. 1 reason children aged 12 years or younger were treated with crisis services and outpatient, inpatient, and day-treatment programs. For adolescent inpatients, it was the chief reason for treatment in the local state children's psychiatric hospital. It was the second most common reason for adolescent admission to private hospitals. It is undoubtedly associated with a longer length of stay in hospitals, referral for special education classes, and multiplicity of foster home placements among young children. It is also a major behavior problem in developmentally disabled children and adults. This symptom cuts across diagnoses, being the major culprit in admissions for acute mania, conduct and oppositional defiant disorder, and attention-deficit hyperactivity disorder. It contributes to the acute problems of agitated depression and schizophrenia. It is stable over time, affects both genders and all races, and leads to morbidity and mortality in all ages. Remarkably, there seems to be little interest in developing psychopharmacologic interventions, if the recent NIMH-sponsored workshop convening scientists, clinicians, Food and Drug Administration officials, drug company representatives, and parent advocates is representative of experts in the field. Perhaps this is a reflection of what may be seen as the political sensitivity to the topic of aggression in general. However, for the young people I have seen who were rejected by peers and family because of their unpredictable outbursts and the remorse and low self-esteem they suffer as a consequence, I have no doubts that they would be grateful if a fairy godmother removed this problem. Because there are no fairy godmothers, leaders in the field will have to substitute.

The changing landscape of health care is likely to add an additional hurdle to the execution of important and sensible research. The gap between clinicians and established researchers is likely to widen. Funded researchers will need to dedicate increasing amounts of time to grant submission and resubmission and will have even less time to be exposed to clinical realities. Conversely, clinically oriented academicians will not have the luxury of sitting on editorial boards, national committees, and study sections (because these activities essentially are not remunerated) to provide the reality check that is often needed.

Much publicity and lip service is given to children and their needs. Emblazoned on all of our minds currently is the photograph of a fireman rescuing a mortally wounded child from the devastation of the bombed government building in Oklahoma City, Okla. However, in a nation that has a chronic "retention-deficit disorder," the long-term mental health and even physical health needs of children are easily forgotten for politically more profitable reasons. A long-term, special-education approach will be needed for a discipline that is chronically fiscally challenged.

Gabrielle A. Carlson, MD
Department of Psychiatry and Behavioral Sciences
State University of New York–Stony Brook
Putnam Hall
Stony Brook, NY 11794-8790

REFERENCES

1. Members of the Committee for the Study of Research on Child and Adolescent Mental Disorders. Report card on the *National Plan for Research on Child and Adolescent Mental Disorders*: the midway point. *Arch Gen Psychiatry.* 1995; 52:715-723.
2. National Institute of Mental Health. *National Plan for Research on Child and Adolescent Mental Disorders: A Report Requested by the US Congress Submitted by the National Advisory Mental Health Council.* Rockville, Md: US Dept of Health and Human Services, Alcohol, Drug Abuse, and Mental Health Administration; 1990. DHHS publication 90-1683.
3. Institute of Medicine. *Research on Children and Adolescents With Mental, Behavioral, and Developmental Disorders.* Washington, DC: National Academy Press; 1989.

Comments on the Report Card From a Services Research Perspective

FROM THE perspective of services delivery and services research, the Institute of Medicine (IOM) report[1] and the "report card" by the IOM Committee for the Study of Research on Child and Adolescent Mental Disorders[2] in this issue of the ARCHIVES reflect a flawed and circumscribed perspective. That perspective needs revision. The original IOM report limited itself to research relating primarily to diagnosable mental disorders. It dealt with phenomena such as drug abuse, teen pregnancy, and dropping out of school as consequences of or risk factors for developing mental disorders.

A POLICY-FOCUSED PERSPECTIVE

Conditions that significantly affect large numbers of lives warrant a high priority. Examples of such conditions are conduct disorder, substance abuse, violence, abuse/neglect, and the use of psychotropic medication in the treatment of children and adolescents. Unfortunately, the attention and resources these prevalent problems receive is meager. Research expenditures per year of potential life lost by violence are 10-fold to 20-fold less than corresponding expenditures for cancer, the acquired immunodeficiency syndrome, or cardiovascular disease.[3]

The current lack of documentation on child and adolescent disorders promotes a failure to appreciate the impact and consequences for our society. Support for research is needed from many agencies, such as the National Institute on Drug Abuse, National Institute on Alcohol Abuse and Alcoholism, Food and Drug Administration, Department of Education, and National Institute of Justice.

The information deficit is appalling. As of February 1995, we could not find a single published controlled-outcome study of treatment for substance abuse in adolescents. Most of the time, children who receive psychotropic medications do so without indications approved by the Food and Drug Administration[4,5] because the research has not been done.

See also pages 715, 724, 729, and 732

The population of children and adolescents is growing. Both the absolute number of births and the birth rate increased substantially from 1975 to 1990.[6] Moreover, the number of children born at elevated risk for psychiatric problems also increased. Very-low-birth-weight children (<1.5 kg) have significantly raised odds of behavioral and neurocognitive problems,[7,8] even after controlling for social risk.[9] The prevalence of very-low-birth-weight infants increased from 11.6 per 1000 live births in 1975 to 12.4 per 1000 live births in 1987.[10] In addition, improved survival for very-low-birth-weight infants is unequivocal throughout the industrialized world.[11]

The rates of problems among children and adolescents are also on the rise. The incidence of adolescent suicide has risen significantly. Once thought to be a phenomenon limited to white male youths,[12] the rise in suicide has spread to African-American male youths.[13] The rate among girls has not risen significantly. Concurrently, the age of onset for violent crime is decreasing.[14] Thus, not only are the absolute numbers of children and adolescents increasing, but per capita disorders and their severity are increasing as well.

Abuse or neglect, the most common reason children enter foster care, increases the risk for psychiatric disorders in childhood and later[15,16] and for aggression toward others.[17] A recent review of the health status of vulnerable populations in the United States concluded,

> the number of children abused by family members or other intimates has burgeoned to an estimated 1.6 to 1.7 million per year, and with the greater use of firearms, intentional acts of violence towards oneself or others are becoming increasingly deadly in their consequences.[18]

The issues cited above necessarily have a great impact on the schools. Seriously emotionally disturbed students have lower grades than any other group of students with disabilities.[19] Only 42% of seriously emotionally disturbed youths graduate from high school as opposed to 50% of all youths with disabilities and 76% of the general population.[19] Twenty percent of seriously emotionally disturbed youths are arrested at least once before they leave school as opposed to 9% of students with other disabilities and 6% of the general school population.

Mental disorders are debilitating, and the presence of students with mental disorders makes many schools less conducive to learning.

There are indirect costs of mental illness other than reduced productivity. There are economic costs to families with a mentally ill family member.[20] Indirect costs also have important implications for policy.

RESPONSE TO OUR INFORMATION DEFICIT

The perspective of the original IOM report was understandable given the shortfalls in knowledge, available methods, personnel, and infrastructure resources. The intent was to remedy these deficits by spurring a significant increase in this area of mental health research. The constrained definition of mental health research was thought to facilitate progress. However, the need for knowledge has grown. Health care costs, consumer expectations, policy needs, and the morbidity and mortality associated with mental illness have increased. We need more research and a broader perspective to guide our research, but increased funding will not be enough.

Even if we had infinite funds for research on childhood mental disorders, we would still have to identify priorities. There is only a limited number of trained investigators in child and adolescent mental health and an even more limited number of trained services researchers. Not only must traditional initiatives be undertaken to ensure that adequate numbers of investigators enter services research but more fundamental training must also occur, especially within child and adolescent psychiatry. We need to move our faculty and our child and adolescent training programs from the realm of personal experience to the realm of rigorous clinical investigation[21] with an emphasis on data and research literacy.

It is important to enlarge the scope of research beyond that traditionally funded by the National Institute of Mental Health to include a larger coalition of interested parties and funding sources. A recent conference[22] in Washington, DC, cosponsored by the National Institute of Mental Health and the Food and Drug Administration was attended by representatives of advocacy groups, foundations, professional organizations, and major pharmaceutical companies; by researchers from other National Institutes of Health; and by experts on bioethical and legal issues concerning children, adolescents, and health care policy. A consensus was established about the need for psychopharmacologic research for children and adolescents, and some necessary steps were identified.

Acknowledging that there are not enough investigators, not enough data, and increasing needs, what is the progress to date? Parity in funding has not been achieved. Outstanding proposals for child and adolescent psychopathologic illness and treatment research go unfunded. Let's be clear about the report card: the letter grade is *F*.

Markus J. P. Kruesi, MD
Boris Astrachan, MD
Department of Psychiatry
Institute for Juvenile Research
University of Illinois–Chicago
M/C 747
907 S Wolcott Ave
Chicago, IL 60612

REFERENCES

1. Institute of Medicine. *Research on Children and Adolescents With Mental, Behavioral, and Developmental Disorders.* Washington, DC: National Academy Press; 1989.
2. Members of the Committee for the Study of Research on Child and Adolescent Mental Disorders. Report card on the *National Plan for Research on Child and Adolescent Mental Disorders:* the midway point. *Arch Gen Psychiatry.* 1995; 52:715-723.
3. Reiss AJ Jr, Roth JA, eds. *Understanding and Preventing Violence.* Washington, DC: National Academy Press; 1993.
4. Jensen PS, Vitello B, Leonard H, Laughren TP. Design and methodology issues for clinical treatment trials in children and adolescents. *Psychopharmacol Bull.* 1994;30:3-8.
5. Zito JM, Craig TJ, Wanderling J. Pharmacoepidemiology of 330 child/adolescent psychiatric patients. *J Pharmacoepidemiol.* 1994;3:47-62.
6. *Statistical Abstract of the United States: 1993.* 113th ed. Washington, DC: US Bureau of the Census; 1993.
7. Breslau N, Klein N, Allen L. Very low birthweight: behavioral sequelae at nine years of age. *J Am Acad Child Adolesc Psychiatry.* 1988;27: 605-612.
8. McCormick MC, Gortmaker SL, Sobol AM. Very low birth weight children: behavior problems and school difficulty in a national sample. *J Pediatr.* 1990;117:687-693.
9. Hack M, Breslau N, Aram D, Weissman B, Klein N, Borawski-Clark E. The effect of very low birth weight and social risk on neurocognitive abilities at school age. *Dev Behav Pediatr.* 1992;13: 412-420.
10. Centers for Disease Control. Low birthweight—United States, 1975-1987. *MMWR Morb Mortal Wkly Rep.* 1990;39:148-151.
11. Bhushan V, Paneth N, Kiely JL. Impact of improved survival of very low birth weight infants on recent secular trends in the prevalence of cerebral palsy. *Pediatrics.* 1993;91:1094-1100.
12. Ryland DH, Kruesi MJP. Suicide among adolescents. *Int Rev Psychiatry.* 1992;4:185-195.
13. Shaffer D, Gould M, Hicks RC. Worsening suicide rates in black teenagers. *Am J Psychiatry.* 1994;151:1810-1812.
14. Tracy P, Wolfgang M, Figlio R. *Delinquency Careers in Two Birth Cohorts.* New York, NY: Plenum Press; 1990.
15. Malinosky-Rummel R, Hansen DJ. Long-term consequences of childhood physical abuse. *Psychol Bull.* 1993;114:68-79.
16. Kendall-Tacket KA, Williams LM, Finkelhor D. Impact of sexual abuse on children: a review and synthesis of recent empirical studies. *Psychol Bull.* 1993;113:164-180.
17. Widom CS. The cycle of violence. *Science.* 1989; 244:160-166.
18. Aday LA. Health status of vulnerable populations. *Annu Rev Public Health.* 1994;15:487-509.
19. *Youth With Disabilities: How Are They Doing? The First Comprehensive Report From the National Transition Study of Special Education Students.* Menlo Park, Calif: Statistical Reference Index; 1991.
20. McGuire TG. Measuring the economic costs of schizophrenia. *Schizophr Bull.* 1991;17:375-388.
21. Goldman L, Cook EF, Orav J, Epstein AM, Komaroff AL, Delbanco TL, Mulley AG, Hiatt HH. Research training in clinical effectiveness: replacing 'in my experience . . .' with rigorous clinical investigation. *Clin Res.* 1990;38:686-93.
22. National Institute of Mental Health Conference on Psychopharmacology in Children and Adolescents: Current Problems, Future Perspectives; January 24-25, 1995; Washington, DC.

Child and Adolescent Mental Disorders Research

Current Directions, Future Needs

LECKMAN, ELLIOTT, and their colleagues[1] have done the field a great service with their clear, in-depth report about research on child and adolescent mental disorders. Their article highlights new approaches and developing technologies that promise to further the understanding of the intricate connections between brain and experiential reality. As the authors point out, although the 152% inflation-adjusted increase in the National Institute of Mental Health (NIMH) research budget from 1987 to 1993 is welcome, it is not nearly enough to sustain the momentum we have achieved. Furthermore, today's intense cost-cutting atmosphere could easily erode this hard-won gain.

The committee's report is intelligent and sophisticated. In addition to lauding its financial analyses, thoughtful observations and suggestions, and legitimate concerns, this communication will raise some issues to further stimulate the meaningful, wide-ranging research that the committee recommends.

THE ISSUES

Should the distinction between child/adolescent and adult disorders be retained? The authors rightly recommend that child and adolescent mental disorders receive a larger share of the total NIMH research budget. Development in childhood is rapid and complex; children's responses to psychopharmacological agents differ from those of adults. But in a way, the division into child/adolescent and adult disorders seems artificial, reflecting primarily the subspecialty status of child and adolescent psychiatry. Child and adolescent disorders become adult disorders, ie, many adult disorders do not truly originate in adulthood. Furthermore, an identified patient of any age may have family members who are profoundly affected by living with, or feeling responsible for, someone with a mental disorder. For example, anyone familiar with a family's efforts to get services for an autistic child has seen the parents' anguish, narcissistic injury, feelings of futility and anger, and the ways siblings and other family members suffer. Mental disorders often cause a conflict between family obligations and demands of the workplace. A national research plan should produce scientific knowledge that helps prevent illness, lessen suffering, and reduce family/workplace conflicts. Therefore, it should be directed at America's *families*, with *all* NIMH funds allocated accordingly.

Services research must focus on the current changes in service provision. One service not mentioned by the Institute of Medicine report[1] was managed care. Medicaid is turning to managed care nationwide; managed care companies may soon be the primary force determining which services and treatments can be offered to children and adolescents with mental disorders and which may not. We need research that analyzes how these companies' decisions are made and what patient needs they fail to meet. Then we will have to marshal both our clinical data and our research findings to make it harder for companies to ignore the needs of children and adolescents with mental disorders.

Foster care is an important mental health service for children and adolescents. In discussing services, the report touched too briefly on foster care and therapeutic foster care. Although foster care is considered part of child welfare, it provides a complete spectrum of mental health services, ranging from preventive and outpatient services to residential treatment facilities for the severely emotionally disturbed. Its financial costs are great. Medicaid recipients use far more mental health services than non-Medicaid recipients. Those in foster care use eight times as many mental health dollars as Medicaid recipients who are not in foster care. Foster care's graduates are overrepresented in both the mental health and criminal justice systems.

See also pages 715, 724, 727, and 732

Mental health expenses have been shifted to child welfare by making foster care's residential facilities "open-air mental hospitals." Almost 50% of their child and adolescent residents have been psychiatric hospital inpatients. As many as 70% of them take a growing array of psychotropic medications. Now therapeutic foster boarding homes are becoming important. Since both Medicaid and managed care companies want to use them as cost-effective alternatives to psychiatric hospitalization and residential treatment, we need far more empirical information about them.

Many children and adolescents with serious mental disorders in themselves and/or in their biological parents spend years in foster care; yet, otherwise excellent research reports almost never consider foster care as a variable. Even research studies, for instance, on the long-term effects of child abuse (and many foster children have been placed because they had been abused and/or neglected), rarely consider foster care placement as a variable in data analysis. But whether the child is removed from his or her biological parents may have a crucial impact on outcome. Perhaps by the next update by Leckman et al, foster care will be considered more often as a variable in research design, and its facilities will train more researchers.

Some issues about the way we do research also need to be considered. We have made progress in developing a new paradigm based on scientific methods. Yet, precisely predesigning every study to include testable hypotheses and possible outcomes can restrict clinical creativity in generating hypotheses and leave researchers less open to serendipitous or intuitive clinical observations.

Biological psychiatry is increasingly, and appropriately, conceptualized as the interaction of organism and environment. Not long ago, biological psychiatry was often seen as a search for biochemical or neurophysiological etiologies for mental disorders in contrast to the environmental, experiential, or intrapsychic causalities that were then considered crucial. The committee report's viewpoint is refreshing. An inclusive consensus is emerging: biology is more fruitfully thought of as the interaction of organism with environment. Brain and experience—the hormonal and the social, temperament and the interpersonal environment—are interdependent. Activity originating in either can alter structure, biochemistry, and physiology, as well as psychology and subjective perceptions. Amblyopia ex anopsia may be a good model. If a neurologically intact eye does not get adequate external stimulation, it will eventually be functionally blind. One wonders whether analogous processes might connect early maternal stimulation and brain development. For instance, might postpartum depression, which can dramatically alter the early mother-child relationship, affect neuropsychological development, activity level, or a child's inner image of the kind of world he or she lives in?

We will continue to need two frames of reference to answer questions about brain and mind. Silbersweig et al[2] have been able to visualize hallucinations on positron emission tomographic scans. That is an astonishing, important bridge between brain and experiential reality. It may herald crucial new understandings that eventually lead to more precise interventions for hallucinatory disorders. Yet, to explain a hallucination's subjective meaning and specificity (eg, a command hallucination telling the person to kill some particular family member) is likely—even if command hallucinations are ultimately localized with positron emission tomographic scans—to continue to require a different frame of reference that addresses questions such as why the hallucinatory command specifies this particular individual and not another relative.

The current research paradigm from writing a proposal to peer review may preclude discovering important, but subjective, psychiatric truths. Contemporary research requires results based on statistical analysis of value. This statistical focus has stimulated great advances and has helped psychiatry reenter medicine. But its strong dependence on measuring specified phenomena can also narrow a researcher's field of vision. Many important psychiatric discoveries require primarily an openness to the unexpected. For instance, the surprising clinical observation that many tuberculous patients given isoniazid to treat the bacillus infection felt euphoric helped stimulate research on antidepressants.

The report proposes we develop methods and measures to capture, among other things, subjective approaches. Were we to do this, psychology would be as scientific as chemistry. But psychology has no table of elements, no agreed upon symbolic language, and no universally accepted vision about what is important in being human. Some things about people cannot be measured accurately, if they can be measured at all. How can a researcher assign a number to feelings, other than to their physiological concomitants? For instance, can an investigator *measure* the sexual feelings one person experiences? If a rise in one person's pulse rate is identical to that in another, are they actually having the same sexual experience? No current method exists to measure the sexually stimulating fantasy's (or experience's) subjective meaning to the person; how it is connected to each individual's early upbringing and unique life experiences; and how good, or disgusting, the excitement felt.

The need to assign a number urges scientific investigators to look at outward, scorable behavior. It tends to discount as too problematic the study of fantasy, mental constructs of reality, and the unique responses that individuals have to circumstances, despite the contributions these may make to mental disorders. While statistics help investigators discover what phenomena or objects have in common, it flattens out differences; it also is poorly suited to approaches that are curious about what makes an individual unique. A treatment like cognitive behavior therapy is easier to evaluate statistically because its easily scored goals are rooted in the same mathematical assumptions that statistics has. Yet that common underpinning may mean that statistical studies that find cognitive behavior therapy more therapeutic are circular. Far more difficult to evaluate statistically are clinical gifts, such as intuition, and methods based on introspection that aim to "restructure the personality." Introspection can be neither validated nor replicated.[3]

This research paradigm may also make funders too cautious. Milton Friedman told a story about Leo Szilard, the famous nuclear physicist. More than 40 years ago, Szilard designed a surefire method of getting research money. He wrote funding requests for research he had already concluded. Then he used the funding to explore what intrigued him. In the next funding cycle, he repeated the process. This approach continued until the funding agency turned down Szilard's proposal for research he had secretly already completed because it was "impossible" to accomplish.

Even carefully designed research cannot entirely do away with the research protocol's impact on the subject. To be "atheoretical"—to use *DSM-III-R* terminology—current research observations are descriptive, usually focusing on easily identifiable behavioral signs and symptoms. Often, they use standardized research interview protocols. But a research interview is also a relationship. If the interviewer is enjoined from having empathic, constructive, human reactions, the subject's (particularly a psychiatric patient's) subsequent actions have to be understood not only as pathology but as a troubled person's response to an interviewer perceived as remote and unemotional.[3(chap3)] In these investigations, good interrater reliability may only mean that this skewing is a systematic error. Yet, a researcher who reacts more spontaneously or intuitively to the subject skews the research data in another direction.

Neutrality that in no way affects research outcome is probably impossible. As social primates, we react to other people. That means that investigators of child and adolescent mental disorders need better ways to deal with subjectivity and the transactional process that research, like all human relationships, entails.

Everyone in this field also ought to pay more attention to what is promulgated publicly and to what is included in cost-benefit analyses: Sometimes, more caution is needed about what research findings are disseminated. The report urges readers to

> convey in appropriate media settings the results of empirical research and the need to take advantage of advances in related scientific disciplines.[1]

Everyone also needs to be vigilant to separate research from premature public debates. Many parents are anxious about their children's emotional health. As experts in mental disorders, child and adolescent mental health clinicians' and researchers' words can have a far-reaching impact. Even well-designed studies of clearly genetic conditions can give misleading results. In 1965, a team of serious researchers suggested that XYY males were more aggressive. That finding was disseminated widely and contributed to a heated debate about behavioral genetics. In 1993, a report from the National Academy of Science dismissed the link as unproven.[4] In those intervening years, many parents were warned about their XYY children's potential for aggressiveness. How many families were hurt because parents worried that their children might grow up to be murderers?

Everyone also needs to be cautious about what "facts" supposedly exist and what interventions, particularly with children, are fundamentally effective. Current clinical research often focuses on observed symptoms, sometimes making a tacit assumption that remediating the disturbing symptom is good. Some hellish roads are paved with good intentions. Cost-benefit ratios are only as good as the considerations factored into the equation. Even remediating frightening symptoms that are inextricably linked to a condition's cause can have unforeseen deleterious effects. For instance, for many years, pediatricians and neurologists treated a child after a first febrile seizure with long-term phenobarbital therapy to prevent further seizures. Seizures were said to cause brain damage. Phenobarbital diminished their frequency. Further research has demonstrated that uncomplicated febrile seizures are relatively innocuous; barbiturates used to treat them can cause hyperactivity, inattentiveness, sleep disturbances, and, possibly, long-term difficulties with cognitive development.

CONCLUSION

The remarkable report by the Institute of Medicine committee[1] is likely a forerunner to research advances that will greatly benefit children, adolescents, and families. The emerging, inclusive synthesis of the physical and the experiential is simultaneously challenging and thrilling. While we likely will never develop a science of the subjective, we need to find ways to broaden the research effort to include approaches that do not easily fit into the statistical universe. And we need scholars who can assimilate the ever-expanding data that we are generating and synthesize them into even more constructive paradigms to guide research, training, and treatment.

Alvin A. Rosenfeld, MD
Director of Psychiatric Services
J.C.C.A. of New York
575 Lexington Ave
New York, NY 10022

The author would like to thank Robert Kavet, PhD, and Dorothy Levine, MD, for their constructive criticism of earlier drafts of this commentary.

Reprint requests to Dr Rosenfeld.

REFERENCES

1. Members of the Committee for the Study of Research on Child and Adolescent Mental Disorders. Report card on the *National Plan for Research on Child and Adolescent Mental Disorders*: the midway point. *Arch Gen Psychiatry.* 1995;52:715-723.
2. Silbersweig D, Stern E, Frith C, Schnorr L, Cahill C, Holmes A, Jones T, Frackowiak RSJ. The functional neuroanatomy of bimodal hallucinations in a drug-naive schizophrenic. *Biol Psychiatry.* 1995;37:631.
3. Bettelheim B, Rosenfeld AA. *The Art of the Obvious: Developing Insight for Psychotherapy and Everyday Life.* New York, NY: Alfred A Knopf Inc; 1993.
4. Mann CC. Behavioral genetics in transition. *Science.* 1994;264:1686-1689.

COMMENTARY

Grading the Progress of Child and Adolescent Mental Health Research

NIMH Perspectives

LECKMAN AND colleagues[1] are to be commended for their "Report Card on the *National Plan for Research on Child and Adolescent Mental Disorders*." This "Report Card" was initiated by the American Academy of Child and Adolescent Psychiatry and has been endorsed by more than 20 national professional and advocacy organizations. Most of these organizations participated in the development of the congressionally mandated blueprint for child and adolescent research at the National Institute of Mental Health (NIMH), the *National Plan for Research on Child and Adolescent Mental Disorders*.[2] Similarly, the principal authors of the Report Card are members of the original Institute of Medicine (IOM) committee that wrote the 1989 report, *Research on Children With Emotional, Behavioral, and Developmental Disabilities*.[3] Because of broad concerns about the lack of progress in child and adolescent research, NIMH commissioned this original IOM report to serve as a springboard for assessing and developing this area of research, and the National Plan was then developed from the recommendations from the 1989 IOM report.

By all accounts, these two original reports have become a remarkable springboard! As documented in the Report Card, this once relatively quiescent field has leaped forward on many fronts. Even the Report Card itself, endorsed by mental health research and clinical communities, bears witness to the activism, dedication, and expansion of this research field.

INTERIM PROGRESS

The Report Card deserves special attention for several reasons. First, it sets an important standard for future NIMH national plans in that it constitutes the first effort to clearly assess interim progress against the yardstick of the goals and objectives set forth in the original document. Leckman and colleagues note that, measured against that yardstick, substantial progress has been made, particularly from 1987 through the first 3 years of the National Plan. Interestingly, some of the most dramatic gains (in terms of percentage increases over baseline funding levels) were made even prior to the release of the National Plan, as NIMH began to redirect internal resources into projects such as the Methodology for Epidemiology in Children and Adolescents (MECA) Study,[4] the first NIMH multisite cooperative agreement in child and adolescent research.

See also pages 715, 724, 727, and 729

Second, the Report Card documents the dramatic gains made in many specific child-related research areas across all NIMH divisions, most notably, services research, prevention research, and other clinical research areas. Not surprisingly, we have been very pleased with the progress made in the child and adolescent research area. Currently, two of NIMH's largest and most influential projects are in this area, namely, the Multimodal Treatment of Attention Deficit Hyperactivity Disorder (MTA) Study[5] and the Services Use, Need, Outcomes, and Costs in Child and Adolescent Populations (UNOCAP) program. Both of these major projects were called for in the 1989 IOM report and envisioned in the National Plan.

Interestingly, when the National Plan was first under development, some individuals were concerned that the child infrastructure would be unable to grow enough to accommodate the infusion of research monies that might come as a result of the National Plan. However, when substantial new monies were made available to NIMH, particularly from 1989 to 1992, a concerted effort from NIMH staff was met with an enthusiastic response from the field, and this research area began to develop and subsequently sustain a remarkable momentum. Most child-related research programs (with exceptions noted in the Report Card) have grown at a rate faster than other NIMH-supported research programs. While there is no means of establishing cause-and-effect relationships between the initial two reports and this overwhelming success, the NIMH staff and researchers in the field worked diligently to carry out the National Plan's recommendations.

The confluence of all of these efforts highlights a third major point illustrated by the Report Card: successful scenarios, such as substantial growth in child and adolescent research, can only occur when internal (ie, NIMH) and external ("the field") factors move in harmony. Simply increasing research dollars in a given area may accomplish no long-term, sustainable growth if the increased monies are not accompanied by substantial development of the research infrastructure and by sustained commitment from the major professional, advocacy, and research communities.

'CHILD CONSORTIUM' ACTIVITIES

The task of coordinating internal NIMH efforts with those in the field is the responsibility of the Consortium for Research in Child and Adolescent Mental Disorders (the so-called "Child Consortium"), established in 1990. Under the guidance of the Acting Director of NIMH (R.W.C.) and working with all NIMH divisions and programs and the larger research field, the Consortium has major responsibilities for implementing the national plan. Through the Consortium, successful examples of field-coordinated, program-building efforts have included the joint sponsorship and planning of technical assistance workshops to help researchers develop new research and research training programs. These efforts, involving several hundred beginning investigators as well as senior scientists, were planned and implemented by NIMH working in concert with its professional and research organization partners. These infrastructure development programs have been very successful, yielding three newly funded institutional research training programs and a growing cadre of new investigators. The success of these efforts clearly depended on cosponsorship by professional organizations. Given the success of past efforts, these workshops will continue, and plans for additional technical assistance workshops are under way. In particular, the career trajectories of those young prospective investigators who receive intensive technical assistance will be evaluated to determine the effectiveness of such technical assistance efforts.

Another example of a systematic effort to coordinate internal and external forces has been the NIMH-sponsored editors' consortium. Each year since the publication of the national plan, the Child and Adolescent Mental Disorders Research Consortium has convened a unique meeting with leading journal editors in the child and adolescent mental disorders field and related areas of developmental psychology, pharmacology, and sociology. The goal of this meeting has been to facilitate research dissemination, to foster interdisciplinary collaboration, and to enable the examination of research paradigms within and across disciplines. This remarkable group of editors has developed common editorials on the topic of "piecemeal publications" and guidelines for the measurement of socioeconomic status. Furthermore, jointly edited, jointly reviewed, and simultaneously published but complementary articles have been printed in several of the participating journals. Future planned topics and possible editorials include issues related to (1) the descriptors used within research publications concerning ethnicity and minority status, (2) the appropriate use of terms related to *risk factors* and *causal factors* (vs *consequences* and *correlates*), and (3) qualitative research methods.

Through the Child and Adolescent Mental Disorders Research Consortium, NIMH has also been active in organizing conferences on critical topics that affect research in child and adolescent mental disorders. For example, in May 1993, NIMH hosted a conference on Ethical and Human Subjects Issues in Mental Health Research With Children and Adolescents. In January 1995, NIMH hosted a conference on Psychopharmacology in Children and Adolescents. Each of these conferences assembled a diverse and expert group of scientists, family advocates, representatives from professional associations, other National Institutes of Health (NIH), the Food and Drug Administration (FDA), the Office for Protection From Research Risks, the Center for Mental Health Services (CMHS), institutional review board associations, and representatives of the pharmaceutical industry. The purposes of the first conference were to address the major ethical challenges involved in research with children and adolescents; to identify the scientific, social, and policy issues that arise in these studies; and to make recommendations for future studies carefully grounded in ethical perspectives. Because there are few guidelines to help investigators balance the rights, safety, and well-being of children with the opportunities for research that can contribute to improved mental health, this conference was seen as a first step both in understanding the complexities of the ethical issues and in identifying possible solutions.

The second conference, cosponsored by NIMH and the Food and Drug Administration, concerned the need for increased research on the safety and efficacy of psychotherapeutic medications for children and adolescents with mental disorders. The 140 participants in the meeting were drawn from the various constituencies around the country that inform, shape, or are affected by research and/or clinical use of these medications. Major recommendations likely to shape the next decade of research in this area were generated. In both of these program-building, consensus-forming conferences, NIMH's goal has been to work with the critical partners who could enable research to proceed in understudied areas.

FUTURE PRIORITIES

The Report Card notes the effect of the significant fiscal constraints experienced over the last few years, which have affected the intramural programs in particular. Also, the Report Card takes NIMH to task because of the need to do more to educate the public about research findings concerning the diagnosis, treatment, and prevention of child and adolescent mental disorders. We agree that these important issues need increased attention, and we plan to examine additional possibilities for activities in this area. Already, NIMH staff have met with their counterparts in the Center for Mental Health Services, with whom we share responsibility for and commitment to dissemination of information. We hope to find ways to work together to increase our research dissemination efforts. Furthermore, jointly sponsored efforts are under way to increase the research knowledge base within *clinical* training programs, with the goal of developing a new generation of practitioners who can readily integrate research findings into clinical practice.

While the Report Card is very well done and represents an even-handed, fair assessment of our progress to date, it brings to our attention (especially during these times of increased fiscal constraint) the need to review our priorities carefully. We must consider how to continue our research programs, develop young investigators, and take advantage of new research opportunities, even while resources are leveling off.

We have had several plans over the last 10 years, including the Schizophrenia Plan, the Decade of the Brain, the National Plan of Research to Improve Services, and most recently, the Prevention Initiative. All of these plans are worthy and require critical support to sustain their programmatic gains.

We are pleased by the sustained interest and growth in child and adolescent research, and we are excited by the prospects for future advances. Although the number of initiatives and the scope of the National Plan initially seemed ambitious, review of our progress to date suggests that the goals were appropriately high and fully in step with the excitement of the field, the public health need, and the levels of growth and expansion witnessed in other NIMH-wide national plans.

This is not a time to compete among ourselves concerning funding for the various national research plans that NIMH and its constituents have set forth. In the current fiscal atmosphere, such infighting or partisan promotion is likely to be both destructive and counterproductive. Further implementation of each of these plans will benefit all of the others. Thus, the *National Plan for Research on Child and Adolescent Mental Disorders* will reap benefits not only for all young people who are or may be afflicted by mental disorders but also for their families and friends. Furthermore, research on the complex origins of child and adolescent mental disorders is likely to clarify the foundations of many mental disorders that primarily affect adults. Efforts at early detection and treatment of psychopathologic conditions in young children, especially through longitudinal studies, may reveal risk factors for and predictors of disorders such as schizophrenia prior to the onset of clinical illness. Similarly, other plans, such as the Decade of the Brain, have already provided and will continue to yield great insights in understanding the development of child and adolescent mental illnesses. It is a privilege to work as public servants on behalf of these noble efforts.

Rex W. Cowdry, MD
Peter S. Jensen, MD
National Institute of Mental Health
5600 Fisher's Ln
Rockville, MD 20857

The opinions and assertions contained in this article are the private views of the authors and are not to be construed as official or as reflecting the views of the Department of Health and Human Services or the National Institute of Mental Health.

REFERENCES

1. Members of the Committee for the Study of Research on Child and Adolescent Mental Disorders. Report Card on the *National Plan for Research on Child and Adolescent Mental Disorders:* the midway point. *Arch Gen Psychiatry.* 1995; 52:715-723.
2. National Institute of Mental Health. *National Plan for Research on Child and Adolescent Mental Disorders: A Report Requested by the U.S. Congress.* Washington, DC: US Dept of Health and Human Services; 1990. Publication ADM 90-1683.
3. Institute of Medicine. *Research on Children and Adolescents With Mental, Behavioral, and Developmental Disorders.* Washington, DC: National Academy Press; 1989. Publication IOM-89-07.
4. Jensen PS, Roper M, Fisher P, Piacentini J, Canino G, Richters J, Rubio-Stipec M, Dulcan M, Goodman S, Davies M, Rae D, Shaffer D, Bird H, Lahey B, Schwab-Stone M. Test-retest reliability of the Diagnostic Interview Schedule for Children (DISC 2.1): parent, child, and combined algorithms. *Arch Gen Psychiatry.* 1995; 52:61-71.
5. Richters J, Arnold LEA, Jensen PS, Abikoff H, Conners CK, Greenhill L, Hinshaw S, Pelham W, Swanson J. The NIMH collaborative multisite, multimodal treatment study of ADHD, I: background and rationale. *J Am Acad Child Adolesc Psychiatry.* In press.

ORIGINAL ARTICLE

Meta-analyses of Studies of Ventricular Enlargement and Cortical Sulcal Prominence in Mood Disorders

Comparisons With Controls or Patients With Schizophrenia

Helio Elkis, MD, PhD; Lee Friedman, PhD; Alexandria Wise; Herbert Y. Meltzer, MD

Background: The findings of ventricular enlargement and increased sulcal prominence are well documented in schizophrenia, but the consistency of similar findings in mood disorders is less well appreciated. Reliable documentation of the presence of these structural abnormalities in mood disorders would require a reassessment of their significance for both schizophrenia and mood disorders. In this article, we meta-analytically review the literature on ventricular enlargement and cortical sulcal prominence in patients with mood disorders compared with controls and patients with schizophrenia.

Methods: Four meta-analytic reviews were conducted, two comparing patients with mood disorders with normal controls on ventricular enlargement (meta-analysis 1) or sulcal prominence (meta-analysis 2) and two comparing patients with mood disorders with schizophrenic patients on these same measures (meta-analyses 3 and 4).

Results: Meta-analyses 1 and 2 revealed statistically significant ($P<.001$) moderate composite effect sizes (d) for the comparisons of patients with mood disorders with controls on both ventricular enlargement (d=0.44) and sulcal prominence (d=0.42). Meta-analysis 3 further revealed that patients with schizophrenia have significantly greater ventricular enlargement than patients with mood disorders (P=.002), but the effect size was small (d=−0.20). There were too few studies comparing these patient groups on sulcal prominence to support a quantitative meta-analysis.

Conclusions: This review documents the presence of ventricular enlargement and increased sulcal prominence in mood disorders. Patients with mood disorders have less ventricular enlargement than patients with schizophrenia, but this effect is small. These results reinforce previous suggestions of the nonspecificity of structural brain changes in schizophrenia and mood disorders.

(Arch Gen Psychiatry. 1995;52:735-746)

IT IS WELL established that patients with schizophrenia have higher rates of ventriculomegaly and/or sulcal widening when compared with normal controls.[1] The finding of ventricular enlargement in schizophrenia has been reviewed extensively and supported by two recent meta-analyses.[2,3] However, the consistency of similar findings in mood disorders is less well appreciated. Reliable documentation of ventricular enlargement and/or cortical sulcal prominence in mood disorders would have significance for the pathophysiology of mood disorders and place similar findings in schizophrenia in perspective.

Excellent narrative reviews of the brain imaging literature in affective disorders have already been published.[4-6] Although such traditional narrative reviews are informative, they frequently are not conclusive. This stems, in part, from the fact that traditional literature reviews typically employ a "vote-counting" method to decide if an effect is present. With this method, each primary study is placed into one of three bins: (1) studies that have statistically significant results in the direction of the hypothesis, (2) studies with nonsignificant results, and (3) studies with significant results opposite to the hypothesis. The bin with the highest tally is considered to best represent the effects reported in the literature. Until recently, little attention has been given to the statistical properties of this commonplace approach. However, Hedges and Olkin[7,8] have evaluated the statistical power of this vote-counting procedure and have come to a surprising and important conclusion: if the true population effect is small to moder-

From the Departments of Psychiatry, University of São Paulo (Brazil) School of Medicine and Hospital do Servidor Publico Estadual, São Paulo (Dr Elkis), and the Department of Psychiatry, Case Western Reserve University School of Medicine, Cleveland, Ohio (Drs Friedman and Meltzer and Ms Wise).

See Methods on next page

METHODS

SELECTION OF STUDIES

To obtain a reasonable sample of studies, we first searched the MEDLINE database using Grateful Med (version 6.0) software (National Library of Medicine, Bethesda, Md). The searches were based on the following medical subject heading (MeSH) categories: Tomography, X-ray Computed or Magnetic Resonance Imaging, and explode Affective Disorders or explode Affective Disorders, Psychotic. The search was conducted in April 1994 and covered the years 1966 to 1994. The April 1994 search was not repeated. Although the potential database of relevant articles would continue to grow, a definite end point for our meta-analyses was required. The search produced about 450 unique articles. The complete references, abstracts (when available), and MeSH categories for each article were printed. Case reports, reviews, and letters were culled from the lists. In a second step, we examined the titles, abstracts, and MeSH categories for each article and selected those studies that were potential candidates for inclusion in the meta-analyses. To be considered a candidate for inclusion, a study had to have compared patients with mood disorders with normal controls or with schizophrenic patients on some measure of ventricular enlargement or cortical sulcal prominence. If, based on the title, abstract, or MeSH categories, it seemed reasonably likely that a study might possibly be appropriate, a reprint of the article was obtained and reviewed. This procedure resulted in the selection of 61 studies. Based on inclusion and exclusion criteria detailed below, these 61 studies were either entered into one or more of the meta-analyses (**Table 1**) or considered to be relevant, but not includable. (Studies that were not included and the reasons for exclusion are available from the authors on request.) All the studies were published between 1978 and 1993.

INCLUSION AND EXCLUSION CRITERIA FOR THE META-ANALYSES

To be included in one or more of the four meta-analyses, a study had to have assessed ventricular enlargement and/or cortical sulcal prominence in patients with mood disorders and compared these data with those from either normal controls and/or patients with schizophrenia. A study had to provide sufficient statistical information for the extraction of an exact effect size. A few studies simply indicated that the differences were not statistically significant and included no other statistical information regarding the effect. Such studies were considered relevant, but not includable, since an exact effect size could not be calculated. Also, the data in a study had to be unique; in several cases the same data were included in more than one published article. In these cases, only one article was chosen, based primarily on the quality and quantity of quantitative statistical and demographic information available. In cases in which a set of subjects was included in a larger set that was published later, the later publication was used. Since it is well established that ventricular enlargement and sulcal prominence both increase with increasing age,[10] we carefully screened articles to determine if the subject groups were matched for age. Only studies that included age-matched samples, or that controlled for age differences in some manner (eg, including age as a covariate in an analysis of covariance or including age as a factor in a factorial analysis of variance [ANOVA]), were included.

According to these criteria, 33 studies[11-43] were included in the meta-analyses (Table 1). Twenty-eight studies[44-71] were considered relevant but were not included in the meta-analyses (table available on request). Six studies had insufficient information to compute effect size, eight studies had insufficient information to determine if subjects were age matched or to compute an age-controlled effect size, seven studies included data that were published elsewhere, two studies were based on relevant but dissimilar dependent measures of brain structure, and the remainder were excluded for miscellaneous reasons.

Four meta-analyses were conducted. Meta-analysis 1 compared patients with mood disorders with controls on measures of ventricular enlargement. Meta-analysis 2 compared patients with mood disorders with controls on measures of cortical sulcal prominence. Meta-analysis 3 compared patients with mood disorders with schizophrenic patients on measures of ventricular enlargement. Meta-analysis 4 compared patients with mood disorders with schizophrenic patients on measures of cortical sulcal prominence.

META-ANALYTIC METHODS

Effect Sizes

The effect size value employed was "Hedges' g,"[9] which is defined as the difference between the mean of the mood disorder group and the mean of the comparison group (controls or schizophrenic patients) divided by their pooled SD. These g values were all corrected for bias due to sample size,[8] with the result expressed as "d." According to Cohen,[72] a large effect size is 0.8, a moderate effect size is 0.5, and a small effect size is 0.2. Although the most straightforward method of effect size computation employed pub-

ate in magnitude (frequently the case in clinical psychiatric research) and if the sample sizes in the individual studies are also moderate (also frequently the case), the vote-counting procedure frequently fails to detect the presence of an effect.

Meta-analysis is a more precise method for quantitatively reviewing a literature, deciding if an effect is present, and estimating the effect size.[8,9] Also, meta-analysis allows one to evaluate the role of possible moderators of effect size, such as the age or gender of the patient group, the method of measurement, and other variables.

A previous meta-analysis[2] has documented the presence of increased ventricular enlargement and cortical sulcal prominence in patients with mood disorders when compared with normal controls. However, only 18 studies were included in that review. We have identified at least 10 additional studies, some of which were published after the previous review. Most important for our purpose, the previous meta-analysis[2] focused on the comparison between patients with mood disorders and controls and did not address the issue of structural abnormalities in patients with mood disorders in comparison with schizophrenic patients.

lished means and SDs, other statistics can be transformed into g. The computation of effect size was performed using the DSTAT software package (Lawrence Erlbaum Associates, Hillsdale, NJ),[73] which provides tools for computation of effect size from means and SDs, *t* tests, F tests, proportions, exact *P* values, and others. The direction of the effect was considered to be positive if the results supported the hypothesis that patients with mood disorders have more ventricular enlargement or more sulcal prominence than the comparison group, be it controls or patients with schizophrenia.

In the overwhelming majority of cases, the computation of effect size was a simple and direct process. In four cases, computation of an age-controlled effect size was somewhat more complicated. In two of these cases, the effect size was based on an F value for diagnosis from a factorial ANOVA with other factors in the model.[23,31] In one case the effect size was calculated using a covariate-adjusted F.[39] In another case, the effect size itself was presented in the article.[42]

A complication arises when a given study includes several subgroups (eg, males and females, patients with unipolar and bipolar illness) that are all measured on the same dependent measure (eg, ventricular-brain ratio [VBR]). In this case, the data from each subgroup was pooled into a single group prior to the computation of the effect size.

A more difficult complication arises when a study includes multiple dependent measures (eg, ventricular volume and ventricular area, or sulcal prominence in the frontal region and in the parietal region). Multiple effect sizes that are calculated from a given study are not statistically independent observations. The effect sizes for all dependent measures relevant to a particular meta-analytic question were integrated (averaged) so that each study would be represented only once in each analysis.

A composite effect size representing all the studies in a meta-analysis was computed as a weighted mean of the effect sizes from each study. For this, each effect was weighted by the reciprocal of its variance.[8,73] Confidence limits around the composite effect size were also calculated. A statistical test of the homogeneity of groups of effect sizes (Q) was computed according to the method of Hedges and Olkin.[8] The power of the average hypothesis test in a meta-analysis was based on the composite effect size and the average sample size.[74]

Potential Moderators of Effect Size

To assess the influence of several potential modifiers of effect size, a series of meta-analytic procedures comparable to ANOVA or correlation analysis in primary-level studies have been developed.[73] Using these methods, we evaluated the influence of the following potential moderators of effect size: (1) the year the study was conducted; (2) the type of control group, ie, if the control subjects were drawn from a community population, a medical population (eg, patients with headaches), or a psychiatric population (eg, patients with personality disorders); (3) the percentage of the patients with mood disorders who were male; (4) the mean age of the patients with mood disorders; (5) the percentage of the patients with mood disorders having a diagnosis of unipolar depression; (6) the imaging modality on which the study was based (computed tomography or magnetic resonance imaging [MRI]); (7) the presence or absence of quantitive data on interrater reliability of measurements; and (8) the complexity or simplicity of effect size extraction. In the "Results" section we present average data for these potential moderators for sets of studies. These averages are across studies (each study weighted equally) rather than weighted by the sample size in a study.

Publication Bias, Funnel Plots, and Fail-Safe N

Publication bias results from the tendency to publish only statistically significant results or results in the direction of the hypothesis. The presence of publication bias can often be detected graphically in a "funnel plot,"[75] which plots the total sample size in each study by its effect size (**Figure**). The law of large numbers predicts that the larger studies will be most representative of the true population effects. Studies with smaller samples should be randomly scattered about the central effect size of the larger studies, with scatter increasing as study size decreases, thus creating an inverted funnel appearance. When publication bias is present, the portion of the funnel near the 0.0 effect size is missing, indicating that small studies with nonsignificant results are not being published. It is certainly possible that nonsignificant studies exist in researchers' files and have not been published. This is referred to as the "file-drawer problem."[76] Orwin[77] has developed a method for determining the number of studies ("fail-safe N") with null effects in file drawers somewhere that would be required to reduce the overall effect size to a negligible level (in the present study, we chose 0.1).

A number of special considerations arose concerning methodological details for several of the studies included in the meta-analyses. A "Special Considerations" table has been prepared and is available from the authors on request.

In the present study, we present four meta-analyses that address the following four questions: (1) Do patients with mood disorders exhibit ventricular enlargement in comparison with controls? (meta-analysis 1); (2) Do patients with mood disorders exhibit increased sulcal prominence in comparison with controls? (meta-analysis 2); (3) Do patients with mood disorders exhibit ventricular enlargement in comparison with schizophrenic patients? (meta-analysis 3); and (4) Do patients with mood disorders exhibit increased sulcal prominence in comparison with schizophrenic patients? (meta-analysis 4).

RESULTS

META-ANALYSIS 1

The studies included in meta-analysis 1, comparing patients with mood disorders with controls on measures of ventricular enlargement, are presented in Table 1 and **Table 2**).

General Description of the Studies

There were 29 studies included in this meta-analysis, making this the largest of the four meta-analyses. The aver-

Table 1. Subject Characteristics of All Studies in the Four Meta-analyses*

Source, y†	Included in Which Meta-analysis?	No. of Patients With Mood Disorder	Patients With Mood Disorder Who Had Unipolar Illness, %	Mean (SD) Age of Patients With Mood Disorder, y
Jacoby and Levy,[11] 1980	1	41	95.1	72.2 (5.9)
Pearlson and Veroff,[12] 1981	1	16	...	...
Nasrallah et al,[13] 1982	1-4	24	0.0	31.8 (7.5)
Tanaka et al,[14] 1982	2	24‡	...	62.8 (6.5)
Weinberger et al,[15] 1982	1-4	23	...	30.3 (10.1)
Kellner et al,[16] 1983	1	10	...	43.5 (14.5)
Scott et al,[17] 1983	1	10	100.0	39.2 (11.4)
Targum et al,[18] 1983	1	38‡	76.3	31.0 (8.8)
Luchins et al,[19] 1984	1, 3	22	63.6	35.2 (11.7)
Pearlson et al,[20] 1984	1, 3	27	0.0	30.8 (6.7)
Shima et al,[21] 1984	1	46	95.6	53.0 (. . .)
Dolan et al,[22] 1985	1	101‡	73.3‡	55.2 (14.3)
Dolan et al,[23] 1986	2	101	73.3	55.2 (14.3)
Kolbeinsson et al,[24] 1986	1, 2	41‡	75.6	54.6 (13.3)
Besson et al,[25] 1987§	1	10	30.0	48.5 (9.5)
Schlegel and Kretzchmar,[26] 1987	1	53	50.9	...
Dewan et al,[27] 1988	1, 2	26	0.0	32.7 (. . .)
Iacono et al,[28] 1988	1-4	34	47.1	24.5 (6.2)
Johnstone et al,[29] 1989§	1, 3	20‡	0.0	38.1 (8.1)
Pearlson et al,[30] 1989	1	26‡	100.0	71.1 (6.3)
Rossi et al,[31] 1989	1, 3	42	100.0	53.2 (9.0)
Abas et al,[32] 1990	1, 2	20‡	80.0	70.4 (6.1)
Andreasen et al,[33] 1990	1, 3	50‡	52.0	36.9 (13.8)
Swayze et al,[34] 1990§	1, 3	48	0.0	33.9 (. . .)
Woods et al,[35] 1990	3	9	0.0	31.0 (15.7)
Beats et al,[36] 1991	1	25	84.0	74.0 (. . .)
Rabins et al,[37] 1991§	1, 2	21	100.0	...
Van den Bossche et al,[38] 1991	1	35‡	100.0	49.6 (14.5)
Lauer et al,[39] 1992	1	24	58.3	39.0 (11.3)
Sacchetti et al,[40] 1992	3	107	50.5	53.0 (10.6)
Coffey et al,[41] 1993§	1, 2	48	91.7	62.4 (16.4)
Raz,[42] 1993	1	16	43.8	35.9 (9.5)
Strakowski et al,[43] 1993§	1	17	0.0	28.4 (6.8)

**C indicates community; M, medical; P, psychiatric; X, mixed; NA, not applicable; and ellipses, missing data.*
†All studies used computed tomography unless otherwise indicated.
‡In a "Special Considerations" table available from the authors on request.
§These studies used magnetic resonance imaging.

age sample size was 31 patients (range, 10 to 101) and 32 controls (range, 10 to 76) per study. There were a total of 912 patients and 932 controls in all the studies. The average age of the patients in these studies was 44.8 years (range, 28.4 to 74.0 years). The majority of patients in most studies were women (average male, 42.9%; range, 19.6% to 100%). The majority of patients in most of the studies had unipolar depression (average, 58.4%; range, 0% to 100%). About half of the studies (15 of 29) used normal controls from the community, and most of the other studies used medical controls (13 of 29). Twenty-three studies were based on computed tomographic data and six studies were based on MRI data. The majority of the studies (20 of 29) used the VBR as a measure of ventricular size, three studies used a rating system, and six used some other quantitative measure of ventricular size. The average VBR for the mood disorder group was 7.08 (average SD, 2.89; range, 3.8 to 11.8) and for the control group it was 5.46 (SD, 2.39; range, 2.9 to 9.1). About one half of the studies (15 of 29) included quantitative interrater reliability data on the brain measure.

Summary of Effects

Twenty-eight (97%) of 29 studies reported effect sizes in the direction of the hypothesis, ie, that patients with mood disorders have a greater degree of ventricular enlargement than controls. Eleven studies reported that the effect was statistically significant ($P<.05$), 15 studies reported that the effect was not statistically significant, and three studies did not indicate statistical significance. Thus, a vote-counting procedure would conclude that there was no significant effect. The smallest effect size was −0.043, and the largest effect size was +1.60. The composite effect size was +0.437 (**Table 3**). This composite was highly statistically significant ($P<.001$). In Cohen's[72] nomenclature this effect size is moderate to small. The set of effect sizes was homogeneous, ie, the test of heterogeneity was not significant. The power of the average hypothesis test (effect size, 0.437; average sample size, 32) was 0.39.

In the set of studies that were relevant to but not included in this meta-analysis, seven[45,46,52,53,55,66,68] reached a useful conclusion regarding the issue in question. Of these, four studies[45,46,52,68] concluded that patients with mood dis-

Male Patients With Mood Disorder, %	No. of Controls	Type of Control Group	Mean (SD) Age of Controls, y	No. of Schizophrenic Patients	Mean (SD) Age of Schizophrenic Patients, y
29.3	50	C	>60.0 (. . .)	NA	NA
. . .	35	P	. . .	NA‡	. . .
100.0	27	M	29.7 (5.8)	55	29.9 (8.2)
25.0	24	M	63.3 (5.7)	NA	NA
34.8	26	M	30.3 (6.9)	17‡	28.3 (9.7)
. . .	12	M	. . .	NA	NA
. . .	10	M	39.9 (11.1)	NA	NA
26.3	26‡	M	30.5 (6.9)	NA	NA
. . .	62	M	33.9 (11.5)	45	29.0 (7.4)
44.4	27	C	30.7 (7.6)	19	28.8 (5.8)
19.6	46	X‡	52.0 (. . .)	NA	NA
. . .	52	C	54.0 (14.6)	NA	NA
. . .	52	C	54.0 (14.6)	NA	NA
22.0	16	C	51.9 (8.0)	NA	NA
20.0	10	C	42.3 (8.9)	NA	NA
34.0	53	M	. . .	NA	NA
73.1	22	M	31.1 (. . .)	NA	NA
58.8	44	C‡	23.2 (5.6)	31	22.8 (5.7)
60.0	21	C	34.4 (5.8)	21	35.9 (6.1)
38.5	31	. . .‡	68.3 (6.7)	NA	NA
59.5	37	M	37.8 (13.4)	36	42.7 (10.3)
45.0	20	C	68.3 (5.6)	NA	NA
46.0	75	C	34.9 (13.7)	108	31.8 (10.4)
60.4	47	C	34.4 (. . .)	54	33.3 (. . .)
66.7	NA	NA	NA	9	24.9 (5.7)
32.0	25	C	. . .	NA	NA
. . .	14	. . .	. . .	NA	NA
25.7	10	M	49.1 (15.7)	NA	NA
50.0	12	M	32.7 (9.7)	NA	NA
40.2	NA	NA	NA	206	26.9 (7.0)
35.4	76	C	61.6 (15.9)	NA	NA
31.3	31	C	28.6 (8.0)	NA	NA
41.2	16	C	30.9 (7.3)	NA	NA

orders have a greater degree of ventricular enlargement compared with controls and three[53,55,66] concluded that there was no difference in ventricle size between these groups.

Potential Moderators of Effect Size

None of the potential moderators of effect size had a statistically significant relationship with effect size (all P values, >.34).

Publication Bias and Fail-Safe N

The funnel plot for this meta-analysis is presented in the Figure, top left. The characteristic inverted funnel appearance is observed. However, the lower left portion of the funnel is missing, suggesting that there is a tendency to not publish studies with results opposite to the hypothesis. The fail-safe N was 98.

META-ANALYSIS 2

The studies included in meta-analysis 2, comparing patients with mood disorders with controls on measures of cortical sulcal prominence, are presented in Table 1 and **Table 4**).

General Description of the Studies

There were 10 studies included in this meta-analysis. The average sample size was 36 patients (range, 19 to 101) and 32 controls (range, 19 to 76) per study. There were a total of 360 patients and 323 controls in all the studies. The average age of the patients in these studies was 49.2 years (range, 31.8 to 70.4 years). About half of the patients in these studies were men (average, 49.3%; range, 35.4% to 100%). The majority of patients in most studies had unipolar depression (average, 58.5%; range, 0% to 100%). Six of 10 studies used normal controls from the community and four studies used medical controls. Eight studies were based on computed tomographic data and two studies were based on MRI data. Sulcal prominence was assessed by rating in all of these studies. One half of the studies included quantitative interrater reliability data on the sulcal prominence rating.

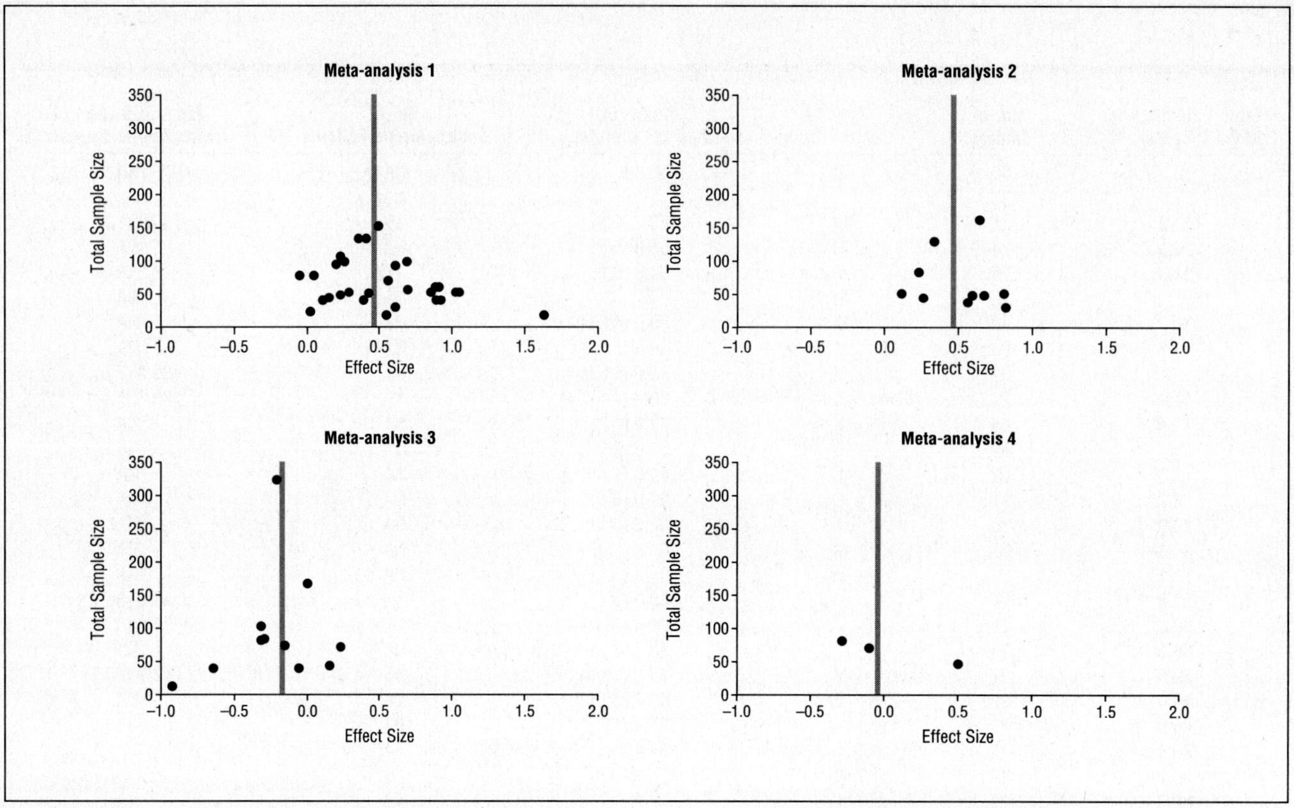

Funnel plots for the four meta-analyses. Each plot relates the effect size to total sample size (both groups). Each solid circle represents the position of a single study. The gray vertical lines indicate the composite effect size.

Summary of Effects

All the studies reported effect sizes in the direction of the hypothesis, ie, that patients with mood disorders have a greater degree of sulcal prominence than controls. However, only three studies reported that the effect was statistically significant ($P<.05$), five studies reported that the effect was not statistically significant, and two studies did not indicate statistical significance. Thus, a vote-counting procedure would once again conclude that there was no significant effect. The smallest effect size was +0.053 and the largest effect size was +0.81. The set of effect sizes was not statistically heterogeneous and the composite effect size was +0.421, which was highly statistically significant ($P<.001$) (Table 3). In Cohen's[72] nomenclature this effect size is moderate to small. The power of the average hypothesis test (effect size, 0.421; average sample size, 34) was 0.40.

In the set of studies that were relevant to but not included in this meta-analysis, five[45,52,68,70,71] reached a useful conclusion regarding the issue in question. Of these, two studies[45,68] concluded that patients with mood disorders have increased sulcal prominence compared with controls and two[52,71] concluded that there was no difference in sulcal prominence or fluid volume between these groups.

Potential Moderators of Effect Size

None of the potential moderators of effect size had a statistically significant relationship with effect size (all P values, >.24).

Publication Bias and Fail-Safe N

The funnel plot for this meta-analysis is presented in the Figure, top right. Notwithstanding the small number of studies, the characteristic inverted funnel appearance is suggested, with no evidence that the lower left portion of the funnel is missing. However, no study with a negative effect size has been published, raising the possibility that there is a tendency to not publish studies with results opposite to the hypothesis. The fail-safe N was 32.

META-ANALYSIS 3

The studies included in meta-analysis 3, comparing patients with mood disorders with schizophrenic patients on measures of ventricular enlargement, are presented in Table 1 and **Table 5**).

General Description of the Studies

There were 11 studies included in this meta-analysis. The average sample size was 37 patients with mood disorders (range, 9 to 107) and 54 patients with schizophrenia (range, 9 to 206) per study. There were a total of 406 patients with mood disorders and 599 patients with schizophrenia in all the studies. The average age of the patients with mood disorder in these studies was 36.3 years (range, 24.5 to 53.2 years). The majority of patients with mood disorder in most studies were men (average, 57.1%; range, 34.8% to 100%). Most of the patients with mood disorders in these studies had bipolar illness (average unipolar, 31.3%; range, 0% to

Table 2. Brain Measure and Effect Size Information for Meta-analysis 1*

Source, y†	QIRR	Ventricular Size, Mean (SD): Patients With Mood Disorder	Ventricular Size, Mean (SD): Controls	Effect Direction and Size, d‡	Our Computed P Value	Reported P Value
Jacoby and Levy,[11] 1980§‖	Absent	NA¶	NA	+0.165	.43	NS
Pearlson and Veroff,[12] 1981	Present	6.5 (3.3)	3.6 (2.6)	+1.01	.001	<.005
Nasrallah et al,[13] 1982	Absent	7.5 (3.2)	4.5 (2.6)	+1.02	.001	<.005
Weinberger et al,[15] 1982	Absent	3.8 (2.9)	2.9 (2.9)	+0.305	.29	.40
Kellner et al,[16] 1983	Absent	5.5 (2.7)	5.5 (2.8)	+0.007	.99	...
Scott et al,[17] 1983	Present	9.5 (3.4)	4.2 (2.9)	+1.60	.002	<.001
Targum et al,[18] 1983	Absent	4.4 (2.8)‖	2.9 (2.9)	+0.522	.04	...
Luchins et al,[19] 1984	Present	4.5 (2.7)	3.0 (2.3)	+0.617	.006	.03
Pearlson et al,[20] 1984	Absent	6.6 (3.4)	4.8 (2.1)	+0.645	.02	<.0125
Shima et al,[21] 1984	Absent	11.2 (3.5)	9.1 (2.4)	+0.694	.001	.001
Dolan et al,[22] 1985	Present	7.24 (3.9)‖	5.6 (2.6)‖	+0.466	.005	<.02
Kolbeinsson et al,[24] 1986	Absent	9.9 (1.8)‖	8.4 (1.5)‖	+0.858	.002	<.01
Besson et al,[25] 1987	Absent	4.5 (0.3)‖	4.3 (0.4)‖	+0.494	.28	NS
Schlegel and Kretzchmar,[26] 1987‖	Absent	7.4 (2.4)	6.9 (2.6)	+0.198	.31	NS
Dewan et al,[27] 1988	Absent	6.9 (2.9)	6.3 (1.9)	+0.240	.41	.20
Iacono et al,[28] 1988	Present	6.3 (2.5)	6.4 (2.8)	−0.043	.85	NS
Johnstone et al,[29] 1989#	Present	0.34 (0.15)‖	0.32 (0.11)‖	+0.128	.68	NS
Pearlson et al,[30] 1989	Present	11.8 (4.3)‖	8.6 (2.8)	+0.881	.002	...
Rossi et al,[31] 1989‖	Present	NA**	NA	+0.055††	.81	NS
Abas et al,[32] 1990	Present	NA‡‡	NA	+0.370	.26	NS
Andreasen et al,[33] 1990	Present	6.8 (3.1)‖	5.8 (2.5)	+0.372	.04	NS
Swayze et al,[34] 1990#	Present	10.8 (5.2)	9.7 (4.2)	+0.232	.26	NS
Beats et al,[36] 1991#	Absent	3.2 (2.0)‖	2.6 (1.1)‖	+0.396	.16	NS
Rabins et al,[37] 1991§‖	Present	1.3 (0.9)	0.50 (0.62)	+0.899	.01	<.05
Van den Bossche et al,[38] 1991‖#	Absent	0.29 (0.05)‖	0.28 (0.05)	+0.164	.58	NS
Lauer et al,[39] 1992‖	Absent	NA§§	NA	+0.922††	.009	<.05
Coffey et al,[41] 1993§‖	Present	NA ‖‖	NA	+0.297	.10	NS
Raz,[42] 1993‖#	Present	NA¶¶	NA	+0.846††	.006	<.01
Strakowski et al,[43] 1993#	Present	9.1 (4.7)	6.7 (3.2)	+0.579	.10	.07

*QIRR indicates quantitative interrater reliability information; NA, not applicable; NS, not significant; and ellipses, missing data.
†All studies used the ventricular-brain ratio (VBR) quantitative measure of ventricular enlargement unless otherwise indicated.
‡Effect type for all studies was simple unless otherwise indicated.
§Used a rating measure of ventricular enlargement.
‖In "Special Considerations" table available from the authors on request.
¶Frequency of abnormal score for patients with mood disorder, 9/40; for controls, 8/50.
#Used a quantitative measure of ventricular enlargement other than VBR.
**Effect size based on an F=0.06.
††Effect type was complex.
‡‡Effect size based on an F=1.36.
§§Effect size based on an F=7.12.
‖‖Frequency of abnormal score for patients with mood disorder, 26/48; for controls, 30/76.
¶¶Effect size was taken from reported "g" value (0.86). (See "Effect Sizes" subsection in the "Methods" section for explanation of g.)

100%). All but two of the studies were based on computed tomographic data. All but one of the 11 studies employed VBR for the assessment of ventricular size. The average VBR for the mood disorder group was 6.23 (average SD, 1.26; range, 3.8 to 7.5) and the average VBR for the schizophrenic patient group was 7.38 (SD, 1.60; range, 6.0 to 10.0). Seven of the 11 studies included quantitative interrater reliability data on the brain measure.

Summary of Effects

Nine (82%) of the 11 studies reported effect sizes in the opposite direction of the hypothesis, indicating that patients with mood disorders have smaller ventricles than patients with schizophrenia. However, all of the studies reported that this comparison was not statistically significant. Thus, a vote-counting procedure would clearly conclude that there was no significant effect. The composite effect size was −0.201, undoubtedly small (Table 3). However, this composite effect was highly statistically significant (P=.002). Thus, the meta-analysis provides evidence for a small, but highly statistically significant effect in support of the notion that patients with schizophrenia have larger ventricles than patients with mood disorders. The effect size was not heterogeneous. The most negative effect size was −0.852 and the most positive effect size was +0.21. The power of the average hypothesis test (effect size, 0.20; average sample size, 45) was 0.15.

In the set of studies that were relevant to but not included in this meta-analysis, there were six[45,46,49,53,61,66] that reached a useful conclusion regarding the hypothesis. Five studies[46,49,53,61,66] concluded that patients with mood disorders do not differ significantly from patients with schizophrenia on measures of ventricular size. The sixth study[45] did not reach a conclusion regarding this question, but our

Table 3. Composite Effect Sizes and Homogeneity Tests for Meta-analyses 1, 2, and 3

Meta-analysis	Composite Effect Size, d	95% Confidence Limits	*P* Value for Composite Effect Size	Homogeneity Test, Q	*P* Value for Homogeneity Test
1	+0.437	+0.34, +0.53	<.001	39.80	.13
2	+0.421	+0.26, +0.58	<.001	9.66	.38
3	−0.201	−0.33, −0.07	.002	9.28	.51

Table 4. Brain Measure and Effect Size Information for Meta-analysis 2*

		Sulcal Prominence Rating, Mean (SD)				
Source, y	QIRR	Patients With Mood Disorder	Controls	Effect Direction and Size, d†	Our Computed *P* Value	Reported *P* Value
Nasrallah et al,[13] 1982‡	Absent	NA§	NA	+0.641‖	.03	<.10
Tanaka et al,[14] 1982‡	Absent	NA¶	NA	+0.177	.54	. . .
Weinberger et al,[15] 1982	Absent	NA#	NA	+0.557	.06	. . .
Dolan et al,[23] 1986‡	Present	NA**	NA	+0.600‖	.00	.001
Kolbeinsson et al,[24] 1986‡	Absent	0.75 (0.76)‡	0.20 (0.40)	+0.808	.003	<.05
Dewan et al,[27] 1988	Absent	1.9 (1.1)	1.9 (1.1)	+0.053	.85	.43
Iacono et al,[28] 1988	Present	1.9 (0.9)	1.8 (0.8)	+0.150	.51	NS
Abas et al,[32] 1990‡	Present	NA††	NA	+0.520	.12	NS
Rabins et al,[37] 1991‡	Present	1.6 (0.6)‡	1.2 (0.2)‡	+0.810	.02	<.05
Coffey et al,[41] 1993‡	Present	NA‡‡	NA	+0.227	.21	NS

*QIRR indicates quantitative interrater reliability information; NA, not applicable; NS, not significant; and ellipses, missing data.
†Effect type for all studies was simple unless otherwise indicated.
‡In "Special Considerations" table available from the authors on request.
§Frequency of abnormal score for patients with mood disorder, 6/24; for controls, 1/27.
‖Effect type was complex.
¶Frequency of abnormal score for patients with mood disorder: frontal, 14/24; temporal, 18/24; parietal, 11/24; and occipital, 6/24. For controls: frontal, 13/24; temporal, 12/24; parietal, 17/24; and occipital, 1/24.
#Frequency of abnormal score for patients with mood disorder, 3/23; for controls, 0/26.
**Effect size based on an F=12.5.
††Effect size based on an F=2.68.
‡‡Frequency of abnormal score for patients with mood disorder, 25/48; for controls, 31/76.

own computation indicates that the differences between the two patient groups were not statistically significant (P>.4). Thus, no single study in our meta-analytic database concluded that there is a statistically significant difference between patients with schizophrenia and patients with mood disorders on measures of ventricular size.

Potential Moderators of Effect Size

None of the potential moderators of effect size had a statistically significant relationship with effect size (all P values, >.41).

Publication Bias and Fail-Safe N

The funnel plot for this meta-analysis is presented in the Figure, bottom left. Notwithstanding the small number of studies, the characteristic inverted funnel appearance is suggested. There is no clear evidence for publication bias, as studies with small N's were published with small positive and negative effect sizes. The fail-safe N was 10.

META-ANALYSIS 4

The studies included in meta-analysis 4, comparing patients with mood disorders with schizophrenic patients on measures of cortical sulcal prominence, are presented in Table 1 and **Table 6**.

General Description of the Studies

There were only three studies that met inclusion criteria for this meta-analysis. This is obviously too small a sample to support a full statistical review or to consider these studies in the aggregate. Therefore, these three studies will be briefly described individually.

Nasrallah et al[13] compared 24 male patients with mood disorders with 55 male schizophrenic patients on cortical atrophy ratings. The mean age of both patient groups was approximately 30 years. The percentage of abnormal ratings was higher in the schizophrenic group (40%) than that in the mood disorders group (25%), although the difference in these proportions was not statistically significant.

Weinberger et al[15] compared 23 patients with mood disorders with 17 schizophrenic patients on cortical atrophy ratings. The mean age for both groups was approximately 30 years. Three of the 23 patients with mood disorders had abnormal ratings, whereas none of the patients with schizophrenia had abnormal ratings. Although a statistical comparison was not provided in the original report, our analysis would indicate that this difference is not statistically significant.

Table 5. Brain Measure and Effect Size Information for Meta-analysis 3*

Source, y†	QIRR	Ventricular Size, Mean (SD): Patients With Mood Disorder	Ventricular Size, Mean (SD): Schizophrenic Patients	Effect Direction and Size, d‡	Our Computed P Value	Reported P Value
Nasrallah et al,[13] 1982	Absent	7.5 (3.2)	8.7 (4.0)	−0.315	.16	NS
Weinberger et al,[15] 1982	Absent	3.8 (2.9)	6.0 (4.2)	−0.615	.06	.17
Luchins et al,[19] 1984	Present	NA§‖	NA‖	+ 0.206	.40	NS
Pearlson et al,[20] 1984	Absent	6.6 (3.4)	6.2 (2.6)	+ 0.127	.67	...
Iacono et al,[28] 1988	Present	6.3 (2.5)	6.7 (2.6)	−0.181	.47	NS
Johnstone et al,[29] 1989	Present	0.34 (0.15)‖	0.35 (0.13)‖	−0.054	.86	NS
Rossi et al,[31] 1989‖	Present	NA¶	NA	−0.339#	.14	.07
Andreasen et al,[33] 1990	Present	6.6 (3.1)‖	6.7 (2.9)	−0.037	.82	NS
Swayze et al,[34] 1990**	Present	10.8 (5.2)	12.7 (5.7)	−0.341	.09	NS
Woods et al,[35] 1990‖	Absent	6.6 (3.8)	10.0 (3.8)	−0.852	.08	<.10
Sacchetti et al,[40] 1992	Present	NA††	NA	−0.237	.04	...

*QIRR indicates quantitative interrater reliability information; NS, not significant; NA, not applicable; and ellipses, missing data.
†All studies used the ventricular-brain ratio (VBR) quantitative measure of ventricular enlargement unless otherwise indicated.
‡Effect type for all, studies was simple unless otherwise indicated.
§Frequency of abnormal score for patients with mood disorder, 4/22; for schizophrenic patients, 5/45.
‖In "Special Considerations" table available from the authors on request.
¶Effect size based on an F=2.27.
#Effect type was complex.
**Used a quantitative measure of ventricular enlargement other than VBR.
††Frequency of abnormal score for patients with mood disorder, 17/107; for schizophrenic patients, 53/206.

Iacono et al[28] compared 34 patients with mood disorders with 31 schizophrenic patients on cortical atrophy ratings. Patients in both groups were in their early 20s. The mean ratings were similar in the two patient groups, and the authors reported that the difference was not statistically significant.

Four studies[45,49,69,71] that were excluded from the meta-analysis were nonetheless relevant. Two[49,69] reported no differences in cortical sulcal appearance between patients with mood disorders and patients with schizophrenia, whereas one article[71] reported that patients with schizophrenia have increased sulcal fluid volume compared with patients with bipolar illness. One article[45] claimed that patients with schizophrenia had more diffuse atrophy than patients with mood disorder.

COMMENT

The four meta-analyses have relevance for two major questions: Do patients with mood disorder have ventricular enlargement or increased sulcal prominence? Is the degree of ventricular enlargement or increased sulcal prominence in patients with mood disorders comparable to or less than that seen in patients with schizophrenia?

MOOD DISORDERS VS NORMAL CONTROLS

Both meta-analyses 1 and 2 yielded highly statistically significant effect sizes, indicating that the published literature, taken as a whole, clearly supports the notion that patients with mood disorders do indeed have increased ventricular enlargement and sulcal prominence when compared with controls. It is noteworthy that the composite effect sizes for both analyses were similar (+0.437 and +0.421) in magnitude. The magnitude of these effects can be described as moderate or moderate to small. On average, the difference between groups of patients with mood disorders and controls on measures of either ventricular enlargement or sulcal prominence is approximately 0.4 SD units. Although there was considerable variability in study results, statistically there was no evidence of heterogeneity in study outcomes. There was no evidence of publication bias against nonsignficant results, since a number of reported effects were nonsignificant. However, there was an indication of a reluctance to publish studies with results opposite to the hypothesis, ie, studies indicating that patients with mood disorders have less ventricular enlargement or sulcal prominence than controls.

None of the methodological factors (imaging modality [computed tomography vs MRI], presence or absence of quantitative interrater reliability data) and none of the subject characteristics (gender, proportion of bipolar vs unipolar subjects, type of control group [medical vs community]) were systematically related to study effect size.

In addition to the evidence of generalized structural abnormalities, a number of recent MRI studies have implicated various specific brain areas in mood disorders. For example, reductions of volume in the frontal lobe,[41] temporal lobe,[78] brain stem, vermis cerebelli,[79] and caudate nuclei[80] have all been reported in patients with mood disorders. However, a number of negative findings have also been reported for most of these regions.[29,43,81,82] The evidence for global abnormalities is more consistent and compelling at this time, although further study is warranted. It is important to note that in the presence of documented global abnormalities, one would expect to find abnormalities in specific brain areas. Parsimony requires that one determines the proportion of the variance accounted for by the volume of a specific brain area after controlling for global structural abnormalities.

Table 6. Brain Measure and Effect Size Information for Meta-analysis 4*

Source, y	QIRR	Sulcal Prominence Rating, Mean (SD): Patients With Mood Disorder	Sulcal Prominence Rating, Mean (SD): Schizophrenic Patients	Effect Direction and Size, d†	Our Computed *P* Value	Reported *P* Value
Nasrallah et al,[13] 1982	Absent	NA‡	NA	−0.314	.17	NS
Weinberger et al,[15] 1982	Absent	NA§	NA	+0.499	.12	...
Iacono et al,[28] 1988	Present	1.9 (0.9)	2.1 (0.9)	−0.137	.58	NS

**QIRR indicates quantitative interrater reliability information; NA, not applicable; NS, not significant; and ellipses, missing data.*
†Effect type for all studies was simple.
‡Frequency of abnormal score for patients with mood disorder, 6/24; for schizophrenic patients, 22/25.
§Frequency of abnormal score for patients with mood disorder, 3/23; for schizophrenic patients, 0/17.

As pointed out by Nasrallah et al,[5] it is not clear if the global structural findings noted in the literature are state-related or stable traits. Reversibility of global structural changes is established in certain conditions, such as alcoholism[83] and anorexia nervosa.[84] However, there is no direct and compelling evidence that ventricular enlargement or sulcal prominence is reversible in depression. Alternatively, the structural abnormalities in mood disorders may reflect hypoplasia, dysplasia, permanent brain damage, or some combination of these.

MOOD DISORDERS VS SCHIZOPHRENIA

The meta-analysis yielded a statistically significant effect size for this comparison, indicating that patients with schizophrenia have greater ventricular enlargement than patients with mood disorders. This meta-analytic result is particularly interesting in light of the fact that no single study in our meta-analytic database reported a statistically significant difference between these two patient groups on VBR. Clearly, a traditional vote-counting procedure would have concluded that there is no effect. Since the effect was small (−0.2), one might be tempted to conclude that it is a chance finding. However, the *P* value associated with the finding was small ($P=.002$). Thus, it appears that patients with schizophrenia have slightly greater ventricular enlargement than patients with mood disorders, but this effect is small and a large sample is required to find such an effect. One interpretation of these findings is that there is a common pathophysiology underlying ventricular enlargement in schizophrenia and mood disorders, but it is more potent in the former. Alternatively, there may be two distinct pathophysiological pathways for ventricular enlargement, with the pathophysiology in schizophrenia leading to increased structural abnormality.

No conclusion can be reached regarding the difference between patients with mood disorders and patients with schizophrenia on cortical sulcal prominence. There were too few studies to support a full quantitative analysis.

A comparison of the effect sizes of meta-analyses 1, 2, and 3, taken together, indicate that, in terms of generalized structural brain abnormalities, patients with mood disorders are less different from patients with schizophrenia than from controls. On review of the brain imaging literature on depression, Jeste et al[4] reached a similar conclusion:

> In every area in which structural abnormalities have been found in neuroradiological studies of schizophrenia, abnormalities of similar magnitude have also been demonstrated in affective disorders.[4]

Thus, the results of the present meta-analysis as well as the review of Jeste et al[4] suggest a commonality between these two major mental disorders.

The potential commonality between psychotic depression, specifically, and schizophrenia has strong face validity and has received considerable attention. Such a commonality is consistent with reports from our laboratory more than 20 years ago. Specifically, early studies by one of us (H.Y.M.) revealed neuromuscular abnormalities (eg, increased serum creatine kinase activity, skeletal muscle fiber abnormalities, and subterminal motor nerve sprouting[85,86]) in patients with psychotic depression as well as patients with schizophrenia. It was proposed that the neuromuscular dysfunction was the result of the loss of neurons, which might be part of a more general loss of neural tissue. On the basis of these findings, it was suggested that schizophrenia was part of a psychotic continuum. The suggestion was that the presence of psychotic symptoms, particularly what are now called positive symptoms, defined a class of patients with shared biological characteristics. This class of patients would encompass individuals who met diagnostic criteria for schizophrenia or mood disorders based on symptoms, clinical course, and customary exclusion criteria. Andreasen and Flaum[87] have discussed the symptom overlap between mood disorders and schizophrenia. Other biological abnormalities have been found to be present in patients with both types of disorders. For example, abnormalities have been noted in both patient groups in hypothalamic-pituitary-adrenal function,[88,89] serum dopamine β-hydroxylase activity,[90] sleep,[91] and evoked potentials.[92] Studies of family history and genetics also support a continuum model of mood disorders and schizophrenia.[93]

It is important to note that ventricular enlargement and/or increased sulcal prominence have been noted in a number of other neurological and psychiatric conditions.[10,94-101] It is not clear at this time whether ventricular enlargement and increased sulcal prominence arise in all of these conditions for the same or different reasons.

CONCLUSION

The meta-analyses provide strong statistical evidence in support of the conclusion that patients with mood disorders have ventricular enlargement and increased cortical sulcal prominence when compared with normal controls. The statistical power of meta-analysis has allowed us to uncover significant evidence for a greater degree of ventricular enlargement in schizophrenia compared with mood disorders. However, this effect is small. In general, the present findings are consistent with a continuum model of mood disorder and schizophrenia.

Accepted for publication May 31, 1995.

This research was supported by grants MH 411684 and MH 415494 from the US Public Health Service (USPHS) (Dr Meltzer), the National Alliance for Research in Schizophrenia and Depression and the Scottish Rite Foundation (Dr Friedman), and the Prentiss Foundation (Dr Meltzer). Dr Meltzer is a recipient of a USPHS Research Career Scientist Development Award (MH 47808) and Dr Elkis was a recipient of a postdoctoral scholarship from CNPq (Brasilia/Brazil).

Reprint requests to Assistant Professor of Psychiatry, Department of Psychiatry, University Hospitals of Cleveland, Hanna Pavilion, First Floor Mail Room, 11100 Euclid Ave, Cleveland, OH 44106-5000 (Dr Friedman).

REFERENCES

1. Shelton RC, Weinberger DR. X-ray computerized tomography studies in schizophrenia: a review and synthesis. In: Nasrallah HA, Weinberger DR, eds. *Handbook of Schizophrenia: The Neurology of Schizophrenia.* New York, NY: Elsevier Science Publishers; 1986;1:207-250.
2. Raz S, Raz N. Structural abnormalities in major psychosis: a quantitative review of the evidences from computerized images. *Psychol Bull.* 1990;108:93-108.
3. Van Horn JD, McManus IC. Ventricular enlargement in schizophrenia: a meta-analysis of studies of the ventricle:brain ratio (vbr). *Br J Psychiatry.* 1992;160:687-697.
4. Jeste DV, Lohr JB, Goodwin FK. Neuroanatomical studies of major affective disorders: a review and suggestions for further research. *Br J Psychiatry.* 1988;153:444-459.
5. Nasrallah HA, Coffman JA, Olson SC. Structural brain-imaging findings in affective disorders: an overview. *J Neuropsychiatry.* 1989;1:21-26.
6. Schlegel S. Computed tomography in affective disorders. In: Hauser P, ed. *Brain Imaging in Affective Disorders.* Washington, DC: American Psychiatric Press; 1991:1-24.
7. Hedges LV, Olkin I. Vote-counting methods in research synthesis. *Psychol Bull.* 1980;88:359-369.
8. Hedges LV, Olkin I. *Statistical Methods for Meta-analysis.* San Diego, Calif: Academic Press; 1985.
9. Cooper H, Hedges LV. *The Handbook of Research Synthesis.* New York, NY: Russell Sage Foundation; 1994.
10. Murphy DGM, DeCarli C, Schapiro MB, Rapoport SI, Horwitz B. Age-related differences in volumes of subcortical nuclei, brain matter, and cerebrospinal fluid in healthy men as measured with magnetic resonance imaging. *Arch Neurol.* 1992;49:839-845.
11. Jacoby RJ, Levy R. Computed tomography in the elderly, 3: affective disorders. *Br J Psychiatry.* 1980;136:270-275.
12. Pearlson GD, Veroff AE. Computerized tomographic scan changes in manic-depressive illness. *Lancet.* 1981;2:370.
13. Nasrallah HA, McCalley-Whitters M, Jacoby CG. Cortical atrophy in schizophrenia and mania: a comparative CT study. *J Clin Psychiatry.* 1982;43:439-441.
14. Tanaka Y, Hazama H, Fukuhara T, Tsutsui T. Computerized tomography of the brain in manic-depressive patients: a controlled study. *Folia Psychiatr Neurolog Jpn.* 1982;36:137-143.
15. Weinberger DR, DeLisi LE, Perman GP, Targun S, Wyatt RJ. Computed tomography in schizophreniform disorder and other acute psychiatric disorders. *Arch Gen Psychiatry.* 1982;39:778-783.
16. Kellner CH, Rubinow DR, Gold PW, Post RM. Relationship of cortisol hypersecretion to brain CT scan alterations in depressed patients. *Psychiatry Res.* 1983;8:191-197.
17. Scott ML, Golden CJ, Ruedrich SL, Bishop RJ. Ventricular enlargement in major depression. *Psychiatry Res.* 1983;8:91-93.
18. Targum SD, Rosen LN, DeLisi LE, Weinberger DR, Citrin CM. Cerebral ventricular size in major depressive disorder: association with delusional symptoms. *Biol Psychiatry.* 1983;18:329-336.
19. Luchins DJ, Lewine RRJ, Meltzer HY. Lateral ventricular size, psychopathology, and medication response in the psychoses. *Biol Psychiatry.* 1984;19:29-44.
20. Pearlson GD, Garbacz DJ, Breakey WR, Ahn HS, DePaulo JR. Lateral ventricular enlargement associated with persistent unemployment and negative symptoms in both schizophrenia and bipolar disorders. *Psychiatry Res.* 1984;12:1-9.
21. Shima S, Shikano T, Kitamura T, Masuda Y, Tsukumo T, Kanba S, Asai M. Depression and ventricular enlargement. *Acta Psychiatr Scand.* 1984;70:275-277.
22. Dolan RJ, Calloway SP, Mann AH. Cerebral ventricular size in depressed subjects. *Psychol Med.* 1985;15:873-878.
23. Dolan RJ, Calloway SP, Thacker PF, Mann AH. The cerebral cortical appearance in the depressed subjects. *Psychol Med.* 1986;16:775-779.
24. Kolbeinsson H, Arnaldsson OS, Petursson H, Skulason S. Computed tomography scans in ECT patients. *Acta Psychiatr Scand.* 1986;73:28-32.
25. Besson JAO, Henderson JG, Foreman EI, Smith FW. An NMR study of lithium-responding manic depressive patients. *Magn Reson Imaging.* 1987;5:273-277.
26. Schlegel S, Kretzchmar K. Computed tomography in affective disorders, I: ventricular and sulcal measurements. *Biol Psychiatry.* 1987;22:4-14.
27. Dewan MJ, Haldipur CV, Lane EE, Ispahani A, Boucher MF, Major LF. Bipolar affective disorder, I: comprehensive quantitative computed tomography. *Acta Psychiatr Scand.* 1988;77:670-676.
28. Iacono WG, Smith G, Moreau M, Beiser M, Fleming JAE, Lin T, Flak B. Ventricular and sulcal size at the onset of psychosis. *Am J Psychiatry.* 1988;145:820-924.
29. Johnstone EC, Owens DG, Crow TJ, Frith CD, Alexandropolous K, Bydder G, Colter N. Temporal lobe structure as determined by nuclear magnetic resonance in schizophrenia and bipolar affective disorder. *J Neurol Neurosurg Psychiatry.* 1989;52:736-741.
30. Pearlson GD, Rabins PT, Kim WS, Speedie LJ, Moberg PJ, Burns A, Bascon MJ. Structural brain CT changes and cognitive deficits in elderly depressives with and without reversible dementia ('pseudodementia'). *Psychol Med.* 1989;19:573-584.
31. Rossi A, Stratta P, di Michelle V, Bolino F, Nistico R, de Leonardis R, Sabatini MD, Casacchia M. A computerized tomographic study in patients with depressive disorder: a comparison with schizophrenic patients and controls. *Acta Psychiatr Belg.* 1989;89:56-61.
32. Abas MA, Sahakian BJ, Levy R. Neuropsychological deficits and CT scan changes in elderly depressives. *Psychol Med.* 1990;20:507-520.
33. Andreasen NC, Swayze VW II, Flaum M, Alliger R, Cohen G. Ventricular abnormalities in affective disorders: clinical and demographic correlates. *Am J Psychiatry.* 1990;147:893-900.
34. Swayze VW II, Andreasen NC, Alliger RJ, Ehrhardt JC, Yuh WT. Structural brain abnormalities in bipolar affective disorder: ventricular enlargement and focal signal hyperintensities. *Arch Gen Psychiatry.* 1990;47:1054-1059.
35. Woods BT, Yurgelun-Todd D, Benes FM, Frankenburg FR, Pope HG, McSparren J. Progressive ventricular enlargement in schizophrenia: comparison to bipolar affective disorder and correlation with clinical course. *Biol Psychiatry.* 1990;27:341-352.
36. Beats B, Levy R, Förstl H. Ventricular enlargement and caudate hyperdensity in elderly depressives. *Biol Psychiatry.* 1991;30:452-458.
37. Rabins PV, Pearlson GD, Aylward E, Kumar AJ, Dowell K. Cortical magnetic resonance imaging changes in elderly in patients with major depression. *Am J Psychiatry.* 1991;148:617-620.
38. Van den Bossche H, Maes M, Brussard C, Schotte C, Cosyns P, De Moor J, De Schepper A. Computed tomography of the brain in unipolar depression. *J Affect Disord.* 1991;21:67-74.
39. Lauer CJ, Wiegand M, Krieg J-C. All-night electroencephalographic sleep and cranial computed tomography in depression. *Eur Arch Psychiatry Clin Neurosci.* 1992;242:59-68.
40. Sacchetti E, Calzeroni A, Vita A, Terzi A, Pollastro F, Cazzullo CL. The brain damage hypothesis of seasonality of births in schizophrenia and major affective disorders: evidence from computerized tomography. *Br J Psychiatry.* 1992;160:390-397.
41. Coffey CE, Wilkinson WE, Weiner RD, Parashos IA, Djang WT, Webb MC, Figiel GS, Spritzer CE. Quantitative cerebral anatomy of depression: a controlled magnetic resonance imaging study. *Arch Gen Psychiatry.* 1993;50:7-16.
42. Raz S. Structural cerebral pathology in schizophrenia: regional or diffuse? *J Abnorm Psychol.* 1993;102:445-452.
43. Strakowski SM, Wilson DR, Tohen M, Woods BT, Douglass AW, Stoll AL. Structural brain abnormalities in first-episode mania. *Biol Psychiatry.* 1993;33:602-609.
44. von Gall M, Becker H. Zur Anwendung der Computertomogtaphie (CT) in der Klinischen Psychiatrie. *Fortschr Neurol Psychiatr.* 1978;46:361-368.
45. Strobl G, Reisner TH, Zeiler K. Die Craniale Computer-Tomographie in der Pscyhiatrie. *Nervenarzt.* 1980;51:36-40.
46. Johnstone EC, Owens DGC, Crow TJ, Jagoe R. A CT study of 188 patients

with schizophrenia, affective psychosis and neurotic illness. In: Perris C, Struwe G, Jansson B, eds. *Biological Psychiatry 1981.* New York, NY: Elsevier/North Holland Biomedical Press; 1981:237-240.
47. Pearlson GD, Veroff AE, McHugh PR. The use of computed tomography in psychiatry: recent applications to schizophrenia, manic-depressive illness and dementia syndromes. *Johns Hopkins Med J.* 1981;149:194-202.
48. Nasrallah HA, McCalley-Whitters M, Jacoby CG. Cerebral ventricular enlargement in young manic males: a controlled CT study. *J Affect Disord.* 1982;4:15-19.
49. Rieder RO, Mann LS, Weinberger DR, van Kammen DP, Post RM. Computed tomographic scans in patients with schizophrenia, schizoaffective, and bipolar affective disorder. *Arch Gen Psychiatry.* 1983;40:735-739.
50. Nasrallah HA, McCalley-Whitters M, Pfohl B. Clinical significance of large cerebral ventricles in manic males. *Psychiatry Res.* 1984;13:151-156.
51. Pearlson GD, Garbacz DJ, Tompkins RH, Ahn HS, Gutterman DF, Veroff AE, DePaulo JR. Clinical correlates of lateral ventricular enlargement in bipolar affective disorders. *Am J Psychiatry.* 1984;141:253-256.
52. Lippman S, Manshadi M, Baldwin H, Drasin G, Wagemaker HW, Rice J, Alrajeh S. Cerebral CAT scan imaging in schizophrenic and bipolar patients. *J Ky Med Assoc.* 1985;83:13-15.
53. Owens DGC, Johnstone EC, Crow TJ, Frith CD, Jagoe JR, Kreel L. Lateral ventricular size in schizophrenia: relationship to the disease process and its clinical manifestations. *Psychol Med.* 1985;15:27-41.
54. Pearlson GD, Garbacz DJ, Moberg PJ, Ahn HS, DePaulo JR. Symptomatic, familial, perinatal and social correlates of computerized axial tomography (CAT) changes in schizophrenics and bipolars. *J Nerv Ment Dis.* 1985;173:42-50.
55. Johnstone EC, Owens DGC, Crow TJ, Colter N, Lawton CA, Jagoe R, Kreel L. Hypothyroidism as a correlate of lateral ventricular enlargement in manic-depressive and neurotic illness. *Br J Psychiatry.* 1986;148:317-321.
56. Kling AS, Metter EJ, Riege WH, Khul DE. Comparison of PET measurement of local brain glucose metabolism and CAT measurement of brain atrophy in chronic schizophrenia and depression. *Am J Psychiatry.* 1986;143:175-180.
57. Rossi A, Stratta P, Petruzzi C, De Donatis M, Nistico R, Casacchia M. A computerized tomographic study in *DSM-III* affective disorders. *J Affect Disord.* 1987;12:259-262.
58. Dewan MJ, Haldipur CV, Boucher M, Major LF. Is CT ventriculomegaly related to hypercortisolemia? *Acta Psychiatr Scand.* 1988;77:230-231.
59. Crow TJ, Colter N, Frith CD, Johnstone EC, Owens DGC. Developmental arrest of cerebral asymmetries in early-onset schizophrenia. *Psychiatry Res.* 1989;29:247-253.
60. Johnstone EC, Owens DGC, Bydder GM, Colter N, Crow TJ, Frith CD. The spectrum of structural brain changes in schizophrenia: age of onset as a predictor of cognitive and clinical impairments and their cerebral correlates. *Psychol Med.* 1989;19:91-103.
61. Clark C, Marbeck R, Li D. An empirical model for analysing and interpreting ventricular measures. *J Neurol Neurosurg Psychiatry.* 1990;53:411-415.
62. Fukushima J, Morita N, Fukushima K, Chiba T, Tanaka S, Yamashita I. Voluntary control of saccadic eye movements in patients with schizophrenic and affective disorders. *J Psychiatr Res.* 1990;24:9-24.
63. Harvey I, Williams M, Toone BK, Lewis SW, Turner SW, McGuffin P. The ventricular-brain ratio (VBR) in functional psychoses: the relationship of lateral ventricular and total intracranial area. *Psychol Med.* 1990;20:55-62.
64. Zubenko GS, Sullivan P, Nelson NP, Belle SH, Huff FJ, Wolf GL. Brain imaging abnormalities in mental disorders of late life. *Arch Neurol.* 1990;47:1107-1111.
65. Lammers C-H, Doraiswamy PM, Husain MM, Figiel GS, Lurie SN, Boyko OB, Ellinwood EH Jr, Nemeroff CB, Krishnan KRR. MRI of corpus callosum and septum pellucidum in depression. *Biol Psychiatry.* 1991;29:295-308.
66. Lewine RRJ, Risch SC, Risby E, Stipetic M, Jewart RD, Eccard M, Caudle J, Pollard W. Lateral ventricle-brain ratio and balance between CSF HVA and 5-HIAA in schizophrenia. *Am J Psychiatry.* 1991;148:1189-1194.
67. Risch SC, Lewine RJ, Kalin NH, Jewart RD, Risby ED, Caudle JM, Stipetic M, Turner J, Eccard M, Pollard W. Limbic-hypothalamic-pituitary-adrenal-axis activity and ventricular-to-brain ratio studies in affective illness and schizophrenia. *Neuropsychopharmacology.* 1992;6:95-100.
68. Shiraishi H, Koizumi J, Hori M, Terashima Y, Suzuki T, Saito K, Mizukami K, Tanaka Y, Yamaguchi N. A computerized tomographic study in patients with delusional and non-delusional depression. *Jpn J Psychiatry Neurol.* 1992;42:99-105.
69. Mulsant BH, Stergiou A, Keshavan MS, Sweet RA, Rifai AH, Pasternak R, Zubenko GS. Schizophrenia in late life: elderly patients admitted to an acute care psychiatric hospital. *Schizopren Bull.* 1993;19:709-721.
70. Krishnan KRR, McDonald WM, Doraiswamy PM, Tupler LA, Husain M, Boyko OB, Figiel GS, Ellinwood EH Jr. Neuroanatomical substrates of depression in the elderly. *Eur Arch Psychiatry Clin Neurosci.* 1993;243:41-46.
71. Harvey I, Persaud R, Ron MA, Barker G, Murray RM. Volumetric MRI measures in bipolars compared with schizophrenics and healthy controls. *Psychol Med.* 1994;4:689-699.
72. Cohen J. *Statistical Power Analysis for the Behavioural Sciences.* 2nd ed. Hillsdale, NJ: Lawrence Erlbaum Associates; 1988.
73. Johnson BT. *DSTAT: Software for the Meta-analytic Review of Research Literature.* Hillsdale, NJ: Lawrence Erlbaum Associates Inc; 1989.
74. Borenstein M, Cohen J. *Statistical Power Analysis: A Computer Program.* Hillsdale, NJ: Lawrence Erlbaum Associates Inc; 1988.
75. Light RJ, Pillemer DB. *Summing Up: The Science of Reviewing Research.* Cambridge, Mass: Harvard University Press; 1984.
76. Rosenthal R. The 'file drawer problem' and tolerance for null results. *Psychol Bull.* 1979;86:638-641.
77. Orwin RG. A fail-safe N for effect size. *J Educ Stat.* 1983;8:157-159.
78. Altshuler LL, Conrad A, Hauser P, Li X, Guze BH, Denikoff K, Tourtellotte W, Post R. Reduction of temporal lobe volume in bipolar disorder: a preliminary report of magnetic resonance imaging. *Arch Gen Psychiatry.* 1991;48:482-483.
79. Shah SA, Doraiswamy PM, Husain MM, Escalona PR, Na C, Figiel GS, Paterson LJ, Ellinwood EH, McDonald WM, Boyko OB, Nemeroff CB, Krishnan KRR. Posterior fossa abnormalities in major depression: a controlled magnetic resonance imaging study. *Acta Psychiatr Scand.* 1992;85:474-479.
80. Krishnan KR, McDonald WM, Escalona PR, Doraiswamy PM, Na C, Husain MM, Figiel GS, Boyko OB, Ellinwood EH, Nemeroff CB. Magnetic resonance imaging of the caudate nuclei in depression: preliminary observations. *Arch Gen Psychiatry.* 1992;49:553-557.
81. Yates WR, Jacoby CG, Andreasen NC. Cerebellar atrophy in schizophrenia and affective disorder. *Am J Psychiatry.* 1987;144:465-467.
82. Raine A, Lencz T, Reynolds G, Harrison G, Sheared C, Medley I, Reynolds LM, Cooper JE. An evaluation of structural and functional prefrontal deficits in schizophrenia: MRI and neuropsychological measures. *Psychiatry Res.* 1992;45:123-137.
83. Ron MA, Acker W, Shaw GK, Lishman WA. Computerized tomography of the brain in chronic alcoholism. *Brain.* 1982;105:497-514.
84. Kohlmeyer K, Lehmkuhl G, Poutska F. Computed tomography of anorexia nervosa. *Am J Neuroradiol.* 1983;4:437-438.
85. Meltzer HY. Skeletal muscle abnormalities in patients with affective disorders. *J Psychiatr Res.* 1973;10:43-57.
86. Meltzer HY. Neuromuscular dysfunction in schizophrenia. *Schizophr Bull.* 1976;2:106-135.
87. Andreasen NC, Flaum M. Schizophrenia: the characteristic symptoms. *Schizophr Bull.* 1991;17:27-49.
88. Carroll BJ, Martin FIR, Davies B. Resistance to suppression by dexamethasone of plasma 11-O.H.C.S. levels in severe depressive illness. *BMJ.* 1968;3:285-287.
89. Kaneko M, Yokoyama F, Hoshino Y, Takahagi K, Murata S, Watanabe M, Kumashiro H. Hypothalamic-pituitary-adrenal axis function in chronic schizophrenia: association with clinical features. *Neuropsychobiology.* 1992;25:1-7.
90. Meltzer HY, Tong C, Luchins DJ. Serum dopamine-beta-hydroxylase activity and lateral ventricular size in affective disorders and schizophrenia. *Biol Psychiatry.* 1984;19:1395-1402.
91. Hudson JI, Lipinski JF, Keck PE Jr, Aizley HG, Vuckovic A, Zierk KC, Pope HG Jr. Polysomnographic characteristics of schizophrenia in comparison with mania and depression. *Biol Psychiatry.* 1993;34:191-193.
92. Wexler BE. Beyond the Kraepelinean dichotomy. *Biol Psychiatry.* 1992;31:539-541.
93. Crow TJ. The continuum of psychosis and its genetic origins: the sixty-fifth Maudsley lecture. *Br J Psychiatry.* 1990;156:788-797.
94. Fazekas F, Alavi A, Chawluk JB, Zimmerman RA, Hackney D, Bilaniuk L, Rosen M, Alves WM, Hurtig HI, Jamieson DG, Kushner MJ, Reivich M. Comparison of CT, MR and PET in Alzheimer's dementia and normal aging. *J Nucl Med.* 1989;30:1607-1615.
95. Burns A, Jacoby R, Philpot M, Levy R. Computerised tomography in Alzheimer's disease: methods of scan analysis, comparison with normal controls, and clinical/radiological associations. *Br J Psychiatry.* 1991;159:609-614.
96. Starkstein SE, Folstein SE, Brandt J, Pearlson GD, McDonnell A, Folstein M. Brain atrophy in Huntington's disease: a CT-scan study. *Neuroradiology.* 1989;31:156-159.
97. Krieg J-C, Backmund H, Pirke K-M. Cranial computed tomography findings in bulimia. *Acta Psychiatr Scand.* 1987;75:144-149.
98. Krieg J-C, Pirke K-M, Lauer C, Backmund H. Endocrine, metabolic, and cranial computed tomographic findings in anorexia nervosa. *Biol Psychiatry.* 1988;23:377-387.
99. Baxter LR Jr. Neuroimaging studies of obsessive-compulsive disorder. *Psychiatr Clin North Am.* 1992;15:871-884.
100. Lader MH, Ron M, Petursson H. Computed axial brain tomography in long-term benzodiazepine users. *Psychol Med.* 1984;14:203-206.
101. Lishman WA. Alcohol and the brain. *Br J Psychiatry.* 1990;156:635-644.

ORIGINAL ARTICLE

Magnetic Resonance Imaging and Mood Disorders

Localization of White Matter and Other Subcortical Abnormalities

Renee M. Dupont, MD; Terry L. Jernigan, PhD; William Heindel, PhD; Nelson Butters, PhD; Kimberly Shafer, MS; Thomine Wilson, MA; John Hesselink, MD; J. Christian Gillin, MD

Background: Recent reports in the literature document an association between focal white matter abnormalities in bipolar as well as unipolar mood disorder. The importance of this finding and other associated anatomic differences is uncertain.

Methods: We examined the volume of abnormal white matter and other brain volumes using quantitative magnetic resonance imaging analysis. We explored the relationship of these variables with diagnosis, cognitive function, and clinical variables in 36 patients with bipolar disorder, 30 patients with unipolar disorder, and 26 control subjects who were free from significant medical and neurologic illness.

Results: Younger patients with bipolar disorder (but not similarly aged patients with unipolar disorder or controls) have an increased volume of abnormal white matter. Data also indicate that the total volume of abnormal white matter may be associated with increased cognitive impairment, increased rate of psychiatric illness in the family, and onset after adolescence.

Conclusion: Patients with bipolar disorder demonstrate a pattern of subcortical brain morphologic abnormalities and cognitive impairment.

(Arch Gen Psychiatry. 1995;52:747-755)

SUBCORTICAL WHITE matter abnormalities may be associated with primary and secondary psychiatric disorders. For example, a relationship between one white matter disease (multiple sclerosis) and depression or mania has been recognized in clinical and epidemiologic studies.[1-3] Moreover, our group,[4,5] Swayze et al,[6] Figiel et al,[7] and Aylward et al[8] have all reported a higher rate of white matter signal hyperintensity in patients with bipolar (BP) disorder than in age-matched control subjects. Patients with depression may also have a higher rate of white matter lesions.[9-14]

To our knowledge, this is the first study in which quantitative magnetic resonance imaging (MRI) analysis was used to compare patients with BP disorder (n=36), patients with unipolar (UP) disorder (n=30), and control subjects (n=26). The purpose of this study was to extend our clinical MRI findings in patients with BP disorder through the use of quantitative image analysis and to include comparison groups of patients with major depressive mood disorder and healthy control subjects. Based on our previous finding of increased prevalence of areas of signal hyperintensity in patients with BP disorder, we predicted an increased volume of abnormal white matter (AWM) in patients with BP disorder compared with age-matched control subjects and patients with UP disorder. Second, prior studies suggest that the abnormalities associated with BP disorder will be located in frontal (cortical or subcortical) and possibly thalamic[15-17] areas. Groups were compared with regard to the volumes of the following cortical and subcortical gray matter structures: caudate, lenticular nucleus, anterior diencephalon, and cortical gray matter, as well as cortical and subcortical fluid. Third, pilot data led us to hypothesize that subcortical cognitive impairment would be associated with an increased volume of AWM.[5]

From the Departments of Psychiatry (Drs Dupont, Jernigan, Butters, and Gillin and Mss Shafer and Wilson) and Radiology (Drs Jernigan and Hesselink), University of California School of Medicine at San Diego, La Jolla; the Psychiatry (Drs Dupont and Gillin) and Psychology (Drs Jernigan and Butters) Services, Department of Veterans Affairs Medical Center at San Diego; and the Department of Psychology, Brown University, Providence, RI (Dr Heindel).

RESULTS

PRESENCE AND VOLUME OF WHITE MATTER ABNORMALITIES

Across all subjects, the number of areas of signal hyperintensity was significantly correlated with the quantitative volume of

See Subjects and Methods on next page

SUBJECTS AND METHODS

SUBJECTS

Healthy control subjects, who themselves and whose first-degree relatives were free of current or past psychiatric diagnoses, as well as patients with UP or BP mood disorder, were recruited through advertisement or physician referral to the University of California at San Diego Mental Health Clinical Research Center, La Jolla. All subjects were screened before the study with use of identical mechanisms, including a structured telephone interview, a standardized psychiatric interview (Schedule for Affective Disorders and Schizophrenia[18] or Structured Clinical Interview for *DSM-III-R*[19]), a physical examination, and laboratory evaluation. Psychiatric interviews were conducted by a trained psychiatry research fellow, psychologist, psychiatric research nurse, or master's level psychology graduate. All medical histories and physical examinations were performed by a psychiatry research fellow. Final diagnoses were made during a weekly consensus conference of all diagnosticians at the Mental Health Clinical Research Center; final application of inclusion and exclusion criteria was made by one of us (R.M.D.). All patients with BP disorder met criteria for BP disorder with at least one full manic episode according to *DSM-III-R.*[20] Information regarding psychiatric disorders in first-degree relatives was gathered from each study participant. All but three patients with BP disorder were outpatients at the time of study. Study participants were told that they might undergo urine toxicology screening as part of the study; this test was administered where clinically indicated to determine reliability.

Medical and neurologic exclusion criteria included any medication known to affect brain volume (eg, steroids), age over 55 years, substantial substance dependence (5 years' duration at any time or meeting criteria for dependence in the 5 years preceding the study), history of intravenous drug abuse, or severe head injury with loss of consciousness lasting more than 5 minutes or with subsequent neurologic sequelae. In addition, subjects who had used amphetamine, cocaine, or methylphenidate more than 10 times were also excluded. Subjects with a medical history of hypertension, seizures, hypoxia, migraine headaches, neurodevelopmental disorders, learning disorders, and other central nervous system disorders that would affect anatomy were excluded.

Two patients with BP disorder who were initially admitted into the study were excluded on the basis of MRI abnormalities: one had an arachnoid cyst and the other had almost total agenesis of the corpus callosum. A single control subject was excluded from the study when MRI assessment revealed a ventricular volume more than 7 SDs larger than normal and blinded clinical evaluation of neuropsychological test results suggested severe cognitive impairment. Eighteen of the subjects with BP disorder and seven of the controls were part of an earlier published study that addressed the clinical assessment of focal abnormalities in MRI scans of patients with BP disorder.[5] All subjects analyzed herein were included in a report on the importance of visually identified focal areas of signal hyperintensity in patients with BP disorder.[21]

As will be explained in the "Results" section, a second control group was selected from the database of the imaging laboratory and matched with the patients with BP disorder on the basis of AWM volume. These controls were generated from a number of studies at the University of California at San Diego and were judged to be medically and psychiatrically healthy before evaluation, but screening and selection criteria were not identical to the entrance criteria of this study. This group was used only for analysis regarding the distribution of AWM.

The data for this study came from 26 control subjects, 36 patients with BP, and 30 patients with UP. Demographic data are shown in **Table 1**. At the time of the study, the mean (±SD) score on the 17-item Hamilton Rating Scale for Depression was 12.5±4.9 for patients with UP disorder, 9.2±6.5 for patients with BP disorder, and 0.6±0.8 for controls. Twenty-two of the 30 patients with UP disorder and six of the 36 patients with BP disorder met criteria for major depression at the time of study entry, while seven patients with BP disorder met criteria for hypomania or mild mania. Data on additional diagnoses and medications for each group can be found in **Table 2** and **Table 3**.

MAGNETIC RESONANCE IMAGING

All subjects underwent MRI with a 1.5-T imager (General Electric, Milwaukee, Wis) according to a standard protocol. Data for quantitative analysis were derived solely from the full axial series (echo time, 25, 70 milliseconds; repetition time, 2000 milliseconds; 5 mm thick; 2.5-mm gap). Partial sagittal series and a full coronal series (used in clinical analyses) were obtained but not used in the quantitative analysis.

All images were blindly rated by a single senior neuroradiologist (J.H.). The instructions to the rater were to identify and localize any and all abnormalities. Areas of signal hyperintensity were defined as areas of increased signal intensity present on the early and late echo images. Ten subjects underwent scanning on two occasions; the results of all ratings were identical on both occasions.

All images were analyzed quantitatively according to previously described methods[22] by a trained operator who did not know the diagnosis of the subject. Briefly, each pixel was classified on the basis of its signal values in both original images (echo time, 25 milliseconds; echo time, 70 milliseconds) as most resembling cerebrospinal fluid (CSF), gray matter, white matter, or signal hyperintensity (tissue abnormality). This was accomplished in two steps: First, two new linear combinations of the pixel values were computed to optimize tissue contrast (CSF/brain, gray matter/white matter). Second, classification criteria that were adjusted separately for each section were applied to these computed values. The full series of axial images was analyzed, beginning at the bottom of the cerebellar hemispheres and extending through the vertex.

Consistently identifiable landmark points and structural boundaries were designated on the pixel-classified images by trained image analysts, as described below. The processed image data were then transformed spatially so that all locations within the brain images could be identified relative to a common anatomic coordinate system. Cerebral regions were then defined relative to this coordinate scheme (ie, stereotactically).

Definition of Subcortical Gray Matter Structures

The operator circumscribed pixels classified as gray matter that were visually identified as caudate nuclei, lenticular nuclei, and diencephalic gray matter structures. A division of anterior from posterior diencephalic structures was made based on a stereotactic coronal dividing plane. The anterior diencephalon was composed of mamillary bodies, hypothalamic gray matter, and septal nuclei. The posterior diencephalon comprised the thalamus. The operators did not trace the edges of the structures but defined polygons that included all gray matter pixels within the structures and excluded those gray matter pixels associated with other structures. In some cases, when the subcortical nuclei were contiguous with other areas classified as gray matter but clearly not in the structures, boundaries were manually constructed with use of the filmed images as a guide. Estimates of the volumes of the subcortical structures were made by summing the designated gray matter pixels across all sections.

Definition of Regions Within the Cerebral Hemispheres

To define anatomically consistent regions, a method was adopted for making subdivisions of the cerebrum relative to the centromedial structural midline and two consistently identifiable (operator-designated) points: the most anterior midline point in the genu and the most posterior midline point in the splenium of the corpus callosum. By calculating estimated rotation angles with use of these landmarks, it was possible to perform a three-dimensional rotation of the images, thus correcting each individual's image data for rotation out of the optimal imaging plane. Regions could then be constructed that resulted in highly consistent placement of regional boundaries relative to gross anatomic landmark (ie, stereotactically).

The division of the cerebrum was based on two major planes: an axial plane, which was perpendicular in orientation to the midsagittal plane and passed through the two corpus callosum points, and a coronal plane, which was defined as perpendicular to the first plane and which passed through the midpoint between the two corpus callosum points. By computing new coordinates for the center point of each voxel relative to these planes, each voxel was assigned to one of four zones: (1) inferior to the axial plane and anterior to the coronal plane; (2) inferior to the axial plane and posterior to the coronal plane; (3) superior to the axial plane and anterior to the coronal plane; and (4) superior to the axial plane and posterior to the coronal plane. Anterior temporal, orbitofrontal, and some dorsolateral and mesial frontal cortex are in the inferior zone. Posterior temporal and inferior occipital cortex are in the inferior posterior zone. Most of the remaining parts of the frontal lobe are in the superior anterior zone, and the superior posterior zone contains primarily parietal and a small portion of the superior occipital cortex.

Measures of White Matter Abnormalities

A global index of signal alterations in the white matter was constructed by summing voxels within the subcortical white matter having signal characteristics meeting criteria for "gray matter" or for areas of "signal hyperintensity," ie, they had longer T_2 relaxation times. These were classified as AWM. Regional measures of signal alteration in the white matter were also computed by summing these voxels separately within each of the eight cerebral regions defined above.

Other Structural and Regional Volumes

The volume of the supratentorial cranium was estimated by summing all supratentorial voxels (including CSF, areas of hyperintensity, and gray and white matter). Eight regional volumes were also computed by summing all supratentorial voxels (including CSF, areas of hyperintensity, and gray and white matter) within each region.

Reliability coefficients (Pearson's r) are available for the following measures from a study of 10 images: cerebral volume (.99), ventricular CSF (.99), cortical CSF (.99), cortical gray matter (.88), caudate (.93), diencephalon (.87), and lenticular nuclei (.73). At the time that interoperator reliability was determined, AWM as expressed herein was not being measured; therefore, reliability coefficients for this measurement are unavailable. Any lack of reliability (noise) in this measurement should serve to decrease group differences, unless it reflects a true (systematic) difference between groups. A discussion of the reliability and validity of this method, as well as factors affecting the outcome of volume measurements, has been published previously.[22]

NEUROPSYCHOLOGICAL ASSESSMENT

All subjects were administered a standard battery of tests for the assessment of attention, learning, memory, and verbal fluency. Performance on tests relevant to the hypothesis that AWM is associated with a pattern of subcortical cognitive impairment are presented, specifically Trails B,[23] letter and category fluency,[24] and learning and memory (the California Verbal Learning Test).[25] A listing of the complete battery is presented in **Table 4**.[26-29]

STATISTICAL ANALYSIS

Analysis of variance (ANOVA) was used to assess the a priori hypothesis that the volume of AWM in patients with BP disorder would be greater than that in patients with UP disorder or controls. Multivariate analysis of variance (MANOVA) was used to explore group volumes on regional white matter differences and other brain structural measurements. When Hotelling's T statistic was significant in the MANOVA, univariate comparisons were performed. Bonferroni's correction for number of comparisons was computed for AWM regional analysis and gray matter structural analyses. Student's-Neuman-Keuls test of significance was used to test for differences between individual groups on post hoc testing. Nonparametric Mann-Whitney U comparisons were used to test differences between groups formed on the basis of AWM volume. Clinical and neuropsychological comparisons across groups were not corrected for the number of comparisons. Pearson's Product-Moment Correlation Coefficients were used to assess the relationship between age at onset and volume of AWM and between lithium use and cognitive impairment.

Table 1. Demographic Characteristics of Subject Groups

	Control Group (n=26)	Bipolar Group (n=36)	Unipolar Group (n=30)	F	P	Post Hoc Tests (Student's-Newman-Keuls)
Mean (SD) age, y	39.1 (9.4)	36.6 (10.8)	38.6 (10.6)	0.54	.5	. . .
Mean (SD) education, y	16.0 (2.2)	15.0 (2.2)	15.0 (1.8)	2.09	.1	. . .
Sex, No. (%)						
M	15 (58)	24 (67)	9 (30)	4.98	.01	Bipolar vs unipolar group; control group vs unipolar group
F	11 (42)	12 (33)	21 (70)			
Handedness, No. (%)						
R	23 (88)	33 (92)	26 (87)	0.21	.8	. . .
L	3 (12)	3 (8)	4 (13)			

Table 2. Additional Diagnoses of Patients With Bipolar and Unipolar Disorders*

Diagnosis	No. of Patients WithBipolar Disorder With Diagnosis	No. of Patients With Unipolar Disorder With Diagnosis
Dysthymia	1	10
Panic disorder with/without agoraphobia	1	6
Agoraphobia without panic	0	1
Bulimia nervosa†	1	1
Somatoform pain disorder	0	1
Social phobia/simple phobia	0	6
Alcohol abuse*	1	1
Cannabis abuse*	1	0
Sedative abuse*	0	1

*No control subject met criteria for any Axis I disorder.
†In remission.

Table 3. Medication Status of Control Subjects and Patients With Bipolar and Unipolar Disorders

Medication(s)*	No. of Patients With Bipolar Disorder Taking Medication(s)	No. of Patients With Unipolar Disorder Taking Medication(s)
Lithium	22	1
Anticonvulsants/calcium channel blockers	4	0
Antidepressants	5	12
Antipsychotics	6	0
Thyroid	6	1
Anticholinergics	2	0

*Ten patients with bipolar disorder, 17 patients with unipolar disorder, and all controls were receiving no medications. Patients may have been taking more than one medication.

AWM (Pearson's r=.38, P<.001). The ANOVA demonstrated a significant difference between groups for the AWM (F[2, 89]=5.5; P<.006), with post hoc tests indicating that the volume of AWM for patients with BP disorder were significantly higher than those for patients with UP disorder or controls (mean AWM volume for patients with BP disorder, 3279±1187 voxels; mean AWM volume for patients with UP disorder, 2803±1147 voxels; and mean AWM volume for controls, 2656±684 voxels). (The relationship between BP disorder and control groups remained significant with use of a nonparametric analysis [Mann-Whitney U, Z=−3.1; P<.002].) An example of the AWM distribution in one patient with BP is shown in **Figure 1**.

The MANOVA for eight white matter regions yielded a significant main effect for group (F[16, 162]=2.08; P<.01); univariate ANOVA (**Table 5**) indicated that significant differences between groups were present for right (F=6.35, P<.003) and left (F=7.84, P<.001) superior anterior, right (F=7.38, P<.001) and left (F=5.44, P<.006) inferior anterior, and right superior posterior (F=3.85, P<.02) regions. Bonferroni's correction for number of comparisons requires a significance level of P<.006 for a result to be considered significant. With use of this conservative assessment, significant differences exist in superior and inferior right and left anterior regions. With use of post hoc Student's-Neuman-Keuls tests, patients with BP disorder had significantly higher AWM volumes than did controls in all four anterior regions and had higher volumes than patients with UP disorder in both superior anterior regions. Patients with UP disorder, although not manifesting an overall increase in volume of AWM, had a larger AWM volume in the right inferior anterior region compared with controls. However, the group×region interaction did not reach significance. When regional white matter abnormalities were analyzed covarying for regional cerebrum size (to correct for any differences in regional cranial volume), the pattern of differences was unchanged.

SPECIFICITY OF PATTERN OF WHITE MATTER ABNORMALITIES

Although the pattern of white matter abnormalities appeared to be different between patients and controls, it is possible that this difference resulted from measurement imprecision or nonspecific factors influencing the distribution of white matter abnormalities (eg, vascular supply). To address the question regarding the specificity of the AWM pattern in patients with BP disorder, a second group of controls was selected from the database of the neuroimaging laboratory based on a previously established age function for the AWM volume.[22] By design, the mean volume of AWM in this control group was very close to that of the patients with BP disorder. The mean age of the second ("older") control group (n=25) was 51.0±6.6 years (15 years older than the patients with BP disorder to whom they were matched for

Table 4. Performance on Cognitive Tests by Volume of White Matter Abnormality in Patients With Bipolar Disorder*

	Low Volume (n=9)†	High Volume (n=25)	P
Age, y	35.8 (11.0)	36.9 (10.9)	...
Education, y	15.6 (1.1)	14.9 (2.5)	...
Trails B (time)	59.0 (14.7)	80.2 (27.1)	.02
Letter fluency	44.1 (9.2)	36.5 (10.1)	.05
Category fluency	53.8 (9.2)	46.1 (9.8)	.04
CVLT List 1-5, total	56.6 (8.2)	49.0 (8.8)	.03
CVLT List B, total	7.7 (1.7)	6.0 (1.7)	.03
List A, Short Delay, free recall	13.0 (2.0)	10.3 (2.9)	.02
List A, Short Delay, cued recall	13.1 (2.3)	10.8 (2.6)	.03
List A, Long Delay, free recall	12.9 (2.6)	10.6 (3.1)	.06
List A, Long Delay, cued recall	13.6 (2.4)	11.3 (3.0)	.06
Discriminability	−0.3 (0.7)	−0.4 (0.6)	...
Semantic cluster	2.7 (0.9)	1.8 (0.9)	.02
Serial cluster	1.2 (0.7)	2.6 (1.4)	.005

*Values are mean (SD) Wilcoxon Mann-Whitney U values.
†Data were missing for two patients and thus are not included. Data from the following tests are not presented: Mattis Dementia Rating Scale,[26] Wechsler Memory Scale–Revised,[27] Logical Memory, Visual Reproduction, Wisconsin Card Sort Test,[28] and Wechsler Adult Intelligence Scale–Revised subtests[29]: Information, Digit Span, Vocabulary, Arithmetic, and Block Design. CVLT indicates California Verbal Learning Test.*

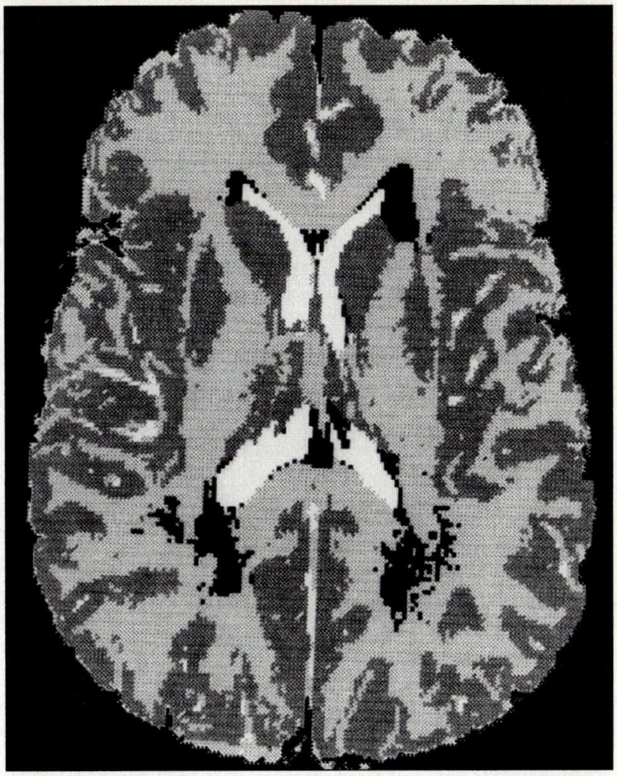

Figure 1. *Segmented magnetic resonance imaging scan showing the distribution of abnormal white matter in a single patient with bipolar disorder. Dark areas represent pixels defined by quantitative image analysis as abnormal white matter.*

AWM volume). As shown in **Figure 2**, the older controls showed elevations compared with younger controls in every region tested. When the Bonferroni correction was applied, however, only the two superior anterior and two posterior inferior regions were significantly different. In contrast, patients with BP disorder demonstrated increases in all frontal regions and no posterior region compared with the younger controls. Nevertheless, the group×region interaction did not reach significance.

The regional pattern suggested that the distribution of AWM in patients with BP disorder may be relatively more frontal than in the healthy older subjects matched for the volume of AWM. Post hoc tests were therefore conducted by comparing groups based on the ratio of anterior AWM volume to total AWM (ie, the proportion of total AWM that is anterior). As a first step to assess whether differences in distribution could be related to differences in total or regional cerebral volume, groups were compared with regard to anterior, posterior, and total cerebral volume and the ratio of anterior to total cerebrum. There were no significant group differences in any of these volumes between groups. The ratio of the frontal to total cerebral volume also did not differ between groups. Given that there were no differences in these relationships, groups were compared with regard to the ratio of frontal to total cerebral AWM. Expressed in percent, the groups differed statistically as follows: patients with BP disorder, 26.3%±5.7%; patients with UP disorder, 23.3%±3.8%; elderly controls, 25.5%±3.5%; and younger controls, 22.8%±4.0% (ANOVA: F=4.035, $P<.009$). Post hoc tests (Student's-Neuman-Keuls) showed that patients with BP disorder had a significantly more anterior distribution of AWM than did younger controls and patients with UP disorder. Older controls were intermediate in the anterior distribution of AWM and did not differ significantly from any other group.

RELATIONSHIP BETWEEN CLINICAL VARIABLES AND VOLUME OF AWM

To explore the relationship of AWM to clinical variables, we divided subjects into groups with high and low volumes of AWM based on the mean of the control subjects. Earlier data on focal signal abnormalities[21] had suggested that AWM in both patients with UP disorder and those with BP disorder was associated with a trend toward an increased rate of familial psychiatric illness. Twelve controls were in the high group (AWM volume, 3154±491 voxels) and 14 were in the low group (AWM volume, 2059±319 voxels); 27 patients with BP disorder were in the high group (AWM volume, 3748±942 voxels) and nine were in the low group (AWM volume, 2247±182 voxels); 17 patients with UP disorder were in the high group (AWM volume, 3517±1033 voxels) and 13 were in the low group (AWM volume, 1869±305 voxels). Nonparametric Mann-Whitney *U* Wilcoxon rank-sum tests were used for comparison of groups with high vs low AWM volume. Because of the number of comparisons, positive post hoc results must be considered highly preliminary. While there was no difference in age within groups between high- and low-volume control or BP groups (control: low volume, 40.2±9.0 years; high volume, 37.8±10.2 years; BP group: low volume,

Table 5. Multivariate Analysis of Variance* and Univariate Analysis of Variance† of the Volume of White Matter Abnormalities by Subcortical Region‡

Region (Side)	Control Group (n=26)	Bipolar Group (n=36)	Unipolar Group (n=30)	F (*df*=2, 89)†	*P*
Superior anterior (R)	249.46 (93.56)	372.31 (180.61)	280.77 (137.11)	6.35	.003
Superior anterior (L)	266.08 (118.05)	404.42 (209.52)	264.00 (144.30)	7.84	<.001
Inferior anterior (R)	49.92 (25.84)	74.39 (33.26)	69.10 (29.25)	7.38	.001
Inferior anterior (L)	49.96 (29.56)	77.25 (47.21)	65.47 (24.81)	5.44	.006
Superior posterior (R)	717.77 (234.63)	884.14 (279.76)	730.57 (285.18)	3.85	.02
Superior posterior (L)	718.42 (212.95)	865.69 (257.46)	787.33 (304.57)	2.41	.10
Inferior posterior (R)	231.54 (111.48)	325.14 (168.74)	295.50 (230.02)	2.10	.13
Inferior posterior (L)	281.92 (109.42)	355.19 (190.82)	310.47 (171.02)	1.56	.22

*For the multivariate analysis of variance, F (16, 162)=2.08, P<.01.
†Univariate analysis of variance.
‡Values are mean (SD) voxels of abnormal white matter.

35.8±11.0 years; high volume, 36.9±10.9 years), patients with UP disorder in the high-volume group were significantly older than those in the low-volume group (32.8±9.7 vs 43.0±9.2 years). In patients with BP disorder and patients with UP disorder, patients in the high AWM volume group had more family members with psychiatric disorders than did patients in the low AWM volume group (BP group: low volume, 0.3±0.5; high volume, 1.7±2.3; *P*<.05; UP group: low volume, 0.8±0.6; high volume, 1.6±1.4). Patients with BP disorder who were receiving lithium showed a nonsignificant trend toward classification in the high AWM volume group (20% in the low-volume group vs 50% in the high-volume group were receiving lithium; *P*<.07). Although this result might suggest that lithium is associated with the presence of AWM, 22% of patients with BP disorder not receiving any medication were also found to have a high volume of AWM. Also in support of this finding is that patients with BP disorder not receiving lithium had more AWM than did control subjects (patients with BP disorder not receiving lithium [n=20]: AWM volume, 3390±1236 voxels; control subjects [n=26]: AWM volume, 2565±684 voxels; *P*<.006).

Because age at the time of study is a significant confounding factor for the presence of AWM[30] (and patients with UP disorder with a higher volume of AWM were significantly older at the time of study), an analysis of covariance (ANCOVA) contrasting high and low AWM volume groups with regard to age at onset, covarying for age at the time of study, was performed. In the patients with BP disorder, but not in those with UP disorder, controlling for age at the time of study revealed a significant partial correlation between age at onset and volume of AWM (in patients with BP disorder, partial *r*=.405; *P*<.008; in those with UP disorder, partial *r*=−.194; *P*<.16). This finding suggests that increased volume of AWM is associated with later age at onset of BP disorder in the age range sampled.

Cerebrovascular risk factors are highly correlated with the incidence of areas of focal white matter signal hyperintensity.[30] Data on cigarette smoking revealed a significant relationship between smoking and AWM volume in patients with UP disorder (*r*=.6, *P*<.001) but not in those with BP disorder or control subjects. Data on smoking duration and amount were available for only a subset of the latter groups (75%). In all groups, the majority had never smoked, and the distribution was skewed (mean pack-years of smoking: patients with BP disorder, 9.9±22.7; patients with UP disorder, 6.8±14.3; control subjects, 9.7±20.1).

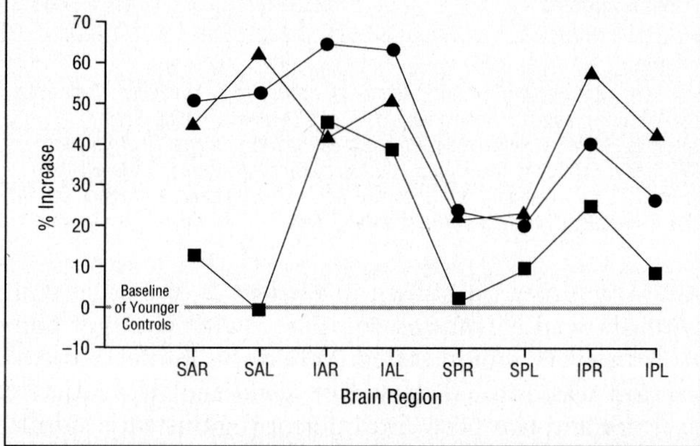

Figure 2. *The distribution of abnormal white matter in patients with bipolar disorder (circles, n=36), patients with unipolar disorder (squares, n=30), and older controls (triangles, n=25) expressed as a percentage increase over the mean of the younger control group. SAR indicates superior anterior right; SAL, superior anterior left; IAR, inferior anterior right; IAL, inferior anterior left; SPR, superior posterior right; SPL, superior posterior left; IPR, inferior posterior right; and IPL, inferior posterior left.*

NEUROPSYCHOLOGICAL CORRELATES OF AWM

Our earlier study[5] had suggested that the presence of focal white matter abnormalities on MRI scans in patients with BP disorder was associated with psychomotor slowing, decreased verbal fluency, and impaired free recall on a test of word list learning. We therefore compared high and low AWM volume groups within diagnoses on tests of these functions (Table 4). Data from two patients with BP disorder are missing owing to failure to complete the testing battery. Groups were compared with use of a nonparametric (Mann-Whitney *U* Wilcoxon rank-sum) test owing to small group size in the low AWM volume BP group. While patients with BP disorder with a high vol-

Table 6. Multivariate Ananysis of Variance* and Univariate Analysis of Variance† of the Volume of Major Brain Regions‡

Region	Control Group (n=26)	Bipolar Group (n=36)	Unipolar Group (n=30)	F (*df*=2, 89)†	*P*
Cerebral volume	193 525.65 (15 901.37)	197 055.61 (15 374.84)	192 060.67 (19 334.80)	0.77	.47
Cortical fluid	15 523.02 (4927.41)	14 510.87 (5466.07)	17 632.82 (5372.94)	2.91	.06
Subcortical fluid	2610.51 (1028.06)	3065.55 (1284.46)	2944.06 (1148.69)	1.17	.32
Caudate nucleus	1806.35 (243.73)	1808.81 (259.72)	1719.17 (245.10)	1.26	.29
Anterior diencephalon	357.77 (111.87)	385.94 (136.89)	355.80 (126.24)	0.58	.56
Posterior diencephalon	1716.85 (293.02)	1904.81 (343.06)	1570.77 (345.89)	8.46	<.001
Lenticular nucleus	1922.77 (299.85)	2030.17 (364.55)	1873.17 (430.86)	1.55	.22
Cortical gray matter	85 494.87 (12 355.46)	89 504.48 (9875.74)	84 691.76 (9631.95)	1.98	.14

For the multivariate analysis of variance, F (16, 162)=1.79, P<.037.

†*Univariate analysis of variance.*

‡*Values are mean (SD) voxels. In pairwise comparisons, values for the bipolar group were greater than those for controls and the unipolar group and values for the unipolar group were greater than those for controls.*

ume of AWM demonstrated significantly more impairment on nine of the 12 scores, with a trend in the same direction on two more, such differences were not found within either control or UP groups. While the pattern of differences is of interest, actual differences between groups were modest and would not be statistically significant if corrected for the number of comparisons performed. In patients with BP disorder, there were no differences between groups on mean Hamilton Depression Rating Scale[31] scores.

Because there was a nonsignificantly higher rate of lithium-treated patients with BP disorder in the high AWM volume group, we performed an ANCOVA to assess the contribution of lithium treatment to cognitive performance (lithium levels were unavailable). The confound between lithium treatment, BP diagnosis, and high AWM volume made the ANCOVA a conservative estimate of non–lithium-related impairment in cognitive function. Specifically, response to lithium therapy and poor cognitive performance could be epiphenomena of a single process. The following variables remained significantly correlated with volume of AWM: Trails B time (r=.411, P<.01), category fluency (r=−.369, P<.02); California Verbal Learning Test List 1 to 5 total (r=.341, P<.03), and List A Short Delay Cued Recall ($r1$=−.360, P<.02). Trends for a relationship remained in Letter Fluency (r=−.257, P<.07) and Long Delay Cued Recall (r=.223, P<.10). Thus, the deficits in the high AWM volume group do not appear to be attributable to lithium treatment. Because of the conservative nature of this analysis, results that are significant at a trend level are presented herein.

ASSOCIATED STRUCTURAL ABNORMALITIES

Because mood disorders have been associated with cortical and subcortical abnormalities, we evaluated measures of supratentorial cranial volume, cortical gray matter volume, cortical and subcortical fluid volume, caudate and lenticular nucleus volume, and anterior and posterior (thalamic) diencephalic volume (**Table 6**).

Our first approach was to assess the relationship between these structural variables and our three diagnostic groups using MANOVA; there was a significant group effect (F[16, 162]=1.79; P<.04). Using ANOVA, we then assessed which of the variables were contributing to this group difference. The only difference between groups was in the volume of the thalamus (posterior diencephalon) (F=8.46, P<.0004), which is significant even with application of Bonferroni's correction for multiple comparisons. Post hoc tests demonstrated a significantly larger thalamus in patients with BP disorder compared with those with UP disorder and controls and a smaller thalamus in the patients with UP disorder compared with those with BP disorder and controls. An increased volume of AWM in the patients with BP and UP disorders was correlated with increased ventricular volume (patients with BP disorder: r=.353, P<.05; patients with UP disorder, r=.581, P<.01).

COMMENT

INCREASED VOLUME OF WHITE MATTER ABNORMALITIES

To our knowledge, this is the first study to use quantitative MRI to compare patients with BP or UP mood disorder and control subjects and to include behavioral (cognitive and clinical) correlates. The major finding was that patients with BP disorder demonstrated a higher volume of AWM than either control subjects or patients with UP disorder. The volume of quantitatively assessed AWM was highly correlated with the number of visually identified areas of focal signal hyperintensity. In addition, for both patients and control subjects, AWM could be identified in locations without visually identified lesions. The quantitative methods appear to delineate a more extensive and diffuse white matter process than that suggested by the small, highly localized areas of signal hyperintensity seen visually. The exact neuropathologic correlates (≥1) of AWM are unknown. That subcortical areas of signal hyperintensity may be related to AWM is suggested (but not proved) by the correlation of AWM volume with the presence of areas of signal hyperintensity. In addition, an earlier report[22] demonstrated a relationship between age and pixels classified as areas of hyperintensity in control subjects. It is possible that the neuropathologic underpinnings of this finding (AWM) are multiple and that they may vary with the location in the brain where AWM is found. Patients with BP disorder with an increased volume of AWM were, on average, more likely to have had a later age at onset than those with low volumes of AWM and to demonstrate a pattern of cognitive impairment suggestive of subcortical dysfunction compared with that of patients with less AWM.

Early research suggested that white matter abnormalities may be related to primary mood disorders.[32] In addition, computed tomographic studies suggest that x-ray attenuation values (the extent to which x-rays fail to be transmitted through a structure) are abnormal in the white matter of patients with BP disorder.[33,34] Moreover, possible state-related change in T_1 relaxation times (suggesting differences in the local proton environment or chemical structure of white matter) have been reported in patients with BP disorder.[35,36] Most recently, as noted previously, there is increasing evidence of white matter abnormalities in patients with UP disorder.[9-14] Our failure to find this relationship is puzzling. However, the exclusion criteria of this study included many risk factors for signal hyperintensities, including hypertension. None of the above studies excluded subjects with hypertension. The age range of the subjects in the present study was relatively limited and did not sample older unipolar subjects.

DISTRIBUTION OF WHITE MATTER ABNORMALITIES

Compared with young controls and similarly aged patients with UP mood disorder, subjects with BP may have had a relatively frontal distribution of AWM. Compared with older controls who are matched for total volume of AWM, our test of the specificity of the frontal pattern was not entirely conclusive. A higher percentage of AWM is found within the frontal lobe in subjects with BP than in any other group, but this difference is not statistically different from the older controls. The fact that one regional pattern is not unique to subjects with BP is not surprising, as even in secondary mood disorders there is not a one-to-one correspondence between lesion location and mood disturbance.

CLINICAL AND NEUROPSYCHOLOGICAL SIGNIFICANCE OF WHITE MATTER ABNORMALITIES

In our study, patients with BP and UP who had higher volumes of AWM had a higher rate of psychiatric disorders among relatives (based on patient-provided history), and subjects with BP in this group had a later age at onset. On first pass, the relationships between AWM, later age at onset, and positive family history in the subjects with BP appears to contrast with the results of Taylor and Abrams,[37] who demonstrated a relationship between younger age at onset and family loading for mood disorder. The majority of our patients, however, would be defined as having "early onset" based on the study of Taylor and Abrams,[37] and only seven (19%) of our subjects had onset after age 29 years, the age cutoff used by Taylor and Abrams to define early vs late onset.

We failed to find a relationship between most clinical variables and structural variables, possibly reflecting the limited sample size, experimental noise, or heterogeneity of the causes of mood disorders. Factors such as treatment effectiveness, duration of illness, medication compliance, and patient symptom reporting bias greatly influence the type of clinical phenomenologic profile of each subject.

The relationship between volume of AWM and impairment on tests of fluency, psychomotor speed, and free recall suggests that this particular structural brain abnormality itself (or a close correlate) mediates trait-related cognitive impairment. Furthermore, the nature of the cognitive impairment seen in the patients with BP disorder is similar to that reported by Junque et al[38] in a study of nonpsychiatric elderly patients with white matter abnormalities seen on MRI scans. The further increase in the incidence of white matter disease with aging may explain why older patients with BP exhibit more cognitive impairment than do age-matched patients with UP disorder, controls, and younger patients with BP disorder.[39]

The presence of white matter signal abnormalities does not necessarily define a group of patients with BP disorder who have "secondary" BP mood disorder. Within the limits of our rather extensive clinical assessment, no patient had a known cause for his or her mood disorder.

OTHER STRUCTURAL ABNORMALITIES ASSOCIATED WITH MOOD DISORDER

Exploratory analysis suggested that the volume of the thalamus was increased in the BP group and decreased in the UP group compared with controls and each other. Like Schlegel and Kretzschmar,[40] we did not find an increase in ventricular fluid volume, as reported by some other investigators,[6,41,42] nor did we find a ventricular size and sex interaction, as reported by Andreasen et al.[43] It is possible that the nature of our patient sample, which included patients with relatively few hospitalizations, a low rate of psychosis, and little substance abuse, is relevant to this outcome, as it is not unreasonable to predict that patients with the most severe symptoms may have the most severe structural anomalies. Finally, these data do not allow conclusions to be drawn regarding the relationship of a particular mood state to structural abnormalities, as these subjects were primarily outpatients and not severely ill. Our earlier report suggests, however, that white matter abnormalities detected on MRI are stable over time.[5] The comorbidity demonstrated in the lifetime diagnoses of the subjects reflects the comorbidity in the general population affected with mood disorders. Results should be interpreted with knowledge of the presence of these comorbid diagnoses, which may themselves or in combination with mood disorder be associated with brain structural changes. Because toxicology screening procedures were not routinely performed, our assessment of substance abuse/dependence reflects information based on patient report and past medical records. One patient was excluded owing to agenesis of the corpus callosum. This finding in a patient with BP disorder is intriguing because it is a relatively rare abnormality hypothesized by Swayze et al[44] to be etiologically related to the development of schizophrenia.

It is conceivable that some of the white matter abnormalities seen in the patients with BP disorder are not a reflection of aging or injury but rather anomalous myelination. The latter process continues throughout adolescence.[45,46] The findings of an absence of volume loss in our patients with BP disorder, combined with increased AWM volume and thalamic volume (similar to thalamic volume found in late adolescent controls[47]), may support the hypothesis that a subset of BP mood disorder results from anomalous neurodevelopment.

Accepted for publication May 31, 1995.

This investigation was supported by grants MH42575, MH30914, MH18399, and RR00827 from the National Institute of Mental Health, Rockville, Md, and a Veterans Affairs merit review grant (Dr Dupont).

Reprint requests to the Department of Psychiatry, 0603, University of California, San Diego, La Jolla, CA 92093-0603 (Dr Dupont).

REFERENCES

1. Garland EJ, Zis AP. Multiple sclerosis and affective disorders. *Can J Psychiatry.* 1991;36:112-117.
2. Rabins PV, Brooks BR, O'Donnell P, Pearlson GD, Moberg P, Jubelt B, Coyle P, Dalos N, Folstein MF. Structural brain correlates of emotional disorder in multiple sclerosis. *Brain.* 1986;109:585-597.
3. Schiffer RB, Wineman M, Weitkamp LR. Association between bipolar affective disorder and multiple sclerosis. *Clin Res Rep.* 1986;143:1:94-95.
4. Dupont RM, Jernigan TL, Gillin JC, Butters N, Delis DC, Hesselink JR. Subcortical signal hyperintensities in bipolar patients detected by MRI. *Psychiatry Res.* 1987;21:357-358.
5. Dupont RM, Jernigan TL, Butters N, Delis D, Hesselink JR, Heindel W, Gillin JC. Subcortical abnormalities detected in bipolar affective disorder using magnetic resonance imaging. *Arch Gen Psychiatry.* 1990;47:55-59.
6. Swayze VW II, Andreasen NC, Alliger RJ, Ehrhardt JC, Yuh WTC. Structural brain abnormalities in bipolar affective disorder. *Arch Gen Psychiatry.* 1990; 47:1054-1059.
7. Figiel GS, Krishnan KRR, Rao VP, Doraiswamy M, Ellinwood EH, Nemeroff CB, Evans D, Boyko O. Subcortical hyperintensities on brain magnetic resonance imaging: a comparison of normal and bipolar subjects. *J Neuropsychiatry Clin Neurosci.* 1991;3:18-22.
8. Aylward EH, Roberts-Twille JV, Barta PE, Kumar AJ, Harris GJ, Geer M, Peyser CE, Pearlson GD. Basal ganglia volumes and white matter hyperintensities in patients with bipolar disorder. *Am J Psychiatry.* 1994;151:687-693.
9. Krishnan KRR, Goli V, Ellinwood EH, France RD, Blazer DG, Nemeroff CB. Leukoencephalopathy in patients diagnosed as major depressive. *Biol Psychiatry.* 1988;23:519-522.
10. Coffey CE, Figiel GS, Djang WT, Weiner RD. Subcortical hyperintensity on magnetic resonance imaging: a comparison of normal and depressed elderly subjects. *Am J Psychiatry.* 1990;147:187-189.
11. Brown FW, Lewine RJ, Hudgins PA, Risch SC. White matter hyperintensity signals in psychiatric and non-psychiatric subjects. *Am J Psychiatry.* 1992; 149:620-625.
12. Coffey CE, Wilkinson WE, Weiner RD, Parashos LA, Djang WT, Webb MC, Figiel GS, Spritzer CE. Quantitative cerebral anatomy in depression. *Arch Gen Psychiatry.* 1993;50:7-16.
13. Krishnan KR, McDonald WM, Doraiswamy PM, Tupler LA, Husain M, Boyko OB, Figiel GS, Ellinwood EH Jr. Neuroanatomical substrates of depression in the elderly. *Eur Arch Psychiatry Clin Neurosci.* 1993;243:41-46.
14. Lesser IM, Miller BL, Boone KB, Hill-Gutierrez E, Mehringer CM, Wong K, Mena I. Brain injury and cognitive function in late onset psychotic depression. *J Neuropsychiatry Clin Neurosci.* 1991;3:33-40.
15. Starkstein SE, Fedoroff P, Berthier ML, Robinson RG. Manic-depressive and pure manic states after brain lesions. *Biol Psychiatry.* 1991;29:149-158.
16. Cummings JL, Mendez MF. Secondary mania with focal cerebrovascular lesions. *Am J Psychiatry.* 1984;141:1084-1087.
17. Binder RL. Neurologically silent brain tumors in psychiatric hospital admissions: three cases and a review. *J Clin Psychiatry.* 1983;44:94-97.
18. Spitzer RL, Endicott J. *Schedule for Affective Disorders and Schizophrenia.* New York, NY: Biometrics Research, Evaluation Section, New York State Psychiatric Institute; 1978.
19. Spitzer RL, Williams JBW, Gibbon M, First MB. *Structured Clinical Interview for* DSM-III-R. *Washington, DC: American Psychiatric Press; 1990.*
20. American Psychiatric Association. *Diagnostic and Statistical Manual of Mental Disorders, Revised Third Edition.* Washington, DC: American Psychiatric Association; 1987.
21. Dupont RM, Butters N, Schafer K, Wilson T, Hesselink J, Gillin JC. Diagnostic specificity of focal white matter abnormalities in bipolar and unipolar mood disorder. *Biol Psychiatry.* In press.
22. Jernigan TL, Press GA, Hesselink JR. Methods for measuring brain morphologic features on magnetic resonance images: validation and normal aging. *Arch Neurol.* 1990;47:27-32.
23. Benton AL. The measurement of aphasic disorders. In: Velasquez AC, ed. *Aspctos Patologicos del Lengage.* Lima, Perru: Centro Neuropsycologico; 1973.
24. Delis DC, Kramer JH, Kaplan E. *California Verbal Learning Test.* New York, NY: Psychological Corp; 1987.
25. Lezak MD. Verbal functions. In: *Neuropsychological Assessment.* 2nd ed. Oxford, England: Oxford University Press; 1983:330-331.
26. Mattis S. Mental status examination for organic mental syndromes in the elderly patient. In: Bellak L, Karasu TB, eds. *Geriatric Psychiatry.* New York, NY: Grune & Stratton; 1976.
27. Wechsler D. *Wechsler Memory Scale–Revised.* New York, NY: Psychological Corp; 1987.
28. Berg EA. A simple objective test for measuring flexibility in thinking. *J Gen Psychol.* 1948;39:15-22.
29. Wechsler D. *WAIS-R Manual.* New York, NY: Psychological Corp; 1981.
30. Gerard G, Weisberg LA. MRI periventricular lesions in adults. *Neurology.* 1986; 36:998-1001.
31. Hamilton M. A rating scale for depression. *J Neurol Neurosurg Psychiatry.* 1960;23:56-62.
32. Elvidge AR, Reed GE. Biopsy studies of cerebral pathologic changes in schizophrenia and manic-depressive psychosis. *Arch Neurol Psychiatry.* 1938;40: 227-268.
33. Schlegel S, Kretzschmar K. Computed tomography in affective disorders, II: brain density. *Biol Psychiatry.* 1987;22:15-23.
34. Coffman JA, Nasrallah HA. Brain density patterns in schizophrenia and mania. *J Affect Disord.* 1984;6:307-315.
35. Rangel-Guerra RA, Perez-Payan H, Minkoff L, Todd LE. Nuclear magnetic resonance in bipolar affective disorders. *AJNR Am J Neuroradiol.* 1983;4:229-231.
36. Dolan RJ, Poynton AM, Bridges PK, Trimble MR. Altered magnetic resonance white-matter T1 values in patients with affective disorder. *Br J Psychiatry.* 1990; 157:107-110.
37. Taylor MA, Abrams R. Early- and late-onset bipolar illness. *Arch Gen Psychiatry.* 1981:38:58-61.
38. Junque C, Pujol J, Vendrell P, Bruna O, Jodar M, Ribas JC, Vinas J, Capdevila A, Marti-Vilalta JL. Leuko-araiosis on magnetic resonance imaging and speed of mental processing. *Arch Neurol.* 1990;47:151-156.
39. Savard RJ, Rey AC, Post RM. Halstead-Reitan category test in bipolar and unipolar affective disorders. *J Nerv Ment Dis.* 1980:168:297-304.
40. Schlegel S, Kretzschmar K. Computed tomography in affective disorders, I: ventricular and sulcal measurements. *Biol Psychiatry.* 1987;22:4-14.
41. Pearlson GD, Garbacz DJ, Breakey WR, Ahn HS, DePaulo JR. Lateral ventricular enlargement associated with persistent unemployment and negative symptoms in both schizophrenia and bipolar disorder. *Psychiatry Res.* 1984;12:1-9.
42. Nasrallah HA, McCalley-Whitters M, Jacoby CG. Cortical atrophy in schizophrenia and mania: a comparative CT study. *J Clin Psychiatry.* 1982;43:439-441.
43. Andreasen NC, Swayze VW II, Flaum M, Alliger R, Cohen G. Ventricular abnormalities in affective disorder: clinical and demographic correlates. *Am J Psychiatry.* 1990;147:893-900.
44. Swayze VW II, Andreasen NC, Ehrhardt JC, Yuh WT, Alliger RJ, Cohen GA. Developmental abnormalities of the corpus callosum in schizophrenia. *Arch Neurol.* 1990;47:805-808.
45. Kinney HC, Brody BA, Kloman AS, Gilles FH. Sequence of central nervous system myelination in human infancy, I: pattern of myelination in autopsied infants. *J Neuropathol Exp Neurol.* 1988;47:217-234.
46. Yakovlev PI, Lecours AR. The myelogenetic cycles of regional maturation of the brain. In: Minkowski A, ed. *Regional Development of the Brain in Early Life.* Boston, Mass: Blackwell Scientific Publications Inc; 1967:3-70.
47. Jernigan TL, Trauner DA, Hesselink JR, Tallal PA. Maturation of human cerebrum observed in vivo during adolescence. *Brain.* 1991;114(pt 5):2037-2049.

ORIGINAL ARTICLE

Risk of Tardive Dyskinesia in Older Patients

A Prospective Longitudinal Study of 266 Outpatients

Dilip V. Jeste, MD; Michael P. Caligiuri, PhD; Jane S. Paulsen, PhD; Robert K. Heaton, PhD; Jonathan P. Lacro, PharmD; M. Jackuelyn Harris, MD; Anne Bailey, MS; Robert L. Fell, MS; Lou Ann McAdams, PhD

Background: Neuroleptic-induced tardive dyskinesia (TD) is a major iatrogenic disorder that is more prevalent among older patients. The objective of this study was to determine the incidence of and risk factors for TD in neuroleptic-treated patients over age 45 years.

Methods: We studied 266 middle-aged and elderly outpatients with a median duration of 21 days of total lifetime neuroleptic exposure at study entry. Most patients were treated throughout the study with either a high-potency or a low-potency neuroleptic and maintained on relatively low doses. The patients were followed up at 1- to 3-month intervals with "blind" assessment of psychopathologic condition, clinically as well as instrumentally (ie, using electromechanical sensors with computerized data reduction, including spectral analysis) evaluated movement disorder, and global cognitive function.

Results: Cumulative incidence of TD was 26%, 52%, and 60% after 1, 2, and 3 years, respectively. The principal risk factors for TD were duration of prior neuroleptic use at baseline, cumulative amount of high-potency neuroleptics, history of alcohol abuse/dependence, borderline or minimal dyskinesia, and tremor on instrumental assessment.

Conclusion: Use of higher amounts of neuroleptics, particularly high-potency ones, should be avoided in older patients, patients with alcohol abuse/dependence, or patients with a subtle movement disorder at baseline; these patients are at a higher risk of developing TD.

(Arch Gen Psychiatry. 1995;52:756-765)

ONE OF the most serious adverse effects of neuroleptic therapy is tardive dyskinesia (TD).[1,2] In a prospective study of more than 850 young adult patients (mean age, 29 years), the cumulative incidence of TD after exposure to neuroleptics was found to be 5% after 1 year, 19% after 4 years, and 26% after 6 years.[3] In a study population that consisted mainly of elderly institutionalized or inpatient subjects,[4] the cumulative incidence of TD was reported as 31% after 43 weeks of neuroleptic treatment.

Despite numerous studies spanning more than three decades, the understanding of risk factors for TD is still incomplete. Aging appears to be the predominant patient-related risk factor for TD.[2,5,6] Other patient-related risk factors, about which there is less evidence in the reported results, include female gender,[7] mood disorders,[4,8,9] alcohol or other substance abuse,[10,11] diabetes mellitus,[12-14] smoking,[15,16] African-American ethnicity,[17,18] and cognitive dysfunction.[19]

In terms of neuroleptic-related risk factors, no significant differences among different types of neuroleptics have been reported. A possible exception is clozapine, which reportedly has a much lower risk of TD.[20] Other suggested medication-related risk factors include a high amount of neuroleptics,[21-23] development of extrapyramidal symptoms (EPS) early in the course of neuroleptic treatment,[3,4,24-26] and use of anticholinergic agents.[27]

In an effort to overcome some of the problems associated with subjective ratings of EPS and to improve our skill at early detection of EPS, we have been using a battery of instrumental assessment procedures.[24,28] Instrumental motor measurement systems yield continuous rather than categorical or ordinal data, produce variables that show a linear positive relationship to the severity of the movement dis-

From the Department of Psychiatry, University of California, San Diego (Drs Jeste, Caligiuri, Paulsen, Heaton, Lacro, Harris, and McAdams, Ms Bailey, and Mr Fell), and San Diego Veterans Affairs Medical Center (Drs Jeste, Caligiuri, Paulsen, Lacro, and Harris).

See Methods and Materials on next page

METHODS AND MATERIALS

Over an approximately 4-year period, 266 consecutive outpatients over the age of 45 years met the following criteria for enrollment into our study: (1) psychiatric diagnoses (based on *DSM-III-R*[33] criteria and confirmed by at least two board-certified psychiatrists) for which neuroleptic therapy was indicated; (2) availability of reliable medical and pharmacological history from the patient, from medical records, and/or from significant others; (3) baseline evaluation prior to or early in the course of neuroleptic treatment; (4) absence of severe physical illness that would preclude study assessments; (5) not meeting criteria for TD (defined below); and (6) willingness to participate and to give informed consent in writing.

Patients were recruited from several sources, the majority coming from the San Diego (Calif) Veterans Affairs Medical Center. The patients' mean (SD) age was 65.5 (12.0) years; education level, 12.4 (3.3) years. Neuroleptics were prescribed to treat psychotic or other severe behavioral symptoms. The median cumulative duration of neuroleptic treatment at baseline was 21 days. We have several ongoing studies of late-onset psychosis, including schizophrenia. Hence, we received a number of referrals of patients over age 45 years who were either starting neuroleptic treatment or in the early stages of neuroleptic treatment. Of the 266 patients, 24.8% were neuroleptic-naive while 45.4% had 1 to 90 days of total lifetime neuroleptic exposure at baseline.

We used the criteria of Schooler and Kane[34,35] to diagnose TD, except that the minimum duration of prior neuroleptic use was 1 month instead of 3 months, given the higher risk and the likelihood of earlier development of TD in older patients.

INITIAL EVALUATION

Medical and Pharmacologic History

We obtained medical and pharmacologic history to record information about pertinent medical illnesses (eg, hyperthyroidism, stroke), alcohol and other substance abuse, smoking, and medications (especially neuroleptics).

Neurological and Other Medical Assessment

A complete neurological and other medical examination was performed to help diagnose "organic" disorders. Appropriate laboratory tests, such as thyroid function tests and computed tomography or magnetic resonance imaging of the brain, were obtained when indicated.

Global Cognitive Assessment

We used the Mini-Mental State Examination (MMSE).[36]

Assessment of Psychopathology

We used the Brief Psychiatric Rating Scale (BPRS)[37] and the Hamilton Depression Rating Scale (HAM-D).[38]

Clinical Assessment of Movement Disorder

We used the Simpson-Angus Scale for early EPS,[39] the Abnormal Involuntary Movement Scale (AIMS),[35] and the Simpson Abbreviated Dyskinesia Rating Scale (ADRS).[40]

Instrumental Assessment of Movement Disorder

Below we describe briefly our methods of evaluating movement or muscle activity using electromechanical sensors with computerized data reduction, including spectral analyses. The details of these procedures have been published previously.[24,41]

Instability. Force instability was used to quantify hand and jaw dyskinesia.[28,42]

Tremor. Postural tremor of the upper extremity was quantified.[43] Spectral amplitudes within the 3- to 7-Hz range have been shown to be reliable indexes of neuroleptic-induced tremor.[24,28,44]

Movement Speed. Bradykinesia was evaluated by measuring the peak instantaneous velocity associated with simple ballistic movements of the wrists.[45]

Rigidity. The procedure for quantifying abnormalities in muscle tone involved measurement of wrist stiffness.[46-48]

Videotaping

A standard procedure was followed to obtain a 10-minute videotape for the AIMS[35] examination.

FOLLOW-UP EVALUATION

The patients were assessed 1 and 3 months after study entry and then every 3 months with review of pharmacotherapy administered since the last assessment, neurological assessment, MMSE,[36] BPRS,[37] HAM-D,[38] Simpson-Angus Scale for early EPS,[39] AIMS,[35] ADRS,[40] instrumental assessment of movement disorder, and videotaping.

The raters were "blind" to other clinical information, including earlier assessments of the same patients. Videotaped recordings of patients' AIMS examinations at various periods were mixed randomly and analyzed at a later date by "blind" evaluators. A high degree of interrater reliability (intraclass correlation coefficient >.84) was established for the AIMS[35] and other rating scales.

TREATMENT

Patients were treated with relatively low doses of neuroleptics, determined individually (often <150 mg/d of chlorpromazine equivalent[6]). Moderate to severe EPS were treated with benztropine mesylate, usually at dosages of 2 mg/d or less.

Our original goal was to randomize every patient entering the study to either haloperidol or thioridazine. We found, however, that this was not possible in patients with a history of allergy to or severe side effects with either medication; or in case of a refusal for randomization by the patient, caregiver, or physician; or in

Continued on next page

patients already receiving neuroleptics who did not wish to be switched to another antipsychotic agent. Similarly, randomization to haloperidol or thioridazine was considered to be contraindicated in patients who were thought to be at a relatively high risk of side effects from either of these medications (eg, patients with severe parkinsonian signs at baseline or those with glaucoma). Additionally, some randomized patients refused to continue the medication prescribed because of side effects, etc. Of the 266 patients entering the study, 107 continued to take haloperidol (n=68) or thioridazine (n=39) for at least a month. Regardless of randomization, we strove to keep every patient in the study on the same medication for the entire duration of the study; failing that, we tried to keep him or her taking only one class of neuroleptics—either high-potency or low-potency. We kept a total of 190 patients taking either high-potency neuroleptics only (n=126) or low-potency neuroleptics only (n=64) throughout the study.

STATISTICAL METHODS

Life-table survival analysis[49] was employed to assess the cumulative incidence of TD for the total sample and for selected subgroups.

The analysis of the data on risk factors for TD was of two types: (1) *Univariable analysis* used either life-table survival analysis[49] or univariable Cox regression analysis.[50] The proportional hazards method (also called survival analysis with covariates or Cox regression) was used to investigate the effects of predictor variables and risk factors on the occurrence of TD.[50] Differences in subgroup survival curves were tested for significance by means of either improvement χ^2 analysis in the Cox regression analysis or the Breslow or Mantel-Cox statistic.[51] (2) The model for *cumulative multivariable analysis* (backward stepwise Cox regression) included more than one significant predictor at a time. Partialing for the effects of other predictors enabled one to assess the unique contribution of a given variable to the risk of TD.

Fixed and Time-Dependent Covariates

The potential risk factors for TD were considered to be either fixed or time-dependent[52] covariates. Fixed covariates were those variables, measured at baseline, that were fixed for the duration of the study (eg, age at intake or gender). Time-dependent covariates were the variables that were reassessed at subsequent visits and whose values could thus change as a function of the survival time (eg, AIMS score). The time-dependent variables for cumulative high-potency and low-potency neuroleptic amount were redefined repeatedly from the baseline visit to the visit at which TD had occurred or, in non-TD patients, from the baseline visit to the last visit; these were the contemporary time-dependent covariates. Thus, to estimate the risk of TD at the 9-month visit, we used a patient's total amount of high-potency neuroleptics received through the 9-month visit as the contemporary time-dependent covariate. All other time-dependent covariates were redefined repeatedly from the baseline value to the value at the visit prior to the occurrence of TD or to the visit prior to the last visit; these were the one-visit-back time-dependent covariates. For example, to estimate the risk of TD at the 9-month visit, we used a patient's MMSE total at the 6-month visit as the one-visit-back time-dependent MMSE covariate.

Cox Regression Analysis

A few continuous variables (eg, cumulative high-potency neuroleptic amount) with large range and skewed distribution of values were subjected to a base 10 logarithmic transformation prior to the Cox regression analysis to obtain useful $\hat{\beta}$ coefficients.[52]

One difficulty encountered in analysis was missing data, the amount of which differed across variables. To maximize the sample size, hence, power, for examining each variable in concert with others, we devised a staged approach to cumulative multivariable Cox regression analysis. We organized the variables into conceptually defined groupings and then ordered them beginning with the set of variables with the largest sample sizes (set 1) and ending with the set of variables with the smallest sample sizes (set 4).

- *Set 1* (N=230 to 266) comprised a basic set of fixed demographic (age, gender, ethnicity, education), fixed diagnostic grouping, fixed health index (history of diabetes, smoking, alcohol abuse/dependence), fixed and time-dependent MMSE score, fixed neuroleptic duration at baseline, and fixed and time-dependent high-potency and low-potency neuroleptic amount variables.
- *Set 2* (N=220 to 266) comprised a set of fixed and time-dependent clinical measures of motor abnormalities (Simpson-Angus EPS scale total score, AIMS global score, and ADRS total score).
- *Set 3* (N=191 to 202) comprised a set of fixed and time-dependent psychopathology rating scale scores (BPRS subscale scores and HAM-D total score).
- *Set 4* (N=153 to 178) comprised a set of fixed and time-dependent instrumental motor measures (instability, tremor, movement speed, and rigidity).

Univariable and cumulative multivariable Cox regression analyses[52,53] were run at each of the four stages corresponding to the four sets of variables. A cumulative multivariable Cox regression was run for the risk factor set corresponding to that stage plus the significant variables from each of the preceding stages. Within a stage, new variables had to meet nominal significance at $\alpha \leq .05$, while previously significant variables had to maintain nominal significance at $\alpha \leq .10$. All the tests for new main effects and new interactions were evaluated at the nominal criterion of $\alpha = .05$.

We also carried out some post hoc analyses, which are described in the "Results" section.

order, and can measure abnormalities below the threshold of human detection.[29] The instruments chosen for the proposed studies are relatively inexpensive, and the testing requires less than 30 minutes.[29]

We undertook the following study to determine the incidence of and risk factors for TD in middle-aged and elderly neuroleptic-treated outpatients because of the paucity of similar work in this population. Furthermore, we wished (1) to include patients prior to or relatively early in the course of their neuroleptic treatment, (2) to assess the subjects at relatively short intervals (1 to 3 months), (3) to employ appropriate rating scales and instrumental motor evaluations, (4) to compare the risk of TD with low-potency vs high-potency neuroleptics given in relatively low dosages, and (5) to analyze the data in ways that would enable us to evaluate the individual and unique contributions of different risk factors for TD. Some of the risk factors reported in the literature are fixed (eg, gender), while others change over time—ie, are time-dependent (eg, cumulative amount of neuroleptics administered). Furthermore, there are varying degrees of associations among certain variables—eg, older age is likely to be associated with a longer duration of therapy and a greater cumulative amount of neuroleptics. Hence, we proposed to undertake univariable and multivariable analyses involving both the fixed and time-dependent variables.

We hypothesized that a number of fixed variables, such as older age, diagnoses of mood disorder and dementia, female gender, and duration of prior neuroleptic use at baseline, as well as time-dependent variables, such as the severity of EPS and cumulative amount of neuoleptics, would be significant univariable predictors of TD. We also hypothesized that older age, longer baseline duration of neuroleptic use, and greater cumulative amount of neuroleptics would emerge as risk factors for TD in the multivariable analysis.

We have previously published data on the 6-month and 1-year cumulative annual incidence of TD and some univariable analyses based on earlier results from the present, ongoing study.[30-32] This report represents our first attempt to examine the cumulative 3-year incidence of TD and risk factors for TD using a larger sample and multivariable as well as univariable data analyses.

RESULTS

At 1 year, the survival rate was 73.9%; hence, the 1-year incidence of TD was 26.1% (95% confidence interval [CI], 19.3% to 32.9%). The cumulative proportion developing TD by the end of 24 months was 51.7% (95% CI, 41.3% to 62.1%) and by the end of 36 months was 59.8% (95% CI, 47.6% to 72.0%) (**Figure 1**). From the life-table analysis we obtained 69 events or cases of TD per 211.9 person-years, or 0.33 events per person-year.

Table 1 shows that the following categorical or artificially dichotomized continuous variables at baseline were significant risk factors for TD: age under 65 years, duration of prior neuroleptic use of greater than 90 days at baseline, history of alcohol abuse/dependence, and baseline AIMS global score greater than 0. Although anticholinergic use was also a significant predictor, the proportion of patients treated with these drugs was small (11%). **Figure 2** shows the incidence of TD in patients with vs without a history of alcohol abuse/dependence.

Table 2 gives the results of univariable analysis using all the time-dependent variables and all the fixed variables for which there were no time-dependent values, but, unlike Table 1, Table 2 does not dichotomize continuous variables (such as age) artificially. The findings are similar to those in Table 1, except for the addition of the following time-dependent variables as significant predictors of the risk of TD: cumulative amount of high-potency neuroleptics, MMSE score, AIMS global score, and ADRS score, with trends for tremor and movement speed on instrumental assessment.

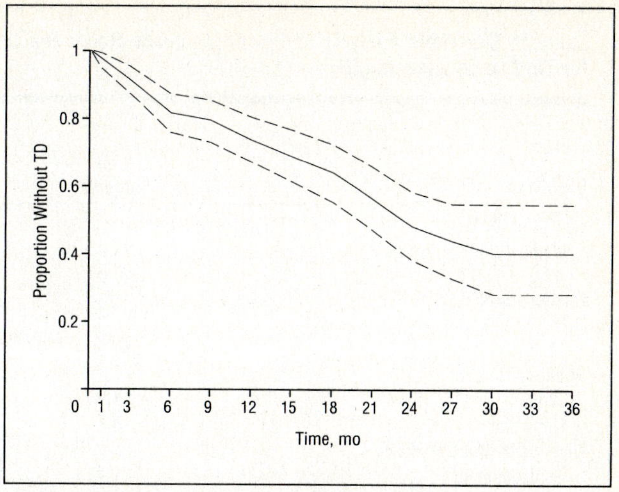

Figure 1. *Survival curve for tardive dyskinesia (TD) onset, with 95% confidence intervals (broken lines) (N=266).*

Table 3 presents the results of cumulative multivariable analysis at four successive stages. The stage 4 analysis may be viewed as the "final" result in that it suggests predictors whose unique contributions to the risk of TD were above and beyond what could be explained by their potential associations with other variables. The five significant predictors that emerged at the final stage were fixed duration of prior neuroleptic use at baseline, time-dependent cumulative amount of high-potency neuroleptics, fixed history of alcohol abuse/dependence, time-dependent AIMS global score, and time-dependent tremor on instrumental assessment. None of the first-order interaction effects among the variables was significant.

INTERPRETATION OF MODEL

From a clinical standpoint, an especially interesting value in Tables 1 through 3 is the risk ratio. Alcohol abuse/dependence may be considered as an example. In Tables 1 and 2 (stage 1), the risk ratio for this variable was 1.7—ie, when considered by itself, a history of alcohol abuse/dependence increased the risk of TD by a factor of 1.7. Table 3 examines the relative impact of the variable on the TD risk, considered in concert with other variables. In stage 1, the risk ratio for alcohol abuse/dependence (as a predictor of TD) was 2.0. In stage 2, the risk ratio for that variable was 1.9, and it remained unchanged in stage 3. In stage 4, the risk ratio for alcohol abuse/dependence was 1.7.

The other predictors identified in Tables 2 and 3 were continuous. Except for age, all the risk ratios for all the continuous variables (Tables 2 and 3) were greater than

Table 1. Life-Table Analysis of 1-Year Incidence Rates and Univariable Cox Regression Risk Ratios for Tardive Dyskinesia (TD)*

Variable	% of Subjects	Life-Table Analysis 1-Year Incidence of TD (95% CI)	Cox Regression Risk Ratio† (95% CI)	Cox Regression *P*‡
Age, y (n=264)				.03
<65	44.0	26.1 (16.1-36.2)	Reference group	
≥65	56.0	25.6 (16.2-34.9)	0.6 (0.4-0.9)	
Gender (n=265)				.36
F	18.5	21.2 (4.2-38.2)	Reference group	
M	81.5	26.6 (19.2-34.1)	1.4 (0.7-3.1)	
Ethnicity (n=265)				.20
White	81.9	23.2 (16.0-30.4)	Reference group	
Nonwhite	18.1	36.8 (19.0-54.7)	1.5 (0.8-2.6)	
Diagnostic group (n=266)				.23
Schizophrenia	21.4	28.6 (14.6-42.5)	1.4 (0.6-3.3)	
Mood disorder	21.1	27.0 (13.2-41.1)	1.0 (0.4-2.4)	
Other nonorganic disorder	16.2	29.3 (6.6-51.9)	Reference group	
Alzheimer's disease	24.4	27.3 (13.7-41.0)	0.7 (0.3-1.6)	
Other organic disorder	16.9	17.5 (3.0-31.9)	0.9 (0.4-2.5)	
Alcohol abuse or dependence (n=266)				.03
No	68.8	20.2 (12.6-27.8)	Reference group	
Yes§	31.2	37.7 (24.6-50.9)	1.7 (1.1-2.9)	
History of smoking (n=230)				.18
No	74.8	26.1 (17.8-34.4)	Reference group	
Yes	25.2	25.0 (11.0-39.1)	1.5 (0.9-2.5)	
Diabetes mellitus (n=266)				.33
No	84.6	25.9 (18.5-33.2)	Reference group	
Yes	15.4	27.6 (9.5-45.7)	1.4 (0.7-2.7)	
Baseline MMSE total (n=257)				.28
<28	57.6	29.5 (17.8-41.2)	Reference group	
≥28	42.4	24.5 (14.4-34.7)	1.3 (0.8-2.1)	
Duration of prior neuroleptic use at baseline, d (n=262)				.001
≤90	70.2	18.8 (11.5-26.1)	Reference group	
>90	29.8	39.7 (26.4-52.9)	2.4 (1.5-3.9)	
Neuroleptic treatment group (n=190)				.11
Low-potency	33.7	24.4 (8.9-39.8)	Reference group	
High-potency	66.3	34.3 (24.0-44.6)	1.7 (0.9-3.4)	
Anticholinergic use (n=147)				.005
No	89.1	20.4 (12.6-28.2)	Reference group	
Yes	10.9	64.4 (38.6-90.2)	3.5 (1.6-7.3)	
Baseline AIMS global score (n=265)				.007
0	67.9	19.8 (12.7-27.0)	Reference group	
>0	32.1	43.2 (27.9-58.6)	2.1 (1.3-3.6)	
Baseline ADRS total (n=244)				.37
<19	59.4	21.8 (13.3-30.3)	Reference group	
≥19	40.6	33.3 (20.9-45.8)	1.3 (0.8-2.2)	

**CI indicates confidence interval; MMSE, Mini-Mental State Examination; AIMS, Abnormal Involuntary Movement Scale; and ADRS, Simpson Abbreviated Dyskinesia Rating Scale.*

†All dichotomous variables were coded 0 and 1. For diagnostic group, four dichotomous variables were coded 0 and 1, with 1 associated with the diagnostic category named.

‡Improvement χ^2 analysis.

§Eleven of these 83 patients were abusing alcohol at baseline; the other 72 patients had a history of only alcohol abuse or dependence.

1; therefore, the higher the value of the continuous variable, the greater the risk of TD.

EVALUATION OF MODEL

Testing the Proportionality Assumption

The only significant categorical predictor of the risk of TD was alcohol abuse/dependence (Tables 1 through 3). Results of the test of the assumption of proportionality for alcohol abuse/dependence were nonsignificant, justifying that assumption.

Testing the Model

The *P* values on global χ^2 analysis for each fixed or time-dependent covariate in univariable Cox regression analysis had to be similar to the backward stepwise improvement χ^2 *P* values for an individual variable to be entered or removed. The *P* values on global χ^2 analysis for both

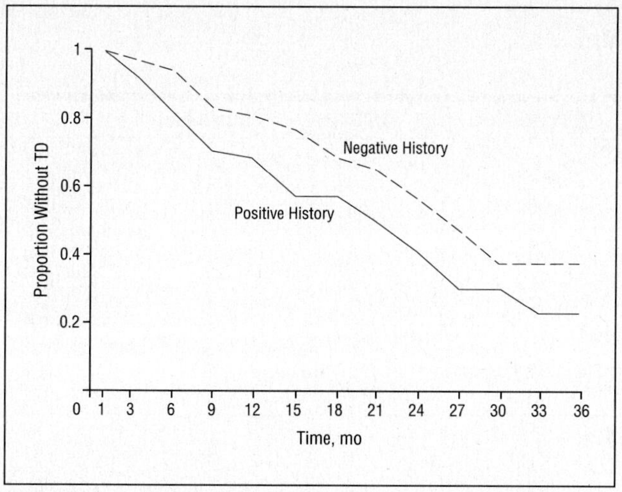

Figure 2. *Survival curves for tardive dyskinesia onset for patients with positive (n=83) vs negative (n=183) history of alcohol abuse or dependence* (P=.01 *by the Breslow test).*

fixed and time-dependent covariates in cumulative multivariable models were all .001 or less.

Assessing Accuracy of the Model

We computed the number of events (occurrences of TD) per predictor variable and compared the obtained ratio with that recommended by Concato et al.[54] The number of events for all cases over the 39-month period of follow-up was 69. We therefore had the recommended minimum ratio of events to predictors.

Assessing Possible Bias in Dropouts

There was an average 20% dropout rate per year. Using univariable Cox stepwise regression survival analysis, the dropouts did not differ from the study completers on any of the final significant predictors of TD except for alcohol abuse/dependence (P=.007). The 1-year dropout rate for nonabusers was 31.7% (95% CI, 24.2% to 39.1%) and for alcohol abusers was 16.3% (95% CI, 7.2% to 25.3%).

Results of Post Hoc Analyses

Diagnosis. Although a diagnosis of schizophrenia had a risk ratio of 1.4 (Table 1), overall psychiatric diagnosis was not a significant predictor of TD in either univariable or multivariable analysis (Tables 1 through 3). The apparently increased risk of TD in patients with schizophrenia was likely to have been secondary to the use of neuroleptics for longer periods and in higher amounts.

Age. Age was correlated significantly with logarithmic cumulative neuroleptic amount (Pearson's $r=-0.24$, df=261, P<.001). Age was a significant predictor of the incidence of TD in the univariable analysis (Tables 1 and 2) but not in the cumulative multivariable analysis (Table 3). This suggested that the apparent effects of age on the risk for TD were secondary to the effects of other significant predictors, such as the cumulative amount of neuroleptics.

AIMS Global Score. Fixed baseline AIMS global score was a significant predictor of TD (Table 1). Patients with a score greater than 0 had a 2.1 times higher risk of developing TD than those with a score of 0. Compared with the patients who had a fixed baseline AIMS global score of 0, those with a score greater than 0 (almost always 1) were significantly younger, were more likely to have schizophrenia or another "nonorganic" disorder, had lower scores on the BPRS positive symptom subscale and HAM-D, had higher scores on the ADRS, and had a longer duration of neuroleptic use at baseline. The cumulative multivariable analysis revealed that the time-dependent AIMS global score (which included the baseline score) was still a significant predictor of TD risk, suggesting that the contribution of AIMS global score to TD incidence was above and beyond what could be explained by other possible predictors (including the duration of neuroleptic use at baseline).

The cumulative incidence of TD for the 165 patients who had an AIMS global score greater than 0 at baseline or at some point during follow-up and who did not concurrently have TD was as follows: 9.9% (95% CI, 4.6% to 15.3%) at 3 months, 31.4% (95% CI, 22.5% to 40.2%) at 6 months, 34.9% (95% CI, 25.7% to 44.1%) at 9 months, and 48.2% (95% CI, 37.5% to 58.9%) at 12 months. The time to occurrence of TD (or dropout or censoring) was measured from the time of the first AIMS global score greater than 0.

Anticholinergic Use. Anticholinergic use was a significant predictor of TD risk in univariable analysis (Table 1) but not in the final stage of the cumulative multivariable analysis (Table 3). This might be in part because only 11% of the patients were receiving anticholinergic therapy. Furthermore, patients receiving anticholinergic therapy had significantly greater mean cumulative logarithmic amounts of high-potency neuroleptics than those not treated with anticholinergics (P<.001, Mann-Whitney U test).

Neuroleptic Potency. The data on neuroleptic potency as a risk factor for TD were analyzed three ways.

1. The 107 patients treated with haloperidol or thioridazine compared with the other 159 patients. The two groups were similar on all the baseline variables except that the haloperidol/thioridazine group was older, had a greater proportion of patients with Alzheimer's disease or other "organic" disorders, had a lower MMSE score, and had a shorter duration of prior neuroleptic use at baseline (P<.001 for all). The two groups did not differ, however, either in the rate of dropouts or in the incidence of TD.

2. Haloperidol-treated (n=68) vs thioridazine-treated (n=39) patients. The two groups did not differ on any of the baseline measures except that the haloperidol-treated group had a greater proportion of patients with Alzheimer's disease or other "organic" disorders and had lower scores on the MMSE and BPRS depression subscale (P<.05 for all). The rate of

Table 2. Univariable Analysis for Several Cox Proportional Hazards Models for Onset of Tardive Dyskinesia for All Cases With Relevant Data*

Variable	Type of Variable†	$\hat{\beta}$ Coefficient	$\hat{\beta}$/SE ($\hat{\beta}$)	Risk Ratio‡	*P*
Stage 1					
Age (y)	f	−0.02	−2.3	1.0	.02
Neuroleptic duration (logarithmic days)	f	0.34	3.6	1.4	<.001
Cumulative high-potency neuroleptic amount (logarithmic mg of CPZE)	t	0.19	2.7	1.2	.004
MMSE total score	t	0.04	2.0	1.0	.04
Alcohol (abuse/dependence)	f	0.52	2.1	1.7	.03
Stage 2					
AIMS global score	t	0.84	4.5	2.3	<.001
ADRS total score	t	0.13	2.7	1.1	.01
Stage 4§					
Tremor (amplitude, dB)	t	0.02	1.8	1.0	.07
Movement speed (velocity, degrees/s)	t	0.14	1.7	1.2	.06

**CPZE indicates chlorpromazine equivalent; MMSE, Mini-Mental State Examination; AIMS, Abnormal Involuntary Movement Scale; and ADRS, Simpson Abbreviated Dyskinesia Rating Scale.*

†*See the section on "Fixed [f] and Time-Dependent [t] Covariates" under "Statistical Methods" for a detailed description of the individual stages and* f *and* t *variables.*

‡*Risk ratio is* $e^{\hat{\beta}}$, *where e is the base of the natural logarithm, 2.72. See the text for a definition of risk ratio.*

§*None of the* t *clinical rating scale scores (set 3: Brief Psychiatric Rating Scale subscale scores or Hamilton Depression Rating Scale total score) was significant at stage 4.*

Table 3. Cumulative Multivariable Analysis for Several Cox Proportional Hazards Models for Onset of Tardive Dyskinesia for All Cases With Relevant Data*

Variable	Type of Variable†	$\hat{\beta}$ Coefficient	$\hat{\beta}$/SE ($\hat{\beta}$)	Risk Ratio‡	*P*
Stage 1§					
Alcohol (abuse/dependence)	f	0.68	2.7	2.0	.008
Neuroleptic duration (logarithmic days)	f	0.34	3.4	1.4	<.001
Cumulative high-potency neuroleptic amount (logarithmic mg of CPZE)	t	0.15	2.2	1.2	.02
Stage 2‖					
AIMS global score	t	0.92	4.9	2.5	<.001
Neuroleptic duration (logarithmic days)	f	0.31	2.9	1.4	.004
Cumulative high-potency neuroleptic amount (logarithmic mg of CPZE)	t	0.12	1.8	1.1	.07
Alcohol (abuse/dependence)	f	0.65	2.6	1.9	.01
Stage 4‖¶					
Tremor (amplitude, dB)	t	0.02	2.6	1.0	.01
Neuroleptic duration (logarithmic days)	f	0.26	2.3	1.3	.02
Cumulative high-potency neuroleptic amount (logarithmic mg of CPZE)	t	0.22	2.2	1.2	.02
Alcohol (abuse/dependence)	f	0.54	1.8	1.7	.08
AIMS global score	t	0.89	4.0	2.4	<.001

**CPZE indicates chlorpromazine equivalent; AIMS, Abnormal Involuntary Movement Scale.*

†*See the section on "Fixed [f] and Time-Dependent [t] Covariates" under "Statistical Methods" for a detailed description of the individual stages and* f *and* t *variables.*

‡*Risk ratio is* $e^{\hat{\beta}}$, *where* e *is the base of the natural logarithm, 2.72. See the text for a definition of risk ratio.*

§*N=216 for the entire basic data set. Since logarithmic neuroleptic duration,* t *logarithmic cumulative high-potency neuroleptic amount, and alcohol (abuse/dependence) were the only significant variables in the multivariable analysis, these three variables were rerun in a backward stepwise Cox regression at their full N=262 to better estimate the three regression coefficients.*

‖*Considerations similar to those described for stage 1 also applied here.*

¶*None of the* t *clinical rating scale scores (set 3: Brief Psychiatric Rating Scale subscale scores or Hamilton Depression Rating Scale total score) was significant at stage 4, individually or in combination with logarithmic neuroleptic duration,* t *logarithmic cumulative high-potency neuroleptic amount, alcohol (abuse/dependence), or* t *AIMS global score.*

dropouts was similar, but the haloperidol group had a higher 1-year cumulative incidence of TD than the thioridazine group (30.3% vs 9.3%; *P*=.05 and *P*=.02 using Breslow and Mantel-Cox statistics, respectively).

3. Total high-potency only (n=126) vs low-potency only (n=64) neuroleptic-treated patients. The high-potency group had a nonsignificantly higher risk of TD (*P*=.10, Breslow test; *P*=.11, Mantel-Cox test). Although the two groups were similar in terms of the rate

of dropouts, the high-potency group received higher time-dependent cumulative amounts of neuroleptics ($P<.001$, Mann-Whitney U test). To sort out the relative contribution of potency vs amount, we dichotomized the high-potency group at its median amount and split it into two subgroups: high-potency/low amount (n=63) and high-potency/high amount (n=63). The former subgroup had a mean daily neuroleptic dose (50.9 mg of chlorpromazine equivalent) comparable to that of the low-potency group (62.5 mg of chlorpromazine equivalent). The high-potency/high-amount group obviously had a much greater daily dose (535.8 mg of chlorpromazine equivalent) ($P<.001$, Kruskal-Wallis analysis of variance) than the other two groups. The three groups were similar in dropout rates. Using life-table analysis, the 1-year cumulative incidence of TD was as follows: low-potency group, 24.4% (95% CI, 8.9% to 39.80%); high-potency/low-amount group, 31.4% (95% CI, 14.8% to 48.0%); and high-potency/high-amount group, 35.8% (95% CI, 22.7% to 49.0%). However, with such small samples, the curves were not significantly different.

COMMENT

We found a distressingly high (26.1%) cumulative annual incidence of TD among psychiatric outpatients with a mean age of 65.5 years who were being treated with relatively low daily doses (average, 150 mg of chlorpromazine equivalent) of neuroleptics. This rate is five to six times that reported in younger adults.[3] Although a number of risk factors were significant in univariable analysis, the final stage of the cumulative multivariable analysis yielded only five significant predictors of TD: fixed baseline duration of prior neuroleptic use, time-dependent cumulative high-potency neuroleptic amount, fixed history of alcohol abuse/dependence, time-dependent AIMS global score, and time-dependent tremor on instrumental assessment.

Two highly significant predictors of TD risk were duration of neuroleptic use at baseline and cumulative neuroleptic amount. Some of the surprising findings can also be explained on the basis of the primacy of neuroleptic use as the most important risk factor for TD. For example, age was negatively and MMSE total score was positively related to the risk of TD—ie, younger (middle-aged) and cognitively less impaired patients had a higher risk of TD than elderly and cognitively more impaired patients. The former group (with higher risk of TD) mainly comprised subjects with schizophrenia and mood disorders, who received greater amounts of neuroleptics than the latter group, which comprised elderly patients with "organic" disorders. With a cumulative multivariable model, neither age nor diagnosis contributed significantly to TD risk, suggesting that these patient-related variables were less important than neuroleptic-related ones as risk factors for TD.

This study had several limitations. Despite our best efforts to obtain as complete information as was possible, we cannot be absolutely certain about the accuracy of neuroleptic history prior to study entry. Similarly, there might have been errors in our calculations of subsequent neuroleptic amounts because of unsuspected noncompliance. Also, there was an approximately 20% annual dropout rate, although the dropouts were similar to the study completers on all the significant predictors of TD risk except for a history of alcohol abuse/dependence. Finally, our findings may not be generalizable to a population under the age of 45 years or to one including predominantly nonveteran or female subjects.

THE FINDING of cumulative high-potency neuroleptic amount as a significant risk factor for TD must be viewed in the context of other limitations of the study. We could not randomize a majority of the patients to haloperidol or thioridazine, as originally planned, for clinical and ethical reasons. More patients were treated with high-potency neuroleptics than with low-potency ones. This might have been partly an artifact of uneven randomization. Also, among the patients not treated with haloperidol or thioridazine, a greater number were receiving high-potency antipsychotics prior to study entry and refused randomization, opting instead to continue receiving the same medications. Furthermore, our patients who were treated only with high-potency antipsychotics received a significantly greater amount of neuroleptics (in milligram chlorpromazine equivalents) than patients treated with low-potency neuroleptics only. The two groups, however, had a similar level of psychopathologic conditions (BPRS and HAM-D scores) at baseline as well as at follow-up visits, suggesting that the doses of medications used were clinically equivalent in reducing psychopathologic conditions to comparable levels. The dosages of medications had been adjusted for individual patients by their respective clinicians. It was not clear why the milligram chlorpromazine equivalent amounts of clinically (therapeutically) equivalent doses were significantly different for high-potency vs low-potency neuroleptics. Several investigators have noted a growing clinical practice in recent years (without clear justification) of using higher dosages of high-potency neuroleptics compared with low-potency agents.[55-57]

Our data suggest that high amounts of high-potency neuroleptics constitute a risk factor for TD. We could not separate out the effects of potency from neuroleptic amount statistically because of inadequate sample sizes in individual subgroups. Nevertheless, these results indicate that high-potency antipsychotics may be more likely to cause TD in at least some older subjects. Our findings may serve to explain some early reports from cross-sectional studies suggesting that drugs such as fluphenazine (a high-potency agent) were associated with a higher prevalence of TD.[26,58,59] A number of researchers have reported early EPS as a risk factor for TD.[3,25,26] This finding could conceivably be related to the patients with early EPS receiving high-potency neuroleptics, which are much more likely than low-potency neuroleptics to produce EPS.

Several possible explanations may be considered regarding why a difference between high-potency and low-potency neuroleptics in their ability to produce TD has not been reported in the past. Cross-sectional studies, which account for most of the literature on TD, cannot determine risk factors for TD. The few published prospective longitudinal studies could not compare different types of neuroleptics because the average duration of neuroleptic use prior to study entry ranged from 9 months to several years. This made it difficult to compute the exact amounts of different medications received in the past. In our investigation the median duration of total lifetime neuroleptic use at study entry was 21 days.

A history of alcohol abuse/dependence was a strong predictor of the risk of TD. Olivera et al[10] and Dixon et al[11] previously reported a higher-than-expected prevalence of TD in subjects with a history of alcohol abuse. The mechanisms underlying possible alcohol-induced susceptibility to TD are presently unknown.

Our finding of tremor (detected using instrumental assessment) prior to development of TD as a predictor of TD risk is consistent with reports linking early EPS to increased incidence of TD.[3,25,26] The clinical ratings of EPS[39] were, however, not significant predictors, possibly suggesting that subclinical motor abnormalities may define the TD risk better. The presence of borderline or minimal abnormal involuntary movements at baseline (AIMS global score >0) as a risk factor for TD indicates that spontaneous or acute neuroleptic-induced dyskinesia could be made worse by continued use of neuroleptics. The finding of time-dependent AIMS global score as a predictor of TD indicates that whenever a patient receiving neuroleptics has an AIMS global score greater than 0, he or she is at a high risk of having TD diagnosed within a few months.

Anticholinergic use is a potentially important risk factor for TD. Because of our policy of avoiding unnecessary medications, 89% of the patients did not receive anticholinergic agents. Nonetheless, the increased incidence of TD in our patients who received anticholinergic agents suggests that caution should be used in prescribing these drugs to older subjects.

Although nonsignificant, two interesting predictors, being nonwhite and having diabetes mellitus, had risk ratios of 1.5 and 1.4, respectively. The role of ethnicity as a risk factor for TD needs further evaluation.[60]

CLINICAL IMPLICATIONS

The observation that a small but significant number of our patients developed TD after less than 3 months of neuroleptic treatment suggests that in older subjects, the research criterion of the minimum length of treatment prior to a diagnosis of TD should be changed from 3 months[34] to 1 month. (This has been done for the clinical diagnosis of TD in *DSM-IV*.[61]) Occurrence of TD with comparable frequency in schizophrenic and nonschizophrenic patients should help put to rest the notion that TD is merely a symptom of schizophrenia. In older patients, neuroleptics are prescribed more frequently for indications other than schizophrenia, mainly by nonpsychiatrist physicians. There is a need for a greater awareness of TD among all clinicians treating older patients. In nonschizophrenic patients, long-term use of neuroleptics should not be undertaken without strong justification. In patients with chronic schizophrenia, neuroleptic discontinuation is associated with a significantly elevated risk of psychotic relapse.[62] Individualized treatment usually aimed at gradually reducing the neuroleptic dose to the lowest effective level is therefore indicated in most patients with schizophrenia.[63]

The frequent assertion that all "typical" neuroleptics are similar in their risk of TD is not based on any large-scale prospective comparison of different types of neuroleptics. We found a higher risk of TD with greater amounts of high-potency neuroleptics. At the same time, there is a well-known risk of anticholinergic toxic effects with low-potency neuroleptics, resulting in confusion, delirium, urinary retention, etc. It is therefore recommended that the use of any type of neuroleptic be restricted to the lowest effective doses. Finally, if the newer serotonin-dopamine antagonists, such as risperidone,[64] olanzapine, sertindole, seroquel, and others, are found to have lower risk of TD, they could significantly change the risk-benefit ratio for neuroleptic treatment.

Accepted for publication May 12, 1995.

This work was supported in part by grants MH43693, MH45131, and MH49671 from the National Institute of Mental Health, Rockville, Md; by the Department of Veterans Affairs; and by a grant from the National Alliance for Research on Schizophrenia and Depression (NARSAD), Chicago, Ill.

Presented in part at the 146th annual meeting of the American Psychiatric Association, San Francisco, Calif, May 24, 1993.

Reprint requests to Director, Geriatric Psychiatry Clinical Research Center, 116A, University of California, San Diego, San Diego Veterans Affairs Medical Center, 3350 La Jolla Village Dr, San Diego, CA 92161 (Dr Jeste).

REFERENCES

1. Baldessarini RJ, Cole JO, Davis JM, Gardos G, Preskorn SH, Tarsy D. *Tardive Dyskinesia: A Task Force Report of the American Psychiatric Association.* Washington, DC: American Psychiatric Association; 1980.
2. Kane JM, Jeste DV, Barnes TRE, Casey DE, Cole JO, Davis JM, Gualtieri CT, Schooler NR, Sprague RL, Wettstein RM. *Tardive Dyskinesia: A Task Force Report of the American Psychiatric Association.* Washington, DC: American Psychiatric Association; 1992.
3. Kane JM. Tardive dyskinesia: epidemiological and clinical presentation. In: Bloom FE, Kupfer DJ, eds. *Psychopharmacology: The Fourth Generation of Progress.* New York, NY: Raven Press Ltd; 1995:1485-1495.
4. Saltz BL, Woerner MG, Kane JM, Lieberman JA, Alvir JMJ, Bergmann KJ, Blank K, Koblenzer J, Kahaner K. Prospective study of tardive dyskinesia incidence in the elderly. *JAMA.* 1991;266:2402-2406.
5. American Psychiatric Association, Task Force on Late Neurological Effects of Antipsychotic Drugs. Tardive dyskinesia: summary of a task force report of the American Psychiatric Association. *Am J Psychiatry.* 1980;137:1163-1172.
6. Jeste DV, Wyatt RJ. *Understanding and Treating Tardive Dyskinesia.* New York, NY: Guilford Press Inc; 1982.
7. Yassa R, Jeste DV. Gender differences in tardive dyskinesia: a critical review of the literature. *Schizophr Bull.* 1992;18:701-715.
8. Friedman LS, Weinrauch LS, D'Elia JA. Metoclopramide-induced neuroleptic malignant syndrome. *Arch Intern Med.* 1987;147:1495-1497.
9. Casey DE. Affective disorders and tardive dyskinesia. *Encephale.* 1988;14:221-226.
10. Olivera AA, Kiefer MW, Manley NK. Tardive dyskinesia in psychiatric patients with substance use disorders. *Am J Drug Alcohol Abuse.* 1990;16:57-66.
11. Dixon L, Weiden PJ, Haas G, Sweeney J, Frances AJ. Increased tardive dys-

kinesia in alcohol-abusing schizophrenic patients. *Compr Psychiatry.* 1992;33: 121-122.
12. Ganzini L, Heintz RT, Hoffman WF, Casey DE. The prevalence of tardive dyskinesia in neuroleptic-treated diabetics: a controlled study. *Arch Gen Psychiatry.* 1991;48:259-263.
13. Woerner MG, Saltz BL, Kane JM, Lieberman JA, Alvir MJ. Diabetes and development of tardive dyskinesia. *Am J Psychiatry.* 1993;150:966-968.
14. Sewell DD, Yoshinobu BH, Caligiuri MP, Jeste DV. Metoclopramide-associated tardive dyskinesia in hemodialysis patients with diabetes mellitus: two case reports. *Gen Hosp Psychiatry.* 1992;14:416-419.
15. Yassa R, Lal S, Korpassy A, Ally J. Nicotine exposure and tardive dyskinesia. *Biol Psychiatry.* 1987;22:67-72.
16. Menza MA, Grossman N, Van Horn M, Cody R, Forman N. Smoking and movement disorders in psychiatric patients. *Biol Psychiatry.* 1991;30:109-115.
17. Sramek J, Roy S, Ahrens T, Pinanong P, Cutler NR, Pi E. Prevalence of tardive dyskinesia among three ethnic groups of chronic psychiatric patients. *Hosp Commun Psychiatry.* 1991;42:590-592.
18. Morgenstern H, Glazer WM. Identifying risk factors for tardive dyskinesia among long-term outpatients maintained with neuroleptic medications: results of the Yale Tardive Dyskinesia Study. *Arch Gen Psychiatry.* 1993;50:723-733.
19. Paulsen JS, Heaton RK, Jeste DV. Neuropsychological impairment in tardive dyskinesia. *Neuropsychology.* 1994;8:2:227-241.
20. Kane JM, Woerner MG, Pollack S, Safferman AZ, Lieberman JA. Does clozapine cause tardive dyskinesia? *J Clin Psychiatry.* 1993;54:327-330.
21. Muscettola G, Pampallona S, Barbato G, Casiello M, Bolini P. Persistent tardive dyskinesia: demographic and pharmacological risk factors. *Acta Psychiatr Scand.* 1993;87:29-36.
22. Gardos G, Cole JO, Haskell D, Marby D, Paine SS, Moore P. The natural history of tardive dyskinesia. *J Clin Psychopharmacol.* 1988;8:31S-37S.
23. Baldessarini RJ, Cohen BM, Teicher MH. Significance of neuroleptic dose and plasma level in the pharmacological treatment of psychosis. *Arch Gen Psychiatry.* 1988;45:79-91.
24. Caligiuri MP, Lohr JB, Bracha HS, Jeste DV. Clinical and instrumental assessment of neuroleptic-induced parkinsonism in patients with tardive dyskinesia. *Biol Psychiatry.* 1991; 29:139-148.
25. Crane GE. Pseudoparkinsonism and tardive dyskinesia. *Arch Neurol.* 1972;27: 426-430.
26. Chouinard G, Annable L, Ross-Chouinard A, Nestoros JN. Factors related to tardive dyskinesia. *Am J Psychiatry.* 1979;136:79-82.
27. Gardos G, Cole O, Haskell DS, Samson JA, Moore P, Boling L. The course of early dyskinesia. In: American Psychiatric Association, ed. *1993 CME Syllabus and Proceedings Summary.* Washington, DC: American Psychiatric Association: 1993:179. Abstract 45c.
28. Wirshing WC, Freidenberg DL, Cummings JL, Bartzokis G. Effects of anticholinergic agents on patients with tardive dyskinesia and concomitant drug-induced parkinsonism. *J Clin Psychopharmacol.* 1989;9:407-411.
29. Lohr JB, Caligiuri MP. Quantitative instrumental measurement of tardive dyskinesia: a review. *Neuropsychopharmacology.* 1992;6:231-239.
30. Harris MJ, Panton D, Caligiuri MP, Krull AJ, Tran-Johnson TK, Jeste DV. High incidence of tardive dyskinesia in older outpatients on low doses of neuroleptics. *Psychopharmacol Bull.* 1992;28:87-92.
31. Jeste DV, Caligiuri MP. Tardive dyskinesia. *Schizophr Bull.* 1993;19:303-315.
32. Jeste DV, Lacro JP, Gilbert PL, Kline J, Kline N. Treatment of late-life schizophrenia with neuroleptics. *Schizophr Bull.* 1993;19:817-830.
33. American Psychiatric Association. *Diagnostic and Statistical Manual of Mental Disorders, Revised Third Edition.* Washington, DC: American Psychiatric Association; 1987.
34. Schooler N, Kane JM. Research diagnoses for tardive dyskinesia. *Arch Gen Psychiatry.* 1982;39:486-487.
35. National Institute of Mental Health. Abnormal Involuntary Movement Scale (AIMS). *Early Clin Drug Eval Unit Intercom.* 1975;4:3-6.
36. Folstein MF, Folstein SE, McHugh PR. Mini-Mental State: a practical method for grading the cognitive state of patients for the clinician. *J Psychiatr Res.* 1975;12:189-198.
37. Overall JE, Gorham DR. The Brief Psychiatric Rating Scale (BPRS): recent developments in ascertainment and scaling. *Psychopharmacol Bull.* 1988;24:97-99.
38. Hamilton M. Development of a rating scale for primary depressive illness. *Br J Soc Clin Psychol.* 1967;6:278-296.
39. Simpson GM, Angus JW. A rating scale for extrapyramidal side effects. *Acta Psychiatr Scand.* 1970;45(suppl 212):11-12.
40. Simpson GM, Lee JH, Zoubok B, Gardos G. A rating scale for tardive dyskinesia. *Psychopharmacology.* 1979;64:171-179.
41. Caligiuri MP, Lohr JB, Jeste DV. Instrumental evidence that age increases motor instability in neuroleptic-treated patients. *J Gerontol.* 1991;46:B197-B200.
42. Caligiuri MP, Lohr JB. Fine force instability: a quantitative measure of neuroleptic-induced dyskinesia in the hand. *J Neuropsychiatry Clin Neurosci.* 1990;2:395-398.
43. Stein RB, Oguztoreli MN. Tremor and other oscillations in neuromuscular systems. *Biol Cybern.* 1976;22:147-157.
44. Alpert M, Diamond R, Friedhoff AJ. Tremographic studies in tardive dyskinesia. *Psychopharmacol Bull.* 1976;12:5-7.
45. Lohr J, Wisniewski A, Jeste DV. Neurological aspects of tardive dyskinesia. In: Nasrallah HA, Weinberger DR, eds. *The Neurology of Schizophrenia.* Amsterdam, the Netherlands: Elsevier Science Publishers; 1986:97-119.
46. Caligiuri MP. Portable device for quantifying parkinsonian rigidity. *Mov Disord.* 1994;9:57-63.
47. Chan HC, Manry MT, Kondraske GV. Classification of resistance to passive motion using minimum probability of error criterion. *Ann Biomed Eng.* 1987; 15:579-590.
48. Kischka U, Mandir AS, Ghika J, Growdon JH. Electrophysiologic detection of extrapyramidal motor signs in Alzheimer's disease. *Neurology.* 1993;43:500-505.
49. Cutler SJ, Ederer F. Maximum utilization of the life table method in analyzing survival. *J Chronic Disord.* 1958;8:669-712.
50. Cox DR. Regression models and life tables. *J R Stat Soc Ser B.* 1972;34:187-220.
51. Breslow NE. A generalized Kruskal-Wallis test for comparing *K* samples subject to unequal pattern of censorship. *Biometrika.* 1970;57:579-594.
52. Dixon WJ, Brown NB, Engleman L, Jennrich RI. *BMDP Statistical Software Manual.* Berkeley: University of California Press; 1990.
53. Collett D. *Modelling Survival Data in Medical Research.* London, England: Chapman & Hall Ltd; 1994.
54. Concato J, Feinstein AR, Holford TR. The risk of determining risk with multivariable models. *Ann Intern Med.* 1993;118:201-210.
55. Baldessarini RJ, Katz B, Cotton P. Dissimilar dosing with high-potency and low-potency neuroleptics. *Am J Psychiatry.* 1984;141:748-752.
56. Zito JM, Craig TJ, Wanderling J, Siegel C. Pharmaco-epidemiology in 136 hospitalized schizophrenic patients. *Am J Psychiatry.* 1987;144:778-782.
57. Reardon GT, Rifkin A, Schwartz A, Myerson A, Siris SG. Changing patterns of neuroleptic dosage over a decade. *Am J Psychiatry.* 1989;146:726-729.
58. Gardos G, Cole JO, LaBrie RA. Drug variables in the etiology of tardive dyskinesia. *Prog Neuropsychopharmacol.* 1977;1:147-154.
59. Smith JM, Oswald WT, Kucharski T, Waterman LJ. Tardive dyskinesia: age and sex differences in hospitalized schizophrenics. *Psychopharmacology.* 1978; 58:207-211.
60. Lacro JP, Jeste DV. The role of ethnicity in the development of tardive dyskinesia. In: Nair NVP, Yassa R, Jeste DV, eds. *Neuroleptic-Induced Movement Disorders.* London, England: Cambridge University Press; 1995:.
61. American Psychiatric Association. *Diagnostic and Statistical Manual of Mental Disorders, Fourth Edition.* Washington, DC: American Psychiatric Association; 1994.
62. Gilbert PL, Harris MJ, McAdams LA, Jeste DV. Neuroleptic withdrawal in schizophrenic patients: a review of the literature. *Arch Gen Psychiatry.* 1995;52:173-188.
63. Jeste DV, Gilbert PL, McAdams LA, Harris MJ. Considering neuroleptic maintenance and taper on a continuum: need for individual rather than dogmatic approach. *Arch Gen Psychiatry.* 1995;52:209-212.
64. Marder SR, Meibach RC. Risperidone in the treatment of schizophrenia. *Am J Psychiatry.* 1994;151:825-835.

Failure of Naltrexone Hydrochloride to Reduce Self-Injurious and Autistic Behavior in Mentally Retarded Adults

Double-blind Placebo-Controlled Studies

Sophie H. N. Willemsen-Swinkels, MS; Jan K. Buitelaar, MD, PhD; Gerard J. Nijhof, MS; Herman van Engeland, MD, PhD

Background: It is hypothesized that self-injurious behavior (SIB) and symptoms of autism may be due to overactivity in some opioid systems in the brain. We examined the efficacy and safety of naltrexone hydrochloride, an opioid antagonist, in the treatment of SIB and autism in mentally retarded adults.

Method: Thirty-three mentally retarded adults with autism and/or SIB participated in double-blind, placebo-controlled crossover studies. Active treatment was first a single 100-mg dose of naltrexone hydrochloride. Subsequently, 19 subjects were treated with 50 mg/d and 14 with 150 mg/d of naltrexone hydrochloride for 4 weeks. The outcome was assessed by means of direct observations (n=11) and on the basis of scores on a list of target behaviors, the Aberrant Behavior Checklist, and the Clinical Global Impression Scale.

Results: Thirty-two subjects (seven with autism, 16 with autism and SIB, and nine with SIB) completed the trial. Naltrexone treatment failed to have therapeutic effects on SIB and autism. On the contrary, naltrexone increased the incidence of stereotypic behavior on the Aberrant Behavior Checklist, and the care staff evaluated the effect of the 50-mg/d treatment as being significantly worse than that of the placebo treatment as measured by the Clinical Global Impression Scale.

Conclusion: Our findings suggest that naltrexone has no clinical value for a broad group of mentally retarded subjects with SIB and/or autism.

(Arch Gen Psychiatry. 1995;52:766-773)

SELF-INJURIOUS behavior (SIB) is a frequent phenomenon in mentally retarded subjects. Prevalence estimates range from 2% to 9% in noninstitutionalized retarded people[1] to 15% to 40% in institutionalized populations.[2] In spite of extensive efforts, no specific and rational pharmacological treatment regimens for SIB are yet available.[3,4] Approximately 70% of all autistic subjects are moderately to severely mentally retarded. The prevalence of autistic disorder in severely mentally retarded subjects is estimated to be 30% to 40%.[5,6] So far, there does not seem to be any really successful treatment for the social impairments of autistic subjects.[7] It has been suggested that opioid antagonists such as naltrexone hydrochloride exert therapeutic effects on SIB and autistic behavior.

According to the pain hypothesis and the addiction hypothesis, opioid mechanisms are involved in the maintenance of high frequencies of SIB.[8,9] The pain hypothesis suggests that SIB does not induce pain because excessive basal activity of the endogenous opioid system has led to an opioid analgesic state. The addiction hypothesis posits that SIB, or more generally stereotypic behavior, stimulates the production and release of endorphins; therefore, chronic maintenance of these behaviors is owing either to addiction to endogenous opiatelike substances or to positive reinforcement brought about by a central release of endorphins that is contingent on the behavior.

Empirical studies on abnormalities of endogenous opioid levels in subjects with SIB are inconclusive.[10-15] Several investigators, however, have described the beneficial effects of opiate receptor–blocking agents. A decrease in SIB has been found in approximately 70% of the patients treated with either naloxone hydrochloride (short-acting antagonist) or naltrexone (longer-acting antagonist).[9,16-20] The naltrexone studies on subjects with SIB[12,21-42] are summarized in **Table 1**. Naltrexone has also been reported to diminish stereotypic

From the Department of Child Psychiatry, Rudolf Magnus Institute for Neurosciences, University of Utrecht (the Netherlands) (Ms Willemsen-Swinkels and Drs Buitelaar and van Engeland), and the Institute for Mental Retardation Eemeroord, Baarn, the Netherlands (Mr Nijhof).

See Subjects and Methods on next page

SUBJECTS AND METHODS

SUBJECTS

All subjects were residents of a public institution for mentally retarded persons (Institute for Mental Retardation Eemeroord in Baarn, the Netherlands, and Sterrenberg in Huis ter Heide, the Netherlands). Informed consent was obtained from the subjects' legally appointed guardians and the management staff of the institutions. The protocol was approved by the ethics committee of Utrecht (the Netherlands) University Hospital. Thirty-three subjects (27 men and six women) participated in this study. Twenty-four subjects were autistic, 17 of whom showed SIB. To be included in the study, two clinicians had to agree that the subject had fulfilled the set of *DSM-III-R*[58] criteria for autistic disorder as a child and still fulfilled them when his or her current behavior in the institution was considered. The social impairment in particular had to be more serious than could be expected on the basis of the level of mental retardation only. In addition, nine subjects without a *DSM-III-R* diagnosis of autistic disorder were included because they had been manifesting moderate to high levels of SIB on a daily basis for a long time.

Ages ranged from 18 to 46 years (mean±SD, 29±6 years); retardation levels ranged from profound to mild. Nine subjects had an additional medical diagnosis (Down syndrome [n=1], congenital hydrocephalus [n=1], Hunter's syndrome [n=1], and congenital anomalies of unknown origin [n=6]). Five subjects had a history of epilepsy and were being treated with antiepileptics. Eleven subjects were receiving neuroleptics. The dosages of all comedications remained fixed during the whole study.

DESIGN

A double-blind, placebo-controlled crossover design was used. Subjects were randomly assigned to a treatment sequence of either naltrexone followed by placebo or placebo followed by naltrexone. The study started with a 2-week single-blind placebo period in which the subjects were trained to accept a capsule once a day. At the beginning and end of this placebo period, a baseline observation took place. At the beginning of week 3, a single dose of either naltrexone hydrochloride, 100 mg, or placebo was administered (8 AM). For the remainder of that week, the subject received a placebo capsule every morning (8 AM). Subsequently, a 4-week treatment of naltrexone or placebo was instituted, followed by a 4-week washout period and a crossover to the other treatment.

Initially, we chose to administer a midrange single dose (naltrexone hydrochloride, 100 mg [mean±SD, 1.61±0.24 mg/kg]; n=33) followed by low-dose long-term treatment (naltrexone hydrochloride, 50 mg [mean±SD, 0.80±0.13 mg/kg]; n=19 [two patients with autism; 11, autism and SIB; and six, SIB]). Because the 50-mg dose had no effect, the long-term dose for the second cohort was changed to 150 mg (mean±SD, 2.45±0.33 mg/kg; n=14 [five patients with autism; six, autism and SIB; and three, SIB).

ASSESSMENTS

For each subject at each assessment point, one set of checklists was rated by a member of the care staff who evaluated the subject's behavior on the ward, and one set of checklists was rated by a workshop staff member who evaluated the subject's behavior during his or her daily program. The set of checklists includedthe Aberrant Behavior Checklist (ABC)[59] and a list of target behaviors. The ABC is a 58-item checklist that measures the factors of irritability, social withdrawal/lethargy, stereotypy, hyperactivity, and excessive speech. It includes three items on SIB. In addition, a checklist was compiled consisting of five target symptoms that were chosen in consultation with the raters and were specific for each subject. The staff were asked to describe the SIB and stereotypic and compulsive behavior of each subject, eg, "face hitting," "self-scratching," and "rocking." The targets had to be rated on a five-point scale. Furthermore, at the end of a treatment period, a consensus about the subject's response to the daily treatment was reached at a staff meeting. The staff rated the subject's behavioral change on the Clinical Global Impression Scale (CGIS).[60] This is a seven-point scale, ranging from "very much improved" to "very much worse."

The behavior of 11 subjects (two with autism, seven with autism and SIB, and two with SIB) from the first cohort (long-term treatment, 50 mg) was observed directly. For practical reasons it was not possible to observe the behavior of all subjects directly. Subjects were observed twice at baseline, 6 and 24 hours after the single-dose administrations, and after 2 and 4 weeks of daily treatment. Each observation was made up of two separate blocks, each consisting of 10 minutes of observation. Subjects were observed during their free time. At least three other residents and one member of the care staff had to be present. The observer was a trained ethology student who recorded 15 behavior elements on a laptop computer by means of the software package The Observer.[61] The behavior elements that were registered included SIB, activities of the subject, and aspects of the interactions between the subject and other individuals. The interrater reliability across two raters was 70% for aspects of social behavior and more than 90% for SIB, stereotypic, and activity behaviors.

Prior to the study, subjects and care staff were familiarized with the assessments. Treatment-emergent adverse effects were assessed by the research team systematically through active questioning of the staff and participants during treatment and at end point. Further, to evaluate the safety of naltrexone administration, liver functions were screened (levels of serum aspartate aminotransferase, serum alanine aminotransferase, alkaline phosphatase, and bilirubin). In addition, we investigated the possible influence of a single dose of naltrexone on plasma β-endorphin and plasma cortisol levels. For these purposes, venipunctures were done 2 weeks prior to and the day after each single dose. Venipunctures were performed in the morning, just after breakfast. Cortisol and β-endorphin levels were assayed with radioimmunoassay procedures.[62,63]

DATA ANALYSIS

The single-dose study was analyzed with repeated measures analysis of variance using SPSS-PC[64] with drug (placebo and naltrexone) as the within-subject factor and diagnosis (autism and SIB without autism) as the between-subject factor. The data relating to the long-term treatment were analyzed in a similar way, but with the additional within-subject factor of time (2 weeks and 4 weeks) and the additional between-subject factor of dose (50 mg and 150 mg). Baseline scores were used as covariates. The Barlett Box-F was used to test for homogeneity of variance. The Box-M was used as a multivariate test for equality of the variance-covariance matrixes. With regard to the ethological and endocrinological data, a logarithmic transformation was necessary to stabilize variances. All testing was two tailed, with α=.05.

Table 1. Studies on the Effect of Naltrexone on Self-Injurious Behavior (SIB)

Reference, y	No. of Subjects	Age, y	Dosage	Design	Effect
Bernstein et al,[21] 1987	1	18	12.5, 25, and 50 mg/d each for 14 d	Double-blind crossover	Dose-dependent decreased SIB
Zelnik et al,[12] 1986; Herman et al,[23] 1989; Herman et al,[22] 1987	3	10-17	0.5, 1.0, 1.5, and 2.0 mg/kg once a week	Single-blind crossover	Dose-dependent decreased SIB up to 1.5 mg/kg (no effect at 2.0 mg/kg)
Szymanski et al,[24] 1987	2	21, 29	50 and 100 mg/d for 3 wk	Double-blind crossover	No effect on SIB
Leboyer et al,[25] 1988	2	10, 12	1-2 mg/kg single dose	Open	Decreased SIB (no effect at 2 mg/kg)
Sandman,[26] 1988; Sandman et al,[27] 1990	4	23-26	25, 50, and 100 mg, each dose twice in 1 wk	Double-blind crossover	Dose-dependent decreased SIB in three patients
Kars et al,[28] 1990	6	15-31	50 mg/d for 3 wk	Double-blind crossover	Half of the subjects showed decreased SIB
Barrett et al,[29] 1989	1	12	50 mg/d for 12 d	Double-blind crossover	Abolished SIB
Lienemann and Walker,[30] 1989	1	27	50 mg/d for more than 1 y	Open	Decreased SIB
Lienemann and Walker,[31] 1989	1	50	50 mg/d for more than 28 d	Open	Decreased SIB
Ryan et al,[32] 1989	1	10	50 mg/d, (12 d) and 100 mg/d (20 d)	Open	Decreased SIB
	1	10	100 mg/d (6 d) and 200 mg/d (8 d)	Double-blind crossover	Decreased SIB, greatest decrease at 200 mg
Knabe et al,[33] 1990	2	27, 46	2.0 mg/kg per day for several days	Open	Decreased SIB
Walters et al,[34] 1990	1	14	1 mg/kg per day for 3 wk	Double-blind crossover	Decreased SIB
Taylor et al,[35] 1991	1	20	0.5, 1.0, and 2.0 mg/kg, each dose twice in 1 wk	Single-blind crossover	Decreased SIB in unstructured setting
Knabe and Bovier,[36] 1992	2	18, 30	1.25 and 1.54 mg/kg per day for more than 2 y	Open	Abolished SIB*
Leboyer et al,[37] 1992	4	4-19	0.5, 1.0, and 2.0 mg/kg per day, each dose for 1 wk	Double-blind crossover	Decreased SIB only for 0.5 and 2.0 mg/kg
Ricketts et al,[38] 1992	1	28	50, 75, and 100 mg/d for several weeks	Open	Decreased SIB†
Zingarelli et al,[39] 1992	8	19-39	50 mg/d for 3 wk	Double-blind crossover	No reduction in maladaptive behavior
Crews et al,[40] 1993	1	28	50 and 75 mg/d for 6 mo each	Open	Decreased SIB
Campbell et al,[41] 1993	23	3-8	0.5 mg/kg (1 wk) and 1.0 mg/kg per day (2 wk)	Double-blind parallel‡	No effect on SIB
Thompson et al,[42] 1994	8	29-41	50 and 100 mg/d for 2 wk each	Double-blind crossover	Decreased SIB

**In combination with sedative neuroleptic and β-adrenoreceptor blocking agent.*
†In combination with other therapy.
‡Forty-one subjects were enrolled.

behavior that is not related to SIB.[43-45] Most reports, however, concern pilot studies that used small numbers of selected subjects and mainly uncontrolled designs. Surprisingly, the study with the largest number of subjects and a carefully controlled design did not demonstrate beneficial effects.[39]

Panksepp and Sahley[46] and Panksepp[47] have postulated that symptoms of early childhood autism may result from excessive brain opioid activity. They claimed that excessive brain opioid activity causes not only a diminished sensitivity to pain, SIB, and stereotypic behavior, but also social withdrawal, inability to convey emotions, reduced crying, attentional dysfunctions, labile affect, and aggressiveness.

Studies concerning endogenous opioid levels in autistic subjects are inconsistent.[48-51] Reports on the effect of naltrexone on autistic behavior* are summarized in **Table 2**. Naltrexone was found to reduce social withdrawal and to increase the verbal output of autistic subjects.[20,37,43-45,52] The only beneficial effect on social behavior reported in two recent double-blind studies was a decrease in nonmeaningful vocalizations.[41,55]

**References 20,25,34,37,41,43-45,50,52-57.*

The present study was designed to assess the therapeutic effect of single-dose as well as long-term naltrexone administration in a large sample of mentally retarded adults with SIB and/or autism. Each subject first received a midrange single dose of naltrexone and subsequently was treated with a low or high dose for 4 weeks. In addition, we wanted to establish whether the effects of the single dose could predict the effects of long-term treatment.

RESULTS

COMPLIANCE AND SIDE EFFECTS

In two women, untoward effects were noticed during the daily treatment with naltrexone hydrochloride, 50 mg. After 2 weeks of naltrexone hydrochloride treatment (50

Table 2. Studies on the Effect of Naltrexone on Autistic Behavior

Reference, y	No. of Subjects Receiving Naltrexone Hydrochloride	Age, y	Dosage	Design	Effect
Herman et al,[50] 1986	5	4-12	0.5, 1.0, 1.5, and 2.0 mg/kg, each once a week	Open	No effect on proximity, eye contact, and uttered words; for parents, increased "enjoys hug"
Leboyer et al,[25] 1988	2	10-12	1.0, 1.5, and 2.0 mg/kg, single-dose	Open	Social behavior improved, reduction of hyperactivity
Campbell et al,[43] 1988; Campbell et al,[44] 1989	10	3-6	0.5, 1.0, and 2.0 mg/kg, single dose	Open	Reduction of withdrawal, increased verbal production (0.5 mg), reduction of sterotypies (2.0 mg)
Walters et al,[34] 1990	1	14	1 mg/kg	Double-blind crossover	Increased social relations
Scifo et al,[52] 1991	12	7-16	0.5, 1.0, and 1.5 mg/kg, every other day, each dose 5 wk	Double-blind crossover	Increased social proximity, improved attention
Panksepp and Lensing,[45] 1991	4	5-21	0.4-0.5 mg/kg for 3 wk and longer	Open	Increased social tendencies, reduction of stereotypies, reduction of aggressive behavior
Leboyer et al,[20] 1990; Leboyer et al,[37] 1992	4	4-19	0.5, 1.0, and 2.0 mg/kg per day, each dose 1 wk	Double-blind crossover	Elevated socialization, restlessness reduced, attentiveness increased
Campbell et al,[41] 1993; Campbell et al,[53] 1990	23	3-8	0.5 for 1 wk, 1.0 mg/kg per day for 2 wk	Double-blind parallel*	Reduction of hyperactivity, no effect on core items of autism
Borghese et al,[54] 1991; Borghese et al,[55] 1993; Herman et al,[56] 1991; Herman et al,[57] 1993	20	3-12	0.5, 1.0, 1.5, and 2.0 mg/kg, single-dose, three times a week	Double-blind crossover	Reduction of hyperactivity, no effect on social behavior and verbal output, decrease of nonmeaningful vocalizations (single dose)

Forty-one subjects were enrolled.

mg/d), a 28-year old woman (with autism and SIB) manifested an acute and severe increase in SIB and acting-out behavior. She had to be isolated for several weeks, and her condition improved only gradually after naltrexone treatment was stopped and lithium treatment was instituted. Since the subject did not finish the trial, her data were excluded from the analysis. The second woman complained of nausea and tiredness. Three subjects were observed to be sedated while being treated daily with naltrexone hydrochloride, 150 mg. Results of liver function profiles for all subjects were normal and did not deviate from the normal range following the administration of naltrexone.

SINGLE DOSE

Neither the questionnaire (sum and subscale scores) nor the observation data revealed significant drug effects in the single-dose study. A separate analysis performed on the items concerning SIB in the ABC questionnaire and the target checklist also did not reveal beneficial effects of naltrexone (data not shown). Naltrexone had no significant effect on plasma β-endorphin levels, but it did significantly increase plasma cortisol levels (mean±SD baseline level, 310±170 nmol/L; following placebo treatment, 300±130 nmol/L; following naltrexone treatment, 360±210 nmol/L; $F[1,29]=8.84$; $P=.006$).

LONG-TERM TREATMENT

The questionnaire and the observation data revealed no significant drug effects during the long-term treatment with naltrexone hydrochloride, 50 and 150 mg, except on the ABC stereotypy subscale. Naltrexone treatment tended to be associated with an increase in stereotypic behavior as rated by the care staff (**Table 3**). This increase was independent of diagnosis or dose (effects of drug-by-dose interaction and drug-by-diagnosis interaction were not significant).

A separate analysis performed on the ABC and target items concerning SIB did not document beneficial effects of long-term naltrexone treatment. The absence of naltrexone treatment effects appeared not to be dependent on the age or sex of the subjects, their level of mental retardation, or their sensitivity to pain.

Figure 1 shows the CGIS ratings given by the staff after 4 weeks of treating subjects with naltrexone hydrochloride, 50 mg, and placebo. Since subjects were sorted according to staff preference, it is immediately clear from Figure 1 that on 12 occasions, the placebo treatment was preferred to the naltrexone treatment, whereas for four subjects the naltrexone treatment was preferred to the placebo treatment. No clear relationship was found between the preference for either treatment and neuroleptic comedication or the presence of SIB. The placebo treat-

Table 3. Pretreatment and Posttreatment Levels of the ABC Stereotypy Factor as Rated by the Care Staff*

Subjects	Placebo Treatment			Naltrexone Treatment		
	Pretreatment	2 Weeks	4 Weeks	Pretreatment	2 Weeks	4 Weeks
With autism	8.3±5.2	8.8±5.0	9.0±4.8	9.7±4.7	10.2±4.6	10.0±4.7
Without autism	8.0±5.0	9.6±2.4	7.7±3.8	8.1±4.3	10.4±4.4	10.9±4.0

*Values are given as mean±SD. ABC indicates Aberrant Behavior Checklist. For drug effect, $F(1,27)=6.33$; $P=.018$.

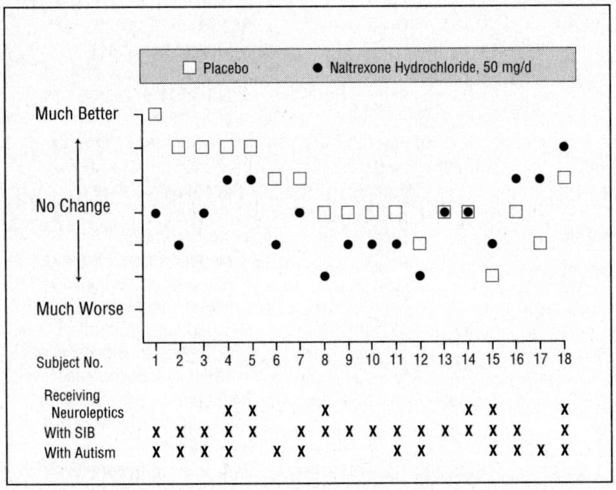

Figure 1. *Graphic display of the Clinical Global Impression Scale ratings for the 18 subjects who completed the course of long-term treatment with naltrexone hydrochloride, 50 mg/d. The staff rated subjects at the end of the 4 weeks of treatment with placebo or naltrexone. Subjects were sorted according to the staff preference. SIB indicates self-injurious behavior; X, subjects who were using neuroleptics during the study, subjects with SIB, and subjects with autism.*

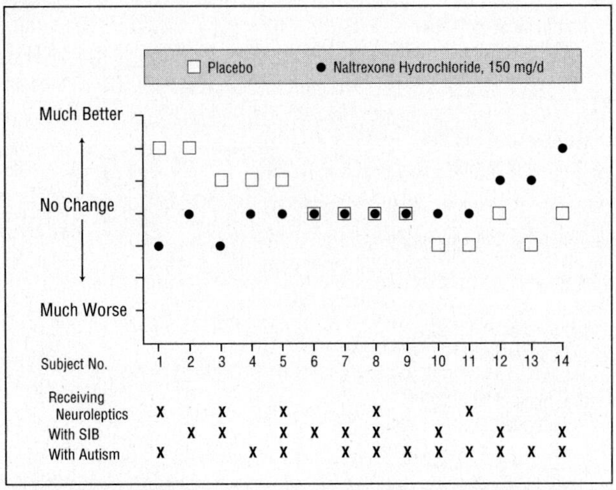

Figure 2. *Graphic display of the Clinical Global Impression Scale ratings for the 14 subjects who completed the course of long-term treatment with naltrexone hydrochloride, 150 mg/d. The staff rated subjects at the end of the 4 weeks of treatment with placebo or naltrexone. Subjects were sorted according to the staff preference. SIB indicates self-injurious behavior; X, subjects who were using neuroleptics during the study, subjects with SIB, and subjects with autism.*

ment turned out to be significantly more successful than the naltrexone treatment (paired *t* test, 2.36; *df*=18; *P*=.03).

The CGIS ratings given by the staff after 4 weeks of treating subjects with naltrexone hydrochloride, 150 mg, and placebo are presented in **Figure 2**. The number of preferences for the placebo treatment is equal to the number of preferences for the naltrexone treatment. The three subjects who were considered "better than usual" during naltrexone treatment were not receiving any neuroleptic comedication.

RELATIONSHIP BETWEEN SINGLE-DOSE AND LONG-TERM TREATMENT

No significant correlations were found between behavioral changes following a single dose of naltrexone hydrochloride, 100 mg, and following a 4-week treatment with naltrexone hydrochloride, 50 or 150 mg. There were no significant correlations between changes in plasma β-endorphin levels after the single dose of naltrexone hydrochloride, 100 mg, and changes in behavior following the single dose or 4 weeks of treatment.

COMEDICATION

Analyses were rerun after the sample had been broken down into subjects with vs subjects without neuroleptic comedication and subjects with vs subjects without any comedication. Naltrexone treatment failed to produce significant therapeutic effects in these further analyses.

COMMENT

To the best of our knowledge, ours is so far the largest sample of mentally retarded adults treated with naltrexone under double-blind, placebo-controlled conditions. We found that neither single-dose (100 mg) nor long-term (50 and 150 mg) naltrexone hydrochloride treatment had any therapeutic effect on the core symptoms of SIB or autism. In fact, according to the CGIS ratings given by the staff, treatment with placebo seemed more beneficial than a 4-week treatment with naltrexone hydrochloride, 50 mg/d. The response to a single dose proved to be of little use for predicting the effect of long-term treatment. The main finding, namely no effect of naltrexone on the primary dependent measures, is in agreement with the results of two other placebo-controlled studies of naltrexone in large samples of subjects with SIB[39] and autism.[41] All studies that have reported therapeutic effects of naltrexone have been seriously flawed from a methodological point of view, owing to factors such as a very small sample size or open-label designs.

There are several possible explanations for our negative findings. The first and most compelling explanation, of course, is that the opioid hypothesis concerning SIB and autism is incorrect. In other words, SIB and autism do not result from excessive activity of the endogenous opioid systems. A second possibility is that excessive brain opioid activity is involved only in the first phase of development of stereotypic patterns of SIB or autism. With regard to SIB, this would fit with data from animal studies. For example, the delay in ceasing the performance of self-biting after the administration of naloxone in tethered sows proved to be positively related to the age of the abnormal behavior.[65] Further, in bank voles, naloxone was found to attenuate the development of captivity-induced jumping stereotypies in the initial phase. After a longer period of captivity, however, induced stereotypic behavior was found to be under the control of dopaminergic systems only.[66] Recent models of stereotypy and self-injury in human subjects also postulate that different mechanisms are involved in the emergence and maintenance phases of the disorder.[67] This possibility suggests that opioid antagonist therapy might be more successful in younger populations of patients with SIB and autism. However, our study in which 20 autistic children aged 3 to 7 years completed a double-blind, placebo-controlled, crossover trial with naltrexone (treatment for 4 weeks) revealed no effects on social and stereotypic behavior.[68]

Third, the discrepancy between the results of case studies and studies with larger samples may also be related to subject selection. Most case studies on SIB have included the most extreme cases in an institution. Although we also included SIB patients who did not respond to therapy in our study, severity of SIB in our patients ranged from moderately to extremely ill on the CGIS.[60] Fourth, it is important to note that both SIB and autism are conditions that are rather heterogeneous with respect to the pattern of symptoms and the underlying biological causes. This is also reflected in the composition of our sample, which consisted of adults with all levels of mental retardation, all kinds of comedications, and a variety of medical diagnoses.

Fifth, several other methodological factors may have had an influence on our results. We administered fixed amounts of naltrexone (multiples of 50 mg) instead of titrating the dose of naltrexone on an individual basis. An individual dosage regimen would certainly have prolonged and complicated the design of the study but might have been more effective. One could also argue that a 4-week treatment of subjects with SIB or autism is much too brief to alter behavioral problems that have existed for years. Other researchers, however, have claimed changes after a single dose of naltrexone or after treatment for only 1 week (Tables 1 and 2). Furthermore, there is much to be said for combining checklist ratings with direct observations of behavior. In this respect, our study had its limitations, since only 11 subjects were directly observed and none received a daily treatment of 150 mg/kg.

Finally, although our study included a relatively large sample of subjects, the power to detect a difference on the checklist data at a level of P=.05 with a medium effect size (0.5) was only 71%.[69] However, because we found a significant *increase* in stereotypic behavior as measured on the stereotypy subscale of the ABC, we can state confidently that naltrexone does not decrease stereotypy. This significant increase suggests that there is some relationship between the opioid system and stereotypic behavior. Further study is needed to investigate the details of this relationship.

Naltrexone had no effect on plasma β-endorphin levels. Since blood samples were not collected until a day after drug administration, it is possible that quick but short-lasting effects of naltrexone were missed. However, we did find a significant increase in cortisol plasma levels after naltrexone administration. Increasing effects of opiate antagonists on plasma cortisol have been reported consistently.[70-72] We found no significant correlations between changes in plasma levels and behavioral changes.

CONCLUSION

This study has evaluated different dosages of naltrexone in different settings with a variety of instruments: checklists, direct observations, and staff discussions. Since no therapeutic effects were found, our data indicate that naltrexone has no clinical usefulness for a broad group of mentally retarded adults with SIB or autism. The findings suggest that naltrexone hydrochloride (in a 50-mg/d dosage) may even aggravate behavior problems. This, of course, is inconsistent with hypotheses that state that excessive endogenous opioid activity plays a role in the pathogenesis of SIB, stereotypic behavior, or deviant social behavior.

Accepted for publication May 31, 1995.

Supported by the Janusz Korczak Foundation, Huizen, the Netherlands.

We wish to thank Tobias Ehlhart, MS, Marianne de Kroon, MS, Florence Weijnen, MS, and the numerous staff members of the Institute for Mental Retardation Eemeroord and Sterrenberg for their assistance with data collection. We are also grateful to Peter Klein, MD, at Du Pont Pharma, Bad Homburg, Germany, who gave us some of the naltrexone.

Reprint requests to Department of Child Psychiatry, University of Utrecht, PO Box 85500, 3508 GA Utrecht, the Netherlands (Dr Buitelaar).

REFERENCES

1. Griffin JC, Ricketts RW, Williams DE, Locke BJ, Altmeyer BK, Stark MT. A community survey of self-injurious behavior among developmentally disabled children and adolescents. *Hosp Community Psychiatry.* 1987;38:959-963.
2. Griffin JC, Williams DE, Stark MT, Altmeyer BK, Mason M. Self-injurious behavior: a state-wide prevalence survey of the extent and circumstances. *Appl Res Ment Retard.* 1986;7:105-116.
3. Verhoeven WMA, Tuinier S, Sijben NES. Biological aspects and pharmacological treatment of self-injurious behavior in persons with mental retardation. In: Fletcher RJ, Dosen A, eds. *Mental Health Aspects of Mental Retardation.* New York, NY: Lexington Books, Free McMillan Inc; 1993:291-323.
4. Buitelaar JK. Self-injurious behaviour in retarded children: clinical phenomena and biological mechanisms. *Acta Paedopsychiatr.* 1993;56:105-111.
5. Gillberg C, Persson E, Grufman M, Themner U. Psychiatric disorders in mildly and severely mentally retarded urban children and adolescents: epidemiological aspects. *Br J Psychiatry.* 1986;149:68-74.
6. Wing L, Gould J. Severe impairments of social interaction and associated ab-

normalities in children: epidemiology and classification. *J Autism Dev Disord.* 1979;9:11-29.

7. Buitelaar JK. Psychopharmacological approaches to childhood psychotic disorders. In: Den Boer JA, Westenberg HGM, Van Praag HM, eds. *Advances in the Neurobiology of Schizophrenia.* New York, NY: John Wiley & Sons Inc; 1995:429-457.
8. Deutsch SI. Rationale for the administration of opiate antagonists in treating infantile autism. *Am J Ment Defic.* 1986;90:631-635.
9. Sandman CA, Datta PC, Barron J, Hoekler FK, Williams C, Swanson JM. Naloxone attenuates self-abusive behavior in developmentally disabled clients. *Appl Res Ment Retard.* 1983;4:5-11.
10. Gillberg C, Terenius L, Lönnerholm G. Endorphin activity in childhood psychosis. *Arch Gen Psychiatry.* 1985;42:780-783.
11. Gillberg C. Plasma beta-endorphin concentrations in autism. *J Autism Dev Disord.* 1992;22:131.
12. Zelnik N, Herman BH, Hammock MK, Arthur-Smith A, Egan J, Chatoor I, Werner A, Boeckx RL. Role of opioid peptides in self-injurious behavior. *Soc Neurosci Abstr.* 1986;12:412.
13. Weizman R, Gil-Ad I, Dick J, Tyano S, Szekely GA, Laron Z. Low plasma immunoreactive beta-endorphin levels in autism. *J Am Acad Child Adolesc Psychiatry.* 1988;27:430-433.
14. Sandman CA, Barron JL, Chicz-DeMet A, DeMet EM. Plasma β-endorphin levels in patients with self-injurious behavior and stereotypy. *Am J Ment Retard.* 1990;95:84-92.
15. Herman BH. A possible role of proopiomelanocortin peptides in self-injurious behavior. *Prog Neuropsychopharmacol Biol Psychiatry.* 1990;14(suppl):S109-S139.
16. Beckwith BE, Couk DI, Schumacher K. Failure of naloxone to reduce self-injurious behavior in two developmentally disabled females. *Appl Res Ment Retard.* 1986;7:183-188.
17. Richardson JS, Zaleski WA. Naloxone and self-mutilation. *Biol Psychiatry.* 1983; 18:99-101.
18. Sandman CA, Barron JL, Crinella FM, Donnelly JF. Influence of naloxone on brain and behavior of a self-injurious woman. *Biol Psychiatry.* 1987;22:899-906.
19. Sandyk R. Naloxone abolishes self-injuring in a mentally retarded child. *Ann Neurol.* 1985;17:520.
20. Leboyer M, Bouvard MP, Lensing P, Launay J, Tabuteau F, Arnaud P, Waller D, Plumet M, Recasens C, Kerdelhue B, Dugas M, Panksepp J. Opioid excess hypothesis of autism: a double-blind study of naltrexone. *Brain Dysfunct.* 1990; 3:285-298.
21. Bernstein GA, Hughes JR, Mitchel JE, Thompson T. Effects of narcotic antagonists on self-injurious behavior: a single case study. *J Am Acad Child Adolesc Psychiatry.* 1987;26:886-889.
22. Herman BH, Hammock MK, Arthur-Smith A, Egan J, Chatoor I, Zelnik N. Naltrexone decreases self-injurious behavior. *Ann Neurol.* 1987;22:550-552.
23. Herman BH, Hammock MK, Egan J, Arthur-Smith A, Chatoor I, Werner A. Role for opioid peptides in self-injurious behavior: dissociation from autonomic nervous system functioning. *Dev Pharmacol Ther.* 1989;12:81-89.
24. Szymanski L, Kedesdy J, Sulkes S, Cutler A, Stevens-Our P. Naltrexone in treatment of self injurious behavior: a clinical study. *Res Dev Disabil.* 1987;8:179-190.
25. Leboyer M, Bouvard MP, Dugas M. Effects of naltrexone on infantile autism. *Lancet.* 1988;26:715.
26. Sandman CA. Beta-endorphin disregulation in autistic and self-injurious behavior: a neurodevelopmental hypothesis. *Synapse.* 1988;2:193-199.
27. Sandman CA, Barron JL, Colman H. An orally administered opiate blocker, naltrexone, attenuates self-injurious behavior. *Am J Ment Retard.* 1990;95:93-102.
28. Kars H, Broekema W, Glaudemans–van Gelderen I, Verhoeven WMA, Van Ree JM. Naltrexone attenuates self-injurious behavior in mentally retarded subjects. *Biol Psychiatry.* 1990;27:741-746.
29. Barrett RP, Feinstein C, Hole WT. Effects of naloxone and naltrexone on self-injury: a double-blind, placebo-controlled analysis. *Am J Ment Retard.* 1989; 93:644-651.
30. Lienemann J, Walker F. Naltrexone for treatment of self-injury. *Am J Psychiatry.* 1989;146:1639-1640.
31. Lienemann J, Walker FD. Reversal of self-abusive behavior with naltrexone. *J Clin Psychopharmacol.* 1989;9:448-449.
32. Ryan EP, Helsel WJ, Lubetsky MJ, Miewald BK, Hersen M, Bridge J. Use of naltrexone in reducing self-injurious behavior: a single case analysis. *J Multihandicapped Person.* 1989;2:295-309.
33. Knabe R, Schulz P, Richard J. Initial aggravation of self-injurious behavior in autistic patients receiving naltrexone treatment. *J Autism Dev Disord.* 1990; 20:591-593.
34. Walters AS, Barrett RP, Feinstein C, Mercurio A, Hole WT. A case report of naltrexone treatment of self-injury and social withdrawal in autism. *J Autism Dev Disord.* 1990;20:169-176.
35. Taylor DV, Hetrick WP, Neri CL, Touchette P, Barron JL, Sandman CA. Effect of naltrexone upon self-injurious behavior, learning and activity: a case study. *Pharmacol Biochem Behav.* 1991;40:79-82.
36. Knabe R, Bovier P. Pharmacological treatment of extreme self-injurious behaviour in autism. *Eur Psychiatry.* 1992;7:297-298.
37. Leboyer M, Bouvard MP, Launay J, Tableau F, Waller D, Kerdelhue B, Lensin P, Panksepp J. Brief report: a double-blind study of naltrexone in infantile autism. *J Autism Dev Disord.* 1992;22:309-319.
38. Ricketts RW, Goza AB, Matese M. Case study: effects of naltrexone and SIBIS on self-injury. *Behav Residential Treatment.* 1992;7:315-326.
39. Zingarelli G, Ellman G, Hom A, Wymore M, Heidorn S, Chicz-DeMet A. Clinical effects of naltrexone on autistic behavior. *Am J Ment Retard.* 1992;97:57-63.
40. Crews WD, Bonaventura S, Rowe FB, Bonsie D. Cessation of long-term naltrexone therapy and self-injury: a case study. *Res Dev Disabil.* 1993;14:331-340.
41. Campbell M, Anderson LT, Small AM, Adams P, Gonzalez NM, Ernst M. Naltrexone in autistic children: behavioral symptoms and attentional learning. *J Am Acad Child Adolesc Psychiatry.* 1993;32:1283-1291.
42. Thompson T, Hackenberg T, Cerutti D, Baker D, Axtell S. Opioid antagonist effects on self-injury in adults with mental retardation: response form and location as determinants of medication effects. *Am J Ment Retard.* 1994;99:85-102.
43. Campbell M, Adams P, Small AM, Tesch LM, Curren EL. Naltrexone in infantile autism. *Psychopharmacol Bull.* 1988;24:135-139.
44. Campbell M, Overall JE, Small AM, Sokol MS, Spencer K, Adams P, Foltz RL, Monti KM, Perry R, Nobler M, Roberts E. Naltrexone in autistic children: an acute open dose range tolerance trial. *J Am Acad Child Adolesc Psychiatry.* 1989;28:200-206.
45. Panksepp J, Lensing P. Brief report: a synopsis of an open-trial of naltrexone treatment of autism with four children. *J Autism Dev Disord.* 1991;21:243-249.
46. Panksepp J, Sahley TL. Possible brain opioid involvement in disrupted social intent and language development of autism. In: Schopler E, Mesibov GB, eds. *Neurobiological Issues in Autism.* New York, NY: Plenum Press; 1987: 357-372.
47. Panksepp J. A neurochemical theory of autism. *Trends Neurosci.* 1979;2: 174-177.
48. Ross DL, Klykylo WM, Hitzemann R. Reduction of elevated CSF beta-endorphin by fenfluramine in infantile autism. *Pediatr Neurol.* 1987;3:83-86.
49. Gillberg C, Terenius L, Hagberg B, Witt-Engerström I, Eriksson I. CSF beta-endorphins in childhood neuropsychiatric disorders. *Brain Dev.* 1990;12: 88-92.
50. Herman BH, Hammock MK, Arthur-Smith A, Egan J, Chatoor I, Zelnik N, Corradine M, Appelgate K, Boeckx RL, Sharp SD. Role of opioid peptides in autism: effects of acute administration of naltrexone. *Soc Neurosci Abstr.* 1986; 12:1172.
51. Sandman CA, Barron JL, Chicz-DeMet A, DeMet EM. Brief report: plasma β-endorphin and cortisol levels in autistic patients. *J Autism Dev Disord.* 1991;21: 83-87.
52. Scifo R, Batticane N, Quattropani MC, Spoto G, Marchetti B. A double-blind trial with naltrexone in autism. Presented at the OASI conference; October 1991; Sicily.
53. Campbell M, Anderson LT, Small AM, Locascio JJ, Lynch NS, Choroco MC. Naltrexone in autistic children: a double-blind and placebo-controlled study. *Psychopharmacol Bull.* 1990;26:130-135.
54. Borghese IF, Herman BH, Asleson G, Chantoor I, Benoit MB, Papero P, McNulty G. Effects of acutely administered naltrexone on social behavior of autistic children. *Soc Neurosci Abstr.* 1991;17:1252.
55. Borghese IF, Herman BH, Anselmi LS, Asleson GS, Lukens E, Benoit MB, Chantoor I, Papero P. Effects of acutely and chronically administered naltrexone on social behavior and language of children with autism. *Soc Neurosci Abstr.* 1993; 19:1785.
56. Herman BH, Asleson GS, Borghese IF, Chantoor I, Benoit MB, Powell A, Papero P, Allen RP, McNulty G. Acute natrexone in autism: selective decreases in hyperactivity. In: *Scientific Proceedings, 38th Annual Meeting of the American Academy of Child and Adolescent Psychiatry.* Washington, DC: AACAP; 1991: 52.
57. Herman BH, Asleson G, Lukens E, Borghese I, Anselmi L, Allen RP, Benoit MB, Chatoor I, Papero P. Acute and chronic naltrexone decreases the hyperactivity of autism. *Soc Neurosci Abstr.* 1993;19:1785.
58. American Psychiatric Association. *Diagnostic and Statistical Manual of Mental Disorders, Revised Third Edition.* Washington, DC: American Psychiatric As-

sociation; 1987.
59. Aman MG, Singh NN, Stewart AW, Field CJ. The Aberrant Behavior Checklist: a behavior rating scale for the assessment of treatment effects. *Am J Ment Defic.* 1985;89:485-491.
60. National Institute of Mental Health. Special feature: rating scales and assessment instruments for use in pediatric psychopharmacology research. *Psychopharmacol Bull.* 1985;21:839-842.
61. Noldus LPJJ. The Observer: a software system for collection and analysis of observational data. *Behav Res Methods Instrum Comput.* 1991;23:415-429.
62. Thijssen JHH, Van den Berg JHM, Adlercreutz J. The determination of cortisol in human plasma: evaluation and comparison of seven assays. *Clin Chim Acta.* 1980;100:39-46.
63. Gispen-De Wied CC, Westerberg HGM, Thijssen JHH. The dexamethasone and cortisol suppression test in depression: β-endorphin as a useful marker. *Psychoneuroendocrinology.* 1987;12:355-366.
64. Nordusis MJ, SPSS Inc. *SPSS/PC+ Advanced Statistics 4.0 for the IBM PC/XT/AT and PC/2.* Chicago, Ill: SPSS Inc; 1990.
65. Cronin GM, Wiepkema PR, Van Ree JM. Endorphins implicated in sterotypies of tethered sows. *Experientia.* 1986;42:198-199.
66. Kennes D, Odberg FO, Bouquet Y, De-Rycke PH. Changes in naloxone and haloperidol effects during the development of captivity-induced jumping stereotypy in bank voles. *Eur J Pharmacol.* 1988;153:19-24.
67. Guess D, Carr E. Emergence and maintenance of stereotypy and self-injury. *Am J Ment Retard.* 1991;96:299-319.
68. Willemsen-Swinkels SHN, Buitelaar JK, Van Engeland H. The effects of chronic naltrexone treatment in young autistic children: a double-blind placebo-controlled crossover study. *Biol Psychiatry.* In press.
69. Cohen J. *Statistical Power Analysis for the Behavioral Sciences.* Hillsdale, NJ: Lawrence Erlbaum Associate Inc; 1988.
70. Judd LJ, Janowsky DS, Zettner A, Huey LY, Takahashi KI. Effects of naloxone-HCL on cortisol levels in patients with affective disorder and normal controls. *Psychiatry Res.* 1981;4:277-283.
71. Blankstein J, Reyes FI, Winter JSD, Faiman C. Effects of naloxone upon prolactin and cortisol in normal women. *Proc Soc Exp Biol Med.* 1980;164:363-365.
72. Pomara N, Stanley M, Rhiew B, Bagne CA, Deptula D, Galloway MP, Tanimoto K, Verebey K, Tamminga CA. Loss of the cortisol response to naltrexone in Alzheimer's disease. *Biol Psychiatry.* 1988;23:726-733.

ORIGINAL ARTICLE

Effects of Alzheimer's Disease and Normal Aging on Cerebrospinal Fluid Norepinephrine Responses to Yohimbine and Clonidine

Elaine R. Peskind, MD; Dane Wingerson, MD; Sharon Murray, RN; Marcella Pascualy, MD; Dorcas J. Dobie, MD; Pascal Le Corre, PharmD, PhD; Roger Le Verge, PharmD, PhD; Richard C. Veith, MD; Murray A. Raskind, MD

Background: The resting cerebrospinal fluid (CSF) norepinephrine concentration is unchanged or even increased in patients with Alzheimer's disease (AD). These in vivo findings appear to be inconsistent with the postmortem locus ceruleus neuronal loss that is reported in patients with AD.

Methods: The effects of AD and advanced age on central nervous system noradrenergic status were estimated by comparing CSF norepinephrine concentrations following the administration of yohimbine hydrochloride, clonidine hydrochloride, and placebo in outpatients with AD and older and young normal subjects. Levels of yohimbine, its metabolite 11-hydroxy-yohimbine, and clonidine were measured in CSF and plasma samples. Behavioral responses were quantified by rating the Tension, Excitement, and Anxiety items on the Brief Psychiatric Rating Scale.

Results: Yohimbine-induced increases of CSF norepinephrine concentrations were greater in both patients with AD and normal older subjects than in normal young subjects. Clonidine-induced decreases of CSF norepinephrine concentrations did not differ among groups. Behavioral arousal following the administration of yohimbine was greater in patients with AD than in the other groups.

Conclusions: Central nervous system noradrenergic responsiveness is enhanced in normal older subjects, and this age effect is retained in patients with AD. Behavioral sensitivity to increased central nervous system noradrenergic activity is enhanced in patients with AD.

(Arch Gen Psychiatry. 1995;52:774-782)

From the Geriatric Research Education and Clinical Center, Seattle (Wash)/American Lake Veterans Affairs Medical Center (Drs Peskind, Pascualy, Dobie, Veith, and Raskind and Ms Murray), the Department of Psychiatry and Behavioral Sciences, University of Washington School of Medicine, Seattle (Drs Peskind, Wingerson, Pascualy, Dobie, Veith, and Raskind and Ms Murray), and the Faculte des Sciences Pharmaceutiques et Biologiques, University of Rennes I (France) (Drs Le Corre and Le Verge).

THE STATUS of central nervous system (CNS) noradrenergic systems in patients with Alzheimer's disease (AD) and the relationship of these systems to behavior in this disorder remain unclear. Studies in living patients are difficult to reconcile with postmortem neurohistologic findings. In postmortem AD brain tissue, a substantial loss of noradrenergic neurons in the locus ceruleus (LC), the major source of CNS noradrenergic innervation,[1] has been consistently demonstrated.[2-4] This loss of LC neurons in patients with AD is much greater than the modest loss of LC neurons that is attributed to normal human aging.[5] In contrast, in vivo studies of CNS noradrenergic activity that have compared resting concentrations of norepinephrine (NE) or its major CNS metabolite 3-methoxy-4-hydroxy-phenylglycol (MHPG) in the cerebrospinal fluid (CSF) among patients with AD, normal older subjects, and normal young subjects have produced unexpected results. The CSF NE concentration is increased in normal older subjects.[6] This age-associated increase in the resting CSF NE concentration is retained in outpatients with AD who have mild or moderate dementia, and it is further increased in patients with AD who have severe dementia.[7,8] Furthermore, the resting CSF MHPG concentration is either unchanged or increased in patients with AD,[7-11] and it may increase with the severity of dementia.[7,12] Thus, as one progressively loses LC noradrenergic neurons with normal aging and through the stages of AD, resting CSF NE and MHPG concentrations paradoxically fail to decline and may actually increase.

Resolving these paradoxical findings has potentially important implications for understanding and treating AD. If the LC neuronal loss that is demonstrated in postmortem tissue accurately reflects a CNS noradrenergic deficiency in

See Subjects and Methods on next page

SUBJECTS AND METHODS

SUBJECTS

This study was approved by the University of Washington Human Subjects Review Committee, Seattle, and informed consent was obtained from all subjects and from the legal representative of the patients with AD. Subjects were 18 normal young men (mean±SEM age, 26.4±0.9 years), 10 older cognitively normal subjects (six men and four women; mean±SEM age, 71.2±1.1 years), and 10 patients with AD (seven men and three women; mean±SEM age, 69.5±2.5 years). Normal older subjects and patients with AD did not differ with respect to age (unpaired t=0.624, P=.54). Most but not all subjects underwent all three study treatment conditions (**Table 1**). The different subject numbers among groups was owing to an additional seven young subjects who participated only in the yohimbine and placebo treatment conditions. These additional young subjects were studied to provide a number that was equivalent to all older subjects (normal older subjects plus patients with AD) to provide adequate power (per a priori estimate) to test our hypothesis of an aging effect on CNS noradrenergic responsiveness to yohimbine.

Subjects were nonsmokers in good general health who had been free of medications for at least 1 month prior to study, were normotensive (<135 mm Hg [systolic pressure] and 90 mm Hg [diastolic pressure]) and were within 125% of their ideal body weight (Metropolitan Life Insurance Tables, 1983). Normal subjects underwent screening with the use of a medical history, semistructured psychiatric interview, physical examination, electrocardiogram, and laboratory evaluation of serum electrolyte and glucose levels, renal and hepatic function, and complete blood cell count. Both young and older normal subjects were free of all past or present major psychiatric disorders, neurologic disorders, renal or hepatic disease, diabetes mellitus, congestive heart failure, and cardiac arrhythmias. Patients with AD met the same criteria with the exception of their AD. Patients with AD met the National Institute of Neurological Disorders and Stroke criteria for probable AD,[31] *DSM-III-R*[32] criteria for primary degenerative dementia of the Alzheimer's type, and other exclusionary criteria as previously described.[33] The mean±SEM Mini-Mental State Examination[34] score in the patients with AD was 14±2. Young and older normal subjects had Mini-Mental State Examination scores of 29 or 30 and no history or evidence of cognitive decline.

PROCEDURES

Studies were performed in a clinical research unit at the Seattle Veterans Affairs Medical Center. The performance of lumbar punctures was separated by at least 1 week. The following three treatment conditions were administered in random order: placebo; clonidine hydrochloride, 5 μg/kg by mouth; and yohimbine hydrochloride, 0.65 mg/kg by mouth. Subjects were blind to the treatment condition. Investigators were aware of the treatment conditions for reasons of subject safety. Subjects fasted from midnight before the start of each study day and were prohibited from the use of caffeine or known stimulants of catecholamine release after midnight to the end of each study day. At approximately 9 AM, subjects assumed a recumbent position, and a 19-gauge plastic catheter was inserted into an antecubital vein. At that time, drug or placebo was administered by mouth. Blood sampling, immediately followed by lumbar puncture, took place 90 minutes following the administration of drug or placebo. Lumbar puncture was performed atraumatically with a 25-gauge spinal needle with the patients in the lateral decubitus position.

SAMPLE COLLECTION AND MEASUREMENT

The CSF NE concentration was measured in the 12th milliliter of the CSF sample that was removed, and blood samples for NE and epinephrine (EPI) determinations were collected into prechilled tubes that contained egtazic acid (ethylene glycol-bis[β-aminoethyl ether]-*N,N*-tetraacetic acid; EGTA) and reduced glutathione. The CSF samples were frozen immediately on dry ice and stored at −70°C until assay. Blood samples were placed on ice and cold-centrifuged within 1 hour of collection; plasma samples were stored at −70°C until assay. The CSF and plasma NE and plasma EPI levels were determined by a sensitive single isotope radioenzymatic assay as previously described.[35] The coefficient of variation within assays was 11% for NE and 12% for EPI. The coefficient of variation between assays was 15% for NE and 35% for EPI. Clonidine concentrations in CSF and plasma samples were measured by using a radioimmunoassay as previously described.[36] The CSF clonidine concentration was measured in the ninth milliliter of a CSF sample that was removed. Yohimbine and 11-hydroxy-yohimbine concentrations in CSF and plasma samples were measured by high-performance liquid chromatography and mass spectral analysis as previously described.[28] The CSF yohimbine and 11-hydroxy-yohimbine concentrations were measured in the 10th and 11th milliliters of the CSF sample that was removed. The results from the two samples were averaged to produce a single value for statistical analysis. If a subject had undetectable CSF concentrations of either yohimbine or clonidine in the respective treatment conditions, data for that subject from that treatment condition were excluded from analysis. Systolic and diastolic blood pressures and heart rate were obtained automatically (Dinamap, Critikon Inc, Tampa, Fla) following blood sampling. The mean arterial pressure (MAP) was calculated with the following formula: MAP=Diastolic+1/3 (Systolic−Diastolic).

BEHAVIORAL RATINGS

Behavioral ratings were performed on all normal older control subjects and patients with AD and on 10 of the normal young subjects at the 90-minute time point just before lumbar puncture. The same experienced psychiatric research nurse (S.M.) rated all subjects in all three treatment conditions by using the Tension, Excitement, and Anxiety items of the Brief Psychiatric Rating Scale. The Mini-Mental State Examination was administered to patients with AD after the lumbar puncture was performed in each condition.

Continued on next page

STATISTICAL ANALYSIS

Variables are expressed as mean±SEM. Differences among groups within the placebo (baseline) treatment condition were evaluated by one-way analysis of variance (ANOVA). Differences between treatment conditions (comparison of yohimbine or clonidine with placebo) within groups were compared by the paired *t* test (two-tailed). Differences (Δ values) between active drug and placebo treatment conditions at the 90-minute time point were calculated for CSF NE, plasma NE, and plasma EPI concentrations, MAP, heart rate, and ratings of Brief Psychiatric Rating Scale items. The significance of differences in the Δ values of these variables among subject groups was evaluated by one-way ANOVA. When a neuroendocrine variable in the placebo treatment condition differed among groups, the difference between placebo and drug treatment conditions among groups also was analyzed as the percent change from the baseline. Post hoc Newman-Keuls tests were used to evaluate differences between specific groups following a significant ANOVA.

patients with AD and normal older persons, pharmacologic enhancement of CNS noradrenergic activity potentially could improve cognitive function.[13,14] Alternatively, if the reported in vivo CSF NE and MHPG findings accurately reflect increased central noradrenergic responsiveness in normal older persons and patients with AD, this phenomenon could contribute to the disruptive hyperactive behavioral problems that frequently complicate AD.[15]

Understanding the status of CNS noradrenergic activity in AD and aging would be enhanced by functional studies that measure CSF NE responses to pharmacologic challenges. Measurements of CSF NE provide an estimate of in vivo CNS noradrenergic activity that does not appear to be influenced by plasma NE released from peripheral sympathetic nervous system (SNS) neurons.[16,17] In contrast to NE, MHPG flows relatively freely across blood-brain and blood-CSF barriers.[16,18-20] The CSF NE concentration therefore provides a more valid measure of CNS noradrenergic activity than does the CSF MHPG concentration, which is influenced by peripheral noradrenergic activity.[21]

The major objective of this study was to evaluate the effect of AD and normal aging on CSF NE responses to the α_2-adrenergic antagonist yohimbine, a drug that stimulates CNS noradrenergic activity by blocking α_2-receptors that mediate NE feedback inhibition of LC neurons.[22] Yohimbine has been used as a pharmacologic probe of CNS noradrenergic responsiveness and of behavioral sensitivity to CNS noradrenergic activation in several psychiatric disorders.[23-25] Based on the findings from our earlier studies,[6,7] we hypothesized increased CNS noradrenergic responsiveness to yohimbine in normal older persons and retention or exaggeration of age-associated–enhanced CNS noradrenergic responsiveness in older persons with AD. We also measured the CSF NE response to the α_2-agonist clonidine hydrochloride, a drug that suppresses CNS noradrenergic activity by α_2-receptor–mediated inhibition of LC neurons.[26] The CSF NE concentrations that were found following these pharmacologic challenges were compared with the CSF NE concentrations that were found following the administration of placebo. We have previously demonstrated that yohimbine increases CSF NE concentrations and clonidine decreases CSF NE concentrations in normal young subjects.[22,27]

The CSF concentrations of yohimbine, its major metabolite 11-hydroxy-yohimbine,[28] and clonidine also were measured. In addition, signs and symptoms that were relevant to the disruptive agitated behaviors often expressed in patients with AD were quantified by using the Tension, Excitement, and Anxiety items of the Brief Psychiatric Rating Scale.[29] These three items have been demonstrated to form an "agitation" factor in geropsychiatric patients.[30] The responses of CSF NE and behavior to yohimbine and clonidine offer an approach to clarifying the functional status of CNS noradrenergic systems in patients with AD and normal older persons and to suggesting relationships of these systems to noncognitive behavioral symptoms in AD.

RESULTS

Catecholamine concentrations and cardiovascular parameters at 90 minutes after the administration of yohimbine and placebo are presented in Table 1. Catecholamine concentrations and cardiovascular parameters at 90 minutes after the administration of clonidine and placebo are presented in **Table 2**. The number of subjects in each group in each treatment condition is presented in the tables. Data from the yohimbine condition in one patient with AD were excluded because he had no detectable CSF yohimbine or 11-hydroxy-yohimbine concentration. Another patient with AD refused participation in the clonidine treatment condition. One young subject was not available for the yohimbine treatment condition.

CSF NE CONCENTRATIONS

The CSF NE concentrations in the placebo (baseline) treatment condition did not differ among groups ($F[2, 37]=0.495$, $P=.61$). The CSF NE concentrations were significantly higher in the yohimbine treatment condition than in the placebo treatment condition in all subject groups. The Δ CSF NE concentrations between the yohimbine and placebo treatment conditions differed significantly among groups ($F[2, 35]=6.11$, $P<.01$). This difference was accounted for by significantly greater ($P<.05$) Δ CSF NE concentrations between the yohimbine and placebo treatment conditions in both patients with AD (1.23±0.27 nmol/L) and normal older subjects (1.05±0.23 nmol/L) compared with that in normal young subjects (0.45±0.08 nmol/L). The Δ CSF NE concentrations between the yohimbine and placebo treatment conditions did not differ between patients with AD and normal older subjects. Clonidine appeared to decrease the CSF NE concentrations in all groups, but dif-

Table 1. CSF NE and Plasma NE and EPI Concentrations, MAP, and Heart Rate at 90 Minutes After Administration of Placebo and Yohimbine Hydrochloride in Normal Young and Older Subjects and Patients With AD*

	Young Subjects		Older Subjects		Patients With AD	
	Placebo (n=18)	Yohimbine (n=17)	Placebo (n=10)	Yohimbine (n=10)	Placebo (n=10)	Yohimbine (n=9)
Concentration						
CSF NE, nmol/L	0.84±0.08	1.31±0.13†	0.97±0.1	2.02±0.19†‡	0.85±0.1	2.02±0.27†‡
Plasma NE, nmol/L	1.03±0.08	2.34±0.21†	1.53±0.18‡	6.69±1.58†‡	1.49±0.16‡	5.12±0.84†‡
Plasma EPI, pmol/L	284±33	497±71†	284±66	535±82†	300±44	409±55
MAP, mm Hg	87±1	92±2†	95±3§	111±5§‖	94±2§	109±4†§
Heart rate, beats/min	61±3	67±3‖	61±3	66±3	63±2	70±3†

*CSF indicates cerebrospinal fluid; NE, norepinephrine; EPI, epinephrine; MAP, mean arterial pressure; and AD, Alzheimer's disease. Data are given as mean±SEM. Significance of differences between yohimbine hydrochloride and placebo treatment conditions within groups analyzed by paired t tests. Significance of these differences among groups determined by one-way analysis of variance, followed by Newman-Keuls post hoc test.
†Greater than that for the placebo treatment condition, P<.01.
‡Greater than that for the young subjects, P<.01.
§Greater than that for the young subjects, P<.05.
‖Greater than that for the placebo treatment condition, P<.05.

ferences between the clonidine and placebo treatment conditions only reached significance in the normal older subjects. The Δ CSF NE concentrations between the clonidine and placebo treatment conditions did not differ among groups (F[2, 29]=0.027, *P*=.97).

PLASMA CATECHOLAMINE CONCENTRATIONS

In contrast to the similar CSF NE concentrations in the placebo treatment condition among groups, the plasma NE concentrations in the placebo treatment condition significantly differed among groups (F[2, 37]=5.29, *P*<.01). This difference was accounted for by a significantly higher plasma NE concentration in the placebo treatment condition both in the normal older subjects compared with that in the normal young subjects (*P*<.05) and in patients with AD compared with that in normal young subjects (*P*<.05). The plasma NE concentration was significantly higher in the yohimbine treatment condition than in the placebo treatment condition in all subject groups. The difference in the plasma NE concentration between the yohimbine and placebo treatment conditions (Δ plasma NE concentration) differed significantly among groups (F[2, 37]=6.7, *P*<.01). This difference was accounted for by a significantly greater Δ plasma NE concentration in the normal older subjects than in the normal young subjects (*P*<.01); patients with AD and normal young subjects did not differ. Because the plasma NE concentration differed among groups in the placebo (baseline) treatment condition and changes in these parameters can be a function of baseline levels, the effects of the pharmacologic challenge on the plasma NE concentration also were calculated as the percent change from the baseline. The percent change of the plasma NE concentration from the placebo to the yohimbine treatment conditions in older subjects (267%±62%), patients with AD (321%±65%), and young subjects (162%±40%) tended to differ among groups (F[2, 37]=2.6, *P*=.09) because of the more modest increase in the younger subjects.

The plasma NE concentration was significantly lower in the clonidine treatment condition than in the placebo treatment condition in normal older subjects (*P*<.01), patients with AD (*P*<.01), and normal young subjects (*P*<.01). Neither the Δ plasma NE concentration between the clonidine and placebo treatment conditions (F[2, 29]=1.39, *P*=.27) nor the percent change of the plasma NE concentration between the clonidine and placebo treatment conditions (F[2, 29]=0.44, *P*=.65) differed among groups.

The plasma EPI concentration in the placebo treatment condition did not differ among groups (F[2, 37] =0.036, *P*=.96). The plasma EPI concentration was higher in the yohimbine treatment condition than in the placebo treatment condition in all groups. These differences were significant in the young (*P*<.01) and older (*P*<.01) normal groups, but not in the group with AD. The plasma EPI concentration was lower in the clonidine treatment condition than in the placebo treatment condition, but differences were significant only in the normal young group (*P*<.01). The Δ plasma EPI concentration between the yohimbine and placebo treatment conditions (F[2, 37]=1.35, *P*=.27) or between the clonidine and placebo treatment conditions (F[2, 29]=1.06, *P*=.36) did not differ among groups.

CARDIOVASCULAR PARAMETERS

The MAP in the placebo treatment condition differed among groups (F[2, 37]=5.26 *P*<.01), with a higher MAP in both the normal older subjects (*P*<.05) and patients with AD (*P*<.05) compared with that in normal young subjects. The MAP was significantly lower in the clonidine treatment condition (*P*<.01) and higher in the yohimbine treatment condition (*P*<.05) than in the placebo treatment condition in all subject groups. The Δ MAP between the yohimbine and placebo treatment conditions differed among groups (F[2, 37]=3.68, *P*<.05) as did the percent change of the MAP (F[2, 37]=3.21, *P*<.05). Although the Δ MAP and the percent change of the MAP between yohimbine and placebo treatment conditions appeared to be greater in normal older subjects and patients with AD than in normal young subjects, post hoc

Table 2. CSF NE and Plasma NE and EPI Concentrations, MAP, and Heart Rate at 90 Minutes After Administration of Placebo and Clonidine Hydrochloride in Normal Young and Older Subjects and Patients With AD*

	Young Subjects		Older Subjects		Patients With AD	
	Placebo (n=18)	Clonidine Hydrochloride (n=11)	Placebo (n=10)	Clonidine Hydrochloride (n=10)	Placebo (n=10)	Clonidine Hydrochloride (n=9)
Concentration						
CSF NE, nmol/L	0.84±0.08	0.69±0.14	0.97±0.1	0.73±0.07†	0.85±0.1	0.69±0.09
Plasma NE, nmol/L	1.03±0.08	0.58±0.07‡	1.53±0.18§	0.77±0.09‡	1.49±0.16§	0.70±0.1‡
Plasma EPI, pmol/L	284±33	191±55‡	284±33	229±38	300±44	267±60
MAP, mm Hg	87±1	75±2‡	95±3‖	73±2‡	94±2‖	75±2‡
Heart rate, beats/min	61±3	59±3	61±3	57±2	63±2	60±1†

**For explanation of the specialized abbreviations, see first footnote to Table 1. Data are given as mean±SEM. Significance of differences between clonidine hydrochloride and placebo treatment conditions within groups analyzed by paired* t *tests. Significance of these differences among groups determined by one-way analysis of variance, followed by Newman-Keuls post hoc test.*

†*Less than that for the placebo treatment condition,* P<.05.

‡*Less than that for the placebo treatment condition,* P<.01.

§*Greater than that for the young subjects,* P<.01.

‖*Greater than that for the young subjects,* P<.05.

analyses did not reveal significant differences between individual groups.

The heart rate in the placebo treatment condition did not differ among groups (F[2, 37]=0.093, *P*=.91). The heart rate was significantly higher in the yohimbine treatment condition than in the placebo treatment condition in the patients with AD (*P*<.01) and normal young subjects (*P*<.05) but not in the normal older subjects. The heart rate was significantly lower in the clonidine treatment condition than in the placebo treatment condition only in the group with AD (*P*<.05). The Δ heart rate between the yohimbine and placebo treatment conditions (F[2, 37]=0.16, *P*=.85) or between the clonidine and placebo treatment conditions (F[2, 29]=0.21, *P*=.81) did not differ among groups.

YOHIMBINE AND CLONIDINE CONCENTRATIONS

Concentrations of yohimbine and clonidine in the CSF and plasma samples are presented in **Table 3**. Yohimbine and 11-hydroxy-yohimbine concentrations were detectable in the CSF samples in all subjects, except for one patient with AD. Data from the yohimbine treatment condition in this one patient with AD therefore were excluded from the analysis. The CSF yohimbine concentrations significantly differed among groups (F[2, 28] =3.51, *P*<.05), with higher CSF yohimbine concentrations in normal older subjects than in normal young subjects (*P*<.05) or patients with AD (*P*<.05). The CSF yohimbine concentrations did not differ between patients with AD and normal young subjects. The CSF 11-hydroxy-yohimbine concentrations also differed among groups (F[2, 28]=7.40, *P*<.01). This difference was accounted for by higher CSF concentrations of 11-hydroxy-yohimbine concentrations in the normal young subjects than in either normal older subjects (*P*<.01) or patients with AD (*P*<.01). Plasma yohimbine concentrations differed significantly among groups (F[2, 30]=3.36, *P*<.05) with higher plasma yohimbine concentrations in normal older subjects than in the normal young subjects or patients with AD (*P*<.05). Plasma 11-hydroxy-yohimbine concentrations differed among groups (F[2, 30]=3.96, *P*<.05) with lower concentrations in normal older subjects than in either normal young subjects (*P*<.05) or patients with AD (*P*<.05). Clonidine concentrations did not differ among groups in either CSF (F[2, 29]=1.24, *P*=.31) or plasma (F[2, 28]=1.80, *P*=.18).

RATINGS OF BEHAVIOR

Ratings of Tension and Excitement in the placebo treatment condition differed significantly among groups (F[2, 28]=5.14, *P*<.05 and F[2, 28]=5.90, *P*<.01, respectively), with significantly higher ratings in the patients with AD (*P*<.01) than in the other groups (**Figure**). Ratings of Tension and Excitement were significantly higher in the yohimbine treatment condition than in the placebo treatment condition in all subject groups. The rating of Anxiety was significantly higher in the yohimbine treatment condition than in the placebo treatment condition in older subjects and patients with AD. Increases in behavioral parameters between the yohimbine and placebo treatment conditions significantly differed among groups (Tension, F[2, 28]=8.16, *P*<.01; Excitement, F[2, 28]=11.03, *P*<.001; Anxiety, F[2, 28]=6.46, *P*<.01), with significantly greater increases in the yohimbine treatment condition in patients with AD than in either normal older (*P*<.05) or young (*P*<.01) subjects. The ratings of Tension and Excitement were significantly lower in the clonidine treatment condition than in the placebo treatment condition in patients with AD (*P*<.05). The Mini-Mental State Examination scores for the patients with AD did not differ among the placebo (13.9±2.2), yohimbine (14.9±2.6), and clonidine (15.3±3.4) treatment conditions.

COMMENT

These results support enhanced CNS noradrenergic responsiveness in normal older persons and patients with AD. Enhanced CSF NE responsiveness to yohimbine is

Table 3. Concentrations of Yohimbine Hydrochloride, 11-Hydroxy-Yohimbine, and Clonidine Hydrochloride in CSF and Plasma at 90 Minutes After Administration in Normal Young (n=10) and Older (n=10) Subjects and Patients With AD (n=9)*

	Young Subjects	Older Subjects	Patients With AD
CSF concentration, ng/mL			
Yohimbine hydrochloride	2.9±0.9	7.7±2.0†	3.3±0.5
11-Hydroxy-yohimbine	7.7±0.7‡	4.6±0.7	4.6±0.4
Plasma concentration, ng/mL			
Yohimbine hydrochloride	167.7±47.3	407.3±112.1†	188.7±36.4
11-Hydroxy-yohimbine	306.2±41.2	189.7±23.9§	307.0±31.5
Clonidine hydrochloride concentration, ng/mL			
CSF	0.50±0.06	0.41±0.05	0.40±0.04
Plasma	0.86±0.14	0.91±0.12	1.16±0.07

For explanation of the specialized abbreviations, see first footnote in Table 1. Data are given as the mean±SEM. One-way analysis of variance, followed by Newman-Keuls post hoc test.

†*Greater than that for the young subjects or patients with AD,* $P<.05$.

‡*Greater than that for the older normal subjects or patients with AD,* $P<.01$.

§*Less than that for the young subjects or patients with AD,* $P<.05$.

retained in older persons with AD despite the extensive LC neuronal loss that has been demonstrated in postmortem studies.[2-4] These data are consistent with findings from postmortem brain tissue studies in which NE and MHPG concentrations have been measured concurrently.[37,38] Brain tissue NE turnover (estimated by the MHPG-NE ratio) in these studies was higher in patients with AD. In one recent study that was notable for obtaining postmortem brain tissue specimens from patients with AD who had not been receiving psychotropic medications before death and for whom postmortem delay to autopsy was brief, the NE concentration in the frontal cortex tended to be higher in patients with AD than in normal older control subjects.[39] The current data and these postmortem neurochemical findings suggest that changes in CNS noradrenergic systems in some brain areas may compensate for the loss of LC neurons in AD.[40,41] Furthermore, the greater Tension, Excitement, and Anxiety scores that were produced by yohimbine in patients with AD than in either young or older normal subjects suggest that CNS noradrenergic changes in AD may be involved in the pathogenesis of agitated behaviors, which are frequent management problems in this disorder.[15]

The CSF yohimbine measurements confirmed that yohimbine gained access to the CNS in all groups. The fact that the CSF yohimbine concentration was higher in normal older subjects than in normal young subjects may have contributed to the difference in the Δ CSF NE concentration between these two groups. This difference in the CSF yohimbine concentrations between these two groups may partially have been compensated for by the higher CSF concentrations of the active yohimbine metabolite (ie, 11-hydroxy-yohimbine) in the normal young subjects than in the normal older subjects. However, 11-hydroxy-yohimbine may not be as potent an α_2-antagonist as yohimbine in CSF. Although yohimbine and 11-hydroxy-yohimbine have approximately equivalent α_2-antagonist activity in solutions with albumin concentrations similar to those in plasma, 11-hydroxy-yohimbine has substantially lower activity than yohimbine in protein-free solutions, which are more comparable with the low albumin concentrations that are found in CSF.[42] Pharmacokinetic factors clearly did not contribute to the greater Δ CSF NE concentrations between the yohimbine and placebo treatment conditions in the patients with AD than in normal young subjects. In fact, combined yohimbine and 11-hydroxy-yohimbine concentrations tended to be lowest in the patients with AD.

The mechanisms underlying the increased CNS noradrenergic responsiveness in aging and AD remain unclear. Previous data from our laboratory suggested a decreased sensitivity of α_2-adrenergic mechanisms that regulate CNS noradrenergic activity with normal aging.[6] The equivalent CSF NE response to clonidine among groups in the present study does not support changes in α_2-noradrenergic sensitivity with aging or AD. We also did not demonstrate higher resting CSF NE concentrations with aging in the present study. These differences between the present study and our earlier study[6] may be attributable to the variability among the small groups of subjects.

A mechanism that might explain the paradoxically increased CSF noradrenergic responsiveness in aging and AD is LC neuronal plasticity. In the rat, LC noradrenergic axons regenerate in response to damage in brain areas that are innervated by the LC.[43,44] Damage to the LC itself stimulates increased NE synthetic capacity[45,46] and an increased firing rate[47] in surviving LC neurons. Similar compensatory responses may occur in patients with AD, but these responses have been difficult to demonstrate directly in brain tissue immunohistochemical[48] or neurochemical[39] studies. Estimating the NE synthetic capacity of LC neurons by quantitating tyrosine hydroxylase messenger RNA and protein in LC neurons would provide useful information with regard to possible compensatory changes in CNS noradrenergic systems in aging and AD.

Although these data failed to demonstrate any further increase of CSF NE responsiveness in patients with AD compared with that in normal older subjects, the results are not unexpected given that patients in the advanced stages of AD were not included in the present protocol. It is only among institutionalized patients in the advanced stages of AD that CSF NE concentrations have been reported to be higher than those of normal older

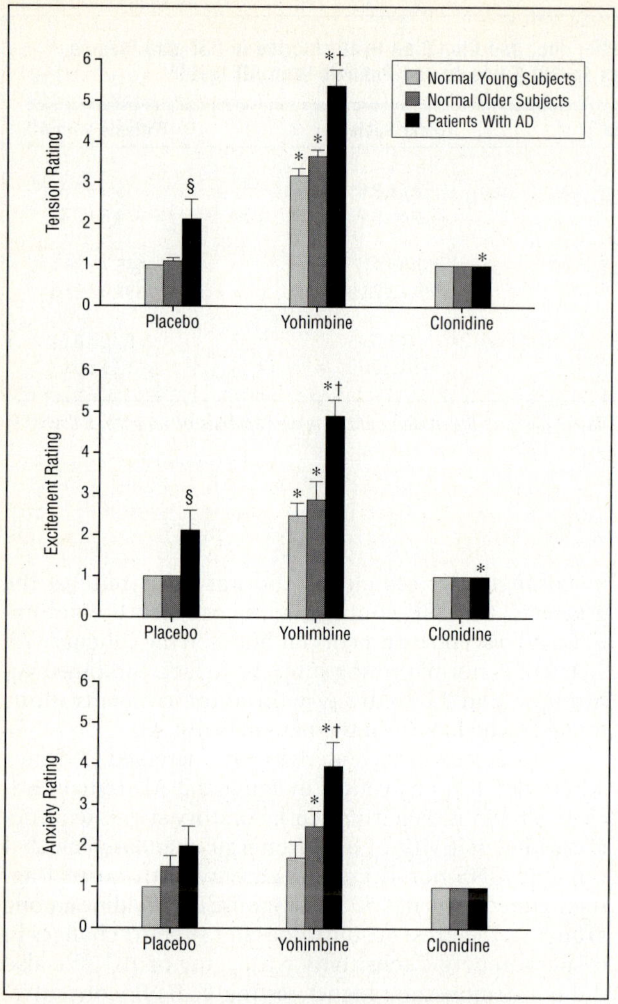

Brief Psychiatric Rating Scale scores for Tension (top), Excitement (center), and Anxiety (bottom) items at 90 minutes following the administration of placebo, yohimbine hydrochloride, or clonidine hydrochloride in normal young subjects (n=11), normal older subjects (n=10), and patients with Alzheimer's disease (AD) (n=9). Asterisk indicates difference from placebo, $P<.05$*; section mark, placebo condition rating greater in patients with AD than in older or young subjects,* $P<.05$*; and dagger, difference between yohimbine or clonidine treatment conditions and placebo treatment condition greater in patients with AD than in older or young subjects,* $P<.01$ *(one-way analysis of variance followed by Newman-Keuls post hoc test).*

persons.[7,8] Functional studies of CNS noradrenergic activity in patients with AD in the more advanced stages of AD would be useful. It is in such patients that disruptive hyperactive behaviors are most common.[15]

The marked arousal and anxiety of the patients with AD following the administration of yohimbine may represent an exaggeration of the mild arousal and anxiety that is produced by yohimbine in normal subjects.[49,50] The greater increase in the Tension, Excitement, and Anxiety ratings in patients with AD compared with that in normal older subjects despite comparable increases in CSF NE concentrations suggests an increased sensitivity to the behavioral effects of CNS noradrenergic activation. Postsynaptic noradrenergic supersensitivity could contribute to the increased behavioral responsiveness to yohimbine. Increased concentrations of presumably postsynaptic β-adrenergic receptors in the prefrontal cortex and hippocampus have been reported in AD.[51]

The high CSF NE responses to yohimbine in AD could have resulted from an increased sensitivity to nonspecific stress. The plasma EPI measurements, which provide some estimate of nonspecific emotional stress,[52] make this possibility unlikely. The basal EPI concentration did not differ between patients with AD and normal subjects, and the increase in the EPI concentration following the administration of yohimbine tended to be lower in the patients with AD than in the other two groups.

The higher plasma NE concentration in the placebo treatment condition in normal older subjects than in normal young subjects is consistent with results of previous reports from our and other laboratories of increased resting SNS activity with human aging.[53,54] The fact that these resting indexes of SNS activity did not differ between outpatients with AD and normal older persons also is consistent with findings from reports of similar plasma NE concentrations in these two groups.[55] To our knowledge, the effects of advanced age and AD on the plasma NE response to yohimbine have not been reported. The enhanced but equivalent NE increases in these two older subject groups compared with those in young subjects, together with a similar sensitivity to clonidine among the three groups, provide support for increased SNS responsiveness with aging as reported by others.[54] Although NE kinetic studies would be necessary to exclude the possibility that the enhanced plasma NE (or CSF NE) response to yohimbine is a function of decreased NE clearance induced by yohimbine in older subjects, this possibility is unlikely. We have previously demonstrated in young normal subjects that the effects of aging on the plasma NE concentration at rest and in response to clonidine,[53] as well as the response of the plasma NE concentration to yohimbine,[56] are predominantly a function of the differential NE appearance rate.

The clear effect of aging on resting plasma NE concentrations, together with the absence of an effect of aging on resting CSF NE concentrations in the subjects in this study, support separate origins for NE in the two compartments. Although both CNS noradrenergic systems and the SNS respond similarly to α_2-regulation[6,22] and to other regulatory stimuli,[57] substantial evidence suggests that CSF NE is derived from CNS noradrenergic neurons and not from the peripheral SNS.[16,18,19] In the rat, chemical sympathectomy has no effect on CSF or brain tissue NE.[17] Furthermore, destruction of the LC substantially reduces the CSF NE concentration, whereas destruction of the superior cervical ganglion (the source of SNS noradrenergic fibers that innervate cerebral vasculature) has no effect on the CSF NE concentration.[58]

The results of the present study demonstrate that CNS noradrenergic changes in patients with AD are complex and that inferences about CNS noradrenergic function in patients with AD that are drawn from postmortem histologic findings alone must be made cautiously. Despite the loss of LC neurons in patients with AD, the remaining noradrenergic neurons appear to be capable of a robust response to the removal of α_2-adrenergic inhibition. The fact that this robust noradrenergic response in patients with AD was associated with behavioral hyperarousal raises the possibility that abnormal sensitivity to CNS noradrenergic activation plays a role in some of the problematic agitation that occurs in the middle and late stages of AD. Anecdotal reports of a therapeutic reduction of agitated behaviors in AD following treatment with the centrally active β-adrenergic antagonist propranolol hydrochloride lend some support to this possibility.[59-62]

Accepted for publication April 26, 1995.

This investigation was supported by the Department of Veterans Affairs, Washington, DC, and by grants AG08419 and AG05136 from the National Institutes of Health, Bethesda, Md.

The authors wish to acknowledge Sally Swedine, MS, for assistance with data management and statistical analyses, Carl Sikkema and Molly Wamble for their technical assistance, and Susan Martin for manuscript preparation.

Reprint requests to Seattle Veterans Affairs Medical Center, GRECC (182B), 1660 S Columbian Way, Seattle, WA 98108 (Dr Peskind).

REFERENCES

1. Loughlin SE, Foote SL, Fallen JH. Locus coeruleus projections to cortex: topography, morphology and collateralization. *Brain Res Bull.* 1982;9:287-294.
2. Bondareff M, Mountjoy CQ, Roth M. Loss of neurons of origin of the adrenergic projection to cerebral cortex (nucleus locus coeruleus) in senile dementia. *Neurology.* 1982;32:164-168.
3. Mann DMA, Lincoln J, Yates PO, Stamp JE, Toper S. Changes in the monoamine containing neurones of the human CNS in senile dementia. *Br J Psychiatry.* 1980;136:533-541.
4. Tomlinson BE, Irving D, Blessed G. Cell loss in the locus coeruleus in senile dementia of the Alzheimer type. *J Neurol Sci.* 1981;49:419-428.
5. Vijayashankar N, Brody H. A quantitative study of the pigmented neurons in the nuclei locus coeruleus and subcoeruleus in man as related to aging. *J Comp Neurol.* 1979;38:490-497.
6. Raskind MA, Peskind ER, Veith RC, Beard JC, Gumbrecht G, Halter JB. Increased plasma and cerebrospinal fluid norepinephrine in older men: differential suppression by clonidine. *J Clin Endocrinol Metab.* 1988;66:438-443.
7. Raskind MA, Peskind ER, Halter JB, Jimerson DC. Norepinephrine and MHPG levels in CSF and plasma in Alzheimer's disease. *Arch Gen Psychiatry.* 1984; 4:343-346.
8. Tohgi H, Ueno T, Takahashi S, Nozaki Y. Concentrations of monoamines and their metabolites in the cerebrospinal fluid from patients with senile dementia of the Alzheimer type and vascular dementia of the Binswanger's type. *J Neural Transm Park Dis Dement Sect.* 1992;4:69-77.
9. Mann JJ, Stanley M, Neophytides A, de Leon MJ, Fems SH, Gershon S. Central amine metabolism in Alzheimer's disease: in vivo relationship to cognitive deficit. *Neurobiol Aging.* 1981;2:57-60.
10. Palmer AM, Sims NR, Bowen DM, Neary D, Palo J, Wikstrom J, Davison AN. Monoamine metabolite concentrations in lumbar cerebrospinal fluid of patients with histologically verified Alzheimer's dementia. *J Neurol Neurosurg Psychiatry.* 1984;47:481-484.
11. Nybäck H, Nyman H, Schalling D. Neuropsychological test performance and CSF levels of monoamine metabolites in healthy volunteers and patients with Alzheimer's dementia. *Acta Psychiatr Scand.* 1987;76:648-656.
12. Blennow K, Wallin A, Gottfries CG, Lekman A, Karlsson I, Skoog I, Svennerholm L. Significance of decreased lumbar CSF levels of HVA and 5-HIAA in Alzheimer's disease. *Neurobiol Aging.* 1991;13:107-113.
13. Bierer LM, Aisen PS, Davidson M, Ryan TM, Stern RG, Schmeidler J, Davis KL. A pilot study of oral physostigmine plus yohimbine in patients with Alzheimer disease. *Alzheimer Dis Assoc Disord.* 1993;7:98-104.
14. Arnsten AFT, Cai JX. Postsynaptic alpha-2 receptor stimulation improves memory in aged monkeys: indirect effects of yohimbine versus direct effects of clonidine. *Neurobiol Aging.* 1993;14:597-603.
15. Raskind MA. Alzheimer's disease: treatment of noncognitive abnormalities. In: Kupfer D, Bloom F, eds. *Psychopharmacology: The Fourth Generation of Progress: American College of Neuropsychopharmacology.* New York, NY: Raven Press; 1995:1427-1435.
16. Ziegler MC, Lake RC, Wood JH, Ebert MH. Norepinephrine in cerebrospinal fluid: basic studies, effects of drugs and disease. In: Wood JH, ed. *Neurobiology of Cerebrospinal Fluid.* New York, NY: Plenum Press; 1980:141-158.
17. Peskind ER, Raskind MA, Wilkinson CW, Flatness DE, Halter JB. Peripheral sympathectomy and adrenal medullectomy do not alter cerebrospinal fluid norepinephrine. *Brain Res.* 1986;367:258-264.
18. Oldendorf WH. Brain uptake of radiolabeled amino amines and hexoses after arterial injection. *Am J Physiol.* 1971;221:1629-1639.
19. Weil-Malherbe H, Axelrod J, Tomchick R. Blood-brain barrier for adrenaline. *Science.* 1959;129:1226-1227.
20. Ziegler MG, Lake CR, Wood JH, Brooks BR, Ebert MH. Relationship between norepinephrine in blood and cerebrospinal fluid in the presence of a blood–cerebrospinal fluid barrier for norepinephrine. *J Neurochem.* 1977;28:677-679.
21. Kopin IJ, Gordon EK, Jimerson DC, Polinksy RG. Relation between plasma and cerebrospinal fluid levels of 3-methoxy-4-hydroxyphenylglycol. *Science.* 1983;219:73-75.
22. Peskind ER, Veith RC, Dorsa DM, Gumbrecht G, Raskind MA. Yohimbine increases cerebrospinal fluid and plasma norepinephrine but not arginine vasopressin in humans. *Neuroendocrinology.* 1989;50:286-291.
23. Guthrie SK, Grunhaus L, Pande AC, Hariharan M. Noradrenergic response to intravenous yohimbine in patients with depression and comorbidity of depression and panic. *Biol Psychiatry.* 1993;34:558-561.
24. Charney DS, Woods SW, Krystal JH, Nagy LM, Heninger GR. Noradrenergic neuronal dysregulation in panic disorder: the effects of intravenous yohimbine and clonidine in panic disorder patients. *Acta Psychiatr Scand.* 1992;86:273-282.
25. Southwick SM, Krystal JH, Morgan CA, Johnson D, Nagy LM, Nicolaou A, Heninger GR, Charney DS. Abnormal noradrenergic function in posttraumatic stress disorder. *Arch Gen Psychiatry.* 1993;50:266-274.
26. Cubeddu LX, Hoffman IS, Davila J, Barbella YR, Ordaz P. Clonidine reduces elevated cerebrospinal fluid catecholamine levels in patients with essential hypertension. *Life Sci.* 1984;35:1336-1341.
27. Peskind ER, Raskind MA, Leake RD, Ervin MG, Ross MG, Dorsa DM. Clonidine decreases plasma and cerebrospinal fluid arginine vasopressin but not oxytocin in humans. *Neuroendocrinology.* 1987;46:395-400.
28. Le Verge R, Le Corre P, Chevanne F. Determination of yohimbine and its two hydroxylated metabolites in humans by high-performance liquid chromatography and mass spectral analysis. *J Chromatogr.* 1992;574:283-292.
29. Overall JE, Gorham DR. The Brief Psychiatric Rating Scale. *Psychol Rep.* 1962; 10:799-812.
30. Overall JE, Beller SA. The Brief Psychiatric Rating Scale (BPRS) in geropsychiatric research, I: factor structure on an inpatient unit. *J Gerontol.* 1983;39: 187-193.
31. McKhann G, Drachman D, Folstein M, Katzman R, Price D, Stadian EM. Clinical diagnosis of Alzheimer's disease: report of the NINCDS-ADRDA Work Group under the auspices of Department of Health and Human Services Task Force on Alzheimer's disease. *Neurology.* 1984;34:939-944.
32. American Psychiatric Association. *Diagnostic and Statistical Manual of Mental Disorders, Revised Third Edition.* Washington, DC: American Psychiatric Association; 1987.
33. Raskind MA, Peskind ER, Lampe TH, Risse SC, Taborsky GJ, Dorsa DM. Cerebrospinal fluid vasopressin, oxytocin, somatostatin and beta-endorphin in Alzheimer's disease. *Arch Gen Psychiatry.* 1986;43:382-388.
34. Folstein MF, Folstein SE, McHugh PR. Mini-Mental State: a practical method for grading the cognitive state of patients for the clinician. *J Psychiatr Res.* 1975;12:189-198.
35. Evans MI, Halter JB, Porte D Jr. Comparison of double- and single-isotope enzymatic derivative methods for measuring catecholamines in human plasma. *Clin Chem.* 1978;24:567.
36. Arndts B, Stahle E, Forster HJ. Development of an RIA for clonidine and its comparison with the reference methods. *J Pharmacol Toxicol Methods.* 1981; 6:285-290.
37. Gottfries C-G, Adolfsson R, Aquilonius S-M, Carlsson A, Eckernas S-A, Nordberg A, Oreland L, Svennerholm L, Wiberg A, Winblad B. Biochemical changes in dementia disorders of Alzheimer type (AD/SDAT). *Neurobiol Aging.* 1983; 4:261-271.
38. Palmer AM, Wilcock GK, Esiri MM, Francis PT, Bowen DM. Monoaminergic innervation of the frontal and temporal lobes in Alzheimer's disease. *Brain Res.* 1987;401:231-238.
39. D'Amato RJ, Zweig RM, Whitehouse PJ, Wenk GL, Singer HS, Mayeux R, Price DL, Snyder SH. Aminergic systems in Alzheimer's disease and Parkinson's disease. *Ann Neurol.* 1987;22:229-246.
40. Bondareff W, Mountjoy CQ. Number of neurons in nucleus locus ceruleus in

demented and nondemented patients: rapid estimation and correlated parameters. *Neurobiol Aging.* 1986;7:297-300.
41. Gottfries CG. Neurochemical aspects of aging and diseases with cognitive impairment. *J Neurosci Res.* 1990;27:541-547.
42. Berlan M, Le Verge R, Galitzky J, Le Corre P. α_2-Adrenoceptor antagonist potencies of two hydroxylated metabolites of yohimbine. *Br J Pharmacol.* 1993; 108:927-932.
43. Madison R, Davis JN. Sprouting of noradrenergic fibers in hippocampus after medial septal lesions: contributions of the central and peripheral nervous systems. *Exp Neurol.* 1983;80:167-177.
44. Nakamura S, Sakaguchi T. Development and plasticity of the locus coeruleus: a review of recent physiological and pharmacological experimentation. *Prog Neurobiol.* 1990;34:505-526.
45. Acheson AL, Zigmund MJ. Short and long term changes in tyrosine hydroxylase activity in rat brain after substantial destruction of central noradrenergic neurons. *J Neurosci.* 1981;1:493-504.
46. Unnerstall JR, Long MM. Induction of tyrosine hydroxylase mRNA in locus coeruleus neurons following 6-hydroxydopamine treatment in young and old Fisher 344 rats. *Soc Neurosci Abstr.* 1993;19:456.
47. Chiodo LA, Acheson AL, Zigmund MJ, Stricker EM. Substantial destruction of central noradrenergic projections increases the firing rate of locus ceruleus neurons. *Brain Res.* 1983;264:123-132.
48. Powers RE, Struble RG, Casanova MF, O'Connor DT, Kitt CA, Price DL. Innervation of human hippocampus by noradrenergic systems: normal anatomy and structural abnormalities in aging and in Alzheimer's disease. *Neuroscience.* 1988; 25:401-417.
49. Goldberg MR, Hollister AS, Robertson D. Influence of yohimbine on blood pressure, autonomic reflexes, and plasma catecholamines in humans. *Hypertension.* 1983;5:772-778.
50. Holmberg G, Gershon S. Autonomic and psychic effects of yohimbine hydrochloride. *Psychopharmacology (Berl).* 1961;2:93-106.
51. Kalaria RN, Andorn AC, Tabaton M, Whitehouse PJ, Harik SI, Unnerstall JR. Adrenergic receptors in aging and Alzheimer's disease: increased β_2-receptors in prefrontal cortex and hippocampus. *J Neurochem.* 1989;53:1772-1781.
52. Dimsdale JE, Moss J. Plasma catecholamines in stress and exercise. *JAMA.* 1980;243:340-342.
53. Featherstone JA, Veith RC, Flatness D, Murburg MM, Villacres EC, Halter JB. Age and alpha-adrenergic regulation of plasma norepinephrine kinetics in humans. *J Gerontol.* 1987;42:271-276.
54. Supiano MA, Linares OA, Smith MJ, Halter JB. Age-related differences in norepinephrine kinetics: effect of posture and sodium-restricted diet. *Am J Physiol.* 1990;259:E422-E431.
55. Vitiello B, Veith RC, Molchan SE, Martinez RA, Lawlor BA, Radcliffe J, Hill JL, Sunderland T. Autonomic dysfunction in patients with dementia of the Alzheimer's type. *Biol Psychiatry.* 1993;34:428-433.
56. Murburg MM, Villacres EC, Ko GN, Veith RC. Effects of yohimbine on human sympathetic nervous system function. *J Clin Endocrinol Metab.* 1991;73:861-865.
57. Elam H, Yao T, Svennson TH, Thoren P. Regulation of locus coeruleus neurons and splanchnic sympathetic nerves by cardiovascular afferents. *Brain Res.* 1984;290:281-286.
58. Mamalaki E, Brady LS, Goldstein D, Herkenham M. Origins of norepinephrine in rat cerebrospinal fluid. *Soc Neurosci Abstr.* 1988;14:1074.
59. Zubenko GS. Biological correlates of clinical heterogeneity in primary dementia. *Neuropsychopharmacology.* 1992;6:77-93.
60. Nielson KA, Shankle WR, Cotman CW. Neurobiological correlates of aggression and agitation in dementia provide bases for effective treatment: a study of propranolol. *Soc Neurosci Abstr.* 1993;19:400.
61. Weiler PG, Mungas D, Bernick C. Propranolol for the control of disruptive behavior in senile dementia. *J Geriatr Psychiatry Neurol.* 1988;1:226-230.
62. Yudofsky S, Williams D, Gorman J. Propranolol in the treatment of rage and violent behavior in patients with chronic brain syndromes. *Am J Psychiatry.* 1981;138:218-220.

Conversions From Système International (SI) Units to Traditional Units (Modified From *The SI Manual in Health Care*)

System	Component	SI Reference Interval*	SI Unit	Conversion Factor (Divide by)	Traditional Reference Interval*	Traditional Unit
Plasma	Epinephrine (radioenzymatic procedure)	170-520 (at rest for 15 min)	pmol/L	5.458	31-95(at rest for 15 min)	pg/mL
Plasma	Norepinephrine (radioenzymatic procedure)	1.27-2.81 (at rest for 15 min)	nmol/L	0.005911	215-475 (at rest for 15 min)	pg/mL

**These reference values are not intended to be definitive since each laboratory determines its own values. They are provided for illustration only.*

Interactions of Serotonin Reuptake Inhibitors With Tricyclic Antidepressants

In the August 1994 issue of the ARCHIVES, Popli et al[1] make several points relevant to the interactions between selective serotonin reuptake inhibitors (SSRIs) and tricyclic antidepressants (TCAs) with which we must take issue. First, we believe it possible to make reasonable predictions of in vivo effects from in vitro data. Second, we believe more care must be taken in drawing conclusions about drug interactions from case reports.

Four research groups, not just one, have made in vitro assessments of the extent to which the SSRIs (and some of their metabolites) inhibit cytochrome P-450 2D6 (CYP2D6).[2-7] We have derived estimates of the corresponding in vivo relevance using the following strategy. All of the published in vitro assessments include a determination of the inhibition constant (K_i) of fluoxetine. If the K_i of each SSRI is normalized to the K_i of fluoxetine in the same study, averaging those relative K_is across studies produces the values shown in the first row of the **Table**.[2-25]

Across studies, the average K_i of fluoxetine was 0.88 μmol/L. Multiplying this by the relative K_i produced estimated K_is for the other SSRIs as shown in the second row of the Table. We then took into account that in vivo effects are a function of both potency and concentration. Steady-state plasma drug levels at the usually effective minimum dose differ by as much as an order of magnitude across SSRIs as shown in the third row of the Table.[8-13] Next, because CYP2D6 inhibition occurs in the liver, the plasma SSRI concentrations were adjusted based on the relative concentration of SSRI in liver relative to plasma. This is described by the liver–water partition ratio given in the fourth row of the Table.[5] Consequently, at the relevant (hepatic) site of action, parent drug levels may be similar to those given in the fifth row. When the K_i from the second row was compared with the probable concentration in the fifth row, we were drawn to the conclusion that, on average, paroxetine and fluoxetine are much more likely than sertraline or fluvoxamine to be present in sufficient quantity to cause clinically relevant inhibition of CYP2D6.

We are well aware that these values are only estimates. Several factors could cause deviation from these estimates. Among them are, first, that certain metabolites of at least three of these SSRIs have themselves been shown to be inhibitors of CYP2D6 with K_is and plasma levels in the same order of magnitude as the parent compound; other SSRI metabolites and their effects are as yet unknown. Second, plasma drug levels vary widely not only across SSRIs but also for each individual SSRI, so average values will not apply to all of the treatment population. Nevertheless, our conclusions regarding the relative in vivo effects are supported by the results of those controlled pharmacokinetic studies that have measured the effects of SSRIs on the CYP2D6-mediated metabolism of desipramine.[8,14-16] All SSRIs increase plasma levels of desipramine as shown in the last two rows of the Table, but, again, paroxetine and fluoxetine are much more likely than sertraline or fluvoxamine to have a clinically significant effect. Even when case reports[17-25] are examined, the rank order of SSRIs is unchanged.

The use of case reports deserves a word of caution. They can suggest hypotheses regarding drug interactions, but they are not a substitute for rigorous studies. For example, in one report[24] to which Popli et al refer, an individual's plasma desipramine levels increased erratically, by 36% over the first 3 days of SSRI coadministration, by only 2% over the next 4 days, and by a further 77% over the next 7 days. These results do not make pharmacokinetic sense and suggest a degree of inaccuracy in the measurements. If that inaccuracy was present in the baseline value, which is the most parsimonious explanation and is consistent with the fact that error in the baseline measurement in an outpatient study is likely and will distort all of the subsequent findings, the true overall elevation in this case might not be so marked.

In a second example of the need for care in interpreting case reports, Popli et al are misleading in their citation of evidence regarding fluvoxamine interactions with TCAs. There is little dispute that, in vitro, this SSRI is only a weak inhibitor of CYP2D6, and the finding is supported in vivo

Inhibition of Cytochrome 450-P 2D6 by Selective Serotonin Reuptake Inhibitors

	Paroxetine	Fluoxetine	Sertraline	Fluvoxamine
Relative K_i[2-7]*	0.4	1.0	5.7	8.7
Estimated K_i, μmol/L	0.35	0.88	5.02	7.66
Plasma concentration, nmol/L[8-13]	135	512	66	164
Liver–water partition ratio[5]	26.2	12.1	12.2	26.6
Liver concentration, μmol/L	3.5	6.2	0.8	4.4
Percentage increase above baseline in desipramine level				
Pharmacokinetic studies[8,14-16]	420	380-640	23-37	14
Case reports[17-25]	No reports	390	100	68

**Inhibition constant (K_i) relative to fluoxetine.*

by a pharmacokinetic study.[16] As evidence for a contrary position, a case report[25] is cited in the letter by Popli et al in which clinical signs of toxic effects developed after the addition of fluvoxamine in two individuals who were receiving desipramine and in two who were receiving imipramine. However, closer examination of the article reveals that the changes in imipramine metabolism were largely due to inhibition of *N*-demethylation. This step involves CYP1A2 and not CYP2D6; fluvoxamine potently inhibits CYP1A2 in vitro.[26] In fact, there were small decreases in the blood level–dose ratio of the metabolite desipramine, which suggests that the inhibition of desipramine clearance (which is primarily dependent on CYP2D6) was less than the inhibition of its formation from imipramine (which is dependent on CYP1A2). In the two individuals receiving desipramine, signs of toxic effects developed, in spite of the fact that the increases in plasma levels were only 54% and 79%, but both patients were already at toxic levels (525 and 415 nmol/L) prior to addition of fluvoxamine and were thus vulnerable to any increase, however slight. The point is that a case report can suggest that an interaction may occur, but it cannot be equated with rigorous, formal, pharmacokinetic studies in terms of establishing the magnitude of the interaction or the mechanism of the interaction.

We would also like to comment on the question of whether individuals who have very rapid clearance of TCAs and hence have low levels on monotherapy are more susceptible to interactions with SSRIs. This concept has been stated previously in regard to both desipramine[27] and paroxetine,[12] drugs that are metabolized by CYP2D6 and that can readily saturate this genetically polymorphic enzyme. The concept is no more than this: poor metabolizers who do not express functional CYP2D6 obviously cannot be affected by CYP2D6 inhibitors, and drugs such as desipramine will be metabolized at the slow rate of alternative enzymes no matter how much inhibitor is present. On the other hand, very rapid metabolism is consistent with the presence of two functional copies of the gene and twice the median complement of enzyme product. Exposure to inhibitor that is sufficient to completely inhibit CYP2D6 will thus cause a greater than average percentage change in blood levels of the drug but should not lead to greater absolute levels than would develop in a poor metabolizer at the same dose. Again, the case report by Barros and Asnis[24] is relevant. The patient in this case at baseline had a desipramine level indicative of either fast extensive metabolism or noncompliance.[28] Other CYP enzymes do not possess the properties of saturability and genetic polymorphism so clearly. Thus, it is not clear that this concept—that individuals who clear TCAs rapidly are more susceptible to drug interactions—can be extended to metabolic pathways (eg, *N*-demethylation of TCAs) that do not involve CYP2D6.

Anne T. Harvey, PhD
Sheldon H. Preskorn, MD
Psychiatric Research Institute
1100 N St Francis, Suite 200
Wichita, KS 67214-2878

1. Popli AP, Baldessarini RJ, Cole JO. Interactions of serotonin reuptake inhibitors with tricyclic antidepressants. *Arch Gen Psychiatry.* 1994;51:666-667.
2. Skjelbo E, Brøsen K. Inhibitors of imipramine metabolism by human liver microsomes. *Br J Clin Pharmacol.* 1992;34:256-261.
3. Crewe HK, Lennard MS, Tucker GT, Woods FR, Haddock RE. The effect of selective serotonin reuptake inhibitors on cytochrome P4502D6 (CYP2D6) activity in human liver microsomes. *Br J Clin Pharmacol.* 1992;34:262-265.
4. von Moltke L, Greenblatt DJ, Harmatz JS, Shader RI. In vitro inhibition of desipramine (DMI) oxidation by fluoxetine (F) and norfluoxetine (NF) is greater than inhibition by sertraline (S) or desmethylsertraline (DS). *Clin Pharmacol Ther.* 1993;53:198. Abstract.
5. von Moltke L, Greenblatt DJ, Court MH, Duan SX, Harmatz JS, Shader RI. Inhibition of alprazolam and desipramine hydroxylation in vitro by paroxetine and fluvoxamine: comparison with other serotonin-reuptake-inhibitor antidepressants. *J Clin Psychopharm.* 1995;15:125-131.
6. Otton SV, Wu D, Joffe RT, Cheung SW, Sellers EM. Inhibition by fluoxetine of cytochrome P450 2D6 activity. *Clin Pharmacol Ther.* 1993;53:401-409.
7. Otton SV, Ball SE, Cheung SW, Inaba T, Sellers EM. Comparative inhibition of the polymorphic enzyme CYP2D6 by venlafaxine (VF) and other 5HT uptake inhibitors. *Clin Pharmacol Ther.* 1994;55:141. Abstract.
8. Preskorn SH, Alderman J, Chung M, Harrison W, Messig M, Harris S. Pharmacokinetics of desipramine coadministered with sertraline or fluoxetine. *J Clin Psychopharmacol.* 1994;14:90-98.
9. Ronfeld RA, Tremaine LM, Wilner KD, Henry EB. Evaluation of the pharmacokinetic properties of sertraline and desmethylsertraline in elderly and young normal volunteers. *Clin Pharmacokinet.* In press.
10. Preskorn SH, Silkey B, Beber J, Dorey C. Antidepressant response and plasma concentrations of fluoxetine. *Ann Clin Psychiatry.* 1991;3:147-151.
11. Lemberger L, Bergstrom RF, Wolen RL, Farid NA, Enas GG, Aronoff GR. Fluoxetine: clinical pharmacology and physiologic disposition. *J Clin Psychiatry.* 1985;46:14-19.
12. Kaye CM, Haddock RE, Langley PF, Mellows G, Tasker TCG, Zussman BD, Greb WH. A review of the metabolism and pharmacokinetics of paroxetine in man. *Acta Psychiatr Scand.* 1989;80(suppl 350):60-75.
13. de Vries MH, Raghoebar M, Mathlener IS, van Harten J. Single and multiple oral dose fluvoxamine kinetics in young and elderly subjects. *Ther Drug Monit.* 1992;14:493-498.
14. Alderman J, Greenblatt DJ, Preskorn S, Harrison W, Chung M. Desipramine pharmacokinetics with the selective serotonin reuptake inhibitors (SSRIs) paroxetine or sertraline. Poster presentation at the Sesquicentennial Celebration, American Psychiatric Association Meeting; May 21-26, 1994; Philadelphia, Pa.
15. Bergstrom RF, Peyton AL, Lemberger L. Quantification and mechanism of the fluoxetine and tricyclic antidepressant interaction. *Clin Pharmacol Ther.* 1992;51:239-248.
16. Spina E, Pollicino AM, Avenoso A, Campo GM, Perucca E, Caputi AP. Effect of fluvoxamine on the pharmacokinetics of imipramine and desipramine in healthy subjects. *Ther Drug Monit.* 1993;15:243-246.
17. Cavanaugh SVA. Drug-drug interactions of fluoxetine with tricyclics. *Psychosomatics.* 1990;31:273-276.
18. Westermeyer J. Fluoxetine-induced tricyclic toxicity extent and duration. *J Clin Psychopharmacol.* 1991;31:388-392.
19. Preskorn SH, Beber JH, Faul JC, Hirschfeld RMA. Serious adverse effects of combining fluoxetine and tricyclic antidepressants. *Am J Psychiatry.* 1990; 147:532.
20. Vaughan DA. Interaction of fluoxetine with tricyclic antidepressants. *Am J Psychiatry.* 1988;145:1478.
21. Bell IR, Cole JO. Fluoxetine induces elevation of desipramine level and exacerbation of geriatric nonpsychotic depression. *J Clin Psychopharmacol.* 1988; 8:447-448.
22. Suckow RF, Roose SP, Cooper TB. Effect of fluoxetine on plasma desipramine and 2-hydroxydesipramine. *Biol Psychiatry.* 1992;31:200-204.
23. Lydiard RB, Anton RF, Cunningham T. Interactions between sertraline and tricyclic antidepressants. *Am J Psychiatry.* 1993;150:1125-1126.
24. Barros J, Asnis G. An interaction of sertraline and desipramine. *Am J Psychiatry.* 1993;150:1751. Correction: *Am J Psychiatry.* 1994;151:300.
25. Spina E, Campo GM, Avenoso A, Pollicino MA, Caputi AP. Interaction between fluvoxamine and imipramine/desipramine in four patients. *Ther Drug Monit.* 1992;14:194-196.
26. Brøsen K, Skjelbo E, Rasmussen BB, Poulsen HE, Loft S. Fluvoxamine is a potent inhibitor of cytochrome P4501A2. *Biochem Pharmacol.* 1993;45: 1211-1214.
27. Brøsen K. Recent developments in hepatic drug oxidation: implications for clinical pharmacokinetics. *Clin Pharmacokinet.* 1990;18:220-239.
28. Preskorn SH. Pharmacokinetics of antidepressants: why and how they are relevant to treatment. *J Clin Psychiatry.* 1993;54(suppl 9):14-34.

In reply

Harvey and Preskorn are to be commended for their efforts to predict the degree of in vivo interaction of SSSRIs with other agents at human hepatic microsomal enzymes of the CYP oxidase family, which is critical for the metabolic clearance of drugs and other xenobiotic molecules. Their models are based on in vitro characterizations of liver–plasma par-

Cytochrome P-450 (CYP) Oxidases and Psychotropic Agents*

Enzyme Type	Reactions Mediated	Representative Substrates†	Inducible‡	CYP Enzyme Inhibitors (SSRIs)
1A2	*N*-demethylation	Tertiary-amine TCAs	Yes	FVX
2C	*N*-demethylation	Diazepam and tertiary-amine TCAs	Unknown	FLX, FVX, SRT
2D6	Ring-hydroxylation	Secondary- and tertiary-amine TCAs and many neuroleptics	No	PRX≥FLX≥NORFLX> SRT≥FVX>>VNX
3A3/4	*N*-demethylation	Tertiary-amine TCAs	Yes	FVX, NFZ, FLX§, SRT§

**Based on recent reviews by De Vane[6] and Preskorn.[8] SSRI indicates selective serotonin reuptake inhibitor; TCA, tricyclic antidepressant; FVX, fluvoxamine; FLX, fluoxetine; SRT, sertraline; PRX, paroxetine, NORFLX, norfluoxetine; VNX, venlafaxine; and NFZ, nefazodone.*

†Secondary-amine TCAs include desipramine and tertiary-amine TCAs include amitryptyline. Neuroleptics include phenothiazines, clozapine, haloperidol, and risperidone.

‡Inducers of increased oxidase activity include carbamazepine.

§Possible CYP enzyme inhibitors.

tition coefficients and normalized K_is of SSRIs and yield plausible results. Nevertheless, several caveats and points of agreement concerning the state of knowledge on this topic need to be reemphasized.

First, we endorse the general proposition that predictions concerning potentially clinically significant drug interactions that arise from laboratory models require extensive verification with various agents and doses in substantial numbers of human subjects, ideally under controlled and quantitative experimental conditions, before firm conclusions can be made. We also concur that clinical data pertinent to relative risks present in interactions of various specific SSRIs with other drugs remain very limited and that case anecdotes without further research can be seriously misleading.

A caveat is that selection or normalization is required for modeling because the K_is of some SSRIs have varied considerably. For example, with the much-studied CYP2D6 isozyme, the K_i for fluoxetine in published reports ranges from 170 to 920 nmol/L and the K_i for sertraline ranges from 700 to 1500 nmol/L.[1-3] In addition, use of a single tissue-partition coefficient to represent a complex in vivo distribution of drugs is a simplification for modeling that may or may not be valid.[4]

A critical clinical study that indicated dissimilar risks of interactions of SSRIs with the TCA desipramine compared a daily dose of 50 mg of sertraline with 20 mg of fluoxetine.[5] This dose of fluoxetine is in the midrange of its usual clinical doses, but that for sertraline is at the low end of its clinical range and may minimize the effects of the more typical higher doses, particularly if given too briefly to attain a steady state.[6]

An additional caveat is that most experimental studies of interactions of psychotropic agents with CYP enzymes have focused on the important 2D6 subtype. However, the number of genetically determined isozymes in the CYP family may exceed 200.[6,7] No doubt, additional drug-drug interactions will be clarified as additional enzymes and agents are considered. For example, the recently introduced SSRI fluvoxamine interacts with the CYP1A subfamily, which is implicated in the N*-demethylation of drugs, including tertiary-amine TCAs.[6] In addition to their well-known inhibitory actions on CYP2D6, fluoxetine and sertraline probably also interact with the 2C and 3A CYP subfamilies.[6] Many of these and other potential interactions remain as in vitro findings of which the potential clinical implications have not been evaluated. Some of our current understanding of the CYP system relevant to psychopharmacology is summarized in the* **Table**.[6,8]

In conclusion, we suggest again that additional clinical studies are required to adequately evaluate the relative safety of the growing list of SSRIs in clinical use, including studies involving clinically realistic doses and duration of exposure. The state of knowledge on this topic provides only a limited basis for preferring one SSRI over another so as to limit the risks of clinically relevant drug-drug interactions.[6,8] A specific hypothesis proposed in our letter remains to be tested: that persons who require relatively high daily doses of a TCA to obtain a nominally therapeutic blood concentration may be at an increased risk of experiencing interactions when an SSRI is added. The critical perspective of Harvey and Preskorn is a valued contribution to this important topic and needs to be pursued vigorously. In the meantime, a clinical suggestion is to approach all combinations of SSRIs with other drugs with caution until the matter of their relative safety is more firmly grounded on adequate clinical research and experience.

Anand Popli, MD
Cleveland Veterans Affairs Medical Center
Psychiatry Service 116A(B)
10000 Brecksville Rd
Brecksville, OH 44141
Ross J. Baldessarini, MD
Jonathan O. Cole, MD
Boston, Mass

1. Crewe HK, Lennard MS, Tucker GT, Woods FR, Haddock RE. The effect of selective serotonin reuptake inhibitors on cytochrome P4502D6 (CYP2D6) activity in human liver microsomes. *Br J Clin Pharmacol.* 1992;34:262-265.
2. Skjelbo E, Brøsen K. Inhibitors of imipramine metabolism by human liver microsomes. *Br J Clin Pharmacol.* 1992;34:256-261.
3. Otton SV, Wu D, Joffe RT, Cheung SW, Sellers EM. Inhibition by fluoxetine of cytochrome P-450-2D6 activity. *Clin Pharmacol Ther.* 1993;53:401-409.
4. von Moltke LL, Greenblatt DJ, Cotreau-Bibbo MM, Duan SX, Harmatz JS, Shader RI. Inhibition of desipramine hydroxylation in vitro by serotonin-reuptake inhibitor antidepressants and by quinidine and ketoconazole: a model system to predict drug interactions in vivo. *J Pharmacol Exp Ther.* 1994;268:1278-1283.
5. Preskorn SH, Alderman J, Chung M, Harrison W, Messig M, Harris S. Pharmacokinetics of desipramine coadministered with sertraline or fluoxetine. *J Clin Psychopharmacol.* 1994;14:90-98.
6. DeVane CL. Pharmacogenetics and drug metabolism of newer antidepressant drugs. *J Clin Psychiatry.* 1994;55(suppl):38-47.
7. Brøsen K. Recent developments in hepatic drug oxidation: implications for clinical pharmacokinetics. *Clin Pharmacokinet.* 1990;18:220-239.
8. Preskorn SH. Update on clinical aspects of cytochrome P-450 mixed function oxidases. *Curr Affect Illness.* 1994;14:5-13.

MANUSCRIPT CRITERIA AND INFORMATION

Submit manuscripts to Jack D. Barchas, MD, Editor, *Archives of General Psychiatry,* Cornell Medical Center, Dept of Psychiatry, Box 171, 525 E 68th St, Room F2315, New York, NY 10021. Manuscripts are received with the understanding that they are not under simultaneous consideration by another publication, have not been published previously, and have the approval of each author. Accepted manuscripts become the permanent property of the ARCHIVES. They may not be republished without permission from the publisher (AMA).

Editing. Copyediting follows AMA style and requires corresponding author approval. The authors are responsible for all statements made in their work, including changes made by the copy editor and authorized by the corresponding author.

Reprints. Forms for ordering are included with the edited typescript sent for approval. Reprints are shipped 6 to 8 weeks after publication.

Cover Letter

- In the cover letter, designate one author as correspondent and provide a complete address and telephone and fax numbers.
- For a manuscript to be reviewed, considered, or edited, the following statement must be signed by *all* authors:

"I have been sufficiently involved in this work to take public responsibility for its validity and final presentation as an original publication. I can and will provide documentation of my work upon reasonable request and I have fulfilled the obligations for full disclosure and authorship as described by *Archives of General Psychiatry*. . . ." This signed statement must conclude with *one* of the two following sentences: "Accordingly, I hereby transfer, assign, or otherwise convey all copyright ownership to the AMA in the event such work is published by the AMA." [OR] "No copyright ownership can be transferred since this work was produced in the course of my official duties as a US government officer or employee."

Manuscript Preparation[1,2]

- Submit an original double-spaced typescript and 7 copies.
- **Manuscripts will not be returned after the review process.** Unpublished manuscripts will be destroyed.
- Type—double-spaced throughout (including references)—on one side only of 8½ × 11-in white bond paper. Number all pages. Do not justify right-hand margins. Use a printer of at least letter quality.
- The length of the text of the manuscript (not including abstract, tables, figures, or references) should be under 5000 words. Include a word count of the text on the title page.
- Titles should be short, specific, and descriptive, emphasizing the main point of the article. Avoid a two-part title, if at all possible. Do not number the title, eg, I or Part I. Title length, including punctuation and spaces, ideally should be under 100 characters and must not exceed 200 characters.
- The title page should list full names, degrees, academic affiliations and their locations, and the name and address to whom reprint requests should be sent. If the paper was presented at a meeting, include the organization, place, and date of presentation. Acknowledgment of grant or drug company support should also be made on this page.
- Include a structured abstract of 250 words or less that states the Background, Methods, Results, and Conclusions in four sections labeled as such.
- Use Système International (SI) measurements throughout the manuscript.
- Use generic names of drugs, unless the specific trade name is directly relevant to the study design or discussion.
- Do not use abbreviations in the title or abstract. Limit their use in the text.
- *Do not use footnotes or appendixes.* Such materials should either be incorporated into the text or offered to interested readers on request.
- Include a statistical analysis section under *Methods* that fully describes the application of each statistical procedure used. If a test is used that is not commonly presented in the ARCHIVES, briefly describe its purpose and how it is to be interpreted. Results should report the test statistic (eg, χ^2, F or *t* value), degrees of freedom, and *P* value. Measures of central tendency (eg, means) should be accompanied by measures of variability (eg, standard deviations). In the cover letter, state the name of your statistical consultant, if appropriate.
- Acknowledge fully any material taken from other publications, and submit written permission from the owner to reprint in any language or form without limitation.
- Tables and figures should provide substantive data and not merely illustrate the text. While the main finding of a table or figure may be discussed in the narrative, the table or figure should not duplicate the text. Although no specific guideline can be applied to all articles, the number and length of tables and figures should be kept to a minimum.

Tables. Double-space on separate sheets of 8½ × 11-in white bond paper. Title each one and number them in the order of their citation in the text. If a table must be continued, repeat the title on a second sheet, followed by "(cont)." Any explanatory notes to be printed with the table must be typed single-spaced beneath the table.

Figures. Once manuscripts are accepted, two sets of professionally prepared, high-resolution color transparencies are required for all color figures. For black and white art, two sets of professionally prepared glossy prints are required. If color figures are necessary, the ARCHIVES may pay part of the expense with the balance to be borne by the author.

- Number figures according to their order in the text. Type the figure number, proper orientation (eg, top), name of the senior author, and an abbreviated title on a gummed label; affix it to the back of the print.
- Double-space legends (maximum length, 40 words) on a separate sheet of 8½ × 11-in paper.

INDEX TO ADVERTISERS

Janssen Pharmaceutica
Risperdal *801-803*

McNeil Pharmaceutical
Haldol Decanoate . . . . *Cover 2-789*

G. D. Searle & Co.
Ambien *796A-B*

Solvay Pharmaceuticals
Lithobid *793-794*
Luvox *874-876*

U.S. Pharmaceuticals Group, Pfizer Inc.
Zoloft . . . . *Covers 3-4*

While every precaution is taken to ensure accuracy, we cannot guarantee against the possibility of an occasional change or omission in the preparation of this index.

THIS MONTH IN
ARCHIVES OF GENERAL PSYCHIATRY

Persons with schizophrenia are impaired on many cognitive tasks that require the integrity of the cerebral cortices, yet the anatomical underpinnings of these deficits are not well established. In a quantitative analysis of over 50 brains, **Selemon et al** (page 805) found that neuronal density is increased in the prefrontal and occipital cortices in schizophrenic brains compared with normal controls. The increased cell packing in the schizophrenic cortex is most likely due to a reduction of intraneuronal neuropil, specifically dendrites and axons. These findings suggest that the anatomical substrate for cortical dysfunction in schizophrenia may be reduction of neuronal processes rather than attrition of neurons.

Patients with schizophrenia sporadically do not retain in short-term memory the spatial location of a target. In two studies, **Park et al** (page 821) report that a significant proportion of otherwise unaffected first-degree relatives of patients with schizophrenia show a similar intermittent failure of spatial working memory. This aspect of memory depends on the integrity of the prefrontal system. These studies strongly suggest that spatial working memory impairment, like smooth pursuit eye movement dysfunction, expresses underlying schizophrenic pathophysiology that is independent of psychotic state. It can also aid in tracing the transmission of schizophrenia in genetic studies.

Recent clinical studies suggest that the symptoms of schizophrenia may result from insufficient stimulation of forebrain glutamate receptors of the *N*-methyl-D-aspartate (NMDA) subtype. **Tsai et al** (page 829) measured several biochemical markers for glutamatergic neurotransmission in brains obtained post mortem from individuals with schizophrenia and from suitable controls. They report an elevation in the level of a neuropeptide that blocks NMDA receptors, reductions in the activity of an enzyme that degrades the neuropeptide, and reductions in glutamate levels in the schizophrenic samples. These alterations were most prominent in the frontal cortex and hippocampal regions. The results provide additional support for a glutamatergic hypothesis for schizophrenia.

Antipsychotics have been used for four decades, but the relationships between their doses (or their blood levels) and effects are unclear. **Volavka et al** (page 837) studied newly admitted schizophrenic and schizoaffective patients. Double-blind haloperidol was administered during two consecutive 3-week experimental periods. Two plasma levels were targeted: low (2 ng/mL) and moderate (10 ng/mL). The subjects were randomly assigned to four treatment sequences (low-low, low-moderate, moderate-moderate, or moderate-low). Moderate plasma levels yielded the best results in the first 3 weeks of treatment. Subsequent lowering of the plasma levels improved negative symptoms.

Several lines of evidence suggest that suicidal behavior may have a genetic basis and may involve altered serotonergic function. Consequently, the gene coding for the rate-limiting enzyme of serotonin, tryptophan hydroxylase (TPH), is a major candidate gene for study. **Abbar et al** (page 846) determined genotype and allele frequencies at a polymorphic TPH site both in suicide attempters and in healthy volunteers. No difference was detected, suggesting that the TPH gene may not be a susceptibility factor for suicidal behavior in the group of patients studied.

Simon et al (page 850) computerized health maintenance organization accounting records to compare health care costs for primary care patients with recognized depression to costs for an age- and gender-matched comparison group. Depressed patients had health care costs approximately 1.8 times as high after adjustment for comorbid medical illness. Specialty mental health costs accounted for only one fifth of cost differences, and large differences persisted for at least 12 months after initiation of depression treatment. While these findings suggest that effective depression treatment could reduce general medical costs, simple recognition of depression is not adequate to realize those savings.

Elevated rates of schizophrenia-related disorders in relatives of schizophrenic probands have been reported in recent family studies using modern, narrow criteria for schizophrenia. **Erlenmeyer-Kimling et al** (page 857) found that rates of narrowly defined schizophrenia were increased in offspring of schizophrenic parents followed up prospectively from midchildhood to adulthood compared with offspring of affectively ill or normal parents. However, the two groups of offspring of mentally ill parents showed no difference in schizoaffective disorder or putative schizophrenia spectrum personality disorders. Future genetic research should focus on distinguishing between the expression of the latter disorders in relatives of schizophrenic vs affectively ill probands.

To detect clinically meaningful effects, a research study must be designed with adequate statistical power. **Leon et al** (page 867) illustrate that statistical power increases when more reliable outcome measures are used. As a consequence of increased power, sample size requirements are reduced and research costs can be decreased. They urge careful consideration of the psychometric properties of outcome measures prior to sample size determination and recommend that effort be devoted to the development and dissemination of psychometrically sound scales.

Correction

Error in Figure. In the article "An In Vivo Study of the Prefrontal Cortex of Schizophrenic Patients at Different Stages of Illness via Phosphorus Magnetic Resonance Spectroscopy" published in the May issue of the ARCHIVES (1995;52:399-406), in Figure 1 on page 402, the lettering of a, b, and c is incorrect. The corrected figure is reprinted below. We regret the error.

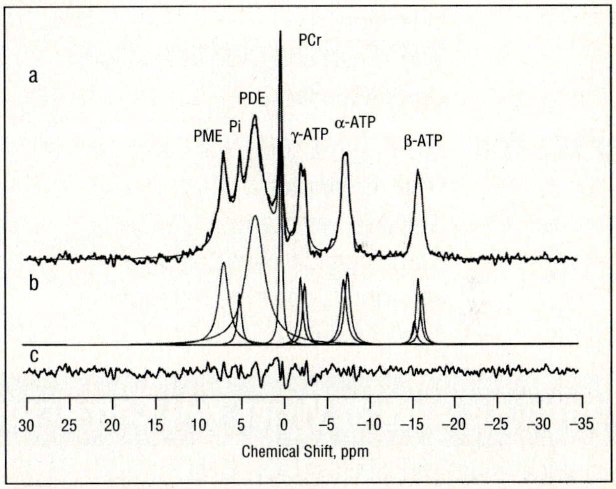

Figure 1. *a, A typical in vivo phosphorus 31 magnetic resonance (^{31}P MR) spectrum (thick line) from the left dorsolateral prefrontal cortex of a control superimposed on the modeled spectrum (thin line). The spectral peaks are phosphomonoester (PME), inorganic orthophosphate (Pi), phosphodiester (PDE), phosphocreatine (PCr), and γ–, α–, and β–adenosine triphosphate (ATP). b, The individual Lorentzian line shapes of the modeled spectrum. c, The difference between the acquired spectrum and the modeled spectrum.*

Archives Interactive

Risperdal® 1-, 2-, 3-, 4-mg tablets
RISPERIDONE

Introducing RISPERDAL ON CALL

A toll-free 800 number that mental healthcare professionals can call for instant access to information about RISPERDAL.

Now You Can Call On Us!

All you need is a touch-tone phone. RISPERDAL ON CALL is available 24 hours a day, 7 days a week. You can access us anytime—anywhere.

Dial 1-800-6R-ON-CALL

Just phone 1-800-6R-ON-CALL (1-800-676-6225), then listen for further instructions to access your choice of information.

PRESS 1 FOR: RISPERDAL PRODUCT INFORMATION
- Clinical Description
- Pharmacokinetics
- Indications
- Side Effects and Drug Interactions
- Quick Mail-Back

PRESS 2 FOR: PHYSICIAN EXCHANGE
- Positive Symptoms
- Negative Symptoms
- Extrapyramidal Symptoms
- Serotonin/Dopamine Antagonism
- Quick Mail-Back

PRESS 3 FOR: CLINICAL REVIEWS
- Abstract Selection
- Abstract Presentation
- Request Full Clinical Paper
- Quick Mail-Back/Quick Fax-Back

PRESS 4 FOR: CONVERSION AND DOSAGE
- From Oral and IM Antipsychotics
- Concomitant Agents
- Switching Strategies
- Dosage
- Quick Mail-Back

A Complete Look at What You Can Access

Here's a quick "map" of RISPERDAL ON CALL:

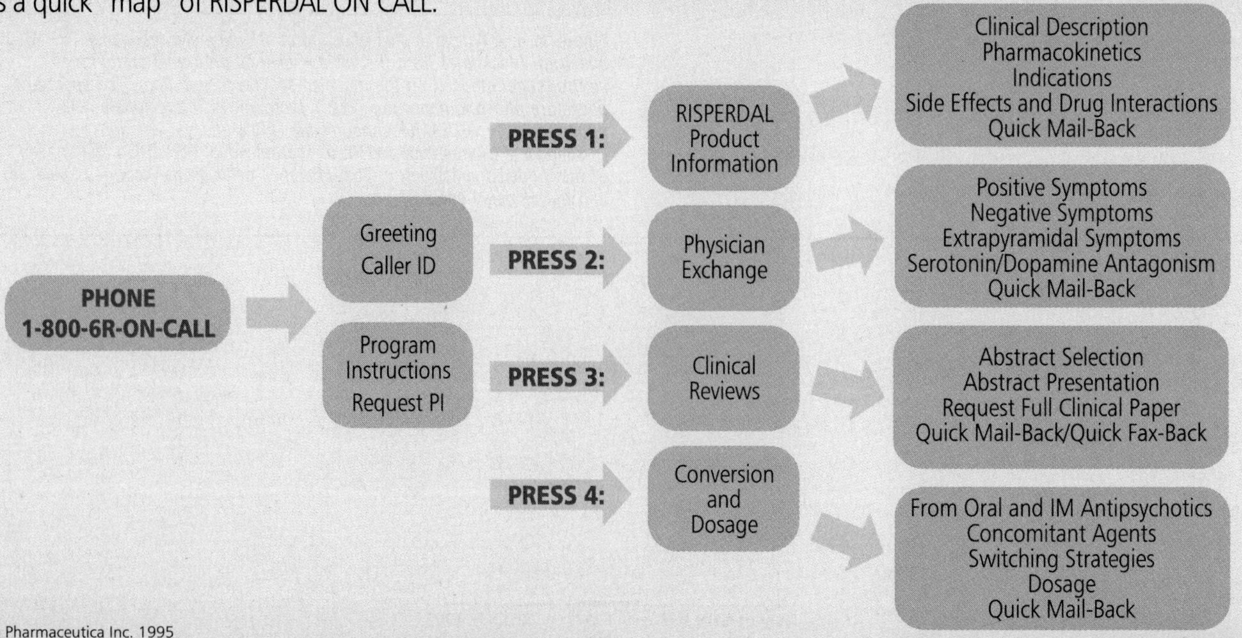

JANSSEN · PHARMACEUTICA · RESEARCH FOUNDATION ·

October 1995 IPI-RS-168

ORIGINAL ARTICLE

Abnormally High Neuronal Density in the Schizophrenic Cortex

A Morphometric Analysis of Prefrontal Area 9 and Occipital Area 17

Lynn D. Selemon, PhD; Grazyna Rajkowska, PhD; Patricia S. Goldman-Rakic, PhD

Background: In the past two decades, gross morphologic changes have been uncovered in the schizophrenic brain, eg, increased ventricular width and decreased cortical volume; however, relatively little is known about the area-specific and laminar density of cells in the schizophrenic cortex, particularly in prefrontal areas.

Method: A direct, three-dimensional counting method was used to determine cell density in 16 brains from patients with schizophrenia, 19 from normal subjects, six from patients with schizoaffective disorder, and nine from patients with advanced-stage Huntington's disease.

Results: Increased neuronal density was found in prefrontal area 9 (17%) and occipital area 17 (10%) in the schizophrenic brains. In area 9, neuronal density was increased in layers III to VI; cell packing of pyramidal and nonpyramidal neurons was elevated. Cortical thickness in the schizophrenic brains was slightly but not significantly reduced in both areas, with a disproportionate reduction in layer V in area 9. In contrast, brains with Huntington's disease exhibited markedly higher glial density (50%) and drastically reduced cortical thickness (28%).

Conclusion: Abnormally high density in the cerebral cortices of schizophrenics suggests that neuronal atrophy is the anatomic substrate for deficient information processing in schizophrenia.

(Arch Gen Psychiatry. 1995;52:805-818)

IT HAS LONG been recognized that many of the symptoms of schizophrenia, such as flattening of affect, looseness of associations, and thought disorder, resemble symptoms exhibited by patients who have frontal lobe damage.[1-6] Moreover, with the advent of neuroimaging techniques that measure blood flow and metabolic activity, Ingvar and Franzen[7] and many subsequent investigators[8-19] have demonstrated a "hypofrontal" pattern of blood flow in schizophrenic patients. More recently, blood flow and metabolic activity have been examined in schizophrenic patients engaged in the Wisconsin Card Sort Task, the Continuous Performance Task, or the Tower of London task, all of which reflect the working memory capacity of the prefrontal cortex.[20] Not only do schizophrenics perform poorly on these tasks but their performance is not accompanied by the increase in blood flow and metabolism that occurs in normal subjects.[21-26]

Despite the prominence of frontal symptoms in the disease, relatively few morphometric studies have been directed to the prefrontal cortex in schizophrenia. Benes et al[27] examined the anterior cingulate cortex, the primary motor cortex, and rostral area 10 in the prefrontal cortex, but significant differences in overall neuronal density were not found in any of these areas, although decreased neuronal density was observed in specific laminae, ie, layer VI of area l0, layer V in the cingulate cortex, and layer III of the motor cortex. Subsequent analysis disclosed a more generalized decrease in nonpyramidal cell density in layers II to VI in the cingulate cortex and an *increase* in pyramidal cell density in layer V of prefrontal area 10.[28] More recently, cell density in area 9 of the schizophrenic brain was measured and no differences from normal were detected.[29]

Previous studies of cell density in the prefrontal cortex in schizophrenics have used traditional, two-dimensional count-

See also page 819

See Materials and Methods on next page

From the Section of Neurobiology, Yale University School of Medicine, New Haven, Conn. Dr Rajkowska is now with the Department of Psychiatry and Human Behavior, University of Mississippi Medical Center, Jackson.

MATERIALS AND METHODS

SOURCES AND DIAGNOSIS OF BRAIN MATERIALS

Schizophrenic and non–neurologically impaired control brains were received from three main sources: the Brain Tissue Resource Center (BTRC) at McLean Hospital, Belmont, Mass, the University of Zagreb (Croatia), and the National Institute of Mental Health at St Elizabeths Hospital in Washington, DC (**Table 1**). One additional control brain was obtained from the Yakovlev collection in Washington, DC; two other control brains were obtained at autopsy from Yale–New Haven (Conn) Hospital. Brains with late-stage (grade 3 or 4) Huntington's disease (HD) were used as a neurologically impaired control group, since patients with HD not only resemble schizophrenics in exhibiting symptoms of frontal lobe dysfunction[32,33] but often undergo similar regimens of neuroleptic treatment and institutionalization. Brains from patients with HD originated from the BTRC with the exception of one brain that was collected from Yale–New Haven Hospital. Brains were excluded from the study if there was evidence of neurologic damage, substantial drug or alcohol abuse during the last year of life (with the exception of one brain from a patient with a secondary diagnosis of alcohol dependency [**Table 2**]), or if there were changes characteristic of Alzheimer's disease in the cortex at autopsy. Only the left hemispheres of brains from individuals younger than 72 years that had postmortem intervals (PMIs) of less than 30 hours were accepted for morphometric analysis (Table 1). The brains used in this study came from subjects of diverse racial and ethnic background, and both men and women were included in the study (Table 1).

The diagnosis of schizophrenia or schizoaffective disorder was made on site at each of these locations by psychiatrists associated with the respective institutes. For the BTRC, the diagnosis was made by Francine Benes, MD, PhD, based on postmortem review of the psychiatric records and application of the Feigner criteria.[34] In one case a brain was accepted from the BTRC for morphometric analysis with a diagnosis of "probable schizophrenia." The Schedule for Affective Disorders and Schizophrenia checklist, which uses Research Diagnostic Criteria , was used by Joel Kleinman, MD, PhD, at St Elizabeths Hospital and by Vera Folnegovic-Smalc, MD, at the University of Zagreb. For case CO237, Dr Folnegovic-Smalc had the additional benefit of a live interview in making the diagnosis of schizophrenia. At St Elizabeths Hospital, Research Diagnostic Criteria were assessed by postmortem review of the medical records. All cases either were assigned the diagnosis of schizophrenia without further specification or were classified into the paranoid or undifferentiated subcategory (Table 2). Schizophrenics from St Elizabeths Hospital were on average older and ill for a longer time than were those from the BTRC or from Zagreb (**Table 3**).

Diagnostic checklists were obtained from the aforementioned sources and medical records were obtained and reviewed thoroughly. Psychiatric symptoms were noted and classified as positive (eg, delusions, hallucinations), negative (eg, flatness of affect, paucity of speech), symptoms that do not fit into either heuristic category (eg, thought disorder, loose associations), or symptoms of depression (eg, decreased appetite, sleep disturbance) (Table 2). In addition, the presence of a family history of schizophrenia was noted, as was previous alcohol or other drug abuse (Table 2). Lifetime intake of neuroleptic medication, as well as other psychiatric drugs, was recorded, and special note was made of those medications in use during the 6 months preceding death. Finally, any anatomic abnormalities that had been documented either before death (eg, frontal atrophy on computed tomographic scan) or at autopsy were listed, and the cause of death also was recorded.

HISTOLOGIC PROCESSING AND CELL COUNTING

Blocks of tissue containing areas 9 and 17 were received in formaldehyde for further processing at Yale–New Haven

ing methods in which extrapolation to three dimensions necessitates the application of an Abercrombie correction factor.[30] Without such a correction, the estimates err in proportion to the size of the cells analyzed, and if cell size is influenced by the disease process, the degree of error in the estimates for the normal and schizophrenic brains is unequal. However, calculation of an Abercrombie correction factor introduces other sources of error because it is based on the relationship between cell diameter and section thickness, with the assumption that cells are nearly spherical. Since the cortex is composed of a heterogeneous population of cells, any assumption about cell size and shape is dubious at best. In addition, variations in section thickness are inescapable in microtome-generated sections and represent another source of error in the correction formula. In the present study, we used a counting method in which cell density is measured directly in an optically defined, precise volume of tissue located entirely within the confines of the section.[31] Because cell density is measured in a three-dimensional space, correction factors are not required. The estimates generated are entirely independent of cell size, cell shape, and section thickness. The sensitivity of this unbiased morphometric approach has enabled us to detect a significant elevation in overall neuronal density in the prefrontal cortex of the schizophrenic brain and, somewhat surprisingly, in the primary visual cortex as well.

RESULTS

QUALITATIVE OBSERVATIONS

We elected to analyze prefrontal area 9 because of our long-standing interest in the dorsolateral prefrontal cortex and because this area exhibited several salient cytoarchitectonic features that made it easy to identify in Nissl-stained sections. In normal brains, area 9 was distinguished by the presence of large pyramidal cells in layers IIIc and Va, a thin layer IV with irregular boundaries caused by the protrusion of pyramidal cells from surrounding layers, and a cell-sparse layer Vb (**Figure 2**, top left).[35] Prefrontal area 9 in schizophrenic and schizoaffective brains did not exhibit any overt abnormalities (Figure 2, top right and bottom left). All six cortical lay-

Hospital. Blocks were embedded in celloidin and sectioned at 40 μm. Sections were Nissl-stained for visualization of cytoarchitectonic structure. Area 9 was identified by means of the morphologic criteria established by Rajkowska and Goldman-Rakic.[35] The extreme rostral and caudal portions of area 9 were excluded because these regions have cytoarchitectonic features that resemble neighboring areas 10 and 8, respectively. Five sections evenly spaced throughout the remainder (midlevels) of area 9 were chosen for analysis (**Figure 1**).[36] Probes were positioned within the section in regions that exhibited clear cytoarchitectonic definition, ie, the plane of cutting was perpendicular to the pial surface, no major tears or artifacts obscured the cortex, and probes were located at a sufficient distance from the cortical convexity and sulcal floor to avoid distortion of cortical laminae. In some of the first brains that were analyzed, six or seven probes were made instead of five. Since the additional probes did not significantly alter the density measured in these cases, only five probes were analyzed in subsequent brains.

Cell density was measured by the direct, three-dimensional counting method of Williams and Rakic[31] by two independent researchers (L.D.S. and G.R.) with the use of two different counting setups, one Macintosh based and the other IBM based. A single vertical probe, consisting of a stack of counting boxes extending from the pial surface to the white matter, was analyzed in each of the five selected sections. Densities from the five probes were averaged to generate a mean density value for each case. Numbers of neurons and glia were recorded separately to generate estimates of neuronal and glial density. Glia were readily distinguished from neurons because they lacked visible cytoplasm and had thicker nuclear membranes and more heterogeneous chromatin. The position of cells with respect to cortical laminae also was noted to provide separate cell density estimates for each of the six cortical layers. In two of the five probes, pyramidal and nonpyramidal neurons were recorded separately to assess the overall and laminar density of these two cell types. Pyramidal neurons were identified as those cells having triangular cell bodies in coronal section, while all other neurons were considered to be nonpyramidal.

STATISTICAL ANALYSIS

A one-way analysis of variance was performed with overall neuronal density in area 9 as the dependent variable and disease group the independent factor. A critical level of .05 was chosen for significance. Post hoc paired comparisons were used to determine which of the diseased groups' means differed significantly from the normal mean with the use of a Bonferroni procedure to arrive at a critical level of .02. Similar analyses were performed for glial density and cortical thickness. A repeated-measures analysis of variance was used to test for differences between schizophrenics and normal subjects in neuronal density in each of the six cortical layers in both areas. In area 9, paired comparisons of schizophrenic and normal values of overall pyramidal density, nonpyramidal density, and pyramidal to nonpyramidal cell ratio, as well as percentage of laminar width for each of the six cortical layers, were performed with Student's *t* test with separate variances. Similarly, in area 17, Student's *t* test was used to test for significance in comparing all variables except laminar neuronal density in schizophrenics and normal subjects. Pearson's correlation matrix was used to determine the interactions among the following variables: neuronal density, glial density, cortical thickness, age, PMI, and time in formaldehyde (TF). Pairwise deletion was used to maximize sample sizes and a Bonferroni correction was applied. In addition, separate correlation analyses were performed on normal and schizophrenic groups to determine whether age selectively influenced the schizophrenic sample, and finally, a possible correlation between duration of illness in the schizophrenics and neuronal density was explored. Multivariate regression analysis was performed to determine the effects of sex and race on neuronal density, glial density, and cortical thickness.

ers were present in the schizophrenic brains, and the laminar patterning did not differ appreciably from that of area 9 in the normal brains. However, in some schizophrenic and schizoaffective brains, cortical sulci were slightly wider than normal, the cortex appeared thinner and denser, and layer IV was more easily distinguished from surrounding pyramidal layers, perhaps because the large pyramidal cells that normally protrude into this layer were less prominent (Figure 2, top right). In certain of the brains from patients with HD, widening of the cortical sulci and thinning of the cortex were obvious. In addition, the relative proportions of the six cortical laminae were shifted such that the supragranular layers occupied a much greater proportion of the total cortical width because of degeneration of infragranular layers V and VI (Figure 2, bottom right). Marked gliosis, particularly of layers IV to VI and in the white matter, was frequently observed in brains from patients with HD as well (Figure 2, bottom right).

In normal brains, area 17 was easily distinguished from surrounding occipital cortices by its wide, stratified layer IV. Sublayers IVa and IVc were densely packed with small granular cells and surrounded sparsely packed sublayer IVb, which contained scattered large neurons. Pyramidal layers III and V, in comparison with prefrontal cortex, were narrower and contained smaller pyramidal neurons. Schizophrenic cortical area 17 exhibited these same cytoarchitectonic features.

SAMPLE OF BRAINS

Nineteen brains of normal subjects, 18 of schizophrenics, six of schizoaffective patients, and nine of patients with HD were originally included this study. Of the 18 schizophrenic brains, two that were assigned intake diagnoses of schizophrenia by the BTRC (B1648 and B1878) and were found to have high neuronal densities in area 9 (60.88/0.001 mm^3 and 57.73/0.001 mm^3, respectively) were later eliminated from the study when sufficient medical records could not be obtained to arrive at a definitive diagnosis of schizophrenia. Area 17 had been analyzed in these cases, and high neuronal densities were found in this area as well (138.04/0.001 mm^3 and 157.68/0.001 mm^3, respectively). Values from these cases are not included in calculations of the means in the following summary or in the accompanying figures.

Table 1. Characteristics of Brains Studied

Case*	Cause of Death	Sex/Race†/Age, y	Postmortem Time	
			Interval, h	In Formaldehyde, mo
		Normal Subjects‡		
A90166	Complications after heart valve surgery	F/W/67	14.0	2.8
A91112§	Myocardial infarction	M/W/59	22.0	1.9
B1638	Heart failure/burns	F/W/34	7.5	2.8
B1824§	Cardiac arrhythmia	M/W/29	24.0	7.5
B1823§	Pulmonary embolism	F/W/40	24.0	26.0
CO133§	Myocardial infarction	M/W/47	12.0	7.5
CO176	Rupture of duodenal ulcer	M/W/33	16.0	13.5
CO188	Myocardial infarction	F/W/71	24.0	5.5
CO189	Blood vessel rupture	M/W/47	18.0	5.0
MU169§	Myocardial infarction	M/W/58	6.0	. . .
N113§	Homicide	M/B/19	13.5	81.0
N129§	Cardiovascular disease	F/B/50	20.0	80.5
N224§	Asphyxia	M/B/32	3.0	151.9
N247	Hypertension	F/B/49	28.0	150.0
N596	Homicide	F/B/29	24.0	158.6
N729§	Cardiovascular disease	M/W/59	20.5	31.7
N730§	Cardiovascular disease	F/B/54	24.0	26.8
N782	Pneumonia	F/B/34	24.5	18.0
N836	Homicide	M/B/20	25.25	. . .
		Schizophrenic Patients‖		
B840§	Suicide, jumping	M/H/22	. . .	45.5
B1138§	Suicide, asphyxiation	M/W/27	8.0	26.0
B1702§	Adenocarcinoma	M/W/62	21.0	2.25
B1932§	Suicide, asphyxiation	M/W/33	9.7	4.5
CO234	Suicide	M/W/23	19.5	10.0
CO237	Suicide, drinking hydrochloric acid	F/W/48	27.0	. . .
N10§	Suicide	M/W/28	3.5	153.1
N12§	Suicide	M/B/28	6.25	166.8
N29	Cardiovascular disease	F/B/55	27.5	70.3
N72	Cardiovascular disease	M/B/46	16.2	76.0
N164§	Tuberculosis	M/B/54	10.0	86.6
N207§	Smoke inhalation	F/W/60	13.5	164.3
N209	Suicide	M/W/25	25.0	166.8
N218	Suicide	M/W/25	21.5	151.0
N313	Pneumonia	M/W/58	23.7	160.2
N371§	Suicide	F/B/48	26.0	136.3
		Schizoaffective Patients		
B1420	Suicide, jumping	M/W/35	6.3	3.0
B1467	Myocardial infarction	M/I/51	15.1	1.0
B1753	Drug overdose anoxia	M/W/37	24.0	. . .
B1972	Suicide, jumping	M/W/29	4.8	15.7
B2002	Suicide, asphyxiation	M/W/24	12.0	5.5
N265	Suicide	M/B/47	18.0	144.0
		Patients With Huntington's Disease		
A9229	. . .	. . ./. . ./. . .	12.5	. . .
B194	Pneumonia	M/W/40	21.25	106.3
B1135	Respiratory arrest	F/W/41	. . .	21.3
B1593	Complications of Huntington's disease	M/W/63	2.5	8.9
B1641	Colitis, sepsis, dehydration	M/W/55	1.9	16.5
B1701	Respiratory arrest, aspiration	M/W/32	4.5	3.0
B1940	Complications of Huntington's disease	F/W/75	15.0	1.0
B1947	Pneumonia	M/W/35	18.5	0.6
B1992	Sepsis	F/W/41	2.5	27.0

**Brain source is coded by the first letter in the case number as follows: A, Yale–New Haven (Conn) Hospital; B, Brain Tissue Resource Center, McLean Hospital, Belmont, Mass; CO, University of Zagreb (Croatia); MU, Yakovlev Collection, Washington, DC; and N, St Elizabeths Hospital of the National Institute of Mental Health, Washington, DC.*

†H indicates Hispanic; I, Asian Indian.

‡Mean±SE age, 46.0±3.3 years; postmortem interval, 18.7±1.7 hours; and time in formaldehyde, 46.8±13.7 months.

§Cases in which area 17 was analyzed.

‖Mean±SE age, 40.1±3.7 years; postmortem interval, 17.2±2.1 hours; and time in formaldehyde, 89.5±17.0 months.

Table 2. Diagnostic Information

Case*	Diagnosis	Age at Onset/ Duration of Illness, y	Symptoms†	Family History	Alcohol and Other Drug History‡	Neuronal Density /0.001 mm³ in Area 9
Schizoaffective Patients						
B1420	Schizoaffective disorder	24/11	1, 3, 4	Manic depressive disorder	M	71.76
B1467	Schizoaffective disorder	17/34	1	No known	None	73.33
B1753	Schizoaffective disorder	20/17	1, 2	Manic depressive disorder	M, D, A	37.55
B1972	Schizoaffective disorder	18/11	1, 2, 3	Unspecified "similar"	M, A	45.60
B2002	Schizoaffective disorder	16/8	1, 2, 4	Manic depressive disorder, depression	M, A	48.75
N265	Schizoaffective disorder	16/21	1, 2, 3, 4	...	None	50.66
Schizophrenic Patients						
B840	Probable	22/<1	1, 2, 3, 4	Epilepsy	M, D	55.87
B1138	Paranoid	24/3	1, 3, 4	No known	M, D?, A	63.75
B1702	Schizophrenia	18/44	1, 2, 3, 4	Unspecified mental illness	None	54.90
B1932	Paranoid	20/13	1, 2	No known	M, A	47.91
C0234	Schizophrenia	21/1	1	...	None	43.22
C0237	Schizophrenia	17/31	1, 3	Schizophrenia	None	58.04
N10	Paranoid	...	1, 4	...	None	52.93
N12	Paranoid	...	1, 3	...	None	56.91
N29	Undifferentiated	26/29	1, 2, 3, 4	...	None	46.41
N72	Undifferentiated	23/24	1, 2, 3, 4	Epilepsy	M, A	60.69
N164	Schizophrenia	20/34	1, 2, 3, 4	...	A§	54.28
N207	Undifferentiated	25/35	1, 3, 4	No known	None	73.32
N209	Undifferentiated	14/11	1, 3	...	...	47.60
N218	Undifferentiated	16/9	1, 2, 3, 4	...	...	56.37
N313	Undifferentiated	23/35	1, 3, 4	Schizophrenia	M	61.30
N371	Schizophrenia	...	...	...	...	58.05

*See Table 1 for explanation of brain source coding.

†1 indicates hallucinations and/or delusions; 2, flat affect; 3, thought disorder; and 4, depression, ie, sleep or appetite loss, hopelessness, social withdrawal, or multiple suicide attempts.

‡A indicates alcohol; D, other street drugs; and M, marijuana.

§Secondary diagnosis of alcohol dependency.

AREA 9: MORPHOMETRIC COMPARISON OF DISEASE GROUPS

The mean (±SE) neuronal density for the normal brains was 47.79±1.65/0.001 mm³ and was higher in the three diseased groups (schizophrenic, 55.72±1.74/0.001 mm³; schizoaffective, 54.61±5.96/0.001 mm³; and HD, 52.48±3.65/0.001 mm³) (**Figure 3**). A one-way analysis of variance indicated that there was no significant effect of disease on neuronal density (*P*=.08). However, post hoc, pairwise comparisons of each of the diseased groups with the normal mean indicated that mean neuronal density was significantly different from normal for the schizophrenic group (*P*=.01). Although the mean for the schizoaffective group was similar to that of the schizophrenic mean, the smaller sample and greater variance in this group precluded a significant finding (*P*=.12; HD, *P*=.21) (**Figure 4**). The Pearson correlation matrix disclosed a significant interaction between neuronal density and cortical thickness (−.624; *P*<.001) and no significant interactions between neuronal density and glial density (*P*=.15), age (*P*=1), PMI (*P*=.09), or TF (*P*=1). Further separate correlation analysis of the effect of age on the normal and schizophrenic groups showed no selective effect of age on either group (normal, *P*=.71; schizophrenic, *P*=.15). No correlation was found between duration of illness in the schizophrenic population and neuronal density (*P*=.27). Likewise, regression analysis showed no effects of sex (*P*=.97) or race (*P*=.08) on neuronal density. Pyramidal and nonpyramidal densities were higher in the schizophrenic brains in comparison with normal brains (pyramidal, *P*=.002; nonpyramidal, *P*=.01) such that the ratio of the two cell types was unchanged (*P*=.16) (**Figure 5**). Neuronal density was elevated in layers III to VI (I, *P*=.40; II, *P*=.12; III, *P*=.04; IV, *P*=.01; V, *P*=.001; VI, *P*=.02), with the largest increases (24%) observed in layers IV and V (**Figure 6**).

Table 3. Data by Source

Source*	Diagnosis	No. of Cases	Age, y	Duration of Illness, y	Neuronal Density /0.001 mm³ in Area 9
BTRC	Normal	3	34.3	...	45.28
	Schizophrenia	4	36.0	15.25	55.61
NIMH	Normal	9	43.1	...	48.54
	Schizophrenia	10	42.7	25.29	56.79
Zagreb	Normal	4	49.5	...	43.11
	Schizophrenia	2	35.5	13.50	50.63

*BTRC indicates Brain Tissue Resource Center at McLean Hospital, Belmont, Mass; NIMH, St Elizabeths Hospital of the National Institute of Mental Health, Washington, DC; and Zagreb, University of Zagreb (Croatia).

When mean neuronal density was computed for controls and schizophrenics sorted by source, neuronal density was higher in each of the three schizophrenic sub-

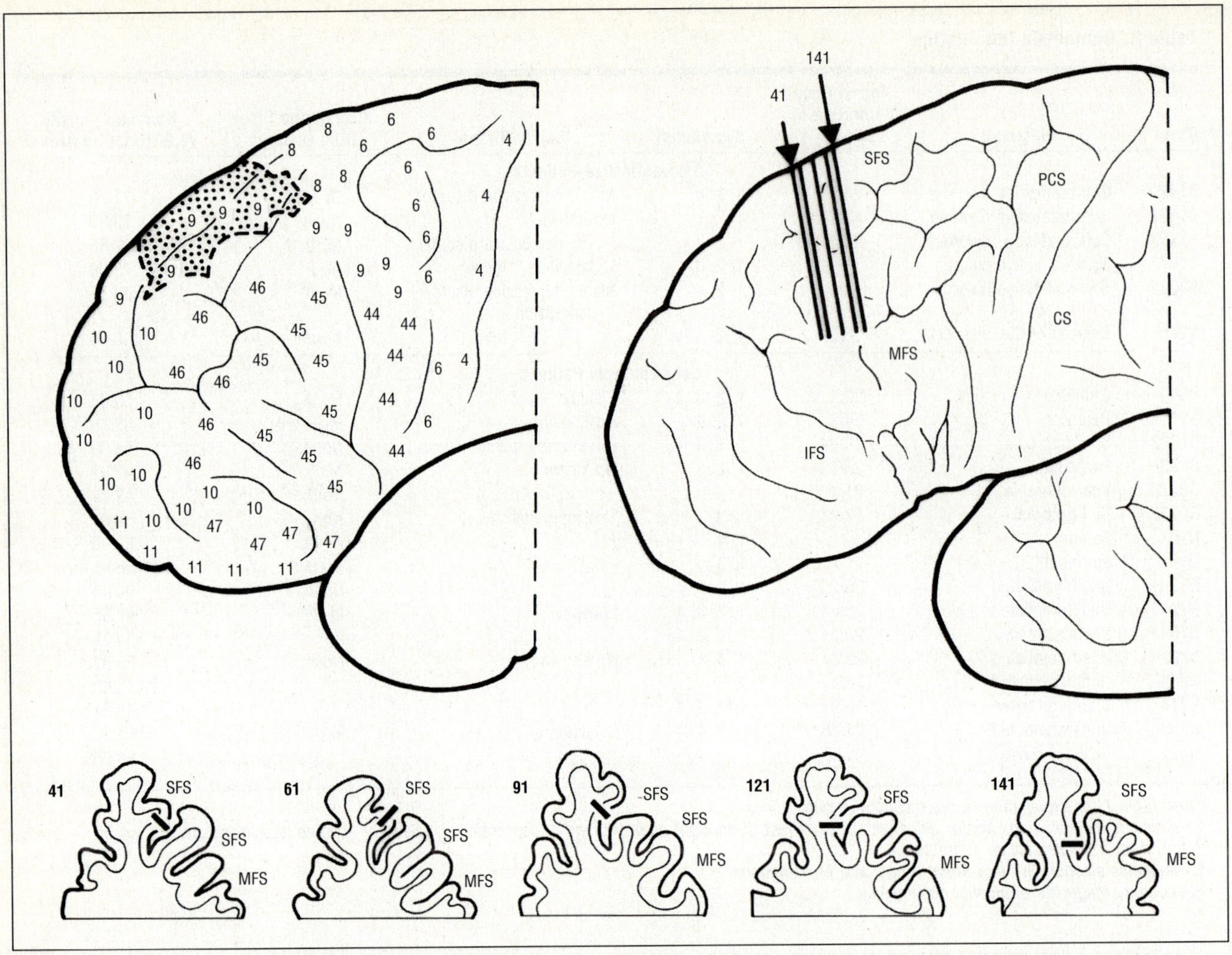

Figure 1. *Top left, Superimposition of area 9 on the Talairach atlas of the human left hemisphere.*[36] *Top right, A lateral view of brain CO189 showing the location of the five coronal sections selected for analysis. Bottom, Drawings of the coronal sections with dark bars indicating the position of each of the five probes on the superior frontal sulcus (SFS) wall. CS indicates central sulcus; IFS, inferior frontal sulcus; MFS, medial frontal sulcus; PCS, precentral sulcus.*

groups in comparison with their respective control populations (Table 3). Moreover, even the lowest of the three schizophrenic means (Zagreb) was higher than the highest of the three control means (National Institute of Mental Health).

The mean (±SE) glial density for the normal brains (71.83±4.13/0.001 mm^3) and schizophrenic brains (69.15±5.84/0.001 mm^3) was similar, slightly elevated in the schizoaffective brains (83.22±9.07/0.001 mm^3), and greatly elevated (50%) in the brains from patients with HD (107.68±13.36/0.001 mm^3) (**Figure 7**). Analysis of variance indicated a significant effect of disease on glial density (P=.003). Subsequent pairwise comparison of each of the diseased groups with the normal mean indicated that the only significant difference was present in the HD group (P=.005; schizophrenic, P=.34; schizoaffective, P=.76). No effects of race (P=.38) or sex (P=.56) were found on regression analysis. The Pearson product moment correlations showed significant interactions between glial density and PMI (−.417; P=.05), TF (−.519; P=.004), and cortical thickness (−.331; $P<.001$). These statistical findings are consistent with our observation that glia were faintly stained and seemed to be sparsely represented in brains obtained from St Elizabeths Hospital that had been stored in formaldehyde for more than 5 years. In an effort to eliminate this confounding factor, an analysis of glial density in schizophrenic and normal brains with TFs of less than 5 years was performed. In this sample of 14 normal, six schizophrenic, six schizoaffective, and eight brains from patients with HD, mean glial density was 22% higher in the schizophrenics (91.63±7.64/0.001 mm^3) relative to the controls (75.06±4.86/0.001 mm^3), although the difference did not reach significance (P=.22). In this same sample, the increase in glial density for the brains from patients with HD (105.45±14.94/0.001 mm^3; P=.02) relative to the normal brains was 40%, compared with 50% in the full sample.

Cortical thickness was shown to vary significantly by group ($P<.001$), with the HD cases (1.75±0.11 mm; $P<.001$) exhibiting the only significant difference from normal subjects (2.41±0.06 mm; $P<.001$) (**Figure 8**). The schizophrenic (2.22±0.06 mm; P=.04) and schizoaffective (2.20±0.15 mm; P=.10) means were also lower than normal, but the difference between schizophrenic and normal brains only approached the significance level of $P<.02$. There were no significant correlations between cortical thickness and age (P=.30), PMI (P=.16), or TF (P=1), and race (P=.34) or sex (P=.45) did not influence cortical thick-

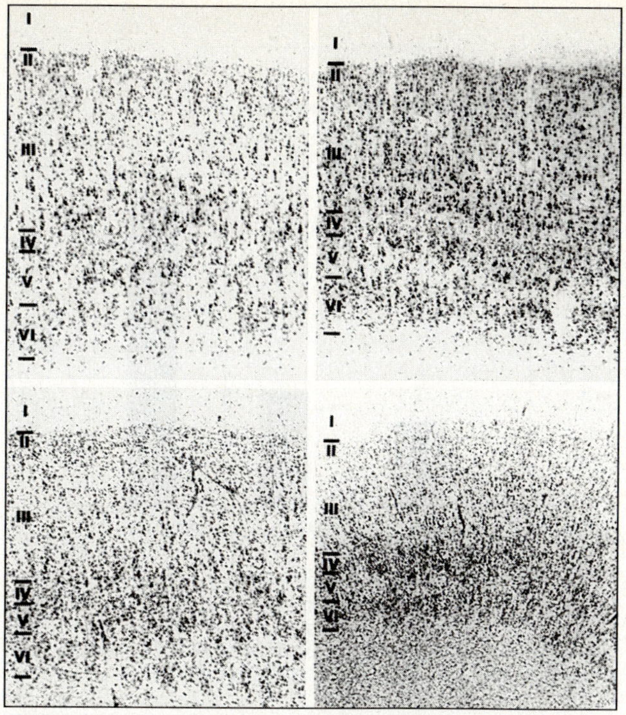

Figure 2. *Nissl-stained coronal sections of area 9 in a normal brain (top left), a schizophrenic brain (top right), a schizoaffective brain (bottom left), and a brain from a patient with Huntington's disease (bottom right). Note that both the schizophrenic and schizoaffective cortices are slightly thinner than normal and that layer IV is more prominent in area 9 in the schizophrenic brain relative to the normal control. In this brain with Huntington's disease, the cortex is greatly reduced in thickness and supragranular layers appear abnormally large because of the drastic reduction in thickness of the infragranular layers (original magnification ×44).*

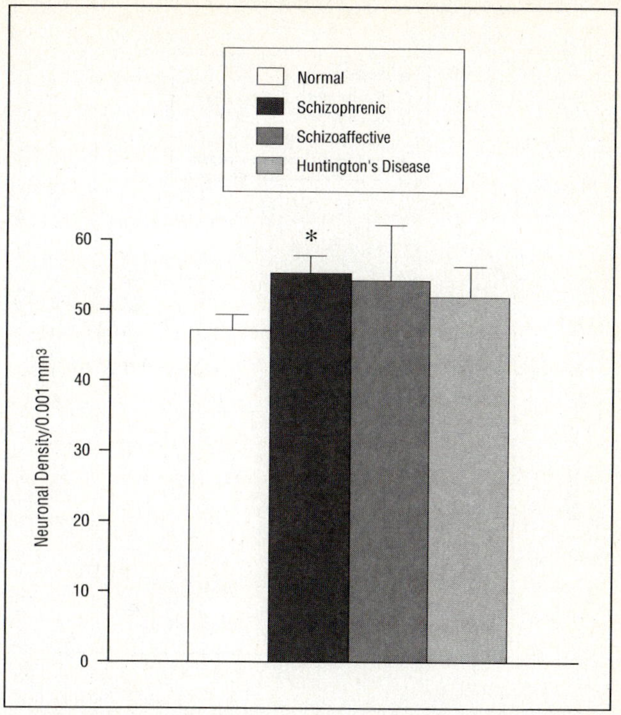

Figure 3. *Mean neuronal density for each of the four disease groups. Neuronal density is significantly elevated above normal levels only for the schizophrenic cohort (asterisk, P<.01).*

ness. Cortical thickness was correlated with neuronal ($P<.001$) and glial ($P<.001$) density. Comparison of the proportion that each cortical layer contributes to total thickness between the schizophrenic and normal groups showed a 7% decrease in percentage of laminar width of layer V ($P<.05$) in the schizophrenic brains, with all other layers showing smaller changes (**Figure 9**).

AREA 17: MORPHOMETRIC COMPARISON OF SCHIZOPHRENIC AND NORMAL BRAINS

Area 17 was analyzed in 10 normal and nine schizophrenic brains, all of which were also included in the morphometric study of area 9 (Table 1). Neuronal density is known to be approximately two times greater in primary visual cortex relative to all other cortical areas, and this was so in our sample. Nonetheless, a 10% increase in neuronal density was found in the schizophrenic brains (136.06±4.90/0.001 mm^3; P=.05) in comparison with normal brains (123.45±3.11/0.001 mm^3) (**Figure 10**). Neuronal density was significantly higher than normal in pyramidal layers III (17%) and V (16%) (I, P=.60; II, P=.28; III, P=.03; IV, P=.17; V, P=.03; VI, P=.13). As in area 9, glial density was not elevated (P=.88) (Figure 10); however, when cases with long TFs were removed, a nonsignificant 15% increase in glial density was observed (P=.27). Only a trend reduction in overall cortical thickness (5%) was detected in the schizophrenic sample (P=.21), and no changes in the proportion of the laminae were found (I, P=.25; II, P=.96; III, P=.22; IV, P=.70; V, P=.97; VI, P=.09). No significant correlations were found among neuronal density, glial density, cortical thickness, age, PMI, and TF.

COMMENT

Neuronal density was significantly higher in our cohort of schizophrenic brains in comparison with a group of non–neurologically impaired control brains. Although brains were obtained from multiple sources, there was a reasonably tight distribution below 50 neurons per 0.001 mm^3 in the normal group and an equally dense banding of schizophrenic brains above this mark (Figure 4). Brains from different sources were interspersed in these distributions, and outliers were as likely to emanate from one source as from another. Thus, a strength of this study is its generality with respect to schizophrenia. If all the schizophrenic brains had been obtained from the BTRC, the result might have indicated that high neuronal density was a feature of young, suicidal schizophrenics, as many of the brains obtained from this source tended to fit in this category. In actuality, the brains of older, more chronically ill patients from St Elizabeths Hospital exhibited the same morphometric abnormalities (see cases N164, N207, and N313 in Tables 1 and 2). Conversely, the higher neuronal density cannot be attributed to long institutionalization, since brains from young schizophrenics who had been treated primarily on an outpatient basis exhibited the same elevated density as those from more chronically ill patients. The absence of significant correlations between sex or race and neuronal density further supports the relevance of these findings to all schizophrenics. Moreover, the present results are compatible with a growing body of evidence indicating

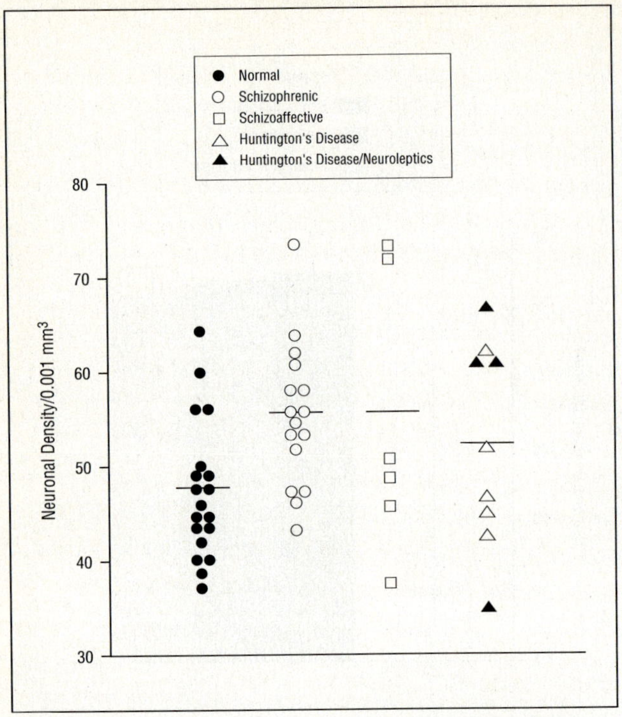

Figure 4. *Neuronal density of individual brains. Note that only four normal brains had neuronal densities above 50/0.001 mm³ in comparison with 12 schizophrenic brains. Neuronal density was much more variable in the schizoaffective and Huntington's disease groups. Solid triangles indicate the brains with Huntington's disease that were exposed to long-term neuroleptic treatment.*

that the frontal lobes are smaller than normal in schizophrenics (to be discussed in detail in a later section).

POSSIBLE CONFOUNDING VARIABLES

Although all of the schizophrenic patients in the present study had undergone treatment with neuroleptic drugs, there are several lines of evidence to suggest that the elevated neuronal density was not caused by medication. First, neuronal density did not correlate with duration of illness, suggesting that the length of neuroleptic exposure did not affect this measure, although this does not discount a plateau effect for drug treatment. Moreover, the brains from two individuals who had limited neuroleptic treatment exhibited high neuronal densities. For example, one schizoaffective patient had refused medication on several occasions in the 2 years before death yet had the third highest neuronal density of any brain in the study. Another young schizophrenic patient who had been ill only 3 years and was not taking neuroleptics because of allergic responses to the drugs had the second highest neuronal density of the schizophrenic group. Finally, one patient with HD who had undergone a similar regimen of neuroleptic treatment exhibited low neuronal density (Figure 4). These observations indicate that increased neuronal density is not associated in any obligatory manner with neuroleptic intake.

Various other factors, including age, PMI, and TF, were evaluated to see if these might account for the elevation in neuronal density. However, neuronal density was not correlated with any of these measures and therefore appears to be specific to the disease state. That neuronal

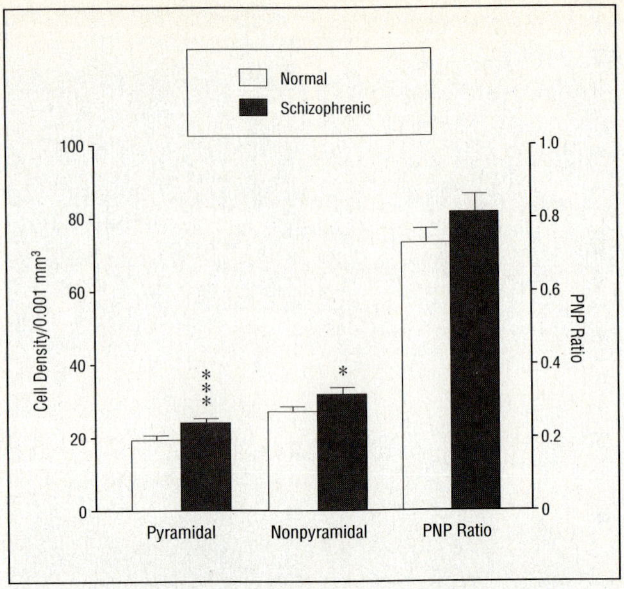

Figure 5. *Pyramidal and nonpyramidal densities in the schizophrenic and normal brains. Because both densities were higher than normal in schizophrenic brains, the pyramidal to nonpyramidal (PNP) ratio was unchanged. Three asterisks indicate* P<*.002; one asterisk,* P<*.01.*

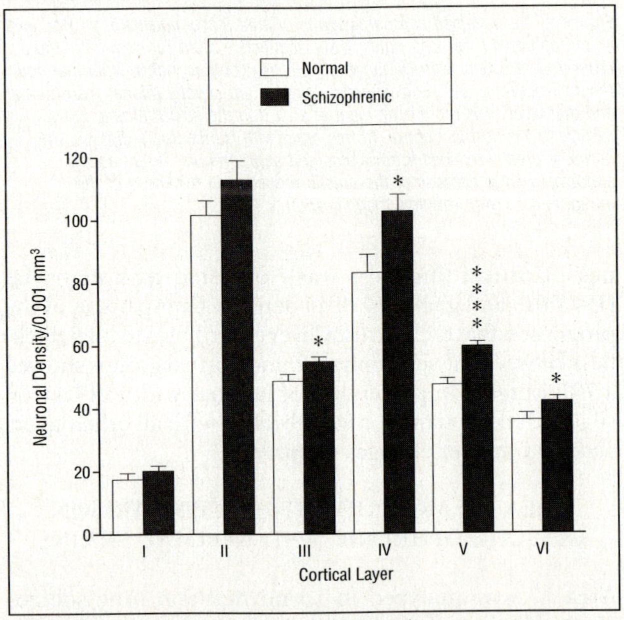

Figure 6. *Neuronal density by cortical layer. Neuronal density was elevated in layers III through VI in the schizophrenic cortex. One asterisk indicates* P<*.05; four asterisks,* P=*.001.*

density was not related to PMI or TF suggests that the higher density is not caused simply by shrinkage. Although it is possible that schizophrenic brains differ from normal brains structurally or chemically in some manner that causes the schizophrenic brains to shrink excessively during processing, differential shrinkage seems to be a highly unlikely explanation for the present results. Moreover, analysis of cell size in a subset of these same schizophrenic brains indicates that only neurons, and not glia, are smaller in the schizophrenic prefrontal cortex.[37] Another indication that shrinkage does not account for the differences between groups is that the cortex was not reduced in thickness uniformly in the schizophrenic brains;

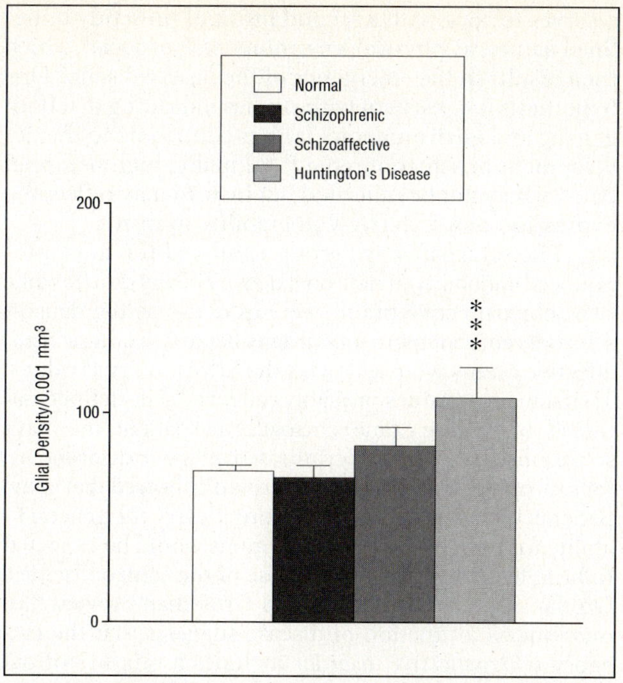

Figure 7. *Mean glial density in the normal, schizophrenic, schizoaffective, and Huntington's disease groups. In the Huntington's disease cortex, glial density was 50% higher than normal (three asterisks,* P=.005*).*

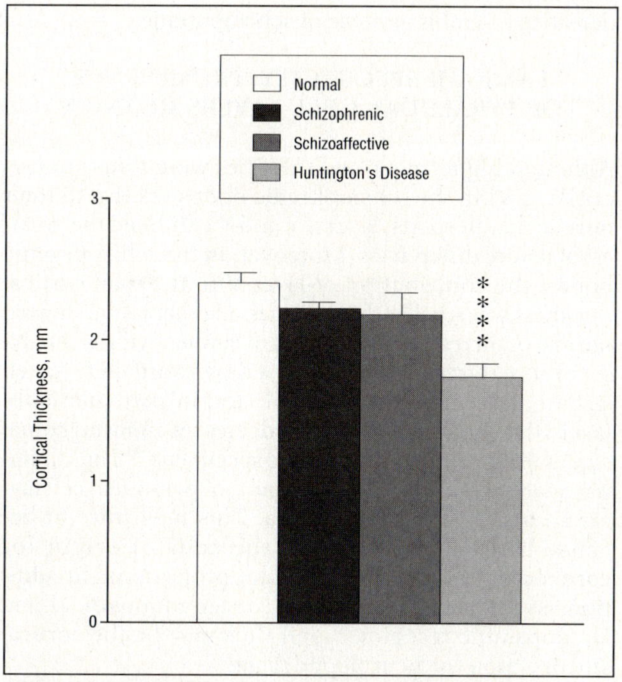

Figure 8. *Mean cortical thickness in the normal, schizophrenic, schizoaffective, and Huntington's disease groups. Cortical thickness was reduced by 8% in the schizophrenic sample and by 28% in the Huntington's disease cohort (four asterisks,* P<.001*) compared with normal brains.*

rather, layer V was reduced more than others, resulting in a change in proportion of the laminae.

Glial density, in contrast to neuronal density, was found to be sensitive to postmortem handling and storage of the brain. Lengthy PMIs and TFs had detrimental effects on glial density. Since the PMIs for the schizophrenic and normal groups were similar and were always less than 30 hours, the effect of PMI can be dismissed entirely in comparing these two groups. Mean TF was greater for the schizophrenic group than for the normal group (Table 1). Thus, an increase in glial density in schizophrenic brains may have been masked by differences in TFs for the two groups. When brains with long TFs were removed from the sample, a 22% increase in glial density was observed, although this difference did not reach significance because of the smaller sample size. It seems likely, therefore, that glial density is elevated in the schizophrenic brains. An increase in glial density would be expected in conjunction with increased neuronal density and loss of cortical volume; unchanged glial density in the schizophrenic brains would imply a loss of glial cells, a result that seems much less probable. However, the increase in density does not necessarily indicate an increase in glial cell number, as discussed below. We also considered whether the large elevation in glial density in the brains from patients with HD may have been exaggerated by the discrepancy in TF between the normal and HD groups, the latter having much shorter TFs. This appears to be so, as the increase in glial density was not quite as marked, although still robust, when brains with high TFs were eliminated from the sample.

Trend reductions were found in cortical thickness in the schizophrenic brains in both areas examined. Studies of human aging have shown that the cortex exhibits thinning with age.[38-40] However, in the present study no significant correlations were found between age and cortical thickness, perhaps because all brains were taken from individuals younger than 72 years. Moreover, age cannot account for the reduced thickness of the schizophrenic cortex in this study because the schizophrenic group was slightly younger than the normal group. Likewise, PMIs were similar between normal and schizophrenic groups, and no significant interaction between PMI or TF and cortical thickness was evident. With regard to HD, the putative effects of age must be considered negligible considering the magnitude of the reduction in thickness.

VARIABILITY IN NEURONAL DENSITY

Overall, neuronal densities for area 9 in schizophrenic brains tended to be higher than comparable densities in normal brains; however, some schizophrenic brains fell within the normal range. Several possible explanations were considered for this variability. First, the diagnosis of schizophrenia is to some degree subjective and therefore imprecise. For example, the schizophrenic brain with the lowest neuronal density in this study (CO234) was obtained from a patient who committed suicide after two brief periods of hospitalization. Had this patient lived several years past the onset of the disease, a more certain diagnosis would have been possible. Other factors relating to the heterogeneity of the disease were weighed as well. These included the duration of the illness, symptoms, presence of a family history, and previous alcohol or other drug use. However, none of these factors exhibited any obvious relationship to neuronal density. One schizophrenic patient (N29) had a computed tomographic scan that showed frontal atrophy. Somewhat surprisingly, neuronal density was not elevated in this case.

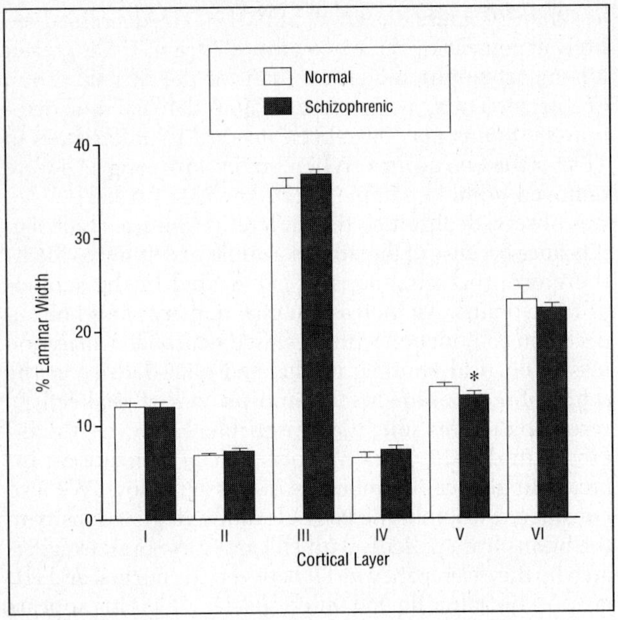

Figure 9. *The relative contributions of each cortical layer to total cortical thickness. Layer V was reduced in the schizophrenic brain (asterisk, P<.05).*

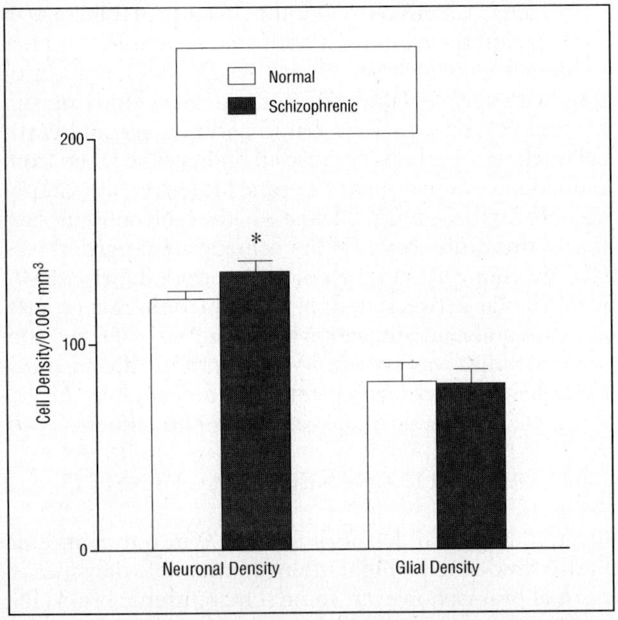

Figure 10. *Glial and neuronal density in normal and schizophrenic brains. In the schizophrenic brains, mean neuronal density was 10% higher in primary visual cortical area 17 (asterisk, P=.05), whereas mean glial density was not different from that of normal subjects.*

However, in the absence of comparable computed tomographic data on the other 15 cases, it is not possible to draw any conclusions from this lack of association.

The wide range of neuronal densities for the normal brains is more difficult to explain, especially the high neuronal densities observed in four allegedly normal brains. One possibility is that neuronal density is a predisposing factor for schizophrenia and other mental illness. Individuals with elevated neuronal density would not necessarily develop schizophrenia, since the presence of tighter cell packing is not in itself the causal factor for disease. However, these individuals might lack the reserves to cope with a second insult of presently undefined nature, ie, physical, environmental, or social, which then results in the emergence of the diseased state. This hypothesis is consistent with studies indicating that both genetic and environmental factors contribute to the development of schizophrenia.[41-43] Finally, high neuronal density may not be inherited but instead may reflect the expression of a selective vulnerability to insult.

The schizoaffective group exhibited the most pronounced variability in neuronal density of any group: while two schizoaffective brains were as dense as the densest schizophrenic brains, neuronal densities in two other schizoaffective brains were as low as the lowest normal values. This schism in values probably reflects the ill-defined nature of this disease. Some schizoaffective patients may have schizophrenia with a superimposed affective disorder, as, for example, Coryell and Zimmerman[44] showed that some patients with schizoaffective disorder carry the genetic liability for both illnesses. These brains would be expected to be at least as abnormal as those of the schizophrenics. On the other hand, Harrow and Grossman's review[45] of outcome as a function of disease suggests that the category *schizoaffective disorder* includes a mixture of patients with schizophrenia and affective disorder, the latter group having a much better clinical outcome than the schizophrenics. This notion fits well with our finding that only a subset of schizoaffective brains had high neuronal densities resembling those of schizophrenics.

LAMINAR SPECIFICITY: PROMINENCE OF PYRAMIDAL CELL LAYERS III AND V

Although higher neuronal densities were found in layers III to VI in the schizophrenic brains relative to their normal counterparts, layers IV and V exhibited the greatest absolute differences. Moreover, in the schizophrenic brains, the contribution of layer V to the total cortical thickness was smaller than normal; all other layers showed normal or increased percentages of laminar widths. Analysis of somal sizes has revealed a downward shift in cell size in all layers, with layer III, and in particular sublayer IIIc, showing significant decreases in mean somal size in these same schizophrenic specimens.[46] Thus, laminar analysis points to a prominence of pyramidal cell layers III and V in schizophrenia. This is of interest because these layers contain the cells of origin for corticocortical and corticostriatal projections. In addition, layer V also contains high concentrations of D1 and D2 dopamine receptors[47] and thus may be the cortical site of action for neuroleptic drugs.

HD: DEGENERATIVE CHANGES AND GLIOSIS

The most conspicuous feature of the HD cortex is its substantial reduction in thickness. In all nine brains from patients with HD, cortical thickness fell below the mean value for normal brains. In the brain with HD that exhibited the most marked degeneration, the cortex was 46% thinner than normal. In addition, in five of nine brains with HD, proliferation of glial cells was evident as indicated by greatly elevated glial density in these brains. Indeed, a remarkable degree of morphologic diversity was found in our cohort of brains with HD. Although all of these brains were from patients with advanced HD (grade 3 or 4) and therefore had suffered severe atrophy of the caudate nucleus,[48] their cortices ranged from nearly normal thickness and normal or even lower than normal cell density in one case, to catastrophically reduced thickness and high neuronal density. Indeed, three of nine brains had abnormally high neuronal densities, much like the schizophrenics. In the eight brains with HD for which PMI data were available, neuronal density was negatively correlated with PMI such that short PMIs (<5 months) were correlated with high neuronal density. Further studies are needed to determine whether this was a chance association. No correlation between PMI and neuronal density was apparent in the remaining sample of 42 brains in this study. If the finding of variable cerebral morphology in brains with advanced HD proves to be valid, it would suggest that progression of the disease in the cortex does not closely parallel the degenerative process in the caudate nucleus. Although the exact sequelae are not clear, the marked differences in integrity of the cortex among brains with late-stage HD indicate that there is ongoing degeneration in the cortex. This contrasts with the seemingly static picture of the cortex in schizophrenics, in which morphometric measures are much more constant across individuals irrespective of duration. Despite the similarity of many cognitive symptoms in schizophrenia and HD, the two diseases are characterized by distinct morphometric profiles. Neuronal density was not elevated in the HD sample, which instead exhibited marked cortical thinning and gliosis. Moreover, cell size analysis indicates that the gliosis observed in HD is accompanied by glial enlargement, which is not present in schizophrenia.[37]

The brains with HD serve as an interesting comparison with respect to corticostriatal involvement. In HD, the infragranular layers atrophy to a much greater extent than the supragranular layers.[49] Thus, HD resembles schizophrenia in involving layer V, the layer that contains corticostriatal cells of origin. However, in many of the HD brains, neuronal density is neither elevated overall nor increased specifically in this layer despite the much larger loss of cortical volume observed in HD relative to that found in schizophrenia. Together, the decreased cortical volume and unchanged neuronal density suggest neuronal loss in HD. Thus, as might be expected based on the catastrophic loss of target neurons in the caudate, there appears to be degeneration of prefrontal corticostriatal neurons in a subset of brains with advanced HD. At what point in the course of the disease such atrophy occurs is an interesting issue for future investigation. In contrast, corticostriatal neurons may be smaller and less viable in schizophrenics relative to normal subjects,[46] but there is currently no evidence to indicate that there are fewer of them in the schizophrenic brain.

HIGH NEURONAL DENSITY: A GLOBAL PROPERTY OF THE CEREBRAL MANTLE IN SCHIZOPHRENIA

We examined neuronal density in area 17 as an internal control, reasoning that since primary visual deficits are not part of the spectrum of symptoms associated with schizophrenia, this region would have a normal morphometric profile. Quite unexpectedly, we found abnormally high neuronal density in this area as well. Although the relative increase above normal levels in area 17 (10%) is not as great as that observed in area 9 (17%), this could result from a ceiling effect, as neuronal packing density is much higher in granular cortices than it is in prefrontal areas. Neuronal density was elevated specifically in layers III and V, suggesting that corticocortical associational connections may be targeted in this area as well.

The elevation in neuronal density in area 17 indicates that abnormally high neuronal density may be a global feature of the cerebral mantle in schizophrenia and may not be confined to regions that are associated with the core symptoms of the disease. Although a few studies have identified abnormalities in visual processing,[50-53] visual dysfunction is not a prominent feature of the schizophrenic spectrum. In this respect, elevated neuronal density seems to be dissociated from the hypofunctional state of the disease. It would be interesting in this regard to determine whether eye tracking deficits in relatives of schizophrenics are correlated with high neuronal density, since poor eye tracking is thought to be associated with a genetic predisposition for schizophrenia.[54,55]

RELEVANCE TO OTHER HISTOPATHOLOGIC STUDIES OF THE FRONTAL LOBE

The initial study by Benes et al[27] of cell density in the anterior cingulate, primary motor, and prefrontal (area 10) cortices failed to uncover differences in overall neuronal density or glial density between schizophrenic and normal brains, although decreased neuronal density was observed in specific layers in each of the three cortices. It seems unlikely that the discrepancy between that study and the present findings can be attributed to regional differences, as we have found abnormally high density in occipital and frontal cortices in our schizophrenic sample. We have also found higher neuronal density in another region of the dorsolateral prefrontal cortex, area 46 (L.D.S., G.R., and P.S.G.-R., unpublished data, December 1993). More probably, the sensitivity of our method coupled with a fairly large and diverse sample of schizophrenics has enabled us to detect significant abnormalities in neuronal density in the schizophrenic cortex. Follow-up studies by Benes et al[28] did uncover increased pyramidal cell density in layer V of prefrontal area 10, although no difference in overall pyramidal cell density in prefrontal or anterior cingulate cortices was observed, and small interneuron density was *decreased* in specific layers in both areas. Benes et al[56] suggested that the decrease in interneuron density might be caused by a loss of γ-aminobutyric acid–ergic cells, since they found increased γ-aminobutyric acid receptor binding in upper cortical layers. However, a more recent study[57] that failed to replicate the decrease in interneuron density but did find a decrease in the density of cells expressing glutamic acid decarboxylase messenger RNA suggests that differences between schizophrenic and normal brains may represent a shift in transmitter expression rather than a loss of nonpyramidal cells. The present results do not support the hypothesis that nonpyramidal cells are de-

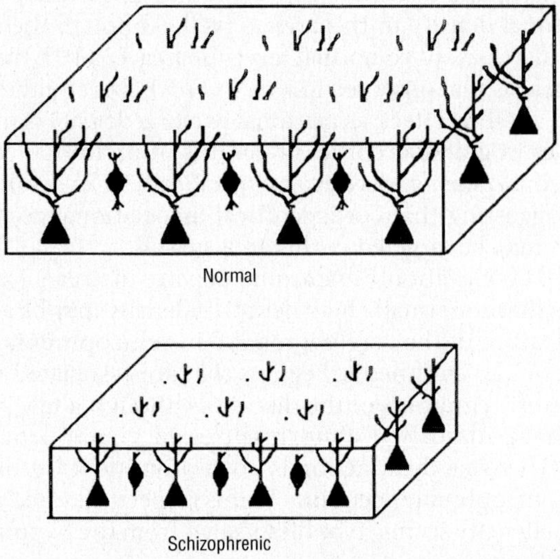

Figure 11. *Schematic diagram of the normal and schizophrenic cortices as regular arrays of pyramidal and nonpyramidal neurons. We postulate that reduction of neuropil, including dendritic arbors and axons, in the schizophrenic cortex results in a thinner cortex with cells that are more densely packed. Note that soma are depicted as being smaller in the schizophrenic cortex relative to the normal cortex, as has been found by Rajkowska et al.[46] Although the same numbers of neurons are shown in both schizophrenic and normal cortices in this figure, increased cell density could also be found in conjunction with increased or decreased cell numbers.*

creased in number, since nonpyramidal and pyramidal neurons exhibited increased density in the schizophrenic prefrontal cortex. Likewise, Daviss and Lewis[58] found increases in the density of two classes of nonpyramidal, γ-aminobutyric acid–ergic cells in the schizophrenic prefrontal cortex. The density of calbindin-stained (50% to 70%) and calretinin-stained (10% to 20%) neurons was elevated above normal levels, although the latter was not statistically significant. On the other hand, Akbarian et al[59] found in layer VI a reduced density of cells histochemically staining for nicotinamide adenine dinucleotide phosphate–diaphorase with an increased density of these cells in the deep white matter. Further studies are needed to determine whether nicotinamide adenine dinucleotide phosphate–diaphorase cells are actually missing from layer VI and perhaps displaced into the white matter, or if in fact the cells are present but contain levels of enzyme below threshold for detection.

A NEW VIEW OF THE NEUROPATHOLOGY OF SCHIZOPHRENIA: ATROPHY, NOT LOSS, OF NEURONS

Measurements of neuronal (or glial) density do not convey any information about whether more or fewer neurons (or glia) are present in the schizophrenic brain. For example, while it is possible that fewer neurons are present in the schizophrenic brain, perhaps because of degenerative processes associated with the disease, this decrease in the number of neurons would have to be coupled with a disproportionately large reduction in neuropil to translate into an increase in density of neurons. At the other extreme, it is possible to imagine a developmental abnormality that could lead to an excess production of neurons, although this scenario is difficult to reconcile with the decrease in cortical thickness. We postulate that the number of neurons does not differ between schizophrenic and normal subjects, and, indeed, Pakkenberg[60] found no difference in total cell number in the frontal lobes or the cerebral cortex as a whole. Rather, increased neuronal density could result from loss of the surrounding neuropil and a consequent shrinkage of the intraneuronal space (**Figure 11**). Our findings of decreased cortical thickness suggest that reduced neuropil is the major deficit in the schizophrenic brain.

This explanation also fits well with a substantial body of literature indicating that the frontal lobes are smaller than normal in schizophrenics. The most thoroughly documented frontal abnormality is enlargement of the anterior horn of the lateral ventricle in schizophrenic subjects.[61,62] Ventricular enlargement implies that there is a corresponding reduction in brain volume, and, in fact, the variable most often measured is ventricular-brain ratio. Although not a universal finding,[63,64] reduced volume of frontal cortex has also been reported in schizophrenic patients, with some studies suggesting that this is accounted for by smaller white-matter volumes and others finding the volumetric deficit in frontal gray matter.[65-69] Other degenerative signs, such as widening of cortical sulci and abnormal cortical markings, have been observed on computed tomographic or magnetic resonance imaging slices of schizophrenic frontal cortex.[70-72] At the molecular level, magnetic resonance spectroscopy has demonstrated a shift in the balance of anabolic and catabolic phosphorus compounds in the dorsal prefrontal cortex of schizophrenics not treated with neuroleptics, as well as chronic schizophrenic patients.[73,74] Indeed, Pettegrew et al[75] speculated that these abnormalities in membrane phospholipid equilibrium could reflect decreased neuropil in the frontal cortex. Furthermore, preliminary analysis of synaptophysin staining in the prefrontal cortex suggests that there are fewer synapses present particularly in supragranular layers in the schizophrenic brain in comparison with normal brains.[76]

Interestingly, morphometric results resembling the present findings in schizophrenic cortex have been reported after lesion studies in cats and primates and in the aged human cortex. For example, Payne et al[77] excised visual areas 17, 18, and 19 in cats and found increased neuronal density in certain layers of a visual associational area, the posteromedial lateral suprasylvian area. In studies of aged human cortex, decreases in cortical volume and cell size are found in conjunction with increased neuronal density.[78,79] These studies suggest that loss of neuropil because of either loss of afferent fibers or shrinkage of dendritic arbors may result in increased neuronal density. Furthermore, x-ray irradiation of fetal monkeys in the first trimester of gestation has been shown to cause cell death in the thalamus and consequent increased neuronal density in the cerebral cortex.[80] The results of this developmental study support the concept that a disturbance early in development may lead to a morphometric picture similar to that found in the schizophrenic cortex, since reduced cell number has been reported in the mediodorsal nucleus of the thalamus[81] and we have now found increased neuronal density in the cortical target of this thalamic nucleus. A recent report[82] of decreased thalamic volume and decreased volume of thalamoprefrontocortical tracts in schizophrenic patients on magnetic resonance images provides additional support for a thalamocortical deficit, although the findings were confined to the right hemisphere. Although it is not possible to determine whether the abnormally high neuronal density found in the schizophrenic cortex is the result of degenerative processes occurring before the onset of disease or secondary to a developmental error, the increase in neuronal density is consonant with a reduction in intraneuronal neuropil including both axons of extrinsic origin and intrinsic neuronal processes.

Accepted for publication February 22, 1995.

This work was supported by grant 44866 from the Center for the Neuroscience of Mental Disorders, National Institute of Mental Health, Rockville, Md.

Presented at the 23rd annual meeting of the Society for Neuroscience, Washington, DC, November 7, 1993.

We thank Joel E. Kleinman, MD, PhD, and Mary M. Herman, MD, of the National Institute of Mental Health Neuroscience Center for procurement of brains from the collection at St Elizabeths Hospital, as well as Dr Kleinman for his expert assistance in ascertaining an accurate diagnosis for these cases. We also acknowledge Edward D. Bird, MD, for the donation of brain specimens from the BRTC (Public Health Service grant MH/NH 31862) in Belmont, Mass, and Francine Benes for diagnosis of these cases. Ivana Delalie, MD, and Elizabeta Radonic, MD, provided valuable assistance in securing medical records for the cases from the University of Zagreb. We are grateful to the late Mahamad Haleem at the Yakovlev collection in Washington, DC, for his expert technical assistance and support for this project. Excellent technical assistance was also provided by JoAnn Coburn, Mary Pappy, John Enwright III, Justin Paquette, and Joe Musco.

Reprint requests to Section of Neurobiology, Yale University School of Medicine, 333 Cedar St, Room C-303 SHM, New Haven, CT 06510 (Dr Selemon).

REFERENCES

1. Kraepelin E; Barclay RM, Robertson GN, trans. *Dementia Praecox and Paraphrenia.* New York, NY: RE Krieger Publishing Co; 1907.
2. Alzheimer A. Beitrage zur pathologischen Anatomie der Dementia Praecox. *Allg Z Psychiatrie.* 1913;70:810-812.
3. Ingvar DH. Abnormal distribution of cerebral activity in chronic schizophrenia: a neurophysiological interpretation. In: Baxter C, Melnechuk T, eds. *Perspectives in Schizophrenia.* New York, NY: Raven Press; 1980:107.
4. Levin S. Frontal lobe dysfunctions in schizophrenia, II: impairments of psychological and brain functions. *J Psychiatry Res.* 1984;18:27-55.
5. Zec RF, Weinberger DR. Brain areas implicated in schizophrenia: a selective overview. In: Nasrallah HA, Weinberger DR, eds. *Handbook of Schizophrenia.* New York, NY: Elsevier Science Publishers BV; 1986;1:175-206.
6. Goldman-Rakic PS. Prefrontal cortical dysfunction in schizophrenia: the relevance of working memory. In: Carroll BJ, Barrett JE, eds. *Psychopathology and the Brain.* New York, NY: Raven Press; 1991:1-23.
7. Ingvar DH, Franzen G. Abnormalities of cerebral blood flow distribution in patients with chronic schizophrenia. *Acta Psychiatr Scand.* 1974;50:425-462.
8. Buchsbaum MS, Ingvar DH, Kessler R, Waters RN, Cappelletti J, van Kammen DP, King AC, Johnson JJ, Manning RG, Flynn RM, Mann LS, Bunney WE Jr, Sokoloff L. Cerebral glucography with positron tomography in normals and in patients with schizophrenia. *Arch Gen Psychiatry.* 1982;39:251-259.
9. Buchsbaum MS, DeLisi LE, Holcomb HH, Cappelletti J, King AC, Johnson J, Hazlett E, Dowling-Zimmerman S, Post RM, Morihisa J, Carpenter W, Cohen R, Pickar D, Weinberger DR, Margolin R, Kessler RM. Anteroposterior gradients in cerebral glucose use in schizophrenia and affective disorders. *Arch Gen Psychiatry.* 1984;41:1159-1166.
10. Ariel RN, Golden CJ, Berg RA, Quaife MA, Dirkson JW, Forsell T, Wilson J, Graber B. Regional cerebral blood flow in schizophrenics. *Arch Gen Psychiatry.* 1883;40:258-263.
11. Farkas T, Wolf AP, Jaeger J, Brodie JD, Christman DR, Fowler JS. Regional brain glucose metabolism in chronic schizophrenia: a positron emission transaxial tomographic study. *Arch Gen Psychiatry.* 1984;41:293-300.
12. Kurachi M, Kobayashi K, Matsubara R, Hiramatsu H, Yamaguchi N, Matsuda H, Maeda T, Hisada K. Regional cerebral blood flow in schizophrenic disorders. *Eur Neurol.* 1985;24:176-181.
13. Chabrol H, Guell A, Bes A, Moron P. Cerebral blood flow in schizophrenic adolescents. *Am J Psychiatry.* 1986;143:130.
14. Guenther W, Moser E, Mueller-Spahn F, von Oefele K, Buell U, Hippius H. Pathological cerebral blood flow during motor function in schizophrenic and endogenous depressed patients. *Biol Psychiatry.* 1986;21:889-899.
15. Volkow ND, Wolf AP, van Gelder P, Brodie P, Overall JE, Cancro R, Gomez-Mont F. Phenomenological correlates of metabolic activity in 18 patients with chronic schizophrenia. *Am J Psychiatry.* 1987;144:151-158.
16. Mathew RJ, Wilson WH, Tant SR, Robinson L, Prakash R. Abnormal resting regional cerebral blood flow patterns and their correlates in schizophrenia. *Arch Gen Psychiatry.* 1988;45:542-549.
17. Wolkin A, Angrist B, Wolf A, Brodie JD, Wolkin B, Jaeger J, Cancro R, Rotrosen J. Low frontal glucose utilization in chronic schizophrenia: a replication study. *Am J Psychiatry.* 1988;145:251-253.
18. Paulman RG, Devous MD, Gregory RR, Herman JH, Jennings L, Bonte FJ, Nasrallah HA, Raese JD. Hypofrontality and cognitive impairment in schizophrenia: dynamic single-photon tomography and neuropsychological assessment of schizophrenic brain function. *Biol Psychiatry.* 1990;27:377-399.
19. Sagawa K, Kawakatsu S, Shibuya I, Oiji A, Morinobu S, Komatani A, Yazaki M, Totsuka S. Correlation of regional cerebral blood flow with performance on neuropsychological tests in schizophrenic patients. *Schizophr Bull.* 1990;3:241-246.
20. Goldman-Rakic PS. Circuitry of the prefrontal cortex and the regulation of behavior by representational memory. In: Plum F, Mountcastle V, eds. *Handbook of Physiology.* Bethesda, Md: American Physiological Society; 1987;5(pt 1):373-417.
21. Devous MD Sr, Raese JD, Herman JH, Paulman RG, Gregory RR, Rush AJ, Chehabi HH, Bonte FJ. Regional cerebral blood flow in schizophrenic patients at rest and during Wisconsin Card Sort tasks. *J Cereb Blood Flow Metab.* 1985; 5(suppl 1):S201-S202.
22. Berman KF, Zec RF, Weinberger DR. Physiological dysfunction of dorsolateral prefrontal cortex in schizophrenia, II: role of neuroleptic treatment, attention, and mental effort. *Arch Gen Psychiatry.* 1986;43:126-135.
23. Weinberger DR, Berman KF, Zec RF. Physiological dysfunction of dorsolateral prefrontal cortex in schizophrenia, I: regional cerebral blood flow (rCBF) evidence. *Arch Gen Psychiatry.* 1986;43:114-124.
24. Weinberger DR, Berman KF, Illowsky BP. Physiological dysfunction of dorsolateral prefrontal cortex in schizophrenia, III: a new cohort and evidence for a monoaminergic mechanism. *Arch Gen Psychiatry.* 1988;45:609-615.
25. Buchsbaum MS, Nuechterlein KH, Haier RJ, Wu J, Sicotte N, Hazlett E, Asarnow R, Potkin S, Guich S. Glucose metabolic rate in normals and schizophrenics during the Continuous Performance Test assessed by positron emission tomography. *Br J Psychiatry.* 1990;156:216-227.
26. Andreasen NC, Rezai K, Alliger R, Swayze VW II, Flaum M, Kirchner P, Cohen G, O'Leary DS. Hypofrontality in neuroleptic-naive patients and in patients with chronic schizophrenia: assessment with xenon 133 single-photon emission computed tomography and the Tower of London. *Arch Gen Psychiatry.* 1992;49:943-958.
27. Benes FM, Davidson J, Bird ED. Quantitative cytoarchitectural studies of the cerebral cortex of schizophrenics. *Arch Gen Psychiatry.* 1986;43:31-35.
28. Benes FM, McSparren J, Bird ED, SanGiovanni JP, Vincent SL. Deficits in small interneurons in prefrontal and cingulate cortices of schizophrenic and schizoaffective patients. *Arch Gen Psychiatry.* 1991;48:996-1001.
29. Akbarian S, Kim JJ, Tafazolli A, Hagman JO, Potkin SG, Bunney WE Jr, Jones EG. Altered neurocellular composition of prefrontal cortex in schizophrenia. *Soc Neurosci Abstr.* 1993;19:200. Abstract.
30. Abercrombie M. Estimation of nuclear population from microtome sections. *Anat Rec.* 1946;94:239-247.
31. Williams RW, Rakic P. Three-dimensional counting: an accurate and direct method to estimate numbers of cells in sectioned material. *J Comp Neurol.* 1988;278: 344-352.
32. Fedio P, Cox CS, Neophytides A, Canal-Frederick G, Chase TN. Neuropsychological profile of Huntington's disease: patients and those at risk. *Adv Neurol.*

1979;23:239-255.
33. Weinberger DR, Berman KF, Iadarola M, Driesen N, Zec RF. Prefrontal cortical blood flow and cognitive function in Huntington's disease. *J Neurol Neurosurg Psychiatry.* 1988;51:94-104.
34. Feigner JP, Robins E, Guze SB, Woodruff RA, Winokur G, Munoz R. Diagnostic criteria for psychiatric research. *Arch Gen Psychiatry.* 1972;26:57-63.
35. Rajkowska G, Goldman-Rakic PS. Cytoarchitectonic definition of prefrontal areas in the normal human cortex, I: remapping of areas 9 and 46 using quantitative criteria. *Cereb Cortex.* 1995;5:307-322.
36. Rajkowska G, Goldman-Rakic PS. Cytoarchitectonic definition of prefrontal areas in the normal human cortex, II: variability in locations of areas 9 and 46 and relationship to the Talairach coordinate system. *Cereb Cortex.* 1995;5:323-337.
37. Rajkowska G, Selemon LD, Goldman-Rakic PS. Reduction in neuronal sizes in prefrontal cortex of schizophrenics and Huntington patients. *Schizophr Res.* 1995;15:31. Abstract.
38. Terry RD, DeTeresa R, Hansen LA. Neocortical cell counts in normal human adult aging. *Ann Neurol.* 1987;21:530-539.
39. Jernigan TL, Press GA, Hesselink JR. Methods for measuring brain morphologic features on magnetic resonance images: validation and normal aging. *Arch Neurol.* 1990;47:27-32.
40. Coffey CE, Wilkinson WE, Parashos IA, Soady SAR, Sullivan RJ, Patterson LJ, Figiel GS, Webb MC, Spritzer CE, Djang WT. Quantitative cerebral anatomy of the aging human brain: a cross-sectional study using magnetic resonance imaging. *Neurology.* 1992;42:527-536.
41. DeLisi LE, Goldin LR, Maxwell ME, Kazuba DM, Gershon ES. Clinical features of illness in siblings with schizophrenia or schizoaffective disorder. *Arch Gen Psychiatry.* 1987;44:891-896.
42. Schulsinger F, Parnas J, Mednick S, Teasdale TW, Schulsinger H. Heredity-environment interaction and schizophrenia. *J Psychiatr Res.* 1987;21:431-436.
43. Cannon TD, Mednick SA, Parnas J, Schulsinger F, Praestholm J, Vestergaard A. Developmental brain abnormalities in the offspring of schizophrenic mothers. *Arch Gen Psychiatry.* 1993;50:551-564.
44. Coryell W, Zimmerman M. The heritability of schizophrenia and schizoaffective disorder: a family study. *Arch Gen Psychiatry.* 1988;45:323-327.
45. Harrow M, Grossman LS. Outcome in schizoaffective disorders: a critical review and reevaluation of the literature. *Schizophr Bull.* 1984;10:87-108.
46. Rajkowska G, Selemon LD, Goldman-Rakic PS. Reduction in neuronal sizes in prefrontal cortex of schizophrenics and Huntington patients. *Soc Neurosci Abstr.* 1994;20:620. Abstract.
47. Goldman-Rakic PS, Lidow M, Gallager DW. Overlap of dopaminergic, adrenergic, and serotinergic receptor and complementarity of their subtypes in the primate prefrontal cortex. *J Neurosci.* 1990;10:2125-2138.
48. Vonsattel J-P, Myers RH, Stevens TJ, Ferrante RJ, Bird ED, Richardson EP Jr. Neuropathological classification of Huntington's disease. *J Neuropathol Exp Neurol.* 1985;44:559-577.
49. Rajkowska G, Selemon LD, Goldman-Rakic PS. Morphometric evidence for prefrontal cellular atrophy in advanced Huntington's disease. *Soc Neurosci Abstr.* 1993;19:838. Abstract.
50. Jibiki I, Takizawa Y, Yamaguchi N. Visual dysfunction in treated schizophrenia suggested by visual evoked potentials from pattern-reversal stimulation. *Eur Psychiatry Clin Neurosci.* 1991;241:61-64.
51. Lewis SW, Ford RA, Syed GM, Reveley AM, Toone BK. A controlled study of ^{99m}Tc-HMPAO single-photon emission imaging in chronic schizophrenia. *Psychol Med.* 1992;22:27-33.
52. Javitt DC, Doneshka P, Zylberman I, Ritter W, Vaughan HG Jr. Impairment of early cortical processing in schizophrenia: an event related potential confirmation study. *Biol Psychiatry.* 1993;33:513-519.
53. Renshaw PF, Yurgellen-Todd DA, Cohen BM. Greater hemodynamic response to photic stimulation in schizophrenic patients: an echo-planar MRI study. *Am J Psychiatry.* 1994;151:1493-1495.
54. Grove WM, Clementz BA, Iacono WG, Katsanis J. Smooth pursuit ocular motor dysfunction in schizophrenia: evidence for a major gene. *Am J Psychiatry.* 1992;149:1362-1368.
55. Holzman PS. Behavioral markers of schizophrenia useful for genetic studies. *J Psychiatry Res.* 1992;26:427-445.
56. Benes FM, Vincent SL, Alsterberg G, Bird ED, SanGiovanni JP. Increased $GABA_A$ receptor binding in superficial layers of cingulate cortex in schizophrenics. *J Neurosci.* 1992;12:924-929.
57. Bunney WE Jr, Akbarian S, Kim JJ, Hagman JO, Potkin SG, Jones EG. Gene expression for glutamic acid decarboxylase is reduced in prefrontal cortex of schizophrenics. *Soc Neurosci Abstr.* 1993;19:199. Abstract.
58. Daviss SR, Lewis DA. Calbindin- and calretinin-immunoreactive local circuit neurons are increased in density in the prefrontal cortex of schizophrenic subjects. *Soc Neurosci Abstr.* 1993;19:201. Abstract.
59. Akbarian S, Bunney WE Jr, Potkin SG, Wigal SB, Hagman JO, Sandman CA, Jones EG. Altered distribution of nicotinamide-adenine dinucleotide phosphate-diaphorase cells in frontal lobe of schizophrenics implies disturbances of cortical development. *Arch Gen Psychiatry.* 1993;50:169-177.
60. Pakkenberg B. Total nerve cell number in neocortex in chronic schizophrenic and controls estimated using optical disectors. *Biol Psychiatry.* 1993;34:768-772.
61. Brown R, Colter N, Corsellis JAN, Crow TJ, Frith CD, Jagoe R, Johnstone EC, Marsh L. Postmortem evidence of structural brain changes in schizophrenia: differences in brain weight, temporal horn area, and parahippocampal gyrus compared with affective disorder. *Arch Gen Psychiatry.* 1986;43:36-42.
62. Shiraishi H, Koizume J, Ofudu K, Suzuki T, Saito K, Hori T, Ikuta T, Kase K, Hori M. Enlargement of the anterior horn of the lateral ventricle in schizophrenic pateints: chronological and morphometrical studies. *Jpn J Psychiatry.* 1990;44:693-702.
63. McCarley RW, Shenton ME, O'Donnell BF, Faux SF, Kikinis R, Nestor PG, Jolesz FA. Auditory P300 abnormalities and left posterior superior temporal gyrus. *Arch Gen Psychiatry.* 1993;50:190-197.
64. Kelsoe JR Jr, Cadet JL, Pickar D, Weinberger DL. Quantitative neuroanatomy in schizophrenia: a controlled magnetic resonance imaging study. *Arch Gen Psychiatry.* 1988;45:533-541.
65. Breier A, Buchanan RW, Elkashef A, Munson RC, Kirkpatrick B, Gellad F. Brain morphology and schizophrenia: a magnetic resonance imaging study of limbic, prefrontal cortex, and caudate structures. *Arch Gen Psychiatry.* 1992;49:921-926.
66. Raine A, Lencz T, Reynolds GP, Harrison G, Sheard C, Medley I, Reynolds LM, Cooper JE. An evaluation of structural and functional prefrontal deficits in schizophrenia: MRI and neuropsychological measures. *Psychiatr Res Neuroimaging.* 1992;45:123-137.
67. Zipursky RB, Lim KO, Sullivan EV, Brown BW, Pfefferbaum A. Widespread cerebral gray matter volume deficits in schizophrenia. *Arch Gen Psychiatry.* 1992; 42:195-205.
68. Friedman L, Knudsen L, Shurell M, Meltzer HY. Prefrontal sulcal prominence is inversely related to response to clozapine. *Biol Psychiatry.* 1993;33:513-519.
69. Andreasen NC, Flashman L, O'Leary DS, Flaum M, Swayze V. Decreased frontal lobe size in schizophrenia measured with volumetric magnetic resonance (MR) imaging. *Soc Neurosci Abstr.* 1994;20:24. Abstract.
70. Shelton RC, Karson CN, Doran AR, Pickar D, Bigelow LB, Weinberger DR. Cerebral structural pathology in schizophrenia: evidence for a selective prefrontal cortical defect. *Am J Psychiatry.* 1988;145:154-163.
71. Doran AR, Boronow J, Weinberger DR, Wolkowitz OM, Breier A, Pickar D. Structural brain pathology in schizophrenia revisited: prefrontal cortex pathology is inversely correlated with cerebrospinal fluid levels of homovanillic acid. *Neuropsychopharmacology.* 1987;1:25-32.
72. Lieberman J, Bogerts B, Degreef G, Ashtari M, Lantos G, Alvir J. Qualitative assessment of brain morphology in acute and chronic schizophrenia. *Am J Psychiatry.* 1992;149:784-794.
73. Pettegrew JW, Keshavan MS, Panchalingam K, Strychor S, Kaplan DB, Tretta MG, Allen M. Alterations in brain high-energy phosphate and membraine phospholipid metabolism in first-episode, drug-naive schizophrenics: a pilot study of the dorsal prefrontal cortex by in vivo phosphorus 31 nuclear magnetic resonance spectroscopy. *Arch Gen Psychiatry.* 1991;48:563-568.
74. Fujimoto T, Nakano T, Takano T, Hokazono Y, Asakura T, Tsuji T. Study of chronic schizophrenics using ^{31}P magnetic resonance chemical shift imaging. *Acta Psychiatr Scand.* 1992;86:455-462.
75. Pettegrew JW, Keshavan MS, Minshew NJ. 31P nuclear magnetic resonance spectroscopy: neurodevelopment and schizophrenia. *Schizophr Bull.* 1993;19:35-53.
76. Glantz LA, Lewis DA. Synaptophysin immunoreactivity is selectively decreased in the prefrontal cortex of schizophrenic subjects. *Soc Neurosci Abstr.* 1993; 19:201. Abstract.
77. Payne BR, Conners C, Cornwell P. Survival and death of neurons in cortical area PMLS after removal of areas 17, 18 and 19 in cats and kittens. *Cereb Cortex.* 1991;1:469-491.
78. Haug H, Kuhl S, Mecke E, Sass N-L, Wasner K. The significance of morphometric procedures in the investigation of age changes in cytoarchitectonic structures of human brain. *J Hirnforschung.* 1984;25:353-374.
79. Haug H, Eggers R. Morphometry of the human cortex cerebri and corpus striatum during aging. *Neurobiol Aging.* 1991;12:336-338.
80. Algan O, Goldman-Rakic PS, Rakic P. Selective laminar and areal deletion of cortical neurons by prenatal x-irradiation in the macaque monkey. *Soc Neurosci Abstr.* 1992;17:1146. Abstract.
81. Pakkenberg B. Pronounced reduction of nerve cell number in mediodorsal thalamic nucleus and nucleus accumbens in schizophrenics. *J Neurol Neurosurg Psychiatry.* 1990;47:1023-1028.
82. Andreasen NC, Arndt S, Swayze V II, Cizadlo T, Flaum M, O'Leary D, Ehrhardt JC, Yuh WTC. Thalamic abnormalities in schizophrenia visualized through magnetic resonance image averaging. *Science.* 1994;266:294-298.

COMMENTARY

Neocortical Abnormalities in Schizophrenia

THE HISTORY of the study of brains of individuals with schizophrenia is replete with novel, fragmentary, and even occasionally enticing findings, if any positive results were obtained at all. Most of these findings have proved to be elusive when replications have been attempted. In fact, the most consistent finding in studies of the brains of persons with schizophrenia is that they are usually not distinguishable from the brains of normal individuals. However, over the last 15

See also page 805

years, a literature has been slowly accumulating in two scientific arenas, structural brain imaging and functional brain imaging. Studies of the structure of schizophrenic brains (via computed tomographic or magnetic resonance imaging scans) have produced a subtle but increasingly reliable set of observations. Such studies have often pointed toward ventricular enlargement, sulcal widening, and cortical atrophy, with occasional suggestions of left temporal lobe, frontal lobe, and thalamic atrophy.[1-4] Functional in vivo imaging studies have demonstrated hypofunction of the prefrontal cortex and other regions of limbic cortex.[5-10] These two lines of noninvasive imaging studies, coupled with dramatic technical improvements in the tools and paradigms for studying the cellular level structure of brain, have recently led to a new generation of histological studies of the brains of schizophrenic individuals.

In the article by Selemon et al in this issue of the ARCHIVES,[11] we see an excellent example of the strategies, methods, and precision needed to begin to appreciate the structural differences between the brains of individuals with schizophrenia and controls. Briefly, these investigators have studied two areas of cortex (Brodmann's areas 9 and 17) using recently developed but labor-intensive three-dimensional quantitative analytic tools to estimate cellular densities in four groups of subjects (patients with schizophrenia, normal subjects, patients with schizoaffective disorder, and those with Huntington's disease). They report that

> increased neuronal density was found in prefrontal area 9 (17%) and occipital area 17 (10%) in schizophrenic brains. In area 9, neuronal density was increased in layers III to IV; cell packing of pyramidal and nonpyramidal neurons was elevated.

Yet they also report a nonsignificant reduction in the thickness of cortex in these schizophrenic brains, "with a disproportionate reduction in layer V in area 9," leading the authors to conclude that "neuronal atrophy is the [possible] anatomic substrate for deficient information processing in schizophrenia."

To restate the authors' observations and conclusions: the density of neurons in cortical areas 9 and 17 is between 10% and 17% higher in brains of schizophrenic subjects than in those of controls, yet in spite of this increased density, the cortical thickness is modestly reduced. How can this be, greater density in less cortex? The answer appears to reside in an understanding of the composition of cortex. The thickness of cortex is the result of all of its cell types (neuron, both pyramidal and nonpyramidal, and glial elements) as well as the fibers that connect neurons—both locally and over large distances. The authors report similar numbers of neurons that are packed more tightly, with a generally thinner cortex. They speculate that the reduction in thickness results from fewer connections between neurons (reduced neuropil), hence allowing cells to be packed more closely together. The actual change in total cortical thickness is modest (7%). Their conclusion that "neuronal atrophy is the anatomic substrate for deficient information processing in schizophrenia" is best understood when one realizes what is atrophied. The authors refer to a reduction in the richness of the dendritic trees, synapses, and axonal ramifications of these cortical neurons, not to a loss of the entire neuron. In effect, they argue that schizophrenia is associated with (or perhaps "caused by"—our words) a "miswired" cortex, a hypothesis that has enjoyed popularity from time to time.[12] The importance of the work by Selemon et al derives from the fact that, for once, such an inference is based on a reasonably solid empirical base. It is not overtly speculative, but grew naturally from the data. Such an inference, and the data it grew from, need both confirmation and expansion. It is unclear what causes this hypothesized cortical miswiring. Is it a defective developmental or genetic signal? Could it be an early viral insult? or a degenerative process? All three types of explanations (genetic-developmental, infectious, or degenerative) are possible.

In our view, the importance of the article by Selemon et al is threefold. (1) It provides potentially important insights in and of itself. It is an excellent example of the care and technical precision required for the productive study of the brains of individuals with schizophrenia. (2) At a broader level, it is representative of an entire set of exciting studies by several groups approaching similar problems in schizophrenia. (3) Finally, it speaks to the nature of the structural and likely biochemical anomalies associated with this disease.

The conclusions of their article are generally supported in other histological and noninvasive imaging studies. Studies of frontal lobe size, blood flow, and metabolic activity are all compatible with the interpretation of a modest decrease in cortical thickness.[9,10,13-15] Estimates of synaptic density (via synaptophysin staining) in the prefontal cortex also suggest that schizophrenic subjects have fewer synapses than controls.[16] Other types of analyses are supportive of a general cortical miswiring in schizophrenia as well. In a series of articles, Benes and her collaborators,[17] have found a decrease in the number of interneurons in cingulate cortex in Brodmann area 10 of schizophrenic prefrontal cortex. Equally suggestive is a set of observations by Akbarian et al,[18] in which nicotinamide-adenine dinucleotide phosphate diaphorase–positive cells are incorrectly located in cortex and are hypothesized to migrate improperly from the cortical subplate into the cortex during development. In a more recent article, Akbarian et al[19] have shown a substantial decrease in the number of glutamic acid decarboxylase messenger RNA–positive neurons throughout schizophrenic cortex. In their work, Akbarian and coauthors tend to support the suggestion that this is a general cortical problem and is not unique to prefrontal areas.

Still, it must be admitted that while these and other studies contribute to a cortical miswiring hypothesis of schizophrenia, none of the work is definitive. Each observation is encouraging, but in no case is there widespread confirmation of the data. It is critical for the acceptance of these studies and the growth of the field of the neuropathology of schizophrenia for investigators to begin to share protocols, samples, and technical expertise. When a substantial set of collaborative studies can confirm this set of cortical findings in schizophrenia and are able to link them to each other, then the field will meet with broader acceptance and a new level of understanding of schizophrenia and the functions of human cortex will have been achieved. We believe the next generation of investigations will begin to meet this need.

Stanley J. Watson, PhD, MD
James H. Meador-Woodruff, MD
Department of Psychiatry and Mental Health Research Institute
University of Michigan
205 Zina Pitcher Pl
Ann Arbor, MI 48109-0720

REFERENCES

1. Shenton ME, Kikinis R, Jolesz FA, Pollak SD, LeMay M, Wible CG, Hokama H, Martin J, Metcalf D, Coleman M, McCarley RW. Abnormalities of the left temporal lobe and thought disorder in schizophrenia: a quantitative magnetic resonance imaging study. *N Engl J Med.* 1992; 327:604-612.
2. Breier A, Buchanan RW, Elkashef A, Munson RC, Kirkpatrick B, Gellad F. Brain morphology and schizophrenia: a magnetic resonance imaging study of limbic, prefrontal cortex, and caudate structures. *Arch Gen Psychiatry.* 1992;49:921-926.
3. Jernigan TL, Zisook S, Heaton RK, Moranville JT, Hesselink J, Braff DL. Magnetic resonance imaging abnormalities in lenticular nuclei and cerebral cortex in schizophrenia. *Arch Gen Psychiatry.* 1991;48:881-890.
4. Harvey I, Ron MA, DuBoulay G, Wicks D, Lewis SW, Murray RM. Reduction of cortical volume in schizophrenia on magnetic resonance imaging. *Psychol Med.* 1993;23:591-604.
5. Berman KF, Illowsky BP, Weinberger DR. Physiological dysfunction of dorsolateral prefrontal cortex in schizophrenia, IV: further evidence for regional and behavioral specificity. *Arch Gen Psychiatry.* 1988;45:616-622.
6. Weinberger DR, Berman KF, Illowsky BP. Physiological dysfunction of dorsolateral prefrontal cortex in schizophrenia, III: a new cohort and evidence for a monoaminergic mechanism. *Arch Gen Psychiatry.* 1988;45:609-615.
7. Tamminga CA, Thaker GK, Buchanan R, Kirkpatrick B, Alphs LD, Chase TN, Carpenter WT. Limbic system abnormalities identified in schizophrenia using positron emission tomography with fluorodeoxyglucose and neocortical alterations with deficit syndrome. *Arch Gen Psychiatry.* 1992; 49:522-530.
8. Friston KJ, Liddle PF, Frith CD, Hirsch SR, Frackowiak RSJ. The left medial temporal region and schizophrenia: a PET study. *Brain.* 1992;115: 367-382.
9. Pettegrew JW, Keshavan MS, Panchalingam K, Strychor S, Kaplan DB, Tretta MG, Allen M. Alterations in brain high-energy phosphate and membrane phospholipid metabolism in first-episode, drug-naive schizophrenics: a pilot study of the dorsal prefrontal cortex by in vivo phosphorus 31 nuclear magnetic resonance spectroscopy. *Arch Gen Psychiatry.* 1991;48:563-568.
10. Fugimoto T, Nakano T, Hokazono Y, Asakura T, Tsuji T. Study of chronic schizophrenics using ^{31}P magnetic resonance chemical shift imaging. *Acta Psychiatr Scand.* 1992;86:455-462.
11. Selemon LD, Rajkowska G, Goldman-Rakic PS. Abnormally high neuronal density in the schizophrenic cortex: a morphometric analysis of prefrontal area 9 and occipital area 17. *Arch Gen Psychiatry.* 1995;52:805-818.
12. Feinberg I. Schizophrenia: caused by a fault in programmed synaptic elimination during adolescence? *J Psychiatr Res.* 1982-83;17:319-334.
13. Andreasen NC, Arndt S, Swayze V II, Cizadlo T, Flaum M, O'Leary D, Ehrhardt JC, Yuh WTC. Thalamic abnormalities in schizophrenia visualized through magnetic resonance image averaging. *Science.* 1994;266:294-298.
14. Zipursky RB, Lim KO, Sullivan EV, Brown BW, Pfefferbaum A. Widespread cerebral gray matter volume deficits in schizophrenia. *Arch Gen Psychiatry.* 1992;49:195-205.
15. Raine A, Lencz T, Reynolds GP, Harrison G, Sheard C, Medley I, Reynolds LM, Cooper JE. An evaluation of structural and functional prefrontal deficits in schizophrenia: MRI and neuropsychological measures. *Psychiatry Res.* 1992;45:123-137.
16. Glantz LA, Lewis DA. Synaptic immunoreactivity is selectively deceased in the prefrontal cortex of schizophrenic subjects. *Soc Neurosci Abst.* 1993; 19:201.
17. Benes FM, McSparren J, Bird ED, Sangiovanni JP, Vincent SL. Deficits in small interneurons in prefrontal and cingulate cortices of schizophrenic and schizoaffective patients. *Arch Gen Psychiatry.* 1991;48:996-1001.
18. Akbarian S, Bunney WE Jr, Potkin SC, Wigal SB, Hagman JO, Sandman CA, Jones EG. Altered distribution of nicotinamide-adenine dinucleotide phosphate-diaphorase cells in frontal lobe of schizophrenics implies disturbances of cortical development. *Arch Gen Psychiatry.* 1993;50:169-177.
19. Akbarian S, Kim JJ, Potkin SG, Hagman JO, Tafazzoli A, Bunney WE Jr, Jones EG. Gene expression for glutamic acid decarboxylase is reduced without loss of neurons in prefrontal cortex of schizophrenics. *Arch Gen Psychiatry.* 1995;52: 258-278.

ORIGINAL ARTICLE

Spatial Working Memory Deficits in the Relatives of Schizophrenic Patients

Sohee Park, PhD; Philip S. Holzman, PhD; Patricia S. Goldman-Rakic, PhD

Background: Studies in nonhuman primates provide evidence that intact spatial working memory depends on the integrity of specific areas in the prefrontal cortex. Patients with schizophrenia have been shown to be impaired on spatial working memory tasks. Relatives of schizophrenic patients show a range of cognitive deficits in the absence of clinical symptoms (eg, thought disorder, eye tracking dysfunctions). We predicted that a significant proportion of relatives of schizophrenic patients would show deficits in working memory as measured by a delayed response task.

Methods: In experiment 1, we tested 18 schizophrenic patients, 15 first-degree relatives of schizophrenic patients, and 18 normal control subjects on an oculomotor delayed response task. In experiment 2, we assessed the performance of another group of 12 first-degree relatives of schizophrenic patients and 16 different normal control subjects on a visual-manual delayed response task.

Results: Relatives of schizophrenic patients showed significant deficits in working memory on both the oculomotor and visual-manual delayed response tasks.

Conclusions: Some relatives of schizophrenic patients are impaired on tasks that tap spatial working memory and that implicate the prefrontal system. The delayed response paradigm may be useful in elucidating the multidimensionality of the schizophrenic phenotype.

(Arch Gen Psychiatry. 1995;52:821-828)

One of the cognitive deficits of schizophrenia is a dysfunction of working memory that leads to a breakdown of behaviors guided by internal representations.[1,2] Neuroanatomical and neurophysiological observations assign an important role to the prefrontal cortex in working memory deficits.[3-6] In the rhesus monkey, lesions in the dorsolateral prefrontal cortex, in particular, the region of the principal sulcus, lead both to severe deficits in spatial working memory, as assessed by various delayed response tasks (DRTs), and to some symptoms that resemble those of schizophrenia, such as distractibility and perseveration.

In an earlier study,[2] we developed a human analogue of the oculomotor delayed response paradigm to test whether schizophrenic patients show spatial working memory deficits. We reported that schizophrenic inpatients were significantly impaired on a memory-guided DRT, whether the sensory modality was visual or haptic, but showed almost no impairment on a sensory-guided DRT. Bipolar inpatients, in contrast, showed no impairments on the memory-guided DRT. We concluded that (1) schizophrenic inpatients have a deficit in the representational guidance of behavior that is independent of the motor system itself and (2) this impairment is not restricted to the oculomotor system. The working memory deficit, as assessed by the memory-guided DRT, is consistent with evidence that implicates prefrontal dysfunction in schizophrenia. Schizophrenic outpatients in remission were also found to have deficits on the oculomotor DRT.[7]

Some of the healthy relatives of schizophrenic patients show some traits related to schizophrenia. For example, a disorder of smooth-pursuit eye movements is present in nearly half of the first-degree relatives of schizophrenic patients in the absence of clinical symptoms of schizophrenia, whereas the prevalence of this eye tracking dysfunction in the normal population is only about 8%.[8,9] Similarly, a significant elevation of thought disorder in about half of the first-degree relatives has also been reported.[10] The existence of eye tracking dysfunction and thought disorder in a substantial proportion of these relatives cannot be attributed to medication effects, to the effects of the illness itself, or to

From the Department of Psychology and Institute of Neuroscience, Northwestern University, Evanston, Ill (Dr Park); the Department of Psychology, Harvard University, Cambridge, Mass, and the Laboratory of Psychology, McLean Hospital, Belmont, Mass (Dr Holzman); and the Section of Neurobiology, Yale University School of Medicine, New Haven, Conn (Dr Goldman-Rakic).

generalized deficit. If relatives of schizophrenic patients also show working memory deficits, it would suggest that these deficits are likely to reflect a behavioral trait rather than an effect of illness or its treatment.

A related approach is to study individuals with schizotypal personality characteristics.[11] Both the study of relatives of schizophrenic patients and the study of people with schizotypic traits address the additional issue of latent liability for schizophrenia, an issue that is relevant to genetic transmission.[12,13]

This study examined whether working memory is impaired in a sample of first-degree relatives of schizophrenic patients. We predicted that, as a group, relatives would perform better than the schizophrenic patients but worse than the normal controls on the spatial DRT but that there would be no impairment on a sensory control task.

Two experiments were carried out to test these predictions. In experiment 1, subjects were tested on both the oculomotor memory and sensory DRT. For experiment 2, a replication, we recruited two new groups of subjects (relatives and controls) and tested them on a visual-manual version of the memory and sensory DRT. If first-degree relatives of schizophrenic patients have a working memory deficit, it should be possible to detect it, regardless of the response modality of the DRT.

EXPERIMENT 1: OCULOMOTOR DRT

Subjects

Fifteen first-degree relatives of schizophrenic patients and 18 outpatients with schizophrenia were recruited from a private psychiatric hospital. The sample of relatives included nine family members of five of the schizophrenic outpatients in this study. Six other relatives were also first-degree relatives of schizophrenic patients (one relative per patient), but these six relatives were not related to the probands in the present study. Results from the schizophrenic outpatients have already been reported[7] and are repeated here only for comparison purposes. Eighteen normal control subjects with no history of schizophrenia, bipolar disorder depression, anxiety disorders, or drug abuse or dependence were also recruited and screened for absence of mental illness (Axis I disorders) in themselves and in their first- and second-degree relatives. All subjects were reimbursed for their participation. The patients met criteria for a *DSM-III-R* diagnosis of schizophrenia, based on a standardized interview (Structured Clinical Interview for *DSM-III-R*[14]) and a review of hospital medical records. None of the relatives of schizophrenic patients had a *DSM-III-R* Axis I diagnosis, as determined from a clinical interview. They were not screened for Axis II conditions. All of the relatives were working full-time. All schizophrenic patients were taking neuroleptic medication. Subjects had no evidence of organic brain damage and were not mentally retarded. The mean (SD) age of the relatives was 35.7 (8.6) years, their mean education was 15.6 (1.9) years, and their mean Wechsler Adult Intelligence Scale (WAIS)–verbal IQ score was 108.0 (1.6). The mean age of the outpatients with schizophrenia was 34.6 (8.7) years, their mean education was 14.2 (2.1) years, and their mean WAIS–verbal IQ score was 105.0 (12.5). The mean age of the normal control subjects was 29.4 (8.6) years, their mean education was 14.7 (2.8) years, and their mean WAIS–verbal IQ score was 112.0 (10.9). There were no statistically significant differences between the three groups in age, WAIS–verbal IQ score, or education level, nor was there any effect of these variables on the principal dependent variables of the DRTs.

Oculomotor DRT

Apparatus. An infrared eye monitoring system (Iscan Inc, Cambridge, Mass), which tracks the difference between the pupil and corneal reflections, was used. An infrared light source was placed in front of the stimulus display monitor, facing the subject. The reflected infrared light from the right eye of the subject was recorded by a video camera with an infrared filter. The video camera was connected to an Iscan RK-426 pupil/corneal reflection tracking system, which recorded the positions of the center of the pupil and a bright corneal reflection moving over the pupil. The spatial difference between the pupil and the corneal reflection gives the direction and magnitude of the eye movement. This method yields a linear representation of the subject's eye position within ±15° of visual angle. Within the linear range, the accuracy is better than 1°.

The pupil/corneal tracking system was connected to a Macintosh II computer, which recorded and stored the eye position information (*x* and *y* coordinates), and to a television monitor, which allowed the experimenter to observe the right eye during the experiment. To take account of small head movements, the pupil/corneal tracker was connected to an Iscan RK-520 Autocalibration System, which calculated the subject's point of regard with respect to the stimulus.

Calibration was performed by asking subjects to fixate on five successive experimenter-defined positions on the stimulus display screen: center, upper left, lower left, upper right, and lower right. We used the autocalibration system, which coordinates the eye position information and calibration position information, to compute the point of regard for subsequent eye movements.

After the calibration, practice trials were performed to ensure that all subjects understood the procedure. Eye movements were monitored on the television screen to ensure that the subject was fixating at the center when each trial began. Further details can be found in previous articles.[2,15]

Procedure. Subjects sat with their heads stabilized by a chin and head rest in front of a stimulus display monitor. A red fixation dot subtending approximately 0.5° of visual angle appeared in the center of the stimulus display screen. The target was a small black circle subtending about 2° of visual angle. The location of the target varied randomly from trial to trial. The distance between the fixation point and any target location was 12° of visual angle.

Subjects were asked to look at the fixation point in the center of the screen. When they were ready to begin, the experimenter clicked a mouse to initiate a trial. In the oculomotor memory DRT, a target (black circle) appeared on the screen for 200 milliseconds in one of the eight possible locations, long enough for it to be seen and identified but too short for an eye movement to be made to it. There were eight possible target locations, equidistant from one another, on the circumference of an imaginary circle. After the presentation of each target, and with the subject continuing to look at the center of the screen, a 10-second delay period followed during which the subject performed a concurrent "category shift" task that forced the subject to shift semantic categories. For example, for the category "animals," animal names (eg, "tiger," "dog") were flashed consecutively, one each second, and occasionally a noncategory word (eg, "car") was flashed, requiring the subject to signal recognition of the noncategory word. A fuller description of the concurrent task is found in Park and Holzman[2] and in Park.[15] This procedure prevented rehearsal and thus circumvented the use of working memory without verbal or other mnemonic mediators and also forced the subjects to fixate in the center of the screen during the delay period. This task does not affect spatial working memory performance.[2,15] After the delay period, the fixation point and eight "reference" circles (empty rather than black) appeared on the screen. Subjects were required to move their eyes to the position that the target circle had occupied; this was a memory-guided eye movement, not a reflexive saccade. If subjects looked at the correct target position, the screen cleared and the red fixation dot replaced the reference circles. The next trial could then begin. If the subject did not look at the correct position, the reference circles remained on the screen until the subject looked at the correct position. The eye positions during this period were recorded every 20 milliseconds. If the subject did not look at the correct location within 10 seconds, the reference circles disappeared and the red fixation point reappeared, indicating that a new trial could begin. Subjects rested after every 16 trials. Eye position was recalibrated after each rest period.

All subjects were also tested on an oculomotor sensory control task. This task was identical to the oculomotor memory task except for one aspect: the target remained on the screen at all times. Subjects were required to move their eyes to the target itself after the delay period. This task required no memory since the target was always present. **Figure 1** shows the schematic plan of the experiment.

The order of presentation of the oculomotor memory and the oculomotor sensory conditions was counterbalanced across subjects. Each task consisted of 64 trials, eight for each target location. All subjects gave written informed consent. There were 16 practice trials before the main testing began.

Measures. Accuracy (percent correct) and response times (in milliseconds) of correct trials were recorded. A response was scored as correct only if an eye movement brought the eye directly to within 1.5° of the center of the correct target position. If the eye moved to a wrong position first and then later moved to the correct target position, the trial was counted as incorrect. Response times were measured from the end of the delay period to the initiation of the first eye movement to a target location. All subsequent eye movements to targets were also recorded with their response times.

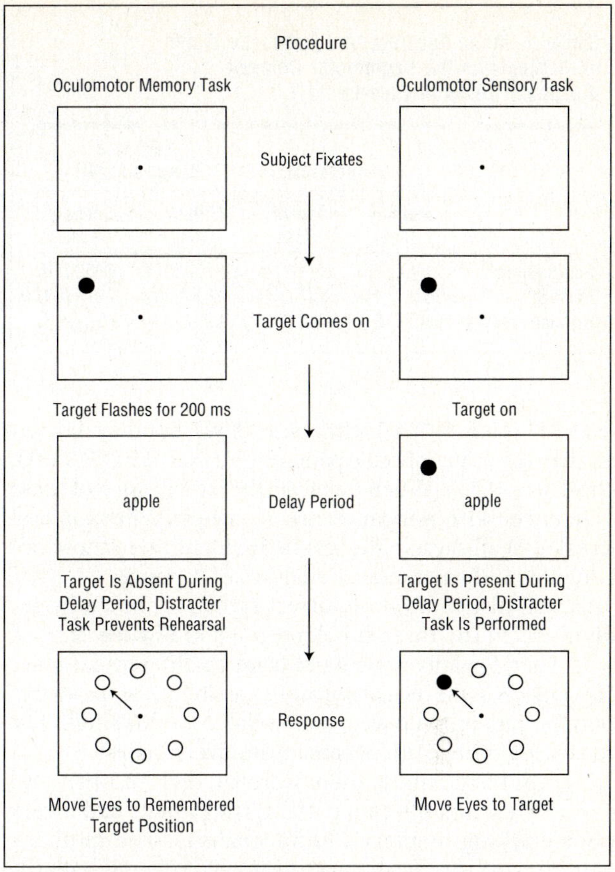

Figure 1. *Oculomotor delayed response memory and sensory tasks.*

Results

Table 1 presents the mean accuracy and response times of the three subject groups for the two DRTs.

Accuracy. In the oculomotor memory task, schizophrenic patients had the lowest percentage of correct scores (mean, 71.4%; SD, 16.0%), normal controls the highest percentage (mean, 95.2%; SD, 4.8%), and relatives fell in between (mean, 86.8%; SD, 7.1%). There were no group differences on the oculomotor sensory task, all groups having scored above 96% correct.

The statistical significance of differences in performance of the groups was compared in a three-way repeated-measures analysis of variance. All subjects, regardless of group, were significantly more accurate on the sensory task than on the memory task, as shown by a main effect of the type of task ($F[1,48]=91.5$; $P<.001$; effect size, 0.81) and a main effect of subject groups ($F[2,48]=16.3$; $P<.001$; effect size, 0.64). The groups differed significantly in accuracy on the memory task ($F[2,48]=21.9$; $P<.001$; effect size, 0.69) but not on the sensory control task ($F[2,48]=0.48$; $P>.60$; effect size, 0.14) (group-by-task interaction: $F[2,48]=22.6$; $P<.001$; effect size, 0.71).

Relatives of schizophrenic patients were less accurate than normal controls on the oculomotor memory task

Table 1. Mean Accuracy and Response Times of Subjects on the Oculomotor Delayed Response Tasks in Experiment 1

	% Correct (SD)		Response Time, ms (SD)	
	Memory Task	Sensory Task	Memory Task	Sensory Task
Schizophrenics	71.4 (16.0)	96.9 (6.4)	1210 (695)	1006 (220)
Relatives	86.8 (7.1)	98.2 (3.6)	767 (239)	781 (269)
Normal controls	95.2 (4.8)	98.2 (2.8)	683 (234)	625 (213)

($F[1,31]=16.5$; $P<.001$; effect size, 0.59), but they did better than the schizophrenic patients ($F[1,31]=11.1$; $P<.003$; effect size, 0.51). When one tests the significance of these differences with nonparametric statistics (Wilcoxon and Kruskal-Wallis tests), the results are identical to those obtained with the parametric analyses of variance.

The distribution of correct scores is shown by individuals in the three subject groups in **Figure 2**.

The 15 relatives were not from 15 different families. Six subjects in the relatives group were siblings of six schizophrenic patients who were not available for this study. The remaining nine relatives came from five families:

From one family, there were a father, mother, and sister of a schizophrenic patient; the patient had a very poor working memory (40.6% correct). The mother's working memory accuracy score was 96.6%, and both the father and the healthy sibling had 84.4% accuracy, which is below the lowest score of the normal group.

From a second family there were two brothers of a schizophrenic patient. The patient and one brother had a very poor working memory (75% and 81.3% accuracy, respectively). The second brother had very few errors on the oculomotor DRT (93.8%).

From a third family there were two relatives, both sisters of a schizophrenic patient. All three members of this family had high numbers of errors on the DRT (84.4% correct for the patient and one sister, 71.9% for the other sister).

There were two families from which one sibling each was tested. In one of these families, the patient had a very poor oculomotor DRT performance (62% correct), but her healthy sister had few errors on the DRT (93.8%). In the second of these two families, the patient had many errors on the DRT (75% correct). His unaffected brother had few errors on the DRT (90.6% correct).

If one selects one random sibling of each schizophrenic patient, the results do not change for these 11 relatives. It therefore appears that the distribution of impaired DRT performance is not unduly weighted by one or two families.

Types of Errors. We grouped the response errors into two kinds, those that are immediately corrected and those that are never corrected during the maximum period allotted for responses (10 seconds). Errors that are immediately corrected are likely to arise from temporary distractions or failures to inhibit irrelevant response tendencies; we labeled these errors E_1. Errors that are never corrected even though subjects make repeated efforts to recall the position of the target are more likely to be caused by a loss of spatial representation of the target during the delay period; we labeled these errors E_n. Park[16] and Park and O'Driscoll[17] reported that these two major types of errors have different distributions in schizophrenic patients, bipolar patients, schizotypic subjects, and normal controls.

The mean (SD) number of E_1 errors for schizophrenic patients in this study was 9.4 (5.8) and the median was 8, while for the normal subjects the mean was 1.8 (1.9) and the median was 1.5, and for the relatives the mean was 2.4 (0.7) and the median was 2.0. The schizophrenic patients made significantly more E_1 errors than did the normal subjects and the relatives ($F[2,48]=21.1$, $P<.001$), but normal subjects and relatives did not differ significantly in the number of E_1 errors. Nonparametric statistical tests (Kruskal-Wallis test) gave identical results. This finding suggests that schizophrenic patients are more susceptible to temporary distractions and to interference by irrelevant response tendencies than are relatives or normal control subjects.

The distribution of E_n errors, however, was quite different. Whereas normal subjects only occasionally made such errors (mean E_n, 1.0; SD, 1.9; median, 1.5), the mean number of E_n errors for the schizophrenic patients was 4.67 (SD, 4.50; median, 2.5), and for the relatives group it was 3.3 (SD, 2.85; median, 4). These differences are statistically significant ($F[2,48]=6.6$, $P<.003$), indicating that the patients and the relatives made significantly more E_n errors than did the normal group. Nonparametric tests of these distributions (Kruskal-Wallis test) gave identical results. The proportion of subjects in each group making more than two E_n errors is instructive: three (17%) of 18 normal subjects (17%) compared with nine (50%) of 18 schizophrenic patients and eight (53%) of 15 relatives. The schizophrenic patients and the relatives did not differ on the number of E_n errors, indicating that they are both prone to loss of memory representation during the delay period.

Response Times. Table 1 shows that the groups differed in response times. The schizophrenic patients were the slowest and the relatives were intermediate between the patients and the normal control subjects. The significance of these differences was tested by a repeated-measures analysis of variance and by a nonparametric test (Kruskal-Wallis test).

The normal subjects were fastest, relatives next, and schizophrenic patients slowest on both the sensory and memory components of the procedure, as reflected in the significant main effect of subject groups ($F[2,48]=11.6$, $P<.001$), but there was no main effect of task type ($F[1,48]=1.9$, $P>.17$), and there was no significant interaction between subject groups and task type ($F[2,48]=1.1$, $P>.34$). Further analyses of simple effects showed that schizophrenic patients were slower than both the normal controls ($F[1,31]=8.6$, $P<.007$) and the relatives ($F[1,31]=6.0$, $P<.03$) on the oculomotor memory task. On the sensory task as well, schizophrenic patients were slower than both the normal controls ($F[1,31]=22.9$, $P<.001$) and the relatives ($F[1,31]=5.7$, $P<.03$). The relatives and the normal controls did not differ significantly in response times. The nonparametric tests gave identical results, except for the difference between normal controls and relatives on the sensory task,

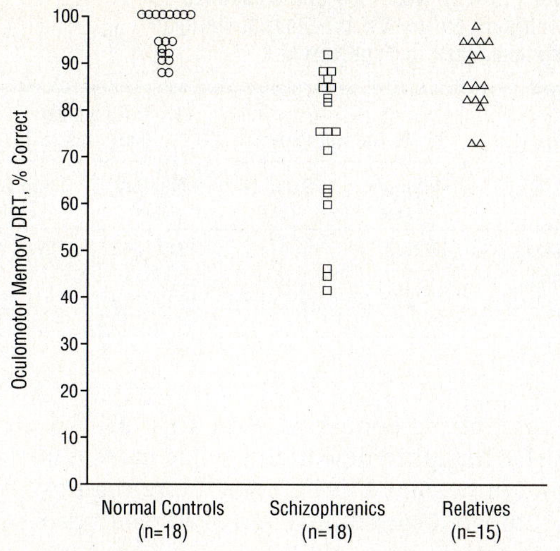

Figure 2. *Scatterplot of accuracy scores of normal controls, schizophrenic patients, and relatives of schizophrenic patients performing the oculomotor memory delayed response task (DRT) in experiment 1.*

where the relatives showed a nonsignificant but borderline tendency to be slower in response time.

Comment

Our data indicate that some first-degree relatives of schizophrenic patients show spatial working memory deficits, as assessed by an oculomotor DRT. We previously reported that schizophrenic inpatients and outpatients show working memory deficits,[2,7] but in those studies it was not possible to rule out the possible effects of medication even though clinical state was shown not to be a decisive factor. In the present experiment, we observed the delayed response deficits in nonpsychotic relatives of schizophrenic patients. It therefore appears that such abnormalities can occur in the absence of any neuroleptic exposure and in the absence of psychotic symptoms. Schizophrenic patients made many E_1 errors, but the normal controls and relatives seldom made this type of error. This type of error may reflect temporary inefficiency, perhaps secondary to state factors. In contrast, both the schizophrenic patients and their relatives made significantly more E_n errors, indicating that both the schizophrenic patients and the relatives are susceptible to loss of spatial representation during the delay period. Because the sample size was small, we conducted a second delayed response experiment using a different sensory modality in new groups of relatives and controls.

EXPERIMENT 2: VISUAL-MANUAL DRT

Results from experiment 1 showed that the first-degree relatives of schizophrenic patients, like schizophrenic patients themselves, are impaired on the oculomotor DRT. In experiment 2, subjects were required to respond with their hands rather than with their eyes. In this version of the DRT, targets were presented visually and the responses were made by hand movements, a procedure that requires a crossmodal transfer of spatial representation. For this experiment we recruited another group of first-degree relatives of schizophrenic patients and another normal control group.

Subjects

We recruited 12 first-degree relatives of schizophrenic patients (seven women), with only one relative per family. None of these subjects had participated in experiment 1. Sixteen normal control subjects (seven women) were recruited from Zürich, Switzerland. The control subjects, none of whom participated in experiment 1, were nurses, clerical workers, or students. They were selected if there was no Axis I *DSM-III-R* psychiatric disorder in any first- or second-degree relative, as determined by a brief psychiatric interview. They had no evidence of organic brain damage and were not mentally retarded. The mean age of the normal control subjects was 36.7 (11.3) years, and their mean education was 14.0 (3.3) years. The mean age of the relatives was 43.4 (14.1) years, and their mean education was 15.4 (3.0) years. There was no significant difference between the two groups in age ($F[1,26]=1.86$, $P>.18$) or education level ($F[1,26]=1.19$, $P>.28$).

Visual-Manual DRT

Procedure and Apparatus. All procedures were identical to those described in experiment 1, except for the modality of response; subjects responded by touching a position on a computer screen rather than by an eye movement.

Subjects sat with their heads steady on a chin and head rest in front of a stimulus display monitor. The stimulus display monitor was fitted with a touch screen (AccuTouch, Ellinor Technology, Berkshire, England). The touch screen consisted of a glass plate covered with a tight-fitting plastic cover sheet. Conductive coatings were applied to the glass plate and the plastic sheet so that light finger pressure caused internal electrical contact at the point of touch. This voltage was then digitized. Position accuracy was better than ±4.6 mm (13 pixels), as measured on a multipoint sampling basis. Calibration procedure involved touching four reference points on the touch screen. Calibration was performed before each subject began the experiment.

Subjects stared fixedly at the center of the screen, and when they were ready to begin, the experimenter clicked a mouse to initiate a trial. In the visual-manual memory task, a target appeared on the screen for 200 milliseconds. Immediately after the target presentation, there was a 10-second delay period, during which the subject performed the category shift task (the distracter task). After the delay period, the fixation point and eight "reference" circles (empty rather than black) appeared on the screen. Subjects were required to touch the screen at the remembered position of the target. If they touched the correct target position, the screen cleared and the next trial could begin. If the subject did not touch the correct position, the reference circles remained on the screen until the subject chose the correct position, or until 10 seconds had elapsed, whichever was sooner.

To control for the sensorimotor component of the visual-manual memory task, a sensory control task was conducted. The sensory control task was identical to the memory task except for one aspect: the target remained on the screen at all times. Subjects were required to touch the target itself after the delay period. This task required no memory since the target was always present.

The order of presentation of the memory and sensory conditions was counterbalanced across subjects. There were 64 trials on the memory task and 64 on the sensory task, eight at each location in both tasks. All subjects gave written informed consent. There were 16 practice trials before the main body of testing began, to ensure that the subjects understood the task.

Measures. Accuracy (percent correct) and response times (in milliseconds) of correct trials were recorded. A response was scored as correct only if the subject touched within 1.5° of the center of the target position and if the finger moved there directly. If the finger moved to a wrong position first and then later moved to the correct target position, this response was counted as incorrect.

Results

Accuracy. Table 2 presents the mean accuracy scores of the two subject groups. Relatives of schizophrenic patients were less accurate than the normal controls on the visual-manual memory DRT (86.5% vs 95.4%) but not the sensory DRT (98.2% vs 99.4%). The differences between the two groups were tested by a repeated-measures analysis of variance. There was a main effect of subject group ($F[1,26]=10.04$; $P<.004$; effect size, 0.53), a main effect of the task type ($F[1,26]=48.3$; $P<.001$; effect size, 0.80), and a subject-by-task interaction ($F[1,26]=12.8$; $P<.002$; effect size, 0.57), indicating that the relatives of schizophrenic patients were significantly less accurate than the normal controls in making the memory-guided hand movements ($F[1,26]=12.86$; $P<.002$; effect size, 0.70), but the two groups did not differ on the sensory-control task ($F[1,26]=1.23$, $P>.27$). The nonparametric tests (Kruskal-Wallis test) gave identical results. **Figure 3** shows the distribution of accuracy scores on the memory-guided DRT for the two subject groups.

Types of Errors. We examined the distributions of the two types of errors, E_1 and E_n errors. The relatives made more E_1 errors than did the normal controls. The mean (SD) number of E_1 errors for the normal control subjects was 1.94 (1.44); for the relatives the mean number of E_1 errors was 6.24 (4.44). This difference is statistically significant ($F[1,26]=14.9$, $P<.001$); a nonparametric test gives a similar significance value. In experiment 2, then, the relatives made more E_1 errors than did the relatives in experiment 1.

The mean number of E_n errors for the normal group was 0.44 (0.73); the mean number of E_n errors for the relatives of schizophrenic patients was 1.42 (1.38). This group difference was statistically significant whether tested by a parametric analysis of variance ($F[1,26]=5.92$, $P=.02$) or a nonparametric Kruskal-Wallis test. Five (31%) of 16 normal controls compared with 15 (94%) of 16 relatives of schizophrenic patients made more than two E_1 errors. No normal control made more than two E_n errors, compared with four (25%) of 16 relatives of schizophrenic patients.

Table 2. Mean Accuracy and Response Times of Subjects on the Visual-Manual Delayed Response Task in Experiment 2

	% Correct (SD)		Response Time, ms (SD)	
	Memory Task	Sensory Task	Memory Task	Sensory Task
Relatives	86.5 (9.1)	98.2 (4.2)	1317 (247)	1311 (251)
Normal controls	95.4 (3.4)	99.4 (1.3)	1120 (156)	1076 (66)

These results are consistent with those obtained in experiment 1. Some relatives of schizophrenic patients perform poorly on tasks that require spatial working memory regardless of the modality of the response.

Response Times. Table 2 shows that the relatives were slower than the normal controls on both the memory and sensory tasks. A repeated-measures analysis of variance reveals that there was a main effect of subject group on the response times ($F[1,26]=13.3$, $P<.001$) but no main effect of the task ($F[1,26]=0.52$, $P>.47$) and no interaction between subject group and the task ($F[1,26]=0.25$, $P>.62$). One-way analysis of variance revealed that the two subject groups differed on the memory task ($F[1,26]=6.67$, $P<.02$) and on the sensory task ($F[1,26]=13.05$, $P<.002$). The relatives were significantly slower than the normal controls on both tasks (1317 and 1311 milliseconds vs 1120 and 1076 milliseconds on the memory and sensory tasks, respectively). This result differs from that found in experiment 1, in which there was no global oculomotor response time difference between the normal controls and the relatives, although there was a trend in the same direction.

Oculomotor and Visual-Manual Spatial Working Memory Performance in the Relatives. We compared the accuracy of the relatives from experiment 1 and experiment 2. There were no differences between the two groups of relatives on the working memory task ($F[1,26]=0.12$, $P>.73$) on the sensory control task ($F[1,26]=0.01$, $P>.91$). As far as accuracy of delayed response is concerned, it does not seem to matter whether the actual test is conducted with the oculomotor paradigm or with the visual-manual paradigm. Similarly, dorsolateral prefrontal lesions in experimental primates induce working memory deficits whether the tasks used to measure these difficulties require oculomotor[5] or manual[18] responses.

We did not directly compare the response times because of the different inherent speed requirements for making an eye movement and a hand movement. Instead, we computed a relative change in the response times

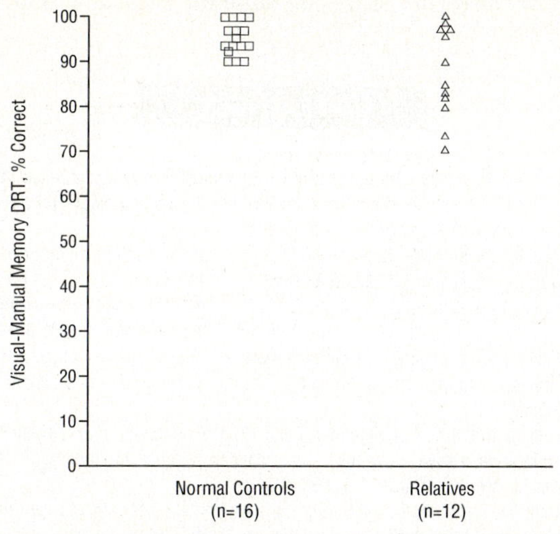

Figure 3. *Scatterplot of accuracy scores of normal controls and relatives of schizophrenic patients performing the visual-manual memory delayed response task (DRT) in experiment 2.*

in the memory-guided task compared with the sensory control task for each subject, as follows:

$$\% \text{ Increase in RT} = [(\text{RT}_{\text{Memory Task}} - \text{RT}_{\text{Sensory Task}}) / (\text{RT}_{\text{Sensory Task}})] \times 100,$$

where RT indicates response time.

On the oculomotor task, relatives had a 6.40% increase in response time, and on the visual-manual task, they had a 2.04% increase in response time. The magnitude of the change in response time was not statistically significant ($F[1,26]=0.21$, $P>.65$).

COMMENT

In this study we examined spatial working memory in first-degree relatives of schizophrenic patients. On the oculomotor working memory task, we observed that a significant number of these relatives had impaired performance. Similarly, on the visual-manual working memory task, the relatives were less accurate than the normal controls.

We classified the types of errors into E_1 and E_n errors. We believe that different psychological processes underlie these two types of errors. In the case of E_1 errors, temporary distractions may be the main source of error. In the case of E_n errors, however, the spatial memory representation is not recoverable, which denotes a failure to maintain the spatial representation in working memory.

In experiment 1, we found that schizophrenic patients made significantly more E_1 errors than did normal subjects or the first-degree relatives. Such evidence of temporary inefficiency is not unexpected in this group. What is noteworthy and thus far not reported, however, is the appearance of large numbers of E_n errors not only among the patients but also among a large proportion of their relatives. This result, found in both experiment 1 and experiment 2, suggests that in some of these otherwise clinically normal relatives, there is a detectable dysfunction in efforts to hold a spatial representation "on line." The patients, as noted above, showed a significant tendency toward temporary inefficiency in experiment 1. This same tendency in the relatives was noted in experiment 2 but not in experiment 1. The normal controls, however, showed no increase in these E_1 errors in experiment 2. It is quite possible that the recruitment of a second response system (hand movement to the target), which introduced a second modality into the response process, complicated the performance for the relatives compared with the simple eye movement response in experiment 1. This hypothesis will be tested in further studies.

One may properly wonder whether the relatives who showed the working memory dysfunction have schizophrenia spectrum disorders. Although systematic examination of the relatives for Axis II disorders, particularly schizotypal personality disorder, was not undertaken, we offer a tentative answer, pending such examination, which is now under way in our laboratory. It is possible that some of the relatives have schizotypal characteristics. For at least two reasons, however, it would be implausible to assume that impaired working memory is a function of schizotypy in this population of relatives. First, the prevalence of schizotypal personality disorder in the first-degree family members of a schizophrenic patient ranges from about 7% to 14%.[19] From these estimates, we would expect at the most two relatives in each of the experiments to have schizotypal personality disorder. In the present experiments, however, six (40%) of 15 relatives in experiment 1 and six (50%) of 12 relatives in experiment 2 had significant working memory impairments (Figures 2 and 3), with "impairment" defined as scores greater than 2 SDs from those of their specific normal population comparison group. It is noteworthy, moreover, that this study examined the working memory of an unselected sample of relatives, who were essentially volunteers. Schizotypal traits, such as interpersonal aversiveness, suspiciousness, social anxiety, guardedness, and lack of motivation, are among those personal qualities that would make it less likely for such people to volunteer for a study such as the present one. The present cohort of relatives thus probably contains even fewer cases than indicated by the cited prevalence of schizotypal personality disorders, although some schizotypal traits may exist in a subgroup of relatives. Since about 40% to 50% of the relatives in experiments 1 and 2 had working memory dysfunction, far greater than the reported prevalence of schizotypal personality disorder in the biological relatives of patients with schizophrenia,[19] we would here opt for a conservative interpretation, maintaining that the majority of the relatives with working memory dysfunction in the present study do not have schizophrenia spectrum disorders.

Second, in a previous study, otherwise normal college students who scored high on an inventory tapping experiences of perceptual aberrations, one of the manifestations of schizotypy,[20,21] made significantly more working memory errors as a group than did those who were selected for having very few or no schizotypal signs. However, only about 25% of these schizotypal students had working memory impairment, and several students with no schizotypal signs also had working memory impairment.

The working memory system may be said to operate like a "mystic writing pad,"[22] providing temporary and limited access to long-term or associative memory; it needs to be wiped clean or updated to be ready to accept new stimuli for temporary storage to guide action. In Baddeley's model,[23,24] the working memory system is supported by modality-specific "slave" or auxiliary systems that allow for focused rehearsals of information in the buffer, such as repeating the telephone number just found in the telephone book or visualizing a spatial array. By employing a distracter task, our experimental paradigm removed the possibility of rehearsals and therefore of the use of these auxiliary aids to working memory and allowed us to detect significant impairments. It is quite possible that the relatives with impaired accuracy on the DRT, who otherwise seem to function adequately, rely on these "subslave" auxiliary systems to mask spatial working memory impairments.

It is noteworthy that a subset of the first-degree relatives of schizophrenic patients show deficits in working memory. These relatives are clinically unaffected and do not manifest any *DSM-III-R* Axis I conditions. Some may, however, have or have had Axis II conditions, and a further study of this possibility is under way. This pool of subjects has generally been neglected for psychobiological investigation. Psychopathologists, and particularly geneticists, have typically focused their attention on the sickest patients and on families with the highest concentrations of morbidity. We have argued that a thorough study of relatives, including those who appear to be well, can offer a richer yield in the search for insights into the disease process, one that penetrates beyond the obvious phenotypic symptoms.[25] In this search, psychology, the neurosciences, and related disciplines have much to contribute in exploring the hidden nature of the phenotype. One of these has been the study of eye tracking dysfunctions in schizophrenia.[8] The present study strongly suggests that spatial working memory dysfunction as measured by the DRT is another behavioral marker that can take its place alongside smooth-pursuit abnormalities as an aid not only in illuminating the pathophysiologic characteristics of schizophrenia but also in characterizing the multidimensional qualities of the schizophrenic phenotype to trace the transmission of schizophrenia-related genes.

Accepted for publication June 7, 1995.

This research was supported in part by a Young Investigator grant from the National Alliance for Research on Schizophrenia and Depression (NARSAD), Chicago, Ill; by a fellowship award from the Stanley Foundation, Arlington, Va; by a long-term fellowship from Human Frontiers of Science, Tokyo, Japan; by a grant from the Swiss National Science Foundation, Zurich (Dr Park); and by grants R01 MH 31340, P05 MH 31154, P50 MH 44866 and K05 MH 01020 from the US Public Health Service, Washington, DC.

We thank Deborah L. Levy, PhD, McLean Hospital, Belmont, Mass; Mark F. Lenzenweger, PhD, Cornell University, Ithaca, NY; Charlotte Simpson, Washington, DC; Clara Lajonchere, Washington University, St Louis, Mo; and Janet Levoff, Watertown, Mass, for their help.

Reprint requests to Department of Psychology, Northwestern University, 2029 Sheridan Rd, Evanston, IL 60208 (Dr Park).

REFERENCES

1. Goldman-Rakic PS. Prefrontal cortical dysfunction in schizophrenia: the relevance of working memory. In: Carroll B, ed. *Psychopathology and the Brain.* New York, NY: Raven Press; 1992:1-23.
2. Park S, Holzman PS. Schizophrenics show spatial working memory deficits. *Arch Gen Psychiatry.* 1992;49:975-982.
3. Funuhashi S, Bruce CJ, Goldman-Rakic PS. Mnemonic coding of visual cortex in monkey's dorsolateral prefrontal cortex. *J Neurophysiol.* 1989;61:331-348.
4. Wilson FAS, Scalaidhe O, Goldman-Rakic PS. Dissociation of object and spatial processing domains in primate prefrontal cortex. *Science.* 1993;260:1955-1958.
5. Funahashi S, Bruce CJ, Goldman-Rakic PS. Dorsolateral prefrontal lesions and oculomotor delayed response performance: evidence for mnemonic 'scotomas.' *J Neurosci.* 1993;13:1479-1497.
6. Goldman-Rakic PS. Circuitry of primate prefrontal cortex and regulation of behavior by representational knowledge. In: Plum F, Mountcastle V, eds. *Handbook of Physiology: The Nervous System V.* Bethesda, Md: American Physiological Society; 1987:373-417.
7. Park S, Holzman PS. Association of working memory deficit and eye tracking dysfunction in schizophrenia. *Schizophr Res.* 1993;11:55-61.
8. Levy DL, Holzman PS, Matthysse S, Mendell NR. Eye tracking dysfunction and schizophrenia: a critical perspective. *Schizophr Bull.* 1993;19:461-536.
9. Holzman PS. Eye movement dysfunction and psychosis. *Int Rev Neurobiol.* 1985;27:179-205.
10. Shenton ME, Solovay MR, Holzman PS, Coleman M, Gale H. Thought disorder in the relatives of psychotic patients. *Arch Gen Psychiatry.* 1989;46:897-901.
11. Lenzenweger MF. Confirming schizotypic personality configurations in hypothetically psychosis-prone university students. *Psychiatry Res.* 1991;37:81-96.
12. Holzman PS, Kringlen E, Matthysse S, Flanagan S, Lipton RB, Cramer G, Levin S, Lange K, Levy DL. A single dominant gene can account for eye tracking dysfunctions and schizophrenia in offspring of discordant twins. *Arch Gen Psychiatry.* 1988;45:641-647.
13. Matthysse S, Holzman PS, Lange K. The genetic transmission of schizophrenia: application of mendelian latent structure analysis to eye tracking dysfunctions in schizophrenia and affective disorder. *J Psychiatr Res.* 1986;20:57-65.
14. Spitzer RL, Williams JDW. *Structured Clinical Interview for* DSM-III-R. New York, NY: Biomedical Research Division, New York State Psychiatric Institute; 1985.
15. Park S. *The Role of Prefrontal Cortex in Spatial Working Memory Deficits of Schizophrenic Patients.* Cambridge, Mass: Harvard University; 1991. Thesis.
16. Park S. Working memory function in schizophrenic patients. In: Spitzer M, Maher BA, eds. *Experimental Psychopathology.* New York, NY: Cambridge University Press. In press.
17. Park S, O'Driscoll G, Components of working memory deficit schizophrenic patients. In: Matthysse S, Levy DL, Kagan J, Benes F, eds. *Psychopathology: Evolution of a New Science.* New York, NY: Cambridge University Press. In press.
18. Goldman PS, Rosvold HE. Localization of function within the dorsolateral prefrontal cortex of the rhesus monkey. *Exp Neurol.* 1979;20:221-226.
19. Kendler KS, Gruenberg AM, Kinney DK. Independent diagnoses of adoptees and relatives as defined by *DSM-III* in the provincial and national samples of the Danish Adoption Study of Schizophrenia. *Arch Gen Psychiatry.* 1994;51:456-468.
20. Holzman PS, Coleman M, Lenzenweger MF, Levy DL, Matthysse S, O'Driscoll G, Park S. Working memory deficits, antisaccades, and thought disorder in relation to perceptual aberration. In: Raine A, Lencz T, Mednick S, eds. *Schizotypal Personality.* New York, NY: Cambridge University Press. In press.
21. Park, S, Holzman PS, Lenzenweger MF. Individual differences in spatial working memory in relation to schizotypy. *J Abnorm Psychol.* 1995;104:355-363.
22. Freud S; Strachey J, trans. A note on the mystic writing pad. In: *The Standard Edition of the Complete Psychological Works of Sigmund Freud.* London, England: Hogarth Press; 1925;19:225-232.
23. Baddeley A. *Working Memory.* New York, NY: Oxford University Press; 1986.
24. Baddeley A. Working memory: the interface between memory and cognition. *J Cogn Neurosci.* 1992;4:281-288.
25. Holzman PS, Matthysse S. The genetics of schizophrenia: a review. *Psychol Sci.* 1990;1:279-286.

ORIGINAL ARTICLE

Abnormal Excitatory Neurotransmitter Metabolism in Schizophrenic Brains

Guochuan Tsai, MD, PhD; Lucius A. Passani, MS; Barbara S. Slusher, PhD; Ruth Carter; Lee Baer, PhD; Joel E. Kleinman, MD, PhD; Joseph T. Coyle, MD

Background: Schizophrenia has been hypothesized to be caused by a hypofunction of glutamatergic neurons. Findings of reduced concentrations of glutamate in the cerebrospinal fluid of patients with schizophrenia and the ability of glutamate-receptor antagonists to cause psychotic symptoms lend support to this hypothesis. *N*-acetylaspartylglutamate (NAAG), a neuropeptide that is highly concentrated in glutamatergic neurons, antagonizes the effects of glutamate at *N*-methyl-D-aspartate receptors. Moreover, NAAG is cleaved to glutamate and *N*-acetylaspartate by a specific peptidase, *N*-acetyl-α–linked acidic dipeptidase (NAALADase). To test the glutamatergic hypothesis of schizophrenia, we studied the NAAG-related glutamatergic variables in postmortem brains from patients with schizophrenia, neuroleptic-treated controls, and normal individuals, with particular emphasis on the prefrontal cortex and hippocampus.

Method: Different regions of frozen brain tissue from three different groups (patients with schizophrenia, neuroleptic-treated controls, and normal controls) were assayed to determine levels of NAAG, *N*-acetylaspartate, NAALADase, and several amino acids, including aspartate and glutamate.

Results: Our study demonstrates alterations in brain levels of aspartate, glutamate, and NAAG and in NAALADase activity. Levels of NAAG were increased and NAALADase activity and glutamate levels were decreased in the schizophrenic brains. Notably, the changes in NAAG level and NAALADase activity in schizophrenic brains were more selective than those for aspartate and glutamate. In neuroleptic-treated control brains, levels of aspartate, glutamate, and glycine were found to be increased.

Conclusions: The changes in levels of aspartate, glutamate, NAAG, and NAALADase are prominent in the prefrontal and hippocampal regions, where previous neuropathological studies of schizophrenic brains demonstrate consistent changes. These findings support the hypothesis that schizophrenia results from a hypofunction of certain glutamatergic neuronal systems. They also suggest that the therapeutic efficacy of neuroleptics may be related to increased glutamatergic activity.

(Arch Gen Psychiatry. 1995;52:829-836)

From the Laboratory of Molecular and Developmental Neuroscience and the Department of Psychiatry, Harvard Medical School, and Massachusetts General Hospital, Boston (Drs Tsai, Slusher, Baer, and Coyle, and Mr Passani and Ms Carter); and the Clinical Brain Disorders Branch, Intramural Research Program, National Institute of Mental Health Neuroscience Center at St Elizabeths Hospital, Washington, DC (Dr Kleinman). Dr Slusher is currently affiliated with Guilford Pharmaceuticals, Baltimore, Md.

OVER A DECADE ago, Kim et al[1] first proposed that schizophrenia may result from a hypofunction of glutamatergic neurons in the brain because of their observation that the concentration of glutamate was reduced in the cerebrospinal fluid of patients with schizophrenia. The hypothesis was not generally accepted until phencyclidine hydrochloride (PCP) was demonstrated to induce a psychotic state that closely resembles schizophrenia.[2,3] Phencyclidine and analogues such as ketamine hydrochloride and dizocilpine maleate induce their neurobehavioral effects[4] by binding to a specific site within the ion channel of *N*-methyl-D-aspartate (NMDA)–receptor complex and acting as noncompetitive antagonists of the NMDA receptors (**Figure 1**). As opposed to amphetamine-induced psychosis, PCP-induced psychosis presents both positive (eg, hallucinations and delusions) and negative (eg, apathy and anhedonia) symptoms. Phencyclidine-induced psychosis also uniquely exhibits the formal thought disorder and some of the neuropsychological deficits associated with schizophrenia.[4] The ability of PCP or ketamine to induce schizophreniform psychosis by inhibiting NMDA-receptor–mediated neurotransmission suggests that endogenous dysfunction or dysregulation of NMDA-receptor–mediated transmission

See Methods on next page

METHODS

Frozen postmortem brain samples from 12 individuals in whom chronic undifferentiated schizophrenia was diagnosed using *DSM-III-R*[21] criteria (nine men and three women), 11 normal controls (eight men and three women), and six neuroleptic-treated controls (four men and two women) were provided by the Neuropathology Section, Clinical Brain Disorders Branch, Intramural Research Program, National Institute of Mental Health, Bethesda, Md. The age, sex, psychiatric diagnosis, and cause of death are presented in **Table 1**.

The diagnosis of schizophrenia had been made ante mortem and was confirmed retrospectively by chart review. All subjects underwent autopsy at the District of Columbia Medical Examiner's Office. All patients with chronic undifferentiated schizophrenia were receiving neuroleptics at the time of death. Normal controls did not have a neurologic or psychiatric disorder and were not receiving psychotropic drugs. The neuroleptic-treated control group was composed of subjects who were receiving neuroleptics for diagnoses other than schizophrenia (organic brain syndrome [n=3], antisocial personality disorder [n=1], and psychotic disorder that was not otherwise specified [n=2]). All had been receiving neuroleptics at the time of death. None of the neuroleptic-treated control or normal control subjects died of suicide. Three of the patients with schizophrenia died of suicide. The three groups did not differ significantly in age or hours elapsed between death and postmortem brain removal. The mean±SD age was similar in patients with schizophrenia, normal controls, and neuroleptic-treated controls (schizophrenia group, 46.6±18.3 years; normal control group, 46.5±14.1 years; and neuroleptic-treated control group, 45.2±12.2 years). Postmortem delay was also not significantly different in the three groups (schizophrenia group, 19.5±12.2 hours; normal control group, 26.3±13.9 hours; and neuroleptic-treated control group, 23.0±12.2 hours).

Sections of gray matter were dissected from eight different regions of brain specimens at autopsy as described in detail.[22,23] The regions sampled included prefrontal cortex, hippocampus, parahippocampus, amygdala, putamen, cerebellum, and parietal and cingulate cortices. Tissue sections of 2 to 3 mm thickness that weighed approximately 20 mg were assayed in duplicate. For amino acid and peptide analyses, the tissues were sonicated in 90% methanol in water (vol/vol) and centrifuged at 10 000g, and aliquots of the supernatant were assayed. For the NAALADase assay, the tissues were sonicated in 1:10 (wt/vol) TRIS hydrochloride buffer containing 0.1% Triton (pH 7.4). All biochemical analyses were performed in a blinded fashion.

NEUROCHEMICAL ANALYSIS

Amino acids were analyzed by *o*-phthalaldehyde precolumn derivatization coupled with reverse-phase C-18 (18-carbon chain) column, high-performance liquid chromatographic separation and fluorescent detection.[24] Absolute concentrations of the amino acids were determined using computer analysis of peak height with internal and external standards. Both NAA and NAAG were assayed by anion-exchange high-performance liquid chromatographic separation and UV detection at the wavelength of 214 nm.[25] Their concentrations were determined by peak height calculation. Activity of NAALADase was measured by the hydrolysis of *N*-acetyl-L-aspartyl-L-[^{3}H]glutamate as described by Slusher et al.[18] Protein was measured by the method of Lowry et al,[26] with bovine serum albumin used as the standard. All results were presented as means±SDs.

STATISTICS

For the a priori research hypotheses that there would be neurochemical changes in prefrontal cortex and hippocampus, we tested at the α=.05 level to protect against a type II error. For all other statistical tests, we used a Bonferroni correction to guard against a type I error. Means were compared with analysis of variance F tests because, in all cases, Bartlett's test for heterogeneity of variance was not significant by a χ^2 analysis (all *P*s>.10).

might occur in schizophrenia and contribute to symptom generation.

A number of postmortem studies also support the notion of glutamatergic dysfunction in schizophrenia. There is a deficit of NMDA-mediated glutamate release from synaptosomes prepared from neocortex of patients with schizophrenia that is partially reversed by preincubation with haloperidol.[5] Glutamate uptake[6] and kainic acid–receptor binding[6,7] are reported to be increased in the prefrontal cortex of patients with schizophrenia, which suggests a decreased synaptic activity in the glutamatergic system. In contrast, kainic acid–receptor binding appears to be decreased in putamen as well as in hippocampus and parahippocampal cortex of patients with schizophrenia.[8,9] There's also a reduction in glutamate uptake[10] and an increase in NMDA receptors in basal ganglia.[11] Together, these findings suggest changes in glutamatergic function in schizophrenia but do not point to a specific direction of the alteration, its anatomical localization, or involvement of the receptor subtype.

At present, the mechanism by which dysfunction and/or dysregulation of glutamatergic function might occur in schizophrenia remains to be determined. In addition to PCP and ketamine, several competitive and noncompetitive antagonists of NMDA receptors have been described. *N*-methyl-D-aspartate receptors are subject to regulation by glycine, polyamines, and specific divalent cations.[12] Endogenous peptides have been described that have PCP-like neurochemical properties and that therefore may act as endogenous psychotogens.[13,14] *N*-acetylaspartylglutamate (NAAG) is a neuropeptide that is highly concentrated in glutamatergic neurons.[15] Physiological and receptor-binding studies have demonstrated that it can act on NMDA receptors as a mixed agonist and antagonist, thereby inhibiting responses to glutamate.[16] Electrical stimulation of a well-characterized glutamatergic neuronal pathway in vivo results in a calcium-

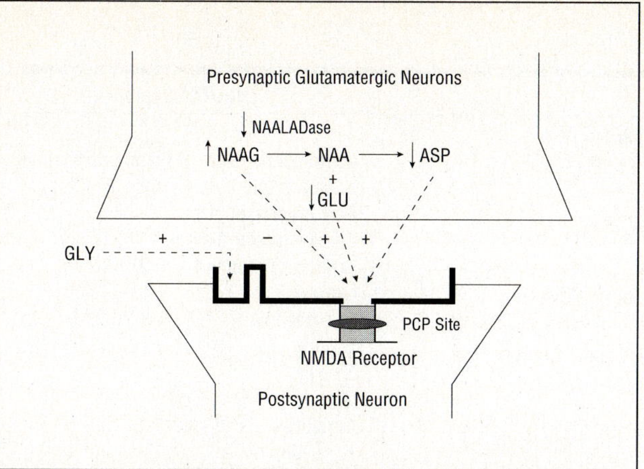

Figure 1. *A glutamatergic nerve ending forming a synapse with a neuron that expresses the* N*-methyl-*D*-aspartate (NMDA) receptor-channel complex. The NMDA receptor has been shown to be regulated by glycine (GLY), which acts on an allosteric site of the receptor (indicated by a plus sign). Phencyclidine hydrochloride (PCP), dizocilpine maleate, and ketamine hydrochloride are noncompetitive antagonists at the channel ionophore. As described in the "Comment" section, increased* N*-acetylaspartylglutamate (NAAG) concentration and decreased* N*-acetyl-α–linked acidic dipeptidase (NAALADase) activity in glutamatergic terminals of schizophrenic brain may result in decreased glutamate (GLU) and aspartate (ASP) concentrations and, thus, may lower postsynaptic NMDA conductance. Alternatively, NAAG may be released directly and act as an antagonist of the NMDA receptor. Increased concentration and release of NAAG may lead to the attenuation of NMDA transmission (indicated by a negative sign). NAA indicates* N*-acetylaspartate.*

dependent release of NAAG.[17] N-methyl-D-aspartate is catabolized to glutamate and *N*-acetylaspartate (NAA) by a specific peptidase, *N*-acetyl-α–linked acidic dipeptidase (NAALADAse).[18] Thus, NAAG may serve as a precursor or storage form for glutamate, in addition to acting as an antagonist of glutamate at NMDA receptors.

Because the limbic system is rich in NAAG-containing neurons, we hypothesized that a reduction in NAALADase activity leading to increased synaptic NAAG levels as well as decreased aspartate and glutamate levels could produce hypoglutamatergic function, accounting for some of the symptoms of schizophrenia, and that these changes would be prominent in the prefrontal cortex and hippocampus, where previous neuropathological and neurophysiological studies demonstrate consistent changes.[19,20] To test this hypothesis, we assayed the concentration of aspartate, glutamate, NAAG, and the activity of NAALADAse in several regions of postmortem brains obtained from patients with schizophrenia, neuroleptic-treated patients without schizophrenia, and normal controls.

RESULTS

Table 2 lists the mean NAAG and amino acid (NAA, aspartate, glutamate, and glycine) content and the enzymatic activity of NAALADase in eight different regions of the brain in the patients with schizophrenia, the normal controls, and the neuroleptic-treated controls. It reveals that most of the changes of excitatory neurotransmitters are localized to the prefrontal cortex and hippocampus (**Figure 2** and Table 2). No statistically significant correlations were observed between age, sex, or postmortem delay and the neurochemical variables. Our results regarding the levels of these variables are comparable with those of other studies.[27,28]

When the schizophrenia group was compared with the normal control group, NAAG content was significantly and markedly elevated in hippocampus (55%) and in prefrontal cortex (63%) of neuroleptic-treated controls (Table 2 and Figure 1). The NAALADase activity was decreased in hippocampus (−28%) and prefrontal cortex (−37%). Glutamate content was significantly decreased in hippocampus (−37%) and prefrontal cortex (−42%). Aspartate content was significantly decreased in hippocampus (−40%). In addition to prefrontal cortex and hippocampus, NAALADase activity had a trend toward a decrease in the parahippocampal cortex (−32%, F=5.67, *P*=.06) (Table 2) but was unchanged in the other five regions assayed and in all the regions assayed from neuroleptic-treated controls when compared with normal controls.

In hippocampus of the schizophrenic brains, there was an inverse correlation between NAALADase activities and NAAG concentrations (r=−.71, P<.004, n=12); glutamate levels increased as NAALADase activities increased (r=.35, P=.22, n=12). A similar, inverse correlation between NAALADase activities and NAAG levels (r=−.52, P=.01, n=12) was observed in prefrontal cortex. Because NAALADase converts NAAG to glutamate, it is not surprising that there would be an inverse correlation between the enzyme activity and NAAG and a positive correlation between the enzyme activity and glutamate.

Levels of NAA were similar in all brain regions from patients with schizophrenia, normal controls, and neuroleptic-treated control subjects. Glycine levels were unchanged in all the regions examined in the patients with schizophrenia. However, when neuroleptic-treated control subjects were compared with normal controls, there was a trend for aspartate, glutamate, and glycine to be increased in several brain regions (Table 2). Aspartate was increased significantly in prefrontal cortex (135%, F=5.63, *P*=.006) and parietal cortex (74%, F=6.24, *P*=.004). Glutamate was significantly elevated in hippocampus (62%, F=5.67, *P*=.006), prefrontal cortex (73%, F=5.67, *P*=.006), and parietal cortex (76%, F=3.25, *P*=.047). Glycine was significantly increased in hippocampus (78%, F=8.08, *P*=.001) and prefrontal (71%, F=3.20, *P*=.049) and parietal (40%, F=3.25, *P*=.047) cortices, but only the increase of glycine in hippocampus survived a Bonferroni correction.

Correlations were found in several brain regions between NAAG and NAALADase, NAAG and NAA, and NAAG and the other amino acids studied when data from all 29 subjects were grouped together (**Table 3**). Significant correlations were found between NAA and aspartate (parahippocampus, r=.44, P<.01; parietal cortex, r=.47, P<.001), NAA and glutamate (parietal cortex, r=.64, P<.001), and NAA and glycine (prefrontal cortex, r=.34, P<.01; parietal cortex, r=.38, P<.005) and between aspartate and glutamate, aspartate and glycine, and glutamate and glycine in various brain regions (Table 3).

Table 1. Patient Characteristics of the Three Sample Groups*

Patient No./Sex/Age, y	*DSM-III-R* Definition	Cause of Death
	Schizophrenic Group	
1/M/34	Undifferentiated	Acute benztropine mesylate intoxication
2/M/54	Undifferentiated	Subarachnoid hemorrhage
3/F/80	Undifferentiated	Accidental asphyxia
4/M/73	Undifferentiated	Cardiovascular disease
5/F/49	Undifferentiated	Chronic obstructive airway disease
6/M/34	Undifferentiated	Unkown
7/M/66	Undifferentiated	Hypothermia
8/M/30	Undifferentiated	Suicide
9/M/25	Undifferentiated	Suicide
10/F/30	Undifferentiated	Suicide
11/M/36	Undifferentiated	Cardiovascular disease
12/M/48	Undifferentiated	Hyponatremia
	Control Group	
13/M/34	NA	Motor vehicle crash
14/M/71	NA	Cardiovascular disease
15/M/33	NA	Multiple blunt force injury
16/F/48	NA	Pulmonary hypertension
17/F/61	NA	Multiple blunt force injury
18/M/57	NA	Cardiovascular disease
19/F/46	NA	Cardiomyopathy
20/M/56	NA	Cardiovascular disease
21/M/25	NA	Homicide
22/M/48	NA	Cardiovascular disease
23/M/33	NA	Arnold-Chiari deformity
	Neuroleptic-Treated Control Group	
24/F/47	Organic brain syndrome	Asthma
25/M/68	Organic brain syndrome	Accidental asphyxia
26/M/34	Organic brain syndrome	Aortic aneurysm
27/M/40	Antisocial personality disorder	Asthma
28/F/37	Psychotic disorder, NOS	Chronic alcoholism
29/M/45	Psychotic disorder, NOS	Cardiovascular disease

**NA indicates not applicable; NOS, not otherwise specified.*

COMMENT

Since Kim et al[1] first reported decreased glutamate concentrations in cerebrospinal fluid from patients with schizophrenia, the findings of subsequent studies have been inconsistent, with several reports of no alteration in cerebrospinal fluid concentrations of glutamate.[2] The results of our study support the hypoglutamatergic hypothesis of schizophrenia. In our study, NAAG levels were increased and aspartate and glutamate levels were decreased, whereas the enzymatic activity of NAALADase, which cleaves NAAG into glutamate and NAA, was decreased in the patients with schizophrenia. The changes in aspartate, glutamate, and NAAG levels and in NAALADase activity were pronounced in the prefrontal cortex and hippocampus regions, where previous neuropathological and neurophysiological studies suggest consistent abnormalities in structure and function in schizophrenia.[19,20] In addition, NAAG concentrations and NAALADase activity were significantly correlated with levels of glutamate, aspartate, and glycine, which are important in glutamatergic transmission (Table 3). Thus, our findings underscore the importance of studying metabolically and physiologically related molecules in addition to glutamate itself.

N-acetylaspartate is a neuronal-specific marker.[29] The fact that the concentrations of NAA are unchanged in several brain regions in schizophrenia argues against cell loss or gliosis as the cause of the changes in excitatory transmitter markers that we observed. It may also reflect the fact that a substantial component of NAA is unrelated to NAAG or glutamatergic neurons but is localized to virtually all neuronal perikarya.

Our study demonstrates alterations in the levels of NAAG, aspartate, and glutamate and in NAALADase activity in schizophrenic brains. Notably, the changes in aspartate, glutamate, and NAAG levels and in NAALADase activity in schizophrenic brains were selective and restricted primarily to prefrontal cortex and hippocampus. The negative results of a previous study of amino acids in postmortem brains of patients with chronic schizophrena may be due to the different brain regions studied.[27] Changes in the size of the parahippocampal gyrus have been reported in both schizophrenic and nonschizophrenic patients who had committed suicide.[23] The small number of subjects who committed suicide (three in the schizophrenia group and none in the other two groups) precluded an analysis of the relationship between suicide and the neurochemical changes that we observed. It would be interesting to know whether nonschizophrenic subjects who committed suicide have similar neurochemical changes in the prefrontal temporal regions.

Table 2. Levels of Excitatory Transmitter Markers in Schizophrenic Brains*

Brain Region and Group	NAAG	NAALADase	Aspartate	Glutamate	NAA	Glycine
Hippocampus, (F, *P*)	(4.30, .01)	(3.67, .03)	(4.41, .02)	(7.45, .002)		(8.08, .001)†
Schizophrenia	8.7±4.5‡	11.6±4.2‡	5.0±2.1‡	29.9±11.1‡	43.9±14.5	13.2±6.2
Normal control	5.6±2.7	16.0±5.6	8.4±3.3	47.3±18.9	42.6±11.9	16.2±7.0
Neuroleptic-treated control	6.2±2.0	12.8±4.9	7.6±2.2	76.8±23.0§	36.2±11.8	28.9±5.1§
Prefrontal cortex, (F, *P*)	(3.74, .03)	(5.59, .006)	(5.63, .006)	(12.81, <.001)		
Schizophrenia	6.1±3.5	5.9±2.1‡	13.4±8.7	39.5±24.9‡	58.8±24.9	19.1±12.8
Normal control	6.5±3.0	9.3±2.7	11.0±6.0	68.6±36.8	56.1±9.3	19.2±9.6
Neuroleptic-treated control	10.6±3.9§	8.3±3.2	25.9±12.7§	118.7±20.6§	46.5±12.7	32.8±7.3
Parahippocampus						
Schizophrenia	5.8±2.1	6.3±1.7	5.4±3.1	28.9±12.1	39.9±12.8	6.3±3.8
Normal control	5.1±2.0	9.2±1.7	3.8±2.0	25.4±14.9	46.8±9.9	9.3±6.3
Neuroleptic-treated control	6.0±2.7	10.6±5.4	4.6±2.9	33.3±23.0	43.2±12.5	5.2±5.6
Putamen						
Schizophrenia	4.3±2.1	12.6±3.8	5.7±2.8	29.8±11.8	43.5±11.4	12.8±6.9
Normal control	5.1±2.7	15.6±3.6	8.5±3.3	37.8±18.9	43.3±7.3	12.9±5.6
Neuroleptic-treated control	6.2±1.5	15.5±4.4	6.3±2.0	46.1±17.1	34.9±11.8	12.2±2.4
Cingulate cortex						
Schizophrenia	4.7±1.7	7.5±3.1	7.7±2.8	50.9±23.2	39.8±8.3	9.9±4.5
Normal control	5.1±2.0	7.7±3.7	9.8±5.0	57.5±21.2	44.3±9.0	10.8±4.6
Neuroleptic-treated control	5.7±3.2	7.2±2.7	9.1±4.7	52.7±22.3	36.3±12.7	8.7±3.4
Amygdala						
Schizophrenia	5.3±4.2	8.1±3.8	9.0±5.5	48.4±15.2	46.0±12.1	13.9±5.9
Normal control	7.2±4.0	11.5±4.6	9.5±4.6	44.2±17.6	45.2±9.6	12.7±4.6
Neuroleptic-treated control	7.2±3.2	10.0±4.2	14.3±3.2	70.6±19.4	46.5±11.3	15.1±3.2
Parietal cortex						
Schizophrenia	4.2±1.0	7.4±2.8	4.9±3.1	21.2±10.0	52.0±14.2	7.9±3.8
Normal control	4.1±1.0	7.8±2.0	5.7±3.0	24.5±12.9	55.5±12.3	9.0±3.0
Neuroleptic-treated control	5.0±0.7	10.9±6.1	9.9±2.2	43.1±15.9	61.9±16.7	12.6±2.7
Cerebellum						
Schizophrenia	13.5±6.2	5.9±3.5	12.0±7.6	41.1±18.0	34.7±7.6	10.9±2.4
Normal control	8.9±4.6	5.9±1.7	13.9±3.6	53.0±8.3	35.0±8.0	13.0±3.6
Neuroleptic-treated control	14.0±4.7	5.8±1.5	18.1±3.9	64.7±18.9	36.6±10.5	14.0±3.2

**Values are mean±SD nanomoles per milligram of protein or picomoles per milligram of protein per hour for* N*-acetyl-α–linked acidic dipeptidase (NAALADase). One-way analyses of variance (ANOVAs) were computed for each molecule in different brain regions. Data originating from a priori hypotheses are presented in the box and were tested at* P<.05. *Post hoc Fisher protected least significant difference (PLSD)* t *test was done only in the regions in which ANOVA found* P<.05. *In regions in which ANOVA found* P<.05, *F(2,28) and* P *values are indicated within parentheses. In the rest of the data groups, we applied Bonferroni-adjusted probability to reduce type I errors. NAAG indicates* N*-acetylaspartylglutamate; NAA,* N*-acetylaspartate.*

†*Passed Bonferroni correction.*

‡*Schizophrenia vs normal control was significant at* P<.05 *by post hoc Fisher PLSD* t *test.*

§*Neuroleptic-treated vs normal control was significant at* P<.05 *by post hoc Fisher PLSD* t *test.*

The region- and group-selective changes argue against the interpretation that the results reflect simply postmortem alterations. Nevertheless, these molecules are involved not only in neurotransmission but also in other metabolic functions. The methods that we applied cannot differentiate the functional localization of these molecules. It awaits detailed neuroanatomical study to delineate the cellular and subcellular localization of the changes. For example, we did not observe any change of the excitatory transmission markers in the cingulate cortex, where an increased density of glutamate-immunoreactive vertical process in superficial laminae has been described.[30] The discrepancy is likely owing to the different cellular resolution of the methods applied and the fact that synaptic glutamate may represent only 10% to 15% of the total pool of glutamate.

Endogenous peptides have been described that have PCP-like neurochemical properties and that therefore may act as endogenous psychotogens.[13,14] *N*-acetylaspartylglutamate acts as a mixed-agonist or antagonist of the NMDA receptors based on its biphasic modulation of norepinephrine release,[16] Mg^{++}-sensitive and 2-amino-5-phosphonovalerate–sensitive electrophysiological effects,[31] and pharmacological blockade of climbing fiber and oocyte responses to glutamate.[32] Immunocytochemical studies demonstrated a widespread congruency of NAA and NAAG with putative glutamatergic pathways, including the corticolimbic structures (Tsai et al[15] and G.T., B. Stauch, PhD, L.A.P., J.T.C., unpublished data, 1995). Increased NAAG concentration can lead to an attenuation of glutamatergic neurotransmission. Alternatively, NAAG also serves as a precursor for the neurotransmitter glutamate. A decrease in NAALADase activity may account for a decreased activity of glutamatergic transmission because less synaptic glutamate would be released from NAAG (Figure 1). It is unclear whether our findings reflect an increased supply of NAAG or a primary defect of NAALADase. Nevertheless, given the PCP/NMDA hypothesis of schizophrenia, the role of NAALADase, NAAG, and glutamate in psychosis in general and in schizophrenia specifically are worthy of further investigation.

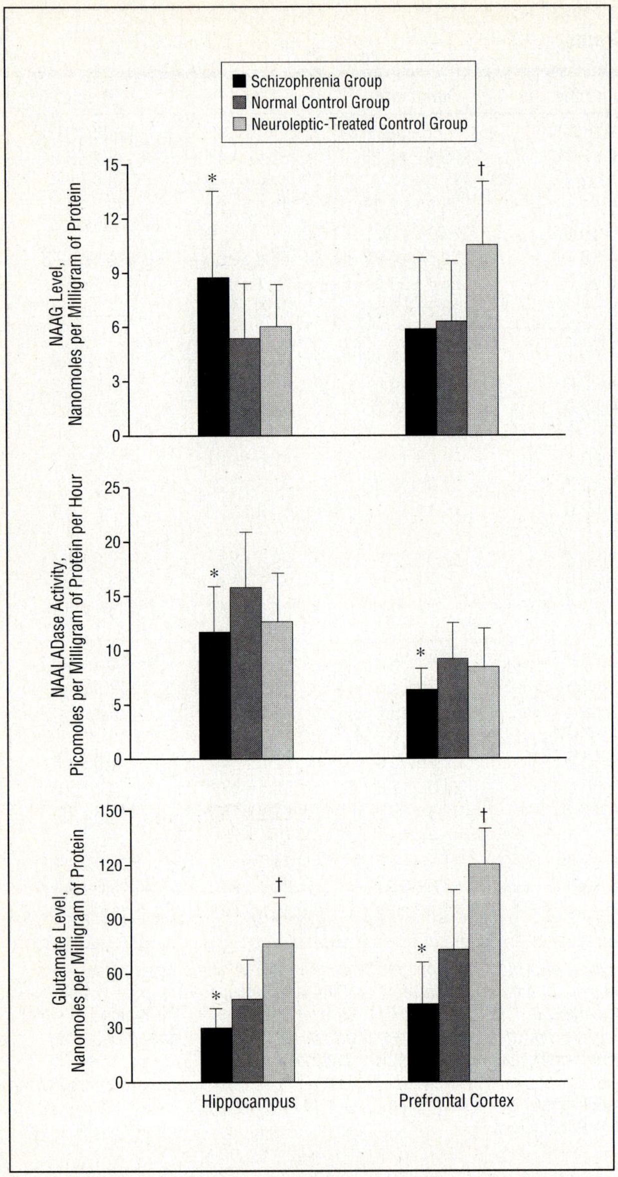

Figure 2. *Mean levels of* N*-acetylaspartylglutamate (NAAG) and glutamate as well as* N*-acetyl-α–linked acidic dipeptidase (NAALADase) activities in hippocampus and prefrontal cortex of schizophrenic patients and normal and neuroleptic-treated controls. One-way analyses of variance (ANOVAs) were computed for each variable in different brain regions. A post hoc Fisher protected least significant difference (PLSD)* t *test was done only in the regions where ANOVAs found* $P<.05$*. Asterisks represent regions in which schizophrenia group vs normal control group was significant (*$P<.05$*) by post hoc Fisher PLSD* t *test; daggers, the regions in which neuroleptic-treated vs normal controls was significant (*$P<.05$*). T-bars represent SD.*

In hippocampus and prefrontal cortex of brains from schizophrenic patients, NAAG concentrations were increased, whereas NAALADase activity was decreased, which is consistent with a reduction in NAAG turnover in these regions. The high cross-correlation among the different molecules that we studied (Table 3) strongly suggests that NAAG and NAALADase play an important role in the metabolism of glutamate and may be relevant to the pathophysiologic processes of schizophrenia. Nevertheless, the relative salience of the interactions between NAAG and other sources of glutamate is unknown. It will be important to study other sources of glutamate as a neurotransmitter, like glutamine, to further delineate the defective pathway(s) of excitatory neurotransmission in schizophrenia.

The precise mechanisms by which NMDA-receptor dysfunction might occur in schizophrenia remain to be determined. *N*-methyl-D-aspartate receptors are sensitive to the effects of glycine, polyamines, and specific divalent cations (eg, Mg^{++} and Zn^{++})[12] in addition to the effects of NAAG and glutamate. Abnormal concentrations of glutamate or of any of these modulators therefore potentially could lead to decreased NMDA-receptor activation. Glycine potentiates NMDA-receptor–mediated neurotransmission (Figure 1).[33] In our study of the brains of patients with schizophrenia, the concentrations of free aspartate and glutamate were found to be decreased. Recently, the NMDA-associated glycine binding site was found to be elevated in schizophrenic brains.[34,35] Taken together with our findings, the elevated NMDA-receptor–linked glycine binding site suggests a hypofunction of NMDA neurotransmission and a compensatory receptor supersensitivity.

Increased concentrations of the neurotransmitters aspartate and glutamate and the neuromodulator glycine in neuroleptic-treated nonschizophrenic brains raise the intriguing possibility that neuroleptics may exert their antipsychotic effects in part by altering glutamatergic neurotransmission. This finding is supported by the report that the cerebrospinal fluid levels of glutamate were higher in the patients who were receiving neuroleptics than in those not receiving neuroleptics.[36] Notably, the levels of markers for the glutamatergic system were not increased in patients with chronic schizophrenia who were exposed to neuroleptics, which suggests a primary defect in the modulation of the glutamatergic system by neuroleptics in this population with chronic schizophrenia. This finding supports the hypothesis of a hypofunction in glutamate-mediated neurotransmission in chronic schizophrenia, which may account for positive and negative symptoms and the neurocognitive deficit in schizophrenia. The changes in the schizophrenic and neuroleptic-treated control groups were in the opposite direction of those in the group of normal controls. This divergence argues against the the notion that the changes in the schizophrenic group are due to the neuroleptic treatment. However, the possibility of a differential neuroleptic dosage or duration effect between the two groups cannot be excluded because information about these factors is difficult to evaluate.

Glutamatergic and dopaminergic systems are closely related in forebrain.[36] The findings in the present study of the postmortem brains of patients with schizophrenia support a hypofunction of glutamatergic neurotransmission as a critical component of this disorder. It is not clear whether the reduced glutamatergic neurotransmission is the primary defect in schizophrenia or a secondary change due to excessive activation of dopamine receptors. Increased dopaminergic activity can inhibit glutamatergic function and could result in a hypoglutamatergic state in schizophrenia.[36] Conversely, overactivity of the dopaminergic system in schizophrenia may be due to a primary defect of glutamatergic transmission.[37]

Table 3. Correlation Coefficients Between Different Acidic Neurotransmitter Markers in Postmortem Human Brain*

	Hippocampus	Prefrontal Cortex	Parahippocampus	Putamen	Cingulate Cortex	Amygdala	Parietal Cortex	Cerebellum
NAAG and NAALADase	.02	.08	.28	.37	.44	.26	.37	.08
NAAG and aspartate	.25	.75†	.15	.17	.23	.78†	.62†	.32
NAAG and glutamate	.18	.67†	.26	.36	.05	.67†	.65†	.12
NAALADase and aspartate	.17	.23	.03	.03	.15	.26	.20	.21
NAALADase and glutamate	.26	.07	.13	.30	.13	.28	.17	.02
Aspartate and glutamate	.40‡	.71†	.61†	.53†	.60†	.80†	.80†	.60†

Correlation coefficients are given between N-acetylaspartylglutamate (NAAG), N-acetylaspartate (NAA), N-acetyl-α-linked acidic dipeptidase (NAALADase), aspartate, and glutamate as indicated in different brain regions (N=29). Data in the "Hippocampus" and "Prefrontal Cortex" columns originate from a priori hypotheses and were tested at P<.05. In the rest of the data groups, Bonferroni-adjusted probability was applied to reduce type I error.

†P<.001.

‡P<.01.

Alternatively, NMDA receptors themselves could be dysfunctional, leading secondarily to changes in presynaptic glutamate markers, as we have observed. Dysfunction of NMDA receptors recently has been suggested to occur in Alzheimer's disease.[38] The NMDA-receptor–bearing cells have an increased risk for apoptosis[39] or degeneration as a result of excitotoxic, ischemic, or hypoglycemic insults.[40] Degeneration of striatal NMDA-receptor–bearing neurons by an excitotoxic mechanism has been hypothesized to account for the pathophysiologic characteristics of Huntington's disease,[41,42] which may present with psychotic symptoms. Indeed, volume reduction and neuronal loss in medial temporal lobe has been reported in the schizophrenic brain.[43] Cortical associational pathways and the perforant pathway from entorhinal cortex to dentate gyrus of hippocampus use excitatory amino acids as their neurotransmitter. The hippocampus is a particularly vulnerable region for excitotoxic insult. The hypoglutamatergic state observed in schizophrenia may be the result of prior glutamate-mediated excitotoxicity or primary disruption of cortical development due to glutamate-receptor dysfunction through the mechanism of apoptosis.[44]

In the last decade, it has become clear that excitatory amino acids play a role in a wide range of neurodegenerative disorders. The evidence is clearest where the degenerative process is acute, such as in ischemia and hypoglycemia, but is strongly circumstantial in slowly progressive neurodegenerative disorders such as amyotrophic lateral sclerosis,[28] Huntington's disease,[41,42] and olivopontocerebellar degeneration.[45] Previous studies have demonstrated alterations in NAAG metabolism and glutamate variables in both ischemia[46] and amyotrophic lateral sclerosis.[28] Interestingly, in contrast to the findings in schizophrenia, levels of NAA and NAAG are decreased and NAALADase activity is increased in both the spinal cord and motor cortex in amyotrophic lateral sclerosis,[28] which is consistent with an overstimulation of glutamate receptors that leads to selective neuronal degeneration. Our findings suggest that NAAG and NAALADase have important roles in the pathological disturbance of glutamatergic neurotransmission, which may be related to the pathophysiologic processes of schizophrenia.

Accepted for publication March 31, 1995.

Supported in part by grant RO1 MH51290-01 from the National Insitute of Mental Health and a Young Investigator Award (Dr Tsai) from the National Alliance for Research on Schizophrenia and Depression, Chicago, Ill.

Presented at the 61st Salmon Lecture, New York, NY, December 2, 1993.

Reprint requests to McLean Hospital, 115 Mill St, Belmont, MA 02178 (Dr Coyle).

REFERENCES

1. Kim JS, Kornhuber HH, Schmid-Burgk W, Holzmuller B. Low cerebrospinal fluid glutamate in schizophrenic patients and a new hypothesis on schizophrenia. *Neurosci Lett.* 1980;20:379-382.
2. Deutsch SI, Mastropaolo J, Schwartz BL, Rosse RB, Morihisa JM. A 'glutamatergic hypothesis' of schizophrenia. *J Clin Psychopharmacol.* 1989;12:1-13.
3. Javitts DC, Zukin SR. Recent advances in the phencyclidine model of schizophrenia. *Am J Psychiatry.* 1991;148:1301-1308.
4. Krystal JH, Karper LP, Seibyl JP, Freeman GK, Delaney R, Brenner JP, Henninger GR, Bowers MB, Charney DS. Subanaesthetic effects of the non-competitive NMDA antagonist, ketamine, in humans: psychotominetic, perceptual, cognitive, and neuroendocrine responses. *Arch Gen Psychiatry.* 1994; 51:199-214.
5. Sherman AD, Davidson AT, Baruah S, Hegwood TS, Waziri R. Evidence of glutamatergic deficiency in schizophrenia. *Neurosci Lett.* 1991;121:77-80.
6. Deakin JFW, Slater P, Simpson MDC, Gilchrist AC, Skan WJ, Royston MC, Reynolds GP, Cross AJ. Frontal cortical and left temporal glutamatergic dysfunction in schizophrenia. *J Neurochem.* 1989;52:1781-1786.
7. Nishikawa T, Takashima M, Toru M. Increased [^{3}H]kainic acid binding in the prefrontal cortex in schizophrenia. *Neurosci Lett.* 1983;40:245-250.
8. Kerwin RW, Patel S, Meldrum BS, Czudek C, Reynolds GP. Asymmetrical loss of glutamate receptors subtype in left hippocampus in schizophrenia. *Lancet.* 1988;1:583-584.
9. Kerwin R, Patel S, Meldrum B. Quantitative autoradiographic analysis of glutamate binding sites in the hippocampal formation in normal and schizophrenic brain post mortem. *Neuroscience.* 1990;39:25-32.
10. Simpson MDC, Slater P, Royston MC, Deakin JFW. Regionally selective deficits in uptake sites for glutamate and gamma-aminobutyric acid in the basal ganglia in schizophrenia. *Psychiatry Res.* 1992;42:273-282.
11. Kornhuber J, Mack-Burkhardt F, Riederer P, Hebenstreit GF, Reynolds GP, Andrews HB, Beckmann H. [^{3}H]MK-801 binding sites in postmortem brain regions of schizophrenic patients. *J Neural Transm Park Dis Dement Sect.* 1989; 77:231-236.
12. Robinson MB, Coyle JT. Glutamate and related acidic excitatory neurotransmitters: from basic science to clinical application. *FASEB J.* 1987;1:446-455.
13. Quirion R, Bayorh MS, Zerbe RL, Pert CV. Evidence for an endogenous peptide ligand for the phencyclidine receptor. *Peptides.* 1984;5:967-973.
14. Zukin SR, Zukin RS, Vale W. An endogenous ligand of the brain s/PCP receptor antagonizes NMDA-induced neurotransmitter release. *Brain Res.* 1987;415: 84-89.

15. Tsai G, Stauch B, Sim L, Coyle JT. Immunocytochemical distribution of *N*-acetylaspartylglutamate in the rat forebrain and glutamatergic pathways. *J Chem Neuroanat.* 1993;6:277-292.
16. Puttfarcken PS, Handen JS, Montgomery DT, Coyle JT, Werling LL. *N*-acetyl-aspartylglutamate modulation of *N*-methyl-D-aspartate stimulated [^{3}H]norepinephrine release from rat hippocampal slices. *J Pharmacol Exp Ther.* 1993; 266:796-803.
17. Tsai G, Stauch B, Vernov J, Deshpondae J, Coyle JT. Selective in vivo release of *N*-acetylaspartylglutamate from rat optic pathway. *Brain Res.* 1990;518:313-316.
18. Slusher BS, Robinson MB, Tsai G, Simmons ML, Richards SS, Coyle JT. Rat brain *N*-acetyl-alpha–linked acidic dipeptidase activity: purification and immunological characterization. *J Biol Chem.* 1990;265:21297-21301.
19. Bogerts B, Ashtari M, Degreef G, Alvir JMJ, Bilder RM, Lieberman JA. Reduced temporal limbic structures volumes on magnetic resonance images in first episode schizophrenia. *Psychiatry Res.* 1990;35:1-13.
20. Weinberger D, Berman KF, Suddath R, Torrey EF. Evidence of dysfunction of a prefrontal-limbic network in schizophrenia: an MRI and rCBF study of discordant monozygotic twins. *Am J Psychiatry.* 1992;149:890-897.
21. American Psychiatric Association. *Diagnostic and Statistical Manual of Mental Disorders, Revised Third Edition.* Washington, DC: American Psychiatric Association; 1987.
22. Korpi ER, Kleinman JE, Goodman SI, Philips I, DeLisi LE, Linnoila M, Wyatt RJ. Serotonin and 5-hydroxyindoleacetic acid in brains of suicide victims: comparison in chronic schizophrenic patients with suicide as cause of death. *Arch Gen Psychiatry.* 1986;43:594-600.
23. Altshuler LL, Casanova MF, Goldberg TE, Kleinman JE. The hippocampus and parahippocampus in schizophrenic, suicide, and control brains. *Arch Gen Psychiatry.* 1990;47:1029-1034.
24. Jones BN. Amino acid analysis by *o*-phthalaldehyde precolumn derivatization and reverse-phase HPLC. In: Shively JE, ed. *Method of Protein Microcharacterization.* Clifton, NJ: Humana Press; 1986:121-151.
25. Koller K, Zaczek R, Coyle JT. *N*-acetyl-aspartyl glutamate: regional levels in rat brain and the effects of brain lesions as determined by a new HPLC method. *J Neurochem.* 1984;43:1136-1142.
26. Lowry OH, Rosebrough NJ, Farr AL, Randall RJ. Protein measurement with Folin phenol reagent. *J Biol Chem.* 1951;193:265-275.
27. Korpi ER, Kleinman JE, Goodman SI, Wyatt RJ. Neurotransmitter amino acids in post-mortem brains of chronic schizophrenic patients. *Psychiatry Res.* 1987; 22:291-301.
28. Tsai G, Slusher BS, Sim L, Hedreen JC, Rothstein JD, Kuncl R, Coyle JT. Reductions in acidic amino acids and *N*-acetylaspartylglutamate in amyotrophic lateral sclerosis CNS. *Brain Res.* 1991;556:151-156.
29. Simmons ML, Frondoza CG, Coyle JT. Immunocytochemical localization of *N*-acetyl-aspartate with monoclonal antibodies. *Neuroscience.* 1991;45:37-45.
30. Benes FM. Neurobiological investigations in cingulate cortex of schizophrenic brain. *Schizophr Bull.* 1993;19:537-549.
31. Sekiguchi M, Okamoto K, Sakai Y. Excitatory action of *N*-acetyl-aspartylglutamate on Purkinje cells in guinea pig cerebellar slices: an intrasomatic study. *Brain Res.* 1987;423:23-33.
32. Sekiguchi M, Okamoto K, Sakai Y. Low concentration *N*-acetyl-aspartylglutamate suppresses the climbing fiber response of Purkinje cells in guinea pig cerebellar slices and the responses to excitatory amino acids of *Xenopus laevis* oocytes injected with cerebellar mRNA. *Brain Res.* 1989;482: 87-96.
33. Thomson AM, Walker VE, Flynn DM. Glycine enhances NMDA-receptor mediated synaptic potentials in neocortical slices. *Nature.* 1989;338:422-424.
34. Ishimaru M, Kurumaji A, Toru M. NMDA-associated glycine binding site increases in schizophrenic brains. *Biol Psychiatry.* 1992;32:379-381.
35. Ishimaru M, Kurumaji A, Toru M. Increases in strychnine-insensitive glycine binding sites in cerebral cortex of chronic schizophrenics: evidence for glutamate hypothesis. *Biol Psychiatry.* 1994;35:84-95.
36. Kotter R. Postsynaptic integration of glutamatergic and dopaminergic signals in the striatum. *Prog Neurobiol.* 1994;44:163-196.
37. Gattaz WF, Gattaz D, Beckmann H. Glutamate in schizophrenics and healthy controls. *Arch Psychiatr Nervenkr.* 1982;231:221-225.
38. Procter AW, Wong EHF, Stratmann GC, Lowe SL, Bowen DM. Reduced glycine stimulation of [^{3}H]MK-801 binding in Alzheimer's disease. *J Neurochem.* 1989;53:698-704.
39. Mitchell IJ, Lawson S, Moser B, Laidlaw SM, Cooper AJ, Walkinshaw G, Waters CM. Glutamate-induced apoptosis results in a loss of striatal neurons in the parkinsonian rat. *Neuroscience.* 1994;63:1-5.
40. Ulas J, Cotman CW. Excitatory amino acid receptors in schizophrenia. *Schizophr Bull.* 1993;19:105-117.
41. Coyle JT, Ferkany JW, Zaczek R. Insights from a neurotoxin into the pathophysiology of Huntington's disease. *Neurobehav Toxicol Teratol.* 1983;5:617-624.
42. Young AB, Greenamyre JT, Hollingsworth A. NMDA receptor losses in putamen from patients with Huntington's disease. *Science.* 1988;241:981-983.
43. Roberts GW. Schizophrenia: a neuropathological perspective. *Br J Psychiatry.* 1991;158:8-17.
44. McDonald JW, Johnston MV. Physiological and pathophysiological roles of excitatory amino acids during central nervous system development. *Brain Res Rev.* 1990;15:41-70.
45. Coyle JT. Excitotoxins. In: Meltzer HY, ed. *Psychopharmacology: The Third Generation of Progress.* New York, NY: Raven Press; 1987:333-340.
46. Deshpande JK, Tsai G, Stauch B, Passani L, Coyle JT. Ischemic changes of excitatory neurotransmitters in rat hippocampus. *Soc Neurosci Abstr.* 1990; 16:1190. Abstract.

Correction

Typographical Error. In the article "Efficacy of Methylphenidate for Attention-Deficit Hyperactivity Disorder in Children With Tic Disorder," which appeared in the June 1995 issue of the ARCHIVES, there was a typographical error in one of the F values. On page 452, the decimal point in the last F value provided in the "Parent Ratings" section was erroneously typeset as a hyphen. The sentence should have read, "A linear function provided a good fit to the data ($F[1,29]=10.66$, $P=.003$)." The ARCHIVES apologizes for its error.

ORIGINAL ARTICLE

Plasma Haloperidol Levels and Clinical Effects in Schizophrenia and Schizoaffective Disorder

Jan Volavka, MD, PhD; Thomas B. Cooper, MA; Pál Czobor, PhD; Morris Meisner, PhD

Background: Plasma haloperidol levels between 5 and 11 ng/mL may be clinically optimal for acutely exacerbated schizophrenia, but the evidence for this therapeutic window has been inconsistent.

Methods: Haloperidol was administered in a double-blind manner during two consecutive 3-week experimental periods to 65 patients with acutely exacerbated schizophrenia or schizoaffective disorder. Two plasma levels were targeted: "low" (2 ng/mL) and "moderate" (10 ng/mL). The subjects were randomly assigned to four treatment sequences (low-low, low-moderate, moderate-moderate, or moderate-low).

Results: In the first 3 weeks, the antipsychotic efficacy of haloperidol increased with plasma levels up to approximately 12 ng/mL. In the second 3 weeks, decrease of plasma levels reduced negative symptoms.

Conclusion: For most patients, plasma levels not exceeding 12 ng/mL yield the best results in the first 3 weeks of treatment. Subsequent lowering of the plasma levels may improve negative symptoms.

(Arch Gen Psychiatry. 1995;52:837-845)

SEVERAL PARADIGMS have been used to elucidate relationships between plasma level and clinical effects of haloperidol. Early studies yielded equivocal results.[1,2] Recent studies used random assignment of subjects to one of several fixed-dose haloperidol treatment regimens. Of the six studies using that design,[3-10] five reported a "therapeutic window"—a range of plasma haloperidol levels that yields optimal therapeutic benefit for most patients.[3-6,9,10]

Four of these six investigations studied patients with acutely exacerbated schizophrenia who had been recently readmitted to a hospital.[3,7,9,10] Three of these four studies indicated a therapeutic window at plasma haloperidol levels of approximately 5 to 11 ng/mL. Levels as low as 5 ng/mL may be effective.[11,12] An additional impetus came from a positron emission tomography study that demonstrated a relationship between plasma levels of haloperidol and dopamine D_2 receptor occupancy in the human striatum.[13] The occupancy increased steeply as a function of the plasma level of haloperidol up to approximately 10 to 15 ng/mL, then it tapered off. These results suggested that the relationship between plasma level and clinical effects of haloperidol might be best defined at levels between 0 and approximately 10 to 15 ng/mL.

Our previous study used fixed plasma levels (instead of fixed doses) of haloperidol in a parallel group trial.[14] Three plasma level ranges were tested: 2 to 13, 13.1 to 24, and 24.1 to 35 ng/mL. No substantial differences in therapeutic efficacy were detected among the three plasma level ranges. We now believe that our previous study (and perhaps other studies as well[7,8]) failed to define a relationship between plasma level and clinical effects because attention was focused at levels that were too high. We present the results of a study focusing on the clinical efficacy of low plasma levels of haloperidol.

From the Nathan S. Kline Institute for Psychiatric Research, Orangeburg, NY, and the Department of Psychiatry, New York (NY) University.

RESULTS

SAMPLE ATTRITION

The actual mean±SD duration of patients' participation in period 1 was 5.9±1.8 days. Overall attrition is presented in **Figure 1**.

See Subjects and Methods on next page

SUBJECTS AND METHODS

A total of 111 patients who gave written consent and met the *DSM-III-R* diagnostic criteria for schizophrenia or schizoaffective disorder were entered into the study. We included only patients with acutely exacerbated conditions, defined by less than 15 days of treatment during the current episode at the time of the patient's entry into the study. Thus, the patients were newly admitted to one of the four participating hospitals: Manhattan (NY) Psychiatric Center; Rockland Psychiatric Center, Orangeburg, NY; Brookdale Memorial Hospital, Brooklyn, NY; or Bellevue Hospital, New York, NY. All subjects were inpatients throughout the study. In 85 patients with adequate data, the mean±SD duration of oral antipsychotic medication taken during the current episode but prior to entry into the study was 6.8±4.2 days; the mean daily dose was 11.4±7.5 mg in haloperidol equivalents. These averages were computed for the current episode rather than the current hospitalization; if the patient was transferred between hospitals during the current episode, the data from these hospitals were combined to obtain the average treatment duration and dose for the episode. Patients who had received an injection of slow-release antipsychotic agent in the preceding month were excluded. Although 1 month after an injection is insufficient to clear the antipsychotic agent from the body,[15] a longer waiting period was not feasible.

PROCEDURES

Experimental Periods 1, 2, and 3

Period 1 was single-blind; all patients received placebo. The planned duration of this period, 1 week, was limited by the deterioration of patients' conditions; the acceptable minimum was 3 days. To qualify for entry into period 2, patients had to meet two criteria at the end of period 1.

The first criterion was based on the absolute level of severity of current psychopathologic symptoms; to enter period 2, the patient had to have a rating of 4 or higher on at least two of the following Brief Psychiatric Rating Scale (BPRS) items: conceptual disorganization, suspiciousness, hallucinatory behavior, and unusual thought content.

The second criterion was based on the reduction of psychopathologic symptoms during the placebo period; to enter period 2, the patient could not have a reduction in the total BPRS score of 50% or more between the beginning and the end of period 1. The 50% criterion was used to enhance the specificity of detection of placebo responders. Both criteria were identical to those used in our previous experiment.[14]

Double-blind haloperidol treatment at randomly assigned low (2 ng/mL) or moderate (10 ng/mL) plasma levels was administered during periods 2 and 3 (3 weeks each). Period 2 was analogous to the published fixed-dose studies.[3-10] Period 3 was added to determine whether patients who did not substantially benefit from treatment with one of the two levels of haloperidol in period 2 would do better when switched to the other level.

Thus, at study entry, each subject was randomly assigned to one of the four plasma haloperidol level treatment sequences to be administered in periods 2 and 3 (low-low, low-moderate, moderate-moderate, or moderate-low). After entry into period 2, the randomly assigned plasma haloperidol level was maintained for 3 weeks. Similar to our previous experiment,[14] those who failed to show at least a 50% reduction in total BPRS score at the end of this period entered period 3 and received haloperidol treatment at the plasma level to which they were assigned. The switch was implemented in half of the eligible patients (the low-moderate and moderate-low sequences); the other half continued at the same plasma haloperidol level as in period 2 (the low-low and moderate-moderate sequences; these groups that were not switched were intended to control for the effects of time).

Dose Management

The initial dose at the beginning of period 2 was determined using the formula, $D=W \times T \times 0.0352$, where D was the daily dose of haloperidol (in milligrams), W was the patient's weight (in kilograms), T was the assigned target plasma level (in nanograms per milliliter; thus, T was either 2 or 10), and 0.0352 was a constant derived empirically from our previous work. As it turned out, this formula resulted in first-week average levels that were slightly below the targets. Adjustments of the dose to keep the plasma levels close to their assigned targets were needed mostly in the first week of periods 2 and 3.

Plasma levels of haloperidol guided the dose adjustments. Plasma levels were determined at the beginning and at the end of the placebo period (period 1) and then at the end of each treatment week during periods 2 and 3. Additional (midweek) samples were drawn during the first week of periods 2 and 3 to facilitate early dose corrections. Each sample was drawn before the morning dose (12 hours after the evening dose) of haloperidol. The sample was assayed by 3 PM, and the result was reported to the principal investigator (or his delegate), who determined what (if any) dose adjustment was needed. Each of the four sites had a (nonblind) psychiatrist who consulted with the principal investigator and adjusted the dose before the evening medication time. The switch from one plasma level to another was accomplished by an appropriate dose change on the last day of period 2 and a subsequent dose adjustment—if needed—depending on the results of the plasma level assays in period 3.

Concomitant Medications

Concomitant medications allowed by the study protocol were benztropine mesylate as needed for extrapyramidal symptoms (during periods 1, 2, and 3), sodium amytal and chloral hydrate as needed for agitation or insomnia (period 1 only), and lorazepam as needed for agitation or insomnia (periods 2 and 3 only).

Assessments

The principal assessments were the BPRS[16] and the Simpson-Angus Scale for extrapyramidal side effects.[17] The BPRS and Simpson-Angus assessments were performed on the same days as the blood sampling (except that the Simpson-Angus midweek ratings were omitted during the first weeks of periods 2 and 3). Patients were rated jointly by two blind raters at weeks 0 (baseline), 1 (period 1), 4 (end of period

2), and 7 (end of period 3). Intermediate ratings (weeks 2, 3, 5, and 6) were done by one of the two raters.

Ratings were performed by 21 trained raters. Intraclass correlation coefficients between raters were computed for each of the 12 pairs of raters who rated jointly at least five times (229 joint ratings); the range was between .87 and .98 for the BPRS total score; 11 of the 12 pairs had coefficients greater than .92.

Haloperidol Assay

Haloperidol levels were determined in plasma using a gas-liquid chromatography procedure[18] modified by the use of chlorohaloperidol as an internal standard. The lower limit of detection was 0.5 ng/mL when 2 mL of plasma was extracted. Separation was achieved using a 1-m, 0.2-mm internal diameter column packed with 1% OV-17 on 80-100 mesh (Supelcoport, Supelco, Bellefonte, Pa). Retention times were 3.4 and 5.8 minutes for haloperidol and chlorohaloperidol, respectively. Quality-control samples were analyzed at three levels with each day's run. Data from 20 consecutive runs at 1.5, 5, and 20 ng/mL showed coefficients of variation of 7.5%, 5.6%, and 3.5%, respectively.

HYPOTHESES AND STATISTICAL ANALYSES

To define improvement as a categorical variable, we selected a cutoff point: reduction of psychopathologic symptoms by 20% or more was considered "improvement." The a priori decision to adopt this cutoff point was based on the literature (see below); it was supported by a post hoc analysis of our data.

Twenty percent has now been customarily accepted as the minimal level of improvement that is clinically significant. Twenty percent improvement has been used either in conjunction with other criteria specifying absolute levels of psychopathologic symptoms[19,20] or as the sole criterion defining "improvers."[20] In a post hoc analysis of our data (receiver operator characteristics, available on request from the authors), we found that the 20% cutoff point was optimal for discrimination between the low and moderate plasma level groups.

Primary Analyses

Our primary analyses tested the following hypotheses separately for positive and negative symptoms and the total BPRS score: (1) Treatment with low and moderate plasma levels of haloperidol will yield similar clinical improvement at the end point of the first 3-week period. (2) Treatment with low and moderate plasma levels of haloperidol will result in improvement that will occur with similar speed at both haloperidol levels. (3) Clinical improvement is related to the change of plasma haloperidol levels in period 3.

Analysis of covariance was the principal method for testing hypothesis 1. Three basic variables were used to define improvement: total BPRS score, positive symptoms, and negative symptoms. The BPRS had 18 items, with scores on each ranging from 1 to 7; thus, the potential total BPRS score range was 18 to 126. The positive symptom score was the sum of the scores on following 10 items: conceptual disorganization, grandiosity, hallucinatory behavior, unusual thought content, tension, mannerisms and posturing, excitement, hostility, suspiciousness, and uncooperativeness. The negative symptom score was the sum of the scores on the following four items: emotional withdrawal, motor retardation, blunted affect, and disorientation.

The three basic variables—total BPRS score, positive symptom score, and negative symptom score—were computed for the baseline (at the end of the placebo period) and at the end of period 2 (the last available data point in period 2). The improvement rate was computed for each patient according to the following formula: $IMP=[(VAR_b-VAR_e)\times 100]/(VAR_b-i)$, where IMP indicates percentage improvement; VAR_b, the three basic variables at baseline; VAR_e, the three basic variables at the end of period 2; and i, the number of BPRS items constituting each of the three basic variables. Since a baseline score of 1 on an individual BPRS item indicates normality (ie, the absence of psychopathologic symptoms), a total score of i on any of the three basic variables implies normality. Hence, the quantity i was subtracted from the baseline because we expressed improvement as the percentage of deviation from normality detected at the baseline.

Analyses of covariance were performed for the improvement of the three basic variables. The independent variable was the plasma level assignment (low or moderate) in period 2; when the dependent improvement variable was total BPRS score, positive symptom score, or negative symptom score, the baseline score of each was used as the covariate. This general procedure was used in analyzing data from the preceding study.[14]

We modeled the relationship between plasma haloperidol level and improvement by the probit transformation.[21-23] The binary dependent variable was improvement by at least 20% compared with the baseline rating. The probability of the improvement was computed as a function of the continuous plasma haloperidol level, specifically, $P=F[b_0+(b_1\times HAL)]$, where HAL indicates the plasma haloperidol level at the end point (concomitant with the BPRS score at the end point) and F indicates the standard normal distribution function.

We used χ^2 analysis to examine whether clinical response was related to the categorical variable, plasma level assignment. Plasma level assignment in period 2 was used as an independent variable. Clinical response at the end point of period 2 was defined as the binary (yes-no) dependent variable, based on the cutoff point of at least 20% improvement. Separate analyses were performed for each of the three improvement measures.

Hypothesis 2 (similar time of onset of the effects of the two treatments) was tested using nonparametric survival analysis (Kaplan-Meier). A nonparametric χ^2 statistic[24] tested equality between the two treatment groups for the probabilities of obtaining 20% improvement. If the findings of this test were not statistically significant, a Wilcoxon test compared the onset time of 20% improvement between these groups. If the χ^2 statistic was significant, the conditional survival distributions (given that improvement occurred) were compared.[25] These tests were run separately for each of the three improvement measures.

Hypothesis 3 concerning the relationship between the change in plasma levels and change in symptom severity between period 2 and period 3 was tested by multiple regression analysis. Change in symptom severity served as the dependent variable; it was defined as a relative (percentage) change in period 3 compared with symptom severity at the end of period 2. Change in plasma levels between the end points of periods 2 and 3 (ie, period 2 minus period 3) was used as an independent variable. Severity at the end point of period 2 served as a covariate. A separate analysis was performed for each of the improvement measures.

Secondary Analyses

Secondary analyses examined the following issues: differential therapeutic effects of the two haloperidol levels on positive and negative symptoms; effects of haloperidol levels on attrition rates, on side effects, and on lorazepam use; and predictability of clinical response using basic demographic variables (age, gender, and age of onset of illness).

Repeated-measures analysis of variance was used to examine differential therapeutic effects of haloperidol on the dependent variables—positive and negative symptoms. Baseline (end of the placebo period) and end point (end of period 2) ratings were used as the repeated measures. Time (baseline or end point) and symptoms (positive or negative) were used as within-subject factors. Interaction between time and symptoms tested differential therapeutic effects of haloperidol on positive and negative symptoms. To facilitate the comparisons between positive and negative symptoms, in this analysis, positive and negative symptom scores (defined as the sums of scores of their constituting items) were divided by the number of items in each.

Additional secondary analyses used analyses of covariance, regression analyses, and χ^2 statistics.

Attrition in Period 1

Thirty-five of the 111 patients who entered period 1 were dropped from the study before entering period 2; an additional 11 patients were excluded from further analyses because their placebo period had to be shortened to less than 3 days for clinical reasons. Among the 35 patients who were dropped from the study, there were eight placebo responders (see above), 10 did not meet the minimal symptom severity criteria required for entry into period 2, eight were dropped because of protocol violations, six withdrew consent, and three were dropped for other reasons.

Attrition in Periods 2 and 3

Of the 65 patients who entered period 2, 30 patients entered period 3 and 35 did not. The reasons for attrition were as follows: improvement by 50% (nine patients in the low plasma level group and seven in the moderate group); withdrawal of consent (five in the low group and four in the moderate group); side effects (none in the low group and two in the moderate group); and other reasons (three in the low group and five in the moderate group). Thus, the total attrition in period 2 was 17 subjects in the low group and 18 in the moderate group.

Data on 54 of the 65 patients who entered period 2 were used in end point data analyses. Data for the remaining 11 patients were not used for the following reasons: seven patients violated the protocol (five cases of noncompliance with medication, one inappropriate breaking of the blind condition, and one rediagnosis), and four additional patients received less than 5 days of their period 2 treatment. Thus, a sample of 54 patients was used in the analyses of period 2. Among these 54 patients, those in the low and moderate plasma level groups spent approximately the same amount of time in period 2 (mean±SD, 2.8±0.5 and 2.7±0.6 weeks in the low and moderate groups, respectively).

Attrition in period 3 had a treatment group distribution to similar to that in period 2.

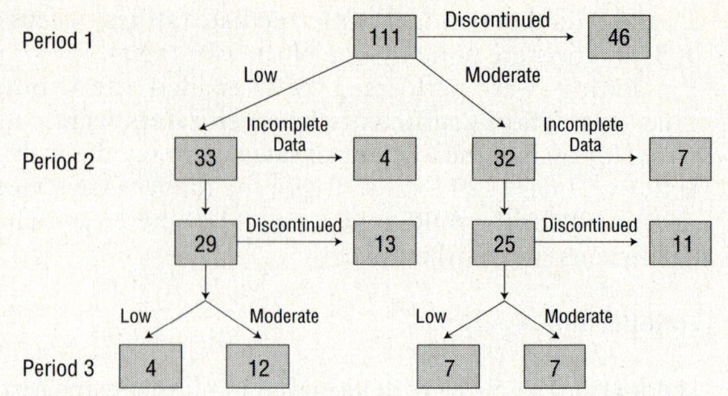

Figure 1. *Number of patients assigned plasma haloperidol levels by experimental period.*

SAMPLE CHARACTERISTICS

The groups assigned to the two plasma levels (low and moderate) were compared univariately on trait characteristics (**Table 1**) as well as on the BPRS measures at baseline (at entry into period 2); no statistically significant differences were detected for gender, diagnosis, age at first symptoms, number of previous hospitalizations, and baseline BPRS measures.

BLOOD LEVELS AND HALOPERIDOL DOSES

Period 2

The patients' plasma levels of haloperidol were generally close to the target levels they were assigned (**Table 2**). Residual haloperidol was detected in plasma at week 0; this demonstrates that the 1-week washout period for oral medications and the 1-month period for the slow-release injectables were too short (see the "Subjects and Methods" section).

There was a linear relationship between the independent variable, daily dose (milligrams per kilogram), and the dependent variable, plasma level (**Figure 2**) (r=.78, y intercept=1.1, slope=23.9, t=8.99, df=53, P<.01). The slope indicated that to accrue an increase of 1 ng/mL requires an increase of daily dose of 0.042 mg/kg of haloperidol under the experimental conditions we described. The relationship between dose and plasma level

Table 1. Characteristics of Patients Entering Experimental Period 2 Used in the Analyses

	Assigned Plasma Haloperidol Level in Period 2*	
	Low (N=29)	Moderate (N=25)
Age, y†	34.8±8.4	33.6±8.5
M/F, No. of patients	24/5	19/6
Black/white/Hispanic, No. of patients	20/8/1	21/4/0
Schizophrenic/schizoaffective, No. of patients	25/4	20/5
Age at first symptoms, y†	19.7±6.4	19.8±6.3
No. of hospitalizations†	13.0±19.2	16.5±26.2
BPRS score at the beginning of period 2†‡		
Total	51.6±9.1	51.2±8.9
Positive symptoms	32.8±6.7	31.3±7.0
Negative symptoms	9.5±3.2	10.1±2.9

*No difference between these two groups was statistically significant.
†Values are mean±SD.
‡BPRS indicates Brief Psychiatric Rating Scale.

Table 2. Plasma Haloperidol Levels in Experimental Period 2

	Mean±SD Plasma Haloperidol Level, ng/mL (No. of Patients)	
Week	Low Group (Target Level, 2 ng/mL)	Moderate Group (Target Level, 10 ng/mL)
0	0.2±0.5 (29)	0.2±0.5 (23)*
1	1.6±0.9 (29)	9.7±5.8 (25)
2	1.9±0.6 (27)†	11.8±4.3 (24)‡
3	2.2±0.8 (25)§	10.5±2.5 (19)‖

*Plasma levels were missing in two patients.
†One patient withdrew consent, and another one was dropped from the study because of clinical deterioration.
‡One patient left without consent.
§One patient withdrew consent, and another one was dropped from the study because of protocol violations.
‖Two patients were discharged or transferred, two patients had missing data, and one patient withdrew consent.

depicted in Figure 2 may not be generalizable to other dose escalation schedules or to other patient populations (see the "Comment" section). Therefore, Figure 2 should not be used by clinicians to determine the dose required to achieve a desired plasma level.

Period 3

At the end of the first week of period 3, the patients who were switched from the low plasma level group (target, 2 ng/mL) to the moderate one (target, 10 ng/mL) achieved a mean plasma level of 10.62±4.89 ng/mL (n=11). The patients switched from the moderate level to the low level achieved a mean plasma level of 2.44±0.99 ng/mL (n=5) at the end of the first week of period 3. These levels were maintained (with very minor deviations) throughout period 3.

The patients who were not switched and were assigned to continue in period 3 on the low and moderate plasma levels had plasma levels at the end of the first week of period 3 of 2.40±0.78 ng/mL (n=4) and 9.67±0.71 ng/mL (n=6), respectively. (Plasma levels in four patients were missing for this time point.)

PRIMARY ANALYSES

Outcome in Period 2

Doses, plasma levels, and effects of the haloperidol treatments on positive symptom scores in individual patients are in **Table 3**. The mean percentage improvements for the group assigned to the low haloperidol level (n=29) were 23.1%±3.8%, 27.5%±34.4%, and 4.5%±65.0% for the total BPRS score, positive symptom score, and negative symptom score, respectively. The analogous means for the group assigned to the moderate haloperidol level (n=25) were 36.8%±26.4%, 40.0%±27.2%, and 16.4%±106.3%, respectively. Thus, the improvement rates were generally smaller in the low group than in the moderate group, but the differences were not statistically significant. Differences in improvement rates among the four participating sites could not be meaningfully tested in view of the low numbers of subjects and their unbalanced distribution across sites.

Probit Transformation for Plasma Levels and Improvement. The results of the sigmoidal probit transformation of positive symptom scores for the range of plasma levels observed in our study are depicted in **Figure 3**. The appropriateness of the model was verified by a goodness-of-fit test (Pearson χ^2=42.3, *df*=40, *P*=.37). Results of the test of the slope parameter of the probit model examining the relationship between plasma level of haloperidol (used as a continuous variable) and the probability of improvement were statistically significant (χ^2=4.3, *df*=1, *P*<.05).

To illustrate the relationship between the computed probability and the actual data, we depicted the probit function jointly with the observed frequencies. For this purpose, the plasma haloperidol level axis was divided into bands that were 3 ng/mL wide (0 to 3 ng/mL, 4 to 6 ng/mL, etc). The relative frequency of improvers (ie, proportion of patients who improved) observed within each band was plotted as a point at the center of the band (Figure 3).

The probability of improvement rose relatively fast at the low levels of haloperidol. The rate of increase of that function slowed down when higher levels were reached. Analogous to the approach of Wolkin et al,[13] we tried to determine the plasma level where the probit curve portrayed in Figure 3 "tapered off," which occurs at 1 SD of a standard normal distribution. That value was the haloperidol level of 11.5 ng/mL, where the probability of improvement is 0.84. Above 11.5 ng/mL, the increase in the chance of improvement is small even when plasma haloperidol levels are increased sharply.

A sigmoidal probit transformation (analogous to that we described for positive symptom score) was obtained for the negative symptom score. The result was similar

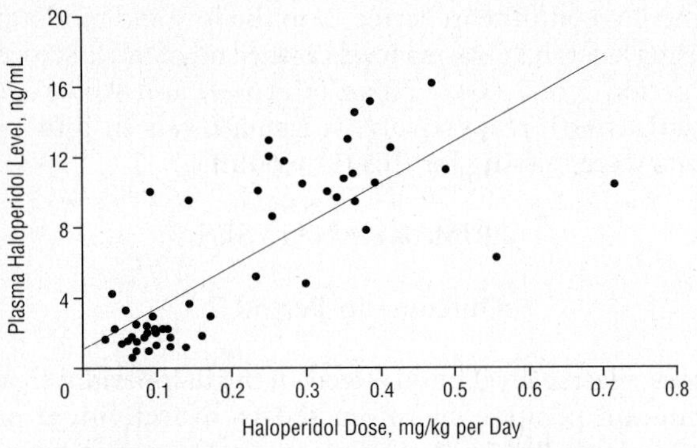

Figure 2. *Plasma level and dose of haloperidol at the end point of experimental period 2.*

to that for the positive symptom score, but the relationship between plasma haloperidol level and improvement was only marginally significant (χ^2=3.73, *df*=1, *P*=.05).

Survival Analysis. For the negative symptom score, the probability of failure to reach 20% improvement differed significantly (χ^2=6.1, *df*=1, *P*<.05) between groups: 28.1% for the low plasma level group and 4.0% for the moderate group. When improvement by 20% occurred, the onset of action occurred before 14 days of treatment in the moderate group and before 21 days of treatment in the low group. No significant group differences were detected for the positive symptom score or the total BPRS score.

χ^2 Analyses for Group Assignment and Improvement. The χ^2 analyses yielded a significant relationship between improvement (categorical, ≥20% improvement at the end of period 2) on positive symptom score and plasma level assignment (n=54, χ^2=5.2, *df*=1, *P*<.05): 55% (n=16) of patients improved in the low plasma level group vs 84% (n=21) in the moderate group.

Analogous analyses for negative symptom score yielded similar results (n=54, χ^2=4.3, *df*=1, *P*<.05), with 48% (n=14) of patients improving in the low plasma level group vs 76% (n=19) in the moderate group.

Outcome in Period 3

The mean percentage improvements for the group assigned to the low haloperidol level in period 3 (n=10 [BPRS scores were missing for one of the 11 patients in this group]) were 9.9%±30.9%, 9.3%±36.3%, and 17.1%±30.6% for the total BPRS, positive symptom score, and negative symptom score, respectively. The analogous means for the group assigned to the moderate haloperidol level (n=18) were 26.1%±22.7%, 23.0%±24.4%, and 10.9%±49.4%, respectively.

The multiple regression analyses used to test hypothesis 3 showed that plasma haloperidol level reduction led to a decrease of negative symptoms, whereas an increase of the plasma level led to an increase of negative symptoms (F=22.6; *df*=1,27; *P*<.01). There were no significant effects for positive symptom score or total BPRS score.

Parkinsonian extrapyramidal side effects as well as depression may confound the assessment of negative symptoms. Therefore, we introduced a measure of extrapyramidal side effects (Simpson-Angus total score) and a measure of depression (anxiety-depression BPRS factor) as covariates in the analyses of negative symptoms described above. These covariates did not affect the outcome of the analyses. These findings do not support the notion that the negative symptoms we observed were secondary to extrapyramidal side effects or depression. However, we cannot exclude the possibility that our ratings of extrapyramidal side effects and depression were not sufficiently sensitive.

SECONDARY ANALYSES

The differential effect of haloperidol on positive and negative symptoms in period 2 was examined by repeated-measures analysis of variance. This analysis showed a significant interaction effect between time and symptoms (F=10.5; *df*=1,52; *P*<.01). The main effects were also significant (time: F=34.4; *df*=1,52; *P*<.01; symptoms: F=35.0; *df*=1,52; *P*<.01). The post hoc analysis of interaction between symptoms and time showed that, whereas there was statistically significant improvement in both the positive symptoms (*t*=7.4, *df*=53, *P*<.01) and the negative symptoms (*t*=3.7, *df*=53, *P*<.01) during period 2, the improvement on positive symptoms was considerably greater. The mean percentage change for positive and negative symptoms was 33.3%±31.2% and 10.0%±86.3%, respectively.

Extrapyramidal side effects measured by the Simpson-Angus Scale showed no significant difference between the two treatments at the end point of period 2. However, the number of patients receiving benztropine was significantly different in the two treatment groups (31% [n=9] in the low group vs 60% [n=15] in the moderate group; χ^2=4.6, *df*=1, *P*<.05).

At least one dose of lorazepam was administered to 52% (n=15) of patients in the low group and 56% (n=13) of patients in the moderate group during period 2. The two groups did not differ in the number of doses or in the total number of milligrams administered.

No relationship was found between therapeutic response (overall percentage improvement on the BPRS) to haloperidol and our basic demographic predictor variables (age, gender, and age of onset of illness).

COMMENT

Plasma levels around 2 ng/mL were significantly less effective against positive symptoms than those around 10 ng/mL in the first 3 weeks of the trial. However, only a small additional chance of improvement can be expected if plasma levels are raised beyond 11.5 ng/mL.

Extrapyramidal side effects, reflected by the increased need for antiparkinsonian medication, were greater in the moderate plasma level group than in the low group. Published data[9] indicate that these side ef-

Table 3. Haloperidol Doses, Plasma Levels, and Positive Symptoms in Experimental Period 2*

Patient No.	Daily Dose† mg	Daily Dose† mg/kg	Plasma Level at End Point, ng/mL	Positive Symptom Score Baseline	Positive Symptom Score End Point	Improvement on Positive Symptoms at End Point‡ Continuous, %	Improvement on Positive Symptoms at End Point‡ Categorical (≥20%)
Low Group (Target Level, 2 ng/mL)							
1	5.3	0.07	0.6	37.5	29.0	30.9	Yes
2	5.0	0.07	1.0	29.5	26.0	17.9	No
3	7.4	0.09	1.0	39.0	13.5	87.9	Yes
4	7.9	0.14	1.2	51.0	26.0	61.0	Yes
5	8.0	0.10	1.3	29.0	22.0	36.8	Yes
6	10.1	0.12	1.3	37.5	26.0	41.8	Yes
7	5.0	0.05	1.4	33.0	36.0	−13.0	No
8	5.0	0.07	1.5	32.0	35.0	−13.6	No
9	6.0	0.06	1.6	34.0	31.0	12.5	No
10	3.6	0.03	1.7	28.0	21.1	38.3	Yes
11	6.0	0.08	1.7	43.5	22.0	64.2	Yes
12	6.0	0.12	1.8	34.5	20.5	57.1	Yes
13	4.0	0.06	1.8	30.5	29.5	4.9	No
14	4.8	0.07	1.8	27.5	19.0	48.6	Yes
15	12.0	0.16	1.9	25.5	27.0	−9.7	No
16	7.6	0.09	2.0	35.0	23.5	46.0	Yes
17	6.0	0.10	2.1	45.5	39.0	18.3	No
18	9.6	0.10	2.3	32.5	39.5	−31.1	No
19	10.0	0.12	2.3	24.5	26.5	−13.8	No
20	7.0	0.11	2.3	28.5	23.0	29.7	Yes
21	2.9	0.04	2.3	28.5	23.0	29.7	Yes
22	5.0	0.09	2.4	27.0	26.0	5.9	No
23	6.0	0.08	2.5	37.5	17.5	72.7	Yes
24	4.0	0.07	2.5	23.0	22.5	3.8	No
25	5.8	0.10	2.9	30.0	18.5	57.5	Yes
26	12.0	0.17	3.0	39.5	17.5	74.6	Yes
27	6.0	0.06	3.3	27.0	14.5	73.5	Yes
28	12.0	0.15	3.7	25.0	32.0	−46.7	No
29	3.9	0.04	4.2	34.5	32.0	10.2	No
Moderate Group (Target Level, 10 ng/mL)							
30	19.9	0.30	4.9	27.5	14.0	77.1	Yes
31	16.0	0.23	5.3	25.0	22.0	20.0	Yes
32	44.0	0.56	6.5	26.5	15.5	66.7	Yes
33	24.3	0.38	8.0	43.5	39.5	11.9	No
34	24.6	0.26	8.7	22.0	16.0	50.0	Yes
35	14.0	0.14	9.6	32.0	24.0	36.4	Yes
36	25.0	0.37	9.6	27.5	17.5	57.1	Yes
37	33.4	0.34	9.8	21.0	18.0	27.3	Yes
38	8.0	0.09	10.1	32.0	14.5	79.5	Yes
39	18.0	0.24	10.2	28.0	33.0	−27.8	No
40	20.7	0.33	10.2	36.5	31.5	18.9	No
41	19.7	0.30	10.6	29.5	25.5	20.5	Yes
42	36.0	0.71	10.7	35.0	24.5	42.0	Yes
43	28.0	0.39	10.7	33.5	26.5	29.8	Yes
44	20.0	0.35	10.9	33.0	27.0	26.1	Yes
45	20.0	0.36	11.2	29.0	22.0	36.8	Yes
46	30.0	0.49	11.5	29.5	13.0	84.6	Yes
47	16.0	0.27	11.9	24.5	14.5	69.0	Yes
48	11.3	0.25	12.2	49.0	38.5	26.9	Yes
49	25.1	0.41	12.7	33.0	35.5	−10.9	No
50	26.0	0.25	13.1	40.5	27.5	42.6	Yes
51	27.9	0.36	13.2	38.3	21.5	59.4	Yes
52	34.0	0.37	14.7	30.0	17.0	65.0	Yes
53	22.1	0.39	15.3	19.5	15.0	47.4	Yes
54	26.0	0.47	16.4	37.5	25.5	43.6	Yes

Analogous tables for negative symptom score and total score on the Brief Psychiatric Rating Scale (BPRS) are available on request from the authors.
†*These doses are the means for the week preceding the end point.*
‡*Improvement on positive symptoms was computed for each patient according to the following formula:* $IMP=[(POS_b-POS_e)\times 100]/(POS_b-i)$, *where IMP indicates percent improvement;* POS_b, *positive symptom score at baseline;* POS_e, *positive symptom score at end point; and i, number of BPRS items constituting the variable POS (n=10) (see the text for further explanation).*

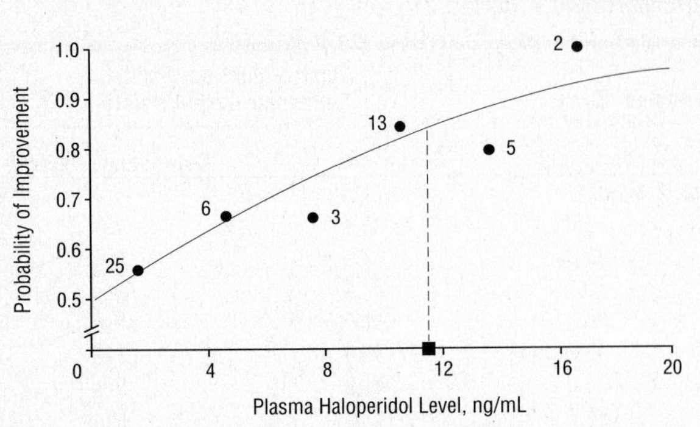

Figure 3. *Probability of improvement (at least a 20% improvement in the positive symptom score on the Brief Psychiatric Rating Scale) at the end point in experimental period 2 as a function of the plasma haloperidol level. The dotted line and square indicate the point (11.5 ng/mL) where the probit curve "tapers off" (ie, 1 SD above the mean). The data points (observed relative frequencies in 3-ng/mL bands; numbers at each point indicate the number of patients in this 3-ng/mL band) displayed (circles) were not used to compute the curve. The portions of the curve below 0.6 ng/mL and above 16.4 ng/mL are extrapolations.*

fects increase significantly when the plasma level exceeds 12 ng/mL.

The time of onset of improvement of positive symptoms appeared independent of the plasma haloperidol level. This negative finding must be interpreted cautiously in view of the small number of subjects and the relatively poor therapeutic response in our sample.

The optimal level for negative symptoms in the first 3 weeks of treatment appears similar to that for positive symptoms. The survival analysis demonstrated a greater rate of improvement of negative symptoms in the moderate plasma level group than in the low group. Additionally, when 20% improvement occurred, the onset of improvement was earlier in the moderate group than in the low group.

Thus, a relationship between plasma haloperidol level and antipsychotic effects is suggested by our data and by most of the evidence obtained in fixed-dose studies. The nature of that relationship has usually been discussed in terms of a "therapeutic window." We now consider the upper and the lower limits of the window.

The upper limit seems to be in the vicinity of 12 ng/mL for patients with acutely exacerbated conditions. Exceeding that limit either tends to reduce antipsychotic activity[3,5,6,9,10] or at least tends to result in no appreciable additional benefit.[7,8,14] There may be an additional cost of increasing plasma levels: extrapyramidal side effects (or the need for anticholinergic treatment to suppress them) may increase.

The existence of a lower limit is in no doubt: a zero plasma level of haloperidol is less effective than a nonzero level. The question is, how low can one go with the plasma level without losing antipsychotic activity? Literature indicates that levels below 4 or 5 ng/mL are not as effective as levels above this limit. Our data suggest a continuous increase of antipsychotic efficacy from levels close to 0 to approximately 12 ng/mL.

Raising the plasma level of haloperidol until a satisfactory antipsychotic effect is obtained or until one reaches the level of approximately 12 ng/mL (whichever occurs first) seems to be a good treatment strategy for the first 3 weeks of treatment. If this treatment strategy is followed, then most patients' plasma levels should be brought up to approximately 8 to 12 ng/mL.

This strategy may not work for all patients; some may require higher plasma levels for antipsychotic effects, others may not tolerate side effects elicited by a haloperidol level of 8 ng/mL. Rather than a "threshold" or a "window" with clearly delineated limits, we see a changing relationship between benefits and risks with changing plasma levels. Therefore, it would be inappropriate to use our suggestion for a treatment strategy for the purposes of quality assurance or litigation.

We found that the changes in plasma haloperidol levels between periods 2 and 3 (caused largely by the switching of level assignments) were associated with changes in negative symptoms: increased plasma levels were associated with deteriorations, whereas decreased levels were associated with improvements in negative symptoms.

These findings appear to be inconsistent with the recent report of exacerbation of negative symptoms after antipsychotic withdrawal.[26] However, in that study, the antipsychotic agents were completely discontinued for 3 weeks (rather than just reduced, as in the present study), and positive symptoms worsened concomitantly with the negative ones (which we did not observe).

The effect of the crossover (in period 3) is consistent with the notion that antipsychotic treatment may cause secondary negative symptoms[27] that improve when the doses are reduced. The implication of this finding for clinical practice is that dose reduction may have beneficial effects after the first 3 weeks of treatment of an acute exacerbation of schizophrenia or schizoaffective disorder.

We studied patients with acutely exacerbated schizophrenia and schizoaffective disorder during the first several weeks after hospitalization. Although their conditions were acutely exacerbated, these patients had been ill for many years and had histories of multiple hospitalizations. Our results may thus be valid only for such a patient population.

In clinical practice, higher doses of haloperidol (eg, 60 mg/d) are still used[28]; some justification for this may exist,[29] but low-dose strategies are more widely accepted.[30,31] Recent evidence indicates that high doses can be reduced in patients with chronic conditions.[32,33] In one of the dose-reduction studies,[32] the optimal plasma level of haloperidol for patients with chronic schizophrenia was found to be 12.4 ng/mL—very close to our findings.

The relationship between dose and plasma level is tenuous. Patients given the same dose of haloperidol show a large interindividual variability of plasma levels; conversely, attempts to achieve any plasma level by giving a group of patients the average daily dose known to produce that level will result in widely scattered levels. To complicate matters further, the average daily dose needed to achieve a given average plasma level may not be the same in all patient populations. Other investigators needed lower doses of haloperidol to achieve plasma levels similar to levels reached in the present study (P. G. Janicak, MD, written communication, June 13, 1994). Furthermore, the relationship between dose and plasma level we report was observed under specific experimental conditions that called for dose adjustments to achieve target plasma levels; the relationship may be different when the doses are held constant for a period sufficient to assure steady state in all subjects. This may take 3 or more weeks.[34,35] Thus, the clinicians who wish to apply our results in clinical practice may prefer to monitor plasma levels in their patients rather than simply relying on the average dose-response relationship we report.

Accepted for publication July 17, 1995.

This study was supported by grants MH41772 and MH42959 from the National Institute of Mental Health, Rockville, Md.

Eugene Laska provided critical comments that improved this report. We thank Istvan Bitter, MD, James Y. Chou, MD, Natarajan Elangovan, MD, Pedro Gaztanaga, MD, Michal Kunz, MD, Jan Libiger, MD, Yar Mohammad, MD, Hana Papezova, MD, Krishniah Ramsetty, MD, Ivan Tuma, MD, and Bertrand Winsberg, MD, for patient evaluations and management. David Allen, Audrey Meister, and Brenda Katof provided expert technical assistance. Jozsef Vitrai, PhD, managed the database. Jane O'Donnell, RN, MA, Jacione Nagel, RN, BSN, Julie E. Scheurer, MD, and Milica Stefanovic, MD, were the study coordinators. We appreciate the cooperation of the administrators and staff at the Rockland Psychiatric Center, Orangeburg, NY; Manhattan (NY) Psychiatric Center; Brookdale Memorial Hospital Medical Center, Brooklyn, NY; and Bellevue Hospital Center, New York, NY.

Reprint requests to Nathan S. Kline Institute for Psychiatric Research, Orangeburg, NY 10962 (Dr Volavka).

REFERENCES

1. Volavka J, Cooper TB. Review of haloperidol blood level and clinical response: looking through the window. *J Clin Psychopharmacol.* 1987;7:25-30.
2. Volavka J, Cooper TB. Plasma levels, clinical effects, and low-dose strategies. In: Lindenmayer JP, Kay SR, eds. *New Biological Vistas on Schizophrenia.* New York, NY: Brunner/Mazel Inc; 1992:273-284.
3. Mavroidis ML, Kanter DR, Hirschowitz J, Garver DL. Clinical response and plasma haloperidol levels in schizophrenia. *Psychopharmacology.* 1981;81:354-356.
4. Potkin SG, Shen Y, Zhou D, Pardes H, Shu L, Phelps B, Poland R. Does a therapeutic window for plasma haloperidol exist? preliminary Chinese data. *Psychopharmacol Bull.* 1985;21:59-61.
5. Santos JL, Cabranes JA, Almoguera I, Ramos JA, Vazquez C, Angeles F. Clinical implications of determination of plasma haloperidol levels. *Acta Psychiatr Scand.* 1989;79:348-354.
6. Santos JL, Cabranes JA, Vasquez C, Fuentenebro F, Almoguera I, Ramos JA. Clinical response and plasma haloperidol levels in chronic and subchronic schizophrenia. *Biol Psychiatry.* 1989;26:381-388.
7. Rifkin A, Doddi SR, Karajgi BM, Borenstein M, Wachspress M. Dosage of haloperidol for schizophrenia. *Arch Gen Psychiatry.* 1991;48:166-170.
8. Doddi S, Rifkin A, Karajgi B, Cooper T, Borenstein M. Blood levels of haloperidol and clinical outcome in schizophrenia. *J Clin Psychopharmacol.* 1994;14:187-195.
9. Van Putten T, Marder SR, Mintz J, Poland RE. Haloperidol plasma levels and clinical response: a therapeutic window relationship. *Am J Psychiatry.* 1992;149:500-505.
10. Palao DJ, Arauxo A, Brunet M, Bernardo M, Haro JM, Ferrer J, Gonzalez-Monclus E. Haloperidol: therapeutic window in schizophrenia. *J Clin Psychopharmacol.* 1994;14:303-310.
11. McEvoy JP, Stiller RL, Farr R. Plasma haloperidol levels drawn at neuroleptic threshold doses: a pilot study. *J Clin Psychopharmacol.* 1986;6:133-138.
12. McEvoy JP, Hogarty GE, Steingard S. Optimal dose of neuroleptic in acute schizophrenia. *Arch Gen Psychiatry.* 1991;48:739-745.
13. Wolkin A, Brodie JD, Barouche F, Rotrosen J, Wolf AP, Smith M, Fowler J, Cooper T. Dopamine receptor occupancy and plasma haloperidol levels. *Arch Gen Psychiatry.* 1989;46:482-483.
14. Volavka J, Cooper T, Czobor P, Bitter I, Meisner M, Laska E, Gastanaga P, Krakowski M, Chou JC-Y, Crowner M, Douyon R. Haloperidol blood levels and clinical effects. *Arch Gen Psychiatry.* 1992;49:354-361.
15. Sampath G, Shah A, Krska J, Soni SD. Neuroleptic discontinuation in the very stable schizophrenic patient: relapse rates and serum neuroleptic levels. *Hum Psychopharmacol.* 1992;7:255-264.
16. Guy W. *ECDEU Assessment Manual for Psychopharmacology.* Rockville, Md: National Institute of Mental Health; 1976.
17. Simpson GM, Angus JWS. A rating scale for extrapyramidal side effects. *Acta Psychiatr Scand Suppl.* 1970;212:11-19.
18. Bianchetti G, Morselli PL. Rapid and sensitive method for determination of haloperidol in human samples using nitrogen-phosphorus selective detection. *J Chromatogr.* 1978;153:203-209.
19. Kane J, Honigfeld G, Singer J, Meltzer H. Clozapine for the treatment-resistant schizophrenic. *Arch Gen Psychiatry.* 1988;45:789-796.
20. Marder SR, Meibach RC. Risperidone in the treatment of schizophrenia. *Am J Psychiatry.* 1994;151:825-835.
21. Bliss CL. The calculation of the dosage-mortality curve. *Ann Appl Biol.* 1935;22:134-167.
22. Engeman RM, Otis DL, Dusenberry WE. Small sample properties of some parametric bioassay estimators of the LD90. *Comput Biomed Res.* 1986;19:588-595.
23. Corbo GM, Foresi A, Morandini S, Valente S, Mattoli S, Ciappi G. Probit analysis applied to the allergen dose-response curve: a method for epidemiologic surveys. *J Allergy Clin Immunol.* 1988;81:41-47.
24. Laska EM, Meisner MJ. Nonparametric estimation and testing in a cure model. *Biometrics.* 1992;48:1223-1234.
25. Laska EM, Siegel C, Sunshine A. Onset and duration: measurement and analysis. *Clin Pharmacol Ther.* 1991;49:1-5.
26. Miller DD, Flaum M, Arndt S, Fleming F, Andreasen NC. Effect of antipsychotic withdrawal on negative symptoms in schizophrenia. *Neuropsychopharmacology.* 1994;11:11-20.
27. Carpenter WT, Jr, Heinrichs DW, Alphs LD. Treatment of negative symptoms. *Schizophr Bull.* 1985;11:440-452.
28. Krakowski MI, Kunz M, Czobor P, Volavka J. Long-term high-dose neuroleptic treatment: who gets it and why? *Hosp Community Psychiatry.* 1993;44:640-644.
29. Brotman AW, McCormick S. A role for high-dose antipsychotics. *J Clin Psychiatry.* 1990;51:164-166.
30. Cohen BM, Benes FM, Baldessarini RJ. Atypical neuroleptics, dose-response relationships, and treatment-resistant psychosis. *Arch Gen Psychiatry.* 1989;46:381-383.
31. Baldessarini RJ, Cohen B, Teicher MH. Significance of neuroleptic dose and plasma level in the pharmacological treatment of psychoses. *Arch Gen Psychiatry.* 1988;45:79-91.
32. Liberman RP, Van Putten T, Marshall BD Jr, Mintz J, Bowen L, Kuehnel TG, Aravagiri M, Marder SR. Optimal drug and behavior therapy for treatment-refractory schizophrenic patients. *Am J Psychiatry.* 1994;151:756-759.
33. Smith RC. Lower-dose therapy with traditional neuroleptics in chronically hospitalized schizophrenic patients. *Arch Gen Psychiatry.* 1994;51:427-429.
34. Campbell A, Baldessarini RJ. Prolonged pharmacologic activity of neuroleptics. *Arch Gen Psychiatry.* 1985;42:637.
35. Hubbard JW, Ganes D, Midha KK. Prolonged pharmacologic activity of neuroleptic drugs. *Arch Gen Psychiatry.* 1987;44:99-100.

Suicidal Behaviors and the Tryptophan Hydroxylase Gene

Mocrane Abbar, MD; Philippe Courtet, MS; Stéphane Amadéo, MD; Yves Caer, MD; Jacques Mallet, PhD; Michel Baldy-Moulinier, MD; Didier Castelnau, MD; Alain Malafosse, MD, PhD

Background: To determine whether the tryptophan hydroxylase gene (ie, the gene that codes for the rate-limiting enzyme in the metabolic pathway of serotonin) may be a susceptibility factor for suicidal behavior.

Methods: Genotypic and allelic frequencies at a polymorphic *Ava* II restriction site were revealed with the use of the complementary DNA tryptophan hydroxylase probe C2-38 in 62 suicide attempters. The psychiatric characteristics of these suicide attempters were determined using the Schedule for Affective Disorders and Schizophrenia–Lifetime version with modification for the study of anxiety disorders, and these characteristics were compared with those in 52 healthy controls.

Results: No association between tryptophan hydroxylase and suicidal behavior was detected.

Conclusion: The tryptophan hydroxylase gene was not a susceptibility factor for suicidal behaviors in the group of suicide attempters in this study.

(Arch Gen Psychiatry. 1995;52:846-849)

THE CURRENT understanding of suicidal behaviors is that such behaviors are multidetermined and result from an interaction between state and trait-related effects.[1] Among the trait-related effects, genetic factors appear to be important, as suggested by the findings of family,[2,3] twin,[4] and adoption studies.[5-7] Whether these genetic factors are similar to those involved in the susceptibility to psychiatric disorders closely related to suicidal behaviors (eg, manic-depressive disorder, schizophrenia, and alcoholism) is unknown. However, a genetic factor of susceptibility to suicide independent of or additive to the genetic transmission of the psychiatric disorders that are related to suicidal behaviors is strongly suggested by the data of the Copenhagen adoption studies[5-7] and a study of Amish families.[8] In this last study, Egeland and Sussex[8] showed that most suicides were clustered in families characterized by heavy loading for affective disorders and suicide. Conversely, there were other pedigrees with heavy loading for affective disorders but without suicide.

Recently, new approaches combining family and population studies have been proposed to identify the genetic component of such complex traits.[9] Association study between genetic markers and a disease phenotype[10] has been successfully applied to several complex diseases (eg, essential hypertension[11] and Alzheimer's disease[12]). Using polymorphic DNA markers, the distribution of alleles can be compared in a sample of unrelated affected individuals and in a control population. There are three possible causes for an association: (1) stratification bias, (2) the associated allele is a cause of the disease, and (3) the associated allele is in linkage disequilibrium with the genetic determinant. Stratification bias has been seen when the selection of patients and controls was inappropriate. In the two remaining situations, use of markers that are close to or within candidate genes increases the likelihood of identifying a true association.[10]

One candidate gene for suicidal behaviors is the tryptophan hydroxylase (*TPH*) gene, which is the first and possibly the rate-limiting enzyme of the metabolic pathway for serotonin (5-hydroxytryptamine).[13] Indeed, altered serotoninergic function in both suicide and suicide attempts has been one of the most replicated findings in modern biological psychiatry.[14-16] The available evidence

From the Department of Psychiatry (Drs Abbar, Amadéo, Caer, and Castelnau and Mr Courtet), University of Montpellier–Nîmes (France), Laboratory of Molecular Genetics of Neurotransmission, Centre National de la Recherche Scientifique (CNRS UMR 9923), Gif-sur-Yvette, France (Dr Mallet), and Institut National de la Santé et de la Recherche Médicale U 249 (CNRS UPR 9008), Montpellier (Drs Baldy-Moulinier and Malafosse). Dr Malafosse is now with the Neuropsychiatry Division, University Hospital of Psychiatry, Geneva, Switzerland.

See Patients and Methods on next page

PATIENTS AND METHODS

Sixty-two case patients who were hospitalized after a serious suicide attempt were included in this study. A serious suicide attempt was defined as the medical condition of a patient who required hospitalization in the intensive care unit of the Montpellier (France) University Hospital. All serious suicide attempters were systematically admitted to the Department of Psychiatry after discharge from the intensive care unit. In the 3 days following their admission, the patients were interviewed by pychiatrists using the Schedule for Affective Disorders and Schizophrenia–Lifetime version with modification for the study of anxiety disorders.[21] Only the following diagnoses were considered: major depressive and bipolar disorders, panic disorder, agoraphobia, social phobia, obsessive-compulsive disorder, alcohol and substance abuse and dependence, antisocial personality disorder, and psychotic disorders. The method used in the suicide attempt was classified as violent or nonviolent according to the criteria proposed by Asberg et al[22] and retained by Träskman et al.[17] Therefore, suicide attempts using methods other than drug overdose were considered serious. Suicide intent and medical seriousness of the attempts were rated according to the six-point scales from the Schedule for Affective Disorders and Schizophrenia–Lifetime version with modification for the study of anxiety disorders.[21]

Fifty-two control patients (28 men and 24 women; mean±SD age, 52.9±18.9 years) with no history of suicidal behaviors were selected from the surgical departments at the Montpellier University Hospital, and these control patients were matched with respect to birthplace. To minimize population heterogeneity, both groups were entirely of Caucasian European origin.

All subjects gave informed consent, and the study protocol was approved by the French Comité National d'Ethique and Commission Nationale Informatique et Liberté.

An *Ava* II restriction fragment length polymorphism at the *TPH* locus was investigated by using the human *TPH* complementary DNA probe C2-38.[23,24] High molecular weight DNA was prepared from blood samples that were obtained from all case and control patients, and it was digested with the restriction endonuclease according to the specifications of the manufacturer, except that 3 U of enzyme was added per microgram of DNA. Electrophoresis, Southern blotting, hybridization, and autoradiography were performed using standard techniques by biologists blind to the diagnosis. Following hybridization and autoradiography, the polymorphism was scored as the presence of bands at 10.5 kilobase (allele A1) and at 7+3.5 kilobase (allele A2).[24] The allelic frequencies (f) in 100 unrelated Caucasian European individuals[24] were f(A1)=0.57 and f(A2)=0.43.

Allelic and genotypic frequencies were determined for case and control patient groups and for subgroups defined by diagnoses that were known to be associated with a high risk for suicide and types of past and present suicide attempts. Categorical variables were compared using a χ^2 test and Yates corrected χ^2 test when necessary.

indicates that low concentrations of 5-hydroxyindoleacetic acid (5-HIAA) (ie, the major catabolite of serotonin that is measured in the cerebrospinal fluid [CSF] of suicide attempters) are related in some way to suicidal behaviors, irrespective of categorical diagnosis. The findings of biological abnormalities in the brains of victims of suicide and in the body fluid of suicide attempters have genetic consequences if these biological changes are trait-dependent. Most studies that have measured 5-HIAA levels in the CSF have not found any temporal relationship between the suicidal gesture and the 5-HIAA level in the CSF.[1] Furthermore, two follow-up studies have found that a low 5-HIAA level in the CSF in suicide attempters is a strong predictor of subsequent suicide attempts or completed suicides.[17,18] Thus, it appears that the 5-HIAA level in the CSF may be a biochemical trait that is predictive of susceptiblity to suicidal behaviors.

In 1992, to our knowledge, we were first to test the association between suicide attempts and the *TPH* gene. We observed no difference between allelic frequencies at the *TPH* locus in case patients and controls in this preliminary case-control study.[19] In a recent report, Nielsen et al[20] found no difference in the allelic distribution at the *TPH* locus between violent offenders with a history of suicidal behaviors and controls. However, these authors suggested that the *TPH* gene is associated with suicidal behaviors because they observed a higher frequency of the rare *TPH* allele in violent offenders without a history of suicidal behaviors than in violent offenders with a history of suicidal behaviors. In the present study, we extend and confirm our preliminary negative results in the ongoing case-control study of suicide attempts and the *TPH* gene.

RESULTS

The demographical and clinical characteristics of the 62 suicide attempters are detailed in **Table 1**. Fifty-one case patients (82%) attempted suicide by drug overdose, and 11 case patients (18%) attempted suicide by violent methods (ie, hanging, shooting, poisoning with gas, and jumping from heights). The proportion of case patients who had used violent methods did not differ significantly between men and women (26% [n=8] vs 10% [n=3], Yates corrected χ^2=1.8). The lifetime comorbidity among the case patients was high: 18 case patients (29%) had one psychiatric disorder (according to the Axis I diagnoses of the *DSM-III-R*), 19 case patients (31%) met the diagnostic criteria for two disorders, and 15 case patients (24%) met the diagnostic criteria for three or more disorders.

The genotypic frequencies of the *Ava* II polymorphic site in the case and control patient groups were not significantly different from those expected for populations in Hardy-Weinberg equilibrium. In **Table 2**, detailed results for the main diagnoses are presented. None of the tests performed for any of the diagnoses that were considered produced statistically significant evidence for an association. The frequency of the *A1A1* genotype was 0.62 in suicide attempters with antisocial personality disorder vs 0.28 in suicide attempters without antisocial personality disorder, but this difference did not reach statistical significance (Yates corrected χ^2=3.43). No significant difference in the frequency of the *A1A1* genotype was observed between the control patients and subgroups defined according to (1) method used for the suicide attempt (violent vs nonviolent as defined above), (2) number of suicide attempts, (3) age at first suicide attempt (before or after 20 years of age), and (4) suicidal intentionality (data not shown).

COMMENT

In this case-control study, we analyzed the *TPH* gene in 62 unrelated case patients with a history of suicide attempts and 52 control patients using a *TPH* restriction fragment length polymorphism (*Ava* II restriction site as revealed by the complementary DNA *TPH* probe C2-38).[24] We found no evidence for an association between a history of suicide attempts and either of the two alleles of the polymorphic *Ava* II restriction site.

This result confirms our preliminary data[19]; however, it is in apparent discrepancy with findings recently reported by Nielsen et al.[20] By using a *TPH* biallelic conformational polymorphism (the allelic variants were labeled U and L),[25] these authors concluded that suicidality is associated with *TPH* on the basis of a difference in the allelic distribution at this locus between violent offenders with and without a history of suicidal behaviors. We disagree; their data showed no difference in *TPH* allelic frequencies between the suicide attempters group (f[U]=0.32) and the control group (f[U]=0.35). Moreover, these frequencies are not significantly different from those previously reported by Nielsen et al[25] in other control populations (families from the Centre d'Etude du Polymorphisme Humain, and Swedes). Thus, they are likely to be the true frequencies consistently observed in the general population among white subjects from different areas.[20] Consequently, there was no significant deviation in the *TPH* allelic frequencies between suicide attempters and control subjects in the study of Nielsen et al.[20] A false interpretation of their data may be explained by the mistake in Table 2 of their article, in which the allelic frequencies have been obviously inverted. Thus, the study by Nielsen et al[20] does not support an association between *TPH* and suicide attempts, and its findings are in agreement with our data.

The absence of a significant difference of *TPH* allelic frequencies between suicide attempters and controls should be interpreted with caution. Indeed, the samples used in both studies (62 suicide attempters in the present study and 36 in the study by Nielsen et al[20]) may not be large enough to detect a true association.[26,27] To exclude the involvement of the *TPH* gene in susceptibility to suicidal behaviors, larger samples will have to be collected. Moreover, because of the sample size required in some circumstances to detect an association,[26] case-control studies may be unable to demonstrate the true effect of a candidate gene. Consequently, other approaches (eg, allele-sharing methods) should be used in combination with association studies.[9]

An explanation for the negative results in the present study may be that the selection of patients only on the basis that they have made a serious suicide attempt is not fully adequate. Indeed, there is some debate as to whether only particular characteristics of suicidal behavior correlate with a low level of 5-HIAA in the CSF.[14-17,22] For example, a violent method has been proposed as a distinguishing characteristic of suicide attempters with a low level of 5-HIAA in the CSF. However, many studies have indicated that the choice of suicide method may depend on the methods avail-

Table 1. Demographical and Clinical Characteristics of the 62 Patients Who Made Suicide Attempts (SAs)

	Men (n=31)	Women (n=31)	Total (N=62)
Age, y*	31.5±11.8	36.1±12.2	33.8±12.2
No. of SAs, No. (%)			
1	17 (55)	10 (32)	**27** (44)
2	8 (26)	7 (23)	**15** (24)
≥3	6 (19)	14 (45)	**20** (32)
Age at 1st SA, y*	28.9±12.2	32.0±12.4	30.5±12.3
Lifetime diagnoses, No. (%)			
Mood disorders	19 (61)	23 (74)	**42** (68)
Major depressive disorders	17 (55)	20 (65)	**37** (60)
Bipolar disorders	2 (6)	3 (10)	**5** (8)
Alcohol abuse and/or dependence	13 (42)	4 (13)	**17** (27)
Substance abuse and/or dependence	8 (26)	1 (3)	**9** (15)
Panic disorder with or without agoraphobia	5 (16)	11 (35)	**16** (26)
Agoraphobia without panic disorder	0	1 (3)	**1** (2)
Social phobia	4 (13)	5 (16)	**9** (15)
Obsessive-compulsive disorder	0	0	0
Antisocial personality disorder	8 (26)	0	**8** (13)
Psychotic disorders	4 (13)	0	**4** (6)

Values are given as mean±SD.

Table 2. Population Association Between *Ava* II/C2-38 Polymorphism at the *TPH* Locus and History of Suicide Attempts*

	History of Suicide Attempts, No. (%)											Control Subjects, No. (%)
	ASPD		MDD		PD		AUD		Gender			
Variable	With	Without	With	Without	With	Without	With	Without	Males	Females	All	
Genotype												
A1A1	5 (63)	15 (28)	11 (30)	9 (36)	5 (31)	15 (33)	7 (41)	13 (29)	11 (35)	9 (29)	20 (32)	18 (35)
A1A2	2 (25)	31 (57)	21 (57)	13 (52)	7 (44)	26 (57)	7 (41)	26 (58)	18 (58)	15 (48)	33 (53)	26 (50)
A2A2	1 (13)	8 (15)	5 (14)	3 (12)	4 (25)	5 (11)	3 (18)	6 (13)	2 (6)	7 (23)	9 (15)	8 (15)
Total	**8**	**54**	**37**	**25**	**16**	**46**	**17**	**45**	**31**	**31**	**62**	**52**
Allele												
A1	12 (75)	61 (56.5)	43 (58)	31 (62)	17 (53)	56 (61)	21 (62)	52 (58)	40 (65)	33 (53)	73 (58.9)	62 (59.6)
A2	4 (25)	47 (43.5)	31 (42)	19 (38)	15 (47)	36 (39)	13 (38)	38 (42)	22 (35)	29 (47)	51 (41.1)	42 (40.4)

**ASPD indicates antisocial personality disorder; MDD, major depressive disorder; PD, panic disorder; and AUD, alcohol use disorder.*

able and on local fashion or personal preference rather than on any biological predisposition.[28-32] Furthermore, we did not select our suicide attempters from violent offenders. It has been suggested that a disturbed serotonin metabolism correlates with abnormalities in aggression and/or impulse control regulation—whatever direction the aggression takes and whatever the psychiatric diagnosis.[14-16] However, the absence of an association with the *TPH* gene in violent offenders with a history of suicide attempts in the study by Nielsen et al[20] suggests that, even in this subgroup of suicide attempters, the *TPH* gene is not a susceptibility gene.

The association reported by Nielsen et al[20] was owing to a significant difference between the allelic frequencies in violent offenders without a history of suicide attempts (f[U]=0.54)and control subjects (f[U]=0.35) (χ^2=4.87, P<.05). If confirmed, this may indicate that *TPH* is a protective gene against suicidal behaviors. Indeed, with violence being a risk factor for suicidal behaviors,[33] the observation reported by Nielsen et al[20] may indicate that violent offenders who have a *TPH* U allele are protected against suicidal behaviors. Further studies that use different independent samples of violent offenders and patients who suffer from psychiatric disorders closely related to suicidal behaviors, with and without a history of suicidal behaviors, are required to confirm this hypothesis.

If *TPH* is not involved in vulnerability to suicidal behaviors, the decreased levels of 5-HIAA in the CSF in subjects with a history of suicidal behaviors reported by most though not all investigators[16] may be associated with *TPH*-independent mechanisms and possibly with abnormalities in other serotoninergic candidate genes (eg, monoamine oxidase genes). Indeed, Buchsbaum et al[34] found that significantly more students with low rather than high monoamine oxidase activity in their blood platelets had a family history of suicidal behavior, and monoamine oxidase A has recently been implicated in severe behavioral disturbances comprising aggression in a large Dutch kindred.[35]

Despite these negative results, association studies that use candidate genes remain one of the methods of choice for studying the genetic component of suicidal behaviors. This approach has shown great power in detecting susceptibility genes for various complex diseases.[9]

Accepted for publication March 31, 1995.

This work was supported by grants from the Centre National de la Recherche Scientifique, Paris, France, and from the Institut National de la Recherche Médicale, Paris.

Reprint requests to Division de Neuropsychiatrie, Institution Universitaire de Psychiatrie de Genève, Chemin du Petit-Bel-Air 2, 1225 Genève, Switzerland (Dr Malafosse).

REFERENCES

1. Mann JJ, Arango V. Integration of neurobiology and psychopathology in a unified model of suicidal behavior. *J Clin Psychopharmacol.* 1992;12:2S-7S.
2. Murphy G, Wetzel R. Family history of suicidal behavior among suicide attempters. *J Nerv Ment Dis.* 1982;170:86-90.
3. Pitts F, Winokur G. Affective disorder, III: diagnostic correlates and incidence of suicide. *J Nerv Ment Dis.* 1964;133:176.
4. Roy A, Segal NL, Centerwall BS, Robinette CD. Suicide in twins. *Arch Gen Psychiatry.* 1991;48:29-32.
5. Schulsinger F, Kety S, Rosenthal D, Wender PH. A family study of suicide. In: Schou M, Stromgren E, eds. *Origins, Prevention, and Treatment of Affective Disorders.* Orlando, Fla: Academic Press Inc; 1979:277-287.
6. Wender P, Kety S, Rosenthal D. Psychiatric disorders in the biological and adoptives families of adopted individuals with affective disorders. *Arch Gen Psychiatry.* 1986;43:923-929.
7. Kety S. Genetic factors in suicide. In: Roy A, ed. *Suicide.* Baltimore, Md: Williams & Wilkins; 1986:chap 3.
8. Egeland JA, Sussex JN. Suicide and family loading for affective disorders. *JAMA.* 1985;254:915-918.
9. Lander ES, Schork NJ. Genetic dissection of complex traits. *Science.* 1994;265: 2037-2048.
10. Gershon ES, Goldin LR, Martinez MM, Hoehe MR. Presidential address: detecting discrete genes for susceptibility to bipolar disorder or schizophrenia. In: Gershon ES, Cloninger CR, eds. *Genetic Approaches to Mental Disorders.* Washington, DC: American Psychiatric Press Inc; 1994:205-231.
11. Zee RY, Lou Y, Griffiths LR, Morris BJ. Association of a polymorphism of the angiotensin I-converting enzyme gene with essential hypertension. *Biochem Biophys Res Commun.* 1992;1:9-15.
12. Corder EH, Saunders AM, Strittmatter WJ, Schmechel DE, Gaskell PC, Small GW, Roses AD, Haines JL, Pericak-Vance MA. Gene dose of apolipoprotein E type 4 allele and the risk of Alzheimer's disease in late-onset families. *Science.* 1993;261:921-923.
13. Cooper JR, Melcer I. The enzymatic oxydation of tryptophan to 5-hydroxytrophan in the biosynthesis of serotonin. *J Pharmacol Exp Ther.* 1961;132:265-268.
14. Stanley M, Mann JJ, Cohen L. Serotonergic receptors in suicide. *Ann N Y Acad Sci.* 1986;487:122-127.
15. Roy A, Linnoila M. Monoamines and suicidal behavior. In: van Praag HM, Plutchik R, Apter A, eds. *Violence and Suicidality.* New York, NY: Brunner/Mazel Inc; 1990:141-183.
16. Apter A, Brown SL, Korn ML, van Praag HM. Serotonergic parameters of aggression and suicide. In: Brown SL, van Praag HM, eds. *The Role of Serotonin in Psychiatric Disorders.* New York, NY: Brunner/Mazel Inc; 1991:284-332.
17. Träskman L, Asberg M, Bertilsson L, Sjöstrand L. Monoamine metabolites in CSF and suicidal behavior. *Arch Gen Psychiatry.* 1981;38:631-636.
18. Roy A, De Jong J, Linnoila M. Cerebrospinal fluid monoamine metabolites and suicidal behavior in depressed patients. *Arch Gen Psychiatry.* 1989;46:609-612.
19. Abbar M, Amadeo S, Malafosse A, Shenk L, Mallet J, Castelnau D. An association study between suicidal behavior and tryptophan hydroxylase markers. *Clin Neuropharmacol.* 1992;15(suppl 1):299.
20. Nielsen DA, Goldman D, Virkkunen M, Tokola R, Rawlings R, Linnoila M. Suicidality and 5-hydroxyindoleacetic acid concentration associated with a tryptophan hydroxylase polymorphism. *Arch Gen Psychiatry.* 1994;51:34-38.
21. Fyer A, Endicott J, Manuzza S, Klein DF. *Schedule for Affective Disorders and Schizophrenia–Lifetime Version Anxiety Version.* New York: Anxiety Disorders Clinic, New York State Psychiatric Institute; 1985.
22. Asberg M, Träskman L, Thorén P. 5-HIAA in the cerebrospinal fluid: a biochemical suicide predictor. *Arch Gen Psychiatry.* 1976;33:1193-1197.
23. Boularand S, Darmon M, Ganem Y, Launay JM, Mallet J. Complete coding sequence of human tryptophan hydroxylase. *Nucleic Acids Res.* 1990;18:4257.
24. Malafosse A, Sabate O, Leboyer M, Laklou H, Abbar M, Amadéo S, Boularand S, Campion D, Canseil O, Castelnau D, D'Amato T, Granger B, Loo H, Poirier MF, Samolyk D, Savoye C, Zarifian E, Feingold J, Mallet J. Association and linkage studies of manic-depressive illness with three polymorphisms in the tryptophan hydroxylase gene. *Am J Med Genet.* In press.
25. Nielsen DA, Dean M, Goldman D. Genetic mapping of the human tryptophan hydroxylase gene on chromosome 11, using an intronic conformational polymorphism. *Am J Hum Genet.* 1992;51:1366-1371.
26. Thompson EA, Deeb S, Walker D, Motulski AG. The detection of linkage disequilibrium between closely linked markers: RFLPs at the AI-CIII apolipoprotein genes. *Am J Hum Genet.* 1988;42:113-124.
27. Lewis G, Pelosi AJ. The case-control study in psychiatry. *Br J Psychiatry.* 1990; 157:197-207.
28. Davidson F, Philippe A. *Suicide et tentatives de suicide aujourd'hui: étude épidémiologique.* Paris, France: Institut National de la Santé et de la Recherche Médicale; 1986.
29. Bill-Brahe U, Jessen G. Suicide in Denmark, 1922-1991: the choice of method. *Acta Psychiatr Scand.* 1994;90:91-96.
30. Markush RE, Bartolucci AA. Firearms and suicide in the United States. *Am J Public Health.* 1984;74:123-127.
31. Oliver RG, Hetzel BS. Rise and fall of suicide rates in Australia: relation to sedative avaibility. *Med J Aust.* 1972;2:919-923.
32. Sloan JH, Rivara FP, Reay DT, Ferris JA, Path MRC, Kellerman AL. Firearms regulation and rates of suicide: a comparison of two metropolitan areas. *N Engl J Med.* 1990;322:369-373.
33. Brown GL, Goodwin FK. Impulsivity, aggression and associated affects: relationship to self-destructive behavior and suicide. In: Maris RW, Berman AL, Maltsberger JT, Yufit RI, eds. *Assessment and Prediction of Suicide.* New York NY: Guilford Press; 1992:586-589.
34. Buchsbaum M, Coursey R, Murphy D. The biochemical high-risk paradigm: behavioral and familial correlates of low platelet monoamine oxidase activity. *Science.* 1976;194:339-341.
35. Brunner HG, Nelen MR, van Zandvoort P, Abeling NGGM, van Gennip AH, Wolters EC, Kuiper MA, Ropers HH, van Oost BA. X-linked borderline mental retardation with prominent behavioral disturbance: phenotype, genetic localization, and evidence for disturbed monoamine metabolism. *Am J Hum Genet.* 1993;52:1032-1039.

Health Care Costs of Primary Care Patients With Recognized Depression

Gregory E. Simon, MD, MPH; Michael VonKorff, ScD; William Barlow, PhD

Background: While an extensive literature documents the influence of depression on general medical services utilization, estimates of the economic burden of depression have focused on the direct costs of depression treatment. Higher use of general medical services may contribute significantly to the true cost of depressive illness.

Methods: Computerized record systems of a large staff-model health maintenance organization (HMO) were used to identify consecutive primary care patients with visit diagnoses of depression (n=6257) and a comparison sample of primary care patients with no depression diagnosis (n=6257). The HMO accounting records were used to compare components of health care costs.

Results: Patients diagnosed as depressed had higher annual health care costs ($4246 vs $2371, $P<.001$) and higher costs for every category of care (eg, primary care, medical specialty, medical inpatient, pharmacy, laboratory). Similar cost differences were observed for each of the subgroups examined (patients treated with antidepressants, those not treated with antidepressants, and those diagnosed at routine physical examination visits). Pharmacy records indicated greater chronic medical illness in the diagnosed depression group, but large cost differences remained after adjustment ($3971 vs $2644). Twofold cost differences persisted for at least 12 months after initiation of treatment.

Conclusions: Diagnosis of depression is associated with a generalized increase in use of health services that is only partially explained by comorbid medical conditions. In the primary care sector, this greater medical utilization exceeds direct treatment costs for depression. The persistence of utilization differences suggests that recognition and initiation of treatment alone are not adequate to reduce utilization differences.

(Arch Gen Psychiatry. 1995;52:850-856)

A LARGE BODY of research over the last decade demonstrates the burden of depressive illness on individuals and on society as a whole.[1] Epidemiologic surveys find that 2% to 5% of community residents[2,3] and 6% to 8% of patients seen in general medical clinics[4] suffer from current major depression. Depressive illness results in significant work loss[5] and is associated with a level of disability comparable to that of major medical illness.[6] Follow-up studies of depressed patients are now showing a significant risk for chronicity and relapse.[7,8] These findings argue for more energetic recognition and more intensive treatment of depressive episodes.[1,9]

Arguments for more intensive treatment of depression come at a time of increasing pressure to control health care costs. In response to cost pressures, insurance coverage of mental health treatment has grown more restrictive during recent years.[10,11] Most proposals to reform health care financing include stricter limits for mental health care than for general medical services.[12] In such a climate, any argument for more comprehensive insurance coverage of depression treatment must consider the overall economic impact of depression on the health care system.

Previous research generally supports an association between depression and increased use of general medical services.[13-21] Using data from the Health Insurance Experiment, Manning and Wells[13] found that high psychological distress and low psychological well-being were associated with greater general medical expenditures even after adjustment for self-

See Methods on next page

From the Center for Health Studies, Group Health Cooperative of Puget Sound, Seattle, Wash.

METHODS

STUDY SETTING

Group Health Cooperative of Puget Sound (GHC) is a large staff-model HMO serving approximately 390 000 residents of western Washington State. The GHC provides comprehensive care on a capitated basis, with members typically receiving GHC coverage through employer-subsidized plans. The GHC enrollment includes approximately 45 000 Medicare members and 22 000 members covered by Medicaid or by Washington's Basic Health Plan (a state program for low-income residents). Members of GHC are similar to Seattle-area residents except for higher educational level and less representation of the high and low extremes of income. Primary care for adults is provided by approximately 360 physicians (full-time and part-time), with each full-time physician responsible for a defined panel of approximately 1600 members. Approximately 80% of adult GHC members make one or more primary care visits in any year, with the average member making approximately four visits. More than 95% of physicians providing primary care to adults are trained in family medicine, with most of the remainder trained in internal medicine. Specialty mental health services are available through either physician-referral or self-referral from six mental health clinics staffed by approximately 20 psychiatrists and 90 nonphysician providers. Specialty mental health clinics emphasize short-term individual psychotherapy, pharmacotherapy, and group therapy. Typical coverage arrangements provide for unlimited psychiatric medication management visits (subject to $5 to $10 visit copayments) and 10 to 20 outpatient psychotherapy visits (subject to $10 to $20 visit copayments). No referral or authorization is required for seeking specialty mental health care, and primary care physicians have no incentive to limit mental health service use. More than 90% of primary care physicians and psychiatrists are certified by appropriate specialty boards. The GHC's computerized information systems include data on all outpatient visits to GHC clinics and all outpatient prescriptions filled at GHC pharmacies. Previous surveys of GHC members have found that more than 95% of prescriptions filled by GHC members (including those for antidepressant drugs) are filled at GHC pharmacies.[26]

SELECTION OF STUDY SAMPLE

Potential subjects were all GHC members 18 years and older receiving an outpatient visit diagnosis of depression from a GHC primary care provider between April 1, 1992, and December 31, 1992. To ensure complete availability of relevant data, the sample was limited to those continuously enrolled in GHC from October 1, 1991, to December 31, 1993. The remaining sample was divided into those beginning new episodes of depression treatment (defined as no visit diagnosis of depression or prescription for antidepressant drugs between October 1, 1991, and April 1, 1992) and those continuing a previously established episode of treatment (ie, those receiving either a visit diagnoses of depression or a prescription for antidepressant drugs between October 1, 1991, and April 1, 1992). For each enrollee, the first visit associated with a diagnosis of depression during the study interval was considered the index visit.

For each patient in the depression sample, a com-

Continued on next page

rated general health status. Epidemiologic surveys document greater use of general medical services by community residents with depression.[14,15] Studies of high users of general medical services find high rates of chronic depressive illness.[16] In medical inpatient samples, depression is associated with longer hospital stays and higher costs.[17]

Recent attempts to estimate the economic impact of depression, however, have typically focused on the direct costs of depression treatment.[22,23] Greenberg and colleagues,[22] for example, considered only the costs of inpatient and outpatient psychiatric care. Because a large portion of depression treatment occurs in the general medical sector,[24] a focus on costs of psychiatric treatment may overestimate the per-case costs of depression treatment and will ignore the costs due to greater use of general medical services. We have previously described patterns of health care utilization in a small sample of primary care patients with depressive and anxiety disorders.[25] Those data showed markedly higher overall service use by psychologically distressed patients and suggested that specific mental health treatment accounted for only a small portion of that higher utilization. Given both the large burden of depressive illness and the significant cost of expanded treatment, more data on the health care costs associated with depression are clearly needed.

This report describes the use of computerized visit-diagnosis data, pharmacy records, and cost accounting data from a large staff-model health maintenance organization (HMO) to estimate the direct health care costs for a large sample of primary care patients with recognized depression. These analyses will address three questions: (1) How do overall health care costs of primary care patients with recognized depression compare with those of other primary care patients? (2) Are any differences in cost explained by differences in the prevalence of chronic medical illness? (3) Do cost differences associated with depression persist over time among patients recognized and treated?

RESULTS

STUDY SAMPLE

The procedures described above identified 6919 GHC members receiving a primary care visit diagnosis of depression between April 1, 1992, and December 31, 1992. Elimination of those not continuously enrolled yielded a sample of 6257 members with recognized depression during this interval. Of that sample, 4915 filled one or more prescriptions for antidepressant medication during the 12 months following the index visit. Selected pa-

parison HMO member was randomly selected from the pool of all GHC members of the same gender and age (±2 years) who met the following criteria: had no visit diagnosis of depression between October 1, 1991, and December 31, 1993; had no prescription for antidepressant medication between October 1, 1991, and December 31, 1993; made a primary care visit during the month of the depressed patient's index visit (this visit was considered the comparison member's index visit); and was continuously enrolled in GHC for the 12 months following the index visit.

For each member in the depression sample and the comparison group, cost data were collected over a 12-month period beginning with study entry. For continuing cases and matched comparison members, the date of study entry was considered to be April 1, 1992. For patients beginning new episodes and the corresponding comparison sample, the date of study entry was the date of the index visit.

CALCULATION OF DIRECT HEALTH CARE COSTS

The GHC computerized cost accounting system organizes detailed cost and utilization for every GHC enrollee since 1989. The GHC utilization and cost system uses data from 15 separate feeder systems to capture various components of utilization (outpatient visits, hospitalizations, pharmacy, laboratory, etc). Each cost center within GHC assigns a cost to each unit of service by allocating actual costs from the general ledger to each unit of service provided. For example, each primary care clinic would allocate its actual monthly costs (facilities, payroll, supplies) over the total number of outpatient visits provided. Overhead costs are fully allocated to patient care departments. Any out-of-plan services reimbursed by GHC are included based on the amount reimbursed.

ADJUSTMENT FOR MEDICAL COMORBIDITY

Ratings of chronic medical morbidity were made using the Chronic Disease Score, a technique developed at GHC for rating chronic medical illnesses using computerized pharmacy records.[27] This method classifies each patient according to the number of medications typically used to treat chronic medical conditions (eg, heart disease, diabetes, hypertension, rheumatoid arthritis, and obstructive lung disease) and is therefore a measure of recognized and treated medical illness. Psychotropic medications and medications used primarily for symptom management (eg, analgesics and nonsteroidal anti-inflammatory drugs) are not included in the index. In prior research in the GHC population, the Chronic Disease Score was correlated with physician ratings of physical disease severity and predicted mortality and was less influenced by current psychological distress than self-report measures of health status.[27]

STATISTICAL ANALYSIS

All statistical analyses were performed with the SAS software package (SAS Institute, Cary, NC). Comparisons of mean values for cost and Chronic Disease Score were made using analysis of variance. Adjustment of mean cost differences for differences in Chronic Disease Score was done by both direct standardization and linear regression. Because of the highly skewed distribution of cost data, tests of statistical significance for cost comparisons were based on log-transformed cost.

tients had a mean age of 46.2 years and 64% were female.

COMPARISON OF ANNUAL HEALTH CARE COSTS

We first compared overall health care costs for primary care patients with recognized depression with those for age- and gender-matched primary care patients with no depression diagnosis. The **Table** displays mean values for total and component costs for depressed primary care patients and the matched comparison group. Total health care costs were markedly higher for depressed patients (mean, $4246) than for the comparison sample (mean, $2371). Specialty mental health care costs (both outpatient and inpatient) accounted for approximately 10% of total costs for depressed patients; the higher specialty mental health care utilization by depressed patients accounted for only approximately one fifth of the difference between depressed and nondepressed patients in total health care costs. For every other category of cost examined, depressed patients had mean annual costs approximately 1.5 times those of the comparison group. Log-transformed costs were significantly higher for depressed patients across all cost categories ($P<.001$ for all comparisons).

A similar pattern was seen for various patient subgroups. Among depressed patients treated with antidepressant drugs (n=4915), the mean total cost was $4371 compared with $2336 for the comparison group (n=4915). While outpatient pharmacy costs were nearly three times as high for depressed patients treated with antidepressant drugs than for comparison enrollees ($632 vs $231), antidepressant drugs accounted for only $194 of the total (or less than half of the difference in pharmacy costs between groups). Among those not receiving antidepressant treatment, the mean total cost for depressed patients (n=1342) was $3785 compared with $2498 for the comparison group (n=1342).

ADJUSTMENT FOR MEDICAL COMORBIDITY AND OTHER POTENTIAL CONFOUNDERS

Our analyses next considered chronic medical illness as a possible confounder of the relationship between depression and health care costs (those with chronic medical conditions might have both higher costs and greater prevalence of depression). When the Chronic Disease Score was used as a measure of treated chronic medical morbidity, patients with recognized depression showed higher levels of treated medical illness than the comparison group. The mean Chronic Disease Score was 2.49 (SD, 2.99) for depressed patients and 1.81 (SD, 2.99) for the comparison group. Adjustment for Chronic Disease Score

Annual Health Care Costs for Health Maintenance Organization (HMO) Primary Care Patients With Depression and Comparison of Age- and Gender-Matched HMO Members

	Mean (SD) Dollars	
Category of Care	Depressed Patients (n=6257)	Comparison Group (n=6257)
Outpatient mental health	356 (859)	29 (172)
Inpatient mental health	85 (925)	1 (59)
Outpatient primary care	799 (709)	446 (403)
Outpatient medical specialty	497 (982)	375 (706)
Emergency department	60 (256)	27 (151)
Outpatient pharmacy	571 (638)	234 (395)
Outpatient laboratory/radiology	309 (535)	216 (378)
Inpatient medical	1066 (4604)	741 (4369)
Total direct health costs	4246 (7156)	2371 (5823)

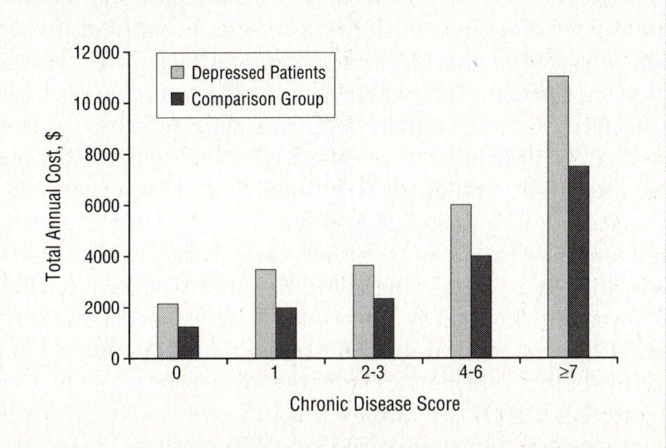

Figure 1. *Mean annual health care costs for primary care patients with recognized depression (n=6257) and comparison group of primary care patients (n=6257), according to level of Chronic Disease Score (a rating of medical morbidity based on medication use).*

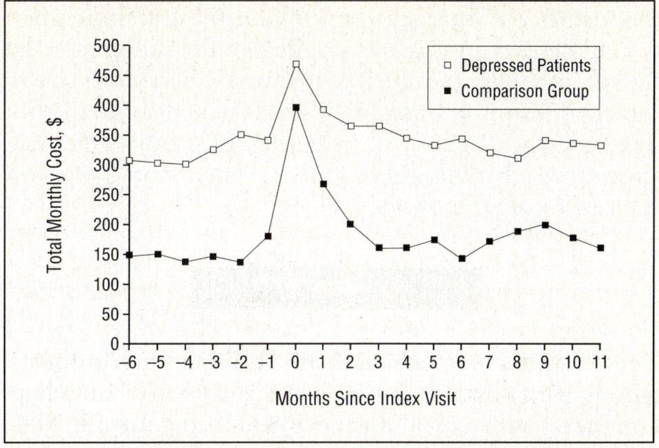

Figure 2. *Mean monthly health care costs for primary care patients with new diagnoses of depression (n=5595) and comparison group of primary care patients (n=5595) for 6 months before and 12 months following the first diagnosis of depression.*

did explain some of the observed cost differences. When costs for the comparison group were standardized to reflect the Chronic Disease Score distribution of depressed patients, the mean total costs for the comparison group increased from $2371 per year to $2880 per year (compared with $4246 per year for depressed patients). As shown in **Figure 1**, depressed patients had markedly higher costs at every level of Chronic Disease Score. Total annual costs were typically 1.5 times those of the comparison group. Adjustment using linear regression yielded similar results: a model containing age, gender, and Chronic Disease Score yielded least-squares mean estimates for a total annual cost of $3972 for depressed patients and $2645 for the comparison group. In a linear model predicting log-transformed total cost, depressed patients had costs 2.1 times as high as the comparison group after adjustment for age and gender. The mean log-transformed cost was 7.74 (SD, 1.06) for depressed patients and 6.98 (SD, 1.17) for the comparison group. The addition of Chronic Disease Score to this model reduced this estimate to a 1.8-fold difference. In this model, no significant interaction was observed between the presence of depression and Chronic Disease Score in predicting log-transformed total cost (ie, depressed patients had costs approximately 1.8 times as high at all levels of treated medical comorbidity). The addition of other potential confounding variables (GHC clinic location, GHC insurance coverage group) did not affect the relationship between depression and overall cost.

As an alternative method for comparing groups with similar levels of medical illness, we restricted the sample of depressed patients to those diagnosed as depressed at the time of a routine physical examination (n=128) and compared this group with a sample of age- and gender-matched primary care patients making a visit for a routine physical examination during the same month. As expected, this subgroup making "well-adult care" visits had lower overall costs, but costs for depressed patients were still more than twice as high: $3157 (SD, $5279) for depressed patients and $1330 (SD, $1488) for the comparison group. Again, depressed patients had higher costs for every category examined, but some of these differences (inpatient mental health costs, inpatient medical costs, outpatient specialty costs) were not statistically significant given large variances and small sample sizes. Mental health treatment costs accounted for less than 20% of the overall difference.

PATTERN OF HEALTH CARE COSTS OVER TIME

We next examined the time course of health care costs before and after initiation of depression treatment. This analysis included only the 5595 patients initiating treatment during the study period (new episodes) along with age- and gender-matched controls. Patients receiving a visit diagnosis of depression or an antidepressant prescription between October 1, 1991, and April 1, 1992 (continuing episodes), were excluded. Results are shown in **Figure 2**. Patients with recognized depression had consistently higher costs than the comparison sample during the period prior to treatment initiation. Utilization in both groups peaked at the time of the index visit, reflecting the requirement that both groups make an outpatient visit during this month. This short-term increase was smaller in the group with treated depression than in the comparison group, and the difference between the two groups was smallest in the index month. By 3 months after the index visit, utilization in both groups returned to approximately the levels seen prior to the index visit. Mean costs for the depressed group remained approximately twice those for the comparison group for the remaining 9 months.

COMMENT

These data demonstrate markedly higher health care costs among HMO patients with recognized depression when compared with age- and gender-matched controls. This increase was seen for every component of health care cost and for each patient subgroup. Adjustment for treated chronic medical illness using pharmacy data reduced the magnitude of cost differences, but costs for depressed patients remained substantially higher. A twofold difference in total cost between those diagnosed as having depression and the comparison group was maintained over 12 months of observation, suggesting a chronic component to utilization differences.

LIMITATIONS AND STRENGTHS

Conclusions from these data are limited by the lack of clinical information on severity or duration of depression. Concurrent research on patients treated for depression by GHC primary care physicians, however, suggests that most meet structured interview criteria for current major depression, with most of the remainder lying near the major depression threshold.[28] Although we may assume that most of the patients in this sample who were treated with antidepressants were significantly depressed, these data lack the clinical detail needed to examine the cross-sectional relationship between clinical severity and utilization or the longitudinal relationship between course of depression and subsequent health care costs.

These data also consider only patients with recognized depression. Epidemiologic studies of depression in primary care indicate a significant portion of depressed patients may go unrecognized and untreated.[29] If costs for unrecognized patients were significantly different from those of recognized patients, these data could misrepresent the true impact of depression on utilization. The presence of members with unrecognized depression in the comparison sample would lead to a negative bias.

We have recently completed similar cost comparisons in a smaller sample of consecutive primary care patients subject to detailed clinical assessment.[25] Those analyses yielded remarkably similar results. Primary care patients satisfying *DSM-III-R* criteria for current major depressive disorder had total health care costs approximately 2.5 times as high as those with no depressive disorder. After adjusting for medical comorbidity, using both primary care physicians' ratings and Chronic Disease Score, depressed patients had total costs approximately 1.5 times as high as the nondepressed group. While that small sample did not permit some of the detailed analyses described in the report, the similarity of results suggests that the absence of detailed clinical data does not seriously compromise these findings.

Given our population-based sampling method, both the group with recognized depression and the comparison group are quite heterogeneous. Consequently, the groups may differ in characteristics likely to influence health care use. While we have matched for age and gender and have attempted to control for overall medical morbidity, important unmeasured confounders may exist. Our secondary analyses of the subsample making well-adult care visits attempt to address such potential confounders by restricting to a more homogeneous group. Similar results in that small sample offer some reassurance about interpretation of the overall results. Analyses stratified by level of treated medical morbidity (Figure 1) found a similar magnitude of difference at all levels of Chronic Disease Score.

Our method for selecting the comparison sample may actually underestimate the true influence of depression on health care utilization. Primary care patients receiving a visit diagnosis of depression were compared with age- and gender-matched members visiting a primary care physician during the same month. By ensuring that all comparison patients also make at least one primary care visit, this method ignores the impact of depression on the likelihood of making the index visit. If depression increases the likelihood of any service use, selecting only service users for the comparison sample may create a conservative bias. This potential bias could be avoided by comparing the health care costs of depressed members with those of similar nondepressed members in a population-based sample (ie, selection not related to use of services). Given the large variation seen in health care cost data, such an epidemiologic survey would require screening of several thousand subjects.

Our data were collected within a single staff-model HMO. Because this capitated system places greater restrictions on the use of specialty care (including medical specialty and mental health care) than do most non-HMO insurance plans, cost data collected here may not generalize to other settings. A strength of this setting, though, is the ability to include all patients recognized as depressed in a large, defined population. Because GHC's cost accounting system incorporates actual operating budgets, these results are based on the costs of providing care rather than on charges.

COMPONENTS OF COST DIFFERENCES

Only a small portion of the cost differences between the group with diagnosed depression and the comparison group appeared directly related to specialty mental health treatment. Specialty mental health treatment costs (inpatient and outpatient) accounted for less than one quarter of the difference in total cost. Even among patients treated with antidepressant drugs, costs of antidepressant prescriptions accounted for less than half of the observed differences in pharmacy cost. Approximately half of the total cost difference was due to a nonspecific increase in the use of outpatient medical and ancillary services. While previous attempts to estimate the economic burden of depression have typically focused on costs of specialty mental health treatment,[22,23] these findings give greater emphasis to the generalized increases in health care use associated with depression. In this 9-month sample of HMO primary patients with recognized depression, depression-related specialty mental health care and antidepressant drugs accounted for approximately $3.8 million, while greater use of general medical services accounted for $8.9 million over 1 year. Policy decisions regarding mental health insurance coverage must consider the full range of health care costs associated with depression.

POSSIBLE EXPLANATIONS

These data demonstrate a strong association between recognized depression and health care utilization, but a number of causal relationships could produce the results described herein.

First, these findings may reflect the direct influence of depression on patients' and physicians' decisions about the use of health services. Depression may amplify patients' experience of pain or other unpleasant physical symptoms and lead to greater use of health care services.[30] Physicians confronted with depressed patients may be more likely to pursue diagnostic evaluations or prescribe treatments in response to patients' physical or psychological distress.

Second, chronic medical conditions may increase the likelihood of depression because of pain, limitations on activity, or direct biological effects (such as with Parkinson's disease or poststroke depression). We have attempted to control for this effect using a measure of treated chronic medical illness based on prescriptions received. That analysis suggests that differences in chronic medical morbidity explain only a portion of the observed cost differences. Potential difficulties remain, however, that could bias results in either direction. Use of an imperfect measure of medical morbidity may "undercontrol" for the effect of medical illness and overstate cost differences associated with depression. Alternatively, use of a medical morbidity measure that is "contaminated" by depression may bias these results against finding a true difference in utilization. Because depressed patients visit medical physicians more frequently, chronic conditions such as diabetes or hypertension may be more often recognized and treated. Increased surveillance might then lead to a greater rate of treated chronic medical illness in depressed patients. In this second case, use of prescription records to adjust cost data for medical morbidity may introduce a conservative bias by overcontrolling for chronic medical conditions. In short, adjustment for medical morbidity is a complex task, and no method can completely exclude error or bias in either direction.

Finally, these results may reflect the greater likelihood that depression will be recognized and treated among patients having frequent contact with health care providers. Among all persons in the population suffering from depression, those making frequent outpatient visits for any reason are more likely than infrequent visitors to receive a depression diagnosis or an antidepressant prescription. This phenomenon could lead to overestimation of the true relationship between depression and use of general medical services. Such an effect may also occur in the opposite direction. As discussed above, depression may increase recognition and treatment of medical conditions or somatic symptoms.

These data do raise questions about what portion of the greater health care costs of depressed patients would be reduced by improved treatment of depression. This observational study cannot address that question. It is likely that each of the causal mechanisms discussed above (direct effects of depression, medical comorbidity, effect of increased surveillance) contributes to the differences observed. If so, only part of the greater cost might respond to more intensive treatment of depression. Estimating the magnitude of such a cost offset effect would require appropriate randomized studies. These data do suggest that simple recognition and initiation of treatment will not necessarily eliminate cost differences. All depressed patients in this sample were recognized and most received antidepressant medication.

TIME COURSE OF COST DIFFERENCES

Cost differences between those with recognized depression and the comparison group were evident prior to the initiation of depression treatment and persisted for at least 1 year despite diagnosis and, in most cases, initiation of antidepressant treatment. Cost differences prior to initiation of treatment suggest at least two explanations. First, recognition of depression may be more likely in those who visit physicians more frequently. In such a scenario, observed cost differences may reflect patients' underlying propensity to use health services rather than a true effect of depression on medical service use. Alternatively, preexisting differences in utilization may reflect the chronic and/or relapsing nature of depressive illness. Patients with treated depression may have had several prior depressive episodes and have likely experienced some level of depressive symptoms prior to initiation of the current treatment episode. Consequently, one might not expect a sample with treated depression to show "normal" patterns of utilization prior to initiation of treatment. As noted above, the narrowing of cost differences around the time of treatment initiation may be partially artifactual. The requirement that members of both the recognized depression group and comparison group make a primary care visit during the index month produced similar utilization rates during the index month. After the first 3 months of follow-up, differences in utilization were remarkably stable. Persistence of higher utilization over time may reflect chronicity of depression. We suspect, however, that most patients in this sample experienced significant decreases in severity of depression over 1 year of follow-up. Data from similar samples of primary care patients[25,28] indicate that more than half of patients initiating treatment for depression experience considerable improvement over the first few months. Given the reasonable assumption of improvement in this sample, these findings suggest that many patients treated for depression continue to use high levels of medical services even after depression improves or resolves.

These findings emphasize the need to understand health care utilization by depressed patients in the context of chronic physical and psychological morbidity. Persistent high utilization even after recognition and initiation of treatment may reflect the low intensity of treatment that many depressed patients receive.[31-33] In this case, more intensive acute treatment might lead to substantial cost savings. Alternatively, chronically high utilization may reflect the complex nature of depression in general medical outpatients. Depressed mood may be only one component of a larger picture including chronic medical illness,[16] functional impairment,[6,34] decreased work productivity,[5] multiple somatic symptoms,[35,36] and a learned pattern of frequent medical visits.[16,18,25] Acute treatment of depressed mood may have limited impact on patterns of medical service use in such multiproblem patients. Cost-effective treatment may require tailoring interventions according to chronicity of depression, presence of medical comorbidity, and level of functional disability. Once potentially effective interventions are defined, experimental studies could estimate the impact of those interventions on overall costs. Given the size of the cost differences described here, such studies are urgently needed.

Accepted for publication June 26, 1995.

Supported by grants MH41739 and MH51338 from the National Institute of Mental Health (NIMH), Rockville, Md.

Presented in preliminary form at the Seventh NIMH International Research Conference on Mental Health Problems in the General Health Care Sector, McLean, Va, September 1993.

Chester Pabiniak assisted with computer programming.

Reprint requests to Center for Health Studies, 1730 Minor Ave, Room 1600, Seattle, WA 98101 (Dr Simon).

REFERENCES

1. Klerman G, Weissman M. The course, morbidity, and costs of depression. *Arch Gen Psychiatry.* 1992;49:831-834.
2. Regier DA, Boyd JH, Burke JD Jr, Rae DS, Myers JK, Kramer M, Robins LN, George LK, Karno M, Locke BZ. One-month prevalence of mental disorders in the United States. *Arch Gen Psychiatry.* 1988;45:977-986.
3. Kessler RC, McGonagle KA, Zhao S, Nelson CB, Hughes M, Eshleman S, Wittchen H-U, Kendler KS. Lifetime and 12-month prevalence of *DSM-III-R* psychiatric disorders in the United States: results from the National Comorbidity Survey. *Arch Gen Psychiatry.* 1994;51:8-19.
4. Katon W, Schulberg H. Epidemiology of depression in primary care. *Gen Hosp Psychiatry.* 1992;14:237-247.
5. Broadhead WE, Blazer DG, George LK, Tse CK. Depression, disability days and days lost from work in a prospective epidemiologic survey. *JAMA.* 1990;264: 2524-2528.
6. Wells KB, Stewart A, Hays RD, Burnam M, Rogers W, Daniels M, Berry S, Greenfield S, Ware J. The functioning and well-being of depressed patients: results from the Medical Outcomes Study. *JAMA.* 1989;262:914-919.
7. Keller MB, Lavori PW, Mueller TI, Endicott J, Coryell W, Hirschfeld RMA, Shea T. Time to recovery, chronicity, and levels of psychopathology in major depression: a 5-year prospective follow-up of 431 subjects. *Arch Gen Psychiatry.* 1992;49:809-816.
8. Wells KB, Burnam M, Rogers WW, Hays R, Camp P. Course of depression for adult outpatients: results from the Medical Outcomes Study. *Arch Gen Psychiatry.* 1992;49:788-794.
9. Regier DA, Hirschfeld RM, Goodwin FK, Burke JD, Lazar JB, Judd LL. The NIMH Depression Awareness, Recognition and Treatment Program: structure, aims, and scientific basis. *Am J Psychiatry.* 1988;145:1351-135.
10. Brady J, Sharfstein S, Muszynski IL. Trends in private insurance coverage for mental illness. *Am J Psychiatry.* 1986;143:1276-1279.
11. Scheidemandel P. *The Coverage Catalog.* Washington, DC: American Psychiatric Association; 1989.
12. Sharfstein S, Stoline AM, Goldman HH. Psychiatric care and health insurance reform. *Am J Psychiatry.* 1993;150:7-18.
13. Manning W, Wells KB. The effects of psychological distress and psychological well-being on use of medical services. *Med Care.* 1992;30:541-553.
14. Kessler LG, Burns BJ, Shapiro S, Tischler GI, George LK, Hough RL, Bodison D, Miller RH. Psychiatric diagnoses of medical service users: evidence from the Epidemiologic Catchment Area program. *Am J Public Health.* 1987;77:18-24.
15. Johnson J, Weissman M, Klerman G. Service utilization and social morbidity associated with depressive symptoms in the community. *JAMA.* 1992;267: 1478-1483.
16. Katon W, VonKorff M, Lin E, Lipscomb P, Russo J, Wagner E, Polk E. Distressed high utilizers of medical care: *DSM-III-R* diagnoses and treatment needs. *Gen Hosp Psychiatry.* 1990;12:355-362.
17. Levenson J, Hamer RM, Rossiter LF. Relation of psychopathology in general medical inpatients to use and cost of services. *Am J Psychiatry.* 1990;147: 1498-1503.
18. Simon G. Psychiatric disorder and functional somatic symptoms as predictors of health care use. *Psychiatr Med.* 1992;10:49-60.
19. Miranda J, Perez-Stable EJ, Munoz RF, Hargreaves W, Henke CJ. Somatization, psychiatric disorder, and stress in utilization of ambulatory medical services. *Health Psychol.* 1991;10:46-51.
20. McFarland BH, Freeborn DK, Mullooly JP, Pope CR. Utilization patterns among long-term enrollees in a prepaid group practice health maintenence organization. *Med Care.* 1985;23:1221-1233.
21. Mechanic D, Cleary PD, Greenley JR. Distress syndromes, illness behavior, access to care and medical utilization in a defined population. *Med Care.* 1982; 20:361-372.
22. Greenberg P, Stiglin LE, Finkelstein SN, Berndt ER. The economic burden of depression in 1990. *J Clin Psychiatry.* 1993;54:405-418.
23. Kind P, Sorensen J. The costs of depression. *Int Clin Psychopharmacol.* 1993; 7:191-195.
24. Regier DA, Narrow WE, Rae DS, Manderscheid RW, Locke BZ, Goodwin FK. The de facto US mental and addictive disorders service system: Epidemiologic Catchment Area prospective 1-year prevalence rates of disorders and services. *Arch Gen Psychiatry.* 1993;50:85-94.
25. Simon G, Ormel J, VonKorff M, Barlow W. Health care costs associated with depressive and anxiety disorders in primary care. *Am J Psychiatry.* 1995;152: 352-357.
26. Saunders K, Stergachis A, VonKorff M. Group Health Cooperative of Puget Sound. In: Strom B, ed. *Pharmacoepidemiology.* New York, NY: John Wiley & Sons; 1994.
27. VonKorff M, Wagner EH, Saunders K. A Chronic Disease Score from automated pharmacy data. *J Clin Epidemiol.* 1992;45:197-203.
28. Katon W, Lin EHB, VonKorff M, Bush T, Walker E, Simon G, Robinson P. Predictors of persistence of affective symptoms in primary care. *J Affect Disord.* 1994;31:81-90.
29. Eisenberg L. Treating depression and anxiety in primary care: closing the gap between knowledge and practice. *N Engl J Med.* 1992;326:1080-1084.
30. Barsky A. Amplification, somatization, and the somatoform disorders. *Psychosomatics.* 1992;33:28-34.
31. Keller MB, Lavori PW, Klerman GL, Andreasen NC, Endicott J, Coryell W, Fawcett J, Rice JB, Hirschfeld RMA. Low levels and lack of predictors of somatotherapy and psychotherapy received by depressed patients. *Arch Gen Psychiatry.* 1986;43:458-466.
32. Katon W, VonKorff M, Lin E, Bush T, Ormel J. Adequacy and duration of antidepressant treatment in primary care. *Med Care.* 1992;30:67-76.
33. Simon G, VonKorff M, Wagner EH, Barlow W. Patterns of antidepressant use in community practice. *Gen Hosp Psychiatry.* 1993;15:399-408.
34. VonKorff M, Ormel J, Katon WJ, Lin EHB. Disability and depression among high utilizers of health care. *Arch Gen Psychiatry.* 1992;49:91-100.
35. Dworkin SF, VonKorff M, LeResche L. Multiple pains and psychiatric disturbance: an epidemiologic investigation. *Arch Gen Psychiatry.* 1990;47:239-244.
36. Simon G, VonKorff M. Somatization and psychiatric disorder in the NIMH Epidemiologic Catchment Area Study. *Am J Psychiatry.* 1991;148:1494-1500.

The New York High-Risk Project

Psychoses and Cluster A Personality Disorders in Offspring of Schizophrenic Parents at 23 Years of Follow-up

L. Erlenmeyer-Kimling, PhD; Elizabeth Squires-Wheeler, PhD; Ulla Hilldoff Adamo, MA; Anne S. Bassett, MD; Barbara A. Cornblatt, PhD; Clarice J. Kestenbaum, MD; Donald Rock, PhD; Simone A. Roberts; Irving I. Gottesman, PhD, FRCPsych(Hon)

Background: We herein present lifetime prevalence rates of psychoses and *DSM-III-R* cluster A personality disorders in sample A of the New York High-Risk Project, a prospective study following offspring of parents with schizophrenia (HRSz subjects) and affective illness (HRAff subjects) and of psychiatrically normal parents (NC subjects) from midchildhood to adulthood.

Methods: We interviewed the offspring in adulthood with the Schedule for Affective Disorders and Schizophrenia, Lifetime Version, for Axis I disorders and the Personality Disorder Examination for Axis II disorders.

Results: Lifetime prevalence rates (±SE) of schizophrenia and unspecified psychosis were 11.1%±4.3% and 5.6%±3.1%, respectively, in the HRSz group and 0% in the HRAff and NC groups. Rates of schizoaffective disorder subclassified as mainly schizophrenic, however, were highest in the HRAff group. Rates of psychotic affective disorders did not differ between the HRSz and other groups. Age-corrected morbidity risks were similar to lifetime prevalence rates. Rates of the three cluster A personality disorders did not differ among the groups, but the combined rate was greater in the HRSz and HRAff groups than in the NC group.

Conclusions: Our data strongly support a specific familial liability to narrowly defined schizophrenia that is not shared by families of probands with affective disorder. Schizoaffective disorder and cluster A personality disorders, however, occur in families of both schizophrenic probands and probands with affective disorder. Psychotic affective disorders, which are not increased in HRSz subjects, do not appear to be an expression of the liability to schizophrenia.

(Arch Gen Psychiatry. 1995;52:857-865)

From the Departments of Medical Genetics (Drs Erlenmeyer-Kimling and Squires-Wheeler and Mss Adamo and Roberts) and Child Psychiatry (Dr Kestenbaum), New York State Psychiatric Institute, the Departments of Psychiatry (Drs Erlenmeyer-Kimling, Squires-Wheeler, and Kestenbaum) and Genetics and Development (Dr Erlenmeyer-Kimling), College of Physicians and Surgeons, Columbia University, and the Department of Psychiatry, Mt Sinai School of Medicine (Dr Cornblatt), New York, NY; Queen Street Mental Health Centre, University of Toronto, Ontario (Dr Bassett); Educational Testing Service, Princeton, NJ (Dr Rock); and the Department of Psychology, University of Virginia, Charlottesville (Dr Gottesman).

FROM THE FIRST family study of schizophrenia conducted by Rüdin[1] early in this century, this illness has been shown to be significantly increased in first-degree relatives of schizophrenic probands,[2-5] compared with a general population expectancy of about 1%. Although the older family studies have been faulted for reasons having to do with diagnosis, sampling, lack of blindness, and other design inadequacies, most studies of contemporary design[6-13] have continued to display a significantly greater aggregation of schizophrenia in families of schizophrenic probands than in families of normal controls. Many of these later studies with comparatively narrow definitions of schizophrenia have also demonstrated an increased risk for certain other psychotic and nonpsychotic (personality) disorders in the relatives of schizophrenic probands,[7-21] thus reinforcing the concept of a spectrum of deviant conditions sharing a common liability.[22-26]

Because of relatively low reproductive rates in schizophrenic individuals,[27] one category of relatives—namely, offspring of schizophrenic parents—often have been sparsely represented in recent family studies. The offspring, however, were the focus of prospective studies started in the 1960s and 1970s with the goal of examining early characteristics of preschizophrenic individuals and the unfolding of the illness itself.[28] Those high-risk studies that have been able to follow the offspring into adulthood[29-32] therefore present an opportunity to expand and update the limited prevalence and morbidity risk data on this group of relatives. Herein, we report lifetime diagnoses of psychoses and *DSM-III-R*[33] cluster A disorders in the New York High-Risk Project

See Subjects and Methods on next page

SUBJECTS AND METHODS

SUBJECT SELECTION

The NYHRP consists of two independent samples of subjects selected in childhood because of their parents' psychiatric diagnoses or lack of psychiatric history as being at high risk for schizophrenia (the HRSz group) or affective disorders (the HRAff group) or at low risk for psychiatric disorders (the normal comparison, or NC, group). The first sample, sample A, entered the study in 1971 to 1972; the second, sample B, in 1977 to 1979. We limit this report to sample A, at the mean (±SE) age of 31.11±1.83 years in 1994.

We selected mentally ill parents by screening consecutive admissions at several state psychiatric facilities in the New York City metropolitan area to identify schizophrenic patients and patients with major affective disorders who (1) were white and English-speaking, (2) had at least one child aged 7 to 12 years, (3) were still married to the other biological parent of the target-age child(ren) at the time of ascertainment, and (4) did not have a diagnosis of chronic alcoholism, other drug addiction, brain trauma, or psychosis of toxic origin. In addition, we required the children to (1) have an IQ above 70, (2) show no overt signs of a major psychiatric disturbance, and (3) have received no treatment for psychiatric problems.

We identified the NC group through two large school districts, having selected the geographical areas for locating NC families to correspond to those in which most of the HRSz families resided. Parents in the NC families had to be free of any psychiatric treatment history and meet the same background and marital criteria as parents in the HRSz and HRAff families. Children in the NC families were in the same age range and met the same inclusion or exclusion criteria as children in the groups at risk.

Table 1 shows the number of children at entry into the study and current follow-up, as well as age and gender compositions of the three groups. The numbers shown for HRSz and HRAff subjects at entry are those applicable after rediagnosis of the parents, as described below.

Informed consent was obtained from the parents for themselves and their minor children at the first contact with the family. Subsequently, informed consent was obtained from each individual participating in the study at each assessment phase.

PARENTS' DIAGNOSES

Initially, two senior psychiatrists independently made *DSM-II*[35] diagnoses from the parents' hospital records, from which hospital diagnoses and medication histories had been removed. Only those patients for whom there was consensus agreement between the two psychiatrists were accepted for study.

Subsequently, at the third round of testing of sample A, all available parents were interviewed with the Schedule for Affective Disorders and Schizophrenia, Lifetime Version (SADS-L),[36] and were given new diagnoses with the Research Diagnostic Criteria (RDC),[37] based on the interview and hospital record materials. All diagnoses were reviewed at a meeting of senior consultants (I.I.G., Leonard L. Heston, MD, John D. Rainer, MD, and Jean Endicott, PhD), and those diagnoses that remained questionable or difficult to decide after applying the RDC rules were resolved by majority agreement. Further details of the initial sampling and the diagnostic procedures appear elsewhere.[32]

Based on the RDC, 24% of the parents originally called schizophrenic received rediagnoses of a major affective disorder; no reclassifications occurred in the opposite direction. Further information about the effects of reclassification of the parental diagnoses is presented in the "Results" section of the text.

DIAGNOSTIC ASSESSMENTS OF THE OFFSPRING

We examined sample A subjects in six evaluation rounds (A-1 through A-6), at mean (±SE) ages of 9.5±1.70, 11.5±1.96, 15±1.94, 20±1.86, 23.5±2.03, and 27.8±1.95 years. Further, throughout the project, staff social workers conducted telephone interviews of the subjects and their parents at least once a year.

Clinical assessments in adolescence were based on results of the Minnesota Multiphasic Personality Inventory[38-40] and a videotaped psychiatric interview rated on the Mental Health Assessment Form.[41,42] Formal diagnostic assessment of *adulthood* disorders—the topic of this report—began in evaluation round A-4 with administration of the SADS-L interview to all subjects aged 18 years or older. In evaluation round A-5, we used an abbreviated version of the SADS-L, covering only the major Axis I disorders, and the Personality Disorder Examination (PDE),[43] a semistructured clinical interview covering all *DSM-III-R* Axis II disorders. Assessments in evaluation round A-6 included both the full SADS-L interview and the revised PDE.[44]

Interviewers were clinical psychologists or psychiatric social workers with previous experience with patients. We gave training workshops and individual supervision in the interview instruments at the beginning of each round. In the latest round (A-6), we also held refresher workshops in midround. The SADS-L workshops were conducted by expert diagnosticians from Dr Endicott's Department of Research Assessment and Training (DRAT) at the New York State Psychiatric Institute, New York City, where the interview schedule and RDC rules originated.[36,37] Throughout the process, the interviewers were blind with respect to parental diagnostic group, but in evaluation round A-6, they learned the RDC diagnoses given the offspring in earlier clinical assessments. At completion of evaluation round A-6, one of us (U.H.A.), who has trained continuously with DRAT in the use of the SADS-L and application of RDC rules, assigned lifetime diagnoses based on the interviews in evaluation rounds A-4 through A-6 and other available clinical materials. In approximately 10% of cases, questions remained concerning differential diagnosis, subtype, or course (chronicity) after this final review. These cases were then referred to DRAT for addi-

(NYHRP),[32] in which we have followed offspring of schizophrenic parents from midchildhood to midadulthood.

The NYHRP and other high-risk studies,[29-31] in which longitudinal data have been collected prospectively in the offspring of schizophrenic probands, provide a "constructive replication"[34] of the usual retrospective and cross-sectional approach to family studies. In addition, because the NYHRP contains as a comparison group the tional review by two senior diagnosticians who have participated in that department's diagnostic and training services for many years; both raters were blind to parental diagnostic group and to the lifetime diagnosis given at the completion of evaluation round A-6. If the two DRAT raters did not fully agree, the case was reviewed by Dr Endicott to reach a final consensus diagnosis.

Reliability between the diagnoses given after evaluation round A-6 and by the DRAT raters was tested using 21 randomly selected cases that had not previously been referred to DRAT. Agreement between both diagnoses was 96% (κ=0.91).

We also used group workshops and supervised reviews to train the interviewers in administration of the PDE. In evaluation round A-6, the group workshops were conducted personally by Armand Loranger, PhD (the principal developer of the instrument).[44] The developers of the PDE reported high interrater reliabilities (intraclass correlations) for dimensional scores and moderately high κs measuring diagnostic agreement; κ=0.80 was reported for schizotypal personality disorder (STPD) but could not be calculated for paranoid and schizoid personality disorders because of their rarity in the sample of Loranger et al.[44] No formal reliability assessment was undertaken in our study. As described in Squires-Wheeler et al,[45] interviews were audiotaped and reviewed by clinical supervisors. The diagnostic algorithm provided in the PDE was used, and the diagnosis of a definite personality disorder was assigned if the subject fullfilled the specified number of features to meet *DSM-III-R* criteria (eg, five or more features for STPD). Results of PDE evaluations in evaluation rounds A-5 and A-6 were combined, so that subjects received a lifetime diagnosis of a definite personality disorder if they met criteria for the given disorder on either or both assessment rounds.

SUBJECTS OF THIS REPORT

Because we have maintained continuous telephone contact with most families in the sample, we have been able to obtain information about the occurrence of major psychiatric disorders in the few subjects whose first episodes took place after evalution round A-6 but prior to April 1994, the closing date for this report. The total number of subjects with data available for lifetime Axis I diagnoses in this report was 188, as shown in Table 1; these subjects represent 86%, 95%, and 93% of the original numbers in the HRSz, HRAff, and NC groups, respectively. Five subjects (two HRSz subjects, one HRAff subject, and two NC subjects) did not have a PDE interview in any round and, thus, could not be assigned Axis II diagnoses.

OFFSPRING DIAGNOSES CONSIDERED IN THIS REPORT

Herein, we report on all diagnoses of psychosis—including schizophrenia, other nonaffective psychotic disorders, and psychotic affective illness—and definite cluster A personality disorders in the offspring. The other nonaffective psychoses are unspecified psychosis and schizoaffective disorder subclassified according to the RDC as mainly schizophrenic (SAS, ie, core schizophrenic symptoms were present for at least 1 week in absence of affective features, or features often associated with schizophrenia were present prior to onset of affective features).[37] The psychotic affective illnesses are bipolar I disorder with psychosis and schizoaffective disorder subclassified according to the RDC as mainly affective (SAA, ie, good premorbid social and occupational adjustment and schizophrenialike features developed simultaneously or followed affective symptoms and were never present for a period of at least 1 week in absence of affective features).[37] The cluster A personality disorders are schizotypal, paranoid, and schizoid.

No subject had more than one psychotic disorder, but several subjects had both a psychosis and one or more cluster A personality disorders. We used a diagnostic hierarchy in which subjects with schizophrenia or schizoaffective disorder were removed from the calculation of the rates of cluster A disorders. Subjects with more than one cluster A disorder were counted only once for the category as a whole.

STATISTICAL METHODS

We mainly present prevalence rates (mean±SE), not corrected for age, in this report. As the ages of the three subject groups fall within the same narrow range (currently 28 to 35 years) in the risk period for psychoses, age correction is not needed for comparisons between the groups. For comparisons with the literature on lifetime morbidity risks in first-degree relatives, however, we also calculated age-corrected morbidity risks using the Kaplan-Meier method.

We used one-tailed tests (treating *P* values of .10 or less as significant) for comparisons when we had a priori directional predictions. These predictions were that schizophrenia, other nonaffective psychotic disorders, and cluster A disorders would occur at higher rates among the HRSz subjects than in the other two groups and that psychotic affective disorders would occur most frequently among the HRAff subjects. We used two-tailed tests (treating *P* values of .05 or less as significant) for all other comparisons. Because we had hypotheses for most comparisons, we did not correct for multiple statistical tests.

For comparison of lifetime prevalences of disorders among the three subject groups, we used logistic regression[46] to calculate odds ratios and their significance. We also calculated χ^2 statistics[47] using Fisher's exact test when cell sizes were small.

We used the Mantel-Cox test of the Kaplan-Meier method of survival analysis[48] for comparison of risk of development of psychoses over time in the three groups. Onset age, defined as the age at which a subject first met criteria for the disorder according to the rules of the RDC, was estimated for all Axis I disorders by one of us (U.H.A.). Agreement between these estimates of age at onset and the estimates made by DRAT raters was 95%, in line with previous calculations of high reliability of onset age estimates based on results of the SADS-L and RDC.[49-51]

offspring of parents hospitalized for major affective disorders, it offers, as have several recent family studies of schizophrenia,[6-8,10,11,15,20] a contrast group of relatives presumably at risk for a different set of disorders. Inclusion of such a group may help to shed light on the specificity of conditions aggregating with schizophrenia and clarify the diagnostic boundaries separating schizophrenic and affective spectra.

Table 1. Number, Age, and Sex Ratio of Subjects at Recruitment and Follow-up

		At Recruitment*			At Follow-up		
Parents' Diagnoses†	Group Label‡	No. of Subjects	Mean (±SD) Age, y	Male-Female Ratio	No. of Subjects	Mean (±SD) Age, y	Male-Female Ratio
Schizophrenia	HRSz	63	9.68±1.65	51:49	54	31.48±1.80	50:50
Major affective disorder (unipolar or bipolar)	HRAff	43	9.30±1.77	40:60	41	31.22±1.84	37:63
No psychiatric disorder identified	NC	100	9.43±1.70	59:41	93	30.84±1.83	57:43
Total	...	**206**	9.48±1.70	52:48	**188**	31.11±1.83	50:50

*Two offspring of a parent with a nonschizophrenic, nonaffective current diagnosis or rediagnosis are excluded. Prior to parents' diagnoses, 83 offspring were in the HRSz group and 25 in the HRAff group.
†Based on Research Diagnostic Criteria.[37]
‡HRSz indicates offspring at high risk for schizophrenic disorders; HRAff, offspring at high risk for affective disorders; and NC, offspring of normal comparison subjects.

We will report on nonpsychotic Axis I disorders in the NYHRP at a future date.

RESULTS

LIFETIME PREVALENCE OF PSYCHOSES AND CLUSTER A DISORDERS

Table 2 presents, for each subject group, the lifetime prevalence rates of the psychoses as a whole and separately and cluster A personality disorders as a whole and separately. The odds ratios and their statistical tests are from the logistic regression analyses.

Psychosis as a Whole

The prevalence of psychosis of any type was greater in the HRSz and HRAff groups than in the NC group, but the two risk groups did not differ from each other.

Schizophrenia-Related Psychoses

As shown in Table 2, combined lifetime prevalences for all schizophrenia-related psychoses (ie, schizophrenia, SAS, and unspecified psychosis) were, again, significantly greater in each risk group than in the NC group but did not differ between risk groups. Both schizophrenia and unspecified psychosis occurred only in the HRSz group. (The single case of completed suicide in this sample occurred in an HRSz subject who had received a diagnosis of schizophrenia.)

On the other hand, SAS occurred in four HRAff subjects (9.8%±4.7%) but in only one subject each in the HRSz and NC groups (1.9%±1.9% and 1.1%±1.1%, respectively). Whereas the SAS rates of the two risk groups were not significantly different, the HRAff and NC groups did differ.

Affective and Other Psychoses

The psychotic affective illnesses—SAA and bipolar I disorder—occurred at low rates in all three subject groups, and acute drug-induced psychosis was diagnosed in one NC subject. There were no group differences in prevalence rates for these disorders.

Cluster A Personality Disorders

For cluster A personality disorders, prevalence rates (shown in Table 2, with subjects with schizophrenia and schizoaffective illnesses removed) were significantly greater in each risk group than in the NC group for the category as a whole but did not differ between groups for any of the component disorders considered separately.

DIAGNOSES IN THE HRAff GROUP AS A FUNCTION OF PARENTAL DIAGNOSES

Table 3 examines the diagnoses of psychotic disorders in HRAff subjects as a function of their parents' diagnoses and their parents' initial classification as having schizophrenia or affective illness. As can be seen, (1) more parents whose initial diagnosis was schizophrenia received a final diagnosis of psychotic disorder (SAA or psychotic bipolar) than parents whose initial diagnosis was affective illness (14/18 vs 3/25, respectively); (2) psychoses were more frequent in the offspring of parents with reclassified diagnoses (4/18) than in offspring of parents whose diagnosis was not changed (2/25); but (3) diagnoses of schizoaffective disorder in offspring did *not* occur in subjects whose parents received—either originally or at reclassification—a diagnosis of SAA.

LIFETIME MORBIDITY RISKS AND KAPLAN-MEIER SURVIVAL CURVES

We estimated cumulative hazard functions for the psychotic disorders using the Kaplan-Meier survival procedures. We found significant differences in the survival curves for the risk for (1) any psychosis (*P*=.007), (2) schizophrenia-related psychoses combined (*P*=.003), and (3) schizophrenia alone (*P*=.001) developing over time (Mantel-Cox test). The survival curves (**Figure**) illustrate the cumulative hazard functions for schizophrenia-related psychoses combined.

Table 2. Lifetime Prevalences of Psychoses and Probable Cluster A Disorders in the Three Subject Groups

Diagnosis	Prevalence, % (± SE)* HRSz (n=54)	HRAff (n=41)	NC (n=93)	*P* HRSz vs HRAff	HRSz vs NC	HRAff vs NC
All psychoses	22.2±5.7	14.6±5.6	2.2±1.5	.35	.001	.01
Schizophrenia-related psychoses	18.5±5.3	9.8±4.7	1.1±1.1	.24	.004	.04
Schizophrenia	11.1±4.3	0.0	0.0	.03	.002	†
Schizoaffective, mainly schizophrenic, disorder	1.9±1.9	9.8±4.7	1.1±1.1	.12	.70	.04
Unspecified functional	5.6±3.1	0.0	0.0	.42	.05	†
Affective and other psychoses	3.7±2.6	4.9±3.4	1.1±1.1	.77	.31	.12
Bipolar I	0.0	2.4±2.4	0.0	.43	†	.31
Schizoaffective, mainly affective	3.7±2.6	2.4±2.4	0.0	.73	.85	.85
Acute drug-induced	0.0	0.0	1.1±1.1	†	<.99	.69
Cluster A disorders‡	15.9±5.6	11.1±5.3	2.2±1.6	.54	.01	.06
Schizotypal	4.5±3.2	2.8±2.8	0.0	.58	.11	.29
Paranoid	6.8±3.8	8.3±4.7	1.1±1.1	.19	.11	.07
Schizoid	6.8±3.8	0.0	1.1±1.1	.16	.10	.71

**HRSz indicates offspring at high risk for schizophrenic disorders; HRAff, offspring at high risk for affective disorders; and NC, offspring of normal comparison subjects.*

†No test was possible because of empty cells.

‡Forty-four subjects were interviewed in the HRSz group, 36 in the HRAff group, and 90 in the NC group. Schizophrenic and schizoaffective subjects were excluded. In addition, five subjects were not interviewed for personality disorders, including two in the HRSz group (one was psychotic), one in the HRAff group (psychotic), and two in the NC group.

The hazard functions complement the prevalence rates and yield an approximate estimate of age-corrected lifetime morbidity risks. The lifetime morbidity risk estimates and SEs were as follows: (1) for all psychoses, 24.4%±7.1% in the HRSz group, 22.5%±11.2% in the HRAff group, and 2.2%±1.5% in the NC group; (2) for schizophrenia, 14.1%±5.3% in the HRSz group and 0% in the HRAff and NC groups; and (3) for schizophrenia-related psychoses combined, 20.5%±6.5% in the HRSz group, 10.8%±5.4% in the HRAff group, and 1.1%±1.1% in the NC group. Thus, for sample A subjects at their current ages, most of the lifetime morbidity risks are very similar to the lifetime prevalences presented in Table 2. However, for psychotic affective disorders, the morbidity risks in the HRAff and NC groups differed at the .04 level, whereas the prevalence rates did not differ.

COMMENT

As expected, both HRSz and HRAff subjects had significantly elevated prevalence rates and age-corrected morbidity risks for psychotic disorders as a whole, compared with NC subjects. Also as expected, schizophrenia occurred at markedly higher rates in the HRSz group than in the other two groups, alone or in combination with unspecified psychosis (11.1%±4.3% and 16.7%±5.1% prevalences, respectively, vs 0% in the HRAff and NC groups). The NYHRP is thus clearly in agreement with contemporary family studies,[6-13] as well as recent reports[30,31] from other longitudinal high-risk studies, in demonstrating that narrowly defined or "classic" schizophrenia aggregates in families of schizophrenic probands and not in families of normal controls. Our findings are also consistent with those of most,[10,11,52,53] although not all,[54] studies that have contrasted schizophrenia risks in relatives of schizophrenic probands vs relatives of probands with affective illness.

The rate of *all* schizophrenia-related psychoses together, however, did not differ between the HRSz and HRAff groups because of the higher rate of SAS in the latter.

Schizoaffective disorder, long recognized as a troublesome diagnosis,[9,55-57] certainly does not present a clear familial pattern in our sample or in many others.[7,9,56,58] We had expected to find a higher prevalence in the HRSz group of a syndrome (SAS) that is mainly schizophrenialike in prominence of symptoms, premorbid functioning, and course and a greater frequency in the HRAff group of a syndrome (SAA) more similar to affective illness. Although earlier analyses using the Minnesota Multiphasic Personality Inventory data in the NYHRP generally supported a commonality between schizophrenia and SAS,[38,39] our present findings are similar to those of other investigators[7,9,56,58] who did not see clear familial relationships for the RDC[37] subclassifications of schizoaffective disorder. In our sample, SAS was less frequent in the HRSz group than in the HRAff group, while SAA occurred at essentially equal prevalence rates in both risk groups.

We explored the possibilities that the parents of our HRAff subjects might represent an atypical group of patients with affective illness or that schizoaffective disorders might occur mainly in the offspring of parents with SAA. Given that we identified HRAff parents through state hospitals and that 40% were psychotic (SAA or bipolar), the group undoubtedly was atypical as to severity, compared with the patients with affective illness identified in many epidemiological studies. The conjecture that schizoaffective disorders occurred chiefly in offspring of parents with schizoaffective diagnoses, however, was not borne out.

Rather than using a distinction between mainly schizophrenic and mainly affective, many investigators have subtyped schizoaffective disorder by polarity.

Table 3. Psychoses in HRAff Subjects by Specific Affective Disorder Diagnoses in Their Parents*

	Offspring (n=43)	
Parental Diagnoses†	No. of Subjects	No. of Psychotic Subjects
Originally classified as affective illness†		
Unipolar, not psychotic	15	2 (SAS)
Bipolar, not psychotic	4	0
Bipolar, psychotic	1‡	...
SAA	2	0
Both parents affective (1 unipolar, 1 bipolar)	3	0
Reclassified from schizophrenia to affective illness‡		
Unipolar, not psychotic	1	0
Bipolar, not psychotic	0	...
Bipolar, psychotic	9	2 (1 SAS, 1 SAA)
SAA	5	0
Both parents affected (1 unipolar, 1 bipolar)	3§	2 (1 Bipolar I, 1 SAS)

*HRAff indicates subjects at high risk for affective disorders; SAS, schizoaffective disorder subclassified as mainly schizophrenic; and SAA, schizoaffective disorder subclassified as mainly affective.
†n=25.
‡n=18.
§One subject was not assessed at follow-up.

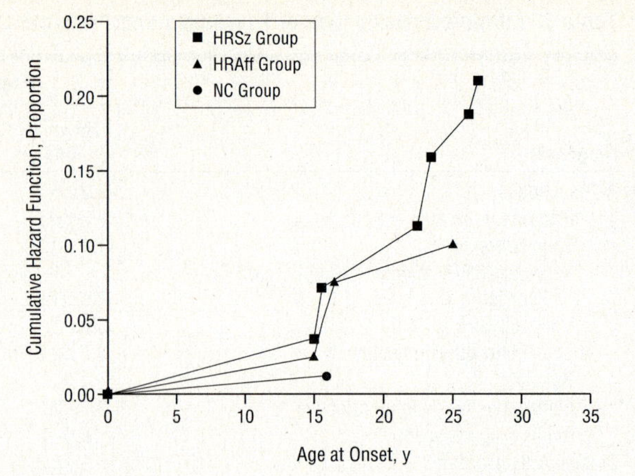

Kaplan-Meier survival curves for the risks for schizophrenia-related psychoses combined (schizophrenia, unspecified functional psychosis, or schizoaffective disorder, subclassified as mainly schizophrenia) developing in the three subject groups. NC indicates offspring of normal comparison subjects; HRSz, offspring of schizophrenic parents; and HRAff, offspring of parents with major affective illness.

Some,[15,59-61] but not all,[56] have reported a familial relationship between unipolar schizoaffective disorder and schizophrenia and between bipolar schizoaffective disorder and affective (especially bipolar) illness. Other studies,[9,10] although partially supporting a familial distinction between unipolar and bipolar schizoaffective disorder, have produced a more mixed picture. Splitting of schizoaffective disorder by polarity did not help to clarify our data: all three subjects with schizoaffective disorder in the HRSz group had the bipolar form and three of five subjects with schizoaffective disorder in the HRAff group had the unipolar form. Also, in a pair of HRAff monozygotic co-twins, one had the unipolar and the other the bipolar form, a complication similar to that noted in a review[57] of genetic relationships among the psychoses. We must, therefore, concur with the conclusion[9] that no method of partitioning schizoaffective disorder to date produces subclasses that are clearly specific to a genetic liability to schizophrenia.

As could be expected, the HRAff group had significantly greater age-corrected risks for psychotic affective illness than the NC group. Neither the low prevalence rates nor age-corrected risks of these disorders differed between the HRSz and NC groups; rates of nonpsychotic major affective disorders also did not differ between the groups. Our findings thus agree with those from the Copenhagen High-Risk Study[30] in showing no excess of psychotic or nonpsychotic affective disorders in offspring of schizophrenic parents. The NYHRP is also consistent with other recent family studies[62] in showing no increase in affective illnesses as a whole among relatives of schizophrenic probands. Our study does not suggest, however, as some others do,[10,11,62] that psychotic affective disorders may be included in the familial liability to schizophrenia.

CLUSTER A PERSONALITY DISORDERS

The Danish adoption studies[14,63] substantiated historical observations[64,65] that, besides schizophrenia, certain subsyndromal traits appear to aggregate in families of schizophrenic probands, thus suggesting expression of the genetic liability in a spectrum of disorders from full-blown manifestations of the illness to milder behavioral aberrations. The cluster A personality disorders proposed in *DSM-III*[66] and subsequent versions were considered to capture the essence of these subsyndromal traits.

Relatives of schizophrenic probands have been reported to show a higher prevalence of cluster A STPD than relatives of normal controls in several,[11,21,30] but not all,[67,68] recent family studies, as well as in the expanded adoption studies.[12,14] Elevated rates of schizotypal personality features and disorder in HRSz compared with NC subjects in analyses combining both samples (A and B) at earlier testing rounds have been previously reported.[45,69] In the present study, examining only sample A and removing subjects in whom schizophrenia had developed, we found a significant difference in HRSz vs NC subjects for cluster A as a whole, but not for STPD alone.

The prevalence of cluster A personality disorder in relatives of probands with affective disorder has been examined in a few studies.[21,70] No differences have been found between the offspring of schizophrenic parents and parents with affective illness in the frequency of cluster A disorders.[45,69] A recent Irish family study[11,70] reported both significantly higher rates of STPD in relatives of schizophrenic probands than in relatives of affectively ill probands and no difference between the latter and relatives of controls. Other investigators, however, have obtained results more similar to ours, showing higher rates of STPD in families of probands with affective disorders than in families of controls[21] and no differences between relatives of schizophrenic or affectively ill probands.[12,25,71] Some investigators, observing an increased frequency of STPD in relatives of probands with nonschizophrenic disorders,[72-75] have concluded that not all cases of STPD are genetically related to schizophrenia,[76-78] a point made some years ago in a discussion of issues associated with defining the "extended" schizophrenia spectrum of disorders.[79]

The NYHRP[80] and others[81] have speculated about alternative constructions of a schizophrenia-spectrum dimension more specifically related to familial aggregation of schizophrenia.[24] One proposal, for example, has been that definitions of STPD limited to certain clinical symptoms (eg, negative features) may enhance specificity in relatives of schizophrenic probands vs relatives of probands with other psychiatric disorders.[81] In another recent exploration of possible heterogeneity in STPD,[76] comorbid disorders were found to differentiate schizotypal relatives of schizophrenic and affective probands. Similarly, the NYHRP[42] has reported differences among the offspring groups in Axis I disorders later expressed by subjects who had schizotypal features in adolescence. Other evidence from the NYHRP also suggests that the accepted criteria for cluster A personality disorders may not be the best for identifying conditions with a familial relationship to schizophrenia. For example, using a latent structure analysis of the PDE data in our NC families, the NYHRP[82] found both STPD and paranoid personality disorder to correlate highly with other personality disorders, indicating that these two conditions are not discrete personality variants. On the other hand, a distinct cluster of personality aberrations assessed by the Minnesota Multiphasic Personality Inventory clearly differentiated the HRSz group (23%) from the HRAff (7%) or NC (2%) groups.[40] Further pursuit of these different approaches to the subsyndromal signs of the familial liability to schizophrenia is needed.

LIMITATIONS AND ADVANTAGES

We note three limitations of this report. First, sample A, at the mean age of 31 years, has not completed the risk period for schizophrenia or other psychoses. It might seem, therefore, that new onsets of these disorders in the future could change the picture now seen in this sample. Important changes are not likely to take place in frequencies of schizophrenia-related psychoses, however, which are already as high in our subjects as previous literature would lead us to expect. In any event, *relative age-corrected* risks among the subject groups would not change.

A second limitation lies in the modest sizes of the two risk groups, which may tend to obscure the significance of differences between them. A positive note, however, is that those group differences that are seen can be considered to be robust. Nevertheless, the statistical power of future analyses of adulthood diagnoses in the NYHRP will be enhanced substantially by inclusion of recently collected Axis I and II diagnoses in our younger sample (sample B) and in the siblings of both samples.

Another important limitation for this and other high-risk or family studies has to do with diagnostic accuracy, given that a "gold standard" is unavailable.[83] Diagnoses of both probands and relatives—parents and offspring in high-risk studies—are subject to fallibility. Because of our unusual, but far from unique,[12,21,25,71-75] lack of difference in rates of cluster A personality disorders between the HRSz and HRAff groups, as well as the mixed picture presented for schizoaffective disorders, one of us (E.S.-W.), along with Andrew Skodal, MD, again reviewed, blind as to information about the offspring, all available clinical material on the parents classified as having affective disorders. No misclassifications of the parents were identified in that review. Nevertheless, as part of the long-term plan for the project, we have begun a painstaking final review of the diagnoses of all parents, who are now between the ages of 50 and 74 years and whose lifetime histories of psychopathology may thus be considered to be completed.

There are at least two advantages of the longitudinal approach used in high-risk studies of psychiatric disorders. First, prospective follow-up, in a developmental genetic study such as the NYHRP, helps to ensure that all cases of emerging psychopathology will be detected in the relatives. Second, the opportunity to carry out repeated assessments at different times during adulthood enhances the possibilities of making accurate differential diagnoses, in contrast to cross-sectional studies with single examinations of the relatives.

Compared with other prospective high-risk studies of schizophrenia, the NYHRP has the added advantages of including a group of relatives of probands with affective illness, thus allowing examination of nosological boundaries between the expressions of familial liability for the two disorders, and of containing an independent sample (B) for added statistical power and confirmatory analyses, as noted above.

CONCLUSIONS

A finding of an increased prevalence of schizophrenia in relatives of schizophrenic probands compared with relatives of the general population is, obviously, not new. It has been demonstrated, using cross-sectional family study methods, by numerous investigators in the past[2-5] with varying definitions of the illness and by several recent investigators[6-13] with narrow definitions and operationalized diagnostic tools. The results of our longitudinal, prospective study of offspring of schizophrenic parents strongly support these later, criterion-based family studies in finding a specific familial liability for narrowly defined schizophrenia.

Our results also clearly show that the offspring of schizophrenic parents and parents with affective illness do not share a liability for the same disorders. First, although rates of schizophrenia and unspecified psychosis are high in the HRSz group, these disorders do not occur at all in the HRAff group. Second, compared with NC subjects, HRAff subjects have an excess of psychotic affective disorders, whereas HRSz subjects do not. The NYHRP, therefore, shows some specificity for schizophrenia limited to offspring of schizophrenic parents and for the psychotic affective disorders limited to offspring of parents with affective illness. The results do not lend support to the hypothesis that these latter disorders are part of the liability to schizophrenia.

Schizoaffective disorder and cluster A personality disorders, however, present less clear boundaries between the two risk groups. Our present data, along with those of others,[62] suggest that schizoaffective disorder shares a liability to both schizophrenia and affective illnesses and that current methods of partitioning schizoaffective disorder are not entirely effective in distinguishing between the two types of familial liability.[9,10] The frequency of cluster A personality disorders, including STPD, also does not differ between offspring of probands with schizophrenia and affective illness, an increasingly common finding in studies comparing relatives of the two types of probands. Several studies[76-78,80] have suggested that STPD observed in relatives of schizophrenic probands and probands with affective illness may not be the same clinical entity, the former being part of the genetic liability to schizophrenia and the latter, not.

Endophenotypic measures (eg, those tapping neurobehavioral functions) may help to discriminate individuals with STPD who have a disorder genetically related to schizophrenia from those whose disorder is not part of the same genetic spectrum.[76] One of the initial goals of high-risk studies such as the NYHRP was to identify endophenotypic "markers" that flag the genetic liability to schizophrenia.[84] There has been considerable progress, both in these studies and in research on other relatives and population groups, toward establishing several such markers.[85-88] In the NYHRP, for example, we have focused heretofore on childhood attentional dysfunctions and their association with certain psychiatric and psychological outcomes in adolescence and young adulthood in the different risk groups.[89] Future analyses of differential associations among early measures of endophenotypic dysfunctions and lifetime diagnoses of specific psychotic or personality disorders in our subject groups may help to distinguish more clearly between adulthood forms of psychopathology that are related to the genetic liability to schizophrenia and those that are not.

Accepted for publication July 27, 1995.

Supported in part by US Public Health Service grant MH19560, National Institute of Mental Health, Rockville, Md (Dr Erlenmeyer-Kimling); the Office of Mental Health of the State of New York, New York City (New York State Psychiatric Institute); and Clinical Research Center grant MH20906, National Institute of Mental Health (New York State Psychiatric Institute).

We especially wish to thank the several interviewers who conducted the clinical interviews over the last several years, as well as Dr Endicott and the diagnostic reviewers (Lawrence Sharpe, MD, and Robert Simon, MA) on her staff of DRAT, and Jeffrey Adamo for reviewing. We are grateful to our social work staff, Rona Silverton, PhD, Maribeth Rourke, MSW, Jane Rotberg Simon, MA, and Karin Wagner, MA, for their tireless efforts in maintaining contact with the research participants in our study. We are grateful also to the many other members of the research staff, in particular Barbara Maminski Shapiro, Mimi Simon, Sky Pape, and Jude Allen, MA, for their many contributions to the project and this article.

Correspondence to Department of Medical Genetics, New York State Psychiatric Institute, 722 W 168th St, Unit 58, New York, NY 10032 (Dr Erlenmeyer-Kimling).

REFERENCES

1. Rüdin E. *Zur Vererbung und Neuentstehung der Dementia Praecox.* New York, NY: Springer-Verlag NY Inc; 1916.
2. Zerbin-Rüdin E. Endogene Psychosen. In: Becker PE, ed. *Humangenetik.* Stuttgart, Germany: Georg Thieme Verlag; 1967;2:446-513.
3. Slater E, Cowie V. *The Genetics of Mental Disorders.* New York, NY: Oxford University Press; 1971.
4. Gottesman II, Shields J. *Schizophrenia: The Epigenetic Puzzle.* New York, NY: Cambridge University Press; 1982.
5. Gottesman II, McGuffin P, Farmer AE. Clinical genetics as clues to the "real" genetics of schizophrenia (a decade of modest gains while playing for time). *Schizophr Bull.* 1987;13:23-47.
6. Tsuang MT, Winokur G, Crowe RR. Morbidity risks of schizophrenia and affective disorders among first-degree relatives of patients with schizophrenia, mania, depression and surgical conditions. *Br J Psychiatry.* 1980;137:497-504.
7. Baron M, Gruen R, Asnis L, Kane J. Schizoaffective illness, schizophrenia and affective disorders: morbidity risk and genetic transmission. *Acta Psychiatr Scand.* 1982;65:253-262.
8. Frangos E, Athanassenas G, Tsitourides S, Katsanou N, Alexandrakou P. Prevalence of *DSM-III* schizophrenia among the first-degree relatives of schizophrenic probands. *Acta Psychiatr Scand.* 1985;142:447-455.
9. Gershon ES, DeLisi LE, Hamovit J, Nurnberger JI, Maxwell ME, Schreiber J, Dauphanais D, Dingman CW, Guroff JJ. A controlled family study of chronic psychoses: schizophrenia and schizoaffective disorder. *Arch Gen Psychiatry.* 1988;45:328-336.
10. Maier W, Lichtermann D, Minges J, Hallmayer J, Heun R, Benkert O, Levinson DF. Continuity and discontinuity of affective disorders and schizophrenia: results of a controlled family study. *Arch Gen Psychiatry.* 1993;50:871-883.
11. Kendler KS, McGuire M, Gruenberg AM, O'Hare A, Spellman M, Walsh D. The Roscommon Family Study, I: methods, diagnosis of probands, and risk of schizophrenia in relatives. *Arch Gen Psychiatry.* 1993;50:527-540.
12. Kety SS, Wender PH, Jacobsen B, Ingraham LJ, Jansson L, Faber B, Kinney DK. Mental illness in the biological and adoptive relatives of schizophrenic adoptees: replication of the Copenhagen Study in the rest of Denmark. *Arch Gen Psychiatry.* 1994;51:442-455.
13. Kendler KS, Gruenberg AM, Kinney DK. Independent diagnoses of adoptees and relatives as defined by *DSM-III* in the provincial and national samples of the Danish Adoption Study of schizophrenia. *Arch Gen Psychiatry.* 1994;51:456-468.
14. Kety SS, Rosenthal D, Wender PH, Schulsinger F. The types and prevalence of mental illness in the biological and adoptive families of adopted schizophrenics. In: Rosenthal D, Kety SS, eds. *Transmission of Schizophrenia.* Elmsford, NY: Pergamon Press; 1968:345-362.
15. Scharfetter C, Nusperli M. The group of schizophrenias, schizoaffective psychoses, and affective disorders. *Schizophr Bull.* 1980;6:586-591.
16. Lowing PA, Mirsky AF, Pereira R. The inheritance of schizophrenic spectrum disorders: a reanalysis of the Danish adoptee study data. *Am J Psychiatry.* 1983;140:1167-1171.
17. Baron M, Gruen R, Rainer JD, Kane J, Asnis L, Lord S. A family study of schizophrenic and normal control probands: implications for the spectrum concept of schizophrenia. *Am J Psychiatry.* 1985;142:447-455.
18. Kendler KS, Gruenberg AM, Tsuang MT. Psychiatric illness in first-degree relatives of schizophrenic and surgical control patients: a family study using *DSM-III* criteria. *Arch Gen Psychiatry.* 1985;42:770-779.
19. Kendler KS, Gruenberg AM, Tsuang MT. A *DSM-III* family study of the nonschizophrenic psychotic disorders. *Am J Psychiatry.* 1986;143:1098-1105.
20. Maj M, Starace F, Pirozzi R. A family study of *DSM-III-R* schizoaffective disorder, depressive type, compared with schizophrenia and psychotic and nonpsychotic major depression. *Am J Psychiatry.* 1991;148:612-616.
21. Maier W, Lichtermann D, Minges J, Heun R. Personality disorders among relatives of schizophrenic patients. *Schizophr Bull.* 1994;20:481-493.
22. Kety SS. Schizotypal personality disorders: an operational definition of Bleuler's latent schizophrenia? *Schizophr Bull.* 1985;11:590-594.
23. Kendler KS. Diagnostic approaches to schizotypal personality disorder: a historical perspective. *Schizophr Bull.* 1985;11:538-553.
24. Ingraham LJ. Family-genetic research and schizotypal personality. In: Raine A, Lencz T, Mednick S, eds. *Schizotypal Personality.* New York, NY: Cambridge University Press. In press.
25. Ingraham LJ, Kety SS. Schizophrenia spectrum disorders. In: Tsuang MD, Simpson JC, eds. *Handbook of Schizophrenia: Nosology, Epidemiology and Genetics of Schizophrenia.* New York, NY: Elsevier Science Publishing Co; 1988;3: 117-137.
26. Webb CT, Levinson DF. Schizotypal and paranoid personality disorder in the relatives of patients with schizophrenia and affective disorders: a review. *Schizophr Res.* 1993;11:81-92.
27. Erlenmeyer-Kimling L. Fertility of psychotics: demography. In: Cancro R, ed. *Annual Review of the Schizophrenic Syndrome, 1976-1977.* New York, NY: Brunner/Mazel; 1978:298-325.

28. Watt NF, Anthony EJ, Wynne LC, Rolf JE, eds. *Children at Risk for Schizophrenia: A Longitudinal Perspective.* New York, NY: Cambridge University Press; 1984.
29. Fish B. Characteristics and sequelae of the neurointegrative disorder in infants at risk for schizophrenia: 1952-1982. In: Watt NF, Anthony EJ, Wynne LC, Rolf J, eds. *Children at Risk for Schizophrenia: A Longitudinal Perspective.* New York, NY: Cambridge University Press; 1984:423-439.
30. Parnas J, Cannon TD, Jacobsen B, Schulsinger H, Schulsinger F, Mednick SA. Lifetime *DSM-III-R* diagnostic outcomes in the offspring of schizophrenic mothers: results from the Copenhagen High-Risk Study. *Arch Gen Psychiatry.* 1993;50:707-714.
31. Ingraham LJ, Kugelmass S, Frenkel E, Nathan M, Mirsky AF. Twenty-five year follow-up of the Israeli High-Risk Study: current and lifetime psychopathology. *Schizophr Bull.* 1995;21:183-192.
32. Erlenmeyer-Kimling L, Cornblatt B. The New York High-Risk Project: a follow-up report. *Schizophr Bull.* 1987;13:451-463.
33. American Psychiatric Association. *Diagnostic and Statistical Manual of Mental Disorders, Revised Third Edition.* Washington, DC: American Psychiatric Association; 1987.
34. Lykken DT. Statistical significance in psychological research. *Psychiatr Bull.* 1968;70:151-159.
35. American Psychiatric Association. *Diagnostic and Statistical Manual of Mental Disorders, Second Edition.* Washington, DC: American Psychiatric Association; 1968.
36. Spitzer RL, Endicott J. *Schedule for Affective Disorders and Schizophrenia, Lifetime Version (SADS-L).* 3rd ed. New York: New York State Psychiatric Institute, Biometrics Unit; 1977.
37. Spitzer RL, Endicott J, Robins E. *Research Diagnostic Criteria (RDC) for a Selected Group of Functional Disorders.* 3rd ed. New York: New York State Psychiatric Institute, Biometrics Unit; 1978.
38. Moldin SO, Gottesman II, Erlenmeyer-Kimling L. Psychometric validation of psychiatric diagnoses in the New York High-Risk Study. *Psychiatry Res.* 1987;22:159-177.
39. Moldin SO, Gottesman II, Erlenmeyer-Kimling L. Searching for the psychometric boundaries of schizophrenia: evidence from the New York High-Risk Study. *J Abnorm Psychol.* 1987;96:354-363.
40. Moldin SO, Gottesman II, Erlenmeyer-Kimling L, Cornblatt B. Psychometric deviance in offspring at risk for schizophrenia, I: initial delineation of a distinct subgroup. *Psychiatry Res.* 1990;32:297-310.
41. Kestenbaum CJ, Bird HR. A reliability study of the Mental Health Assessment Form for school-age children. *J Am Acad Child Adolesc Psychiatry.* 1978;17:338-347.
42. Squires-Wheeler E, Skodol AE, Erlenmeyer-Kimling L. The assessment of schizotypal features over two points in time. *Schizophr Res.* 1992;6:75-85.
43. Loranger AW, Susman VL, Oldham JM, Russakoff LM. The Personality Disorder Examination: a preliminary report. *J Pers Disord.* 1987;1:1-13.
44. Loranger AW. The impact of *DSM-III* on diagnostic practice in a university hospital: a comparison of *DSM-II* and *DSM-III* in 10 914 patients. *Arch Gen Psychiatry.* 1990;47:672-675.
45. Squires-Wheeler E, Skodol AE, Adamo UH, Bassett AS, Gewirtz GR, Honer WG, Cornblatt BA, Roberts SA, Erlenmeyer-Kimling L. Personality features and disorder in the subjects in the New York High-Risk Project. *J Psychiatr Res.* 1993;27:379-393.
46. Logistic regression. In: *SPSS Reference Guide.* Chicago, Ill: SPSS Inc; 1990:312-322.
47. Crosstabs. In: *SPSS Reference Guide.* Chicago, Ill: SPSS Inc; 1990:98-108.
48. Life tables and survivor functions. In: Dixon WJ, ed. *BMDP Statistical Software Manual.* Berkeley, Calif: University of California Press; 1992;2:795-824.
49. Andreasen NC, Grove WM, Shapiro RW, Keller MB, Hirschfeld RM, McDonald-Scott P. Reliability of lifetime diagnosis: a multicenter collaborative perspective. *Arch Gen Psychiatry.* 1981;38:400-405.
50. Egeland JA, Blumenthal RL, Nee J, Sharpe L, Endicott J. Reliability and relationship of various ages of onset criteria for major affective disorder. *J Affect Disord.* 1987;12:159-165.
51. Blumenthal RL, Egeland JA, Sharpe L, Nee J, Endicott J. Age of onset in bipolar and unipolar illness with and without delusions or hallucinations. *Compr Psychiatry.* 1987;28:547-554.
52. Maier W, Hallmayer J, Minges J, Lichtermann D. Affective and schizoaffective disorders: similarities and differences. In: Marneros A, Tsuang MT, eds. *Morbid Risks in Relatives of Affective, Schizoaffective and Schizophrenia Patients: Results of a Family Study.* New York, NY: Springer-Verlag NY Inc; 1990:201-207.
53. Onstad S, Skre I, Edvardsen J, Torgersen S, Kringlen E. Mental disorders in first-degree relatives of schizophrenics. *Acta Psychiatr Scand Suppl.* 1991;83:463-467.
54. Taylor MA, Berenbaum SA, Jampala VC, Cloninger CR. Are schizophrenia and affective disorder related? preliminary data from a family study. *Am J Psychiatry.* 1993;150:278-285.
55. Angst J, Felder W, Lohmeyer B. Schizoaffective disorders: results of a genetic investigation, I. *J Affect Disord.* 1979;1:139-153.
56. Angst J, Felder W, Lohmeyer B. Are schizoaffective psychoses heterogeneous? results of a genetic investigation, II. *J Affect Disord.* 1979;1:155-165.
57. Propping P. Genetic relationship between the psychoses: implications for genetic modeling. In: Marneros A, Tsuang MT, eds. *Affective and Schizoaffective Disorders.* New York, NY: Springer-Verlag NY Inc; 1990:195-200.
58. Kendler KS, McGuire M, Gruenberg AM, Spellman M, O'Hare A, Walsh D. The Roscommon Family Study, II: the risk of nonschizophrenic nonaffective psychoses in relatives. *Arch Gen Psychiatry.* 1993;50:645-652.
59. Rice JP, Reich T, Andreasen NC, Endicott J, Van Eerdewegh M, Fishman P, Hirschfeld RMA, Klerman GL. The familial transmission of bipolar illness. *Arch Gen Psychiatry.* 1987;44:441-447.
60. Andreasen NC, Rice J, Endicott J, Coryell W, Grove WM, Reich T. Familial rates of affective disorder: a report from the National Institute of Mental Health Collaborative Study. *Arch Gen Psychiatry.* 1987;44:461-469.
61. Maier W, Lichtermann D, Minges J, Heun R, Hallmeier J, Benkert O. Schizoaffective disorder and affective disorder with mood-incongruent psychotic features: keep separate or combine? evidence from a family study. *Am J Psychiatry.* 1992;49:1666-1673.
62. Kendler KS, McGuire M, Gruenberg AM, O'Hare A, Spellman M, Walsh D. The Roscommon Family Study, IV: affective illness, anxiety disorders, and alcoholism in relatives. *Arch Gen Psychiatry.* 1993;50:952-960.
63. Kety SS, Rosenthal D, Wender PH, Schulsinger F, Jacobsen B. Mental illness in the biological and adoptive families of adopted individuals who have become schizophrenic: a preliminary report. In: Fieve RR, Rosenthal D, Brill H, eds. *Genetic Research in Psychiatry.* Baltimore, Md: Johns Hopkins University Press; 1975:147-165.
64. Kraepelin E; Barclay RM, trans. *Dementia Praecox.* Edinburgh, Scotland: E & S Livingstone; 1919.
65. Bleuler E; Zinkin J, trans. *Dementia Praecox or the Group of Schizophrenias.* New York, NY: International Universities Press Inc; 1950.
66. American Psychiatric Association. *Diagnostic and Statistical Manual of Mental Disorders, Third Edition.* Washington, DC: American Psychiatric Association; 1980.
67. Coryell W, Zimmerman M. The heritability of schizophrenia and schizoaffective disorder: a family study. *Arch Gen Psychiatry.* 1988;45:323-327.
68. Ritsner M, Karas S, Ginath Y. Relatedness of schizotypal personality to schizophrenic disorders: multifactorial threshold model. *J Psychiatr Res.* 1993;27:27-38.
69. Squires-Wheeler E, Skodol A, Friedman D, Erlenmeyer-Kimling L. The specificity of *DSM-III* schizotypal personality traits. *Psychol Med.* 1988;18:757-765.
70. Kendler KS, McGuire M, Gruenberg AM, O'Hare A, Spellman M, Walsh D. The Roscommon Family Study, III: schizophrenia-related personality disorders in relatives. *Arch Gen Psychiatry.* 1993;50:781-788.
71. Ingraham LJ, Kety SS. Schizophrenia spectrum disorders: exclusively related to schizophrenia? In: Schulz SC, Tamminga CA, eds. *Schizophrenia: Scientific Progress.* New York, NY: Oxford University Press; 1989.
72. Schulz PM, Schulz SC, Goldberg SC, Ettigi P, Resnick RJ, Friedel RO. Diagnoses of the relatives of schizotypal outpatients. *J Nerv Ment Dis.* 1986;174:457-463.
73. Dahl AA. The personality disorders: a critical review of family, twin and adoptive studies. *J Pers Disord.* 1993;7(suppl):86-99.
74. Silverman JM, Siever LH, Horvath TB, Coccaro EF, Klar H, Davidson M, Pinkham L, Apter SH, Mohs RC, Davis KL. Schizophrenia-related and affective personality disorder traits in relatives of probands with schizophrenia and personality disorders. *Am J Psychiatry.* 1993;150:435-442.
75. Yeung AS, Lyons MJ, Waternaux CM, Faraone SV, Tsuang MT. A family study of self-reported personality traits and *DSM-III-R* personality disorders. *Psychiatry Res.* 1993;48:243-255.
76. Lyons MJ, Toomey R, Faraone SV, Tsuang MT. Comparison of schizotypal relatives of schizophrenia versus affective probands. *Am J Med Genet.* 1994;54:279-285.
77. Thaker G, Moran M, Casidy S. Normal smooth pursuit eye-movements in volunteer subjects meeting schizotypal personality disorder criteria. *Am J Psychiatry.* 1991;148:1096-1097.
78. Siever LJ, Keefe R, Bernstein DP. Dr Siever and colleagues reply. *Am J Psychiatry.* 1991;148:1097.
79. Shields J, Heston LL, Gottesman II. Schizophrenia and the schizoid: the problem for genetic analysis. In: Fieve RR, Rosenthal D, Brill H, eds. *Genetic Research in Psychiatry.* Baltimore, Md: Johns Hopkins University Press; 1975:167-197.
80. Squires-Wheeler E, Skodol A, Bassett A, Erlenmeyer-Kimling L. *DSM-III-R* schizotypal personality traits in offspring of schizophrenic disorder, affective disorder, and normal control parents. *J Psychiatr Res.* 1989;23:229-239.
81. Torgersen S, Onstad S, Skre I, Edvarsen J, Kringlen E. 'True' schizotypal personality disorder: a study of co-twins and relatives of schizophrenic probands. *Am J Psychiatry.* 1993;150:1661-1667.
82. Moldin S, Rice J, Erlenmeyer-Kimling L, Squires-Wheeler E. Latent structure of *DSM-III-R* Axis II psychopathology in a normal sample. *J Abnorm Psychol.* 1994;103:259-266.
83. Faraone SV, Tsuang MT. Measuring diagnostic accuracy in the absence of a 'gold standard.' *Am J Psychiatry.* 1994;151:650-657.
84. Erlenmeyer-Kimling L, Cornblatt B. High-risk research in schizophrenia: a summary of what has been learned. *J Psychiatr Res.* 1987;21:401-411.
85. Erlenmeyer-Kimling L. Biological markers for the lability to schizophrenia. In: Helmchen H, Fenn FA, eds. *Biological Perspectives of Schizophrenia: Dahlem Konferenzen.* New York, NY: John Wiley & Sons; 1987:33-56.
86. Matthysse S, Levy DL, Kinney D, Deutsch D, Lajonchere C, Yurgelun-Todd D, Woods B, Holzman PS. Gene expression in mental illness: a navigation chart to future progress. *J Psychiatr Res.* 1992;26:461-473.
87. Moldin S, Erlenmeyer-Kimling L. Measuring liability to schizophrenia. *Schizophr Bull.* 1994;20(special issue):25-29.
88. Erlenmeyer-Kimling L, Cantoni G, Kety S. Genetics and gene expression in mental illness. *J Psychiatr Res.* 1992;26(special issue):221-224.
89. Erlenmeyer-Kimling L, Cornblatt B. A summary of attentional findings in the New York High-Risk Project. *J Psychiatr Res.* 1992;26:405-426.

More Reliable Outcome Measures Can Reduce Sample Size Requirements

Andrew C. Leon, PhD; Peter M. Marzuk, MD; Laura Portera

In the design of a clinical trial, considerations of statistical power primarily involve the evaluation of prospective sample sizes. Another strategy for increasing statistical power that is rarely used focuses on the selection of the outcome measure. When an outcome measure is selected, its reliability and validity must be carefully evaluated. Here the relationship between reliability and statistical power is explored empirically. We show that as the number of *related* items in an outcome scale increases, the internal consistency reliability of the scale also increases. As a consequence, the within-group variability decreases and, in turn, the between-group effect size increases and sample size requirements decrease. As a result, sample size requirements can be reduced and research costs decreased. We recommend careful consideration of the psychometric properties of outcome measures prior to sample size determination in any statistical power analyses.

(Arch Gen Psychiatry. 1995;52:867-871)

A fundamental concern in the design of a randomized clinical trial is to ensure that if a treatment difference exists, it is detected. For that reason much consideration is devoted to determining sample sizes that afford adequate statistical power. Although there is always a trade-off between sample size and the feasibility and cost of a clinical trial, it is essential that a trial be designed with the statistical power necessary to detect clinically meaningful treatment effects.

There are essentially two ways of increasing the power of a test, either by increasing sample size or by increasing effect size. The typical strategy used is to increase the sample size at a cost of additional time and expense. An alternative strategy to increase power that does not require larger samples has been widely overlooked. It shifts the initial focus from sample size determination to the evaluation of instruments that are considered as possible outcomes in the trial. An investigator can increase statistical power merely by employing an outcome measure that has less measurement error. To do so, the investigator must examine the psychometric properties of the scales considered for use in a trial. Certainly the validity of an outcome is absolutely essential, where validity, loosely defined, concerns the accuracy with which a construct is measured. However, by selecting the most highly reliable among available outcome measures, measurement error is reduced and, in turn, statistical power is increased.

Reliability refers to the *precision* or *replicability* of an assessment, including internal consistency among multiple items used in a scale, consistency among multiple observers using the same measure at the same time (interobserver reliability), and consistency within a subject over a period during which the construct does not change (test-retest reliability). Among these three sources of error (instrumental, observer, subject inconsistency), typically the weakest is instrumental. In the following we will be manipulating instrumental error (internal inconsistency) by changing the number of items on the instrument to show the effects of such manipulation. However, it should be remembered that this illustrates the much stronger effects that could be obtained by manipulating the number of observers to

From the Department of Psychiatry, Cornell University Medical College, New York, NY.

increase interobserver reliability, or by manipulating the number of time points at which a subject is observed to increase test-retest reliability.

BACKGROUND

In classical test theory, one of several test theory models, reliability refers to the proportion of variability in an instrument that represents *true* differences between subjects.[1] Such theory posits that an individual's score on a scale, the *observed score*, consists of two components: true score and error. The true score, which is defined as a population mean of multiple assessments per subject, is unknowable, but can be estimated by averaging a large number of assessments (multiple items, multiple observers, multiple retests) for each subject. The difference between the true score and that observed by the investigator is referred to as "measurement error," or simply, "error."

An approach for assessing that component of reliability of a scale related to internal consistency considers scale items as multiple observations of a single attribute at a single point of time. Coefficient alpha, which was introduced by Cronbach,[2] is an index of such internal consistency among the multiple items of the scale. It is an estimate of the proportion of variance in a scale that is not attributable to internal inconsistency among multiple items of the scale.

METHODS

Subjects

Data are from the 8th week of a randomized double-blind clinical trial of active medication (alprazolam or imipramine hydrochloride) and placebo.[3] Subjects met *DSM-III-R*[4] criteria for both panic disorder and depression and were assessed with the 24-item Hamilton Rating Scale for Depression (HRSD).[5,6] There were 72 subjects in the active medication group and 30 subjects in the placebo group.

Procedure

To illustrate the relationship between reliability and statistical power with existing clinical trial data, scales of various length were examined. Twenty separate subscales were derived, ranging in length from four to 23 HRSD items, in the following manner. First, four HRSD items were randomly selected (using a random number table) to compose a "four-item HRSD" subscale. The subscale score was the sum of its component items divided by the number of items. This was done five times to create a set of five subscales, each consisting of four randomly selected HRSD items. The subscale among the five evaluated that was most highly correlated with the 24-item HRSD total was then designated as the "four-item HRSD subscale" for subsequent analyses. In the same manner, scales consisting of five through 23 HRSD items were derived. For comparative purposes we included the complete 24-item HRSD in the analyses presented below. Note that these scales were derived for illustrative purposes and not to find a better HRSD. We selected the best subset of items, rather than merely selecting the first random subset of items, because we sought to carefully choose the best measure of depression, as defined by the 24-item HRSD and to minimize the chance of choosing an outlier. However, even then, there is a certain amount of chance variance in the choice of a subscale that is much greater with shorter subscales than with larger subscales. This produces instability in the results with shorter subscales.

Statistical Analyses

Description of Subscales. The group means and pooled SDs were computed for each of the newly constructed subscales. The difference between group means was also computed. Under classical test theory, which assumes that all items are measured on the same scale, the means and the mean differences should be constant over subscales. This is not usually true; the instability of means and mean differences is more likely with short than with long subscales. Under the classical model, the product of the length of the scale and its variance should increase linearly with the length of the scale. The larger the individual differences among the subjects in the construct being measured and the more uncorrelated the measurement errors of individual items, the more rapid the increase.

Scale Length and Internal Consistency. The relationship between scale length and reliability was explored by calculating Cronbach's coefficient alpha for each of the 20 HRSD subscales and the 24-item total. Under the classical model, alpha will increase with the length of the scale, asymptoting at 1.0 if the measurement errors are uncorrelated and at some lower value if there is such correlation.

Scale Internal Consistency, Effect Size, and Statistical Power. The relationship between reliability and statistical power was then explored. Recall that power is a function of sample size and effect size. For this reason, the between-group effect size, which is a ratio of the group mean difference to the pooled SD, was calculated for each of the 20 HRSD subscales and the 24-item HRSD total. Under the classical model, effect size will increase in a curvilinear fashion with the length of a scale; the rate of increase is greater with larger individual differences among the subjects on the construct being measured and more uncorrelated the measurement errors of individual items. The value of the asymptote here indicates the upper limit of what can be achieved by manipulating internal consistency. Any further increase would have to be achieved by increasing the number of observers and the number of retests per subject.

Next, power calculations were conducted for each HRSD subscale to provide estimates of the sample size per group that would be required to achieve statistical power of 0.80 for two-tailed t tests with an α level of .05.[7,8] (For simplicity, these calculations assume an equal number of subjects per group.) Under the classical model, the sample size would be curvilinearly related to length of the scale, with an asymptote that would be determined by individual differences and correlation of measurement errors of individual items. Further re-

Subscales of Hamilton Rating Scale for Depression Items

No. of Items in Subscale	Placebo Group Mean	Active Medication Group Mean	Group Mean Difference	Pooled SD	Between-Group Effect Size
4	0.63	0.42	0.21	0.42	0.50
5	0.81	0.47	0.34	0.52	0.66
6	0.77	0.50	0.27	0.46	0.57
7	0.59	0.40	0.19	0.37	0.50
8	0.59	0.37	0.22	0.36	0.62
9	0.58	0.34	0.24	0.37	0.65
10	0.60	0.37	0.23	0.35	0.66
11	0.65	0.40	0.25	0.41	0.61
12	0.55	0.35	0.20	0.34	0.58
13	0.67	0.46	0.21	0.39	0.55
14	0.56	0.36	0.20	0.34	0.59
15	0.64	0.41	0.23	0.37	0.63
16	0.58	0.37	0.21	0.37	0.57
17	0.55	0.33	0.22	0.34	0.66
18	0.53	0.32	0.21	0.32	0.64
19	0.59	0.37	0.22	0.34	0.64
20	0.57	0.35	0.22	0.33	0.66
21	0.57	0.36	0.21	0.33	0.64
22	0.55	0.35	0.20	0.32	0.62
23	0.55	0.35	0.20	0.33	0.63
24	0.53	0.34	0.19	0.31	0.63

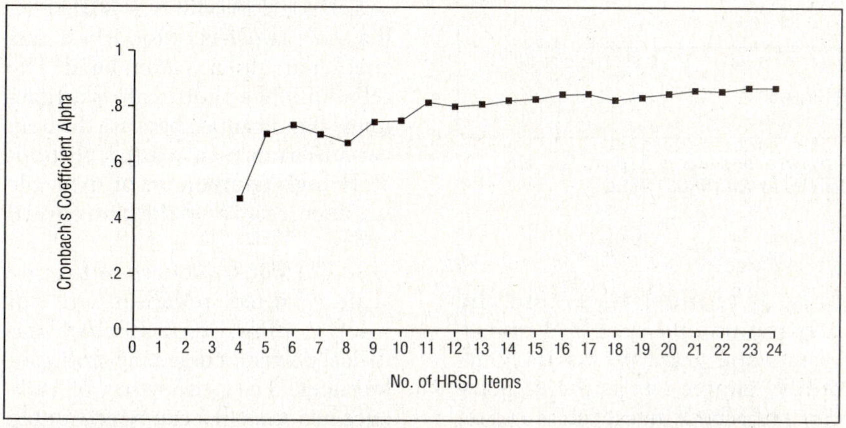

Figure 1. *Scale length and internal consistency reliability, using Hamilton Rating Scale for Depression (HRSD) items.*

duction in necessary sample size could be achieved by increasing the number of observers and the number of retests per subject.

RESULTS

Subscales of the HRSD items were constructed, consisting of four through 23 HRSD items. The descriptive statistics of these subscales and the 24-item HRSD total are presented in the **Table**, stratified by treatment. The SDs indicate that there is a general trend of decreasing within-group variability as the number of items in a subscale increases. This is because each subscale score is an estimate of the same population parameter. As the subscale length increases, the estimates are more precise, resulting in reduced within-group variability. The group mean difference and pooled SD are also presented, as is their ratio, the between-group effect size. These are discussed below.

Scale Length and Internal Consistency

Figure 1 illustrates that as scale length increases, internal consistency reliability increases. The results are similar for the active treatment and placebo groups. Therefore, for ease of presentation we chose not to present coefficient alpha for each group but, instead, the mean alpha for the subscales of each length. The mean alpha, rather than the pooled alpha, is presented because the latter includes between-group variability. An increase in the number of items comprising a subscale results in more reliable subscales, and thus less measurement error due to internal inconsistency. For example, the alpha coefficients range from below .50 for the four-item subscale to .88 for the complete 24-item HRSD. In sum, as the number of *related* items in a scale increases, the internal consistency reliability increases.

Scale Reliability, Effect Size, and Statistical Power

Figure 2 illustrates the relationship between reliability and effect size. As the reliability of the subscales increases, the between-group effect size increases. Here, the effect sizes range from about 0.50 to 0.66. These are considered "medium" effect sizes based on the criteria presented by Cohen.[7]

In turn, as a result of the increased effect size, the statistical power increases. **Figure 3** illustrates that the sample size required for statistical power of 0.80, in a two-tailed t test with an α level of .05, is reduced as the subscales are increased in length. The sample size requirements range from 72 subjects per group for the four-item HRSD subscale to less than 50 subjects per group for each of the subscales with more than 16 HRSD items. For simplicity, these calculations assume an equal number of subjects per group.

COMMENT

This report illustrates the relationship between the reliability of an outcome measure and sample size requirements in a clinical trial. As the number of related items in a scale increases, the internal consistency increases and the within-group variability decreases. As a result, the between-group effect size and statistical power increase. Most important, the sample size requirements

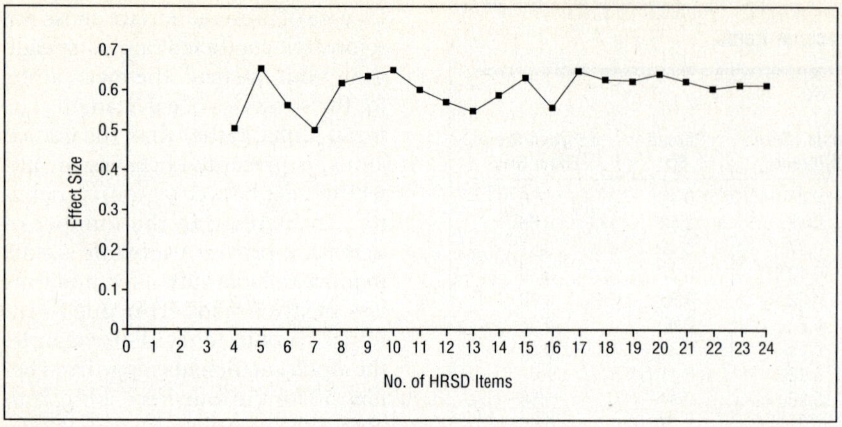

Figure 2. *Scale length and effect size, using Hamilton Rating Scale for Depression (HRSD) items.*

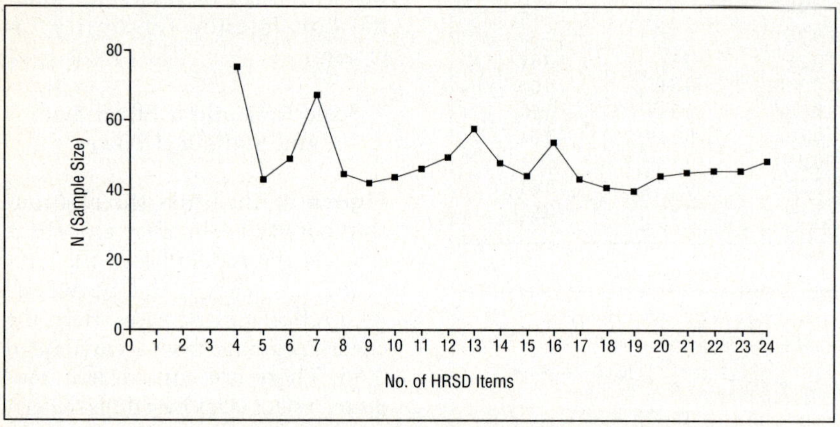

Figure 3. *Scale length and sample size requirements (N required for power of 0.80 in* t *test with two-tailed* α *level of .05), using Hamilton Rating Scale for Depression (HRSD) items.*

are reduced through the use of a more reliable outcome measure, holding statistical power constant. Of course, a reduction in sample size corresponds to a decrease in research costs.

We have chosen to demonstrate the relationship between reliability and statistical power through an empirical examination of scales with varying levels of internal consistency reliability. Internal consistency was used because we could easily manipulate it with existing clinical trial data. Nevertheless, statistical power is attenuated by other sources of unreliability (eg, across raters or over time). Had we also been able to manipulate interobserver and test-retest reliability, the relationship between reliability and sample size requirements would have been more dramatic.

The relationship between reliability and statistical power has important implications for the planning of clinical trials and the preparation and review of manuscripts and grant proposals. Currently, sample size is the primary concern of both investigators and reviewers regarding statistical power. We recommend that prior to estimating sample size requirements, investigators carefully select research instruments on the basis of the psychometric properties of the instruments (ie, internal consistency, interobserver reliability, test-retest reliability, and construct validity). Statistical power analyses that are conducted for studies that propose to use outcomes with limited reliability will suggest large sample size requirements that may be unnecessary and more costly.

Undoubtedly, there are problems that investigators will face in making informed choices among outcome measures. Psychometric properties of an instrument can vary from one population of subjects to another, or from one group of raters to another. For instance, the psychometric properties of a scale designed to assess symptomatology (eg, the HRSD) in psychiatric inpatients could be very different from those of the same scale administered to outpatients enrolled in a clinical trial. The same scale used by clinicians may be quite different from that used by researchers, even for the same population.

To improve reliability of instruments, consider reasons for a low internal consistency reliability.[9-11] First, coefficient alpha is low if there is little heterogeneity among subjects' responses to individual items. Adding items to a scale that have little variability, and thus little sensitivity to the individual differences among the subjects, actually decreases the reliability of a scale. Second, if the errors of measurement are correlated (ie, if essentially the same question is asked repeatedly), alpha will be low. Finally, if a scale consists of too few items, coefficient alpha is attenuated. The reliability of a short scale is artifactually handicapped because the item variances represent a disproportionately high component of the scale variance, relative to the item covariances.

The consequences of using a scale with low reliability are not solely confined to inadequate statistical power for detecting group differences. The proportion of variance in a scale that can be accounted for by explanatory variables (eg, diagnosis, baseline illness severity, or other prognostic factors) is attenuated by the unreliability of that scale. Thus, an examination of determinants of treatment response, for instance, is hampered by the unreliability of one or the other outcome measures. Furthermore, the relationship between reliability and sample size extends beyond clinical trials to other designs used in psychiatric research.

Kraemer[12] considers several strategies for improving statistical power without increasing the sample size based solely on theoretical considerations. They include matching, stratification, multiple ratings, and intensive designs as well as the use of reliable outcomes. We closely examined the last issue based on empirical data. Clinical trials will benefit by incorporating each of the strategies that is feasible.

In general, we have shown that increasing the scale length of an instrument may increase reliability, but several caveats should be mentioned. The mere addition of unrelated items to increase scale length will not improve statistical power; scale items must be measures of the same underlying construct and should have relatively independent errors of measurement. Moreover, even when additional related items are used in the scale, there is a point of diminishing return. In the example presented herein, the improvement in statistical power was slight when subscales consisting of more than about 11 items were used. Kraemer[12] showed that the gain in statistical power was limited once test-retest reliability reached 0.80. Costs of increased scale length include patient compliance and administration time and expense. At some point a more lengthy assessment procedure becomes a burden to the patient and more cumbersome for data entry and management. Thus, the researcher should seek to balance the benefits of increasing scale length with the burden of administering a long instrument.

One solution to the problem of outcomes with excessive measurement error is to develop new scales that have been constructed to optimize psychometric properties. The use of such scales would undoubtedly result, in the long run, in reduced research costs. Unfortunately, the development of scales is itself costly and time consuming and must compete for funding with, for example, proposals for the same randomized clinical trials for which the scales are being developed. Moreover, investigators and reviewers are often wary of new scales and prefer to use the tried-and-true instruments, however suboptimal they may be. Furthermore, if the outcome measures are unfamiliar to other investigators, the results will not be interpretable. Nevertheless, effort should be devoted to the development and dissemination of psychometrically sound scales.

In conclusion, outcome measures should be selected on the basis of their psychometric properties. As Fleiss states, "The most elegant design of a clinical study will not overcome the damage caused by unreliable or imprecise measurement."[13] Of course, a comprehensive examination of rating scales does not supplant the need to evaluate sample size when planning a clinical trial. Rather, these should be considered sequential steps of statistical power analyses.

Accepted for publication June 7, 1995.

This work was supported, in part, by research grants for Protocol 4443 from The Upjohn Company, Kalamazoo, Mich.

Presented as a poster at the American College of Neuropsychopharmacology Annual Meeting, Honolulu, Hawaii, December 13, 1993.

The authors thank Helena Chmura Kraemer, PhD, for her critique of an earlier version of the manuscript when it was presented as a poster at the American College of Neuropsychopharmacology Annual Meeting. The authors also acknowledge the helpful comments of Kenneth Tardiff, MD, and an anonymous reviewer. Joy Pelayo assisted in manuscript preparation.

Reprint requests to Department of Psychiatry, Box 147, Cornell University Medical College, 525 E 68th St, New York, NY 10021 (Dr Leon).

REFERENCES

1. Lord FM, Novick MR. *Statistical Theories of Mental Test Scores.* Reading, Mass: Addison-Wesley Publishing Company Inc; 1968.
2. Cronbach LJ. Coefficient alpha and the internal structure of tests. *Psychometrika.* 1951;16:297-334.
3. Keller MB, Lavori PW, Goldenberg IM, Baker LA, Pollack MH, Sachs GS, Rosenbaum JF, Deltito JA, Leon AC, Shear KS, Klerman GL. Influence of depression on the treatment of panic disorder with imipramine, alprazolam and placebo. *J Affect Disord.* 1993;28:27-38.
4. American Psychiatric Association. *Diagnostic and Statistical Manual of Mental Disorders, Revised Third Edition.* Washington, DC: American Psychiatric Association; 1987.
5. Hamilton M. A rating scale for depression. *J Neurol Neurosurg Psychiatry.* 1960;23:56-62.
6. Hamilton M. Development of a rating scale for primary depressive illness. *Br J Soc Clin Psychol.* 1967;6:278-296.
7. Cohen J. *Statistical Power Analysis for the Behavioral Sciences.* 2nd ed. Hillsdale, NJ: Lawrence Erlbaum Associates; 1988.
8. Kraemer HC, Thiemann S. *How Many Subjects? Statistical Power Analysis in Research.* Newbury Park, Calif: Sage Publications; 1987.
9. Kerlinger FN. *Foundations of Behavioral Research.* 2nd ed. New York, NY: Holt Rinehart & Winston; 1973.
10. Nunnally JC. *Psychometric Theory.* New York, NY: McGraw-Hill International Book Co; 1978.
11. Pedhazur EJ, Schmelkin LP. *Measurement, Design and Analysis: An Integrated Approach.* Hillsdale, NJ: Lawrence Erlbaum Associates; 1991.
12. Kraemer HC. To increase power in randomized clinical trials without increasing sample size. *Psychopharmacol Bull.* 1991;27:217-224.
13. Fleiss JL. *The Design and Analysis of Clinical Experiments.* New York, NY: John Wiley & Sons; 1986.

Child and Adolescent Mental Disorders and the Search for an NIMH Director

Quo Vadis?

SIX YEARS ago, James Leckman, MD, of Yale University, New Haven, Conn, and Glen Elliott, MD, PhD, of the University of California–San Francisco, spearheaded a review of the needs and opportunities for research in mental disorders of children and adolescents. This effort, sponsored by the Institute of Medicine of the National Academy of Sciences, Washington, DC, was an extraordinary enterprise that included experts in fields such as genetics, epidemiology, and behavioral development. The original report[1] noted that substantive progress had been made in understanding illnesses that cause enormous hardship and pain to the afflicted children, their families, and society. The report laid out a research agenda while highlighting how little money was being spent on either basic or applied research in this area.

In last month's issue of the ARCHIVES, many of the contributors to the original report prepared an update[2]—a report card on the recent funding and a blueprint for new research opportunities. These concerned scholars and clinicians have given us their best judgment of the current situation. The outlook is mixed. We can be optimistic because in many areas the science base is primed. For example, we now have tools in genetics that may unlock the mysteries of autism.[3] We also have the capacity to study the complex behavioral development of infants.[4] At the same time, we can only continue to despair about the limited resources that are being allocated to study these disorders.

All of which take us to the search for a director of the National Institute of Mental Health (NIMH) (Bethesda, Md) and the implications of this appointment for advancing the knowledge base in urgent areas of mental health. As of this writing, the selection still has not been made. The first search committee, which was a highly capable group, proposed a list of impressive candidates, several of whom may have been genuinely interested in the position. That no one was eventually selected makes a powerful statement on the selection process rather than on the individual candidates.

Now the search committee has been restocked with new members and recharged. The new committee is also an excellent group. We would hope, however, that in their deliberations, the scholarly field of the candidate will not be made a litmus test for selecting the new director.

The needs of our field transcend any single discipline. In fact, we anticipate that some of the most important and exciting work of the 21st century will come from cross-disciplinary efforts, notably in the field of behavioral neurobiology.[5] Therefore, we would hope that the individual who is selected will have the broad vision to see the interconnectedness of a variety of scientific approaches, such as genetics, molecular biology and pharmacology, epidemiology, developmental psychology, and cognitive and behavioral methods.

Our fundamental point about the NIMH is that the individual who heads this country's effort on mental disorders must be committed to a variety of approaches.[6] The report again spearheaded by Leckman and Elliott[2] and the four commentaries[7-10] on the state of research in child and adolescent mental disorders underscore how important it is for the selection committee not to narrow their focus too sharply. The director must have the judgment to define priorities and the ability to bring people together to work toward common goals regardless of their own backgrounds. Such a director can leave a profound legacy on the development of new cross-disciplinary approaches to solving research problems in our field. At the same time, the director must be a compelling advocate for research who can give both scientists and nonscientists a sense of the importance, relevance, and drama of our new advances. The tragic premature death of Roland Ciaranello, MD, a gifted molecular neurobiologist and child psychiatrist and a leading candidate for the NIMH directorship, deprived us all of an individual with these talents.

At a time when the political landscape has changed and when the morale of scientists is flagging, we hope that the new director will have the vision to see our field from different vantages, the energy to lead, the judgment to make fair assessments, the willingness to take needed risks, and the courage to make critical decisions.

Jack D. Barchas, MD
Peter M. Marzuk, MD

REFERENCES

1. Institute of Medicine. *Research on Children and Adolescents With Mental, Behavioral, and Developmental Disorders.* Washington, DC: National Academy Press; 1989.
2. Committee for the Study of Research on Child and Adolescent Mental Disorders. Report Card on the *National Plan for Research on Child and Adolescent Mental Disorders. Arch Gen Psychiatry.* 1995;52:715-723.
3. Ciaranello RD. Molecular and linkage genetics of infantile autism. In: Watson SJ, ed. *Biology of Schizophrenia and Affective Disease.* New York, NY: Elsevier Science Publishing Co Inc. In press.
4. Stern DN. *The Motherhood Constellation.* New York, NY: Basic Books; 1995.
5. Bloom FE, Kupfer DJ, eds. *Psychopharmacology: the Fourth Generation of Progress.* New York, NY: Raven Press; 1995.
6. Barchas JD, Marzuk PM. Some issues for the new director of NIMH. *Arch Gen Psychiatry.* 1994;51:998-1000.
7. Carlson GA. The report card: progress report or final grade? *Arch Gen Psychiatry.* 1995;51:724-726.
8. Cowdry RW, Jensen PS. Grading the progress of child and adolescent mental health research: NIMH perspectives. *Arch Gen Psychiatry.* 1995;51:732-734.
9. Kruesi MJP, Astrachan B. Comments on the report card from a services research perspective. *Arch Gen Psychiatry.* 1995;51:727-728.
10. Rosenfeld AA. Child and adolescent mental disorders research: current directions, future needs. *Arch Gen Psychiatry.* 1995;51:729-731.

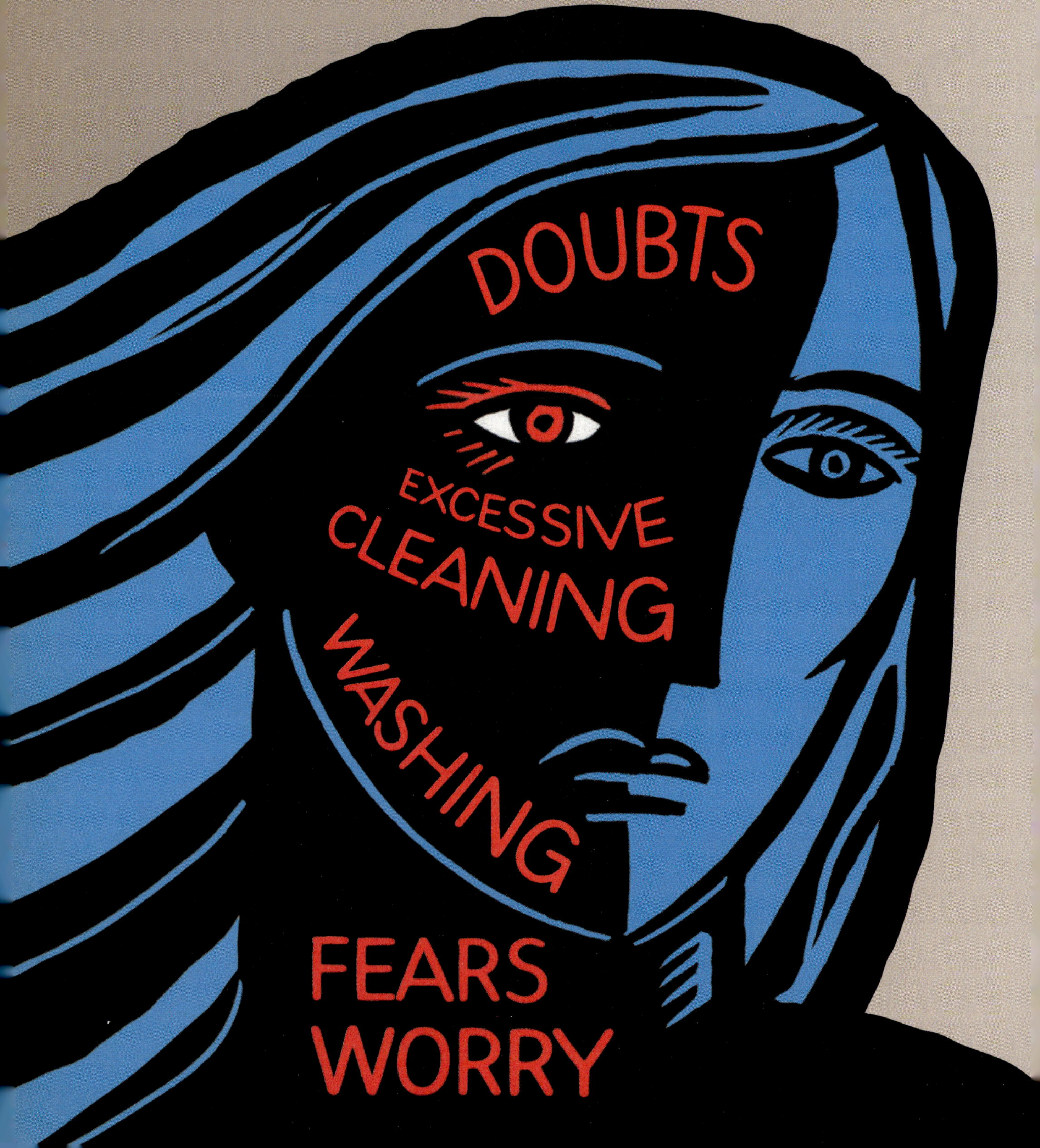
DOUBTS
EXCESSIVE
CLEANING
WASHING
FEARS
WORRY

Clozapine-Induced Increase in Plasma Levels of Soluble Interleukin-2 Receptors

Increased levels of soluble interleukin-2 receptor (SIL-2R) have been reported in schizophrenia and are thought to indicate prior or current activation of T lymphocytes.[1,2] Clozapine is an antipsychotic drug known for an associated high risk for agranulocytosis, and immunological processes have been suggested as possible pathophysiological factors (for an overview see the article by Alvir et al[3]). Recently, it has been reported that long-term clozapine treatment of highly variable duration (33 to 194 days) increased plasma SIL-2R levels.[4] A single dose of the typical neuroleptic haloperidol, on the other hand, did not influence plasma SIL-2R levels of this cytokine receptor in healthy controls.[5]

We report herein on the time course of plasma SIL-2R levels evaluated prospectively during 6 weeks of treatment with clozapine. Ten patients (three women and seven men; mean±SD age, 31.8±5.5 years) who fulfilled *DSM-III-R*[6] criteria for a schizophrenic disorder and who had responded insufficiently to classical neuroleptic medication or had shown severe side effects were treated with clozapine. Only one patient had ever received clozapine (more than 1 year prior to this investigation). Six had been without any psychotropic medication for at least 4 weeks, and one each had been treated with haloperidol, perphenazine, lorazepam, or risperidone. None of the patients required any medication in addition to clozapine. In addition, a control group of eight schizophrenic patients (two women and six men; mean±SD age, 35.1±12.4 years) who were drug free for at least 1 year prior to the investigation and who were receiving monotherapy with haloperidol was studied. None of these patients had ever received clozapine.

Leukocyte, granulocyte, and lymphocyte counts, rectal temperature, and plasma levels of SIL-2R were assessed between 8 and 9 AM prior to treatment and 1, 2, and 6 weeks after treatment was initiated. In the clozapine-treated subjects, mean±SD doses were 188±89, 285±138, and 343±169 mg/d at 1, 2, and 6 weeks, respectively. In the patients receiving haloperidol, mean±SD dosages were 6.9±2.9, 6.9±2.9, and 5.5±2.7 mg/d at weeks 1, 2, and 6, respectively. Levels of SIL-2R were measured by an enzyme-linked immunosorbent assay (Biermann Diagnostica, Bad Nauheim, Germany) (sensitivity, 16 U/mL; interassay and intra-assay coefficients of variation, <8%; mean plasma level in 51 healthy blood donors, 523 U/mL; range, 85 to 961 U/mL [according to the supplier]). Time courses were statistically analyzed by analysis of variance for repeated measures; post hoc comparisons were done using paired Student's *t* tests.

The results summarized in the **Table** show that SIL-2R levels were significantly elevated 2 and 6 weeks after the initiation of treatment with clozapine, whereas they remained constant throughout in haloperidol-treated subjects. Nine of the 10 patients treated with clozapine showed increased SIL-2R levels at the end of the second and sixth weeks of treatment. Neither clozapine nor haloperidol treatment significantly influenced granulocyte and lymphocyte counts or rectal temperature (data not shown).

Influence of Clozapine and Haloperidol Treatment on Plasma SIL-2R Levels*

	Clozapine (n=10)	Haloperidol (n=8)
Mean±SD SIL-2R level, U/mL		
Baseline	285±115	213±73
1 wk	351±121	232±73
2 wk	456±165†	225±61
6 wk	392±131†	247±74
ANOVA for repeated measures		
df	3, 27	3, 21
F	4.08	1.79
P	.02	.18

**SIL-2R indicates soluble interleukin-2 receptor; ANOVA, analysis of variance.*
†P<.05 vs baseline.

Soluble interleukin-2 receptor is shed into plasma by activated T cells and is therefore thought to indicate immunoactivation.[7] In addition, B cells[8] and macrophages[9] can probably release this receptor molecule on appropriate stimulation. The results presented herein are therefore compatible with the idea that clozapine but not the typical antipsychotic drug haloperidol activates those immunocompetent cells directly or indirectly, and, hence, further investigations of clozapine's immunological properties are warranted. Future studies should also address whether there might be any relationship between clozapine-induced immunoactivation (for example, its time course or its extent) and agranulocytosis. Finally, it should be kept in mind that clozapine treatment may influence the results of studies investigating illness-related abnormalities of immune function in schizophrenia.

Thomas Pollmächer, MD
Dunja Hinze-Selch, MD
Janet Mullington, PhD
Florian Holsboer, MD, PhD
Max Planck Institute of Psychiatry
Clinical Institute
Kraepelinstrasse 10
Munich, Germany D-80804

1. Ganguli R, Rabin BS. Increased serum interleukin 2 receptor concentration in schizophrenic and brain-damaged subjects. *Arch Gen Psychiatry.* 1989;46:292.
2. Rapaport MH, McAllister CG, Pickar D, Nelson DL, Paul SM. Elevated levels of soluble interleukin 2 receptors in schizophrenia. *Arch Gen Psychiatry.* 1989;

46:291-292.
3. Alvir JMJ, Lieberman JA, Safferman AZ, Schwimmer JL, Schaaf JA. Clozapine-induced agranulocytosis. *N Engl J Med.* 1993;329:162-167.
4. Maes M, Meltzer HY, Bosmans E. Immune-inflammatory markers in schizophrenia: comparison to normal controls and effects of clozapine. *Acta Psychiatr Scand.* 1994;89:346-351.
5. Rapaport MH, Doran AR, Nelson DL, McAllister C, Magliozzi JR, Paul SM. Haloperidol and soluble interleukin-2 receptors. *Biol Psychiatry.* 1991;30:1063-1064.
6. American Psychiatric Association. *Diagnostic and Statistical Manual of Mental Disorders, Revised Third Edition.* Washington, DC: American Psychiatric Association; 1987.
7. Robb RJ, Kutny RM. Structure-function relationships for the IL-2 receptor system, IV: analysis of the sequence and ligand-binding properties of soluble tac protein. *J Immunol.* 1987;139:855-862.
8. Rubin LA, Nelson DL. The soluble interleukin-2 receptor: biology, function, and clinical application. *Ann Intern Med.* 1990;113:619-627.
9. Crispino S, Lissoni P, Ardizzoia A, Rovelli F, Perego MS, Grassi MG, Barni S, Pittalis S, Tancini G. Effects of granulocyte-macrophage colony stimulating factor on soluble interleukin-2 receptor serum levels and their relationship to neopterin and tumor necrosis factor–alpha in cancer patients. *J Biol Regul Homeost Agents.* 1993;7:92-94.

In reply

We would like to comment on the report by Pollmächer et al as well as present some data on patients at our center. The results reported by Pollmächer et al reveal an interesting trend. The levels of SIL-2R began to increase immediately, peaking at about 2 weeks. This is followed by a decrease that is noted at the end of the 6 weeks of observation. It is thus conceivable that the levels of SIL-2R may in fact return to baseline with continuing clozapine treatment; however, they did not measure SIL-2R levels beyond 6 weeks of treatment.

In view of these interesting results, we examined the relationship between SIL-2R levels in groups of patients who were being treated with different antipsychotic drugs to see whether patients treated on a long-term basis with clozapine had higher SIL-2R levels than did patients receiving long-term treatment with other antipsychotics. Levels of SIL-2R were measured in freshly separated serum collected from subjects after an overnight fast using a commercially available IL-2 receptor test kit (CELLFREE, T Cell Diagnostics Inc, Cambridge, Mass). We compared the SIL-2R levels of patients who met DSM-III-R[1] *criteria for schizophrenia who were treated with clozapine with those of patients treated with conventional neuroleptic agents. We only examined patients who had been treated with these medications for at least 6 months. To reduce the variability that may result from different neuroleptic agents, only those patients treated with haloperidol or fluphenazine were used for comparison (clozapine, n=12, mean±SD SIL-2R level, 604±386.5 U/mL; haloperidol, n=30, mean±SD SIL-2R level, 575.1±500.6 U/mL; fluphenazine, n=52, mean±SD SIL-2R level, 471.7±234.5 U/mL).*

There were no statistically significant differences in the mean SIL-2R level in any of the three medication groups (analysis of variance: F=1.15; df=2,91; *P=.32). The mean SIL-2R level in patients treated with clozapine did not differ from the mean SIL-2R level of the haloperidol and fluphenazine groups combined (n=82; mean±SD SIL-2R level, 509.5±356.2; Student's* t*=0.85; P=.40).*

The mechanism of clozapine-induced agranulocytosis is poorly understood. It has been suggested that cytokines may mediate the agranulocytosis-producing effects of clozapine.[2] The transient increase of cytokine SIL-2R levels observed by Pollmächer et al is also consistent with the observation that the risk of clozapine-induced agranulocytosis decreases dramatically after the first 6 months of treatment.[3] If the transient rise in SIL-2R level following the initiation of treatment with clozapine occurs in only a few and not all patients, the relationship between the early activation of immunocompetent T cells and the subsequent development of agranulocytosis should be examined.

Rohan Ganguli, MD
Jaspreet S. Brar, MD, MPH
Bruce S. Rabin, MD, PhD
Departments of Psychiatry and Pathology
University of Pittsburgh School of Medicine
Western Psychiatric Institute and Clinic
3811 O'Hara St
Pittsburgh, PA 15213-2593

1. American Psychiatric Association. *Diagnostic and Statistical Manual of Mental Disorders, Revised Third Edition.* Washington, DC: American Psychiatric Association; 1987.
2. Sperner-Unterweger B, Gaggl S, Fleischhacker WW, Barnas C, Herold M, Geissler D. Effects of clozapine on hematopoiesis and the cytokine system. *Biol Psychiatry.* 1993;38:536-543.
3. Alvir JM, Lieberman JA, Safferman AZ, Schwimmer JL, Schaaf JA. Clozapine-induced agranulocytosis: incidence and risk factors in the United States. *N Engl J Med.* 1993;329:162-167.

Complicating Factors in the Analysis of Acute Drug-Induced Akathisia

The detailed and interesting report of Sachdev and Kruk[1] in the December 1994 issue of the ARCHIVES itemizes many of the complexities involved in the assessment of acute neuroleptic-induced akathisia. There are several issues, however, that merit comment.

An important oversight in the article is the lack of attention to the use of benzodiazepines by the patients being studied. Benzodiazepine medication is a well-recognized treatment for acute neuroleptic side effects, including akathisia.[2,3] Even the occasional use of benzodiazepines for bedtime sedation could confuse matters because it might result in suppression of the akathisia the following morning when assessments were carried out. Although the inclusion criteria for the study specified "freedom from nonneuroleptics known to sometimes cause or modify akathisia," benzodiazepines were not among the four categories of medications listed in this connection. Given the wealth of other details provided in the article, including alcohol consumption and smoking habits, one would have expected some explicit attention to the potentially confounding influence of benzodiazepines on the incidence and clinical manifestations of akathisia.

Another unmentioned factor that can complicate the analysis is the effect of benzodiazepine withdrawal. The clinical features of benzodiazepine withdrawal, including restlessness, agitation, and subjective dysphoria, bear more than a casual resemblance to those of akathisia. Furthermore, as we have noted elsewhere,[2] withdrawal of benzodiazepine medication may predispose patients to late-onset neuroleptic-induced side effects. It would be useful to know in this connection how many of the patients in the present series had been taking benzodiazepines in the

2 weeks prior to admission and whether these medications were withdrawn after admission to hospital.

Also deserving consideration is the possibility of diurnal variation in the expression of akathisia. It has been our experience that neuroleptic-induced akathisia, like acute dystonia, is more likely to occur in the afternoon and evening.[4,5] Assessments limited to the morning hours may underestimate the frequency and severity of akathisia.

A potential complicating factor in any study of acute neuroleptic side effects is prior exposure to neuroleptic medication. A large majority of patients in the study by Sachdev and Kruk had previously received neuroleptics for a mean of 19.3 months. The potential for neuroleptics to produce lasting changes in basal ganglia function is underlined by the well-known observation that tardive dyskinesia, tardive dystonia, and tardive akathisia can persist in some patients for months or even years following the withdrawal of neuroleptics. Even in those without overt tardive syndromes, it seems likely that subclinical changes persist after neuroleptic withdrawal and affect the susceptibility to acute reactions, including akathisia, on subsequent neuroleptic exposures. It therefore cannot be assumed that the 2-week washout period used in the study by Sachdev and Kruk is sufficient to return the brain to a neuroleptic-naive state. We have recently found that an 8-week course of haloperidol administration followed by a 2-week washout period resulted in a 32% to 46% reduction ($P<.01$) of dopamine neurons in the rat substantia nigra, as identified by tyrosine hydroxylase immunohistochemistry.[6] Subclinical changes of this magnitude in humans would be expected to predispose patients to neuroleptic-induced parkinsonism, which may partially explain why the extrapyramidal side effects score correlated with the development of akathisia in the study by Sachdev and Kruk.

One of most interesting results of the study was an inverse correlation between baseline serum iron levels and the subsequent development of akathisia. This potentially important contribution to the literature on iron and neuroleptic side effects[7-10] receives relatively little attention in the article. We would have appreciated more detail concerning the iron data and some discussion relating these findings to Sachdev and Loneragan's earlier report,[10] which suggested a lack of relationship between serum iron levels and acute drug-induced akathisia.

These comments are not intended to diminish the achievement of Sachdev and Kruk, who have provided an important and thorough analysis of this most elusive and difficult-to-describe neuroleptic side effect. We recognize the difficulty of carrying out a study of this sort. It is because their study is so complete that we chance to offer these suggestions for potential refinement of the analysis.

Patricia I. Rosebush, MScN, MD, FRCPC
Michael F. Mazurek, MD, FRCPC
McMaster University Medical Centre
1200 Main St W
Hamilton, Ontario, Canada L3N 3Z5

Dr Mazurek is a Career Scientist of the Ontario Ministry of Health.

1. Sachdev P, Kruk J. Clinical characteristics and predisposing factors in acute drug-induced akathisia. *Arch Gen Psychiatry*. 1994;51:963-974.
2. Rosebush PI, Mazurek MF. Do benzodiazepines modify the incidence of neuroleptic-induced dystonia? *Am J Psychiatry*. 1993;150:528.
3. Fleischhacker WW, Roth SD, Kane JM. The pharmacologic treatment of neuroleptic-induced akathisia. *J Clin Psychopharmacol*. 1990;10:12-21.
4. Rosebush PI, Mazurek MF. Acute neuroleptic-induced dystonic reactions have a circadian pattern. *Can J Neurol Sci*. 1994;21(suppl):S28.
5. Rosebush PI, Hildebrand A, Mazurek MF. Neuroleptic-induced akathisia in older patients: a prospective study. Presented at the 194th Annual Meeting of the American Psychiatric Association; May 21-26, 1994; Philadelphia, Pa.
6. Parkinson disease–like changes in substantia nigra following short-term haloperidol treatment in the rat. In: Abstracts of the 15th Washington International Spring Symposium: Neurodegenerative Diseases '95: Molecular and Cellular Mechanisms and Therapeutic Advances; May 15-17, 1995; Washington, DC. Abstract 89.
7. Brown KW, Glen SE, White T. Low serum iron status and akathisia. *Lancet*. 1987;1:1234-1236.
8. Barton A, Bowie J, Ebmeier K. Low plasma iron status and akathisia. *J Neurol Neurosurg Psychiatry*. 1990;53:671-674.
9. Rosebush PI, Mazurek MF. Serum iron and neuroleptic malignant syndrome. *Lancet*. 1991;338:149-151.
10. Sachdev P, Loneragan C. Acute drug-induced akathisia is not associated with low serum iron status. *Psychopharmacology*. 1991;103:138-139.

In reply

Rosebush and Mazurek are correct in acknowledging the complexities involved in an investigation of akathisia; these complexities are such that all aspects of the disorder cannot be addressed in one study. Because acute akathisia usually occurs in patients who also have acute psychosis, the management of psychosis and the control of behavior assume priority over demands made by a fastidious researcher. I, therefore, accept certain deficiencies in our research, some of which we have already acknowledged in our article.[1]

The issue of the use of benzodiazepines is extremely relevant, and we did not disregard it. In our study protocol, the use of a benzodiazepine at bedtime on an "as required" basis (which was decided by the resident physician) was permitted. The majority (56%) received such medication in the first 3 days, and fewer (10%), subsequently. In five patients, the use of a benzodiazepine was consistent throughout the 2 weeks of investigation and may have had an impact on the development of akathisia. Akathisia did develop in one of these five, as was noted, on days 7 and 14. We do not, therefore, believe that benzodiazepines were likely to have altered considerably the reported incidence figures. None of our subjects had received benzodiazepines on more than one occasion in the 2 weeks prior to inclusion into the study, thus making it unlikely that benzodiazepine withdrawal was a confounding factor.

It is well recognized that the subjective and motor manifestations of akathisia are variable throughout the day,[2] *but to my knowledge, a definite diurnal pattern has not been described. It is our clinical observation that akathisia is less obvious for a short period after the patient wakes up, and this may be due to the markedly ameliorating effect of sleep on akathisic movements.*[3,4] *Because our assessments were carried out in midmorning, it is unlikely that we missed any patients who had definite akathisia. Our assessment scales were supplemented with information from interviews with the subjects as well as with the nursing staff, thus ensuring that akathisia did not go unrecognized.*

Previous exposure to neuroleptics complicates any study of acute neuroleptic-related side effects. Practical constraints make it difficult, if not impossible, to recruit only never-medicated subjects. Prior exposure to neuroleptics may, as Rosebush and Mazurek point out, increase the vulnerability to extrapyramidal side effects and akathisia. On the other hand, it can be argued that the effect may in fact be the reverse. A nonsignificant trend was observed in our data[1] that suggested that previous exposure to neuroleptics may reduce the likelihood of akathisia developing. An important feature of our study was to ensure that the subjects did not have akathisia at baseline owing to previous neuroleptic use. We interpreted the association between extrapyramidal side effects and akathisia to indicate a common vulnerability to these side effects, as we have previously stated.[1]

Studies of the relationship between akathisia and serum iron level status have produced inconsistent results, and I have reviewed this elsewhere.[2,5] Our investigation[1] suggested that a low serum iron level perhaps does make a small contribution to akathisia. An earlier analysis of these data[6] resulted in the reported lack of an association. The main difference from the previous analysis was that akathisia was defined differently in our recent publication,[1] which led to some reclassification of subjects, and we used a logistic regression analysis with P=.15 for inclusion rather than a t test between groups. The difference in the results reflects the fact that they are extremely sensitive to the methods and choice of statistical analysis, and this may also explain the other conflicting reports in the literature. I believe that the role of iron should be explored further, and this should include more representative indexes of brain iron level status as well as the impact of iron supplementation on akathisia.

Finally, I thank Rosebush and Mazurek for their perceptive criticism of our work and hope that their concerns have been adequately addressed.

Perminder Sachdev, MD, PhD, FRANZCP
Neuropsychiatric Institute
The Prince Henry Hospital
PO Box 233, Matraville
Sydney, Australia NSW 2036

1. Sachdev P, Kruk J. Clinical characteristics and predisposing factors in acute drug-induced akathisia. *Arch Gen Psychiatry.* 1994;51:963-974.
2. Sachdev P. *Akathisia and Restless Legs.* New York, NY: Cambridge University Press; 1995.
3. Walters AS, Hening WA, Rubinstein M, Chokroverty S. A clinical and polysomnographic comparison of neuroleptic-induced akathisia and the idiopathic restless syndrome. *Sleep.* 1991;14:339-345.
4. Lipinski JF, Hudson JI, Cunningham SL, Aizley HG, Keck PE Jr, Mallya G, Aranow RB, Lukas SE. Polysomnographic characteristics of neuroleptic-induced akathisia. *Clin Neuropharmacol.* 1991;5:413-419.
5. Sachdev P. The neuropsychiatry of brain iron. *J Neuropsychiatry Clin Neurosci.* 1993;5:18-29.
6. Sachdev P, Loneragan C. Acute drug-induced akathisia is not associated with low serum iron status. *Psychopharmacology.* 1991;103:138-139.

THIS MONTH IN ARCHIVES OF GENERAL PSYCHIATRY

Understanding how families influence the development of early and later antisocial behavior is important. **Lyons et al** (page 906) examined antisocial behavior before and after 15 years of age in twins who served in the military during the Vietnam era. The family environment exerted a much greater influence on juvenile compared with adult antisocial behavior, whereas genetic factors exerted a much greater influence on adult compared with juvenile antisocial behavior. The family environment, while the individual is living in it, has a powerful influence. However, once the individual leaves the family and other aspects of the environment shared with his twin, the shared environment's strong influence seems to diminish.

Aggressivity and conduct disorder contribute significantly to public health problems such as substance abuse and delinquency. In an adoption study, **Cadoret et al** (page 916) report that genetically inherited factors from antisocial biologic parents interact with an adverse adoptive home environment to affect adoptee outcome. In the presence of a biologic background of antisocial parentage, an adverse adoptive environment resulted in increased aggressivity and conduct disorders in adoptees; however, the same environmental factor did not affect conduct disorder or aggressivity in the absence of the antisocial biologic background. The finding of significant gene-environment interaction has important practical implications for prevention and intervention in conditions such as delinquency or substance abuse.

Recent studies of child development suggest that pathologic development is sensitive mainly to those environmental influences that differ for children in the same family. These influences have been labeled as "nonshared." Such studies have not directly observed children's environments to determine what specific nonshared factors might account for development. **Reiss et al** (page 925) observed 720 families in the home and found that antisocial behavior and depressive symptoms could be accounted for by conflictual parental behavior directed specifically at the adolescent. In addition, when harsh parenting was directed toward one sibling, antisocial behavior in the other sibling was reduced.

Commentaries by Dr Kenneth S. Kendler on genes and environment and by Dr Elliot S. Gershon on antisocial behavior are included in this issue (pages 895 and 900).

The availability of plasma L-trytophan (L-TRP), the precursor of serotonin (5-HT), determines, in part, the synthesis of 5-HT in the brain. A lowered activity of serotonergic neurons may underlie the pathophysiology of depression and (violent) suicide. **Maes et al** (page 937) found a significant seasonal variation in the availability of L-TRP to the brain, with troughs in spring and fall. There was a highly significant inverse relationship between the seasonal variation in plasma L-TRP levels and the seasonal pattern of violent suicide in the local population. The authors suggest that the seasonal variation in plasma L-TRP availability to the brain, with a possibly altered central 5-HT activity in spring and fall, could put suicide-prone subjects at higher risk and could be related to an increased incidence of depression or an increase in severity of depression observed in these seasons.

The long-term pattern of mood variation in normal and outpatient bipolar subjects was evaluated by **Gottschalk et al** (page 947) and revealed that bipolar mood variation is quantitatively less complex than that of normal subjects and does not exhibit the periodicities see in earlier short-term observations of hospitalized bipolar patients. Their findings support the hypothesis that the mood variation of bipolar disorder originates from a deterministic, chaotic source, as opposed to a purely cyclic or random one. They discuss how the exploitation of these findings could lead to new methods for predicting and controlling pathologic mood.

A commentary by Dr Cindy L. Ehlers on mood and behavior is included in this issue (page 960).

INDEX TO ADVERTISERS

Bristol-Myers Squibb
Buspar 972-974

Janssen Pharmaceutica
Ⓒ *Risperdal* 903-905

McNeil Pharmaceutical
Haldol Decanoate . . . . Cover 2-885

Solvay Pharmaceuticals
Lithobid 965-966
Luvox 890-892

U.S. Pharmaceuticals Group, Pfizer Inc
Zoloft . . . . Covers 3-4

While every precaution is taken to ensure accuracy, we cannot guarantee against the possibility of an occasional change or omission in the preparation of this index.

COMMENTARY

Genetic Epidemiology in Psychiatry

Taking Both Genes and Environment Seriously

THIS ISSUE of the ARCHIVES contains three articles that examine diverse aspects of the genetic epidemiology of psychiatric illness.[1-3] These articles attest to the vibrancy of this field, which represents a hybrid discipline, combining features of traditional medical genetics and epidemiology. While medical genetics has generally focused on classic, rare, Mendelian disorders where the genetic signal is so powerful that environmental effects are irrelevant, genetic epidemiology examines common, familial disorders where an inherited vulnerability interacts with environmental risk factors in often complex and uncertain ways.[4,5]

As demonstrated by these articles, the field of the genetic epidemiology of psychiatric illness has been maturing rapidly. As little as a decade ago, most publications focused solely on the assessment of the familial or genetic transmission of psychiatric disorders. Although these questions are fundamental, they represent only the beginning rather than the conclusion of the endeavor.

Each article examines a critical issue in the genetic epidemiology of psychiatric illness: development, gene-environment interaction, and clarification of the nature of the familial environment. Let me examine these issues and the specific articles in turn.

DEVELOPMENT

Genetic and environmental risk factors act in time on developing and senescent organisms.[6] From the perspective of development, genetic epidemiology can pose the following two critical questions: (1) Does the relative importance of genetic vs environmental risk factors change across the life span? and (2) Do the same genetic and environmental risk factors have an impact on risk throughout life?

The first question addresses the relative magnitude of risk factors over time; the second examines their continuity or discontinuity. Turning to the first question, the human life cycle contains varying developmental stages, the environmental contexts of which differ rather dramatically. In infancy and early childhood, the social environment is largely restricted to the family of origin. In adolescence, this environment begins to expand beyond the family, giving individuals an opportunity to actively select their own friends and social activities. The school environment, usually shared by an individual with siblings and peers, remains quite important. In early adult life, individuals typically leave the parental home, select an occupation and a mate, and create much of their own work, family, and social environments.

From this developmental perspective, it would be surprising if, for many traits, the importance of environmental factors shared within families (sometimes called common environment) did not change over the life course. In early childhood, children are largely passive recipients of their social world. In later childhood, they can begin to create their own network of friends but still share with each other most of their social world in the context of their family and school. In adulthood, by contrast, as individuals leave the parental home, they are largely free to make their own way.

The results of Lyons et al,[1] obtained within the large-sample Vietnam Era Twin Registry, fit well within this model. They found that twin resemblance for juvenile antisocial (AS) traits, retrospectively reported in adulthood, was largely due to the familial environment, with genetic factors making only a slight contribution. The picture was reversed when adult AS traits were examined: twin resemblance was almost entirely genetic, with the familial environment having only a very modest impact.

See also pages 900, 906, 916, and 925

This pattern (a strong impact of family environment during childhood and adolescence that attenuates in adulthood) may be a common one for human behavioral characteristics.[7] Although family environment can be a potent source of individual differences, its effect on some traits may be largely contemporaneous and may decrease in importance dramatically as the individual leaves the home of origin. There is another piece to this pattern: a modest impact of genes in childhood that increases substantially as the individual enters adulthood.

The second question asks, regardless of whether the overall importance of genetic and environmental risk factors for a given trait is stable or variable over time: Are the same or different risk factors acting? We know that genes can turn "on" and "off" throughout the life cycle, influencing the timing of a range of temporal traits, including type of β-globin chain, puberty, and blood pressure and plasma lipid changes in late adult life.[8-11] Some environmental risk factors such as stressful life events in adulthood, which can have quite a strong impact on risk for illness, may act only over a short period.[12-14]

The bivariate twin modeling of Lyons et al[1] addresses the question of the continuity or discontinuity of genetic and environmental risk factors on AS traits from adolescence to adulthood. The results of their best-fitting model are particularly intriguing. No new genetic or familial environmental risk factors for AS traits came "online" between adolescence and adulthood. That is, the risk factors present in early adolescence endured into adulthood. However, as noted above, the familial environmental risk factors diminished in importance, while the genetic factors became much stronger.

HOW CAN WE understand this result? Antisocial acts are often committed in and encouraged by a individual's social environment. In childhood, the ability of individuals to select their environment is limited. However, in adulthood, the genes that predispose to AS traits become amplified; not only can they have a direct impact on the probability of committing any AS acts, but they can indirectly increase the probability of self-selection into a social environment that further encourages AS traits. Let me give an example. Assume that an individual, partly because of his genetic endowment, has high levels of sensation seeking and impulsivity and low levels of empathy. He is born into a religiously observant household, and his childhood peers are from the local school and church, which share his parents' highly negative views toward "acting out" behaviors. While he has one or two problems (eg, fighting on the playground), his temperament in childhood has only limited room for expression. However, his high school contains children from more varied social backgrounds, and he begins to socialize with individuals who, like himself, enjoy rebellious, risk-taking activities. This trend becomes even greater over time, as he eventually finds and joins a group of like-minded individuals who use drugs extensively, steal first for kicks and later to support drug habits, and engage in a range of other AS behaviors. Partly via his self-selection into a predisposing social environment, his genetically influenced temperament has now reached fuller expression, while the early family environmental influences have attenuated.

This important article[1] is not without methodologic limitations, two of which are noteworthy. First, information about juvenile AS acts was retrospectively reported in adulthood. The impact of the filter of recollection (and the associated social desirability biases) is unknown, but it could be substantial. Several longitudinal studies of twins from childhood through adolescence or adulthood are now in progress, and it will be of great interest to see if, using prospective data, they obtain this same pattern of findings. Second, the study did not assess how often the twins, in childhood and adulthood, socialized with one another or committed their AS acts together. This may be an important source of "sibling resemblance" for AS traits.[15,16] While the interpretation of such data is not straightforward (is resemblance in the twins the cause or the effect of greater social contact?), it may provide some important insights into the origins of AS traits. The authors[1] do note that a sibling interaction model (where the interaction effect is inferred from patterns of twin variance and covariance) does not improve their explanation of the data. However, the power to detect environmental effects is probably much greater when they are directly measured than when their presence is inferred from patterns of twin resemblance.[17]

GENE-ENVIRONMENT INTERACTION

In considering the contributions of genetic and environmental risk factors to the causes of psychiatric disorders, most individuals initially consider what we have termed the "additive" model.[18] That is, an individual's overall vulnerability to a psychiatric disorder can be considered as simply the sum of the impact of genetic and environmental risk factors.

A bit of reflection, however, indicates the limitations of this approach. One has already been discussed above. Genes and environment may be correlated, as genes may influence the selection of individuals into high-risk environments. The additive model also assumes that the impact of a pathogenic environment is independent of genotype. That is, this model predicts that the increase in risk for illness associated with a pathogenic environmental experience is the same for individuals with low-risk and high-risk genotypes.

However, the plant and animal kingdoms are full of examples of "genetic control of sensitivity to the environment."[18,19] That is, genes can modify the vulnerability of the organism to the disease-predisposing effects of the environment. Examples of such a mechanism in humans, which is also termed "gene-environment interaction," have been increasing.[20] Genes have been shown to control the hypertensive response to dietary sodium,[21] the degenerative effect of environmental neurotoxins,[22] the impact of chronic smoking on lung function,[23] and the plasma lipid response to changes in fat and cholesterol consumption.[24]

An illustration might help. If we selected 100 genetically diverse individuals and took them on a "love-boat" cruise in which all of their needs (eg, entertainment, food, and love) were met, we would find, I predict, both low levels of anxiety and depression and very little variability. Almost everybody would be happy. Suppose, however, that we then expose these same 100 individuals to a highly stressful experience, such as combat. The average levels of anxiety and depression would increase but, more important, so would the variability. Some individuals who are good at coping would deal effectively with the adversity and demonstrate few psychiatric symptoms. Others, with poorer coping abilities, would become very symptomatic.

I would further predict that the heritability of psychiatric symptoms would increase after combat exposure. New genes that influence the capacity to cope with adversity (which were quiescent on the love boat) would come on-line when the population was exposed to severe stress. Consistent with this prediction, we have recently shown that genetic factors influence the probability of development of major depression after a severe stressful life event.[25] The difference in risk for major depression between those with low and high genetic vulnerability *substantially increased* after exposure to stress.

Cadoret et al[2] use an adoption design to examine the important question of gene-environment interaction in the etiology of aggression, conduct disorder, and AS behaviors. Biological parent diagnoses of AS personality (ASP) or substance abuse and/or dependency made from prison and hospital records are used as measures of genetic risk. Environmental risk is assessed by a summary measure reflecting marital, legal, or psychiatric problems in the adoptive family.

The results are best illustrated in Figures 2 through 4 from their article.[2] Consistent with previous work by Cadoret and others,[26] three of the four adoptee outcomes (childhood aggressivity, adolescent aggressivity, and conduct disorder) displayed the pattern predicted for genetic control of sensitivity to the environment. That is, individuals at high genetic risk are more sensitive to the pathogenetic effects of an adverse adoptive home environment than individuals at low genetic risk. In fact, for all three variables, individuals at low genetic risk seemed to be virtually unaffected by stress in the adoptive home.

Why such an interaction was not seen for adult ASP behavior is not clear. One might predict, from the data of Lyons et al,[1] that this might be due to a diminished overall impact of rearing environment on adult outcome variables. However, the impact of an adverse adoptive home on adult ASP behavior in the study of Cadoret et al[2] was highly significant and as strong as, if not stronger than, that seen for the childhood and adolescent outcomes. These results are, in this regard, not fully consistent with the findings by Lyons et al.[1]

While this study[2] uses a powerful design to produce intriguing results, it is not without limitations, some of which are inherent in the use of adoption data, at least in the United States. Biological parents were not interviewed. Few false-positive findings are likely to occur when relying on prison and hospital data, but false-negative findings are more likely. However, this should reduce, rather than augment, their power to detect effects. The refusal rate from adoptive families was over 50%. Previous survey results suggest that the psychiatric status of the adoptive family and the adoptee probably differed in the cooperative and noncooperative families.[27,28] With refusal rates this high, moderate differences might significantly bias results. Parental report was used for one of their major outcome measures (childhood aggression)[2] and also appears to have been a source of data for the other outcomes. If parents who had more marital or psychiatric problems were also more sensitive to behavior problems in their adoptive child, such a rater-bias effect could artificially induce evidence of an association between parental problems and childhood aggression. Such an association, however, would more likely appear as a main effect of adoptive environment, rather than a gene-environment interaction.

Finally, in these kinds of retrospective designs that attempt to relate environmental variables to psychiatric outcomes, there is an inherent problem of the direction of effects. While a disturbed adoptive home environment might cause AS and aggressive symptoms in the adoptee, an adoptee with high levels of aggression and/or AS traits might certainly also cause disruption in the adoptive home. In a noteworthy attempt to address this important methodologic issue, Cadoret et al[2] compared the distribution of adverse adoptive environments in adoptive families containing adoptees at high and low genetic risk (Table 5). No significant difference was seen. As noted by the authors, these results make the child-to-environment model (disturbed child behavior causing difficult home environment) considerably less plausible than the environment-to-child model.

One final methodologic point. As noted in introductory quantitative genetics texts,[19,29] the detection of gene-environment interaction (as any other statistical interaction) is sensitive to the scale of measurement. For most but not all interactions with continuous measures, some transformation of the measure can be found that eliminates the interaction. (Of note, the interaction seen by Cadoret et al[2] seemed, intriguingly, to be quite insensitive to the effects of transformations.) Even worse, reducing continuous data to dichotomies (often done when making "psychiatric diagnoses") can make the detection of interactions particularly difficult. Our statistical models are, on average, much more sensitive to main effects than to interactions.[30] Researchers interested in the important issue of genetic control of sensitivity to the environment need to be aware that large sample sizes and careful attention to issues of statistical analysis are needed to examine for gene-environment interactions.

THE NATURE OF FAMILY ENVIRONMENT

The article by Reiss and coworkers[3] differs in important respects from the other two reviewed herein. Although oversimplified, the reports by Lyons et al[1] and Cadoret et al[2] incorporate environmental measures into primarily genetic studies. The major goal of Reiss et al,[3] by contrast, is to understand the nature of the environmental effects of the family. They use a genetic design to aid them in that task. The design they use in this quest—studying families with monzygotic and dizygotic twins and similarly aged full siblings, half siblings and stepsiblings—is a potentially powerful one, but that remains in the background in this article. Instead, the spotlight is on differential parenting—differences in the ways in which individual parents treat their offspring.

A brief historical note is in order. During the days of psychoanalytic dominance of the mental health field, many considered the family to be the essential crucible that, depending on its functioning, forged individuals for a life of either mental well being or illness. Imbedded in this construct was the implicit assumption that children growing up in the same family would have the same set of health-promoting or pathogenic experiences. Contrary to the predictions of this theory, a large body of behavior genetic studies in the last two decades of both normal variation (eg, personality) and psychopathology have found little or no effect of the familial (or common) environment.[31,32] That is, resemblance among relatives was found to be entirely or largely due to genetic effects. While the environment was usually found to be quite important, it was the unique or individual-specific environment that individuals *did not share* with family members.

Two different conclusions could be drawn from these findings. Either the family had no substantial impact on psychological functioning, or the family was important but most of its effects were not shared by members of the same family. Reiss and colleagues,[3] suspecting that the second position was closer to the truth, turned their attention to differential parenting.

The analytic methods used by these authors[3] are somewhat complex and likely to be unfamiliar to many readers. A brief exposition may be helpful. They begin by focusing on the following two broad domains of adolescent functioning, measured on a continuous scale: depressive symptoms and AS behavior. Next, they take a wide range of self-reported and observational assessments of parenting behavior and reduce them to three dimensions, termed "conflict-negativity," "warmth-support," and "monitoring-control." Finally, they ask three key questions about the relationship between parenting behavior and their outcome measures. These can be most easily described with a fictional family with a mother and two male offspring: Tim and Billy. These three questions are (1) How similarly does Mom treat Tim and Billy? (2) Controlling for how Mom treats Tim, how strongly correlated is Mom's treatment of Billy with *Billy*'s symptoms? and (3) Controlling for how Mom treats Tim, how strongly correlated is Mom's treatment of Billy with *Tim*'s symptoms?

Question 1 is straightforward and assesses the similarity of parental treatment of their offspring. Question 2, the key one for these authors,[3] assesses differential parenting. For example, controlling for Mom's warmth toward Tim, how much does Mom's warmth toward Billy correlate with Billy's level of depression? Assume that, on average, warm parents make for less depressed children. However, if Moms are just generally warm and loving or cold and distant with *all* of their children, then Mom's warmth will have no *specific* effect on Billy, once we have taken account of how warm she is toward Billy's brother Tim. However, if mothers do not treat all their children the same, but rather form unique relationships with each of them, then Mom's warmth directed specifically toward Billy could have a specific impact on Billy's symptoms.

Question 3 is probably the hardest to understand. If siblings are highly sensitive to differential treatment, it could be that, regardless of the specific level of warmth Mom shows to Billy, if Billy sees Mom being *even more* loving to Tim, that makes Billy depressed ("Mom always did love you more"). Alternatively, even if Mom is generally angry at her kids, when Billy sees her being even meaner to Tim than she is to him, this makes Billy feel better.

The authors' main results are presented in Tables 4 and 5.[3] While parental treatment of their children (question 1) is similar, it is far from perfectly correlated. The highest correlations were found for parental monitoring-control, suggesting that on this parenting dimension, parents do treat their children very similarly. The authors find much evidence of differential parenting (question 2) for conflict-negativity and warmth-support, but much less for monitoring-control. That is, the specific level of conflict-negativity or warmth-support directed toward one offspring substantially correlates with that offspring's depressive symptoms and AS behavior.

What about question 3? This contrast effect was only sporadically significant in their data and was most noticeable for two components of their conflict-negativity dimension: disagreement and punitiveness. With some consistency using these measures, a high level of conflict directed toward one sibling is associated with a reduction in levels of both depression and AS behavior in the other sibling.

In sum, these findings are consistent with the hypothesis that families are important for mental health. However, much of their importance appears to reside in the unique features of individual parent-child relationships rather than in some generic familial environment. These results hold an important message for behavior geneticists. While modeling latent measures of the family environment is easy and elegant, a real understanding of the impact of families on mental illness is likely to require much more effort, like that taken by Reiss et al.[3]

As pointed out by the authors,[3] this article must be interpreted in the light of an important methodologic limitation. Like Cadoret et al,[2] these authors, using only cross-sectional data, have limited ability to infer causal relationships. Although one might be inclined to assume that parental conflict-negativity cause AS behavior in children or that unloving parents cause depression in adolescents, two other interpretations are plausible. First, the main effects may flow from child to parent rather than parent to child. An impulsive, angry, acting-out adolescent may cause conflicted and negative parent-child relationships. A withdrawn, sulky, underachieving teenager may be hard to treat lovingly. Second, the relationship between parental and child behavior may be mediated by genetic and not environmental factors. All major personality traits appear to be at least moderately heritable.[33] The same personality type, such as a predisposition to irritability and impulsivity accompanied by low levels of agreeableness, could predispose parents to negative and conflicted parent-child relationships and children to AS behavior. High levels of neuroticism and emotional instability may produce low levels of warmth in parents and depression in their adolescent children.

A useful illustration of this last point has arisen in our own research. In a twin-family study with female-female adult twins, childhood parental loss is strongly correlated with alcoholism in adulthood in the twins.[34] One might conclude from this that disruption of the parent-child bond predisposes to the development of alcoholism. However, one of the strongest predictors of childhood parental loss is parental alcoholism. In particular, alcoholic fathers are often divorced by the twins' mothers. Maybe parental loss is an index of the level of parental liability to alcoholism, which is then genetically transmitted to their children. In this scenario, the association between childhood parental loss and alcoholism is not causal, but is instead mediated through genetic factors. Using a twin-family design that incorporates the environmental measure of parental loss, we were able to evaluate these two contrasting hypotheses.[34] Of interest, *both* were true. While the larger part of the relationship between parental separation and later alcoholism in their children was truly environmental, a significant portion was indirect and attributable to genetic factors.

Reiss and colleagues[3] are collecting longitudinal data on their unique cohort. Using multiwave data in conjunction with their genetic design, they possess powerful means to address the critical questions about the nature of the causal pathways linking parenting behavior and child psychiatric outcome. We should look forward to these analyses with anticipation.

CONCLUSIONS

Geneticists in general and psychiatric geneticists in particular have the reputation for being interested in genetic factors only; the environment is a nuisance variable—something that gets in the way of gene expression. As indicated by the three articles in this issue of the ARCHIVES, this reputation is ill founded—at least for a sizable minority in the field. A conviction is growing, which I strongly share, that the untangling of the common complex psychiatric conditions such as major depression, the anxiety disorders, ASP, and substance abuse and dependence will require an integration of genetic and epidemiologic strategies.

This is an exciting time for those working in the genetic epidemiology of psychiatric disorders. Propelled by increasingly rapid advances in molecular biology, the field is making major efforts to locate and eventually clone susceptibility genes for psychiatric disorders. At the same time as we pursue this powerful reductionist biological agenda, we reach out to incorporate environmental measures in our etiologic models. Nature will not, I think, surrender her secrets easily. From both a genetic and an environmental perspective, the causes of psychiatric and substance use disorders are likely to be particularly complex, and unraveling them will be especially challenging.

Kenneth S. Kendler, MD
Departments of Psychiatry
PO Box 980710
Medical College of Virginia
Richmond, VA 23298-0710

Supported by grants MH-494928 and AA-09095 and Research Scientist Award MH-01277, National Institutes of Health, Bethesda, Md.

REFERENCES

1. Lyons MJ, True WR, Eisen SA, Goldberg J, Meyer JM, Faraone SV, Eaves LJ, Tsuang MT. Differential heritability of adult and juvenile antisocial traits. *Arch Gen Psychiatry.* 1995;52:906-915.
2. Cadoret RJ, Yates WR, Troughton E, Woodworth G, Stewart MA. Genetic-environmental interaction in genesis of aggressivity and conduct disorders. *Arch Gen Psychiatry.* 1995;52:916-924.
3. Reiss D, Hetherington EM, Plomin R, Howe GW, Simmens SJ, Henderson SH, O'Connor TJ, Bussell DA, Anderson ER, Law T. Genetic questions for environmental studies: differential parenting and psychopathology in adolescence. *Arch Gen Psychiatry.* 1995;52:925-936.
4. Khoury MJ, Beaty TH, Cohen BH. *Fundamentals of Genetic Epidemiology.* New York, NY: Oxford University Press Inc; 1993.
5. Weiss KM. *Genetic Variation and Human Disease: Principles and Evolutionary Approaches.* New York, NY: Cambridge University Press; 1993.
6. Eaves LJ, Long J, Heath AC. A theory of developmental change in quantitative phenotypes applied to cognitive development. *Behav Genet.* 1986; 16:143-162.
7. Scarr S, McCartney K. How people make their own environments: a theory of genotype×environment effects. *Child Dev.* 1983;54:424-435.
8. Paigen K. Temporal genes and other developmental regulators in mammals. In: Leighton T, Loomis WF, eds. *The Molecular Genetics of Development.* Orlando, Fla: Academic Press Inc; 1980:419-470.
9. Treloar SA, Martin NG. Age at menarche as a fitness trait: nonadditive genetic variance detected in a large twin sample. *Am J Hum Genet.* 1990;47:137-148.
10. Colletto GMDD, Cardon LR, Fulker DW. A genetic and environmental time series analysis of blood pressure in male twins. *Genet Epidemiol.* 1993;10:533-538.
11. Jarvik GP, Austin MA, Fabsitz RR, Auwerx J, Reed T, Christian JC, Deeb S. Genetic influences on age-related change in total cholesterol, low density lipoprotein-cholesterol, and triglyceride levels: longitudinal apolipoprotein E genotype effects. *Genet Epidemiol.* 1994;11:375-384.
12. Brown GW, Harris TO. *Social Origins of Depression: A Study of Psychiatric Disorder in Women.* London, England: Tavistock; 1978.
13. Thoits PA. Dimensions of life events that influence psychological distress: an evaluation and synthesis of the literature. In: Kaplan HB, ed. *Psychosocial Stress: Trends in Theory and Research.* Orlando, Fla: Academic Press Inc; 1983: 33-103.
14. Kendler KS, Neale MC, Kessler RC, Heath AC, Eaves LJ. A longitudinal twin study of 1-year prevalence of major depression in women. *Arch Gen Psychiatry.* 1993;50:843-852.
15. Rowe DC, Gulley B. Sibling effects on substance use and delinquency. *Criminology.* 1992; 30:217-233.
16. Carey G. Sibling imitation and contrast effects. *Behav Genet.* 1986;16:319-341.
17. Kendler KS, Neale MC, Kessler RC, Heath AC, Eaves LJ. Childhood parental loss and adult psychopathology in women: a twin study perspective. *Arch Gen Psychiatry.* 1992;49:109-116.
18. Kendler KS, Eaves LJ. Models for the joint effect of genotype and environment on liability to psychiatric illness. *Am J Psychiatry.* 1986;143: 279-289.
19. Mather K, Jinks JL. *Biometrical Genetics: The Study of Continuous Variation.* 3rd ed. London, England: Chapman & Hall; 1982.
20. Wachs TD, Plomin R, eds. *Conceptualization and Measurement of Organism-Environment Interaction.* Washington, DC: American Psychological Association; 1991.
21. John SWM, Krege JH, Oliver PM, Hagaman JR, Hodgin JB, Pang SC, Flynn TG, Smithies O. Genetic decreases in atrial natriuretic peptide and salt-sensitive hypertension. *Science.* 1995;267: 679-681.
22. Barbeau A, Roy M, Paris S, Cloutier T, Plasse L, Poirier J. Ecogenetics of Parkinson's disease: 4-hydroxylation of debrisoquine. *Lancet.* 1985;2: 1213-1216.
23. Khoury MJ, Beaty TH, Newill CA, Bryant S, Cohen BH. Genetic-environmental interactions in chronic airways obstruction. *Int J Epidemiol.* 1986; 15:65-72.
24. Boerwinkle E, Hallman DM. Genotype-by-environment interaction: it's a fact of life. In: Sing CF, Hanis CL, eds. *Genetics of Cellular, Individual, Family, and Population Variability.* New York, NY: Oxford University Press Inc; 1993:93-105.
25. Kendler KS, Kessler RC, Walters EE, MacLean CJ, Sham PC, Neale MC, Heath AC, Eaves LJ. Stressful life events, genetic liability and onset of an episode of major depression in women. *Am J Psychiatry.* 1995;152:833-842.
26. Cadoret RJ, Cain CA, Crowe RR. Evidence for gene-enviroment interaction in the development of adolescent antisocial behavior. *Behav Genet.* 1983;13:301-310.
27. Allgulander C. Psychoactive drug use in a general population sample, Sweden: correlates with perceived health, psychiatric diagnoses, and mortality in an automated record-linkage study. *Am J Public Health.* 1989;79:1006-1010.
28. Kessler RC, Little RJA, Groves RM. Advances in strategies for minimizing and adjusting for survey nonresponse. *Epidemiol Rev.* 1995;17:192-204.
29. Falconer DS. *Introduction to Quantitative Genetics.* 3rd ed. New York, NY: John Wiley & Sons Inc; 1989.
30. McCall RB. So many interactions, so little evidence: why? In: Wachs TD, Plomin R, eds. *Conceptualization and Measurement of Organism-Environment Interaction.* Washington, DC: American Psychological Association; 1991:142-161.
31. Plomin R, Daniels D. Why are children in the same family so different from each other? *Behav Brain Sci.* 1987;10:44-54.
32. Reiss D, Plomin R, Hetherington EM, Howe GW, Rovine M, Tryon A, Hagan MS. The separate worlds of teenage siblings: an introduction to the study of the nonshared environment and adolescent development. In: Hetherington EM, Reiss D, Plomin R, eds. *Separate Social Worlds of Siblings: The Impact of Nonshared Environment on Development.* Hillsdale, NJ: Lawrence Erlbaum Associates; 1994:63-109.
33. Loehlin JC. *Genes and Environment in Personality Development.* Newbury Park, Calif: Sage Publications; 1992.
34. Kendler KS, Neale MC, Prescott CA, Kessler RC, Heath AC, Corey LA, Eaves LJ. Childhood parental loss and alcoholism in women: a causal analysis using a twin-family design. *Psychol Med.* In press.

Antisocial Behavior

THE MODERN debate on the causes of human behavioral differences goes back to the last century, when Francis Galton originated the phrase "nature vs nurture." He came down solidly on the side of "nature" as he understood it, which in retrospect is most unfortunate since he was acting on prejudice rather than evidence, and went on to be a proponent of eugenics and racism.[1] Today, a generation after the Nazi mass murders with a pseudoscientific justification based on inherited "nature," it is understandable that genetics of behavior is not an acceptable variable in American political and social discourse.

Yet there is evidence for genetic factors in behavior, including mental illnesses and antisocial behavior, and it is timely that this evidence be examined and made use of by behavioral scientists. For antisocial behavior, adoption and twin studies since the 1970s have consistently implied a genetic factor, as reviewed elsewhere.[2] The excellent series of articles in this issue of the ARCHIVES[3-5] enhance the behavioral epidemiologic data on this topic, and further buttress the evidence that there is a genetic factor playing a measurable role in the observed behavioral outcomes.

See also pages 895, 906, 916, and 925

In the current era of molecular genetics, one must distinguish between the term *genetic* as applied to a specific gene (such as a disease mutation or a disease linkage) and "genetic" in the very broad sense of a characteristic whose transmission is not correlated solely with environment of rearing. One may conclude that there is a genetic influence on traits that are more highly correlated in identical (monozygotic) than in fraternal (dizygotic) twins, with the assumption that the degree of environmental sharing by a twin pair is not determined by whether they are monozygotic or dizygotic. Similarly, with the assumption of unbiased sampling of adoptees, and random placement on adoption, one can conclude that genetic influences contribute to observed correlations between adoptees and their biological relatives.

As important as the conclusion of genetic influence may be for theorists of social deviance, it is imprecise. Early environmental events, which discriminate between monozygotic and dizygotic twins, may be confounded with true genetic events in family-behavioral studies. The observed phenotype may be an end product far removed from its genes, even when the observed correlation is in fact due to genes and not to prenatal environment or biased sampling. This point is particularly pertinent to the general implication of the articles by Cadoret et al[3] and Lyons et al[5] that there are genetic components of antisocial behavior. For example, the "genetic" variables in the adoption study of Cadoret et al are antisocial personality or alcoholism in the biological parent observed and the use of alcohol during pregnancy. It would be a mistake to conclude that this is a claim that there is an antisocial gene, or that antisocial behavior is evidence of defective genes. These authors do not make this mistake, but the history of eugenics in the first part of this century is replete with such facile (and grossly incorrect) generalizations.

In other words, detecting a genetic influence in an epidemiological design is an important hint that particular genes may later become detectable, but in itself does not lead directly to a biological understanding or a diagnostic test usable in individuals. Furthermore, until genes are identified, the possibility of intrauterine and other early environmental influences producing apparently genetic events is not entirely excluded.

RESULTS OF GENETIC ANALYSIS OF ANTISOCIAL BEHAVIOR

Two of the articles in this issue[3,5] have genetic analyses, in the sense of analyzing correlations between relatives based on the degree of genetic and environmental relationship. These are in broad agreement that there is a detectable heritable component to adolescent and adult antisocial behavior, as well as a shared-environment component. These studies add to a growing body of research, which makes inescapable the conclusion that some important part of some very undesirable behavior is heritable, in the sense used here (see the review by Mednick et al[2]).

The proportion of variance that is heritable is modest in some of the analyses, and the precise estimates of the magnitude of each component of behavioral variance are not the same in each article. These differences do not undermine the social, political, and theoretical challenges posed by the overall conclusion. The challenge is this: if behavioral differences between individuals are "constitutional," how can they be dealt with in the political and social arena.

An enormous public controversy erupted over these questions in 1992, when a grant was awarded by the Ethical Legal and Social Issues group of the National Center for Human Genome Research for a conference on "Genetic Factors in Crime." There were numerous newspaper editorials and letters to editors attacking this conference, of which Dorothy Gilliam's column in the *Washington Post*, on July 29, 1992, was representative. She wrote about the conference and about genetic research on the topic:

> "There are no known genetic factors in crime," said Peter Breggin, director of Bethesda's Center for the Study of Psychiatry, who calls the conference ludicrous and wants it cancelled. [Breggin] says the promotion of such a conference now reconfirms the National Institute of Mental Health's "racist intentions."

Gilliam continued with her own comments:

> It is difficult for scientists to separate themselves from society; they are as prone to the same prejudices, bigotry and stereotypical thinking as other Americans are. Even without impugning the motives of health officials or conference planners, it is obvious that stereotypical thinking went into formulating some hypotheses. And it is wrong when, in the name of science, they promote stereotypes and attempt to give them a validity they neither have nor deserve. For when they allow these things to go unchallenged and enter what is supposed to be a scientific inquiry, they taint not only the inquiry but also society.

So one response to the challenge of genetic evidence is to discredit it because it can be misused. This is a know-nothing response and easily countered by the unfortunate history of this century, when racial, ethnic, and class persecutions occurred with the flimsiest of rationalizations, whether or not there were supporting scientists. It is reasonable, then, to consider what this knowledge might lead to and how it could be applied in a positive way.

HOW MIGHT KNOWLEDGE OF PREDISPOSITION BE APPLIED?

The key development, which may eventually result from research into predisposition, is that at some point it may be possible to prospectively categorize individuals at risk for antisocial behavior, rather than whether the individual differences are associated with genes or other events such as perinatal trauma. It is not unreasonable to expect that individually tailored interventions could be developed, applied with due concern for rights of the individuals, based on medical models. This is not to say that a medical model of criminal behavior is appropriate but that issues such as disability and informed consent could be resolved by reference to the way in which they are handled in medical settings.

When predisposing genes become detectable in individuals, one would expect that not all cases would have a heritable component, that heritable components will be overwhelming in a few cases (as in the recent report of monoamine oxidase A mutations in violent persons in one family[6]), and that genetic predisposition does not mean that positive intervention is hopeless (as in the medical experience with inherited disease).

The issue of genetic connection to race is an entirely spurious holdover from an earlier era; races do not have genes, individuals do. This point is addressed rather nicely at the end of the article by Lyons et al, who point out that their evidence is on individual differences and not group differences.

WHAT GENES?

It is time to advance beyond behavioral epidemiology and begin looking for genes that predispose to antisocial behavior in males, with due distinction between adult and adolescent antisocial behavior. Genetic linkage methods could well be applied, given the advances in linkage mapping, including knowledge of correct family sampling for quantitative traits,[7] the improved human genetic linkage map, and semi-automated methods for large-scale genotyping. Very large samples of sibling-pairs may be needed. Collection of these samples may be the major obstacle to execution of this research.

From these studies, we would hope to understand the nature and physiological role of particular genes, which constitute important biological underpinnings of an entire range of human behaviors. The ultimate benefits of such knowledge would extend far beyond men with antisocial behavior.

PREVENTION BY ABORTION?

In another context, that of our ongoing genetic study of homosexual men, I have been asked if the goal is to abort or otherwise eliminate what we may consider deviance. Anybody working in genetics nowadays has to share this concern—that genetic tests could be misused to abort fetuses for ideological reasons. Based on what is now known about the genetics of human behavior, and specifically of male antisocial behavior, it does not appear that this work will lead to a test that would be widely used for abortion. There are several reasons for this opinion. Like many other complex human behaviors, we expect multiple genes to be involved in antisocial behavior. There may turn out to be rare single-gene causes of severe antisocial behavior, as the monoamine oxidase A mutation appears to be, but we would do not expect these *in toto* to amount to more than a tiny fraction of antisocial men. In a complex trait, a single-gene changes the probability of showing the trait by only a small amount. Counseling experience suggests that parents with a desired pregnancy will rarely choose to abort for reasons that *may* occur in adolsecence or adulthood. Putting all this together, I would not expect prenatal genetic tests for a complex late-onset behavior to be offered prenatally in the forseeable future.

Elliot S. Gershon, MD
Intramural Research Program
National Institute of Mental Health
10 Center Dr, MSC 1274
Bethesda, MD 20892-1274

REFERENCES

1. Freeman D. *Margaret Mead and Samoa: The Making and Unmaking of an Anthropological Myth.* Cambridge, Mass: Harvard University Press; 1983.
2. Mednick SA, Brennan P, Kandel E. Predisposition to violence. *Aggressive Behav* 1988;14:25-33.
3. Cadoret RJ, Yates WR, Troughton E, Woodworth G, Stewart MA. Gene-environment interaction in the genesis of aggressivity and conduct disorders. *Arch Gen Psychiatry.* 1995;52:916-924.
4. Reiss D, Hetherington EM, Plomin R, Howe GW, Simmens SJ, Henderson SH, O'Connor TJ, Bussell DA, Anderson ER, Law T. Genetic questions for environmental studies. *Arch Gen Psychiatry.* 1995;52:925-936.
5. Lyons MJ, True WR, Eisen SA, Goldberg J, Meyer JM, Faraone SV, Eaves LJ, Tsuang MT. Differential heritability of adult and juvenile antisocial traits. *Arch Gen Psychiatry.* 1995;52:906-915.
6. Brunner HG, Nelen M, Breakefield XO, Ropers HH, van Oost BA. Abnormal behavior associated with a point mutation in the structural gene for monoamine oxidase A. *Science.* 1993;262:578-580.
7. Eaves L, Meyer J. Locating human quantitative trait loci. *Behav Genet.* 1994;24:443-456.

Archives Interactive

Risperdal® 1-, 2-, 3-, 4-mg tablets
RISPERIDONE

Introducing RISPERDAL ON CALL

A toll-free 800 number that mental healthcare professionals can call for instant access to information about RISPERDAL.

Now You Can Call On Us!

All you need is a touch-tone phone. RISPERDAL ON CALL is available 24 hours a day, 7 days a week. You can access us anytime — anywhere.

Dial 1-800-6R-ON-CALL

Just phone 1-800-6R-ON-CALL (1-800-676-6225), then listen for further instructions to access your choice of information.

PRESS 1 FOR: RISPERDAL PRODUCT INFORMATION
- Clinical Description
- Pharmacokinetics
- Indications
- Side Effects and Drug Interactions
- Quick Mail-Back

PRESS 2 FOR: PHYSICIAN EXCHANGE
- Positive Symptoms
- Negative Symptoms
- Extrapyramidal Symptoms
- Serotonin/Dopamine Antagonism
- Quick Mail-Back

PRESS 3 FOR: CLINICAL REVIEWS
- Abstract Selection
- Abstract Presentation
- Request Full Clinical Paper
- Quick Mail-Back/Quick Fax-Back

PRESS 4 FOR: CONVERSION AND DOSAGE
- From Oral and IM Antipsychotics
- Concomitant Agents
- Switching Strategies
- Dosage
- Quick Mail-Back

A Complete Look at What You Can Access

Here's a quick "map" of RISPERDAL ON CALL:

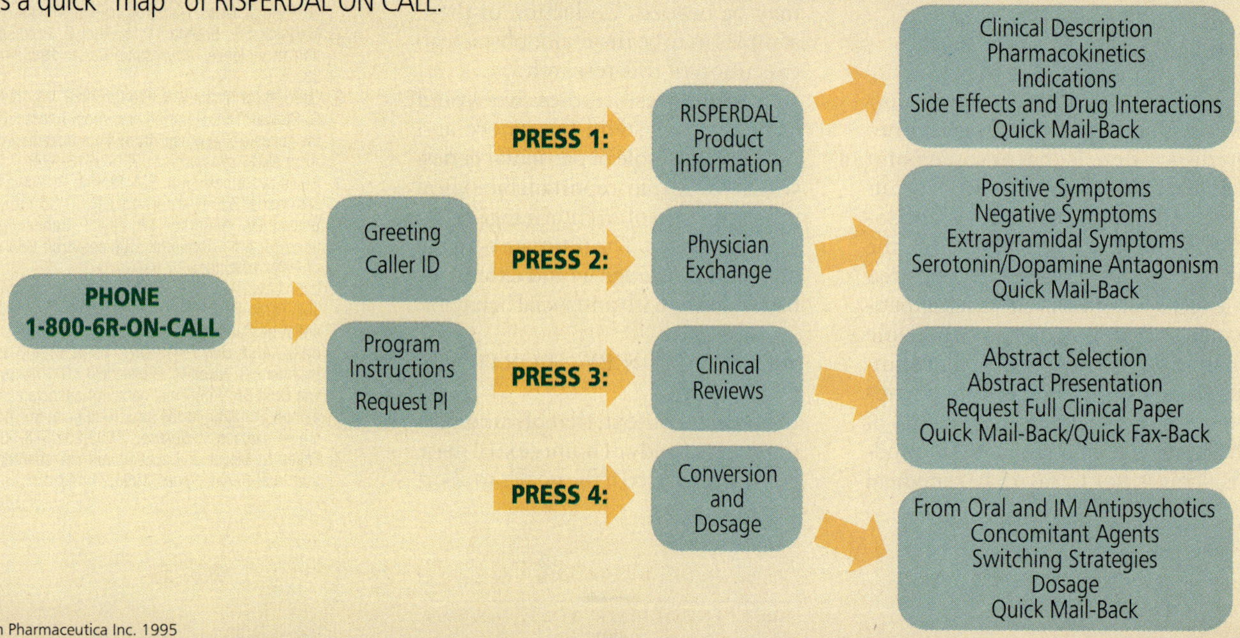

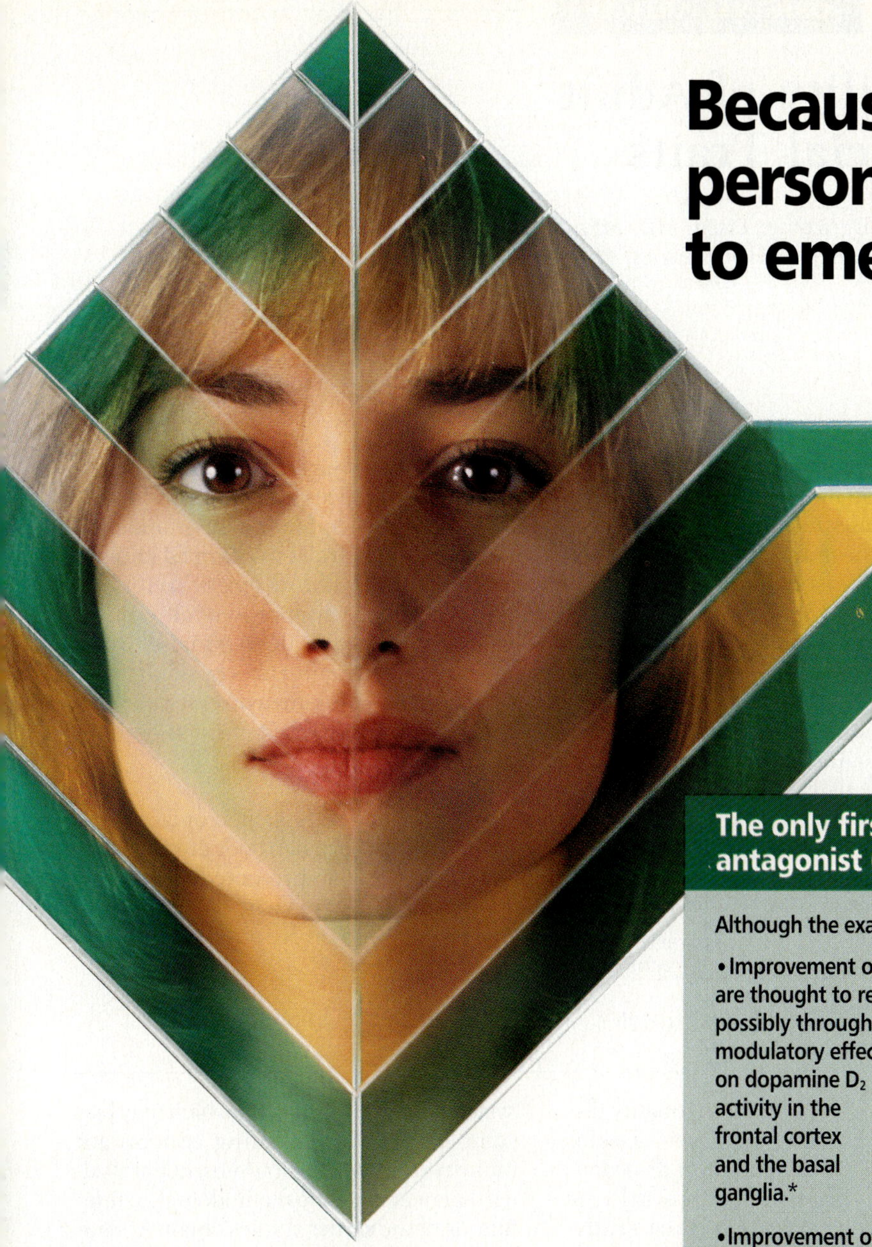

Because a whole person is waiting to emerge.

The only first-choice serotonin/dopamine antagonist (SDA).

Although the exact mechanism of action is unknown:

- Improvement of negative symptoms and lessened risk of EPS are thought to result from blockade of serotonin 5-HT_2 receptors, possibly through a modulatory effect on dopamine D_2 activity in the frontal cortex and the basal ganglia.*
- Improvement of positive symptoms is thought to result from blockade of dopamine D_2 receptors in the limbic system.*

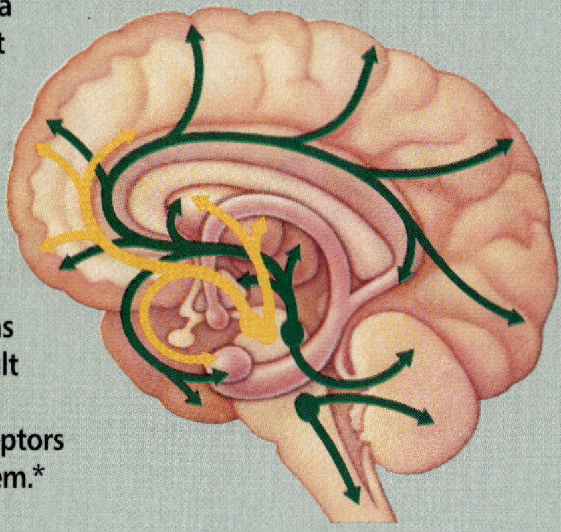

1-, 2-, 3-, 4-mg tablets

Risperdal®
RISPERIDONE

A first choice in psychosis.

*Ereshefsky L, Lacombe S. Pharmacological profile of risperidone. *Can J Psychiatry.* 1993;38(Suppl 3):S80-S88.

Please see the brief summary of Prescribing Information adjacent to this ad.

JANSSEN · PHARMACEUTICA · RESEARCH FOUNDATION · SmithKline Beecham Pharmaceuticals

ORIGINAL ARTICLE

Differential Heritability of Adult and Juvenile Antisocial Traits

Michael J. Lyons, PhD; William R. True, PhD; Seth A. Eisen, MD, MSc; Jack Goldberg, PhD; Joanne M. Meyer, PhD; Stephen V. Faraone, PhD; Lindon J. Eaves, PhD, DSc; Ming T. Tsuang, MD, PhD, DSc

Background: Studies of adult antisocial behavior or criminality usually find genetic factors to be more important than the family environment, whereas studies of delinquency find the family environment to be more important. We compared *DSM-III-R* antisocial personality disorder symptoms before vs after the age of 15 years within a sample of twins, rather than comparing across studies.

Methods: We administered the Diagnostic Interview Schedule Version III–revised by telephone to 3226 pairs of male twins from the Vietnam Era Twin Registry. Biometrical modeling was applied to each symptom of antisocial personality disorder and summary measures of juvenile and adult symptoms.

Results: Five juvenile symptoms were significantly heritable, and five were significantly influenced by the shared environment. Eight adult symptoms were significantly heritable, and one was significantly influenced by the shared environment. The shared environment explained about six times more variance in juvenile antisocial traits than in adult traits. Shared environmental influences on adult antisocial traits overlapped entirely with those on juvenile traits. Additive genetic factors explained about six times more variance in adult vs juvenile traits. The juvenile genetic determinants overlapped completely with genetic influences on adult traits. The unique environment (plus measurement error) explained the largest proportion of variance in both juvenile and adult antisocial traits.

Conclusions: Characteristics of the shared or family environment that promote antisocial behavior during childhood and early adolescence also promote later antisocial behavior, but to a much lesser extent. Genetic causal factors are much more prominent for adult than for juvenile antisocial traits.

(Arch Gen Psychiatry. 1995;52:906-915)

Antisocial personality disorder (APD) is a relatively common disorder[1]; in the Epidemiologic Catchment Area study, 4.5% of males and 0.8% of females were diagnosed as having APD at some time during their lives.[2] There is a substantial overlap between APD and criminality, with prevalence rates for APD as high as 75% reported among incarcerated criminals.[3] Data that address the causes of criminal behavior may have relevance for understanding the cause of APD. Findings from reviews of adoption studies support the significance of genetic influences on criminal behavior[4,5] and suggest that genetic factors may be more important for property crimes than for violent crimes.

Early twin studies provided consistent evidence for genetic influences on criminality, but these studies have been criticized for methodological shortcomings (eg, "nonblind" diagnosis and nonsystematic ascertainment), which may bias samples toward including concordant monozygotic (MZ) pairs. Subsequent studies that overcame the methodological limitations of the earlier studies obtained similar findings. Gottesman and Goldsmith[5] reviewed twin studies that were carried out in North America, Germany, Japan, Norway, and Denmark since 1931. The pooled pairwise concordance rate for male MZ pairs was 51.5% compared with a 23.1% concordance rate among male-male dizygotic (DZ) pairs, indicating a substantial genetic influence. Centerwall and Robinette[6] studied the National Academy of Sciences–National Research Council World War II Veteran Twin Registry that contained 15 924 twin pairs. The MZ concor-

The affiliations of the authors appear in the "Acknowledgment" section at the end of the article.

See Subjects and Methods on next page

SUBJECTS AND METHODS

SUBJECTS

The VET Registry consists of male twin pairs in which both twins served in the military during the Vietnam era (May 1965 to August 1975). Information about the method of assembling the registry has been detailed elsewhere.[15] Zygosity was evaluated by using a series of questions on twin similarity and limited blood group typing obtained from military records.[16] This method has achieved 95% accuracy.[16] Of the twin pairs in the total registry, 43.8% were identified as DZ and 53.5% as MZ; 2.7% could not be classified and were excluded. The relative overrepresentation of MZ pairs is owing to the absence of opposite-sex DZ pairs.

Of 10 300 eligible individuals (5150 pairs), 47 were deceased or incapacitated. Of the remaining subjects, 8039 (78.4%) were successfully interviewed. The 3226 pairs in which both members responded to every APD item are the subject of this report (number of MZ pairs, 1788; number of DZ pairs, 1438). The mean age of the respondents was 44.6 years (SD, ±2.8; age range, 36 to 55 years); 90.4% were non-Hispanic white, 4.9% were African American, 2.7% were Hispanic, 1.3% were Native American or Alaskan Native, and 0.7% were "other"; 33.3% were high school graduates, and 38.6% were college graduates; 92.6% were employed full-time, and 1.8% were employed part-time. The response rate was higher for non-Hispanic white twins than for any other group and resulted in their relative overrepresentation among respondents compared with that of all veterans of the Vietnam era. Seventy-five percent were married at the time of a 1987 survey, 11% were never married, and 77% had fathered at least one child.

DATA COLLECTION

Subjects were interviewed by using a computed version of the National Institute of Mental Health Diagnostic Interview Schedule Version III–revised[17] that was administered by telephone. Data were collected by the Institute for Survey Research, Temple University, Philadelphia, Pa, by trained and experienced interviewers. Training of the interviewers was conducted by one of the investigators (M.J.L.). Their supervisor attended a training course at Washington University, St Louis, Mo, that was conducted by the developers of the interview. It was not feasible to conduct face-to-face interviews because of the nationally distributed nature of the sample.

Subjects were sent a letter that explained the purpose of the study and informed them that they would be receiving a telephone call from an interviewer; 1 to 2 weeks later, an interviewer called the subject, explained the procedure, and solicited his consent to participate.

Summary scores were calculated for each subject to determine the total number of juvenile and adult diagnostic criteria present. Krueger et al[18] pointed out several advantages of summing the total number of antisocial criteria (what they called the "variety" score) in comparison with measures of frequency of specific acts. The summary score is typically less skewed than frequency scores. This summing procedure gives equal weight to all included antisocial behaviors, rather than disproportionately reflecting minor acts that may be committed frequently. For example, the use of frequency counts might lead to the overrepresentation of minor violations (eg, truancy) that occur frequently compared with more serious behaviors (eg, sexual assault that is likely to be less frequent). Krueger et al[18] found that self-reported delinquency correlated significantly with reports of informants, official records of police contacts, and official records of court convictions. Robins[19] also reported that the extent of involvement in different types of antisocial behaviors was highly predictive of future antisocial outcomes.

DATA ANALYSIS

Univariate Analyses

The twin method compares the degree of similarity within MZ pairs with the degree of similarity within DZ pairs. One method for quantifying similarity is the concordance rate. However, the concordance rate does not use all available information because only pairs in which at least one member is affected are included in its calculation. The tetrachoric correlation, calculated from the 2×2 contingency table, is an alternative approach for dichotomous outcomes that uses all available information within pairs because pairs that are concordant for being unaffected, as well as affected, are also included in its computation. The tetrachoric correlation is also known as the correlation of liability.[20]

The second step tests whether additive genetic effects or family environmental effects alone are responsible

Continued on next page

dance rate for dishonorable discharge was 14.9%, and the DZ concordance rate was 1.6%, indicating a genetic influence.

According to the *DSM-III-R,* APD is the only mental disorder that requires the presence of certain symptoms in childhood and early adolescence and the presence of different symptoms after the age of 15 years. This

See also pages 895, 900, 916, and 925

allows the assessment of whether the determinants of childhood antisocial behavior are the same as those for adult antisocial behavior. McGuffin and Gottesman[7] reported a significantly higher MZ than DZ concordance rate for adult criminality across the studies that they reviewed, indicating a genetic influence. However, concordance rates for MZ and DZ pairs were similar for juvenile delinquency (MZ concordance rate of 87% vs DZ concordance rate of 72%), suggesting that the family or shared environment, rather than genetic factors, is primarily responsible for familial resemblance in juvenile delinquency. The twin studies of Rosanoff et al[8] and Shields[9] provided two of the earliest observations that juvenile delinquency was more strongly influenced by the shared environment and adult criminality was more influenced by genetic factors.[10,11] However, Rowe[12] and Rowe and Osgood[13] reported significant heritability, as well as a significant influence from the shared environment for

for observed familial similarity. The analysis fits univariate structural equation models to the 2×2 contingency tables separately for MZ and DZ twin pairs. These models explain the twin similarity for liability (ie, the tetrachoric correlations) in terms of additive genetic effects (heritability or h^2), common, shared, or family environmental effects (c^2), and unique or nonshared environmental effects (e^2). Parameters are estimated by the method of maximum likelihood by using a publicly available software package (MX Software, Virginia Commonwealth University, Richmond).[21] The process begins with a full model, including the effects of additive genes (A), common or shared environment (C), and unique environment (E). The term E reflects influences that are specific to individuals rather than the pair and random error; these influences promote dissimilarity within pairs. The full or ACE model is compared with reduced models that delete either additive genes (a CE model) or common environment (an AE model). Models *without* additive genetic effects test whether the twin correlation is due solely to common environmental influences; alternately, models *without* common environmental effects test whether familial aggregation is due solely to additive genetic effects. Models that include only E test for an absence of family resemblance. Models with E only are not presented, because all analyses demonstrated familial resemblance. Models that included a sibling interaction parameter were also fit to the data.[22] To assess whether a submodel (without A, C, or sibling interaction) fits the data worse than the full model, a χ^2 difference test is used. This test evaluates the difference in the χ^2 of the full vs the reduced model and is distributed as the χ^2 with df equal to $df_{reduced}$ minus df_{full}. If this test statistic is not significant, the reduced model is accepted.

The summary measures of juvenile and adult traits were also analyzed. For these analyses, polychoric correlations are computed from discrete ordinal data (in this case, the number of symptoms) that are assumed to have resulted from multiple thresholds that are imposed on an underlying multivariate normal distribution.[22] Parameters are estimated by the method of weighted least squares, by using the inverse of the asymptotic variances of the correlations as the weights. The commercially available software packages PRELIS and LISREL[23] were used for these analyses. Juvenile antisocial traits in one twin are correlated with juvenile antisocial traits in his sibling, and adult antisocial traits in one twin are correlated with adult antisocial traits in his sibling.

Bivariate Analyses

When two phenotypes (ie, adult and juvenile antisocial traits) are correlated, as in this study, additional bivariate models are fit to the traits jointly to assess the determinants of the observed phenotypic correlation of these variables. Bivariate structural equation modeling[21] permits assessment of whether genetic and environmental effects on two variables correlate. The following correlations are computed for each zygosity group: two within-variable, cross-twin correlations (juvenile traits–juvenile traits and adult traits–adult traits, TWIN1 with TWIN2); two within-twin, cross-variable correlations (juvenile traits–adult traits, TWIN1 with TWIN1 and TWIN2 with TWIN2); and two cross-twin, cross-variable correlations (juvenile traits–adult traits, TWIN1 with TWIN2 and TWIN2 with TWIN1). The MZ cross-twin, cross-variable correlations that are no lower than the within-twin, cross-variable correlations indicate that unique environmental factors do not contribute to the juvenile-adult correlation. If, in addition, the MZ cross-twin, cross-variable correlations are approximately twice those of DZ twins, a genetic influence on the cross-variable correlation is suggested. Conversely, if the MZ cross-twin, cross-variable correlations are equal to those of the DZ twin pairs, a common environmental influence on the correlation between the two traits is indicated.

Correlated genetic and environmental effects on juvenile and adult antisocial traits are tested statistically by comparing the fit of the full bivariate model (that includes all of these effects, ie, the ACE model for juvenile traits, the ACE model for adult traits and parameters that are shared by adult and juvenile traits) with that of reduced models that delete all or a subset of effects. These estimates were determined by using structural equation modeling that was implemented with the LISREL software package[23] and the method of weighted least squares.[22] The inverse of the asymptotic variances of the correlations are used as weights. A χ^2 difference test is used to determine whether a reduced model fits the data significantly worse than the full model. The "best-fitting" model is selected on the basis of parsimony (ie, the model with the fewest included parameters) from among the submodels that do not fit the data significantly worse than the full model.

adolescent antisocial behavior, based on the results of their twin studies. Grove et al,[14] in a study of 32 sets of MZ twins who were reared apart, found a nonsignificantly higher heritability for juvenile antisocial criteria (heritability, 0.42) vs adult criteria (heritability, 0.29).

To date, twin studies on APD have not used *DSM-III-R* criteria. Furthermore, few studies have examined juvenile and adult diagnostic criteria in the same subjects. The present study was carried out by using a systematically ascertained twin registry; thus, it avoided problems associated with samples that were identified on the basis of clinical or criminal status. Twins from the Vietnam Era Twin (VET) Registry were used to evaluate the role of genetic and environmental factors in the origin of antisocial behaviors. We capitalized on the *DSM-III-R* distinction between conduct disorder symptoms that occurred before the age of 15 years and irresponsible and antisocial behavior that occurred after the age of 15 years to investigate whether they shared the same determinants. Our design permitted the examination of change in the relative contributions of genetic and environmental factors to earlier vs later antisocial behavior.

RESULTS

Table 1 contains the frequency of each symptom of APD according to the *DSM-III-R*. A total score was computed separately for the juvenile and adult criteria by adding the number of criteria present. Scores on the juvenile total ranged from 0 to 8, with a mean (±SD) of 0.78 (±1.04). Scores on the adult total ranged from 0 to 9, with a mean (±SD) of 1.57 (±1.51). Since so few sub-

Table 1. Prevalence of Juvenile and Adult *DSM-III-R* APD Criteria, Tetrachoric Correlations, and Variance Components for 6452 MZ and DZ Twins*

DSM-III-R/ *DIS-III-R* Criteria	Prevalence, %	Tetrachoric Correlations r_{mz}	r_{dz}	Variance Components, %† Genetic (A)	Shared Environment (C)	Unique Environment (E)
The juvenile criteria (before the age of 15 y)						
Often truant‡	13.6	.26	.19	28	...	72
Initiates fights‡	5.0	.37	.18	37	...	63
Used weapon‡	1.3	.39	.22	40	...	60
Ran away§‖	1.9	.47	.78	...	55	45
Forced sex¶	0	...	...	...	...	...
Cruel to animals‡	8.6	.21	.11	21	...	79
Cruel to people§‖	6.1	.10	.28	...	18	82
Damage property§	5.4	.26	.37	...	32	68
Starts fires§	5.7	.38	.47	...	41	59
Lies often‡	9.9	.38	.27	41	...	59
Steals, no confrontation§	29.4	.46	.36	...	41	59
Steals, with confrontation¶	0.3	...	...	...	...	...
Adult criteria (since the age of 15 y)						
Inconsistent work#	16.1	.34	.15	34	...	66
Fails to conform to social norms#	20.5	.49	.32	52	...	48
Aggressive#	38.5	.50	.27	50	...	50
Fails to honor financial obligations‡	5.1	.39	.20	38	...	62
Impulsive‡	7.0	.41	.23	41	...	59
No regard for truth**	2.7	.15	.28	...	77	23
Reckless#	47.8	.47	.31	48	...	52
Irresponsible parent¶	1.2	.22	...	...	...	...
Never monogamous‡	4.2	.30	.19	31	...	69
Lacks remorse‡	4.0	.22	.14	22	...	78

**APD indicates antisocial personality disorder; MZ, monozygotic; DZ, dizygotic; and* DIS-III-R, National Institute of Mental Health Diagnostic Interview Schedule Version III–revised.

†*Best-fitting model. In no cases did a model with sibling interaction and additive genetic, shared environmental, unique environmental effects provide a better fit to the data than a model without sibling interaction. In all cases, a model with only unique environmental influences on the phenotype was rejected by a goodness-of-fit* χ^2.

‡*Neither an AE or a CE model was rejected against the full ACE model. However, the goodness-of-fit* χ^2 *of the AE model was less than that of the CE model.*

§*The CE model was not rejected against the full model, while the AE model was rejected.*

‖*However, the goodness-of-fit* χ^2 *of the CE model has a* $P<.05$. *The poor fit of this model reflects the fact that the DZ twin correlation is less than the MZ twin correlation.*

¶*A tetrachoric correlation could not be computed because of an empty cell.*

#*The AE model was not rejected against the full model, while the CE model was rejected.*

***Neither an AE nor a CE model was rejected against the full ACE model. However, the goodness-of-fit* χ^2 *of the CE model was less than that of the AE model.*

jects had a score of 9 on the adult scale, these subjects were combined with subjects with a score of 8 for the purposes of calculating polychoric correlations. **Table 2** contains the percentage of respondents at each level of the total number of symptoms. The MZ and DZ twin pairs are presented separately, but they did not differ significantly on the number of adult or juvenile symptoms. Approximately 8.8% of subjects exceeded the *DSM-III-R* threshold for symptoms before the age of 15 years, and approximately 9.1% of subjects exceeded the threshold after the age of 15 years.

To assess the possibility that nonrespondents might differ from respondents in their level of antisocial traits, we compared the mean number of juvenile and adult symptoms for respondents whose co-twin did not respond with one randomly selected twin from each pair concordant for response. The respondents from response-discordant pairs had a slightly, but statistically significantly, higher number of juvenile (approximately 0.08 SD units) and adult (approximately 0.12 SD units) symptoms than did respondents from response-concordant pairs. This suggests that nonrespondents are likely to have a somewhat higher number of both juvenile and adult antisocial symptoms compared with that of the subjects included in this report who were all members of response-concordant pairs.

Table 1 also includes the tetrachoric correlations for the MZ and DZ twins for each symptom, along with the results of biometrical model fitting. Tetrachoric correlations could not be computed for variables if the 2×2 contingency table contained any empty cells, as was the case for the diagnostic criteria of forcing sex, stealing with confrontation of the victim, and being an irresponsible parent. For five juvenile symptoms, neither an AE or a CE model was rejected against the full ACE model. However, the χ^2 goodness of fit of the AE model was less than that of the CE model. For five other juvenile symptoms, the CE model was not rejected against the full model, while the AE model was rejected. For two symptoms in which the DZ correlation was greater than the MZ correlation (ran away and cruel to people), the goodness of fit of the CE model had a $P < .05$, indicating a relatively poor fit of the model to the data. For four adult symptoms, the AE model was not rejected against the full model, while the CE model was rejected. For four adult symptoms, neither an AE or a CE model was rejected against the full ACE model. However, the χ^2 goodness of fit of the AE model was less than that of the CE model. For one adult symptom, neither an AE or a CE model was rejected against the full ACE model, but the goodness of fit of the CE model was less than that of the AE model. The sibling interaction parameter was not significant for any of the juvenile or adult variables.

Table 3 contains the MZ and DZ polychoric correlations for the total number of juvenile and adult antisocial traits. The threshold model provided an adequate fit to the data (range of *P* values, .14 to .96). The MZ cross-twin correlation for juvenile antisocial traits was .39, and the DZ correlation was .33. The cross-variable, cross-twin correlations of juvenile antisocial traits with adult antisocial traits were .33 and .23 and .22 and .19 for MZ and DZ pairs, respectively. The within-twin pair, cross-variable correlations of juvenile antisocial traits with adult antisocial traits were higher in the MZ pairs than in the DZ pairs, suggesting a sharing of additive genes between juvenile and adult traits.

Table 4 contains the results of univariate biometrical modeling for juvenile and adult antisocial traits. Results are from the best-fitting models and indicate that the heritability of juvenile antisocial traits is rather low, with a much larger contribution from the shared or family environment. The converse was found for adult antisocial traits, with a substantial genetic contribution, and a modest influence from the shared or family environment.

Bivariate structural equation models that describe the shared and specific effects of additive genes, common environment, and unique environment on juvenile and adult antisocial traits were fitted to the MZ and DZ correlations. **Table 5** contains the parameter estimates for the full model in which all nine parameters are included. The comparison of the full model with the data produced a goodness-of-fit χ^2 that was slightly below 0.05. The fit of the full model is mildly degraded by the inclusion of a nonsignificant parameter (specific adult C [the letters A, C, and E refer to the same in the "Univariate Analyses" subsection above]). With such a large sample, relatively small differences yield statistical significance. Table 5 also contains the χ^2 values for a series of submodels. The first three submodels delete the parameters adult common E, adult common C, and adult common A, respectively. The poor fit of all three of these submodels indicates that the covariation between adult and juvenile antisocial traits reflects genetic, shared environmental, and unique environmental influences that are common to both. The next two submodels that delete adult-specific C and adult-specific A test whether the overlap in genetic and shared environmental influences on the adult and juvenile phenotypes is complete. Both of these models provide a good fit to the data. The final submodel, namely, the model that provides the best fit to the data, deletes both adult-specific C and A. This is the most parsimonious submodel (ie, the model with the fewest included parameters) that does not differ significantly from the full model (χ^2=12.7, *df*=7, *P*=.08). This model suggests that there are no additive genetic and shared environmental effects on adult antisocial traits that

Table 2. Percentage of Subjects With Each Number of Juvenile and Adult Symptoms*

No. of Symptoms	Juvenile Symptoms, % MZ	Juvenile Symptoms, % DZ	Adult Symptoms, % MZ	Adult Symptoms, % DZ
0	52.52	47.53	29.56	28.64
1	27.57	29.91	31.01	29.72
2	11.86	12.93	19.66	21.55
3	5.38	5.46	10.93	10.67
4	1.72	2.61	4.95	5.28
5	0.53	1.08	2.27	2.47
6	0.24	0.17	1.09	0.73
7	0.13	0.21	0.25	0.45
8	0.05	0.10	0.25	0.32
9	...	...	0.03	0.17

**MZ indicates monozygotic; DZ, dizygotic.*

Table 3. Twin Polychoric Correlations for Adult and Juvenile Antisocial Traits Derived From the 'Best-Fitting' Model*

	MZ Twins				DZ Twins			
	Juvenile Traits		Adult Traits		Juvenile Traits		Adult Traits	
Traits	Twin 1	Twin 2	Twin 1	Twin 2	Twin 1	Twin 2	Twin 1	Twin 2
Juvenile traits Twin 1	1.0				1.0			
Juvenile traits Twin 2	*.39*	1.0			*.33*	1.0		
Adult traits Twin 1	**.43**	.23	1.0		**.44**	.19	1.0	
Adult traits Twin 2	.33	**.46**	*.47*	1.0	.22	**.39**	*.27*	1.0

**MZ indicates monozygotic (n pairs=1788); DZ, dizygotic (n pairs=1438); italic numbers, cross-twin same-trait correlations; and bold-faced numbers same-twin cross-trait correlations.*

do not also influence juvenile traits and vice versa (ie, we cannot discern whether effects are specific to adult or juvenile traits). This model indicates that the phenotypic correlation between adult and juvenile antisocial traits (r=.44) is owing to genes, shared experiences, and unique or nonshared experiences that influence both outcomes. Genetic influences that are common to both adult and juvenile phenotypes account for 28% of the correlation between the two outcomes. Influences of the environment that are shared by members of the twin pair account for 35% of the correlation between adult and juvenile phenotypes. Aspects of the environment that are not shared by members of the twin pairs are responsible for 37% of the correlation between adult and juvenile antisocial traits. In addition to the analyses reported in Table 5, we carried out a parallel series of analyses in which the outcome was meeting the *DSM-III-R* threshold number of symptoms for juvenile (three or more symptoms) or adult (four or more symptoms) diagnoses. The results of these analyses were similar to those reported in Table 5 for the continuous trait scores. The best-fitting model was the same for both the continuous traits and the diagnostic thresholds, and none of the parameter estimates contained in Table 5 differed by more than .05 for the diagnostic thresholds. The models based on diagnostic thresholds provided a somewhat better fit to the data because the dichotomous variables had larger SEs than the more precise trait scores.

The **Figure** illustrates that the effects of the shared or family environment that influence adult antisocial traits overlap entirely with those that influence juvenile traits. Juvenile genetic determinants overlap completely with genetic influences on adult traits. The unique or nonshared environment (plus measurement error) explains the largest proportion of variance in both juvenile and adult antisocial traits. A portion of the unique or nonshared environment influences both juvenile and adult antisocial traits.

Table 4. Estimates of the Effects of Genetic and Environmental Factors on Juvenile and Adult Antisocial Traits*

Antisocial Traits	h^2 (Heritability)	c^2 (Common Environment)	u^2 (Unique Environment)
Juvenile	0.07	0.31	0.62
Adult	0.43	0.05	0.52

**Monozygotic pairs (n=1788); dizygotic pairs (n=1438).*

COMMENT

The pattern of results for individual criteria suggests that, in general, shared environmental influences are relatively more important for individual juvenile symptoms while genetic influences are relatively more important for individual adult symptoms. There is a strong influence of the environment that is shared by twins on the summary measure of juvenile antisocial traits, but only a modest genetic influence. Conversely, there is a strong genetic influence on the summary measure of adult antisocial traits, but only a modest influence from the shared environment. Characteristics of the shared environment, which could include peers common to both twins and the home environment, that promote antisocial behavior during childhood and early adolescence also promote later antisocial behavior, but much less potently. The environment that is shared by the twins, while the individual is living in it, has a powerful influence on the individual's behavior. However, once the individual leaves the family and other aspects of the environment that are shared with his twin, the shared environment's strong influence seems to "evaporate." The lack of persistence of the shared environment on traits that are measured during adulthood is not unique to the current investigation of antisocial traits.

Table 5. Bivariate Biometrical Modeling of Juvenile and Adult Antisocial Traits*

	Common											
	Juvenile			Adult			Specific Adult			Fit of Model		
Type of Model	A	C	E	A	C	E	A	C	E	χ^2	*df*	*P*
Full model	.36	.51	.78	.43	.25	19	.47	.07	.71	11.8	5	.04
Tests of any covariations between traits†	✓	✓	✓	✓	✓	. . .	✓	✓	✓	63.4	6	<.01
	✓	✓	✓	✓	. . .	✓	✓	✓	✓	20.4	6	<.01
	✓	✓	✓	. . .	✓	✓	✓	✓	✓	25.1	6	<.01
Tests of complete covariation between traits‡	✓	✓	✓	✓	✓	✓	✓	. . .	✓	11.8	6	.07
	✓	✓	✓	✓	✓	✓	. . .	✓	✓	12.4	6	.05
"Best-fitting" model§	.26	.56	.79	.66	.21	.19	. . .	. . .	.70	12.7	7	.08

**The check mark indicates that parameter is included in the model.*
†Models with deletion of common A, C, and E test whether the adult and juvenile phenotypes share the influence of each of these determinants.
‡Models with deletion of specific A and C test whether adult and juvenile phenotypes have the same genetic and common environmental determinants.
§The model with the best fit to the data deletes specific influences on A and C.

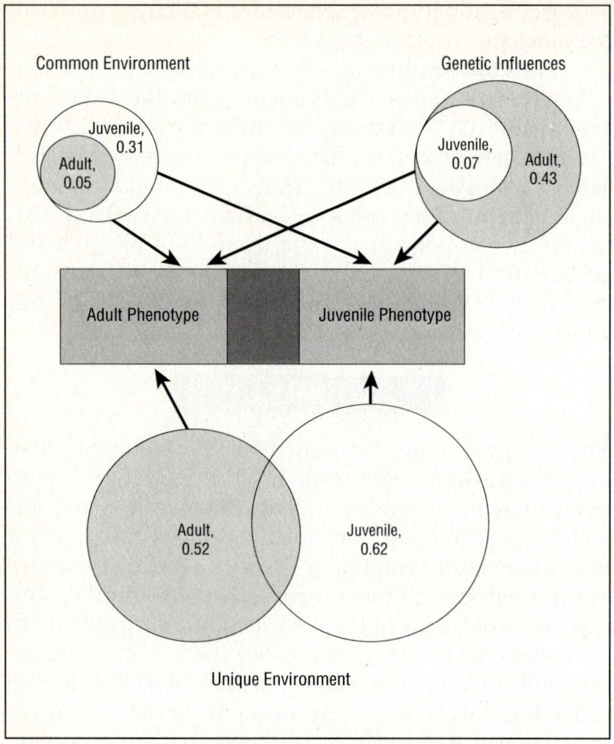

Boxes represent the juvenile and adult phenotypes; circles, latent variables that are the sources of genetic and environmental variance in the phenotypes (the area of each circle is roughly proportional to the amount of variance that it explains in the phenotype); the numbers within the circles labeled "Genetic Influences," h^2 (proportion of variance attributable to additive genetic influences); the numbers within the circles labeled "Common Environment," c^2 (proportion of variance due to the shared or common environment); and the numbers within the circles labeled "Unique Environment," e^2 (proportion of variance due to the unique environment). The overlap of the rectangles reflects the fact that juvenile and adult antisocial traits (ie, phenotypes) share about 18.5% of their variance, as determined by the square of the phenotypic correlation.

RELATIONSHIP OF JUVENILE TO ADULT TRAITS

DiLalla and Gottesman[24,25] delineated three subgroups of antisocial children: *continuous antisocials* are juvenile delinquents who become adult criminals, *transitory delinquents* are youths who do not become adult criminals, and *late bloomers* are nondelinquent youths who become adult criminals. The moderate phenotypic correlation between juvenile and adult antisocial traits, observed in our study, is consistent with their view that some individuals are consistently antisocial, and some "outgrow" their antisocial behavior, while still others seem to "grow into" their antisocial behavior. DiLalla and Gottesman[24] concluded that among adolescent delinquents, genetic factors were most prominent among those who went on to become criminals. In contrast, among all juvenile delinquents, shared environmental factors were a more prominent cause of delinquent behavior.[26] Achenbach[27] suggested a taxonomy of two conduct disorder syndromes, characterized by either delinquent or aggressive behavior; Achenbach[27] cited twin research that found a high heritability for the aggressive behavior syndrome, but not the delinquent behavior syndrome.[28,29]

Results reported here are consistent with the conclusion of McGuffin and Gottesman[7]; in their review, they found that delinquent behavior was more influenced by the shared or family environment, and adult criminal or antisocial behavior was more heritable. Scarr and McCartney[30] suggested that aging allows the individual to have greater control over his or her environment. Environments that promote genetically influenced predilections are more likely to be sought out and experienced in adulthood than childhood. With regard to antisocial traits, the child's parents may provide an environment that correlates with the relevant genes that they share with their child. When the individual can select his or her own environment, it may be one that is more closely matched to the degree of "antisociality" that is inherent in the individual's genotype. This is an example of a genotype-environment correlation. Consistent with this view, Robins[31] found that individuals who had been antisocial in childhood experienced more unemployment, marital breakdown, and lack of social support in adulthood.

Other studies have found that certain adult characteristics are more heritable than childhood ones. Plomin[32] reported that the correlation for cognitive abilities between biologically unrelated adoptive siblings is about .25 during childhood, but later in life, it approaches 0. McGue[33] reviewed data from twin studies of intelligence at various ages; McGue[33] found that the heritability of intelligence consistently increased from 4 to 6 years of age to adulthood, while the variance attributable to the family environment decreased from approximately 38% to 0% during the same period. McCartney et al[34] also found that the heritability of intelligence increased over time. Pedersen et al[35] found that general cognitive abilities that were assessed in later life (mean age of their sample, 65 years) demonstrated a substantially higher heritability (80%) than general cognitive ability that was assessed earlier in life (heritability, approximately 50%). Scarr and McCartney[30] and McGue[33] suggested that part of the environmental influence on intelligence is a genotype-environment correlation.

Compared with data on intelligence, there is less information available about changes in the heritability of personality over time.[36] However, a number of investigators have found that genetic influences on some personality variables may be stronger earlier in life. Eaves et al[37] compared the genetic influence on extraversion and neuroticism in three age cohorts, and they found that the youngest twin pairs demonstrated the greatest genetic variance. In a longitudinal study of the Multidimensional Personality Questionnaire by McGue and colleagues,[38] they found greater heritability for baseline assessments compared with that for follow-up studies an average of 10 years later. Viken et al,[39] using a combined cross-sectional and longitudinal approach, found that the heritabilities of neuroticism and extraversion decreased from late adolescence to the late 20s. For extraversion, but not neuroticism, there was a smaller additional decrease at about the age of 50 years.

MODELS OF APD

The *DSM-III-R* defines APD in terms of characteristic *behaviors* that occur during childhood and after the age of 15 years. This approach has been criticized because its emphasis on observable behavior, although providing good reliability, fails to include traditional psychological aspects of psychopathy (eg, selfishness, egocentricity, callousness, manipulativeness, and lack of empathy).[40] Hare et al[40] suggested that although all individuals who fulfill *DSM-III-R* criteria for APD may be antisocial, they may differ substantially with regard to psychological characteristics (eg, capacity for empathy, remorse, guilt, etc). Also, overt behavior can reflect more than one personality trait.[41] In the present study, we treated APD as a continuous trait, rather than as a discrete, dichotomous diagnostic entity. Our approach is predicated on the assumption that there are underlying continuously distributed dimensions of juvenile and adult antisocial traits. Although the individual *DSM-III-R* diagnostic criteria for APD, for the most part, refer to behaviors rather than psychological characteristics, clearly, there are not genes that cause one to carry out some specific antisocial behavior. Rather, we assume that the behaviors described in the *DSM-III-R* diagnostic criteria reflect a latent trait that influences probabilistically the likelihood of carrying out certain behaviors. We hypothesize that there are psychological characteristics (eg, sensation-seeking and impulsivity) that mediate the relationship between genes and observable antisocial behavior. Supporting our view that *DSM-III-R* diagnostic criteria for APD relate to personality characteristics, Krueger et al[18] found that the personality traits of constraint and negative emotionality were strongly associated with self-reported delinquent behavior, indicating that delinquent adolescents were more impulsive, danger-seeking, and rejecting of conventional values than were nondelinquent adolescents. Gottesman and Goldsmith[5] found that anger, inhibitory control, high pleasure (thrill- and adventure-seeking), and impulsivity are heritable in children and are related to externalizing or undercontrolled behavior.

LIMITATIONS

One limitation of this study is that only males were included. Therefore, these findings cannot be generalized to females. There are several factors that could reduce the level of antisocial traits among the subjects who were included here compared with that among the general population. The VET Registry may have failed to include some of the most antisocial individuals who were not eligible for military service because of a criminal record, but there was still a substantial range of antisocial behavior in our sample.

The influence of the shared environment on juvenile antisocial traits that was observed may reflect, at least in part, the mutual influence of siblings on one another. Rowe and Gulley[42] found that the correlation of nontwin siblings for delinquent behavior was influenced by the degree of contact between them; the correlation of delinquent behaviors between brothers who reported a close relationship was three times higher than that of brothers who reported a distant relationship. Carey[43] also found evidence for a reciprocal twin influence on twin similarity for registered criminality. The influence of the twins on each other may constitute an important aspect of the shared or family environment. It should be noted that Carey[43] suggested the MZ twins may imitate one another more than the DZ twins, and this phenomenon could lead to an overestimation of heritability. However, corroborating evidence from adoption studies and twins who were reared apart demonstrates that heritability estimates derived from twin studies cannot simply reflect imitation effects.[5] Moreover, we fitted models that included sibling interaction for each of the juvenile and adult symptoms. In no case did a model with sibling interaction and additive genetic, shared environmental, and unique environmental effects provide a better fit to the data than a model without sibling interaction.

In about 63% of the pairs, both twins responded to our interview and were therefore included in the sample reported here. We could not include pairs in which one or both twins could not be located or refused participation. Comparisons of twins from pairs that were discordant for response with pairs that were concordant for response revealed slightly more antisocial behavior among twins whose co-twins did not respond. It is likely that pairs in which neither twin responded had higher levels of antisocial behavior than pairs in which one or both twins responded. Thus, nonresponse appeared to have resulted in a usable sample that was somewhat lower in antisocial traits than the population from which they were drawn. This situation corresponds to what Neale and Eaves[44] referred to as "soft selection." In soft selection, there is no absolute threshold that determines which subjects are excluded; rather, the probability of selection varies over the range of the trait. Small correlations are reduced by soft selection by about the same amount as large correlations, which may reduce the proportion of variance attributed to the shared environment. However, it is unlikely that the reduction in the mean level of antisocial traits in the pairs that were included in this study would significantly alter the primary conclusions of this article. Neale and Eaves[45] provided formulas to correct estimates of heritability for volunteer bias; however, such an approach would be computationally intensive and difficult to implement on the data in this study. It is possible that the exact values of the estimated parameters might be somewhat different with a 100% response rate. However, these values are relativistic and do not represent a concrete "amount" of some entity.

In our study, all subjects were exposed to a military environment for some period of their early adulthood—most often for 2 to 4 years. Estimates of the influence of genetic and environmental factors are sensitive to the degree of variability among the included individuals. To the extent that military service experienced by everyone in our sample created more homogeneous adult environments for individuals in our sample compared with those for the general population, estimates of heritable influences on observed individual differences during adulthood might be increased. Virtually all of our subjects were educated in American primary and secondary schools, and we suspect that the heterogeneity of these educational settings is probably not much more or less than that for military settings. We do not believe that the adult environments experienced by our twins were more homogeneous than their childhood environments.

Our data about juvenile antisocial traits required

adults to recall behaviors from childhood and adolescence. Thus, differences between juvenile and adult traits could have been influenced by differences in the length of the recall period. Although little is known about the validity of retrospective reports of child antisocial behavior by using the National Institute of Mental Health Diagnostic Interview Schedule Version III–revised, recent work has demonstrated the validity of such reports for a variety of psychiatric diagnoses.[46,47] From our own data, we also note that an increased error of measurement due to recall effects would have been evident in larger contributions of the unique environment for juvenile traits. Although variance that was attributed to the unique environment was somewhat higher for juvenile compared with adult traits (E=0.62 compared with E=0.52), the most robust differences between the two were observed for heritability and common environment. Also, previous studies of delinquency that did not rely on adult recall demonstrated similar results.[7]

It is important to consider whether the telephone interview format may have produced different results than would have been obtained from face-to-face interviews. Several comparisons of telephone vs face-to-face interviews for drug use[48,49] have found somewhat higher rates among subjects who were interviewed face-to-face compared with subjects who were interviewed by telephone. However, a number of empirical studies suggest that the results of telephone interviews are generally comparable with those of face-to-face interviews.[50-53]

CONCLUSIONS

Although these data strongly support the role of genetic factors in the origin of antisocial behavior, they are also consistent with an important role for the environment. As Plomin[32] pointed out, it is no longer the case that environmental influences are the default assumption about the source of individual differences in behavior. These data suggest that the most important aspects of the environment for adult APD traits are those that operate on the individual, rather than both members of the twin pair. This may sharpen the focus of investigations of specific environmental factors. The data reported here suggest that adult antisocial traits may actually be more familial (ie, h^2+c^2, the total variance contributed by additive genes and the shared environment) than are juvenile antisocial traits; 62% of the variance in juvenile traits is explained by nonfamilial influences, whereas 52% of the variance in adult antisocial traits is explained by nonfamilial influences. However, this difference may also reflect differences in the reliability of self-reported adult vs juvenile behavior owing to a greater interval of time from the behavior to the time of data collection. To the extent that the unreliability of measurement attenuates the resemblance observed within twin pairs, greater influence will be attributed to the unique environment. Considerably more of the family influence on adult antisocial traits is owing to genes rather than to the environment. The estimates of the contribution of genes and environment to antisocial behavior are relativistic and reflect the genotypes and environments of the included subjects. In certain times and places (eg, high-crime economically disadvantaged neighborhoods), the relative influence of environmental vs genetic factors could be different from that observed in the present study. It is also important to keep in mind that the findings reported here address the sources of *individual differences* (as opposed to *group differences*) in juvenile and adult antisocial traits. To the extent that groups may differ on some characteristic (eg, antisocial traits), it is mistaken to assume that the source of variation within a group is also the source of differences between groups. Genetic factors might be most important for explaining why individuals within a group differ from one another with regard to antisocial behavior. However, environmental factors might be most important for explaining why members of one group differ from members of another group.

Accepted for publication June 26, 1995.

From the Department of Psychology, Boston (Mass) University (Dr Lyons); the Harvard Institute of Psychiatric Epidemiology and Genetics, and the Harvard Medical School Department of Psychiatry, Brockton (Mass)/West Roxbury Department of Veterans Affairs Medical Center (Drs Lyons, Faraone, and Tsuang); the Department of Epidemiology, Harvard School of Public Health (Dr Tsuang), and the Harvard Medical School Department of Psychiatry, Massachusetts Mental Health Center (Dr Tsuang), Boston; the School of Public Health, St Louis (Mo) University (Dr True); the Research and Medical Service, St Louis Department of Veterans Affairs Medical Center (Drs True and Eisen); the Department of Medicine, Washington University, St Louis (Dr Eisen); the Department of Epidemiology, University of Illinois School of Public Health, Chicago (Dr Goldberg); the Hines (Ill) Center for Cooperative Studies in Health Services (Drs Goldberg and Meyer); and the Department of Human Genetics, Medical College of Virginia, Richmond (Drs Meyer and Eaves).

This study was supported by grant DA04604 from the National Institute on Drug Abuse, Washington, DC (Dr Tsuang), and by the Department of Veterans Affairs, Health Services Research and Development Service, Cooperative Studies in Health Services, Hines, Ill (Study 992 [investigators: Drs Tsuang, Lyons, Eisen, Goldberg, Eaves, and True]).

Presented in part at the 146th Annual Meeting of the American Psychiatric Association, San Francisco, Calif, May 26, 1993.

We acknowledge the work of the following groups of people: (1) Hines Center for Cooperative Studies in Health Services—William G. Henderson, PhD, VET Registry director; Jack Goldberg, PhD, epidemiologist; Ken Bukowski, registry programmer; Mary Ellen Vitek, coordinator; and Mary Lou White, survey consultant; (2) VET Registry Advisory Committee, Hines—Alexander G. Bearn, MD (past); Gary Chase, ScD (past) (past *refers to individuals who previously occupied the role); Theodore Colton, ScD; Walter E. Nance, MD, PhD; Ralph A. Paffenbarger, Jr, MD, DrPH; Myrna M. Weissman, PhD; and Roger R. Williams, MD; (3) Health Services Research and Development Service, Department of Veterans Affairs Central Office, Washington, DC—Daniel Deykin, MD, director; and Shirley Meehan, MBA, PhD, deputy director; and (4) Cooperative Studies in Health Services, Washington—Charles Welch III, PhD, program manager; and Janet Gold, administrative officer. The authors acknowledge the contribution of Mary Ann Ausetts, MA, and the interviewers at Temple University. Irving Gottesman, PhD, and Jag Khalsa, PhD, also made important contributions to the success of this study. Most importantly, the authors gratefully acknowledge the continued cooperation and participation of the members of the VET Registry; without their contribution, this research would not have been possible.*

Reprint requests to Department of Psychology, Boston University, 64 Cummington St, Boston, MA 02215 (Dr Lyons).

REFERENCES

1. Lyons MJ. Epidemiology of personality disorders. In: Tohen M, Zahner G, Tsuang MT, eds. *Textbook in Psychiatric Epidemiology.* New York, NY: John Wiley & Sons Inc; 1995:407-436.
2. Robins LN, Tipp J, Prszybeck T. Antisocial personality. In: Robins L, Regier D, eds. *Psychiatric Disorders in America: The Epidemiologic Catchment Area Study.* New York, NY: Free Press; 1991:258-290.
3. Correctional Service of Canada. A mental health profile of federally sentenced offenders. *Forum Correct Res.* 1990;2:7-8.
4. Brennan PA, Mednick SA, Gabrielli WF. Genetic influences and criminal behavior. In: Tsuang M, Kendler K, Lyons M, eds. *Genetic Issues in Psychosocial Epidemiology.* New Brunswick, NJ: Rutgers University Press; 1991:231-246.
5. Gottesman II, Goldsmith HH. Developmental psychopathology of antisocial behavior: inserting genes into its ontogenesis and epigenesis. In: Nelson CA, ed. *Threats to Optimal Development: Integrating Biological, Psychological, and Social Risk Factors.* Hillsdale, NJ: Erlbaum; 1994:69-104.
6. Centerwall BS, Robinette CD. Twin concordance for dishonorable discharge from the military: with a review of the genetics of antisocial behavior. *Compr Psychiatry.* 1989;30:442-446.
7. McGuffin P, Gottesman II. Genetic influences on normal and abnormal development. In: Rutter M, Hersov L, eds. *Child and Adolescent Psychiatry: Modern Approaches.* Boston, Mass: Blackwell Scientific Publications Inc; 1985:17-33.
8. Rosanoff AJ, Handy LM, Plesset IR. The etiology of child behavior difficulties, juvenile delinquency, and adult criminality with special reference to occurrence in twins. In: *Psychiatric Monograph (California) No. 1.* Sacramento, Calif: Department of Institutions; 1941.
9. Shields J. Some delinquent twins. Presented at the meeting of the British Society of Criminology; June 12, 1963.
10. Cowie J, Cowie V, Slater E. *Delinquency in Girls.* London, England: Heinemann Medical Books Ltd; 1968.
11. Slater E, Cowie V. *The Genetics of Mental Disorders.* New York, NY: Oxford University Press Inc; 1974.
12. Rowe DC. A biometrical analysis of perceptions of family environment: a study of twin and singleton sibling kinships. *Child Dev.* 1983;54:416-423.
13. Rowe DC, Osgood DW. Sociological theories of delinquency and heredity: a reconsideration. *Am Sociol Rev.* 1984;49:526-540.
14. Grove WM, Elke ED, Heston L, Bouchard TJ Jr, Segal N, Lykken DT. Heritability of substance abuse and antisocial behavior: a study of monozygotic twins reared apart. *Biol Psychiatry.* 1990;27:1293-1304.
15. Eisen S, True W, Goldberg J, Henderson W, Robinette CD. The Vietnamese Era Twin (VET) Registry: method of construction. *Acta Genet Med Gemellol (Roma).* 1987;36:61-66.
16. Eisen S, Neuman R, Goldberg J, Rice J, True W. Determining zygosity in the Vietnam Era Twin Registry: an approach using questionnaires. *Clin Genet.* 1989;35:423-432.
17. Robins LN, Helzer JE, Cottler L, Godlring E. *National Institute of Mental Health Diagnostic Interview Schedule Version III–revised.* St Louis, Mo: Department of Psychiatry, Washington University; 1988.
18. Krueger RF, Schmutte PS, Caspi A, Moffitt TE, Campbell K, Silva PA. Personality traits are linked to crime among men and women: evidence from a birth cohort. *J Abnorm Psychol.* 1994;103:328-338.
19. Robins LN. Etiological implications in childhood histories relating to antisocial personality In: Hare RD, Schalling D, eds. *Psychopathic Behavior: Approaches to Research.* New York, NY: John Wiley & Sons Inc; 1978:255-272.
20. Falconer DS. The inheritance of liability to certain diseases, estimated from incidence among relatives. *Ann Hum Genet.* 1965;29:51-76.
21. Neale MC. *MX Software.* Richmond, Va: Virginia Commonwealth University; 1994.
22. Neale MC, Cardon LR. *Methodology for Genetic Studies of Twins and Families.* Norwell, Mass: Kluwer Academic Publishers; 1992.
23. SPSS. *SPSS LISREL 7 and PRELIS: User's Guide and Reference.* Chicago, Ill: SPSS Inc; 1990.
24. DiLalla LF, Gottesman II. Heterogeneity of causes for delinquency and criminality: lifespan perspectives. *Dev Psychopathol.* 1989;1:339-349.
25. DiLalla LF, Gottesman II. Biological and genetic contributors to violence—wisdom's untold tale. *Psychol Bull.* 1991;109:125-129.
26. LaBuda MC, Gottesman II, Pauls DL. Usefulness of twin studies for exploring the etiology of childhood and adolescent psychiatric disorder. *Am J Med Genet Neuropsychiatric Genet.* 1993;48:47-59.
27. Achenbach TM. Taxonomy and comorbidity of conduct problems: evidence from empirically based approaches. *Dev Psychopathol.* 1993;5:51-64.
28. Ghodsian-Carpey J, Baker LA. Genetic and environmental influences on aggression in 4- to 7-year-old twins. *Aggress Behav.* 1987;13:173-186.
29. Edelbrock C, Rende R, Plomin R, Thompson LA. Genetic and environment effects on competence and problem behavior in childhood and early adolescence. *J Child Psychol Psychiatry.* In press.
30. Scarr S, McCartney K. How people make their own environments: a theory of genotype environment effects. *Child Dev.* 1983;54:424-435.
31. Robins LN. *Deviant Children Grow Up: A Sociological and Psychiatric Study of Sociopathic Personality.* Baltimore, Md: Williams & Wilkins; 1966.
32. Plomin R. Environment and genes: determinants of behavior. *Am Psychol.* 1989;44:105-111.
33. McGue M. From proteins to cognitions: the behavioral genetics of alcoholism. In: Plomin R, McClearn GE, eds. *Nature, Nurture and Psychology.* Washington, DC: American Psychological Association; 1993:245-268.
34. McCartney K, Bernieri F, Harris MJ. Growing up and growing apart: a developmental meta-analysis of twin studies. *Psychol Bull.* 1990;107:236-237.
35. Pedersen NL, Plomin R, Nesselroade JR, McClearn GE. A quantitative genetic analysis of cognitive abilities during the second half of the life span. *Am Psychol Sci.* 1992;3:346-352.
36. Brody N. Intelligence and the behavioral genetics of personality. In: Plomin R, McClearn GE, eds. *Nature, Nurture and Psychology.* Washington, DC: American Psychological Association; 1993:161-178.
37. Eaves LJ, Eysenck HJ, Martin NG. *Genes, Culture, and Personality: An Empirical Approach.* Orlando, Fla: Academic Press Inc; 1989.
38. McGue M, Bacon S, Lykken DT. Personality stability and change in early adulthood: a behavioral genetic analysis. *Dev Psychol.* 1993;29:96-109.
39. Viken RJ, Rose RJ, Kaprio J, Koshenvuo M. A developmental genetic analysis of adult personality: extraversion and neuroticism from 18 to 59 years of age. *J Pers Soc Psychol.* 1994;66:722-730.
40. Hare RD, Hart SD, Harpur TJ. Psychopathy and the *DSM-IV* criteria for antisocial personality disorder. *J Abnorm Psychol.* 1991;100:391-398.
41. Widiger TA, Frances AJ, Trull TJ. Personality disorders. In: Craig RJ, ed. *Clinical and Diagnostic Interviewing.* New York, NY: J Aronson; 1989:221-236.
42. Rowe DC, Gulley B. Sibling effects on substance use and delinquency. *Criminology.* 1992;30:217-233.
43. Carey G. Twin imitation for antisocial behavior: implications for genetics and family research. *J Abnorm Psychol.* 1992;101:18-25.
44. Neale MC, Eaves LJ, Kendler KS, Hewitt JK. Bias in correlations from selected samples of relatives: the effects of soft selection. *Behav Genet.* 1989;19:163-170.
45. Neale MC, Eaves LJ. Estimating and controlling for the effects of volunteer bias with pairs of relatives. *Behav Genet.* 1993;23:271-277.
46. Biederman J, Faraone SV, Spencer T, Wilens T, Norman D, Lapey KA, Mick E, Lehman BK, Doyle A. Patterns of psychiatric comorbidity, cognition, and psychosocial functioning in adults with attention deficit hyperactivity disorder. *Am J Psychiatry.* 1993;150:1792-1798.
47. Biederman J, Faraone SV, Spencer T, Wilens T, Mick E, Lapey KA. Gender differences in a sample of adults with attention deficit hyperactivity disorder. *Psychiatry Res.* 1994;53:13-29.
48. Gfroerer JC, Hughes AL. The feasibility of collecting drug abuse data by telephone. *Public Health Rep.* 1991;106:384-383.
49. Johnson TP, Hougland JG, Clayton RR. Obtaining reports of sensitive behavior: a comparison of substance use reports from telephone and face-to-face interviews. *Soc Sci Q.* 1989;70:174-183.
50. Sobin C, Weissman MM, Goldstein R, Adams P, Wiekramaratne P, Warner V, Lish JD. Diagnostic interviewing for family studies: comparing telephone and face-to-face methods for the diagnosis of lifetime psychiatric disorders. *Psychiatr Genet.* 1993;3:227-233.
51. Wells KB, Burnam A, Leake B, Robins L. Agreement between face-to-face and telephone administered versions of the depression section of the NIMH Diagnostic Interview Schedule. *J Psychiatr Res.* 1988;22:207-220.
52. Paulsen AS, Crowe RR, Noyes R, Pfohl B. Reliability of the telephone interview in diagnosing anxiety disorders. *Arch Gen Psychiatry.* 1988;45:62-63.
53. Zimmerman M, Coryell WH. Diagnosing personality disorders in the community: a comparison of self-report and interview measures. *Arch Gen Psychiatry.* 1990;47:527-531.

ORIGINAL ARTICLE

Genetic-Environmental Interaction in the Genesis of Aggressivity and Conduct Disorders

Remi J. Cadoret, MD; William R. Yates, MD; Ed Troughton; George Woodworth, PhD; Mark A. Stewart, MD

Background: The purpose of this study was to determine the effect of an adverse adoptive home environment on adoptee conduct disorder, adult antisocial behavior, and two measures of aggressivity, all of which are behaviors that contribute to adult antisocial personality disorder and that also are associated with increased vulnerability to drug abuse and/or dependence.

Methods: The study used an adoption paradigm in which adopted offspring who were separated at birth from biologic parents with documented (by prison and hospital records) antisocial personality disorder and/or alcohol abuse or dependence were followed up as adults. They and their adoptive parents were interviewed in person. These adoptees were compared with controls whose biologic background was negative for documented psychopathologic behavior. Subjects were 95 male and 102 female adoptees and their adoptive parents.

Results: Multiple regression analysis was used to measure separately genetic and environmental effects. It showed that (1) a biologic background of antisocial personality disorder predicted increased adolescent aggressivity, conduct disorder, and adult antisocial behaviors, and (2) adverse adoptive home environment (defined as adoptive parents who had marital problems, were divorced, were separated, or had anxiety conditions, depression, substance abuse and/or dependence, or legal problems) independently predicted increased adult antisocial behaviors. Adverse adoptive home environment interacted with biologic background of antisocial personality disorder to result in significantly increased aggressivity and conduct disorder in adoptees in the presence of but not in the absence of a biologic background of antisocial personality disorder.

Conclusions: Environmental effects and genetic-environmental interaction account for significant variability in adoptee aggressivity, conduct disorder, and adult antisocial behavior and have important implications for the prevention and intervention of conduct disorder and associated conditions such as substance abuse and aggressivity.

(Arch Gen Psychiatry. 1995;52:916-924)

A NUMBER of studies have suggested that genetic factors interacting with the environment are etiologic in the genesis of childhood and adolescent conduct disorder and adult antisocial personality disorder.[1-3] Recently, Cadoret and colleagues demonstrated that, in both male and female adoptees, conduct disorder and aggressivity acted as important intervening variables in the relation between biologic parents with antisocial personality disorder and adoptee outcome for drug abuse and/or dependence (Cadoret et al[4] and R.J.C., W.R.Y., E.T., C. Cutrona, PhD, G.W., M.A.S., unpublished data, 1995). These studies showed evidence of two genetic factors leading to drug abuse. One factor, from alcoholic biologic parentage, correlated directly with drug abuse; the second factor, from biologic parents with antisocial personality disorder, led to conduct disorder, adolescent aggressivity, and then to adult antisocial personality disorder and drug abuse. It is this second genetic factor and its relationship to conduct disorder, aggressivity, and antisocial personality disorder that will be addressed in this article.

In both male and female adoptees, environmental variables defined by a variety of psychiatric and other problems in adoptive parents (alcoholism, anxiety conditions, depression, and marital problems, including separation

See Methods on next page

From the Departments of Psychiatry (Drs Cadoret, Yates, and Stewart, and Mr Troughton), Statistics (Dr Woodworth), and Preventive Medicine (Dr Woodworth), the University of Iowa, Iowa City.

METHODS

Details of the methods are available in Cadoret et al.[4] This section outlines the essentials of the methods only.

SUBJECT SELECTION

Subjects for this study were recruited from four adoption agencies: Lutheran Social Services of Iowa, Des Moines; Catholic Charities of the Archdiocese of Dubuque (Iowa), Hillcrest Family Services, Cedar Rapids, Iowa; and the Iowa Department of Human Services, Des Moines. Adoptees and their adoptive parents were selected on the basis of whether the adoptee had a biologic parent with alcohol or other drug abuse and/or dependence or antisocial personality disorder (experimental group) or whether there was no evidence from available records of biologic parent psychopathologic conditions (control group). Controls were matched to patients in the experimental group by agency, sex, age, and age of the biologic mother at the time of the adoptee's birth. All adoptees in the study had to have been separated at birth or within a few days from the biologic parent, placed with nonrelatives, and eventually adopted successfully by nonrelatives. Adoptees were further selected to be between 18 and 47 years of age at the time of the study.

Adoptive parents were initially contacted by the agency that handled the adoption. If these parents agreed to be contacted by the investigators, a research assistant explained the project and obtained written permission from both the adoptive parents and the adoptee to participate in the study. The contact procedure and permission request were designed to protect the confidentiality of adoptive families and were approved by the Human Subjects Internal Review Board of the University of Iowa College of Medicine, Iowa City.

DIAGNOSIS OF BIOLOGIC PARENTS

A method was devised to locate hospital and prison records of biologic parents in such a way that the names of parents were not revealed. Many institutional records did not contain enough information to make a diagnosis of antisocial personality disorder or substance abuse and/or dependence, eg, an emergency department visit for acute gastroenteritis. In those cases, subjects were not used in the study. Only when a diagnosis was made was that subject used in the study. Diagnoses were made as follows: institutional records were read independently by three psychiatrists (R.J.C., W.R.Y., and M.A.S.), and psychiatric diagnoses were made according to *DSM-III-R*[9] criteria. The κ statistics for diagnoses of substance abuse and antisocial personality disorder were satisfactory and ranged from 0.66 to 0.84 for biologic parent alcohol abuse and/or dependence and from 0.67 to 0.79 for antisocial personality disorder. Disagreements about diagnoses were settled by conference between the three judges. When agreement was not possible, these cases were discarded and not used in the study.

SUBJECT ATTRITION AND SELECTION BIAS

The overall refusal rate was 54%. There was no evidence that biologic parent status (control or experimental) was correlated with refusal.[4] The final sample consisted of 95 male and 102 female adoptees.

STUDY INSTRUMENTS AND THEIR ADMINISTRATION

All interviews were administered in person by a research assistant who was blind to the biologic background of the adoptee. The adoptive parent interview was administered to adoptive parents to gather information about adoptee physical health, temperament, development, and school achievement from infancy to adulthood. The interview also inquired into substance use and/or abuse in family members. Because the previous adoption study of Cadoret et al[10] found correlations between drug abuse and family disturbances such as separations, divorce, and psychiatric problems, the adoptee and adoptive parent interviews sought evidence of such problems as well as emotional or psychiatric problems in the adoptive household members, including the exposure of the adoptee to these situations. To further specify adoptive parent psychiatric problems, each parent was administered the Diagnostic Interview Schedule Screening Interview by computer. This screening instrument was used to minimize time commitments from subjects yet allow a psychiatric diagnosis to be made on the basis of a structured, self-administered instrument. Robins and Marcus[11] have shown sensitivities for diagnoses between the Diagnostic Interview Schedule Screening Interview and the *NIMH Diagnostic Interview Schedule, Version III, Revised.*[12] Diagnoses such as alcohol abuse, drug abuse, and antisocial personality disorder have sensitivities of greater than 95%. Only two diagnoses had sensitivities less than 75%: cognitive impairment and somatization disorder. Remaining diagnoses such as depression had intermediate sensitivities.

Adoptees received the *NIMH Diagnostic Interview Schedule, Version III, Revised* described by Robins et al.[12] Additional demographic data was collected from adoptees as well as information about the adoptive environment, including behavior or psychiatric problems in sibs and parents.

DIAGNOSIS OF ADOPTEE OUTCOME

DSM-III-R criteria were used to characterize adoptee psychiatric outcome. Aggressivity in the adoptee was measured by a scale devised by Loney et al.[13] An additional five items were added to this scale.[4] Aggressivity was measured by the sum of these items. Adolescent conduct disorder was defined by the sum of endorsed items from Robins,[2] such as truancy, school expulsion, lying, and stealing. These items from Robins had been used in the *DSM-III*[14] as criteria that had to occur prior to age 15 years to make an adult diagnosis of antisocial personality disorder. Four adoptee outcome variables were used for this study to characterize the conduct disorder path. These were defined as follows: (1) childhood aggression, the sum of 16 items from the parent interview detailing aggressive behaviors during the preschool and grade school years; (2) adolescent aggressivity, the sum of the items in the modified scale from Loney et al[13] described above; (3) conduct disorder, the sum of the items from Robins[2] described above; and (4) adult antisocial behavior, the sum of *DSM-III* adult behavior criterion items for the diagnosis of antisocial personality disorder.

Continued on next page

ASSESSMENT OF ENVIRONMENTAL FACTORS

Both sources of information, the parent interview and the adoptee interview, were used to determine the presence of a substance abuse problem or an anxiety or depression diagnosis in adoptive parents or siblings. The presence of a marital problem, including divorce or separation, or serious physical health problems in family members was also determined from the adoptee and adoptive parent interviews.

Diagnosis of potentially adverse adoptive parent conditions made from interviews, including the Diagnostic Interview Schedule Screening Interview, included such factors as anxiety conditions (phobias, general anxiety disorder, panic disorder, and agoraphobia), depression, marital problems (including separation and divorce), legal problems, and alcohol and other drug problems. Adverse adoptive home environment factor was equivalent to the total number of the following conditions that were met: presence of a marital problem in adoptive parents; divorce or separation of adoptive parents; alcohol or other drug abuse and/or dependence in a parent; depression in a parent; anxiety condition in a parent (eg, panic disorder and generalized anxiety disorder); other psychopathologic condition in a parent (eg, conduct disorder and somatization); and legal problems in a parent.

The distribution of this composite variable is shown in **Table 1**. This is the same variable that was found to predict adult antisocial personality disorder as a main effect in log-linear analyses in this sample.[4]

STATISTICAL METHODS

The purpose of this study was to examine more closely for genetic-environmental interaction the conduct disorder pathway between a biologic parent with antisocial personality disorder and adoptee outcome variables (conduct disorder and aggressivity), which lead to substance abuse and adult antisocial personality disorder. The original analysis had used log-linear methods to construct models. To focus on the conduct disorder path and to have more power to detect interaction by using ordinal or interval variables, a series of linear multiple regression models was developed to assess the influence of genetic factors, environmental factors, and their interactions.

The basic multiple regression model started with biologic variables of parent with antisocial personality disorder (X_1) or alcoholism (X_2) as independent variables. There were 21 alcoholic biologic mothers in the data who had a record of drinking during the pregnancy of adoptees in this study. Thus, the environmental factor of drinking during pregnancy was confounded with biologic parent alcoholism. To control for this confound, a separate independent variable was added to model 1 as X_3, biologic mother who used alcohol during adoptee pregnancy. Four measures of adoptee outcome (aggressivity as a child, aggressivity as an adolescent, conduct disorder, and adult antisocial behavior) were included as dependent variables (Y_1 to Y_4), resulting in model 1:

$$(1) \qquad Y_n = C + B_1X_1 + B_2X_2 + B_3X_3,$$

where C represents a constant, and B, the regression coefficient.

From model 1, the importance of the genetic factors (including the antenatal exposure to alcohol, which was largely confounded with alcoholism in biologic mothers) could be determined as measured by the R^2 of the model. The second step involved adding environmental factors to model 1. Accordingly, the composite variable of the adverse adoptive home environment conditions (E) was added to the basic model, resulting in model 2:

$$(2) \qquad Y_n = C + B_1X_1 + B_2X_2 + B_3X_3 + B_eE.$$

Environmental effects were assessed both by differences in R^2 or proportion of variance accounted for in the dependent variables by the addition of the environmental variable and by the significance level of the individual regression coefficient of the environmental variable.

Another measure of environmental effect is the genetic-environmental interaction, or the change in manifestation of an environmental factor determined by the presence or absence of a genetic factor. To assess genetic-environmental interaction, three additional terms were added to model 2, consisting of cross products of each genetic factor with the environmental factor ($X_1 \times E$, $X_2 \times E$, and $X_3 \times E$) resulting in model 3:

$$(3) \qquad Y_n = C + B_1X_1 + B_2X_2 + B_3X_3 + B_eE + B_{i1}(X_1 \times E) + B_{i2}(X_2 \times E) + B_{i3}(X_3 \times E),$$

where B_{i1} through B_{i3} are regression coefficients associated with the interaction terms. Again, the R^2 of each of these models can be compared with the corresponding R^2 from model 2 to assess the significance of adding the terms measuring interaction.

Regression analysis was used to assess the significance of the fit of each model, to determine the significance of each separate term's contribution to the model, to determine the improvement in fit from one model to another, and to determine the effect of sex of adoptee on the four outcome measures. Probability for individual terms in each model were computed on the basis that each variable was the last to be entered into the model. In this way, the presence of all other factors in the model was controlled.

and divorce) increased the probability of development of adoptee conduct disorder as well as a related condition, adoptee aggressivity (Cadoret et al[4] and R.J.C., W.R.Y., E.T., C. Cutrona, PhD, G.W., M.A.S., unpublished data, 1995). This effect was independent of the genetic influence of biologic parents with alcoholism or antisocial personality disorder. The finding of significant environmental factors influencing adoptee conduct disorder and aggressivity in the pathway from biologic parent with antisocial personality disorder to adoptee drug abuse and/or dependence raised the question of the role of genetic-environmental interaction as an additional factor. This interaction is the focus of this article.

Literature from previous adoption studies indicates that the genetic-environmental interaction is of importance in the genesis of antisocial behavior. Relevant to the present study are the findings from three independent earlier adoption studies.[5] Two of these studies[6,7] showed a genetic-environmental interaction between a

Table 1. Distribution of Count for the Variable Adverse Adoptive Home Environment

Adverse Factors Present, No.	No. (%) of Families
0	58 (29.4)
1	54 (27.4)
2	41 (20.8)
3	23 (11.7)
4	13 (6.6)
5	5 (2.5)
6	3 (1.5)

genetic background of alcoholic and/or antisocial behavior and an adverse adoptive home environment (defined as a psychiatric or behavioral problem in adoptive parent or sib or adoptive parents who experience marital separation or divorce). The nature of the interaction was such that an adverse adoptive home environment in the presence of a genetic factor contributed by a parent with alcoholism and/or antisocial personality disorder produced a much higher number of adolescent conduct disorder symptoms than would be predicted by either genetic or environmental factors acting independently. The third study showed a significant interaction between adoptee age at the time of adoptive placement and a genetic background of alcoholism and/or antisocial personality disorder.[5] Later age at placement in the adoptive home in the presence of the genetic diathesis for alcoholism and/or antisocial personality disorder resulted in a significant increase in conduct disorder behaviors in adolescence.

A later adoption study[8] from a different agency also showed a significant genetic-environmental interaction between genetic diatheses for alcoholism and/or antisocial personality disorder and psychiatric or alcohol problems in the adoptive family for adoptee conduct disorder behaviors. Again the adverse adoptive home environment produced a much higher number of conduct behaviors in the presence of the genetic diathesis.

See also pages 895, 900, 906, and 925

Thus, at least four independent adoption studies[5,6] have demonstrated a significant genetic-environmental interaction in the genesis of adolescent conduct disorder behavior. One of the studies has suggested sex differences in the genetic and environmental factors important to conduct disorder,[6] but these studies characterized the biologic parents only through adoption agency records, which did not allow an unequivocal diagnosis of biologic backgrounds such as alcoholism or antisocial personality disorder. Only one of the studies[7] used prison records of biologic parents and was able to thereby diagnose antisocial personality disorder. That study showed the interaction between a parent with antisocial personality disorder and the adverse adoptive home environment variable described above.

The present study was able to use hospital and prison records of biologic parents to diagnose substance abuse and antisocial personality disorder. Adoptive home environment was better characterized by the use of multiple informants and by the administration of a structured psychiatric interview to the adoptive parents. This article will describe the evidence for genetic-environmental interaction found between biologic factors of antisocial personality disorder and alcoholism and adverse home environment in the genesis of conduct disorder, aggressivity, and adult antisocial behaviors, which contribute to vulnerability to drug and alcohol abuse and to adult antisocial personality disorder.

RESULTS

A regression analysis fitting the three models using the total data set of male and female adoptees showed that there were no significant male-female differences in genetic, environmental, or genetic-environmental interaction effects. In this analysis, a sex term, sex by genetics, sex by environment, and a triple interaction term, sex by genetics by environment, were included in the model tested. None of the added interaction terms were significant. The sex term was significant, as would be expected, because men generally rate higher on aggressivity, conduct disorder, and antisocial behavior. However, inclusion of a sex term in models involving the total sample did not change the estimate of the significance of the individual terms (genetic, environmental, and genetic-environmental) in the models, and, in the analyses that follow, results are presented for the total sample across sex of adoptee.

Linear regression was used on untransformed dependent variables for these analyses. Examination of the dependent variables showed a J-shaped distribution for each, with the modal value at zero, a distribution commonly found with psychopathologic variables. This intrinsic skewing cannot be transformed to normality, but the regressions were rerun using logarithmic transformation, log $(Y+1)$; the logarithmic-logarithmic transformation, log [log $(Y+1) + 1$]; and the inverse transformation, $-1/(Y+1)$, and the same pattern of significant interactions occurred. As an additional check, the models were fit using ordinal logistic regression, and, in this analysis, the pattern of significant interaction was the same as the linear regression analyses with untransformed variables. Although transformation of the dependent variable in some cases may reduce or eliminate mild interactions, it typically has little effect on strong interactions, so that it is not at all paradoxical that the same interactions may appear under several transformations of the dependent variable. Accordingly, we will present the linear regression analyses with untransformed variables herein.

Table 2 shows the results of fitting model 1 to the four behavioral outcome variables. The significance of the overall fit of the model is given in the first column, the R^2 value, and, as expected, the results reflect the correlations reported from the log-linear analyses. Significant individual effects are limited largely to the genetic factor of parent with antisocial personality disorder (X_2), as expected from the log-linear models described previously (Cadoret et al[4] and R.J.C., W.R.Y., E.T., C. Cutrona, PhD, G.W., M.A.S., unpublished data, 1995). A heretofore unreported effect is the significant correlation between having a biologic mother who was known to drink alcohol during her pregnancy (Table 2) and conduct disorder and adult antisocial behavior. The direction of the effect is for maternal drinking during pregnancy to be associated with an increase in these types of behaviors as indicated by the positive regression coefficients shown in Table 2.

Table 3 presents the results of fitting model 2 to the four behavioral outcomes variables. The main feature shown by the R^2 values is a general improvement in fit accomplished through the addition of the environmental factor of adoptive homes with adverse parental conditions. This is shown graphically in **Figure 1**. Two of the four models show a significant improvement in dependent variable prediction: conduct disorder and adult antisocial behavior. The direction of effect, as shown in Table 3 (last column), is for increased amount of psychopathologic conditions to be associated with an increased number of adverse adoptive home environment factors. Thus, the results support the conclusion of a significant environmental effect, which was demonstrated by the log-linear modeling (Cadoret et al[4] and R.J.C., W.R.Y., E.T., C. Cutrona, PhD, G.W., M.A.S., unpublished data, 1995). The next step in the analysis was to add genetic-environmental interaction terms to model 2.

Table 4 shows the results of adding the three genetic-environmental interaction terms to model 2. Three of the four genetic-environmental interaction terms for biologic parent with antisocial personality disorder by adverse adoptive home environment are significant ("$X_2 \times E$" column), and overall, the addition of genetic-environmental interaction terms increases R^2 significantly for the same three dependent variables: childhood aggressivity, adolescent aggressivity, and conduct disorder (Figure 1). The nature of these interactions is clarified by **Figure 2** through **Figure 4**, in which the interaction is graphed by plotting predicted outcome, eg, aggressivity, against increasing adverse adoptive home environment factors for adoptees with and without a biologic background of a parent with antisocial personality disorder. All three figures show that in the absence of a biologic parent with antisocial personality disorder, there is no correlation between adoptee outcome and adverse adoptive home environment (broken line, Figures 2 through 4). In contrast, the adverse adoptive home environment–outcome relationship is significant only for adoptees with a biologic parent with antisocial personality disorder (solid line, Figures 2 through 4).

Table 2. Genetic-Environmental Factors in Behavior Disorder Pathway to Drug Abuse: Model 1*

Dependent Variable	R^2	Alcoholic Biologic Parent (X_1)	Biologic Parent With Antisocial Personality Disorder (X_2)	Prenatal Alcohol Exposure (X_3)
Childhood aggressivity	.02	−.01	.15†	.02
Adolescent aggressivity	.09‡	.05	.26§	.06
Conduct disorder	.07§	0	.19‖	.15‖
Adult antisocial behavior	.10‡	.01	.10	.28‡

Values are R^2 values (column 1) and standardized regression coefficients (columns 2 through 4).
†*Significant at P=.10.*
‡*Significant at P=.001.*
§*Significant at P=.01.*
‖*Significant at P=.05.*

COMMENT

The findings of genetic-environmental interaction in these studies confirm the importance of such interactions in the genesis of conduct disorder and aggressivity. Adult antisocial behavior does not show the genetic-environmental effect demonstrated by aggression and conduct disorder (Table 4) but does show a main effect for environment, the adverse adoptive home environment factor. The lack of genetic-environmental interaction is also apparent from the R^2s of the three models predicting adult antisocial behavior (Figure 1). Reasons for failure to demonstrate a role for the genetic-environmental interaction in adult antisocial behaviors are not apparent. There are many possible explanations, such as other environmental (or genetic) factors operating in early adulthood to modify the conduct disorder trajectory. For example, the finding in these data that prenatal exposure to alcohol was a factor in significantly increasing adult antisocial symptoms (Tables 1 through 3) demonstrates the operation of other factors modifying adult behavior.

The variable of adverse adoptive home environment is similar to that of previous studies detailed in the intro-

Table 3. Genetic-Environmental Factors in Behavior Disorder Pathway to Drug Abuse: Model 2*

Dependent Variable	R^2	Alcoholic Biologic Parent (X_1)	Biologic Parent With Antisocial Personality Disorder (X_2)	Prenatal Alcohol Exposure (X_3)	Adverse Adoptive Home Environment (E)
Childhood aggressivity	.04	−.04	.16†	.01	.14‡
Adolescent aggressivity	.13§	.01	.28§	.05	.19‖
Conduct disorder	.13§	−.04	.22‖	.12†	.25§
Adult antisocial behavior	.15§	−.03	.13†	.26§	.23§

Values are R^2 values (column 1) and standardized regression coefficients (columns 2 through 5).
†*Significant at P=.05.*
‡*Significant at P=.10.*
§*Significant at P=.001.*
‖*Significant at P=.01.*

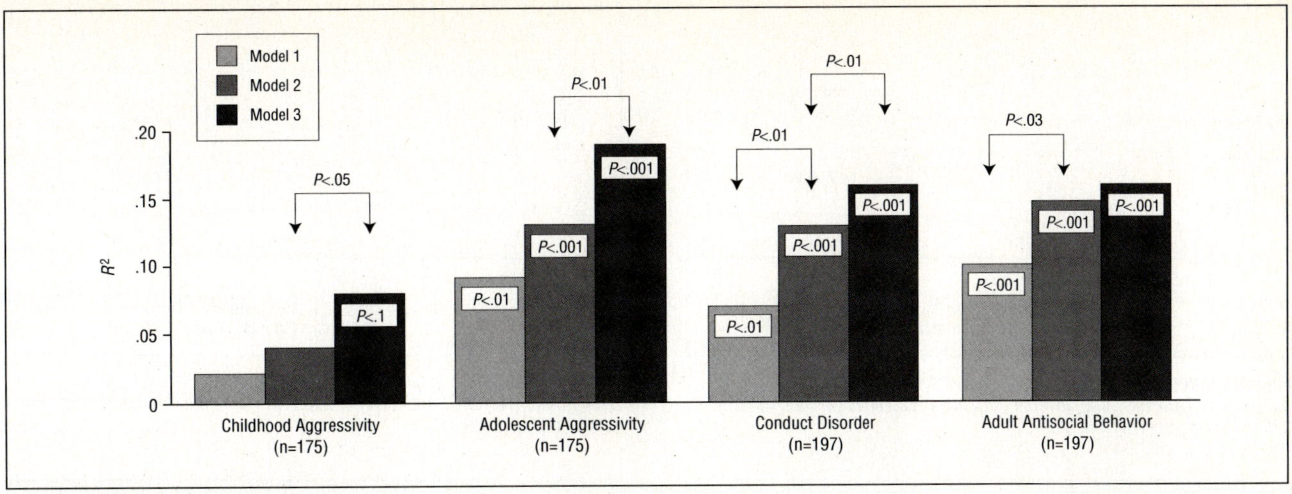

Figure 1. *Amount of variance in behavior disorders controlled by three different models of genetic-environmental factors. For an explanation of the three models, see the "Statistical Methods" subsection of the "Methods" section. The probability for the null hypothesis that $R^2=0$ is indicated in the box in each significance bar.*

Table 4. Genetic-Environmental Factors and Their Interaction in the Behavior Disorder Pathway: Model 3*

Dependent Variable	R^2	Alcoholic Biologic Parent (X_1)	Biologic Parent With Antisocial Personality Disorder (X_2)	Prenatal Alcohol Exposure (X_3)	Adverse Adoptive Home Environment (E)	Interactions ($X_1 \times E$)	Interactions ($X_2 \times E$)	Interactions ($X_3 \times E$)
Childhood aggressivity	.08†	0	.15†	−.03	.33‡	−.07	.22‡	.09
Adolescent aggressivity	.19§	.04	.27§	.03	.23	−.10†	.31§	−.12
Conduct disorder	.16§	−.02	.21‖	.08	.44§	−.06	.23‖	.09
Adult antisocial behavior	.16§	−.03	.13†	.24‖	.32‡	.06	.08	.05

**Values are R^2 values (column 1) and standardized regression coefficients (columns 2 through 8).*
†*Significant at P=.10.*
‡*Significant at P=.05.*
§*Significant at P=.0001.*
‖*Significant at P=.01.*

duction.[5,6] In this study, it was possible to specify the genetic background more exactly through the use of prison and hospital records and to separate the genetic factors associated with alcohol abuse from those contributing to antisocial personality disorder. The results herein show that it is the genetic diathesis for antisocial personality disorder, not that for alcoholism, that interacts with the adverse adoptive home environment to produce a significant increase in conduct disorder and aggressivity in adoptees. A previous independent adoption study by Crowe[7] found a similar interaction between biologic parent with antisocial personality disorder (diagnosed by prison records) and adverse adoptive home environment (reviewed in Cadoret et al[5]). In the remaining previously studied samples reported by Cadoret et al,[5,8] interaction was reported in both men and women and for the combination of biologic backgrounds of alcohol and of antisocial personality disorder. However, in those studies, biologic parent diagnosis was determined from adoption agency records only, so there is more uncertainty as to the validity of the distinction in those studies between genetic diatheses for alcoholism and antisocial personality disorder.

In the log-linear models that were fit to these data (Cadoret et al[4] and R.J.C., W.R.Y., E.T., C. Cutrona, PhD, G.W., M.A.S., unpublished data, 1995), no evidence of genetic-environmental interaction was found. In part, this failure to detect interactions in the log-linear modeling reflects the fact that information is lost in the formation of dichotomous variables in the log-linear situation. In the linear regression models herein, both the dependent variables and the adverse home environment factor were used in their full range of values, thus providing more information and increased power to detect interaction.

In two of the studies described in the introduction,[15,16] there was evidence for an environmental effect of adoptee age at the time of adoptive home placement on adolescent conduct disorder: adoptees who were older at placement showed more conduct disorder symptoms during adolescence. In one of these studies (reviewed in Cadoret et al[5]), there was a significant genetic-environmental interaction, with biologic parent with alcoholism and/or antisocial personality disorder and age of placement resulting in an increased number of conduct disorder behaviors. In the present study, no environmental or genetic-environmental effect was found involving age of adoptee at placement in the adoptive home. Reasons for this failure at replication are not clear.

Many variables affect the variability of age at placement. For example, in the early studies reported by Cadoret and Cain,[6,15] more adoptees were adopted after hav-

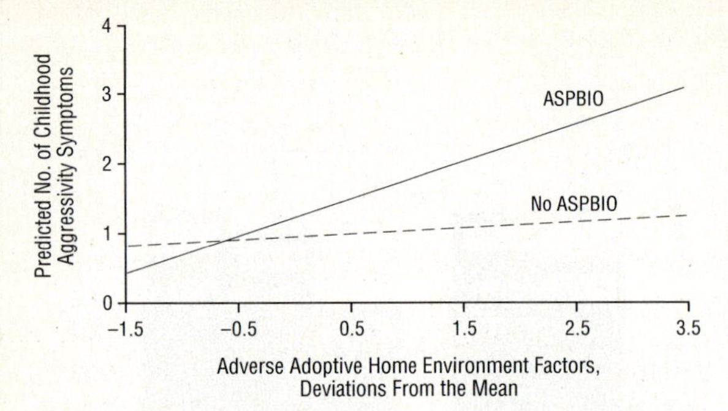

Figure 2. *Interaction between antisocial personality disorder biologic background (ASPBIO) and adverse adoptive home environment: effect on childhood aggressivity (n=175).*

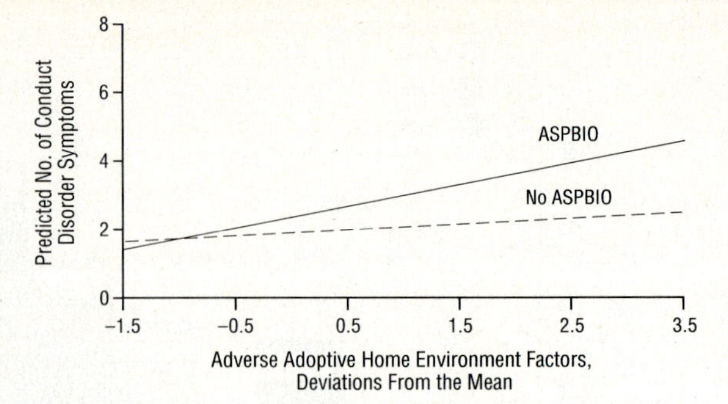

Figure 4. *Interaction between antisocial personality disorder biologic background (ASPBIO) and adverse adoptive home environment: effect on conduct disorder (n=197).*

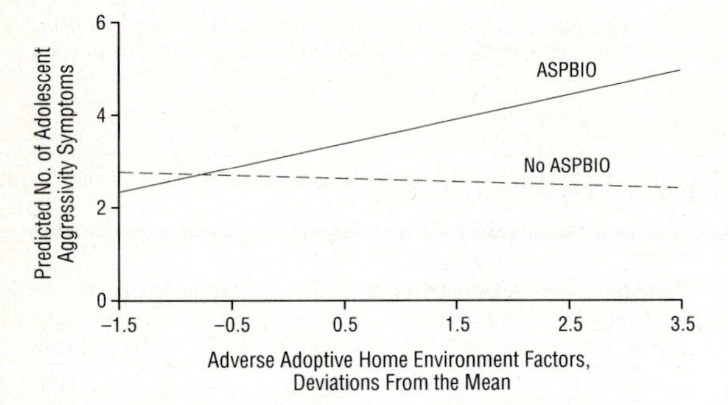

Figure 3. *Interaction between antisocial personality disorder biologic background (ASPBIO) and adverse adoptive home environment: effect on adolescent aggressivity (n=175).*

Table 5. Score Distribution for Adverse Adoptive Home Environment in Adoptees With and Without a Background of Antisocial Personality Disorder

	Antisocial Personality Disorder Background*	
Score	Yes	No
0	15 (27)	43 (30.3)
1	17 (31)	37 (26.1)
2	14 (26)	27 (19.0)
3	4 (7)	19 (13.4)
4	4 (7)	9 (6.3)
5	0	5 (3.5)
6	1 (2)	2 (1.4)

*Values are No. (%) of adoptees. Percentages are based on column totals.

ing spent their first 6 months in foster care or in home management homes on a college campus where they were cared for by a number of undergraduate students enrolled in a home economics course. This experience was associated with several behavioral manifestations later in life: increased affective symptoms[17] and increased conduct disorder symptoms.[8] Adoptees in the present study were not involved in the home management situation, and more were placed directly with adoptive families, thus bypassing foster care and later placement and generally resulting in earlier placement.

One of the factors in the model that showed a significant effect on outcome (Tables 2 through 4, "Prenatal Alcohol Exposure" column) is having a biologic mother who was drinking while pregnant with the proband adoptee. There were 21 of these mothers in the sample, most of whom also had diagnoses of alcohol abuse and/or dependence. Thus, the observed effect could be environmental (due to alcohol intake during pregnancy or some other associated adverse factor such as smoking, poor diet, or use of other drugs) or could be considered a genetic-environmental interaction. It is not likely to represent a purely genetic factor because alcoholic biologic parents did not produce this effect in their offspring when controlling for maternal drinking (Tables 2 through 4). In support of the effect being related to maternal drinking during pregnancy (or other variables such as associated smoking, other drug use, and poor nutrition) is the fact that the offspring of these 21 drinking mothers had significantly lower birth weights than the remaining sample of adoptees.[4] The results suggest that prenatal exposure to alcohol could represent an additional vulnerability to adult antisocial behavior and ultimately to drug abuse and/or dependence in offspring.

One interpretation of the adoptee outcomes–adverse adoptive home environment correlation would suggest that aggressive, conduct disorder behaviors in adoptees causes increased parental distress, which would manifest as a higher number of adverse home environment factors. This interpretation, however, is inconsistent with the findings that show that the score distribution of the adverse home environment factor is the same when comparing families with adoptees from backgrounds of antisocial personality disorder with those families whose adoptees do not have a parent with antisocial personality disorder. This similarity of score distribution is shown in **Table 5**. There is no evidence that biologic parents with antisocial personality disorder caused an increase in the number of adverse adoptive home environment factors. This finding is also an argument against a selective placement hypothesis, which would claim that children from a biologic background of antisocial personality disorder are more likely to be placed into more disturbed families. Figures 2 through 4 show that in the absence of a biologic background of antisocial personality disorder, there is essentially a zero slope relating the number of adverse home environment factors and aggressivity or conduct disorder. This is compatible with a direction of effect from parent to adoptee rather than adoptee to parent. Thus, the evidence from the genetic-environmental interaction data is consistent with the interpretation that the adverse home environment factors result in increased aggressive and conduct disorder behaviors in the presence of a biologic background of antisocial personality disorder.

The environmental effects and their interaction reported herein are important for the prevention of conduct disorders, aggressivity, and associated substance abuse. The interaction results show that antisocial behaviors and aggressivity are increased in the presence of predisposing genetic factors. These adverse environments are ubiquitous but are likely to be especially increased in families of persons with antisocial personality disorder, where marital problems and substance abuse are extremely common.[1-3] The environment in the present study as defined by adverse home environment factors is undoubtedly less extreme than would be the case for individuals exposed to parents with antisocial personality disorder. We would predict more marked environmental effects in that situation. These considerations would lead to action to protect genetically predisposed individuals from these adverse environments. In child psychiatry, aggressivity and conduct disorder combine in the clinical entity of the unsocialized aggressive child.[18] Aggressivity has been shown to lead to less improvement in children with conduct disorder.[19] The present finding relating both aggressivity and conduct disorder to a biologic background of antisocial personality disorder is compatible with findings from family studies associating aggressive conduct disorder with parents with antisocial personality disorder.[20]

In addition to aggressive conduct disorder, behaviors of aggressivity and conduct disorder are of special importance in predicting drug abuse.[21-23] Childhood and adolescent aggression have been implicated as risk factors in the transition from moderate to heavy use of drugs[24] and in the transition both from no drug use to drug use and from drug use to abuse.[25] There is suggestive evidence that aggressivity predicts substance abuse independently of such variables as hyperactivity[26,27] and conduct disorder.[28] Conduct disorder is well documented as a factor in drug abuse and/or dependence in both men and women.[28-30] The present adoption study is compatible with the role of aggressivity and conduct disorder in substance abuse described above but reports for the first time to our knowledge the importance of both genetic and environmental factors acting in an interactive fashion, so that the environmental factor depends on the presence of a particular genetic background for its effect. The adverse home environment factor described herein as interacting with the biologic background of antisocial personality disorder could have influenced the adoptee through such influences as altered parental affection, availability, and involvement, which are parental behaviors that have been reported to have an effect on both aggressivity and drug use.[31] The present data would suggest that such parental effects act through genetic-environmental interaction.

Examples of genetic-environmental interaction rarely have been described in human behavior and may just reflect the fact that very few adoption studies are available to measure such effects directly. One study of adopted offspring of criminal parents did look at the effect of criminal adoptive parents on criminality and was unable to find evidence for a genetic-environmental interaction,[32] although there was evidence for genetic transmission of criminality. However, a recent adoption study of schizophrenia from Finland has reported a genetic-environmental interaction: disturbed adoptive families were more likely to produce disturbed adoptees if the latter were offspring of schizophrenic mothers.[33] Subjects with a genetic predisposition for schizophrenia appeared to be more vulnerable to a disturbed adoptive family environment, an interaction similar to the type described herein with conduct disorder and aggressivity.

Genetic-environmental interaction has also been reported in a previous Iowa adoption study. Cutrona et al[34] reported an interaction between family conflict and adoptive family psychopathologic conditions and a biologic background of alcoholism. Among women with at least one alcoholic biologic parent, the presence of conflict (reported by the adoptive parents) or adoptive family psychopathologic conditions increased the chance of adoptee alcohol abuse and/or dependence. No evidence for similar interactions were found for men.

In a similar vein, there is little direct evidence in the literature for genetic inheritance of aggressivity. A recent review of 12 published twin studies of aggressiveness showed that eight were consistent with a genetic effect.[35] An additional twin study from Iowa found a significant heritability in both boys (78%) and girls (36%) for aggressivity.[36] While, to our knowledge, no adoption study relates aggressivity in biologic parents to aggressivity in offspring, one study that correlated psychiatric disorders in adoptive and biologic parents of adoptees with aggressive conduct disorder in children found a significant increase of biologic fathers with antisocial personality disorder among the biologic parents of the adoptees with conduct disorder.[37] This result is compatible with the present data and suggests inheritance of aggressiveness from a parent with antisocial personality disorder because antisocial personality disorder is associated with increased aggressivity.[38]

The finding of nonadditive effects as shown in Figures 2 through 4 for aggressivity and conduct disorder raises the question of what genetic mechanism could account for these results. Kendler and Eaves[39] present three major models for the joint effect of genes and environment on the liability to psychiatric illness. Their first model of simple additivity of genetic and environmental factors is rejected by these findings. Their second model is compatible with these data and proposes a genetic control of sensitivity to effects of the environment. The third model proposed by Kendler and Eaves is not compatible with these data. This third model proposes that there is genetic control of an individual's exposure to the environment as, for example, an individual whose personality traits lead him or her to experience stressful events, which in turn precipitate psychiatric illness. In the present situation, adoptees are not in a position to seek out disturbed parents, who occur with equal frequency in adoptees from control as well as alcoholic biologic backgrounds. It appears that the differential sensitivity model is closer to the present facts.

Knowledge that genetic-environmental interaction is

important in aggressivity and conduct disorder could be of importance in the current efforts to link human behaviors with biologic factors in molecular genetics. In these studies, efforts are made to correlate behavioral outcome with the presence of certain genomes. Interaction effects could be important in the analysis of genetic association studies in which correlations are sought between clinical conditions and the presence of a particular allele of a candidate gene or in linkage studies or other genetic analyses such as segregation analyses.[40] Thus, the interaction findings of this study are of relevance to both basic science, eg, in correlating behavior with molecular genetic factors, and applied social science, for example, in determining high-risk populations that are especially vulnerable to common environmental factors, such as adverse parenting, for the purpose of intervention and prevention. Awareness that genetic-environmental interaction occurs with such common conditions as described in this article should also lead to important changes in mathematical models used in behavior genetics, which sometimes assume that there is no genetic-environmental interaction to simplify model fitting.[41]

Accepted for publication March 29, 1995.

This work was supported by grant RO1 DA05821 from the National Institute on Drug Abuse, Rockville, Md.

We wish to acknowledge the cooperation of the following individuals and agencies in making this study possible: James Yeast, Catholic Charities of the Archdiocese of Dubuque; Craig Mosher, PhD, and Nancylee Ziese, Hillcrest Family Services; Paul Loeffelholz, MD, Iowa Department of Corrections, Des Moines; Marge Corkery, Iowa Department of Human Services; and Leonard Larson, PhD, Lyn Lienhard, and Louise Koch, Lutheran Social Service of Iowa. We thank the following individuals who performed data collection for this study: Michelle Appel, Alberta Conrad, Nancy Copeland, Donna Davis, Rebecca Hansel, Roxane Moller, Carol Moss, Scott Murray, Helen Peck, Chris Richards, Jody Speer, Sommai Ung, and Angela Wright.

Reprint requests to University of Iowa Hospitals and Clinics, 200 Hawkins Dr, No. 2887 JP, Iowa City, IA 52242-1057 (Dr Cadoret).

REFERENCES

1. Glueck S, Glueck E. *Delinquents and Nondelinquents in Persepctive.* Cambridge, Mass: Harvard University Press; 1968.
2. Robins LN. *Deviant Children Grown Up.* Baltimore, Md: Williams & Wilkins; 1966.
3. West DJ, Farrington DP. *The Delinquent Way of Life.* London, England: Heinemann Medical Books; 1977.
4. Cadoret RJ, Yates WR, Troughton E, Woodworth G, Stewart MA. Adoption study demonstrating two genetic pathways to drug abuse. *Arch Gen Psychiatry.* 1995;52:42-52.
5. Cadoret RJ, Cain CA, Crowe RR. Evidence for gene-environment interaction in the development of adolescent antisocial behavior. *Behav Genet.* 1983;13:301-310.
6. Cadoret RJ, Cain CA. Environmental and genetic factors in predicting adolescent antisocial behavior in adoptees. *Psychiatr J Univ Ottawa.* 1981;6:220-225.
7. Crowe RR. An adoption study of antisocial personality. *Arch Gen Psychiatry.* 1974;31:785-791.
8. Cadoret RJ. Genes, environment and their interaction in the development of psychopathology. In: Sakai T, Tsuboi T, eds. *Genetic Aspects of Human Behavior.* Tokyo, Japan: Igaku-Shoin; 1985:165-175.
9. American Psychiatric Association. *Diagnostic and Statistical Manual of Mental Disorders, Revised Third Edition.* Washington, DC: American Psychiatric Association; 1987.
10. Cadoret RJ, Troughton E, O'Gorman TW, Heywood E. An adoption study of genetic and environmental factors in drug abuse. *Arch Gen Psychiatry.* 1986;43:1131-1136.
11. Robins LN, Marcus SC. The diagnostic screening procedure writer: a tool to develop individualized screening procedures. *Med Care.* 1987;25:5106-5122.
12. Robins L, Helzer J, Cottler L, Goldring E. *NIMH Diagnostic Interview Schedule, Version III, Revised (DIS-III-R).* St Louis, Mo: Washington University School of Medicine; 1989.
13. Loney J, Langhorne JE, Paternite CE, Whaley-Klahn M, Blair-Broeker CT, Hacker M. The Iowa habit: hyperkinetic/aggressive boys in treatment. In: Sells SB, Crandall R, Roff M, Strauss JS, Pollin W, eds. *Human Functioning in Longitudinal Perspective.* Baltimore, Md: Williams & Wilkins; 1980.
14. American Psychiatric Association. *Diagnostic and Statistical Manual of Mental Disorders, Third Edition.* Washington, DC: American Psychiatric Association; 1980.
15. Cadoret RJ, Cain CA. Sex differences in predictors of antisocial behavior in adoptees. *Arch Gen Psychiatry.* 1980;37:1171-1173.
16. Cadoret R, Cunningham L, Loftus R, Edwards J. Studies of adoptees from psychiatrically disturbed biological parents, II. *J Pediatrics.* 1975;87:301-306.
17. Cadoret RJ, Troughton E, Merchant LM, Whitters A. Early life psychosocial events and adult affective symptoms. In: Robins L, Rutter M, eds. *Straight and Devious Pathways from Childhood to Adulthood.* New York, NY: Cambridge University Press; 1990:300-313.
18. Stewart MA. Aggressive conduct disorder: a brief review. *Aggressive Behav.* 1985;11:323-331.
19. Stewart MA, Behar D. Subtypes of aggressive conduct disorder. *Acta Psychiatr Scand.* 1983;68:178-185.
20. Stewart MA, Leone L. A family study of unsocialized aggressive boys. *Biol Psychiatry.* 1978;13:107-117.
21. Kellam SG, Brown CH, Rubin BR, Ensminger ME. Paths leading to teenage psychiatric symptoms and substance use: developmental epidemiological studies in Woodlawn. In: Guze SB, Barrett JE, eds. *Childhood Psychopathology and Development.* New York, NY: Raven Press; 1983:17-47.
22. Kandel DB. *Longitudinal Research on Drug Use.* Washington, DC: Hemisphere Publishing Corp; 1978.
23. Penning M, Barnes GE. Adolescent marijuana use: a review. *Int J Addict.* 1982;17:749-791.
24. Brook JS, Cohen P, Whiteman M, Gordon AS. Psychosocial risk factors in the transition from moderate to heavy use or abuse of drugs. In: Glantz M, Pickens R, eds. *Vulnerability to Drug Abuse.* Washington, DC: American Psychological Association; 1992:359-388.
25. Cadoret RJ. Genetic and environmental factors in initiation of drug use and the transition to abuse. In: Glantz M, Pickens R, eds. *Vulnerability to Drug Abuse.* Washington, DC: American Psychological Association; 1992:99-113.
26. Loney J, Kramer J, Milich R. The hyperactive child grows up: predictors of symptoms, delinquency and achievement at follow-up. In: Gadow K, Loney J, eds. *Psychosocial Aspects of Drug Treatment for Hyperactivity.* Boulder, Colo: Westview Press; 1981:381-415.
27. Halikas JA, Meller J, Morse C, Lyttle MD. Predicting substance abuse in juvenile offenders. *Child Psychiatry Hum Dev.* 1990;21:49-55.
28. Henn FA, Bardwell R, Jenkins R. Juvenile delinquents revisited: adult criminal activity. *Arch Gen Psychiatry.* 1980;37:1160-1163.
29. Robins LN. The consequences of conduct disorder in girls. In: Olweus D, Yarrow MR, eds. *Development of Antisocial and Prosocial Behavior.* Orlando, Fla: Academic Press Inc; 1985:385-414.
30. Robins LN, McEvoy L. Conduct problems as predictors of substance abuse. In: Robins LN, Rutter M, eds. *Straight and Devious Pathways from Childhood to Adulthood.* New York, NY: Cambridge University Press; 1990:182-204.
31. Brook JS, Whiteman M, Brook DW, Gordon AS. Sibling influences on adolescent drug use. *J Am Acad Child Adolesc Psychiatry.* 1991;30:958-966.
32. Mednick SA, Moffitt T, Gabriellei W, Hutchings B. Genetic factors in criminal behavior: a review. In: Olweus D, Block J, Radke-Yarrow M, eds. *Development of Antisocial and Prosocial Behavior: Research, Theories, and Issues.* Orlando, Fla: Academic Press; 1985:33-50.
33. Tienari P. Interaction between genetic vulnerability and family environment. *Acta Psychiatr Scand.* 1991;84:460-465.
34. Cutrona CE, Cadoret RJ, Suhr JA, Richards CC, Troughton E, Schutte K, Woodworth G. Interpersonal variables in the prediction of alcoholism among adoptees: evidence for gene-environment interactions. *Compr Psychiatry.* 1994;35:171-179.
35. Plomin R, Nitz K, Rowe D. Behavioral genetics and aggressive behavior in childhood. In: Lewis M, Miller SM, eds. *Handbook of Developmental Psychopathology.* New York, NY: Plenum Press; 119-133.
36. Poole ED. *Relations of Aggression to Shared and Nonshared Environments of Twins.* Iowa City: Dept of Psychology, University of Iowa; 1992. Thesis.
37. Jary ML, Stewart MA. Psychiatric disorder in the parents of adopted children with aggressive conduct disorder. *Neuropsychobiology.* 1985;13:7-11.
38. Robins LN. *Deviant Children Grown Up.* Baltimore, Md: Williams & Wilkins; 1966.
39. Kendler K, Eaves L. Models for the joint effect of genotype and environment on liability to psychiatric illness. *Am J Psychiatry.* 1986;143:279-289.
40. Cadoret RJ, Wesner RB. Use of the adoption paradigm to elucidate the role of genes and environment and their interaction in the genesis of alcoholism. In: Cloninger CR, Begleiter H, eds. *Genetics and Biology of Alcoholism.* Cold Spring Harbor, NY: Cold Spring Harbor Laboratory Press; 1990:31-42.
41. Wachs TD. The use and abuse of environment in behavior-genetic research. *Child Dev.* 1983;54:396-407.

ORIGINAL ARTICLE

Genetic Questions for Environmental Studies

Differential Parenting and Psychopathology in Adolescence

David Reiss, MD; E. Mavis Hetherington, PhD; Robert Plomin, PhD; George W. Howe, PhD; Samuel J. Simmens, PhD; Sandra H. Henderson, PhD; Thomas J. O'Connor, PhD; Danielle A. Bussell, PhD; Edward R. Anderson, PhD; Tracy Law, PhD

Background: Recent genetic evidence suggests that the most important environmental influences on normal and pathologic development are those that are not shared by siblings in the same family. We sought to determine the relationship between differences in parenting styles and depressive symptoms and antisocial behavior in adolescence, and to compare the influence of these nonshared experiences with genetic influences.

Methods: We studied 708 families with at least two same-sexed adolescent siblings who were monozygotic twins (93 families), dizygotic twins (99 families), ordinary siblings (95 families), full siblings in step families (181 families), half siblings in step families (110 families), and genetically unrelated siblings in step families (130 families). Data on parenting style were collected by questionnaire and by video recording of interaction between parents and children.

Results: Almost 60% of variance in adolescent antisocial behavior and 37% of variance in depressive symptoms could be accounted for by conflictual and negative parental behavior directed specifically at the adolescent. In contrast, when a parent directed harsh, aggressive, explosive, and inconsistent parenting toward the *sibling*, we found *less* psychopathologic outcome in the adolescent.

Conclusions: Parenting behavior directed specifically at each child in the family is a major correlate of symptoms in adolescents. Furthermore, harsh parental behavior directed at a sibling may have protective effects for adolescents, a phenomenon we call the "sibling barricade."

(Arch Gen Psychiatry. 1995;52:925-936)

From the Center for Family Research, Department of Psychiatry and Behavioral Sciences, George Washington University School of Medicine and Health Sciences, Washington, DC (Drs Reiss, Howe, Simmens, and Bussell); Department of Psychology, University of Virginia, Charlottesville (Drs Hetherington, Henderson, O'Connor, and Law); The College of Health and Human Development, Pennsylvania State University, University Park (Dr Plomin); and the Department of Human Development and Family Studies, Texas Tech University, Lubbock (Dr Anderson).

RECENT GENETIC studies have suggested that siblings raised in the same family differ on a broad range of measures of competence and psychopathologic outcome. Whatever similarities siblings show mostly result from shared genes rather than common family environments.[1,2] These findings from genetic studies have posed two questions to researchers of the family environment. First, are siblings treated differently by their parents or do they experience themselves as being treated differently? Second, do these differences play an important role in the development of either competence or psychopathologic outcome?

The term *nonshared environment* refers to those environmental factors that produce different developmental outcomes for each sibling in a family. Examples of shared environmental influences are social class, neighborhood decay, and maternal depression. Examples of nonshared environment are differential treatment of the siblings by the parents, highly discrepant life experience within any sibship, and differences in the quality of marriage of two siblings when they become adults.

To estimate the importance of the nonshared environment in depression and antisocial behavior, some investigators have examined variations in dimensions of depressive symptoms and antisocial behavior in nonclinical populations. In studies of depressive symptoms in adults[3] and child twins,[4] environmental influence is predominantly of the nonshared type. Studies of antisocial behavior[5-8] showed a more equal influence of shared and nonshared influences. With clinical populations, adoption studies of conduct disorders and antisocial personality disorder yield little evidence of shared environmental influences,[9] but twin studies show a substantial effect.[10] For diagnosed affective disorders, the evidence of the importance of nonshared environmental factors, in sharp

See Subjects and Methods on next page

SUBJECTS AND METHODS

TYPES OF FAMILIES STUDIED

The sample included families in two broad classes. The first class consisted of those with no divorce after the birth of the oldest child in our sample (nondivorced families); thus, both children were biologic offspring of both parents. This class had three groups: 93 families with identical (monozygotic) twins, 99 with fraternal (dizygotic) twins, and 95 with full nontwin siblings. Eighty-five of the families with monozygotic twins, 87 of those with dizygotic twins, and 90 full-sibling families had no history of marriage before the current one for the mothers, and 85, 81, and 87 families, respectively, had no history of previous marriage for the fathers. Twin zygosity was determined by the research staff interviewer and parent report of physical similarity by means of a modified form of a questionnaire designed to determine zygosity in adolescent twins.[21] This questionnaire, when compared with blood tests of single-gene markers, is accurate in greater than 90% of cases. Zygosity could not be determined in 6% of the twins with this questionnaire, a rate comparable with that in other studies.

The second class included step families, also divided into three groups: 181 families with full siblings, brought into the current marriage by the mother from a previous marriage (sibling pairs share approximately 50% of their genes); 110 families with half siblings in which the mother brought one child from a previous marriage and had the second child with her current spouse (sibling pairs share approximately 25% of their genes); and 130 families with genetically unrelated siblings in which the father and mother each brought a child to the current family from a previous marriage. In our total sample, 70% of the families had one or more other siblings, with the total number of children from those families ranging from three to 10. In 238 families (33%), the siblings tested were the only two children in the family, in 272 (38%) there were only younger children than those tested, in 141 (20%) there were only older children, and in 69 (10%) there were both younger and older children. (Twelve twin pairs were excluded from analysis because of uncertain zygosity.)

Each family, to be included in the sample, must have had two children of the same gender, no more than 4 years apart in age and no younger than 10 years or older than 18 years. To be sure that none of the step families were in the early stages of family formation, the current marriage had to be of at least 5 years' duration. The tested siblings in each family had to be residents in the household at least half of each week.

According to the 1980 Current Population Survey, only 0.04% of households met our sampling requirements for unrelated siblings, and 0.12% met requirements for half siblings.[22] Thus, we screened 675 000 households, by means of a combination of random digit dialing and market panels, to meet the minimum sample size of 100 families of blended and unrelated siblings.

All remarried families of unrelated siblings and of half siblings drawn from the market panels were approached, since these were the rarest types. The participation rates were 44% and 48%, respectively. This rate compares favorably with sampling procedures in other family studies that have used community or national registers and that required three or four members of a family to be recruited for joint testing and assessment (30.5%[23] and 41%).[24] We do not have enough information on nonparticipant families to estimate the bias in our test sample, if any. Both families of twins and remarried families of full siblings were sampled until a targeted group size was reached, with some attempt to select families that matched those of unrelated siblings and half siblings with respect to age and age spacing of children. Families of twins were also sampled until a targeted group size was reached. Since we did not approach all eligible families in these groups, no true response rate can be computed. Nondivorced families of full siblings were obtained by the random digit dialing procedure.

The mean age of children in the sample was 13.8 years; the mean age for mothers and fathers was 38.1 and 41.0 years, respectively. As a consequence of their identical age, the older twin in the twin families was younger than the older siblings in other families, whereas the younger twin was older than the younger siblings in other families. There were few differences in demographic variables across the six groups. The mean duration of marriage was, as expected, significantly greater for the nondivorced sample (18.4 years) than it was for the step families (8.9 years). Again, as expected, the families with half siblings had a longer mean (±SD) duration of marriages (13.2±2.76 years) than did the full (7.5±2.76 years) or unrelated-sibling (7.2±2.7 years) step families. The mean number of years of education was 13.6 for mothers and 14.0 for fathers, with families of half siblings showing significantly lower scores, for both, in comparison with the other five groups. Family income (mean for the total sample ranged between $25 000 and $35 000) was also significantly lower in the half-sibling families. The Hollingshead four-factor indicator of socioeconomic status showed that step families were significantly lower than the nondivorced families. Ninety-four percent of the women and 93% of the men were white, with the remainder consisting of other ethnic groups. The relatively high proportion of whites in our sample of families with long marital duration reflects their lower divorce and higher remarriage rates, when compared with African Americans and nonwhite Hispanics.[25]

Our sample scored approximately the same on several measures of psychopathologic outcome as other nonpsychiatric samples of children of approximately the same age.[4,26-28]

PROCEDURE

Families were studied during a 15-month period in all states, with the exception of South Dakota, Alaska, and Hawaii. Thirty-seven interviewer teams, unaware of the study's hypotheses and under the supervision of four full-time field managers, conducted all interviews in the families' homes. Most interviews were conducted by two member teams, but for some families with older children, they were conducted by single interviewers. Data were collected in two 3-hour sessions in the home no more than 2 weeks apart. Family members also completed simple questionnaires between the two sessions. Interview teams collected videotaped family interaction during the interviews, about half from each of the two sessions. These consisted of nine 10-minute interactions of each parent with each of the two siblings. Each dyad discussed and attempted to resolve a problem they had previously selected as a problem for them.

MEASURES OF DEPRESSIVE SYMPTOMS AND ANTISOCIAL BEHAVIOR

We measured depressive symptoms and antisocial behavior as continuous variables rather than making categorical distinctions between "cases" and "noncases." This strategy was more likely to yield analyzable distributions in an ordinary-risk population. It has been used to predict concurrent adaptive functioning in adolescents,[22,29-31] to make concurrent distinctions between cases and noncases[32] as well as more specific syndromes,[26] and to assess adolescents' risk for adult psychopathologic development and maladaptive functioning.[33]

We used three measures of depressive symptoms in the adolescents: the Child Depression Inventory[26] (27 symptom items, including feelings of loneliness, sadness, poor appetite and sleep, and thoughts about suicide during the past 2 weeks) and a comparable parent version of the Child Depression Inventory[34]; the Behavior Problems Index[35] (adapted from the Child Behavior Checklist,[36] this is a 32-item scale that covers a full range of psychopathologic development during the past 3 months with six items concerning depression); and the Behavior Events Inventory.[17,20] This last measure asked each parent and both children to report the presence or absence of specific depressive behaviors, such as "cried" or "been withdrawn" during the past week.

Antisocial behavior was measured by a six-item scale from the Behavior Problems Index and nine items from the Behavior Events Inventory, such as "stole," "lied or cheated," or "skipped school." In addition, coders rated videotapes of the child's interaction with both parents, on a single five-point scale, for antisocial behavior, including instances of disruptive, rude, coercive, and aggressive behavior. Weighted κ for the reliability of this coding judgment was 0.77,[37] and the intraclass correlation coefficient between coders was .86. Separate coders were always used for each of the two children in a family.

The Child Depression Inventory and Behavior Events Inventory were administered twice at least a week apart. Thus, combined scores are less likely to reflect transient mood or behavioral disturbances.

MEASURES OF PARENTING

Three domains of parenting were measured by means of coding of videotaped interaction and self-report questionnaires: conflict/negativity; warmth/support; and monitoring/control.[17] Twenty-one undergraduate and graduate students served as coders of parenting measures. We used 21 global scales from the Global Coding System.[17] Each rating required judging a 10-minute videotaped segment of interaction on a five-point scale. Coders were trained until they reached a criterion level of 60% exact agreement with a criterion coder. After they met that criterion, an average of 48% of all subsequent coding was checked for reliability. Where reliability fell below 60% perfect agreement, coding was redone.

The self-report and observer rating scales used to assess parenting are summarized in **Table 1**.[38]

ANALYTIC STRATEGY

Operationalizing Differential Parenting Effects

We framed hypotheses concerning differential parenting in two ways. First, we examined certain patterns of simple correlations between parenting and adolescent symptoms. The relationships between these patterns and our hypotheses concerning differential parenting are summarized in **Table 2**. When parenting and outcome were substantially correlated for each child, but parenting toward each of the children was not correlated, then the lack of sibling correlation of symptom patterns was likely to result in part from differential parenting for this particular parenting variable. To test for this pattern, the relevant correlations were estimated for the three parenting domains and the two sets of outcomes, antisocial behavior and depressive symptoms.

Second, it seemed likely that most findings would not necessarily fit exactly any of the cells in Table 1. For example, it is possible that the correlation between parenting toward the adolescent and parenting toward the sibling would be moderate, but the correlation between parenting and outcome could still reflect effects specific to each adolescent. Regression analyses were used to test this hypothesis, by estimating parameters reflecting the relationship between parenting toward an adolescent and that adolescent's outcome while controlling for the level of parenting directed toward that adolescent's sibling. In this case the effects of differential parenting are measured directly, as indicated by this coefficient. We refer to this as the *specific effect*, since only variance in parenting that is specific to the child is related to variance in that child's symptoms. **Figure 1** presents a path diagram depicting these regression analyses.

Aggregating Symptom Measures

Seven aggregate measures of symptoms for each child in a family were used. These reflect depressive symptoms as reported by mother, father, and child, and antisocial behavior as reported by mother, father, child, and observer. Aggregation was accomplished in the following way. First, each measure administered twice over the set of interviews was averaged across the two administrations. (The correlations between session 1 and session 2 on all measures of psychopathologic outcome were invariably high.) Next, each measure from each respondent or source was standardized across all 1440 siblings in all families. Finally, all standardized measures of depressive symptoms and antisocial behavior from a particular respondent were averaged.

Composting Measures of Parenting

We examined patterns of intercorrelations among all measures of parenting to verify that each measure was properly assigned to its correct domain. First, for the self-report scales, we performed a confirmatory factor analysis with the use of a three-factor solution on all parenting scales from the oldest child's report of the mother's parenting. Scales were constrained to load only on one factor. The same analysis was repeated for each child's report of parenting toward the mother, each child's report of parenting

Continued on next page

toward the father, and each parent's report of his or her parenting toward each child. All eight analyses achieved a satisfactory fit, with Bentler's[39] nonnormed fit index ranging from 0.79 to 0.88 across all analyses. That is, our hypotheses about three parenting variables—conflict/negativity, warmth/support, and monitoring/control—fit the observed correlations among the 14 measures of parenting for each reporter and each parent.

We used the same approach to test the dimensionality of the observer ratings. Four analyses were done on four different sets of ratings, reflecting the mother's observed behavior toward her oldest and youngest child and the father's observed behavior toward his oldest and youngest child (Bentler's nonnormed fit index, 0.89 to 0.92).

These findings justified aggregating measures within dimensions for each respondent. Each measure was standardized across all 1440 children, and standardized measures were averaged to create an index of each parenting domain as reported by each respondent and by observers. This resulted in 18 variables: three domains of parenting (conflict/negativity, warmth/support, and monitoring/control) for each parent (mother and father) as reported by that parent, by the child, and by observers.

TESTING HYPOTHESES CONCERNING DIFFERENTIAL PARENTING

Dealing With Response Bias

Preliminary analyses indicated that simple aggregation across respondents (parent, child, and observer) might introduce biases into analyses testing hypotheses about the link between parenting and child symptoms. For example, mothers may consistently see their parenting as less conflictual and negative than it really is. Moreover, this reporting bias may also influence reports of outcome variables, such that mothers who see their own parenting as less negative may also report their children as less depressed than they actually are.

Thus, we used structural equation modeling techniques that allow for aggregation of such reports independent of respondent bias. This algebraic procedure fits an observed set of correlations among many variables with a model of how those variables might be related.[40] The two components of the model are (1) a "measurement model," which specifies that certain measured variables are all indicators of an underlying or "latent variable," and (2) a specified set of relationships among the latent variables. In these analyses, measures of each parenting domain are considered as indicators of the underlying latent variable for that domain. Similarly, measures of each set of symptoms are considered as indicators of latent variables reflecting that symptom group.

We can also specify a relationship between the errors of measurement of two or more of the measured variables. If we expect errors of measurement from the same respondent (eg, the mother) to be correlated between her report of parenting and her report of her children's psychopathologic outcome, this is similar to partialing these errors or biases from our estimate of the relationship between the latent variable of parenting and of psychopathologic outcome (**Figure 2**).[41]

Correlation and Regression Analyses

With the use of all 1440 children, structural equation models with correlated errors were used to calculate the correlations between latent variables reflecting parenting toward a child, parenting toward his or her sibling, and symptoms reported for a child and for the sibling (Table 2). Data concerning each child were entered twice, once to represent the parenting toward that child and once to represent that child as the sibling of the other child in the family. This required us to restrict our model by (1) constraining the path "parenting toward adolescent" and path "parenting toward sibling" to be equal and (2) adjustment of the *df* for each analysis because of the redundancy introduced by including data from all individual children in measuring each latent variable.

Regression analyses (Figure 1) were conducted in a similar fashion. The only difference involved a respecification of the structural model such that both parenting variables (parenting toward adolescent and parenting toward sibling) were included as exogenous variables predicting each of the outcomes (symptoms for adolescent and symptoms for sibling).

contrast to shared environmental factors, is clear. For example, twin studies show concordance well below 100%,[10-12] and adoption studies show little difference between the adopting parents of depressed or manic-depressed patients and the adopting parents of index subjects without affective disorders.[10-13]

Unfortunately, these genetic studies cannot specify which specific nonshared environmental factors are important. These factors may be biologic (such as toxins or intrauterine viruses) or social. Furthermore, they may not be general influences: influential differences may be unique for each family. Recent preliminary studies have directly measured specific nonshared factors in the family environment by sampling families with two or more children and have studied the effects of differential parenting or other sibling differences in family and social factors. Dunn et al[14] showed that children who received more maternal affection and less maternal control than their siblings showed less internalizing symptoms. Siblings who received more control showed more externalizing behavior.[15] Other investigators have shown that more parental punishment is associated with more suicidal ideation and oppositional behavior.[16]

See also pages 895, 900, 906, and 916

More conventional studies, involving only one child per family, suggest that parental warmth and support buffers children against externalizing and antisocial behavior[17] and is positively associated with a child's self-esteem.[18] Conflictual and coercive parenting is positively associated with externalizing, including disruptive and deceitful behavior, in general[17] and with more narrowly defined antisocial behavior in particular.[19,20] However, where parents can track the behavior of their children—both inside and outside the home—and can exert effective disci-

Table 1. Measures of Parenting and Their Reliabilities

Domains and Scales	Focus of Measurement	Coefficient α Child	Coefficient α Parent	Intraclass
	Conflict/Negativity			
Self-report				
Parent-child disagreement	Frequency of disagreements on specific issues (eg, telephone use)	.78-.91	.83-.85	...
Punitiveness	Frequency of yelling and punishing	.89-.90	.89-.91	...
Yielding to coercion	Surrendering to concompliant and disruptive behavior	.57-.61	.63-.73	...
Verbal aggression[38]	Swearing, threatening, stomping out of room	.72-.75	.73-.74	...
Open conflict	Frequency of severe conflict and fights	.70-.72	.70-.78	...
Observer ratings				
Anger and rejection	Verbal and nonverbal criticism and denigration	...	...	.81
Coercion	Manipulative control, including whining and threat	...	...	.78
Transactional conflict	Reciprocated and escalated argument and conflict	...	...	.79
	Warmth/Support			
Self-report				
Closeness and rapport	Pleasure in closeness and involvement	.90-.92	.85-.90	...
Expression of affection	Overt signs of affection and pleasures in joint activity	.69-.85	.73-.88	...
Observer ratings				
Warmth and support	Positive feelings, affection	...	...	.79
Assertiveness	Positive expressions of needs; self-confidence and patience	...	...	.75
Communication	Ability to listen, explain, and elicit other's view	...	...	.62
Involvement	Own initiative and encouraging other's participation	...	...	.68
	Monitoring/Control			
Self-report				
Knowledge	Information about child's activities	.88-.90	.90-.91	...
Attempted control	Efforts to control child's activities	.92-.93	.91-.91	...
Actual control	Successes in controlling child's activities	.95-.94	.93-.94	...
Observer ratings				
Child monitoring	Parent knows about child's activities	...	...	.64
Influence	Parent attempt at control	...	...	.68
Parental authority	Successful influences on child's behavior and opinions	...	...	.64

Table 2. Interpreting the Possible Patterns of Correlations Among Parenting and Adolescent Outcome Variables

Correlation Between Parenting and Outcome	Correlation Between Parenting Toward Child X and Child Y	Interpretation
Low	Low	Parenting is different for the 2 children and is also unrelated to outcome
Low	High	Parenting of the 2 children is highly correlated and is unrelated to outcome
High	Low	Clearest indication of nonshared effects: parenting is both different for each child and highly associated with outcome
High	High	Parenting is correlated for both children and strongly associated with outcome; nonshared parenting effects are impossible to detect

pline, the risk of antisocial behavior in children and adolescents is reduced.[19,20] These findings suggest that three domains of parental behavior influence adolescent depression and antisocial behavior: (1) warmth/support, (2) conflict and coercion, and (3) monitoring/control. The present study seeks to assess whether parents treat their children differently and, if they do, whether these differences are associated with offspring psychopathologic development. Subsequent reports will detail the role of genetic factors in these associations.

RESULTS

CONFLICT/NEGATIVITY

Data concerning parents' engagement in conflict/negativity were analyzed at three levels. At the most general level, all conflict/negativity measures reporting behavior of both mother and father were used as indicators of a general conflict/negativity latent variable. We saw this latent variable as reflecting the general atmosphere of parenting as directed toward a particular adolescent by both parents. This seemed reasonable, since structural equations that included separate mother and father latent variables reflecting conflict/negativity indicated a high correlation between these two (r=.85, SE=.19). At the next lower level, the measures for mother's and father's behavior were analyzed separately. Finally, we repeated our analyses for each particular measure of conflict/negativity for each parent, to clarify our more general findings.

Table 3 summarizes findings from the regression models for general parental conflict/negativity in relation to antisocial behavior and depressive symptoms. Since

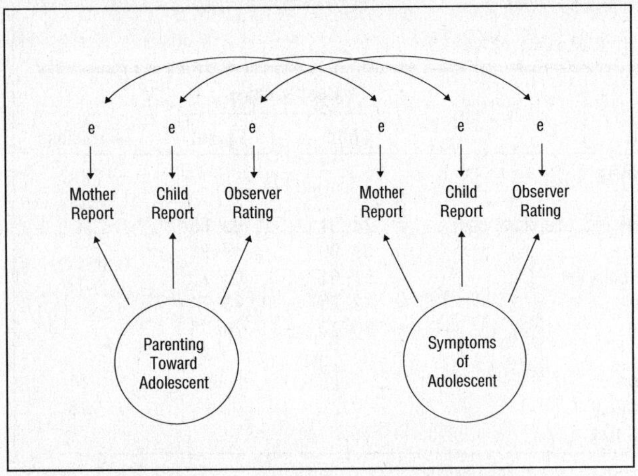

Figure 1. *Path diagram of regression analyses for testing specific relationships between parenting and outcome, the* specific effects *as well as the relationship of parenting to siblings on the outcomes for the adolescents, the* cross-sibling effects.

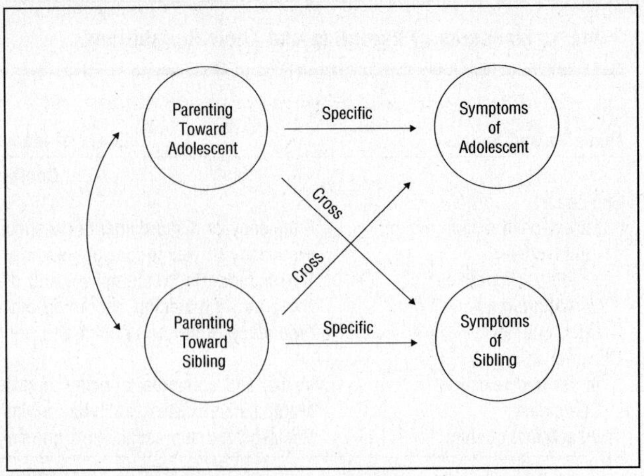

Figure 2. *Partial structural equation model showing correlated error method of eliminating respondent bias effects.*

this table format will be used to present data from most analyses, we will discuss Table 3 in some detail.

In Table 3, row 1 provides an estimate of the correlation of general parental conflict/negativity directed toward each child with general parental conflict/negativity directed toward his or her sibling. This is equivalent to an intraclass correlation coefficient. Estimates for this correlation, for any parenting variable, should be equal in all models; the slight differences in these tables result from minor fluctuations in the estimation procedures used. These correlations address our first primary question: how similarly do parents treat two children of the same gender close in age? These data demonstrate a substantial correlation between sibling environments as measured by parental conflict/negativity.

Row 2 of Table 3, labeled "specific," reports the standardized regression coefficient estimating the relationship between parental conflict/negativity toward each child adjusted for the level of conflict/negativity toward each child's sibling. As noted earlier, we consider this regression coefficient to provide an adjusted estimate of the association of parenting specific to a child with that child's symptoms. The regressions in Table 2 suggest that this effect is substantial for parental conflict/negativity, as it has an association with antisocial behavior and depressive symptoms in adolescents. This provides strong support for the interpretation that parental conflict/negativity specific to each child, as indexed by this partialing approach, is strongly associated with adolescent antisocial behavior and depressive symptoms.

Row 3, labeled "cross," contains the standardized regression coefficient estimating unique cross-sibling effects. That is, these measure the indirect association of parenting toward a sibling with outcomes in the adolescent. While the cross correlations, not shown in Table 3, are significant for antisocial behavior (0.39) and depressive symptoms (0.21), the regression coefficients (which are adjusted for the level of parental conflict/negativity toward the adolescent whose symptoms are being predicted) are small, suggesting that the simple cross correlations are attributable mostly to the strong correlation between siblings on this parenting variable.

Table 3. Relationships Between Parental Conflict/Negativity, Depression, and Antisocial Behavior for Mothers and Fathers Combined*

Relationship of Conflict/Negativity	Antisocial Behavior Coefficient±SE	Depression Coefficient± SE
Between parenting toward adolescent and sibling	0.56±0.08	0.55±0.07
Between parenting and outcome, *specific*	0.79±0.06	0.62±0.05
Between parenting and outcome, *cross*	−0.05±0.03	−0.14±0.04
χ^2/df	309/63	236/53
Bentler's NNFI	0.89	0.90

**See Figure 1 for illustration of notation. NNFI indicates nonnormed fit index.*

Rows 4 and 5 provide summary statistics for the structural equation models used to estimate the correlations in this table. These indicate that the fit between model and data are good. Correlations among errors estimated by the model are not reported herein to conserve space, but in general most of these correlations were substantial, indicating that much of the variance in our measures involved observer bias and providing strong support for the need to remove this variance by means of this method of modeling.

Table 4 presents data on antisocial behavior and depressive symptoms separately for mothers and fathers. Coefficients for mothers and fathers were similar and did not differ greatly from those in analyses of general parental conflict/negativity. Regression coefficients estimating unique cross-sibling effects were negligible for fathers but showed a small but significant negative relationship for mothers.

Table 5 reports results of separate scales used as indicators of parental conflict/negativity for antisocial behavior and depressive symptoms. The regression coefficients are reported in Table 5. In an occasional instance in this table, as well as others, we display regression co-

Table 4. Relationship Between Conflict/Negativity, Warmth/Support, and Monitoring/Control and Antisocial Behavior or Depressive Symptoms*

	Coefficient±SE					
	Conflict/Negativity		Warmth/Support		Monitoring/Control	
Relationships	Mother	Father	Mother	Father	Mother	Father
Antisocial Behavior						
Between parenting toward adolescent and sibling	0.52±0.05	0.61±0.10	0.61±0.06	0.67±0.04	0.80±0.04	0.89±0.03
Between parenting and outcome, *specific*	0.75±0.06	0.82±0.07	−0.30±0.05	−0.37±0.05	−0.12±0.05	−0.15±0.07
Between parenting and outcome, *cross*	−0.04±0.04	−0.04±0.05	−0.03±0.05	0.10±0.05	−0.09±0.05	−0.04±0.06
χ^2/df	139/30	157/30	131/30	115/30	62/30	89/30
Bentler's NNFI	0.91	0.89	0.89	0.91	0.97	0.95
Depressive Symptoms						
Between parenting toward adolescent and sibling	0.50±0.07	0.57±0.11	0.60±0.06	0.66±0.04	0.79±0.04	0.88±0.03
Between parenting and outcome, *specific*	0.56±0.05	0.64±0.06	−0.26±0.06	−0.37±0.06	−0.03±0.06	−0.17±0.08
Between parenting and outcome, *cross*	−0.12±0.04	0.01±0.04	0.10±0.06	0.20±0.05	−0.09±0.06	0.09±0.09
χ^2/df	97/22	150/22	85/22	75/22	59/22	78/22
Bentler's NNFI	0.91	0.84	0.91	0.93	0.95	0.94

See Figure 1 for illustration of notation. NNFI indicates nonnormed fit index.

efficients that are greater than 1.0 and/or SEs that are very high. These are the results of very high correlations of measures of parenting toward the adolescent with measures of parenting toward the sibling. The very high coefficients or SEs reflect uncertainty in the estimation procedure and are interpreted as nonsignificant findings.

Five of these scales involve self-report measures. Since each was completed by the parent and the child about that parent, structural equation modeling with latent variables and correlated errors to remove respondent bias effects could be used. However, this is not true for the observer coding of parental conflict/negativity, which was based on only one reporter, the coder. Thus, comparisons of coefficients are valid across the five self-report measures but must be somewhat tentative when these measures are compared with the observer data.

Correlations between parenting toward adolescent and that toward sibling (row 1) showed striking differences among the scales. Yielding to coercion showed much higher correlations than did symbolic aggression or conflict, particularly for fathers. Standardized regression coefficients reflecting the specific effects of parenting all tended to be similar across measures (row 2). These findings again support the interpretation that parental conflict/negativity specific to a particular child has a strong relationship with that child's antisocial behavior.

Punitiveness, for mothers and fathers, showed moderate levels of unique cross-sibling effects as reflected in standardized regression coefficients. These data suggest that the *greater* the parental punitiveness that is shown to the sibling, the *less* antisocial behavior that is shown by the adolescent.

Observer measures of parental conflict/negativity show lower correlations between parenting toward adolescent and toward sibling, and lower correlations between parental conflict/negativity and child antisocial behavior, in correlational and regression analyses. Although muted, these data show general patterns similar to those of self-report data, with specific conflict/negativity being significantly associated with adolescent behavior and cross-sibling regression coefficients showing little or no effect. Patterns of coefficients for analyses involving depressive symptoms, reported in Tables 4 and 5, were similar to those found for antisocial behavior, except that cross-sibling effects were more frequent.

WARMTH/SUPPORT

Structural equations including separate mother and father latent variables reflecting warmth/support indicated only a moderate correlation between these two (r=.50, SE=.14). For this reason, analyses were not conducted for general parental warmth/support, but only for mothers and fathers separately.

Table 4 reports the results of structural equation estimates of regression coefficients relating parental warmth/support to adolescent antisocial behavior and depressive symptoms. Considering the correlation between sibling environments on the dimension of parental warmth/support, these data were similar to those for conflict/negativity, showing substantial correlations for parental warmth/support. However, regression coefficients between parental warmth/support and both types of symptoms were smaller, although still significant. As Table 4 shows, this pattern was generally true for the standardized regression coefficients reflecting the specific effects of parental warmth toward a particular child. These data provide support for the importance of parental warmth/support specific to each child, but the effects appear to be much lower than those found for conflict/negativity. The cross-sibling effects in Table 4 also show that the *more* warmth/support that is shown to the sibling, the *more* the adolescent shows depressive symptoms.

We examined, in greater detail, the four component measures of warmth/support. The following spe-

Table 5. Relationship of the Six Component Scales of Conflict/Negativity and Antisocial Behavior or Depressive Symptoms*

	Disagreement		Punitiveness	
Relationship	Mother	Father	Mother	Father
Between parenting toward adolescent and sibling	0.53±0.09	0.52±0.12	0.67±0.10	0.73±0.13
Between parenting and outcome, *specific*	0.70±0.06	0.74±0.08	0.71±0.09	0.80±0.14
Between parenting and outcome, *cross*	0.00±0.04	0.02±0.07	−0.21±0.08	−0.28±0.13
χ^2/df	90/22	83/22	83/22	92/22
Bentler's NNFI	0.93	0.93	0.93	0.92
Between parenting toward adolescent and sibling	0.52±0.08	0.52±0.11	0.60±0.10	0.64±0.12
Between parenting and outcome, *specific*	0.49±0.06	0.54±0.07	0.56±0.07	0.62±0.10
Between parenting and outcome, *cross*	−0.15±0.05	−0.16±0.06	−0.21±0.06	−0.18±0.08
χ^2/df	65/12	62/12	63/12	53/12
Bentler's NNFI	0.90	0.90	0.91	0.92

**See Figure 1 for illustration of notation. NNFI indicates nonnormed fit index.*

cific regressions were significant for the components of warmth/support and antisocial behavior: mother's and father's closeness and rapport (−0.27; −0.34), mother's and father's expressive affection (−0.27; −0.27), and mother's observed warmth (−0.14). The following were significant for depressive symptoms: mother's and father's closeness and rapport (0.33; −0.26) and father's instrumental affection (−0.20). None of the cross-sibling regressions were significant.

MONITORING/CONTROL

Structural equations including separate mother and father latent variables reflecting monitoring/control indicated a strong correlation between these mothers and fathers (r=.75, SE=.27). Because of high correlations, as shown in Table 4, between parents' scores, we report analyses only for mothers and fathers separately. These tables also show that the effects of specific parental monitoring/control on adolescent symptoms were not significant. Cross-sibling regression coefficients also show low or no significant effects.

Analyses of the specific scales from the monitoring/control composites, presented in **Table 6**, essentially replicated these findings in the case of depressive symptoms, with one exception: the regression coefficient for maternal control attempts was significant, indicating that attempts specific to a particular adolescent are related to increased depressive symptoms. A more interesting picture emerges for antisocial behavior: knowledge and actual control appear to have the predicted effect; they are inversely related to antisocial behavior. Control attempts, which may reflect ineffective monitoring, are positively related to antisocial behavior. These contrasting effects are almost certainly responsible for the null findings, shown in Table 3, when all four measures of monitoring/control are aggregated.

Cross-sibling correlations provide evidence that *higher* father's knowledge of sibling activities is significantly associated with *lower* antisocial behavior in the other adolescent. However, *higher* father's successful control of the sibling is associated with *higher* antisocial behavior in the other adolescent.

INFLUENCE OF GENDER, SOCIAL CLASS, AND AGE OF CHILDREN

We compared the effects of sibship genders for all the models presented in Tables 3 through 6. We estimated statistical significance by comparing models in which the two genders were constrained to have equal coefficients with those in which the models were free to vary.[39] There were no gender differences for any of the specific effects. We also examined the effects of social class, mean education level of the parents, and mean age of the two children by recomputing the regressions shown in Table 4 after controlling for these variables. Of the 36 regressions shown in these tables, only two were changed by more than 0.10 (father's warmth/support, specific association with depressive symptoms, −0.26; father's warmth/support, cross-sibling regression with depressive symptoms, 0.08). At this level, where scale scores are aggregated, there were no more effects than would be expected by chance, so we did not examine these effects on the component scales of the three main parenting variables.

COMMENT

LIMITATIONS

At the outset, the reader should be aware of two major limitations. First, direction of effects cannot be estimated: variation among adolescents in symptoms may lead to variation in correlated parental response, or the reverse relationship may hold. The literature using the traditional single-sibling design indicates that, for families of preadolescents and adolescents, either is possible.[17,20,39,42,43] We recently collected a second panel of data from this sample; this will help to resolve which of these influences are most important and will explore between-group differences—if any—in causal direction.

Coefficient±SE							
Yielding to Coercion		Symbolic Aggression		Conflict		Observer Coding Coefficient	
Mother	Father	Mother	Father	Mother	Father	Mother	Father
Antisocial Behavior							
0.75±0.31	0.96±0.23	0.45±0.10	0.39±0.14	0.36±0.11	0.51±0.14	0.39±0.03	0.41±0.03
0.66±0.37	1.92±6.9	0.57±0.07	0.63±0.09	0.61±0.07	0.68±0.08	0.26±0.03	0.22±0.03
−0.26±0.37	−1.63±7.1	−0.01±0.05	0.04±0.08	0.00±0.06	−0.08±0.07	0.10±0.03	0.03±0.03
69/22	89/22	68/22	64/22	93/22	95/22	38/10	46/10
0.93	0.91	0.94	0.94	0.91	0.91	0.95	0.94
Depressive Symptoms							
0.51±.42	0.92±0.20	0.40±0.11	0.35±0.14	0.36±0.11	0.44±0.14	0.39±0.03	0.41±0.03
0.27±0.09	1.17±2.6	0.54±0.07	0.56±0.08	0.46±0.07	0.49±0.07	0.10±0.03	0.12±0.03
0.10±0.09	−1.04±2.5	−0.03±0.06	0.10±0.07	−0.12±0.06	−0.04±0.06	0.04±0.03	0.01±0.03
56/12	54/12	58/12	48/12	74/12	59/12	49/10	41/10
0.89	0.90	0.89	0.91	0.87	0.91	0.91	0.93

Second, the mechanisms linking parenting practices and psychiatric symptoms may not be purely psychosocial. There may be a substantial influence of heritable characteristics of the child on parenting practices.[44] Moreover, our outcome measures—depressive symptoms and antisocial behavior—also show significant heritabilities; for antisocial behavior, h^2=0.55, and for depressive symptoms, h^2=0.44. Where independent and dependent measures are heritable, genetic influences common to both may explain part or all of any associations observed.[45] Using other data in this study, we are currently testing models to parse out these common genetic influences.

SPECIFIC ASSOCIATION BETWEEN PARENTING AND ADOLESCENT ADJUSTMENT

Conflict/negativity showed strong associations with antisocial behavior and, to a lesser extent, with depressive symptoms. These associations were roughly the same in magnitude for mothers and fathers. Furthermore, all five subscales for the self-report measures showed strong associations with psychopathologic outcome. It is not simply aggressiveness or punitiveness by the parent that plays a role, but also the parent's yielding to coercion by the child. Thus, what may lie at the core here is a toxic combination of sustained negative and disruptive affect and inconsistency in parental authority and direction. As such, our findings may relate to those single-child family studies of both Baumrind,[46] who reported the importance of parental consistency for competent adolescent adjustment, and Elder,[47] who reported the disruptive effects of emotionally explosive parental behavior.

The large magnitude of these effects, particularly for conflict/negativity, is notable. For antisocial behavior, this variable accounted for 56% of variance for fathers and 69% for mothers. For depressive symptoms, it accounted for 31% for fathers and 41% for mothers. The multiagent, multimethod measurement strategy permits a more reliable estimate of an underlying true score for independent and dependent measures and thus may increase variance explained. Studies using somewhat comparable research strategies and analytic methods with adolescents, parenting measures, and antisocial behaviors have produced large effect sizes of 21% to 27%,[17] 30% to 40%,[20] and 42% to 53%, respectively.[30] However, the latter two studies used a broader band of parenting measures and for this reason probably showed large effect sizes. It is fair to say that our results account for nearly twice as much variance as those of previous studies of a single domain of parenting variables and antisocial behavior.

Thus, some factor other than our statistical and measurement procedure must be responsible for the large effect sizes. The presence of a second sibling in our design does not fully account for these unusual effect sizes. While informative, the unique cross correlations were, for the most part, small and did not alter the specific effect sizes much. Thus, it might be argued that the unique, specific effects are those that could have been measured in any study that used the conventional one-child-per-family design if a researcher concentrated on just those parenting behaviors that were directed at the child in question. However, as noted, one-child studies have not shown effect sizes this large. It is possible that, in our study, inclusion of two siblings in the research design was usefully reactive. The central feature of this research design may alert parents and children that the research team is interested in contrasts and comparisons. Indeed, many of our self-report measures for parents regularly asked the parents to rate their behavior toward one child on a large number of items and then rate the second child on the same items, a procedure that must call attention to contrasts and comparisons. Children are asked to compare directly how they are treated by each parent with the treatment received by the other child by means of a unique instrument called the Sibling Inventory of Differential Experience.[48] These explicit techniques, plus the welter of demand characteristics, may act to bring out in the open those contrasting environmental experiences whose validity is confirmed by their predictable association with outcome variables.

Table 6. Relationship Between the Four Components of Monitoring/Control and Antisocial Behavior or Depressive Symptoms*

Relationships	Knowledge: Mother	Knowledge: Father	Control Attempts: Mother	Control Attempts: Father	Actual Control: Mother	Actual Control: Father	Observer Coding Coefficient: Mother	Observer Coding Coefficient: Father
	Coefficient ±SE							
Antisocial Behavior								
Between parenting toward adolescent and sibling	0.86±0.21	0.85±0.19	0.80±0.22	0.81±0.18	0.79±0.24	0.85±0.20	0.30±0.03	0.42±0.03
Between parenting and outcome, *specific*	−0.30±0.10	−0.16±0.07	0.21±0.08	0.18±0.07	−0.21±0.05	−0.40±0.11	−0.02±0.02	0.04±0.03
Between parenting and outcome, *cross*	−0.09±0.09	−0.17±0.07	−0.22±0.07	−0.20±0.07	0.01±0.04	0.22±0.11	−0.01±0.03	0.01±0.03
χ^2/df	65/22	71/22	48/22	47/22	65/22	59/22	37/10	46/10
Bentler's NNFI	0.95	0.96	0.97	0.98	0.95	0.96	0.95	0.93
Depressive Symptoms								
Between parenting toward adolescent and sibling	0.83±0.16	0.86±0.17	0.81±0.22	0.80±0.16	0.78±0.22	0.82±0.17	0.30±0.03	0.42±0.03
Between parenting and outcome, *specific*	−0.12±0.10	−0.15±0.08	0.22±0.10	0.09±0.07	−0.16±0.06	−0.10±0.07	0.04±0.03	0.07±0.03
Between parenting and outcome, *cross*	0.01±0.09	0.09±0.09	−0.29±0.08	−0.13±0.07	0.02±0.05	0.01±0.05	0.01±0.03	−0.01±0.03
χ^2/df	53/12	45/12	36/12	43/12	39/12	42/12	43/10	45/10
Bentler's NNFI	0.93	0.96	0.96	0.96	0.95	0.95	0.92	0.92

**See Figure 1 for illustration of notation. NNFI indicates nonnormed fit index.*

In contrast, the relatively small associations between observed parenting and adolescent symptoms may, as noted, result from one or more of a set of factors. First, we observed only a brief 10 minutes of interaction between a parent and each child. Second, there is only one type of observer—by definition and design—in observer coding, so we cannot correct for observer bias. Third, observer coding may be examining a different domain of parenting than do the self-report scales. The correlation among all self-report scales, within a domain, were high. However, those between self-report and observer ratings, within a domain, ranged from only 0.11 ($P<.01$) to 0.27 ($P<.001$).

Findings for warmth/support show a different pattern. The associations of parental warmth/support specific to each child with outcome measures are much lower for parental warmth/support. Where it does show significant associations, it is inversely related to psychopathologic outcome as predicted. Warmth/support is more strongly and positively associated with positive outcomes in adolescents, particularly social responsibility.[49]

Data on monitoring/control show yet another pattern. Parenting behavior toward the siblings is much more highly correlated. This allows less opportunity for specific effects to emerge (Table 2). Nonetheless, this domain shows an interesting difference among the component subscales. Two measures, the parents' knowledge about the adolescents and their behavior and the parents' successful control of that behavior, show modest negative correlations with antisocial behavior as predicted. These two domains of monitoring may be thought of as competent monitoring. However, the scale measuring attempted control probably reflects attempts that fail; if this is the case, it is not surprising that it shows modest positive associations with antisocial behavior.

The correlation between antisocial behavior and depressive symptoms in our data was .43 and was consistent with previous findings.[50-52] Thus, it is not surprising that we did not find specific family correlates for each.

EFFECTS OF PARENTING TOWARD SIBLINGS ON ADOLESCENT SYMPTOMS

For the aggregated variables shown in Table 4, the unique cross correlations are small, suggesting that—at the aggregated level—there are virtually no indirect effects of parenting, via treatment of the sibling, on adolescent antisocial behavior or depressive symptoms.

However, analysis of the component scales of conflict/negativity shows an interesting pattern: for punitiveness, the *more* conflict/negativity is aimed at the sibling, the *less* antisocial behavior is shown by the adolescent. A similar effect is apparent for disagreement and punitiveness and for depressive symptoms. The effect sizes for some of these unique cross correlations are comparable with the specific effects for warmth/support and antisocial and depressive symptoms. In other words, an adolescent is less likely to show antisocial behavior and depressive symptoms as much by having his or her sibling be the focus of parent conflict/negativity as by being the direct recipient of parental warmth/support.

The cross correlations of the monitoring/control scales add a dimension to this pattern. The *more* control attempts and knowledge of sibling behavior is directed at the sibling, the *less* likely that the adolescent will show abnormal behavior. If we can read the father's knowledge of sibling behavior as signifying his preoccupation with the sibling, all of the significant cross correlations fall into a pattern. The *more* harsh, aggressive, explosive, inconsistent, ineffective, and preoccupied behavior is shown toward the sibling, the *less* psychopathologic outcome is seen in the adolescent.

Apparently, adolescents are least likely to show antisocial behavior or depressive symptoms if they receive little conflict/negativity and much warmth directly from their parents *and* their sibling receives a good deal of problematic parenting. We may refer to this profile of effects as a *sibling barricade*. Evidence of a sibling barricade as a socialization phenomenon cannot be obtained in an ordinary single-child design.

The possible connection between sibling barricade and conflict/negativity is supported by the correlation between mothers and fathers for conflict/negativity, which was the highest of three domains of parenting ($r_{c/n}$=.84, SE=.19; $r_{w/s}$=.50, SE=.14; and $r_{m/c}$=.74, SE=.27, where c/n indicates conflict/negativity; w/s, warmth/support; and m/c, monitoring/control). In families in which an adolescent is receiving high levels of conflict/negativity, he or she is getting it more or else equally from both parents. Furthermore, we found that conflict/negativity from both parents is equally associated with the child's symptoms. Other studies suggest that it is likely that there is considerable conflict between husbands and wives in those families in which at least one child is the recipient of parental conflict/negativity.[17,30,53,54] Whether the child's behavior is cause or effect, the data suggest a tangled triad of family members—mother, father, and the child who is the target of problematic parenting. This triad show relationships filled with tension, aggression, inconsistency, and ineffectiveness. A child who is not protected by the barricade gets a double dose of conflict/negativity from both parents, who also may be in a state of war with one another. It becomes more understandable, therefore, why a child who is, for whatever reason, barricaded from this troubled family subsystem may be much less likely to show symptoms.

CORRELATION OF PARENTING TOWARD ADOLESCENT WITH THAT TOWARD SIBLING

These correlations form the hub for subsequent searches for nonshared effects. It has not been known whether parents treat same-sex, similar-aged children alike. If their treatment is similar, then it is unlikely that parenting is a source of nonshared environmental influence. As already suggested, it is critical to understand who is reporting these differences: parents, children, or observers. For example, parents may be biased by a strong desire to treat both children equally. Children, on the other hand, may be exquisitely sensitive to differences in how they and siblings are treated; this may start early in the second year of life.[15] In our study, for conflict/negativity, parents were most likely to report that they treat children similarly. The mean correlation across all the component scales for parent reports was .64. On the other hand, the correlation between the adolescent and siblings on their reports on the same parent was only .23 averaged across all scales and both parents. Observer ratings were midway between the parents' and children's' reports; for conflict/negativity, the correlation was .30. Similarly, findings have been reported in previous studies.[55]

The striking contrasts between parents' and children's perceptions of parenting have two implications for family systems and the impact of uncorrelated experiences on development. First, the differing parental and child sensitivities may—in healthy families—operate to keep actual differences in parenting relatively low. The parents' bias toward reporting consistency may reflect their investment in maintaining equity. Thus, while they may be relatively blind to actual inconsistencies across children, they would be sensitive to complaints about it. Children, probably from the earliest ages, develop capacities not only to observe these differences but also to complain about them.[56] This two-generational dipole may function to keep actual differences to a relative minimum. We previously reported that the magnitude of these differences is associated with maladjustment in adolescent siblings.[22]

Second, the high level of children's sensitivities to differences may mean that relatively small differences—as detected by either parents or casual outsiders—may make a big difference in the psychological life of children. Indeed, this generational dipole directs our attention to differences among children in how they perceive family process; these differences may play a large role in their psychological development.

Taken together, these data represent an early effort, using sensitive measures of psychosocial process, to explore a hypotheses generated by research on behavioral genetics. The genetic data, without direct measures of environmental data, suggested that environments specific for each sibling in the family have the biggest impact on normal and pathologic psychological development. The findings reported herein, using a broad range of direct measures of the environment, support this environmental hypothesis derived from genetic studies.

Accepted for publication June 19, 1995.

This research was supported by grant 5-RO1-MH43373 from the National Institute of Mental Health, Rockville, Md, and by a grant from the William T. Grant Foundation, New York, NY.

Reprint requests to Department of Psychiatry and Behavior, George Washington University, Division of Research, 2300 Eye St NW, Ross Hall #613, Washington, DC 20037 (Dr Reiss).

REFERENCES

1. Plomin R, Daniels D. Why are children in the same family so different from one another? *Behav Brain Sci.* 1987;10:1-16.
2. Plomin R, Emde RN, Braungart JM, Campos J, Corley R, Fulker DW, Kagan J, Reznick JS, Robinson J, Zahn-Waxler C, DeFries JC. Genetic change and continuity from fourteen to twenty months: the MacArthur Longitudinal Twin Study. *Child Dev.* 1994;64:1354-1376.
3. Kendler KS, Heath A, Martin NG, Eaves LJ. Symptoms of anxiety and depression in a volunteer twin population. *Arch Gen Psychiatry.* 1986;43:213-221.
4. Wierzbicki M. Similarity of monozygotic and dizygotic child twins in level and lability of subclinically depressed mood. *Am J Orthopsychiatry.* 1987;57:33-40.
5. Rowe DC. Biometrical genetic models of self-reported delinquent behavior: twin study. *Behav Genet.* 1983;13:473-489.
6. Rowe DC. Genetic and environmental components of antisocial behavior: a study of 255 twin pairs. *Child Dev.* 1986;54:473-489.
7. Rowe DC, Rodgers JL, Meseck-Bushey S, St John C. Sexual behavior and non-

sexual deviance: a sibling study of their relationship. *Dev Psychol.* 1989;23: 61-69.

8. Plomin R, Chipuer HH, Neiderhiser J. Behavioral genetic evidence for the importance of the nonshared environment. In: Hetherington EM, Reiss D, Plomin R, eds. *Separate Social Worlds of Siblings: Impact of the Nonshared Environment on Development.* Hillsdale, NJ: Lawrence Erlbaum Associates; 1993:1-33.
9. Cadoret RJ, O'Gorman TW, Troughton E, Heywood E. Alcoholism and antisocial personality: interrelationships, genetic and environmental factors. *Arch Gen Psychiatry.* 1986;42:161-167.
10. Cloninger CR, Gottesman II. Genetic and environmental factors in antisocial behavior disorders. In: Mednick S, Moffitt T, Stack S, eds. *The Causes of Crime.* New York, NY: Cambridge University Press; 1987:92-109.
11. Bertelsen A, Harvald B, Hauge M. A Danish twin study of manic-depressive disorder. *Br J Psychiatry.* 1977;130:330-351.
12. Nurnburger JI, Gershon ES. Genetics of affective disorders. In: Friedman E, ed. *Depression and Antidepressants: Implications for Course and Treatment.* New York, NY: Raven Press; 1981:23-39.
13. Wender PH, Kety SS, Rosenthal D, Schulsinger F, Ortmann J, Lunde I. Psychiatric disorders in the biological and adoptive families of adopted indivduals with affective disorders. *Arch Gen Psychiatry.* 1986;43:923-929.
14. Dunn J, Stocker C, Plomin R. Nonshared experiences within the family: correlates of behavioral problems in middle childhood. *Dev Psychopathol.* 1990; 2:113-126.
15. Dunn J, McGuire S. Young children's nonshared experiences: a summary of studies in Cambridge and Colorado. In: Hetherington EM, Reiss D, Plomin R, eds. *Separate Social Worlds of Siblings: Impact of the Nonshared Environment on Development.* Hillsdale, NJ: Lawrence Erlbaum Associates; 1993:111-128.
16. Tejerina-Allen M, Wagner B, Cohen P. A comparison of across-family and within-family parenting predictors of adolescent psychopathology and suicidal ideation. In: Hetherington EM, Reiss D, Plomin R, eds. *Separate Social Worlds of Siblings: Impact of the Nonshared Environment on Development.* Hillsdale, NJ: Lawrence Erlbaum Associates;1994:143-158.
17. Hetherington EM, Clingempeel WG. Coping with marital transitions: a family systems perspective. *Mongr Soc Res Child Dev.* 1992;57(serial no. 227).
18. Bell DC, Bell LG. Parental validation and support in the development of adolescent daughters. In: Grotevant HD, ed. *Adolescent Development in the Family.* San Francisco, Calif: Jossey Bass Inc; 1983:27-42.
19. Patterson G. *Coercive Family Process: A Social Learning Approach.* Eugene, Ore: Castalia; 1982.
20. Patterson GR, DeBaryshe BD, Ramsey E. A developmental perspective on antisocial behavior. *Am Psychol.* 1989;44:329-335.
21. Nichols RC, Bilbro WC. The diagnosis of twin zygosity. *Acta Genet.* 1966;16: 265-275.
22. Reiss D, Plomin R, Hetherington EM, Howe G, Rovine M, Tryon A. The separate social worlds of teenage siblings. In: Hetherington EM, Reiss D, Plomin R, eds. *Separate Social Worlds of Siblings: Impact of the Nonshared Environment on Development.* Hillsdale, NJ: Lawrence Erlbaum Associates; 1993:63-109.
23. Fisher L, Ransom DC, Terry HW, Lipkin M, Weiss R. The California family health project, I: introduction and description of family health. *Fam Process.* 1992; 31:231-250.
24. Olson DH, McCubbin H, Barnes HL, Larsen AS, Muxen MJ, Wilson MA. *Families: What Makes Them Work.* Beverly Hills, Calif: Sage Publishers Inc; 1989.
25. Sweet JA, Bumpass LL. *American Families and Their Households.* New York, NY: Russell Sage Foundation; 1987.
26. Kovacs M. The Children's Depression Inventory (CDI). *Psychopharmacol Bull.* 1985;21:995-998.
27. Glyshaw K, Cohen LH, Towbes LC. Coping strategies and psychological distress: prospective analyses of early and middle adolescence. *Am J Community Psychol.* 1989;17:607-623.
28. Peterson JL, Zill N. Marital disruption, parent-child relationships and behavior problems in children. *J Marr Fam.* 1986;48:295-307.
29. Faust J, Baum CG, Forehand R. An examination of the association between social relationships and depression in early adolescence. *J Appl Dev Psychol.* 1985;6:291-297.
30. Fauber R, Forehand R, Thomas AM, Wierson M. A mediational model of the impact of conflict on adolescent adjustment in intact and divorced families: the role of disrupted parenting. *Child Dev.* 1990;61:1112-1123.
31. Slotkin J, Forehand R, Fauber R, McCombs A, Long N. Parent-completed and adolescent-completed CDIs: relationship to adolescent social and cognitive functioning. *J Abnorm Child Psychol.* 1988;16:207-217.
32. Achenbach TM, Edelbrock C. Behavioral problems and competencies reported by parents of normal and disturbed childred aged four to sixteen. *Mongr Soc Res Child Dev.* 1981;46(serial no. 188).
33. Kandel DH, Davies M. Adult sequelae of adolescent depressive symptoms. *Arch Gen Psychiatry.* 1986;43:255-262.
34. Panak WF, Garber J, Schwartz D. Parent report on the Child Depression Inventory: reliability and validity. Presented at the American Psychological Association Annual Meeting; August 11-15, 1989; New Orleans, La.
35. Zill N. *Behavior Problems Scale Developed for the 1981 Child Health Supplement to the National Health Interview Survey.* Washington, DC: Child Trends Inc; 1985.
36. Achenbach TM, Edelbrock C. *Manual for the Child Behavior Checklist and Revised Child Behavior Folder.* Burlington, Vt: University of Vermont; 1983.
37. Cohen J. Weighted kappa nominal scale agreement with provision for scaled disagreement or partial credit. *Psychol Bull.* 1968;70:213-222.
38. Straus MA. Measuring intrafamily violence and conflict: the Conflict Tactics (CT) Scale. *J Marr Fam.* 1979;41:75-85.
39. Bentler PM. *EQS Structural Equations Program Manual.* Los Angeles, Calif: BMDP Statistical Software Inc; 1989.
40. Loehlin JC. *Latent Variable Models: An Introduction to Factors, Path and Structural Analysis.* Hillsdale, NJ: Lawrence Erlbaum Associates; 1987.
41. Bank L, Dishion T, Skinner M, Patterson GR. Method variance in structural equation modeling: living with 'glop.' In: Patterson GR, ed. *Depression and Aggression in Family Interaction.* Hillsdale, NJ: Lawrence Erlbaum Associates; 1990:247-279.
42. Gjerde PF, Block J, Block JH. The preschool family context of 18 year olds with depressive symptoms: a prospective study. *J Res Adolesc.* 1991;1:63-92.
43. Patterson GR, Capaldi D, Bank L. An early starter model for predicting delinquency. In: Pepler DJ, Rubin KH, eds. *The Development and Treatment of Childhood Aggression.* Hillsdale, NJ: Lawrence Erlbaum Associates; 1991:139-168.
44. Plomin R, Reiss D, Hetherington EM, Howe G. Nature and nurture: genetic influence on measures of family environment. *Dev Psychol.* 1994;30:32-43.
45. Plomin R, Bergeman CS. The nature of nurture: genetic influence on 'environmental' measures. *Brain Behav Sci.* 1991;14:373-427.
46. Baumrind D. The influence of parenting style on adolescent competence and substance abuse. *J Early Adolesc.* 1991;11:56-95.
47. Elder GH Jr. Problem behavior and family relationships: life course and intergenerational themes. In: Sorensen AM, Weinert FE, Sherrod LR, eds. *Human Development and the Life Course: Multidisciplinary Perspectives.* Hillsdale, NJ: Lawrence Erlbaum Associates; 1986:293-342.
48. Daniels D, Dunn J, Furstenberg F, Plomin R. Environmental differences within the family and adjustment differences within pairs of adolescent siblings. *Child Dev.* 1985;56:764-774.
49. Anderson E, Reiss D, Plomin R, Hetherington EM. The effects of differential parental treatment on personality development during adolescence. *J Fam Psychol.* 1994;8:303-320.
50. Geller B, Chestnut EC, Miller MD, Price DT, Yates E. Preliminary data on *DSM III* associated features of major depressive disorders in children and adolescents. *Am J Psychiatry.* 1985;142:643-644.
51. Puig-Antich J. Major depression and conduct disorder in prepuberty. *J Am Acad Child Psychiatry.* 1982;21:118-128.
52. Woolston JL, Rosenthal SL, Riddle MA, Sparrow SS, Cicchetti D, Zimmerman LD. Childhood comorbidity of anxiety/affective disorders and behavior disorders. *J Am Acad Child Adolesc Psychiatry.* 1989;28:707-713.
53. Capaldi DM. Co-occurrence of conduct problems and depressive symptoms in early adolescent boys, I: familial factors and general adjustment at grade 6. *Dev Psychopathol.* 1991;3:277-300.
54. Conger RD, Conger KJ, Elder GH Jr, Lorenz FO, Simons RL, Whitbeck LB. A family process model of economic hardship and adjustment of early adolescent boys. *Child Dev.* 1992;63:526-541.
55. Daniels D, Plomin R. Differential experiences of siblings in the same family. *Dev Psychol.* 1985;21:747-760.
56. Dunn J, Munn P. Development of justification in disputes with mother and sibling. *Dev Psychol.* 1987;23:791-798.

Seasonal Variation in Plasma L-Tryptophan Availability in Healthy Volunteers

Relationships to Violent Suicide Occurrence

Michael Maes, MD, PhD; Simon Scharpé, PhD; Robert Verkerk, RT; Peter D'Hondt, MD; Dirk Peeters, MD; Paul Cosyns, MD; Paul Thompson, PhD; Frans De Meyer, PhD; Annick Wauters, MS; Hugo Neels, PhD

Objective: To investigate the seasonal variation in levels of plasma L-tryptophan and competing amino acids (CAAs) in healthy humans in relation to climatic variables, total serum protein levels, and violent suicide occurrence.

Methods: Twenty-six healthy volunteers (13 men and 13 women; mean [±SD] age, 38.7±13.4 years) had monthly blood samplings for assays of L-tryptophan, valine, leucine, isoleucine, tyrosine, and phenylalanine during 1 calendar year.

Results: Significant annual rhythms were detected in L-tryptophan, the L-tryptophan/CAA ratio, phenylalanine, valine, and leucine, and semiannual rhythms in L-tryptophan values and in L-tryptophan/CAA ratios. Plasma L-tryptophan and the L-tryptophan/CAA ratio were significantly lower in the spring than in the other seasons. The peak-trough differences in the yearly variation expressed as a percentage of the mean were 17.1% and 16.1% for L-tryptophan values and L-tryptophan/CAA ratios, respectively. The amplitude of the yearly variation in all CAAs was low, ie, less than 7%. An important part of the variance in L-tryptophan availability (ie, 12% to 14%) could be explained by the composite effects of present and past climatic factors; higher ambient temperature and relative humidity in the face of lower air pressure are the most important predictors of low L-tryptophan availability. Important and positive time relationships were noted between total serum protein level and all amino acid concentrations, and a significant time relationship was also noted between the seasonal variation in L-tryptophan availability and the occurrence of violent suicide in Belgium.

Conclusion: Our results show a bimodal seasonal pattern in the availability of plasma L-tryptophan that matches seasonal patterns in the prevalence of violent suicide in the local population and depression in other studies.

(Arch Gen Psychiatry. 1995;52:937-946)

TOTAL OR free plasma L-tryptophan levels and the ratio of L-tryptophan to the sum of amino acids known to compete for the same cerebral uptake mechanism, or competing amino acids (CAAs), ie, valine, leucine, isoleucine, phenylalanine, and tyrosine, are indicators of the availability of L-tryptophan to the brain[1,2] and, consequently, for serotonin (5-hydroxytryptamine [5-HT]) synthesis in the brain.[3] The plasma levels of L-tryptophan and CAAs are subject to an important biological variation.[2] However, the components of biologic variation in these plasma amino acids have not yet been established. It is known that levels of plasma L-tryptophan and CAAs may change in association with eating, eg, protein-rich meals may increase plasma CAAs and L-tryptophan levels, while lowering brain L-tryptophan and 5-HT contents.[2]

Recent reviews[4,5] have provided some evidence that among the biologic factors predisposing toward depressive mood and major depression, alterations in presynaptic 5-HT activity, including decreased plasma total L-tryptophan levels, may be of special interest. Several published reports have claimed that plasma total L-tryptophan levels and the L-tryptophan/CAA ratio are significantly lower in depressed subjects than in healthy controls.[4,6-9] It has been reported that a low L-tryptophan/CAA ratio is related to a favorable clinical response to 5-HT precursors and selective 5-HT reuptake inhibitors.[10,11] Recent studies suggest that a short-term reduction in dietary L-tryptophan intake causes a rapid lowering of mood in healthy humans[12,13] and a rapid, clinically important return of de-

Affiliations of the authors are given in the acknowledgment section at the end of the article.

See Subjects and Methods on next page

SUBJECTS AND METHODS

SUBJECTS

The geographic coordinates for this study were 51.2°N and 4.5°E around Antwerp, Belgium. White volunteers participated in this study. Inclusion criteria were (1) the willingness to undergo monthly blood samplings and (2) physical and psychological health. Subjects were screened for past history of psychiatric and personality disorders by means of the Semi-Structured Clinical Interview of the *DSM-III-R*.[40,41] None of the subjects suffered from Axis I or Axis II disorders. All had scores below 40 on the Zung Anxiety and Depression Inventories and below 9 on the Beck Depression Inventory. All subjects were free of medical (eg, endocrine, immune, or metabolic) disorders. All volunteers reported that they were not taking any drugs (including contraceptives). Subjects with drug (alcohol and any other drugs of dependence) use or abuse were not included. (3) The subjects had to live in an area less than 30 km from the Meteorological Station, Royal Meteorological Institute, Deurne, Antwerp, Belgium. (4) A stable, settled lifestyle was also required for inclusion in the study. Subjects regularly taking international flights and subjects with unusual sleep patterns were excluded. Subjects who travel a lot, such as commercial travelers, were also excluded from this study. No specific instructions were given to the subjects about sleep schedules. (5) Subjects were required to have normal results of blood tests, such as complete blood count and levels of blood urea, nitrogen, electrolytes, liver enzymes (alanine aminotransferase, aspartate aminotransferase, and γ-glutamyltransferase), hemoglobin, and hematocrit, as well as erythrocyte sedimentation rate and thyroid function (basal thyroid-secreting hormone, free thyroxine, and free triiodothyronine levels). (6) Women of childbearing potential were only included if they were willing not to become pregnant during the study.

Exclusion criteria for subjects were (1) acquired immunodeficiency syndrome, (2) premenstrual syndrome, and (3) tobacco use amounting to more than five cigarettes a day. Subjects were excluded during the study span if (1) a new medical illness occurred, except a common cold or oropharyngitis; (2) medications were started during the study period, except occasional use of an over-the-counter drug, such as aspirin; and (3) important negative life events occurred during the study span. The subjects were evaluated every 4 weeks by one of us (D.P. or P.D., who are physicians and psychiatry residents) to check the medical and psychological condition of the subjects. During the study period, subjects were not allowed to spend more than 1 week in a geographic area other than the province of Antwerp or to travel outside an area more than 250 km from Antwerp. After a vacation in an area other than the province of Antwerp, blood was sampled at least 7 days following the return to Antwerp. Use of over-the-counter drugs, such as aspirin, was prohibited for at least 2 days before blood sampling.

Twenty-six volunteers (13 men and 13 women; mean [±SD] age, 38.7±13.4 years; range, 23 to 69 years) participated in this study. All controls were known to one or more of us and gave informed consent to participate in this study in accordance with the ethical standards of the Ethical Committee of the University of Antwerp. All control subjects had the socioeconomic status of the middle-class Belgian population and a mean net monthly income between $1500 and $2500. Subjects were all urbanized persons with a comparable rest-activity schedule.

There are basically three different ways to examine (seasonal) variation over time: (1) the longitudinal study design, (2) the transversal study design, and (3) the hybrid longitudinal-transversal study design.[38] We followed the transversal study design, ie, several individuals are studied during a single period (1 year) to detect whether seasonal rhythms, such as annual rhythms or the harmonics (ie, rhythms of 366 days), are expressed as a group phenomenon.

The study span extended from December 11, 1991, until December 25, 1992. Sixteen subjects had their first blood sampling in December 1991; the other 10 started in January 1992. Seasons were defined by their respective solstices and equinoxes (ie, winter, December 21 through March 20; spring, March 21 through June 20; summer, June 21 through September 20; and fall, September 21 through December 20). Cross-seasons were defined as the periods between (1) November 6 and February 5, (2) February 6 and May 5, (3) May 6 and August 5, and (4) August 6 and November 5.

METHODS

The preparation of the subjects before blood collection was carefully controlled, and the blood collection itself was performed under standardized conditions to minimize sources of preanalytic variation. Blood was always sampled after an overnight fast. An intravenous cannula was inserted at 8 AM (±30 minutes) into the antecubital vein of the subjects. Multiple serum and plasma samples, ie, 65 mL of blood in total, were obtained during a 30-minute period. A total of 50 μL of plasma was stored at −70°C until thawed for assay of the amino acids. The same two phlebotomists (P.D. and D.P.) performed all blood samplings. Each phlebotomist was allocated to the same subjects, so that each subject was always treated by the same investigator. Each subject had 12 monthly blood samplings. Blood samplings in premenopausal women were always performed 5 to 10 days after the first day of the menstrual cycle. There were, during the study period, 59 days on which blood was sampled. The blood sampling procedures were kept constant throughout the study period. All blood samples of each subject (ie, 12 monthly samples) were always assayed in the same run. Blood samples of all subjects were determined in four runs. To compute the intra-assay analytic coefficient of variation (CVa) values, 18 control samples were run and assayed in duplicate. The interassay CVa values were computed on these 36 determinations across the four runs. The amino acids were determined by means of a high-performance liquid chromatography method, as previously described by us.[16] Total serum protein was assayed by means of an automated clinical chemistry analyzer (Kodak Ektachem Analyzer, Kodak, Rochester, NY); the interassay CVa during the study period in our laboratory was 2.89%. The total intraindividual coefficient of variation (CVti) variability (ie, 4.8%=intraindividual+analytic interassay variability) was significantly ($P<.01$) greater than the interassay CVa.

Weather data for the vicinity were taken at the Royal

Meteorological Station of Deurne, which is situated in the eastern part of Antwerp. These data included mean daily atmospheric pressure, air temperature, relative humidity, and wind speed, together with minutes of sunlight and daily precipitation. The daily weather data reflect measurements obtained from midnight to midnight. Therefore, it could be argued that the daily weather measurements from midnight to midnight predominantly reflect weather conditions obtained after blood was sampled (at 8 AM). However, weather variables are known to exhibit a highly positive autocorrelation of a 1-day lag; during the study period, we found positive autocorrelations for air pressure (r=.84, P<.001), light-dark span (r=.55, P<.001), ambient temperature (r=.94, P<.001), humidity (r=.64, P<.001), wind speed (r=.59, P<.001), and rainfall (r=.22, P<.001). Therefore, it may be assumed that weather conditions measured from midnight to midnight reflect the climatic condition around the time that blood samples were obtained.

STATISTICS

Repeated-measures analyses of variance (ANOVAs) were used to investigate the interindividual variability with sex and age (<35 years vs ≥35 years) effects; intraindividual variability with seasonal, cross-seasonal, or monthly differences; and two- or three-way interactions between time×age, time×sex, and time×sex×age. Multiple comparisons among treatment means (eg, seasons) were assessed with the Dunn test.

Variation over time was ascertained by means of least-squares spectral analysis of a single time series or a group of time series and by means of multiple regression and cosinor fit analysis.[42] For a comprehensive review of the theoretical backgrounds of the procedures used in our present study, see De Meyer and Vogelaere.[42] The statistical methods described by De Meyer and Vogelaere are, in part, based on those described in previous publications.[43-46] When the study period contains nonuniformly sampled observations, nonequidistant time intervals, or some missing data, the traditional methods of power spectrum estimation cannot be applied, and use of least-squares amplitude spectrum is advocated.[42]

Spectral analysis identifies the significant rhythms by relatively sharp peaks rising above a continuous background. The only guarantee that these peaks correspond to real physical mechanisms is a significant signal-to-noise ratio in the spectral peaks. F statistics are generated as indicators of the signal-to-noise ratio for each of the rhythms investigated and are listed in a periodogram or F spectrum. In the present study, up to 100 frequencies (rhythms) were scanned during a period of 2 to 366 days. Spectral analyses of single time series were performed on the pooled time series of the 26 healthy subjects after normalization of the amino acid data relative to the yearly mean of the monthly measurements in each of the subjects. This normalization is performed to eliminate all interindividual variability in the data. This study used all significant seasonal rhythms (ie, the annual rhythms and/or the harmonics), which were found in the time series by means of spectral analysis, to compute a multiple-component model. Thus, the total amount of variance in the amino acid data explained by the significant rhythms is estimated by means of multiple regression analysis, ie, time series of amino acids as the dependent variable and the significant rhythms as explanatory variables.[20,23] This procedure allows the delineation of a multiple-component model with estimates of orthophase and range from peak to trough values in a time series with different rhythmic components, as well as the relative contribution of each of the significant rhythms in explaining the variance in the raw data.[20,23] The predicted values are used as an index of the estimated cyclic signal in the time series.[23] These values are, subsequently, extrapolated to all the days in the study period to display the cyclic signal in the raw data. Results of multiple regression analyses on time series are checked for autocorrelation by means of the Durbin-Watson statistic.[47]

Relationships between the amino acids and other explanatory variables were investigated by the following techniques: (1) bivariate or group cosinor or spectral analysis[42] with the assessment of coherence between time series (checked with F statistics) and (2) regression analyses, which considered the amino acids as dependent variables and were pooled over the time series of the 26 healthy subjects (to minimize interindividual variability). Meteorotropism (relationships with climatic variables) was investigated by means of stepwise (step-up), multiple regression analyses pooled over the time series of the 26 healthy subjects; the climatic data were entered as explanatory variables. When evaluating the possible impact of the weather condition on plasma variables, it may be assumed that the latter may respond to a set of climatic variables that work in concert rather than individually and that it takes time (eg, some weeks) for some climatic factors to affect plasma constituents (memory effect). To investigate these possible synergistic and memory effects, a multiple regression model is used whereby present together with lagged climatic data are entered as explanatory variables. Time lags of 1 to 4 weeks of the climatic variables are entered in multiple regression analyses as additional explanatory variables.[23] Thus, 30 present and lagged climatic variables are used as explanatory variables. To prevent multicollinearity, we performed multiple regression analyses whereby (1) the climatic variables are entered in a forward stepwise (step-up) automatic inclusion method (with an F to enter of P=.05) with inspection of the determinant and (2) the first 26 principal components, subtracted from the 30 past and present climatic data by means of factor analysis, are entered as explanatory variables. Relationships between the time series of L-tryptophan availability and violent or nonviolent suicide, alone and together, were investigated by means of regression analyses. The weekly mean number of suicides for all of Belgium was computed by averaging the data of 9 consecutive years, ie, 1979 to 1987.[24]

The total variability (CVt), and total interindividual (ie, analytic and interindividual [CVtg]) and intraindividual (ie, analytic and intraindividual [CVti]) variability, was computed from the sum of squares derived by ANOVA and expressed as CVs.[48-51] The intraindividual (CVi) and interindividual (CVg) values were estimated from the CVti, CVtg, and CVa values according to the following formulas: $CVi^2 = CVti^2 - CVa^2$ and $CVg^2 = CVtg^2 - CVa^2$, where CVa indicates the intra-assay and interassay CVa values, respectively.[48-51] The index of individuality (I index), ie, the CVi/CVg ratio, describes the relationship between CVg and CVi and may be used to evaluate the usefulness of conventional population-based reference values.[50]

Table 1. Seasonal Differences in Plasma Amino Acid Concentrations*

Season	Tryptophan	Tyrosine	Phenylalanine	Valine	Isoleucine	Leucine	L-Tryptophan/CAA Ratio, ×100
Fall	67 (12)	73 (16)	60 (7)	235 (36)	71 (15)	136 (24)	11.9 (2.0)
Winter	69 (16)	72 (15)	59 (8)	232 (36)	72 (15)	132 (24)	12.3 (2.8)
Spring	64 (15)	69 (14)	58 (8)	230 (37)	69 (15)	129 (23)	11.6 (2.5)
Summer	67 (12)	73 (13)	60 (7)	238 (38)	71 (13)	134 (21)	11.8 (2.3)
F (*P*)†	5.1 (.002)	2.9 (.03)	3.2 (.02)	1.6 (.2)	1.1 (.3)	3.0 (.03)	2.2 (.08)
t (*P*)‡	3.8 (<.001)	2.9 (.004)	2.7 (.008)	...	...	2.5 (.01)	2.0 (.04)

*Values are mean (SD) and $\times 10^{-6}$ mol/L.

†Results of repeated-measures analyses of variance (for all, df=3, 274, except tryptophan and tryptophan/competing amino acid [CAA] ratio, for which df=3, 273).

‡Results of Dunn tests for spring vs all other seasons.

pressive symptoms in patients whose depression has remitted.[14,15] Anorexia, anergy, sleep disorders, cognitive disturbances, and depressed mood were shown to be psychopathologic correlates of lower L-tryptophan or L-tryptophan/CAA ratios in depression.[16,17] These findings suggest that lower plasma L-tryptophan availability plays a role in the serotonergic pathophysiology of mood disturbances and major depression.[5]

Numerous studies have reported that there is a seasonal variation in various phenomena, such as mood, depression, feeding behavior, and suicide, that may be related to alterations in central and peripheral 5-HT activity.[2,4] In healthy humans, a seasonal variation is observed in mood, restlessness, appetite, and sleep[18,19]; the seasonal multifrequency time structure in these features is related to multiple cyclic subunits with periodicities around 52 (annual), 26 (semiannual), and 8 (bimensual) weeks.[20,21] Depression and hospital admission rates for depressive disorders have been reported to be more common in spring and autumn.[22,23] In depressed patients, significant annual rhythms are detected in self-rated severity of depression, while peak values in severity of depression are found in the spring.[24] It has long been recognized that some individuals regularly experience depressive episodes annually, ie, recurrent summer and winter depression.[25] The latter is characterized by a distinctive constellation of symptoms, such as carbohydrate craving and overeating, and is labeled seasonal affective disorder.[25] Several studies have reported that suicide occurrence peaks in spring and summer, with lows in fall and winter.[26-28]

Reports also suggest a seasonal variation in various peripheral and central aspects of 5-HT function, eg, tritiated imipramine and tritiated paroxetine binding to platelets, 5-HT levels in the hypothalamus, 5-hydroxyindoleacetic acid concentrations in cerebrospinal fluid, and neuroendocrine responses to 5-HT agonists.[29-36] Some reports have cited a possible seasonal variation in plasma L-tryptophan levels.[29,36,37] Moreover, it has been suggested that the seasonal variation in serotonergic markers, such as plasma L-tryptophan and platelet imipramine-binding sites, parallels the seasonal variation in psychopathologic phenomena, such as the violent suicide rate.[28] The above findings led us to suggest that the yearly variation in psychopathologic phenomena possibly related to 5-HT function, such as violent suicide, may result from yearly rhythms in brain 5-HT metabolism that may underlie a changing susceptibility to various psychosocial loads.[28] However, to our knowledge, no chronoepidemiologic research has investigated the putative time relationships between the seasonal variation in clinical phenomena and 5-HT markers.

Circadian and circannual rhythms in many human physiologic functions are probably related to genetically fixed processes (endogenous rhythms), ie, these rhythms continue after removal of all periodic environmental inputs.[38,39] Although rhythms may be genetically determined, they are continuously modulated and adjusted in time by periodic events in the environment, eg, cycles in light-dark span, ambient temperature, and the activity-rest pattern.[38,39] Thus, the latter serve as entraining agents or synchronizers for endogenous rhythms and determine their timing, ie, they may modulate rhythm parameters, such as acrophase, mesor, or amplitude.[38,39]

The aims of our present study were to (1) quantify the components of biological variation, including seasonality, in levels of plasma L-tryptophan and CAAs, and (2) examine possible relationships between plasma L-tryptophan availability and climatic variables, total serum protein levels, and the occurrence of violent suicide.

RESULTS

ANALYSES OF VARIANCE

Table 1 lists the mean amino acid values in the four seasons. Seasonal differences are shown because these are more significant than the cross-seasonal differences. L-tryptophan values were significantly lower in spring than in the other seasons. By means of repeated-measures ANOVA, significant differences between the study months were found in plasma L-tryptophan concentrations (F=3.3; *df*=11,265; *P*<.001). **Figure 1** shows the mean L-tryptophan values in the 12 study months. Table 1 shows that tyrosine, phenylalanine, and leucine levels were significantly lower in spring than in the other seasons. No seasonal differences were found for valine or isoleucine levels. No monthly (F=1.3; *df*=11,266; *P*=.2) or cross-seasonal (F=1.2; *df*=3,274; *P*=.3) differences were found for plasma valine level. No significant monthly (F=0.7; *df*=11,266; *P*=.7) or cross-seasonal (F=1.6; *df*=3,274; *P*=.2) differences were found for isoleucine levels. The L-tryptophan/CAA ratio was significantly lower in spring than

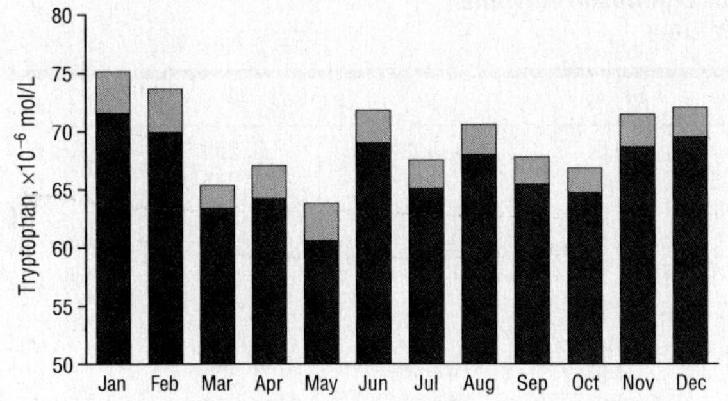

Figure 1. *Monthly mean (darker shading) (SEM [lighter shading]) L-tryptophan values in 26 healthy volunteers.*

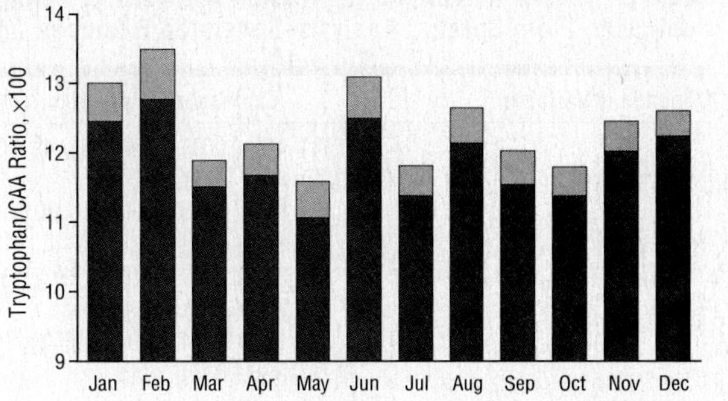

Figure 2. *Monthly mean (darker shading) (SEM [lignter shading]) values for the L-tryptophan/competing amino acids (CAAs) ratio in 26 healthy volunteers.*

in the other seasons; the monthly differences in the L-tryptophan/CAA ratio were significant (F=3.3; *df*=11,265; *P*<.001). **Figure 2** shows the mean L-tryptophan/CAA ratios for the 12 months. No significant time×age, time×sex, or time×sex×age interactions were observed for any of the amino acids.

COSINOR AND SPECTRAL ANALYSIS OF AMINO ACID DATA

Cosinor analyses were performed on the pooled time series of the normalized amino acid values to detect annual or semiannual rhythms. Significant annual rhythms were detected for L-tryptophan (*P*=.009), valine (*P*=.04), phenylalanine (*P*=.002), and leucine (*P*=.003) levels; a trend toward significant annual rhythms was found for isoleucine level (*P*=.07) and the L-tryptophan/CAA ratio (*P*=.09). Significant semiannual rhythms were found for L-tryptophan values (*P*<.001) and L-tryptophan/CAA (*P*=.005) ratios.

Table 2 lists the results of multiple regression analyses, which were performed on the pooled time series of the normalized amino acid data and considered the significant seasonal rhythms subtracted by means of spectral analysis (the rhythms with peak F values in the F spectra) as explanatory variables. We found that 9.8% of the variance in plasma L-tryptophan levels could be explained by three seasonal rhythms, ie, 169 (semiannual), 359 (annual), and 49 days (the latter rhythm corresponds to the eighth harmonic of the annual rhythm); 9.1% of the variance in the L-tryptophan/CAA ratio was explained by three seasonal rhythms, ie, 169 (semiannual), 28, and 57 days (the latter two rhythms correspond to the 14th and seventh harmonics of the annual rhythm, respectively). A small part of the variance in phenylalanine, valine, and leucine values (4% to 6.7%) was explained by annual and some higher-frequency rhythms.

By means of group spectral analysis, a significant annual rhythm (F=3.1, *P*<.05; coherence: F=0, *df*=3,1811; *P*=.99) was found in the time series of the normalized L-tryptophan, valine, tyrosine, phenylalanine, isoleucine, and leucine data (all in *z* transformation). Significant annual rhythms were also detected in the grouped time series of the aromatic amino acids, L-tryptophan, tyrosine, and phenylalanine (F=4.0, *P*<.05; coherence: F=0.7; *df*=2,905; *P*=.5), and in those of the five CAAs (F=3.7, *P*<.05; coherence: F=0; *df*=4,1510; *P*=.99). **Figure 3** and **Figure 4** show the cyclic signals in L-tryptophan levels and L-tryptophan/CAA ratios, computed as the experimental values minus the residualized values obtained from the multiple regression analyses shown in Table 2. Peaks in plasma L-tryptophan level were observed in December to January, troughs were found in March to April to May, and September to October. The peak-trough difference in L-tryptophan values expressed as a percentage of the mean was 17.1%. The differences between winter and spring in Table 1, on the other hand, were only 7.5%. Indeed, as we have explained previously,[24] the computation of differences between seasons (or months) largely underestimates the true variability over time that may exist in a time series. Troughs in the L-tryptophan/CAA ratio were observed in March to April to May and in September to October; peaks were observed in December to January and in June to July to August. The peak-trough difference expressed as a percentage of the mean was 16.1%. There was a highly significant time relationship between plasma L-tryptophan level and L-tryptophan/CAA ratio (pooled *r*=.72; F=329; *df*=1,300; *P*<.001). Bivariate cosinor analysis showed a significant annual rhythm in the time series of L-tryptophan level and L-tryptophan/CAA ratio (F=3.2, *P*<.05; coherence: F=2.6; *df*=1,602; *P*=.1).

An alternative hypothesis is that the yearly variation observed in plasma L-tryptophan levels and in those of the other amino acids could be related to an interaction between a putative circadian variation and changes back and forth between the standard and daylight sampling times. Therefore, we reanalyzed the results of Table 2 (regressions with the significant rhythms index) with the differences between standard and daylight times as additional explanatory variables (entered as a dummy variable). No significant standard vs daylight time effects were found in any of the regression analyses listed in Table 2, eg, for L-tryptophan (F=1.1, *P*=.3) or the L-tryptophan/CAA ratio (F=0.05, *P*=.8).

METEOROTROPISM

Table 2 shows the relationships between the amino acid data and climatic variables. Regression 2 (regressions with the 26 principal components index) shows that an im-

Table 2. Results of Multiple Regression Analyses of Amino Acid Data on Significant Rhythms Subtracted From Spectral Analysis–Generated F Spectra and on Climatic Data

Dependent Variable	Explanatory Variables, (*P*)*	R^2, %	F	*df*	*P*
Tryptophan	(1) 169 (.001); 359 (.03); 49 (.05)	9.8	5.3	6, 295	<.001
	(2) First 26 PCs	12.5	1.5	26, 275	.05
	(3) −T0 (<.001); −H3 (.001)	6.5	10.4	2, 299	<.001
Phenylalanine	(1) 366 (.01); 23.8 (.07)	5.9	4.7	4, 298	.001
Valine	(1) 344 (.03); 13 (.03); 28 (.03)	6.7	3.5	6, 296	.002
	(2) First 26 PCs	14.0	1.7	26, 276	.02
	(3) −R0 (.001); −W2 (.003); −P3 (.02)	6.2	6.6	3, 299	<.001
Leucine	(1) 366 (.002)	4.0	6.3	2, 300	.003
	(2) First 26 PCs	13.0	1.6	26, 276	.04
	(3) −P3 (.02); −R0 (.03); −W2 (.04)	3.6	3.7	3, 299	.01
Tryptophan/competing amino acid ratio	(1) 169 (.002); 28 (.02); 57 (.03)	9.1	4.9	6, 295	<.001
	(2) First 26 PCs	14.1	1.7	26, 275	.02
	(3) −T0 (<.001); −H3 (.003); +P0 (.02)	7.4	7.9	3, 298	<.001

Listed are the results of 13 multiple regression analyses with the following explanatory variables: (1) the significant rhythms (in days) subtracted from the spectral analysis–generated F spectra; (2) the first 26 principal components (PCs) subtracted from the past and present climatic data; and (3) past and present climatic data and T indicates ambient temperature; H, relative humidity; R, rainfall; W, wind speed; P, air pressure; 0, 1, 2, and 3, the time lag (in weeks) by which the climatic variables were entered in the analyses; and plus or minus sign, the sign of the explanatory variables in the regression equation.

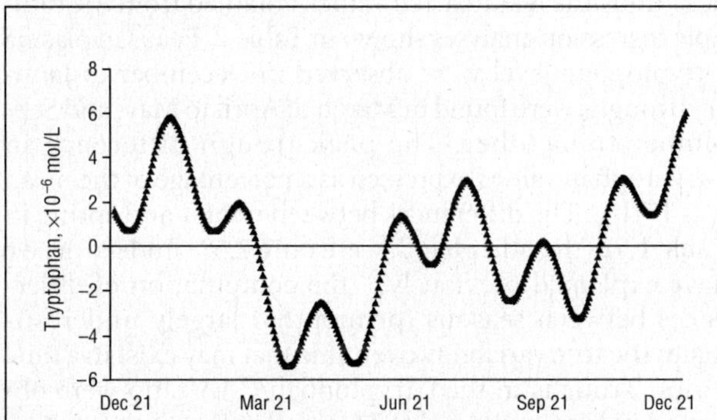

Figure 3. *Seasonal variation in plasma L-tryptophan concentrations. This chronogram shows the cyclic signal in plasma L-tryptophan values subtracted by means of spectral analysis on the pooled time series of the normalized L-tryptophan data (ie, normalized relative to the yearly mean values in each subject).*

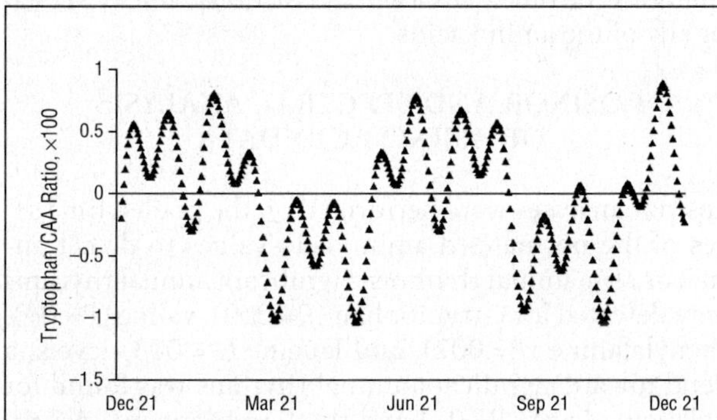

Figure 4. *Seasonal variation in the L-tryptophan/competing amino acids (CAAs) ratio. This chronogram shows the cyclic signal in the L-tryptophan/CAAs ratio subtracted by means of spectral analysis on the pooled time series of the normalized L-tryptophan/CAAs data (ie, normalized relative to the yearly mean values in each subject).*

portant part of the variance (>10%) in L-tryptophan, valine, and leucine values and the L-tryptophan/CAA ratio could be explained by the first 26 principal components subtracted from the 30 current and lagged climatic data. No significant time relationships were found between the climatic data and phenylalanine, tyrosine, or isoleucine values. By means of step-up multiple regression analyses pooled over the time series of the 26 healthy subjects, we determined which climatic variables correlated with the amino acid values. Lower temperature and humidity (memory effect of 3 weeks) explained part of the variance in L-tryptophan values. The same variables together with air pressure explained part of the variance in the L-tryptophan/CAA ratios. Valine and leucine levels were, in part, predicted by rainfall, air pressure, and wind speed (all negatively loaded in the regression analysis).

RELEVANT RELATIONSHIPS

Correlation analyses pooled over the time series of the 26 healthy subjects (which assess the within-subject variability in the amino acid data and, thus, the time relationships) showed significant and positive correlations between all amino acids (all *P*<.001). The within-subject variability in the L-tryptophan/CAA ratio was significantly related to L-tryptophan level (positive) and negatively to valine, isoleucine, and leucine levels (all *P*<.001). No significant time relationships were found between the ratio and tyrosine and phenylalanine levels.

Correlation analyses pooled over the time series of the 26 subjects showed significant and positive correlations between total serum protein and L-tryptophan (*r*=.28, *P*<.001), tyrosine (*r*=.21, *P*<.001), phenylalanine (*r*=.26, *P*<.001), valine (*r*=.17, *P*=.004), isoleucine (*r*=.13, *P*=.02), and leucine (*r*=.25, *P*<.001) values. Group spectral analysis showed a significant annual rhythm in total serum protein and L-tryptophan, valine, tyrosine, phenylalanine, isoleucine, and leucine values (F=4.5, *P*<.05; coherence: F=0; *df*=6,2117; *P*=.99).

There were significant relationships between the time series of plasma L-tryptophan levels and the weekly number of total suicides (*r*=−.49, *P*<.001) and violent sui-

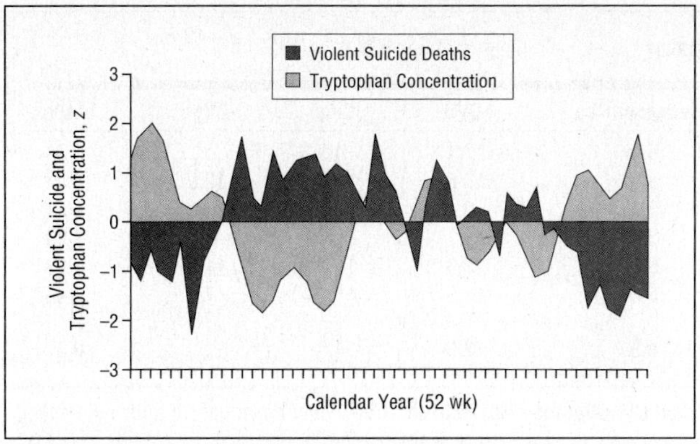

Figure 5. *Time relationship between plasma L-tryptophan concentrations in 26 healthy volunteers and the incidence of violent suicide (mean weekly values from 1979 to 1987) for the local population (both variables are in z transformation). Lightly shaded area indicates tryptophan concentrations; heavily shaded area, deaths.*

cides ($r=-.61$, $P<.001$) but not the number of nonviolent suicides ($r=.08$, $P=.6$). **Figure 5** shows the time series of plasma L-tryptophan levels and number of violent suicides in Belgium. After *P* value correction (*P* level adjusted for multiple tests: $P=.008$) and correction for autocorrelation, a trend toward a significant and negative correlation ($r=-.32$, $P=.02$) between the L-tryptophan/CAA ratio and the weekly number of violent suicides was detected. The acrophases of the annual rhythm in violent suicide and L-tryptophan levels were 161.4° (or 23.3 weeks) and 339.2° (or 49 weeks), respectively. Consequently, the phase difference between the annual rhythms in both time series equals 178°. This shows that the annual rhythms in both time series are ±180° out of phase with respect to each other, which is in correspondence with the significant inverse relationship between both factors (see also Figure 4). Therefore, bivariate cosinor analysis was performed on the time series of violent suicide and L-tryptophan levels after rotation of the latter by 180°. A highly significant common annual rhythm was detected in the time series of violent suicide and plasma L-tryptophan levels ($F=36.6$, $P<.001$; coherence: $F=0$; $df=1,102$; $P=.95$). The common peak and nadir values of violent suicide and L-tryptophan levels, respectively, occurred at 23.2 weeks (160.5°).

COMPONENTS OF BIOLOGICAL VARIATION

Table 3 shows the CVa values and the components of biological variation in the amino acid data expressed as CV values. Listed are total CVt, intra-assay and interassay CVa, intraindividual CVi, interindividual CVg, and the I index. Because significant sex effects (men showed higher plasma concentrations) were detected for tyrosine ($F=7.5$; $df=1,23$; $P=.01$), phenylalanine ($F=5.2$; $df=1,23$; $P=.03$), valine ($F=12.4$; $df=1,23$; $P=.002$), isoleucine ($F=13.2$; $df=1,23$; $P=.002$), and leucine ($F=17.4$; $df=1,23$; $P<.001$), the CVg values of those amino acids were adjusted for sex effects. The I index was computed on those sex-adjusted CVg values. It can be seen that for each amino acid and the L-tryptophan/CAA ratio, the intra-assay CVa values were significantly ($P<.01$) lower than the CVi values. For most variables, except L-tryptophan values and L-tryptophan/CAA ratios, the I index was greater than 1; for phenylalanine and leucine values, the I index was greater than 1.4.

COMMENT

The major findings of our study are that the availability of plasma L-tryptophan to the brain shows a significant seasonal variation in healthy humans and that it is related to climatic variables, total serum protein level, and the occurrence of violent suicide. The findings are discussed below.

SEASONAL VARIATION IN PLASMA TRYPTOPHAN AVAILABILITY

The major finding of our study is that the availability of L-tryptophan to the brain exhibits a significant seasonal variation in healthy persons and that it is expressed as a group phenomenon (Figures 3 and 4). It was found that a significant part of the variance (±10%) in L-tryptophan values and L-tryptophan/CAA ratios could be explained by seasonal rhythms, such as annual and semiannual rhythms. The peak-trough differences in the yearly variation expressed as a percentage of the mean L-tryptophan values and L-tryptophan/CAA ratios were 17.1% and 16.1%, respectively. The yearly variation in the CAAs, on the other hand, was less pronounced, although significant annual rhythms were found for valine, phenylalanine, and leucine. Overall, there was a trend for the plasma CAA levels to be lower in spring, but the amplitude of the seasonal changes was very low. In this respect, L-tryptophan values showed significant time relationships with all other amino acids. The variability over time in the L-tryptophan/CAA ratio appeared to be determined by changes in L-tryptophan, valine, leucine, and isoleucine values, but not by changes in tyrosine or phenylalanine levels. Most important, the six amino acids showed significant and positive time relationships with total serum protein level. This may suggest that the seasonal variation in L-tryptophan availability is, in part, related to changes in protein homeostasis.

Comparison of our results and those of previous reports on seasonal variation in the availability of L-tryptophan[29,36,37] is hampered by the following. First, the delineation of "seasonal variation" should rely on the detection of seasonal rhythms (ie, annual rhythms or derivatives thereof, such as the harmonics) in the time series of the variables under consideration.[20,23,28] Least-squares spectral analysis in conjunction with cosinor fit and multiple regression analysis are most suited to identify all significant (seasonal) rhythms that may exist in a time series and estimate their relative contribution to the variance in the time series.[20,23,28,42] These methods allow the computation of a multiple component cosine model with estimates of orthophase and the range of change from low to peak values in a time series with different rhythmic components.[20,23,28] Most previous studies on "seasonal variation" in 5-HT–related functions, including plasma L-tryptophan levels, have often computed the monthly or bimonthly means and have analyzed these data by ANOVA or Student's *t* tests. Because these meth-

Table 3. Components of Biological Variation in Plasma Amino Acid Data*

Variables	CVt	Intra-assay CVa	Interassay CVa	CVi	CVg	CVg[1]	I Index
Tryptophan	20.8	4.1	5.8	13.4	14.3	...	0.94
Tyrosine	20.6	2.7	3.9	13.8	14.6	12.9	1.07
Phenylalanine	13.1	2.9	5.3	9.1	7.1	6.0	1.52
Valine	16.0	1.3	3.4	11.1	11.0	8.6	1.29
Isoleucine	21.1	3.2	5.8	13.6	14.7	11.2	1.21
Leucine	17.5	3.2	5.8	11.3	11.5	7.8	1.45
Tryptophan/competing amino acid ratio	20.1	4.4	4.8	12.5	14.3	...	0.87

**CVt indicates total coefficient of variation (CV); CVa, analytic CV; CVi, intraindividual CV; CVg, interindividual CV; CVg[1], interindividual CV after subtracting the effects of sex; and I index, index of individuality. Values are CVs in percentages.*

ods do not allow proof of seasonal rhythms, these studies only suggest that there are differences in the variables across the months or seasons rather than providing conclusive evidence for seasonal "variation." Second, study design and analytic assays should be performed according to a rigid protocol.[52] Thus, a series of specimens is taken from ostensibly healthy individuals, the specimen handling procedures are kept constant throughout the study period to minimize preanalytic variation, and each set of specimens from an individual should be analyzed in a single run.[52] In addition, the magnitude of the intra-assay CVa values should be compared with that of the intraindividual CVi values to ascertain that the intraindividual, including seasonal, variation is detectable with the analytic assay used. Most previous studies reporting "seasonal variation" in 5-HT–related functions did not adequately describe the study design or analytic procedures. None of the above studies has presented data on CVi values, while CVa values were sometimes not even mentioned. Third, previous research has examined fewer subjects in prospective studies or performed cross-sectional studies. From our results, it is clear that seasonal variation in L-tryptophan availability may be difficult to detect in cross-sectional studies owing to the large interindividual variability and the lower percentage of the intraindividual variability explained by seasonal effects. Fourth, accurate high-performance liquid chromatography assays to determine amino acid levels were not always used in previous studies. Fifth, differences in geographic coordinates of the studies may explain differences between studies examining biologic functions. Indeed, the specific genetic constellation of the European population and the specific environmental and climatic factors in this part of Belgium may have produced a seasonal variation in L-tryptophan variability that is specific to this part of Europe.

Although the results of our study clearly show that the availability of L-tryptophan to the brain is organized along a multifrequency seasonal time structure, they do not provide further information on the nature of this variation. Indeed, there are two possibilities: (1) the rhythms observed herein are due to a seasonal variation in the daily mean availability of L-tryptophan and (2) the findings are due to a putative seasonal modulation of putative circadian rhythms in plasma L-tryptophan availability. Circadian rhythms in plasma L-tryptophan have been observed in humans by some but not all authors.[53-55] Seasonal modulation of circadian rhythms has been observed in some other human functions organized along a daily and seasonal time structure, eg, immune functions.[56] The results of our study show that further investigation of a putative seasonal modulation of circadian rhythms in L-tryptophan availability may be limited to some time points during the calendar year, ie, January, May, June, and September (ie, those periods with maximal changes, or with peaks and troughs in L-tryptophan availability).

PLASMA TRYPTOPHAN AVAILABILITY, WEATHER VARIABLES, AND TOTAL SERUM PROTEIN LEVEL

Our study showed that an important part of the variance in L-tryptophan availability (ie, 12.5% to 14.1%) could be explained by present and past (ie, memory effect) climatic factors. Higher ambient temperature and increased relative humidity in the face of lower air pressure appeared to be related to lower L-tryptophan availability. The lack of a significant relationship between the light-dark span and plasma L-tryptophan values is important in light of the extensive literature on the relationships between light (changes in light-dark span as well as phototherapy) and recurrent winter depression.[25] Sarrias et al,[36] on the other hand, were unable to find any relationship between total L-tryptophan levels and ambient temperature or photoperiod. However, these authors did not investigate the synergistic and memory effects of the climatic data on L-tryptophan availability. Multiple regression analysis with inclusion of present and lagged climatic data as explanatory variables and pooled over the time series of the subjects should be used to evaluate the effects of short-term changes in atmospheric activity on the availability of L-tryptophan to the brain. In any case, our findings support the view that environmental factors, such as weather conditions, may modulate the seasonal time structure of L-tryptophan availability. Future research should investigate whether there is a time relationship between the seasonal variation in tryptophan availability and factors that are known to modulate L-tryptophan or protein homeostasis and to act as putative messenger molecules transducing environmental signals to the body, eg, glucocorticoids[57] and catecholamines.[58]

Our results suggest that part of the intraindividual variability in levels of all amino acids, including

L-tryptophan, is related to total serum protein level. These findings could suggest that the seasonality in L-tryptophan availability may, in part, be a reflection of a seasonal rhythm in dietary habits, especially because there is some evidence of a progressive increase in energy intake as well as in protein intake from spring to winter.[59] Other authors, however, reported that food intake is higher in autumn and winter than in spring and summer,[60] while Debry et al[61] observed a maximum of protein intake in spring and autumn in 4- to 5-year-old children. It has been suggested that the seasonal variation in protein (and food) intake is, in part, endogenously determined and that it is a function of nutritional requirements.[59] Moreover, it is believed that the annual changes in photoperiod and periodic variations in lifestyle (rest-activity level) may be synchronizers for these rhythms in protein homeostasis.[59]

PLASMA TRYPTOPHAN AVAILABILITY AND PSYCHOPATHOLOGIC PHENOMENA

The results of our study show a bimodal seasonal pattern in the availability of plasma L-tryptophan that matches seasonal patterns in the prevalence of depression and suicide in other studies and the prevalence of violent suicide in the local population. Thus, the findings may be considered to be consistent with the literature on recurrent winter and summer depression in that these types of depression typically begin in late fall and late spring, respectively,[25] the times of low L-tryptophan availability. Increased risk for violent suicide,[28] increased admission rates to psychiatric hospitals,[23] and increased severity of self-rated depression in depressed subjects[24] in Belgium also typically occur during March to May or September to October, the times of low L-tryptophan availability. Moreover, we found a significant inverse relationship between the time series of L-tryptophan availability and the occurrence of violent suicide in the local population, suggesting that there is an inverse relationship between the availability of L-tryptophan to the brain and increased risk for violent suicide. There is some evidence that dysfunctional 5-HT activity is related to depression, suicide, violent suicide, or impulsivity.[4,5,62-64] Therefore, it may be hypothesized that the seasonal variation in plasma L-tryptophan availability to the brain with possibly altered central 5-HT activity (see the introductory portion of this article) in spring and fall could put suicide-prone subjects at higher risk and could be related to an increased incidence of depression or an increase in severity of depression in these seasons.

COMPONENTS OF BIOLOGICAL VARIATION

Data on biological variation are required for the interpretation of changes in serial results and for the evaluation of the desirable standards of analytic performance and population-based reference ranges.[52] The computation of the interindividual (CVg) and intraindividual (CVi) CVs showed that the index of individuality (CVi/CVg ratio) for phenylalanine and leucine was greater than 1.4. Therefore, population-based reference ranges for these two amino acids may be used for the correct interpretation of amino acid measurements.[50,52] The index of individuality for the other amino acids was between 1.0 and 1.4, and for L-tryptophan and L-tryptophan/CAA ratios was even less than 1.0. Thus, population-based reference ranges for L-tryptophan levels and the L-tryptophan/CAA ratio have less clinical relevance for the correct interpretation of the data: individuals may have values that are unusual for them but that still fall within the population-based reference limits. Comparison of test results with those obtained previously in the same individuals are of more interest.[50] From the computed CVi values, it may also be deduced that the analytic goals for acceptability[50] of the imprecision of a L-tryptophan assay should be less than 6.75% and that of the L-tryptophan/CAA ratio should be less than 6.25%.[50] In our laboratory, the intra-assay CVa for L-tryptophan was 3.2% and for the L-tryptophan/CAA ratio was 5.0%.

CONCLUSIONS

Our results show a significant seasonal variation in the availability of plasma L-tryptophan to the brain, with low levels occurring in spring. The availability of plasma L-tryptophan to the brain was, in part, related to climatic factors, such as ambient temperature, air pressure, and relative humidity, and to total serum protein level. The seasonal pattern in plasma L-tryptophan level was inversely related to the seasonal variation in the occurrence of violent suicide in the local population.

Accepted for publication March 13, 1995.

From the University Department of Psychiatry, Clinical Research Center–Mental Health, Antwerp, Belgium (Dr Maes); the Department of Psychiatry (Dr Maes) and the Data Center (Dr Thompson), Case Western Reserve University, Cleveland, Ohio; the Departments of Clinical Biochemistry (Dr Scharpé) and Medical Biochemistry (Mr Verkerk), University of Antwerp (Belgium); the Department of Psychiatry, University Hospital of Antwerp (Drs Maes, D'Hondt, Peeters, and Cosyns); the Department of Geophysics and Statistics, Royal Meteorological Institute, Brussels, Belgium (Dr De Meyer); and the Laboratory of Clinical Biology, Middelheim Ziekenhuis, Antwerp (Mr Wauters and Dr Neels).

This research was supported in part by the American Suicide Foundation, the Michael Kaplen Investigator Award (Dr Maes), the Nationaal Fonds voor Wetenschappelijk Onderzoek, and the University of Antwerp (Belgium) Program.

The secretarial assistance of Carine Maes, RN, and Lee Mason is greatly appreciated.

Reprint requests to Clinical Research Center–Mental Health, Department of Psychiatry, AZ Stuivenberg, 267 Lange Beeldekensstraat, 2060 Antwerp, Belgium (Dr Maes).

REFERENCES

1. Fernstrom JD. Tryptophan availability and serotonin synthesis in rat brain: effects of experimental diabetes. In: Schlossberger HG, Kochen W, Linzen B, Steinhart H, eds. *Progress in Tryptophan and Serotonin Research.* Berlin, Germany: Walter de Gruyter; 1984:161-172.
2. Acworth IA, During MJ, Wurtman RJ. Processes that couple amino acid availability to neurotransmitter synthesis and release. In: Huether G, ed. *Amino Acid*

Availability and Brain Function in Health and Disease. New York, NY: Springer-Verlag NY Inc; 1988:117-136.
3. Moir ATB, Eccleston D. The effect of precursor loading in the cerebral metabolism of 5-hydroxyindoles. *J Neurochem.* 1968;15:1093-1108.
4. Meltzer HY, Lowy MT. The serotonin hypothesis of depression. In: Meltzer HY, ed. *Psychopharmacology: The Third Generation of Progress.* New York, NY: Raven Press; 1987:513-526.
5. Maes M, Meltzer HY. The serotonin hypothesis of depression. In: Bloom FE, Kupfer DJ, eds. *Psychopharmacology: The Fourth Generation of Progress.* New York, NY: Raven Press; 1995:933-944.
6. Maes M, De Ruyter M, Hobin P, Suy E. Relationship between the dexamethasone suppression test and the L-tryptophan/competing amino acids ratio in depression. *Psychiatry Res.* 1987;21:323-335.
7. Maes M, Jacobs M-P, Suy E, Minner B, Leclercq C, Christiaens F, Raus J. Suppressant effects of dexamethasone on the availability of plasma L-tryptophan and tyrosine in healthy controls and in depressed patients. *Acta Psychiatr Scand.* 1990;81:19-23.
8. Maes M, Jacobs M-P, Suy E, Vandewoude M, Minner B, Raus J. Effects of dexamethasone on the availability of L-tryptophan and on the insulin and FFA concentrations in unipolar depressed patients. *Biol Psychiatry.* 1990;27:854-862.
9. Cowen PJ, Parry-Billings M, Newsholme EA. Decreased plasma tryptophan levels in major depression. *J Affect Disord.* 1989;16:27-31.
10. MHoller SE. Tryptophan to competing amino acids ratio in depressive disorder: relation to efficacy of antidepressive treatments. *Acta Psychiatr Scand Suppl.* 1985;72:1-30.
11. Møller SE, Bech P, Bjerrum H, Bøjholm S, Butler B, Folker H, Gram LF, Larsen JK, Lauritzen L, Loldrup D, Munk-Andersen E, Odum K, Rafaelsen OJ. Plasma ratio tryptophan/neutral amino acids in relation to clinical response to paroxetine and clomipramine in patients with major depression. *J Affect Disord.* 1990; 18:59-66.
12. Young SN, Smith SE, Pihl R, Ervin FR. Tryptophan depletion causes a rapid lowering of mood in normal males. *Psychopharmacology.* 1985;87:173-177.
13. Smith SE, Pihl RO, Young SW, Ervin FR. A test of possible cognitive and environmental influences on the mood lowering effect of tryptophan depletion in normal males. *Psychopharmacology.* 1987;91:451-457.
14. Delgado PL, Charney DS, Price LH, Landis H, Heninger GR. Neuroendocrine and behavioral effects of dietary tryptophan restriction in healthy subjects. *Life Sci.* 1990;45:2323-2332.
15. Heninger GR, Delgado PL, Charney DS, Price LH, Aghajanian GK. Tryptophan-deficient diet and amino acid drink deplete plasma tryptophan and induce a relapse of depression in susceptible patients. *J Chem Neuroanat.* 1992;5:347-348.
16. Maes M, Maes L, Schotte C, Vandewoude M, Martin M, D'Hondt P, Blockx P, Scharpé S, Cosyns P. Clinical subtypes of unipolar depression; III: quantitative differences in various biological markers between the cluster analysis-generated non-vital and vital depression classes. *Psychiatry Res.* 1990;34:59-75.
17. Maes M, Maes L, Suy E. Symptom profiles of biological markers in depression: a multivariate study. *Psychoneuroendocrinology.* 1990;15:29-37.
18. Kasper S, Wehr TA, Bartko JJ, Gaist PA, Rosenthal NE. Epidemiological findings of seasonal changes in mood and behavior. *Arch Gen Psychiatry.* 1989; 46:823-833.
19. Haggag A, Eklund B, Linaker O, Gotestam KG. Seasonal mood variation: an epidemiological study in northern Norway. *Acta Psychiatr Scand.* 1990;81:141-145.
20. Maes M, De Meyer F, Peeters D, Meltzer H, Cosyns P, Schotte C. Seasonal variation and meteotropism in various self-rated psychological and physiological features of a normal couple. *Int J Biometeorol.* 1992;36:195-200.
21. Barnston AG. The effect of weather on mood, productivity, and frequency of emotional crisis in a temperate continental climate. *Int J Biometeorol.* 1988; 32:134-143.
22. Eastwood MR, Peacocke J. Seasonal patterns of suicide, depression and electroconvulsive therapy. *Br J Psychiatry.* 1976;129:472-475.
23. Maes M, De Meyer F, Peeters D, Meltzer HY, Schotte C, Scharpé S, Cosyns P. Seasonality and meteotropism in psychiatric psychopathology: the periodicities in and biometeorological relationships with the number of patients admitted to an acute psychiatric ward. *Int J Biometeorol.* 1993;37:78-82.
24. Maes M, Meltzer HY, Suy E, De Meyer F. Seasonality in severity of depression: relationships to suicide and homicide occurrence. *Acta Psychiatr Scand.* 1993; 88:156-161.
25. Wehr TA, Rosenthal NE. Seasonality and affective illness. *Am J Psychiatry.* 1989;146:829-839.
26. Barraclough BM, White SJ. Monthly variation of suicidal, accidental and undetermined poisoning deaths. *Br J Psychiatry.* 1978;132:279-282.
27. Souetre E, Salvati E, Belugou JL, Douillet P, Braccini T, Darcourt G. Seasonality of suicides: environmental, sociological and biological covariations. *J Affect Disord.* 1987;13:215-225.
28. Maes M, Cosyns P, Meltzer HY, De Meyer F, Peeters D. Significant seasonality in violent suicide occurrence but not in non-violent suicide or homicide occurrence. *Am J Psychiatry.* 1993;150:1380-1385.
29. Swade C, Coppen A. Seasonal variations in biochemical factors related to depressive illness. *J Affect Disord.* 1980;2:249-255.
30. Carlsson A, Svennerholm L, Winblad B. Seasonal and circadian monoamine variations in human brains examined post mortem. *Acta Psychiatr Scand Suppl.* 1979;280:75-85.
31. Brewerton TD. Seasonal variation of serotonin function in humans: research and clinical implications. *Ann Clin Psychiatry.* 1989;1:153-164.
32. Brewerton TD, Berrettini W, Nurnberger J, Linnoila M. An analysis of seasonal fluctuations of CSF monoamines and neuropeptides in normal controls: findings with 5-HIAA and HVA. *Psychiatr Res.* 1988;23:257-265.
33. Klompenhouwer JL, Fekkes D, van Hulst AM, Moleman P, Pepplinkhuizen L, Mulder PGH. Seasonal variations in binding of ^{3}H-paroxetine to blood platelets in healthy volunteers: indications for a gender difference. *Biol Psychiatry.* 1990;28:509-517.
34. Arora RC, Meltzer HY. Seasonal variation of imipramine binding in the blood platelets of normal controls and depressed patients. *Biol Psychiatry.* 1988;23:217-226.
35. DeMet EM, Reist C, Bell KM, Gerner RH, Chicz-DeMet A, Warren S, Wu J. Decreased seasonal mesor of platelet ^{3}H-imipramine binding in depression. *Biol Psychiatry.* 1991;29:427-440.
36. Sarrias MJ, Artigas F, Martinez E, Gelpi E. Seasonal changes of plasma serotonin and related parameters: correlations with environmental measures. *Biol Psychiatry.* 1989;26:695-706.
37. Wirz-Justice A, Ritcher R. Seasonality in biochemical determinations: a source of variance and a clue to the temporal incidence of affective illness. *Psychiatr Res.* 1979;1:53-60.
38. Haus E, Touitou Y. Chronobiology in laboratory medicine. In: Touitou Y, Haus E, eds. *Biologic Rhythms in Clinical and Laboratory Medicine.* New York, NY: Springer-Verlag NY Inc; 1992:673-708.
39. Haus E, Touitou Y. Principles of clinical chronobiology. In: Touitou Y, Haus E, eds. *Biologic Rhythms in Clinical and Laboratory Medicine.* New York, NY: Springer-Verlag NY Inc; 1992:6-34.
40. American Psychiatric Association. *Diagnostic and Statistical Manual of Mental Disorders, Revised Third Edition.* Washington, DC: American Psychiatric Association; 1987.
41. Spitzer RL, Williams JBW, Gibbon MSW, First MB. *Structured Clinical Interview According to* DSM-III-R. Washington, DC: American Psychiatric Press Inc; 1990.
42. De Meyer F, Vogelaere P. Spectral resolution of cardio-circulatory variations in men measured by autorhythmometry over 2 years. *Int J Biometeorol.* 1991; 34:105-121.
43. Nelson W, Tong YL, Lee J, Halberg F. Methods for cosinor rhythmometry. *Chronobiologia.* 1979;6:305-323.
44. Bingham C, Arbogast B, Cornelissen G, Lee JK, Halberg F. Inferential statistical methods for estimating and comparing cosinor parameters. *Chronobiologia.* 1982;9:397-439.
45. Blackman RB, Tukey JW. *The Measurement of Power Spectra.* New York, NY: Dover Publications Inc; 1959.
46. Vanicek P. Approximate spectral analysis by least-squares fit. *Astrophys Space Sci.* 1969;4:387-391.
47. Ostrom CW. The time series analysis: regression techniques. In: Sullivan JL, Niemi RG, eds. *Quantitative Applications in the Social Sciences.* London, England: Sage Publications; 1988.
48. Fraser CG, Harris EK. Generation and application of data on biological variation in clinical chemistry. *Crit Rev Clin Lab Sci.* 1989;27:409-437.
49. Fraser CG. Biological variation. In: *Interpretation of Clinical Chemistry Laboratory Data.* Boston, Mass: Blackwell Scientific Publications Inc; 1986:111-135.
50. Libeer J-P. *External Quality Assessments in Clinical Laboratories: European Perspectives, Today and Tomorrow.* Antwerp, Belgium: University of Antwerp; 1993. Doctoral Thesis.
51. Fraser CG. Biological variation in clinical chemistry: an update: collected data, 1988-1991. *Arch Pathol Lab Med.* 1992;116:916-923.
52. Fraser CG. Data on biological variation: essential prerequisites for introducing new procedures? *Clin Chem.* 1994;40:1671-1673.
53. Malatino L, Fiore CE, Costa M, Calandra C, Petrone G, Cacciola S. Circadian rhythm of plasma tryptophan in clinically healthy subjects and patients with endogenous depression. *Chronobiologia.* 1981;9:13-20.
54. Birkmayer W, Linauer W. Storung des Tyrosin und Tryptophan Metabolismus bei Depression. *Arch Psychiatr Nervenkr.* 1970;213:377-387.
55. Tagliamonte A, Gessa R, Biggio G, Vargiu L, Gessa GL. Daily changes of free serum tryptophan in humans. *Life Sci.* 1974;14:349-354.
56. Lévi F, Canon C, Touitou Y, Reinberg A, Mathé G. Seasonal modulation of the circadian time structure of circulating T and natural killer lymphocyte subsets from healthy subjects. *J Clin Invest.* 1988;81:407-413.
57. Agrimonti F, Angeli A, Frairia R, Fazzari AM, Tamagnone C, Fornaro D, Ceresa F. Circannual rhythmicalities of cortisol levels in the peripheral plasma of healthy adult subjects. *Chronobiologia.* 1982;9:107-114.
58. Keatinge WR, Coleshaw SRK, Cotter F, Mottoie M, Murphy M, Chelliah R. Increases in platelet and red cell counts, blood viscosity and arterial pressure during mild surface cooling: factors in mortality from coronary and cerebral thrombosis in winter. *BMJ.* 1984;289:1405-1408.
59. Mejean L, Kolopp M, Drouin P. Chronobiology, nutrition, and diabetes mellitus. In: Touitou Y, Haus E, eds. *Biologic Rhythms in Clinical and Laboratory Medicine.* New York, NY: Springer-Verlag NY Inc; 1992:375-385.
60. Sargent F. Season and the metabolism of fat and carbohydrate: a study of vestigal physiology. *Meteorol Monogr.* 1954;2:68-80.
61. Debry G, Bleyer R, Reinberg A. Circadian, circannual and other rhythms in spontaneous nutrient and caloric intake of healthy four year olds. *Diabetes Metab Rev.* 1975;1:91-99.
62. Lidberg L, Tuck JR, Asberg M, Scalia-Tomba GP, Bertilsson L. Homicide, suicide and CSF 5-HIAA. *Acta Psychiatr Scand.* 1985;71:230-236.
63. Asberg M, Traskman L, Thoren P. 5-HIAA in the cerebrospinal fluid. *Arch Gen Psychiatry.* 1976;33:1193-1197.
64. Linnoila M, Virkkunen M, Scheinin M. Low cerebrospinal fluid 5-hydroxyindoleacetic acid concentration differentiates impulsive from nonimpulsive violent behaviour. *Life Sci.* 1983;33:2609-2614.

ORIGINAL ARTICLE

Evidence of Chaotic Mood Variation in Bipolar Disorder

Allan Gottschalk, MD, PhD; Mark S. Bauer, MD; Peter C. Whybrow, MD

Background: Using long-term daily mood records obtained from patients with bipolar disorder and normal subjects, we sought to determine the temporal pattern of mood in bipolar disorder.

Methods: Time series of 1.0 to 2.5 years from seven rapid-cycling patients with bipolar disorder and 28 normal controls were obtained. These were evaluated with several techniques to identify whether the temporal pattern of mood originates from a periodic, a random, or a deterministic source.

Results: True cyclicity was not apparent in the power spectra of either the normal subjects or the patients with bipolar disorder. Instead, spectra with a broadband "1/f" shape were observed in both groups, and these spectra were significantly flatter in normal subjects ($P=.02$). Correlation dimension estimates are a measure of nonlinear deterministic structure, and convergent estimates could be obtained for six of the seven patients with bipolar disorder and none of the normal subjects ($P<.001$). Additional findings are consistent with these results.

Conclusions: These studies indicate that mood in patients with bipolar disorder is not truly cyclic for extended periods. Nonetheless, self-rated mood in bipolar disorder is significantly more organized than self-rated mood in normal subjects and can be characterized as a low-dimensional chaotic process. This characterization of the dynamics of bipolar disorder provides a unitary theoretical framework that can accommodate neurobiologic and psychosocial data and can reconcile existing models for the pathogenesis of the disorder. Furthermore, consideration of the dynamical structure of bipolar disorder may lead to new methods for predicting and controlling pathologic mood.

(Arch Gen Psychiatry. 1995;52:947-959)

DEVELOPING AN appropriate model to describe the pattern of mood instability in bipolar disorder is important because a given model leads to the pursuit of specific neurobiologic investigations and treatment strategies. Chief among the *current* models for bipolar disorder are the biologic rhythms model and the kindling model. The biologic rhythms model is based on the observation of 48-hour mood cycles in patients with bipolar disorder and the tendency of periods of mania to follow periods of depression with what some have suggested is an intrinsic periodicity.[1-4] It has been proposed that these findings result from some abnormality of endogenous, perhaps circadian, rhythms.[2,4-6] The kindling model is based on the observations that episodes may become more frequent as bipolar disorder progresses and that later episodes appear to be spontaneous while earlier episodes appear to be stressor-associated.[7,8] This pattern resembles the course of kindled seizures, in which the seizures are initially stimulus-elicited but later become spontaneous.[7,8]

The biologic rhythms model is based on relatively short-term observations,[1-4] whereas the clinical application of the kindling model is based on tracking data generated from signal events, such as hospitalizations or major mood episodes, over a period of years. Each of these models provides a powerful conceptual framework for understanding the longitudinal course of bipolar disorder. However, it is difficult to invoke either of these models to explain the irregular pattern of mood fluctuation often seen in long-term daily mood records obtained from outpatients under naturalistic conditions (eg, **Figure 1**, top, and **Figure 2**). Specifically, inspection of such

From the Departments of Anesthesia (Dr Gottschalk) and Psychiatry (Dr Whybrow), Hospital of the University of Pennsylvania, Philadelphia; and Department of Psychiatry and Human Behavior, Brown University School of Medicine and Department of Veterans Affairs Medical Center, Providence, RI (Dr Bauer).

See Subjects and Methods on next page

SUBJECTS AND METHODS

SUBJECT SELECTION

All patients (**Table 1**) met criteria for bipolar disorder or bipolar disorder not otherwise specified by *DSM-III-R* criteria.[11] Mood records were kept as part of prospective assessment of symptoms in a mood disorders research clinic. Each patient who enrolled in the research clinic was requested to keep a mood record, and all of the 43 enrolled patients with at least 12 consecutive months of mood recording at the time data analysis was initiated were included in this study. No other selection criteria were used. The patients maintained daily mood records for 1.0 to 2.5 years on a 100-mm analogue scale, with "best I ever felt" to "worst I ever felt" used as the anchor points and with the midpoint anchored as "normal." Patients were instructed to complete the scale each evening by placing an *X* at the point on the line that best reflected their mood in relation to the anchor points, giving the average mood for the previous 24 hours. For each patient, deviation from normal was well correlated with physician ratings of global psychopathology by means of the Brief Psychiatric Rating Scale (r=.56±.06).[12] Each of the patients included in this study had a rapid-cycling course, ie, they had experienced by definition a minimum of four affective episodes in the preceding 12 months, which characterizes approximately 15% of patients with bipolar disorder.[13,14] Characteristics of the patients with bipolar disorder are summarized in Table 1.

Controls were recruited by newspaper advertisement or word of mouth. Normal controls (**Table 2**) without current or earlier history of psychiatric disorder, and who tested negative for bipolar or unipolar traits by the General Behavior Inventory,[15] rated themselves twice daily on a 24-point scale with anchor points identical to those for the patients with bipolar disorder. They were instructed to complete the mood record each morning and evening, with the rating reflecting their average mood since the last rating. Twenty-eight of the 73 subjects initially recruited provided at least 300 days of mood recording and were included in this study, without further selection for any clinical or demographic characteristics and without additional consideration of their mood records.

DATA ANALYSIS

All time series were initially examined with plots of mood as a function of time. Autocorrelation functions[16] and power spectra were examined next. After linear trend and the mean were removed, power spectra were estimated by use of the raw periodogram,[16] normalized with respect to the maximal value of each spectrum, and plotted in log-log coordinates. For estimation of the power spectrum, and at the step just before computing of the Fourier transform, each time series was extended by adding zeroes until the length of the time series reached the next power of two.[16] For the purpose of computing the power spectra *only*, missing values were replaced by the mean of the time series after linear trend was first removed.

Each power spectrum was fitted in the minimum mean square sense to the pair of lines that represent the spectrum obtained from the sum of a process with a "white" (flat) spectrum and one with a $1/f^{\alpha}$ spectrum. In a log-log coordinate system, a process with a $1/f^{\alpha}$ spectrum will be displayed as a straight line of which the negative slope is α. For each spectrum, α and the frequency at which the lines representing the two processes intersected were recorded, and the differences in α between patients with bipolar disorder and normal subjects were compared.

Time series of mood represent the output of a single variable from a multidimensional system. To perform certain types of analysis, it is necessary to generate a multidimensional phase space from time series of a single variable. This is done by performing a time-delay embedding with the original time series.[17] A time-delay embedding is generated by starting with the original time series and delaying it T units of time for each additional dimension. Thus, the original time series is a one-dimensional embedding. Collectively, the pairs of points formed by the time series and the same time series delayed by T units of time form a two-dimensional embedding, and the use of $M-1$ delays of T units of time would result in an M-dimensional embedding space. This technique is a necessary first step for techniques that will be described below and include estimation of the correlation dimension, phase space reconstruction, and generation of recurrence plots. Missing values in the time series resulted in missing values in the embedding space, since missing values in the time series were not filled in by any type of interpolation or estimation technique. When the embedding space is formed, any value of the delay T can theoretically be used. However, some values of T are practically more useful than others. One simple means of obtaining a reasonable value of the delay T is by examining the autocorrelation function and using for T the location of the first minimum or zero crossing.[18]

The correlation dimension D was computed as described by Grassberger and Procaccia[19,20] without any previous filtering or data processing. Briefly, the correlation sum $C(r)$ is computed as a function of the separation distance r for a given embedding dimension.

$$C(r) = \frac{1}{N^2}\sum_{i=1}^{N}\sum_{j=1}^{N}\Theta(r-|X_i-X_j|)$$

$$\Theta(\alpha) = \begin{cases} 0 & (\alpha \leq 0) \\ 1 & (\alpha > 0) \end{cases}$$

Here, $|X_i-X_j|$ is the distance function used in the embedding space, which is euclidean in what follows, and N is the number of points in the embedding space of embedding dimension M. Since $C(r)$ is approximately equal to r^D in an appropriate linear scaling region, D is estimated by plotting $\log C(r)$ vs $\log r$ and examining the slope of these curves in the linear scaling region. This is done for progressively higher values of the embedding dimension M until there is no further increase in D for an increase in M. Such convergence is not always achieved, and the amount of data limits the size of the

records provides evidence that truly cyclic mood patterns are uncommon and, when they do occur, are short-lived (see bracketed region of Figure 1, top). In addition, there does not appear to be an orderly progression in severity of mood fluctuations that would support a kindling model. However, visual inspection of these records suggests that mood patterns in bipolar disorder, although aperiodic, may be more organized than those of normal subjects (see Figure 1 and contrast Figure 2 and **Figure 3**). These qualitative observations led us to hypothesize that long-term embedding dimension that can be used in this calculation. The size of the linear scaling region and the convergence of the correlation dimension estimate can sometimes be improved by modifying the estimation process to account for relationships between adjacent points in the time series.[21,22] To demonstrate the robustness of the correlation dimension estimates with respect to the size of the delay *T* used in forming the time-delay embedding space, the correlation dimension was also estimated as a function of the delay *T* for a fixed embedding dimension.

To visualize the attractor, sequential points in the two- and three-dimensional phase space formed by time-delay embedding were plotted and connected by a line for various choices of delay.[17] These phase space reconstructions could be examined in greater detail by rotation on a computer screen.

Nonstationarity of a time series implies that the properties of the time series are a function of the time at which it is obtained. One dynamic tool that is useful for addressing issues of nonstationarity is the recurrence plot.[23] For a given embedding dimension and distance criterion, this type of plot is a grid that considers the distance between all possible pairs of points in the given embedding space of embedding dimension *M* and blackens the corresponding grid location if two points in the space are within the specified distance criterion of one another. In practice, the distance criterion varies for each point in the embedding space and is chosen so that it is sufficiently large that a specified number of other points in the embedding space lie within that radius of the specified point. Thus, the number of points to contain within the calculated distance is specified a priori, and the distance criterion becomes a function of which point in the embedding space is being examined. Consequently, recurrence plots are not necessarily symmetric. To help interpret the recurrence plot, the fraction of possible points along each diagonal (lower left to upper right) is plotted at the bottom. The large value for the central diagonal is not shown so that structure in the periphery is apparent.

Several types of surrogate data sets were used to test the null hypothesis that convergent estimates of the correlation dimension could be obtained from a stochastic source with statistical properties similar to the original time series, and to seek evidence of additional structure in the time series from which convergent estimates of the correlation dimension could not be obtained.[24] To use the surrogate data sets in this manner, correlation dimension estimates are made for the original and surrogate time series, and the correlation dimension vs embedding dimension curves are compared. Since the surrogate time series are formulated to eliminate the deterministic structure present in the original time series, the finding of identical convergence properties in the surrogate time series and in the originals would suggest that the original correlation dimension estimates were artifactual. Surrogate data can also be used to obtain evidence of nonlinear deterministic structure, even when convergence of the correlation dimension estimate cannot be obtained for the original time series. When the correlation dimension vs embedding dimension curves for the original and surrogate time series are compared, the observation that the curve from the original time series converges to a greater extent than that of the surrogate time series is evidence of nonlinear deterministic structure in the original time series.

Three distinct types of surrogate data sets were generated. The simplest retained the amplitude distribution of the original time series and little else. This type of surrogate was obtained by randomly shuffling the original time series. The next type of surrogate data set has as its null hypothesis that the original time series originates from a linear stochastic source. If this is the case, then randomizing the phases of the time series in the frequency domain so that the power spectrum of the time series is unchanged should not change the correlation dimension estimates. For the generation of these surrogate time series, missing values of the original time series were replaced by the mean value of the original time series. Because the original data sets were extended with zeroes to the next power of two, these types of surrogate data sets contain a corresponding number of additional points. In addition, linear trend was not removed from the time series when the surrogates were generated to avoid potentially confounding differences between the processing of the surrogate and original time series. We note that the original time series was not extended with zeroes before the correlation dimension estimates that were to be compared with those of the corresponding surrogate time series were generated. The third type of surrogate data assumes as its null hypothesis that the time series originates from a linear stochastic source and is further transformed by a static monotonic nonlinearity (eg, squaring, cubing, log). The resulting surrogate time series is a well-defined reordering of the original time series. Missing values from the original time series were replaced by the mean value of the original time series for the purpose of computing the new position of each member of the time series in the new surrogate time series. However, in computing the appropriate embedding space from the surrogate, the corresponding points were treated as missing data points. For each time series, we generated three realizations of each surrogate and determined the correlation dimension as a function of embedding dimension for each of these. The mean (±SD) estimate of the correlation dimension is plotted for each time series and type of surrogate and compared with the correlation dimension estimates from the original time series.

The effects of extending the time series with zeroes and linear trend removal in the context of generating the surrogate data sets were examined by using several shorter data sets that did not require extension with zeroes to reach a power of two in length, and by comparing the effects of linear trend removal on the power spectra of the time series.

mood records of patients with bipolar disorder might be described in terms of chaotic dynamics, rather than as a primarily periodic or progressively accelerating process.

Although, in general parlance, *chaos* implies disorder, it is also a term used to describe *apparently* random behavior by a deterministic system.[9] One important implication of this distinction is that complex-appearing chaotic behavior can originate from deterministic systems that have simple mathematical descriptions.[10] Such behavior contrasts with genuinely random phenomena be-

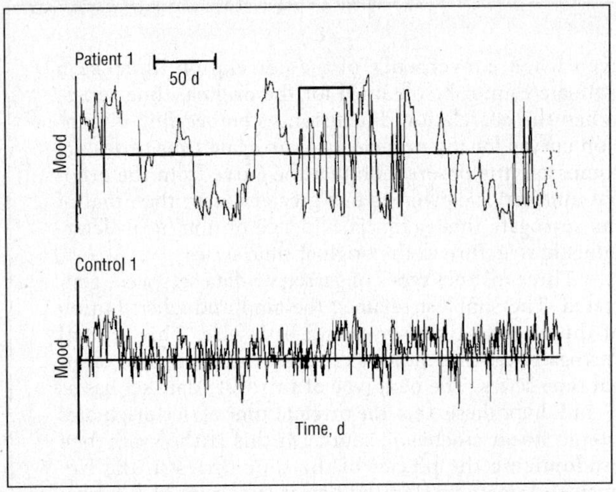

Figure 1. *One year of the time series from a patient with bipolar disorder (top) and a normal control (bottom). The figures have been scaled to make the horizontal distances correspond to the same amount of time, and so that the full range of possible moods is shown vertically. The bracketed portion of the patient's series illustrates the presence of "pseudocycles," which, if observed separately, would suggest a periodic component to the mood in bipolar disorder. Note the distinct and typical qualitative differences in the mood record of the patient compared with the control. Additional details can be found in Tables 1 and 2 and Figures 2 and 3.*

cause the dynamics of a chaotic process can be described with a finite number of dimensions and are confined to an attracting region within that finite dimensional space. Random processes are not confined to an attractor, and their description requires an infinite number of dimensions. Thus, the ability to represent the behavior of a process with a low number of dimensions is a feature of low-dimensional chaotic attractors, whereas

See also page 960

the inability to do so suggests that the observed behavior originates from a random process or a high-dimensional deterministic one with extraordinarily complex dynamics. These differences between random and chaotic systems are exploited in the present study to obtain evidence of a chaotic attractor in bipolar disorder.

RESULTS

Time series from seven patients with bipolar disorder and 28 normal controls were available for analysis. Portions of typical mood records for a patient and a control are shown in detail in Figure 1. Times series of the entire set of patients with bipolar disorder are displayed in Figure 2, and those of the first seven of 28 normal controls are shown in Figure 3. The time scale is the same for all the time series in Figures 2 and 3. In addition, the vertical scale spans the anchor points appropriate for the given time series and is of the same physical dimension in Figures 2 and 3. As noted in the introduction, brief segments of the patient time series (see bracketed portion of Figure 1, top) display characteristics of periodic activity, as expected from previous studies.[1-4] However, as can be seen in the remainder of Figure 1, top, and Figure 2, such patterns are not sustained. The absence of significant periodic activity is demonstrated quantitatively in

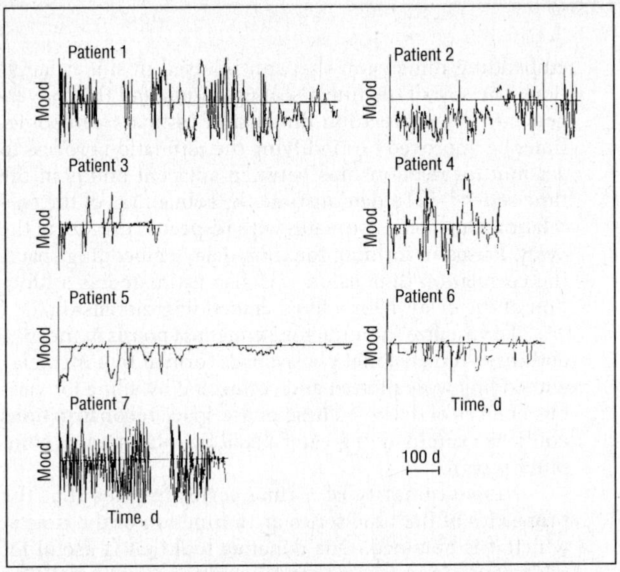

Figure 2. *Entire time series of mood from the seven patients with bipolar disorder. The same horizontal time scale in days is used for each of these time series and those from the normal controls in Figure 3. The vertical scale spans the entire range between the two anchor points used to obtain the bipolar mood ratings and is adjusted to be the same physical dimension as the scale that spans the anchor points for the normal controls in Figure 3. The time series for patient 1 in Figure 1, top, is shown in its entirety here. The order of presentation of the time series in this figure corresponds with that of Table 1. Although patients 3 and 6 met diagnostic criteria for bipolar disorder by history, during the study period the manic component of their cycle had responded to treatment. However, they continued to experience episodic depression.*

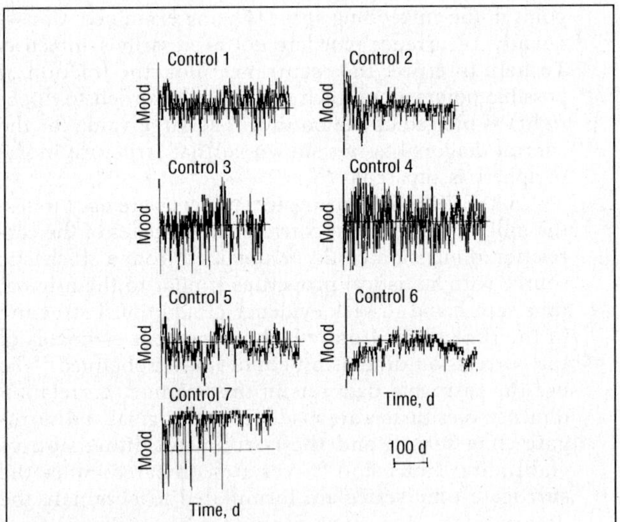

Figure 3. *Entire time series of mood from the first seven of 28 normal controls. The same horizontal time scale in days is used for each of these time series and those from the patients with bipolar disorder in Figure 2. The vertical scale spans the entire range between the two anchor points used to obtain the mood ratings in normal subjects and is adjusted to be the same physical dimension as the scale that spans the anchor points in Figure 2. The time series for control 1 in Figure 1, bottom, is shown in its entirety here. The only distinguishing feature in this sample is that the time series in control 6 produced a value of α=1.07, which was the largest value of α observed in the power spectra from normal controls and was significantly different than that observed over the entire data set. However, a convergent estimate of the corresponding correlation dimension still could not be obtained.*

Table 1. Patient Characteristics

Patient No./ Age, y/Sex	Length of Time Series, d	No. of Observations	Correlation Dimension	α
1/40/F	870	709	3.8	1.02
2/45/F	600	504	3.8	0.93
3/32/F	400	227	1.1	1.44
4/30/F	358	320	2.9	1.28
5/58/F	922	855	2.5	1.58
6/64/F	500	439	4.8	1.17
7/36/F	520	444	>7.8	0.26
Mean±SD*	596±220	499±217	3.2±1.3†	1.10±0.43‡

*The mean± SD age was 44± 13 years.
†The mean for the correlation dimension does not include patient 7, whose estimate of the correlation dimension did not converge.
‡The mean and SD for α includes the value of α for the bipolar patient for whom the correlation dimension did not converge. If this is not included, the mean would be 1.24± 0.25.

Table 2. Characteristics of Controls

No. of subjects	28
Age, y*	45.6±14.8
Sex, % F	79
Length of time series, d*	378.5±35.0
No. of observations in each time series*	735.4±82.5
Value of α*	0.69±0.16

*Values are mean± SD.

Figure 4 by means of the power spectra of the mood records of the patient and control in Figure 1. In these and the remaining power spectra of the patients and controls, there is no evidence of well-defined spectral peaks that would indicate a predominantly periodic process. However, in no case for either the patients or controls is the spectrum completely flat. When plotted in a log-log coordinate system, the spectra manifest an approximately linear increase in power with decreasing frequency. Spectra for which the power is proportional to $1/f^{\alpha}$ will produce a straight line in log-log coordinates for the region of 1/f behavior, and such spectra are often associated with chaotic processes.[25,26] Each spectrum was assumed to be composed of a 1/f region and a region of white noise the spectrum of which is flat (Figure 4). The frequency where these two regions cross and the negative slope α of the 1/f region that best fit each spectrum in the minimum mean square sense were determined. The slope information, summarized in Tables 1 and 2, indicates that the slopes for the patients with bipolar disorder are significantly steeper than those for the normal controls (P=.02). Whether or not linear trends were removed before the power spectrum was estimated did not significantly affect the mean value of α for either the patients with bipolar disorder or the normal controls. To help ensure that the different sampling rates used for the patients with bipolar diorder (once per day) and the normal controls (twice per day) were not responsible for the observed differences in α, the above analysis was repeated with the time series from the normal controls being sampled at the same rate as the bipolar time series (once per day). Under these conditions, the mean value of α (0.57±0.22) was lower than that obtained with the original sampling rate and was still significantly different from that obtained from the patients with bipolar disorder (P=.009).

To quantitate further the dynamical features of these time series, we obtained estimates of their correlation dimension.[19,20] The process of obtaining a convergent estimate of the correlation dimension for a patient and a normal control is described in the "Subjects and Methods" section and illustrated in **Figure 5** for the subjects in Figure 1, and demonstrates the dynamical differences between the patients with bipolar disorder and the normal controls. Examples of the correlation sum vs separation distance from which the curves of Figure 5 were generated are shown in **Figure 6**. Convergent estimates of the correlation dimension could be obtained for six of the seven patients with bipolar disorder and were relatively low (Table 1), indicating that the important dynamical features of these time series can be represented in a low-dimensional phase space. In contrast, for all of the normal controls, reliable convergent estimates of the correlation dimension were not obtainable, and the estimation process produced only a lower bound on the correlation dimension. For several normal controls, some evidence of convergence to a correlation dimension of 8 to 10 was observed, which is still substantially greater than that for the patients with bipolar disorder. However, the scaling regions for these subjects with high correlation dimension estimates were extremely small and marginally linear. Use of an estimation procedure for the correlation dimension that accounts for the relationship between adjacent points in the time series[21,22] can improve the length of the scaling regions for some time series from patients with bipolar disorder and from normal controls. However, these improvements in the length of the scaling region did not result in instances where the convergence properties of a given time series were altered or the value of a correlation dimension estimate substantially changed. Consequently, all correlation dimension estimates presented herein were obtained by the procedure of Grassberger and Procaccia.[19,20] The proportion of patients with bipolar disorder who exhibited a convergent correlation dimension estimate of their mood records (six of seven) is significantly greater than that of normal controls (none of 28) (Fisher's exact test, P<.001). The only distinguishing feature of the one patient for whom a convergent correlation dimension could not be obtained was that her mood reflected the greatest degree of clinical improvement among the subjects studied. For the six patients with bipolar disorder for whom a convergent estimate of the correlation dimension could be obtained,

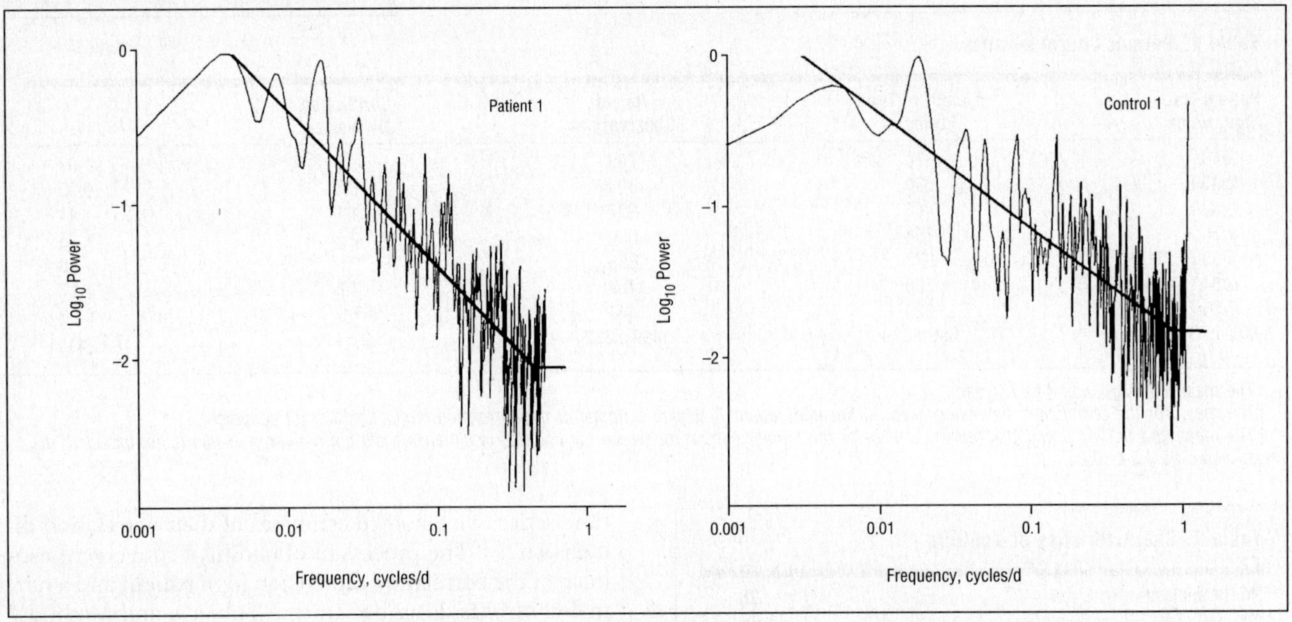

Figure 4. *Power spectral densities[16] for patient 1 and control 1. Power, normalized with respect to the maximum, and frequency are both plotted on a logarithmic scale. In neither case is there a well-defined spectral peak. Each spectrum is shown along with the pair of lines that best describes the spectrum as the combination of a "white" (flat) and a 1/f$^\alpha$ process. The steeper slope of the spectrum in patient 1 is consistent with observations in other biologic systems.[27] For these illustrations, the spectra were filtered with a nine-point triangular filter[16] and linear trend was removed from the time series before estimation of the power spectrum.*

the resulting estimates were not significantly correlated (*P*>.05) with the slope α of the 1/f region of the corresponding power spectrum.

To ensure that our choice of delay in the generation of the embedding space for any of the above calculations did not exert extensive influence on the outcome of these calculations, we computed estimates of the correlation dimension as a function of the lag *T* used to construct the embedding space. These estimates were made for a fixed value of the embedding dimension that was the level of embedding dimension at which saturation of the correlation dimension was observed. An example of these results is shown in **Figure 7** for the bipolar time series of Figure 1. When correlation dimension was plotted as a function of delay for a fixed embedding dimension, four of the six patients with bipolar disorder had a *single* point that lay close to an integer value. Therefore, an integer correlation dimension cannot be completely excluded in all patients with bipolar disorder.

One potentially confounding aspect of our study is the nonuniformity of treatment among patients with bipolar disorder during the course of the study. To assess whether changes in treatment confounded results, we investigated the patients' time series for nonstationarity by the technique of recurrence plots.[23] An example of a recurrence plot is shown in **Figure 8**, top, for the patient time series shown in Figure 1, top. Nonstationarity would be indicated by a fading out of the plot when moving from the diagonal that is present to either the upper left or lower right corner. This can be evaluated more quantitatively, as shown in Figure 8, bottom, where the fraction of possible points for each diagonal is plotted as a function of position from the central diagonal. In no case was there evidence of marked nonstationarity in the time series from the patients with bipolar disorder. In addition, for some of the longer bipolar time

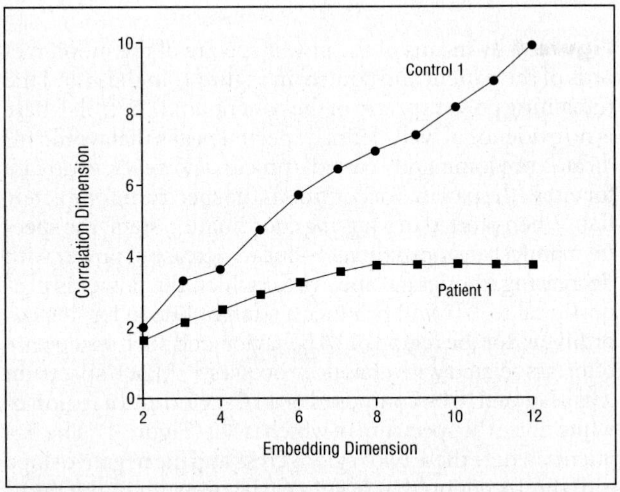

Figure 5. *Estimate of the correlation dimension as a function of embedding dimension for patient 1 and control 1. Convergence of the estimates from the patient time series, marked by asymptotic flattening of the curve, indicates that no new information is provided by the additional dimensions. Failure to achieve convergence in the estimates from the normal time series demonstrates that each additional dimension supplies additional information as might occur with a high dimensional attractor or noise.*

series, we obtained estimates of the correlation dimension for segments of the original time series and did not observe substantial differences.

One means of visualizing the chaotic attractor of bipolar disorder is to reconstruct its trajectory in phase space.[17] This is done by plotting mood for a given day as a function of mood on a previous day for all points in the time series and connecting each successive coordinate with a line. This type of plot can be constructed for two or more dimensions and for a lag of 1 or more days. The phase space trajectories

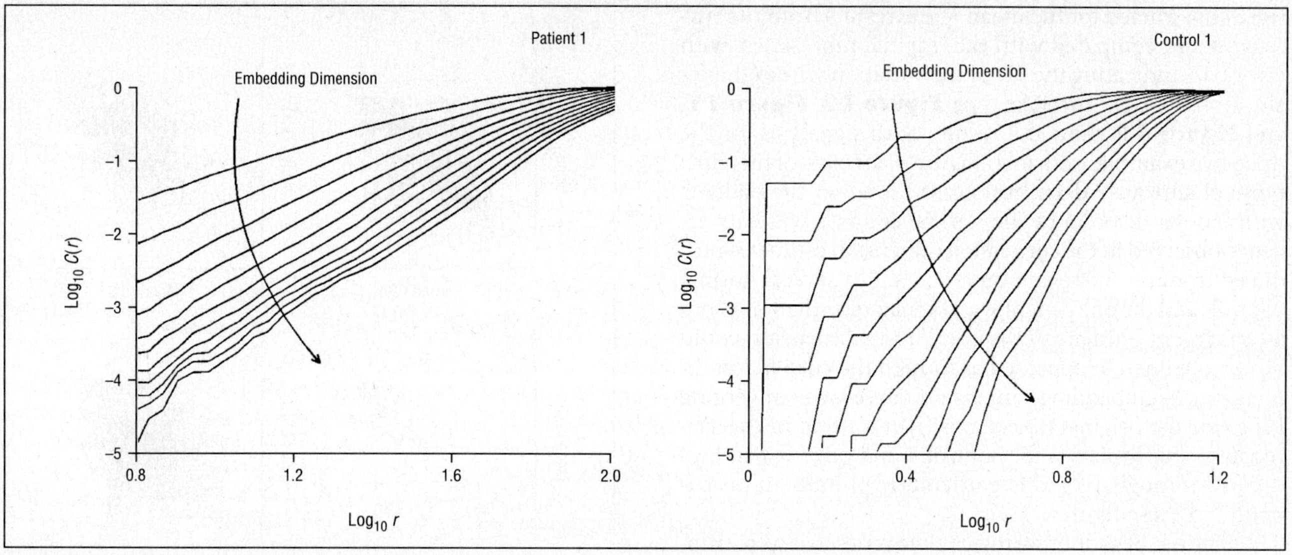

Figure 6. *Log-log plot of the correlation sum C(r) vs separation distance r for patient 1 and control 1 for embedding dimensions 2 through 12, and where the time delay embedding was constructed for each by means of a lag of 5 days. As shown in Figure 5, the correlation dimension is estimated by measuring the slope of the best linear scaling region for each embedding dimension and examining the slope vs embedding dimension for convergence. In this figure, convergence would be indicated by curves that become more parallel in a linear scaling region as the embedding dimension increases. This is seen for patient 1 but not for control 1, where the slopes of these curves are steeper than for patient 1 and do not become parallel with increasing embedding dimension, and linear scaling regions are difficult to appreciate.*

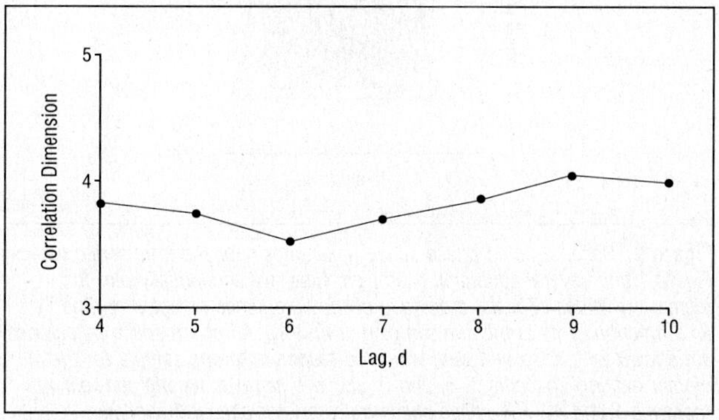

Figure 7. *Correlation dimension estimate as a function of the lag T in days for a fixed embedding dimension for the time series from patient 1. Here, the embedding dimension used was the first value where the correlation dimension converged, and the correlation dimension was estimated from the same scaling region for each value of the lag. Because one point does approach an integer value, for this patient it cannot be completely ruled out that the correlation dimension estimate is an integer. This is true of four of the six patients with bipolar disorder for whom convergent estimates of the correlation dimension could be obtained.*

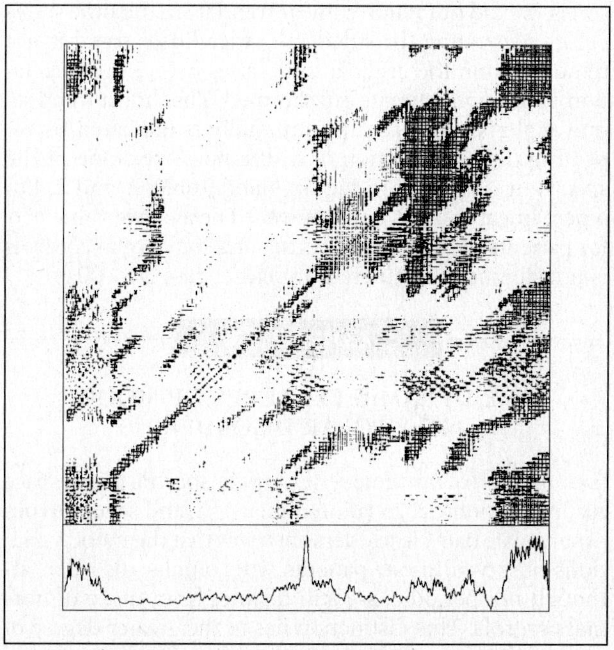

Figure 8. *Top, Recurrence plot for patient 1 for an embedding dimension of 8, a lag of 5 days, and a distance criterion that finds the 100 points in the embedding space that are closest to the point under examination. Bottom, Fraction of the number of possible points along each diagonal of the recurrence plot. The value for the central diagonal is not shown, to permit better illustration of the values for the peripheral diagonals. The persistence of structure over the entire plot indicates that the time series is stationary. Similar results were observed for all bipolar patients. Some open space in the recurrence plot is the consequence of points that are missing from the embedding space.*

for the time series in Figure 1 and several additional examples are shown in **Figure 9** for a phase space of two dimensions and a lag of 1 day. Few additional features were observed with higher-dimensional phase spaces or at lags greater than 1 day. Figure 9 helps to illustrate how much structure is present in the time series of patients with bipolar disorder compared with those of normal controls. All patients with bipolar disorder and normal controls had phase space trajectories similar to the representative examples in Figure 9, with the exception of the patient with bipolar disorder for whom a convergent estimate of the correlation dimension could not be obtained (patient 7). The phase space trajectory for this bipolar time series (Figure 9, patient 7) is similar but not identical to one from a normal control.

For each patient with bipolar disorder and each normal control, three surrogates of each of the three types of surrogate time series were generated. These were analyzed by the same methods as already described for the original time series. With the use of all of the three surrogate time series for a given type of surrogate data, plots of correlation dimension as a function of embedding dimension were constructed for the mean of the results from the surrogates and compared with the original time series, with error bars indicating the SD of the variation within the realizations of each surrogate type. **Figure 10**, **Figure 11**, and **Figure 12** show the results of this analysis for the same five examples shown in Figure 9, for each of the three types of surrogate data. In no case for either the patients with bipolar disorder or the normal controls was convergence observed in the correlation dimension estimates produced from the surrogate time series. For several normal controls and the one patient with bipolar disorder for whom a convergent estimate of the correlation dimension could not be obtained, it appeared as though the correlation dimension vs embedding dimension curve was converging faster for the original time series than for that of the surrogates. This is shown for control 4 and patient 7 in Figures 10 through 12 and is particularly prominent for patient 7 in these figures.

The use of shorter surrogate time series that were truncated to a length that is a power of two did not result in any demonstrable change in the results of Figures 10 through 12, and consequently we present results that reflect the use of the entire time series, the length of which was extended by the addition of zeroes to the next power of two. For the purpose of generating the surrogate time series, we did not remove linear trend from the time series before generating the surrogate, since linear trend is not removed from the original time series before the correlation dimension estimate is performed. That linear trend removal alters the spectrum minimally is indicated by repeating the computation of α, the negative slope of the spectrum, as shown in Figure 4 and Tables 1 and 2, but where linear trend is not removed. The average value of α for patients with bipolar disorder and for normal controls is not significantly different for either case ($P<.001$).

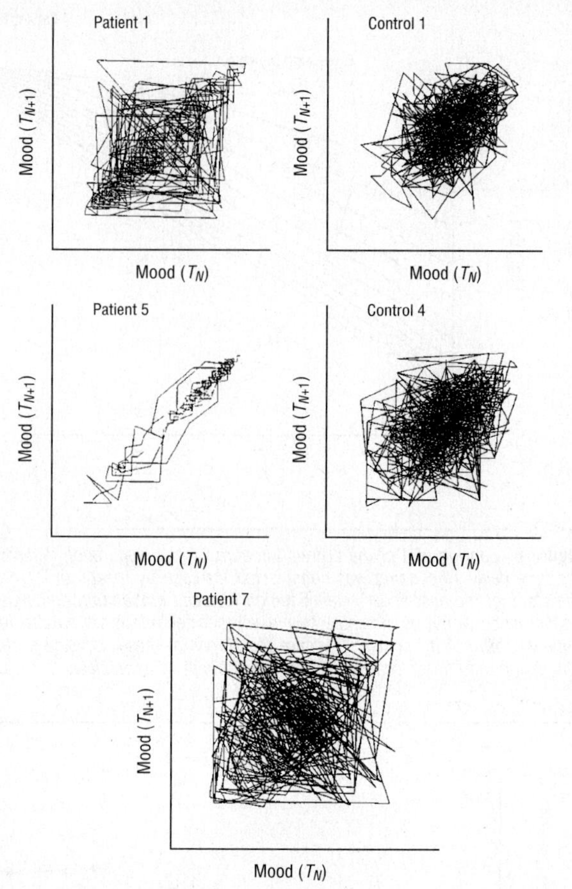

Figure 9. *Reconstructed phase space trajectories[17] for the time series in Figure 1 and several additional examples. Here, we sequentially plot for increasing values of N the amplitude of the time series sampled at time T_{N+1} as a function of its amplitude sampled at time T_N. All phase space trajectories are shown with a lag of 1 day, which corresponds to one sample for the bipolar patients (patients 1, 5, and 7) and two samples for the controls (controls 1 and 4). The phase space trajectory for patient 1 exhibits considerably more structure than one from control 1. The corresponding bipolar time series was shown to have a correlation dimension of 3.8 and a spectrum with an α of 1.02, whereas control 1 produced a spectrum with an α of 0.75 without producing a convergent estimate of the correlation dimension. Mood records were shown to have a correlation dimension of 2.5 and an α of 1.58 in patient 5; in control 4, the value of α was 0.65, and a convergent estimate of the correlation dimension could not be obtained. The highly organized phase space trajectory seen for patient 5 is more typical of our bipolar patients than the somewhat less organized attractor shown for patient 1. With the exception of patient 7, for whom a convergent estimate of the correlation dimension could not be found, all bipolar and normal subjects could be correctly classified by examination of their trajectories in phase space. The phase space trajectory of patient 7 has a value of α of 0.26. See Figures 2 and 3 for the bipolar time series from which the phase space trajectories were generated.*

COMMENT

THE DYNAMIC FEATURES OF MOOD IN BIPOLAR DISORDER

Examination of raw time series, power spectra, phase space reconstructions, correlation dimension, and several types of surrogate data clearly demonstrates that the mood variations observed in our patients with bipolar disorder, although not periodic, are still distinct from those of normal controls. This distinction lies in the greater degree of organization that is present in the time series from the patients with bipolar disorder. This relative degree of organization is indicated by the appearance of the raw time series, by the corresponding phase space reconstructions and their power spectra, and by the fact that we obtained convergent estimates of the correlation dimension for all but one of the patients with bipolar disorder and for none of the normal controls.

Although short segments of some of the bipolar time series displayed periodic-appearing segments, such as that highlighted in Figure 1, top, sustained periodic-appearing behavior was not observed in the patients with bipolar disorder or the normal controls. This was examined more quantitatively using estimates of the power spectra obtained from each of the time series. In no case was a well-defined spectral peak observed in either the patients with bipolar disorder or the normal controls, indicating that long-term mood variations are not periodic in either group. However, the broadband nature of the spectra and the region of 1/f behavior observed in both groups are consistent with chaotic behavior.[25,26] The properties of these spectra are sufficient to enable patients with bipolar disorder and normal controls to be distinguished by examination of the slope of the 1/f region of the spectrum, where it was demonstrated that the absolute value of the slope (α) was significantly greater in the patients with bipolar

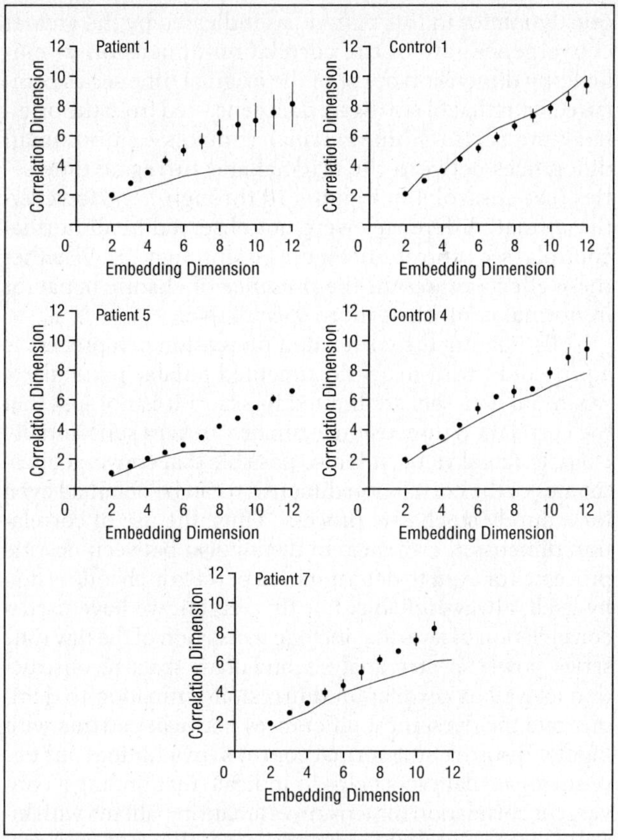

Figure 10. *Correlation dimension vs embedding dimension for the time series in Figure 9 (solid line) and surrogates (solid circles) obtained by shuffling the original time series. Each point from the surrogate data represents the mean of three surrogates, and the error bars indicate the SD. Note that the curves from the surrogate data do not converge. However, for patient 7, the original time series converges faster than the surrogate time series, suggesting the presence of some nonlinear deterministic structure in the original time series that is not present in the surrogate time series. A similar but smaller effect may also be present for control 4.*

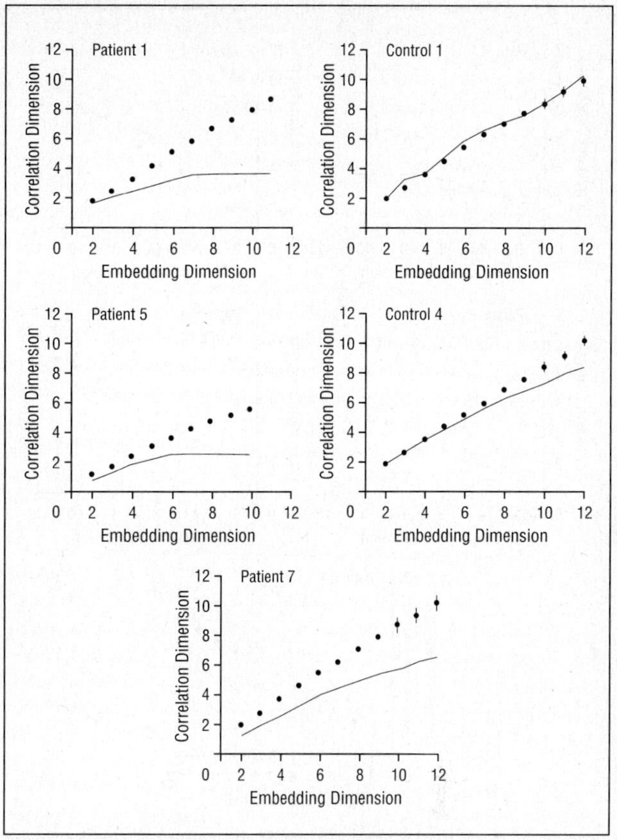

Figure 11. *Same as Figure 10, but the surrogate data were obtained from surrogates whose power spectral density exactly matched that of the original time series. Thus, the surrogates represent the null hypothesis that the time series was generated from a linear stochastic source.*

disorder than in the normal controls. This observation from the slopes of the power spectra of mood variability in patients with bipolar disorder and normal controls is consistent with observations about heart rate variability in that the greater the absolute value of the slope of the 1/f region, the greater the extent of the underlying pathologic features.[27] Here, the presence of additional power in the lower-frequency portion of the spectrum (increased α; increased absolute value of slope) is consistent with the process becoming organized over a longer time scale.

To quantitate further the dynamic features of the time series from the patients with bipolar disorder and normal controls, we estimated the correlation dimension of these time series. The correlation dimension is a measure of the structure in chaotic time series, and the finding of a noninteger correlation dimension strongly supports the presence of chaotic dynamics.[28] Although other techniques exist for quantitating the dynamical features of chaotic time series, the correlation dimension may be the only technique that permits reasonable estimates with data sets of the length available in this study.[21,29]

We were able to obtain convergent estimates of the correlation dimension for all but one of the patients with bipolar disorder. This contrasts significantly with our results with the time series from the normal controls, where convergent estimates of the correlation dimension could not be obtained, and only a lower bound on the correlation dimension was produced by the estimation process. The patient with bipolar disorder for whom a convergent estimate of the correlation dimension could not be obtained did not stand out with respect to any clinical or demographic characteristic, except that she showed the greatest degree of clinical improvement during the study. Thus, the time series from the patients with bipolar disorder are substantially more organized than those obtained from normal controls, and this organization appears to reflect the emergence of a low-dimensional chaotic attractor in bipolar disorder.

Failure to achieve convergence in the estimates of the correlation dimension in normal controls may result from the large magnitude of the attractor dimension, if the system is chaotic, or from the fact that no deterministic structure is present. In the former case, the attractor dimension may be sufficiently high and the process sufficiently complex that convergent estimates of the attractor dimension cannot be obtained with the available data, and only a lower bound on the correlation dimension is produced. Alternatively, failure to obtain convergence of the correlation dimension in the normal controls may reflect the fact that the time series originate from a stochastic source. It is also conceivable that a low-dimensional chaotic attractor, if present, could be hidden by the stochastic component of the time series.

The use of surrogate data serves as an important

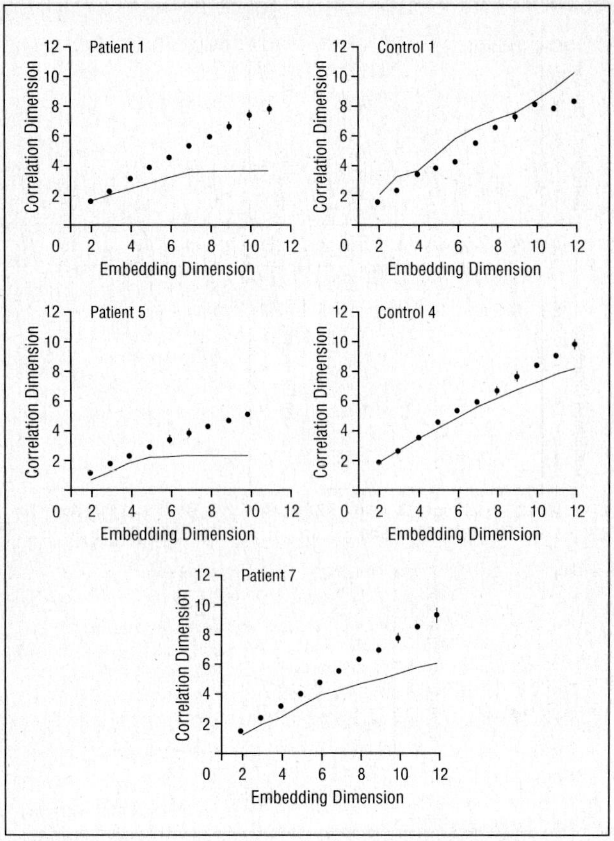

Figure 12. *Same as Figure 10, but the surrogate data were obtained by assuming as the null hypothesis that the time series was generated by a linear stochastic source whose output is operated on by a static nonlinearity.*

check on the process of estimating and interpreting the correlation dimension.[24] Convergence of the correlation dimension estimate was not observed for any of the surrogate data sets generated from the patients with bipolar disorder for whom a convergent estimate of the correlation dimension could be obtained (see patients 1 and 5 in Figures 10 through 12). This indicates that the estimation process did not artifactually produce a convergent estimate of the correlation dimension.

The examination of surrogate data is also useful for evaluating the presence of nonlinear deterministic structure in a time series when convergent estimates of the correlation dimension cannot be obtained.[24] If the correlation dimension vs embedding dimension curves of the original time series converge at a faster rate than those of the corresponding surrogate time series, this suggests that higher-dimensional chaotic dynamics may be responsible for the patterns of mood variation present in the original time series. The one patient with bipolar disorder for whom a convergent estimate of the correlation dimension could not be obtained was also the patient with bipolar disorder with the best functional status, and this patient does exhibit some evidence of nonlinear deterministic behavior when the original time series is compared with surrogates (see patient 7 in Figures 10 through 12). Thus, the failure to achieve convergence of the correlation dimension estimate for one of the patients with bipolar disorder does not rule out the presence of chaotic dynamics in this patient, as indicated by the greater convergence rate of the correlation dimension vs embedding dimension curve of the original time series compared with that of surrogate data generated from the original time series. Some normal controls exhibit small differences between the original and surrogate time series (see control 4 in Figures 10 through 12). However, these small differences were not observed in all normal controls (see control 1 in Figures 10 through 12). Whether these effects represent the presence of chaotic behavior in normal controls is more speculative.

Estimating the correlation dimension of a process is a procedure with many documented pitfalls, particularly when the data sets are limited in size.[22] It is not just that the correlation dimension estimate can vary substantially from its actual value, it is also possible that convergent estimates of the correlation dimension can be obtained even for a purely stochastic process. Thus, the use of correlation dimension estimates to distinguish between chaotic processes or even to determine if a process is chaotic is not, by itself, always reliable. For this reason, we have used a constellation of tests that include inspection of the raw time series, power spectral analysis, and phase space reconstruction as well as correlation dimension estimation to demonstrate the dynamical differences between patients with bipolar disorder and normal controls. In addition, our use of surrogate data sets helps to indicate that finding a convergent correlation dimension estimate in patients with bipolar disorder and not in normal controls is not spurious. In this work, we have used the fact that convergent correlation dimension estimates could be obtained for all but one patient with bipolar disorder and for none of the normal controls. Although reliable correlation dimension estimates can be made from small data sets,[21,29] we have been reluctant to use the specific numeric values of the correlation dimension that were obtained in the estimation process because of the potential limitations of the data set and the estimation procedure. No aspect of the hypothesis tested in this work depends critically on obtaining an accurate estimation of the correlation dimension, and the above limitations probably proscribe the association of a specific value of the correlation dimension with the dynamics of bipolar disorder.

Several features of our data may limit the application of our findings to all patients with bipolar disorder. First, our patients with bipolar disorder were drawn from an outpatient population. Next, treatment was not standardized. Finally, the patients in our study were all women with a rapid-cycling course. It is entirely conceivable that our findings may not be applicable to hospitalized patients with bipolar disorder. However, as discussed in the next section, the paradigm of chaotic dynamics offers a ready explanation for some of the differences between our findings in outpatients and those obtained by others from hospitalized patients. Although treatment was not controlled over the period in which our data were obtained, we found no differences among smaller data segments where treatment had been uniform. Ideally, one would like to determine the long-term dynamical effects of various treatment regimens and compare them with the untreated state. However, this might not be ethically tolerable given the lethality of untreated or inadequately treated bipolar disorder.[30] Although bipolar disorder with a rapid-cycling course represents only about 15% of patients with bipolar disorder,[13,14] patients with this variant of bipolar disorder have been the subjects in many studies, particularly studies that have suggested that bipolar disorder is a disease with an intrinsic rhythmicity.[1-4] Consequently, a population of patients with bipolar disorder with a rapid-cycling course is a reasonable population to study when questions of rhythmicity are being addressed, as they are in the present study. The extent to which our findings can be generalized to non–rapid-cycling bipolar disorder awaits definitive investigation.

IMPLICATIONS FOR INVESTIGATING NEUROBIOLOGIC AND PSYCHOSOCIAL FACTORS IN BIPOLAR DISORDER

Although the increased degree of organization of mood in bipolar disorder with respect to normal controls may seem counterintuitive, these data fit an increasingly apparent pattern in biology. In these instances, the normal state is characterized by a high-dimensional process that is not necessarily chaotic, while pathophysiologic states are marked by increasing degrees of organization[31] that reflect the emergence of a low-dimensional chaotic process. Examples of this pattern in humans include electroencephalographic (EEG) activity in epilepsy[32-34] and the pattern of heart rate variability.[35] For the waking EEG, the correlation dimension is sufficiently high that it is difficult to obtain, even when large time series are available. However, during non–rapid eye movement sleep, the correlation dimension of the EEG is more readily estimated, and it decreases with increasing depth of non–rapid eye movement sleep. Furthermore, the correlation dimension of the EEG is lowest during seizure activity.[32] The heart rate of healthy humans is extremely variable and possibly chaotic, while ambulatory recordings of the electrocardiogram document the loss of heart rate variability before cardiac arrest.[35] In addition, the loss of fetal heart rate variability is an important and well-used clinical indicator of fetal distress.[36]

Perhaps the most important implication of the findings of the present study is that a relatively simple mechanism may be responsible for the complex mood variations in bipolar disorder, a possibility anticipated in part by earlier theoretical arguments.[37,38] Whether our findings represent a neural process that is latent in normal controls and becomes dominant in bipolar disorder or whether they represent the emergence of a new qualitatively distinct process cannot be determined from our analysis. In either case, any process that alters the coupling between elements of the central nervous system or that alters coupling of endogenous[2,39] to exogenous circadian[4,5] or circannual[4,6,40] rhythms could be responsible.

It is therefore conceivable that, although we did not observe periodic behavior in our bipolar time series, biologic rhythms[1-4] may still be involved in the pathogenesis of the complex mood variations that characterize bipolar disorder. Specifically, circadian rhythms are frequently modeled by systems of differential equations, such as the van der Pol oscillator.[41] It is well established that such oscillators can generate chaotic dynamics when interacting with other oscillatory systems.[42] Therefore, an abnormally coupled or configured internal circadian oscillator involved in mood regulation could be driven to chaotic behavior by exogenous oscillations, such as the light-dark or seasonal cycles. In this case, a chaotic rather than a cyclic pattern of mood could result.[43]

The complex relationship of external stressors to mood in bipolar disorder[44] may also be accounted for by a model that describes the pattern of mood in bipolar disorder as originating from a low-dimensional chaotic attractor. Specifically, there are many mathematical examples in which a well-timed input of the appropriate amplitude can result in a chaotic transient or sustained chaotic dynamics.[42] Thus, an appropriately timed psychosocial stressor may exacerbate symptoms by driving the pathologically configured system to a region of its phase space where transient or sustained pathologic dynamics are generated. In this way, a stressor may produce long-lasting effects on mood, producing many episodes apparently unlinked to any stressor, rather than being linked in a simple stimulus-response fashion to a single episode. This may also explain why it is more difficult to associate later episodes in bipolar disorder with discrete, identifiable stressors, which is an important assumption for the kindling model.[7,8]

Power spectral analysis of the time series from patients with bipolar disorder and normal controls failed to disclose any well-defined spectral peaks, and this finding must be reconciled with the findings of earlier studies[1-4] that support the concept that bipolar disorder manifests itself in a largely rhythmic fashion. Such reconciliation is possible when the properties that distinguish time series in this study from those of earlier studies are examined from the point of view of chaotic dynamics. The bipolar time series in this study differ from those of earlier studies in their longer duration and their acquisition under naturalistic conditions in an outpatient setting. Thus, although we did observe occasional brief episodes of periodiclike behavior, these were clearly not sustained in these time series. When such patterns did appear, they were similar to the short time series obtained from hospitalized patients in earlier studies. Since many types of behavior are present, power spectral estimates of the *entire* time series will not necessarily demonstrate a well-defined spectral peak. In addition, periodic-appearing data like those of earlier studies or as in the example of Figure 1, top, will not necessarily produce a well-defined peak when the power spectrum of that time series is estimated. Such broadband behavior emerges because each cycle is not a perfect copy of the preceding one, differing somewhat in amplitude and duration. Examples of time series that appear periodic but have a broad spectrum and can be shown to be chaotic are known.[32,45] Thus, the previous observation of segments of periodiclike activity in time series from patients with bipolar disorder is not inconsistent with the presence of a low-dimensional chaotic attractor.

Other features of the respective data sets may help to account for the apparent differences in the degree of rhythmicity. Hospitalization implies a level of dysfunction the severity of which exceeds that seen in our sample of outpatients. Results of this study, which are consistent with findings in other pathophysiologic systems, indicate that some type of organization accompanies the pathologic features of bipolar disorder. Thus, the degree to which mood is organized may reflect the severity of the patients' bipolar disorder. For example, the most functional bipolar subject in this study exhibited the least organized mood record of all the bipolar subjects. The more cyclic-appearing data obtained from hospitalized patients in earlier studies may thus reflect an even greater degree of mood organization compared with our sample of bipolar outpatients. We speculate that the degree of mood organization varies inversely with functional status, and that the degree of mood organization could potentially be assessed by correlation dimension estimates or from the 1/f properties of the corresponding power spectrum (α).

IMPLICATIONS FOR TREATMENT OF BIPOLAR DISORDER

Aspects of current treatment for bipolar disorder are also consistent with the concept that pathologic states are characterized by a high degree of organization relative to normal. For example, some drugs that are efficacious in the treatment of seizure disorders, which is the central nervous system state that produces the most highly organized EEG,[32] are also effective mood stabilizers in patients with bipolar disorder.[46-49] It is, therefore, conceivable that the antiepileptic drugs are effective in the treatment of seizure disorders and bipolar disorder because their administration results in a similar alteration in the dynamical structure of the central nervous system.

Furthermore, the existence of chaotic dynamics in bipolar disorder may have important implications for generating new treatment strategies. Although the presence of chaotic dynamics implies an unassailable barrier to long-term prediction, recent work demonstrates that the presence of chaotic dynamics can be exploited to improve prediction from time series originating from a chaotic attractor.[50] Regardless of its origin, the organization observed in the mood records of the patients with bipolar disorder studied here implies an ability to predict mood in patients with bipolar disorder to a far greater extent than in normal controls. Thus, many techniques from time series analysis could prove to be useful tools for predicting the affective course of these patients, and it has yet to be established whether techniques that assume the presence of a low-dimensional chaotic attractor are superior.

Finally, experimental work in mechanical[51] and biologic[52,53] systems indicates that the chaos in these systems can be controlled with an appropriate signal derived from observation of the trajectory of the system in an empirically determined phase space. Importantly, this body of experimental work now indicates how to take a chaotic system and induce periodicity, or how to convert a highly organized but chaotic system to one that is less organized. This latter strategy could be important in bipolar disorder, where our data indicate that mood is far more organized than in the normal state. Thus, observing mood fluctuations and applying pulsatile or phasic treatment in an anticipatory manner (eg, short courses of medication, electroconvulsive therapy, or phototherapy) may offer additional opportunities for the treatment of bipolar disorder. Whether such dynamically oriented strategies are feasible or efficacious in any aspect of bipolar disorder remains an issue for future investigation.

IMPLICATIONS FOR OTHER PSYCHIATRIC DISORDERS

It is reasonable to speculate on the extent to which concepts from chaotic dynamics might be applicable to other psychiatric disorders. For example, a model of the central dopaminergic neuronal system exhibits chaotic dynamics for certain choices of model parameters.[54] This theoretical study was proposed as an explanation for the marked variability in the behavior of schizophrenics. Data that document greater variance in the mood of patients with unipolar depression[55] are consistent with the emergence of a low-dimensional chaotic attraction, since it is known that EEG signals with an increased variance are associated with lower correlation dimension estimates.[56] Whether chaotic dynamics are present in other disorders that are associated with rhythmic processes, such as premenstrual syndrome, remains open to speculation.

CONCLUSIONS

These data indicate that long-term mood in bipolar disorder, although not cyclic, is still highly organized compared with that of normal controls and can be characterized by the presence of a low-dimensional chaotic attractor. These results are consistent with evidence from other biologic processes in which the pathologic state is characterized by increased levels of organization through the emergence of a low-dimensional chaotic attractor. Traditional steady-state or simple oscillatory models of mood disorders cannot account for these findings. Consequently, the study of more dynamically complex oscillatory systems will be necessary to understand the relevant pathogenic mechanisms and may result in new dynamically oriented treatment strategies.

Accepted for publication March 31, 1995.

This work was supported in part by funds from the National Alliance for Research on Schizophrenia and Depression, Chicago, Ill; by grants MH00720 and MH44210 from the National Institute for Mental Health, Rockville, Md; and by funds from the Fowler Fund for Psychiatric Research, Hanover, NH.

Presented in part at the 45th Annual Convention and Scientific Program of the Society of Biological Psychiatry, New York, NY, May 11, 1990, and at the Dynamical Systems in the Neurosciences Multiscale Time and Space Coherence in Brain Function Satellite Symposium of the 23rd Annual Meeting of the Society for Neuroscience, Washington, DC, November 13, 1993.

We thank A. Mandell, MD, for his comments and Kurt A. E. Geitz, MS, for his comments on and assistance with some of the software used in the data analysis.

Reprint requests to Department of Anesthesia, Hospital of the University of Pennsylvania, 3400 Spruce St, Philadelphia, PA 19104 (Dr Gottschalk).

REFERENCES

1. Jenner FA, Gjessing LR, Cox JR, Davies-Jones A, Hullin R, Hanna S. A manic depressive psychotic with a persistent forty-eight hour cycle. *Br J Psychiatry.* 1967;113:895-910.
2. Wehr TA, Goodwin FK. Rapid cycling in manic depressives induced by tricyclic antidepressants. *Arch Gen Psychiatry.* 1979;36:555-559.
3. Kukopulus A, Reginaldi D, Laddomada P, Floris G, Serra G, Tondo L. Course of the manic-depressive cycle and changes caused by treatment. *Pharmacopsychiatry.* 1980;13:156-167.
4. Wehr TA, Goodwin FK, Wirz-Justice A, Breitmaier J, Craig C. 48-hour sleep-wake cycles in manic-depressive illness: naturalistic observations and sleep deprivation experiments. *Arch Gen Psychiatry.* 1982;39:559-565.
5. Wehr TA, Sack D, Rosenthal N, Duncan W, Gillin JC. Circadian rhythm disturbances in manic-depressive illness. *Fed Proc.* 1983;42:2809-2814.
6. Lewy AJ, Wehr TA, Goodwin FK, Newsome DA, Rosenthal NE. Manic-depressive patients may be supersensitive to light. *Lancet.* 1981;1:383-384.
7. Post RM, Rubinow DR, Ballenger JC. Conditioning, sensitization, and the longitudinal course of affective illness. *Br J Psychiatry.* 1986;149:191-201.
8. Post RM, Rubinow DR, Ballenger JC. Conditioning, sensitization, and kindling: implications for the course of affective illness. In: Post R, Ballenger J, eds. *Neurobiology of Mood Disorders.* Baltimore, Md: Williams & Wilkins; 1985: 432-466.
9. Li TY, Yorke JA. Period three implies chaos. *Am Math Mon.* 1985;82:985-992.
10. May RM. Simple mathematical models with very complicated dynamics. *Nature.* 1976;261:459-467.
11. American Psychiatric Association Committee on Nomenclature and Statistics. *Diagnostic and Statistical Manual of Mental Disorders, Revised Third Edition.* Washington, DC: American Psychiatric Press; 1987.
12. Overall JE, Gorham DR. The brief psychiatric rating scale. *Psychol Rep.* 1962; 10:799-812.
13. Bauer M, Whybrow P. Validity of rapid cycling as a modifier for bipolar disorder in *DSM-IV. Depression.* 1993;1:11-19.
14. Bauer M, Calabrese J, Dunner D, Post R, Whybrow P, Gyulai L, Tay L, Younkin S, Bynum D, Lavori P, Price RA. Multi-site data reanalysis: rapid cycling as a modifier for bipolar disorder in *DSM-IV. Am J Psychiatry.* 1994;151:506-515.
15. Depue RA, Slater JF, Wolfstetter-Kausch H, Klein D, Goplerud E, Farr D. A behavioral paradigm for identifying persons at risk for bipolar depressive disorder: a conceptual framework and five validation studies. *J Abnorm Psychol.* 1981;90:381-437.
16. Jenkins GM, Watts DG. *Spectral Analysis and Its Applications.* San Francisco, Calif: Holden-Day; 1968.
17. Takens F. Detecting strange attractors in turbulence. In: Rand DA, Young LS, eds. *Dynamical Systems and Turbulence.* New York, NY: Springer-Verlag; 1981; 898:366-381. Springer Lecture Notes in Mathematics.
18. Fraser AM, Swinney HL. Independent coordinates for strange attractors from mutual information. *Phys Rev A.* 1986;33:1134-1140.
19. Grassberger P, Procaccia I. On the characterization of strange attractors. *Phys Rev Lett.* 1983;50:346-349.
20. Grassberger P, Procaccia I. Measuring the strangeness of strange attractors. *Physica D.* 1983;9:189-208.
21. Havstad JW, Ehlers CL. Attractor dimension of nonstationary dynamical systems from small data sets. *Phys Rev A.* 1989;39:845-853.
22. Theiler J. Spurious dimension from correlation algorithms applied to limited time-series. *Phys Rev A.* 1986;34:2427-2432.
23. Eckmann JP, Oliffson Kamphorst S, Ruelle D. Recurrence plots of dynamical systems. *Europhys Lett.* 1987;4:973-977.
24. Theiler J, Galdrikian B, Longtin A, Eubank S, Farmer JD. Using surrogate data to detect nonlinearity in time series. In: Casdagli M, Eubank S, eds. *Nonlinear Modeling and Forecasting.* Reading, Mass: Addison-Wesley Publishing Co; 1992: 163-188.
25. Glass L, Mackey MC. *From Clocks to Chaos.* Princeton, NJ: Princeton University Press; 1988.
26. Shlesinger MF. Fractal time and 1/f noise in complex systems. *Ann N Y Acad Sci.* 1987;504:214-228.
27. Goldberger AL, West BJ. Applications of nonlinear dynamics to clinical cardiology. *Ann N Y Acad Sci.* 1987;504:195-213.
28. Grassberger P. Estimating the fractal dimensions and entropies of strange attractors. In: Holden AV, ed. *Chaos.* Princeton, NJ: Princeton University Press; 1986:291-311.
29. Abraham NB, Albano AM, Das B, De Guzman G, Young S, Gioggia RS, Puccioni GP, Tredicce JR. Calculating the dimension of attractors from small data sets. *Phys Lett.* 1986;114A:217-221.
30. Department of Health, Education, and Welfare Medcial Practice Project. *A State-of-the-Science Report for the Office of the Assistant Secretary of the US Department of Health, Education, and Welfare.* Baltimore, Md: Policy Research; 1979.
31. Degn H, Holden AV, Olsen LF, eds. *Chaos in Biological Systems.* New York, NY: Plenum Press; 1987.
32. Babloyantz A, Destexhe A. Low-dimensional chaos in an instance of epilepsy. *Proc Natl Acad Sci U S A.* 1986;83:3513-3517.
33. Basar E, ed. *Chaos in Brain Function.* New York, NY: Springer-Verlag; 1990.
34. Ehlers CL, Havstad JW, Garfinkel A, Kupfer DJ. Nonlinear analysis of EEG sleep states. *Neuropsychopharmacology.* 1991;5:167-176.
35. Goldberger AL, West BJ. Chaos in physiology: health or disease? In: Degn H, Holden AV, Olsen LF, eds. *Chaos in Biological Systems.* New York, NY: Plenum Press; 1987:1-4.
36. Paul RH, Suidan AK, Yeh SY, Schifrin BS, Hon EH. Clinical fetal monitoring, VII: the evaluation and significance of intrapartum baseline FHR variability. *Am J Obstet Gynecol.* 1975;123:206-210.
37. Mandell A, Knapp S, Ehlers C, Russo P. The stability of constrained randomness: lithium prophylaxis at several neurobiologic levels. In: Post R, Ballenger J, eds. *Neurobiology of Mood Disorders.* Baltimore, Md: Williams & Wilkins; 1985:744-776.
38. Sabelli HC, Carlson-Sabelli L, Javaid JI. The thermodynamics of bipolarity: a bifurcation model of bipolar illness and bipolar character and its psychotherapeutic applications. *Psychiatry.* 1990;53:346-368.
39. Extein I, Potter WZ, Wehr TA, Goodwin FK. Rapid mood cycles after a noradrenergic but not a serotonergic antidepressant. *Am J Psychiatry.* 1979;136: 1602-1603.
40. Ehlers C, Frank E, Kupfer D. Social zeitgebers and biological rhythms: a unified approach to understanding the etiology of depression. *Arch Gen Psychiatry.* 1988;45:948-952.
41. Wever RA. Toward a mathematical model of circadian rhythmicity. In: Moore-Ede MC, Czeisler CA, eds. *Mathematical Models of the Circadian Sleep-Wake Cycle.* New York, NY: Raven Press; 1984:17-79.
42. Guckenheimer J, Holmes P. *Nonlinear Oscillations, Dynamical Systems, and Bifurcations of Vector Fields.* New York, NY: Springer-Verlag; 1983:87.
43. Geitz KAE, Bauer MS, Gottschalk A. Modeling mood with a forced van der Pol oscillator. Read before the Dynamical Systems in the Neurosciences, Multiscale Time and Space Coherence in Brain Function, Satellite Symposium of the 23rd Annual Meeting of the Society for Neuroscience; Washington, DC; November 13, 1993.
44. Ellicott A, Hammen C, Gitlin M, Brown G, Jamison K. Life events and the course of bipolar disorder. *Am J Psychiatry.* 1990;147:1194-1198.
45. Olsen LF, Schaffer WM. Chaos versus noisy periodicity: alternative hypotheses for childhood epidemics. *Science.* 1990;249:499-504.
46. Post RM. *Psychopharmacology: The Third Generation of Progress.* New York, NY: Raven Press; 1987:567-576.
47. Post RM, Weiss SR. Sensitization, kindling, and anticonvulsants in mania. *J Clin Psychiatry.* 1989;50:23-30.
48. Emrich HM, Dose M, von Zerssen D. The use of sodium valproate, carbamazepine and oxcarbazepine in patients with affective disorders. *J Affect Disord.* 1985;8:243-250.
49. Calabrese J, Delucchi G. Spectrum of efficacy of valproate in 55 patients with rapid-cycling bipolar disorder. *Am J Psychiatry.* 1990;147:431-434.
50. Casdagli M. Nonlinear prediction of chaotic time series. *Physica D.* 1989;35: 335-356.
51. Ditto WL, Rauseo SN, Spano ML. Experimental control of chaos. *Phys Rev Lett.* 1990;65:3211-3214.
52. Garfinkel A, Spano ML, Ditto WL, Weiss JN. Controlling cardiac chaos. *Science.* 1992;257:1230-1235.
53. Schiff SJ, Jerger K, Duong DH, Chang T, Spano ML, Ditto WL. Controlling chaos in the brain. *Nature.* 1994;370:615-620.
54. King R, Barchas JD, Huberman BA. Chaotic behavior in dopamine neurodynamics. *Proc Natl Acad Sci U S A.* 1984;81:1244-1247.
55. Hall DP, Sing HC, Romanoski AJ. Identification and characterization of greater mood variance in depression. *Am J Psychiatry.* 1991;148:1341-1345.
56. Babloyantz A. Estimation of correlation dimensions from single and multichannel recordings: a critical review. In: Basar E, ed. *Chaos in Brain Function.* New York, NY: Springer-Verlag; 1990:83-91.

Chaos and Complexity

Can It Help Us to Understand Mood and Behavior?

When a disaster such as the bombing of the federal building in Oklahoma City occurs, many people wonder why psychiatrists, law officials, friends, and relatives are not more capable of accurately predicting human behavior. Not only during periods of disaster but also in day-to-day practice, psychiatrists are constantly faced with life-defining decisions based on the accurate prediction of behavior. One of the most common and important decisions facing psychiatrists treating very ill patients is predicting if or when patients will be dangerous to themselves or to others. While great strides have been made in the diagnosis and treatment of severe mental illness, few models have directly addressed the issue of predictability of behavior. Gottschalk et al[1] address this issue from a new theoretical approach. The article, in part, challenges us to question whether the laws governing complex physical systems may help us better predict the fluctuations in mood states associated with bipolar disorder.

The article artfully tackles some intuitively powerful but technically challenging issues in nonlinear dynamics. In such an article, it is always difficult for the authors to provide enough background to make their argument technically convincing without losing the general reader. In this case, the authors have done an admirable job. The same problem exists in preparing a Commentary on this topic. Thus, for those unfamiliar with the topic, I will provide a short overview of some principles of nonlinear dynamics. Informed readers can skip this section and go directly to the "Comments."

CAN THE BEHAVIOR OF COMPLEX SYSTEMS BE ACCURATELY PREDICTED?

The natural behavior of many physical systems is highly predictable. As an example, eclipses can be predicted accurately thousands of years in advance. Many natural phenomena, such as earthquakes, tornadoes, and hurricanes, however, have unpredictable aspects. What makes the motion of the planets in our solar system so much easier to predict than the earth's atmospheric movements, the shifting of the earth's crust, or the behavior of humans?

Until somewhat recently, it was believed that phenomena such as the weather could be precisely predicted if enough simultaneous information were known about the system over sufficient time. This viewpoint dramatically changed in the 1960s with the emerging science of chaos. Chaos, one style of behavior of complex systems, has the characteristic of appearing random and is unpredictable at certain scales but retains a highly defined and overall predictable form. The discovery of chaos has led to a new approach to the measurement and modeling of physical systems such as the atmosphere and turbulent fluids. On one hand, the existence of chaos implies that many seemingly random processes could be more predictable than previously thought; however, it also implies that there are limits to exact predictability.

Recently, attempts have been made to apply these principles to better the understanding of complex behavior in biological systems, and a new discipline is emerging called the science of complexity. The theory of chaos and complexity has been applied to the study of the heart,[2-4] brain waves,[5-8] enzymes,[9] and neurotransmitters.[10] In recent years, some excellent reviews have been written in attempts to describe chaos to nonphysicists[2,11-17] and to apply chaos to issues relevant to psychiatry.[18-25] Chaos is only one principle within a field called nonlinear dynamics. Nonlinear dynamics offers new tools with which to quantify, model, and attempt to predict the behavior of complex biological systems. One of its seductive properties is that it also offers a new way of *thinking* about the behavior of complex systems: a so-called metaphysics of chaos. The principles of chaos provide powerful metaphysical analogies that are useful in postulating and designing experiments as well as formulating theories.

See also page 947

The potential importance of the principles of nonlinear dynamics to psychiatry may be best explained through an example of how nonlinear behavior might be modeled. The behavior of a bird in flight will be used for illustrative purposes. The first step in model building might be to develop a model based on the known laws of fluid dynamics that describe the airflow through which the bird flies. However, problems can arise when we try to apply simple models to biological systems. For instance, one problem is that birds do not have just one style of flight but have several *modes* of flying behavior that depend on the physical environment (ie, changes in air currents, air velocity, etc) as well as motivational factors (eg, to catch prey, migration). Some examples of these modes of flying include fixed-wing soaring, slow flapping of wings, fast flapping of wings, cruising (some soaring and some wing flapping), hovering (ultrahigh-frequency wing flapping), and takeoffs and landings. Some of these modes of behavior are rhythmic and some are not. The bird can also abruptly switch from one of these modes to another depending on wind currents and what the bird wishes to do. This general phenomenon that occurs in complex systems is called a *critical phase transition.* There are many examples of these phenomena occurring in physical as well as biological systems; for example, consider the transition from the solid to the liquid state or from the liquid to the gaseous state. In biological systems, consider the transition between sleeping and waking and the "switch phenomena" in bipolar disorder as poignant examples.

How might such a system actually be modeled? In the early 1960s, it would have been virtually impossible. However, a meteorologist from the Massachusetts Institute of Technology, Edward N. Lorenz, was struggling with a similar problem in the physics of weather prediction.[26] He started by using a model that consisted of a truncation of the standard equations for airflow and fluid flow. As he let the model run, he realized that it simulated complex, near-periodic patterns of winds and temperatures that repeated themselves but never in the same way. Lorenz had been the first to discover chaos in the behavior of the weather patterns observed in his model. Lorenz discovered another cardinal feature of nonlinear systems called *sensitive dependence on initial conditions.* Crutchfield et al[13] have described an analogy of this phenomenon. Imagine a rock poised at the top of a hill. If the rock is placed at a slightly different spot or given a tiny push one way or another, it will tumble down widely differing paths. What this concept means to our bird model is that it is impossible to predict *exactly* when the bird is going to flap its wings during flight, because something, such as a change in thermal updrafts, might alter its flight unpredictably.

In practice, how does one actually model or measure the dynamics of such nonlinear systems? A set of general techniques to evaluate properties of nonlinear systems has been developed over the last 10 years.[27] These techniques were also used in part by Gottschalk et al[1] to evaluate the dynamics of mood ratings. To better understand these methods, it is important to see that a dynamical system generally consists of two essential parts (see Crutchfield et al[13] for further descriptions). The first is the *state,* which is the information necessary to describe a system, and the second is the *dynamic,* which is a rule that describes how the state of the system is going to change over time. A dynamical system can be represented in *state space.* State space is an abstract construct whose coordinates are the components of state. The coordinates of a particular *portrait* of state space depend on the actual system and the dynamic that is to be represented. For instance, in a mechanical system, the components might be position and velocity. In a neuronal system, the state space coordinates might represent the amount of neuronal activity over a specified period. In bipolar disorder, the coordinates might be a mood scale rating sampled at different intervals, as used by Gottschalk et al.

A state space portrait can consist of the behavior of a dynamical system in a geometric form. When these geometric forms appear they are called *attractors* because the behavior of the system appears to be "attracted" into certain modes. Lorenz observed that the attractor in his system, which modeled weather, was not simple. It had an overall definable shape that was near-periodic but could not be described by a series of oscillators. The behavior of his system was *deterministic* and could be described by a few key variables but still was not completely predictable. The behavior of the weather in Lorenz's model appeared to be strange; for this reason, attractors that display chaotic behavior have been termed *strange attractors.* This collective behavior observed in nonlinear systems is more generally termed *self-organization.* A system is generally called self-organizing if it takes on a functional, spatial, or temporal structure without outside interference.[28] The process of self-organization can be observed in several systems in the natural world, such as the spiral arms of a galaxy, the organized funnel structure of a hurricane or tornado, or eddies (whirlpools) in fluid flows.

Nonlinear processes, with their chaotic behavior, have been found to occur in many physical systems and are in the process of being described and quantified in biology and physiology. Gottschalk et al[1] attempt to identify and quantitate nonlinear behavior in the mood ratings of patients with bipolar disorder and controls.

COMMENTS ON 'EVIDENCE OF CHAOTIC MOOD VARIATION IN BIPOLAR DISORDER'

The goal of the study by Gottschalk et al[1] was "to determine the temporal pattern of mood in bipolar disorder." To accomplish this goal, they used two methods: conventional power spectral analyses and a method to evaluate nonlinear properties of complex systems. By inspecting the power spectra, Gottschalk et al surmised that neither the control nor patient group displayed any significant linear rhythmicity, as evidenced by the fact that there were no prominent spectral peaks at any frequency. What they found instead was a broadband spectral profile with a 1/f shape (a relationship between the amplitude of a particular wave and its frequency, ie, the lower the frequency of the signal, the more likely it will have a higher amplitude). What does this mean? First, it suggests that simple linear rhythmicity does not exist in the mood ratings of the patients studied. Second, it suggests that a nonlinear system may be present, as many nonlinear complex systems display these kinds of spectra.[29] For instance, the attractor described by Lorenz has a

1/f spectral distribution. This relationship is also observed in several complex biological systems, such as electroencephalographic waves during sleep. Delta waves (slow waves of sleep) have the highest amplitude and the lowest frequency, while beta waves have the highest frequency and the lowest amplitude. In their study, however, Gottschalk et al found that the control subjects had significantly flatter power spectral distributions than the patients ($P<.02$). These data suggest that there is more evidence for periodicity of some type in the mood ratings of the patients than in those of the controls.

To EXPLORE further the fluctuations in mood states of patients with bipolar disorder, the authors used a measure that has been developed over the last 10 years to detect and quantify nonlinear systems, namely, dimension. Measures of dimension are computationally demanding and not easily applied to experimental systems.[30] Grassburger and Procaccia[31] developed the most commonly used algorithm for estimation of dimension. Dimension can be thought of as a measure of the information required to describe the behavior of a system, the number of degrees of freedom, or any single measure of a system's complexity. Dimension is actually estimated by collecting data about a particular system over time or space and then sampling the data so that the state of the system can be represented as an attractor in state space. Some simple attractors actually have easily estimated dimensions. The estimation of the dimension of more complex strange attractors, however, is more difficult and remains controversial.[14,32-35] Applications of efficient algorithms by several investigators, mostly to electroencephalographic data, have resulted in a number of publications suggesting that attractors may be present in brain electrical activity. In addition, some investigators have presented data to suggest that certain clinical groups can be distinguished from controls based on differences in attractor dimension.[36,37] However, these data have recently been put under some scrutiny based on the growing recognition that methods of nonlinear dynamical analyses can be misapplied and can produce spurious conclusions.[34]

Recently, a new procedure of nonlinear dynamical analysis has been introduced, namely, the method of surrogate data.[38,39] This procedure has become essential in nonlinear analyses if performed with care.[40] In this method, the original data set is shuffled (usually a phase randomization is performed and a Gaussian distribution is applied to the amplitudes) in such a way as to destroy the nonlinear structure present in the original time series (the data points represented as a function of time). This procedure generates a so-called *surrogate time series*. A comparison of the original and surrogate time series using several measures of nonlinear structure can help to secure one's suspicion that the system actually contains some nonlinear deterministic structure.[41] Gottschalk et al[1] used this method and present convincing evidence that their data set actually has nonlinear structure. They go on to estimate the dimension of the original time series (mood ratings over time) for seven patients with bipolar disorder and 28 normal controls. They found that dimension could be estimated for six of the seven patients with bipolar disorder and for none of the normal controls ($P<.001$). Statistically, this finding of differences in the ability to estimate dimension in the patients vs the controls may be more robust than measures of the power spectra in the two groups. The fact that a low dimensional estimate combined with 1/f power spectra is found in the patient group suggests that mood ratings in patients with bipolar disorder may be quasiperiodic and may be described by a strange attractor. The authors find no evidence to suggest that fluctuations in mood ratings in normal controls have any deterministic structure. Whether higher-dimensional nonlinear structure may eventually be detected in the mood ratings of normal subjects by methods other than dimension estimates is not now known.

Gottschalk et al[1] state that "perhaps the most important implication of the findings of the present study is that a relatively simple mechanism may be responsible for the complex mood variations in bipolar disorder." The authors speculate that a model that is abnormally coupled or configured, such as the van der Pol oscillator, may account for such a mechanism. They also suggest that "an appropriately timed psychosocial stressor may exacerbate symptoms by driving the pathologically configured system to a region of its phase space where transient or sustained pathologic dynamics are generated."

A simple model may help to explain how such pathological dynamics may be generated in a nonlinear system. Several authors have proposed simple mathematical models with very complicated dynamics in which changes in the delay and/or sensitivity of a regulated system can produce oscillations (eg, pathological dynamics).[42] Such a system may be represented theoretically by a person performing on a driving simulator, such as those present at a video arcade. When the operator turns the wheel, the video car moves a proportional amount. The goal of such a game is to win a road race without crashing into other cars or running off the road. Now, let us introduce a delay into the system between the turning of the steering wheel and the movement of the player's car on the video screen. The delay does not need to be very long to cause the operator to overcompensate. Imagine that the delay is fairly long and that at some point in the race the driver must quickly move the car to the right to stay on the road. Although the driver steers to the right quickly, the car does not respond rapidly, so the driver overcompensates. When the car eventually moves, it careens to the right, so the driver must compensate by quickly turning the wheel to the left. Thus, the delay causes the car to weave from side to side on the road (ie, pathological dynamics). A biological example of such a phenomenon has been suggested in the case of alcohol intoxication.[23] Alcohol at higher doses can slow reaction time, perhaps by causing a delay in the ability of a person to process information and subsequently perform a task, such as driving. The higher the dose of alcohol, at least theoretically, the longer the delay in performance. Such a model could explain the appearance of weaving when a drunk person attempts to drive a car or the appearance of staggering when a severely intoxicated person tries to walk.

A similar model can be constructed in which the parameter that is changed is not delay but the sensitivity of the system to some environmental condition. Such models have been successfully used in biological systems, including neuronal dynamics and psychological processes.[43-45] Such a model might be applied to the "emergence" of lower-dimensional quasiperiodic behavior observed in the patients with bipolar disorder studied by Gottschalk et al.[1] Lewy et al[46] have suggested that patients with bipolar disorder may be supersensitive to light and thus could be more sensitive to phase shifts. In addition, it has been demonstrated that phase shifts induced by transmeridian flight can actually precipitate affective episodes in patients with bipolar disorder, with the direction of flight predicting the prominence of manic vs depressive symptoms.[47] Thus, patients with bipolar disorder may be particularly sensitive to factors that disrupt their systems, particularly their biological rhythms. Social or physical factors that disrupt biological rhythms are called *zeitstörers*.[48] It may be that patients with bipolar disorder are supersensitive to such disrupters, and further disruption of their systems may induce near-periodic oscillations (eg, pathological dynamics).

Gottschalk et al[1] also state that "the existence of chaotic dynamics in bipolar disorder may have important implications for generating new treatment strategies." They point out that some drugs used for seizure disorders are also effective in the treatment of bipolar disorder and that, over time, both seizure states and mood patterns are characterized by a higher degree of organization than normal. Thus, antiepileptic drugs may be useful in both disorders because they may effect similar changes in the "dynamical structure of the central nervous system." They further suggest that "applying pulsatile or phasic treatment in an anticipatory manner (eg, short courses of medication, electroconvulsive therapy, or phototherapy) may offer additional opportunities for the treatment of bipolar disorder." While such treatments have proved interesting in experimental manipulations in cardiac tissue,[4] such extrapolation to mood disorders, while provocative and interesting, may be premature. First, not all aspects of bipolar disorder appear to be more organized than control conditions. For instance, the sleep of bipolar patients has similar characteristics to the sleep of patients with unipolar depression, with clear disruption of the normal quasiperiodic fluctuations between sleep states.[49-51] Thus, there may be more low-dimensional chaos in the mood fluctuations of patients with bipolar disorder, but certain physiological processes, such as sleep, may in fact be less organized in patients with bipolar disorder than in controls. In suggesting dynamic-based treatment for bipolar disorder, should one treat the patients' mood dynamic or their physiological dynamic?

Goodwin and Jamison[52] argue that an "instability model" may account for the fundamental dysfunction in manic-depressive illness. According to this model, affective episodes may emerge from such factors as drug noncompliance, stressful life events, and disruptions in social rhythms. Frank and colleagues[53] have drawn from such theories to develop a therapeutic intervention called *interpersonal and social rhythm therapy*. One part of this therapy focuses on lifestyle alteration, attempting to institute more stable social rhythms through behavioral techniques such as self-monitoring, realistic goal setting, graded task assignment, and cognitive restructuring. In dynamical terms, such therapy may produce prophylaxis against or protection from people or events that might have detrimental impact on a system that may be more sensitive or unstable in the face of perturbation.

The simple models presented in this Commentary serve to explain some of the principles of nonlinear dynamics. While the actual application of these principles to complex biological systems will require further development, the potential existence of chaos in biological systems, as demonstrated by Gottschalk et al[1] in mood states, has several implications. It undermines the views of reductionists, who believe that a system can ultimately be understood by breaking that system down into its constituent parts and studying each piece in isolation. The "cause" of bipolar disorder must be considered multilevel and multideterminate. As suggested by Abraham,[43] the study of nonlinear dynamics and complexity "is emerging as the metalanguage, the metaparadigm of science." Not all researchers, however, are enthusiastic about the emergence of the metaphysics of chaos. In his recent, somewhat unreasonably critical article in *Scientific American*, Horgan[54] cites Philip Anderson, a condensed-matter physicist and Nobel laureate at Princeton (NJ) University: "I don't think there is a theory of everything. . . . I think there are basic principles that have very wide generality . . . but you mustn't give in to the temptation that when you have a good general principle at one level it's going to work at all levels." Horgan also quotes Santa Fe (NM) Institute researcher James Crutchfield, one of the early pioneers in chaos: "If a theory applies to everything, it may really apply to nothing . . . you need not only statistics but also mechanisms."

Despite these cautions, nonlinear modeling can now offer a broader, more holistic approach to the study of mental illness. The article by Gottschalk et al[1] pioneers application of the method and theory of nonlinear systems to the study of mental illness. While the study may be criticized for the attempt to generalize from seven patients with bipolar disorder to an entire population, the collection of over 1 year's worth of mood ratings is an extremely formidable process that deserves commendation. The authors have also used sophisticated and technically demanding analysis techniques skillfully. They make the important point that both biological and psychological variables that influence mood and behavior can be introduced into nonlinear models. The use of nonlinear models does not in any way negate important theories such as the biological rhythm disruption[55] and kindling[56,57] models, but in fact adds explanatory power to those theories. In the future, nonlinear dynamics may provide some new measures by which to quantify and improve the prediction of human behavior.

Cindy L. Ehlers, PhD
The Scripps Research Institute
CVN-14
10666 N Torrey Pines Rd
La Jolla, CA 92037

This work was supported in part by grants AA 00098 and AA 09652 from the National Institute of Alcoholism and Alcohol Abuse, Bethesda, Md.

REFERENCES

1. Gottschalk A, Bauer MS, Whybrow PC. Evidence of chaotic mood variation in bipolar disorder. *Arch Gen Pscyhiatry.* 1995;52:947-959.
2. Goldberger AL, Rigney DR, West BJ. Chaos and fractals in human physiology. *Sci Am.* February 1990;262:42-49.
3. Mackey MC, Glass L. Oscillation and chaos in physiological control systems. *Science.* 1977;6: 287-289.
4. Garfinkel A, Spano ML, Ditto WL, Weiss JN. Controlling cardiac chaos. *Science.* 1992;257:1230-1235.
5. Rapp PE, Bashore TR, Martinerie JM, Albano AM, Zimmerman ID, Mees AI. Dynamics of brain electrical activity. *Brain Topogr.* 1989;2:99-119.
6. Ehlers CL, Havstad JW, Garfinkel A, Kupfer DJ. Nonlinear analysis of EEG sleep states. *Neuropsychopharmacology.* 1991;5:167-176.
7. Jansen BH. Quantitative analysis of electroencephalograms: is there chaos in the future? *Int J Biomed Comput.* 1991;27:95-123.
8. Pritchard WS, Duke DW. Measuring chaos in the brain: a tutorial review of nonlinear dynamical EEG analysis. *Int J Neurosci.* 1992;67:31-88.
9. Mandell AJ. Non-equilibrium behavior of some brain enzyme and receptor systems. *Annu Rev Pharmacol Toxicol.* 1984;24:237-274.
10. King R, Barchas JD, Huberman BA. Chaotic behavior in dopamine neurodynamics. *Proc Natl Acad Sci U S A.* 1984;81:1244-1247.
11. Garfinkel A. A mathematics for physiology. *Am J Physiol.* 1983;245:R455-R466.
12. Schuster HG. *Deterministic Chaos.* 2nd ed. Weinheim, Germany: Physik Verlag; 1988.
13. Crutchfield JP, Farmer JD, Packard NH, Shaw RS. Chaos. *Sci Am.* December 1986;46:46-57.
14. Theiler J. Estimating the fractal dimension of chaotic time series. *Lincoln Lab J.* 1990;3:63-86.
15. Rapp PE. A guide to dynamical analysis. *Integr Physiol Behav Sci.* 1994;29:311-327.
16. Gleick J. *Chaos: Making a New Science.* New York, NY: Penguin Books; 1987.
17. Waldrop MM. *Complexity: The Emerging Science at the Edge of Order and Chaos.* New York, NY: Simon & Schuster; 1992.
18. Skarda CA, Freeman WJ. Chaos and the new science of the brain. *Concepts Neurosci.* 1990;1: 275-285.
19. Rapp PE, Jimenez-Montano MA, Langs RJ, Thomson L, Mees AI. Toward a quantitative characterization of patient-therapist communication. *Math Biosci.* 1991;105:207-227.
20. Freeman WJ. Chaos in psychiatry. *Biol Psychiatry.* 1992;31:1079-1081.
21. Mandell AJ, Selz KA. Dynamical systems in psychiatry: now what? *Biol Psychiatry.* 1992;32: 299-301.
22. Globus GG, Arpia JP. Psychiatry and the new dynamics. *Biol Psychiatry.* 1993;35:352-364.
23. Ehlers CL. The new physics of chaos: can it help us to understand the effects of alcohol? *Alcohol Health Res World.* 1992;16:267-272.
24. Lipsitz LA, Goldberger AL. Loss of 'complexity' and aging: potential applications of fractals and chaos theory to senescence. *JAMA.* 1992;267: 1806-1809.
25. Rapp PE, Theiler JM. Reexamination of the evidence for low-dimensional and non-linear structure in the human electroencephalogram. *Electroencephalogr Clin Neurophysiol.* In press.
26. Lorenz EN. Deterministic nonperiodic flow. *J Atmospher Sci.* 1963;20:130-141.
27. Abraham RH, Shaw CD. *Dynamics: The Geometry of Behavior.* Santa Cruz, Calif: Aerial Press; 1982-1988. Parts 1-4.
28. Haken H. *Information and Self-organization: A Macroscopic Approach to Complex Systems.* Berlin, Germany: Springer-Verlag; 1988. Springer Series in Synergetics.
29. Farmer D, Crutchfield J, Froehling H, Packard N, Shaw R. Power spectra and mixing properties of strange attractors. *Ann N Y Acad Sci.* 1980; 357:453-472.
30. Farmer JD, Ott E, Yorke JA. The dimension of chaotic attractors. *Physica.* 1983;7D:153-180.
31. Grassburger P, Procaccia I. Measuring the strangeness of strange attractors. *Physica.* 1983;9D: 189-208.
32. Theiler J. Spurious dimension from correlation algorithms applied to limited time series. *Phys Rev A.* 1986;34:2427-2433.
33. Havstad JW, Ehlers CL. Attractor dimension of non-stationary dynamical systems from small data sets. *Physical Rev.* 1989;39:845-853.
34. Rapp PE. Chaos in the neurosciences: cautionary tales from the frontier. *Biologist.* 1993;40: 89-94.
35. Rapp PE, Albano AM, Schmah TI, Farwell LA. Filtered noise can mimic low-dimensional chaotic attractors. *Phys Rev E.* 1993;47:2289-2297.
36. Roschke J, Aldenhoff JB. Estimation of the dimensionality of sleep-EEG data in schizophrenics. *Eur Arch Psychiatry Clin Neurosci.* 1993; 242:191-196.
37. Ehlers CL, Havstad JW, Schuckit MA. EEG dimension in the sons of alcoholics. *Alcohol Clin Exp Res.* In press.
38. Theiler J, Galdrikian B, Longtin A, Eubank S, Farmer JD. Using surrogate data to detect nonlinearity in time series. In: Casdagli M, Eubank S, eds. *Nonlinear Modeling and Forecasting.* Reading, Mass: Addison-Wesley Publishing Co; 1992: 163-188.
39. Pritchard D, Theiler J. Generating surrogate data for time series with several simultaneously measured variables. *Phys Rev Lett.* 1994;73:951-954.
40. Rapp PE, Albano AM, Zimmerman ID, Jimenez-Montano. Phase-randomized surrogates can produce spurious identifications of non-random structure. *Phys Lett A.* 1994;192:27-33.
41. Theiler J. On the evidence for low-dimensional chaos in an epileptic electroencephalogram. *Phys Lett A.* 1994;196:335-341.
42. May RM. Simple mathematical models with very complicated dynamics. *Nature.* 1976;261:459-467.
43. Abraham FD. *A Visual Introduction to Dynamical Systems Theory for Psychology.* Santa Cruz, Calif: Aerial Press; 1991.
44. Skarda CA, Freeman WJ. How brains make chaos in order to make sense of the world. *Behav Brain Sci.* 1987;10:161-195.
45. Glass L, Mackey MC. *From Clocks to Chaos: The Rhythms of Life.* Princeton, NJ: Princeton University Press; 1988.
46. Lewy AJ, Wehr TA, Goodwin FK, Newsome DA, Rosenthal NE. Manic-depressive patients may be supersensitive to light. *Lancet.* 1981;1:383-384.
47. Jauhar P, Weller MPL. Psychiatric morbidity and time zone changes: a study of patients from Heathrow Airport. *Br J Psychiatry.* 1982;140:231-235.
48. Ehlers CL, Kupfer DJ, Frank E, Monk TH. Biological rhythms and depression: the role of Zeitgebers and Zeitstörers. *Depression.* 1994;1: 285-293.
49. Hudson JI, Lipinski JF, Frankenburg FR, Grochocinski VJ, Kupfer DJ. Electroencephalographic sleep in mania. *Arch Gen Psychiatry.* 1988;45: 267-273.
50. Hudson JI, Lipinski JF, Frankenburg FR, Tohen M, Kupfer DJ. Effects of lithium on sleep in mania. *Biol Psychiatry.* 1989;25:665-688.
51. Hudson JI, Lipinski JF, Keck PE Jr, Aizley HG, Lukas SE, Rothschild AJ, Waternaux CM, Kupfer DJ. Polysomnographic characteristics of young manic patients: comparison with unipolar depressed patients and normal control subjects. *Arch Gen Psychiatry.* 1992;49:378-383.
52. Goodwin FK, Jamison KR. *Manic-Depressive Illness.* London, England: Oxford University Press; 1990.
53. Frank E, Kupfer DJ, Ehlers CL, Monk TH, Cornes C, Carter S, Frankel D. Interpersonal and social rhythm therapy for bipolar disorder: integrating interpersonal and behavioral approaches. *Behav Ther.* 1994;17:143-149.
54. Horgan J. From complexity to perplexity. *Sci Am.* June 1995;272:104-109.
55. Wehr TA, Sack D, Rosenthal N, Duncan W, Gillin J. Circadian rhythm disturbances in manic-depressive illness. *Fed Proc.* 1983;42:2809-2814.
56. Post R, Rubinow D, Ballenger J. Conditioning, sensitization and kindling: implications for the course of affective illness. In: Post R, Ballenger J, eds. *Neurobiology of Mood Disorders.* Baltimore, Md: Williams & Wilkins; 1985:432-466.
57. Post R, Rubinow D, Ballenger J. Conditioning, sensitization and longitudinal course of affective illness. *Br J Psychiatry.* 1986;149:191-201.

EDITORIAL

Managed Care in *JAMA* and the *Archives* Journals

A Call for Papers for Coordinated Theme Issues

MANAGEMENT IS the recognition, harnessing, and channeling of all available appropriate forces and resources toward meeting defined goals and objectives. What is "managed" in managed care? How a physician practices, among other things. Managed care is the application of management principles in a comprehensive, prepaid health care delivery system that controls input and output to optimize efficiency and effectiveness with the prior consent of providers and patients. In 1982, 10 million Americans were in managed care; in 1992, 90 million—a megatrend that continues to expand.

Victor Cohn of the *Washington Post* says, "If you've seen one managed care plan you've seen one managed care plan." The alphabet soup of managed care includes IPA (independent practice association), HMO (health maintenance organization), PPO (preferred provider organization), POS (point-of-service plan), PGP (prepaid group practice), and the beat goes on.

The principles and practices of managed care are hardly new. The first group practice in the United States was established in 1887 at the Mayo Clinic and the first capitated plan was set up in Elk City, Okla, in 1929. The Kaiser plan began in 1933 for employees and went public in 1947 as the first group-model HMO. By 1995, 56 million Americans were registered in HMOs, half of these in IPA-HMOs. Managed care has been touted as a savior and as an evil as well as a helpful component of our evolving health care system.

The editors and editorial boards of *JAMA*, the 10 AMA *Archives* journals, and *American Medical News* used our annual Delphi vote process to identify managed care as the subject to be dealt with by all 12 of our publications at a common date in 1996. We invite research papers, critical reviews, clinical reports, and commentaries for consideration at *JAMA*, the entire *Archives* family, and *American Medical News*. Manuscripts should be sent to the publication of first choice, although all submissions are subject to entering our AMA Editorial Consortium as well. We are particularly interested in the subject of managed care in relation to physicians, clinical research, graduate medical education, medical schools, academic health centers, quality of care, medical ethics, conflict resolution, patient-physician relationships, and mental health.

Please craft your manuscripts according to the Instructions for Authors in each of our journals. Understand that, although these papers are invited, they are all subject to our usual rigorous peer review and will be accepted on the basis of quality and priority. Manuscripts received by February 15, 1996, have the best chance for publication. Articles that are accepted for each journal may appear in the dedicated theme issue or they may be scheduled for issues before or after that date.

Times are changing rapidly and managed care is part of that change. We welcome your best offerings.

George D. Lundberg, MD

Dr Lundberg is Editor of JAMA.

Reprint requests to JAMA, *515 N State St, Chicago, IL 60610 (Dr Lundberg).*

Make Archives of Internal Medicine your first choice for staying on the leading edge of clinical knowledge

Timely information applicable to everyday practice

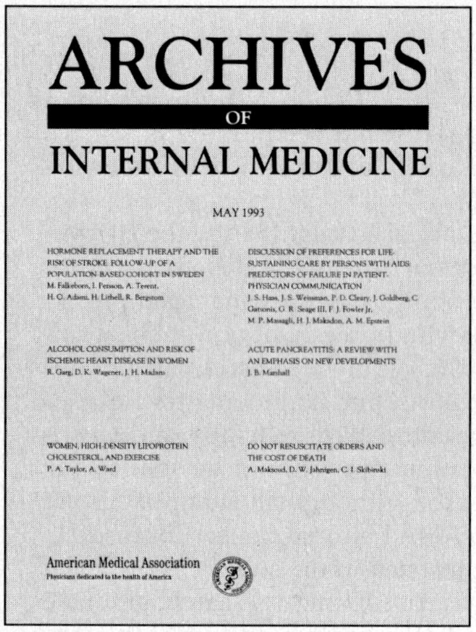
ARCHIVES OF INTERNAL MEDICINE

MAY 1993

HORMONE REPLACEMENT THERAPY AND THE RISK OF STROKE: FOLLOW-UP OF A POPULATION-BASED COHORT IN SWEDEN
M. Falkeborn, I. Persson, A. Terent, H. O. Adami, H. Lithell, R. Bergstrom

DISCUSSION OF PREFERENCES FOR LIFE-SUSTAINING CARE BY PERSONS WITH AIDS: PREDICTORS OF FAILURE IN PATIENT-PHYSICIAN COMMUNICATION
J. S. Haas, J. S. Weissman, P. D. Cleary, J. Goldberg, C. Gatsonis, G. R. Seage III, F. J. Fowler Jr, M. P. Massagli, H. J. Makadon, A. M. Epstein

ALCOHOL CONSUMPTION AND RISK OF ISCHEMIC HEART DISEASE IN WOMEN
R. Garg, D. K. Wagener, J. H. Madans

ACUTE PANCREATITIS: A REVIEW WITH AN EMPHASIS ON NEW DEVELOPMENTS
J. B. Marshall

WOMEN, HIGH-DENSITY LIPOPROTEIN CHOLESTEROL, AND EXERCISE
P. A. Taylor, A. Ward

DO NOT RESUSCITATE ORDERS AND THE COST OF DEATH
A. Maksoud, D. W. Jahnigen, C. I. Skibinski

American Medical Association
Physicians dedicated to the health of America

Selected recent topics from Archives of Internal Medicine

- Antioxidants and the Prevention of Coronary Heart Disease
- Influenza and Pneumococcal Vaccines
- Dialysis Discontinuation
- Preconceptional Counseling and Intervention
- Influence of Blood Culture Results in the Treatment of Bacteremia
- Adherence to Aspirin in the Prevention of Myocardial Infarction
- Ambulatory Electrocardiography

Twice each month, the Archives helps you keep pace with internal medicine and the subspecialties. Its relevant, clinically-focused articles represent the latest thinking in all aspects of this multi-specialty discipline.

An authoritative clinical approach

Archives of Internal Medicine's peer-reviewed, original articles are a vital information resource. High editorial standards and a rigorous review process result in breakthrough research studies, articles on recent clinical advances and thorough coverage of illnesses frequently encountered in clinical practice.

New, reader-friendly design

The Archives' new design emphasizes practicality and readability. Concise, structured abstracts guide you to the key points of primary source articles. And the journal's twice-monthly frequency means you stay current with the very latest information.

Find out for yourself why Archives of Internal Medicine is the journal you need to keep up with all aspects of the discipline.

SUBSCRIBE TODAY!

American Medical Association
Physicians dedicated to the health of America

Yes! Please enter my one-year subscription (23 issues) to Archives of Internal Medicine for $115.

☐ My check made payable to the AMA is enclosed.

Please charge my subscription to:

☐ Visa ☐ MasterCard ☐ American Express

Card #

Exp. / Signature

Name (Please Print)

☐ MD/DO ☐ Other (Please Specify)

Address

City/State/Zip

Institution rate is $135. Individual rate does not apply if payment is made through an institution. Washington, DC residents add 6% sales tax. Canada residents add 7% GST (R 126 225 556). An airmail delivery surcharge of $35 for individual orders ($45 surcharge for institution orders) will be applied to all orders outside the US. Rates subject to change.

Mail to: **American Medical Association**
P.O. Box 10945
Chicago, IL 60610 USA

For fast service, call toll-free 1-800-AMA-2350 or fax your order to 312-464-5831 today!

P5FA3

Pindolol, 5-Hydroxytryptamine, and Antidepressant Augmentation

I read with interest the letter by Howland[1] in the February issue of the ARCHIVES on the use of pindolol to augment antidepressant effects.[2] Howland argues that pindolol could be acting through β-adrenergic receptors to potentiate the effects of 5-hydroxytryptamine (5-HT) reuptake inhibitors and monoamine oxidase inhibitors. Based on the augmentation of antidepressant effects induced by buspirone hydrochloride,[3] a partial 5-HT_{1A} agonist, he also found it difficult to reconcile the fact that agonists and antagonists of the same receptors may produce the same effect. It is important to clarify this issue because it may be critical to understanding the mode of action of pindolol and other potentially useful 5-HT_{1A} antagonists.

The 5-HT_{1A} receptors are anatomically and pharmacologically heterogeneous. They are localized on the soma and dendrites of serotonergic neurons in the raphe nuclei (presynaptic or somatodendritic location) or on other cell types, in limbic, cortical, and hypothalamic areas.[4-7] Regarding pharmacological differences, 5-HT and 5-HT_{1A} agonists, like 8-hydroxy-2-(di-*R*-propylamino) tetralin (8-OH-DPAT) or ipsapirone hydrochloride, are equally effective at the somatodendritic 5-HT_{1A} receptor, whereas 5-HT is more effective at hippocampal postsynaptic receptors.[8] Also, 5-HT_{1A} antagonists (BMY 7378, SDZ 216525, and NAN 190) easily block postsynaptic effects but display partial agonistic properties at the somatodendritic receptors.[9-11] By contrast, spiperone preferentially blocks the presynaptic responses.[12] Some of these differences may result from the receptor reserve in the raphe,[13,14] which would enhance the efficacy of partial agonists (although this would not explain the responses of spiperone and 5-HT). Furthermore, chemically dissimilar 5-HT_{1A} agonists elicit different behavioral effects mediated by postsynaptic 5-HT_{1A} receptors,[15] raising the possibility of the existence of different subtypes. It is unclear whether these differences have a molecular origin or are simply due to posttranscriptional modifications. Three different bands of the messenger RNA encoding this receptor subtype have been found,[16] but attempts to subdivide the 5-HT_{1A} receptor by molecular biology techniques have proven to be unsuccessful.

Howland[1] also commented on the difficulty of reconciling a potential therapeutic effect of 5-HT_{1A} antagonists with the reported subsensitivity of 5-HT_{1A} receptors in major depression.[17,18] So far, there is no solid proof showing that hypothermia caused by 5-HT_{1A} agonists is a presynaptic response in humans. On the contrary, recent findings suggest that buspirone-induced hypothermia is not attenuated by tryptophan depletion.[19] This suggests a postsynaptic mediation of the hypothermic response because tryptophan depletion impairs 5-HT release.[20] In rats, the initial views suggesting the involvement of presynaptic 5-HT_{1A} receptors in the hypothermia induced by 5-HT_{1A} agonists[21] have been seriously challenged.[22-24]

New evidence has appeared in recent months that indicates that pindolol blocks the inhibitory effects of 5-HT on somatodendritic 5-HT_{1A} receptors. It reversed the suppressive effects of citalopram and paroxetine, two 5-HT reuptake inhibitors, on the release and firing of serotonergic neurons of the dorsal raphe nucleus.[25,26] On the contrary, it did not block hyperpolarizing effects on CA_3 pyramidal cells of the hippocampus[26] (although it blocks other postsynaptic responses, even at lower doses[27]). Accordingly, pindolol potentiated the 5-HT–enhancing effects of citalopram and paroxetine in the striatum[28] (an area receiving serotonergic afferents exclusively from the dorsal raphe) and those of fluoxetine hydrochloride in hypothalamus.[29]

Thus, the available data support the conclusion that pindolol blocks presynaptic but not some postsynaptic 5-HT_{1A} responses. In this way, it enhances presynaptic serotonergic function by preventing self-inhibitory actions of 5-HT on the firing and release of serotonergic neurons and does not hinder postsynaptic hippocampal responses that contribute to the antidepressant effect.[30] Within this conceptual framework, it may be predicted that the combination of a full 5-HT_{1A} agonist (ie, one that acts on presynaptic and postsynaptic receptors) plus a selective antagonist of presynaptic 5-HT_{1A} receptors (eg, pindolol) would have rapid antidepressant effects. Pindolol would prevent the initial suppression of serotonergic cell firing induced by 5-HT_{1A} agonists in the raphe while permitting full responses at postsynaptic 5-HT_{1A} receptors in hippocampus (and perhaps in other limbic and cortical areas).

One important point regarding pindolol effects in depressed patients is the dose, which is much lower than that used in the above animal studies. The affinity of pindolol for human 5-HT_{1A} receptors is not known, despite extensive studies.[31] Recent results show that iodine 125–labeled iodocyanopindolol, which is used to label β-adrenergic receptors in human brain, recognizes a population of 5-HT_{1A} receptors in the human dorsal raphe nucleus and hippocampus with very high (down to nanomoles per liter) affinity.[32] The determination of whether the high affinity of iodocyanopindolol for human (and not rat) 5-HT_{1A} receptors is also shared by its parent compound must await further studies (cyanopindolol labels 5-HT_{1B}, but not 5-HT_{1A} receptors in the rat[33]).

Despite all the above, the possibility remains that pindolol may exert a certain effect through β-adrenergic receptors. Yet, this effect should be small because the dose used to potentiate antidepressant response is lower than that used to treat cardiovascular diseases.[34] At the dose given (2.5 mg, three times a day), pindolol did not alter pulse rate or arterial pressure, which suggests little blockade of β-adrenergic receptors.[35] Also, the use of β-adrenergic receptor blockers has been associated with a higher prevalence of depression.[36]

Many antidepressants, particularly nonselective compounds like the tricyclic antidepressants and monoamine oxidase inhibitors, down-regulate β-adrenergic receptor responses.[37] This is not a universal effect because some 5-HT reuptake inhibitors (eg, paroxetine and citalopram) and selective inhibitors of norepinephrine and 5-HT uptake, like milnacipran, are without such effect.[38-42] Positive and negative results have been reported for fluoxetine.[42-44] As suggested by Howland,[1] an interesting study to discern the degree of involvement of β-adrenergic receptors in pindolol augmentation would be to compare the effects of pindolol with those of other β-adrenergic receptor blockers without affinity for 5-HT_{1A} receptors. Also, the theory that pindolol operates through a serotonergic mechanism would be indirectly proven if pindolol did not potentiate the effects of selective norepinephrine uptake inhibitors.

Certainly, much more experimental work is needed to clarify the complex interplay between serotonergic and noradrenergic systems. The notion that the blockade of both aminergic transporters is more effective in the treatment of depression than is the blockade of 5-HT alone is becoming increasingly clear.[45,46] Interestingly, recent observations[47] show that imipramine hydrochloride may be more effective than 5-HT reuptake inhibitors in increasing the extracellular concentration of 5-HT in cortex, despite the lower affinity of the former for the 5-HT transporter. Yet, in the absence of new data supporting an adrenergic component of the action of pindolol in depressed patients, available clinical and preclinical evidence suggests the involvement of serotonergic mechanisms.

Francesc Artigas, PhD
Department of Neurochemistry
Consejo Superior de Investigaciones Científicas
Jordi Girona 18-26
Barcelona E-08034, Spain

Supported by the Fondo de Investigación Sanitaria, Madrid, Spain (grant 95/266).

1. Howland RH. Biochemical effects of antidepressant augmentation. *Arch Gen Psychiatry.* 1995;52:156.
2. Artigas F, Perez V, Alvarez E. Pindolol induces a rapid improvement of depressed patients treated with serotonin reuptake inhibitors. *Arch Gen Psychiatry.* 1994;51:248-251.
3. Jacobsen FM. Possible augmentation of antidepressant response by buspirone. *J Clin Psychiatry.* 1993;54:269-271.
4. Pazos A, Palacios JM. Quantitative autoradiographic mapping of serotonin receptors in the rat brain, I: serotonin-1 receptors. *Brain Res.* 1985;346:205-230.
5. Vergé D, Daval G, Marcinkiewicz M, Patey A, El Mestikawy S, Gozlan H, Hamon M. Quantitative autoradiography of multiple 5-HT receptor subtypes in the brain of control and 5,7-dihydroxytryptamine-treated rats. *J Neurosci.* 1986;6:3474-3482.
6. Sotelo C, Cholley B, El Mestikawy SE, Gozlan H, Hamon M. Direct immunohistochemical evidence of the existence of 5-HT autoreceptors on serotonergic neurons in the midbrain raphe nuclei. *Eur J Neurosci.* 1990;2:1144-1154.
7. Pompeiano M, Palacios JM, Mengod G. Distribution and cellular localization of mRNA coding for 5-HT_{1A} receptor in the rat brain: correlation with receptor binding. *J Neurosci.* 1992;12:440-453.
8. Sprouse JS, Aghajanian GK. Responses of hippocampal pyramidal cells to putative serotonin 5-HT_{1A} and 5-HT_{1B} agonists: a comparative study with dorsal raphe neurons. *Neuropharmacology.* 1988;27:707-715.
9. Hjorth S, Sharp T. Mixed agonist/antagonist properties of NAN-190 at 5-HT_{1A} receptors: behavioural and in vivo brain microdialysis studies. *Life Sci.* 1990; 46:955-963.
10. Sharp T, Backus LI, Hjorth S, Bramwell SR, Grahame-Smith DG. Further investigation of the in vivo pharmacological properties of the putative 5-HT_{1A} antagonist, BMY 7378. *Eur J Pharmacol.* 1990;176:331-340.
11. Sharp T, Mcquade R, Fozard JR, Hoyer D. The novel 5-HT(1A)–receptor antagonist, SDZ 216-525, decreases 5-HT release in rat hippocampus in vivo. *Br J Pharmacol.* 1993;109:699-702.
12. Blier P, Lista A, de Montigny C. Differential properties of presynaptic and postsynaptic 5-hydroxytryptamine(1A) receptors in the dorsal raphe and hippocampus, I: effect of spiperone. *J Pharmacol Exp Ther.* 1993;265:7-15.
13. Meller E, Goldstein M, Bohmaker K. Receptor reserve for 5-hydroxytryptamine–mediated inhibition of serotonin synthesis: possible relationship to anxiolytic properties of 5-hydroxytriptamine agonists. *Mol Pharmacol.* 1990; 37:231-237.
14. Cox RF, Meller E, Waszczak BL. Electrophysiological evidence for a large receptor reserve for inhibition of dorsal raphe neuronal firing by 5-HT(1A) agonists. *Synapse.* 1993;14:297-304.
15. Scott PA, Chou JM, Tang H, Frazer A. Differential induction of 5-HT(1A)–mediated responses in vivo by three chemically dissimilar 5-HT(1A) agonists. *J Pharmacol Exp Ther.* 1994;270:198-208.
16. Albert PR, Zhou QY, Van Tol HHM, Bunzow JR, Civelli O. Cloning, functional expression, and mRNA tissue distribution of the rat $5\text{-hydroxytryptamine}_{1A}$ receptor gene. *J Biol Chem.* 1990;265:5825-5832.
17. Lesch KP, Mayer S, Disselkamp Tietze J, Hoh A, Schoellnhammer G, Schulte HM. Subsensitivity of the $5\text{-hydroxytryptamine}_{1A}$ (5-HT_{1A}) receptor–mediated hypothermic response to ipsapirone in unipolar depression. *Life Sci.* 1990;46:1271-1277.
18. Cowen PJ, Power AC, Ware CJ, Anderson IM. 5-HT_{1A} receptor sensitivity in major depression: a neuroendocrine study with buspirone. *Br J Psychiatry.* 1994;164:372-379.
19. Blier P, Seletti B, Young SN, Benkelfat C, De Montigny C. Serotonin_{1A} receptor activation and hypothermia: evidence for a postsynaptic mechanism in humans. *Neuropsychopharmacology.* 1994;10(suppl 3):92S.
20. Artigas F, Bel N, Ferrer A, Cortés R. Increased cortical extracellular 5-HT after repeated, but not acute, treatment with low doses of antidepressants: reduction after tryptophan depletion. *Soc Neurosci Abstr.* 1993;19:297. Abstract.
21. Green AR, Goodwin GM. The pharmacology of the hypothermic response of rodents to 8-OH-DPAT administration and the effects of psychotropic drug administration on this response. In: Dourish CT, Ahlenius S, Hutson PH, eds. *Brain 5-HT_{1A} Receptors.* Chichester, England: Ellis Horwood Ltd; 1987: 161-176.
22. Hutson PH, Donohoe TP, Curzon G. Hypothermia induced by the putative 5-HT_{1A} agonists LY 165163 and 8-OH-DPAT is not prevented by 5-HT depletion. *Eur J Pharmacol.* 1987;143:221-228.
23. O'Connell MT, Sarna GS, Curzon G. Evidence for postsynaptic mediation of the hypothermic effect of 5-HT_{1A} receptor activation. *Br J Pharmacol.* 1992; 106:603-609.
24. Bill DJ, Knight M, Forster EA, Fletcher A. Direct evidence for an important species difference in the mechanism of 8-OH-DPAT-induced hypothermia. *Br J Pharmacol.* 1991;103:1857-1864.
25. Artigas F, Romero L, Celada P, Bel N. 5-HT_{1A} antagonists and terminal 5-HT release: effects of the combined treatment with 5-HT uptake inhibitors. *Soc Neurosci Abstr.* 1994;20:1541. Abstract.
26. Blier P, Seletti B, Bouchard C, Artigas F, De Montigny C. Functional evidence for the differential responsiveness of pre- and postsynaptic 5-HT_{1A} receptors in the rat brain. *Soc Neurosci Abstr.* 1994;20:1540. Abstract.
27. Aulakh CS, Wozniak KM, Haas M, Hill JL, Zohar J, Murphy DL. Food intake, neuroendocrine and temperature effects of 8-OHDPAT in the rat. *Eur J Pharmacol.* 1988;146:253-259.
28. Bel N, Romero L, Celada P, De Montigny C, Blier P, Artigas F. Neurobiological basis for the potentiation of the antidepressant effect of 5-HT reuptake inhibitors by the 5-HT_{1A} antagonist pindolol. In: Louilot A, Durkin T, Spampinato U, Cador M, eds. *Monitoring Molecules in Neuroscience: Proceedings of the 6th International Conference of In Vivo Methods.* Bordeaux, France: University of Bordeaux; 1994:209-210.
29. Wong DT, Dreshfield LJ, Perry KW, Engleman EA. Augmentation of fluoxetine-induced elevation of extracellular 5-HT levels by pindolol, an antagonist at 5-HT_{1A} receptors. In: *The 33rd Annual Meeting of the American College of Neuropsychopharmacology.* Nashville, Tenn: ACNP Secretariat; 1994; 102.
30. Blier P, De Montigny C. Current advances and trends in the treatment of

depression. *Trends Pharmacol Sci.* 1994;15:220-226.
31. Palacios JM, Pazos A, Hoyer D. Characterization and mapping of 5-HT$_{1A}$ sites in the brain of animals and man. In: Dourish CT, Ahlenius S, Hutson PH, eds. *Brain 5-HT$_{1A}$ Receptors.* Chichester, England: Ellis Horwood Ltd; 1987: 67-81.
32. Pazos A, Gonzalez-Gil J, Castillo MJ. Increased affinity of beta-blockers for 5-HT$_{1A}$ receptors in the human brain: an autoradiographic study. *IUPHAR Satellite Meeting Serotonin.* 1994;3:99.
33. Hoyer D, Engel G, Kalkman HO. Characterization of the 5-HT$_{1B}$ recognition site in rat brain: binding studies with (-)(^{125}I)iodocyanopindolol. *Eur J Pharmacol.* 1985;118:1-12.
34. Martindale. *The Extra Pharmacopoeia.* 30th ed. London, England: Pharmaceutical Press; 1993.
35. Blier P, Bergeron R. Effectiveness of pindolol with selected antidepressant drugs in the treatment of major depression. *J Clin Psychopharmacol.* 1995; 15:217-221.
36. Avorn J, Everitt DE, Weiss D. Increased antidepressant use in patients prescribed β-blockers. *JAMA.* 1986;255:357-360.
37. Sulser F, Vetulani J, Mobley PL. Mode of action of antidepressant drugs. *Biochem Pharmacol.* 1978;27:257-261.
38. Assie MB, Charvern M, Palmier C, Puozzo C, Moret C, Briley M. Effects of prolonged administration of milnacipran, a new antidepressant, on receptors and monoamine uptake in the brain of the rat. *Neuropharmacology.* 1992; 31:149-155.
39. Dechant KL, Clissold SP. Paroxetine: a review of its pharmacodynamic and pharmacokinetic properties, and therapeutic potential in depressive illness. *Drugs.* 1991;41:225-253.
40. Hyttel J, Overo KF, Arnt J. Biochemical effects and drug levels in rats after long-term treatment with the specific 5-HT-uptake inhibitor, citalopram. *Psychopharmacology (Berl).* 1984;83:20-27.
41. Nalepa I, Vetulani J. Enhancement of the responsiveness of cortical adrenergic receptors by chronic administration of the 5-hydroxytryptamine uptake inhibitor citalopram. *J Neurochem.* 1993;60:2029-2035.
42. Palvimaki EP, Laakso A, Kuoppamaki M, Syvalahti E, Hietala J. Upregulation of beta(1)-adrenergic receptors in rat brain after chronic citalopram and fluoxetine treatments. *Psychopharmacology (Berl).* 1994;115:543-546.
43. Peroutka SJ, Snyder SH. Long-term antidepressant treatment decreases spiroperidol-labeled serotonin receptor binding. *Science.* 1980;210:88-90.
44. Byerley WF, McConnell EJ, McCabe RT, Dawson TM, Grosser BI, Wamsley JK. Decreased beta-adrenergic receptors in rat brain after chronic administration of the selective serotonin uptake inhibitor fluoxetine. *Psychopharmacology.* 1988;94:141-143.
45. Nelson JC, Mazure CM, Bowers MB, Jatlow PI. A preliminary open study of the combination of fluoxetine and desipramine for rapid treatment of major depression. *Arch Gen Psychiatry.* 1991;48:303-307.
46. Danish University Antidepressant Group. Paroxetine: a selective serotonin reuptake inhibitor showing better tolerance but weaker antidepressant effect than clomipramine in a controlled multicenter study. *J Affect Disord.* 1990;18:289-299.
47. Bel N, Artigas F. Acute and chronic effects of imipramine on serotonergic function: microdialysis studies in conscious rats. In: *Eighth Congress of the European College of Neuropsychopharmacology*. October 1995; Venice, Italy. In press.

UNITED STATES POSTAL SERVICE™

Statement of Ownership, Management, and Circulation

(Required by 39 U.S.C. 3685)

1. Publication Title	2. Publication No.	3. Filing Date
Archives of General Psychiatry	0 2 9 - 6 4 0	9-30-95
4. Issue Frequency	**5. No. of Issues Published Annually**	**6. Annual Subscription Price**
Monthly	12	$95.00

7. Complete Mailing Address of Known Office of Publication *(Street, City, County, State, and ZIP+4) (Not Printer)*

515 N. State Street, Chicago, Cook, IL 60610

8. Complete Mailing Address of Headquarters or General Business Office of Publisher *(Not Printer)*

515 N. State Street, Chicago, Cook, IL 60610

9. Full Names and Complete Mailing Addresses of Publisher, Editor, and Managing Editor *(Do Not Leave Blank)*

Publisher *(Name and Complete Mailing Address)*

American Medical Association, 515 N. State Street, Chicago, IL 60610

Editor *(Name and Complete Mailing Address)*

Jack D. Barchas, M.D., 515 N. State Street, Chicago, IL 60610

Managing Editor *(Name and Complete Mailing Address)*

None

10. Owner *(If owned by a corporation, its name and address must be stated and also immediately thereafter the names and addresses of stockholders owning or holding 1 percent or more of the total amount of stock. If not owned by a corporation, the names and addresses of the individual owners must be given. If owned by a partnership or other unincorporated firm, its name and address as well as that of each individual must be given. If the publication is published by a nonprofit organization, its name and address must be stated.) (Do Not Leave Blank.)*

Full Name	Complete Mailing Address
American Medical Association	515 N. State Street, Chicago, IL 60610

11. Known Bondholders, Mortgagees, and Other Security Holders Owning or Holding 1 Percent or More of Total Amount of Bonds, Mortgages, or Other Securities. If none, check here. ☒ None

Full Name	Complete Mailing Address
None	

12. For completion by nonprofit organizations authorized to mail at special rates. The purpose, function, and nonprofit status of this organization and the exempt status for federal income tax purposes: *(Check one)*
☒ Has Not Changed During Preceding 12 Months
☐ Has Changed During Preceding 12 Months
(If changed, publisher must submit explanation of change with this statement)

PS Form **3526**, October 1994 *(See Instructions on Reverse)*

13. Publication Name	14. Issue Date for Circulation Data Below
Archives of General Psychiatry	9/95

15. Extent and Nature of Circulation	Average No. Copies Each Issue During Preceding 12 Months	Actual No. Copies of Single Issue Published Nearest to Filing Date
a. Total No. Copies *(Net Press Run)*	10/94 9/95 30326	29226
b. Paid and/or Requested Circulation (1) Sales Through Dealers and Carriers, Street Vendors, and Counter Sales *(Not Mailed)*	546	525
(2) Paid or Requested Mail Subscriptions *(Include Advertisers' Proof Copies/Exchange Copies)*	27395	27151
c. Total Paid and/or Requested Circulation *(Sum of 15b(1) and 15b(2))*	27941	27676
d. Free Distribution by Mail *(Samples, Complimentary, and Other Free)*	0	0
e. Free Distribution Outside the Mail *(Carriers or Other Means)*	0	0
f. Total Free Distribution *(Sum of 15d and 15e)*	0	0
g. Total Distribution *(Sum of 15c and 15f)*	27941	27676
h. Copies Not Distributed (1) Office Use, Leftovers, Spoiled	2385	1550
(2) Return from News Agents	0	0
i. Total *(Sum of 15g, 15h(1), and 15h(2))*	30326	29226
Percent Paid and/or Requested Circulation *(15c / 15g x 100)*	100%	100%

16. This Statement of Ownership will be printed in the 11/95 issue of this publication. ☐ Check box if not required to publish.

17. Signature and Title of Editor, Publisher, Business Manager, or Owner — [signature], Publisher — Date 9/25/95

I certify that all information furnished on this form is true and complete. I understand that anyone who furnishes false or misleading information on this form or who omits material or information requested on the form may be subject to criminal sanctions *(including fines and imprisonment)* and/or civil sanctions *(including multiple damages and civil penalties).*

Instructions to Publishers

1. Complete and file one copy of this form with your postmaster on or before October 1, annually. Keep a copy of the completed form for your records.
2. Include in items 10 and 11, in cases where the stockholder or security holder is a trustee, the name of the person or corporation for whom the trustee is acting. Also include the names and addresses of individuals who are stockholders who own or hold 1 percent or more of the total amount of bonds, mortgages, or other securities of the publishing corporation. In item 11, if none, check box. Use blank sheets if more space is required.
3. Be sure to furnish all information called for in item 15, regarding circulation. Free circulation must be shown in items 15d, e, and f.
4. If the publication had second-class authorization as a general or requester publication, this Statement of Ownership, Management, and Circulation must be published; it must be printed in any issue in October or the first printed issue after October, if the publication is not published during October.
5. In item 16, indicate date of the issue in which this Statement of Ownership will be printed.
6. Item 17 must be signed.

Failure to file or publish a statement of ownership may lead to suspension of second-class authorization.

PS Form **3526**, October 1994 *(Reverse)*

THIS MONTH IN ARCHIVES OF GENERAL PSYCHIATRY

Schizophrenia is a complex illness, characterized by serious disturbances in thinking, perception, emotions, and behavior. Based on several lines of evidence, **Olney and Farber** (page 998) propose that a combined dysfunction of the glutamatergic and dopaminergic transmitter systems can account for major features of this baffling disorder (ie, developmental brain changes, age at onset, neuroleptic resistance, and secondary neurodegenerative and cognitive changes). They discuss the etiological, theoretical, and treatment implications of the proposed model and suggest several potential avenues for research. Three commentaries discuss this article.

The reliability of Axis II diagnosis has improved with the use of structured interviews, but questions about validity remain. **Pilkonis et al** (page 1025) examined the validity of two of the most commonly used interviews for personality disorders using a "best-estimate" consensus diagnosis as the validity standard. The validity of the interviews was modest, even when analyses were limited to patients with "marked" personality disorders. For identifying cases of personality disorder, researchers should consider the use of continuous data and methods adapted from signal detection theory as well as conventional categorical data.

Lidz et al (page 1034) examined patients' perceptions of coercion during admission to psychiatric hospitals, and found that these perceptions may contribute to patients' hostility to subsequent community care. Perceptions of procedural justice (patients' sense of fair, respectful and empathetic inclusion in decision-making processes) and legal status were most closely associated with perceived coercion, while force and threats were more weakly associated with it. The study suggests that clinicians may be able to improve subsequent cooperation with outpatient treatment, even among those involuntarily committed, by attending more closely to procedural justice at admission.

While classical ego-defense mechanisms have been empirically verified, the categories are not generally applied in all schools of evaluation and treatment. In an effort toward integration, **Horowitz et al** (page 1040) have attempted to revise defensive control processes theory. They measured observable signs of efforts to stifle as well as express emotion during treatment sessions. They also measured changes in focus of attention during talk about personal topics. A new, quantitative, computer-based paradigm was used in a way that was analogous to how clinicians work. This design led to empirical results that may inform clinical practice.

Kessler et al (page 1048) present findings from the first national survey to assess the general population prevalence and correlates of posttraumatic stress disorder (PTSD). Lifetime PTSD is estimated to be 10% among women and 5% among men, to be highly comorbid with other psychiatric disorders, and to persist in many cases for years. The traumas most often associated with PTSD are sexual assault among women and combat exposure among men.

The clinical presentation of schizophrenia is heterogeneous, and differences in symptoms may relate to differences in regional brain pathology. In one of the largest studies to date, **Turetsky et al** (page 1061) found selective volume reductions in left temporal and right frontal lobe regions in schizophrenic patients. However, reduced left temporal lobe volume was observed only for patients subtyped as deficit, and correlated with severity of negative symptoms. Right frontal lobe abnormality, in contrast, correlated with duration of illness but was not related to specific symptoms. The findings suggest that temporal rather than frontal lobe pathology may underlie negative schizophrenic symptomatology.

This year saw the passing of many great members of the psychiatric community whose contributions to the field will endure for years to come. Included in this issue are obituaries of Roland Ciaranello, Helen Singer Kaplan, James W. Maas, Samuel W. Perry III, Eli Robins, John Romano, and Joseph Wortis.

REVIEWERS FOR 1995

Few of our readers and authors recognize the enormous contributions that reviewers make to the process of publishing articles in the journal. These women and men give unselfishly, without compensation, of their time, effort, and consideration to the analysis, judgment, and evaluation of the multitude of manuscripts that are submitted to us each year. This is the only public opportunity that we have to commend and thank them. Listed below are those reviewers active from December 1994 through December 1995.

Our special appreciation is extended to all persons on this list for their efforts on behalf of our readers, authors, and editorial staff.—ED.

Amir Abdul-Jalil
Larry Abel
James L. Abelson
Richard Abrams
Robert F. Ackermann
Lawrence E. Adler
W. Stewart Agras
Saeed Ahmed
Schahram Akbarian
Hagop S. Akiskal
Anne Marie Albano
Marilyn Albert
Georgios Alexopoulos
John S. Allen
Christer Allgulander
Margaret Altemus
Arthur Alterman
Lori Altshuler
Jose Alvir
Donna Ames
Thomas Anders
Barbara Anderson
George Anderson
Jessie C. Anderson
Gavin Andrews
Douglas H. Anglin
Adrian Angold
Burton Angrist
Jules Angst
Lawrence Annable
James C. Anthony
Ray Anton
Paul Appelbaum
Josephine Arendt
Mark Armstrong
Stephan Arndt
Robert Asarnow
Boris Astrachan
M. Atkins
Elizabeth Aylward
Thomas Babor
Judith A. Badner
Lee Baer
Susan Baker
James C. Ballenger
Isaac Barchas
David Barlow
Miron Baron
Herbert Barry III
Arthur Barsky
John J. Bartko
George Bartzokis
Lance Bauer
Mark Bauer
Andrew Baum
Lewis Baxter
Charles M. Beasley
Aaron T. Beck
Helmut Beckmann
Henri Begleiter
Allan Beigel
Alan S. Bellack
Elisa Benedek
Francine Benes
Chawki Benkelfat
Neal Benowitz
Kathleen Benson
Leonard Berkowitz
Karen Faith Berman
Wade Berrettini
Tahir Bhatti
Joseph Biederman
Robert Bilder
Eric Bing
Edward Bird
Hector Bird
Donald Black
Jack Blaine
R. Clifford Blair
Jack Blanchard
Dan G. Blazer
Floyd E. Bloom
Arthur G. Blouin
Susan Blumenthal
Michael Bond
William Bondareff
G. E. Bonney
Michael Borenstein
Lisa Borg
Jonathan Borus
Gilbert Botvin
Nashant Boutrus
Dana Bovbjerg
David Braff
Devra L. Braun
Alan Breier
David Brent
Naomi Breslau
Timothy D. Brewerton
Jonathan Brodie
Evelyn Bromet
David Brook
Judith S. Brook
George W. Brown
Joe Brown
Walter Armin Brown
Gerard E. Bruder
Stephen Bryant
Robert W. Buchanan
Kathy Bucholz
Monte Buchsbaum
Benjamin S. Bunney
William E. Bunney
Jack D. Burke
Greg Burkhardt
Audrey Burnam
Nelson Butters
Daniel Buysse
Alexander Bystritsky
John Cacciola
Remi Cadoret
Eric Caine
Joseph Callicott
Oliver G. Cameron
Scott Campbell
Robert Cancro
Dennis Cantwell
Gabrielle Carlson
Dorit Carmelli
Bernard J. Carroll
Kathleen M. Carroll
Rosland Cartwright
Manuel Casanova
Daniel E. Casey
Nicholas Casken
Regina Casper
Ned Cassem
F. Xavier Castellanos
Carol Caton
Aravinda Chakravarti
John Chappel
Dennis S. Charney
Michael Chase
Thomas N. Chase
Harry Chugani
Roland D. Ciaranello
Ted Cizadlo
Camellia Clark
John Clarkin
M. David Clayson
Paula Clayton
Emil Coccaro
C. Edward Coffey
Carl I. Cohen
Donald Cohen
Lisa Cohen
Robert Cohen
D. Jackson Coleman
Gregory Collins
David E. Comings
Ruth Condray
P. Michael Conneally
John Constantino
Brian Cook
Edwin H. Cook
James Cooper
Richard Coppola
William Coryell
Jane Costello
Eric Courchesne
David Cox
Paul Crits-Christoph
Tim Crow
Raymond Crowe
Thomas Crowley
John Csernansky
Joseph Cubells
Jeffrey Cummings
Charles Czeisler
Pal Czobor
Mary F. Dallman
Antonio R. Damasio
Jean-Marie Danion
Jonathan Davidson
Lucy Davidson
Michael Davidson
John M. Davis
Kenneth Davis
Michael Davis
Claude De Montigny
Lynn DeLisi
Jose deLeon
Joseph A. Deltito
Kevin Delucchi
Edward Demet
Lakshimi Demi
Richard Depue
John R. DeQuardo
Mary Amanda Dew
Barbara Dickey
Steven Dilsaver
Bill Dixon
John Docherty
Bruce Dohrenwend

Edward F. Domino
Robert Dorwart
Alan Douglass
Wayne Drevets
David Dunner
Renee Dupont
Mary Durham
Felton Earls
Charmane Eastman
William Eaton
Michael Ebert
James Eberwine
Craig Edelbrock
Robert H. Edwards
John Efron
Cindy L. Ehlers
Burr Eichelman
Everett H. Ellinwood
Robert Emde
Jean Endicott
Jane Erb
Javier Escobar
Christopher Evans
David W. Evans
Dwight Evans
John L. Fahey
Christopher Fairburn
Stephen Faraone
Lars Farde
Kym Faull
Jan Fawcett
Fawzy I. Fawzy
Irwin R. Feinberg
Wayne S. Fenton
John D. Fernstrom
Steven Ferris
Sheila K. Fifer
Max Fink
Marion Fischman
Barbara Fish
Baruch Fishman
Michael Flaum
Kenneth Fletcher
Edna B. Foa
Susan Folkman
Marshal F. Folstein
Judith Ford
Steven Forman
David Foulkes
Allen Frances
Ellen Frank
Richard Frank
Frances Frankenburg
Alan Frazer
Robert Freedman
Betty J. Freeman
Nelson Freimer
Arnold J. Friedhoff
Edward S. Friedman
Howard S. Friedman
Richard A. Friedman
C. D. Frith
Gary R. Gaffney
G. Galbaud du Fort
Christopher Gallen
Marc Gallanter
Rohan Ganguli
David M. Garner
Constantine Gatsonis
Frank Gawin
Alan Gelenberg
Joel Gelernter
M. George
Elliot Gershon
Sam Gershon
Mark Geyer
Robert D. Gibbons
Christopher Gillberg
T. Conrad Gilliam
J. Christian Gillin
Alfred Gilman
Sander Gilman
Michael Gitlin
Alexander Glassman
William Glazer
Ira D. Glick
James Gold
Mark Gold
Phillip W. Gold
Terry E. Goldberg
Robert Golden
Lyn Goldin
Jacqueline M. Golding
Morris Goldman
Patricia Goldman-Rakic
Avram Goldstein
Jill Goldstein
Rise B. Goldstein
Daniel Goodman
Wayne Goodman
Donald Goodwin
Enoch Gordis
David Gorenberg
Irving Gottesman
David K. Grandy
Igor Grant
Ann M. Graybiel
John Greden
Alan I. Green
Bonnie L. Green
Michael Green
David Greenblatt
Paul Greengard
Lawrence Greenhill
Joel Greenhouse
Steven Greenwalk
John H. Greist
Roland Griffiths
John Gruzelier
John G. Gunderson
Raquel Gur
Ruben Gur
Hugh M. Gurling
Thomas Gutheil
Donald Guthrie
Sally K. Guthrie
Barry Guze
Samuel Guze
Gretchen Haas
Fady Hajal
Angelos Halaris
Uriel Halbreich
Martica Hall
Joachim Hallmayer
Katherine Halmi
Susan Hamburger
Constance Hammen
Gregory L. Hanna
Josette Harris
Wilma Harrison
Martin Harrow
Elizabeth Hart
Richard Hauger
Jim Haustad
Don Hedecker
Larry Hedges
Martti Heikkinen
John E. Helzer
Robert Hendren
Hugh Hendrie
George Heninger
Jack E. Henningfield
Markus Henriksson
Tracy Herbert
Magaret Hertzig
Victor Hesselbrock
Len Heston
Ian Hickie
Stephen T. Higgins
J. D. Higley
Elizabeth Hill
Shirley Hill
Melissa Hines
Robert Hirschfeld
Carolyn Hoch
Susan Hodge
Sheilagh Hodgins
Rudolf Hoehn-Saric
Myron Hofer
Randi Hoff
Andrea Hoffman
Diane C. Hoffman
Ralph Hoffman
Gerard E. Hogarty
Ann Hohmann
Lowell E. Hokin
Theodore Holford
Jimmie C. Holland
Eric Hollander
Florian Holsboer
David Holtzman
Philip Holzman
Rebecca Howland
Robert Howland
John Hughes
Stephen Hurt
Steven Hyman
Marco Iacoboni
William G. Iacono
Thomas R. Insel
Michael Irwin
Goran B. Isaacson
Erik Isometsa
Assen Jablensky
Jerome H. Jaffe
Kay Jamison
Philip G. Janicak
David M. Janowsky
Lissy Jarvik
Murray Jarvik
Daniel C. Javitt
Terry Jernigan
Dilip Jeste
Tong Joh
Robin Johnson
Barry Jones
Edward Jones
Peter Jones
Reese Jones
Peter R. Joyce
Lewis L. Judd
Bruce Kagan
Jerome Kagan
Rene S. Kahn
Tatsu Kakuma
Anthony Kales
Kyle Kampman
Denise Kandel
John Kane
Hooshang Kangarloo
Gurmeet Kanwal
Bert Kaplan
Marvin Karno
Craig Karson
Javad H. Kashani
Leon Kass
Wayne Katon
Charles Kaelber
Claudia Kawas
Walter Kaye
Samuel Keith
Kelly Kelleher
Adrienne Keller
Martin Keller
John Kelsoe
Margaret Kemeny
Kenneth Kendler
Matcheri Keshavan
Ronald Kessler
K. Ketter
Seymour Kety
Kenneth Kidd
Joel Killen
Kathleen Kim
Bryan King
Raymond King
Brian Kirkpatrick
Herbert D. Kleber
Rachel G. Klein
Arthur Kleinman
Joel Kleinman
James H. Kocsis
Harold W. Koenigsberg
Lorrin Koran
Thomas Kosten
Maria Kovacs
Rachel Kramer
Henry Richard Kranzler
Mary Jane Kreek
William S. Kremen
Marcus Kruesi
John Krystal
Michael J. Kuhar
Sanjiv Kumar
Samuel Kuperman
Asenath LaRue
Ben Lahey
H. Richard Lamb
Douglas R. Langbehn
Philip Lavori
William B. Lawson
James Leckman

Julian Leff
Robert J. Lefkowitz
Tony Lehman
Ellen Leibenluft
Robert Lenox
Andrew C. Leon
Lynna Lesko
Ira M. Lesser
Andrew Leuchter
Bennett Leventhal
Harvey S. Levin
Robert A. Levine
Douglas F. Levinson
Deborah Levy
Richard Lewine
David Lewis
Lisa Lewis
Alfred Lewy
Robert Liberman
Peter F. Liddle
Jeffrey A. Lieberman
Michael Liebowitz
Keh-Ming Lin
Marsha Linehan
Walter Ling
Markku Linnoila
Jennifer D. Lish
Robert E. Litman
James Lohr
Peter T. Loosen
Armand Loranger
R. Bruce Lydiard
Charles J. MacLean
James MacMurray
Richard Maddock
Bertha K. Madras
Michael Maes
Nigel Maidment
Wolfgang Maier
George Makari
Alain Malafosse
Kevin Malone
Husseini K. Manji
J. John Mann
Willard Manning
Thomas D. Marcotte
Joseph Marcus
Stephen Marder
John C. Markowitz
Isaac Marks
Laura Marsh
Frederick Marsteller
Ronald Martin
Mauri Marttunen
Roy J. Mathew
Jeff Mattes
Steven Matthysse
Marlin Mattson
Matig Mavissakalian
John Mazziotta
P. Anne McBride
Una McCann
Robert W. McCarley
Joan McCord
James T. McCracken
Barbara S. McCrady
Christopher McDougle
Bruce S. McEwen
Thomas P. McGlashan
Peter McGuffin
Michael McGuire
Jack McIntyre
James McKay
R. Craig McKenna
Guy M. McKhann
A. Thomas McLellan
Sarnoff Mednick
Paul E. Meehl
Ivan Mefford
Herbert Y. Meltzer
David B. Menkes
Kathleen Merikangas
Roger Meyer
James L. Meyerhoff
Barnett Meyers
Robert Michels
David Miklowitz
Andrew H. Miller
Bruce Miller
Del Miller
Frank T. Miller
Robert B. Millman
Mark J. Mills
Jim Mintz
Olga Mintzer
Steven Mirin
Steven Moldin
Margaret Moline
Perry Molinoff
John Monahan
John J. Mooney
Hal Morgenstern
John Morley
Robert Morse
Eve K. Moscicki
Sukdeb Mukherjee
Dennis Murphy
George Murphy
Jane Murphy
Robin M. Murray
Bengt Muthen
James L. Myerhoff
Henry A. Nasrallah
J.Craig Nelson
Charles Nemeroff
John Newcomer
David A. Nielsen
Ernest Noble
Eric Nofzinger
Thomas Noga
Thomas Nordahl
Russell Noyes
Keith Nuechterlein
Edward Nunes
John I. Nurnberger
David Nutt
Stephanie O'Malley
Daniel Offer
David R. Offord
Mark Olfson
J. Ormel
Edward Ornitz
David Oslin
Jurg Ott
Michael Otto
John E. Overall
A. J. Pakstis
G. N. Pandey
Morris Parloff
Barbara Parry
Oscar Parsons
Jayendra K. Patel
Thomas L. Patterson
Steven M. Paul
David Pauls
Eugene Paykel
Godfrey D. Pearlson
Victor Peralta
Stephen J. Peroutka
T. Peters
Jay Pettegrew
Helen Pettinati
Richard Petty
Cynthia Pfeffer
Adolf Pfefferbaum
Bruce Pfohl
David Phillips
Eric Phillips
David Pickar
Carl F. Pieper
Teresa Pigott
Bruce Pike
Paul Pilkonis
Harold Pincus
Daniel Pine
Michael Pogue-Geile
Russell Poland
John Polich
Simcha Pollack
Bruce Pollock
Harrison G. Pope
Michael Popkin
Michael Posner
Robert Post
Steve Potkin
Nicholas Potts
Arthur Prange
Sheldon H. Preskorn
Lawrence H. Price
Robert Prien
Holly Prigerson
Robert Proctor
Frank Putnam
Robert Pynoos
Bruce Quinn
Frederic Quitkin
Bruce S. Rabin
Peter Rabins
Judith Rabkin
Richard Rada
George K. Radda
Marcus E. Raichle
Adrian Raine
Michael J. Raleigh
Stanley Rapoport
Murray Raskind
Rebecca Rausch
Darrel Regier
Theodore Reich
Walter Reich
Seymour Reichlin
Eric Reiman
Alan Reiss
Richard Rende
Victor I. Reus
Charles F. Reynolds
Howard Rhoades
George Ricaurte
John P. Rice
Charles Rich
John Richters
Karl Rickels
Arthur Rifkin
Craig Risch
Edward Ritvo
Rosalinda Roberts
Marjorie Robertson
Lee Robins
Delbert Robinson
Robert Robinson
Joseph Rochford
Howard P. Roffwarg
Barbara Rohland
Jed Rose
Robert Rose
John Rosecrans
Jerrold Rosenbaum
Charles Rosenberg
Davis Rosenberg
Norman E. Rosenthal
Christopher Ross
Helen E. Ross
Thomas Roth
Walton T. Roth
Bruce Rounsaville
Peter Roy-Byrne
John Rubenstein
Robert Rubin
David Rubinow
Mathew Rudorfer
A. John Rush
Mark Russ
Andrew T. Russell
James T. Russell
Megan Rutherford
Michael Rutter
Neal D. Ryan
Perminder Sachdev
Robert Sack
Harold Sackeim
Bruce Sales
Carl Salzman
Elaine Sanders-Bush
James R. Sands
Paul Satz
Andrew Saykin
Carla Schatz
Ursula Scheffel
Arnold Scheibel
Susan Schenk
Donald J. Scherl
Joseph Schildkraut
Franklin Schneier
Nina Schooler
Marc Schuckit
Susan K. Schultz
S. Charles Schulz
Charles R. Schuster
Jeffrey Schwartz
Goran Sedvall
Phillip Seeman
Erich Seifritz

Edward M. Sellars
Edward C. Senay
Sally Severino
David Shaffer
Mohammed Shafii
Theodore Shapiro
Steven S. Sharfstein
Rajiv Sharma
Katherine Shear
David V. Sheehan
Richard Shelton
Martha Shenton
Patrick E. Shrout
Marc Shuckit
Carol Siegel
Larry Siever
Soren Sigvordsson
Linmarie Sikich
David Silbersweig
Jeremy Silverman
George Simpson
J. Sines
Cliff Singer
Andrew Skodol
William Sledge
Gary Small
Joyce Small
G. Richard Smith
Robert C. Smith
Solomon Snyder
Susan Solomon
Steven Southwick
Cynthia Spanier
M. Anne Spence
Tom Spencer
David Spiegel
Herbert Spiegel
Robert L. Spitzer
Herbert Spohn
Stephen M. Stahl
Jeff A. Stanley
Larry Stark
R. Dennis Staton
Marvin Stein
Murray B. Stein
Martin Steiner
Emily Stern
Yaakov Stern
Janice R. Stevens
Mark A. Stewart
Maxine Stitzer
C. A. Stockmeier
David Stoff
Peter Stokes
Robert Stout
Richard E. Straub
Robert E. Straub
John Strauss
Michael Strober
Albert J. Stunkard
Brian Suarez
E. Sullivan
Fridolin Sulser
Suzanne Sunday
Ezra Susser
Suzanne Sutherland
Susan Swedo
John Sweeney
Charles Swenson
Neil Swerdlow
Martin Szuba
Carol Tamminga
Peter E. Tanguay
Kenneth Tardiff
Pierre Tariot
C. Barr Taylor
Eric Taylor
Stephan F. Taylor
Laurence Tecott
Christopher Tennant
Michael Terman
Leonore Terr
Gunvant Thaker
Anita Thapar
Michael E. Thase
Allen Tien
Richard D. Todd
Svenn Torgersen
E. Fuller Torrey
Paul Trautman
Richard E. Tremblay
Ming T. Tsuang
L. Lee Tynes
Thomas Uhde
George R. Uhl
E. H. Uhlenhuth
George Vaillant
Karen Valentino
Daniel Van Kammen
Herman Van Praag
Milton Viederman
Veronica Vieland
Benedetto Vitiello
Gerald Vogel
Jan Volavka
Nora Volkow
Joseph R. Volpicelli
Mark Von Zastrow
John L. Waddington
Jerene Waite
C. J. Wallace
B. Timothy Walsh
Royce W. Waltrip II
Susan Warren
Christine Waternaux
Tom Wehr
Daniel Weinberger
Roger D. Weiss
Avery Weissman
Michael Welch
David Wellisch
Charles Wells
Kenneth Wells
Paul H. Wender
Robert Wesner
Lennart Wetterberg
Nancy Wexler
Maureen Whittal
Peter Whybrow
Priya Wickmaratne
Janet B. W. Williams
R. B. Williams
Marilyn Winkleby
Andrew Winokur
Anna Wirz-Justice
Sandra Witelson
Steven J. Wolf
Peter Wolff
Tanya Wolfson
Susan Wolk
Adam Wolkin
Owen Wolkowitz
Robert L. Wolski
Dean F. Wong
Dona Wong
Catherine Woodman
Scott Woods
Steven H. Woodward
George Woody
Richard J. Wurtman
Richard Jed Wyatt
Joel Yager
William R. Yates
Jerome A. Yesavage
Anne Young
Robert Yu
James P. Zacny
Theodore Zahn
Alan Zametkin
Vincent Zarcone
Deborah A. Zarin
Ming Dong Zhang
Zhongxin Zhang
Mark Zimmerman
Robert Zipursky
Sidney Zisook
George Zubenko
Stephen R. Zukin

Archives Interactive

Risperdal 1-, 2-, 3-, 4-mg tablets® RISPERIDONE

Introducing RISPERDAL ON CALL

A toll-free 800 number that mental healthcare professionals can call for instant access to information about RISPERDAL.

Now You Can Call On Us!

All you need is a touch-tone phone. RISPERDAL ON CALL is available 24 hours a day, 7 days a week. You can access us anytime—anywhere.

Dial 1-800-6R-ON-CALL

Just phone 1-800-6R-ON-CALL (1-800-676-6225), then listen for further instructions to access your choice of information.

PRESS 1 FOR: RISPERDAL PRODUCT INFORMATION
- Clinical Description
- Pharmacokinetics
- Indications
- Side Effects and Drug Interactions
- Quick Mail-Back

PRESS 2 FOR: PHYSICIAN EXCHANGE
- Positive Symptoms
- Negative Symptoms
- Extrapyramidal Symptoms
- Serotonin/Dopamine Antagonism
- Quick Mail-Back

PRESS 3 FOR: CLINICAL REVIEWS
- Abstract Selection
- Abstract Presentation
- Request Full Clinical Paper
- Quick Mail-Back/Quick Fax-Back

PRESS 4 FOR: CONVERSION AND DOSAGE
- From Oral and IM Antipsychotics
- Concomitant Agents
- Switching Strategies
- Dosage
- Quick Mail-Back

A Complete Look at What You Can Access

Here's a quick "map" of RISPERDAL ON CALL:

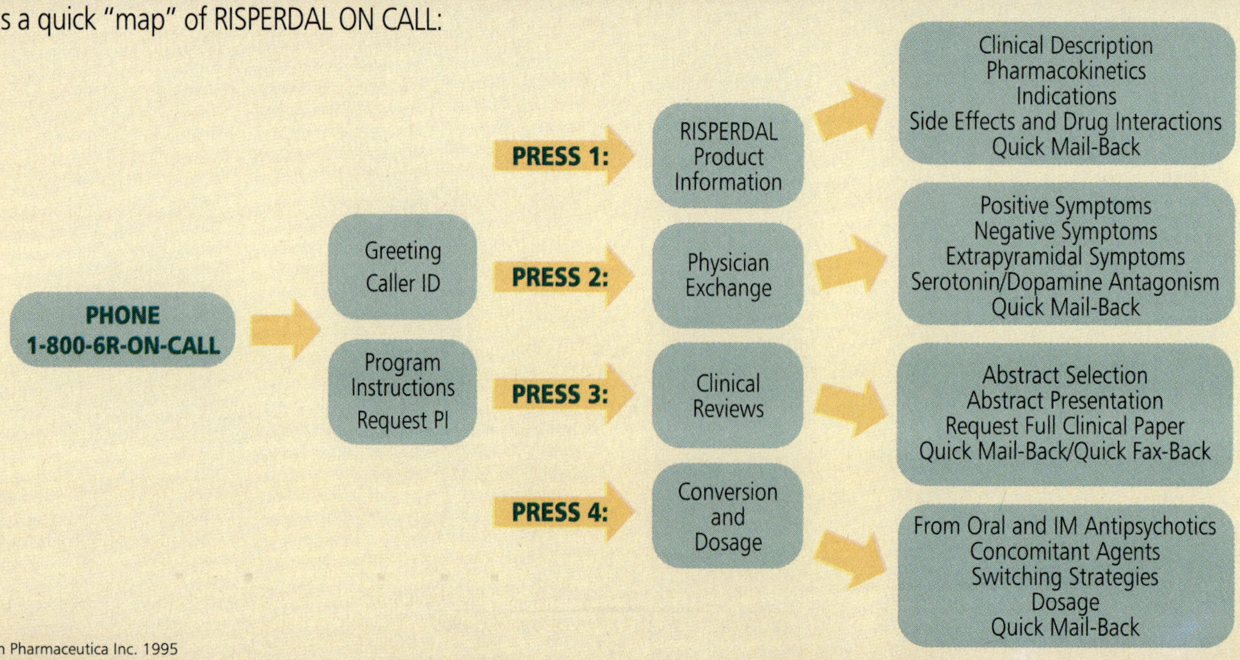

October 1995 IPI-RS-168

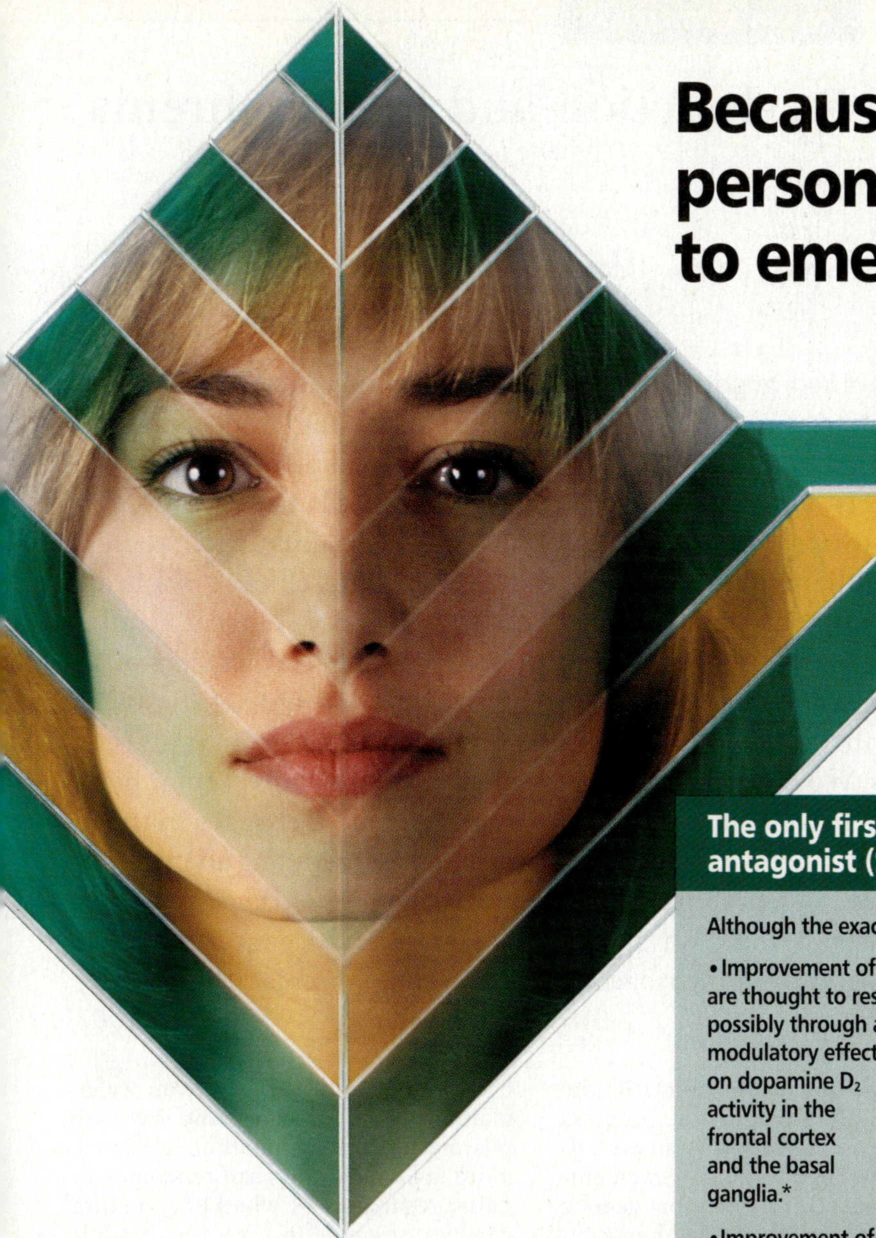

Because a whole person is waiting to emerge.

The only first-choice serotonin/dopamine antagonist (SDA).

Although the exact mechanism of action is unknown:

- Improvement of negative symptoms and lessened risk of EPS are thought to result from blockade of serotonin 5-HT_2 receptors, possibly through a modulatory effect on dopamine D_2 activity in the frontal cortex and the basal ganglia.*
- Improvement of positive symptoms is thought to result from blockade of dopamine D_2 receptors in the limbic system.*

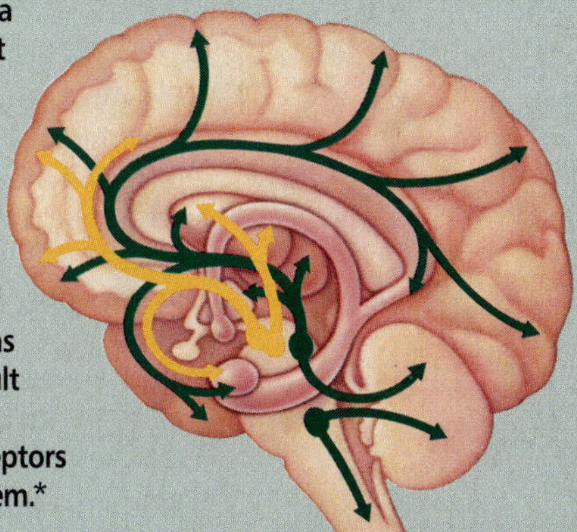

Dopaminergic system   Serotoninergic system

1-, 2-, 3-, 4-mg tablets

Risperdal®
RISPERIDONE

A first choice in psychosis.

*Ereshefsky L, Lacombe S. Pharmacological profile of risperidone. *Can J Psychiatry.* 1993;38(Suppl 3):S80-S88.

Please see the brief summary of Prescribing Information adjacent to this ad.

JANSSEN · PHARMACEUTICA · RESEARCH FOUNDATION ·   SB SmithKline Beecham Pharmaceuticals

NEWS AND VIEWS

Glutamate Receptor Dysfunction and Schizophrenia

John W. Olney, MD, Nuri B. Farber, MD

In this article, we advance a unified hypothesis pertaining to combined dysfunction of dopamine and N-methyl-D-aspartate glutamate receptors that highlights N-methyl-D-aspartate receptor hypofunction as a key mechanism that can help explain major clinical and pathophysiological aspects of schizophrenia. The following fundamental features of schizophrenia are accommodated by this hypothesis: (1) the occurrence of structural brain changes during early development that have the potential for producing subsequent clinical manifestations of schizophrenia, (2) a quiescent period in infancy and adolescence before clinical manifestations are expressed, (3) onset in early adulthood of psychotic symptoms, (4) involvement of dopamine (D_2) receptors in some cases but not others that would explain why some but not all patients are responsive to typical neuroleptic therapy, and (5) ongoing neurodegenerative changes and cognitive deterioration in some patients. We propose that since N-methyl-D-aspartate receptor hypofunction can cause psychosis in humans and corticolimbic neurodegenerative changes in the rat brain, and since these changes are prevented by certain antipsychotic drugs, including atypical neuroleptic agents (clozapine, olanzapine, fluperlapine), a better understanding of the N-methyl-D-aspartate receptor hypofunction mechanism and ways of preventing its neurodegenerative consequences in the rat brain may lead to improved pharmacotherapy in schizophrenia.

(Arch Gen Psychiatry. 1995;52:998-1007)

Despite a prodigious effort to clarify the pathogenesis of schizophrenia, progress has been modest and definitive answers to the most pressing questions remain elusive. It is generally accepted that genetic factors play an important role,[1] but accumulating evidence from monozygotic twin studies[2] suggests that nongenetic prenatal or perinatal factors may be powerful determinants of whether the schizophrenic genotype will be expressed.

Accumulating evidence suggests that structural changes in cerebrocortical and limbic brain regions are characteristic of the disorder,[3-15] and there is a growing belief that these changes may originate in utero.[16-21] However, if the structural changes occur in utero, why are symptoms not expressed until early adulthood?[22] Why do some victims of the disease show a progressive downhill course suggestive of ongoing pathological brain changes in adulthood? How can we explain evidence[23,24] suggesting that early pharmacological intervention results in a more favorable long-term outcome? Finally, regardless of whether structural changes originate in early life or adulthood (or both), what is the mechanistic basis for these structural changes, and how do specific structural changes in diverse anatomical locations relate to specific signs and symptoms of the disease?

Several transmitter systems have been implicated, but the primary focus has been on the dopamine (DA) system[25,26] because of evidence that most drugs that ameliorate psychotic symptoms in patients with schizophrenia are DA receptor blockers. However, attempts to explain the disease solely in terms of an aberrantly overactive dopaminergic transmitter system leave many aspects of the riddle unsolved.

Recently, it has been suggested that combined dysfunction of the DA and glutamate (Glu) transmitter systems may be

From the Department of Psychiatry, Washington University School of Medicine, St Louis, Mo.

a mechanism worth considering. We agree with this view, but we believe that the concept, particularly with respect to the potential role of Glu receptor dysfunction, has not been adequately developed. In this article, we present a more fully developed conceptual framework that is empirically derived and that views schizophrenia as a complex multinetwork disturbance in which hypofunction of a specific subtype of Glu receptor, the *N*-methyl-D-aspartate (NMDA) receptor, may play a particularly important role.

NMDA RECEPTOR HYPOFUNCTION HYPOTHESIS

Hypofunction of the Glu transmitter system was first proposed as a causal mechanism in schizophrenia by Kim et al[27] based on their finding of low concentrations of Glu in cerebrospinal fluid samples from schizophrenic patients. Because subsequent attempts to confirm this finding were not successful,[28] the Glu hypofunction hypothesis, as originally formulated, did not gain many adherents. However, several

See also pages 1008, 1011, 1015, and 1019

authors[29-34] have generated new versions of the hypothesis based largely on the important discovery by Lodge and colleagues[35,36] that phencyclidine, a psychotomimetic drug known popularly as PCP or angel dust, noncompetitively blocks the ion channel of the NMDA subtype of Glu receptor (**Figure 1**). Recent evidence, reviewed herein, strengthens this hypothesis and justifies viewing NMDA receptor hypofunction (NRH) as a type of transmitter disturbance that, if present in the brain of a schizophrenic patient, could explain the following major features of this disorder: (1) the full range of symptoms (positive, negative, and disorganized) that typify the disorder; (2) onset of symptoms in early adulthood; (3) structural brain changes; and (4) cognitive deterioration.

NRH Is Psychotogenic

The NRH hypothesis, as initially formulated,[29-31] held that since blockade of NMDA receptor function by phencyclidine is associated with schizophrenia-like psychotic symptoms, NRH per se may be psychotogenic and may be viewed as a candidate mechanism to explain schizophrenia. There now is new evidence confirming that NRH per se is psychotogenic. Three competitive NMDA antagonists (CPP, CPP-ene, CGS 19755) that block NMDA receptors by acting at the NMDA (rather than phencyclidine) recognition site (Figure 1) have now been administered to human subjects, and each was found in low dosage to induce a phencyclidine-like psychotic reaction.[37-39] Therefore, the phenomenon known for decades as "PCP psychosis" is not a phencyclidine receptor–specific phenomenon; rather, it is a phenomenon that results from effective blockade of the NMDA receptor–ionophore complex (ie, effective induction of NRH).

Schizophrenomimetic Quality of NRH-Induced Psychosis

Three decades ago, phencyclidine was introduced into clinical medicine as an anesthetic agent, but it was soon withdrawn because it caused a high incidence of psychotic "emergence" reactions. Researchers in this era were impressed by the schizophrenomimetic quality of the psychosis that was induced by phencyclidine in normal subjects; they were also impressed with the ability of phencyclidine to trigger a prolonged recrudescence of the acute psychotic state in stabilized chronic schizophrenic patients.[40-45] During the past 30 years, illicit use of phencyclidine has resulted in countless drug abusers being admitted to psychiatric hospitals with a psychotic illness that is difficult to distinguish from schizophrenia in acute, subacute, or (sometimes) chronic manifestations.[46-48]

Ketamine, a short-acting dissociative anesthetic agent with phencyclidine receptor–binding properties, also produced emergence reactions,[49,50] but it gained acceptance as an anesthetic agent in human medicine because these untoward reactions could be suppressed by benzodiazepines[49,51] or prevented by barbiturates.[52] The psychotic reaction induced by ketamine is similar to that induced by phencyclidine, and most authors agree that these drugs, more faithfully than other psychotomimetic agents, mimic the range of symptoms seen in patients with schizophrenia.[34,48,53-58]

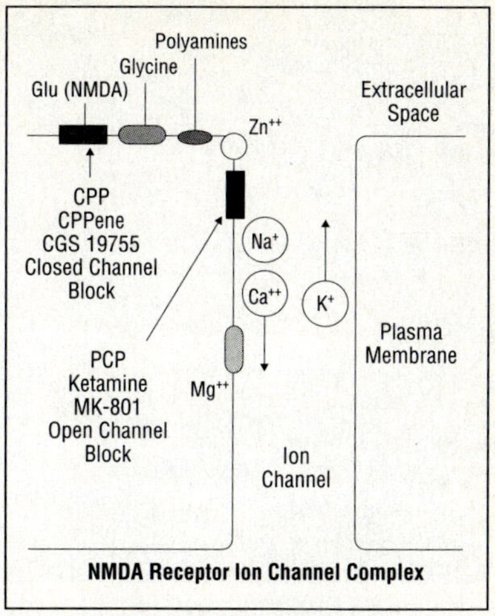

Figure 1. *Associated with the* N*-methyl-*D*-aspartate (NMDA) receptor complex are multiple recognition sites through which receptor channel function is modulated. Currently, it is recognized that NMDA receptor hypofunction (NRH) results in psychosis in humans and cerebrocortical damage in rats regardless of whether the NRH is induced by agents acting at the phencyclidine (PCP) site to perform an open channel block (PCP, ketamine, MK-801) or by agents acting at the NMDA-specific glutamate (Glu) site to perform a closed channel block (CPP, CPPene, CGS 19755).*

NRH Produces Brain Damage

In recent years, it has been shown that various NMDA antagonists, both competitive and noncompetitive, that cause psychotic reactions in humans cause neurodegenerative changes in corticolimbic regions of the rat brain.[59-61] A single low subcutaneous dose acutely injures neurons in the posterior cingulate and retrosplenial (PC/RS) cortex; the injured neurons display a vacuole reaction (**Figure 2**, B) detectable 4 hours after treatment, and this reaction is followed by an abnormal expression of 72-kd heat shock protein that is most conspicuous 24 hours after treatment (Figure 2, C) but remains detectable for up to 2 weeks.[60,62,63] A higher dose causes an extensive heat shock protein reaction (Figure 2, D to F) that is followed over a 4-day period by a neuron-necrotizing reaction that

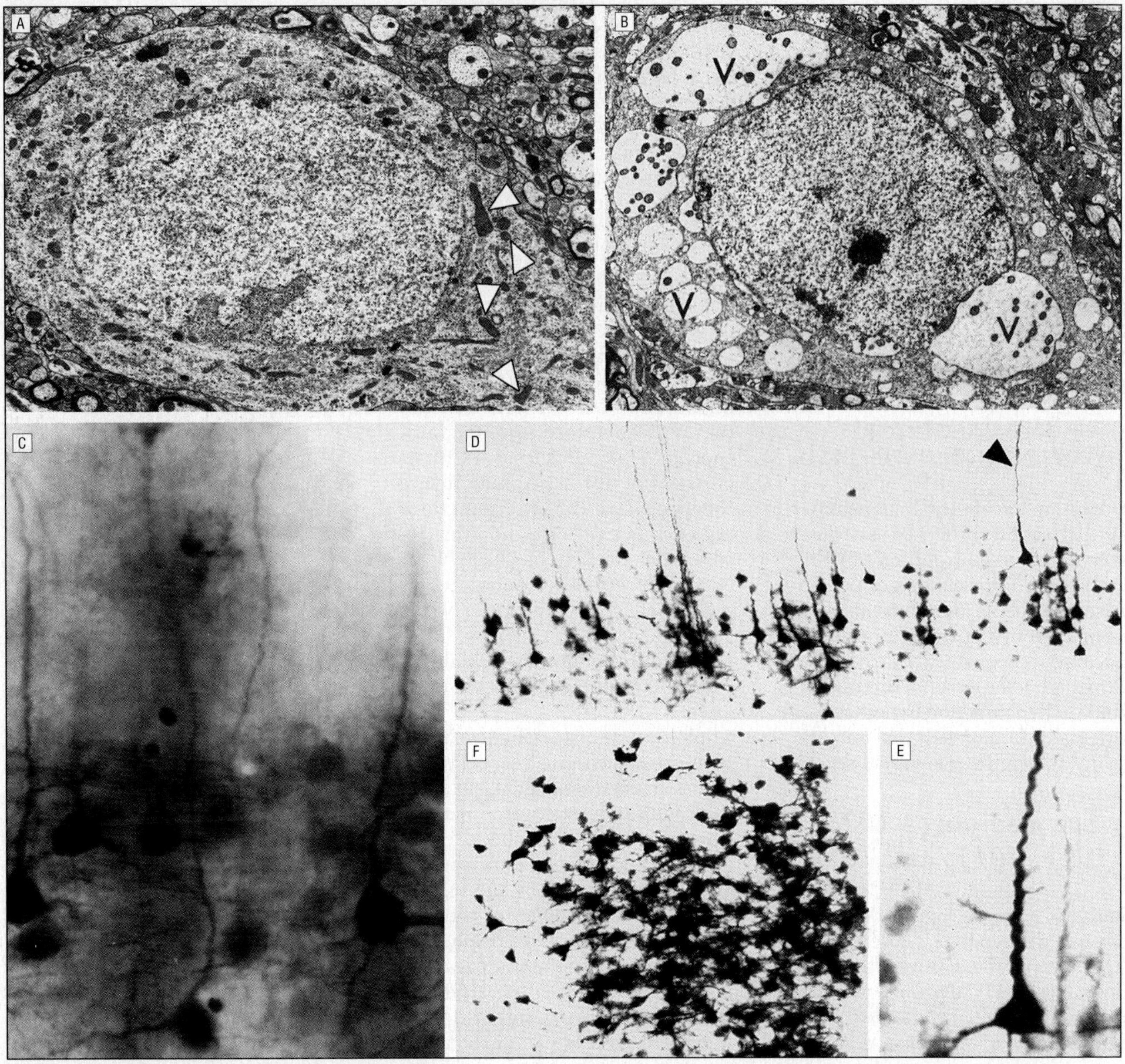

Figure 2. *A, Electron micrograph depicts a pyramidal posterior cingulate cortical neuron from the brain of a normal, untreated rat. The cytoplasm of this neuron contains many normal-appearing mitochondria (arrowheads), and there are no abnormal vacuoles (×7000). B, A pyramidal posterior cingulate cortical neuron from a rat treated subcutaneously with phenyclidine, 5 mg/kg, 4 hours earlier. Few normal mitochondria are evident in the cytoplasm, but many vacuoles (V) are present (×7000). C, Pyramidal neurons in the rat posterior cingulate cortex labeled immunocytochemically by a monoclonal antibody directed against 72-kd heat shock protein (HSP). These neurons show abnormal expression of HSP as a sign of injury 24 hours after intraperitoneal injection of MK-801, 0.5 mg/kg (×360). D, Pyramidal neurons in the rat parietal cortex show abnormal expression of HSP 24 hours after intraperitoneal injection of phencyclidine, 50 mg/kg (×150). E, A magnified view of an injured neuron (see arrowhead in D) shows a corkscrew appearance of the apical dendrite, suggesting cytoskeletal changes associated with the injurious process (×340). F, A large cluster of injured neurons in the rat amygdala showing abnormal expression of HSP 24 hours after intraperitoneal injection of phencyclidine, 50 mg/kg (×150).*

spreads beyond the PC/RS cortex to involve neurons in several additional neocortical and limbic brain regions (**Figure 3**), including the anterior cingulate, parietal, temporal, piriform, and entorhinal cortices, hippocampus, amygdala, and taenia tecta.[64-69] Moreover, repeated treatment with an NMDA antagonist during a 3- to 4-day period induces a pattern of neurodegenerative changes that is distributed over several of the above corticolimbic brain regions.[70-73] These findings signify that persistent suppression of NMDA receptor function (ie, persistent NRH) for only a few days can result in relatively subtle but permanent structural changes that are distributed over the neocortical and limbic brain regions in a pattern roughly similar to the pattern of structural changes that has been reported in schizophrenia.[15]

Pharmacological Manipulation of NRH-Induced Brain Damage

During the past several years, we have intensively studied underlying mechanisms and methods of preventing NRH-induced brain damage. The basic strategy used in most experiments was to administer an NMDA antagonist systemically to adult female rats in a dose sufficient to induce a fully developed acute vacuolar reaction in

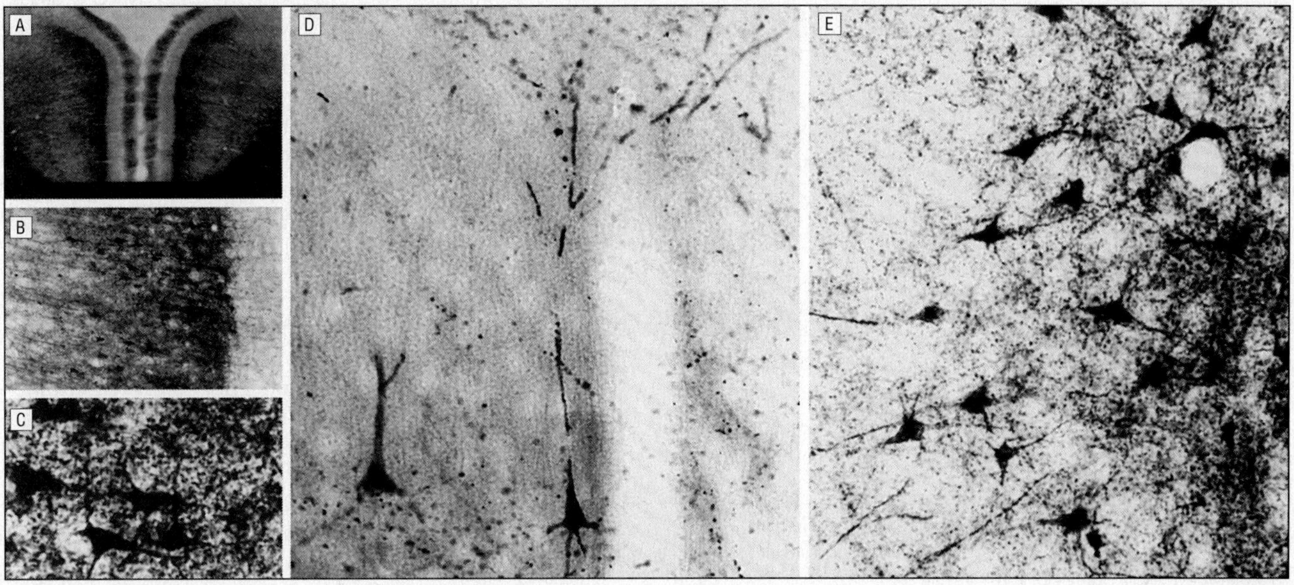

Figure 3. *Scenes from the adult rat brain stained by the de Olmos silver impregnation method to show degenerating neurons 4 days following treatment with an* N*-methyl-*D*-aspartate antagonist. A, Posterior cingulate cortex from a rat treated intraperitoneally with MK-801, 5 mg/kg. Degenerating nerve cell bodies and processes are visible as dark bands in layers III and IV (primarily cell bodies) and layer I (processes) (×40). B and C, Progessively magnified views from layers III and IV (×90 [B], ×200 [C]). D, Pyramidal neurons in the parietal cortex of a rat treated intreperitoneally with phencyclidine, 50 mg/kg. Severe fragmentation of the dendritic arbor in both the apical and basilar fields signifies an advanced stage of irreversible degeneration (×220). E, Multipolar neurons in the amygdala of a rat treated intraperitoneally with phencyclidine, 50 mg/kg. These neurons are in an advanced stage of degeneration, as evidenced by fragmentation of their dendritic processes (×220).*

neurons of the PC/RS cortex, and simultaneously, a neuroactive drug with specificity for a given transmitter system was injected intraperitoneally or directly into certain brain regions in an attempt to block the neurotoxic reaction. In some experiments, we injected various agents directly into the PC/RS cortex in an effort to reproduce the vacuolar reaction by activation of specifically identified proximal mechanisms. Four hours after pharmacological treatment(s), the animals were killed, and the brains were evaluated quantitatively for the number of vacuolated neurons in the PC/RS cortex.

From experiments in which all agents were administered systemically, it was found [60,74-80] that several classes of drugs effectively block the neurotoxic effects of NMDA antagonists in the PC/RS cortex, including (1) muscarinic receptor antagonists; (2) $GABA_A$ (γ-amino-butyric acid) receptor facilitators (benzodiazepines and barbiturates); (3) sigma receptor ligands; (4) non-NMDA Glu receptor antagonists; (5) α_2-adrenergic receptor agonists; (6) certain typical antipsychotic agents (haloperidol, thioridazine, loxapine); and (7) atypical antipsychotic agents (clozapine, fluperlapine, olanzapine).

Evidence from additional experiments, some of which involved intracranial injections,[79,81] suggests that the circuit that mediates the neurotoxic reaction in the PC/RS cortex involves neurons not only in the PC/RS cortex but also in the thalamus, basal forebrain, and brain stem. In addition, it appears that several transmitter pathways must be activated simultaneously for the reaction in the PC/RS cortex to occur. In one set of experiments, this was demonstrated by injecting a muscarinic agonist (carbachol), a sigma agonist ([+]SKF 10,047), and a non-NMDA Glu agonist (kainic acid) into the PC/RS region as single-drug injections or as a combination cocktail. We found that injection of only one or any two of these agents did not reproduce the vacuolar reaction, but injection of all three faithfully did reproduce the full reaction. In another set of experiments, we found that injection of an antagonist of any one of the three receptors (muscarinic, sigma, kainic acid) into the PC/RS cortex of rats treated systematically with the powerful NMDA antagonist, MK-801, prevented the toxic reaction in the PC/RS cortex. These results suggest that the proximal mechanism responsible for this neurotoxic reaction is simultaneous hyperactivation of three receptors on the pyramidal neuron in the PC/RS cortex.

Proposed Circuitry to Explain NRH-Induced Neuronal Injury and Dysfunction

In **Figure 4**,[82-86] we present a circuit diagram that is consistent with our several findings and that can explain NRH-induced neurodegeneration in terms of a complex disinhibition principle. We propose that Glu acting through NMDA receptors on GABAergic and noradrenergic neurons maintains tonic inhibitory control over multiple excitatory pathways that convergently innervate the neurons in the PC/RS cortex. In addition, the PC/RS neuron regulates its own firing rate through a recurrent collateral circuit in which the inhibitory drive is provided by Glu acting at NMDA receptors on GABAergic neurons. The implications of this wiring diagram are that systemic administration of an NMDA antagonist (or NRH produced by any other mechanism) would simultaneously abolish inhibitory control over multiple excitatory inputs to neurons in the PC/RS cortex, while also abolishing the negative feedback mechanism by which the PC/RS neuron normally monitors and restrains its own discharge activity. This would create chaotic disruption among multiple intracellular second-messenger systems and could cause severe derangement of psy-

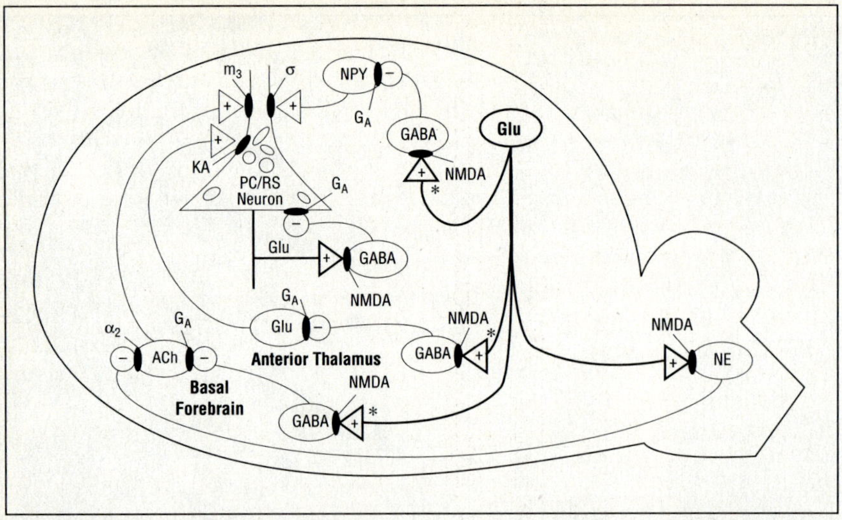

Figure 4. *Proposed circuitry to explain how hypofunction of the* N*-methyl-*D*-aspartate (NMDA) receptor system can induce dysfunction and injury of neurons in the posterior cingulate and retrosplenial (PC/RS) cortex by a disinihibition principle. Glutamate (Glu) acting at NMDA receptors on γ-aminobutyric acid (GABA) and norepinephrine (NE) neurons maintains tonic inhibition over three excitatory inputs (plus signs) to the PC/RS neuron. All three excitatory inputs are subject to disinhibition when NMDA receptors are blocked. In addition, the PC/RS neuron uses Glu as transmitter and gives off a recurrent collateral that terminates at an NMDA receptor on a GABAergic neuron; through this collateral circuit, the PC/RS neuron regulates its own firing. An NMDA antagonist would abolish inhibition in this collateral circuit, thereby removing inhibitory restraint over firing of the PC/RS neuron at the same time that the PC/RS neuron is being hyperstimulated through three disinhibited excitatory pathways. Asterisks indicate the postulated sites where dopamine inputs may presynaptically regulate Glu release. The proposed circuitry is speculative with regard to certain details, but in broad outline and basic concept it is grounded in empirical data generated by the authors[60,74-79,81] and others.[80,82-86] Minus sign indicates inhibitory input; ACh, acetylcholine; NPY, neuropeptide Y; σ, sigma receptor; α_2, α_2 subtype of adrenergic receptor; G_A, $GABA_A$ subtype of GABA receptor; m_3, m_3 subtype of muscarinic cholinergic receptor; KA, kainic acid subtype of Glu receptor; and NMDA, NMDA subtype of Glu receptor.*

chological functions subserved by the afflicted neurons, as well as eventual degeneration of these neurons.

Age Dependency of NRH-Induced Phenomena

Farber and colleagues[87,88] have shown that fetal rats and postnatal rats younger than 1½ months (roughly puberty in the rat) are totally insensitive to the cerebrocortical neurotoxic action of NMDA antagonists. Between puberty (age, 1½ months) and full adulthood (ages, 3 and 4 months), rats gradually become fully sensitive to this toxic mechanism and remain so until at least 10 months of age. Similarly, the incidence of emergence reactions associated with ketamine-induced anesthesia is age-dependent, with the reaction occurring rarely, if ever, in prepubertal children but manifesting in nearly 50% of young to middle-aged adults.[89] For this reason, ketamine is currently used much more frequently in pediatric than adult medicine. Case reports that have indicated a lack of susceptibility of children to the psychotic effects of phencyclidine[90,91] suggest a similar age-dependency profile for this entire class of psychotogenic agents. Thus, rats have a gradual onset of susceptibility to NRH-induced neuronal injury in late adolescence just as humans become susceptible to NRH (ketamine or phencyclidine)-induced psychosis and to the symptomatic expression of schizophrenia in late adolescence.

IMPLICATIONS OF THE NRH MODEL

Implications for the Developmental Hypothesis of Schizophrenia

It logically follows from the above age-dependency information that a lesion that has NRH potential could be present in the developing human brain at birth, and this would not trigger psychopathological or neuropathological processes until late adolescence, at which time it presumably would spontaneously begin to trigger schizophrenia-like psychotic symptoms. An in utero structural lesion that has a latent NRH psychotogenic potential that remains quiescent until late adolescence would be consistent with current speculation[16-21] that in utero structural brain changes occur in schizophrenia and with the fact that psychotic symptoms potentially attributable to such structural changes do not begin to manifest until late adolescence.[22]

The pathogenic potential of NRH is based on a disinhibition principle. If NMDA receptors in certain circuits are hypofunctional, GABAergic inhibitory control over the activity of corticolimbic neurons is impaired. We postulate that these circuits normally mature and form their adult connections in late adolescence. At this time, if either the NMDA receptors or the GABAergic neurons that possess these receptors are missing or are impaired (because of an earlier developmental lesion), the newly formed circuits would be dysfunctional (uninhibited) and would allow unmodulated stimulatory activity to flood corticolimbic brain regions—a process that could produce psychotic symptoms initially and ongoing structural changes eventually if the NRH condition remains severe and unremitting. It is worth emphasizing that the NRH condition might be induced during development by any mechanism that impairs the functional status of NMDA receptors *or that impairs or destroys specific GABAergic neurons through which the function of these receptors is expressed.* In other words, loss of these specific GABAergic neurons would represent an NRH-equivalent condition. Highly relevant to this point is the fact that Benes et al[12] have reported a specific defect in the cerebral cortex of schizophrenic patients, consisting of a loss of GABAergic neurons.

Accumulating evidence suggests that structural changes in cerebrocortical and limbic brain regions constitute a characteristic of schizophrenia; however, opinions vary concerning whether such changes occur during development or in adulthood. The NRH hypothesis holds that both may be the case in that it posits structural changes of two different types: one with latent NRH potential that would occur during development, and another that would occur during adulthood and would represent the delayed pathological expression of the NRH potential of the earlier structural change. This is a compound unifying hypothesis that avoids the either-or impasse and accommodates several lines of evidence and speculation from both the experimental animal and human clinical literature.

There are many possible mechanisms by which NMDA receptor–bearing GABAergic neurons might be destroyed in the developing brain. There is evidence[92-94] that excitotoxic neuronal degeneration in the developing central nervous system is primarily mediated by NMDA receptors and that different groups of NMDA receptor–bearing neurons may be hypervulnerable to excitotoxic degeneration at different times in development (vulnerability of any given neuronal group being based on having NMDA receptors that are at peak sensitivity to excitotoxic stimulation at the time of insult). It is possible that GABAergic neurons that are destined to be innervated by Glu via NMDA receptors in the adult central nervous system may express NMDA receptors in utero that reach peak sensitivity to excitotoxic stimulation at some relatively early (perhaps midtrimester) stage of pregnancy. If so, an excitotoxic insult at this stage of pregnancy might selectively delete NMDA receptor–bearing GABAergic neurons, and this would set the stage for expression of an NRH syndrome in early adulthood. In utero viral infection has been proposed as the basis for schizophrenogenic damage to the developing brain,[20] and Andersson et al[95] have reported that the measles virus induces damage in the mouse brain that can be prevented by NMDA antagonists. Thus, viruses provide an excellent example of agents that are not themselves excitotoxins but that, after infecting the developing brain, can recruit an excitotoxic mechanism to kill NMDA receptor–bearing neurons.

Implications for Structural Changes Reported in Schizophrenia

How does the type of brain damage predicted by the NRH hypothesis compare with histological changes that have been described in the brains of schizophrenic patients? The NRH hypothesis predicts that some schizophrenic patients may be subject to two different brain-damaging processes: one based on an excitotoxic or other mechanism that damages NMDA receptors and/or GABAergic neurons in prenatal life, and one that becomes operative in young adulthood based on a process by which circuits that are subject to NRH incur self-inflicted damage that may be a progressive process causing cognitive deterioration over the years if not effectively arrested. The postulated prenatal lesion affecting GABAergic neurons fits the description of the type of lesion that Benes et al[12] have reported in the cerebral cortex of schizophrenic patients. The distribution of neuronal degeneration induced by NRH in the adult rat brain is roughly similar to the distribution of abnormalities that have been reported in the brains of schizophrenic patients; this distribution includes the cingulate cortex,[96] hippocampus,[7,9,11,14,16,97] parahippocampal gyrus,[8,14] and entorhinal cortex.[10,17]

It has been argued that a relative lack of glial scarring in damaged regions of the schizophrenic brain signifies that the damage occurred prenatally. It is noteworthy that when NRH-induced degeneration of cerebrocortical neurons occurs in the adult rat brain, it is accompanied by a mild microglial and astroglial reaction that is not conspicuous and not persistent for more than a few weeks or months after the neurodegenerative event.[98] If NRH were responsible for neurodegeneration as an ongoing process in schizophrenia, it would perhaps not entail a conspicuous glial reaction, and the residual tissue changes might be interpreted with some ambiguity from one laboratory to another.

Implications for the Gating Hypothesis of Schizophrenia

A long-standing concept in schizophrenia research is that a sensorimotor gating disturbance may underlie psychotic symptom formation. In general, the concept is that an inhibitory filter or gating mechanism is operative in sensorimotor circuits that normally prevents receptive centers from being flooded with unmodulated information. For example, a filter is presumed to be present at the level of the thalamus that gates sensory inputs to the cortex. Recently, Andreasen et al[99] reported neuroimaging evidence of structural changes in the thalamus of schizophrenic patients that might be viewed as morphological evidence for a damaged thalamic filter. The NRH hypothesis is consistent with this concept, but it includes the added complexity that several inputs to the cerebral cortex, only one of which is thalamocortical, simultaneously lose their gating competence (become disinhibited) and flood cortical neurons convergently via multiple-signal transduction pathways with unmodulated stimulatory activity. Moreover, the NRH mechanism is further complicated by failure of recurrent inhibition at the cerebrocortical level.

Implications for the Dopaminergic Hyperactivity Hypothesis of Schizophrenia

Traditionally, the most widely held hypothesis to explain positive schizophrenic symptoms has been the DA hyperactivity hypothesis. The most compelling evidence for the DA hypothesis of schizophrenia is the fact that DA receptor antagonists are at least partially effective in ameliorating positive symptoms in many patients with schizophrenia. Any hypothesis of schizophrenia that does not explain this observation is a weak hypothesis. It is possible to improve the explanatory power of either the DA or Glu hypothesis by incorporating the former into the latter. For example, since one action of DA receptors is to inhibit Glu release,[100-105] a primary defect in the DA system that causes DA hyperactivity could result in excessive suppression of Glu release at NMDA receptors, with consequent hypofunction of the NMDA receptor system (NRH) as the basis for schizophrenic symptoms. Amelioration of schizophrenic symptoms by DA receptor blockers could be explained in terms of the DA receptor blockade disinhibiting Glu release, thereby correcting Glu hypofunction (see Figure 4 for the suggested sites where DA receptor blockers might act to relieve NRH). If the postulated defect in the DA system were congenital or genetic in origin and, therefore, were present from birth, it would not be expected to produce psychotic symptoms until early adulthood since secondary induction of NRH is the mechanism by which DA hyperactivity would produce symptoms and, as discussed above, NRH does not trigger psychotic symptoms until early adulthood.

To explain cases of schizophrenia that are not responsive to DA receptor blockers, we propose that this may represent an etiologically different form of the disease in which NRH is present as a primary pathogenic factor in the absence of a primary disturbance in the DA system. To explain evidence that clozapine blocks NMDA antagonist neurotoxicity and is particularly effective in treating schizophrenic patients who manifest negative symptoms and who are resistant to typical neuroleptic therapy, whereas typical neuroleptic agents are primarily effective in treating positive symptoms, we propose that more than one neural network and more than one type of DA receptor may be involved; however, in all networks, NRH may be an operative mechanism (since phencyclidine and ketamine, which induce NRH, mimic both negative and positive symptoms of schizophrenia).

Implications for Therapeutic Approaches in Schizophrenia

If it can be shown that NRH is an operative mechanism that contributes to all or even some cases of schizophrenia, the pharmacotherapeutic implications are not trivial. A potentially important implication is that if the degree of NRH is severe, early pharmacological intervention and continuous maintenance therapy may be necessary to prevent cognitive deterioration, since permanent brain damage is a potential consequence of persistent NRH. Therefore, it is important to consider whether medications currently being used in treating patients with schizophrenia would be expected to reduce the risk of NRH-induced neurodegeneration and whether research guided by the NRH hypothesis can lead to new and improved treatments for patients with schizophrenia.

Theoretically, in cases of schizophrenia in which NRH occurs secondary to a primary DA hyperactivity defect, typical neuroleptic agents that block DA receptors should correct the NRH and prevent NRH-induced neurodegeneration. On the other hand, it is possible that NRH induces some schizophrenic symptoms through one neural network and other symptoms through another, and structural brain changes might be induced through one or the other, or even through a third and different network. Assuming that multiple relevant networks do exist, and that both dopaminergic and NRH mechanisms are involved in each, it is possible that D_2 receptors modulate only one network, and other DA receptor subtypes modulate the other(s). If so, typical neuroleptic agents that act primarily at D_2 receptors would be effective in preventing structural brain changes only if these changes are induced through the specific network that is modulated by D_2 receptors. In view of evidence that negative symptoms may correlate with structural brain changes and cognitive deterioration,[4,106-109] and the clinical observation that typical neuroleptic agents are only equivocally effective in treating negative symptoms, there is a basis for concern that typical neuroleptic medications may not be useful in reducing the risk of NRH-induced neurodegeneration. Although certain typical neuroleptic agents (haloperidol and thioridazine) block NRH-linked neurodegeneration in the rat, this could be explained by their sigma or muscarinic blocking activity, which might be relatively weak at doses used in human neuroleptic therapy. Thus, at the doses used in treating humans, these drugs may act on a network relevant to positive symptoms but may have little influence on the network(s) relevant to negative symptoms and structural brain damage. While there is evidence[23,24] that early pharmacological intervention results in a more favorable long-term outcome in patients with schizophrenia, it is difficult to sort out the role of typical neuroleptic vs antimuscarinic agents in this long-term outcome (see below).

Clozapine and its analogues olanzapine and fluperlapine are effective in preventing NRH-linked neurodegeneration in rats, and clozapine is effective in treating both negative and positive symptoms in schizophrenic patients, including those who are resistant to treatment with typical neuroleptic agents.[110,111] This suggests that a clozapine-sensitive network may exist through which NRH can induce both negative symptoms and pathomorphological brain changes, and that another network may exist that is sensitive to both atypical and typical neuroleptic agents, through which NRH induces primarily positive symptoms but may not induce brain damage. Further animal research aimed at clarifying the specific circuitry and receptor systems through which clozapine and its analogues act to prevent NRH-linked neurodegeneration may provide clues to the mechanism(s) by which clozapine ameliorates negative symptoms of schizophrenia, and it will be interesting in future clinical research to determine whether clozapine and olanzapine prove to be effective in preventing not only negative symptoms but also structural brain changes and cognitive deterioration.

It would be predicted from the NRH model that Glu agonists might be effective in ameliorating positive or negative symptoms of schizophrenia. Clearly, if a specific defect in NMDA receptor–mediated neurotransmission were identified, therapy aimed at compensating for that specific defect would be indicated. Current efforts to treat schizophrenic patients with glycinergic agents are based on this principle.[32,112] Theoretically, Glu agonists might also be useful for treating patients in whom DA hyperactivity is the basic defect and NRH occurs secondarily because of excessive inhibition of Glu release at certain NMDA receptors. Introduction of a selective agonist that can act at these NMDA receptors would correct the Glu hypofunctional state even though the DA hyperactivity would not be corrected. However, other forms of therapy based on the NRH model should be considered first since these might be less treacherous than using an agonist of Glu receptors that might have excitotoxic side effects in some brain regions, while correcting Glu tone in other regions. Pharmacotherapies aimed at increasing Glu release or inhibiting

Glu uptake would be subject to the same drawback.

The NRH model suggests that activation of GABA receptors may be therapeutic. While a positive response to benzodiazepine treatment has been reported in a few studies that used high doses or that investigated the catatonic subtype of schizophrenia or negative aspects of the illness, most studies have shown little or no value of benzodiazepines over placebo in the treatment of schizophrenia (see Wolkowitz and Pickar[113] and Hollister et al[114] for reviews). These results are perhaps consistent with our finding that diazepam provides only partial protection against NRH-induced neurodegeneration,[60] which in turn is consistent with the knowledge that benzodiazepines do not by themselves open the GABA chloride ion channel. They act only to potentiate the action of GABA, and under NRH conditions, GABAergic neurons are inactivated so that in the synaptic cleft there is little GABA to potentiate. Certain barbiturates (eg, those referred to as anesthetic barbiturates) directly open the GABA chloride ion channel and, therefore, would theoretically be more effective in treating patients with schizophrenia. However, they would probably not be of practical value because at doses required to open the GABA chloride ion channel, they are sedative hypnotic agents.

According to the NRH model, antimuscarinic agents might be therapeutically beneficial in treating patients with schizophrenia. Some students of schizophrenia have maintained that cholinergic dysfunction plays an important role in the disease[115,116]; more specifically, it has been maintained that negative schizophrenic symptoms are caused by excessive muscarinic activity. It has been reported that antimuscarinic drugs relieve negative symptoms and increase sociability,[117,118] and that schizophrenic patients have a strong tendency to abuse antimuscarinic drugs in a quest for self-relief from negative symptoms.[119,120] If, as posited above, there is a network through which NRH induces negative symptoms and structural brain changes, several classes of drugs that block NRH-linked neurodegeneration in the rat (eg, muscarinic antagonists, sigma antagonists, α_2-adrenergic agonists, and non–NMDA Glu antagonists) might be expected to block negative symptoms, structural brain changes, and cognitive deterioration in patients with schizophrenia. We are not aware of any appropriately designed studies aimed at determining whether any of these classes of drugs, if administered in appropriate dosage at the onset of schizophrenia and continuously thereafter, would prevent negative symptoms, structural brain changes, and cognitive deterioration. Antimuscarinic agents have been used extensively in treating patients with schizophrenia, but not in the absence of neuroleptic agents. Therefore, it is reasonable to propose that the ability of early pharmacological intervention to improve the long-term outcome in patients with schizophrenia[23,24] might be explained by the fact that antimuscarinic agents were undoubtedly included in the treatment regimen of these studies. It is also reasonable to propose that the powerful antimuscarinic action of clozapine might contribute not only to its lack of extrapyramidal side effects but also to its efficacy in blocking negative symptoms; if future research reveals that clozapine prevents not only negative symptoms but also structural brain changes and cognitive deterioration, its antimuscarinic action would be a prime candidate to help explain these therapeutic benefits.

CONCLUSIONS

In this article, we have advanced a unified hypothesis that pertains to the combined dysfunction of DA and NMDA Glu receptors and that highlights NRH as a key mechanism that can help explain several fundamental features of schizophrenia. The hypothesis derives credibility from evidence that drug-induced NRH triggers schizophrenia-like psychotic reactions in adult humans and neuronal degeneration in several cerebrocortical and limbic brain regions in adult rats. We postulate that NRH might be induced in early human ontogenesis—perhaps by an excitotoxic event; once induced, it becomes a permanent condition in the brain that can serve as a latent mechanism that can become active and spontaneously trigger psychotic symptoms and neurodegenerative changes. However, the postulated NRH condition cannot trigger neuropsychopathological effects until early adulthood in view of recent evidence that, until early adulthood, the brain is not sensitive to the mechanism by which NRH induces neuropsychopathological effects. The NRH hypothesis of schizophrenia is easily integrated with the DA hypothesis in that a primary disturbance early in life that causes hyperactivity of the DA system is one possible mechanism by which NRH might occur. Schizophrenia that is caused by this mechanism would have age of onset in early adulthood and would be responsive to neuroleptic (DA antagonist) therapy, whereas other forms of schizophrenia that involve NRH in the absence of DA hyperactivity would have the same symptomatic manifestations and the same age of onset but would be resistant to typical neuroleptic therapy. We conclude that the explanatory power of the DA hypothesis of schizophrenia is markedly enhanced by factoring the NRH concept into the equation.

Accepted for publication April 20, 1995.

This work was supported in part by grants DA 06454, DA 05072, DA 07261, and AG 05681, by Research Scientist Award MH 33894 (Dr Olney) and by Scientist Development Award DA00290 (Dr Farber) from the National Institutes of Health, Bethesda, Md; by an Established Investigator Award (Dr Olney) from the National Alliance for Research on Schizophrenia and Depression (NARSAD), Chicago, Ill; by a research award (Dr Farber) from the Schizophrenia Research Program of the Scottish Rite Benevolent Foundation, New Haven, Conn; and by a training grant from the National Institute of Drug Abuse, Bethesda, Md.

Reprint requests to Department of Psychiatry, Washington University School of Medicine, 4940 Children's Pl, St Louis, MO 63110 (Dr Olney).

REFERENCES

1. Kendler KS, Diehl SR. The genetics of schizophrenia: a current genetic-epidemiologic perspective. *Schizophr Bull.* 1993;19:261-285.
2. Stabenau JR, Pollin W. Heredity and environment in schizophrenia, revisited: the contribution of twin and high-risk studies. *J Nerv Ment Dis.* 1993;181:290-297.
3. Stevens JR. An anatomy of schizophrenia? *Arch Gen Psychiatry.* 1973;29:177-189.
4. Johnstone EC, Crow TJ, Frith CD, Husband J,

Kreel L. Cerebral ventricular size and cognitive impairment in chronic schizophrenia. *Lancet.* 1976;2:924-926.
5. Weinberger DR, Torrey EF, Neophytides AN, Wyatt RJ. Lateral cerebral ventricular enlargement in chronic schizophrenia. *Arch Gen Psychiatry.* 1979;36:735-739.
6. Scheibel AB, Kovelman JA. Disorientation of the hippocampal pyramidal cell and its processes in the schizophrenic patient. *Biol Psychiatry.* 1981;16:101-102.
7. Bogerts B, Meertz E, Schonfeldt-Bausch R. Basal ganglia and limbic system pathology in schizophrenia: a morphometric study of brain volume and shrinkage. *Arch Gen Psychiatry.* 1985; 42:784-791.
8. Brown R, Colter N, Corsellis JAN, Crow TJ, Frith CD, Jagoe R, Johnstone EC, Marsh L. Postmortem evidence for structural brain changes in schizophrenia: differences in brain weight, temporal horn area and parahippocampal gyrus width as compared with affective disorder. *Arch Gen Psychiatry.* 1986;43:36-42.
9. Falkai P, Bogerts B. Cell loss in the hippocampus of schizophrenics. *Eur Arch Psychiatry Neurol Sci.* 1986;236:154-161.
10. Falkai P, Bogerts B, Rozumek M. Limbic pathology in schizophrenia: the entorhinal region—a morphometric study. *Biol Psychiatry.* 1988;24:515-521.
11. Jeste D, Lohr JB. Hippocampal pathologic findings in schizophrenia. *Arch Gen Psychiatry.* 1989; 46:1019-1024.
12. Benes FM, McSparren J, San-Giovanni JP, Vincent SL. Deficits in small interneurons in cingulate cortex of schizophrenic and schizoaffective patients. *Arch Gen Psychiatry.* 1991;48: 996-1001.
13. Stevens JR. Abnormal reinnervation as a basis for schizophrenia: a hypothesis. *Arch Gen Psychiatry.* 1992;49:238-243.
14. Shenton ME, Kikinis R, Jolesz FA, Pollak, SD, LeMay M, Wible CG, Hokama H, Martin J, Metcalf D, Coleman M, McCarley RW. Abnormalities of the left temporal lobe and thought disorder in schizophrenia: a quantitative magnetic resonance imaging study. *N Engl J Med.* 1992;327:604-612.
15. Bogerts B. Recent advances in the neuropathology of schizophrenia. *Schizophr Bull.* 1993; 19:431-445.
16. Kovelman JA, Scheibel AB. A neurohistological correlate of schizophrenia. *Biol Psychiatry.* 1984;191:1601-1621.
17. Jakob H, Beckman H. Prenatal developmental disturbances in the limbic allocortex in schizophrenics. *J Neural Transm.* 1986;65:303-326.
18. Murray RM, Lewis SW. Is schizophrenia a neurodevelopmental disorder? *BMJ.* 1987;95:681-682.
19. Weinberger DR. Implications of normal brain development for the pathogenesis of schizophrenia. *Arch Gen Psychiatry.* 1987;44:660-669.
20. Mednick SA, Machon RA, Huttunen MO, Bonett D. Adult schizophrenia following prenatal exposure to an influenza epidemic. *Arch Gen Psychiatry.* 1988;45:189-192.
21. Benes FM. Myelination of cortical-hippocampal relays during late adolescence. *Schizophr Bull.* 1989;15:585-593.
22. DeLisi LE. The significance of age of onset for schizophrenia. *Schizophr Bull.* 1992;18:209-215.
23. Wyatt RJ. Neuroleptics and the natural course of schizophrenia. *Schizophr Bull.* 1991;17:325-351.
24. Loebel AD, Lieberman JA, Alvir JM, Mayerhoff DI, Geisler SH, Szymanski SR. Duration of psychosis and outcome in first-episode schizophrenia. *Am J Psychiatry.* 1992;149: 1183-1188.
25. Carlsson A. Antipsychotic drugs, neurotransmitters and schizophrenia. *Am J Psychiatry.* 1978;135:165-173.
26. Carlsson A. The current status of the dopamine hypothesis of schizophrenia. *Neuropsychopharmacology.* 1988;1:179-186.
27. Kim JS, Kornhuber HH, Schmid-Burgk W, Holzmuller B. Low cerebrospinal fluid glutamate in schizophrenia patients and a new hypothesis on schizophrenia. *Neurosci Lett.* 1980; 20:379-382.
28. Perry TL. Normal cerebrospinal fluid and brain glutamate levels in schizophrenia do not support the hypothesis of glutamatergic neuronal dysfunction. *Neurosci Lett.* 1982;28:81-85.
29. Olney JW. Endogenous excitotoxins and neuropathological disorders. In: Lodge D, ed. *Excitatory Amino Acids in Health and Disease.* Chichester, England: John Wiley & Sons Ltd; 1988:337-351.
30. Olney JW. Excitatory transmitters and neuropsychiatric disorders. In: Ferrendelli JA, Collins RC, Johnson EM, eds. *Neurobiology of Amino Acids, Peptides, and Trophic Factors.* Boston, Mass: Kluwer Academic Publishers; 1988: 51-61.
31. Olney JW. Excitatory amino acids and neuropsychiatric disorders. *Biol Psychiatry.* 1989;26: 505-525.
32. Deutsch SI, Mastropaolo J, Schwartz BL, Rosse RB, Morihisa JM. A 'glutamatergic hypothesis' of schizophrenia: rationale for pharmacotherapy with glycine. *Clin Neuropharmacol.* 1989; 12:1-13.
33. Carlsson M, Carlsson A. Schizophrenia: a subcortical neurotransmitter imbalance syndrome? *Schizophr Bull.* 1990;16:425-432.
34. Javitt DC, Zukin SR. Recent advances in the phencyclidine model of schizophrenia. *Am J Psychiatry.* 1991;148:1301-1308.
35. Lodge D, Anis NA. Effects of phencyclidine on excitatory amino acid activation of spinal interneurons in the cat. *Eur J Pharmacol.* 1982; 77:203-204.
36. Lodge D, Aram JA, Church J, Davies SN, Martin D, O'Shaughnessy CT, Zeman S. Excitatory amino acids and phencyclidine-like drugs. In: Hicks TP, Lodge D, McLennan H, eds. *Excitatory Amino Acid Transmission.* New York, NY: Alan R Liss Inc; 1987:83-90.
37. Kristensen JD, Svensson B, Gordh T. The NMDA-receptor antagonist CPP abolishes neurogenic 'wind-up pain' after intrathecal administration in humans. *Pain.* 1992;51:249-253.
38. Herrling PL. D-CPPene (SDZ EAA 494), a competitive NMDA antagonist: results from animal models and first results in humans. *Neuropsychopharmacology.* 1994;10(No. 3S):591S.
39. Grotta J. Safety and tolerability of the glutamate antagonist CGS 19755 in acute stroke patients. *Stroke.* 1994;25:255.
40. Luby ED, Cohen BD, Rosenbaum G, Gottlieb JS, Kelley R. Study of a new schizophrenomimetic drug—Sernyl. *Arch Neurol Psychiatry.* 1959;81:363-369.
41. Rosenbaum G, Cohen BD, Luby ED, Gottlieb JS, Yelen D. Comparison of Sernyl with other drugs: simulation of schizophrenic performance with Sernyl, LSD-25, and amobarbital (Amytal), I: attention, motor function, and proprioception. *Arch Gen Psychiatry.* 1959;1: 651-656.
42. Davies BM, Beech HL. The effect of 1-arylcyclohexylamine (Sernyl) on twelve normal volunteers. *J Ment Sci.* 1960;106:912-924.
43. Bakker C, Amini F. Observations on the psychotomimetic effects of Sernyl. *Compr Psychiatry.* 1961;2:269-280.
44. Ban TA, Lohrenz JJ, Lehmann HE. Observations on the action of Sernyl—a new psychotropic drug. *Can Psychiatr Assoc J.* 1961;6: 150-157.
45. Cohen BD, Rosenbaum G, Luby ED, Gottlieb JS. Comparison of phencyclidine hydrochloride (Sernyl) with other drugs: simulation of schizophrenic performance with phencyclidine hydrochloride (Sernyl), lysergic acid diethylamide (LSD-25), and amobarbital (Amytal) sodium, II: symbolic and sequential thinking. *Arch Gen Psychiatry.* 1962;6:395-401.
46. Luisada PV, Brown BL. Clinical management of phencyclidine psychosis. *Clin Toxicol.* 1976;9: 539-545.
47. Allen RM, Young SJ. Phencyclidine-induced psychosis. *Am J Psychiatry.* 1978;135:1081-1084.
48. Erard R, Luisada PV, Peele R. The PCP psychosis: prolonged intoxication or drug-precipitated functional illness? *J Psychedelic Drugs.* 1980;12:235-245.
49. Reich DL, Silvay G. Ketamine: an update on the first twenty years of clinical experience. *Can J Anaesth.* 1989;36:186-197.
50. White PF, Way WL, Trevor AJ. Ketamine—its pharmacology and therapeutic uses. *Anesthesiology.* 1982;56:119-136.
51. Korttila K, Levanen J. Untoward effects of ketamine combined with diazepam for supplementing conduction anaesthesia in young and middle-aged adults. *Acta Anaesthesiol Scand.* 1978;22:640-648.
52. Magbagbeola JAO, Thomas NA. Effect of thiopentone on emergence reactions to ketamine anaesthesia. *Can J Anaesth.* 1974;21:321-324.
53. Luby ED, Gottlieb JS, Cohen BD, Rosenbaum G, Domino EF. Model psychoses and schizophrenia. *Am J Psychiatry.* 1962;119:61-67.
54. Garey RE. PCP (phencyclidine): an update. *J Psychedelic Drugs.* 1979;11:265-275.
55. Domino E, Luby E. Abnormal mental states induced by phencyclidine as a model of schizophrenia. In: Domino E, ed. *PCP (Phencyclidine): Historical and Current Perspectives.* Ann Arbor, Mich: NPP Books; 1981:401-418.
56. Krystal JH, Karper LP, Seibyl JP, Delaney R, Bremner JD, Bowers MB, Charney DS. Dose-related effects of the NMDA antagonist, ketamine, in healthy humans. *Schizophr Res.* 1993; 9:240-241.
57. Krystal JH, Karper LP, Seibyl JP, Freeman GK, Delaney R, Bremner JD, Heninger GR, Bowers MB, Charney DS. Subanesthetic effects of the noncompetitive NMDA antagonist, ketamine, in humans: psychotomimetic, perceptual, cognitive and neuroendocrine responses. *Arch Gen Psychiatry.* 1994;51:199-214.
58. Lahti AC, LaPorte DJ, Mokriski B, Tamminga CA. Effects of the NMDA antagonist ketamine in schizophrenic patients. *Soc Neurosci Abstr.* 1993;19:1351.
59. Olney JW, Labruyere J, Price MT. Pathological changes induced in cerebrocortical neurons by phencyclidine and related drugs. *Science.* 1989; 244:1360-1362.
60. Olney JW, Labruyere J, Wang G, Sesma MA, Wozniak DF, Price MT. NMDA antagonist neurotoxicity: mechanism and protection. *Science.* 1991;254:1515-1518.
61. Hargreaves RJ, Rigby M, Smith D, Hill RG, Iversen LL. Competitive as well as uncompetitive NMDA receptor antagonists affect cortical neuronal morphology and cerebral glucose metabolism. *Neurochem Res.* 1993;18:1263-1269.
62. Sharp FR, Jasper P, Hall J, Noble L, Sagar SM. MK-801 and ketamine induce heat shock protein HSP72 in injured neurons in posterior cingulate and retrosplenial cortex. *Ann Neurol.* 1991; 30:801-809.
63. Sharp FR, Butman M, Aardalen K, Nakki R, Koistinaho J, Massa S, Sagar SM. Phencyclidine induces the HSP70 heat shock gene in injured cortical neurons via multiple receptors: disinhibition as a mechanism of injury. *Soc Neurosci Abstr.* 1993;19:1697.
64. Allen HL, Iversen LL. Phencyclidine, dizocilpine and cerebrocortical neurons. *Science.* 1990; 247:221.
65. Fix AS, Horn JW, Wightman KA, Johnson CA, Long GC, Storts RW, Farber NB, Wozniak DF, Olney JW. Neuronal vacuolization and necrosis induced by the noncompetitive *N*-methyl-D-aspartate (NMDA) antagonist MK(+)801 (dizocilpine maleate): a light and electron microscopic

evaluation of the rat retrosplenial cortex. *Exp Neurol.* 1993;123:204-215.
66. Fix AS, Wozniak DF, Truex LL, McEwen M, Miller JP, Olney JW. Quantitative analysis of factors influencing neuronal necrosis induced by MK-801 in the rat posterior cingulate/retrosplenial cortex. *Brain Res.* In press.
67. Wozniak DF, McEwen M, Sesma MA, Olney JW, Fix AS. MK-801 induces extensive neuronal necrosis in posterior cingulate/retrosplenial cortices. *Soc Neurosci Abstr.* 1993;19:1770.
68. Corso TD, Wozniak DF, Sesma MA, Olney JW. Neuron necrotizing properties of phencyclidine. *Soc Neurosci Abstr.* 1994;20:1531.
69. Sharp FR, Butman M, Koistinaho J, Aardalen K, Nakki R, Massa SM, Swanson RA, Sagar SM. Phencyclidine induction of the *hsp70* stress gene in injured pyramidal neurons is mediated via multiple receptors and voltage gated calcium channels. *Neuroscience.* 1994;62:1079-1092.
70. Corso T, Neafsey EL, Collins M. Ethanol-induced degeneration of dentate gyrus, entorhinal cortex and other olfactory related areas in rat: effects of co-administration of MK-801, DNQX, or nimodipine. *Soc Neurosci Abstr.* 1992; 18:540.
71. Horvath Z, Buzsaki G. MK-801-induced neuronal damage in normal rats. *Soc Neurosci Abstr.* 1993;19:354.
72. Ellison G, Switzer RC. Dissimilar patterns of degeneration in brain following four different addictive stimulants. *Neuroreport.* 1993;5:17-20.
73. Ellison G. Competitive and non-competitive NMDA antagonists induce similar limbic degeneration. *Neuroreport.* 1994;5:2688-2692.
74. Olney JW, Sesma MA, Wozniak DF. Glutamatergic, cholinergic, and GABAergic systems in posterior cingulate cortex: interactions and possible mechanisms of limbic system disease. In: Vogt BA, Gabriel M, eds. *Neurobiology of Cingulate Cortex and Limbic Thalamus.* Boston, Mass: Birkhäuser; 1993:557-580.
75. Olney JW, Farber NB. Efficacy of clozapine compared to other antipsychotics in preventing NMDA antagonist neurotoxicity. *J Clin Psychiatry.* 1994; 55(suppl B):9.
76. Farber NB, Price MT, Labruyere J, Nemnich J, St Peter H, Wozniak DF, Olney JW. Antipsychotic drugs block phencyclidine receptor–mediated neurotoxicity. *Biol Psychiatry.* 1993; 34:119-121.
77. Farber NB, Price MT, Labruyere J, Nemnich J, St Peter H, Olney JW. Protection against NMDA antagonist neurotoxicity by clozapine and related analogs correlates with antipsychotic efficacy. *Soc Neurosci Abstr.* 1993;19:384.
78. Farber NB, Foster J, Olney JW. Clozapine and related analogs block NMDA antagonist neurotoxicity: implications for schizophrenia. *Schizophr Res.* 1995;15:57-58.
79. Farber NB, Foster J, Duhan NL, Olney JW. A_2-Adrenergic agonists prevent MK-801 neurotoxicity. *Neuropsychopharmacology.* 1995;12:347-349.
80. Sharp FR, Butman M, Wang S, Koistinaho J, Graham SH, Sagar SM, Noble L, Berger P, Longo FM. Haloperidol prevents induction of the hsp70 heat shock gene in neurons injured by phencyclidine (PCP), MK-801, and ketamine. *J Neurosci Res.* 1992;33:605-616.
81. Price MT, Farber NB, Labruyere J, Foster J, Olney JW. Tracing the circuitry that mediates NMDA antagonist neurotoxicity. *Soc Neurosci Abstr.* 1994;20:1532.
82. Bolden C, Cusack B, Richelson E. Antagonism by antimuscarinic and neuroleptic compounds at the five cloned human muscarinic cholinergic receptors expressed in Chinese hamster ovary cells. *J Pharmacol Exp Ther.* 1992;260:576-580.
83. Monnet FP, Debonnel G, Junien JL, De Montigny C. *N*-methyl-D-aspartate–induced neuronal activation is selectively modulated by sigma receptors. *Eur J Pharmacol.* 1990;179:441-445.
84. Monnet FP, Debonnel G, De Montigny C. In vivo electrophysiological evidence for a selective modulation on *N*-methyl-D-aspartate–induced neuronal activation in rat CA_3 dorsal hippocampus by *sigma* ligands. *J Pharmacol Exp Ther.* 1992;261:123-130.
85. Gue M, Junien JL, Del Rion C, Bueno L. Neuropeptide Y and sigma ligand (JO 1784) suppress stress-induced colonic motor disturbances in rats through sigma and cholecystokinin receptors. *J Pharmacol Exp Ther.* 1992;261: 850-855.
86. Riviere PJM, Pascaud X, Junien JL, Porreca F. Neuropeptide Y and JO 1784, a selective sigma ligand, alter intestinal ion transport through a common, haloperidol-sensitive site. *Eur J Pharmacol.* 1990;187:557-559.
87. Farber NB, Price MT, Labruyere J, Fuller TA, Olney JW. Age dependency of NMDA antagonist neurotoxicity. *Soc Neurosci Abstr.* 1992; 18:1148.
88. Farber NB, Wozniak DF, Price MT, Labruyere J, Huss J, St Peter H, Olney JW. Age specific neurotoxicity in the rat associated with NMDA receptor blockade: potential relevance to schizophrenia? *Biol Psychiatry.* In press.
89. Marshall BE, Longnecker DE. General anesthetics. In: Goodman LS, Gilman A, Rall TW, Nies AS, Taylor P, eds. *The Pharmacological Basis of Therapeutics.* Elmsford, NY: Pergamon Press Inc; 1990:285-310.
90. Karp HN, Kaufman ND, Anand SK. Phencyclidine poisoning in young children. *J Pediatr.* 1980; 97:1006-1009.
91. Welch MJ, Correa GA. PCP intoxication in young children and infants. *Clin Pediatr (Phila).* 1980; 19:511-514.
92. McDonald JW, Silverstein FS, Johnston MV. Neurotoxicity of *N*-methyl-D-aspartate is markedly enhanced in developing rat central nervous system. *Brain Res.* 1988;459:200-203.
93. Ikonomidou C, Price MT, Mosinger JL, Frierdich G, Labruyere J, Shahid Salles K, Olney JW. Hypobaric-ischemic conditions produce glutamate-like cytopathology in infant rat brain. *J Neurosci.* 1989;9:1693-1700.
94. Ikonomidou C, Mosinger JL, Shahid Salles K, Labruyere J, Olney JW. Sensitivity of the developing rat brain to hypobaric/ischemic damage parallels sensitivity to *N*-methyl-aspartate neurotoxicity. *J Neurosci.* 1989;9:2809-2818.
95. Andersson T, Schwarcz R, Löve A, Kristensson K. Measles virus–induced hippocampal neurodegeneration in the mouse: a novel, subacute model for testing neuroprotective agents. *Neurosci Lett.* 1993;154:109-112.
96. Benes FM, Davidson J, Bird ED. Quantatative cytoarchitectural studies of the cerebral cortex of schizophrenics. *Arch Gen Psychiatry.* 1986; 43:31-35.
97. Bogerts B, Falkai P, Tutsch J. Cell numbers in the pallidum and hippocampus of schizophrenics. In: Shagass C, Josiassen RC, Bridger WH, Weiss KJ, Stoff D, Simpson GM, eds. *Biological Psychiatry.* Amsterdam, the Netherlands: Elsevier Science Publishers; 1986;7:1178-1180.
98. Fix AS, Wightman KA, O'Callaghan JP. Reactive gliosis induced by MK-801 in the rat posterior cingulate/retrosplenial cortex: GFAP evaluation by sandwich ELISA and immunocytochemistry. *Neurotoxicology.* 1995;16:229-239.
99. Andreasen NC, Arndt S, Swayze V, Cizadlo T, Flaum M, O'Leary D, Ehrhardt JC, Yuh WTC. Thalamic abnormalities in schizophrenia visualized through magnetic resonance image averaging. *Science.* 1994;266:294-298.
100. Schwarcz R, Creese I, Coyle JT, Snyder SH. Dopamine receptors localized on cerebral cortical afferents to rat corpus striatum. *Nature.* 1978; 271:766-768.
101. Rowlands GC, Roberts PJ. Activation of dopamine receptors inhibits calcium-dependent glutamate release from cortico-striatal terminals in vitro. *Eur J Pharmacol.* 1980;62:241-247.
102. Kornhuber J, Kornhuber ME. Presynaptic dopaminergic modulation of cortical input to the striatum. *Life Sci.* 1986;39:699-774.
103. Maura G, Giardi A, Raiteri M. Release-regulating D-2 dopamine receptors are located on striatal glutamatergic nerve terminals. *J Pharmacol Exp Ther.* 1988;247:680-684.
104. Maura G, Carbone R, Raiteri M. Aspartate-releasing nerve terminals in rat striatum possess D-2 dopamine receptors mediating inhibition of release. *J Pharmacol Exp Ther.* 1989;251:1142-1146.
105. Maura G, Barzizza A, Lottero P, Raiteri M. The excitatory amino acid–releasing nerve terminals in rat striatum possess D-2 dopamine receptors mediating inhibition of release. *Neurochem Int.* 1990;16(suppl 1):53.
106. Weinberger DR, Bigelow LB, Kleinman JE, Klein ST, Rosenblat JE, Wyatt RJ. Cerebral ventricular enlargement in chronic schizophrenia: an association with poor response to treatment. *Arch Gen Psychiatry.* 1980;37:11-13.
107. Andreasen NC, Olsen SA, Dennert JW, Smith MR. Ventricular enlargement in schizophrenia: relationship to positive and negative symptoms. *Am J Psychiatry.* 1982;139:297-302.
108. Pearlson GD, Garbacz DJ, Breakey WR, Ahn HS, DePaulo JR. Lateral ventricular enlargement associated with persistent unemployment and negative symptoms in both schizophrenia and bipolar disorder. *Psychiatry Res.* 1984;12:1-9.
109. Pogue-Geille MF, Harrow M. Negative symptoms in schizophrenia: their longitudinal course and prognostic importance. *Schizophr Bull.* 1985; 11:427-439.
110. Kane J, Honigfeld G, Singer J, Meltzer H. Clozapine for the treatment-resistant schizophrenic: a double-blind comparison with chlorpromazine. *Arch Gen Psychiatry.* 1988;45:789-796.
111. Meltzer HY. Clozapine: pattern of efficacy in treatment-resistant schizophrenia. In: Meltzer HY, ed. *Novel Antipsychotic Drugs.* New York, NY: Raven Press; 1992:33-46.
112. Javitt DC, Zylberman I, Zukin SR, Heresco-Levy U, Lindenmayer JP. Amelioration of negative symptoms in schizophrenia by glycine. *Am J Psychiatry.* 1994;151:1234-1236.
113. Wolkowitz OM, Pickar D. Benzodiazepines in the treatment of schizophrenia: a review and reappraisal. *Am J Psychiatry.* 1991;148:714-726.
114. Hollister LE, Müller-Oerlinghausen B, Rickels K, Shader RI. Clinical use of benzodiazepines. *J Clin Psychopharmacol.* 1993;13(suppl 1):1S-169S.
115. Tandon R, Greden JF. Cholinergic hyperactivity and negative schizophrenic symptoms. *Arch Gen Psychiatry.* 1989;46:745-753.
116. Tandon R, Shipley JE, Greden JF, Mann NA, Eisner WH, Goodson J. Muscarinic cholinergic hyperactivity in schizophrenia: relationship to positive and negative symptoms. *Schizophr Res.* 1991;4:23-30.
117. Fayen M, Goldman MB, Moulthrop MA, Luchins DJ. Differential memory function with dopaminergic versus anticholinergic treatment of drug-induced extrapyramidal symptoms. *Am J Psychiatry.* 1988;145:483-486.
118. Tandon R, Greden JF, Silk KR. Treatment of negative schizophrenic symptoms with trihexiphenidyl. *J Clin Psychopharmacol.* 1988;8:212-215.
119. Fisch RJ. Trihexiphenidyl abuse: therapeutic implications for negative symptoms of schizophrenia. *Acta Psychiatr Scand.* 1987;75:91-94.
120. Wells BG, Marken PA, Richman LA, Brown CS, Hamann G, Grimmig J. Characterizing anticholinergic abuse in community mental health. *J Clin Psychopharmacol.* 1989;9:431-435.

The NMDA Receptor as a Site for Psychopathology

Primary or Secondary Role?

THE ARTICLE by Olney and Farber[1] elaborates a hypothesis concerning the role of decreased *N*-methyl-D-aspartate (NMDA) receptor function as an etiological factor in schizophrenia. The novel feature of this hypothesis is that the postulated structural lesion, due to attenuated NMDA receptor function, can potentially reconcile the age of onset data[2] with the hypothesis that early neurodevelopmental disturbances underlie schizophrenic symptom production.[3,4] The fact that the psychotic phase of the disorder is usually initially manifest in the early adult years is at variance with the hypothesis that the lesion leading to psychosis may occur as early as the second trimester of pregnancy. A potential solution is suggested through results of animal studies reported by Farber et al,[5] showing that structural damage due to NMDA antagonists such as phencyclidine hydrochloride (PCP) is not found experimentally until after puberty. These results and the psychotomimetic effect of PCP prompted Olney and Farber[1] to put forward the hypothesis that a prenatal injury to the inhibitory inputs controlling excitation of corticolimbic neurons may occur, giving rise to an apparent NMDA receptor inactivation and resulting in postpubertal structural lesions that can manifest as schizophrenic symptoms. This elegant mechanism allows one to explain many aspects of schizophrenia, including the role of dopamine antagonists in treating psychosis and the possibility of cognitive decline in the course of the disease process as elaborated by the authors.[1]

Among the issues that need to be addressed is that of specificity, with regard to both illness and the role of glutamate. Recent exciting and provocative hypotheses have suggested that alcoholism,[6] depression,[7] and now schizophrenia all may have a basis in NMDA receptor dysfunction. This may of course be the case, but it provides some grounds for thought when one considers the leading role of the catecholamines in hypotheses concerning mental disorders at a time when the understanding of these transmitter or modulator systems initially became possible. As fluorescence staining allowed the definition of amine pathways, hypotheses concerning their role in a variety of illnesses sprang up. These have been fruitful and heuristic but have not led to a clear biological understanding of any psychiatric disorder. With the development of receptor assays and molecular cloning techniques, a much clearer picture of excitatory neurotransmission has emerged, and with it, increased interest in glutamate's role in disease.

See also pages 998, 1011, 1015, and 1019

The acidic amino acids glutamate and aspartate are the major transmitters mediating fast excitatory transmission in the central nervous system (CNS). They act through both the opening of specific ion channels and the inositol second messenger system. The action on cation channels appears to be the major route for excitatory transmission throughout the CNS. These systems have been identified in cortex, subcortical circuits, cerebellum, primary sensory afferent projections, and the brain stem.[8] Recent molecular studies have provided a clue as to how such a widely distributed system might achieve some measure of chemical specificity. The glutamate receptor family is extremely complex and heterogeneous. In addition to the two receptor types, ion-gated channels and metabolic, there are multiple differing subunits that confer differing specificity at the receptor level. The ion-gated channels consist of NMDA receptors that interact preferentially with NMDA, kainate receptors that preferentially bind kainate, and AMPA (α amino-3-hydroxy-5-methylisoxazole-4-propionic acid) receptors that preferentially bind AMPA. The receptor that concerns us in this hypothesis is the NMDA receptor, which appears to be the site of action of PCP and MK-801, specific NMDA antagonists binding inside the cation channel in a noncompetitive fashion. That is, they cannot be displaced by glutamate. The psychotomimetic effect of these compounds is the major piece of evidence implicating this receptor in schizophrenia.[9] The NMDA receptor comes in differing configurations consisting of various combinations of subunits. This receptor is normally in the closed configuration with magnesium ions, blocking the cation channel. A partial depolarization releases magnesium ions and allows the flow of calcium ions and sodium ions. The receptor also has a modulatory site that requires an obligatory facilitator in the form of glycine for activation.

A further property of glutamate is the potential for a toxic action on neurons when it is present in high concentrations. This excitotoxic effect has been well documented by Rothman and Olney[10] and has been postulated to play a role in a variety of degenerative conditions, including stroke and ischemic insults. This toxic action is a widespread, nonlocalized reaction mediated, as described by Olney and Farber,[1] by the interaction of several transmitter systems. Thus the glutamate system is seen to be the most widespread excitatory transmitter system in the brain, with different toxic consequences when it is either too active or underactive. It is clear that such a widespread system is probably involved in the mediation of most CNS activity. Given the range of excitatory connections, it is almost certain that any complex behavioral change will involve an alteration in the glutamate system. What needs to be established is specifically where the system is altered and whether the alteration is primary or secondary.

The unique feature in the proposal of Olney and Farber[1] is that they have a mechanism, a primary alteration in inhibitory input occurring prenatally, with which they can explain the age of onset of schizophrenia. This is one of the two critical points supporting their hypothesis. An examination of this issue suggests there are other possibilities that will need to be distinguished. Lipska and Weinberger[11] have presented a model of neonatal excitotoxic damage to the ventral hippocampus, which also demonstrates onset of genetically mediated behavioral alterations post puberty. Feinberg[12] has suggested that psychosis may emerge after puberty due to synaptic reductions that occur at that point in time. Thus, several mechanisms appear capable of beginning with a developmental lesion and only showing psychotic symptoms after puberty. Evidence of an early lesion appears to be getting stronger,[13,14] but there is no clear evidence at present as to the nature of the lesion.

The second central piece of evidence offered by Olney and Farber[1] is the similarity of PCP psychosis to schizophrenia. Phencyclidine clearly produces a psychotic reaction with disorganized thinking,[9] but does it really mimic the chronic negative symptoms such as poverty of speech, anhedonia, and asocial behavior? This is not clear, and it is not clear that the typical PCP reaction has a course consistent with the typical schizophrenic reaction. One of the hallmarks of PCP psychosis is unpredictability and occasional violence.[15] This appears somewhat atypical when looking at typical schizophrenic behavior, although it clearly can occur in selected cases. In addition, evidence that patients with chronic schizophrenia have lesions that continue to develop with cell loss is questionable, and, if this process occurs at all, it is subtle and seen only in a minority of patients.

In looking at a model of psychosis and thinking about issues of specificity, one is forced to consider the question of definition. What is schizophrenia? Is it one illness or a group of disorders? The most compelling argument is that schizophrenia is the name for a collection of diverse etiological diseases[16] that share a variety of symptoms. This is a situation that we clearly see in other CNS disorders, as exemplified by the dementias. Alzheimer's disease, which involves clear phenomenology including cognitive decline, and even has a moderately well-defined neuropathological basis, can be subdivided into several etiologically distinct disorders. Clinically this can be done on the basis of age of onset and genetic analysis, which has defined three chromosomes and at least four sites, all potentially leading to the disease picture identified as Alzheimer's disease. In the case of schizophrenia, this etiological diversity appears a most likely result as well. Although we have no evidence of clear-cut pathology, phenomenologically there are clues that several disorders may be involved. For example, the paranoid forms of the disease, with preserved affect and good medication response, differ from the disorganized chronic forms of the disease, which show affective changes. Late-onset schizophrenia, involving mainly postmenopausal women,[17] is another category that may be a special case. These observations provide suggestive evidence that we are not dealing with a unitary condition. What the current hypothesis is attempting to do is explain all early adult-onset schizophrenic illnesses with a single hypothesis. That may be overextended. A psychosis that appears to be predominantly mediated by the dopamine system, is illustrated by a late-onset paranoid psychosis responsive to dopamine antagonists, and does not lead to altered affect or a downhill course would be a form of illness that might not require the prenatal involvement of the glutamate system. On the other hand, a patient with a chronic illness with disorganized thinking, anhedonia, and poverty of speech could well be addressed by this hypothesis.

Finally, how might we test this hypothesis? First we need evidence of prenatal or developmental problems that could result in hypofunctional NMDA receptor function. There are two possibilities in the literature. First are the findings of Benes et al[18,19] of decreased small neurons utilizing γ-aminobutyric acid (GABA) in specific cortical layers. Second are the findings of Akbarian et al[20] of decreased messenger RNA levels for glutamic acid decarboxylase in prefrontal cortex. These two groups disagree about the loss of cells but agree that GABA function may be impaired in prefrontal cortex. This would be a mechanism consistent with a disordered function involving overstimulation of cortical neurons and leading to subsequent degeneration. This scenario would be expected to lead to altered NMDA receptor levels, and these are beginning to be reported in schizophrenia.[21] We would also expect decreased cell numbers in the cortex, and that was not seen in two recent studies.[22,23]

The implications for psychopharmacological improvements in treating schizophrenia are especially important in suggesting that we consider ways of improving outcome and preventing deterioration. Further work is required in evaluating the effectiveness of early treatment in modifying course. The specific treatment suggestions are interesting in that, in every case, data derived from blocking muscarinic receptors,[24] stimulating GABA receptors with benzodiazepines,[25] and enhancing glutamate transmission with glycine[26] provide suggestions of some effects, but in no case are there powerful effects on the order of those seen with neuroleptics.

In summary, this hypothesis adds to our ways of thinking about the biological basis of postpubertal psychotic disorders. It could well provide both a conceptual framework to test neurodevelopmental causes more closely using animal models and a sharper focus to postmortem studies. Particularly interesting is the documentation of widespread subtle effects in many parts of the CNS due to an initial insult in one brain area. This appears an important reminder that the connectivity of the nervous system may come into play in defining a lesion as well as transmitting information. The work of Olney and coworkers over a 20-year period in defining the toxic capacity of the glutamate sytem is a clear indication of how systematic investigations can lead to informative results in entirely unexpected areas.

Fritz A. Henn, PhD, MD
Department of Psychiatry
Central Institute of Mental Health
J5
Mannheim D-68159
Germany

REFERENCES

1. Olney JW, Farber NB. Glutamate receptor dysfunction and schizophrenia. *Arch Gen Psychiatry.* 1995;52:998-1007.
2. DeLisi LE. The significance of age of onset for schizophrenia. *Schizophr Bull.* 1992;18:209-215.
3. Kovelman JA, Scheibel AB. A neurohistological correlate of schizophrenia. *Biol Psychiatry.* 1984; 191:1601-1621.
4. Jakob H, Beckmann H. Prenatal developmental disturbances in the limbic allocortex in schizophrenia. *J Neural Transm.* 1986;65:303-326.
5. Farber N, Wozniak DF, Price MT, Labruyere J, Huss J, Peter H, Olney JW. Age-specific neurotoxicity in rat associated with NMDA receptor blockade: potential relevance to schizophrenia? *Biol Psychiatry.* In press.
6. Tsai G, Gastfriend DR, Coyle JT. The glutaminergic basis of human alcoholism. *Am J Psychiatry.* 1995;152:332-340.
7. Nowak G, Paul IA, Popik P, Young A, Skolnick O. Ca^{++} antagonists effect an antidepressant-like adaptation of the NMDA receptor complex. *Eur J Pharmacol.* 1993;247:101-102.
8. Cotman CW, Monaghan DT. Chemistry and anatomy of excitatory amino acid systems. In: Meltzer HY, ed. *Psychopharmacology: The Third Generation of Progress.* New York, NY: Raven Press; 1987:197-211.
9. Allen RM, Young SJ. Phencyclidine-induced psychosis. *Am J Psychiatry.* 1978;135:1081-1084.
10. Rothman SM, Olney JW. Excitotoxicity and the NMDA receptor. *Trends Neurosci.* 1987;10:299-302.
11. Lipska B, Weinberger D. Phenotypic variations in responses to neonatal excitotoxic hippocampal damage. *Abstr Am Coll Neuropsychopharmacol.* 1994;178.
12. Feinberg I. Schizophrenia: caused by a fault in programmed synaptic elimination during adolescence? *J Psychiatr Res.* 1982;17:319-334.
13. Walker E, Lewine RJ. Prediction of adult-onset schizophrenia from childhood home movies of the patients. *Am J Psychiatry.* 1990;147:1052-1056.
14. Fish B, Marcus J, Hans SL, Auerbach JG, Perdue S. Infants at risk for schizophrenia: sequelae of a genetic neurointegrative defect: a review and replication analysis of pandysmaturation in the Jerusalem Infant Development Study. *Arch Gen Psychiatry.* 1992;49:221-235.
15. Luisada PV, Brown BL. Clinical management of phencyclidine psychosis. *Clin Toxicol.* 1976;9: 539-545.
16. Carpenter WT, Buchanan RW. Schizophrenia. *N Engl J Med.* 1994;330:681-690.
17. Häfner H, Maurer K, Löffler W, Riecher-Rössler A. The influence of age and sex on the onset and early course of schizophrenia. *Br J Psychiatry.* 1993;162:80-86.
18. Benes FM, Vincent SL, Alsterberg G, Bird ED, SanGiovanni JP. Increased $GABA_A$ receptor binding in superficial layers of cingulate cortex in schizophrenics. *J Neurosci.* 1992;12:924-929.
19. Benes FM, McSparren J, Bird ED, SanGiovanni JP, Vincent SL. Deficits in small interneurons in prefrontal and cingulate cortices of schizophrenic and schizoaffective patients. *Arch Gen Psychiatry.* 1991;48:996-1001.
20. Akbarian S, Kim JJ, Potkin SG, Hagman JO, Tafazzoli A, Bunney WE, Jones EG. Gene expression for glutamic acid decarboxylase is reduced without loss of neurons in prefrontal cortex of schizophrenics. *Arch Gen Psychiatry.* 1995; 52:258-266.
21. Beckwith JP, Stefanis NC, McLaughlin DP, Kerwin RW. The expression of NMDA receptor subunits in schizophrenic post-mortem hippocampus. *Schizophr Res.* 1995;15:54.
22. Selemon LD, Rajkowska G, Goldman-Rakic PS. Cytologic abnormalities in area 9 of the schizophrenic cortex. *Soc Neurosci Abstr.* 1993;19: 200.
23. Pakkenberg B. Total nerve cell number in neocortex in chronic schizophrenics and controls estimated using optical disectors. *Biol Psychiatry.* 1993;34:768-772.
24. Tandon R, Greden JF, Silk KR. Treatment of negative schizophrenic symptoms with trihexyphenidyl. *J Clin Psychopharmacol.* 1988;8:212-215.
25. Wolkowitz OM, Pickar D. Benzodiazepines in the treatment of schizophrenia: a review and reappraisal. *Am J Psychiatry.* 1991;148:714-726.
26. Javitt DC, Zylberman I, Zukin SR, Heresco-Levy U, Lindenmayer JP. Amelioration of negative symptoms in schizophrenia by glycine. *Am J Psychiatry.* 1994;151:1234-1236.

Constraints on Concepts of Pathogenesis

Language and the Speciation Process as the Key to the Etiology of Schizophrenia

OLNEY AND Farber[1] present a "unified hypothesis" based on N-methyl-D-aspartate (NMDA) receptor hypofunction, which they claim accounts for "major clinical and pathophysiological aspects of schizophrenia." Although, as I shall show, there are elements of interest in this hypothesis, it is flawed in that it depends on an erroneous account of etiology, predicts neurological symptoms that are not present in schizophrenia, and is inconsistent with the known epidemiological characteristics of the disease. A comparison of this hypothesis with previous hypotheses of the same type ("neurohumoral" theories) and with two other classes of hypotheses of pathogenesis ("focal damage" and "connectionist" theories) in their ability to explain known drug effects, phenomenological characteristics, brain changes, and epidemiological characteristics, reveals constraints on the type of theory that we may entertain and a pattern of strengths and weaknesses that points the way to a more incisive theory.

See also pages 998, 1008, 1015, and 1019

THE NEED FOR AN EVOLUTIONARY THEORY

The central problem of etiology arises from two epidemiological findings:

1. Relative constancy of incidence across societies was demonstrated in the World Health Organization Ten Country Study[2]: "schizophrenic illnesses are ubiquitous, appear with similar incidence in different cultures, and have clinical features that are more remarkable by their similarity across cultures than by their difference."

In this respect, schizophrenia may differ from other common somatic illnesses, eg, heart disease and diabetes, and therefore may be more intrinsic, ie, genetic, in origin. Perhaps schizophrenia in this sense is inseparable from human populations, ie, "a disease of humanity."

2. Onsets occur throughout the reproductive, ie, the most healthy, phase of life,[3] a fact that acquires particular significance in view of the associated biological disadvantage, ie, decrease in fecundity.[4,5]

These facts require an evolutionary theory of etiology, an explanation of why the predisposing genes are not selected out of the population, and a concordant theory of pathogenesis.

THEORIES OF PATHOGENESIS

Neurohumoral Theories and Psychotomimesis

Neurohumoral theories (**Table**, columns 2 through 5),[6-9] popular since the discovery of hallucinogenic compounds and chlorpromazine, attempt to account for psychotomimesis and the antipsychotic effects of neuroleptic drugs. They have the attraction of explaining the lability (eg, onset and recovery) of what was previously described as a "functional" psychosis in terms of the chemical physiology of the nervous system.[10] However, they do not predict the presence of structural brain changes or intellectual impairment, nor do they account for the singularity of the epidemiological characteristics.

Olney and Farber[1] argue that the NMDA receptor theory is particularly good at explaining the psychotic manifestations of schizophrenia, but it is not clear that it is better in this respect than models based on the psychoses related to the amphetamines, which clearly can induce nuclear symptoms, or LSD, which (although variably) provokes a range of symptoms sometimes seen in schizophrenic illnesses. On present evidence, the theory appears less good at explaining the antipsychotic effects of neuroleptic drugs than the dopamine hypothesis.[7] Olney and Farber claim that NMDA receptor–mediated damage could account for intellectual impairment and deterioration, but this claim reveals a difficulty for their theory. Why should not NMDA receptors throughout the nervous system be affected, and patients present with symptoms attributable to cerebellum and spinal cord as well as cerebral damage?

Focal Damage and Exogenous Pathogens

The most serious weakness of neurohumoral theories is in the relationship between pathogenesis and etiology. What could cause a selective deviation of neurotransmission? Olney and Farber postulate "in utero excitotoxic events and viral infections," but the evidence that they cite for the latter is fraught with inconsistencies and contradictions,[11] and, insofar as it is supposed that either factor represents an exogenous influence, this appears implausible in terms of the known epidemiological characteristics. What exogenous toxin or virus could be exerting a uniformly deleterious effect on

Theories of Pathogenesis of Schizophrenia*

	Neurohumoral				
	5-HT	DA	NA	NMDA	Focal Damage
Exemplars	Woolley and Shaw[6]	Randrup and Munkvad[7]	Stein and Wise[8]	Olney and Farber[1] and Carlsson and Carlsson[9]	Torrey and Peterson,[12] Mednick et al,[13] Murray et al,[14] Hillbom,[15] Dohan,[16] Crow[17]
Putative causative agent	Toxins?				Viruses, trauma, toxins
					Explanatory
Neuropharmacologic characteristics					
Psychotomimesis	+	+	0	+	0
Antipsychotic effect	0	+	0	?	0
Selectivity to higher functions	0	0	0	0	0
Psychopathologic characteristics					
Positive	+	+	0	+	?
Negative	0	?	++	?	?
Thought disorder	?	?	0	?	0
Affective change	Depression?	Elation?	Depression?	?	0
Brain changes					
Ventricular enlargement	0	0	0	0	+
Decreased cortical mass	0	0	0	0	?
Loss of asymmetry	0	0	0	0	0
Epidemiologic characteristics					
Universal distribution	0	0	0	0	0
Age of onset	0	0	0	0	??
Sex difference	0	0	0	0	0
Episodicity	0	0	0	0	0
Population dynamics					
Persistence	0	0	0	0	0
Origins of genetic diversity	0	0	0	0	0

*5-HT indicates 5-hydroxytryptamine; DA, dopamine; NA, noradrenaline; NMDA, N-methyl-D-aspartate; HMAC, heteromodal association cortex; DLPFC, dorsolateral prefrontal cortex; +, explains; 0, does not explain; ?, possibly explains; ++, explains well; and ??, doubtfully explains.

pregnancies across the world? Similar objections apply to the second class of theories (Table, column 6)[12-17]: these postulate some form of focal damage to the nervous system, although not necessarily before birth. Such theories are as dependent on, and have invoked a wider range of, hypothetical environmental pathogens, but are less specific than neurohumoral theories about the mechanism of their effect. Their empirical support is weakened by failure to find evidence of gliosis in postmortem studies[18] or of focal impairments in cognitive investigations.[19] These theories account only arbitrarily for the pattern of symptoms, and although it appears that onset in adult life might be explained by an exogenous insult, this interpretation is undermined by evidence from affected sibling pairs.[20]

Connectionist Theories and the Nature of the Symptoms

While neither neurohumoral deviation nor focal damage is able to account readily for the relative selectivity of the impairments to higher aspects of nervous system function, theories that invoke dysfunction in specific sets of cortical connections (defined in terms of either anatomical[21-27] [Table, columns 7 through 10] or physiological[28-33] [Table, columns 11 through 13] functions) do somewhat better. Thus, negative symptoms are plausibly accounted for by a disturbance of dorsolateral[27] or orbital[29] prefrontal cortex, or of cortical projections to the amygdala,[29] and some positive symptoms (including thought disorder) are plausibly accounted for by deviations in language-related areas (eg, asymmetrically distributed or connected systems).[21-23,26,34] The general notion[21,25,35] that it is the structures that are latest evolved and most specific to *Homo sapiens* that are the most vulnerable explains the apparent functional selectivity of the disease process. Since these phylogenetically recent systems are also those that develop latest in an individual organism, the anatomical connectionist theories provide an explanation (although only in general terms) of age of onset and might also be relevant to universal incidence.[2]

Some theories have attempted to account for onset in terms of deviations in specific processes, eg, synaptic pruning,[36] myelination,[27] or random corticocortical interconnection,[37] although why deviations should continue to occur (at constant rates in different populations) is unexplained.

The functions that are most characteristic of primate species are complex social abilities, including facial recognition, and, in man above all, language. These functions have evolved (as in the theory of mind[38] and the concept of Machiavellian intelligence[39]) in the context of the need to negotiate a path to survival and procreation in an environment (both cooperative *and* competitive) increasingly dominated by members of the same species. The notion that these

Connectionist						
Anatomical				Physiological		
Left Brain	Corpus Callosum	HMAC	DLPFC	Facial Recognition	Social Brain	Language Lateralization
Southard,[21] Flor-Henry,[22] McCarley et al[23]	Beaumont and Dimond[24]	Miskolczy[25] and Pearlson et al[26]	Weinberger[27]	Grusser[28]	Brothers[29]	Crow[30-33]
Diverse or unspecified toxins, viruses, or injuries; variant genes?				Unspecified	Unspecified	Variant genes
Power						
0	0	0	0	0	0	0
0	0	0	0	0	0	0
+	+	++	++	+	++	++
+	+	+	0	0	++	+
?	0	?	++	+	++	?
+	?	+	0	0	0	++
0	0	?	+	?	+	?
?	?	?	?	0	0	+
+	+	+	+	0	?	+
+	?	+	0	0	0	+
++	+	++	++	++	++	++
+	+	++	++	++	++	++
??	+	??	??	?	?	+
0	0	0	0	0	0	0
0	0	0	0	0	0	+
0	0	0	0	0	0	Selection for language competence

functions are most vulnerable is a cogent explanation of some features of psychosis,[29,30,40] eg, the Capgras syndrome, morbid jealousy, affective flattening, and social withdrawal.

THE MEANING OF THE STRUCTURAL BRAIN CHANGES

Three anatomical changes are fairly consistently established in the recent literature—a degree of ventricular enlargement,[41] a reduction in cortical or brain mass,[42-44] and loss of or reduction in asymmetry.[34,45] The change in each case is small, and there is substantial overlap with the normal population but no evidence of bimodality within the patient group. It seems that these changes must be related and that schizophrenia in some sense is a disorder of brain size or brain shape. The changes must be, at least in part, developmental, but which type of theory of pathogenesis can account for all three? Neurohumoral theories account for none, and focal damage for no more than ventricular enlargement. Only some version of connectionist theory that includes asymmetrically disposed cortical components appears able to account for all three anatomical changes. Loss of asymmetry and its morphological concomitants is perhaps the most direct pointer we have to the nature of the disease process.[34]

A GENE FOR LANGUAGE UNDER SELECTIVE PRESSURE

Although connectionist theories as a group look more promising as explanations of universal incidence and age of onset, only one theory provides an account of the persistence of schizophrenia in the face of a biological disadvantage, ie, the decrease in fecundity. If the condition is intrinsic, ie, genetic, why is this variation retained in the population? What is the function of the relevant gene or genes? The answer, it seems, is that the gene must be still under selection and that this is apparently so in all human populations. The gene must therefore be relevant to the human condition, and from this deduction the conclusion appears to follow that it is the gene that separates us from the great apes, ie, the gene by which *Homo sapiens* has speciated.[30-33]

Language has evolved by a process of increasing hemispheric specialization,[46,47] and this process, it has been suggested, could have taken place under the influence of a gene that, with persisting interindividual variation, biased one hemisphere to develop along a slightly different trajectory from the other. Annett[46] proposed that the persisting diversity associated with this gene arises from a heterozygote advantage for cognitive ability, and this is supported by data on relative hand skills at age 11 years in a cohort study (T.J.C., L. R. Crow, D. J. Done, PhD, unpublished results, 1995). Although such a simple genetic mechanism cannot account for the genetics of psychosis (eg, the risk to first-degree relatives and rates of concordance in monozygotic twins), there is an a priori case that the variation associated with this determinant of cerebral dominance is relevant to predisposition to psychosis. An association between sex and handedness within families[48] is consistent with the possibility that this gene is in the recently described (and evolutionarily labile) class represented in homologous form on X and Y chromosomes.[49] Such a gene could account for a sexual dimorphism, such as is present with respect to cerebral asymmetry.[31] If there is a mean difference between the two sexes in the relative rates of development of the hemispheres, this might account for the sex difference in age of onset of schizophrenia.

EPISODICITY AND THE NEUROHUMORAL COMPONENT

No theory (including the language/asymmetry hypothesis) explains episodicity. Perhaps this requires the isolation of the gene itself. Connectionist theories, which otherwise provide the best account of selectivity to higher functions, of phenomenological features, and of the singular epidemiological characteristics, cannot explain psychotomimesis or the antipsychotic effect. Perhaps these latter features can be explained on the basis of the assumption that as the result of an aberrant and genetically determined developmental program, some relatively localized imbalance (corticocortical or corticosubcortical) between transmitter systems is revealed, and it is this, rather than a generalized disturbance of a single transmitter system or a primary abnormality at the receptor, that contributes the drug-sensitive component. According to this concept, the selectivity of the disease process is conferred not by an exogenous toxin or virus but by a dyssynchrony in hemispheric development that represents a component of the persisting diversity of *Homo sapiens*.

T. J. Crow, MD
Department of Psychiatry
University of Oxford
Warneford Hospital
Headington
Oxford OX3 7JX, England

REFERENCES

1. Olney JW, Farber NB. Glutamate receptor dysfunction and schizophrenia. *Arch Gen Psychiatry.* 1995;52:998-1007.
2. Jablensky A, Sartorius N, Ernberg G, Anker M, Korten A, Cooper JE, Day R, Bertelsen A. Schizophrenia: manifestations, incidence and course in different cultures: a World Health Organization Ten Country Study. *Psychol Med.* 1992;22 (suppl 20):1-97.
3. Penrose LS. Survey of cases of mental illness. *Eur Arch Psychiatry Clin Neurosci.* 1991;240:315-324.
4. MacSorley K. An investigation into the fertility rates of mentally ill patients. *Ann Hum Genet.* 1964;27:247-256.
5. Haverkamp F, Propping P, Hilger T. Is there an increase in reproductive rates in schizophrenics? I: critical review of the literature. *Arch Psychiatrie Nervenkrankh.* 1982;232:439-450.
6. Woolley DW, Shaw E. A biochemical and pharmacological suggestion about certain mental disorders. *Proc Natl Acad Sci U S A.* 1954;40:228-231.
7. Randrup A, Munkvad I. Stereotyped activities produced by amphetamine in several animal species and man. *Psychopharmacologia.* 1967;11:300-310.
8. Stein L, Wise CD. Possible etiology of schizophrenia: progressive damage to the noradrenergic reward system by 6-hydroxydopamine. *Science.* 1971;171:1032-1036.
9. Carlsson M, Carlsson A. Schizophrenia: a subcortical neurotransmitter imbalance syndrome? *Schizophr Bull.* 1990;16:425-434.
10. Crow TJ. *Disorders of Neurohumoural Transmission.* Orlando, Fla: Academic Press Inc; 1983.
11. Crow TJ. Prenatal exposure to influenza as a cause of schizophrenia: there are inconsistencies and contradictions in the evidence. *Br J Psychiatry.* 1994;164:588-592.
12. Torrey EF, Peterson MR. Slow and latent viruses in schizophrenia. *Lancet.* 1973;2:22-24.
13. Mednick SA, Machon RA, Huttunen MO, Bonett D. Adult schizophrenia following prenatal exposure to an influenza epidemic. *Arch Gen Psychiatry.* 1988;45:189-192.
14. Murray RM, Lewis SW, Reveley AM. Towards an aetiological classification of schizophrenia. *Lancet.* 1985;1:1023-1026.
15. Hillbom E. After-effects of brain injuries. *Acta Psychiatr Scand.* 1960;35(suppl 142):1-195.
16. Dohan FC. Genetic hypothesis of idiopathic schizophrenia: its exorphin connection. *Schizophr Bull.* 1988;14:489-493.
17. Crow TJ. Is schizophrenia an infectious disease? *Lancet.* 1983;1:173-175.
18. Roberts GW, Colter N, Lofthouse R, Johnstone EC, Crow TJ. Is there gliosis in schizophrenia? investigation of the temporal lobe. *Biol Psychiatry.* 1987;22:1459-1468.
19. Blanchard JJ, Neale JM. The neuropsychological signature of schizophrenia: generalized or differential deficit? *Am J Psychiatry.* 1994;151:40-48.
20. Crow TJ, Done DJ. Age of onset of schizophrenia in siblings: a test of the contagion hypothesis. *Psychiatry Res.* 1986;18:107-117.
21. Southard EE. On the topographical distribution of cortex lesions and anomalies in dementia praecox, with some account of their functional significance. *Am J Insanity.* 1915;71:603-671.
22. Flor-Henry P. *Cerebral Basis of Psychopathology.* Boston, Mass: John Wright–PSG Inc; 1983.
23. McCarley RW, Shenton ME, O'Donnell BF, Faux SF, Kikinis R, Nestor PG, Jolesz FA. Auditory P300 abnormalities and left posterior superior temporal gyrus volume reduction in schizophrenia. *Arch Gen Psychiatry.* 1993;50:190-197.
24. Beaumont JG, Dimond SJ. Brain disconnection and schizophrenia. *Br J Psychiatry.* 1973;123:661-662.
25. Miskolczy D. Über das anatomische Korrelat der Schizophrenie. *Z Neurol.* 1933;147:509-544.
26. Pearlson GD, Barta PE, Schlaepfer TE, Petty RG, Tien AY, McGilchrist IK. Heteromodal association cortex in schizophrenia: grey matter changes and clinical correlates. *Schizophr Res.* 1995;15:1-2.
27. Weinberger DR. The pathogenesis of schizophrenia: a neurodevelopmental theory. In: Nasrallah HA, Weinberger DR, eds. *Handbook of Schizophrenia, I: The Neurology of Schizophrenia.* Amsterdam, the Netherlands: Elsevier Science Publishers; 1986;1:397-406.
28. Grusser OJ. Impairment of perception and recognition of faces, facial expression and gestures in schizophrenic children and adolescents. In: Eggers C, ed. *Schizophrenia and Youth.* Berlin, Germany: Springer-Verlag; 1991:100-118.
29. Brothers L. The social brain: a project for integrating primate behavior and neurophysiology in a new domain. *Concepts Neurosci.* 1990;15:27-51.
30. Crow TJ. Origins of psychosis and 'The Descent of Man.' *Br J Psychiatry.* 1991;159(suppl 14):76-82.
31. Crow TJ. Sexual selection, Machiavellian intelligence and the origins of psychosis. *Lancet.* 1993;342:594-598.
32. Crow TJ. Origins of psychosis and the evolution of human language and communication. In: Langer S, Mendlewicz J, Racagni J, eds. *New Generation of Antipsychotic Drugs: Novel Mechanisms of Action.* Basel, Switzerland: S Karger AG; 1993:39-61.
33. Crow TJ. A Darwinian approach to the origins of psychosis. *Br J Psychiatry.* 1995;167:12-25.
34. Crow TJ. Temporal lobe asymmetries as the key to the etiology of schizophrenia. *Schizophr Bull.* 1990;16:433-443.
35. Parfitt DN. The neurology of schizophrenia. *J Ment Sci.* 1956;102:671-718.
36. Feinberg I. Schizophrenia: caused by a fault in programmed synaptic elimination during adolescence? *J Psychiatr Res.* 1983;17:319-334.
37. Randall PL. Schizophrenia, abnormal connection, and brain evolution. *Med Hypotheses.* 1983;10:247-280.
38. Leslie AM. Pretense and representation: the origins of 'theory of mind.' *Psychol Rev.* 1987;94:412-426.
39. Byrne R, Whiten A, eds. *Machiavellian Intelligence: Social Expertise and the Evolution of Intellect in Monkeys, Apes and Humans.* Oxford, England: Clarendon Press; 1988.
40. Frith CD. *The Cognitive Neuropsychology of Schizophrenia.* Hillsdale, NJ: Lawrence Erlbaum Associates Inc Publishers; 1992.
41. Daniel DG, Goldberg TE, Gibbons RD, Weinberger DR. Lack of a bimodal distribution of ventricular size in schizophrenia: a Gaussian mixture analysis of 1056 cases and controls. *Biol Psychiatry.* 1991;30:886-903.
42. Bruton CJ, Crow TJ, Frith CD, Johnstone EC, Owens DG, Roberts GW. Schizophrenia and the brain: a prospective clinico-neuropathological study. *Psychol Med.* 1990;20:285-304.
43. Brown R, Colter N, Corsellis JAN, Crow TJ, Frith CD, Jagoe R, Johnstone EC, Marsh L. Post-mortem evidence of structural brain changes in schizophrenia. *Arch Gen Psychiatry.* 1986;43:36-42.
44. Pakkenberg B. Postmortem study of chronic schizophrenic brains. *Br J Psychiatry.* 1987;151:744-752.
45. Crow TJ, Ball J, Bloom SR, Brown R, Bruton CJ, Colter N, Frith CD, Johnstone EC, Owens DG, Roberts GW. Schizophrenia as an anomaly of development of cerebral asymmetry: a postmortem study and a proposal concerning the genetic basis of the disease. *Arch Gen Psychiatry.* 1989;46:1145-1150.
46. Annett M. *Left, Right, Hand and Brain.* Hillsdale, NJ: Lawrence Erlbaum Associates Inc Publishers; 1985.
47. Corballis MC. *The Lopsided Ape: Evolution of the Generative Mind.* New York, NY: Oxford University Press; 1991.
48. Corballis MC, Lee K, McManus IC, Crow TJ. Location of the handedness gene on the X and Y chromosomes. *Neuropsychiatry Genet.* In press.
49. Lambson B, Affara NA, Mitchell M, Ferguson-Smith MA. Evolution of DNA sequence homologies between the sex chromosomes in primate species. *Genomics.* 1992;14:1032-1040.

COMMENTARY

Altered Glutamatergic and GABAergic Mechanisms in the Cingulate Cortex of the Schizophrenic Brain

THE ARTICLE in this issue of the ARCHIVES entitled "Glutamate Receptor Dysfunction and Schizophrenia" by Olney and Farber[1] presents a provocative hypothesis concerning the role of *N*-methyl-D-aspartate (NMDA)–mediated glutamatergic dysfunction in the pathophysiology of schizophrenia. The ideas have evolved out of Dr Olney's studies of phencyclidine (PCP)-induced neurotoxicity in the cingulate and retrosplenial cortices of the rat brain and his subsequent efforts to elucidate the neuropharmacological characteristics of this effect. It is timely that the authors have brought together this body of work and that they have used it to model several key questions concerning schizophrenia. Toward this end, the article focused primarily on animal investigations to support the details of the model circuit they presented in Figure 4. It is noteworthy that other data from postmortem studies can corroborate several aspects of the Olney and Farber model, particularly the central idea that there may be key neuropathological changes in the glutamate and γ-aminobutyric acid (GABA) systems within the cingulate gyrus of schizophrenics,[2-7] where PCP-induced neurotoxicity has been primarily identified.

THE CINGULATE GYRUS AND SCHIZOPHRENIA

At the outset, it is pertinent to ask whether the cingulate gyrus represents a logical region to implicate in the pathophysiology of schizophrenia. Broca[8] was the first to emphasize that this region is a key component of the "great limbic lobe," which includes the parahippocampal gyrus, hippocampal formation, and amygdala. Based in part on the observation that these structures have retained a remarkably similar location and relative size throughout mammalian evolution, Paul MacLean[9] has postulated that the cingulate gyrus may have evolved in relation to the appearance of maternal nurturance, separation behaviors, and play, which are characteristic of mammalian species. Much earlier, however, Papez[10] emphasized that this region may play a fundamental role in the integration of emotion with higher cognitive functions, and a variety of studies now point to the anterior portions of the cingulate gyrus being a pivotal component in a larger corticolimbic system that mediates motivation, selective attention, social interactiveness, and logical processing,[11,12] functions that are centrally disturbed in schizophrenia.[11]

The connections of the anterior cingulate region with subcortical and cortical limbic structures that directly mediate visceral activity, such as the amygdala, septal nuclei, periaqueductal grey matter, lower brain stem, and spinal cord,[13] as well as with associative neocortical regions, such as the prefrontal cortex and inferior parietal lobe,[14] provide the anterior cingulate region with a unique capability to integrate affective experience with cognitive activity. Consistent with this idea, bilateral infarction of the cingulate gyrus is associated with a unique syndrome, called *akinetic mutism*,[12] in which a loss of movement and speech is associated with the simultaneous loss of emotion and motivation.[15] There are also documented cases of cingulate seizures in which changes in facial expression, affective outbursts, and either fixed or intermittent psychoses occur in relation to ictal activity.[16]

Taken together, these various basic and clinical observations suggest that the cingulate gyrus should be considered in the pathophysiology of schizophrenia. It is important to point out, however, that the Olney-Farber model is based on studies conducted in the posterior portion of the cingulate gyrus, where connectivity and functional specialization are quite different from those in the anterior portion of the gyrus. Given the relevance of these findings to schizophrenia, it is pertinent to know whether the PCP-induced changes observed in the posterior cingulate region are also found in the anterior cingulate region.

POSTMORTEM EVIDENCE FOR ALTERATIONS OF CINGULATE CIRCUITRY IN SCHIZOPHRENIA

According to the model of the cingulate gyrus presented by Olney and Farber, NMDA-sensitive glutamate receptors on GABAergic interneurons could be responsible for loss or impairment of inhibitory modulation in the cingulate cortex and other subcortical regions of patients with schizophrenia. Consistent with this, reduction in the density of interneurons[5] and up-regulation of $GABA_A$ receptor binding activity[7] have been

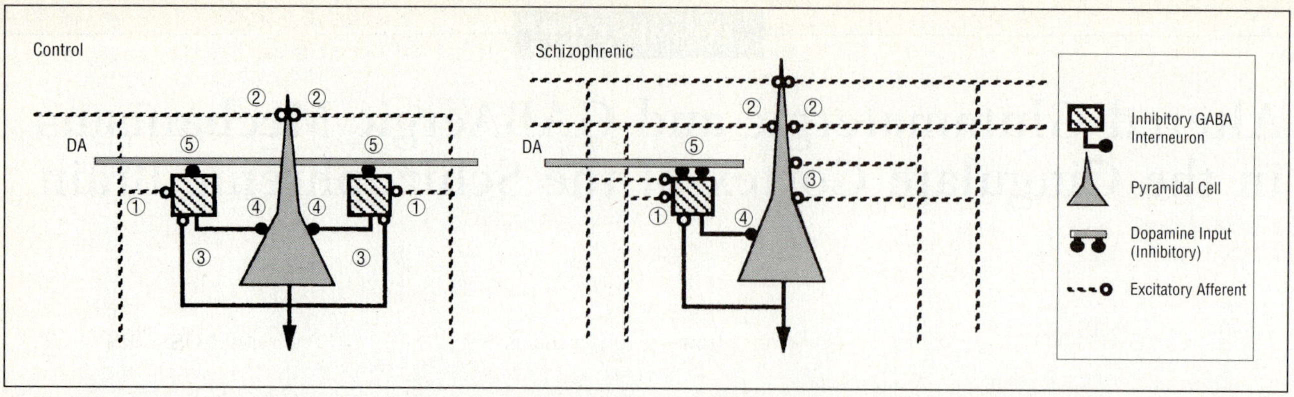

This diagram derived from postmortem studies depicts how the intrinsic circuitry in layer II of the anterior cingulate cortex may be altered in schizophrenia. GABA indicates γ-aminobutyric acid. (1) The schizophrenic circuit shows increased numbers of vertical, glutamatergic axons (see Benes et al[6]), and these give off increased numbers of collateral branches that provide an excitatory input to GABAergic interneurons. (2) Distal portions of the pyramidal cell dendrite in layer I also receive this increased excitatory input from these same vertical fibers. (3) With the increased inflow of activity to the distal portions of apical dendrites of pyramidal neurons, increased outflow of activity from this same pyramidal cell would also feed into the GABAergic cell via a collateral branch. (4) A reduced number of GABAergic cells and/or activity could be excitotoxically induced in the schizophrenic circuit by the convergence of both extrinsic (vertical axon) and intrinsic (pyramidal cell) collateral axons (see Benes[17]). (5) Dopamine (DA) projections to the cortex have been found to form direct appositions with GABAergic cells, and a relative increase in the number of such contacts could arise if there is a loss and/or a decrease in the activity of these GABAergic interneurons (see Benes[11,17]).

demonstrated in the upper cortical laminae of the cingulate region of schizophrenic subjects.

A model developed independently, from postmortem studies of the anterior cingulate region of schizophrenic subjects,[6,7] shows some striking similarities to the model proposed by Olney and Farber (**Figure**), although the model derived from studies of schizophrenics is based on a preponderance of abnormalities noted in layer II of the anterior cingulate region (see Benes[11,17] for a review). According to the model, loss or impairment of GABA cells in layer II may be triggered, at least in part, by excessive glutamatergic inputs that pass through this layer.[4,6] Interestingly, the highest density of NMDA-sensitive glutamate receptors also occurs in the superficial cortical laminae, consistent with the Olney-Farber hypothesis that this receptor subtype may play a role in GABAergic dysfunction within the cingulate area. To date, data concerning glutamate receptor abnormalities in schizophrenia have been confusing and at times contradictory (for a comprehensive review, see Shapiro[18]); however, increases in PCP receptor binding activity have been observed in the cortex[19] and hippocampal formation[20] of schizophrenics.

It is pertinent to ask whether supersensitivity of PCP receptors might contribute to neuronal toxicity in the upper laminae. With the information that is currently available, it is not possible to interpret these findings with respect to the Olney-Farber model, although an increase of PCP binding in schizophrenia is consistent with the possibility of supersensitivity of PCP receptors. It is not possible to say at this time whether such supersensitivity might be associated with loss and/or impairment of GABAergic interneurons, particularly those in layer II.

See also pages 998, 1008, 1011, and 1019

Olney and Farber also postulate that there might be a reduction of GABAergic activity in the anterior nucleus of the thalamus and possibly other subcortical regions projecting to the cingulate cortex. In support of this idea, Gavin Reynolds and colleagues[21] have reported a reduction of GABA uptake in the hippocampus and a smaller, nonsignificant decrease in the amygdala, a region known to send a massive projection to layer II of the cingulate cortex,[13] where, as indicated above, the evidence for loss of GABAergic neurons and/or activity seems quite compelling. Thus, it seems plausible that there is impairment of GABAergic modulation both in the cingulate gyrus and possibly also in other key subcortical regions projecting to it. Accordingly, a subtle decrease of GABAergic activity in the amygdala (or thalamus) would tend to cause an increase of glutamatergic activity, and this in turn could result in increased outflow of excitatory activity from the projection neurons of this region to layer II of the cingulate cortex.

As represented in the model (Figure), at least two studies have now provided anatomic evidence in support of an increase in the density of glutamate-immunoreactive vertical axons that are believed to be excitatory afferent inputs to layers I and II of the cingulate cortex.[4,6] More recently, it has been suggested that these fibers may originate in the basolateral nucleus of the amygdala,[22] where the projection cells show particularly intense immunoreactivity to glutamate,[23] similar to that seen in the vertical axons in layer II of the cingulate region. Although the amygdala is currently believed to be the source of these fibers,[22] the thalamus must still be considered a candidate region, because a reduction of interneurons has been found there as well.[24] This issue is complicated by the complex projections the anterior cingulate region receives from the anterior, dorsomedial, ventral anterior, and reuniens thalamic nuclei and, to a lesser extent, from several other midline thalamic nuclei.[25] In any case, as suggested by the Olney-

Farber model, it is conceivable that increased flow of non–NMDA-mediated glutamatergic activity into the cingulate cortex from either the amygdala or the thalamus could contribute to some of the alterations observed in layer II of the anterior cingulate region.[3-7]

THE DOPAMINE SYSTEM AND ALTERED CINGULATE CIRCUITRY IN SCHIZOPHRENIA

Olney and Farber consider how the dopamine system might interplay with their model; they correctly assert that "Any hypothesis of schizophrenia that does not explain" why "DA [dopamine] receptor antagonists are at least partially effective in ameliorating positive symptoms in many patients with schizophrenia . . . is a weak hypothesis." They propose that the dopaminergic inputs to the cingulate cortex may act to disinhibit pyramidal cell firing in at least some schizophrenics; however, recent evidence has demonstrated that both pyramidal cells and GABAergic interneurons may be subject to nonsynaptic dopaminergic modulation at the level of the cell body.[26] If, as the authors propose, there is loss or impairment of GABAergic interneurons in schizophrenia, a relative hyperdopaminergic state could occur with respect to these cells, even in the absence of any absolute increase in the activity of the dopamine system.[11] A similar model has been independently proposed for the amygdala.[21]

Indeed, apart from increased D_2 receptor binding activity,[27] little evidence exists for a primary defect in the dopamine system of the schizophrenic brain. In support of the idea that the dopamine system modulates GABAergic activity in the cortex, interneurons appear to have D_1 and, in many cases, D_2 receptor binding activity,[28,29] and long-term administration of haloperidol to rats is associated with an increase of GABAergic terminal staining on pyramidal neuron cell bodies.[30] The Olney-Farber model predicts that a neuroleptic-induced increase of GABAergic activity could potentially help to suppress increases of both non–NMDA-mediated excitatory effects originating in the amygdala or thalamus and NMDA-mediated effects originating in the cortex itself.

THE ONSET OF SCHIZOPHRENIA DURING LATE ADOLESCENCE AND EARLY ADULTHOOD

Olney and Farber also tackled the question of how a disorder that is postulated to involve a prenatal or perinatal insult could have a characteristic onset during late adolescence. One of the mechanisms they invoke to explain the age of onset of symptoms in this disorder is the formation of mature connections between glutamatergic and GABAergic neuronal elements. While experimental studies in rodents or primates have not yet defined such late maturational changes between these two cortical transmitter systems, other ontogenetic changes that influence glutamatergic transmission could be relevant to schizophrenia. For example, a late postnatal increase in the myelination of the superior medullary lamina has been noted in the parahippocampal gyrus during the second decade of life.[31,32] Since this lamina probably contains distal portions of the cingulum bundle, an overall increase in the conduction of action potentials from the cingulate gyrus toward the hippocampal formation could play a role in the onset of schizophrenia during late adolescence, although the myelination in this lamina occurs sooner in females and schizophrenia has an earlier onset in males. Even so, changes of this type visible on gross examination are likely accompanied by other, more subtle alterations in the local circuitry of the cingulate cortex and hippocampal formation, and changes of this type could play a more proximate role in the onset of schizophrenia. For example, dopamine projections to the cortex have been reported to increase into the adult period.[33,34] Since dopamine fibers were recently found to interact not only with pyramidal cells[35] but also with GABAergic neurons,[26] and since both cell types seem to have dopamine receptor binding activity,[28,29] it does seems plausible that the onset of symptoms in schizophrenia could be explained by direct or indirect changes in the dopaminergic modulation of an impaired population of GABAergic cells.[16] Though this might seem to contradict some of the assertions put forth by Olney and Farber, such a neurodevelopmental mechanism is nevertheless compatible with the model of schizophrenia they have presented.

CONCLUSIONS

In sum, Olney and Farber have offered a hypothesis of schizophrenia predicated on the idea that there is dysregulation of intrinsic cortical circuitry in the cingulate gyrus of schizophrenics. As discussed above, ample empiric evidence from recent postmortem studies has provided support not only for this idea but also for the possibility that the GABA and glutamate systems may be abnormally integrated within the cingulate gyrus and possibly other regions, such as the hippocampus and amygdala. Though it is not specifically addressed by this model, the dopamine system can be conceived of as contributing not only to the onset of schizophrenia during late adolescence but also to the therapeutic effects of neuroleptic drugs. The model presented by Olney and Farber, while based almost entirely on animal investigations, shows considerable overlap with another model derived primarily from postmortem findings in the cingulate gyrus of schizophrenic subjects.[5-7,12,16] It is both gratifying and reassuring to witness a convergence of evidence from widely divergent studies conducted in rats and in actual schizophrenic subjects. The apparent differences in these two emerging models will undoubtedly prompt more intensive investigations of this problem.

Francine M. Benes, MD, PhD
Laboratory for Structural Neuroscience
McLean Hospital
115 Mill St
Belmont, MA 02178

Dr Benes is supported by grants MH00423, MH42261, and MH31154 from the National Institute of Mental Health, Rockville, Md, and by an award from the Stanley Foundation, Arlington, Va.

REFERENCES

1. Olney JW, Farber NB. Glutamate receptor dysfunction and schizophrenia. *Arch Gen Psychiatry.* 1995;52:998-1007.
2. Benes FM, Davidson J, Bird ED. Quantitative cytoarchitectural studies of cerebral cortex of schizophrenics. *Arch Gen Psychiatry.* 1986;43:31-35.
3. Benes FM, Bird ED. An analysis of the arrangement of neurons in the cingulate cortex of schizophrenic patients. *Arch Gen Psychiatry.* 1987;44:608-616.
4. Benes FM, Majocha R, Bird ED, Marotta CA. Increased vertical axon numbers in cingulate cortex of schizophrenics. *Arch Gen Psychiatry.* 1987;44:1017-1021.
5. Benes FM, McSparren J, Bird ED, SanGiovanni JP, Vincent SL. Deficits in small interneurons in prefrontal and anterior cingulate cortices of schizophrenic and schizoaffective patients. *Arch Gen Psychiatry.* 1991;48:996-1001.
6. Benes FM, Sorensen I, Vincent SL, Bird ED, Sathi M. Increased density of glutamate-immunoreactive vertical processes in superficial laminae in cingulate cortex of schizophrenic brain. *Cereb Cortex.* 1992;2:502-512.
7. Benes FM, Vincent SL, Alsterberg G, Bird ED, SanGiovanni JP. Increased GABA-A receptor binding in superficial layers of cingulate cortex in schizophrenics. *J Neurosci.* 1992;12:924-929.
8. Broca P. Anatomie comparée des circonvolutions cérébrales: le grand lobe limbique et la scissure limbique dans la série des manmiferes. *Rev Anthropol.* 1878;1:385-498.
9. MacLean PD. *The Triune Brain.* New York, NY: Plenum Press; 1990:242-243.
10. Papez JW. A proposed mechanism of emotion. *Arch Neurol Psychiatry.* 1937;38:725-743.
11. Benes FM. Relationship of cingulate cortex to schizophrenia and other psychiatric disorders. In: Vogt BA, Garbiel M, eds. *Neurobiology of Cingulate Cortex and Limbic Thalamus.* Boston, Mass: Birkhauser; 1993:581-605.
12. Devinsky O, Morrell MJ, Vogt BA. Contributions of anterior cingulate cortex to behaviour. *Brain.* 1995;118:279-306.
13. Neafsey EJ, Terreberry RR, Hurley KM, Ruit KG, Frysztak RJ. Anterior cingulate cortex in rodents: connections, visceral control functions and implications for emotion. In: Vogt BA, Gabriel M, eds. *Neurobiology of Cingulate Cortex and Limbic Thalamus.* Boston, Mass: Birkhauser; 1993:206-223.
14. Van Hoesen GW, Morecraft RJ, Vogt BA. Connections of the monkey cingulate cortex. In: Vogt BA, Gabriel M, eds. *Neurobiology of Cingulate Cortex and Limbic Thalamus.* Birkhauser: Boston, Mass; 1993:249-284.
15. Damasio AR, Van Hoesen GW. Emotional disturbances associated with focal lesions of the limbic frontal lobe. In: Heilman KM, Satz P, eds. *Neuropsychology of Human Emotion.* New York, NY: Guilford Press; 1983:85-110.
16. Mazars G. Criteria for identifying cingulate epilepsies. *Epilepsia.* 1970;11:41-47.
17. Benes FM. Is there a neuroanatomic basis for schizophrenia? *Neuroscientist.* 1995;1:112-120.
18. Shapiro RM. Regional neuropathology in schizophrenia: where are we? where are we going? *Schizophr Res.* 1993;10:187-239.
19. Simpson MD, Slater P, Royston MC, Deakin JFW. Alterations in phencyclidine and sigma binding sites in schizophrenic brains. *Schizophr Res.* 1992;6:41-48.
20. Toru M, Watanabe S, Shibuya H, Nishikawa T, Noda K, Mitshushio H, Ichikawa H, Kurumaji A, Takashima M, Mataga N, Ogawa A. Neurotransmitters, receptors and neuropeptides in postmortem brains of chronic schizophrenic patients. *Acta Psychiatr Scand.* 1988;78:121-137.
21. Reynolds GP, Czudek C, Andrews H. Deficit and hemispheric asymmetry of GABA uptake sites in the hippocampus in schizophrenia. *Biol Psychiatry.* 1990;27:1038-1044.
22. Benes FM. The role of glutamate in the pathophysiology of schizophrenia. In: Conti F, Hicks TP, eds. *Excitatory Amino Acids and the Cerebral Cortex.* Cambridge, Mass: MIT Press. In press.
23. MacDonald AJ, Beitz AJ, Larson M, Kuriyama R, Sellitto C, Madl JE. Co-localization of glutamate and tubulin in putative excitatory neurons of the hippocampus and amygdala: an immunohistochemical study using monoclonal antibodies. *Neuroscience.* 1989;30:405-421.
24. Dom R. Neostriatal and thalamic interneurons: their role in the pathophysiology of Huntington's chorea, Parkinson's disease and catatonic schizophrenia. *Acta Psychiatr Scand Suppl.* 1976;265:103-123.
25. Vogt BA, Sikes RW, Vogt LJ. Anterior cingulate cortex and the medial pain system. In: Vogt BA, Gabriel M, eds. *Neurobiology of Cingulate Cortex and Limbic Thalamus.* Boston, Mass: Birkhauser Press; 1993:313-344.
26. Benes FM, Vincent SL, Molloy R. Dopamine-immunoreactive axon varicosities form nonrandom contacts with GABA-immunoreactive neurons in rat medial prefrontal cortex. *Synapse.* 1993;15:285-295.
27. Carlsson A. The current status of the dopamine hypothesis of schizophrenia. *Neuropsychopharmacology.* 1988;1:179-186.
28. Vincent SL, Khan Y, Benes FM. Cellular distribution of dopamine D_1 and D_2 receptors in rat medial prefrontal cortex. *J Neurosci.* 1993;13:2551-2561.
29. Vincent SL, Khan Y, Benes FM. Cellular colocalization of dopamine D_1 and D_2 receptors in rat medial prefrontal cortex. *Synapse.* 1995;19:112-120.
30. Vincent SL, Adamec E, Sorensen I, Benes FM. The effects of chronic haloperidol administration on GABA-immunoreactive axon terminals in rat medial prefrontal cortex. *Synapse.* 1994;17:26-35.
31. Benes FM. Myelination of cortical-hippocampal relays during late adolescence: anatomical correlates to the onset of schizophrenia. *Schizophr Bull.* 1989;15:585-594.
32. Benes FM, Turtle M, Khan Y, Farol P. Myelination of a key relay zone in the hippocampal formation occurs in human brain during childhood, adolescence and adulthood. *Arch Gen Psychiatry.* 1994;51:477-484.
33. Verney C, Berger B, Adrien J, Vigny A, Gay M. Development of the dopaminergic innervation of the rat cerebral cortex: a light microscopic immunocytochemical study using anti–tyrosine hydroxylase antibodies. *Dev Brain Res.* 1982;5:41-52.
34. Kalsbeek A, Voorn P, Buijs RM, Pool CW, Uylings HB. Development of the dopaminergic innervation in the prefrontal cortex of rat. *J Comp Neurol.* 1988;269:58-72.
35. Goldman-Rakic PS, Leranth C, William SM, Mons N, Geffard M. Dopamine synaptic complex with pyramidal neurons in primate cerebral cortex. *Proc Natl Acad Sci U S A.* 1989;86:9015-9019.

Response to Commentaries and to the Challenge of Building a Perfect Theory to Explain Schizophrenia

RESPONSE TO DR BENES' COMMENTARY

When we wrote our original article we felt constrained to limit speculation to a bare minimum. In developing our response to the commentaries of Benes, Henn, and Crow, it became evident that such constraint would be inappropriate. Their insightful, challenging, and sometimes provocative comments, especially those of Dr Crow, inspired us to expand our hypothesis well beyond its empirical base. Accordingly, our response reflects an effort to expand our hypothesis in speculative directions necessary to make it competitive with other theories (reviewed by Crow) dedicated to the worthy but elusive goal of explaining all aspects of schizophrenia.

See also pages 998, 1008, 1011, and 1015

Benes[1] examines potential parallels between the schizophrenia model we have developed based on animal studies[2] and a model she has developed based on postmortem histological examination of the brains of schizophrenic patients. We agree that there are some striking similarities between the two models and, of course, some differences. Both models focus on the cingulate gyrus, but, as Benes points out, her model revolves around the anterior and ours around the posterior division of the cingulate gyrus (which include retrosplenial cortex). Therefore, Benes asks whether phencyclidine (PCP)-induced changes can be found in the anterior as well as the posterior cingulate cortex. The answer is yes, PCP can damage neurons in the anterior as well as posterior cingulate cortex; the parietal, piriform, entorhinal, perirhinal, and insular cortices; and the amygdala, hippocampus, and tenia tecta; but the posterior cingulate is far more sensitive than any of these other regions. However, it is important to distinguish between PCP, a tool, and *N*-methyl-D-aspartate (NMDA) receptor hypofunction (NRH), the mechanism by which the tool exerts its effects. Even though the posterior cingulate is the region in the rat brain most sensitive to damage induced by PCP, the fact that the anterior cingulate and many other corticolimbic brain regions can be damaged when subjected to NRH produced by PCP signifies that NRH is a candidate mechanism for triggering neuronal dysfunction (at a minimum) or neuronal injury and death (at a maximum) in any of these regions. Thus, in schizophrenia, it is possible that NRH is present in specific circuits referable to the anterior cingulate and not the posterior cingulate, or it might be present in circuits referable to both or to any of the brain regions listed above. Since loss of GABAergic neurons in the anterior cingulate would create an NRH equivalent condition in that brain region, Benes' finding of GABAergic neuron loss in the anterior cingulate is entirely consistent with our hypothesis. However, a finding of GABAergic neuron loss in any of a number of other brain regions would also be consistent with our hypothesis. Therefore, we would ask Benes whether a careful search has been made for GABAergic neuron loss in the posterior cingulate or in various other regions where our model would predict that such losses might be found in the schizophrenic brain. If not, we hope that our hypothesis will stimulate an interest in searching meticulously for such losses.

Benes recognizes the potential importance of our model for explaining age at onset in schizophrenia but notes a lack of specific evidence for late maturational changes between glutamate and GABAergic neuronal elements. It would be consistent with our circuit diagram (Figure 4 in our original article[2]) if the late maturational changes occurred between other constituents, for example between GABAergic and cholinergic neurons or between the GABAergic neuron and the cingulate neuron that it regulates by a recurrent inhibitory mechanism. A process such as synaptic pruning, which occurs during adolescence in monkeys,[3] might play a role, ie, a GABAergic system that is already impaired due to a pathological event in utero might be further weakened beyond a critical threshold by the synaptic pruning process.

Returning to the theme that PCP is our tool but NRH is our mechanism, we would like to stress that PCP causes NRH throughout the central nervous system (CNS) and therefore demonstrates the full pattern of dysfunction and damage that can be triggered by the NRH mechanism. However, we do not necessarily propose that in schizophrenia all the NMDA receptors in the CNS are in a hypofunctional state (although this is one possibility). Rather, we favor the proposal that only some portion of the NMDA receptor system is dysfunctional in the brain of a given schizophrenic patient. For example, a pathological event during development may destroy GABAergic neurons or the NMDA receptors on their surface within certain circuits, and this would provide a restricted pathological substrate for triggering psychotic symptoms in adulthood. The psychotic symptoms would result from disinhibition in only the specific circuits damaged during development. Other circuits throughout the CNS would have NMDA receptors and GABAergic neurons that function normally. The severity and qualitative characteristics of the schizophrenic syndrome would depend on how many and which circuits are damaged. In this sense, the hypothesis is very broad and flexible—it can explain various clinical syndromes conventionally subsumed under the heading of the schizophrenias and perhaps various other psychotic states as well. In addition, it is flexible with respect to etiology (**Figure**). Instead of (or in addition to) a pathological event during development, there could be a genetic defect involving a specific subtype of NMDA or GABA receptor that would limit the dysfunction to only those circuits served by the defective receptor subtype.

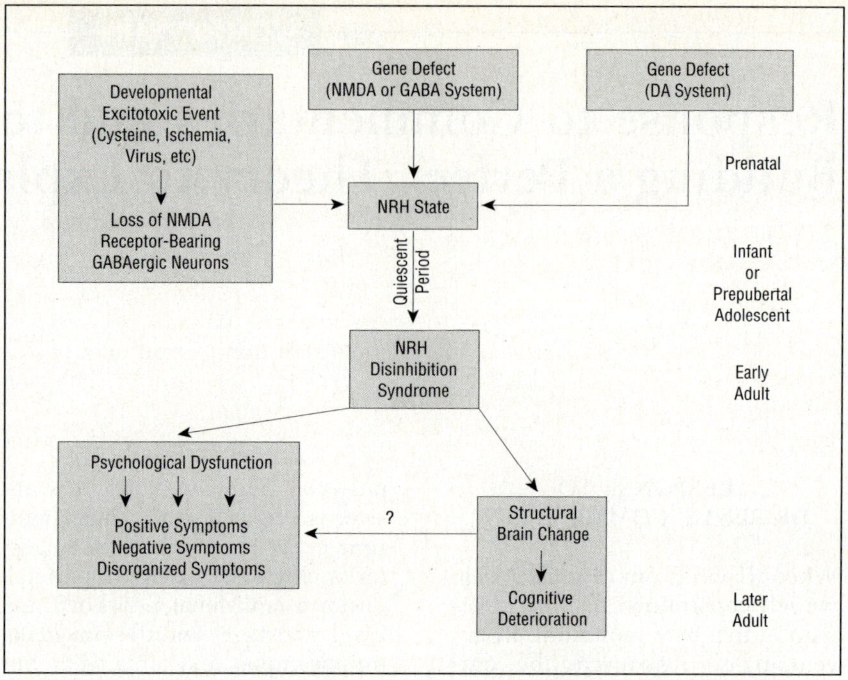

The N-methyl-D-aspartate (NMDA) receptor hypofunction (NRH) hypothesis in expanded form to accommodate genetic and epidemiological features of schizophrenia. A genetic defect involving the dopamine (DA) system is depicted as a separate pathway to emphasize that schizophrenia induced through this pathway would be responsive to typical neuroleptic (dopamine antagonist) therapy, whereas schizophrenia induced through the other genetic pathway would be resistant to such therapy. Cysteine is listed as a potential cause of a developmental excitotoxic event because it is an NMDA receptor–specific excitotoxin to which the fetus is naturally exposed, and it penetrates both placental and blood-brain barriers. In addition to being an environmental excitotoxin, cysteine is synthesized in the body and qualifies as an endogenous pathogen to which the fetal brain might be exposed in abnormal amounts owing to a genetic metabolic defect, as explained in more detail elsewhere.[23] All causal factors have the potential to produce the NRH state. The genetic and environmental factors are not mutually exclusive; they can act independently or in concert to induce the NRH state. Once it is induced, the stage is set for late maturational events to trigger a disinhibition syndrome that potentially can cause both psychological dysfunction and structural brain changes. Multiple arrows in the psychological dysfunction box indicate the possibility that dysfunction in different neural pathways may be responsible for different symptom clusters. GABA indicates γ-aminobutyric acid.

We agree with Benes that dysfunction of circuits subserving the cingulate gyrus is an excellent candidate mechanism for explaining symptoms of schizophrenia, and we think that both the posterior and anterior portions of the cingulate gyrus should be included in the equation. The functional roles of these two cortical areas are different but complementary and reflect a relationship that is seen throughout the CNS in which areas derived from the dorsal part of the neural tube perform "sensory" evaluative functions while ventrally derived areas engage in "motor" output tasks. The posterior cingulate as a "dorsal" sensory area probably combines sensory information from diverse sensory cortical areas with "emotional" information. This compilation is then sent via the cingulum (the projection pathway that links the anterior and posterior cingulate) to the anterior cingulate, where the appropriate motor output (based on emotional considerations) is generated and passed along to other areas.[4,5] Thus, dysfunction of either the anterior or posterior cingulate is a prime candidate to explain the pathophysiological aspects of schizophrenia.

The similarities that Benes finds between her model and ours are perhaps all the more striking when one considers the many potential confounders that render such comparisons difficult. We propose that the pattern of neuronal dysfunction induced by PCP in the rat brain may be analogous to the pattern of neuronal dysfunction occurring in the human brain during PCP intoxication and, because the human manifestations of this dysfunction pattern include schizophrenialike symptoms, the PCP dysfunction pattern in either rat or human brain may have relevance to schizophrenia. However, we do not know whether the dysfunction pattern that PCP induces in the human brain primarily involves the same circuits and neuronal groups as are involved in the rat brain. We consider it likely that in the human brain, as in the rat brain, there are NMDA receptors on GABAergic neurons through which glutamate regulates inhibitory tone, and we propose that dysfunction (disinhibition) of this regulatory mechanism may play an important role in both the psychosis induced by PCP and the psychosis observed in schizophrenia. However, it is possible that owing to differences in the wiring of the rat and human brains, PCP induces a dysfunction pattern that is maximally expressed in the posterior cingulate cortex of rat brain and in some other region (possibly the anterior cingulate cortex) of the human brain. Therefore, it will be important to determine which regions of the human brain are primarily perturbed by PCP, and these are the regions to focus on for correlating the disinhibition type of mechanism we are studying in rat brain with either the human psychosis induced by PCP or the human psychosis observed in schizophrenia.

RESPONSE TO DR HENN'S COMMENTARY

In his introductory paragraph, Henn[6] clearly summarizes the basic thrust and some of the more important implications of our glutamate receptor dysfunction hypothesis. We are heartened that he found substantial strengths and no serious weaknesses in our hypothesis. We will respond to points raised by Henn that can benefit from further discussion.

Henn discusses briefly the paradoxical observation that the NMDA receptor system possesses neurotoxic potential that can be released by either hyperactivation or hypoactivation of this system. This is an important point on which we would like to elaborate. We and many other neuroscientists have intensively studied glutamate as a Jekyll-Hyde molecule that serves many beneficial functions in the CNS but also harbors enormous neurotoxic (excitotoxic) potential that can rapidly destroy CNS neurons. In addition to this conventional view of glutamate as an excitant and excitotoxin, we are now beginning to view glutamate as a master regulator of inhibitory tone in the CNS, and we propose that disruption of this inhibitory tone is a mechanism that mediates the schizophrenia-like psychotic reactions induced by NMDA antagonist drugs and that could also explain idiopathic psychoses such as schizophrenia. Thus, although our NRH hypothesis emphasizes the role of NMDA receptors in schizophrenia, the emphasis could just as well be placed on inhibition failure, because the primary gist of our hypothesis is that the signs and symptoms of schizophrenia are due to impairment of mechanisms by which glutamate (via NMDA receptors on inhibitory neurons) ordinarily holds major excitatory circuits under inhibitory restraint. The general proposal that inhibition failure may be involved in the pathophysiology of schizophrenia is not new; various gating hypotheses rest on this premise. However, identifying the glutamate excitatory system as a major driving force behind CNS inhibition is novel and potentially important for therapeutic purposes in that it invites attention to a number of specific mechanisms by which inhibition failure might occur, eg, (1) by a decreased amount of glutamate being released at NMDA receptors (see "Implications in Relation to the Dopaminergic Hyperactivity Hypothesis of Schizophrenia" in our primary article[2]); (2) by impairment or loss of NMDA receptors; and (3) by impairment or loss of GABAergic (or other) inhibitory neurons driven by NMDA receptors.

Henn questions whether PCP faithfully mimics negative symptoms such as poverty of speech, anhedonia, and asocial behavior, whether the typical PCP reaction has a course consistent with the typical schizophrenic reaction, and whether patients with chronic schizophrenia characteristically have lesions that continue to develop. We think that the similarities between a PCP reaction and schizophrenia are quite striking, bearing in mind that one would not expect an acute drug reaction to perfectly mirror every feature of a chronic disease process. The PCP reaction, as seen in humans, is an acute reaction induced by a single exposure to a drug that induces the NRH state in the brain for a circumscribed period of time. In contrast, we propose that in schizophrenia the NRH state may be maintained persistently at low-grade intensity over a period of weeks, months, or years. We can manipulate the PCP reaction in rats by administering a dose that transiently causes mild behavioral symptoms and no pathomorphological brain changes; one that causes slightly more severe behavioral symptoms and reversible pathomorphological brain changes; or one that causes a profound dissociative anesthetic state for several days, accompanied by irreversible brain damage in several corticolimbic brain regions. This suggests a range of possibilities for schizophrenic patients. If the NRH state is persistent but of mild intensity, it may cause psychotic symptoms without brain damage; if persistent and of greater intensity, it might begin to cause brain damage that might be subtle and result in a change in the symptom complex, perhaps with an increased display of negative symptoms; with greater chronicity and escalating intensity, it might cause a more severe case of structural damage and cognitive deterioration, which we agree is seen only in a minority of patients. However, this raises the interesting question of whether a deteriorative course has always been a rarity among schizophrenic patients or has become a rarity because modern treatment methods are more effective than we realize in modifying the pathological process responsible for progressive deterioration.[7,8] If modern treatment regimens do prevent progressive deterioration, what component of the treatment regimen possesses such magic? Do typical neuroleptics have this capability, or should we begin seriously considering the possibility that anticholinergics, which are routinely administered together with neuroleptics, might have neuroprotective potential (as would be predicted by the NRH hypothesis)?

Henn points out that certain treatment approaches predicted by our hypothesis to be beneficial in schizophrenia have been reported to have some effects, but not on the order of magnitude of those seen with neuroleptics. This is certainly true, but it must be kept in mind that the dramatic effects of typical neuroleptics are effects largely limited to positive symptoms and only to some patients. Our hypothesis is currently in its infancy, and we are not sure how it may have to be modified to maximally accommodate the pathophysiology and treatment of positive symptoms. Eventually, as new information is acquired, we may be able to modify our circuit diagram to include specific pathways that are linked to dopamine mechanisms and relate primarily to positive symptoms, whereas other pathways may prove more relevant to negative symptoms. We propose that the pathways linked to negative symptoms may also prove relevant to cognitive deterioration. Based on this proposal, we would expect that certain drugs, eg, antimuscarinics, if administered from the beginning of the illness and continuously thereafter, might prevent or alleviate negative symptoms and prevent deteriorative changes. Tandon and colleagues[9] have reported that antimuscarinics do alleviate negative symptoms. There are no studies addressing the important question of whether antimuscarinics or other treatments that our hypothesis predicts can be beneficial in schizophrenia would prevent deteriorative changes if treatment were begun early in the illness and were continued on a long-term basis thereafter.

Also, it bears mentioning that atypical antipsychotic drugs, including clozapine and olanzapine, are among the most effective agents we have identified for preventing the neurotoxic effects of NMDA antagonists.[10] Therefore, these agents are at the top of the list of drugs that our hypothesis (developed independently of human clinical research) predicts can be beneficial in schizophrenia. Today we are witnessing a revolutionary period in pharmacotherapy for schizophrenia, in which atypical antipsychotic agents are proving to be more effective than typical neuroleptics, and schizophrenologists have yet to decipher the mechanistic basis for the therapeutic efficacy of these wonder drugs. We expect that by further careful study, we will be able to specify the mechanistic basis for the efficacy of clozapine and olanzapine in preventing the neurotoxic side effects of NMDA antagonists. Whether the results of our analysis will help elucidate the basis for therapeutic efficacy of these agents in schizophrenia remains to be seen.

There are additional subtle points regarding the therapeutic implications of our hypothesis that warrant discussion. In a series of studies aimed at establishing the minimum requirements for inducing brain damage by the NRH mechanism (see "Pharmacological Manipulation of NRH-Induced Brain Damage" in our article[2]), we have learned that it is necessary for at least three transmitter pathways to be disinhibited simultaneously for the brain damage to occur. Therefore, if NRH is present in the brain of a schizophrenic patient but only affects one or two of the three pathways required for producing brain damage, this patient would not be at risk for brain damage. However, we assume that NRH in only one or two pathways may be sufficient to trigger psychotic symptoms. If so, then the amount of brain damage that would have to occur during development to provide the substrate for NRH-induced psychosis in adulthood would be relatively slight, ie, a disinhibition syndrome in just one or two pathways would be sufficient. This analysis has the following interesting implications:

1. It requires a relatively complex developmental lesion to provide the substrate for subsequent onset of a deteriorative schizophrenic syndrome in adulthood, ie, a syndrome that entails ongoing neurodegenerative events in adulthood. Therefore, such a syndrome is likely to be a relatively infrequent occurrence, which signifies that only a small percentage of schizophrenic patients would require continuous long-term treatment to prevent ongoing brain damage and cognitive deterioration. Moreover, the treatment required to prevent ongoing brain damage may be quite simple, in that blockade of only one of the deranged pathways is sufficient. For example, long-term treatment with an antimuscarinic would be a good choice.

2. Therapeutic measures aimed at controlling psychotic symptoms may not be so simple. If psychotic symptoms can be triggered by disinhibition of just one pathway, then finding the right treatment will be more complicated, ie, a given patient may have involvement of just one pathway or two or three, and if it is just one pathway, the clinician does not know which one. If two or three pathways are involved, all two or three must be addressed therapeutically to relieve the disinhibition syndrome.

3. Examination of our circuit diagram (Figure 4 of our article[2]) suggests that it may be possible to treat one deranged pathway at a time, or, if therapy is directed at certain points in the circuitry, it may be possible to treat several pathways at once.

4. Since our circuit diagram at present is in its infancy, it may be possible with further research to specify additional relevant pathways and additional relevant treatment strategies for the control of mechanisms giving rise to either the deteriorative process or the psychotic process in schizophrenia.

We agree with Henn that schizophrenia may be an etiologically heterogeneous condition. Accordingly, our flow diagram (Figure) shows how multiple etiologic factors could act, either alone or in concert, through a final common pathway (NRH-linked disinhibition) and result in various clinical syndromes that have enough similarities to warrant collectively calling them "the schizophrenias." We recognize that the odds are against a single hypothesis explaining all cases of schizophrenia or all forms of psychosis. However, if it turns out that our hypothesis does lead to a better understanding and better treatment for even a single subpopulation of schizophrenic patients, that would represent an important step forward in solving the schizophrenia puzzle.

RESPONSE TO DR CROW'S COMMENTARY

According to Crow,[11] our hypothesis is flawed because it "depends on an erroneous account of etiology, predicts neurological symptoms that are not present in schizophrenia, and is inconsistent with the known epidemiological characteristics of the disease." As a comment on our hypothesis, we find Crow's Commentary flawed because, instead of identifying and evaluating the strengths and weaknesses of our position, he misconstrues our position and describes flaws that pertain to his misconstruance rather than to our position.

In his quest for the perfect theory to explain all aspects of schizophrenia, including etiologic and epidemiologic aspects, Crow patches together a "connectionist, physiologic, variant gene" theory that he judges to be superior to all other hypotheses pertaining to schizophrenia. Our approach is very different from that of Crow in that we have restricted ourselves to an empirical base and have not attempted to explain every feature of schizophrenia. When Crow faults us for giving an "erroneous account of etiology," we are surprised, because we did not think we had given an account of etiology. In our article,[2] we briefly alluded to pathophysiological mechanisms that might give rise to developmental brain changes, but we did not intend this to be taken as our "account" of etiology. However, if challenged to speculate beyond our data, we can expand our hypothesis so that it will qualify as both a neurohumoral and "connectionist physiological" hypothesis and one that assumes that "variant genes" play a prominent etiological role. Indeed, a primary genetic defect altering neurotransmission in the dopamine, NMDA, or GABA system would be at the top of our list for explaining the etiology of schizophrenia (Figure). On the other hand, the substantial rate of discordance for schizophrenia among monozygotic twins suggests the involvement of nongenetic factors to explain some cases of schizophrenia. For this reason, we have suggested that in some cases a pathological event may occur during development, and we consider it likely that an excitotoxic mechanism might underlie the pathological event. Crow erroneously assumes that the pathological event could only be mediated by an environmental toxin or virus and downgrades our hypothesis on the basis of this assumption. He is apparently unaware that glutamate is an *endogenous* agent whose excitotoxic wrath can be unleashed in the fetal brain by circumstances as common as ischemia, and that ischemia can be induced in the fetal brain by a mechanism as simple as transient compression of the umbilical cord. If the perfect theory Crow is seeking requires a toxin that can exert "a uniformly deleterious effect on pregnancies across the world," glutamate is an excellent candidate. Therefore, with regard to either etiology or epidemiology, we believe our hypothesis (Figure) has at least as much explanatory power as Crow's hypothesis, and ours is nowhere near as vague, elusive, and nontestable as his.

Crow faults our hypothesis for predicting "neurological symptoms that are not present in schizophrenia." Since our hypothesis does not predict any neurological symptoms (other than cognitive deterioration), we do not know what Crow is talking about. At one point, he leaps to the conclusion that a defect involving NMDA receptors would have to be expressed throughout the CNS and therefore would cause damage in the spinal cord and cerebellum as well as cerebrum. If this prediction is what Crow means when he says that our hypothesis "predicts neurological symptoms that are not present in schizophrenia," we would point to the evidence in our article that when PCP is administered in doses that block all NMDA receptors in the CNS, it results in pathomorphological changes selectively affecting specific neurons in specific corticolimbic regions of the brain and does not cause such changes anywhere else. Moreover, if NMDA receptor hypofunction is a mechanism operative in schizophrenia, as we hypothesize, we assume it would most likely be a mechanism expressed only through some subcomponent of the NMDA receptor system. Again, the flaw appears to lie in Crow's version of our hypothesis and not in the hypothesis itself.

In a section addressing structural brain changes, Crow focuses on three categories of such changes and asserts that "neurohumoral theories account for none" of these changes, whereas connectionist theory accounts for all three. In support of this conclusion, Crow speculates in his Commentary[11] that "loss of asymmetry and its morphological concomitants is perhaps the most direct pointer we have to the nature of the disease process" and cites another article[12] to that effect. We find it difficult to follow Crow's logic, but he apparently is maintaining that NMDA receptor hypofunction that causes obvious structural brain changes in animal brain cannot account for brain changes in schizophrenia, whereas a speculative hypothesis of Crow's that does not identify any mechanism capable of causing brain changes is the best explanation for brain changes in schizophrenia.

Crow expresses several opinions that run counter to a large body of evidence that he arbitrarily ignores. For example, numerous researchers in the schizophrenia field have carefully studied the psychotic symptoms typically induced by PCP or its analogues. This includes symptoms induced in normal human volunteers, in drug abusers intoxicated with PCP, and in schizophrenic patients experimentally exposed to various hallucinogenic drugs (eg, PCP, lysergic acid diethylamide [LSD], and amphetamines) for the specific purpose of making an empirical comparison. The latter experiments were performed in an era when such human experimentation was more freely allowed than it is today. There is an excellent consensus among researchers[13-18] that the symptoms induced by PCP closely mimic the spectrum of symptoms seen in schizophrenia, whereas the symptoms induced by amphetamines, at best, only resemble a narrow category of such symptoms. Lysergic acid diethylamide induces a psychedelic syndrome consisting primarily of visual hallucinations, whereas PCP-induced hallucinations are usually auditory.[15] Of particular interest, PCP caused stable patients with chronic schizophrenia to have an acute exacerbation of their illness for up to several weeks.[19,20] In contrast, LSD triggered a brief psychedelic episode that was not more prolonged or more severe in schizophrenic patients than in normal volunteers.[20-22] Crow disregards all these empirical observations by researchers in this field and, without citing any specific evidence, asserts his opinion that the PCP-based NMDA receptor hypothesis is no better at explaining the psychotic manifestations of schizophrenia than amphetamine or LSD models, all of which he rejects on the basis of his opinion that neurohumoral hypotheses are inherently deficient in explanatory power.

Crow shows very little inclination to study our hypothesis and think through its implications. For example, when he asserts that amphetamines (the dopamine hypothesis) can explain psychotic manifestations as well as PCP (the NMDA hypothesis) and believes that he is effectively refuting our hypothesis, he is simply demonstrating that he has not made a serious effort to understand our hypothesis. According to our hypothesis, the psychotic manifestations elicited by amphetamines could be due to NRH occurring secondary to the dopamine hyperfunctional state induced by the amphetamines. Since amphetamine treatment would not be a very efficient means of inducing NRH, this would explain why the psychotic syndrome induced by amphetamines is decidedly less impressive than the syndrome induced by PCP.

In a section dealing with focal damage and exogenous pathogens, Crow cites his own evidence regarding lack of gliosis as basis for rejecting the hypothesis that focal brain damage might play a role in the pathophysiology of schizophrenia. There are two problems with Crow's position. First, in this section, he appears to be talking about structural damage during development. Those who argue for focal damage during development base their argument on the assumption that such damage would occur without causing gliosis. Thus, failure of Crow to find gliosis adds strength, not weakness, to their hypothesis. Second, in our article,[2] we propose that two types of brain damage might occur in schizophrenia. One type would be a developmental lesion that would not be expected to cause gliosis; the other type would occur during adulthood as a result of an NRH state. We have pointed out in our article[2] and cited empirical evidence that this is a kind of brain damage in which neurons are selectively deleted from various corticolimbic regions *of the adult brain* with little or no residual gliosis. Again, Crow's Commentary does not give much indication that he has carefully read our manuscript and attempted, with an open mind, to evaluate its strengths and weaknesses.

Crow has a fixed concept of neurohumoral hypotheses and, for ease of discounting such hypotheses, he assumes that all of them merely posit a "generalized disturbance of a single transmitter system." This allows him to depict his connectionist theory as superior to any neurohumoral hypothesis on grounds that, by invoking "dysfunction in specific sets of cortical connections," he can "account readily for the relative selectivity of the impairments to higher aspects of nervous system function." Our hypothesis (Figure) is not as limited or impoverished as Crow infers. We postulate a basic defect that can give rise to dysfunction (disinhibition) in multiple transmitter pathways, ie, in multiple "sets of cortical connections." The disinhibition process could be initiated by a defect in any of at least three transmitter systems (dopamine, NMDA glutamate, or GABA), and when such a defect becomes operative, it has the same implications for brain function as a connectionist defect. In fact, it is a connectionist defect involving failure of certain sets of synaptic connections that normally hold excitatory systems under inhibitory restraint. Perhaps if we would rename our hypothesis the "connectionist, variant gene, inhibition failure" hypothesis, Crow would study our hypothesis more closely and give it better marks.

John W. Olney, MD
Nuri B. Farber, MD
Department of Psychiatry
Washington University
School of Medicine
4940 Children's Pl
Campus Box 8143
St Louis, MO 63110-1093

REFERENCES

1. Benes FM. Altered glutamatergic and GABAergic mechanisms in the cingulate cortex of the schizophrenic brain. *Arch Gen Psychiatry.* 1995; 52:1015-1018.
2. Olney JW, Farber NB. Glutamate receptor dysfunction and schizophrenia. *Arch Gen Psychiatry.* 1995;52:998-1007.
3. Lewis DA, Anderson SA, Rosenberg DR, Lund JS, Conde F. Postnatal refinements of prefrontal cortical circuitry and schizophrenia. *Schizophr Res.* 1995;15:29-30.
4. Baleydier C, Mauguiere F. The duality of the cingulate gyrus in monkey: neuroanatomical study and functional hypothesis. *Brain.* 1980;103:525-554.
5. Van Hoesen GW, Morecraft RJ, Vogt BA. Connections of the monkey cingulate cortex. In: Vogt BA, Gabriel M, eds. *Neurobiology of Cingulate Cortex and Limbic Thalamus.* Boston, Mass: Birkhäuser; 1993:249-284.
6. Henn FA. The NMDA receptor as a site for psychopathology: primary or secondary role? *Arch Gen Psychiatry.* 1995;52:1008-1010.
7. Wyatt RJ. Neuroleptics and the natural course of schizophrenia. *Schizophr Bull.* 1991;17:325-351.
8. Loebel AD, Lieberman JA, Alvir JM, Mayerhoff DI, Geisler SH, Szymanski SR. Duration of psychosis and outcome in first-episode schizophrenia. *Am J Psychiatry.* 1992;149: 1183-1188.
9. Tandon R, Greden JF, Silk KR. Treatment of negative schizophrenic symptoms with trihexiphenidyl. *J Clin Psychopharmacol.* 1988;8:212-215.
10. Farber NB, Foster J, Olney JW. Clozapine and related analogs block NMDA antagonist neurotoxicity: implications for schizophrenia. *Schizophr Res.* 1995;15:57-58.
11. Crow TJ. Constraints on concepts of pathogenesis: language and the speciation process as the key to the etiology of schizophrenia. *Arch Gen Psychiatry.* 1995;52:1011-1014.
12. Crow TJ. Temporal lobe asymmetries as the key to the etiology of schizophrenia. *Schizophr Bull.* 1990;16:433-443.
13. Domino EF. Neurobiology of phencyclidine (Sernyl): a drug with an unusual spectrum of pharmacological activity. *Int Rev Neurobiol.* 1964;6: 303-347.
14. Domino E, Luby E. Abnormal mental states induced by phencyclidine as a model of schizophrenia. In: Domino E, ed. *PCP (Phencyclidine): Historical and Current Perspectives.* Ann Arbor, Mich: NPP Books; 1981:401-418.
15. Erard R, Luisada PV, Peele R. The PCP psychosis: prolonged intoxication or drug-precipitated functional illness? *J Psychedelic Drugs.* 1980; 12:235-245.
16. Garey RE. PCP (phencyclidine): an update. *J Psychedelic Drugs.* 1979;11:265-275.
17. Javitt DC, Zukin SR. Recent advances in the phencyclidine model of schizophrenia. *Am J Psychiatry.* 1991;148:1301-1308.
18. Snyder SH. Phencyclidine. *Nature.* 1980;285: 355-356.
19. Luby ED, Cohen BD, Rosenbaum G, Gottlieb JS, Kelley R. Study of a new schizophrenomimetic drug: Sernyl. *Arch Neurol Psychiatry.* 1959;81: 363-369.
20. Ban TA, Lohrenz JJ, Lehmann HE. Observations on the action of Sernyl—a new psychotropic drug. *Can Psychiatr Assoc J.* 1961;6:150-157.
21. Rosenbaum G, Cohen BD, Luby ED, Gottlieb JS, Yelen D. Comparison of Sernyl with other drugs: simulation of schizophrenic performance with Sernyl, LSD-25, and amobarbital (Amytal) sodium, I: attention, motor function, and proprioception. *Arch Gen Psychiatry.* 1959;1:651-656.
22. Cohen BD, Rosenbaum G, Luby ED, Gottlieb JS. Comparison of phencyclidine hydrochloride (Sernyl) with other drugs: simulation of schizophrenic performance with phencyclidine hydrochloride (Sernyl), lysergic acid diethylamide (LSD-25), and amobarbital (Amytal) sodium, II: symbolic and sequential thinking. *Arch Gen Psychiatry.* 1962;6:395-401.
23. Olney JW. Excitotoxicity and ischemic brain damage in infancy and adulthood. In: Krieglstein J, Oberpichler H, eds. *Pharmacology of Cerebral Ischemia 1990.* Stuttgart, Germany: Wissenschaftliche Verlagsgesellschaft mbH; 1990:153-167.

ORIGINAL ARTICLE

The Reliability and Validity of Two Structured Diagnostic Interviews for Personality Disorders

Paul A. Pilkonis, PhD; Carol L. Heape, RN, MSN; Joseph M. Proietti, MS; Suzan W. Clark, MEd; Joshua D. McDavid, MD; Timothy E. Pitts, MEd

Background: The reliability and validity of Axis II diagnoses were investigated in a sample of 108 patients with nonpsychotic Axis I disorders.

Methods: Patients were assessed for personality disorders (PDs) with either the Personality Disorder Examination (PDE) or the Structured Interview for *DSM-III-R* Personality (SIDP-R). Validity was examined by comparing interview diagnoses with "best-estimate" consensus diagnoses assigned by a panel of judges.

Results: Interrater reliabilities were excellent when using continuous data (eg, total or cluster scores; intraclass correlation coefficients, .82 to .92); they were lower with categorical diagnoses (eg, any PD vs no PD; κ=0.55 and 0.58 with the two interviews). Validity coefficients (ie, κ values reflecting agreement between the interviews and the consensus diagnosis) for the decision of any PD vs no PD were 0.18 (56% agreement) with the PDE and 0.37 (75% agreement) with the SIDP-R; validity coefficients for identifying cases of "marked" PD were 0.21 (62% agreement) with the PDE and 0.24 (60% agreement) with the SIDP-R.

Conclusions: There have been important advances in the development of structured interviews for Axis II diagnoses, but the findings suggest a continued need to be thoughtful about their strengths and weaknesses before accepting their results as definitive diagnostic tests. The findings also demonstrated some of the advantages of continuous vs categorical data.

(Arch Gen Psychiatry. 1995;52:1025-1033)

THE DIAGNOSIS of personality disorders (PDs) remains controversial because of concerns about both the adequacy of the *DSM-III-R*,[1] now the *DSM-IV*, in defining such categories[2,3] and the reliability and validity of alternative methods for making such diagnoses, even given the current classification "rules."[4-9] In traditional epidemiological approaches, there are three methods used to define "caseness": clinical diagnosis (ie, people seeking treatment are cases when the physician says they deserve a diagnosis); research diagnosis (which usually relies on a structured assessment, often administered by a clinician); and self-reports on a screening measure.[10]

Each of these methods has different advantages and disadvantages, and none can claim to be a gold standard. The advent of structured interviews for diagnosing psychiatric disorders is usually hailed, however, as the most important recent advance for studies of classification, largely on the basis of the improved reliability that such interviews provide. Systematic inquiry about the symptoms and signs of Axis I disorders is now an accepted part of any clinical research endeavor. Similar approaches have been applied to the diagnosis of Axis II disorders, and this extrapolation has, indeed, led to improved reliability.

Three interviews have received the largest share of research attention: the Personality Disorder Examination (PDE),[11-13] the Structured Interview for *DSM-III-R* Personality (SIDP-R),[14,15] and the Structured Clinical Interview for *DSM-III-R* Personality Disorders.[16] The range of interrater reliabilities (κ coefficients) for assessing the presence vs absence of any PD with these structured approaches is 0.41 to 0.89.[9,13,15,17-20] In our earlier work, we reported reliabilities of 0.76 to 0.84 with the second developmental version of the PDE.[7]

From the Department of Psychiatry, Western Psychiatric Institute and Clinic, University of Pittsburgh (Pa) School of Medicine.

See Subjects and Methods on next page

SUBJECTS AND METHODS

SAMPLE

The present report describes the findings from 108 patients who provided complete data and received a best-estimate Axis II diagnosis at intake. Patients from 21 to 60 years old were solicited from open-treatment inpatient and outpatient programs within the Mood Disorders Module at Western Psychiatric Institute and Clinic, Pittsburgh, Pa. Patients with psychotic disorders, organic mental disorders, and mental retardation were excluded, as were patients with major medical illnesses that influence the central nervous system and might be associated with organic personality changes (eg, Parkinson's disease, cerebrovascular disease, insulin-dependent diabetes, seizure disorders).

Outpatients were required to have had no treatment (including psychotropic medication) within the previous 3 months; given the longitudinal component of the study, treatment outcome will be examined as an important measure of predictive validity. Therefore, an effort was made to ensure that outpatients were equivalent in beginning a new treatment episode. For the same reason, it was required, with inpatients, that the current hospitalization be the only inpatient stay for the present Axis I episode. Patients were not preselected on the basis of a suspected PD (since the goal was to assess both positive and negative cases), and they were told that the assessment protocol was focused on "getting to know you better as a person" when informed consent was solicited.

To assure a range of severity of psychopathology and functional impairment, approximately one inpatient (n=31, 29%) was accepted for every three outpatients (n=77, 71%). The average age of the group was 35.6 years (SD=9.4); 62 of the patients were women (57%); 93 were white (86%); 14 were black (13%), and one was Asian (1%). In terms of marital status, 54 patients (50%) were single and never married, 33 (31%) had suffered some marital disruption (ie, they were separated, divorced, or remarried), and 21 (19%) were stably married. Among these 108 patients, 77 (71%) nominated a significant other (SO) to serve as an informant; 65 of these SOs (87% of those eligible) completed the assessment. Thus, 60% (65/108) of the assessments included collateral information from a spouse, relative, or good friend.

During the first assessment session (see the "Procedures" section below), all patients were administered the Structured Clinical Interview for *DSM-III-R* (SCID)[29] to identify Axis I diagnoses. The tabulation below summarizes those best-estimate consensus diagnoses at intake (N=108).

Diagnosis	No. (%) of Patients
Affective disorders only	36 (33.3)
Anxiety disorders only	6 (5.6)
Substance abuse disorders only	6 (5.6)
Affective and anxiety disorders	23 (21.3)
Affective and substance abuse disorders	11 (10.2)
Anxiety and substance abuse disorders	3 (2.8)
Affective, anxiety, and substance abuse disorders	5 (4.6)
Other diagnoses (eg, eating and somatoform disorders)	11 (10.2)
None (V-codes or past diagnoses only)	7 (6.5)

As shown above, the most prevalent current diagnoses were affective disorders alone and comorbid affective and anxiety disorders.

PROCEDURES

The method had several specific steps.

1. Following a referral, one member of the research team was designated the primary interviewer for each patient and became responsible for soliciting consent, scheduling appointments, presenting the patient's case at diagnostic conferences, and maintaining contact with the patient during the 12-month follow-up. All assessments were conducted with two interviewers present if scheduling constraints allowed; if a backup interviewer was unavailable, the assessment was videotaped for later review by another member of the research team. The use of two interviewers for every evaluation allowed a systematic assessment of interrater reliability throughout the study. With this method, the primary interviewer was present for every assessment (providing consistency over time and across informants), whereas the secondary interviewer was allowed to vary (providing an opportunity for as many members of the research team as possible to have direct contact with the patient).

2. Assessments at intake required three sessions with every patient, with each session lasting approximately 2 hours, for a total of 6 to 7 hours of face-to-face contact with all subjects. Session 1 included the administration of the SCID and the Hamilton Rating Scales for Depression and Anxiety.[30,31] Session 2 included the taking of a detailed social and developmental history using a semistructured interview, the Interpersonal Relations Assessment (IRA), developed for this purpose.[32] The IRA focuses on the lifetime history of relations with first-degree relatives and other important attachment figures, and also includes information about school achievement, work history, and other social relationships. During this session, a brief life-events interview was also conducted so that the patient could recount the major occurrences of the past year. During session 3, one or the other of two structured interviews for Axis II diagnosis was given randomly to patients: the PDE (n=55) or the SIDP-R (n=53). It was regarded as too great a burden for patients to receive both interviews in a test-retest format, especially given the other lengthy portions of the assessment battery.

Potential differences between the two groups receiving the PDE vs the SIDP-R were examined with regard to demographic (age, gender, race, marital status) and clinical variables (symptomatic status, presence and severity of Axis II diagnoses) at intake. There were no statistically significant differences in any of these comparisons.

These two interviews were selected for several reasons: they provide comprehensive coverage of all personality features included in the *DSM-III-R* (ie, there are no "skipouts"), they have received the most attention in the research literature to date, and they can be administered without knowing if the patient will score above threshold on any specific disorder since they are organized around areas of functioning (eg, interpersonal relations, work, affect regulation) rather than individual PDs. This last reason was especially important because consensus diagnostic conferences were conducted with judges still blinded to the specific results from the Axis II interviews. The general themes that patients endorsed on the interviews were discussed, but judges were unaware if patients had formally met criteria for a diagnosis using the current scoring conventions. Patients were paid $25 at the completion of the intake evaluation.

3. Following the patient assessment, an interview with the patient's SO was performed. The SO was given the same Axis II interview that was administered to the patient (the PDE or SIDP-R), but the interview was done in the third person to solicit the SO's reports about the patient's characteristic personality features. This information was also integrated into the clinical consensus decision.

4. Following the SO evaluation, the primary interviewer presented the case at a 2-hour diagnostic conference, with four judges required for a quorum. All available data (historical and concurrent) were reviewed and discussed at the conference, and each clinician voted independently on the presence or absence of a PD. For each judge, the primary task was to make an overall yes-vs-no decision on the presence of any Axis II disorder; decisions about specific disorders were left to the group as a whole, reviewing the entire set of *DSM-III-R* criteria (see below).

Judges were given access to all the data that had been collected (current and lifetime Axis I information, symptomatic status, social and developmental history, life events, personality features, and SO reports about personality and functioning) and were asked to integrate this information, with a particular emphasis on functional impairment (eg, difficulties in major social roles, problems in interpersonal relationships) and longitudinal consistency (eg, chronic difficulties not restricted to episodes of Axis I problems, markers of persistent social disability). Since there is often uncertainty about how to disentangle Axis I vs Axis II impairment and how to integrate discrepant information from patients and SOs, these questions were posed with each case and debated until judges were prepared to vote.

JUDGES

All six members of the research team participated as both interviewers and judges in the consensus process. Thus, the diagnostic conferences included participants with a mix of firsthand and secondhand knowledge and more vs less interpersonal distance from each patient, a procedure that ensured alternative perspectives in every case formulation. Judges also varied in discipline and experience, with one having a PhD degree in psychology, one with an MD degree, three master's-level clinicians trained in psychology or counseling, and one master's-level nurse. Years of experience (in working in psychiatric settings) ranged from 3 to 21, with a mean of 9 years.

CONSENSUS DATA

There were several measures that emerged from the best-estimate consensus. The most critical was the overall decision about the presence vs absence of a PD on clinical grounds. Individual votes about the presence vs absence of a PD were tallied, however, and in cases of disagreement, a majority rule was used to assign the clinical diagnosis.

Following the yes/no decision, all features of all PDs were reviewed for every subject by the group as a whole. Each feature was noted as present and clinically significant; probable, less significant, or occurring at a subclinical level; or absent. This discrimination made it possible to assign a *DSM-III-R* diagnosis at two levels: a "conservative" level at which only major, clinically significant features were used, and a "liberal" level at which both definite and probable markers were incorporated. An overall rating of severity of the Axis II disorder was also done by consensus on a 100-point scale (an analog to the Global Assessment Scale[33]) developed for this purpose. The scale was segmented into quintiles, with associated descriptive anchors. For example, the range from 61 to 80 was labeled "significant to marked personality pathology associated with chronic impairment and definite personality disorder." Individual interviewers also made ratings of Axis II severity following their assessments and prior to the consensus conference; the reliability (intraclass correlation) of these ratings was .78.

On the basis of severity, patients were grouped into three categories: no PD vs PD of moderate severity (a rating of 61 to 69 on the 100-point scale) vs PD of marked severity ($\geq$70). Finally, each patient was assigned to one (and only one) of the three *DSM-III-R* clusters on the basis of the predominant features and clinical formulation characterizing each case; given the number of mixed and multiple diagnoses that emerged (see below), it was necessary to make such a mutually exclusive decision rather than relying on the diagnoses alone.

STRUCTURED INTERVIEWS

The PDE

The third (and definitive) version of the PDE[11] was used in the present study. In this form, the PDE contains 126 items (corresponding to the features used to define *DSM-III-R* Axis II disorders) to be rated by the interviewer on the basis of both subjects' responses to direct questioning and their nonverbal behavior during the interview. Items are rated on a three-point scale, ranging from 0 (absent) to 2 (present and clinically significant), using a manual that details the criteria for scores at each level for each item. Only items scored 2 are included in the scoring algorithms for categorical diagnoses. The algorithms allow diagnosis at the "definite" and "probable" levels, and for all analyses reported herein, diagnoses at both these levels were combined into a single "PD present" category. "Mixed" (or not otherwise specified [NOS]) diagnoses are assigned at the probable level if 10 to 14 criteria are scored 2 without the patient's qualifying for any specific disorder and at the definite level if 15 or more criteria are endorsed without any other diagnosis.

The SIDP-R

The SIDP-R[14] is an instrument with a similar structure. Questions referring to aspects of different PDs are used to elicit information that is integrated by the clinician into three-point ratings (again ranging from 0 to 2) on each of the *DSM-III-R* criteria for Axis II disorders. On the SIDP-R, levels 0, 1, and 2 have brief descriptive phrases as anchors on

Continued on next page

each item. The anchors for ratings of 1 tend to indicate probable to definite presence of the marker ("moderately present"), and the anchors for ratings of 2 indicate definite to severe features ("severely present"). Thus, the intervals on the three-point rating scales are not equivalent for the SIDP-R and the PDE, and the categorical scoring algorithms for the SIDP-R are more liberal: items scored either 1 *or* 2 count toward a diagnosis. No probable diagnoses are assigned with the SIDP-R, and a mixed (NOS) diagnosis is assigned when two or more disorders are just one criterion short of diagnostic thresholds.

As mentioned above, there is some difference between the interviews in their approach to temporal stability. Given the definition of PDs, both interviews encourage the clinician to identify features that had an early onset and have been long-standing. At a minimum, the PDE requires the presence of personality features throughout the entire past 5 years, whereas the SIDP-R focuses on the personality that has predominated for the greatest amount of time during the same interval. Finally, questions about the same features are phrased in different ways on the interviews, introducing another source of variability.

RELIABILITY TRAINING

The study began with a reliability substudy. Members of the research team reviewed all the assessment measures (SCID, IRA, PDE, and SIDP-R), discussed their contents, and had some initial practice with each other and with pilot cases. To calibrate all judges, it was required that members of the team rate the first several interviews done with each Axis II instrument: seven patients and four SOs with the PDE; six patients and five SOs with the SIDP-R. (The SCIDs and IRAs for these patients were also seen by all raters.) These interviews were conducted in person by the primary and secondary interviewers and reviewed on videotape by all of the other raters. To prevent drift, all the judges viewed all (three or four) parts of the evaluation for approximately 10% of all remaining cases, randomly selected (total n for the complete reliability subsample: 12 patients and eight SOs with the PDE and 11 patients and six SOs with the SIDP-R). Again, these interviews were conducted in person by the primary and secondary interviewers and reviewed on videotape by all of the other raters.

Validity, however, is a more problematic issue. The definition of Axis II disorders[1(p335)] describes an inferred or "latent" construct reflected in a longitudinal history of dysfunction, lack of flexibility, subjective distress, and impairment in major social roles, as well as a specific personality style. Ideally, the measurement of such a latent construct will incorporate "manifest" indicators in each of these areas. Nonetheless, the interviews developed for Axis II diagnoses tend to rely heavily on inquiry about the traits that characterize the personality style alone, with secondary inquiry about specific behavioral examples, personal estimates of impairment and distress, or both. The PDE is most stringent in this regard, requiring examples and a consistent, 5-year history to support each positive response, with the SIDP-R "intermediate" in stringency, and the Structured Clinical Interview for *DSM-III-R* Personality Disorders the most "lenient." One can endorse this approach as a necessary first step, but it is important to acknowledge that there is limited assessment of the functional severity of the disorder, only partial information about the social and developmental history that puts the clinical material in a longitudinal perspective, and no simple antidote for the distortions introduced by social desirability response biases. These limitations may constrain validity, and, again, to cite our own earlier findings, agreement between a carefully derived clinical consensus diagnosis and the PDE was modest (κ=0.28 at intake and 0.29 at a 6-month follow-up evaluation).[7]

To be fair to the interviews, however, it may be less their form or content that is problematic and more the ways in which they are currently scored. Whatever their limitations, they can be considered "tests" for which alternative methods of case identification may have different utilities. A continuing task is to identify appropriate ways to extract useful information from them: ". . . the results of structured interviews are being accepted as valid without explicit consideration of the consequences of choosing specific case definition strategies based on these instruments."[21(p204)] Given the excellent reliabilities of continuous scores derived from structured interviews, the moderate-to-good categorical reliabilities, and the poor-to-adequate validity coefficients with categorical decision rules (see below), the use of continuous scores rather than categorical diagnoses may prove to be more useful.

In further attempts at validation, we have continued to refine a method that relies heavily on comprehensive clinical assessment, integrated into a consensual decision-making process. The method combines elements of different "best-estimate" diagnostic procedures discussed in the literature.[22-26] Clinical judgment can be faulted as arbitrary, subjective, or biased in the direction of seeing illness when identified patients are used as research subjects, but an effort was made to limit these influences by aggregating across judges and over time.[27] In the current work, patients were assessed at three points: intake into treatment, and 6 and 12 months after intake (although only intake data are reported here). Multiple judges were used, careful attention was paid to reliability among these judges, and there was a consensus system of checks and balances, ie, there was no single expert but rather a panel (all of us) that provided alternative perspectives on the same patient.

Another complication that must be considered in any work on diagnostic classification is the influence of base rates on the operating characteristics of different assessment tools and on the stability of quantitative indicators for assessing reliability and validity (eg, κ coefficients, corrected for chance agreement, which is substantial when base rates are extremely high or low; positive and negative predictive values).[28] The current work, done in a tertiary care facility where base rates of Axis II disorders are high, must be introduced and interpreted in this context.

RESULTS

PREVALENCE AND TYPES OF PDs

The prevalence of PDs in the sample was high. According to the best-estimate consensus, 85 (79%) of 108 cases were diagnosed as having PDs. When using the trichotomy based on Axis II severity, 44 patients were judged to have marked PDs (41% of the overall sample and 52% of all patients with PDs), and 41 patients were rated as having moderate PDs (38% of the overall sample and 48% of all patients with PDs). Thus, the yes/no decisions produced approximately an 80/20 split, and the trichotomy of marked/moderate/no PDs produced about a 40/40/20 split. Eighty-four (78%) of the 108 yes/no decisions were unanimous, producing a κ of 0.64 across the binary votes of the six judges.

When using conservative thresholds on the *DSM-III-R* criteria (ie, including only those Axis II features that were definitely present and clinically significant), the most frequent diagnosis was mixed PD (n=45; 53%) or more technically, PD NOS. Eleven patients (13%) received multiple diagnoses. The remaining 29 patients with Axis II diagnoses (34% of the PD patients) had only a single diagnosis, with 17 of these coming from cluster C, 11 from cluster B, and one labeled "self-defeating," a provisional category.

When liberal thresholds were used (combining definite and probable features), the balance shifted from mixed diagnoses (n=7; 8%) to multiple diagnoses (n=59 PD patients, with a range of two to six Axis II diagnoses; 69%). Nineteen patients (22%) had a single diagnosis: 10 from cluster C, seven from cluster B, one from cluster A, and one labeled "sadistic" (also a provisional category). Since mixed and multiple diagnoses were more common than individual diagnoses when applying the descriptive criteria of the *DSM-III-R*, mutually exclusive decisions about cluster membership were made on clinical grounds; by this measure, six cases belonged to cluster A (7% of all PD patients), 55 cases (65%) fell into cluster B, and 24 cases (28%) were assigned to cluster C. Thus, in this nonpsychotic sample (unrestricted in terms of other Axis I disorders), there was an approximate 10/60/30 split across clusters A, B, and C.

STRUCTURED INTERVIEWS

Interrater Reliability

Excellent and equivalent results were obtained with both interviews when reliabilities were computed as intraclass correlation coefficients[34] using continuous measures, ie, total scores summed either across the entire interview or limited to one of the three clusters. These reliabilities ranged from .85 to .92 on the PDE and from .82 to .90 on the SIDP-R. In all instances, the data were taken from intake assessments with the patient version of the Axis II interviews as rated by the primary and secondary interviewers. When reliabilities were calculated from the subsample of cases rated by the entire panel of judges, the same intraclass correlation coefficients ranged from .76 to .92 on the PDE and .81 to .89 on the SIDP-R.

Reliabilities decreased when agreement about categorical decisions (the presence vs absence of any PD) was examined. Given the present sample in which the majority of patients showed some-to-marked personality disorder, the introduction of a categorical threshold is likely to decrease reliability by separating judges (whose continuous scores may be similar) onto opposite sides of the yes/no distinction. On the PDE, interrater reliability (κ) for two judges scoring any PD vs no PD was 0.55 (78% agreement); with the SIDP-R, the same κ was 0.58 (81% agreement). With the subsample of patients rated by all of the judges, the corresponding κ values were 0.55 with the PDE and 0.52 with the SIDP-R. Again, the two interviews did not differ significantly.

These categorical reliability coefficients were somewhat lower than those obtained in our earlier work where κ values ranged from 0.76 to 0.84.[7] While investigating these results further, we were impressed with the number of cases in which interview protocols were close to the thresholds at which diagnoses are assigned. Therefore, every protocol was reexamined to identify those in which a change in a *single* diagnostic criterion (eg, moving from a score of 1 to 2 on an individual PDE item, or vice versa; changing from a score of 0 to 1 on a single SIDP-R item, or vice versa) could change the overall decision of any PD vs no PD. On the PDE and SIDP-R, 31% and 15%, respectively, of the interviews scored by the two primary judges met this criterion. Best- and worst-case analyses were then performed, adjusting the scoring on the protocols that could be changed by altering a single item, to maximize or minimize agreements between the judges. On the PDE, the best- and worst-case agreements produced κ values of 0.88 and 0.05, respectively; with the SIDP-R, best- and worst-case κ's were 0.91 and 0.31. These striking results demonstrate the powerful impact of small changes in scoring procedures when categorical algorithms are used in a sample in which many cases are near the diagnostic threshold.

Validity

We have emphasized validity as a major concern. Thus, a central issue was the extent to which diagnoses from the structured interviews matched the best-estimate clinical diagnoses. In general, agreement was fair to moderate. Kappa coefficients were computed comparing the interview diagnosis from the primary rater's protocol and the best-estimate consensus. Again, to maximize sample size, only data from intake interviews with patients alone were used. Kappa was 0.18 with the PDE and 0.37 with the SIDP-R. These κ's were not significantly different when compared using the method proposed by Cohen.[35(p44)]

Both interviews underdiagnosed in comparison with the consensus: the percentage of agreements with

Table 1. Operating Characteristics of the Axis II Interviews*

Diagnosis	P	Q	Agreement, %	κ	Sensitivity	Specificity	PPV	NPV
			Personality Disorder Examination (n=55)					
Any PD	0.76	0.44	56	0.18	0.50	0.77	0.88	0.32
Any marked PD	0.38	0.44	62	0.21	0.57	0.65	0.50	0.71
Any cluster A disorder	0.13	0.02	89	0.23	0.14	1.00	1.00	0.89
Any cluster B disorder	0.36	0.07	67	0.15	0.15	0.97	0.75	0.67
Histrionic	0.22	0.04	82	0.24	0.17	1.00	1.00	0.81
Narcissistic	0.15	0.02	87	0.20	0.13	1.00	1.00	0.87
Borderline	0.15	0.04	82	−0.06	0.00	0.96	0.00	0.85
Any cluster C disorder	0.49	0.22	62	0.23	0.33	0.89	0.75	0.58
Avoidant	0.26	0.13	80	0.37	0.36	0.95	0.71	0.81
Dependent	0.16	0.06	82	0.09	0.11	0.96	0.33	0.85
Obsessive-compulsive	0.15	0.06	91	0.51	0.38	1.00	1.00	0.90
Passive-aggressive	0.24	0.02	78	0.11	0.08	1.00	1.00	0.78
PD not otherwise specified	0.09	0.27	64	−0.16	0.00	0.70	0.00	0.88
			Structured Interview for *DSM-III-R* Personality (n=53)					
Any PD	0.81	0.68	75	0.37	0.77	0.70	0.92	0.41
Any marked PD	0.43	0.68	60	0.24	0.83	0.43	0.53	0.76
Any cluster A disorder	0.17	0.17	77	0.20	0.33	0.86	0.33	0.86
Paranoid	0.09	0.15	79	0.04	0.20	0.85	0.13	0.91
Any cluster B disorder	0.60	0.38	66	0.35	0.53	0.86	0.85	0.55
Histrionic	0.42	0.25	75	0.46	0.50	0.94	0.85	0.73
Narcissistic	0.40	0.17	74	0.39	0.38	0.97	0.89	0.70
Antisocial	0.09	0.04	91	0.25	0.20	0.98	0.50	0.92
Borderline	0.34	0.21	75	0.40	0.44	0.91	0.73	0.76
Any cluster C disorder	0.57	0.40	75	0.52	0.63	0.91	0.90	0.66
Avoidant	0.17	0.26	83	0.51	0.78	0.84	0.50	0.95
Dependent	0.30	0.13	83	0.52	0.44	1.00	1.00	0.80
Obsessive-compulsive	0.11	0.06	91	0.40	0.33	0.98	0.67	0.92
Passive-aggressive	0.32	0.19	79	0.47	0.47	0.95	0.80	0.79
Self-defeating	0.09	0.08	94	0.64	0.60	0.60	0.75	0.96

**Individual disorders are included in the table when there was a minimum of five cases diagnosed, either by the (liberal) diagnostic consensus or the interview. P indicates prevalence of the disorder by the diagnostic consensus; Q, level of the test; PPV, positive predictive value; NPV, negative predictive value; and PD, personality disorder.*

the PDE was 56% (31 of 55 patients; 21 true positives, 10 true negatives), with the majority of disagreements (21/24; 88%) being false negatives; with the SIDP-R, the percentage of agreements was 75% (40 of 53 patients; 33 true positives, seven true negatives), and again the most frequent disagreements were false negatives (10/13; 77%). With this high base-rate sample, the SIDP-R produced more agreements because the "level" of this test[36] in diagnosing PDs (68%) was higher than that of the PDE (44%), more nearly matching the base rate. We assume that this higher level is a result of the more liberal intervals developed for the three-point scale used to rate each item and the categorical scoring rules (using both ratings of 1 and 2) associated with this method. It seems likely that the results would change, perhaps even reverse, if the alternative scoring rules were applied to each interview.

Best- and worst-case analyses were also performed with the validity coefficients, using every protocol from the primary rater in which changing a single diagnostic criterion altered the overall decision on the presence or absence of a PD. Agreements between the primary rater's protocol and the consensus were then maximized and minimized: the best and worst agreements with the PDE produced κ values of 0.53 (80% agreement) and 0.03 (47% agreement), respectively; with the SIDP-R, best and worst agreements resulted in κ values of 0.43 (79% agreement) and 0.26 (68% agreement), respectively.

The same analyses were repeated using only the marked PD cases (with a lower base rate of 41%) as true positives. In these analyses, equivalent results were again obtained with the two interviews. Kappa reflecting agreement between the interview and the clinical consensus was 0.21 (62% agreement; 12 true positives, 22 true negatives) with the PDE and 0.24 (60% agreement; 19 true positives, 13 true negatives) with the SIDP-R. The best- and worst-case agreements with the PDE produced κ's of 0.49 (75% agreement) and −0.13 (42% agreement), respectively; with the SIDP-R, best and worst agreements resulted in κ's of 0.41 (70% agreement) and 0.21 (58% agreement), respectively, for cases of marked PD.

The data were also inspected at the level of individual disorders, comparing liberal consensus diagnoses (incorporating all probable and definite features) and interview diagnoses. Liberal rather than conservative consensus diagnoses were used because only the former produced sufficient prevalences of specific PDs; as described above, the latter produced a majority of mixed (NOS) diagnoses. We examined all disorders in which a minimum of five cases (approximately 10% of

Table 2. Diagnostic Thresholds for Any Personality Disorder: Quality Receiver Operating Characteristics Analyses*

Interview	Threshold	P	Q	Quality of Sensitivity	Quality of Efficiency	Quality of Specificity
Personality Disorder Examination (n=55)	≥15	0.76	0.82	0.48†	0.40	0.34
	≥25	0.76	0.67	0.35	0.42†	0.54
	≥35	0.76	0.36	0.14	0.24	0.79†
Structured Interview for *DSM-III-R* Personality (n=53)	≥13	0.81	0.81	0.51†	0.51	0.51
	≥17	0.81	0.72	0.42	0.53†	0.72
	≥29	0.81	0.47	0.21	0.34	1.00†

**Thresholds identifying the maximum quality of sensitivity, efficiency, and specificity are included and identified by daggers. P indicates the prevalence of any personality disorder by the diagnostic consensus; Q, the level of the test at each threshold.*

Table 3. Diagnostic Thresholds for Any Marked Personality Disorder: Quality Receiver Operating Characteristics Analyses*

Interview	Threshold	P	Q	Quality of Sensitivity	Quality of Efficiency	Quality of Specificity
Personality Disorder Examination (n=55)	≥15	0.38	0.82	1.00†	0.24	0.14
	≥26	0.38	0.65	0.86	0.42†	0.28
	≥45	0.38	0.20	0.23	0.32	0.56†
Structured Interview for *DSM-III-R* Personality (n=53)	≥13	0.43	0.81	1.00†	0.30	0.18
	≥33	0.43	0.40	0.57	0.61†	0.66
	≥41	0.43	0.25	0.37	0.51	0.86†

**Thresholds identifying the maximum quality of sensitivity, efficiency, and specificity are included and identified by daggers. P indicates the prevalence of any marked personality disorder by the diagnostic consensus; Q, the level of the test at each threshold.*

the patients receiving each interview) were diagnosed, either by the consensus or the interview. This constraint restricted the analysis primarily to cluster B and C disorders. The range of κ values for agreement on individual disorders was −0.16 to 0.51 (median=0.16) with the PDE and 0.04 to 0.64 (median=0.43) with the SIDP-R. Agreement at the level of any cluster A, B, or C diagnosis ranged from 0.15 to 0.23 with the PDE and 0.20 to 0.52 with the SIDP-R across the three clusters.

The statistical significance of the differences between the κ's with the two interviews was computed for all possible comparisons. Despite the apparent differences in the magnitude of some of the κ values, only one comparison approached significance: the agreement between interview and best-estimate consensus for the presence of any cluster C diagnosis (κ=0.52 [SIDP-R] vs κ=0.23 [PDE]) ($P<.10$). **Table 1** provides a summary of all the validity results, with additional information about the operating characteristics (sensitivity, specificity, positive predictive value, and negative predictive value) of both interviews at various levels of resolution (ie, any PD, any marked PD, cluster diagnosis, and specific PD diagnosis).

THRESHOLDS FOR CONTINUOUS SCORES

Given the excellent reliabilities of continuous scores from the interviews, thresholds on total scores from the PDE and the SIDP-R were examined as an alternative way of making categorical decisions about the presence of any PD or any marked PD. For this purpose, signal detection analyses were performed, using the quality receiver operating characteristics (QROC) method developed by Kraemer.[36] The QROC method provides "quality" measures of sensitivity, efficiency, and specificity that weight the impact of false negatives, any misses, and false positives (respectively) and that take into account the level of a test relative to the "true" prevalence of the disorder being diagnosed. These quality indices can be understood as weighted (in the case of sensitivity and specificity) and unweighted (in the case of efficiency) κ coefficients.

For these analyses, the average total score (ie, the sum of all item scores) across all judges available was used to maximize reliability. The range of these total scores on the PDE was 4.2 to 88.5 and on the SIDP-R, 1.0 to 79.0. Results from the QROC analyses are summarized in **Tables 2** and **3**. Scores of 25 or higher on the PDE (κ=0.42, 76% agreement) and 17 or higher on the SIDP-R (κ=0.53, 83% agreement) were the most efficient thresholds for identifying any PD. Total scores of 26 or higher on the PDE (κ=0.42, 69% agreement) and 33 or higher on the SIDP-R (κ=0.61, 81% agreement) were the most efficient thresholds for identifying any marked PD. Correlations between the consensus clinical judgment of Axis II severity and total scores on the PDE and SIDP-R were 0.50 and 0.66, respectively (both significant at $P<.01$). Again, there were no statistically significant differences between the interviews.

COMMENT

Among the most striking findings in the present sample were (1) the large prevalence of PDs (79% by our best-estimate diagnoses) and (2) the "blended" forms that such disorders took. With more conservative diagnostic criteria, the largest proportion of patients received mixed (or NOS) diagnoses, whereas with more liberal criteria, the largest proportion received multiple diagnoses that spanned the *DSM-III-R* clusters. These results are consistent with earlier work on the frequency of multiple diagnoses when assessing Axis II disorders,[5] and they continue to raise questions about the discriminant validity of the individual disorders in the current nosology. The large overall prevalence of Axis II diagnoses may have been inflated somewhat by the nature of the clinical research setting in which we work. Before "filtering" down to open-treatment settings at Western Psychiatric Institute and Clinic, many patients are screened for research protocols requiring "purer" manifestations of Axis I affective and anxiety problems, uncomplicated by substance abuse or marked personality disorder. Nonetheless, the results argue that one should be aware of the potentially important influence of Axis II disorders in samples ascertained in university-based tertiary care facilities.

Another theme that deserves emphasis is the relative advantages of continuous vs categorical data for personality assessment. Excellent reliabilities can be obtained with continuous measures; reliability is lessened by the imposition of categorical decision rules, especially in samples in which many cases are likely to be near the categorical threshold. Kraemer[37] provides a similar example of this phenomenon in a different context; in her data set, an intraclass correlation coefficient of .59 was deflated to a κ of 0.05 when a positive-vs-negative threshold was imposed on the data. Consistent with Kraemer's observation, our results illustrate the potential importance of determining reliability and validity for "tests" when used in new settings rather than relying on historical data alone. This caveat is especially relevant for signal detection analyses and other diagnostic operating characteristics (sensitivity, specificity, positive predictive value, and negative predictive value) influenced by differences in base rates.

In interpreting the results, an important ceiling effect must be acknowledged. The κ coefficient reflecting agreement among our yes/no votes at the diagnostic conference was 0.64, and this reliability coefficient constrains validity, ie, one cannot expect another judge, method, or instrument (PDE or SIDP-R) to agree more highly with our gold standard than we agreed among ourselves. Given this constraint, the QROC results for efficiency (0.42 with the PDE and 0.53 with the SIDP-R) take on a more positive cast. In any case, the use of continuous data analytic strategies (eg, signal detection analyses for determining diagnostic thresholds, regression approaches with total PD scores as a predictor, analyses of covariance with PD scores as a covariate) may be preferable to categorical strategies (eg, the use of personality diagnosis as a grouping variable, contingency table analyses) by virtue of greater reliability and enhanced power.

In summary, the results demonstrate that even with structured diagnostic techniques, reliability can be strongly influenced by characteristics of different samples. Structured interviews provide guides to diagnosis with the promise of more uniform case identification, but data generated by them should be considered carefully in terms of optimal case identification strategies for the purpose at hand. Applying the *DSM-III-R* decision rules, as operationalized by the developers of the instruments, may serve some purposes but not others.

Most important, the use of structured interviews should be linked to some external validator and not rely on face validity alone: " . . . explicit definition of the external validator being used would represent a marked improvement over current practice."[21(p204)] In the present case, the external validator was a clinical consensus diagnosis, and the agreement between the two methods was modest, probably because our clinical decisions were most swayed by historical variables and reports of social and interpersonal impairment, whereas the interviews focused more on reports about personality styles. Obviously, the use of a consensus diagnosis can be criticized as a validity standard, but the larger principle of using some external measure of criterion validity (eg, biological or genetic markers, family history, significant life outcomes, social role performance, response to alternative treatments) remains. One shortcoming in the use of structured interviews is that their applications expand on the basis of face validity alone, a limited approach to improving classification and taxonomy.

Finally, it should be pointed out that the issues we have emphasized are not unique to Axis II disorders. To cite only two examples (but examples that are especially relevant, given the concerns raised above), there have been thoughtful discussions of the difficulties involved in establishing the external validity of Axis I diagnoses[38] and in establishing accurate lifetime prevalence rates for Axis I disorders.[39]

Accepted for publication April 19, 1995.

This research was supported by grant MH44672 from the National Institute of Mental Health, Rockville, Md.

Joan Hick and Nicole LeViere scored the Axis II interviews and assisted with data entry.

Reprint requests to Western Psychiatric Institute and Clinic, 3811 O'Hara St, Pittsburgh, PA 15213 (Dr Pilkonis).

REFERENCES

1. American Psychiatric Association. *Diagnostic and Statistical Manual of Mental Disorders, Revised Third Edition.* Washington, DC: American Psychiatric Association; 1987.
2. Livesley WJ, Jackson DN. Guidelines for developing, evaluating, and revising the classification of personality disorders. *J Nerv Ment Dis.* 1992;180:609-618.
3. Morey LC. The categorical representation of personality disorder: a cluster analysis of *DSM-III-R* personality features. *J Abnorm Psychol.* 1988;97:314-321.
4. Miller HR, Streiner DL, Parkinson A. Maximum likelihood estimates of the ability of the MMPI and MCMI personality disorder scales and the SIDP to identify personality disorders. *J Pers Assess.* 1992;59:1-13.
5. Oldham JM, Skodol AE, Kellman HD, Hyler SE, Rosnick L, Davies M. Diagnosis of *DSM-III-R* personality disorders by two structured interviews: patterns of comorbidity. *Am J Psychiatry.* 1992;149:213-220.
6. Perry JC. Problems and considerations in the valid assessment of personality disorders. *Am J Psychiatry.* 1992;149:1645-1653.

7. Pilkonis PA, Heape CL, Ruddy J, Serrao P. Validity in the diagnosis of personality disorders: the use of the LEAD standard. *Psychol Assess J Consult Clin Psychol.* 1991;3:46-54.
8. Renneberg B, Chambless DL, Dowdall DJ, Fauerbach JA, Gracely EJ. The Structured Clinical Interview for *DSM-III-R*, Axis II and the Millon Clinical Multiaxial Inventory: a concurrent validity study of personality disorders among anxious outpatients. *J Pers Disord.* 1992;6:117-124.
9. Zimmerman M. Diagnosing personality disorders: a review of issues and research methods. *Arch Gen Psychiatry.* 1994;51:225-245.
10. Goldberg D. A classification of psychological distress for use in primary care settings. *Soc Sci Med.* 1992;35:189-193.
11. Loranger AW. *Personality Disorder Examination (PDE) Manual.* Yonkers, NY: DV Communications; 1988.
12. Loranger AW, Lenzenweger MF, Gartner AF, Susman VL, Herzig J, Zammit GK, Gartner JD, Abrams RC, Young RC. Trait-state artifacts and the diagnosis of personality disorders. *Arch Gen Psychiatry.* 1991;48:720-728.
13. Loranger AW, Susman VL, Oldham JM, Russakoff LM. The Personality Disorder Examination: a preliminary report. *J Pers Disord.* 1987;1:1-13.
14. Pfohl B, Blum N, Zimmerman M, Stangl D. *Structured Interview for* DSM-III-R *Personality (SIDP-R).* Iowa City: University of Iowa, Dept of Psychiatry; 1989.
15. Stangl D, Pfohl B, Zimmerman M, Bowers W, Corenthal C. A structured interview for the *DSM-III* personality disorders: a preliminary report. *Arch Gen Psychiatry.* 1985;42:591-596.
16. Spitzer RL, Williams JBW, Gibbon M, First MB. *Structured Clinical Interview for* DSM-III-R *Personality Disorders (SCID-II, 9/1/89 version).* New York, NY: Biometrics Research Dept, New York State Psychiatric Institute; 1989.
17. Arntz A, van Beijsterveldt B, Hoekstra R, Hofman A, Eussen M, Sallaerts S. The interrater reliability of a Dutch version of the Structured Clinical Interview for *DSM-III-R* Personality Disorders. *Acta Psychiatr Scand.* 1992;85: 394-400.
18. Brent DA, Zelenak JP, Bukstein O, Brown RV. Reliability and validity of the Structured Interview for Personality Disorders in adolescents. *J Am Acad Child Adolesc Psychiatry.* 1990;29:349-354.
19. O'Boyle M, Self D. A comparison of two interviews for *DSM-III-R* personality disorders. *Psychiatry Res.* 1990;32:85-92.
20. Standage K, Ladha N. An examination of the reliability of the Personality Disorder Examination and a comparison with other methods of identifying personality disorders in a clinical sample. *J Pers Disord.* 1988;2:267-271.
21. Zarin DA, Earls F. Diagnostic decision making in psychiatry. *Am J Psychiatry.* 1993;150:197-206.
22. Leckman JF, Sholomskas D, Thompson WD, Belanger A, Weissman MM. Best estimate of lifetime psychiatric diagnosis: a methodological study. *Arch Gen Psychiatry.* 1982;39:879-883.
23. Kosten TA, Rounsaville BJ. Sensitivity of psychiatric diagnosis based on the best estimate procedure. *Am J Psychiatry.* 1992;149:1225-1227.
24. Spitzer RL. Psychiatric diagnosis: are clinicians still necessary? *Compr Psychiatry.* 1983;24:399-411.
25. Skodol AE, Rosnick L, Kellman D, Oldham JM, Hyler SE. Validating structured *DSM-III-R* personality disorder assessments with longitudinal data. *Am J Psychiatry.* 1988;145:1297-1299.
26. Skodol AE, Oldham JM, Rosnick L, Kellman D, Hyler SE. Diagnosis of *DSM-III-R* personality disorders: a comparison of two structured interviews. *Int J Methods Psychiatr Res.* 1991;1:13-26.
27. Overholser JC. Aggregation of personality measures: implications for personality disorder research. *J Pers Disord.* 1992;6:267-277.
28. Widiger TA, Hurt SW, Frances A, Clarkin JF, Gilmore M. Diagnostic efficiency and *DSM-III. Arch Gen Psychiatry.* 1984;41:1005-1012.
29. Spitzer RL, Williams JBW, Gibbon M, First MB. *Structured Clinical Interview for DSM-III-R: Patient Edition With Psychotic Screen (SCID-P w/Psychotic Screen, 9/1/89 version).* New York, NY: Biometrics Research Dept, New York State Psychiatric Institute; 1989.
30. Hamilton M. The assessment of anxiety states by rating. *Br J Med Psychol.* 1959;32:50-55.
31. Hamilton M. A rating scale for depression. *J Neurol Neurosurg Psychiatry.* 1960;23:56-62.
32. Pilkonis PA, Heape CL, Proietti JM, Smith K. Prototypes of adult attachment styles: reliability of clinical judgments and validity in predicting treatment outcomes in depression. Presented at the Meeting of the Society for Psychotherapy Research; July 21, 1991; Lyons, France.
33. Endicott J, Spitzer RL, Fleiss JL, Cohen J. The Global Assessment Scale: a procedure for measuring overall severity of psychiatric disturbance. *Arch Gen Psychiatry.* 1976;33:766-771.
34. Fleiss J. *The Design and Analysis of Clinical Experiments.* New York, NY: John Wiley & Sons Inc; 1986.
35. Cohen J. A coefficient of agreement for nominal scales. *Educ Psychol Measurement.* 1960;20:37-46.
36. Kraemer HC. *Evaluating Medical Tests: Objective and Quantitative Guidelines.* Newbury Park, Calif: Sage Publications; 1992.
37. Kraemer HC. Measures of agreement. In: Kotz S, Johnson NL, Read CB, eds. *Encyclopedia of Statistical Sciences.* New York, NY: John Wiley & Sons Inc; 1985;5:389-391.
38. Kendler KS. Toward a scientific nosology: strengths and limitations. *Arch Gen Psychiatry.* 1990;47:969-973.
39. Parker G. Are the lifetime prevalence estimates in the ECA study accurate? *Psychol Med.* 1987;17:275-282.

Perceived Coercion in Mental Hospital Admission

Pressures and Process

Charles W. Lidz, PhD; Steven K. Hoge, MD; William Gardner, PhD; Nancy S. Bennett, MA; John Monahan, PhD; Edward P. Mulvey, PhD; Loren H. Roth, MD, MPH

Background: Patients' perceptions of coercion in admission may affect their attitude toward subsequent treatment, including their inclination to adhere to treatment plans. This study looks at the determinants of patients' perceptions of coercion.

Methods: A sample of 157 patients admitted to a rural Virginia state hospital and a Pennsylvania community hospital were interviewed within 48 hours of admission about their experience of coming to the hospital. All subjects were 17 years or older. Diagnoses were diverse, and 42% were involuntarily committed. The interview gathered an open-ended description of the admission experience followed by a structured interview that included several measures.

Results: Perceptions of being respectfully included in a fair decision-making process ("procedural justice") and legal status were most closely associated with perceived coercion, and a significant relationship was found with perceived negative pressures, ie, force and threats. However, only procedural justice was related to the perception of coercion at both sites and with both voluntary and involuntary patients.

Conclusions: Patients' feelings of being coerced concerning admission appears to be closely related to their sense of procedural justice. It may be that clinicians can minimize the experience of coercion even among those legally committed by attending more closely to procedural justice issues.

(Arch Gen Psychiatry. 1995;52:1034-1039)

PERHAPS NO issue in mental health law and policy has been so controversial as the use of coercion to assure that people with mental illness receive treatment. At least since Pinel unchained asylum inmates, many have believed that coercion is an undesirable way to treat people with mental illnesses. Nevertheless, there has been a consistent public demand that enforced treatment be available for dealing with some persons with mental illness.[1]

Modern psychiatric care is far from Pinel's era, but mental hospitalization against the expressed wishes of a patient continues to be controversial. Patient advocates and libertarians have often pressed for the abolition of commitment or, failing that, a narrowing of the criteria for involuntary hospitalization.[2-4] The mental health professions and family groups have with equal fervor and, in recent years with more success, lobbied that civil commitment be maintained, often with broadened criteria.[5-8]

Most research on coercion has assumed that being coerced is identical to having the legal status "involuntarily committed." Because the debate has largely focused on the legitimacy of involuntary commitment, this appears reasonable. However, several studies suggest that equating coercion with involuntary commitment may prevent us from seeing other coercive pressures that come to bear on patients when they are hospitalized.[9,10]

The pathbreaking study by Gilboy and Schmidt[11] described the variety of coercive pressures that came to bear on "voluntary patients" in Cook County, Illinois.

> In a majority of cases in which voluntary admission procedures were used, the individuals were already under some form of official custody and were faced with the threat of involuntary commitment proceedings as the principal alternative to voluntary admission.

See Methods on next page

From the Department of Psychiatry, Western Psychiatric Institute and Clinic, University of Pittsburgh (Pa) (Drs Lidz, Gardner, Mulvey, and Roth); the School of Law, University of Virginia, Charlottesville (Drs Hoge and Monahan). Ms Bennett resides in Bronx, NY.

METHODS

SAMPLE

Between June and December 1991, 157 patients were recruited. All the subjects were interviewed within 48 hours after being admitted to a psychiatric hospital. The sample was selected consecutively except when a large number of patients were admitted and could not be interviewed within the time limit or when patients' involvement with treatment precluded their taking time for the interview. Patients with diagnoses of dementia or more than mild mental retardation were excluded because of difficulties completing the interview. All the subjects gave informed consent and were paid $10 for the interview; a small number refused. Most (102 [65%]) of these subjects entered a community-based general psychiatric facility in Pennsylvania; 55 (35%) entered a rural state hospital in Virginia. The two facilities differed both as to the types of patients and the hospital's admission procedures. However, both served as the primary inpatient facility for their geographic areas. Two interviewers in Pennsylvania and one in Virginia were trained together, including observing each others' interviews and periodically reviewing audiotapes of each others' interviews.

Table 1 describes the samples at the two sites. Pennsylvania patients were more likely to be African American ($\chi^2[1]=29.14$, $P=.001$) and less likely to be diagnosed with schizophrenia ($\chi^2[4]=14.53$, $P=.001$). In the overall sample, 42% of the patients were involuntarily committed; 87% of the Virginia state hospital patients were involuntarily committed compared with only 18% of the Pennsylvania community hospital patients ($\chi^2[1]=74.56$, $P=.001$).

When compared with data for all patients at their respective sites, the samples were similar except that the Virginia sample underrepresented African Americans ($\chi^2[1]=14.27$, $P<.001$) and the Pennsylvania sample overrepresented African Americans ($\chi^2[1]=6.72$, $P<.01$). The Pennsylvania sample also had a mean age that was about 3 years younger than the site as a whole ($t[1501]=2.93$, $P<.01$), probably reflecting the exclusion of older, demented patients.

MEASURES

Each patient was administered the MacArthur Admission Experience Interview,[16] a semistructured interview that focused on the patients' perceptions of (1) coercion in the decision to be admitted, (2) the nature of any pressures brought to bear on them to be hospitalized, and (3) the ways they were treated by others during the process of coming to the hospital and being admitted.

The initial part of the interview was open-ended. In it, patients were encouraged to describe their experiences of coming to the hospital. The second part of the interview included structured questions in which the patient chose from predetermined answer sets. This interview yielded several scores reflecting the above aspects of the admission process.

Perceived Coercion

In a previous article,[16] we reported psychometric analyses of four questions in the MacArthur Admission Experience Interview that compose the MacArthur Perceived Coercion Scale. These questions focus on influence ("What had more influence on your being admitted: what you wanted or what others wanted?"), control ("How much control did you have . . . ?"), choice ("You chose?" or "someone made you?"), and freedom ("How free did you feel to do what you wanted . . . ?"). These questions were weighted using a principal components analysis to yield a 1-to-5 scale of perceived coercion, with higher values indicating more perceived coercion (mean=1.75, SD=2.07).

Pressures

We also asked patients about the occurrence of four different ways in which others might have tried to influence the decision about hospitalization ("pressures"). The pressures were persuasion ("Did anyone try to talk you into going to the hospital or being admitted?"), inducement ("Did anyone offer or promise you something?"), threats ("Did anyone threaten you?"), and force ("Did anyone try to force you?"). All of these questions had dichotomous yes/no answers. If the patient answered yes, he or she was asked which person or persons had used the pressures.

Procedural Justice

Finally, to measure the patients' views of the procedural justice of the admission, we asked the patients four questions about how they were treated by particular persons involved in the admission and two questions about their perceptions of the admission process as a whole.

First, for every person whom the patient named as being involved in any way with the decision, we asked four procedural justice questions about his or her involvement. These questions involved motivation ("To what extent did s/he do what s/he did out of concern for you?—very much, mostly, a little, not at all"), respect ("How much respect did s/he treat you with?—very, some, a little, none"), validation ("How seriously did s/he consider what you had to say?—very, some, a little, none"), and fairness ("How fairly did s/he treat you?—very fair, mostly fair, mostly unfair, very unfair"). Because there were different numbers of participants in different cases, for each question we averaged across the identified participants to generate case-level values for motivation, respect, validation, and fairness shown by others toward the patient. The sample means and SDs of these case-level scores were as follows: motivation (mean=1.64, SD=0.78), respect (mean=1.53, SD=0.66), validation (mean=1.73, SD=0.88), and fairness (mean=1.63, SD=0.79).

We also asked two general questions reflecting aspects of procedural justice: voice ("How much of a chance did you have to say what you wanted to about being admitted to the hospital?—very, some, a little, none") (mean=1.97, SD=1.19) and deception ("Did anyone try to trick you, lie to you, or fool you into coming into the hospital?"—yes/no) (80.8%, no).

STATISTICAL ANALYSIS

Principal components analysis was used to create a summative scale from the six questions related to procedural justice. Multiple regression analysis was used to assess the degree to which procedural justice and other variables were associated with perceived coercion. All *t* tests are based on separate variance estimates.[28]

Table 1. Demographic and Diagnostic Characteristics of the Sample by Site

	Virginia (n=55)	Pennsylvania (n=102)	Total Sample (N=157)
Mean age, y	34.2	31.7	32.5
Gender, % male	67.3	53.9	58.6
% Currently married	14.5	11.8	12.2
Mean education, y	12.0	12.3	12.2
Race, % African American	12.7	54.9	40.1*
Diagnosis, %†			
Schizophrenia	23.4	6.9	12.1
Affective disorder	12.8	19.6	17.4
Substance abuse	25.5	54.9	45.7
Personality disorder	4.3	12.8	10.1
Other disorder	34.0	5.9	14.8‡
% Involuntarily committed	87.3	17.8	42.0§

*χ^2 [1]=26.45, P<.001.
†All diagnoses are admission diagnoses based on DSM-III-R.
‡χ^2 [4]=29.75, P<.001.
§χ^2 [3]=75.21, P<.001.

Their study has since been replicated.[12] As Brakel et al[13] comment, "the voluntary-involuntary distinction is in application quite blurred."

Several other studies suggest that patients' perceptions of coercion do not always correspond with legal status. We have shown elsewhere (S.K.H. et al, unpublished data) that a significant portion of formally committed patients did not feel coerced and that a somewhat smaller proportion of the legally voluntary patients felt coerced. Others have found that many legally involuntary patients do not report the negative experiences usually associated with coercion. Bradford et al[14] reported that, interviewed 1 week after admission, almost two thirds of a sample of committed patients stated that they would recommend hospitalization to a mentally ill friend. Candefjord[15] reports similar findings from Sweden. In summary, patients' perceptions of coercion do not always match their legal status.[16]

Perceived coercion, however, is not simply important for its own sake. Several writers have argued that people with mental illness would be more likely to stay involved with treatment if they did not feel coerced.[3,4] Thus, if the perception of coercion could be diminished, even if the number of involuntary commitments could not be decreased, some of the negative effects of coercion might be minimized. Unfortunately, research toward this goal has been hindered by the absence of a conceptually distinct measure of patients' perceptions of coercion that is more than a proxy for legal status. Recently we have reported the development of a psychometrically consistent measure of patients' perceptions of coercion,[17] which we have used in this research.

If we accept the premise that it is the patient's perception of coercion rather than only the patient's formal legal status that needs to be understood, then one important task is to determine how different aspects of a patient's experience, including legal status, contribute to the feeling of being coerced. There are three factors that might contribute to a perception of coercion. The first is actions by others that are intended to influence the subject to enter the hospital, which we will call "pressures."[4,18] For example, it may be that people who are admitted under a legally voluntary status, but who have been threatened by others with negative consequences if they do not enter, feel that the choice about admission is a false one.

A second possibility is that individuals from different demographic and/or cultural groups experience hospitalization and commitment differently so that the differences in perceived coercion are partially differences in interpretations of the experience. For example, some current theorists of gender might hypothesize that women experience commitment more as a threat to their interpersonal relationships, whereas men might see it largely as a threat to their autonomy.[19] Similarly, different geopolitical areas have different legal and administrative procedures for hospitalization[13,20] that may be related to feelings about coercion among people with mental illness in different areas.

Finally, some critics argue that patients feel coerced because they are not listened to, they are treated disrespectfully, and their views are ignored.[3] In support of this view, Shannon[21] found that patients who felt coerced were much less likely to think that the staff would be helpful or that they needed and would get treatment. Patients reported negative perceptions about deception and not having a "say in what was happening to them."[21] We have reported elsewhere that, in open-ended interviews, patients often seemed as concerned about the motives and intentions of those with whom they interacted as they were with their legal status or what pressures were placed on them.[22] Following the work of Thibaut and Walker[23] and others,[24-27] who have shown that there are strong procedural components to our perceptions of justice and fairness, we will call these "procedural justice" issues.

This study describes the degree to which each of these sets of variables is associated with patients' reports of coercion.

RESULTS

PROCEDURAL JUSTICE SCALE

Correlations among the six questions concerning procedural justice (the four averaged values and the two general questions) ranged between .37 and .77. A principal components analysis yielded a single factor with an eigenvalue greater than 1, accounting for 64% of the variance in these questions. A procedural justice scale was calculated by summing the weighted standardized scores for the above questions to yield a score ranging between 1 and 5, with the higher scores indicating more procedural justice.

PRESSURES

Many patients reported little pressure to admit themselves. Almost half of the patients (46%) reported no pressures of any type. However, 38% reported persuasion and

Table 2. Correlation Matrix of Predictor Variables

	Age	Procedural Justice	Legal Status	Negative Pressures	Positive Pressures	Race	Gender	Site
Procedural justice	.140							
Legal status	.034	−.496*						
Negative pressures	−.102	−.596*	.344*					
Positive pressures	−.097	.121	−.150	.046				
Race	−.083	.169†	−.231‡	−.148†	.083			
Gender	−.063	−.021	.123	.084	−.083	−.083		
Site	−.127	.337*	−.659*	−.202‡	.197†	.394*	−.141	
Perceived coercion	−.060	−.720*	.621*	.555*	−.038	−.200‡	.052	−.314*

*$P \leq .01$ level (two tailed).
†$P \leq .05$ level.
‡$P \leq .01$ level.

19% reported force. Since only 9% reported threats and 4% reported inducements, we collapsed together, for analytic purposes, persuasion and inducements into "positive" pressures and threats and force into "negative" pressures. Pressure was positive when someone sought to show that a patient would be better off if he or she was admitted. Pressure was negative when someone either indicated that a patient would be worse off if the patient resisted admission or removed the choice from the patient altogether. The tabulation below shows the frequencies of these pressures.

Pressures	No. (%) of Cases
None	72 (45.9)
Positive only	49 (31.2)
Negative only	19 (12.1)
Both positive and negative	17 (10.8)
Total	**157 (100)**

Of course, patients did not report just one type of pressure or one instance of the same pressure. Some cases involved several people placing pressures on them and some people used more than one type of pressure. Patients reported a mean of 0.99 (SD=1.37) pressures per case, including a mean of 0.62 (SD=0.95) positive pressures per case and 0.37 (SD=0.83) negative pressures. Nonetheless, both positive and negative pressures are measured dichotomously (present/absent) in subsequent analyses since no significant information appears to be added by more complex measures.

DETERMINANTS OF PERCEIVED COERCION

The primary goal of this analysis was to describe the association of the perceived coercion scale with case characteristics other than legal status, ie, demographic variables, pressures, and procedural justice. We will begin by describing the bivariate relationships between these case characteristics and perceived coercion.

Perceived coercion was not related to gender (mean for males=1.84, SD=2.00; mean for females=1.62, SD=2.19) ($t[155]=-0.64$, $P=.53$). The correlation for age was −.060 with perceived coercion, which is not significant. Site was significantly related to perceived coercion, with the Virginia state hospital perceived as more coercive than the Pennsylvania community hospital (Virginia: mean=2.69, SD=2.32; Pennsylvania: mean=1.24, SD=1.74) ($t[155]=4.41$, $P<.001$). Race was related to perceived coercion. The mean score for whites (mean=2.11, SD=2.21) was higher compared with African Americans (mean=1.21, SD=1.73) ($t[155]=2.73$, $P<.007$). However, when site is entered into an analysis of variance with race, only the main effect for site is significant and there is no significant interaction between the variables.

Table 2 presents a correlation matrix of the predictors of perceived coercion with each other and with perceived coercion. Clearly, procedural justice, negative pressures, site, and legal status are all strongly related to perceived coercion and to each other. Therefore, we did three separate regression analyses to assess the unique contributions to perceived coercion of three different variables: negative pressures, positive pressures, and procedural justice. For the three regressions, we first entered patients' legal status, demographic variables, site, and two of the three variables of interest (negative pressures, positive pressures, and procedural justice). We then tested whether the third variable of interest explained any of the remaining variance in perceived coercion by entering the specific variable of interest for that regression. This procedure shows that procedural justice makes a significant unique contribution ($t[143]=6.89$, $P<.001$) and adds 11% to the proportion of the variance explained with the other variables controlled. Negative pressures also contribute a significant amount of unique variance to the equation ($t[143]=2.37$, $P<.02$) and add 1% to the unique variance explained with the other variables controlled. Positive pressures do not uniquely contribute significantly to the equation ($t[143]=1.00$, $P<.40$). Clearly, when demographic variables and legal status are controlled, procedural justice is by far the strongest predictor of perceived coercion. Negative pressures were also substantially related to perceived coercion but less strongly than procedural justice; positive pressures were not related at all.

PERCEIVED COERCION, SITE, AND LEGAL STATUS

Because site and legal status were substantially related to each other and some of the predictors as well as to perceived coercion, a fourth regression was done to exam-

Table 3. Regression Analysis of Perceived Coercion With Interaction Terms Included*

Variables in Final Step	β	t	P
Procedural justice	−0.65	−6.23	.001
Site	−0.63	−2.72	.007
Negative pressures	−0.44	−1.99	.05
Legal status	0.10	0.82	.41
Legal status/negative pressures interaction	0.35	3.06	.003
Legal status/site interaction	0.31	3.31	.001
Procedural justice/site interaction	0.60	2.89	.005
Procedural justice/negative pressures interaction	0.35	2.36	.02
Procedural justice/legal status interaction	−0.06	−0.21	.83
Site/negative pressures interaction	−0.07	−0.59	.56

*R^2=.68, df=148.

Table 4. Regression Analysis of Perceived Coercion by Patient Status

Variables in Final Step	β	t	P
Voluntary Patients*			
Site	−0.05	0.46	.65
Negative pressures	0.05	0.47	.64
Procedural justice	−0.26	−2.34	.02
Involuntary Patients†			
Site	0.26	3.28	.002
Procedural justice	−4.78	−4.51	.001
Negative pressures	0.33	2.89	.002

*R^2=.07, df=87.
†R^2=.61, df=62.

ine whether the association of procedural justice and negative pressures varied across legal status or site. We entered all the significant variables from the previous analysis: procedural justice, site, legal status, and negative pressures along with interaction terms for all possible combinations of those variables. **Table 3** shows the final step of this regression. As in the prior analyses, procedural justice, site, and negative pressures were associated with perceived coercion. However, legal status is not significant when the interaction between legal status and site is entered into the equation. The strong association between legal status and site, as seen in the bivariate *r* of −.659 (Table 1), makes it quite difficult to disentangle their respective impacts on perceived coercion.

To clarify these interaction effects, we repeated the regressions separately for the voluntary and involuntary patients (**Table 4**) and for Pennsylvania and Virginia patients (**Table 5**). In the regression equation for involuntary patients, procedural justice, negative pressures, and site were all significant and accounted for 60.7% of the variance. The regression for voluntary patients, in contrast, accounted for only 7% of the variance and only procedural justice contributed significantly. Neither site nor negative pressures are significantly related to perceived coercion after the variance for procedural justice is removed. The weakness of the relationship between the predictors and perceived coercion in this regression results from the lack of variance

Table 5. Regression Analysis of Perceived Coercion by Patient Site

Variables in Final Step	β	t	P
Pennsylvania Patients*			
Legal status	0.61	8.69	.001
Negative pressures	0.10	1.44	.15
Procedural justice	−0.22	−3.00	.003
Virginia Patients†			
Legal status	0.07	0.81	.42
Procedural justice	−4.78	−4.42	.001
Negative pressures	0.33	2.84	.007

*R^2=.64, df=98.
†R^2=.66, df=51.

among the voluntary patients in perceived coercion (s^2 [voluntaries]=1.04, s^2 [involuntaries]=4.61) and the predictor variables (procedural justice: s^2 [voluntaries]=0.23, s^2 [involuntaries]=1.41; negative pressures: s^2 [voluntaries]=0.09, s^2 [involuntaries]=0.22). By and large, the voluntary patients perceived themselves as autonomous decision makers who were treated justly.

Pennsylvania patients' perceptions of coercion were significantly predicted by both procedural justice and legal status (Table 5, top). These two variables accounted for 64.1% of the variance. Procedural justice was also a significant component of the equation that predicted 65.7% of the variance in the Virginia patients, as were negative pressures (Table 5, bottom). Legal status, however, was not predictive because of the lack of variance in legal status (Table 1).

COMMENT

These findings clarify how patients experience their admission to a mental hospital. First, there was wide variation in patients' perceptions of the level of coercion in the hospitalization process. These perceptions were independent of age, sex, and race (when site was controlled for). Indeed, it is somewhat surprising the demographic factors do not appear to be related to patients' perceptions of coercion in any way.

Another surprising finding is that while legal status was strongly related to perceived coercion on a bivariate basis, at the Virginia site, legal status was not predictive of perceived coercion. Do the data suggest that legal status is not related to coercion? Not at all. At the Pennsylvania site, where most patients were voluntary and described themselves as not coerced, legal status was a strong predictor of which patients described themselves as coerced. At the Virginia site, it was not a useful predictor because, while there was considerable variability of perceived coercion, there was little variance in legal status. This suggests that legal status may be a reasonable measure of patients' perceptions of coercion in some sites but not in others and that it should be used as such only with considerable care.

In contrast, the procedural justice aspect of admission was related to patients' perceptions of coercion in all of our analyses. This was true for no other variable. Consistent with the literature on procedural justice,[22-26] the way a person felt that he or she was treated in terms of respect, validation, voice, and related aspects of the interaction was consistently associated with the perception of coercion. It is interesting, however, that procedural justice had such a substantial impact on the perception of coercion of the involuntary patients. This suggests that the use of legal commitment can be at least partially accepted by some people with mental illness *if* they feel that they have been treated with respect, concern, and fairness in the process.

Positive pressures (persuasion and inducement) were not related to perceptions of coercion. Efforts to persuade or induce patients may have bothered or annoyed patients but they apparently do not produce feelings of coercion. However, among involuntary patients, negative pressures were predictive of perceived coercion. Involuntarily committed patients appear to relate their perceptions of coercion to things other than just legal status.

Several limitations of this study should be kept in mind in its interpretation. First, the sample is relatively small. Some relationships that do not appear significant might appear so in a larger sample. Second, it is based on only two sites and there were substantial differences among them. Clearly, studies of more sites would be advantageous. Third, this study describes how patients thought about the experience of hospitalization and the role of coercion in it. Because all the data we have discussed came from one-time interviews with patients, we can see only the ways in which they describe their experience. We cannot know whether the patients reported the facts about the process of admission nor can we treat the associations in these data as causal. To achieve more certainty about what happened would require a triangulation of documentary evidence of coercion with the reports of other parties involved in the decision making about hospitalization, such as family members and hospital staff.[29]

In spite of the above concerns, we note that how involuntary patients were dealt with during their admission had a major impact on their perceptions about coercion. This strongly suggests that clinicians would be well advised to attend to the manner in which they admit patients, particularly those admitted involuntarily. Those patient activists who have suggested that the process of admission does not validate and respect patients may be surprised by our findings that many patients feel good about the process of admission. However, our findings provide considerable support for the contention by such advocates that admitting patients with respect and dignity can affect patients' assessments of the admission experience.[2-4]

It is important to remember that the consequences of coercion are not the only concern and that many believe that coercion is wrong because it violates inherent human rights. Nonetheless, by opening up the process of the admission to the patient's point of view and being respectful and attentive to his or her suggestions and concerns, some of the negative consequences of coercion might be mitigated.

Accepted for publication August 2, 1995.

We are grateful for the support of this research by the John D. and Catherine T. MacArthur Foundation Research Network on Mental Health and the Law.

Reprint requests to Department of Psychiatry, University of Pittsburgh School of Medicine, Western Psychiatric Institute and Clinic, 3811 O'Hara St, Pittsburgh, PA 15213 (Dr Lidz).

REFERENCES

1. McCandless P. Liberty and lunacy: the Victorians and wrongful confinement. In: Scull A, ed. *Madhouses, Mad Doctors and Madmen.* Philadelphia: University of Pennsylvania Press; 1981.
2. Morse S. A preference for liberty: the case against involuntary commitment of the mentally disordered. *Calif Law Rev.* 1988;70:54-106.
3. Blanch A, Parrish J. Alternatives to involuntary interventions: perspectives of consumers/survivors. *Psychiatr Rehabil Community Support Monogr.* 1990;1:17-34.
4. Parrish J. Involuntary use of interventions: pros and cons. *Innovations Res.* 1993;2:15-21.
5. Hoge SK, Appelbaum P, Geller J. Involuntary treatment. In: Tasman A, Hales RE, Frances AJ, eds. *American Psychiatric Press: Annual Review of Psychiatry.* Washington, DC: American Psychiatric Press; 1989;8:432-450.
6. Geller J. Rx: a tincture of coercion in outpatient treatment. *Hosp Community Psychiatry.* 1991;42:678-679.
7. Group for the Advancement of Psychiatry: Committee on Government Policy. *Forced Into Treatment.* Washington, DC: American Psychiatric Press; 1994. Report No. 137.
8. Appelbaum PS. *Almost a Revolution.* New York, NY: Oxford University Press; 1994.
9. Hiday V. Coercion in civil commitment: processes, preferences and outcome. *Int J Law Psychiatry.* 1992;15:359-377.
10. Lidz CW, Mulvey EP, Arnold RM, Bennett NS, Kirsch MA. Coercive interactions in a psychiatry emergency room. *Behav Sci Law.* 1993;11:269-280.
11. Gilboy J, Schmidt J. 'Voluntary' hospitalization of the mentally ill. *Northwestern Univ Law Rev.* 1971;66:452.
12. Lewis D, Goets E, Schoenfield M, Gordon A, Griffin E. The negotiation of involuntary civil commitment. *Law Society Rev.* 1984;18:629-949.
13. Brakel J, Parry J, Weiner B. *The Mentally Disabled and the Law.* 3rd ed. Chicago, Ill: American Bar Foundation; 1985:50.
14. Bradford B, McCann S, Mersky H. A survey of involuntary patients attitudes toward their commitment. *Psychiatr J Univ Ottawa.* 1986;11:162-165.
15. Candefjord T-L. Studier av psykiatrisk vård, särskilt tvångsvård i tvårdsvenska län. De psykiatiska patienternas upplevelse av tvångsvård. *Nord Psykiatr Tidsskr.* 1989;43:353-356.
16. Monahan J, Hoge SK, Lidz CW, Roth LH, Bennett NS, Gardner WP, Mulvey EP. Coercion and commitment: understanding involuntary mental hospital admission. *Int J Law Psychiatry.* 1995;18:1-15.
17. Gardner W, Hoge SK, Bennett N, Roth LH, Lidz CW, Monahan J, Mulvey EP. Two scales for measuring coercion during mental hospital admission. *Behav Sci Law.* 1993;11:307-322.
18. Rogers A. Coercion and 'voluntary' admission: an examination of psychiatric patient views. *Behav Sci Law.* 1993;11:259-268.
19. Tannen D. *You Just Don't Understand: Men and Women in Conversation.* New York, NY: Ballantine Books; 1990.
20. Reicher-Rossler A, Rossler W. Compulsory admission of psychiatric patients: an international comparison. *Acta Psychiatr Scand.* 1993;87:231-236.
21. Shannon P. Coercion and compulsory hospitalization: some patient attitudes. *Med J Aust.* 1976;2:798-800.
22. Bennett NS, Lidz CW, Monahan J, Mulvey EP, Hoge SK, Roth LH, Gardner WP. Inclusion, motivation and good faith: the morality of coercion in mental hospital admission. *Behav Sci Law.* 1993;11:295-306.
23. Thibaut J, Walker L. *Procedural Justice: A Psychological Analysis.* Hillsdale, NJ: Lawrence Erlbaum Associates; 1975.
24. Tyler T. *Why People Obey the Law.* New Haven, Conn: Yale University Press; 1990.
25. Tyler T. The psychological consequences of judicial procedures: implications for civil commitment hearings. *South Methodist Univ Law Rev.* 1992;46:433-445.
26. Lind E, Kanfer R, Early P. Voice, control and procedural justice: instrumental and noninstrumental concerns in fairness judgments. *J Pers Soc Psychol.* 1990; 20:952-959.
27. Lind E, Tyler T. *The Social Psychology of Procedural Justice.* New York, NY: Plenum Press; 1988.
28. Wilcox R. *New Statistical Procedures for the Social Sciences.* Hillsdale, NJ: Lawrence Erlbaum Associates; 1987:120.
29. Hoge SK, Lidz CW, Mulvey EP, Roth LH, Bennett NS, Siminoff LA, Arnold RM, Monahan J. Patient, family and staff perceptions of coercion in mental hospital admission: an exploratory study. *Behav Sci Law.* 1993;11:281-294.

ORIGINAL ARTICLE

Signs of Defensive Control Locate Conflicted Topics in Discourse

Mardi J. Horowitz, MD; Constance Milbrath, PhD; Charles H. Stinson, MD

Background: Psychodynamic clinicians cite defensive actions observed in evaluation and treatment as a source of important information. Empirical support for such assertions has seldom been based on objective study of recorded psychotherapy. A quantitative study of the association of signs of defensive control with disclosure of conflicted beliefs was undertaken.

Methods: Brief dynamic psychotherapies of two patients with pathological grief reactions were recorded and reviewed by independent judges. Periods of heightened defensive control of verbal and nonverbal communication were quantified using operational definitions. Reliably scored defensive episodes were algorithmically selected by computer programs. The people and topics discussed by patients were independently scored.

Results: Highly defensive periods contained disproportionately more frequent instances of patient discourse about people involved in conflict and unresolved topics.

Conclusions: The findings support the psychodynamic hypothesis that observation of defensive behaviors may locate times of communication about conflicted themes.

(Arch Gen Psychiatry. 1995;52:1040-1047)

From the Department of Psychiatry, University of California, San Francisco.

PSYCHODYNAMIC approaches emphasize observation for signs of defensive avoidance that might occur more frequently near those moments when conflicted topics are partially expressed and partially hidden. Cognitive-behavioral approaches attend to the patient's patterns of noncompliance with the therapist's suggestions.[1] Such noncompliance, especially noncompliance with instructions to provide frank discourse of beliefs, may be similar to psychodynamic observations of defensiveness. Issues of defense could be integrated in a combined psychodynamic and cognitive-behavioral perspective. We have approached that integration empirically by developing methods for assessing communication signs that signal defensive control processes.

Psychodynamic research on defensiveness takes two primary approaches. One defines and assesses categories of defensive mechanisms,[2,3] and the other observes multiple features of communication to define signs of resistance in the treatment processes.[4] In the immediacy of clinical sessions, such signs include verbal and nonverbal actions. We hypothesized that the quantitative location of such signs of defensive control processes would locate times when patients were more likely to partially express unresolved topics. Empirical evidence for this hypothesis would in turn support a theoretical construct of defensiveness and set aside one obstacle to the integration of psychodynamic and cognitive-behavioral theories.

BACKGROUND

Measures based on defense mechanisms theory are reliable and valid.[2-5] For example, Bloch and colleagues[6] scored video records of entire clinical sessions for the types of defense mechanisms in use and found significant differences in which levels of defense mechanisms were used by dysthymic and nondysthymic patients. We studied discourse about topics related to recent stressor events and noted state-dependent shifts in whether memories and

See Methods on next page

METHODS

DESIGN

Two subjects with pathological grief were selected because the relationship with the deceased and other loss-related topics would be expected to be conflictual. Brief therapies were videotaped. Quantitative methods for identifying when signs of defensive control were high were applied to these records. Separately, communication was categorically scored in units of discourse in terms of which people and topics were discussed by the patient. Three measures of defensive control were combined into an algorithm and used to locate 5-minute segments in each session that were high, medium, and low in such signs. We then could statistically determine if segments high in signs of defensive control contained disproportionately more discourse on conflicted people and topics.

SUBJECTS

We recruited and evaluated individuals with pathological grief responses characterized by the symptoms of stress response syndromes, ie, continuing intrusions and avoidances with prolonged absence of behavioral adaptation to life changes. We selected one man and one woman for intensive research study in the context of videotaped psychotherapy. Both subjects were treated by one experienced psychotherapist. All participants gave written informed consent.

PROCEDURE

The treatments followed a procedure for brief dynamic psychotherapy of stress response syndromes.[42] Therapy sessions were videotaped with time codes. Audiotapes of the sessions were transcribed following defined standards.[43] Transcriptions were segmented by thematic units: a unit that varies in size from one to a few clauses and expresses a single idea.[44] Video-based measures were scored on time intervals; text-based measures were scored on thematic units. Different sets of judges were used for each of the different measures.

MEASURES

Objects and Topics of Discourse

While linguists have identified topics through an analysis of shifts signaled by specific markers in the discourse,[45] this type of analysis does not usually classify the content of discourse. Finding topics that are salient to an individual case is a special problem in psychotherapy research. Accordingly, we asked judges first to define the important objects and topics of discourse, and then to go back and rate each thematic unit for these emergent categories.[46] The *objects* of discourse were the persons referenced in the talk; the *topics* were related propositions.

Dyselaboration

Judges followed a manual[12] to score every thematic unit of transcribed discourse for five categorized levels of dyselaboration, from none to most dyselaborative (levels 3 to 5) as follows: (1) none (the absence of dyselaboration); (2) filler speech that stalls disclosure by insertion of pauses, sounds, and words with low meaning; hedging phrases that minimize or blunt the impact of speech; (3) peripheral speech that moves away from the heart of emotional topics; jitter speech that takes alternative perspectives on a topic in a way that disconnects meanings rather than linking and comparing them; (4) distortion of a statement's significance by disavowal, misattribution, misunderstanding, or ignoring; and (5) abrupt shifts in theme when the theme is still clearly under discussion. For the purposes of the algorithm, higher levels of dyselaboration (levels 3 through 5) were combined to form a single category called "obscuring dyselaboration." The proportion of obscuring dyselaboration in a 30-second segment was calculated by counting the number of thematic units with it as numerator and the number of thematic units without it as denominator.

States

Raters independently viewed every 30-second interval of videotape, assigning a single category for the predominant state during that interval.[47,48] These four categories are distinguished by the individual's apparent degree of control over emotional expression: well modulated, in which an individual appears well regulated and harmonious in revealing ideas and feelings; undermodulated, in which a person appears to lose self-regulation; overmodulated, in which the person successfully stifles emotion and feigns poise at the expense of appearing rigid and wooden; and shimmering, in which an individual has discordant features of both expressing and stifling emotion.

Continued on next page

fantasies about such events were suppressed, repressed, denied, or disavowed.[7] As we studied the phenomena of denial, disavowal, suppression, and repression, we developed a classification theory of defensive control processes that could lead to these outcomes.[8,9] In particular, we examined observable signs of avoidance, obscurity, retraction, and disinformation in communication.[8,9] We then constructed quantitative measures.[10-12] Their reliability enabled us to conduct the present study to test the hypothesis that signs of defensive control processes would locate times when a person was talking about conflicted, unintegrated, or unresolved topics.

Our methods rest on clinical observations of how patients use vague metaphors, juggle topics, and give contradictory verbal and nonverbal signals to dampen how they experience and communicate emotions.[13-16] Some patients ward off discussions of conflictual matters by keeping their talk focused at the periphery of a topic rather than going to its heart; others go to the heart of a topic's emotional meaning but then retract or contradict what they say.[17-19] Weintraub and Aronson[20-23] and Weintraub[24] combined extralinguistic and grammatical parameters of speech to define a multicategory system for rating verbal signs of defense. They found that the fre-

Nonverbal Warding Off

A system[11,12] for scoring NVWO behaviors evolved from prior work that associated nonverbal behaviors with heightened anxiety,[49] disclosure,[50] deceptions and emotion,[36,51] and regulation of emotional experience.[37] The NVWO facial signs scored included shifting gaze patterns, mouth movements that suggest withholding or avoidance (eg, rapid recomposure or pressing the lips together), head movements that suggest shaking off or dismissal (eg, shaking or jerking of the head), and attempts to cover or hide the face with hands or by neck movements.

Raters viewed session videotapes with the sound turned off. Scores for a 30-second segment were determined either by a proportion of occurrence of positively rated in 5-second blocks (numerator) and the number of 5-second blocks without ratings (denominator).

ALGORITHM FOR CLIP SELECTION

Defensive moments were defined algorithmically by a combination of the three measures: obscuring dyselaboration, shimmering states of mind, and NVWO. For each 30-second interval, each variable was assigned a value of 3 for high, 2 for medium, and 1 for low. High values for each variable were defined as "present" for shimmering, and for dyselaboration and NVWO as proportions at or above the 10% highest values for the entire therapy. Low values for each variable were defined as absence of shimmering, and at or below the 10% lowest value for the entire therapy for dyselaboration and NVWO proportions. Scores for each measure in a 30-second interval were added, resulting in a range from 3 to 9 for each 30-second interval. These combination scores were summed over a moving 5-minute window, yielding a defensiveness value ranging from 30 to 90 for each overlapping 5-minute segment of each session. Using these 5-minute segment scores, a computer program then identified three "clips" for each session of therapy: one high, one medium, and one low. The "high clip" was the 5-minute segment that had the highest defensiveness score for that session. The "low clip" was the 5-minute segment with the lowest defensiveness score, and the "medium clip" was one with the median defensiveness score for the session. In case of a tie, the earliest segment in the session was selected.

STATISTICAL PROCEDURES

Independent sets of judges were systematically trained in scoring each measure (11 judges total). There were four teams, one for each measure: (1) objects and topics of discourse (two judges), (2) dyselaboration (four judges), (3) states (three judges), and (4) NVWO behaviors (two judges). Each judge within a team first made his or her judgments independent of the others. The team then came together to determine a consensus rating. Statistical analyses for testing the hypothesis used the consensus ratings.

Reliabilities were calculated on the independent judgments before consensus. The two judges rating the objects and topics of discourse were reliable with a κ of 0.7.[52] The four judges rating dyselaboration were reliable with a κ of 0.7. The three judges rating state were reliable with a κ of 0.8. The two judges rating NVWO behaviors were reliable with a κ of 0.8.

Proportions of objects and topics of discourse were determined for each 5-minute clip. During each 5-minute segment, the numerator of the proportion was the number of thematic units that the patient devoted to discourse on the specific object or topic; the denominator was the total number of thematic units in the segment. These proportions are expressed as percentages in the figures (proportion$\times$100).

The probability of significant differences in object or topic of discourse between high, medium, and low defensiveness clips was calculated using the Wilcoxon matched pairs signed ranks test, a nonparametric analog of the matched pairs *t* test. The pairs used on the Wilcoxon ranking were the object or topic of discourse values in the high clips and the pooled object or topic of discourse values of both low and medium clips. A one-sided test was used for power because we predicted the direction of results (more conflictual objects and topics in high clips).

T values of the Wilcoxon test should not be read as parametric *t* values. The equations leading to the Wilcoxon T are such that when the sample size is held constant, small T values are more significant in terms of probability values than larger T values. Ties, however, reduce sample size and our sample sizes vary depending on the number of ties in a comparison.

quent use of negatives related to a habitual use of denial. Gottschalk and Gleser[25] also developed reliable content analysis scales for the quantification of verbal signs of warded-off anxiety and hostility. A variety of their important findings supported the validity of measuring defense-related variables on verbal communication.[26-29] Extralinguistic aspects of communication have been used as another quantitative method for detecting conflict between expressive and defensive aims.[29-33] We condensed leads from such research into a measure of verbal defensiveness called *dyselaboration.*[12]

Dyselaboration consists of verbal efforts to avoid disclosure or, if a disclosure has already occurred, to retract, obscure, or purposely dilute and distort its meaning. This can include hedging phrases, movement into a less vital and more peripheral aspect of meaning to draw attention away from central issues, and efforts to disavow or misattribute ideas and feelings that have already been stated. Unlike the methods of Gottschalk and Gleser,[25] dyselaboration is defined primarily by form rather than by reference to potential affective contents. Like the measure of Weintraub and Aronson,[20-23] and that of Mahl[32] or Dibner,[29] dyselaboration reflects a count of mannerisms over a small portion of transcribed text, which can locate a specific moment in the time of discourse on specific topics.

In addition to linguistic and extralinguistic verbal signs, the importance of nonverbal cues as indices of defenses has been emphasized.[34] Ekman and Friesen[35,36] developed a system for the coding of facial muscle actions, the Facial Action Coding, and, recently, Ekman defined actions that may reveal efforts to deceive others about emotions.[37,38] These signs include exaggerating, minimizing, neutralizing, and masking feelings by presenting facial expressions incompatible with the concealed emotion. Izard[39] also emphasized such facial signs. We built on these efforts to develop simpler measures of nonverbal cues of defensive control.

The first measure was *state analysis*. We concentrated specifically on displays of emotion and attempts to stifle its communication, rather than on efforts to categorize specific emotions.[40,41] We defined four categories: (1) *overmodulated states*, which successfully conceal emotional expression; (2) *shimmering states*, which partially but unsuccessfully stifle emotional displays; (3) *undermodulated states*, which present seemingly uncontrolled emotional expressions; and (4) *well-modulated states*, which express harmonious medleys of verbal and nonverbal signs. These four categories allow for the simple scoring of any segment of a videotape.

Shimmering states are most relevant to our present study. They contain a rapid oscillation of signs of different intentions to express an emotion and to cancel or mask that expression. Examples would be to show a facial expression that signaled affect such as disgust and then to mask it by a rigid, feigned smile. Central to the definition of shimmering states is quickly switching back and forth between emotional signals that carry contradictory implications. Judges can observe the discordant features that "shimmer" together.

The second nonverbal measure was a video-based method for scoring nonverbal warding-off (NVWO) behaviors.[10,11] Signs scored included covering the face, pursing the lips, and shutting or squinting down the eyes—all movements that mask or reduce the muscle changes that display and convey emotions and affective intensity.

In preliminary work, we studied elementally the association of dyselaboration, NVWO behaviors, shimmering states, and other communication variables to topical content.[10,11] In the current study, we developed an algorithm for the combination of these variables. This algorithm permitted computer review of the variables as scored on all the time of discourse throughout the entirety of brief psychotherapies. The computer programming was done in such a way that we could select 5-minute segments (10% of a 50-minute session) for intense quantitative and qualitative scrutiny. We were then in the position to test the hypothesis that moments high in signs of defensive control might signal unresolved themes of discourse during psychotherapy.

RESULTS

CASE 1

Woman With a Pathological Reaction to Loss

Mrs C was in her early 40s when she experienced the sudden death of her husband, Mr C. At the time of evaluation, over a year later, she complained of prolonged symptoms, including unbidden intrusive images, uncontrollable crying, nightmares, sleep disturbance, irritability, anxiety, demoralization, and depression. She felt she was not progressing through mourning. On evaluation, she met criteria for *DSM-III-R*[53] diagnoses of both posttraumatic stress disorder and major depressive disorder.

Table 1. Objects of Discourse for Female Patient in Psychotherapy for Pathological Grief Reaction*

Persons Rated by Judges as Objects of Discourse	Amount of Discourse, %
Self	**23.8**
Miscellaneous other(s)	11.8
New intimacy	11.2
A woman friend	8.4
Daughter	6.8
Mother	5.3
New intimate and self	4.3
Father	4.1
Friends	4.0
A child	3.4
Deceased husband	**3.3**
Children	2.7
Family as a group	2.1
Deceased and new intimate	**1.6**
Siblings	1.3
Own parents	1.0
Deceased and self	**1.0**
Mother of new intimate	1.0
Family of deceased	0.9
Future project	0.8
Therapist	0.5
Family of new intimate	0.4
Self and therapist	0.2
Official	0.1

**Objects of discourse are listed in order by amount of discourse in the entire therapy; those present disproportionately more frequently in the highly defensive segments are boldfaced.*

Mrs C and Mr C had a secure marriage and healthy children. The death was unexpected and violent. For months afterward, Mrs C felt numbed, dazed, and as if she were "just going through the motions" of life. She engaged in many distracting activities, but avoided dating for a year. Then, shortly before the beginning of therapy, she began seeing Mr S. She felt confused when her feelings deepened for this man. Formulation suggested that the death of Mr C had led to a sense of disrupted identity not yet resolved by new schematizations of herself as a widow and Mr C as dead.[54] The pleasure of being with Mr S was diminished by shame and guilt over "leaving" Mr C and by concerns that she would become too dependent rather than evolve a sense of independence.

Her individual brief therapy consisted of 28 50-minute sessions. During sessions, Mrs C tried to maintain control over her emotions, often avoiding painful topics by declaring resolutely that it was now "over with." With the therapist's help, Mrs C gradually was able to relinquish avoidance, and mourning did proceed. She had a good treatment outcome with a resolution of both disorders.

Relation of Heightened Defensive Control to Objects of Discourse

In the list of 24 people scored as objects of discourse, four were disproportionately present during the clips

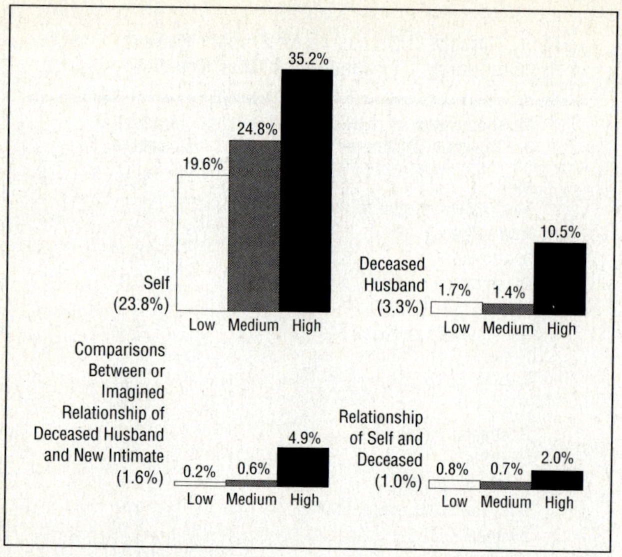

Figure 1. *Percentages of some objects of discourse in 5-minute segments from each session that were high, medium, and low in signs of defensiveness in a female patient treated with psychotherapy for a pathological grief reaction.*

Table 2. Topics of Discourse for Female Patient in Psychotherapy for Pathological Grief Reaction*

Topics of Discourse Rated by Judges	Amount of Discourse, %
Nonconflicted caretaking	19.2
Conflict in new relationship	**16.6**
Conflict in caretaking	15.9
Death of spouse	**11.2**
Conflicted self-development	**9.7**
Filler talk	7.4
Nonconflicted relationship	5.0
Therapy process	4.3
Nonconflicted self-development	3.7
Overburdened self	3.2
Other deaths	2.6
Idealizing/normalizing	1.1

**Topics of discourse are listed in order by amount of discourse in the entire therapy; those present disproportionately more frequently in the highly defensive segments are boldfaced.*

that were high in signs of defensive control processes (**Table 1**). These four objects were judged clinically to be conflictual: herself (self), her dead husband (deceased), the comparison of Mr C with Mr S (deceased and new intimate), and her relationship with Mr C (deceased and self). The relative amounts of discourse about these four objects in the high, medium, and low clips are shown in **Figure 1**.

Statistical analyses compared the proportions of discourse on these objects for the high clips to the proportions found in the low and medium clips combined. High clips had significantly more discourse about self (high clip mean proportion=0.35, SD=0.22; low+medium clips mean proportion=0.22, SD=0.13; Wilcoxon T=86; n=28 [no ties]; $P<.003$); deceased husband (high clip mean proportion=0.11, SD=0.15; low+medium clips mean proportion=0.01, SD=0.03; Wilcoxon T=13; n=20 [due to ties]; $P<.001$); deceased and new intimate (high clips mean proportion=0.05, SD=0.11; low+medium clips mean proportion=0.00, SD=0.01; Wilcoxon T=6; n=11 [due to ties]; $P<.007$); and deceased and self (high clips mean proportion=0.02, SD=0.04; low+medium clips mean proportion=0.01, SD=0.01; Wilcoxon T=19; n=12 [due to ties]; $P<.06$).

We then performed a similar analysis on the 12 topics of her discourse (**Table 2**). Of these, three (in boldface) were disproportionately frequent in the defensively high clips. Clinically, these were viewed as the most unresolved topics: her conflicts about developing a relationship with Mr S (conflict in new relationship), the events surrounding the death of Mr C (death of spouse), and conflicts about her own direction of personal development (conflicted self-development). These topics interrelated. If she were to pursue affiliation with Mr S, she would feel disloyal to Mr C. If she remained loyal to Mr C, she would have no current intimate attachment. Were she to pursue affiliation with Mr S, she feared she would reduce her chance to develop herself as a fully independent woman. Her conflicts on developing herself as independent dealt with how to balance caretaking, intimate relations, and career activities. She was not nearly so conflicted over issues of taking care of her children. She sometimes dismissed problems in a generalized way by statements that idealized and normalized life, which avoided contradictory intentions altogether.

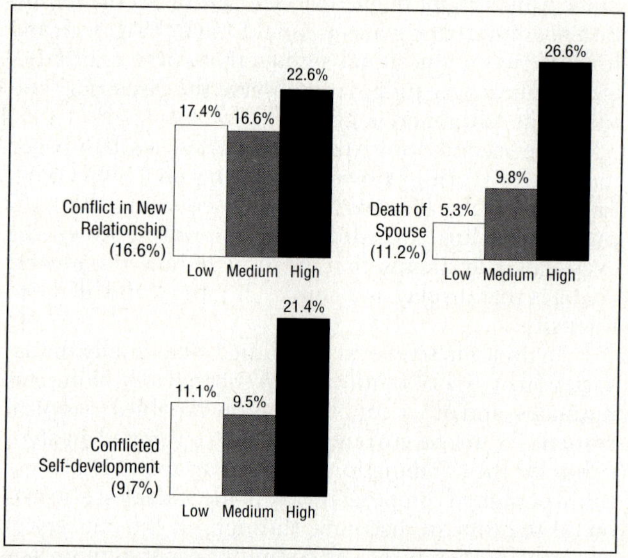

Figure 2. *Percentage of some topics of discourse in 5-minute segments from each session that were high, medium, and low in signs of defensiveness in a female patient treated with psychotherapy for a pathological grief reaction.*

The relative amounts of discourse on the unresolved topics in defensively high, medium, and low clips are shown in **Figure 2**. The *P* values, calculated with the Wilcoxon test, were significant for the events surrounding the death of spouse (high clips mean proportion=0.27, SD=0.25; low+medium clips mean proportion=0.08, SD=0.11; Wilcoxon T=17; n=23 [due to ties]; $P<.001$).

Table 3. Objects of Discourse for Male Patient in Psychotherapy for Pathological Grief Reaction*

Persons Rated by Judges as Objects of Discourse	Amount of Discourse, %
Self	26.4
Deceased brother	**9.8**
Generalized "others"	7.4
Miscellaneous people	7.2
Current intimate	6.8
Friends	4.8
Ms A	4.6
Work associates	4.3
Family members	4.2
Self and intimate	3.9
Parents	3.4
Mother	3.2
Work assistants	3.1
Self and brother	**1.9**
Therapist	**1.8**
Self and therapist	1.7
Father	1.3
Previous intimate	1.1
Sisters	0.7
Mr C	0.6
Self and previous intimate	0.6
Brothers	0.6
People associated with death	0.6
Official	0.2
Ms B	0.2

Objects of discourse are listed in order by amount of discourse in the entire therapy; those present disproportionately more frequently in the highly defensive segments are boldfaced.

CASE 2

Man With a Pathological Reaction to Loss

Mr D, a young professional man, reported experiencing continued problems in adapting to the sudden, unexpected death of his older brother from a homicide more than a year earlier. He felt preoccupied with intrusive thoughts and images of the deceased, and these were often accompanied by surges of remorse, guilt, and feelings of lost opportunity. In an attempt to control his emotions, he avoided reminders of the deceased, but subsequently found himself sapped of motivation for doing his work. He felt distant from all other people and felt trapped in a dissatisfying and exploitative, intimate relationship with a man.

He met *DSM-III-R* diagnostic criteria for adjustment disorder. He was formulated as a person who habitually used strongly avoidant coping maneuvers to avoid emotions present in a maladaptive but repetitive interpersonal pattern of ambivalent relationships at work and in intimacies. The subject reported that, as a boy, he had been sexually abused by the deceased. For many years afterward, the relationship went through cycles in which he would act with warmth and friendship toward his brother, with anger at his brother's exploitation of him, with hostile remarks to others about his brother, and with cold rejection to his brother's overtures for friendship. Eventually after feeling lonely and guilty at the rejection and hostility, Mr D would resume a friendly relationship and the cycle would begin again. Just prior to the loss, he considered having another reconciliation, but did not make any attempt to do so. The research-based therapy was completed after 35 50-minute sessions with a good result.

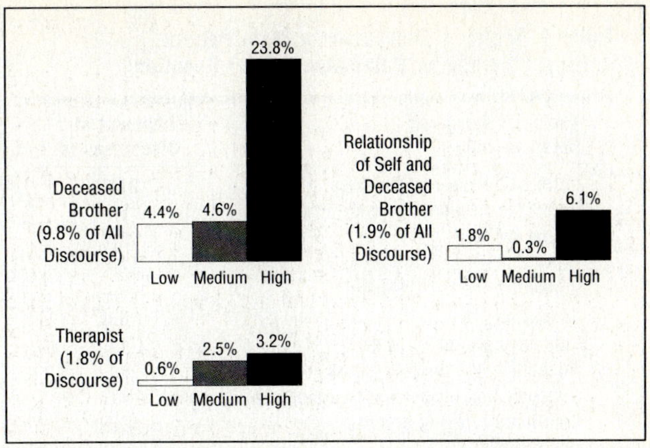

Figure 3. *Percentages of some objects of discourse in 5-minute segments from each session that were high, medium, and low in signs of defensiveness in a male patient treated with psychotherapy for a pathological grief reaction.*

Relation of Heightened Defensive Control to Objects of Discourse

Twenty-five objects of discourse emerged from judgments of Mr D's narratives (**Table 3**). Of these, three of the clinically most conflicted objects were disproportionately more frequent in the discourse of highly defensive 5-minute segments. As boldfaced in Table 3, these were his deceased brother, his relationship with the brother (self and brother), and the therapist. **Figure 3** shows the relative percentages of discussing these target objects in the segments high, medium, and low in defensiveness.

Statistical analyses compared the proportions of discourse on various objects during highly defensive clips with the proportion of discourse on such people during the low and medium clips combined. The *P* values, calculated with the Wilcoxon test, were significant for discourse about his deceased brother (high clips mean proportion=0.24, SD=0.30; low+medium clips mean proportion=0.05, SD=0.11; Wilcoxon T=36; n=24 [due to ties]; $P<.001$) and nearly significant for his relationship with his brother (high clips mean proportion=0.05, SD=0.16; low+medium clips mean proportion=0.01, SD=0.05; Wilcoxon T=20; n=12 [due to ties]; $P<.07$).

Analyses by quartiles of therapy indicated that the clip selection algorithm located his deceased brother as a distinctive conflictual object of discourse most frequently in the highly defensive segments of the first, third, and fourth quarters of the treatment. The therapist as an object of discourse was most frequent in the highly defensive clips during the last quarter of treatment.

Twelve topics were obtained from Mr D's therapy discourse (**Table 4**). Four were disproportionately more frequent in the highly defensive segments: events surrounding his intimate sexual relationship, the death of

Table 4. Topics of Discourse for Male Patient in Psychotherapy for Pathological Grief Reaction*

Topics of Discourse Rated by Judges	Amount of Discourse, %
Intimate sexual relationships	**21.3**
Conflicted relationships with others	15.5
Death events	**12.7**
Nonconflicted self-development	12.7
Conflicted self-development	11.2
Sexual identity	**6.6**
Conflicted therapy process	5.6
Nonconflicted therapy process	4.8
Nonconflicted relationships with others	4.6
Conflicted grieving process	**3.5**
Other deaths	1.0
Nonconflicted grieving process	0.6

**Topics of discourse are listed in order by amount of discourse in the entire therapy; those present disproportionately more frequently in the highly defensive segments are boldfaced.*

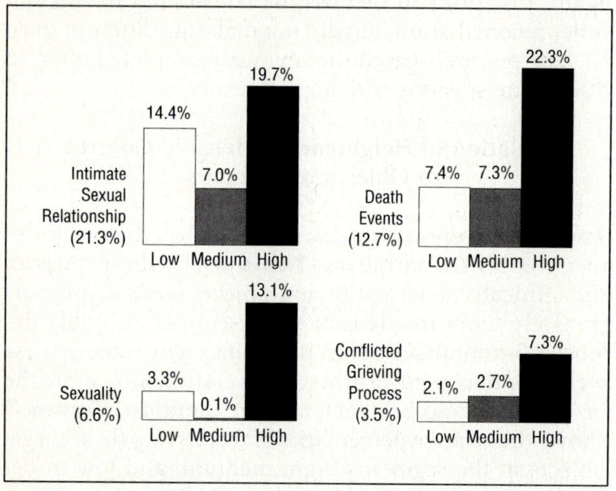

Figure 4. *Percentages of some topics of discourse in 5-minute segments from each session that were high, medium, and low in signs of defensiveness in a male patient treated with psychotherapy for a pathological grief reaction.*

his brother (death events), sexual identity, and conflicted grieving process. The percentages of these in each type of clip are shown in **Figure 4**. The Wilcoxon test was significant for death events (high clips mean proportion=0.22, SD=0.34; low+medium clips mean proportion=0.07, SD=0.15; Wilcoxon T=54; n=22 [no ties]; $P<.009$) and sexuality (high clips mean proportion=0.13, SD=0.25; low+medium clips mean proportion=0.02, SD=0.10; Wilcoxon T=12; n=12 [due to ties]; $P<.02$).

COMMENT

These results support the hypothesis that in both cases, increased signs of defensive control processes occurred when conflictual or unresolved themes were being communicated. Observing for such signs of defensiveness may be a useful way to identify what issues are unresolved.

The advantage of selecting cases with pathological grief reactions was the known clinical centrality of persons and topics connected to the loss event. However, based on this same premise, it would be premature to generalize from such a specific sampling of cases. The hypothesis, while supported, is not proved. Generalization of the hypothesis will require replication of the study with larger groups, including cases without prior clear stressor events.

For purposes of empirical research, this study involved different judges for different measures. During clinical teaching sessions of psychiatry and psychotherapy using videotape, we use less arduously equivalents of these measures. While watching a videotape, verbal dyselaboration and facial signs of stifling emotion can be observed to wax and wane. Moments of intense presence of such signs are noted by the observer looking at the time stamp on the videotape. These times lead to the selection of a highly defensive 5-minute segment. These selected segments are then repeatedly reviewed to decipher communicated meanings and sequences of ideas and emotions to infer motivational conflicts.

Using this process, trainees can learn how keen observation of clinical evidence yields ingredients for case formulation and how microanalytic formulations relate to larger scale, macroanalytic case formulations.[54] Inferences drawn from microanalysis of a 5-minute segment in one session can also be treated as predictions to be checked by similar review of segments from subsequent sessions with the patient.

CONCLUSION

We chose subjects with unresolved grief after a major loss to capitalize on face validity for what themes of discourse are likely to be conflictual. Signs of defensive control of communication were operationally defined and reliably scored by independent judges. The objects and topics of discourse were also rated by independent judges for all segments of all therapy sessions. From each session, episodes high, medium, and low in signs of defensive control were algorithmically selected. The highly defensive segments contained disproportionately more of what were clinically deemed to be conflictual and unresolved themes. The results suggest the validity of (1) observing patients for defensive behaviors and (2) using observable signs of heightened defensiveness as a way of locating conflictual topics.

Accepted for publication July 19, 1995.

This research was supported by the Program on Conscious and Unconscious Mental Processes of the John D. and Catherine T. MacArthur Foundation.

Mary Ewert, DMH, Steve Reidbord, MD, and Rebecca Bauknight, PhD, made important contributions to the behavioral variables definitions and measurements; Norman Mages, MD, Alan Skolnikoff, MD, Michael Windholz, PhD, and Bram Fridhandler, PhD, made valuable clinical and qualitative contributions; and Clyde Sugahara, PhD, the University of California, San Francisco, devised the statistical analyses with important contributions in computational algorithms from James Stewart.

Reprint requests to Director, Center on Stress and Personality, Department of Psychiatry, University of California, 401 Parnassus, San Francisco, CA 94143 (Dr Horowitz).

REFERENCES

1. Persons JB. *Cognitive Therapy in Practice.* New York, NY: WW Norton & Co Inc; 1989.
2. Bond M, Perry JC, Gautier M, Goldenberg M, Oppenheimer J, Semand J. Validating the self-report of defensive styles. *J Pers Disord.* 1989;3:101-112.
3. Vaillant GE. *Ego Mechanisms of Defense: In Clinical Practice and in Empirical Research.* Washington DC: American Psychiatric Press; 1992.
4. DePaulis D, Fridhandler BM, Hayes S. Psychological defense: contemporary theory and research. In: Briggs SR, Hogan R, Jones W, eds. *Handbook of Personality Research.* New York, NY: Academic Press; 1992.
5. Perry JC, Cooper SH. Empirical studies of defense mechanisms. In: Michels R, Cavenar JO, eds. *Psychiatry.* New York, NY: JB Lippincott and Basic Books; 1987:1-19.
6. Bloch AL, Shear M, Markowitz JC, Leon AC. An empirical study of defense mechanisms in dysthymia. *Am J Psychiatry.* 1993;150:1194-1198.
7. Horowitz MJ. Stress response syndromes: character style and brief psychotherapy. *Arch Gen Psychiatry.* 1974;31:768-781.
8. Horowitz MJ, Stinson CH. Consciousness and processes of control. *J Psychother Pract Res.* 1995;4:123-139.
9. Horowitz MJ, Znoj HJ, Stinson CH. Defensive control processes: use of theory in research, formulation and therapy of stress response syndromes. In: Zeidner M, Endler N, eds. *Handbook of Coping.* New York, NY: John Wiley & Sons. In press.
10. Horowitz MJ, Stinson CH, Curtis D, Ewert M, Redington D, Singer JL, Bucci W, Mergenthaler E, Milbrath C, Hartley D. Topics and signs: defensive control of emotional expression. *J Consult Clin Psychol.* 1993;61:1-10.
11. Horowitz MJ, Milbrath C, Jordan D, Stinson CH, Ewert M, Redington DJ, Fridhandler B, Reidbord SP, Hartley D. Expressive and defensive behavior during discourse on unresolved topics: a single case study. *J Pers.* 1994;62:527-563.
12. Horowitz MJ, Milbrath C, Reidbord SP, Stinson CH. Elaboration and dyselaboration: measures of expression and defense in discourse. *Psychother Res.* 1993; 3:278-293.
13. Salzman L. *Treatment of Obsessive Personality.* New York, NY: J Aronson; 1980.
14. Nagera H. *Obsessional Neuroses.* New York, NY: J Aronson; 1976.
15. Salzman L. *The Obsessive Personality.* New York, NY: Science House; 1968.
16. Freud A. *The Ego and Mechanisms of Defense.* New York, NY: International Universities Press; 1936.
17. Darby JK, ed. *Speech Evaluation in Psychiatry.* New York, NY: Grune & Stratton Inc; 1981.
18. Shapiro D. *Neurotic Styles.* New York, NY: Basic Books; 1965.
19. Perry JC, Cooper SH. What do cross-sectional measures of defense mechanisms predict? In: Vaillant GE, ed. *Empirical Studies of Ego Mechanisms of Defense.* Washington, DC: American Psychiatric Press; 1986:32-46.
20. Weintraub W, Aronson H. The application of verbal behavior analysis to the study of psychological defense mechanisms: methodology and preliminary report. *J Nerv Ment Dis.* 1963;134:169-181.
21. Weintraub W, Aronson H. The application of verbal behavior analysis to the study of psychological defense mechanisms, II: speech pattern associated with impulsive behavior. *J Nerv Ment Dis.* 1964;139:75-82.
22. Weintraub W, Aronson H. The application of verbal behavior analysis to the study of psychological defense mechanisms, III: speech pattern associated with delusional behavior. *J Nerv Ment Dis.* 1965;141:172-179.
23. Weintraub W, Aronson H. The application of verbal behavior analysis to the study of psychological defense mechanisms, IV: speech pattern associated with depressive behavior. *J Nerv Ment Dis.* 1967;144:23-28.
24. Weintraub W. *Verbal Behavior: Adaptation and Psychopathology.* New York, NY: Springer Publishing Co Inc; 1981.
25. Gottschalk LA, Gleser GC. *The Measurement of Psychological States Through the Content Analysis of Verbal Behavior.* Berkeley: University of California Press; 1969.
26. Gottschalk LA. Some psychoanalytic research into the communication of meaning through language: the quality and magnitude of psychological states. *Br J Med Psychol.* 1971;44:131-148.
27. Gottschalk LA, Lolas F, Viney LL, eds. *Content Analysis of Verbal Behavior: Significance in Clinical Medicine and Psychiatry.* Berlin, Germany: Springer-Verlag; 1986.
28. Gottschalk LA, Uliana RL. Further studies in the relationship of nonverbal to verbal behavior. In: Freedman N, Grand S, eds. *Communicative Structures and Psychic Structures.* New York, NY: Plenum Publishing Corp; 1977:311-330.
29. Dibner AS. Cue-counting: a measure of anxiety in interviews. *J Consult Psychol.* 1956;20:475-478.
30. Eldred SH, Price DB. The linguistic evaluation of feeling states in psychotherapy. *Psychiatry.* 1958;21:115-121.
31. Mahl GF. Disturbances and silences in the patient's speech in psychotherapy. *J Abnorm Soc Psychol.* 1956;53:1-15.
32. Mahl GF. Everyday disturbances of speech. In: Russell RL, ed. *Language in Psychotherapy: Strategies of Discovery.* New York, NY: Plenum Press; 1987: 213-269.
33. Rice LN, Wagstaff AK. Client voice quality and expressive style as indexes of productive psychotherapy. *J Consult Psychol.* 1967;31:557-563.
34. Waxer PH. Nonverbal cues for anxiety: an examination of emotional leakage. *J Abnormal Psychol.* 1977;86:306-314.
35. Ekman P, Friesen WV. *The Facial Action Coding System (FACS): A Technique for the Measurement of Facial Action.* Palo Alto, Calif: Consulting Psychologists Press; 1978.
36. Ekman P, Friesen WV. *Unmasking the Face: A Guide to Recognizing Emotions From Facial Clues.* Englewood Cliffs, NJ: Prentice-Hall; 1975.
37. Ekman P, Friesen WV. Felt, false, and miserable smiles. *J Nonverbal Behav.* 1982;6:238-252.
38. Ekman P, Friesen WV, O'Sullivan M. Smiles when lying. *J Pers Soc Psychol.* 1988;54:414-420.
39. Izard CE. *The Face of Emotion.* New York, NY: Appleton-Century-Crofts; 1971.
40. Horowitz MJ. *States of Mind: Configurational Analysis of Individual Psychology.* 2nd ed. New York, NY: Plenum Publishing Corp; 1987.
41. Horowitz MJ, Milbrath C, Ewert M, Sonneborn D, Stinson CH. Cyclical patterns of states of mind in psychotherapy. *Am J Psychiatry.* 1994;151:1767-1770.
42. Horowitz MJ. *Stress Response Syndromes.* 2nd ed. Northvale, NJ: J Aronson; 1986.
43. Mergenthaler E, Stinson CH. Psychotherapy transcription standards. *Psychother Res.* 1992;2:125-142.
44. Stinson CH, Milbrath C, Reidbord SP, Bucci W. Thematic segmentation of psychotherapy transcripts for convergent analysis. *Psychotherapy.* 1994;31:36-48.
45. Brown G, Yule G. *Teaching the Spoken Language: An Approach Based on the Analysis of Conversational English.* Cambridge, England: Cambridge University Press; 1983.
46. Milbrath C, Bauknight R, Horowitz MJ, Amaro R, Sugahara C. Sequential analysis of topics in the psychotherapy discourse of a single case. *Psychother Res.* 1995;5:199-217.
47. Horowitz MJ, Wilner N, Marmar C. Research applications. In: Horowitz MJ, ed. *States of Mind: Configurational Analysis of Individual Psychology.* 2nd ed. New York, NY: Plenum Publishing Corp; 1987:185-194.
48. Horowitz MJ, Ewert M, Milbrath C. States of mind: assessing control of emotion during psychotherapy. *J Psychother Pract Res.* In press.
49. Shreve EG, Harrigan JA, Kues JR, Kagas DK. Nonverbal expressions of anxiety in physician patient interactions. *Psychiatry.* 1988;51:378-384.
50. Davis M, Hadiks D. Nonverbal behavior and client state changes during psychotherapy. *J Clin Psychol.* 1990;46:340-351.
51. Ekman P, Friesen W, Ellsworth P. *Emotion in the Human Face.* New York, NY: Pergamon Press Inc; 1972.
52. Light RL. Measures of response agreement for qualitative data: some generalizations and alternatives. *Psychol Bull.* 1971;76:365-377.
53. American Psychiatric Association. *Diagnostic and Statistical Manual of Mental Disorders, Revised Third Edition.* Washington, DC: American Psychiatric Association; 1987.
54. Horowitz MJ, Stinson CH, Fridhandler B, Ewert M, Milbrath C, Redington D. Pathological grief: an intensive case study. *Psychiatry.* 1993;56:356-374.

ORIGINAL ARTICLE

Posttraumatic Stress Disorder in the National Comorbidity Survey

Ronald C. Kessler, PhD; Amanda Sonnega, PhD; Evelyn Bromet, PhD; Michael Hughes, PhD; Christopher B. Nelson, MPH, PhD

Background: Data were obtained on the general population epidemiology of *DSM-III-R* posttraumatic stress disorder (PTSD), including information on estimated lifetime prevalence, the kinds of traumas most often associated with PTSD, sociodemographic correlates, the comorbidity of PTSD with other lifetime psychiatric disorders, and the duration of an index episode.

Methods: Modified versions of the *DSM-III-R* PTSD module from the Diagnostic Interview Schedule and of the Composite International Diagnostic Interview were administered to a representative national sample of 5877 persons aged 15 to 54 years in the part II subsample of the National Comorbidity Survey.

Results: The estimated lifetime prevalence of PTSD is 7.8%. Prevalence is elevated among women and the previously married. The traumas most commonly associated with PTSD are combat exposure and witnessing among men and rape and sexual molestation among women. Posttraumatic stress disorder is strongly comorbid with other lifetime *DSM-III-R* disorders. Survival analysis shows that more than one third of people with an index episode of PTSD fail to recover even after many years.

Conclusions: Posttraumatic stress disorder is more prevalent than previously believed, and is often persistent. Progress in estimating age-at-onset distributions, cohort effects, and the conditional probabilities of PTSD from different types of trauma will require future epidemiologic studies to assess PTSD for all lifetime traumas rather than for only a small number of retrospectively reported "most serious" traumas.

(Arch Gen Psychiatry. 1995;52:1048-1060)

IT HAS LONG been known that pathologic stress response syndromes can result from exposure to war,[1] sexual assault,[2] and other types of trauma.[3-6] The codification of diagnostic criteria for these responses in *DSM-III*[7] under the diagnosis of posttraumatic stress disorder (PTSD) stimulated a considerable amount of research on these responses. A number of traumas have been studied in detail since that time, including criminal victimization,[8,9] sexual assault,[10,11] exposure to natural disaster,[12-14] and combat exposure.[15-18] The empiric information and conceptual refinements[19] generated by this research have importantly advanced our understanding of traumatic stress responses and led to revisions of the diagnostic criteria for PTSD in *DSM-III-R*. These require (A) exposure to a traumatic event that is "outside the range of usual human experience"; (B) reliving the experience in nightmares, flashbacks, or intrusive thoughts; (C) numbing or avoidant symptoms; and (D) hypersensitivity, either as indicated by general signs and symptoms of autonomic arousal or by hypersensitivity to cues reminiscent of the trauma. These symptoms must persist for at least 1 month.[20] Despite a growing body of work on the extent to which PTSD is associated with specific traumas, limited epidemiologic data are available that describe the population prevalence of PTSD, the kinds of traumas most strongly associated with PTSD, the demographic correlates of PTSD, the comorbidity of PTSD with other disorders, and the typical course of PTSD. The purpose of this article is to present findings of this sort from the National Comorbidity Survey (NCS), the first nationally representative face-to-face general population survey to assess a broad range of *DSM-III-R* disorders that includes PTSD.

From the Institute for Social Research (Drs Kessler and Sonnega) and the Department of Sociology (Dr Kessler), University of Michigan, Ann Arbor; Department of Psychiatry and Behavioral Science, State University of New York at Stony Brook (Dr Bromet); Department of Sociology, Virginia Polytechnic Institute and State University, Blacksburg, Va (Dr Hughes); and Max Planck Institute of Psychiatry—Clinical Institute, Munich, Germany (Dr Nelson).

See Patients and Methods on next page

PATIENTS AND METHODS

SAMPLE

The data come from the NCS, a survey designed to study the distribution, correlates, and consequences of psychiatric disorders in the United States. The survey is based on a stratified, multistage area probability sample of persons aged 15 to 54 years in the noninstitutionalized civilian population in the 48 contiguous states, including a supplemental sample of students living in campus group housing, selected from a clustered sample of 1205 block-level segments in 176 counties throughout the country. A special nonresponse survey was carried out to ascertain and then statistically adjust for nonresponse bias.[37] Interviews were administered by the staff of the Survey Research Center at the University of Michigan, Ann Arbor, between September 14, 1990, and February 6, 1992. The 158 interviewers who participated in the NCS had an average of 5 years of previous interviewing experience with the Survey Research Center. Interviewers went through a 7-day study-specific training program in the use of the Composite International Diagnostic Interview (CIDI)[38] and were closely monitored throughout the data collection period. The response rate was 82.4%. A total of 8098 respondents participated in the survey.

The NCS was administered in two parts, each of which took somewhat more than 1 hour to complete. Part 1 included the core diagnostic interview, a brief risk factor battery, and an inventory of sociodemographic information. Part 2 included a much more detailed risk factor battery and secondary diagnoses, including PTSD, that were not included in the core diagnostic interview. Part 1 was administered to all 8098 respondents. Budgetary constraints required that we administer part 2 to only a subsample of respondents consisting of all those aged 15 to 24 years (99.4% of whom completed part 2), all others who screened positive for any lifetime diagnosis in part 1 (98.1% of whom completed part 2), and a random subsample of other respondents (99% of whom completed part 2). A total of 5877 respondents completed part 2. More details about the design of the NCS are presented elsewhere.[37]

DIAGNOSTIC ASSESSMENT

The diagnostic interview in the NCS was a modified version of the CIDI.[38,39] The CIDI is a fully structured interview developed collaboratively by the World Health Organization and the US Alcohol, Drug, and Mental Health Administration to foster cross-cultural epidemiologic research by producing diagnoses according to the definitions and criteria of both *DSM-III-R*[20] and the Diagnostic Criteria for Research of the *International Classification of Diseases, 10th Revision*.[40] The modifications of the CIDI developed at the University of Michigan for the NCS consisted largely of changes in question order to improve flow and the introduction of clarifications to some of the more complex probe questions.[37]

The NCS disorders used to study comorbidity with PTSD included affective disorders (major depressive disorder, dysthymia, bipolar disorder), anxiety disorders (generalized anxiety disorder, panic disorder, phobia), antisocial personality disorder, and substance use disorders (alcohol abuse without dependence, alcohol dependence, drug abuse without dependence, drug dependence). All these diagnoses were based on *DSM-III-R* criteria. Diagnoses were generated by the use of the CIDI diagnostic program[41] for all disorders other than antisocial personality disorder. The latter was assessed with the antisocial personality disorder module from the DIS because this disorder was not part of the CIDI field trials. The field trials documented acceptable reliability and validity for all the CIDI diagnoses used herein.[42]

Posttraumatic stress disorder was assessed with a modified version of the Revised DIS[26] to be consistent with the assessment used in recent US epidemiologic surveys of PTSD.[26,29] In addition to the Revised DIS symptom questions, additional questions were asked about how soon the symptoms began after the trauma and how long the symptoms continued "at least a few times a week." Responses to the latter question were used as the basis for studying speed of recovery.

We also made four modifications to the Revised DIS PTSD section. The first involved the method for inquiring about traumatic stressors. Unlike the Revised DIS, which asks a single question about the lifetime occurrence of a list of traumatic events to oneself and a second question about traumas to others, the NCS asked 12 questions, one for each of 12 types of trauma, in an effort to focus memory search. Eleven questions were about events and experiences that qualify as traumas in *DSM-III-R* (**Figure 1**). A 12th question was an open-ended question about "any other terrible experience that most people never go through." Open-ended responses to this 12th question were subsequently coded as either qualifying under criterion A (eg, discovering a dead body) or not qualifying under criterion A (eg, normal bereavement). Responses that did not refer to specific events, were vague, or were confounded with PTSD (eg, biologic depression) were eliminated. In each case of the 12 events, we asked whether the event had ever occurred. For experiences 1, 9, and 10, that was the only

Continued on next page

PREVALENCE

The two earliest community prevalence studies of PTSD were carried out as part of the Epidemiologic Catchment Area (ECA) Program in St Louis, Mo,[21] and North Carolina.[22] Using *DSM-III* criteria as operationalized in the Diagnostic Interview Schedule (DIS),[23] these studies found lifetime prevalences of 1.0% in St Louis and 1.3% in North Carolina. A lifetime prevalence of 2.6% was subsequently found in the control sample of a case-control study of the Mount St Helens volcanic eruption[24] with the use of the same diagnostic instrument and criteria as the ECA study. Two recent studies that used *DSM-III-R* criteria reported much higher rates. In a national telephone survey of women, Resnick et al[25] found that 12.3% of respondents (17.9% of those exposed to trauma) question asked. For the others, we also asked the age at which the experience first occurred. Additional probe questions were also asked for some traumas, but are not included in the following analyses.

Second, based on evidence that respondents are sometimes reluctant to admit the occurrence of embarrassing and stigmatizing traumas, such as rape and sexual abuse, the 12 traumatic experiences were presented to respondents in a booklet. Interviewers asked about these experiences by number (eg, "Did you ever experience event number 1 on the list?" "How old were you when event number 1 first happened?") rather than by name.

The third modification is that we evaluated criteria B through D for the "most upsetting" event whether or not that event met the requirement in criterion A that it be outside the range of usual human experience. This allowed us to determine the extent to which the estimated prevalence of PTSD changed when criterion A was relaxed. The standard DIS symptom questions were used to evaluate criteria B through D, and standard DIS coding rules for criteria B through D were used to arrive at a diagnosis of PTSD according to the *DSM-III-R* criteria.

The fourth modification is that we evaluated criteria B through D only for one event per respondent. When a respondent reported the occurrence of more than one type of event, he or she was asked to nominate one of these as "most upsetting" for purposes of this evaluation. The Revised DIS, in comparison, evaluates these symptoms for up to three events. This restriction was imposed because of time and budget constraints in the NCS and with the recognition that only a small number of respondents who fail to meet PTSD diagnostic criteria for their "most upsetting" event are likely to meet these criteria for any other event (Naomi Breslau, PhD, oral communication, 1994).

The failure to obtain a complete trauma history and to assess PTSD for each lifetime trauma, a limitation not only of the NCS but of all previous community epidemiologic surveys of PTSD, means that estimates of lifetime prevalence are lower-bound estimates. It also means that the NCS and other community epidemiologic surveys of PTSD are unable to obtain unbiased data on either age-at-onset distributions or variation across events in the conditional probability of PTSD after trauma exposure. We will return to these limitations in the "Comment" section.

A small validation survey of the NCS PTSD module was conducted in which a probability sample of 29 NCS respondents who reported the occurrence of a lifetime trauma in the NCS were reinterviewed by trained clinical interviewers with a modified version of the PTSD module from an instrument that includes items from both the Structured Clinical Interview for *DSM-III-R*–Patient Version[43] and the Schedule for Affective Disorders and Schizophrenia–Lifetime Version.[44] This combined instrument was developed by researchers at the Harvard-Brown Anxiety Disorders Research Program.[45,46] Respondents who were diagnosed as having PTSD in the NCS (n=18) were oversampled compared with those diagnosed as being noncases (n=11). Interviewers were unaware of the NCS diagnoses. A weighted analysis that took this oversampling into consideration led to an estimated cross-sectional κ of 0.75, with an SE of .11. Positive predictive value was 1.0 and negative predictive value was 0.88, indicating that the NCS procedures somewhat underdiagnose PTSD.

ANALYSIS PROCEDURES

The NCS data were weighted to adjust for variation in within-household and between-household probabilities of selection and differential nonresponse. We also used a weight to adjust for differential nonresponse based on the nonrespondent survey and a comparison of the part 1 data reported by the small number of part 1 respondents who refused to complete part 2 vs those who did complete part 2. Respondents in the part 2 subsample were also weighted by the inverse of their probability of selection into part 2 to make the part 2 sample representative of the total population. Finally, the part 2 data were poststratified by means of an iterative procedure to approximate the national population distributions of the cross-classification of age, sex, race or ethnicity, marital status, education, living arrangements, region, and urbanicity as defined by the 1989 US National Health Interview Survey.[47] As shown in **Table 1**, the part 2 sample is representative of the total US population aged 15 to 54 years on a variety of sociodemographic characteristics. The weighted part 2 sample is used as the basis of the analyses reported in this article, and sample distributions reported reflect the weighted number of respondents (rounded to the nearest whole number).

Most of the results reported below are presented in the form of prevalences and zero-order odds ratios (ORs). The latter were obtained by exponentiating the regression coefficients from logistic models. The speed of recovery curve for the index episode was obtained by means of the Kaplan-Meier method for estimating survival curves. Because of the complex sample design, estimates of SEs of prevalences were obtained by the Taylor series linearization method.[48] The PSRATIO program in the OSIRIS software package[49] was used to make these calculations. Estimates of SEs of logistic regression coefficients were obtained by the method of balanced repeated replication[50,51] in 44 design-based balanced subsamples. The LOGISTIC program in the SAS software package[52] was used to estimate the parameters in each replicate, and an SAS macro was used to calculate the balanced repeated replication estimates of the variances of these parameter estimates across replicates. The speed of recovery curve was estimated by means of the SURVIVAL procedure in the SPSS software package.[53]

had a lifetime history of *DSM-III-R* PTSD. Breslau et al[26] administered the revised version of the DIS for *DSM-III-R* to a sample of young adults enrolled in a health maintenance organization in Detroit, Mich, and found that 11.3% of women (equivalent to 30.7% of those exposed to trauma) and 6% of men (equivalent to 14% of those exposed to trauma) had a lifetime history of PTSD.

Multiple factors might be involved in the much higher prevalences in the *DSM-III-R* vs *DSM-III* studies, including differences in diagnostic criteria, assessment procedures, and other sample characteristics.[27,28] Resnick et al[25] noted that the anonymity of telephone interviews may have contributed to the fact that so many women in their study reported traumatic experiences. Breslau et al[26] noted that recall bias might have been minimized in their study because of the young age of their respon-

Did Any of These Events Ever Happen to You?

1. You had direct combat experience in a war
2. You were involved in a life-threatening accident
3. You were involved in a fire, flood, or natural disaster
4. You witnessed someone being badly injured or killed
5. You were raped (someone had sexual intercourse with you when you did not want to by threatening you or using some degree of force)
6. You were sexually molested (someone touched or felt your genitals when you did not want them to)
7. You were seriously physically attacked or assaulted
8. You were physically abused as a child
9. You were seriously neglected as a child
10. You were threatened with a weapon, held captive, or kidnapped
11. Other ("any other terrible experience that most people never go through")
12. You suffered a great shock because one of the events on this list happened to someone close to you

Figure 1. *Questions about events and experiences that qualified as traumas according to* DSM-III-R.

dents, and that this could have played an important part in explaining why their prevalence estimate was higher than in previous studies.

TYPES OF TRAUMA

Only limited information is available on the types of traumatic experiences most strongly associated with PTSD. Many of the traumas identified as likely to cause PTSD are common,[9,29] and so the stipulation in criterion A of *DSM-III-R* that the trauma must be outside the range of usual human experience is difficult to defend.[30] Yet, ignoring this stipulation and allowing people with intrusive recollections of any stressful event to be evaluated as potential cases could dilute the meaning of PTSD as a stress-response syndrome.[31] One way of investigating this issue more carefully is to obtain base rates of exposure to specific traumas and to study variation in conditional probabilities of PTSD across different traumas. Data of this sort are presented below.

COMORBIDITY

Another important consideration in understanding PTSD is the high rate of comorbidity. Kulka et al[18] reported that 98.8% of Vietnam theater veterans with PTSD had a history of some other DIS *DSM-III-R* disorder, compared with 40.6% of those without PTSD. Helzer et al[21] and Breslau et al[26] reported that close to 80% of respondents with PTSD had experienced other psychiatric disorders, compared with about 30% and 44.3%, respectively, of those without PTSD. Rates of comorbidity between 62%[22] and 92%[24] have been reported in other population-based surveys of PTSD. Research in both treatment samples[32,33] and population-based samples[29] has used information on age at onset to show that history of other psychiatric disorders is associated with increased risk of subsequent PTSD. It is not clear, however, how large a proportion of all PTSD cases are primary vs secondary. This issue is examined in the present report.

Table 1. National Health Interview Survey (NHIS)*–National Comorbidity Survey (NCS) Part II Demographic Comparisons (n=5877)

	US Population (NHIS), %*	NCS Weighted, %	NCS Unweighted, %
Sex			
Male	49.1	47.8	48.2
Female	50.9	52.2	51.8
Race			
White	75.0	76.3	76.5
Black	11.9	11.4	11.3
Hispanic	8.6	9.0	8.9
Other	4.5	3.3	3.2
Education, y			
0-11	22.5	23.2	20.6
12	36.8	36.7	32.4
13-15	21.2	21.7	26.9
≥16	19.5	18.3	20.1
Marital status			
Married	59.8	62.1	49.3
Separated/widowed/divorced	10.1	9.7	15.3
Never married	30.1	28.2	35.3
Region			
Northeast	20.0	20.2	19.3
Midwest	24.6	25.2	26.3
South	33.7	34.2	33.3
West	21.7	20.4	21.2
Age, y			
15-24	25.5	25.9	29.9
25-34	30.8	30.8	30.4
35-44	25.9	27.4	24.9
≥45	17.8	15.9	14.9
Urbanicity†			
MSAs ≥250 000	71.2	68.1	69.7
MSAs <250 000	8.1	7.3	6.3
Not MSA	20.7	24.6	24.0
Total No.	65 244	5877	5877

*National Health Interview Survey, 1989, *US Department of Health and Human Services, National Center for Health Statistics.*[47]
†*MSA indicates Metropolitan Statistical Area.*

CHRONICITY

Finally, we consider the issue of chronicity. The *DSM-III-R* requires a 1-month duration of symptoms as a criterion for PTSD. The sub–work group on PTSD for *DSM-IV* suggested that PTSD that endures for 3 months should be considered chronic based on evidence from several prospective studies of trauma victims that the number of people with PTSD symptoms decreases substantially within 3 months[34] and on evidence that people whose symptoms persist beyond 3 to 6 months have a high probability of becoming chronic cases.[21,24,32,35] Although much of this evidence comes from treatment samples in which chronicity would be expected to be worse, Breslau and Davis[36] found that 57% of PTSD cases in their sample had a duration of more than 1 year. We present data herein on the persistence of an index episode of PTSD in a nationally representative general population sample to investigate whether PTSD does, in fact, become chronic if symptoms last beyond 3 months.

Table 2. Lifetime Prevalence of Posttraumatic Stress Disorder by Age, Sex, and Marital Status

	% (SE)							
	Married		Previously Married		Never Married		Total	
Age, y	Male	Female	Male	Female	Male	Female	Male	Female
15-24	9.6 (5.0)	16.4 (2.6)	12.6 (9.4)	10.4 (5.3)	1.7 (0.5)	7.9 (1.3)	2.8 (0.7)	10.3 (1.2)
25-34	6.0 (1.7)	9.9 (1.5)	11.1 (5.2)	20.5 (5.9)	2.9 (0.9)	10.0 (2.8)	5.6 (1.0)	11.2 (1.3)
35-44	5.1 (1.7)	8.1 (1.7)	7.0 (2.0)	25.8 (4.9)	1.1 (0.8)	16.3 (6.7)	5.0 (1.4)	10.6 (1.6)
45-54	7.1 (2.1)	8.3 (1.9)	10.2 (5.4)	11.6 (3.8)	4.6 (1.9)	11.8 (7.3)	7.6 (2.0)	8.9 (1.7)
Total	6.1 (0.9)	9.6 (0.8)	9.4 (2.8)	18.9 (3.0)	1.9 (0.4)	8.9 (1.4)	5.0 (0.6)	10.4 (0.8)

RESULTS

PREVALENCE OF PTSD

The estimated lifetime prevalence of *DSM-III-R* PTSD in the total sample was 7.8% (with an SE of 0.5%). This estimate increased only modestly, to 8.4% (SE, 0.5%), when nonqualifying events were included, so the remainder of the analysis was based only on qualifying events. Lifetime prevalence estimates within the cells of the three-way cross-classification of age, sex, and marital status are reported in **Table 2**. As shown there, women were more than twice as likely overall as men to have lifetime PTSD (10.4% vs 5.0%, z=5.4, P<.05). Gender differences were apparent in all birth cohorts with lifetime prevalence significantly greater among older birth cohorts for men but not women. Lifetime prevalence was higher among the previously married (separated, divorced, or widowed) than the currently married, but this was significant only among women (18.9% vs 9.6%, z=3.0, P=.004, compared with 9.4% vs 6.1%, z=1.3, P=.17 among men). Prevalence was also higher among the married than the never married, but this was significant only among men (6.1% vs 1.9%, z=4.3, P=.001, compared with 9.6% vs 8.9%, z=0.4, P=.37 among women).

PREVALENCE OF TRAUMA EXPOSURE

Estimates of the lifetime prevalence of trauma exposure are presented in **Table 3** separately for men and women; 60.7% of men and 51.2% of women reported at least one traumatic event (z=3.8, P=.001). Consistent with previous research,[9] the majority of people with some type of lifetime trauma actually experienced two (14.5%/60.7%=23.9% of men with a lifetime trauma, 13.5%/51.2%=26.4% of women with a lifetime trauma), three (9.5%/60.7%=15.7% of men with a lifetime trauma, 5.0%/51.2=9.8% of women with a lifetime trauma), or more (10.2%/60.7%=16.8% of men with a lifetime trauma, 6.4%/51.2%=12.5% of women with a lifetime trauma) types of trauma. The types of trauma experienced by the largest proportions of people were witnessing someone being badly injured or killed (35.6% of men and 14.5% of women), being involved in a fire, flood, or natural disaster (18.9% of men and 15.2% of women), and being involved in a life-threatening accident (25% of men and 13.8% of women). A significantly higher proportion of men than women reported experiencing each of these three as well as physical attacks, combat experience, and being threatened with a weapon, held captive, or kidnapped. A significantly higher proportion of women than men, in comparison, reported rape, sexual molestation, childhood parental neglect, and childhood physical abuse.

Table 3. Lifetime Prevalence of Trauma Experience

	Lifetime Prevalence of Trauma					
	Men (n=2812)*			Women (n=3065)*		
Trauma	%	(SE)	No.	%	(SE)	No.
Rape	0.7†	(0.2)	19	9.2	(0.8)	281
Molestation	2.8†	(0.5)	78	12.3	(1.0)	376
Physical attack	11.1†	(1.0)	313	6.9	(0.9)	210
Combat	6.4†	(0.9)	179	0.0	...	0
Shock	11.4	(1.1)	320	12.4	(1.1)	381
Threat with weapon	19.0†	(1.3)	535	6.8	(0.6)	208
Accident	25.0†	(1.2)	703	13.8	(1.1)	422
Natural disaster with fire	18.9†	(1.4)	532	15.2	(1.2)	467
Witness	35.6†	(2.0)	1002	14.5	(0.7)	445
Neglect	2.1†	(0.4)	58	3.4	(0.5)	105
Physical abuse	3.2†	(0.4)	91	4.8	(0.6)	146
Other qualifying trauma	2.2	(0.5)	61	2.7	(0.4)	83
Any trauma	60.7†	(1.9)	1707	51.2	(1.9)	1570
No. of traumas						
1	26.5	(1.5)	745	26.3	(1.7)	806
2	14.5	(0.9)	407	13.5	(0.9)	415
3	9.5†	(0.9)	268	5.0	(0.6)	154
4	10.2†	(0.8	287	6.4	(0.6)	195

**Sample distributions reflect the weighted number of respondents rounded to the nearest whole number.*

†Sex difference significant at the .05 level, two-tailed test.

DIFFERENCES ACROSS TRAUMAS IN PROBABILITY OF PTSD

As described above, the NCS assessed PTSD either for the respondent's only lifetime trauma or, in the case of respondents who experienced more than one trauma type, for the one lifetime trauma nominated as "most upsetting." As shown in **Table 4**, the probability of a trauma being the basis for the assessment of PTSD (P1 in the table) varied substantially across trauma types. This variation was a complex function of differences in the distribution of the joint occurrences of multiple traumas and the likelihood that some types of trauma are generally more distressing than others. Among men and women alike, rape was the listed trauma with the highest conditional probability of

Table 4. Conditional Probabilities of Specific Traumas Being the Basis for the Assessment of Posttraumatic Stress Disorder (PTSD) and, Once Selected for Assessment, for Being Associated With PTSD*

	Lifetime Prevalence of PTSD					
	Men			Women		
Trauma	P1 (SE)	P2 (SE)	n_t	P1 (SE)	P2 (SE)	n_t
Rape	62.1 (11.6)	65.0 (15.6)	12	74.4 (4.1)	45.9 (5.9)	209
Molestation	26.9 (6.2)	12.2† (5.3)	21	61.4 (2.8)	26.5 (4.0)	231
Physical attack	35.7 (5.1)	1.8† (0.9)	112	42.0 (7.7)	21.3 (7.3)	88
Combat	57.7 (6.7)	38.8† (9.9)	103	. . .	. . .	0
Shock	44.8 (4.7)	4.4† (1.4)	144	55.4 (4.0)	10.4 (2.0)	211
Threat with weapon	32.9 (3.0)	1.9† (0.8)	176	36.4 (4.8)	32.6 (7.8)	76
Accident	44.6 (3.6)	6.3 (1.8)	314	44.5 (4.1)	8.8 (4.3)	188
Natural disaster with fire	35.9 (2.8)	3.7 (1.8)	191	44.4 (4.4)	5.4 (3.8)	207
Witness	52.4 (2.7)	6.4 (1.2)	524	47.1 (4.2)	7.5 (1.7)	209
Neglect	27.8 (5.8)	23.9 (10.3)	16	28.1 (5.8)	19.7 (7.7)	30
Physical abuse	50.4 (4.7)	22.3† (5.2)	46	37.0 (5.0)	48.5 (9.5)	54
Other qualifying trauma	77.6 (7.8)	12.7† (4.8)	48	80.8 (5.0)	33.4 (8.0)	67
Any trauma	. . .	8.1 (1.0)	1707	. . .	20.4 (1.5)	1570

**P1 indicates the probability that a respondent who reported the lifetime occurrence of a particular trauma type will have this be the basis for the assessment of PTSD (ie, that this trauma will either be the respondent's only lifetime trauma or the nominated "most upsetting" trauma); P2, the probability that a particular trauma type, once selected as the basis for the assessment of PTSD, will be associated with PTSD; and n_t, the weighted number of respondents (rounded to the nearest whole number) with a particular "only or most upsetting" trauma type who were diagnosed as having lifetime PTSD.*

†Sex difference significant at the .05 level, two-tailed test.

being the basis for the assessment of PTSD, while sexual molestation and childhood neglect had the lowest conditional probabilities for men and women, respectively.

Consistent with previous research reviewed by March[31] and by Kilpatrick and Resnick,[9] the columns in Table 4 labeled P2 show that the proportion of respondents with a trauma who met criteria for PTSD varied significantly by type of most upsetting trauma. The trauma of this sort most likely to be associated with PTSD among men and women alike was rape. Sixty-five percent of men and 45.9% of women who reported this as their most upsetting trauma developed PTSD. Other most upsetting listed traumas associated with a high probability of PTSD included combat exposure, childhood neglect, and childhood physical abuse among men (with probabilities of developing PTSD of 38.8%, 23.9%, and 22.3%, respectively) and sexual molestation, physical attack, being threatened with a weapon, and childhood physical abuse among women (with probabilities of developing PTSD of 26.5%, 21.3%, 32.6%, and 48.5%, respectively).

A comparison of the results in Tables 3 and 4 shows that, although men were more likely than women to experience at least one trauma overall, women were more likely than men to experience a trauma associated with a high probability of PTSD. While 44.6% of men with a lifetime trauma reported that their most upsetting trauma was one of those associated with high probability of PTSD among men (ie, rape, combat exposure, childhood neglect, or childhood physical abuse), a significantly higher percentage of women (67.6%; z=11.5, P=.001) with a lifetime trauma reported that their most distressing trauma was one of those associated with a high probability of PTSD among women (ie, rape, sexual molestation, physical attack, being threatened with a weapon, or childhood physical abuse). Furthermore, for all most upsetting traumas other than rape and childhood neglect, a higher proportion of women than men met criteria for PTSD. The combination of these influences—greater exposure to high-impact traumas and greater likelihood of developing PTSD once exposed—led to the finding that women exposed to a trauma were more than twice as likely as men to develop PTSD (20.4% of women compared with 8.2% of men, z=6.7, P=.001).

DISTRIBUTION OF MOST UPSETTING TRAUMAS AMONG PEOPLE WITH PTSD

The probabilities of having each type of most upsetting trauma in the subsample of respondents with lifetime PTSD are presented in **Table 5**. The traumas most commonly associated with PTSD among men were combat exposure, which was the nominated most upsetting trauma for 28.8% of men with PTSD, and witnessing someone being badly injured or killed, which was the nominated trauma for 24.3% of men. Combat exposure was a fairly uncommon event (6.4% lifetime prevalence among men) associated with a high probability of PTSD when it was nominated as most upsetting (38.8%). Witnessing, in comparison, was a much more common event (35.6% lifetime prevalence among men) associated with a low probability of PTSD when it was nominated as most upsetting (6.4%).

Among women, the events most commonly associated with PTSD were rape, which was nominated as most upsetting for 29.9% of women with PTSD, and sexual molestation, which was the nominated event for 19.1% of female cases. Together, rape and molestation were the nominated events for 49% of women with PTSD. These events are both common in the general population of women (9.2% of women in the NCS reported lifetime rape and 12.2% reported molestation) and associated with high probabilities of PTSD when nominated as most upsetting (45.9% for rape and 26.5% for molestation).

Table 5. Those With Posttraumatic Stress Disorder (PTSD) Reporting Each Most Upsetting Trauma Type by Sex

	Men (n=139)*		Women (n=320)*	
Trauma	% (SE)	No.*	% (SE)	No.*
Rape	5.4† (2.8)	8	29.9 (3.4)	96
Molestation	1.8† (0.7)	3	19.1 (3.1)	61
Physical attack	1.4† (0.6)	2	5.9 (1.6)	19
Combat	28.8 (6.1)	40	...	0
Shock	4.5 (1.4)	6	6.8 (1.2)	22
Threat with weapon	2.5† (1.1)	3	7.7 (2.2)	25
Accident	12.1 (3.4)	20	5.1 (2.4)	16
Natural disaster with fire	5.2 (2.5)	7	3.5 (2.3)	11
Witness	24.3† (4.8)	30	4.9 (1.1)	16
Neglect	2.8 (1.1)	4	1.8 (0.7)	6
Physical abuse	7.4 (2.0)	10	8.2 (2.9)	26
Other qualifying trauma	3.8 (1.6)	6	7.0 (2.1)	22
Any trauma	100.0 (. . .)	139	100.0 (. . .)	320

*Sample distributions reflect the weighted number of respondents rounded to the nearest whole number.

†Sex difference significant at the .05 level, two-tailed test.

DEMOGRAPHIC CORRELATES OF PTSD

Multiple logistic regression analyses were carried out to describe the sociodemographic correlates of lifetime PTSD. Sex, age, marital status, and the interactions of age with sex and sex with marital status were all found to be significant predictors of lifetime PTSD. Once these significant predictors were controlled, there were no significant residual associations of PTSD with race, education, urbanicity, or region of the country.

The ORs under model 1 in **Table 6** describe the significant associations of age, sex, and marital status with PTSD. The results in the rest of the table decompose these total associations into components resulting from the relationships of these predictors with exposure to at least one lifetime trauma (model 2), with PTSD in the subsample of respondents exposed to at least one lifetime trauma (model 3), and with PTSD in the subsample of respondents exposed to at least one lifetime trauma after controlling for differences in most upsetting trauma type (model 4). If the association of a particular demographic variable with PTSD results from its being associated with higher-impact traumas, the OR for that variable under model 3 will be larger than the OR under model 4.

Sex

Consistent with our earlier results, Table 6 shows that women had a significantly higher lifetime prevalence of PTSD than men. The coding of the variables in Table 6, however, is such that the OR of 4.87 for women under model 1 is for the comparison between never-married women and never-married men aged 15 to 24 years. A substantial sex difference in PTSD existed in this subsample despite the finding under model 2 that a lower proportion of women than men in this subsample reported ever experiencing a trauma (OR=0.82). As shown under model 3, women in this subsample who had been exposed to at least one trauma had a much higher odds than comparable men of developing PTSD (OR=6.13). The OR is smaller under model 3 than model 4, which means that this greater vulnerability partly results from the fact that the most upsetting traumas nominated by women were associated with a higher probability of PTSD than those nominated by men (assuming, for purposes of this analysis, that there was no sex difference in the probability of PTSD among men and women who nominated the same most upsetting event). However, the fact that the OR under model 4 remained significant shows that these women were significantly more vulnerable than men even when we controlled for sex differences in the types of most upsetting trauma. This sex difference might be explained by detailed aspects of trauma exposure, such as age at exposure and/or previous trauma history, but we were unable to investigate this possibility because PTSD was not assessed for a random trauma.

Age

Because the relationship between age and lifetime prevalence of PTSD differed by sex, the ORs associated with age were estimated separately for men and women in Table 6. Among men, there was no consistent association between age and PTSD (model 1), controlling for marital status. The results under model 2, however, show that lifetime trauma exposure was significantly and positively associated with age, while the results under models 3 and 4 showed a counterbalancing, but not statistically significant, negative association between age and probability of PTSD given exposure. Among women, in comparison, there was a nonsignificant trend for lifetime PTSD to be negatively associated with age (model 1), controlling for marital status. This is because the increasing prevalence of trauma exposure with age was much less pronounced among women than men, while the same general pattern of a modestly decreasing probability of PTSD among the exposed with increasing age held for women as well as men.

Marital Status

Lifetime PTSD was significantly more prevalent among the previously married (separated, divorced, or widowed) than the currently married for both men and women, controlling for age. Furthermore, among men but not women, PTSD was significantly more prevalent among the currently married than the never married, controlling for age. These associations resulted largely from a combination of significantly elevated probabilities of PTSD among the exposed (models 3 and 4) rather than differential lifetime probabilities of trauma exposure.

LIFETIME COMORBIDITY BETWEEN PTSD AND OTHER DISORDERS

Estimates of the lifetime prevalences of 11 *DSM-III-R* disorders are reported in **Table 7** separately for men and women with and without a lifetime history of PTSD. The ORs show a consistently significant cross-sectional relationship between lifetime PTSD and these other disor-

Table 6. Sociodemographic Correlates of Lifetime Posttraumatic Stress Disorder (PTSD)*

	OR (95% Confidence Interval)			
	Model 1: Risk of PTSD	Model 2: Risk of Trauma	Model 3: Risk of PTSD in Trauma Subsample	Model 4: Risk of PTSD in Trauma Subsample Controlling Trauma Type
Sex				
Male	1.00 (. . .)	1.00 (. . .)	1.00 (. . .)	1.00 (. . .)
Female	4.87† (2.92-8.12)	0.82 (0.65-1.04)	6.13† (3.59-10.46)	4.05† (2.48-6.63)
Age (males), y				
15-24	1.00 (. . .)	1.00 (. . .)	1.00 (. . .)	1.00 (. . .)
25-34	0.87 (0.36-2.07)	1.25 (0.92-1.70)	0.85 (0.36-1.99)	0.81 (0.32-2.09)
35-44	0.66 (0.21-2.10)	1.46† (1.00-2.13)	0.58 (0.18-1.88)	0.31 (0.09-1.10)
45-54	0.96 (0.34-2.72)	1.76† (1.02-3.05)	0.81 (0.28-2.29)	0.57 (0.17-1.95)
Age (females), y				
15-24	1.00 (. . .)	1.00 (. . .)	1.00 (. . .)	1.00 (. . .)
25-34	0.89 (0.60-1.31)	1.06 (0.78-1.43)	0.83 (0.52-1.32)	0.82 (0.51-1.33)
35-44	0.81 (0.49-1.35)	1.45† (1.00-2.10)	0.61 (0.36-1.03)	0.58 (0.37-1.05)
45-54	0.64 (0.36-1.30)	1.05 (0.72-1.53)	0.55 (0.31-1.00)	0.59 (0.35-1.01)
Marital status (males)				
Never married	1.00 (. . .)	1.00 (. . .)	1.00 (. . .)	1.00 (. . .)
Married	3.82† (1.64-8.87)	1.14 (0.79-1.63)	3.56† (1.62-7.82)	3.21† (1.43-7.86)
Previously married	6.00† (1.73-20.79)	1.60 (0.87-2.93)	5.11† (1.39-18.71)	3.47 (0.96-15.04)
Marital status (females)				
Never married	1.00 (. . .)	1.00 (. . .)	1.00 (. . .)	1.00 (. . .)
Married	1.27 (0.77-2.10)	1.02 (0.73-1.42)	1.33 (0.78-2.26)	1.20 (0.76-1.91)
Previously married	2.86† (1.48-5.53)	1.35 (0.83-2.21)	2.93† (1.14-6.08)	2.59† (1.33-5.06)

**The coefficients are based on multivariate logistic regression models in which age, sex, marital status, age × sex, and marital status × sex are predictors of the outcome. The outcome in the first model is PTSD. The outcome in the second model is trauma. The outcome in the third model is the same as in the first, with the exception that the model is estimated in the subsample of respondents who experienced trauma. The outcome in the fourth model is the same as in the third and in the same subsample, with the exception that the model includes controls for trauma type. The interaction between age and sex (3 dfs) is significant in each of the four models, with Wald χ^2 values (adjusted for design effects) ranging between 10.6 and 16.7. The interaction between marital status and sex (2 dfs) is also significant in all models, with Wald χ^2 (again adjusted for design effects) ranging between 13.1 and 17.5. More detailed modeling failed to find any significant age × sex or age × sex × marital status interactions.*

†The odds ratio (OR) is significantly different at the .05 level (two-tailed) from the reference category value of OR=1.0.

ders among both men and women. A lifetime history of at least one other disorder was present in 88.3% of the men with lifetime PTSD and 79% of the women with lifetime PTSD.

The relative magnitudes of the ORs in Table 7 are worth noting in light of observations by previous commentators that comorbidity with PTSD would be expected for some disorders because of overlap in symptom criteria.[54,55] In particular, several of the criteria C and D symptoms of PTSD (eg, diminished interest, restricted range of affect, sleep difficulties, difficulty concentrating) overlap with symptoms of depression, while several criterion C symptoms of PTSD (eg, irritability, hypervigilance, startle) overlap with symptoms of generalized anxiety disorder, and criterion D6 (physiologic reactivity) could create an overlap with social phobia, simple phobia, and panic disorder. The cross-sectional results in Table 7 show that PTSD does, in fact, have substantial comorbidities with all of these disorders.

Absence of a complete PTSD assessment for all lifetime traumas made it impossible to determine unequivocally how often comorbid PTSD was a primary disorder in the sense of having an earlier age at onset than other comorbid conditions. It is possible, however, to place upper and lower bounds on this estimate. The upper bound is the percentage of patients with comorbidity who had no other NCS/*DSM-III-R* disorder as of the age at their earliest lifetime trauma. The lower bound is the percentage of patients with comorbidity who had no other NCS/*DSM-III-R* disorder as of the age at their most upsetting trauma. These upper and lower bound estimates are reported in **Table 8**. The results suggest that PTSD was primary more often than not with respect to comorbid affective disorders and substance use disorders and, among women, with respect to comorbid conduct disorder (range, 52.7% to 84.3%). Posttraumatic stress disorder was less likely to be primary with respect to comorbid anxiety disorders and, among men, comorbid conduct disorder, although even in these cases the percentage of cases in which PTSD was primary was substantial (range, 30.3% to 61.4%). We estimate that PTSD was primary with respect to all other comorbid disorders between 29.3% and 51.3% of the time among men and between 40.8% and 57.6% of the time among women.

PERSISTENCE OF PTSD

As noted earlier, NCS respondents who met criteria for PTSD were asked how many weeks, months, or years after onset of their index episode they continued to have symptoms at least a few times a week. Survival curves based on these retrospective reports are presented in **Figure 2** separately for respondents who ever sought pro-

Table 7. Comorbidity of Posttraumatic Stress Disorder (PTSD) With Other Disorders in the Total Sample*

	PTSD		No PTSD		
	% (SE)	No.†	% (SE)	No.†	OR (95% CI)
Men					
Affective disorders					
MDE	47.9 (5.5)	67	11.7 (0.8)	314	6.90‡ (4.36-10.92)
Dysthymia	21.4 (4.5)	30	4.4 (0.4)	117	5.95‡ (3.18-11.13)
Mania	11.7 (3.5)	16	1.3 (0.3)	34	10.41‡ (4.20-25.76)
Anxiety disorders					
GAD	16.8 (4.5)	23	3.3 (0.4)	89	5.89‡ (2.59-13.38)
Panic disorder	7.3 (2.3)	10	1.9 (0.4)	52	4.11‡ (1.60-10.11)
Simple phobia	31.4 (6.0)	44	6.0 (0.5)	161	7.14‡ (4.13-12.35)
Social phobia	27.6 (4.9)	38	11.3 (0.7)	302	2.99‡ (1.77-5.04)
Agoraphobia	16.1 (4.7)	22	4.1 (0.5)	109	4.53‡ (1.88-10.92)
Substance use disorders					
Alcohol abuse/dependence	51.9 (6.7)	72	34.4 (1.2)	919	2.06‡ (1.14-3.70)
Drug abuse/dependence	34.5 (6.9)	48	15.1 (1.0)	403	2.97‡ (1.52-5.79)
Other disorder					
Conduct disorder	43.3 (4.9)	60	19.5 (1.2)	521	3.15‡ (2.12-4.69)
Any disorder§					
No other diagnosis	11.7 (3.0)	67	45.2 (1.9)	1476	0.16‡ (0.07-0.35)
1 diagnoses	14.9 (2.8)	49	24.4 (1.1)	515	2.36 (0.99-5.64)
2 diagnoses	14.4 (3.9)	59	14.7 (1.1)	341	3.80‡ (1.37-10.58)
≥3 diagnoses	59.0 (5.2)	144	15.7 (0.9)	414	14.51‡ (6.65-31.66)
Women					
Affective disorders					
MDE	48.5 (3.4)	155	18.8 (0.9)	516	4.07‡ (3.08-5.39)
Dysthymia	23.3 (3.3)	75	6.8 (0.6)	187	4.14‡ (2.74-6.25)
Mania	5.7 (1.7)	18	1.3 (0.4)	37	4.45‡ (1.74-11.41)
Anxiety disorders					
GAD	15.0 (2.5)	48	5.9 (0.7)	162	2.81‡ (1.60-4.95)
Panic disorder	12.6 (2.3)	40	4.3 (0.5)	119	3.18‡ (1.89-5.37)
Simple phobia	29.0 (2.9)	93	14.5 (1.2)	397	2.42‡ (1.66-3.51)
Social phobia	28.4 (3.1)	91	14.1 (1.2)	387	2.42‡ (1.71-3.43)
Agoraphobia	22.4 (2.8)	72	7.8 (0.7)	214	3.42‡ (2.40-4.88)
Substance use disorders					
Alcohol abuse/dependence	27.9 (3.6)	90	13.5 (1.1)	372	2.48‡ (1.78-3.45)
Drug abuse/dependence	26.9 (3.4)	86	7.6 (0.7)	209	4.46‡ (3.11-6.39)
Other disorder					
Conduct disorder	15.4 (2.0)	49	5.9 (0.7)	163	2.88‡ (1.98-4.18)
Any disorder§					
No other diagnosis	21.0 (3.7)	16	53.8 (2.2)	1209	0.23‡ (0.14-0.37)
1 diagnosis	17.2 (2.2)	20	20.4 (1.4)	522	2.17‡ (1.35-3.48)
2 diagnoses	18.2 (3.1)	9	11.7 (0.8)	398	3.98‡ (2.11-7.50)
≥3 diagnoses	43.6 (3.8)	93	14.1 (1.4)	544	7.91‡ (4.82-12.96)

**OR indicates odds ratio; CI, confidence interval; MDE, major depressive episode; and GAD, generalized affective disorder. n=139 and 2673 for men with and without PTSD, respectively; n=320 and 2745 for women with and without PTSD, respectively.*
†Sample distributions reflect the weighted number of respondents rounded to the nearest whole number.
‡Odds ratio significant at the .05 level, two-tailed test.
§Odds ratios for one, two, and three or more disorders from a multivariate model.

fessional treatment for a mental problem and those who did not. The survival curves decreased most steeply in the first 12 months after the onset of symptoms in both subsamples. The curves continued to decline with a more gradual slope for approximately 6 years after symptom onset. The median time to remission was 36 months among the respondents who ever sought professional treatment (n=266) and 64 months among those who did not (n=193). Statistical analysis based on the Lee-Desu χ^2 test[56] showed that these two survival curves were significantly different (χ^2=5.0, *df*=1, *P*=.02), although absence of data on the timing of treatment made it impossible to interpret this difference as resulting from the effects of treatment. Perhaps of more interest than the difference between the two curves was the consistent finding that PTSD failed to remit in somewhat more than one third of persons even after many years not only in the subsample of respondents who did not receive professional treatment but also in the treatment subsample.

COMMENT

PREVALENCE

The results reported herein are based on data that require lifetime recall of traumas and the symptoms associated with them. It is likely that there was some recall failure in respondent reports, leading to underestimation of the lifetime prevalences of both traumatic experiences and PTSD. In addition, PTSD was assessed for only one event per respondent, which could have led to additional underestimation of PTSD. Furthermore, the clinical validation study of the NCS diagnostic assessment showed that PTSD was somewhat underdiagnosed.

Even with these biases toward underreporting, however, the results show that PTSD is a highly prevalent disorder. A full 7.8% of respondents (5% of men and 10.4% of women) were estimated to have a lifetime history of PTSD. Similar prevalence estimates were reported by Breslau et al[26] (6% among men and 11.3% among women) and Resnick et al[25] (12.3% among women) in the two previous epidemiologic surveys of PTSD that used *DSM-III-R* criteria. These are much higher than the 1% to 3% prevalence estimates found in the ECA study[21,22] and in a subsequent study that used the same methods as the ECA.[24]

It is unclear why the results of recent studies differ so dramatically from those of the earlier ECA studies. Differences in diagnostic criteria, sampling frames, years of administration, or administrative procedures could all be involved. There are also differences across studies in the kinds of events that were counted as fulfilling criterion A. For example, Davidson et al,[22] in their analysis of the North Carolina ECA data, included among the qualifying events such things as mother's illness and death and anaphylactic reaction to medication as qualifying events, while Helzer et al,[21] in their analysis of the St Louis ECA data, included having a miscarriage and Shore et al[24] included husband's illness and death and wife's seizures. Our reading of *DSM-III-R* suggests that none of these is a qualifying event and, as a result, open-ended reports of such events by NCS respondents were not counted in estimating PTSD. At the same time, some of the events that we included might not have been included by previous investigators. Because of these differences, it is difficult to make rigorous comparisons across the different community surveys of PTSD.

The estimated prevalence of PTSD did not increase much when we relaxed criterion A to include nonqualifying events reported in response to an open-ended question about "any other terrible experiences that most people never go through." It is important to recognize, though, that we did not systematically attempt to elicit information about nonqualifying events by asking explicit questions about such things as chronic illness, job loss, or marital difficulties, and we have no way of knowing how often these experiences are associated with PTSD-like symptoms. It would be useful for subsequent research to conduct a more broad-based investigation of this sort to determine which types of nonqualifying life events are most likely to provoke such symptoms and to facilitate research on individual differences in vulnerability aimed at explaining why some people develop PTSD-like symptoms in response to events that are not normally considered traumatic.[9,31] This would be especially useful in light of the substantial changes introduced into *DSM-IV* concerning the definitions of qualifying events.[57]

Table 8. Proportions of Comorbid Lifetime Posttraumatic Stress Disorder That Are Primary Disorders

	Men, % (SE)		Women, % (SE)	
	Upper Bound	Lower Bound	Upper Bound	Lower Bound
Any affective disorder	76.8 (6.1)	53.0 (8.1)	78.4 (3.5)	57.9 (4.9)
Any anxiety disorder	50.0 (7.4)	30.3 (6.2)	56.1 (4.9)	37.3 (4.1)
Conduct disorder	61.4 (8.1)	45.9 (7.9)	72.7 (8.8)	56.3 (9.4)
Any alcohol or substance disorder	65.3 (5.9)	52.7 (6.8)	84.3 (2.7)	65.1 (4.2)
Any disorder	51.3 (5.0)	29.3 (4.6)	57.6 (3.6)	40.8 (3.5)

EXPOSURE TO TRAUMATIC EXPERIENCES

The results concerning the types of traumatic experiences that are associated with PTSD are also relevant to a controversy concerning criterion A in *DSM-III-R*, which stipulates that the trauma must be outside the range of usual human experience and of a type that would be markedly distressing to almost anyone. The NCS results are consistent with recent research in showing that virtually all of the qualifying events for PTSD are quite common[9] and that none is such that virtually everyone exposed to it develops PTSD. There is also enormous

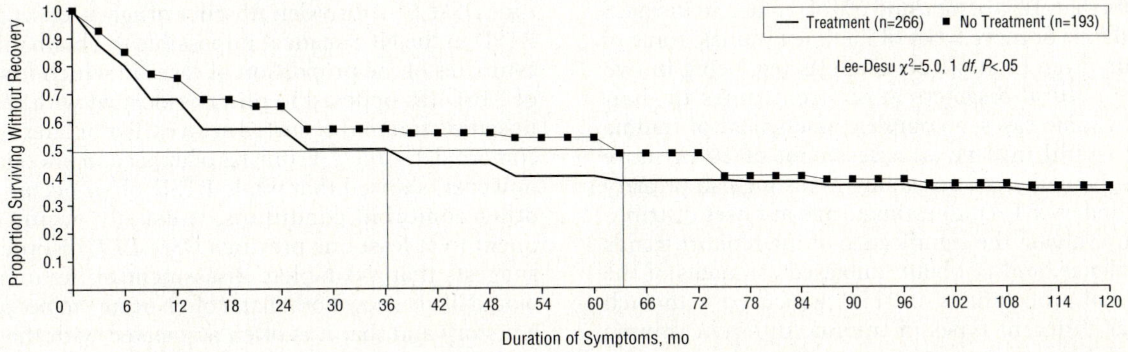

Figure 2. *Survival curves based on duration of symptoms for respondents who did and did not receive treatment for posttraumatic stress disorder.*

variability across nominated most distressing traumatic events in the probability of PTSD. Furthermore, events that are traumatic in one sector of the population may not be traumatic in another. For example, men in the NCS were nearly twice as likely as women to report being seriously physically attacked or assaulted (11.1% vs 6.9%, z=3.2, P=.002). Yet, this type of event, when nominated as most upsetting, was more than 15 times as likely to be associated with PTSD among women as men (21.3% vs 1.8%, z=2.6, P=.01). Such subgroup differences make it difficult to categorize stressful events neatly into those that are traumatic and those that are not traumatic.[31]

In evaluating the results concerning the types of traumatic experiences associated with PTSD, it is important to remember that the NCS assessed criteria B through D for only one event per person. As a result, the event-specific analyses focus on the subsample of events that were rated most upsetting by respondents who had two or more lifetime trauma types. This creates the potential for an overestimation of the associations of particular events with PTSD. For example, while 65% of the subsample of men who reported that being raped was either their only or their most upsetting lifetime trauma developed PTSD after that event, a much smaller percentage (46.4%) of the larger group of all men who reported being raped (whether or not it was their only or most upsetting trauma) reported lifetime PTSD associated with their most upsetting trauma. The most plausible way to interpret this discrepancy is to assume that the rapes nominated as most upsetting shared some objective features that made them more traumatizing than the rapes not nominated as most upsetting. If this is the case, it would be a mistake to assume that "typical" traumas are associated with probabilities of PTSD as high as those found herein.

The only way to correct this problem and obtain unbiased estimates of the extent to which traumas of particular types are likely to lead to PTSD is to obtain data on "typical" traumas rather than "most upsetting" traumas. This could be done, in simplest form, by carrying out a survey in which an enumeration of all lifetime traumas was obtained from each respondent and a randomly selected trauma or subset of traumas from this list was assessed for PTSD. A complete assessment of trauma history and whether PTSD occurred after each lifetime trauma would provide much better information. However, this would be a substantial task. The results in Table 3 show that more than 10% of men and 6% of women in the NCS reported four or more types of lifetime traumas, some of which involved multiple occurrences (eg, being in two or more natural disasters at different times in their lives). In some cases, a complete assessment of trauma history would involve an assessment of 20 or more traumas. Nonetheless, our ability to distinguish primary and secondary PTSD, to estimate age-at-onset distributions, to evaluate the significance of intercohort trends in prevalence, and to obtain unbiased estimates of the conditional probabilities of PTSD associated with such things as different types of trauma, different trauma ages, and different trauma histories all require complete assessments of this sort. This should be a goal of future epidemiologic research on PTSD.

SOCIODEMOGRAPHIC CORRELATES OF PTSD

The NCS found that PTSD was approximately twice as prevalent among women as men. This is consistent with the findings of Breslau et al[26] in a community survey of young adults, but inconsistent with the results of two reports from the ECA study, neither of which found a sex difference in PTSD.[21,22] Both the NCS and Breslau et al[26] found that women exposed to a trauma are significantly more likely than men exposed to a trauma to develop PTSD and that this is the main reason for the sex difference in PTSD. This evidence of greater vulnerability among women is inconsistent with studies of people exposed to a single trauma that found conflicting results concerning whether men and women exposed to the same trauma differ significantly in the probability of PTSD.[13,58-60]

The NCS findings concerning different patterns of PTSD with age among men and women could reflect sex differences in substantive age effects, in substantive cohort effects, in methodologic artifacts caused by differential recall failure or differential sample attrition, or in some combination of these processes. There is no way to distinguish these possibilities with the data available to us. The situation is especially difficult in that we have no way of establishing age at onset of first PTSD because PTSD was assessed only for a single lifetime trauma.

The NCS found that lifetime PTSD was significantly more prevalent among respondents who were previously married than those who were married at the time of interview and, among men, more prevalent among the currently married than the never married. The only other general population study of PTSD that examined similar associations was that of Davidson et al[22] in the North Carolina ECA, who found an elevated but nonsignificant prevalence of PTSD among married respondents vs others in the sample. Results concerning the effects of marital status in studies of particular traumas are inconsistent.[18,61,62]

COMORBIDITY

The NCS results concerning comorbidity are consistent with previous research[21,22,24,32,33,35] in showing that the relative odds of other lifetime disorders are significantly elevated among people with lifetime PTSD and that the vast majority of these people also have at least one other lifetime *DSM-III-R* disorder. Absence of age-at-onset data for PTSD in the NCS made it impossible to obtain unbiased estimates of the proportion of cases in which first onset of PTSD (as opposed to onset associated with the most upsetting trauma) occurred at an earlier or later age than comorbid disorders. Estimates of upper and lower bounds, however, showed that while PTSD often occurs before other comorbid conditions, it usually occurs subsequent to at least one previous *DSM-III-R* disorder. This suggests that a complete assessment of lifetime PTSD would likely show both that it often occurs to people with a history and that it is often associated with the subsequent onset of yet other disorders. Further research is needed to investigate these issues. In the ideal case, this would be done prospectively to avoid the retrospective recall bias that clouds the interpretation of this part of the NCS analysis.

It was noted above that previous commentators have argued that comorbidity with PTSD would be expected for some disorders because of overlap of several criteria C and D symptoms of PTSD with symptoms of depression, of several criterion C symptoms of PTSD with symptoms of generalized anxiety disorder, and of criterion D6 of PTSD with social phobia, simple phobia, and panic disorder.[54,55] It would be useful for future research to determine whether comorbidity of PTSD with these other disorders remains if the definition of PTSD were based on the more distinctive criterion B symptoms concerning flashbacks and reactions to reexposure.

DURATION OF THE INDEX EPISODE

Our analysis of the duration of PTSD symptoms associated with the most upsetting lifetime trauma, finally, yielded several important results. First, we found that the average duration of symptoms was shorter in the subsample of people who ever obtained treatment (36 months) than in the subsample of people who did not obtain treatment (64 months). Although this difference cannot be taken as definitive evidence of the effectiveness of treatment because of differential selection into treatment and the possibility that error in recall of symptom duration is correlated with treatment, it suggests that treatment may be effective in reducing the duration of PTSD. Second, we found that more than one third of persons with PTSD never fully remit even after many years and irrespective of whether they were in treatment. In addition, consistent with the results of several previous prospective and retrospective studies,[21,22,32,36,37] we found that the survival curve decreased most steeply in the first 12 months after the onset of symptoms. We also found that the curve continues to decline with a more gradual slope for approximately 6 years after symptom onset. This part of the pattern is inconsistent with the suggestion of the sub–work group on PTSD for *DSM-IV* that people whose symptoms persist beyond 3 months rarely recover without professional treatment. Indeed, these results suggest that even after 2 years, the average person with PTSD who has not been in treatment still has a 50% chance of eventual remission.

CONCLUSION

The results reported herein show that PTSD is a highly prevalent lifetime disorder that often persists for years. The qualifying events for PTSD are also common, with many respondents reporting the occurrence of quite a few such events during their lifetimes. Although there is great variability in the associations of these different events with PTSD, none is such that virtually everyone exposed to it develops the disorder. Future research should assess PTSD for each respondent's full lifetime trauma history to resolve uncertainties concerning age at onset, cohort effects, the relative risk of PTSD associated with different precipitating events, the impact of previous disorders on subsequent PTSD, and the impact of PTSD on subsequent secondary disorders.

Accepted for publication June 7, 1995.

The NCS is supported by the US Alcohol, Drug Abuse, and Mental Health Administration (grants MH46376 and MH49098) with supplemental support from the W. T. Grant Foundation (grant 90135190). Preparation of this report was also supported by a Research Scientist Development Award to the first author (grant 1 K01 MH00507).

Dr Kessler is the principal investigator in the NCS. Collaborating NCS sites and investigators are as follows: The Addiction Research Foundation, Toronto, Ontario (Robin Room, PhD); *Duke University Medical Center, Durham, NC* (Dan Blazer, MD, Marvin Swartz, MD); *Johns Hopkins University, Baltimore, Md* (James Anthony, PhD, William Eaton, PhD, Richard Frank, PhD, Philip Leaf, PhD); *the Max Planck Institute of Psychiatry–Clinical Institute, Munich, Germany* (Hans-Ulrich Wittchen, PhD); *the Medical College of Virginia, Richmond* (Kenneth Kendler, MD); *the University of Michigan, Ann Arbor* (Lloyd Johnston, PhD, Ronald Kessler, PhD); *New York (NY) University* (Patrick Shrout, PhD); *State University of New York at Stony Brook* (Evelyn Bromet, PhD); *The University of Toronto (Ontario)* (R. Jay Turner, PhD); *and Washington University School of Medicine, St Louis* (Linda Cottler, PhD).

We thank Jonathon Davidson, Mardi Horowitz, and the anonymous reviewers for helpful comments, and Naomi Breslau and Gabrielle Carlson for help in classifying events as either qualifying or nonqualifying according to criterion A of DSM-III-R. *Special thanks go to Helena Kraemer, who read multiple drafts and offered sage advice on the special difficulties introduced by the fact that PTSD was not assessed for all lifetime traumas. A complete list of NCS publications can be obtained by writing to the address below. The text of this and other NCS publications, working papers, and instruments can be obtained from the Internet by (1) ftping 141.211.207.206; (2) NAME=anonymous; (3) PASSWORD=(your Internet e-mail address); (4) reading the INSTRUCTIONS to download NCS documents. A public access NCS data file can be obtained from the Internet by (1) ftping ftp.icpsr.umich.edu; (2) NAME=anonymous; (3) PASSWORD=(your Internet e-mail address); (4) reading the INSTRUCTIONS to download NCS data.*

Reprint requests to Institute for Social Research, University of Michigan, Box 1248, Ann Arbor, MI 48106-1248 (Dr Kessler).

REFERENCES

1. Freud S. *Introduction to the Psychology of the War Neuroses.* Standard Edition, 18. London, England: Hogarth Press; 1919.
2. Burgess AW, Holstrum L. The rape trauma syndrome. *Am J Psychiatry.* 1974; 131:981-986.
3. Grinker K, Spiegel S. *Men Under Stress.* Philadelphia, Pa: Blakiston; 1945.
4. Horowitz MJ. *Stress Response Syndromes.* New York, NY: Jason Aronson Inc; 1976.
5. Lindemann E. Symptomology and management of acute grief. *Am J Psychiatry.* 1944;101:141-148.
6. Parad H, Resnick H, Parad Z. *Emergency Mental Health Services and Disaster Management.* New York, NY: Prentice Hall; 1976.
7. American Psychiatric Association, Committee on Nomenclature and Statistics. *Diagnostic and Statistical Manual of Mental Disorders, Third Edition.* Washington, DC: American Psychiatric Association; 1980.
8. Kilpatrick DG, Saunders BE, Veronen LJ, Best CL, Von JM. Criminal victim-

ization: lifetime prevalence, reporting to police, and psychological impact. *Crime Delinquency.* 1987;33:479-489.
9. Kilpatrick DG, Resnick HS. Posttraumatic stress disorder associated with exposure to criminal victimization in clinical and community populations. In: Davidson JRT, Foa EB, eds. *Posttraumatic Stress Disorder:* DSM-IV *and Beyond.* Washington, DC: American Psychiatric Press; 1992.
10. Frank E, Anderson BP. Psychiatric disorders in rape victims: past history and current symptomatology. *Compr Psychiatry.* 1987;28:77-82.
11. Pynoos RS, Nader K. Children who witness the sexual assaults of their mothers. *J Am Acad Child Adolesc Psychiatry.* 1988;27:567-572.
12. Green BL, Grace ML, Gleser CG. Identifying survivors at risk: long-term impairment following the Beverly Hills Supper Club fire. *J Consult Clin Psychol.* 1985;53:672-678.
13. Madakasira S, O'Brien KF. Acute posttraumatic stress disorder in victims of a natural disaster. *J Nerv Ment Dis.* 1987;53:672-678.
14. Wilkinson CB. Aftermath of a disaster: the collapse of the Hyatt Regency Hotel skywalks. *Am J Psychiatry.* 1983;140:1134-1139.
15. Blanchard EB, Kolb LC, Pallmeyer TP, Gerardi RJ. The development of a psychophysiological assessment procedure for posttraumatic stress disorder in Vietnam veterans. *Psychiatr Q.* 1982;54:220-229.
16. Egendorf A, Kashudin C, Laufer RS, Rothbart G, Sloan L. *Legacies of Vietnam: Comparative Adjustment of Veterans and Their Peers.* New York, NY: Center for Policy Research; 1981;5.
17. Keane TM, Malloy PF, Fairbank JA. Empirical development of an MMPI subscale for the assessment of combat-related posttraumatic stress disorder. *J Consult Clin Psychol.* 1984;52:888-891.
18. Kulka RA, Schlenger WE, Fairbank JA, Hough RL, Jordan BK, Marmar CR, Weiss DS. *Trauma and the Vietnam War Generation.* New York, NY: Brunner/Mazel; 1990.
19. Brett EA, Ostroff R. Imagery and posttraumatic stress disorder: an overview. *Am J Psychiatry.* 1985;142:417-424.
20. American Psychiatric Association, Committee on Nomenclature and Statistics. *Diagnostic and Statistical Manual of Mental Disorders, Revised Third Edition.* Washington, DC: American Psychiatric Association; 1987.
21. Helzer JE, Robins LN, McEvoy L. Post-traumatic stress disorder in the general population. *N Engl J Med.* 1987;317:1630-1634.
22. Davidson JRT, Hughes D, Blazer D, George LK. Posttraumatic stress disorder in the community: an epidemiological study. *Psychol Med.* 1991;21:1-19.
23. Robins LN, Helzer JE, Cottler LB, Goldring E. *The Diagnostic Interview Schedule, Version IIIR.* St Louis, Mo: Washington University School of Medicine; 1988.
24. Shore JH, Vollmer WM, Tatum EI. Community patterns of posttraumatic stress disorders. *J Nerv Ment Dis.* 1989;177:681-685.
25. Resnick HS, Kilpatrick DG, Dansky BS, Saunders BE, Best CL. Prevalence of civilian trauma and posttraumatic stress disorder in a representative national sample of women. *J Consult Clin Psychol.* 1993;61:984-991.
26. Breslau N, Davis GC, Andreski P, Peterson E. Traumatic events and posttraumatic stress disorder in an urban population of young adults. *Arch Gen Psychiatry.* 1991;48:216-222.
27. Koss MP. The scope of rape: implications for the clinical treatment of victims. *Clin Psychol.* 1983;36:88-91.
28. Croyle RT, Loftus EF. Improving episode memory performance of survey respondents. In: Tanur JM, ed. *Questions About Questions: Inquiries Into the Cognitive Bases of Surveys.* New York, NY: Russell Sage Foundation; 1992.
29. Resnick HS, Kilpatrick DG, Lipovsky JA. Assessment of rape-related posttraumatic stress disorder: stressor and symptom dimensions. *J Consult Clin Psychol.* 1991;3:561-572.
30. Solomon S, Canino G. Appropriateness of the *DSM-III-R* criteria for posttraumatic stress disorder. *Compr Psychiatry.* 1990;31:227-237.
31. March JS. What constitutes a stressor? The 'criterion A' issue. In: Davidson JRT, Foa EB, ed. *Posttraumatic Stress Disorder:* DSM-IV *and Beyond.* Washington, DC: American Psychiatric Press; 1992.
32. Mellman TA, Randolph CA, Brawan-Mintzer O, Flores LP, Milanes FJ. Phenomenology and course of psychiatric disorders associated with combat-related posttraumatic stress disorder. *Am J Psychiatry.* 1992;149:1568-1574.
33. Davidson JRT, Kudler HS, Saunders WB, Smith SD. Symptom and morbidity patterns in World War II and Vietnam veterans with posttraumatic stress disorder. *Compr Psychiatry.* 1990;31:162-170.
34. Rothbaum BO, Foa EB. Subtypes of posttraumatic stress disorder and duration of symptoms. In: Davidson JRT, Foa EB, eds. *Posttraumatic Stress Disorder: DSM-IV and Beyond.* Washington, DC: American Psychiatric Press; 1992.
35. McFarlane AC. The longitudinal course of posttraumatic morbidity. *J Nerv Ment Dis.* 1988;1976:30-39.
36. Breslau N, Davis GC. Posttraumatic stress disorder in an urban population of young adults: risk factors for chronicity. *Am J Psychiatry.* 1992;149:671-675.
37. Kessler RC, McGonagle KA, Zhao S, Nelson CB, Hughes M, Eshleman S, Wittchen H-U, Kendler KS. Lifetime and 12-month prevalence of *DSM-III-R* psychiatric disorders in the United States: results from the National Comorbidity Survey. *Arch Gen Psychiatry.* 1994;51:8-19.
38. World Health Organization. *Composite International Diagnostic Interview.* Version 1.0. Geneva, Switzerland: World Health Organization; 1990a.
39. Robins LN, Wing J, Wittchen H-U, Helzer JE. The Composite International Diagnostic Interview: an epidemiologic instrument suitable for use in conjunction with different diagnostic systems and in different cultures. *Arch Gen Psychiatry.* 1988;45:1069-1077.
40. World Health Organization. *The* ICD-10 *Classification of Mental and Behavioral Disorders: Diagnostic Criteria for Research.* Geneva, Switzerland: World Health Organization; 1993.
41. World Health Organization. *Composite International Diagnostic Interview Computer Programs.* Version 1.1. Geneva, Switzerland: World Health Organization; 1990b.
42. Wittchen H-U. Reliability and validity studies of the WHO-Composite International Diagnostic Interview (CIDI): a critical review. *J Psychiatr Res.* 1994;28:57-84.
43. Spitzer RL, Williams JBW, Gibbon M, First MD. *Structured Clinical Interview for* DSM-III-R—*Patient Version (SCID-P).* New York, NY: New York State Psychiatric Institute, Biometrics Research Division; 1989.
44. Endicott J, Spitzer RL. A diagnostic interview: the Schedule for Affective Disorders and Schizophrenia. *Arch Gen Psychiatry.* 1978;35:837-844.
45. Keller MB, Lavori PW, Nielsen E. *SCALUP (SCID Plus SADS-L).* Providence, RI: Department of Psychiatry, Butler Hospital; 1987.
46. Warshaw MG, Fierman E, Pratt L, Hunt M, Yonkers KA, Massion AO, Keller MB. Quality of life and dissociation in anxiety disorder patients with histories of trauma or PTSD. *Am J Psychiatry.* 1993;150:1512-1516.
47. US Dept of Health and Human Services. *National Health Interview Survey, 1989.* Hyattsville, Md: National Center for Health Statistics; 1992. Computer file.
48. Woodruff RS, Causey BD. Computerized method for approximating the variance of a complicated estimate. *J Am Stat Assoc.* 1976;71:315-321.
49. *OSIRIS VII.* Ann Arbor, Mich: Institute for Social Research, University of Michigan; 1981.
50. Kish L, Frankel MR. Balanced repeated replications for standard errors. *J Am Stat Assoc.* 1970;65:1071-1094.
51. Koch GG, Leneshow S. An application of multivariate analysis to complex sample survey data. *J Am Stat Assoc.* 1972;67:780-782.
52. SAS Institute. *SAS 6.03.* Cary, NC: SAS Institute Inc; 1988.
53. Norusis MJ. *SPSS Advanced Statistics User's Guide.* Chicago, Ill: SPSS Inc; 1990.
54. Davidson JRT, Foa EB. Diagnostic issues in posttraumatic stress disorder: considerations for the *DSM-IV. J Abnorm Psychol.* 1991;100:346-355.
55. Southwick SM, Krystal JH, Morgan A, Johnson D, Nagy LM, Nicholaou A, Heninger GR, Charney DS. Abnormal noradrenergic function in posttraumatic stress disorder. *Arch Gen Psychiatry.* 1993;50:266-274.
56. Lee E, Desu M. A computer program for comparing k samples with right censored data. *Comput Programs Biomed.* 1972;2:315-321.
57. American Psychiatric Association, Committee on Nomenclature and Statistics. *Diagnostic and Statistical Manual of Mental Disorders, Revised Fourth Edition.* Washington, DC: American Psychiatric Association; 1994.
58. Green BL, Lindy JD, Grace MC, Gleser GC, Leonard AC, Korol M, Winget C. Buffalo Creek survivors in the second decade stability of stress symptoms. *Am J Orthopsychiatry.* 1990;60:45-54.
59. Smith EM, North CS. *Aftermath of a Disaster: Psychological Response to the Indianapolis Ramada Jet Crash.* Boulder, Colo: Natural Hazards Research and Application Information Center; 1988. Quick Response Research Report No. 23.
60. Steinglass P, Gerrity E. Natural disaster and post-traumatic stress disorder: short-term versus long-term recovery in two disaster-affected communities. *J Appl Soc Psychol.* 1990;20:1746-1765.
61. Card JJ. Epidemiology of PTSD in a national cohort of Vietnam veterans. *J Clin Psychol.* 1987;43:6-17.
62. Solomon Z, Mikulincer M, Freid B, Wosner Y. Family characteristics and posttraumatic stress disorder: a follow-up of Israeli combat stress reaction casualties. *Fam Process.* 1987;26:383-394.

ORIGINAL ARTICLE

Frontal and Temporal Lobe Brain Volumes in Schizophrenia

Relationship to Symptoms and Clinical Subtype

Bruce Turetsky, MD; Patricia E. Cowell, PhD; Ruben C. Gur, PhD; Robert I. Grossman, MD; Derri L. Shtasel, MD; Raquel E. Gur, MD, PhD

Background: Quantitative magnetic resonance imaging (MRI) studies demonstrate reduced brain volumes in schizophrenics, but specific structural abnormalities have not been clearly delineated. The structural abnormalities of this disorder are likely to be heterogeneous, consistent with its diverse clinical presentation. To investigate the relationship between structural abnormality and clinical symptoms, we examined regional brain and cerebral spinal fluid (CSF) volumes in a large sample of schizophrenic patients and controls, with patients aggregated into clinical subtypes.

Methods: Right and left hemisphere frontal and temporal lobe brain and CSF volumes were quantified from 5-mm axial spin-echo MRIs for 71 schizophrenic patients and 77 age- and sex-matched controls. The following four standardized rating scales were used to assess symptom severity: Negative Symptoms, Disorganization, Schneiderian Delusions and Hallucinations, and Suspicion-Hostility. Patients were also subtyped as either deficit or nondeficit on the basis of enduring negative symptoms.

Results: Schizophrenic patients overall exhibited abnormal brain asymmetry, with selective decrease in brain volume in the left temporal and right frontal regions. Left temporal lobe parenchymal volume reduction and CSF volume increase were correlated with the severity of negative symptoms. Consistent with this, the subtype analysis revealed abnormal temporal lobe asymmetry for the deficit subgroup only. Right frontal lobe volume reduction correlated with the duration of illness, independent of symptom severity or schizophrenic subtype.

Conclusions: Abnormal lateral asymmetry suggests selective structural deficits in schizophrenia, rather than diffusely undifferentiated CNS abnormalities. The pattern of regional abnormalities is related to clinical symptoms, with negative symptoms being associated with left temporal lobe rather than frontal lobe abnormality. This is consistent with suggestions of a temporolimbic prefrontal network abnormality in schizophrenia. Further longitudinal studies are warranted, using higher-resolution MRI technology and gray matter–white matter segmentation to confirm and extend these findings.

(Arch Gen Psychiatry. 1995;52:1061-1070)

From the Departments of Psychiatry (Drs Turetsky, Cowell, R. C. Gur, Shtasel, and R. E. Gur) and Radiology (Dr Grossman), University of Pennsylvania, Philadelphia.

EARLY NEUROIMAGING studies reported global structural abnormalities in schizophrenia, manifested by enlarged ventricles and increased sulcal cerebral spinal fluid (CSF) volume.[1-4] More recent efforts have focused on assessing regional brain abnormalities and the relationship between neuroanatomic parameters and clinical measures. Quantitative high-resolution magnetic resonance imaging (MRI) has been used to examine specific brain regions hypothesized as salient to the neurobiological features of schizophrenia. Volumetric deficits have been reported for both frontal and temporal lobes,[5,6] temporal lobe gray matter,[7,8] and, more selectively, the superior temporal gyrus, parahippocampal gyrus, hippocampus, and amygdala.[9-11] Volume reduction of the left superior temporal gyrus has been correlated with severity of auditory hallucinations[9] and thought disorder[11] in patients. Results, however, remain equivocal. Structural abnormalities have been inconsistently lateralized, and some studies have failed to find selective regional deficits or have reported diffuse changes rather than specific regional abnormalities.[4,12,13]

Schizophrenia is heterogeneous in its clinical presentation, and it is possible that its associated pathophysiologic features are also variable. Furthermore, discrepant anatomic findings may be owing, in part, to relatively small sample sizes, differences in

See Subjects and Methods on next page

SUBJECTS AND METHODS

Unless otherwise indicated, data are given as mean±SD.

SUBJECTS

Subjects were 71 patients with a *DSM-III-R*[16] diagnosis of schizophrenia (44 men and 27 women) and 77 healthy controls (48 men and 29 women). These are a subset of the sample for whom whole-brain volumetric data have been presented.[15] Ten patients and four control subjects included in the whole-brain analysis were excluded because movement artifact or head tilt impeded reliable reslicing and region-of-interest determination from MRIs. Patient age was 29.7±3.2 years (range, 18 to 48 years), education was 12.7±2.2 years, and paternal and maternal education were 12.4±3.1 and 12.0±2.4 years, respectively. Control group age was 28.0±7.3 years (range, 18 to 48 years), paternal education was 12.9±3.2 years, and maternal education was 12.8±2.4 years, with no significant differences between patients and controls. As expected, control subjects attained a higher education level (14.6±2.1 years) than patients ($t[146]=5.6$, $P<.001$).

Patients received medical, neurologic, and psychiatric evaluations, including the Structured Clinical Interview for *DSM-III-R*–Patient Version.[17,18] To ensure diagnostic accuracy, they underwent clinical reassessment at 6-month intervals following initial intake. Availability of follow-up data ranged from 6 months to 12 years and 2 months, with a mean follow-up period of 44.0±28.1 months. There was no history of any other disorder or event, except for schizophrenia, that could potentially affect brain function. Age of onset of psychotic symptoms associated with functional decline was 23.2±5.9 years (range, 11 to 41 years; men, 22.2±5.1 years; women, 24.9±6.7 years); duration was no more than 2 years for 22 patients (nine men and 13 women) and 9.1±4.7 (range, 3 to 22 years; men, 9.1±4.1 years; women, 9.2±6.2 years) for the remaining 49. Fifty-one patients were enrolled in the study while hospitalized in an acute psychiatric inpatient unit; 20 patients were enrolled as outpatients. For 25 patients (12 men and 13 women), enrollment was during their first hospitalization; the number of previous hospitalizations for the remainder was 4.2±5.1 (range, 1 to 25; men, 4.3±5.4; women, 4.1±4.6). Twenty-two patients had never been exposed to antipsychotic medications. All remaining subjects had not received neuroleptics for a minimum of 2 weeks prior to study. Only right-handed subjects were included.[19] Weight and height were 77.4±11.6 kg and 176.0±9.1 cm, respectively, for men and 66.0±13.0 kg and 162.6±7.4 cm, respectively, for women.

Healthy controls were recruited by advertisement and underwent medical, neurologic, and psychiatric (with the Structured Clinical Interview for *DSM-III-R*–Nonpatient Version) evaluation.[20,21] Weight and height were 73.4±10.5 kg and 176.3±7.4 cm, respectively, for men and 62.5±12.1 kg and 165.4±7.6 cm, respectively, for women. Informed consent was obtained prior to participation in the study.

CLINICAL RATINGS AND TYPOLOGY

The Brief Psychiatric Rating Scale (BPRS),[22] the Scale for the Assessment of Negative Symptoms (SANS),[23] the Scale for the Assessment of Positive Symptoms (SAPS),[24] and the Strauss-Carpenter Outcome Scale[25] were administered on admission to the protocol. Ratings were completed by investigators trained to a reliability of .90 (intraclass correlation coefficient). A statistical approach was used to derive the fewest separable symptom dimensions from these ratings.[15] The following three tentative symptom categories were formed based on prior findings[26,27] and clinical judgment: negative symptoms, disorganization, and delusions and hallucinations. Next, two of us (B.T. and D.L.S.) independently assigned SANS, SAPS and BPRS items to these categories. After pooling these item-category assignments, the procedure attempted to maximize the coefficient α[28] by adding or subtracting items with high or low correlations with category totals. Items that correlated with more than one category were excluded to maximize scale independence. Items that did not correlate with any of the candidate scales were free to form new scales. This method relates to other scale construction approaches, such as factor analysis, but generally produces superior results.[29] The method confirmed the three "seed" categories but indicated that suspicion-hostility (including paranoid delusions) was an independent category. This was owing to lack of significant intercorrelation of the paranoid items with Schneiderian delusions and hallucinations. Thus, our procedure yielded four summary symptom dimension scales: Negative Symptoms, Disorganization, Schneiderian Delusions and Hallucinations, and Suspicion-Hostility. Item compositions of these scales and their item-scale correlations have been presented elsewhere.[15] All scales have adequate reliabilities (Cronbach's αs, .94, .88, .90, and .75) and are statistically independent of each other (intercorrelation coefficients ranging from −.16 to .15 [differences were not significant]). Final scores were expressed as the average of individual items in each scale (with BPRS items rescaled to be equivalent to SANS and SAPS items prior to averaging). Scale scores thus retained the original 1 to 5 metric of the SANS and SAPS item ratings.

Patients were also classified into deficit and nondeficit categories (subgroups) following the criteria of Carpenter et al.[30] This yielded 21 patients in the deficit subgroup (18 men and three women) and 49 in the nondeficit subgroup (26 men and 23 women) patients, and one patient without sufficient longitudinal data to permit classification. While gender distribution was uneven, there was no difference in age between the two subtypes. **Table 1** presents mean clinical rating scale scores for patients by gender and by deficit-nondeficit categorization.

MRI MEASUREMENT

Magnetic resonance images were acquired on a 1.5-tesla scanner (General Electric Co, Milwaukee, Wis). Transaxial images were obtained parallel to the orbitomeatal line. Each slice was 5 mm thick, with no interslice gaps. A multiecho acquisition sequence was used (repetition time, 3000 milliseconds; echo time, 30 and 80 milliseconds). This allowed for measurement of the two independent properties of proton density and T_2-weighted value.

Images were realigned in three dimensions and resliced into transaxial images parallel to the anterior/posterior commissure axis to standardize for differences in head tilt during image acquisition. The borders of the frontal and temporal lobes were drawn on these resliced images by investigators (B.T. and P.E.C.) working with a neuroradiologist (R.I.G.), using operationally standardized boundary criteria.[31] While frontal and temporal lobe borders are most clearly delineated on coronal images, the 5-mm resolution of our transaxial images did not permit reslicing in the coronal plane without excessive degradation of the interpolated images. Relatively minor realignment of the transaxial images to conform to the anterior/posterior commissure line did not reduce image quality.

In inferiormost slices, the temporal lobe did not share common lateral or anterior borders with other structures and was easily outlined. The posteriomedial temporal lobe border was formed by the pons and cerebellum (**Figure 1**, A). At the level of the midbrain, borders of the frontal lobe were drawn along the interhemispheric fissure and followed the middle cerebral artery through the suprasellar cistern (Figure 1, B). The temporal lobe was separated from adjacent frontal regions by the sylvian fissure. The amygdala and hippocampus were included within the temporal lobe, and midbrain structures were excluded. The posterior temporal lobe was defined by a line extending from the anterior tip of the contralateral cerebral peduncle to the anteromedial tip of the cerebellum (dashed line in Figure 1, B).

Above the mamillary bodies, the posterior border of the frontal lobe was defined by a horizontal line that extended from the anteromedial aspect of the sylvian fissure to the midline (Figure 1, C). The medial borders of the temporal lobe were the sylvian fissure and diencephalon structures (Figure 1, C and D). A horizontal line from the posterior tip of the posterior fossa to the lateral cortical perimeter delineated the posterior temporal lobe (Figure 1, C). The posterior border of the frontal lobe, for remaining superior slices, was delineated on the slice immediately inferior to the splenium of the corpus callosum (Figure 1, D). The horizontal line defined by the anterior aspect of the caudate was projected from this slice onto all superior slices to form the posterior boundary. This slice also denoted the superior extent of the temporal lobes.

Figure 2 depicts the anterolateral and posterolateral aspects of the three-dimensional reconstruction of these brain regions, as defined by the above boundary criteria. While some loss of image resolution occurs with reconstruction from 5-mm images, it is still apparent that the frontal region, as we have defined it, is exclusively prefrontal and that the temporal lobe, although generally well encompassed, may include small edges of inferior frontal and parieto-occipital cortexes.

A segmentation program with established reliability and validity[32] was applied to the resliced images, to separate brain parenchyma from surrounding CSF within the operator-defined regions of interest. The segmentation program isolates proton density and T_2-weighted values of each pixel within a "feature space" plot, permitting identification of discrete clusters of pixels representing brain and CSF. Phantom studies have shown that, even when shading artifacts distort cluster shape, the ability to separate CSF from brain is preserved, and valid quantitation is achieved despite the partial volume effects inherent in 5-mm MRI slices. Also, analysis of both original and realigned images of the same brain indicate that reslicing images along the anterior/posterior commissure line does not introduce errors into the segmentation process. Following segmentation, brain parenchymal and CSF volumes were computed separately for left temporal, right temporal, left frontal, and right frontal lobes by summing pixel counts for each tissue type within each region, scaling appropriately for pixel size, and combining these area measures across slices.

RELIABILITY OF REGIONAL VOLUMETRIC MEASUREMENTS

A sample of 10 randomly selected scans was analyzed by two of us (B.T. and P.E.C.), and one (B.T.) reanalyzed these same scans 1 year after the initial analysis. Interrater and intrarater reliabilities were computed as intraclass correlations for each regional brain and CSF volume. Reliabilities of brain measures, both within and across raters, were above .85. Reliabilities of CSF measures were somewhat lower but still acceptable (**Table 2**). Remaining scans were then analyzed by a single rater (either B.T. or P.E.C.). All image analysis was conducted with raters blind to subject status as either patient or control.

DATA PROCESSING AND ANALYSIS

Previous work in our laboratory has shown, in normal controls, interactive effects of age and sex on these lobar measures.[31] Patient-control differences in total cranial volume, related to specific patient symptoms, have also been found.[15] Therefore, these regional analyses were performed on measures corrected for age, sex, age-sex interaction, and total cranial volume. To remove the effects of these variables, coefficients were generated based on the regression of age, sex, age-sex interaction, and cranial volume on each anatomic measure within the healthy comparison sample. A predicted score for each anatomic variable was then computed for each subject, using these normative regression coefficients. These predicted values were subtracted from the actual measures, and the residuals were added to the mean control sample scores to produce corrected lobar volumes that were not influenced by age, sex, age-sex interaction, or differences in overall cranial volume.[33]

Repeated-measures analyses of variance (ANOVAs) were conducted with region (frontal vs temporal), hemisphere (right vs left), and tissue (CSF vs brain parenchyma) as within-subject factors. The initial analysis compared the entire schizophrenic sample with healthy controls, with gender and diagnosis as between-subjects factors. Based on observed hemisphere interaction effects, measures of lateral asymmetry (defined as [left hemisphere − right hemisphere]/[left hemisphere + right hemisphere]) were computed for each patient from the adjusted lobar brain and CSF volumes. Correlative analyses were employed to examine the relationship, within the schizophrenic sample, of the lobar volume and asymmetry measures to clinical symptom scale scores and measures of illness duration and onset.

Following the whole-sample analysis, a subtype analysis was conducted with subgroup (deficit vs nondeficit) as between-subjects factor. Significant effects were followed by planned contrasts between each subgroup and the normal control group.

Table 1. Clinical Rating Measures*

Variables	Patient Gender: Male (n=44)	Patient Gender: Female (n=27)	Patient Subgroups†: Deficit (n=21)	Patient Subgroups†: Nondeficit (n=49)
Age at onset of illness, y	22.2 (5.1)	24.9 (6.7)‡	22.8 (4.1)	23.2 (6.3)
Duration of illness, y	7.4 (5.0)	5.0 (6.3)	8.6 (6.1)	5.7 (5.1)§
Clinical rating scale scores				
BPRS (total)	51.3 (10.7)	51.5 (9.8)	54.5 (11.2)	50.2 (9.5)
SANS (total)	56.9 (26.1)	50.3 (23.9)	71.3 (22.4)	47.2 (23.4)‖
SAPS (total)	52.0 (22.1)	48.2 (20.5)	47.5 (21.9)	52.8 (20.5)
Symptom dimension scale scores¶				
Negative Symptoms	2.3 (1.1)	2.0 (1.1)	3.0 (1.1)	1.9 (1.1)‖
Disorganization	1.7 (0.9)	1.5 (0.8)	1.8 (1.1)	1.6 (0.8)
Schneiderian Delusions and Hallucinations	1.7 (1.2)	1.8 (1.0)	1.4 (0.9)	1.9 (1.1)
Suspicion-Hostility	2.5 (1.0)	2.4 (1.1)	2.3 (1.1)	2.5 (1.0)

**Data are given as mean±SD. BPRS indicates Brief Psychiatric Rating Scale; SANS, Scale for the Assessment of Negative Symptoms; and SAPS, Scale for the Assessment of Positive Symptoms.*
†One patient could not be classified.
‡P=*.07*
§P=*.05.*
‖P<.001.
¶Symptom dimension scales are described in the "Clinical Ratings and Typology" subsection of the "Subjects and Methods" section of the text.

subject selection criteria, and differences in the amount of brain tissue included in the analysis. Correlational studies of neuroanatomic and phenomenological features of schizophrenia also employ multiple clinical measures and risk excessive type I error. Clarification of underlying structural abnormalities and their associated clinical phenomenological features requires the study of larger samples of patients, with assessment of the specificity of findings to schizophrenic subtypes defined by symptom profiles. In a previous study in our laboratory of 59 patients with schizophrenia,[14] a relationship between the severity of negative symptoms and left hemisphere prominence of CSF-to-cranial ratios was observed. In an expanded study of 81 patients and 81 healthy controls,[15] subtype differences in whole-brain volume and ventricle-to-brain and sulcal-to-brain volume ratios were also reported. Patients with primarily negative symptoms had a global reduction of brain volume and proportional increase in CSF volume. In contrast, patients with Schneiderian symptoms (prominent hallucinations and bizarre delusions) showed reduced cranial and brain volumes without proportionate increase in CSF volumes, whereas patients with isolated symptoms of suspicion and hostility had normal cranial, brain, and ventricular CSF volumes.

We now investigate regional differences in brain abnormalities by assessing left and right temporal and frontal lobe volumes in a large sample of schizophrenic patients and sociodemographically balanced control subjects. The sample size permits us to consider the relationship of structural deficits to schizophrenic subtypes and to symptom dimensions.

RESULTS

Table 3 presents temporal and frontal brain and CSF volumes (uncorrected) for male and female schizophrenic patients and controls. The ANOVA of uncorrected data revealed significant effects of gender on regional MRI measures. Women had smaller parenchymal volumes than men, more pronounced for the temporal than the frontal lobes (gender-region interaction, $F[1,144]=7.97$; $P=.005$). Men, however, showed a greater hemisphere difference (right greater than left), independent of region (gender-hemisphere interaction, $F[1,144]=8.37$; $P=.004$). These findings replicate previous results in our laboratory from a normative sample.[31] However, gender and diagnosis did not interact ($F[1,144]=0.40$; $P=.53$), and therefore gender was not included as a between-subjects factor in subsequent analyses. Patients showed a rather consistent pattern of smaller regional brain volumes and concomitantly greater CSF volumes, but the diagnosis-tissue interaction was not statistically significant across anatomic regions ($F[1,146]=3.10$; $P=.08$). Rather, there was a four-way interaction of diagnosis, region, hemisphere, and tissue ($F[1,146]=4.89$; $P=.03$), indicating that patient-control differences were not global, but instead were lateralized, regional, and tissue specific. Correcting for the generic effects of age, sex, and total cranial volume increased, rather than diminished, the significance of this four-way interaction ($F[1,146]=5.68$; $P=.02$). No other significant group effects were observed. All subsequent analyses reported refer to these adjusted volume measures.

Separate post hoc analyses for the individual tissue types revealed a three-way interaction of diagnosis, region, and hemisphere for brain parenchyma ($F[1,146]=4.19$; $P=.04$). This is illustrated in **Figure 3**, which presents corrected brain and CSF volume and asymmetry measures. While schizophrenic patients and controls had similar brain volumes across all regions, schizophrenic patients showed abnormalities of brain asymmetry. Controls had asymmetric frontal lobes, right larger than left, and relatively symmetric temporal lobes. Patients, in contrast, had asymmetric temporal volumes, the left being smaller, and diminished frontal asymmetry.

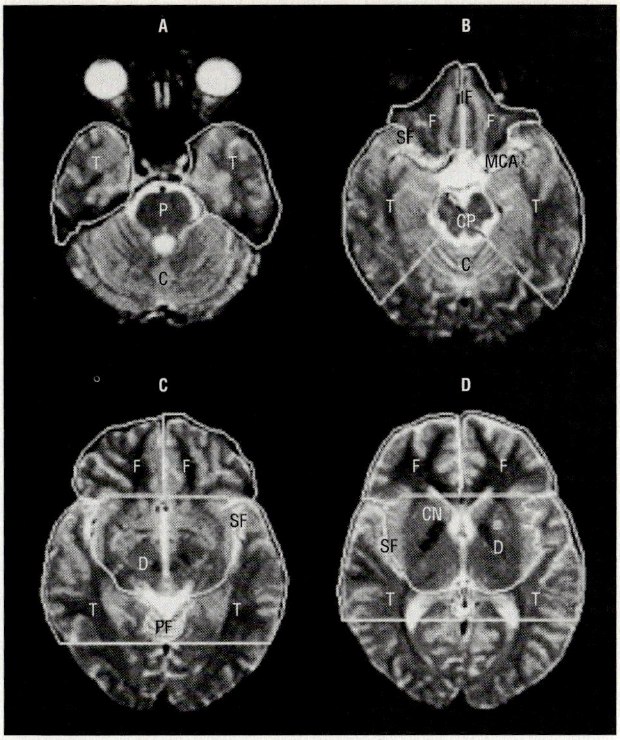

Figure 1. *Temporal and frontal lobe regions as drawn on four representative slices of a 5-mm axial T_2-weighted image, following realignment with the anterior/posterior commissure line. Selected slices depict sequential 1-cm steps from inferior to superior. A, Temporal lobe boundary as delimited for all inferior slices. B, The line used to delineate the posterior temporal border is depicted with dashes from the anteriormost tip of the contralateral cerebral peduncle to the anteromedialmost tip of the cerebellum. C, Posterior frontal lobe boundary defined by anteromedial aspect of sylvian fissure. Posterior temporal boundary is defined by posterior point of posterior fossa. D, All frontal regions superior to this used the same posterior boundary defined by anterior point of head of caudate. C indicates cerebellum; CN, caudate nucleus; CP, cerebral peduncle; D, diencephalon; F, frontal region; IF, interhemispheric fissure; MCA, middle cerebral artery; P, pons; PF, posterior fossa; SF, sylvian fissure; and T, temporal region.*

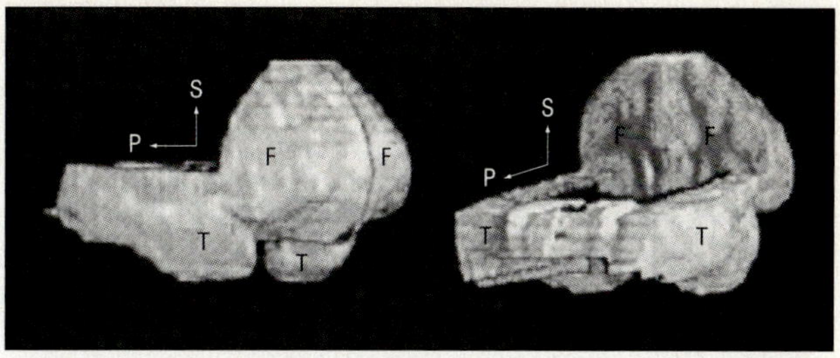

Figure 2. *Three-dimensional reconstruction of frontal and temporal lobes, defined by regions drawn on axial images as in Figure 1. Left, anterolateral image; right, posterolateral image. F indicates frontal region; P, posterior; S, superior; and T, temporal region.*

Table 2. Reliability of Regional Volumetric Measurements*

	Interrater Measurements		Intrarater Measurements	
Region	Brain	CSF	Brain	CSF
Left temporal	.89	.73	.88	.77
Right temporal	.86	.69	.85	.71
Left frontal	.91	.88	.93	.91
Right frontal	.90	.81	.93	.93

**Data are presented as intraclass correlation coefficients (r). CSF indicates cerebral spinal fluid.*

The pattern of group differences for CSF measurements was not the same as that seen for brain measurements. The diagnosis-region-hemisphere interaction was not evident in the CSF data (F[1,146]=0.98; *P*=.32). Schizophrenic patients had more CSF than controls in the temporal lobes bilaterally (F[1,146]=5.84; *P*=.02), and there was no difference between patients and controls in CSF volume in the frontal lobes (F[1,146]=0.38; *P*=.54) (Figure 3).

We considered the possibility that these findings were merely reflective of the whole-brain ventricular-cranial and sulcal-cranial abnormalities reported previously for this patient sample.[15] Within the schizophrenic group, left and right hemisphere sulcal CSF-cranial ratios were correlated with all adjusted regional CSF measures and inversely correlated with both left and right frontal brain volumes (all correlations between .52 and .62; *P*<.001). However, sulcal CSF-cranial ratios were not related to measures of temporal lobe brain volume, and ventricular CSF-cranial ratios were not correlated with any of the regional measures. Moreover, ventricular and sulcal CSF-cranial ratios were insensitive to the abnormalities of regional asymmetry.

RELATIONSHIP TO CLINICAL SYMPTOM SCALE SCORES AND CHRONICITY

To examine the association between anatomic abnormality and clinical symptom severity, adjusted lobar volume and asymmetry measures were correlated with scores on the SANS, SAPS, BPRS, and each of the four clinical dimension scales. These revealed a significant association only between temporal lobe asymmetry and the SANS and Negative Symptoms scales. Patients with more severe negative symptoms deviated most from controls, exhibiting the largest relative decrease in left temporal lobe parenchymal volume (*r*=−.30; *P*=.01) and the largest relative increase in left temporal lobe CSF asymmetry (*r*=.28; *P*=.02) (**Figure 4**). Ratings on the SAPS, BPRS, Disorganization, Schneiderian Delusions and Hallucinations, and Suspicion-Hostility scales were unrelated to anatomic volume measures.

Duration of illness was correlated with abnormal frontal lobe brain asymmetry (*r*=.26; *P*=.03) (Figure 4). Covarying for differences on clinical symptom scales had virtually no effect on this relationship. Patients with longer-term illness had greater relative decreases in right frontal lobe volume, irrespective of the extent or specific character of their clinical symptoms. Age at onset of illness, in contrast, while inversely correlated with illness duration, was unrelated to brain asymmetry when adjusted for actual age. Other demographic variables, including education and parental education, were similarly unrelated to MRI measures.

Given the association with illness duration, we considered whether our subsample of first-episode patients (n=24) differed anatomically from the schizophrenic subsample with more long-standing illness (n=47). How-

Table 3. Frontal and Temporal Lobe Brain Parenchymal and CSF Volumes*

Regions	Brain Volume: Schizophrenic Patients	Brain Volume: Controls	CSF Volume: Schizophrenic Patients	CSF Volume: Controls
Men				
Left frontal	101.0±14.4	103.8±12.8	10.7±5.0	10.6±5.2
Right frontal	103.2±14.2	107.1±12.9	12.0±5.9	12.0±6.0
Left temporal	110.4±14.0	115.5±13.4	7.6±2.8	6.6±2.1
Right temporal	113.4±14.2	117.2±14.4	7.1±2.8	6.3±2.3
Women				
Left frontal	90.3±12.4	92.5±10.6	9.2±6.6	8.0±5.0
Right frontal	91.1±11.3	94.2±11.6	10.3±6.5	8.5±6.0
Left temporal	96.1±11.6	98.0±15.3	5.7±4.3	4.8±1.6
Right temporal	96.4±11.8	97.1±15.2	5.4±3.2	4.4±1.6

Data are presented as mean±SD, in milliliters. CSF indicates cerebral spinal fluid.

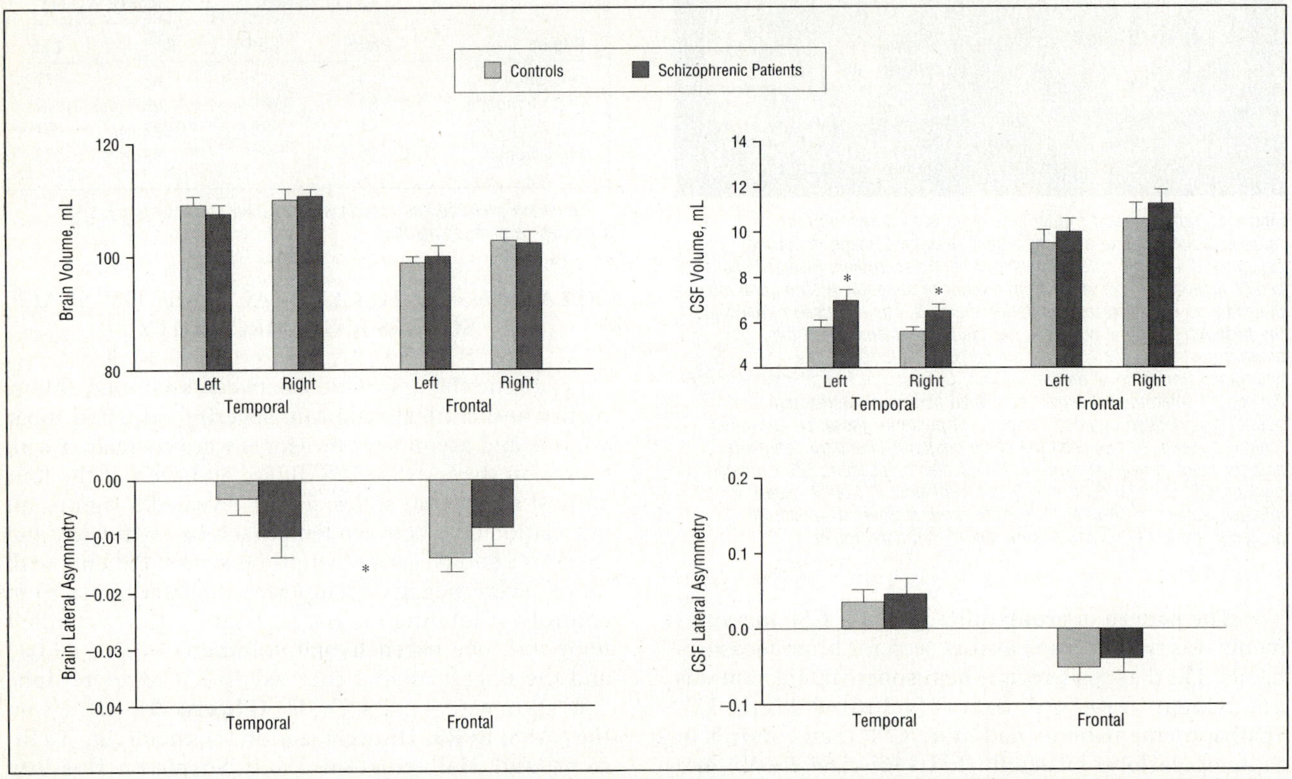

Figure 3. *Regional brain and cerebral spinal fluid (CSF) volumes of schizophrenic patients (n=71) and normal controls (n=77). Top, Lobar measures corrected for age, sex, and total cranial volume. Bottom, Hemisphere asymmetry measures ([left hemisphere − right hemisphere]/[left hemisphere + right hemisphere]). Schizophrenic patients exhibit abnormal asymmetry, with relatively smaller left temporal and right frontal brain volumes (diagnosis-region-hemisphere interaction). Asterisk indicates* $P<.05$*, patients vs controls.*

ever, there were no significant differences between these two groups, and it is primarily those patients with the longest history of illness (eg, greater than 10 years) who show abnormal frontal lobe asymmetry (Figure 4).

CLINICAL SUBTYPE ANALYSIS

Deficit-nondeficit contrasts revealed a group-hemisphere-tissue interaction ($F[1,68]=3.96$; $P=.05$), reflecting a significant group-hemisphere interaction for CSF volume ($F[1,68]=16.28$; $P<.001$) and an insignificant effect for brain volume (**Figure 5**). Post hoc contrasts within individual regions revealed that the deficit subgroup had significantly greater left temporal lobe CSF volume than the nondeficit subgroup ($t[68]=2.70$; $P<.01$) but did not differ on other measures. Similarly, when contrasted with normal controls, the deficit subgroup had greater left temporal lobe CSF volume ($t[96]=4.15$; $P<.001$) and no significant differences on other regional measures. Parallel analyses contrasting the nondeficit subgroup and controls revealed no significant regional differences and particularly no difference in left temporal CSF volume ($t[124]=1.08$; $P=.28$). Moreover, the diagnosis-region-hemisphere interaction for brain parenchyma, observed

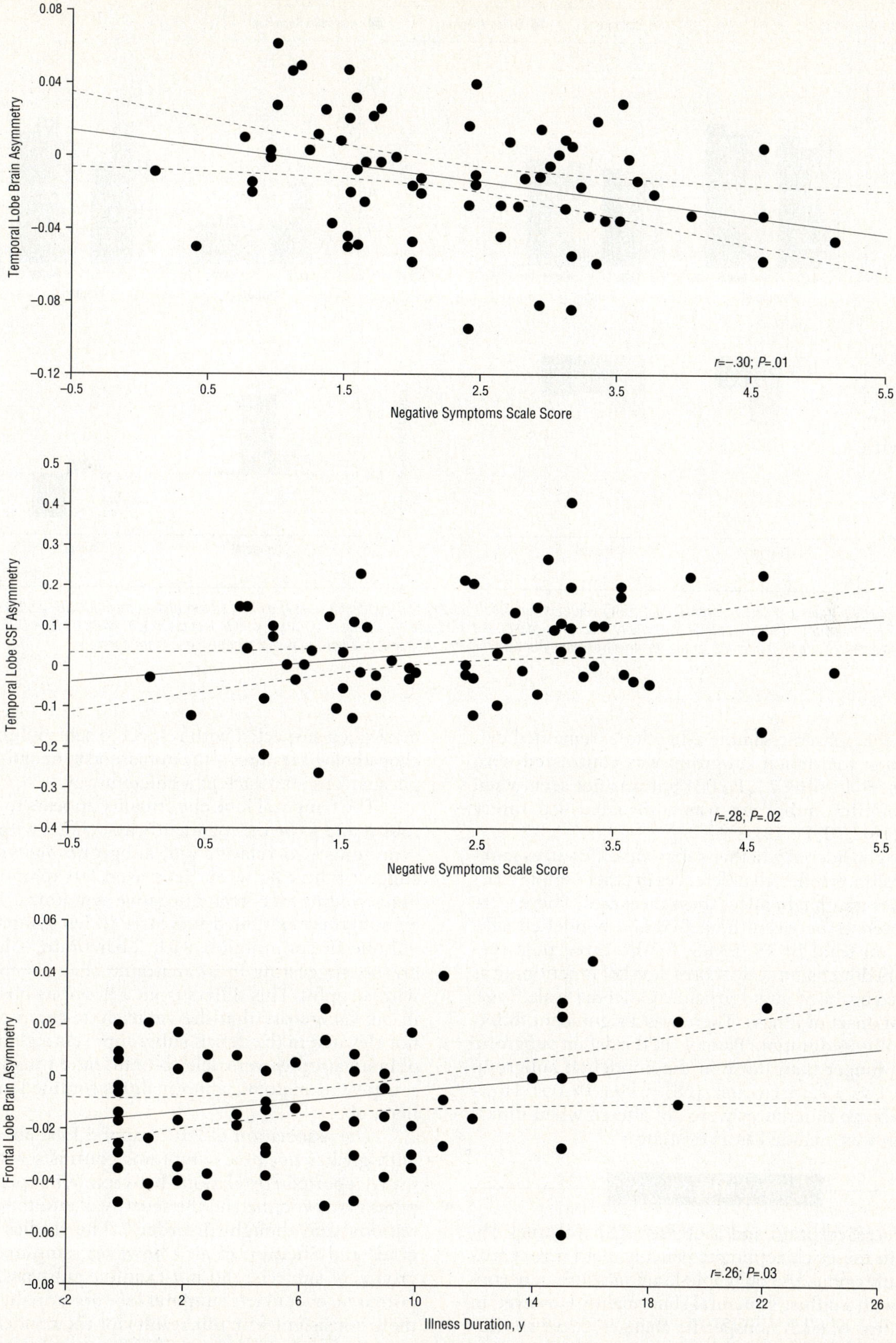

Figure 4. *Relationships between regional asymmetry measures and clinical variables. Asymmetry measure is described in Figure 3. Positive scores therefore indicate that the left hemisphere is greater than the right. Negative scores indicate that the right hemisphere is greater than the left. Negative Symptoms Scale is described in the "Clinical Ratings and Typology" subsection of the "Subjects and Methods" section of the text. CSF indicates cerebrospinal fluid.*

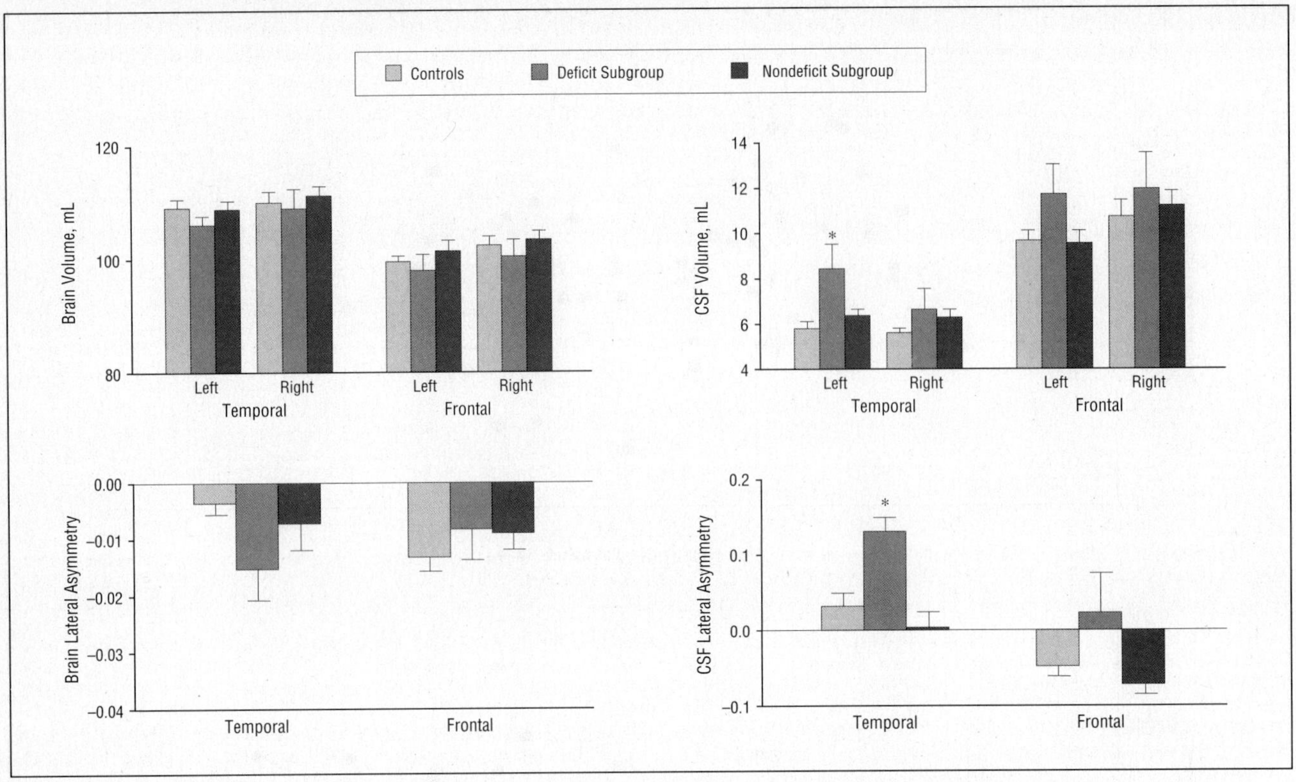

Figure 5. *Regional brain and cerebral spinal fluid (CSF) volumes for deficit (n=21) and nondeficit (n=49) patient subgroups, compared with controls. Top, Corrected lobar measures. Bottom, Lateral asymmetry measures (described in Figure 3). Deficit subgroup exhibits increased left temporal lobe CSF volume (asterisk indicates* $P<.001$*) in addition to the observed parenchymal asymmetry. Nondeficit subgroup is indistinguishable from controls.*

in the schizophrenic sample as a whole, remained evident when the deficit subgroup was contrasted with controls ($F[1,96]=4.74$; $P=.03$) but was not seen when the nondeficit subgroup was contrasted separately ($F[1,124]=2.70$; $P=.15$).

We considered whether subgroup differences in regional volumes reflected differences in other sample characteristics that might affect these measures. There were no differences between the deficit and nondeficit subgroups on total BPRS, SAPS, or the three positive-symptom dimension scale scores, level of functioning as measured by the Strauss-Carpenter Outcome Scale,[25] age, or age at onset of illness. There was a significant difference in illness duration. Patients in the deficit subgroup were ill longer than those in the nondeficit subgroup (8.6 ± 6.1 vs 5.7 ± 5.1 years; $t(68)=1.993$; $P=.05$). However, subtype differences were not altered when illness duration was included as a covariate.

COMMENT

The decreased brain and increased CSF volumes observed in these schizophrenic patients, both across anatomic subregions and on whole-brain measures, are consistent with a diffuse structural abnormality. However, in the context of such nonspecific changes, there are further regionally selective neuroanatomic abnormalities. Specifically, differences in lateral asymmetry imply structural deficits, in schizophrenia, that are greatest in the left temporal and right frontal regions. Thus, the two regions most often suspected with respect to schizophrenic psychopathologic features—the frontal and temporal—are implicated here, but each in a different way.

The temporal lobe abnormality appears to be more robust and to be independently associated with clinical symptoms. Correlative and subgroup analyses both suggest a link between decreased left temporal lobe brain volume and greater negative symptoms. The deficit subgroup exhibited increases in left temporal CSF volume in conjunction with lobar brain volume decrease, suggesting focal anatomic changes consistent with atrophy. This differs from a previous observation in our laboratory that the ventricle-to-brain ratio was not elevated in the deficit subgroup.[15] As a global index of brain atrophy, ventricle-to-brain ratio thus seems insensitive to anatomic abnormalities confined to a single hemilobe.

The association of left temporal lobe abnormality with greater negative symptoms contrasts with previously reported correlations between left superior temporal gyrus volume and the severity of auditory hallucinations[9] and thought disorder.[11] The studies of Barta et al[9] and Shenton et al,[11] however, employed small groups of subjects, did not examine subtypes, and reported no overall left temporal lobe abnormality. This is more consistent with our results for the nondeficit subgroup, who showed more prominent auditory hallucinations and no overall abnormality of the left temporal lobe. This subgroup may have abnormalities of selected temporal lobe structures that are not discernible from our lobar measures, and higher-resolution MRI scans may now provide unambiguous quantitation of focal cortical and subcortical regions of interest. However, clarification of this issue requires additional analyses, larger samples to permit patient subtyping, and more refined segmentation algorithms to discriminate gray from white matter.

These findings also question the presumptive role of frontal lobe abnormalities in the production of negative symptoms.[34] Insults to the frontal lobes can clearly produce behavioral syndromes reminiscent of negative-type schizophrenia,[35] and Andreasen and colleagues[36] and others[37] have reported a correlation between negative symptoms and reduced frontal lobe blood flow. However, the relationship between structure and function is not necessarily straightforward, and no associations were found between negative symptoms and frontal lobe size.[38,39] The existence of dispersed neural networks raises the possibility, instead, that structural abnormalities in one area might alter functional relationships in other regions. We are reminded, in this regard, of J. Hughlings Jackson's admonition[40] that a lesion does not simply produce a loss of those functions intrinsic to the damaged region but alters functional relationships within the remaining intact brain as it attempts to function in the absence of the lesioned area.

Recent animal data illuminate this point, with perhaps special relevance for the pathophysiologic features of negative symptoms in schizophrenia. Normal development was observed in rats receiving ventral hippocampal lesions as neonates, until early adulthood, when they began to exhibit behavioral abnormalities reminiscent of those seen in adult rats after lesions, not of the ventral hippocampus, but of the medial prefrontal cortex.[41,42] This suggests that early hippocampal lesions can affect the functional integrity of other brain areas, such as the prefrontal cortex, that continue to develop into adulthood.[43]

Human data from the same laboratory[44] provide further support for this idea of a pathologic disturbance of a distributed neocortical-limbic neural network. In a study of monozygotic twin pairs discordant for schizophrenia, abnormal prefrontal physiologic activation in the affected twin was strongly correlated with decreased hippocampal volume, relative to that of the unaffected twin.[44] Similarly, the negative symptoms observed in some schizophrenic patients in association with decreased prefrontal cortical activation may be linked to anatomic abnormalities of temporal lobe structures.

This is not to suggest that temporal lobe structural abnormalities are of etiologic significance in schizophrenia. The direction of causality need not project solely from a primary anatomic abnormality to a secondary loss of function. Conceivably, increased neuronal activation could produce both behavioral abnormalities of hyperarousal and hypervigilance in schizophrenia and also lead to secondary changes in cerebral volume. Consistent with this, resting positron emission tomography glucose metabolic data from our laboratory have suggested that patients with prominent negative symptoms, whom we found herein to have reduced left temporal lobe volumes, also exhibit relative increases in left midtemporal metabolism.[45] Clarification of the temporal relationship between these structural and functional abnormalities requires serial longitudinal assessment of both physiologic and anatomic measures in the same cohort of patients.

The apparent relationship between relative right frontal lobe volume decrement and duration of illness raises the possibility of a regional neuroanatomic correlate to the often-cited "downhill course" of schizophrenia. It is perhaps notable, in this regard, that normative effects of male aging also appear to be most evident in the right frontal lobe.[31] This region may be especially sensitive to the protracted effects of physiologic dysfunction or, alternatively, to the long-term effects of pharmacotherapy. However, to establish an unambiguous association between illness duration and progressive regional brain changes would require, again, repeated MRI scanning in a large patient cohort.

The current study has indicated a heterogeneous substrate of neuroanatomic abnormalities underlying two clinical subtypes of schizophrenia. A subtyping strategy is one approach to the question of whether biological heterogeneity underlies observed clinical heterogeneity. The idea that clinical variability may be related to biological differences *within* the patient group is, in the broadest sense, merely an extension of the notion that biological differences underlie observed behavioral differences between patients and controls. Whether schizophrenic phenomenology and neuropathology actually represent multiple discrete disease processes or constitute a unitary phenomenon with gradients of abnormality along one or more dimensions is unknown. It is possible for a single disease process to produce highly variable signs and symptoms, reflecting premorbid individual differences in neuroanatomy, neurophysiology, genetics, or psychology. It is premature at this point to presume one or another of these disease models. Empirical studies of the biological heterogeneity of schizophrenia must, at this stage, be considered exploratory and are likely to employ broad analytic strategies. In this study, the focal difference in left temporal lobe volume between deficit and nondeficit subgroups is consistent with a distinct pathologic process affecting only the deficit subgroup. At the same time, the correlation between temporal lobe asymmetry and negative symptoms in the total sample argues for disease expression along a continuum. The data do not permit us to distinguish between these two models. However, the convergence of results with the use of two different analytic strategies strengthens the principal finding of an association between focal left temporal lobe abnormality and negative symptoms in schizophrenia.

Accepted for publication July 27, 1995.

Presented in part at the annual meeting of the Society for Biological Psychiatry, Philadelphia, Pa, May 21, 1994.

Reprint requests to Neuropsychiatry Program, Department of Psychiatry, 10th Floor, Gates Building, University of Pennsylvania, Philadelphia, PA 19104 (Dr Turetsky).

REFERENCES

1. Pfefferbaum A, Zipursky RB, Lim KO, Zatz LM, Stahl SM, Jernigan TL. Computed tomographic evidence for generalized sulcal and ventricular enlargement in schizophrenia. *Arch Gen Psychiatry.* 1988;45:633-640.
2. Gur RE, Mozley PD, Resnick SM, Shtasel D, Kohn M, Zimmerman R, Herman G, Atlas S, Grossman R, Erwin R, Gur RC. Magnetic resonance imaging in schizophrenia, I: volumetric analysis of brain and cerebrospinal fluid. *Arch Gen Psychiatry.* 1991;48:407-412.
3. Pearlson GD, Kim WS, Kubos KL, Moberg PJ, Jayaram G, Bascom MJ, Chase GA, Goldfinger AD, Tune LE. Ventricle-brain ratio, computed tomographic density, and brain area in 50 schizophrenics. *Arch Gen Psychiatry.* 1989;46:690-697.
4. Kelsoe JR, Cadet JL, Pickar D, Weinberger DR. Quantitative neuroanatomy in schizophrenia: a controlled magnetic resonance imaging study. *Arch Gen Psychiatry.* 1988;45:533-541.
5. Andreasen NC, Nasrallah HA, Dunn V, Olson SC, Grove WM, Ehrhardt JC, Coffman JA, Crossett JHW. Structural abnormalities in the frontal system in schizophrenia: a magnetic resonance imaging study. *Arch Gen Psychiatry.* 1986; 43:136-144.
6. Dauphinais D, DeLisi LE, Crow TJ, Alexandropoulos K, Colter N, Tuma I, Gershon ES. Reduction in temporal lobe size in siblings with schizophrenia: a magnetic resonance imaging study. *Psychiatry Res Neuroimaging.* 1990;35: 137-147.
7. Suddath RL, Casanova MF, Goldberg TE, Daniel DG, Kelsoe JR, Weinberger DR. Temporal lobe pathology in schizophrenia. *Am J Psychiatry.* 1989;1146: 464-472.
8. Suddath RL, Christison GW, Torrey EF, Casanova MF, Weinberger DR. Anatomical abnormalities in the brains of monozygotic twins discordant for schizophrenia. *N Engl J Med.* 1990;322:789-794.
9. Barta PE, Pearlson GD, Powers RE, Richards SS, Tune LE. Auditory hallucinations and smaller superior temporal gyral volume in schizophrenia. *Am J Psychiatry.* 1990;147:1457-1462.
10. Bogerts B, Ashtari M, Degreet G, Alvir JM, Bilder RM, Lieberman JA. Reduced temporal limbic structure volumes on magnetic resonance images in first episode schizophrenia. *Psychiatry Res Neuroimaging.* 1990;35:1-13.
11. Shenton ME, Kikinis R, Jolesz FA, Pollak SD, LeMay M, Wible CG, Hokama H, Martin J, Metcalf D, Coleman M, McCarley RW. Abnormalities of the left temporal lobe and thought disorder in schizophrenia: a quantitative magnetic resonance imaging study. *N Engl J Med.* 1992;327:604-612.
12. DeLisi LE, Hoff AL, Schwartz JE, Shields GW, Halthore SN, Gupta SM, Henn FA, Anand AK. Brain morphology in first-episode schizophrenic-like psychotic patients: a quantitative magnetic resonance imaging study. *Biol Psychiatry.* 1991; 29:159-175.
13. Zipursky RB, Lim KO, Sullivan EV, Brown BW, Pfefferbaum A. Widespread cerebral gray matter volume deficits in schizophrenia. *Arch Gen Psychiatry.* 1992; 49:195-205.
14. Mozley PD, Gur RE, Resnick SM, Shtasel DL, Richards J, Kohn M, Grossman R, Herman G, Gur RC. Magnetic resonance imaging in schizophrenia: relationship with clinical measures. *Schizophr Res.* 1994;12:195-203.
15. Gur RE, Mozley PD, Shtasel DL, Cannon TD, Gallacher F, Turetsky B, Grossman R, Gur RC. Clinical subtypes of schizophrenia: differences in brain and CSF volume. *Am J Psychiatry.* 1994;151:343-350.
16. American Psychiatric Association. *Diagnostic and Statistical Manual of Mental Disorders, Revised Third Edition.* Washington, DC: American Psychiatric Association; 1987.
17. Spitzer RL, Williams JBW, Gibbon M. *Structured Clinical Interview for* DSM-III-R*–Patient Version (SCID-P).* New York, NY: New York State Psychiatric Institute; 1986.
18. Shtasel DL, Gur RE, Gallacher F, Heimberg C, Cannon TD, Gur RC. Phenomenology and functioning in first-episode schizophrenia. *Schizophr Bull.* 1992; 18:449-462.
19. Gur RE. Motoric laterality imbalance in schizophrenia: a possible concomitant of left hemisphere dysfunction. *Arch Gen Psychiatry.* 1977;34:33-37.
20. Spitzer RL, Williams JBW, Gibbon M. *Structured Clinical Interview for* DSM-III-R*–Nonpatient Version (SCID-NP).* New York, NY: New York State Psychiatric Institute; 1987.
21. Shtasel DL, Gur RE, Mozley PD, Richards J, Taleff MM, Heimberg C, Gallacher F, Gur RC. Volunteers for biomedical research: recruitment and screening of normal controls. *Arch Gen Psychiatry.* 1991;48:1022-1025.
22. Overall JR, Gorham DR. The Brief Psychiatric Rating Scale. *J Operat Psychiatry.* 1980;11:48-64.
23. Andreasen NC. *The Scale for the Assessment of Negative Symptoms (SANS).* Iowa City, Iowa: The University of Iowa; 1983.
24. Andreasen NC. *The Scale for the Assessment of Positive Symptoms (SAPS).* Iowa City, Iowa: The University of Iowa; 1984.
25. Strauss JS, Carpenter WT. Characteristic symptoms and outcome in schizophrenia. *Arch Gen Psychiatry.* 1974;30:429-434.
26. Liddle PF. The symptoms of chronic schizophrenia: a re-examination of the positive-negative dichotomy. *Br J Psychiatry.* 1987;151:145-151.
27. Arndt S, Alliger RJ, Andreasen NC. The positive and negative distinction: failure of the two-dimensional model. *Br J Psychiatry.* 1991;158:317-322.
28. Cronbach LJ. Coefficient alpha and the internal structure of tests. *Psychometrika.* 1951;16:297-234.
29. Hase HD, Goldberg LR. Comparative validity of different strategies of constructing personality inventory scales. *Psychol Bull.* 1967;67:231-248.
30. Carpenter WT, Heinrichs DW, Wagman AMI. Deficit and nondeficit forms of schizophrenia: the concept. *Am J Psychiatry.* 1988;145:578-583.
31. Cowell PE, Turetsky B, Gur RC, Grossman RI, Shtasel DL, Gur RE. Sex differences in aging of the human frontal and temporal lobes. *J Neurosci.* 1994; 14:4748-4755.
32. Kohn MI, Tanna NK, Herman GT, Resnick SM, Mozley PD, Gur RE, Alavi A, Zimmerman RA, Gur RC. Analysis of brain and CSF volumes from magnetic resonance imaging: methodology, reliability and validation. *Radiology.* 1991; 178:115-122.
33. Saykin AJ, Gur RC, Gur RE, Mozley DP, Mozley LH, Resnick SM, Kester DB, Stafiniak P. Neuropsychological function in schizophrenia: selective impairment in memory and learning. *Arch Gen Psychiatry.* 1991;48:618-624.
34. Bogerts B. Recent advances in the neuropathology of schizophrenia. *Schizophr Bull.* 1993;19:431-445.
35. Fuster JM. *The Prefrontal Cortex.* New York, NY: Raven Press; 1989.
36. Andreasen NC, Rezai K, Alliger R, Swayze VW, Flaum P, Kirchner P, Cohen G, O'Leary DS. Hypofrontality in neuroleptic-naive patients and in patients with chronic schizophrenia: assessment with xenon 133 single-photon emission computed tomography and the Tower of London. *Arch Gen Psychiatry.* 1992;49: 943-958.
37. Liddle PF, Friston KJ, Frith CD, Hirsch SR, Jones T, Frackowiak RSJ. Patterns of cerebral blood flow in schizophrenia. *Br J Psychiatry.* 1992;60:179-186.
38. Andreasen NC, Nasrallah HA, Dunn V, Olson SC, Grove WM, Ehrhardt JC, Coffman JA, Crossett JHW. Structural abnormalities in the frontal system in schizophrenia: a magnetic resonance imaging study. *Arch Gen Psychiatry.* 1986; 43:136-144.
39. Andreasen NC, Ehrhardt JC, Swayze VW, Alliger RJ, Yuh WTC, Cohen G, Ziebell S. Magnetic resonance imaging of the brain in schizophrenia: the pathophysiologic significance of structural abnormalities. *Arch Gen Psychiatry.* 1990; 47:35-44.
40. Jackson JH. On the anatomical and physiological localization of movements in the brain. *Lancet.* 1873;1:84-85, 162-164, 232-234.
41. Lipska BK, Weinberger DR. Delayed effects of neonatal hippocampal damage on haloperidol-induced catalepsy and apomorphine-induced stereotypic behaviors in the rat. *Dev Brain Res.* 1993;75:213-222.
42. Lipska BK, Jaskiw GE, Weinberger DR. Postpubertal emergence of hyperresponsiveness to stress and to amphetamine after neonatal excitotoxic hippocampal damage: a potential animal model of schizophrenia. *Neuropsychopharmacology.* 1993;9:67-75.
43. Kalsbeek A, Voorn P, Buijs RM, Pool CW, Vylings HBM. Development of the dopaminergic innervation in the prefrontal cortex of the rat. *J Comp Neurol.* 1988;269:56-72.
44. Weinberger DR, Berman KF, Suddath R, Torrey EF. Evidence of dysfunction of a prefrontal-limbic network in schizophrenia: a magnetic resonance imaging and regional cerebral blood flow study of discordant monozygotic twins. *Am J Psychiatry.* 1992;149:890-897.
45. Gur RE, Mozley PD, Resnick SL, Mozley LH, Shtasel DL, Gallacher F, Arnold SE, Karp JS, Alavi A, Reivich M, Gur RC. Resting cerebral glucose metabolism in first-episode and previously treated patients with schizophrenia relates to clinical features. *Arch Gen Psychiatry.* 1995;52:657-667.

Conversions From Clozapine to Other Antipsychotic Drugs

Conversions between dissimilar antipsychotic agents can be problematic. Agents of low potency present risks of central depressant and autonomic side effects, whereas agents of high potency carry a higher risk of inducing acute extrapyramidal effects. Conversions between clozapine and other more typical antipsychotic drugs, including the new agent risperidone,[1] are increasingly common and may cause special problems. For example, over a dozen cases of worsening of psychotic symptoms after abrupt withdrawal from clozapine therapy have been reported[2-7] and at least five additional similar cases have been observed recently at our centers (D.M.G and R.J.B., unpublished data, June 1995). These reactions often evolved over several days and so were much more rapid than relapses after stopping treatment with standard agents, which average 50% risk over a 3- to 4-month period.[8,9] Moreover, several case reports[6,10,11] and cases observed at our centers (by D.M.G., D.L.G., and R.J.B. May 1995) suggest that risperidone may fail to protect fully from the withdrawal of clozapine treatment as well as risking acute extrapyramidal reactions.

The incidence of such reactions to removal of clozapine treatment, risk factors that might predict them, and their pharmacodynamic basis are not clear. Clinical worsening and lack of protection by switching to treatment with other agents might simply reflect superior clinical efficacy of clozapine. A contributing factor may be its relatively rapid clearance from tissue (plasma elimination half-life, circa 12 hours in man) compared with other neuroleptic drugs.[12,13] Elimination from brain tissue, at least in the rat, is even more rapid (elimination half-life, circa 1.5 hours) and much faster than other typical neuroleptic drugs such as fluphenazine or haloperidol.[13,14]

An alternative hypothesis is that rapid removal of clozapine and substitution of a more typical neuroleptic with potent antagonistic activity at D_2 dopamine receptors and autoreceptors may lead to a relative excess of activation of D_4 receptors in limbic, cortical, or other nonextrapyramidal areas of the forebrain. Clozapine is reported to be the most selective antagonist for D_4 over D_2 receptors of any clinically employed antipsychotic agent.[12,15-18] In addition, the product of its typical daily doses to its selectivity for D_4 receptors might be an indication of its impact on the D_4 dopamine receptor system. This index (over 2000) is the highest of any reported antipsychotic agent (**Table**). While several other neuroleptic drugs are also reported to have rather high affinity for D_4 receptors (eg, trifluoperazine ≥ haloperidol ≥ risperidone), they also have high D_2 affinity and are typically administered in much lower daily doses than clozapine (Table). The antagonistic effects of typical neuroleptic drugs at D_2 receptors and autoreceptors probably stimulate acute compensatory increases in presynaptic production and release of dopamine.[19] Moreover, the increased turnover and release of dopamine have been found in rat forebrain after abruptly interrupting repeated treatment with clozapine, but not a typical neuroleptic drug.[5,20] If prolonged exposure to clozapine induces up-regulation and supersensitivity at D_4 receptors, its rapid removal may have a particularly great impact. Switching from clozapine treatment to treatment with an agent with prominent D_2 antagonist activity is likely to increase availability of dopamine while leaving D_4 receptors relatively unprotected.[20] We hypothesize that these effects might contribute to rapid exacerbation of psychotic symptoms when switching from clozapine to another antipsychotic agent.

Among available antipsychotic agents that have been evaluated, thioridazine has moderate affinity at D_2 dopamine receptors but its D_4 affinity is even higher than that of clozapine and it has an unusually high product of dose and D_4 selectivity (>100) as well as low potency. These characteristics suggest that thioridazine might be preferable to high-potency neuroleptic drugs such as haloperidol or risperidone when removing clozapine, even though some high-potency neuroleptic drugs have substantial D_4 affinity (Table). The prominent antimuscarinic actions of thioridazine also may limit autonomic ef-

Relative Dopamine Receptor Affinities and Doses of Antipsychotic Agents

	Affinity (K_i),* nmol/L				
Agent	D_2	D_4	D_4 vs D_2 Preference†§	Typical Dose, mg/d	D_4-Over-D_2 Preference ×Dose‡§
Clozapine	193	25	7.72	300	2316
S-(−)-sulpiride	9.2	52	0.18	1000	180
Thioridazine	3.3	12	0.28	400	112
Chlorpromazine	2.2	32	0.07	500	34
Trifluoperazine	1.2	3.0	0.40	15	6.0
Risperidone	6.6	11	0.59	6	3.6
Haloperidol	2.4	7.4	0.30	10	3.0
Fluphenazine	0.5	46	0.01	10	0.1

Affinities are averages of previously reported values;[13,16-18] unpublished data on clozapine and risperidone kindly provided by J. E. Leysen, PhD, Janssen Research Institute, Beerse, Belgium, as well as unpublished data by N. S. Kula, MD; R. J. B.; J. W. Kebabian, PhD; and J. L. Neumeyer, PhD.

†*D_4 vs D_2 receptor preference =(K_i D_2/K_i D_4).*

‡*D_4-over-D_2 preference times typical daily antipsychotic dose is intended as an index of potential impact on central D_4 receptors.*

§*The ratios provided are only approximations since there is substantial variability in receptor affinity determinations (eg, coefficient of variation for K_i averaged 58% for clozapine, the most extensively studied agent).*

fects of rapid removal of the strongly anticholinergic agent clozapine.[12] These considerations lead to testable hypotheses. For example, replacement of clozapine with thioridazine may be better tolerated than other alternatives, with respect to early relapse and withdrawal-associated adverse effects.

Without direct evidence to support such speculations, it may be safest clinically to manage the removal of clozapine by gradual discontinuation with simultaneous addition of increasing doses of an alternative agent. Such crossed and overlapping conversions between clozapine and risperidone can be managed with little risk of rapid clinical worsening and without substantial increase of side effects over those associated with use of the individual agents (D.M.G., R.J.B., Jose Benzo, MD, Carlos Zarate Jr, MD, and Mauricio Tohen, MD, DrPH, unpublished data, June 1995). In general, gradual removal and discontinuation of therapy with various psychotropic agents may tend to minimize iatrogenic risks of early recurrences of illness associated with abrupt removal of ongoing treatment.[9,21]

Ross J. Baldessarini, MD
Mailman Research Center 316
McLean Hospital
115 Mill St
Belmont, Mass 02178
David M. Gardner, BSPharm
Toronto, Ontario
David L. Garver, MD, PhD
Dallas, Tex

This study was supported, in part, by grants MH-31154 and MH-47370 from the National Institute of Mental Health, Washington, DC, and by the Bruce J. Anderson Foundation, Boston, Mass, and the Vivian M. Temte Fund, McLean Hospital.

1. Marder SR, Meibach RC. Risperidone in the treatment of schizophrenia. *Am J Psychiatry*. 1994;151:825-835.
2. Ekblom B, Eriksson K, Lindstrom LH. Supersensitivity psychosis in schizophrenic patients after sudden clozapine withdrawal. *Psychopharmacology*. 1984; 83:293-294.
3. Perenyi A, Kuncz E, Bagdy G. Early relapse after sudden withdrawal or dose reduction of clozapine. *Psychopharmacology*. 1986;86:244.
4. Eklund K. Supersensitivity and clozapine withdrawal. *Psychopharmacology*. 1987;90:135.
5. Alphs LD, Lee HS. Comparison of withdrawal of typical and atypical antipsychotic drugs: a case study. *J Clin Psychiatry*. 1991;52:346-348.
6. Parsa MA, Al-Lahham YH, Ramirez JF, Meltzer HY. Prolonged psychotic relapse after abrupt clozapine withdrawal. *J Clin Psychopharmacol*. 1993;13:154-155.
7. Abuzzahab FS, Gillund JM. Clozapine and risperidone in schizophrenia. In: *ACNP Annual Meeting Abstracts*. Nashville, Tenn: American College of Neuropsychopharmacology; 1994;33:225.
8. Gilbert PL, Harris MJ, Jeste DV. Neuroleptic withdrawal in schizophrenic patients: a review of the literature. *Arch Gen Psychiatry*. 1995;52:173-188.
9. Baldessarini RJ, Viguera AC. Neuroleptic withdrawal in schizophrenic patients. *Arch Gen Psychiatry*. 1995;52:189-192.
10. Dickson R, Williams R, Dalby JT. Dystonic reaction and relapse with clozapine discontinuation and risperidone initiation. *Can J Psychiatry*. 1994;39:184.
11. Mok H, Yatham LN. Response to clozapine as a predictor of risperidone response in schizophrenia. *Am J Psychiatry* 1994;151:1393-1394.
12. Baldessarini RJ, Frankenburg FR. Clozapine: a novel antipsychotic agent. *N Engl J Med* 1991;324:746-754.
13. Cohen BM, Tsuneizumi T, Baldessarini RJ, Campbell A, Babb SM. Differences between antipsychotic drugs in persistence of brain levels and behavioral effects. *Psychopharmacology*. 1992;108:338-344.
14. Baldessarini RJ, Centorrino F, Flood JG, Volpicelli SA, Huston-Lyons D, Cohen BM. Tissue concentrations of clozapine and its metabolites in the rat. *Neuropsychopharmacology*. 1993;9:117-124.
15. Van Tol HHM, Bunzow JR, Guan H-C, Sunahara RK, Seeman P, Niznik HB, Civelli D. Cloning of the gene for a human dopamine D_4 receptor with high affinity for the antipsychotic clozapine. *Nature*. 1991;350:610-614.
16. O'Malley KL, Harmon S, Tang L, Todd RD. The rat D_4 receptor: sequence, gene structure, and demonstration of expression in the cardiovascular system. *New Biologist*. 1992;4:137-146.
17. Kimmel SE, Calabrese JR, Woyshville MJ, Meltzer HY. Clozapine in treatment-refractory mood disorders. *J Clin Psychiatry*. 1994;55(suppl B):91-93.
18. Leysen JE, Janssen PMF, Megens AAHP, Schotte A. Risperidone: a novel antipsychotic with balanced serotonin-dopamine antagonism: receptor occupancy profile and pharmacologic activity. *J Clin Psychiatry*. 1994;55(suppl 5):5-12.
19. Wolf ME, Roth RH. Autoreceptor regulation of dopamine synthesis. *Ann N Y Acad Sci*. 1990;604:323-342.
20. Ichikawa J, Meltzer HY. Differential effects of repeated treatment with haloperidol and clozapine and dopamine release and metabolism in the striatum and the nucleus accumbens. *J. Pharmacol Exp Ther*. 1991;256:348-357.
21. Suppes T, Baldessarini RJ, Faedda GL, Tondo L, Tohen M. Discontinuation of maintenance treatment in bipolar disorder: risks and implications. *Harvard Rev Psychiatry*. 1993;1:131-144.

Correction

Incomplete Reference Citation. In the article titled "Report Card on the *National Plan for Research on Child and Adolescent Mental Disorders:* The Midway Point," published in the September ARCHIVES (1995;52:715-723), on page 723 in the "References" section, the name of the author and the title of the article, respectively, should have read as follows: Depression Guideline Panel. *Clinical Practice Guideline: Depression in Primary Care: Treatment of Major Depression.* We regret the formatting error.

Helen Singer Kaplan, MD, PhD
February 6, 1929, to August 17, 1995

Dr Helen Singer Kaplan, educator, master clinician, and innovator in the field of sex therapy, died August 17, 1995, in her Manhattan, NY, home after a long fight with breast cancer. Clinical professor of psychiatry at Cornell University, New York, NY, since 1970, she was the founder and director of the first medical school–based clinic for sexual disorders, the Human Sexuality Program at the Payne Whitney Clinic of New York Hospital. This program provided postgraduate training courses in sex therapy for physicians and other mental health professionals. The centerpiece of the program was the always well-attended Wednesday seminar conducted by Dr Kaplan and structured around a videotaped case presentation, followed by a discussion of the dynamics of the problem, the course of treatment, and any relevant medical issues. In addition to being a training facility, the Human Sexuality Program was also an outpatient clinic for evaluation and treatment of psychosexual disorders, which in turn provided clinical cases for trainees. It also served as a major source of the voluminous data that fueled Dr Kaplan's contributions to the field.

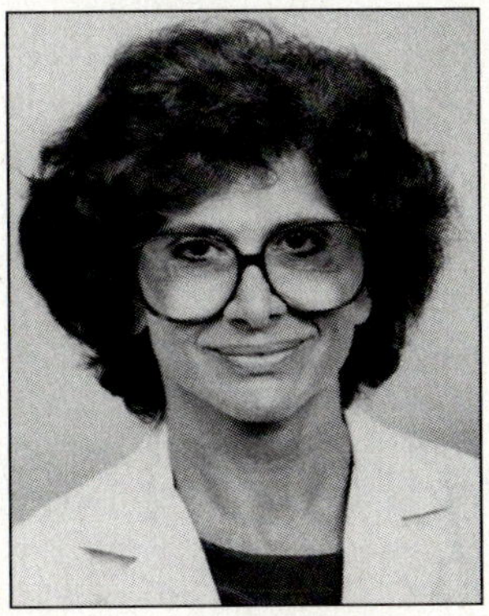

Helen Singer Kaplan, MD, PhD

It is for her important theoretical contributions that Dr Kaplan will likely be best remembered. Chief among these was her insight that Masters' and Johnson's model for sexual dysfunction—predicated on the idea of a two-phase sexual response consisting of excitement and orgasm—while groundbreaking in its day, was not all-encompassing. A large number of Dr Kaplan's own patients suffered not from any impairment of performance but rather from disorders of desire. Therefore, she proposed a three-phase sequence to the sexual response system: desire, excitement, and orgasm. Specific problems were referable to each phase, each requiring different treatment strategies and interventions.

Dr Kaplan's insight into the origins of different inhibitory feelings (eg, anxiety, guilt, shame, and rage) informed her treatment plans. She distinguished two kinds of precipitating causes of anti-sexual feelings: the sometimes superficially induced negative feelings that occur at the inception of lovemaking and the deeper intrapsychic and interactional predispositions. Depending on the cause of the patient's presenting problem, her treatment plan invoked some combination of structured behavioral interventions and psychodynamically oriented insight therapy. She was able to weave together treatments combining cognitive therapy, couples therapy, brief psychodynamic therapy, and psychopharmacology. She was one of the few psychiatrists able to fully integrate biological, psychological, and psychosocial approaches to psychiatric disorders.

Born in Vienna, Austria, February 6, 1929, Helen Singer and her family became Holocaust refugees and emigrated to the United States in 1940. She was educated in public school in New York, attended the High School of Music and Art, and graduated magna cum laude from the Syracuse College of Fine Arts in 1951. She went on to earn a master's degree in psychology at Columbia University in 1952, and a PhD degree in 1955, and, finally, an MD degree from the New York Medical College in 1959. It was there that she also trained in psychoanalysis. She did her psychiatric training at Bellevue Hospital and then at New York Medical College–Metropolitan Hospital Center.

It was at the New York Medical College–Metropolitan Hospital Center that Helen first established herself as a teacher, developing and coordinating a basic behavioral science program for psychiatric residents and a course for freshman medical students as well. By that time she had achieved a mastery of psychopharmacology and taught a course in that subject. She was an associate professor of psychiatry at New York Medical College until 1970 when she moved to Cornell, and from 1970 until 1976 she was in charge of medical student teaching of psychiatry at the New York Hospital.

Although Helen retained no trace of an accent, her roots in Europe were very strong. She attributed part of her interest in sexuality to the fact that Europeans—particularly women—did not stigmatize sex to the same degree as Americans and were freer to enjoy it. But at the same time, her outrage at the atrocities of World War II made her adamant against returning to or speaking in Austria, a reluctance she only overcame when she delivered a major address in the German language in Vienna in 1992.

Helen's publications number well over 100. Several of her books are classics, including *New Sex*

Therapy: Active Treatment of Sexual Dysfunctions (Random House, 1974), a book that integrated behavioral and psychodynamic treatment interventions, and *Disorders of Sexual Desires and Other New Concepts and Techniques in Sex Therapy* (Brunner-Mazel, 1979). And surely her posthumously published *The Sexual Desire Disorders: Dysfunctional Regulation of Sexual Motivation* (Brunner-Mazel, 1995) will also become a classic. Her undaunted spirit and ability to cope with adversity found its way into some of her later papers in which she addressed the damage to sexuality in patients with breast cancer as a side effect of chemotherapy and assessed possible remedies.

Helen participated in many professional associations. She was a fellow of the American Academy of Psychoanalysis and the American Psychiatric Society and a member of the American Society of Sex Educators and Counselors and the American Association of Marriage and Family Therapy. In addition, she was the editor of the *Journal of Sex and Marital Therapy*.

Helen's creativity was not confined to her professional life. Her artistic temperament was evident in the drawing she began to engage in in early childhood and she continued to paint, sculpt, and work with acrylics until shortly before her death. Some of her paintings are haunting, echoing the horrors of the Holocaust, others erotic. Her self-portraits are remarkable. Several artists have voiced the opinion that had she chosen to pursue a career in art she might well have become one of the modern masters. Her keen visual sense extended to a passionate affair with gardening, horticulture, the growing of orchids, and devoted attention to the beauty of her city and country homes.

Helen Singer Kaplan also achieved great happiness in her personal life. She is survived by her beloved and loving husband of 15 years, Charles Lazarus; her well-loved sons and daughter, Phillip Kaplan, MD, Peter Kaplan, MD, and Jennifer Kaplan-D'Addio; and two grandsons.

Ethel Person, MD
Department of Psychiatry
Columbia University
New York, NY

Roland D. Ciaranello, MD
February 27, 1943, to December 14, 1994

ROLAND D. CIARANELLO, MD, was a leader in the effort to bring developmental biology and molecular neuroscience knowledge to child psychiatry and clinical problems. His premature and unexpected death of a heart disorder on December 14, 1994, while attending a meeting of his favorite scientific association, the American College of Neuropsychopharmacology, deprived psychiatry of one of its strongest figures at the prime of his career. At Stanford University he held the Nancy Friend Pritzker Professorship, was the Director of the Nancy Pritzker Laboratory of Developmental Neurobiology, and was the Director of the Division of Child Psychiatry.

Shortly before he died, Roland wrote of his career:

> "My scientific work has been dominated by a long-standing fascination with the regulation of biochemical processes, and a desire to understand them in the context of central nervous system disorders. This interest links my work in genetic control of the catecholamine synthetic enzymes, begun over 20 years ago, with my current work on regulation of genes . . . controlling serotonin receptors, genetic control of neuronal developmental and the genetics of infantile autism."

In each of these areas he was a pioneer and made substantial contributions to scientific knowledge.

Born in Schenectady, NY, on February 27, 1943, Roland David Ciaranello attended Union College before coming to the Stanford Medical School. He immediately started research in the Department of Psychiatry. His first studies dealt with the formation and metabolism of epinephrine in the brain. He was a corecipient of the A. E. Bennett Award from the Society of Biological Psychiatry for those studies.

Particularly noteworthy was the work that Roland accomplished on genetic processes. He was especially interested in neurotransmitters and neuromodulators and, with his coauthors, coined the term "neuroregulators" to describe chemicals that fit into those broad categories. He used the regulation of the enzymes that are involved with the formation of catecholamines (dopamine, norepinephrine, and epinephrine) as a model to study genetic processes and molecular controls that relate to behavior. The study of those regulatory steps has profound implications for improving our understanding of individual vulnerability to stress and mental disorders. Roland may have been the first to recognize that genetic processes can and do control each step in the formation and action of neuroregulators. His important contributions in this line of inquiry over the years constitute one part of his enduring legacy.

Julius Axelrod, PhD had a profound impact on Roland. In a 3-year postdoctoral with the Nobelist at the National Institutes of Mental Health in Bethesda, Md, Roland became intensely interested in the fundamental processes controlling regulatory steps. Those processes ranged from hormones to the enzymes (proteases) that metabolize the synthetic enzymes involved in the formation of neuroregulators.

Roland returned to Stanford to train in child psychiatry. It was highly unusual in the early 1970s for a person with his background to enter that clinical arena; however, he saw it as a natural extension. He believed, with the passion, alacrity, zest, and determination that all who knew him saw repeatedly, that the developmental disorders, such as autism, were a clinical area that could be approached from a biochemical and genetic perspective.

Roland's concerns were not only with science—he felt deeply about the pain and difficulty of such disorders for patients and their families. He initiated an important study of the genetics of autism, with great attention to the clinical components of the problem. That study was just bearing fruit at the time of his death. So another part of his enduring legacy was the establishment of a precedent: the significance of developmental biology for child psychiatry.

At Stanford, Roland established an independent laboratory that became known for the quality of its science and training. A series of superb individuals were trained in his program, another legacy of his career. Dona Wong, PhD, a molecular pharmacologist and the head of a section in the Pritzker laboratory, extended the regulatory studies on epinephrine formation, while Roland's interests turned toward the regulation of receptors. He was unusual among psychiatrists in that much of his work was published in the most rigorous of basic science journals. His studies were marked by care and elegance. He published about 160 papers and several monographs and had hoped to be involved in a revision of a highly successful textbook of psychopharmacology.

A special pleasure for Roland was derived from working with students. He was key to the establishment at Stanford of one of the first research-oriented residency programs in the country—the first to have more than half of its trainees in research tracks. The Stanford program placed a special emphasis on those students entering psychiatry with combined MD/PhD training. Roland was particularly sensitive to the need to individualize the experience of talented trainees, and he was able to use the unique qualities of Stanford to achieve that goal. He was fabled for his recruiting, not only for the Stanford residency but also for the University's athletic programs, particularly the football and women's basketball teams. He loved advising students and helping them develop their careers. His advising went the full range from high school students interested in possible careers in medicine or research to undergraduates, medical students, residents, doctoral candidates, and postdoctoral fellows.

Roland had stunning capacities as a lecturer. His science was complex and he relished the art of explaining it. He was active in undergraduate teaching at Stanford and had a rare capacity to communicate with students regardless of their knowledge level or background. He was also outstanding in his ability to explain science to nonscientists.

In addition to the Bennett Award, Roland received the highest research commendation of the American College of Neuropsychopharmacology, the Daniel Effron Award. His receipt of the Distinguished Mentor Award of the American Academy of Child and Adolescent Psychiatry was particularly appropriate to his values.

At a personal level, Roland was deeply involved with his family. He shared with his father a great love for classical music, particularly that of Mozart. His daughter, Andrea, as a Harvard undergraduate, worked in the laboratory as a student research assistant and was coauthor of a paper with him. His wife, Nancy, was involved in special education. Always an athlete and in superb physical condition, Roland had been a star high-school football player, was an assertive player in intramural "lab" baseball at Stanford, was an avid runner and skier, and was active in the Ski Patrol. Apart from science, music, and athletics, he had a deep interest in the German language and in modern European history.

Roland was an institution builder, strengthening whatever he touched. His activities at Stanford covered every aspect of the school (he served terms as President of the Faculty Senate and as Chair of the Budget Committee) and the department of which he was a member. His interest in institution building, recruitment, and the application of basic science knowledge to the clinical arena led to his being a cofounder, with his friend Tom Barton, an attorney, and other scientists, of one of the first neuroscience companies, Neurex. He was active in the Scottish Rite Schizophrenia Foundation. He served in many capacities for the American College of Neuropsychopharmacology and became the co-editor of its superb journal, *Neuropsychopharmacology*. Despite the demands of that position, he was also extremely helpful to the ARCHIVES. He played a role held by only a few others—what Dan Freedman used to call the "Solomon" reviewer, brought in to help resolve decisions about manuscripts about which there were sharply differing reviews. His decisions were clear, penetrating, and incisive. They were also scrupulously fair and constructive.

Roland left us all a legacy of lasting value: his personal attributes, his scientific accomplishments, his professional leadership, and his authentic inspiration. At the time of his death, Roland was widely viewed as the leading candidate to become the Director of the National Institutes of Mental Health, the most significant position in the entire field of psychiatry. His sense of the importance of science in its many directions as well as his broad concerns for the field and interests in the development of young people would have shown him to be truly spectacular in that role.

Jack D. Barchas, MD, Editor

Stanley J. Watson, MD, PhD
University of Michigan
Ann Arbor

David A. Hamburg, MD
Carnegie Corp
New York, NY

John Romano, MD
November 20, 1908, to June 19, 1995

JOHN ROMANO, MD, age 86, died on June 19, 1995, a few days after an acute stroke. He was a Distinguished University Professor of Psychiatry Emeritus. He was still an active participant in department, school, and university projects. John's wife of 56 years, Miriam, died in 1989.

He was born November 20, 1908, and received his undergraduate and medical training at Marquette University. He had postgraduate training in neurology and psychiatry at Yale, the University of Colorado, and Harvard. During this time he worked with many outstanding physicians who went on to become leaders in American medicine and with whom he maintained a close ring of friendship. He worked and wrote on a number of topics during this period, including autonomic disorders, alcoholism and its complications, electroencephalography, and schizophrenia.

In 1942, at the age of 34, Dr Romano became chair of psychiatry at the University of Cincinnati. He developed an outstanding department and a coterie of fine investigators such as George Engel, MD, and others. They worked on many projects, and their team made observations on the physiological changes accompanying decompression, a topic of interest to the military.

Dean George Whipple successfully recruited him as the founding chair of psychiatry at the University of Rochester in 1946. As a relatively new medical school, there was very little instructional activity in this area. Dr Romano not only had to recruit his faculty, but he had to plan and design the structure for the clinic, inpatient area, and laboratories. The department flourished, and many of the trainees went on to head their own programs and to become prominent in clinical and research areas. His own clinical and research interest became centered on schizophrenia. However, more and more of his time and talents was spent on topics of medical education. Dr Romano was a leader both locally and nationally in assessing the goals of education and in devising means to attain these goals. He emphasized the importance of education by his own devotion to student and trainee teaching. He held the position of chair for 25 years and then remained active in teaching and research.

The period after he relinquished administrative responses was, in many ways, quite fulfilling for Dr Romano. He became a wise counselor to many of his colleagues. He could indulge his broad interests in art and literature. His greatest joy was visiting and traveling with his son, David; his daughter-in-law, Irene; and his three granddaughters, Katherine, Elizabeth, and Sarah. The yearly report of his activities and writings were chronicles of diverse interests reflecting his great energy and insatiable curiosity. He was the consummate dinner companion—always showing an interest in the other person's family, activities, and interests. Dr Romano was a frequent visitor at the state psychiatric center, where the patients succeeded in having one of their housing units named after him. There were many people, at all stations of life, who could recite some special gift from him, remembrance of him, or thoughtful act of him.

He was an engaging teacher, always emphasizing the importance of keeping the focus on the patient. Dr Romano was a keen observer and was indefatigable in bringing out pertinent details of a patient's history. His approach to disease permeated the educational and patient care programs of the medical students, house staff, and faculty at Rochester. He looked upon his advancement of patient-centered medical care as his greatest achievement.

Dr Romano served on the original National Advisory Mental Health Council and helped fashion the government's participation in patient care, training, and research. This was a crucial time for medicine, as the government was now taking a major role in areas they had neglected in the past. He was chair of the Research Study Section, and he worked successfully to get funding for psychiatric research. His broad view of medicine and wide knowledge led to many important committee and consultant appointments. He was an articulate and witty speaker and delivered many of the important lectures in the field of psychiatry. His talk, "The Battered Chairman Syndrome,"[1] was a classic observation of what befalls the academic administrator. Dr Romano believed strongly that psychiatrists should be grounded in general medicine and reacted strongly when the medical internship was eliminated as part of psychiatric training. His article, "The Elimination of the Internship--an Act of Regression"[2] was his impassioned response, followed by "Is There a Stethoscope in the House (and Is It Used)?"[3]

He was the recipient of many honors. A particularly prized one was an honorary degree from his alma mater. He was honored at the 150th anniversary of the founding of the American Psychiatric Association and cited as "the most influential voice in psychiatric education in this century." In the book, *The Healer's Tale: Transforming Medicine and Culture*,[4] he was designated as particularly influential in shaping modern psychiatry in this century.

Dr Romano was always awed by the privilege of being a doctor. He once said, "You have a relationship, indeed a covenant, with another person that is unlike any other. You have the ability to reach out and touch what is human in another person that no one else ever has. I am still excited every time I speak with a patient."

Robert J. Joynt, MD, PhD
Professor of Neurology
Rochester, NY

REFERENCES

1. Romano J. The battered chairman syndrome. *Arch Gen Psychiatry.* 1991;48: 371-374.
2. Romano J. The elimination of the internship—an act of regression. *Am J Psychiatry.* 1970;126:1565-1576.
3. McIntyre J, Romano J. Is there a stethoscope in the house (and is it used)? *Arch Gen Psychiatry.* 1977;34:1147-1151.
4. Kaufman SR. *The Healer's Tale: Transforming Medicine and Culture.* Madison, Wis: University of Wisconsin Press; 1994.

Joseph Wortis, MD
October 2, 1906, to February 22, 1995

JOSEPH WORTIS, MD, the founding editor of *Biological Psychiatry* and for the subsequent 23 years until 1992 the chief editor of that journal, died February 22, 1995, of complications from prostatic cancer. With his direction, *Biological Psychiatry* grew from a quarterly to bimonthly publication and developed a major influence on the field of psychiatry.

Joe Wortis was regarded by many as the consummate editor. He had a broad intellectual background and diverse interests and was curious and knowledgeable about every aspect of publishing.

As the first-generation immigrant son of a Ukrainian Jewish father and a mother from the Jewish community of Alsace-Lorraine in France, he grew up in a family where Russian, Yiddish, French, and German were familiar languages. His writing ability received early recognition when he was made editor of the literary paper of the Eastern District High School in Brooklyn, NY. Supported by New York State and college scholarships, Joe received a bachelor's degree in English with honors in 1927 from New York University. He was admitted to Yale University Medical School, but opted to study medicine in Vienna, Munich, and Paris and graduated from Vienna Medical College in 1932. Following an internship at Bellevue Hospital in New York City, Joe received a privately funded fellowship (1934-1941) through the National Science Council to study sexual psychology under the joint guidance of Havelock Ellis, MD, and Aldolf Meyer, MD. Under the auspices of this fellowship, Wortis undertook a didactic analysis with Sigmund Freud in Vienna for 5 months (1934-1935). At that time he also observed Manfred Sakel's use of insulin shock treatment for schizophrenia, and on returning to the United States in 1935, he introduced this treatment, subsequently translating Sakel's monograph. For the next 3 years, Wortis focused on studying and refining this treatment at Bellevue Psychiatric Hospital. In 1938 to 1939 he was an assistant in psychiatry at The Johns Hopkins Medical School, Baltimore, Md, and thereafter an instructor and assistant professor in psychiatry at New York University Medical College until 1952. During World War II, Wortis was assigned to the Ellis Island Marine Hospital and was honorably discharged from the US Public Health Service in 1945 with the rank of lieutenant commander.

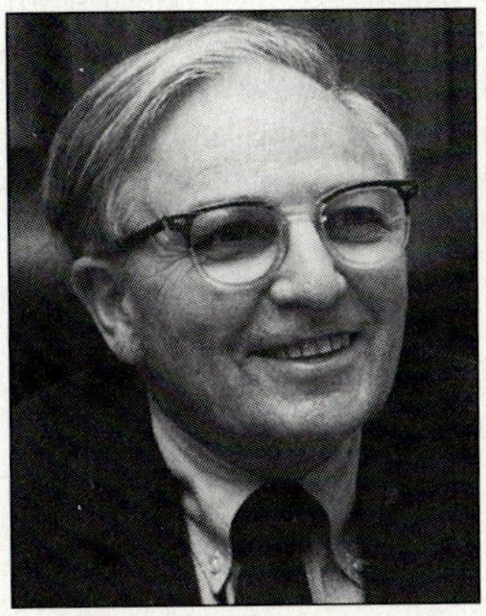

Joseph Wortis, MD

During the 1930s and 1940s, Wortis had a steady flow of publications on insulin shock, both clinical treatment and basic brain mechanism studies. For the latter, he collaborated with Harold Himwich, PhD, a well-known physiologist. They were among the first to study lactic acid and brain oxidation.[1] During this period, Wortis expressed his skepticism of psychoanalysis as a scientific means for studying psychology and as an effective treatment.[2] However, *Fragments of an Analysis With Freud*,[3] the account of his didactic analysis, was not published until 1954. In his studies of human sexuality, Wortis repeatedly emphasized the importance of social and environmental influences on conditioning sexual behavior.[4]

Wortis came under the scrutiny of the Senate Internal Security Subcommittee in 1953 as part of an investigation of purported Communist infiltration of education. His book *Soviet Psychiatry*[5] had aroused their interest. This experience did not cause him to waver in his lifelong commitment to socialism and political activities devoted to peace and civil rights.

As the director of the division of pediatric psychiatry at the Jewish Hospital of Brooklyn (1950-1967), Wortis established a highly regarded developmental evaluation clinic. For many years he edited "Mental Retardation and Developmental Disabilities–An Annual Review" in addition to publishing in this area. He continued with this field of interest at Maimonides Medical Center in Brooklyn, 1967 to 1973, and in his final appointment as professor of psychiatry, State University of New York at Stony Brook.

Wortis maintained his strong interest in international science throughout his life. For 6 years he was editor of the *International Behavioral Sciences Series*, which published English-language translations of foreign-language scientific articles. As editor of *Biological Psychiatry* he developed a plan to distribute that journal to Third World countries and had as one of his associate editors someone from a foreign country.

Joe's zest for life, sense of humor, mental and physical energy, and diverse interests were apparent in his editorials. His model for good writing was George Bernard Shaw. "Hard writing makes for easy reading," he would say as he meticulously crafted his editorials to a high level of clarity and lucidity. Titles of his editorials—"Psychiatric Tidbits From Teratopogi," "Data Is Plural," "The Medieval Garden," "Privatization," "Struwwelpter Heinrich Hoffman," and "Venus and Adonis: An Early Account of Sexual Harassment"—reflect Joe's broad intellectualism.

Two months before his death Joe was writing the talk on Freud that he was invited to give (January 16, 1995) at the Verein fur Psychiatrie und Neurologie, one of the oldest psychiatric societies, founded in Vienna the mid-19th century. He was not to have that pleasure. This was the conclusion of his talk:

> At the present time I would say that Freud made his historical contribution by humanizing psychiatry at a time when it was grossly neglecting developmental psychology and social influences, broadened the range of interest far beyond the prior limitations to the major psychoses, and stimulated a lot of thinking on the complexities of psychodynamics. On the negative side, many of his basic views were mistaken and scientific methodology almost non-existent.
>
> If he regarded himself as a novelist, let us accept him on his own terms, read him with interest, and profit as we read Schnitzler, Thomas Mann, or Hemingway, praise him for his insights and reject what seems incorrect or unsound. I regard him as an interesting cultural phenomenon, sometimes with harmful influence, but he is not a good example of a principled scientist, bound to his data, using careful methodology to interpret their meaning. If he remains one of Vienna's most famous sons, let us remember that he was especially proud of the Goethe prize, awarded to him by the city of Frankfurt. It was a prize for literature.

Jeffery Lieberman, MD, a clinical research scientist, wrote to me,

> I was deeply saddened to learn of Joe's death. Although he was an octogenarian, he was such a bright and important figure in the firmament of academic and biological psychiatry that we thought (hoped) that he would remain with us forever. His courtly manner combined with his impressive erudition were refreshing qualities that are all too rare in this era of boisterous and intemperate behavior. I will particularly miss the anecdotes—and have for some time missed the personal notes that he would send as editor of *Biological Psychiatry*.

Katherine Ann Halmi, MD
Professor of Psychiatry
The New York Hospital–Cornell Medical Center
21 Bloomingdale Rd
White Plains, NY 10605

REFERENCES

1. Wortis J, Bowman KM, Goldfarb W, Fazekas JF, Himwich HE. Availability of lactic acid for brain oxidations. *J Neurophysiol.* 1941;4:243-249.
2. Wortis J. How progressive is psychoanalysis? *New Masses.* October 2 and 9, 1945.
3. Wortis J. *Fragments of an Analysis With Freud.* New York, NY: Simon & Schuster; 1954.
4. Wortis J. Sex taboos, sex offenders and the law. *Am J Orthopsychiatry.* 1939; 9:554-564.
5. Wortis J. *Soviet Psychiatry.* Baltimore, Md: Williams & Williams; 1950.

Samuel Wesley Perry III, MD
December 10, 1940, to March 15, 1994

Dr Samuel Wesley Perry III, "the scion of generations of physicians" as the *New York Times* noted, died of pancreatic cancer on March 15, 1994, at the age of 53 years. He graduated from Princeton (NJ) University, received his medical training at Columbia University College of Physicians and Surgeons in New York, NY, and completed his psychoanalytic training at the Columbia Psychoanalytic Center where he became a training and supervising analyst. He was married for 28 years to Anna, and they had three children.

Dr Perry completed 2 years as an Air Force Captain in Biloxi, Miss, as the psychiatric coordinator of prisoner of war returnees, and then was an instructor in the department of psychiatry at Columbia University for 4 years. Since 1977, he was a full-time faculty member of the department of psychiatry at Cornell University Medical College in New York City where he rose from assistant professor to Professor and Associate Chairman for Research in 15 years. He served on several national committees and advisory councils, including the Human Immunodeficiency Virus Infection (HIV) Prevention Advisory Board at the National Institute of Mental

Health (NIMH). His appointment to the Editorial Board of the *Archives of General Psychiatry* was pending at the time of his death. During these years as teacher, clinician, and scientist, he was always involved with his family and in life outside the university walls. He was an athlete, and at the time of his cancer diagnosis, he was training for a triathlon. He was a terrific poker player, as many of his friends learned to their misfortune, and a superb raconteur.

During his years at Cornell, he played multiple and central roles as scientist, teacher, and director of the medical student mental health service, which one of his former chairmen considered "the most important clinical responsibility in the whole department." He taught residents and medical students in formal roles within the consultation/liaison division, and he taught everyone else who came within his sphere, including his patients and his colleagues, about doing well at work and in life. As another of his chairmen noted, "he could help the most junior person or the most experienced . . . he was a man who could suffer fools and convert them to a higher life form." In truth, his central identity was as a "helper" to us all. He was direct, he was candid, but he also so clearly enjoyed helping others that one did not take offense or feel diminished even when he was forthright in disagreement or criticism. Despite his impeccable pedigree and academic credentials, or maybe because of them, he was "Sam" to everyone.

Sam made major contributions to teaching and mentoring the research careers of members of his own department. He also held major positions in the field of psychiatry nationally, from editorial positions on six journals, to membership in 12 professional organizations, ranging from the American Psychoanalytic Association to the American Burn Association. He played an active role in the evolution of the NIMH Office on AIDS [acquired immunodeficiency syndrome], and served on its review committee for several years.

But it is as a scientist that Sam made what is perhaps his most enduring intellectual contributions to the field of psychiatry and the care of patients, more generally. His first area of study was burn patients, from which his interest in pain and pain recognition and management naturally evolved. His first grant from the National Institutes of Health was for the study of analgesia for burn patients, starting in 1979. He wrote extensively about management of pain in burn patients, the associated trauma for the patients, and also the attending staffs on the burn unit. He was a true pioneer in documenting and calling attention to the fact that pain in burn patients and in other conditions is undertreated. In a series of articles, he kept focusing and refining this message, and he offered original psychodynamic explanations for why physicians and nurses tend to limit the amount of analgesia they give to their patients. Embedded in his scientific writing is a sense of the humanity of the patients and the deep sympathy of the writer. He taught staff to empathize with patients, rather than over-identify or become too detached, as many tended to do. Over the years he joined with other pain specialists in a persistent effort to address the problem of undermedication of pain through research, education, and persuasion. As a result, thousands of people around the world have suffered less pain because of his pioneering research and writing.

Sam was one of the first mental health professionals to be caught up in the plague of our times, AIDS. By 1985 he was already engaged in funded research on psychological responses to HIV antibody testing. An early and significant contribution of his research was the finding that, despite fears to the contrary, most people were able to handle the news of HIV seropositivity with relative competence after brief systematic counseling and that such news did not lead to elevated levels of significant distress or psychiatric disorders in the following months. He studied and wrote extensively about neuropsychiatric effects of HIV infection, and continually emphasized the fact that most people with HIV illness do surprisingly well emotionally. A major issue to which he made significant contributions is the question of whether stress and depression hasten progression of HIV illness. He found no evidence of such psychoimmune effects, which is somewhat jarring in terms of the general societal conviction that stress is bad for your health. Not only did he publish this research in the ARCHIVES (1992;49:396-401), but he and one of us (B.F.) wrote an influential editorial in *JAMA* (1993;270:2609-2610) to this effect. On the day he died, a letter he wrote on this topic (coauthored by the other of us, J.R.) appeared in the ARCHIVES (1994;51:247), pursuing this matter. He continued to emphasize that, despite the innate appeal of the notion that stress and depression are unhealthy, the field of psychoimmunology and HIV illness has so far not produced any evidence to this effect. On the other hand, he always emphasized that depression in patients with HIV infection is a disorder that can and must be treated, rather than a common, "normal" reaction.

Sam was respected, he was loved, and he is missed by all who knew him and worked with him. He was a scholar, a role model for students, a kind and skilled clinician with patients, and a dearly valued friend. Those who knew him considered themselves fortunate for this opportunity.

Judith Rabkin, PhD
College of Physicians and Surgeons
Columbia University
722 W 168th St
New York, NY 10032
Baruch Fishman, MD
New York, NY

Eli Robins, MD
February 22, 1921, to December 21, 1994

Eli Robins, MD, professor of psychiatry, and from 1963 to 1975 head of the department, died on December 21, 1994, of multiple sclerosis. He was born in Houston, Tex, on February 22, 1921, and was raised in the small town of Rosenberg, Tex. His parents had come to this country from Russia. Eli's exceptional intellect and energy were evident early. He received his bachelor's degree from Rice University in Houston at age 19 years and his medical degree from Harvard University at age 22 years. He was trained in both psychiatry and neurology in Boston, at the Massachusetts General Hospital, the McLean Hospital, and Pratt Diagnostic Hospital. He left a scientific legacy unmatched in psychiatry. He was a pivotal player in establishing American psychiatry as a scientific discipline.

He had said that from early in his career it was his aim to find the open sesame that would bring to light the hidden connections between brain dysfunctions and psychiatric illnesses. He recognized that before that was possible there was need for a reliable classification system in psychiatry, a field dominated at the time by untestable theories in which diagnostic classification was not taken seriously. Eli's first published clinical research, with Mandel Cohen, MD, at Harvard University in 1951, delineated the criteria for the diagnosis of hysteria. These criteria have stood the test of time for four decades, their predictive validity confirmed in follow-up studies. From that beginning, Eli built a body of literature based on descriptive, follow-up, and family studies that encompassed all psychopathological conditions then amenable to systematic classification. This work, in which Lee Robins, PhD, Samuel Guze, MD, and George Winokur, MD, were his chief collaborators, culminated in the diagnostic system in current worldwide use in psychiatry. It is taken for granted today that explicit diagnostic criteria for psychiatric disorders, validated by follow-up and family studies, must be employed if clinical, epidemiological, and pathophysiological studies of psychiatric illnesses are to be sound. This has become part of the scientific foundation of the field, largely because of work done at Washington University, St Louis, Mo, of which Eli was the chief architect. It is an enduring monument to him.

Early in his career, Eli recognized that the ultimate key to understanding psychiatric disorders lay at the cellular level, to be found through chemical, physiological, and anatomic studies of the central nervous system. He sought out a position at Washington University in 1949 because the head of the department of psychiatry, Edwin Gildea, MD, had established a reputation for studying biological correlates of mental diseases. He started as a fellow in the laboratory of Oliver Lowry, MD, PhD, learning the then-new microtechniques for the study of brain chemistry. He continued biological as well as clinical research throughout his career. His interests stayed in the forefront of the field, with his most recent involvement in positron emission tomography scanning as an avenue to understanding the bridge between brain function and the symptoms of psychiatric disorders. Early on, he conducted biochemical studies of the brains of people who had committed suicide. That work fit in appropriately with his pioneering clinical studies on suicide, another area where his writings have been of lasting significance. He initiated the retrospective psychobiological reconstruction in suicide, the so-called psychological autopsy, that moved the field from speculation to replicable data. The schedule-driven interview he devised for that inquiry proved to be the forerunner of the diagnostic and sociobiological interview schedules now in wide use in psychiatry and epidemiology.

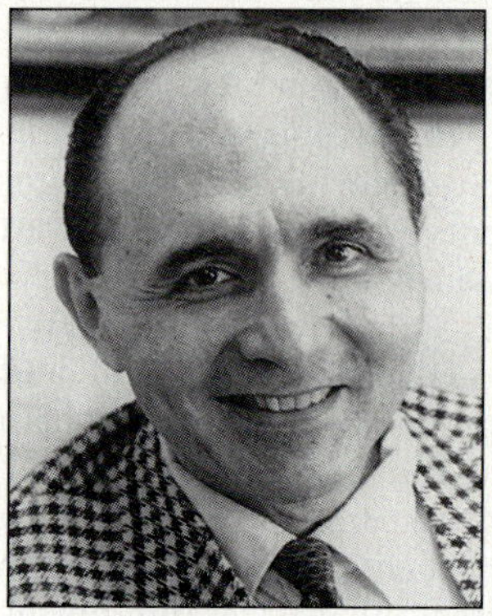

Eli Robins, MD

Eli was an exceptional teacher. He had a breadth of knowledge and interests that encompassed the arts as well as sciences beyond his own field. He was gifted in his ability to see to the essentials of clinical and laboratory problems, to not be distracted by red herrings. He was skeptical of any theoretical claims unless evidence supported them, and he was an articulate enemy of nonsense. The many scores of us who were fortunate enough to be his students and junior colleagues found him amazingly accessible, consistently kind and helpful in his criticism of our research and writing, and possessed of warm humor and mellow wisdom even during the worst of times for him. We owe him so much for nurturing our careers and caring about how we turned out, as well as about the quality of our work. He inspired a special affection in us all.

Eli had the first symptoms of multiple sclerosis in 1961, 2 years before he became head of the psychiatry department. It was a cruel irony that this particular disease afflicted a man whose very essence was rapid mobility of mind and body. Early in the course of the illness, before it was diagnosed with certainty, he was advised to rest and was taking medications that sedated him. He stayed home for several months then, carrying out his duties there. That approach did not help; so for the next 30 years, until shortly before his death, he went to his office every day. His teaching, research, departmental leadership, all the works for which he received international recognition and honors, were carried out under the cloud of multiple sclerosis. In his last years as he became more infirm, he continued to accept with stubborn grace the necessary ministrations of his caregivers. He simply never gave up, though one by one the things he loved to do were taken from him by the illness. He maintained his humor and sweetness of manner throughout. Eli was especially skeptical of hyperbole, even more so if it was applied to him, so he never thought of himself as a hero. But he certainly was.

Richard W. Hudgens, MD
George E. Murphy, MD
Washington University School of Medicine
4940 Children's Pl
St Louis, MO 63110

James W. Maas, MD
October 26, 1929, to January 14, 1995

JAMES W. MAAS, MD, was described in *Science* in 1981 as one of the "founding fathers" of a new field of psychiatric chemistry. He was honored later for his studies of biogenic amine metabolism in depressed patients and for being one of the first to exploit the measuring of 3-methoxy-4-hydroxyphenylglycol (MHPG) concentration in body fluids to provide a biochemical index of norepinephrine metabolism in the brain. He was best known for applying these techniques to studies of depression and anxiety. But he will be remembered as much for his style, the uncommon capacity to move back and forth between animal and human research. He had a unique blend of talents and skills. A trained psychoanalyst and a first-rate biochemist, he was that rare scientist in our field who could bring the approach and findings of basic research to the clinical investigation of the "whole" patient.

Jim Maas graduated from the Washington University School of Medicine, St Louis, Mo, in 1954 and completed his psychiatric residency at the Cincinnati General Hospital. From 1960 to 1966 he was at the National Institute of Mental Health (NIMH) as Chief of the Section on Psychosomatic Medicine and from 1963 to 1964, as Acting Chief of the Adult Psychiatry Branch. In 1966 he was a fellow at the Institute of Animal Physiology in Cambridge, England. Later that year he became the director of research at the Illinois State Psychiatric Institute and professor at the University of Illinois Medical School. In 1972 he joined Yale University as professor of psychiatry where he remained until 1982. He later accepted the post of Professor of Psychiatry and Pharmacology at the University of Texas Health Sciences Center at San Antonio. In 1986 he was appointed to the Hugo A. Auler Professorship, which was his post when he died on January 14, 1995.

Jim Maas began research on the neurochemistry of mental disorders at the NIMH in 1960. His studies of the neurochemical differences between two strains of mice and their relationships to behavior were published in *Science* and *Nature*. During this period he began a lifelong interest in the relationship of norepinephrine to the emotions and to depressive illness by refining new techniques for assaying the kinetics of norepinephrine metabolism in the central nervous system. He was the first to conclusively demonstrate that a significant proportion of plasma MHPG is derived from brain in human subjects. Moving forward, he and other investigators began measuring the concentrations of certain neurotransmitters and their metabolites in urine, blood, and cerebrospinal fluid in depressed patients. The information would later assist in the diagnosis of mental disease, the prediction of response to antidepressants, and the monitoring of the proper medication for therapy.

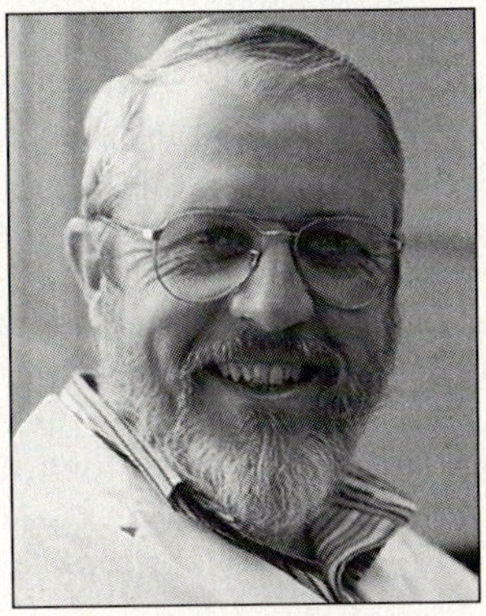

James W. Maas, MD

This research heralded a new era of biological psychiatry. The face of psychiatric science was changed in the 1950s by the discovery of new effective chemical treatments for the mental disorders and the pioneering research on the metabolism of catecholamines in the brain. Psychiatric investigators now needed to be expert in a biological science and in the phenomena of mental disorders. Jim Maas was one of a few young investigators who helped establish a sound scientific base for the new discipline.

Jim spent much of his future career trying to bridge basic research and clinical practice. He was a prime mover in the NIMH Collaborative Study of the Psychobiology of Depression initiated in 1971. Earlier hypotheses about the neurochemical bases of depression were derived from limited studies conducted in clinical settings. The Collaborative Study would definitively test these early hypotheses by using the most advanced biochemical technology, examining two or more biological systems concurrently, and assembling a sufficiently large and diverse sample of reliably diagnosed depressed patients. This unprecedented collaborative experiment to test basic hypotheses helped to clarify the strengths and limitations of current thinking about the biochemical bases of depression. One of the major findings was a clarification of the differences in the biochemical predictors of response to tricyclic antidepressants in patients with unipolar and bipolar illness. It provided further evidence that the biochemical disturbance underlying depression in these two subtypes was different. It enabled the field to move beyond oversimplified hypotheses of "too much or too little" of a neurotransmitter. The Program was directly responsible for the development of a scientific approach to diagnosis and laid the foundation for the modern *DSM*.

As the chairman of the biological study, Jim was the intellectual "force" that kept the group united and focused. He was dedicated to determining the validity of these earlier hypotheses so that the field could be freed up to proceed in new directions.

In Texas in 1982, Jim started a new phase of studies on the psychobiology of schizophrenia. These studies contributed to assessing the role of dopamine and its relationship to atrophic brain change. They also confirmed our conclusion from the Collaborative Study that to link biological factors and psychopathology it was more effective to work directly with the components of pathology than with the entity of schizophrenia itself.

Jim published some 200 scientific papers. In 1973 he was honored by the Anna-Monika Stiftung for his work on the "neurobiological bases of depressive illness" and in 1994, toward the end of his career, for his "breadth and excellence" in psychiatry, by the Texas Society of Psychiatric Physicians.

In an editorial in *Biological Psychiatry* in 1993 he expressed his frustration about the fact that more than 30 years after the discovery of the drugs, the field had still not established a reliable biological marker for any of the mental disorders. In a 1994 article in *Neuropsychopharmacology*, he and I concluded that the research model followed in these studies of biochemical causation and mechanisms of drug action was probably wrong. We drew on what was learned from the Collaborative Program and proposed a new model. He took pride in the fact that we could suggest a new path, not simply criticize the old.

Those of us who knew Jim were also inspired by his other lives. On the day of his death he was returning from a visit to his ranch in San Antonio. At the age of 50 years, he left a Yale professorship to pursue cattle ranching in Montana. It was only a moderate success but it brought him tremendous pleasure to have followed that lifetime dream. Jim was a sportsman and hunter, which made his 1987 stroke that much more devastating. He was not expected to survive. When I visited him in the hospital, Jim brushed away the small talk and insisted on discussing strategy for our next grant proposal. On his recovery he would not remember that conversation. To all who were close to him, that incident reflected his characteristic tenacity, a battling spirit that infused his and our lives. Following the stroke that left him partially paralyzed, Jim went on in 1992 to win an NIMH research grant enabling him to continue his studies of schizophrenia.

Jim Maas, with characteristic modesty, once described himself to a colleague as simply a "worker in the vineyard." Those of us who were privileged to know him, his colleagues at NIMH, at Illinois, at Yale, at Texas, and in the Collaborative Group, remember him more as one of the overseers, a "force" who helped guide psychiatric research through its most creative and productive era. His students and friends will continue that work.

He is survived by his wife Marilyn, his daughter Elizabeth, and his sons, Jimmy and Jonathan.

Martin M. Katz, PhD
Department of Psychiatry
Albert Einstein College of Medicine–Montefiore Medical Center
New York, NY

I would like to thank Malcolm Bowers, MD, Peter Stokes, MD, Robert Roth, MD, Gene Redmond, MD, Stephen Koslow, PhD, Rosalyn Barclay, PhD, Nancie Katz, and Marilyn Maas, PhD, for their contributions to this article.

MANUSCRIPT CRITERIA AND INFORMATION

Submit manuscripts to Jack D. Barchas, MD, Editor, *Archives of General Psychiatry,* Cornell Medical Center, Dept of Psychiatry, Box 171, 525 E 68th St, Room F2315, New York, NY 10021. Manuscripts are received with the understanding that they are not under simultaneous consideration by another publication, have not been published previously, and have the approval of each author. Accepted manuscripts become the permanent property of the ARCHIVES. They may not be republished without permission from the publisher (AMA).

Editing. Copyediting follows AMA style and requires corresponding author approval. The authors are responsible for all statements made in their work, including changes made by the copy editor and authorized by the corresponding author.

Reprints. Forms for ordering are included with the edited typescript sent for approval. Reprints are shipped 6 to 8 weeks after publication.

Cover Letter

- In the cover letter, designate one author as correspondent and provide a complete address and telephone and fax numbers.
- For a manuscript to be reviewed, considered, or edited, the following statement must be signed by *all* authors:

"I have been sufficiently involved in this work to take public responsibility for its validity and final presentation as an original publication. I can and will provide documentation of my work upon reasonable request and I have fulfilled the obligations for full disclosure and authorship as described by *Archives of General Psychiatry*. . . ." This signed statement must conclude with *one* of the two following sentences: "Accordingly, I hereby transfer, assign, or otherwise convey all copyright ownership to the AMA in the event such work is published by the AMA." [OR] "No copyright ownership can be transferred since this work was produced in the course of my official duties as a US government officer or employee."

Manuscript Preparation[1,2]

- Submit an original double-spaced typescript and 7 copies.
- **Manuscripts will not be returned after the review process.** Unpublished manuscripts will be destroyed.
- Type—double-spaced throughout (including references)—on one side only of 8½ × 11-in white bond paper. Number all pages. Do not justify right-hand margins. Use a printer of at least letter quality.
- The length of the text of the manuscript (not including abstract, tables, figures, or references) should be under 5000 words. Include a word count of the text on the title page.
- Titles should be short, specific, and descriptive, emphasizing the main point of the article. Avoid a two-part title, if at all possible. Do not number the title, eg, I or Part I. Title length, including punctuation and spaces, ideally should be under 100 characters and must not exceed 200 characters.
- The title page should list full names, degrees, academic affiliations and their locations, and the name and address to whom reprint requests should be sent. If the paper was presented at a meeting, include the organization, place, and date of presentation. Acknowledgment of grant or drug company support should also be made on this page.
- Include a structured abstract of 250 words or less that states the Background, Methods, Results, and Conclusions in four sections labeled as such.
- Use Système International (SI) measurements throughout the manuscript.
- Use generic names of drugs, unless the specific trade name is directly relevant to the study design or discussion.
- Do not use abbreviations in the title or abstract. Limit their use in the text.
- *Do not use footnotes or appendixes.* Such materials should either be incorporated into the text or offered to interested readers on request.
- Include a statistical analysis section under *Methods* that fully describes the application of each statistical procedure used. If a test is used that is not commonly presented in the ARCHIVES, briefly describe its purpose and how it is to be interpreted. Results should report the test statistic (eg, χ^2, F or *t* value), degrees of freedom, and *P* value. Measures of central tendency (eg, means) should be accompanied by measures of variability (eg, standard deviations). In the cover letter, state the name of your statistical consultant, if appropriate.
- Acknowledge fully any material taken from other publications, and submit written permission from the owner to reprint in any language or form without limitation.
- Tables and figures should provide substantive data and not merely illustrate the text. While the main finding of a table or figure may be discussed in the narrative, the table or figure should not duplicate the text. Although no specific guideline can be applied to all articles, the number and length of tables and figures should be kept to a minimum.

Tables. Double-space on separate sheets of 8½ × 11-in white bond paper. Title each one and number them in the order of their citation in the text. If a table must be continued, repeat the title on a second sheet, followed by "(cont)." Any explanatory notes to be printed with the table must be typed single-spaced beneath the table.

Figures. Once manuscripts are accepted, two sets of professionally prepared, high-resolution color transparencies are required for all color figures. For black and white art, two sets of professionally prepared glossy prints are required. If color figures are necessary, the ARCHIVES may pay part of the expense with the balance to be borne by the author.

- Number figures according to their order in the text. Type the figure number, proper orientation (eg, top), name of the senior author, and an abbreviated title on a gummed label; affix it to the back of the print.
- Double-space legends (maximum length, 40 words) on a separate sheet of 8½ × 11-in paper.

References. References should be carefully selected to acknowledge previous work or to document a specific point. They should not be exhaustive. Number references in the order they are mentioned in the text; do *not* alphabetize. In text, tables, and legends, identify references with superscript arabic numbers. Double-space, follow AMA style and abbreviate names of journals according to *Index Medicus*. List all authors and/or editors. Citation accuracy is the responsibility of the author.

Examples:

1. DuBois RN, Lazenby AJ, Yardley JH, Hendrix TR, Bayless TM, Giardiello FM. Lymphocytic enterocolitis in patients with 'refractory sprue.' *JAMA*. 1989;262:935-937.

2. Ritchie JM, Greene NM. Local anesthetics. In: Gilman AG, Goodman LS, Rall TW, Murad F, eds. *The Pharmacological Basis of Therapeutics*. 7th ed. New York, NY: Macmillan Publishing Co Inc; 1985:309-310.

Informed Consent and Confidentiality. A statement of informed consent for human investigation should be made. Authors must ensure that patient confidentiality is in no way breached. Do not use real names, initials, or disclose information that might identify a particular subject.

Obligations for Full Disclosure and Authorship[3,4]

Previous Publications. Manuscripts that are submitted must not have been previously published in *whole* or *substantial part* and must not be simultaneously under consideration elsewhere. This policy applies to the essential contents, tables, or figures, but does not apply to abstracts. Authors must disclose in their cover letters if the submitted manuscript contains any data or material that have already been published or are in press, submitted, or nearly submitted. Copies of closely related manuscripts should be submitted to the Editor for examination.

Financial Disclosure. At the time of initial submission, each author should disclose any financial arrangement he or she has with companies who either have products featured in the manuscript or with companies that produce competing products. These arrangements include, but are not limited to, company support, consultantships, patent rights, stock ownership, or other equity interests. Such arrangements do not constitute grounds for automatic rejection of the manuscript. Financial information will be held in confidence. If the manuscript is accepted for publication, the Editor and the author(s) will confer about the way this information will be communicated to the readers. Reviewers are also expected to notify the Editor of their own financial arrangements involving companies whose products (or competing products) are featured in the manuscripts they agree to review.

Other Disclosures. Authors should disclose to the Editor at the time of submission any special circumstances, vested interests, or sources of bias that might affect the integrity of the reported information. These disclosures also apply to referees.

Authorship does not require expertise in every aspect of the work. It does mean that each author within his or her own limits has exerted sufficient reasonable effort to vouch for the validity of the entire work and to bear public accountability for maintaining the integrity of the scientific information communicated. Each author must have had enough substantial involvement in generating and formulating the published product to bear such accountability. More than six authors requires a statement of justification in the cover letter.

Letters to the Editor

Letters to the Editor will be considered for publication if they are accompanied by a cover letter stating they are "for publication." Their purpose should be to comment on articles published in the ARCHIVES or to provide significant news that can be conveyed in a short format. The Editor reserves the right to edit the material prior to publication.

Letters intended for publication *must* follow manuscript preparation guidelines (eg, double-spaced, copyright transfer). They generally should not exceed 750 words. Include 3 copies. Illustrative material is not usually accepted; brief tables may occasionally be considered. Authors will receive only a brief acknowledgment of acceptance or rejection.

Review Process

A submitted manuscript will be acknowledged by postcard and assigned a manuscript number, which is to be used in all further correspondence. Manuscripts are reviewed and given a priority based upon their originality, scientific merit, appropriateness of statistical analyses, importance of their findings, significance for the field, lucidity, interest to readers, suitability for publication, and the journal's current portfolio. All reviewers remain anonymous and are expected to maintain the curtain of strict confidentiality. After the review process has been completed, authors will be informed by mail of the Editor's decision.

References

1. Iverson CL, Dan BB, Glitman P, et al. *American Medical Association Manual of Style*. 8th ed. Baltimore, Md: Williams & Wilkins; 1988.

2. International Committee of Medical Journal Editors. Uniform requirements for manuscripts submitted to biomedical journals. *Ann Intern Med*. 1988;108:258-265.

3. Freedman DX. The meaning of full disclosure. *Arch Gen Psychiatry*. 1988;45:689-691.

4. Freedman DX. Megamultiple authorship. *Arch Gen Psychiatry*. 1982;39:351.

Checklist

____ (1) Cover letter including all information deemed necessary for the editor's review.

____ (2) Statement on copyright and authorial responsibility, signed by *all* authors.

____ (3) Corresponding author identified and address and telephone and fax numbers provided.

____ (4) Original manuscript (including structured abstract, references, legends, tables, and figures) plus 7 copies.

____ (5) Word count of text only (not including abstract, tables, references) on the title page.

____ (6) Right-hand margin unjustified.

____ (7) Copies of publications considered to be helpful for the review process or that bear on any possible overlap of published data.

ARCHIVES
OF
GENERAL PSYCHIATRY

Index to

Volume 52

January through December 1995

Editor
Jack D. Barchas, MD
New York, NY

Assistant to Editor
Peter M. Marzuk, MD
New York, NY

Editorial Administrator
Angela McGregor
New York, NY

In this index in alphabetical order are listed names of authors of all articles and letters. Full citation is given under first author only; reference is made from joint authors. Names which begin with a prefix are entered under the prefix. The month is given as a two-letter notation in parentheses.

A

Abnormalities
Developmental brain abnormalities in schizophrenia: contributions of genetic and perinatal factors (letter) [Vita] (reply) [Cannon] 157 (Fe)
Magnetic resonance imaging and mood disorders: localization of white matter and other subcortical abnormalities [Dupont] 747 (Se)
Prefrontal cortex and schizophrenia: a quantitative magnetic resonance imaging study [Wible] 279 (Ap)
Activities of Daily Living
Functioning and well-being outcomes of patients with depression compared with chronic general medical illnesses [Hays] 11 (Ja)
Adaptation, Psychological
Role-relationship models for case formulation [Horowitz] 625 (Au)
Adenosine Diphosphate
Low levels of pertussis toxin adenosine diphosphate ribosylation in the schizophrenic brain (letter) [Okada] 319 (Ap)
Adenosine Diphosphate Ribose
Guanine nucleotide-binding proteins in bipolar affective disorder: effects of long-term lithium treatment [Manji] 135 (Fe)
Adolescence
Child and adolescent mental disorders and the search for an NIMH director: quo vadis? [Barchas] 873 (Oc)
Child and adolescent mental disorders research: current directions, future needs [Rosenfeld] 729 (Se)
Comments on the report card from a services research perspective [Kruesi] 727 (Se)
Genetic questions for environmental studies: differential parenting and psychopathology in adolescence [Reiss] 925 (No)
Grading the progress of child and adolescent mental health research: NIMH perspectives [Cowdry] 732 (Se)
Report card on the *National Plan for Research on Child and Adolescent Mental Disorders:* the midway point [Members of the Committee for the Study of Research on Child and Adolescent Mental Disorders] 715 (Se); correction, 1072 (De)
Report card: progress report or final grade? [Carlson] 724 (Se)
Adoption
Adoption study demonstrating two genetic pathways to drug abuse [Cadoret] 42 (Ja)
Genetic-environmental interaction in the genesis of aggressivity and conduct disorders [Cadoret] 916 (No)
Adrenal Glands
Adrenal gland volume in major depression: increase during the depressive episode and decrease with successful treatment [Rubin] 213 (Mr)
Adrenergic Antagonists
Biochemical effects of antidepressant augmentation (letter) [Howland] 156 (Fe)
Adrenocorticotropic Hormone
Adrenal gland volume in major depression: increase during the depressive episode and decrease with successful treatment [Rubin] 213 (Mr)
Depression in patients with cancer: diagnosis, biology, and treatment [McDaniel] 89 (Fe)
Effects of the menstrual cycle on dependent variables in mood disorder research [Leibenluft] 51:761 (Oc); correction, 52:144 (Fe)
Adult
Double-blind, crossover comparison of methylphenidate and placebo in adults with childhood-onset attention-deficit hyperactivity disorder [Spencer] 434 (Je)
Failure of naltrexone hydrochloride to reduce self-injurious and autistic behavior in mentally retarded adults: double-blind placebo-controlled studies [Willemsen-Swinkels] 766 (Se)
Affect
Chaos and complexity: can it help us to understand mood and behavior? [Ehlers] 960 (No)
Evidence of chaotic mood variation in bipolar disorder [Gottschalk] 947 (No)
Pharmacotherapy of impaired affect in recovering schizophrenic patients [Hogarty] 29 (Ja)
Premenstrual dysphoric disorder and response to cholecystokinin-tetrapeptide (letter) [Le Melledo] 605 (Jy)
Structure and course of positive and negative symptoms in schizophrenia [Eaton] 127 (Fe)
Affective Disorders
Effects of the menstrual cycle on dependent variables in mood disorder research [Leibenluft] 51:761 (Oc); correction, 52:144 (Fe)
Family study of early-onset dysthymia: mood and personality disorders in relatives of outpatients with dysthymia and episodic major depression and normal controls [Klein] 487 (Je)
Family study of manic-depressive (bipolar I) disease: is it a distinct illness separable from primary unipolar depression? [Winokur] 367 (My)
Guanine nucleotide-binding proteins in bipolar affective disorder: effects of long-term lithium treatment [Manji] 135 (Fe)
In quest of identifying vulnerability markers for psychiatric disorders by all-night polysomnography [Lauer] 145 (Fe)
Magnetic resonance imaging and mood disorders: localization of white matter and other subcortical abnormalities [Dupont] 747 (Se)
Meta-analyses of studies of ventricular enlargement and cortical sulcal prominence in mood disorders: comparisons with controls or patients with schizophrenia [Elkis] 735 (Se)
New York High-Risk Project: psychoses and cluster A personality disorders in offspring of schizophrenic parents at 23 years of follow-up [Erlenmeyer-Kimling] 857 (Oc)
Premenstrual dysphoric disorders, anxiety, and depressions: vulnerability traits or comorbidity (letter) [Halbreich] 606 (Jy)
Schizotypal symptoms and signs in the Roscommon Family Study: their factor structure and familial relationship with psychotic and affective disorders [Kendler] 296 (Ap)
Suicidal behaviors and the tryptophan hydroxylase gene [Abbar] 846 (Oc)
Switching from 'unipolar' to bipolar II: an 11-year prospective study of clinical and temperamental predictors in 559 patients [Akiskal] 114 (Fe)
Tryptophan depletion in stable lithium-treated patients with bipolar disorder in remission (letter) [Benkelfat] 154 (reply) [Delgado] 155 (Fe)
Affective Psychosis, Bipolar see Bipolar Disorder
Age Factors
Prevalence and correlates of drug use and dependence in the United States: results from the National Comorbidity Survey [Warner] 219 (Mr)
Age of Onset
Double-blind, crossover comparison of methylphenidate and placebo in adults with childhood-onset attention-deficit hyperactivity disorder [Spencer] 434 (Je)
Mitogen-stimulated interleukin-2 production in never-medicated, first-episode schizophrenic patients: the influence of age at onset and negative symptoms [Ganguli] 668 (Au)
Aged
Duration of neuroleptic treatment and prevalence of tardive dyskinesia in late life [Sweet] 478 (Je)
Prevalence of dementia and depression in the elderly community in a southern European population: the Zaragoza study [Lobo] 497 (Je)
Quality of care for depressed elderly patients hospitalized in the specialty psychiatric units or general medical wards [Norquist] 695 (Au)
Risk of tardive dyskinesia in older patients: a prospective longitudinal study of 266 outpatients [Jeste] 756 (Se)
Aggression
Efficacy of methylphenidate for attention-deficit hyperactivity disorder in children with tic disorder [Gadow] 444 (Je); correction, 836 (Oc)
Genetic-environmental interaction in the genesis of aggressivity and conduct disorders [Cadoret] 916 (No)
Report card: progress report or final grade? [Carlson] 724 (Se)
Aging
Effects of Alzheimer's disease and normal aging on cerebrospinal fluid norepinephrine responses to yohimbine and clonidine [Peskind] 774 (Se)
Increased rate of P300 latency prolongation with age in schizophrenia: electrophysiological evidence for a neurodegenerative process [O'Donnell] 544 (Jy)
Agoraphobia
Is the comorbidity between social phobia and panic disorder due to familial cotransmission or other factors? [Horwath] 574 (Jy)
Specificity in familial aggregation of phobic disorders [Fyer] 564 (Jy)
Agranulocytosis
Clozapine-induced increase in plasma levels of soluble interleukin-2 receptors (letter) [Pollmächer] 877 (reply) [Ganguli] 878 (Oc)
Akathisia see Psychomotor Agitation
Alcohol Abuse see Alcoholism
Alcoholism
Adoption study demonstrating two genetic pathways to drug abuse [Cadoret] 42 (Ja)
Generalized social phobia: reliability and validity [Mannuzza] 230 (Mr)
Mental illness and suicide: a case-control study in east Taiwan [Cheng] 594 (Jy)
Risk of tardive dyskinesia in older patients: a prospective longitudinal study of 266 outpatients [Jeste] 756 (Se)
Structure of the genetic and environmental risk factors for six major psychiatric disorders in women: phobia, generalized anxiety disorder, panic disorder, bulimia, major depression, and alcoholism [Kendler] 374 (My)
Alzheimer's Disease
Effects of Alzheimer's disease and normal aging on cerebrospinal fluid norepinephrine responses to yohimbine and clonidine [Peskind] 774 (Se)
Prevalence of dementia and depression in the elderly community in a southern European population: the Zaragoza study [Lobo] 497 (Je)
Risk of Alzheimer's disease in first-degree relatives (letter) [Heun] 317 (reply) [Silverman] 318 (Ap)
Amino Acids
Abnormal excitatory neurotransmitter metabolism in schizophrenic brains [Tsai] 829 (Oc)
Seasonal variation in plasma L-tryptophan availability in healthy volunteers: relationships to violent suicide occurrence [Maes] 937 (No)
Anorexia Nervosa
Prospective study of outcome in bulimia nervosa and the long-term effects of three psychological treatments [Fairburn] 304 (Ap)
Anticholinergic Agents see Parasympatholytics
Antidepressants, Tricyclic see Antidepressive Agents, Tricyclic
Antidepressive Agents
Pharmacotherapy of impaired affect in recovering schizophrenic patients [Hogarty] 29 (Ja)
Pindolol, 5-hydroxytryptamine, and antidepressant augmentation (letter) [Artigas] 969 (No)
Switching from 'unipolar' to bipolar II: an 11-year prospective study of clinical and temperamental predictors in 559 patients [Akiskal] 114 (Fe)
Tryptophan depletion in stable lithium-treated patients with bipolar disorder in remission (letter) [Benkelfat] 154 (reply) [Delgado] 155 (Fe)
Antidepressive Agents, Tricyclic
Interactions of serotonin reuptake inhibitors with tricyclic antidepressants (letter) [Harvey] 783 (reply) [Popli] 784 (Se)
Antipsychotic Agents
Clozapine-associated postoperative ileus: case report and review of the literature (letter) [Erickson] 508 (Je)
Clozapine-induced increase in plasma levels of soluble interleukin-2 receptors (letter) [Pollmächer] 877 (reply) [Ganguli] 878 (Oc)
Complicating factors in the analysis of acute drug-induced akathisia (letter) [Rosebush] 878 (reply) [Sachdev] 879 (Oc)
Considering neuroleptic maintenance and taper on a continuum: need for individual rather than dogmatic approach [Jeste] 209 (Mr)
Conversions from clozapine to other antipsychotic drugs (letter) [Baldessarini] 1071 (De)
Duration of neuroleptic treatment and prevalence of tardive dyskinesia in late life [Sweet] 478 (Je)
Early course of schizophrenia and long-term maintenance neuroleptic therapy [Nuechterlein] 203 (Mr)
In reply [Akbarian] 277 (Ap)
Mitogen-stimulated interleukin-2 production in never-medicated, first-episode schizophrenic patients: the influence of age at onset and negative symptoms [Ganguli] 668 (Au)
Neuroleptic withdrawal in schizophrenic patients [Baldessarini] 189 (Mr)
Neuroleptic withdrawal in schizophrenic patients: a review of the literature [Gilbert] 173 (Mr)
Neuroleptic withdrawal in schizophrenic patients: an idea whose time has come [Meltzer] 200 (Mr)
Pharmacotherapy of impaired affect in recovering schizophrenic patients [Hogarty] 29 (Ja)
Risk of tardive dyskinesia in older patients: a prospective longitudinal study of 266 outpatients [Jeste] 756 (Se)

Risks of withdrawing antipsychotic medications [Wyatt] 205 (Mr)
Why neuroleptic withdrawal in schizophrenia? [Carpenter] 192 (Mr)

Antisocial Personality Disorder
Adoption study demonstrating two genetic pathways to drug abuse [Cadoret] 42 (Ja)
Antisocial behavior [Gershon] 900 (No)
Differential heritability of adult and juvenile antisocial traits [Lyons] 906 (No)
Genetic-environmental interaction in the genesis of aggressivity and conduct disorders [Cadoret] 916 (No)

Anxiety
Behavioral vs biochemical prediction of clinical stability following haloperidol withdrawal in schizophrenia [van Kammen] 673 (Au)
Double-blind, crossover comparison of methylphenidate and placebo in adults with childhood-onset attention-deficit hyperactivity disorder [Spencer] 434 (Je)
Is hyperarousal essential to obsessive-compulsive disorder? diminished physiologic flexibility, but not hyperarousal, characterizes patients with obsessive-compulsive disorder [Hoehn-Saric] 688 (Au)
Positron emission tomographic study of simple phobic symptom provocation [Rauch] 20 (Ja)
Premenstrual dysphoric disorder and response to cholecystokinin-tetrapeptide (letter) [Le Melledo] 605 (Jy)
Premenstrual dysphoric disorders, anxiety, and depressions: vulnerability traits or comorbidity (letter) [Halbreich] 606 (Jy)

Anxiety Disorders
Specificity in familial aggregation of phobic disorders [Fyer] 564 (Jy)
Structure of the genetic and environmental risk factors for six major psychiatric disorders in women: phobia, generalized anxiety disorder, panic disorder, bulimia, major depression, and alcoholism [Kendler] 374 (My)

ARCHIVES OF GENERAL PSYCHIATRY
Reviewers for 1995 [Abdul-Jalil] 990 (De)
Some thoughts about the *Archives* [Barchas] 313 (Ap)

Arousal
Is hyperarousal essential to obsessive-compulsive disorder? diminished physiologic flexibility, but not hyperarousal, characterizes patients with obsessive-compulsive disorder [Hoehn-Saric] 688 (Au)

Attention
Role of methylphenidate in psychiatry [Klein] 429 (Je)
Structure and course of positive and negative symptoms in schizophrenia [Eaton] 127 (Fe)
Symptoms of schizophrenia: methods, meanings, and mechanisms [Andreasen] 341 (My)

Attention Deficit Disorder With Hyperactivity
Double-blind, crossover comparison of methylphenidate and placebo in adults with childhood-onset attention-deficit hyperactivity disorder [Spencer] 434 (Je)
Efficacy of methylphenidate for attention-deficit hyperactivity disorder in children with tic disorder [Gadow] 444 (Je); correction, 836 (Oc)
Family-environment risk factors for attention-deficit hyperactivity disorder: a test of Rutter's indicators of adversity [Biederman] 464 (Je)
Role of methylphenidate in psychiatry [Klein] 429 (Je)

Attention Deficit Hyperactivity Disorder see Attention Deficit Disorder with Hyperactivity

Autism
Failure of naltrexone hydrochloride to reduce self-injurious and autistic behavior in mentally retarded adults: double-blind placebo-controlled studies [Willemsen-Swinkels] 766 (Se)

B

Baboons see Papio

Basal Ganglia
Reduced caudate nucleus volume in obsessive-compulsive disorder [Robinson] 393 (My)

Basal Ganglia Diseases
Neuroleptic withdrawal in schizophrenic patients: a review of the literature [Gilbert] 173 (Mr)

Behavior
Effects of Alzheimer's disease and normal aging on cerebrospinal fluid norepinephrine responses to yohimbine and clonidine [Peskind] 774 (Se)
Risks of withdrawing antipsychotic medications [Wyatt] 205 (Mr)
Role-relationship models for case formulation [Horowitz] 625 (Au)
Schizotypal symptoms and signs in the Roscommon Family Study: their factor structure and familial relationship with psychotic and affective disorders [Kendler] 296 (Ap)
Structure and course of positive and negative symptoms in schizophrenia [Eaton] 127 (Fe)
Symptoms of schizophrenia: methods, meanings, and mechanisms [Andreasen] 341 (My)

Behavior Therapy
Cingulotomy for intractable obsessive-compulsive disorder: prospective long-term follow-up of 18 patients [Baer] 384 (My)
Double-blind parallel comparison of three dosages of sertraline and placebo in outpatients with obsessive-compulsive disorder [Greist] 289 (Ap)
Prospective study of outcome in bulimia nervosa and the long-term effects of three psychological treatments [Fairburn] 304 (Ap)

Behavior Therapy, Cognitive see Cognitive Therapy

Benzodiazepines
Complicating factors in the analysis of acute drug-induced akathisia (letter) [Rosebush] 878 (reply) [Sachdev] 879 (Oc)

Benztropine
Pharmacotherapy of impaired affect in recovering schizophrenic patients [Hogarty] 29 (Ja)

Binding Proteins see Carrier Proteins

Binding Sites
Is methylphenidate like cocaine? studies on their pharmacokinetics and distribution in the human brain [Volkow] 456 (Je)

Biofeedback (Psychology)
Critical review of psychosocial interventions in cancer care [Fawzy] 100 (Fe)

Biological Markers
Depression in patients with cancer: diagnosis, biology, and treatment [McDaniel] 89 (Fe)

Biological Psychiatry
Child and adolescent mental disorders research: current directions, future needs [Rosenfeld] 729 (Se)

Bipolar Disorder
Chaos and complexity: can it help us to understand mood and behavior? [Ehlers] 960 (No)
Evidence of chaotic mood variation in bipolar disorder [Gottschalk] 947 (No)
Family study of early-onset dysthymia: mood and personality disorders in relatives of outpatients with dysthymia and episodic major depression and normal controls [Klein] 487 (Je)
Family study of manic-depressive (bipolar I) disease: is it a distinct illness separable from primary unipolar depression? [Winokur] 367 (My)
Guanine nucleotide-binding proteins in bipolar affective disorder: effects of long-term lithium treatment [Manji] 135 (Fe)
In quest of identifying vulnerability markers for psychiatric disorders by all-night polysomnography [Lauer] 145 (Fe)
In vivo D_2 dopamine receptor density in psychotic and nonpsychotic patients with bipolar disorder [Pearlson] 471 (Je)
Signal transduction pathways: molecular targets for lithium's actions [Manji] 531 (Jy)
Switching from 'unipolar' to bipolar II: an 11-year prospective study of clinical and temperamental predictors in 559 patients [Akiskal] 114 (Fe)
Tryptophan depletion in stable lithium-treated patients with bipolar disorder in remission (letter) [Benkelfat] 154 (reply) [Delgado] 155 (Fe)

Blood Platelets
Guanine nucleotide-binding proteins in bipolar affective disorder: effects of long-term lithium treatment [Manji] 135 (Fe)

Blood Pressure
Is hyperarousal essential to obsessive-compulsive disorder? diminished physiologic flexibility, but not hyperarousal, characterizes patients with obsessive-compulsive disorder [Hoehn-Saric] 688 (Au)

Body Temperature
Effects of the menstrual cycle on dependent variables in mood disorder research [Leibenluft] 51:761 (Oc); correction, 52:144 (Fe)

Brain
Abnormal excitatory neurotransmitter metabolism in schizophrenic brains [Tsai] 829 (Oc)
Developmental brain abnormalities in schizophrenia: contributions of genetic and perinatal factors (letter) [Vita] (reply) [Cannon] 157 (Fe)
Is methylphenidate like cocaine? studies on their pharmacokinetics and distribution in the human brain [Volkow] 456 (Je)
Low levels of pertussis toxin adenosine diphosphate ribosylation in the schizophrenic brain (letter) [Okada] 319 (Ap)
Prefrontal cortex and schizophrenia: a quantitative magnetic resonance imaging study [Wible] 279 (Ap)
Reduced caudate nucleus volume in obsessive-compulsive disorder [Robinson] 393 (My)

Brain Damage, Chronic
Considering neuroleptic maintenance and taper on a continuum: need for individual rather than dogmatic approach [Jeste] 209 (Mr)

Breast Feeding
Treatment of postpartum depression with interpersonal psychotherapy (letter) [Stuart] 75 (reply) [Weissman] 76 (Ja)

Breathing Exercises
Critical review of psychosocial interventions in cancer care [Fawzy] 100 (Fe)

Bulimia
Prospective study of outcome in bulimia nervosa and the long-term effects of three psychological treatments [Fairburn] 304 (Ap)
Structure of the genetic and environmental risk factors for six major psychiatric disorders in women: phobia, generalized anxiety disorder, panic disorder, bulimia, major depression, and alcoholism [Kendler] 374 (My)

Buspirone
Biochemical effects of antidepressant augmentation (letter) [Howland] 156 (Fe)

C

Calcium-Binding Proteins
Neural circuitry of the prefrontal cortex in schizophrenia [Lewis] 269 (Ap)

Carrier Proteins
Guanine nucleotide-binding proteins in bipolar affective disorder: effects of long-term lithium treatment [Manji] 135 (Fe)
In reply [Akbarian] 277 (Ap)
Low levels of pertussis toxin adenosine diphosphate ribosylation in the schizophrenic brain (letter) [Okada] 319 (Ap)

Case-Control Studies
Mental illness and suicide: a case-control study in east Taiwan [Cheng] 594 (Jy)

Catecholamines
Effects of Alzheimer's disease and normal aging on cerebrospinal fluid norepinephrine responses to yohimbine and clonidine [Peskind] 774 (Se)

Cathartics
Prospective study of outcome in bulimia nervosa and the long-term effects of three psychological treatments [Fairburn] 304 (Ap)

Cations, Monovalent
Signal transduction pathways: molecular targets for lithium's actions [Manji] 531 (Jy)

Caudate Nucleus
Reduced caudate nucleus volume in obsessive-compulsive disorder [Robinson] 393 (My)

Cell Count
Abnormally high neuronal density in the schizophrenic cortex: a morphometric analysis of prefrontal area 9 and occipital area 17 [Selemon] 805 (Oc)
Neocortical abnormalities in schizophrenia [Watson] 819 (Oc)

Cell Density see Cell Count

Cell Membrane
In vivo study of the prefrontal cortex of schizophrenic patients at different stages of illness via phosphorus magnetic resonance spectroscopy [Stanley] 399 (My); correction, 799 (Oc)

Central Nervous System
Effects of Alzheimer's disease and normal aging on cerebrospinal fluid norepinephrine responses to yohimbine and clonidine [Peskind] 774 (Se)
In pursuit of the molecular neuropathology of schizophrenia [Trojanowski] 274 (Ap)

Cerebral Cortex
Abnormally high neuronal density in the schizophrenic cortex: a morphometric analysis of prefrontal area 9 and occipital area 17 [Selemon] 805 (Oc)
Magnetic resonance imaging and mood disorders: localization of white matter and other subcortical abnormalities [Dupont] 747 (Se)
Neocortical abnormalities in schizophrenia [Watson] 819 (Oc)
Positron emission tomographic study of simple phobic symptom provocation [Rauch] 20 (Ja)

Cerebral Ventricles
Developmental brain abnormalities in schizophrenia: contributions of genetic and perinatal factors (letter) [Vita] (reply) [Cannon] 157 (Fe)
Reduced caudate nucleus volume in obsessive-compulsive disorder [Robinson] 393 (My)

Cerebrospinal Fluid
Clozapine therapy and increases in homovanillic acid (letter) [Risch] 244 (Mr)
Effects of Alzheimer's disease and normal aging on cerebrospinal fluid norepinephrine responses to yohimbine and clonidine [Peskind] 774 (Se)

Chaos Theory see Nonlinear Dynamics

Chemotherapy see Drug Therapy

Child
Child and adolescent mental disorders and the search for an NIMH director: quo vadis? [Barchas] 873 (Oc)
Child and adolescent mental disorders research: current directions, future needs [Rosenfeld] 729 (Se)
Comments on the report card from a services research perspective [Kruesi] 727 (Se)
Grading the progress of child and adolescent mental health research: NIMH perspectives [Cowdry] 732 (Se)
Report card on the *National Plan for Research on Child and Adolescent Mental Disorders:* the midway point [Members of the Committee for the Study of Research on Child and Adolescent Mental Disorders] 715 (Se); correction, 1072 (De)
Report card: progress report or final grade? [Carlson] 724 (Se)
Test-retest reliability of the Diagnostic Interview Schedule for Children (DISC 2.1): parent, child, and combined algorithms [Jensen] 61 (Ja); correction, 312 (Ap)

Child Abuse
Comments on the report card from a services research perspective [Kruesi] 727 (Se)
Child Behavior Disorders
Efficacy of methylphenidate for attention-deficit hyperactivity disorder in children with tic disorder [Gadow] 444 (Je); correction, 836 (Oc)
Genetic-environmental interaction in the genesis of aggressivity and conduct disorders [Cadoret] 916 (No)
Report card: progress report or final grade? [Carlson] 724 (Se)
Child Neglect see Child Abuse
Child of Impaired Parents
New York High-Risk Project: psychoses and cluster A personality disorders in offspring of schizophrenic parents at 23 years of follow-up [Erlenmeyer-Kimling] 857 (Oc)
Cholecystokinin-Tetrapeptide see Tetragastrin
Chronic Disease
Functioning and well-being outcomes of patients with depression compared with chronic general medical illnesses [Hays] 11 (Ja)
Ciaranello, Roland D. (1943-1994)
Roland D. Ciaranello, MD, February 27, 1943 to December 14, 1994 [Barchas] 1074 (De)
Classification
'Richly complex' but needs an emotion theory [Dahl] 649 (Au)
Clinical Trials
More reliable outcome measures can reduce sample size requirements [Leon] 867 (Oc)
Clomipramine
Cingulotomy for intractable obsessive-compulsive disorder: prospective long-term follow-up of 18 patients [Baer] 384 (My)
Double-blind parallel comparison of three dosages of sertraline and placebo in outpatients with obsessive-compulsive disorder [Greist] 289 (Ap)
Efficacy and tolerability of serotonin transport inhibitors in obsessive-compulsive disorder: a meta-analysis [Greist] 53 (Ja)
Clonidine
Effects of Alzheimer's disease and normal aging on cerebrospinal fluid norepinephrine responses to yohimbine and clonidine [Peskind] 774 (Se)
Clozapine
Clozapine therapy and increases in homovanillic acid (letter) [Risch] 244 (Mr)
Clozapine-associated postoperative ileus: case report and review of the literature (letter) [Erickson] 508 (Je)
Clozapine-induced increase in plasma levels of soluble interleukin-2 receptors (letter) [Pollmächer] 877 (reply) [Ganguli] 878 (Oc)
Conversions from clozapine to other antipsychotic drugs (letter) [Baldessarini] 1071 (De)
Neuroleptic withdrawal in schizophrenic patients: an idea whose time has come [Meltzer] 200 (Mr)
Cocaine
Is methylphenidate like cocaine? studies on their pharmacokinetics and distribution in the human brain [Volkow] 456 (Je)
Role of methylphenidate in psychiatry [Klein] 429 (Je)
Coercion
Perceived coercion in mental hospital admission: pressures and process [Lidz] 1034 (De)
Cognition Disorders
Event-related potentials in the study of psychiatric disorders [Pfefferbaum] 559 (Jy)
Family-environment risk factors for attention-deficit hyperactivity disorder: a test of Rutter's indicators of adversity [Biederman] 464 (Je)
Impaired mismatch negativity generation reflects widespread dysfunction of working memory in schizophrenia [Javitt] 550 (Jy)
Magnetic resonance imaging and mood disorders: localization of white matter and other subcortical abnormalities [Dupont] 747 (Se)
Cognitive Therapy
Are case formulations useful for outcomes research? [Clarkin] 645 (Au)
Prospective study of outcome in bulimia nervosa and the long-term effects of three psychological treatments [Fairburn] 304 (Ap)
Commitment of Mentally Ill
Perceived coercion in mental hospital admission: pressures and process [Lidz] 1034 (De)
Comorbidity
Double-blind, crossover comparison of methylphenidate and placebo in adults with childhood-onset attention-deficit hyperactivity disorder [Spencer] 434 (Je)
Generalized social phobia: reliability and validity [Mannuzza] 230 (Mr)
Health care costs of primary care patients with recognized depression [Simon] 850 (Oc)
Is the comorbidity between social phobia and panic disorder due to familial cotransmission or other factors? [Horwath] 574 (Jy)
Mental illness and suicide: a case-control study in east Taiwan [Cheng] 594 (Jy)
Posttraumatic stress disorder in the National Comorbidity Survey [Kessler] 1048 (De)
Premenstrual dysphoric disorders, anxiety, and depressions: vulnerability traits or comorbidity (letter) [Halbreich] 606 (Jy)
Trial of the effect of a standardized psychiatric consultation on health outcomes and costs in somatizing patients [Smith] 238 (Mr)
Conduct Disorders, Child see Child Behavior Disorders
Conflict (Psychology)
Personality theory: clinical practice, social development, and the biology of individual differences [Reiss] 633 (Au)
Signs of defensive control locate conflicted topics in discourse [Horowitz] 1040 (De)
Constipation
Clozapine-associated postoperative ileus: case report and review of the literature (letter) [Erickson] 508 (Je)
Controlled Clinical Trials
Efficacy and tolerability of serotonin transport inhibitors in obsessive-compulsive disorder: a meta-analysis [Greist] 53 (Ja)
CORRECTIONS
Effects of the menstrual cycle on dependent variables in mood disorder research [Leibenluft] 51:761 (Oc); correction, 52:144 (Fe)
Efficacy of methylphenidate for attention-deficit hyperactivity disorder in children with tic disorder [Gadow] 444 (Je); correction, 836 (Oc)
In vivo study of the prefrontal cortex of schizophrenic patients at different stages of illness via phosphorus magnetic resonance spectroscopy [Stanley] 399 (My); correction, 799 (Oc)
Report card on the *National Plan for Research on Child and Adolescent Mental Disorders:* the midway point [Members of the Committee for the Study of Research on Child and Adolescent Mental Disorders] 715 (Se); correction, 1072 (De)
Test-retest reliability of the Diagnostic Interview Schedule for Children (DISC 2.1): parent, child, and combined algorithms [Jensen] 61 (Ja); correction, 312 (Ap)
Corticotropin see Adrenocorticotropic Hormone
Corticotropin-Releasing Factor see Corticotropin-Releasing Hormone
Corticotropin-Releasing Hormone
Depression in patients with cancer: diagnosis, biology, and treatment [McDaniel] 89 (Fe)
Cortisol see Hydrocortisone
Cost-Benefit Analysis
Multiple-family groups and psychoeducation in the treatment of schizophrenia [McFarlane] 679 (Au)
Costs and Cost Analysis
Trial of the effect of a standardized psychiatric consultation on health outcomes and costs in somatizing patients [Smith] 238 (Mr)
Counseling
Prospective study of outcome in bulimia nervosa and the long-term effects of three psychological treatments [Fairburn] 304 (Ap)
Cytochrome P-450
Interactions of serotonin reuptake inhibitors with tricyclic antidepressants (letter) [Harvey] 783 (reply) [Popli] 784 (Se)

D

Dangerous Behavior
Chaos and complexity: can it help us to understand mood and behavior? [Ehlers] 960 (No)
Defense Mechanisms
Signs of defensive control locate conflicted topics in discourse [Horowitz] 1040 (De)
Delusions
In pursuit of the molecular neuropathology of schizophrenia [Trojanowski] 274 (Ap)
Longitudinal study of symptom dimensions in schizophrenia: prediction and patterns of change [Arndt] 352 (My)
Structure and course of positive and negative symptoms in schizophrenia [Eaton] 127 (Fe)
Symptoms of schizophrenia: methods, meanings, and mechanisms [Andreasen] 341 (My)
Dementia
Prevalence of dementia and depression in the elderly community in a southern European population: the Zaragoza study [Lobo] 497 (Je)
Risk of Alzheimer's disease in first-degree relatives (letter) [Heun] 317 (reply) [Silverman] 318 (Ap)
Dementia, Multi-infarct
Prevalence of dementia and depression in the elderly community in a southern European population: the Zaragoza study [Lobo] 497 (Je)
Depression
Treatment of postpartum depression with interpersonal psychotherapy (letter) [Stuart] 75 (reply) [Weissman] 76 (Ja)
Depression, Bipolar see Bipolar Disorder
Depressive Disorder
Adrenal gland volume in major depression: increase during the depressive episode and decrease with successful treatment [Rubin] 213 (Mr)
Depression in patients with cancer: diagnosis, biology, and treatment [McDaniel] 89 (Fe)
Double-blind, crossover comparison of methylphenidate and placebo in adults with childhood-onset attention-deficit hyperactivity disorder [Spencer] 434 (Je)
Family study of early-onset dysthymia: mood and personality disorders in relatives of outpatients with dysthymia and episodic major depression and normal controls [Klein] 487 (Je)
Family study of manic-depressive (bipolar I) disease: is it a distinct illness separable from primary unipolar depression? [Winokur] 367 (My)
Functioning and well-being outcomes of patients with depression compared with chronic general medical illnesses [Hays] 11 (Ja)
Generalized social phobia: reliability and validity [Mannuzza] 230 (Mr)
Health care costs of primary care patients with recognized depression [Simon] 850 (Oc)
In quest of identifying vulnerability markers for psychiatric disorders by all-night polysomnography [Lauer] 145 (Fe)
Is the comorbidity between social phobia and panic disorder due to familial cotransmission or other factors? [Horwath] 574 (Jy)
Mental illness and suicide: a case-control study in east Taiwan [Cheng] 594 (Jy)
Meta-analyses of studies of ventricular enlargement and cortical sulcal prominence in mood disorders: comparisons with controls or patients with schizophrenia [Elkis] 735 (Se)
Premenstrual dysphoric disorders, anxiety, and depressions: vulnerability traits or comorbidity (letter) [Halbreich] 606 (Jy)
Prevalence of dementia and depression in the elderly community in a southern European population: the Zaragoza study [Lobo] 497 (Je)
Quality of care for depressed elderly patients hospitalized in the specialty psychiatric units or general medical wards [Norquist] 695 (Au)
Structure of the genetic and environmental risk factors for six major psychiatric disorders in women: phobia, generalized anxiety disorder, panic disorder, bulimia, major depression, and alcoholism [Kendler] 374 (My)
Switching from 'unipolar' to bipolar II: an 11-year prospective study of clinical and temperamental predictors in 559 patients [Akiskal] 114 (Fe)
Tryptophan depletion in stable lithium-treated patients with bipolar disorder in remission (letter) [Benkelfat] 154 (reply) [Delgado] 155 (Fe)
Desipramine
Interactions of serotonin reuptake inhibitors with tricyclic antidepressants (letter) [Harvey] 783 (reply) [Popli] 784 (Se)
Pharmacotherapy of impaired affect in recovering schizophrenic patients [Hogarty] 29 (Ja)
Tryptophan depletion in stable lithium-treated patients with bipolar disorder in remission (letter) [Benkelfat] 154 (reply) [Delgado] 155 (Fe)
Dexamethasone
Dose-response changes in plasma cortisol and lymphocyte glucocorticoid receptors following dexamethasone administration in combat veterans with and without posttraumatic stress disorder [Yehuda] 583 (Jy)
Diabetes Mellitus
Duration of neuroleptic treatment and prevalence of tardive dyskinesia in late life [Sweet] 478 (Je)
Functioning and well-being outcomes of patients with depression compared with chronic general medical illnesses [Hays] 11 (Ja)
Diagnosis
Diagnosis, assessment, and individual complexity [Emde] 637 (Au)
Longitudinal study of symptom dimensions in schizophrenia: prediction and patterns of change [Arndt] 352 (My)
Personality theory: clinical practice, social development, and the biology of individual differences [Reiss] 633 (Au)
Progress on case formulation [Crits-Christoph] 639 (Au)
Reliability and validity of two structured diagnostic interviews for personality disorders [Pilkonis] 1025 (De)
Role-relationship models for case formulation [Horowitz] 625 (Au)
Signs and symptoms: what can they tell us about the clinical course and pathophysiologic processes of schizophrenia? [Lieberman] 361 (My)
Symptoms of schizophrenia: methods, meanings, and mechanisms [Andreasen] 341 (My)
Test-retest reliability of the Diagnostic Interview Schedule for Children (DISC 2.1): parent, child, and combined algorithms [Jensen] 61 (Ja); correction, 312 (Ap)
Diagnostic Imaging
Event-related potentials in the study of psychiatric disorders [Pfefferbaum] 559 (Jy)
Diagnostic Interview Schedule for Children
Test-retest reliability of the Diagnostic Interview Schedule for Children (DISC 2.1): parent, child, and combined algorithms [Jensen] 61 (Ja); correction, 312 (Ap)
Diphenhydramine
In vivo D_2 dopamine receptor density in psychotic and nonpsychotic patients with bipolar disorder [Pearlson] 471 (Je)

Disease Progression
Early course of schizophrenia and long-term maintenance neuroleptic therapy [Nuechterlein] 203 (Mr)
In vivo study of the prefrontal cortex of schizophrenic patients at different stages of illness via phosphorus magnetic resonance spectroscopy [Stanley] 399 (My); correction, 799 (Oc)
Increased rate of P300 latency prolongation with age in schizophrenia: electrophysiological evidence for a neurodegenerative process [O'Donnell] 544 (Jy)
Longitudinal study of symptom dimensions in schizophrenia: prediction and patterns of change [Arndt] 352 (My)
Signs and symptoms: what can they tell us about the clinical course and pathophysiologic processes of schizophrenia? [Lieberman] 361 (My)
Disease Susceptibility
Developmental brain abnormalities in schizophrenia: contributions of genetic and perinatal factors (letter) [Vita] (reply) [Cannon] 157 (Fe)
Risk of Alzheimer's disease in first-degree relatives (letter) [Heun] 317 (reply) [Silverman] 318 (Ap)
Schizotypal symptoms and signs in the Roscommon Family Study: their factor structure and familial relationship with psychotic and affective disorders [Kendler] 296 (Ap)
Disease Transmission
Is the comorbidity between social phobia and panic disorder due to familial cotransmission or other factors? [Horwath] 574 (Jy)
Dopamine
Is methylphenidate like cocaine? studies on their pharmacokinetics and distribution in the human brain [Volkow] 456 (Je)
Dopamine D2 Receptors see Receptors, Dopamine D2
Dopamine Receptors see Receptors, Dopamine
Dose-Response Relationship, Drug
Dose-response changes in plasma cortisol and lymphocyte glucocorticoid receptors following dexamethasone administration in combat veterans with and without posttraumatic stress disorder [Yehuda] 583 (Jy)
Plasma haloperidol levels and clinical effects in schizophrenia and schizoaffective disorder [Volavka] 837 (Oc)
Double-Blind Method
Double-blind, crossover comparison of methylphenidate and placebo in adults with childhood-onset attention-deficit hyperactivity disorder [Spencer] 434 (Je)
Double-blind parallel comparison of three dosages of sertraline and placebo in outpatients with obsessive-compulsive disorder [Greist] 289 (Ap)
Failure of naltrexone hydrochloride to reduce self-injurious and autistic behavior in mentally retarded adults: double-blind placebo-controlled studies [Willemsen-Swinkels] 766 (Se)
Drive
Symptoms of schizophrenia: methods, meanings, and mechanisms [Andreasen] 341 (My)
Drug Abuse see Substance Abuse
Drug Interactions
Interactions of serotonin reuptake inhibitors with tricyclic antidepressants (letter) [Harvey] 783 (reply) [Popli] 784 (Se)
Drug Therapy
Critical review of psychosocial interventions in cancer care [Fawzy] 100 (Fe)
Pharmacotherapy of impaired affect in recovering schizophrenic patients [Hogarty] 29 (Ja)
Treatment of postpartum depression with interpersonal psychotherapy (letter) [Stuart] 75 (reply) [Weissman] 76 (Ja)
Drug Tolerance
Efficacy and tolerability of serotonin transport inhibitors in obsessive-compulsive disorder: a meta-analysis [Greist] 53 (Ja)
Drug Withdrawal Symptoms see Substance Withdrawal Syndrome
DSM-III-R
Generalized social phobia: reliability and validity [Mannuzza] 230 (Mr)
Multiple-family groups and psychoeducation in the treatment of schizophrenia [McFarlane] 679 (Au)
Premenstrual dysphoric disorder and response to cholecystokinin-tetrapeptide (letter) [Le Melledo] 605 (Jy)
Prevalence of dementia and depression in the elderly community in a southern European population: the Zaragoza study [Lobo] 497 (Je)
Specificity in familial aggregation of phobic disorders [Fyer] 564 (Jy)
DSM-IV
Diagnosis, assessment, and individual complexity [Emde] 637 (Au)
Personality theory: clinical practice, social development, and the biology of individual differences [Reiss] 633 (Au)
'Richly complex' but needs an emotion theory [Dahl] 649 (Au)
Role-relationship model configurations: a summation [Horowitz] 654 (Au)
Dyskinesia, Drug-Induced
Considering neuroleptic maintenance and taper on a continuum: need for individual rather than dogmatic approach [Jeste] 209 (Mr)
Duration of neuroleptic treatment and prevalence of tardive dyskinesia in late life [Sweet] 478 (Je)
Early course of schizophrenia and long-term maintenance neuroleptic therapy [Nuechterlein] 203 (Mr)
Long-term treatment for lifetime disorders? [Greden] 197 (Mr)
Neuroleptic withdrawal in schizophrenic patients: a review of the literature [Gilbert] 173 (Mr)
Risk of tardive dyskinesia in older patients: a prospective longitudinal study of 266 outpatients [Jeste] 756 (Se)
Risks of withdrawing antipsychotic medications [Wyatt] 205 (Mr)
Why neuroleptic withdrawal in schizophrenia? [Carpenter] 192 (Mr)
Dyskinesia, Tardive see Dyskinesia, Drug-Induced
Dysthymic Disorder see Depressive Disorder
Dystonia
Why neuroleptic withdrawal in schizophrenia? [Carpenter] 192 (Mr)

E

Eating Disorders
Prospective study of outcome in bulimia nervosa and the long-term effects of three psychological treatments [Fairburn] 304 (Ap)
Economics, Medical
Health care costs of primary care patients with recognized depression [Simon] 850 (Oc)
Educational Status
Prevalence of dementia and depression in the elderly community in a southern European population: the Zaragoza study [Lobo] 497 (Je)
Elderly see Aged
Electroencephalography
Event-related potentials in the study of psychiatric disorders [Pfefferbaum] 559 (Jy)
Increased rate of P300 latency prolongation with age in schizophrenia: electrophysiological evidence for a neurodegenerative process [O'Donnell] 544 (Jy)
Electromyography
Is hyperarousal essential to obsessive-compulsive disorder? diminished physiologic flexibility, but not hyperarousal, characterizes patients with obsessive-compulsive disorder [Hoehn-Saric] 688 (Au)
Emotions
Longitudinal study of symptom dimensions in schizophrenia: prediction and patterns of change [Arndt] 352 (My)
'Richly complex' but needs an emotion theory [Dahl] 649 (Au)
Symptoms of schizophrenia: methods, meanings, and mechanisms [Andreasen] 341 (My)
Environment
Antisocial behavior [Gershon] 900 (No)
Differential heritability of adult and juvenile antisocial traits [Lyons] 906 (No)
Family-environment risk factors for attention-deficit hyperactivity disorder: a test of Rutter's indicators of adversity [Biederman] 464 (Je)
Genetic epidemiology in psychiatry: taking both genes and environment seriously [Kendler] 895 (No)
Genetic questions for environmental studies: differential parenting and psychopathology in adolescence [Reiss] 925 (No)
Genetic-environmental interaction in the genesis of aggressivity and conduct disorders [Cadoret] 916 (No)
Structure of the genetic and environmental risk factors for six major psychiatric disorders in women: phobia, generalized anxiety disorder, panic disorder, bulimia, major depression, and alcoholism [Kendler] 374 (My)
Epidemiology
Genetic epidemiology in psychiatry: taking both genes and environment seriously [Kendler] 895 (No)
Prevalence of schizophrenia in Ireland: readdressing the enigma (letter) [Waddington] (reply) [Walsh] 509 (Je)
Europe
Prevalence of dementia and depression in the elderly community in a southern European population: the Zaragoza study [Lobo] 497 (Je)
Evoked Potentials
Event-related potentials in the study of psychiatric disorders [Pfefferbaum] 559 (Jy)
Impaired mismatch negativity generation reflects widespread dysfunction of working memory in schizophrenia [Javitt] 550 (Jy)
Increased rate of P300 latency prolongation with age in schizophrenia: electrophysiological evidence for a neurodegenerative process [O'Donnell] 544 (Jy)
Extrapyramidal Tracts
Pharmacotherapy of impaired affect in recovering schizophrenic patients [Hogarty] 29 (Ja)
Eye Movements
Spatial working memory deficits in the relatives of schizophrenic patients [Park] 821 (Oc)

F

Family
Family study of early-onset dysthymia: mood and personality disorders in relatives of outpatients with dysthymia and episodic major depression and normal controls [Klein] 487 (Je)
Family study of manic-depressive (bipolar I) disease: is it a distinct illness separable from primary unipolar depression? [Winokur] 367 (My)
Family-environment risk factors for attention-deficit hyperactivity disorder: a test of Rutter's indicators of adversity [Biederman] 464 (Je)
Risk of Alzheimer's disease in first-degree relatives (letter) [Heun] 317 (reply) [Silverman] 318 (Ap)
Spatial working memory deficits in the relatives of schizophrenic patients [Park] 821 (Oc)
Feces, Impacted
Clozapine-associated postoperative ileus: case report and review of the literature (letter) [Erickson] 508 (Je)
Financing, Government
Child and adolescent mental disorders and the search for an NIMH director: quo vadis? [Barchas] 873 (Oc)
Comments on the report card from a services research perspective [Kruesi] 727 (Se)
Grading the progress of child and adolescent mental health research: NIMH perspectives [Cowdry] 732 (Se)
Report card: progress report or final grade? [Carlson] 724 (Se)
5-Hydroxytryptamine see Serotonin
Fluoxetine
Cingulotomy for intractable obsessive-compulsive disorder: prospective long-term follow-up of 18 patients [Baer] 384 (My)
Efficacy and tolerability of serotonin transport inhibitors in obsessive-compulsive disorder: a meta-analysis [Greist] 53 (Ja)
Interactions of serotonin reuptake inhibitors with tricyclic antidepressants (letter) [Harvey] 783 (reply) [Popli] 784 (Se)
Fluvoxamine
Efficacy and tolerability of serotonin transport inhibitors in obsessive-compulsive disorder: a meta-analysis [Greist] 53 (Ja)
Interactions of serotonin reuptake inhibitors with tricyclic antidepressants (letter) [Harvey] 783 (reply) [Popli] 784 (Se)
Follow-Up Studies
New York High-Risk Project: psychoses and cluster A personality disorders in offspring of schizophrenic parents at 23 years of follow-up [Erlenmeyer-Kimling] 857 (Oc)
Foster Home Care
Child and adolescent mental disorders research: current directions, future needs [Rosenfeld] 729 (Se)
Frontal Lobe
Abnormally high neuronal density in the schizophrenic cortex: a morphometric analysis of prefrontal area 9 and occipital area 17 [Selemon] 805 (Oc)
Frontal and temporal lobe brain volumes in schizophrenia: relationship to symptoms and clinical subtype [Turetsky] 1061 (De)
In pursuit of the molecular neuropathology of schizophrenia [Trojanowski] 274 (Ap)
Reciprocal lateralization of frontal lobe functions (letter) [Goldberg] (reply) [Rauch] 159 (Fe)

G

GABA
Altered glutamatergic and GABAergic mechanisms in the cingulate cortex of the schizophrenic brain [Benes] 1015 (De)
Gene expression for glutamic acid decarboxylase is reduced without loss of neurons in prefrontal cortex of schizophrenics [Akbarian] 258 (Ap)
In reply [Akbarian] 277 (Ap)
Neural circuitry of the prefrontal cortex in schizophrenia [Lewis] 269 (Ap)
Reduced inhibitory capacity in prefrontal cortex of schizophrenics [Lee] 267 (Ap)
GABA Receptors see Receptors, GABA
gamma-Aminobutyric Acid Receptors see Receptors, GABA
Gender see Sex
Gene Expression
Gene expression for glutamic acid decarboxylase is reduced without loss of neurons in prefrontal cortex of schizophrenics [Akbarian] 258 (Ap)
Reduced inhibitory capacity in prefrontal cortex of schizophrenics [Lee] 267 (Ap)
Signal transduction pathways: molecular targets for lithium's actions [Manji] 531 (Jy)
Genetics
Antisocial behavior [Gershon] 900 (No)
Differential heritability of adult and juvenile antisocial traits [Lyons] 906 (No)
Genetic epidemiology in psychiatry: taking both genes and environment seriously [Kendler] 895 (No)
Genetic questions for environmental studies: differential parenting and psychopathology in adolescence [Reiss] 925 (No)
Genetic-environmental interaction in the genesis of aggressivity and conduct disorders [Cadoret] 916 (No)
Genetics, Biochemical
Signal transduction pathways: molecular targets for lithium's actions [Manji] 531 (Jy)

Genetics, Medical
Adoption study demonstrating two genetic pathways to drug abuse [Cadoret] 42 (Ja)
Genotype
Suicidal behaviors and the tryptophan hydroxylase gene [Abbar] 846 (Oc)
Gliosis
Abnormally high neuronal density in the schizophrenic cortex: a morphometric analysis of prefrontal area 9 and occipital area 17 [Selemon] 805 (Oc)
Glucocorticoid Receptors see Receptors, Glucocorticoid
Glucose
Resting cerebral glucose metabolism in first-episode and previously treated patients with schizophrenia relates to clinical features [Gur] 657 (Au)
Glutamate Receptors see Receptors, Glutamate
Glutamates
Abnormal excitatory neurotransmitter metabolism in schizophrenic brains [Tsai] 829 (Oc)
Glutamic Acid
Gene expression for glutamic acid decarboxylase is reduced without loss of neurons in prefrontal cortex of schizophrenics [Akbarian] 258 (Ap)
In reply [Akbarian] 277 (Ap)
Neural circuitry of the prefrontal cortex in schizophrenia [Lewis] 269 (Ap)
Reduced inhibitory capacity in prefrontal cortex of schizophrenics [Lee] 267 (Ap)
Glycine
Abnormal excitatory neurotransmitter metabolism in schizophrenic brains [Tsai] 829 (Oc)
Glycopyrrolate
Pharmacotherapy of impaired affect in recovering schizophrenic patients [Hogarty] 29 (Ja)
Grief
Signs of defensive control locate conflicted topics in discourse [Horowitz] 1040 (De)
Group Therapy see Psychotherapy, Group
Guanine Nucleotides
Guanine nucleotide-binding proteins in bipolar affective disorder: effects of long-term lithium treatment [Manji] 135 (Fe)
Signal transduction pathways: molecular targets for lithium's actions [Manji] 531 (Jy)
Guanosine Triphosphate
Low levels of pertussis toxin adenosine diphosphate ribosylation in the schizophrenic brain (letter) [Okada] 319 (Ap)
Gyrus Cinguli
Altered glutamatergic and GABAergic mechanisms in the cingulate cortex of the schizophrenic brain [Benes] 1015 (De)
Cingulotomy for intractable obsessive-compulsive disorder: prospective long-term follow-up of 18 patients [Baer] 384 (My)
Response to commentaries and to the challenge of building a perfect theory to explain schizophrenia: response to Dr Benes' commentary [Olney] 1019 (De)

H

Hallucinations
In pursuit of the molecular neuropathology of schizophrenia [Trojanowski] 274 (Ap)
Longitudinal study of symptom dimensions in schizophrenia: prediction and patterns of change [Arndt] 352 (My)
Structure and course of positive and negative symptoms in schizophrenia [Eaton] 127 (Fe)
Symptoms of schizophrenia: methods, meanings, and mechanisms [Andreasen] 341 (My)
Haloperidol
Behavioral vs biochemical prediction of clinical stability following haloperidol withdrawal in schizophrenia [van Kammen] 673 (Au)
Clozapine therapy and increases in homovanillic acid (letter) [Risch] 244 (Mr)
Complicating factors in the analysis of acute drug-induced akathisia (letter) [Rosebush] 878 (reply) [Sachdev] 879 (Oc)
In vivo D_2 dopamine receptor density in psychotic and nonpsychotic patients with bipolar disorder [Pearlson] 471 (Je)
Neuroleptic withdrawal in schizophrenic patients: a review of the literature [Gilbert] 173 (Mr)
Plasma haloperidol levels and clinical effects in schizophrenia and schizoaffective disorder [Volavka] 837 (Oc)
Health Care Costs
Health care costs of primary care patients with recognized depression [Simon] 850 (Oc)
Health Maintenance Organizations
Health care costs of primary care patients with recognized depression [Simon] 850 (Oc)
Health Services Research
Child and adolescent mental disorders research: current directions, future needs [Rosenfeld] 729 (Se)
Comments on the report card from a services research perspective [Kruesi] 727 (Se)
Grading the progress of child and adolescent mental health research: NIMH perspectives [Cowdry] 732 (Se)
Health Status
Functioning and well-being outcomes of patients with depression compared with chronic general medical illnesses [Hays] 11 (Ja)
Heart Failure, Congestive
Functioning and well-being outcomes of patients with depression compared with chronic general medical illnesses [Hays] 11 (Ja)
Heart Ventricle
Meta-analyses of studies of ventricular enlargement and cortical sulcal prominence in mood disorders: comparisons with controls or patients with schizophrenia [Elkis] 735 (Se)
Hereditary Diseases
Antisocial behavior [Gershon] 900 (No)
Developmental brain abnormalities in schizophrenia: contributions of genetic and perinatal factors (letter) [Vita] (reply) [Cannon] 157 (Fe)
Differential heritability of adult and juvenile antisocial traits [Lyons] 906 (No)
Family study of early-onset dysthymia: mood and personality disorders in relatives of outpatients with dysthymia and episodic major depression and normal controls [Klein] 487 (Je)
Family study of manic-depressive (bipolar I) disease: is it a distinct illness separable from primary unipolar depression? [Winokur] 367 (My)
Family-environment risk factors for attention-deficit hyperactivity disorder: a test of Rutter's indicators of adversity [Biederman] 464 (Je)
Genetic epidemiology in psychiatry: taking both genes and environment seriously [Kendler] 895 (No)
Genetic questions for environmental studies: differential parenting and psychopathology in adolescence [Reiss] 925 (No)
In quest of identifying vulnerability markers for psychiatric disorders by all-night polysomnography [Lauer] 145 (Fe)
Is the comorbidity between social phobia and panic disorder due to familial cotransmission or other factors? [Horwath] 574 (Jy)
Magnetic resonance imaging and mood disorders: localization of white matter and other subcortical abnormalities [Dupont] 747 (Se)
New York High-Risk Project: psychoses and cluster A personality disorders in offspring of schizophrenic parents at 23 years of follow-up [Erlenmeyer-Kimling] 857 (Oc)
Risk of Alzheimer's disease in first-degree relatives (letter) [Heun] 317 (reply) [Silverman] 318 (Ap)
Schizotypal symptoms and signs in the Roscommon Family Study: their factor structure and familial relationship with psychotic and affective disorders [Kendler] 296 (Ap)
Spatial working memory deficits in the relatives of schizophrenic patients [Park] 821 (Oc)
Specificity in familial aggregation of phobic disorders [Fyer] 564 (Jy)
Structure of the genetic and environmental risk factors for six major psychiatric disorders in women: phobia, generalized anxiety disorder, panic disorder, bulimia, major depression, and alcoholism [Kendler] 374 (My)
Hippocampus
Abnormal excitatory neurotransmitter metabolism in schizophrenic brains [Tsai] 829 (Oc)
In pursuit of the molecular neuropathology of schizophrenia [Trojanowski] 274 (Ap)
In reply [Akbarian] 277 (Ap)
Low levels of pertussis toxin adenosine diphosphate ribosylation in the schizophrenic brain (letter) [Okada] 319 (Ap)
Prefrontal cortex and schizophrenia: a quantitative magnetic resonance imaging study [Wible] 279 (Ap)
Homovanillic Acid
Behavioral vs biochemical prediction of clinical stability following haloperidol withdrawal in schizophrenia [van Kammen] 673 (Au)
Clozapine therapy and increases in homovanillic acid (letter) [Risch] 244 (Mr)
Hospitalization
Multiple-family groups and psychoeducation in the treatment of schizophrenia [McFarlane] 679 (Au)
Perceived coercion in mental hospital admission: pressures and process [Lidz] 1034 (De)
Quality of care for depressed elderly patients hospitalized in the specialty psychiatric units or general medical wards [Norquist] 695 (Au)
Huntington's Disease
Abnormally high neuronal density in the schizophrenic cortex: a morphometric analysis of prefrontal area 9 and occipital area 17 [Selemon] 805 (Oc)
Hydrocortisone
Adrenal gland volume in major depression: increase during the depressive episode and decrease with successful treatment [Rubin] 213 (Mr)
Dose-response changes in plasma cortisol and lymphocyte glucocorticoid receptors following dexamethasone administration in combat veterans with and without posttraumatic stress disorder [Yehuda] 583 (Jy)
Hydroxyindoleacetic Acid
Behavioral vs biochemical prediction of clinical stability following haloperidol withdrawal in schizophrenia [van Kammen] 673 (Au)
Clozapine therapy and increases in homovanillic acid (letter) [Risch] 244 (Mr)
Hypertension
Functioning and well-being outcomes of patients with depression compared with chronic general medical illnesses [Hays] 11 (Ja)
Hypnosis
Critical review of psychosocial interventions in cancer care [Fawzy] 100 (Fe)
Hypotension, Orthostatic
Neuroleptic withdrawal in schizophrenic patients: a review of the literature [Gilbert] 173 (Mr)
Hypothalamus
Depression in patients with cancer: diagnosis, biology, and treatment [McDaniel] 89 (Fe)

I

Ileus see Intestinal Obstruction
Immune Function
Depression in patients with cancer: diagnosis, biology, and treatment [McDaniel] 89 (Fe)
Immunoassay
Low levels of pertussis toxin adenosine diphosphate ribosylation in the schizophrenic brain (letter) [Okada] 319 (Ap)
Immunohistochemistry
Guanine nucleotide-binding proteins in bipolar affective disorder: effects of long-term lithium treatment [Manji] 135 (Fe)
Immunolabeling Techniques see Immunohistochemistry
Impulsive Behavior
Role of methylphenidate in psychiatry [Klein] 429 (Je)
In Situ Hybridization
Gene expression for glutamic acid decarboxylase is reduced without loss of neurons in prefrontal cortex of schizophrenics [Akbarian] 258 (Ap)
In pursuit of the molecular neuropathology of schizophrenia [Trojanowski] 274 (Ap)
In reply [Akbarian] 277 (Ap)
Neural circuitry of the prefrontal cortex in schizophrenia [Lewis] 269 (Ap)
Information Processing, Human see Mental Processes
Informed Consent
Considering neuroleptic maintenance and taper on a continuum: need for individual rather than dogmatic approach [Jeste] 209 (Mr)
Institute of Medicine (US)
Comments on the report card from a services research perspective [Kruesi] 727 (Se)
Grading the progress of child and adolescent mental health research: NIMH perspectives [Cowdry] 732 (Se)
Report card: progress report or final grade? [Carlson] 724 (Se)
Interleukin-2
Mitogen-stimulated interleukin-2 production in never-medicated, first-episode schizophrenic patients: the influence of age at onset and negative symptoms [Ganguli] 668 (Au)
Interpersonal Relations
Are case formulations useful for outcomes research? [Clarkin] 645 (Au)
Between the past and the future of psychotherapy research [Akhtar] 642 (Au)
Diagnosis, assessment, and individual complexity [Emde] 637 (Au)
Personality: psychodynamic perspectives [Shapiro] 651 (Au)
Personality theory: clinical practice, social development, and the biology of individual differences [Reiss] 633 (Au)
Progress on case formulation [Crits-Christoph] 639 (Au)
'Richly complex' but needs an emotion theory [Dahl] 649 (Au)
Role-relationship model configurations: a summation [Horowitz] 654 (Au)
Role-relationship models: are they useful for research and practice? [Jones] 646 (Au)
Role-relationship models for case formulation [Horowitz] 625 (Au)
Treatment of postpartum depression with interpersonal psychotherapy (letter) [Stuart] 75 (reply) [Weissman] 76 (Ja)
Interviews
Reliability and validity of two structured diagnostic interviews for personality disorders [Pilkonis] 1025 (De)
Risk of Alzheimer's disease in first-degree relatives (letter) [Heun] 317 (reply) [Silverman] 318 (Ap)
Intestinal Obstruction
Clozapine-associated postoperative ileus: case report and review of the literature (letter) [Erickson] 508 (Je)
Ireland
Prevalence of schizophrenia in Ireland: readdressing the enigma (letter) [Waddington] (reply) [Walsh] 509 (Je)
Islet-Activating Protein see Pertussis Toxins
Isocarboxazid
Biochemical effects of antidepressant augmentation (letter) [Howland] 156 (Fe)
Isoenzymes
Signal transduction pathways: molecular targets for lithium's actions [Manji] 531 (Jy)

Isozymes see Isoenzymes

J

JOURNAL OF THE AMERICAN MEDICAL ASSOCIATION
Managed care in *JAMA* and the *Archives* journals: a call for papers for coordinated theme issues [Lundberg] 967 (No)

K

Kaplan, Helen Singer (1929-1995)
Helen Singer Kaplan, MD, PhD, February 6, 1929, to August 17, 1995 [Person] 1073 (De)

L

Language
Constraints on concepts of pathogenesis: language and the speciation process as the key to the etiology of schizophrenia [Crow] 1011 (De)
Laterality
Reciprocal lateralization of frontal lobe functions (letter) [Goldberg] (reply) [Rauch] 159 (Fe)
Laxatives see Cathartics
Learning Disorders
Family-environment risk factors for attention-deficit hyperactivity disorder: a test of Rutter's indicators of adversity [Biederman] 464 (Je)
Leukocytes, Mononuclear
Guanine nucleotide-binding proteins in bipolar affective disorder: effects of long-term lithium treatment [Manji] 135 (Fe)
Lithium
Guanine nucleotide-binding proteins in bipolar affective disorder: effects of long-term lithium treatment [Manji] 135 (Fe)
Signal transduction pathways: molecular targets for lithium's actions [Manji] 531 (Jy)
Tryptophan depletion in stable lithium-treated patients with bipolar disorder in remission (letter) [Benkelfat] 154 (reply) [Delgado] 155 (Fe)
Lithium Carbonate
Pharmacotherapy of impaired affect in recovering schizophrenic patients [Hogarty] 29 (Ja)
Longitudinal Studies
Risk of tardive dyskinesia in older patients: a prospective longitudinal study of 266 outpatients [Jeste] 756 (Se)
Lumbar Puncture see Spinal Puncture
Lymphocytes
Dose-response changes in plasma cortisol and lymphocyte glucocorticoid receptors following dexamethasone administration in combat veterans with and without posttraumatic stress disorder [Yehuda] 583 (Jy)

M

Maas, James W. (1929-1995)
James W. Maas, MD, October 26, 1929, to January 14, 1995 [Katz] 1081 (De)
Magnesium
In vivo study of the prefrontal cortex of schizophrenic patients at different stages of illness via phosphorus magnetic resonance spectroscopy [Stanley] 399 (My); correction, 799 (Oc)
Magnetic Resonance Imaging
Adrenal gland volume in major depression: increase during the depressive episode and decrease with successful treatment [Rubin] 213 (Mr)
Increased rate of P300 latency prolongation with age in schizophrenia: electrophysiological evidence for a neurodegenerative process [O'Donnell] 544 (Jy)
Magnetic resonance imaging and mood disorders: localization of white matter and other subcortical abnormalities [Dupont] 747 (Se)
Prefrontal cortex and schizophrenia: a quantitative magnetic resonance imaging study [Wible] 279 (Ap)
Reduced caudate nucleus volume in obsessive-compulsive disorder [Robinson] 393 (My)
Resting cerebral glucose metabolism in first-episode and previously treated patients with schizophrenia relates to clinical features [Gur] 657 (Au)
Magnetic Resonance Spectroscopy see Nuclear Magnetic Resonance
Managed Care Programs
Managed care in *JAMA* and the *Archives* journals: a call for papers for coordinated theme issues [Lundberg] 967 (No)
Manic-Depressive Psychosis see Bipolar Disorder
Manuscripts, Medical
Managed care in *JAMA* and the *Archives* journals: a call for papers for coordinated theme issues [Lundberg] 967 (No)
Marital Status
Generalized social phobia: reliability and validity [Mannuzza] 230 (Mr)
Marriage
Family-environment risk factors for attention-deficit hyperactivity disorder: a test of Rutter's indicators of adversity [Biederman] 464 (Je)
Medicaid
Child and adolescent mental disorders research: current directions, future needs [Rosenfeld] 729 (Se)
Medical Research see Research
Melatonin
Effects of the menstrual cycle on dependent variables in mood disorder research [Leibenluft] 51:761 (Oc); correction, 52:144 (Fe)
Memory
Impaired mismatch negativity generation reflects widespread dysfunction of working memory in schizophrenia [Javitt] 550 (Jy)
Memory Disorders
Spatial working memory deficits in the relatives of schizophrenic patients [Park] 821 (Oc)
Menstrual Cycle
Effects of the menstrual cycle on dependent variables in mood disorder research [Leibenluft] 51:761 (Oc); correction, 52:144 (Fe)
Premenstrual dysphoric disorder and response to cholecystokinin-tetrapeptide (letter) [Le Melledo] 605 (Jy)
Premenstrual dysphoric disorders, anxiety, and depressions: vulnerability traits or comorbidity (letter) [Halbreich] 606 (Jy)
Mental Disorders
Child and adolescent mental disorders and the search for an NIMH director: quo vadis? [Barchas] 873 (Oc)
Child and adolescent mental disorders research: current directions, future needs [Rosenfeld] 729 (Se)
Comments on the report card from a services research perspective [Kruesi] 727 (Se)
Diagnosis, assessment, and individual complexity [Emde] 637 (Au)
Event-related potentials in the study of psychiatric disorders [Pfefferbaum] 559 (Jy)
Grading the progress of child and adolescent mental health research: NIMH perspectives [Cowdry] 732 (Se)
Mental illness and suicide: a case-control study in east Taiwan [Cheng] 594 (Jy)
Report card on the *National Plan for Research on Child and Adolescent Mental Disorders:* the midway point [Members of the Committee for the Study of Research on Child and Adolescent Mental Disorders] 715 (Se); correction, 1072 (De)
Report card: progress report or final grade? [Carlson] 724 (Se)
Mental Processes
Between the past and the future of psychotherapy research [Akhtar] 642 (Au)
Event-related potentials in the study of psychiatric disorders [Pfefferbaum] 559 (Jy)
Impaired mismatch negativity generation reflects widespread dysfunction of working memory in schizophrenia [Javitt] 550 (Jy)
Role-relationship models: are they useful for research and practice? [Jones] 646 (Au)
Mental Retardation
Failure of naltrexone hydrochloride to reduce self-injurious and autistic behavior in mentally retarded adults: double-blind placebo-controlled studies [Willemsen-Swinkels] 766 (Se)
Messenger RNA see RNA, Messenger
Meta-analysis
Meta-analyses of studies of ventricular enlargement and cortical sulcal prominence in mood disorders: comparisons with controls or patients with schizophrenia [Elkis] 735 (Se)
Neuroleptic withdrawal in schizophrenic patients: a review of the literature [Gilbert] 173 (Mr)
Metabolism
Abnormal excitatory neurotransmitter metabolism in schizophrenic brains [Tsai] 829 (Oc)
Resting cerebral glucose metabolism in first-episode and previously treated patients with schizophrenia relates to clinical features [Gur] 657 (Au)
Methylphenidate
Double-blind, crossover comparison of methylphenidate and placebo in adults with childhood-onset attention-deficit hyperactivity disorder [Spencer] 434 (Je)
Efficacy of methylphenidate for attention-deficit hyperactivity disorder in children with tic disorder [Gadow] 444 (Je); correction, 836 (Oc)
Is methylphenidate like cocaine? studies on their pharmacokinetics and distribution in the human brain [Volkow] 456 (Je)
Role of methylphenidate in psychiatry [Klein] 429 (Je)
Mianserin
Biochemical effects of antidepressant augmentation (letter) [Howland] 156 (Fe)
Middle Age
Risk of tardive dyskinesia in older patients: a prospective longitudinal study of 266 outpatients [Jeste] 756 (Se)
Mini-Mental State Examination
In vivo D_2 dopamine receptor density in psychotic and nonpsychotic patients with bipolar disorder [Pearlson] 471 (Je)
Prevalence of dementia and depression in the elderly community in a southern European population: the Zaragoza study [Lobo] 497 (Je)
Mitogens
Mitogen-stimulated interleukin-2 production in never-medicated, first-episode schizophrenic patients: the influence of age at onset and negative symptoms [Ganguli] 668 (Au)
Molecular Genetics see Genetics, Biochemical
Mononuclear Leukocytes see Leukocytes, Mononuclear
Mood see Affect
Morphometric Analysis
Abnormally high neuronal density in the schizophrenic cortex: a morphometric analysis of prefrontal area 9 and occipital area 17 [Selemon] 805 (Oc)
Reduced caudate nucleus volume in obsessive-compulsive disorder [Robinson] 393 (My)
Muscle Relaxation
Critical review of psychosocial interventions in cancer care [Fawzy] 100 (Fe)
Myocardial Infarction
Functioning and well-being outcomes of patients with depression compared with chronic general medical illnesses [Hays] 11 (Ja)

N

Naltrexone
Failure of naltrexone hydrochloride to reduce self-injurious and autistic behavior in mentally retarded adults: double-blind placebo-controlled studies [Willemsen-Swinkels] 766 (Se)
National Comorbidity Survey
Prevalence and correlates of drug use and dependence in the United States: results from the National Comorbidity Survey [Warner] 219 (Mr)
National Institute of Mental Health (US)
Child and adolescent mental disorders and the search for an NIMH director: quo vadis? [Barchas] 873 (Oc)
Child and adolescent mental disorders research: current directions, future needs [Rosenfeld] 729 (Se)
Grading the progress of child and adolescent mental health research: NIMH perspectives [Cowdry] 732 (Se)
Report card: progress report or final grade? [Carlson] 724 (Se)
Neoplasms
Critical review of psychosocial interventions in cancer care [Fawzy] 100 (Fe)
Depression in patients with cancer: diagnosis, biology, and treatment [McDaniel] 89 (Fe)
Nerve Degeneration
Increased rate of P300 latency prolongation with age in schizophrenia: electrophysiological evidence for a neurodegenerative process [O'Donnell] 544 (Jy)
Nervous System
Positron emission tomographic study of simple phobic symptom provocation [Rauch] 20 (Ja)
Neuroanatomy
Reciprocal lateralization of frontal lobe functions (letter) [Goldberg] (reply) [Rauch] 159 (Fe)
Neuroleptic Malignant Syndrome
Why neuroleptic withdrawal in schizophrenia? [Carpenter] 192 (Mr)
Neuroleptics see Antipsychotic Agents
Neurons
Abnormally high neuronal density in the schizophrenic cortex: a morphometric analysis of prefrontal area 9 and occipital area 17 [Selemon] 805 (Oc)
Gene expression for glutamic acid decarboxylase is reduced without loss of neurons in prefrontal cortex of schizophrenics [Akbarian] 258 (Ap)
In pursuit of the molecular neuropathology of schizophrenia [Trojanowski] 274 (Ap)
In reply [Akbarian] 277 (Ap)
Neocortical abnormalities in schizophrenia [Watson] 819 (Oc)
Neural circuitry of the prefrontal cortex in schizophrenia [Lewis] 269 (Ap)
Reduced inhibitory capacity in prefrontal cortex of schizophrenics [Lee] 267 (Ap)
Neuropsychological Tests
Magnetic resonance imaging and mood disorders: localization of white matter and other subcortical abnormalities [Dupont] 747 (Se)
Neurotransmitters
Abnormal excitatory neurotransmitter metabolism in schizophrenic brains [Tsai] 829 (Oc)
Effects of the menstrual cycle on dependent variables in mood disorder research [Leibenluft] 51:761 (Oc); correction, 52:144 (Fe)
Signal transduction pathways: molecular targets for lithium's actions [Manji] 531 (Jy)
New York
New York High-Risk Project: psychoses and cluster A personality disorders in offspring of schizophrenic parents at 23 years of follow-up [Erlenmeyer-Kimling] 857 (Oc)
N-Methyl-D-Aspartate Receptors see Receptors, N-Methyl-D-Aspartate
Nomenclature
Role-relationship model configurations: a summation [Horowitz] 654 (Au)
Nonlinear Dynamics
Chaos and complexity: can it help us to understand mood and behavior? [Ehlers] 960 (No)
Evidence of chaotic mood variation in bipolar disorder [Gottschalk] 947 (No)

Norepinephrine
Biochemical effects of antidepressant augmentation (letter) [Howland] 156 (Fe)
Effects of Alzheimer's disease and normal aging on cerebrospinal fluid norepinephrine responses to yohimbine and clonidine [Peskind] 774 (Se)
Nuclear Magnetic Resonance
In vivo study of the prefrontal cortex of schizophrenic patients at different stages of illness via phosphorus magnetic resonance spectroscopy [Stanley] 399 (My); correction, 799 (Oc)

O

OBITUARIES
Roland D. Ciaranello, MD, February 27, 1943 to December 14, 1994 [Barchas] 1074 (De)
Samuel Wesley Perry III, MD, December 10, 1940, to March 15, 1994 [Rabkin] 1078 (De)
Helen Singer Kaplan, MD, PhD, February 6, 1929, to August 17, 1995 [Person] 1073 (De)
James W. Maas, MD, October 26, 1929, to January 14, 1995 [Katz] 1081 (De)
Eli Robins, MD, February 22, 1921, to December 21, 1994 [Hudgens] 1080 (De)
John Romano, MD, November 20, 1908 to June 19, 1995 [Joynt] 1076 (De)
Joseph Wortis, MD October 2, 1906, to February 22, 1995 [Halmi] 1077 (De)
Obsessive-Compulsive Disorder
Cingulotomy for intractable obsessive-compulsive disorder: prospective long-term follow-up of 18 patients [Baer] 384 (My)
Double-blind parallel comparison of three dosages of sertraline and placebo in outpatients with obsessive-compulsive disorder [Greist] 289 (Ap)
Efficacy and tolerability of serotonin transport inhibitors in obsessive-compulsive disorder: a meta-analysis [Greist] 53 (Ja)
Is hyperarousal essential to obsessive-compulsive disorder? diminished physiologic flexibility, but not hyperarousal, characterizes patients with obsessive-compulsive disorder [Hoehn-Saric] 688 (Au)
Reciprocal lateralization of frontal lobe functions (letter) [Goldberg] (reply) [Rauch] 159 (Fe)
Reduced caudate nucleus volume in obsessive-compulsive disorder [Robinson] 393 (My)
Occipital Lobe
Abnormally high neuronal density in the schizophrenic cortex: a morphometric analysis of prefrontal area 9 and occipital area 17 [Selemon] 805 (Oc)
Oculomotor Muscles
Spatial working memory deficits in the relatives of schizophrenic patients [Park] 821 (Oc)
Office Visits
Health care costs of primary care patients with recognized depression [Simon] 850 (Oc)
Outcome Assessment (Health Care)
Are case formulations useful for outcomes research? [Clarkin] 645 (Au)
Between the past and the future of psychotherapy research [Akhtar] 642 (Au)
Functioning and well-being outcomes of patients with depression compared with chronic general medical illnesses [Hays] 11 (Ja)
More reliable outcome measures can reduce sample size requirements [Leon] 867 (Oc)
Prospective study of outcome in bulimia nervosa and the long-term effects of three psychological treatments [Fairburn] 304 (Ap)
Quality of care for depressed elderly patients hospitalized in the specialty psychiatric units or general medical wards [Norquist] 695 (Au)
Trial of the effect of a standardized psychiatric consultation on health outcomes and costs in somatizing patients [Smith] 238 (Mr)
Outcomes Research see Outcome Assessment (Health Care)
Outpatients
Double-blind parallel comparison of three dosages of sertraline and placebo in outpatients with obsessive-compulsive disorder [Greist] 289 (Ap)
Family study of early-onset dysthymia: mood and personality disorders in relatives of outpatients with dysthymia and episodic major depression and normal controls [Klein] 487 (Je)

P

Panic Attacks see Panic Disorder
Panic Disorder
Is the comorbidity between social phobia and panic disorder due to familial cotransmission or other factors? [Horwath] 574 (Jy)
Premenstrual dysphoric disorder and response to cholecystokinin-tetrapeptide (letter) [Le Melledo] 605 (Jy)
Premenstrual dysphoric disorders, anxiety, and depressions: vulnerability traits or comorbidity (letter) [Halbreich] 606 (Jy)
Relationship of panic disorder to posttraumatic stress disorder (letter) [Safadi] 76 (reply) [Southwick] 77 (Ja)
Specificity in familial aggregation of phobic disorders [Fyer] 564 (Jy)
Structure of the genetic and environmental risk factors for six major psychiatric disorders in women: phobia, generalized anxiety disorder, panic disorder, bulimia, major depression, and alcoholism [Kendler] 374 (My)
Suicidal behaviors and the tryptophan hydroxylase gene [Abbar] 846 (Oc)
Papio
Is methylphenidate like cocaine? studies on their pharmacokinetics and distribution in the human brain [Volkow] 456 (Je)
Parasympatholytics
Risk of tardive dyskinesia in older patients: a prospective longitudinal study of 266 outpatients [Jeste] 756 (Se)
Parenting
Family-environment risk factors for attention-deficit hyperactivity disorder: a test of Rutter's indicators of adversity [Biederman] 464 (Je)
Genetic questions for environmental studies: differential parenting and psychopathology in adolescence [Reiss] 925 (No)
Parents
Efficacy of methylphenidate for attention-deficit hyperactivity disorder in children with tic disorder [Gadow] 444 (Je); correction, 836 (Oc)
Test-retest reliability of the Diagnostic Interview Schedule for Children (DISC 2.1): parent, child, and combined algorithms [Jensen] 61 (Ja); correction, 312 (Ap)
Pargyline
Role of methylphenidate in psychiatry [Klein] 429 (Je)
Paroxetine
Interactions of serotonin reuptake inhibitors with tricyclic antidepressants (letter) [Harvey] 783 (reply) [Popli] 784 (Se)
Parvalbumins
Neural circuitry of the prefrontal cortex in schizophrenia [Lewis] 269 (Ap)
Patient Admission
Perceived coercion in mental hospital admission: pressures and process [Lidz] 1034 (De)
Patient Compliance
Failure of naltrexone hydrochloride to reduce self-injurious and autistic behavior in mentally retarded adults: double-blind placebo-controlled studies [Willemsen-Swinkels] 766 (Se)
Multiple-family groups and psychoeducation in the treatment of schizophrenia [McFarlane] 679 (Au)
Why neuroleptic withdrawal in schizophrenia? [Carpenter] 192 (Mr)
Patient Education
Critical review of psychosocial interventions in cancer care [Fawzy] 100 (Fe)
Patient Outcome Assessment see Outcome Assessment (Health Care)
Peer Review
Child and adolescent mental disorders research: current directions, future needs [Rosenfeld] 729 (Se)
Pemoline
Role of methylphenidate in psychiatry [Klein] 429 (Je)
Periodicals
Some thoughts about the *Archives* [Barchas] 313 (Ap)
Perry, Samuel Wesley III, (1940-1994)
Samuel Wesley Perry III, MD, December 10, 1940, to March 15, 1994 [Rabkin] 1078 (De)
Personality
Switching from 'unipolar' to bipolar II: an 11-year prospective study of clinical and temperamental predictors in 559 patients [Akiskal] 114 (Fe)
Personality Disorders
Are case formulations useful for outcomes research? [Clarkin] 645 (Au)
Between the past and the future of psychotherapy research [Akhtar] 642 (Au)
Diagnosis, assessment, and individual complexity [Emde] 637 (Au)
Family study of early-onset dysthymia: mood and personality disorders in relatives of outpatients with dysthymia and episodic major depression and normal controls [Klein] 487 (Je)
New York High-Risk Project: psychoses and cluster A personality disorders in offspring of schizophrenic parents at 23 years of follow-up [Erlenmeyer-Kimling] 857 (Oc)
Personality: psychodynamic perspectives [Shapiro] 651 (Au)
Personality theory: clinical practice, social development, and the biology of individual differences [Reiss] 633 (Au)
Progress on case formulation [Crits-Christoph] 639 (Au)
Reliability and validity of two structured diagnostic interviews for personality disorders [Pilkonis] 1025 (De)
'Richly complex' but needs an emotion theory [Dahl] 649 (Au)
Role-relationship model configurations: a summation [Horowitz] 654 (Au)
Role-relationship models: are they useful for research and practice? [Jones] 646 (Au)
Role-relationship models for case formulation [Horowitz] 625 (Au)
Personnel Recruitment see Personnel Selection
Personnel Selection
Child and adolescent mental disorders and the search for an NIMH director: quo vadis? [Barchas] 873 (Oc)
Pertussis Toxins
Guanine nucleotide-binding proteins in bipolar affective disorder: effects of long-term lithium treatment [Manji] 135 (Fe)
Low levels of pertussis toxin adenosine diphosphate ribosylation in the schizophrenic brain (letter) [Okada] 319 (Ap)
Pharmacokinetics
Is methylphenidate like cocaine? studies on their pharmacokinetics and distribution in the human brain [Volkow] 456 (Je)
Phenothiazines
Clozapine-associated postoperative ileus: case report and review of the literature (letter) [Erickson] 508 (Je)
Neuroleptic withdrawal in schizophrenic patients: a review of the literature [Gilbert] 173 (Mr)
Phobia, Social see Phobic Disorders
Phobias see Phobic Disorders
Phobic Disorders
Generalized social phobia: reliability and validity [Mannuzza] 230 (Mr)
Is the comorbidity between social phobia and panic disorder due to familial cotransmission or other factors? [Horwath] 574 (Jy)
Positron emission tomographic study of simple phobic symptom provocation [Rauch] 20 (Ja)
Specificity in familial aggregation of phobic disorders [Fyer] 564 (Jy)
Structure of the genetic and environmental risk factors for six major psychiatric disorders in women: phobia, generalized anxiety disorder, panic disorder, bulimia, major depression, and alcoholism [Kendler] 374 (My)
Phosphoinositides
Signal transduction pathways: molecular targets for lithium's actions [Manji] 531 (Jy)
Phospholipids
In vivo study of the prefrontal cortex of schizophrenic patients at different stages of illness via phosphorus magnetic resonance spectroscopy [Stanley] 399 (My); correction, 799 (Oc)
Phosphorus
In vivo study of the prefrontal cortex of schizophrenic patients at different stages of illness via phosphorus magnetic resonance spectroscopy [Stanley] 399 (My); correction, 799 (Oc)
Pindolol
Biochemical effects of antidepressant augmentation (letter) [Howland] 156 (Fe)
Pindolol, 5-hydroxytryptamine, and antidepressant augmentation (letter) [Artigas] 969 (No)
Pituitary-Adrenal System
Depression in patients with cancer: diagnosis, biology, and treatment [McDaniel] 89 (Fe)
Placebos
Double-blind parallel comparison of three dosages of sertraline and placebo in outpatients with obsessive-compulsive disorder [Greist] 289 (Ap)
Failure of naltrexone hydrochloride to reduce self-injurious and autistic behavior in mentally retarded adults: double-blind placebo-controlled studies [Willemsen-Swinkels] 766 (Se)
Plasma
Clozapine-induced increase in plasma levels of soluble interleukin-2 receptors (letter) [Pollmächer] 877 (reply) [Ganguli] 878 (Oc)
Effects of Alzheimer's disease and normal aging on cerebrospinal fluid norepinephrine responses to yohimbine and clonidine [Peskind] 774 (Se)
Plasma haloperidol levels and clinical effects in schizophrenia and schizoaffective disorder [Volavka] 837 (Oc)
Platelets see Blood Platelets
Polymorphism, Restriction Fragment Length
Suicidal behaviors and the tryptophan hydroxylase gene [Abbar] 846 (Oc)
Polysomnography
In quest of identifying vulnerability markers for psychiatric disorders by all-night polysomnography [Lauer] 145 (Fe)
Positron-Emission Tomography see Tomography, Emission-Computed
Postoperative Complications
Clozapine-associated postoperative ileus: case report and review of the literature (letter) [Erickson] 508 (Je)
Postpartum Period see Puerperium
Posttraumatic Stress Disorders see Stress Disorders, Post-traumatic
Prefrontal Cortex
Abnormal excitatory neurotransmitter metabolism in schizophrenic brains [Tsai] 829 (Oc)
Abnormally high neuronal density in the schizophrenic cortex: a morphometric analysis of prefrontal area 9 and occipital area 17 [Selemon] 805 (Oc)
Gene expression for glutamic acid decarboxylase is reduced without loss of neurons in prefrontal cortex of schizophrenics [Akbarian] 258 (Ap)
Impaired mismatch negativity generation reflects wide-

spread dysfunction of working memory in schizophrenia [Javitt] 550 (Jy)
In pursuit of the molecular neuropathology of schizophrenia [Trojanowski] 274 (Ap)
In reply [Akbarian] 277 (Ap)
In vivo study of the prefrontal cortex of schizophrenic patients at different stages of illness via phosphorus magnetic resonance spectroscopy [Stanley] 399 (My); correction, 799 (Oc)
Neocortical abnormalities in schizophrenia [Watson] 819 (Oc)
Neural circuitry of the prefrontal cortex in schizophrenia [Lewis] 269 (Ap)
Prefrontal cortex and schizophrenia: a quantitative magnetic resonance imaging study [Wible] 279 (Ap)
Reduced caudate nucleus volume in obsessive-compulsive disorder [Robinson] 393 (My)
Reduced inhibitory capacity in prefrontal cortex of schizophrenics [Lee] 267 (Ap)
Spatial working memory deficits in the relatives of schizophrenic patients [Park] 821 (Oc)

Pregnancy Outcome
Developmental brain abnormalities in schizophrenia: contributions of genetic and perinatal factors (letter) [Vita] (reply) [Cannon] 157 (Fe)

Premenstrual Syndrome
Premenstrual dysphoric disorder and response to cholecystokinin-tetrapeptide (letter) [Le Melledo] 605 (Jy)
Premenstrual dysphoric disorders, anxiety, and depressions: vulnerability traits or comorbidity (letter) [Halbreich] 606 (Jy)

Primary Health Care
Health care costs of primary care patients with recognized depression [Simon] 850 (Oc)

Prolactin
Effects of the menstrual cycle on dependent variables in mood disorder research [Leibenluft] 51:761 (Oc); correction, 52:144 (Fe)

Protein Kinase C
Signal transduction pathways: molecular targets for lithium's actions [Manji] 531 (Jy)

Psychiatric Department, Hospital
Quality of care for depressed elderly patients hospitalized in the specialty psychiatric units or general medical wards [Norquist] 695 (Au)

Psychometrics
More reliable outcome measures can reduce sample size requirements [Leon] 867 (Oc)

Psychomotor Agitation
Complicating factors in the analysis of acute drug-induced akathisia (letter) [Rosebush] 878 (reply) [Sachdev] 879 (Oc)

Psychopathology
NMDA receptor as a site for psychopathology: primary or secondary role? [Henn] 1008 (De)

Psychotherapy
Are case formulations useful for outcomes research? [Clarkin] 645 (Au)
Between the past and the future of psychotherapy research [Akhtar] 642 (Au)
Critical review of psychosocial interventions in cancer care [Fawzy] 100 (Fe)
Personality: psychodynamic perspectives [Shapiro] 651 (Au)
Personality theory: clinical practice, social development, and the biology of individual differences [Reiss] 633 (Au)
Progress on case formulation [Crits-Christoph] 639 (Au)
'Richly complex' but needs an emotion theory [Dahl] 649 (Au)
Role-relationship model configurations: a summation [Horowitz] 654 (Au)
Role-relationship models: are they useful for research and practice? [Jones] 646 (Au)
Signs of defensive control locate conflicted topics in discourse [Horowitz] 1040 (De)
Treatment of postpartum depression with interpersonal psychotherapy (letter) [Stuart] 75 (reply) [Weissman] 76 (Ja)

Psychotherapy, Group
Critical review of psychosocial interventions in cancer care [Fawzy] 100 (Fe)
Depression in patients with cancer: diagnosis, biology, and treatment [McDaniel] 89 (Fe)
Multiple-family groups and psychoeducation in the treatment of schizophrenia [McFarlane] 679 (Au)

Psychotic Disorders
Abnormally high neuronal density in the schizophrenic cortex: a morphometric analysis of prefrontal area 9 and occipital area 17 [Selemon] 805 (Oc)
Longitudinal study of symptom dimensions in schizophrenia: prediction and patterns of change [Arndt] 352 (My)
Neocortical abnormalities in schizophrenia [Watson] 819 (Oc)
New York High-Risk Project: psychoses and cluster A personality disorders in offspring of schizophrenic parents at 23 years of follow-up [Erlenmeyer-Kimling] 857 (Oc)
Plasma haloperidol levels and clinical effects in schizophrenia and schizoaffective disorder [Volavka] 837 (Oc)
Schizotypal symptoms and signs in the Roscommon Family Study: their factor structure and familial relationship with psychotic and affective disorders [Kendler] 296 (Ap)

Psychotropic Drugs
Prevalence and correlates of drug use and dependence in the United States: results from the National Comorbidity Survey [Warner] 219 (Mr)

Publication Bias
Meta-analyses of studies of ventricular enlargement and cortical sulcal prominence in mood disorders: comparisons with controls or patients with schizophrenia [Elkis] 735 (Se)

Publishing
Some thoughts about the *Archives* [Barchas] 313 (Ap)

Puerperium
Treatment of postpartum depression with interpersonal psychotherapy (letter) [Stuart] 75 (reply) [Weissman] 76 (Ja)

Putamen
Low levels of pertussis toxin adenosine diphosphate ribosylation in the schizophrenic brain (letter) [Okada] 319 (Ap)

Q

Quality of Health Care
Quality of care for depressed elderly patients hospitalized in the specialty psychiatric units or general medical wards [Norquist] 695 (Au)

Quality of Life
Cingulotomy for intractable obsessive-compulsive disorder: prospective long-term follow-up of 18 patients [Baer] 384 (My)

Questionnaires
Risk of Alzheimer's disease in first-degree relatives (letter) [Heun] 317 (reply) [Silverman] 318 (Ap)

R

Reaction Time
Spatial working memory deficits in the relatives of schizophrenic patients [Park] 821 (Oc)

Receptors, Dopamine
Low levels of pertussis toxin adenosine diphosphate ribosylation in the schizophrenic brain (letter) [Okada] 319 (Ap)

Receptors, Dopamine D2
In vivo D_2 dopamine receptor density in psychotic and nonpsychotic patients with bipolar disorder [Pearlson] 471 (Je)

Receptors, GABA
Gene expression for glutamic acid decarboxylase is reduced without loss of neurons in prefrontal cortex of schizophrenics [Akbarian] 258 (Ap)
In reply [Akbarian] 277 (Ap)

Receptors, Glucocorticoid
Dose-response changes in plasma cortisol and lymphocyte glucocorticoid receptors following dexamethasone administration in combat veterans with and without posttraumatic stress disorder [Yehuda] 583 (Jy)

Receptors, Glutamate
Abnormal excitatory neurotransmitter metabolism in schizophrenic brains [Tsai] 829 (Oc)
Altered glutamatergic and GABAergic mechanisms in the cingulate cortex of the schizophrenic brain [Benes] 1015 (De)
Glutamate receptor dysfunction and schizophrenia [Olney] 998 (De)

Receptors, Interleukin-2
Clozapine-induced increase in plasma levels of soluble interleukin-2 receptors (letter) [Pollmächer] 877 (reply) [Ganguli] 878 (Oc)

Receptors, N-Methyl-D-Aspartate
Constraints on concepts of pathogenesis: language and the speciation process as the key to the etiology of schizophrenia [Crow] 1011 (De)
NMDA receptor as a site for psychopathology: primary or secondary role? [Henn] 1008 (De)
Response to commentaries and to the challenge of building a perfect theory to explain schizophrenia: response to Dr Benes' commentary [Olney] 1019 (De)

Recurrence
Behavioral vs biochemical prediction of clinical stability following haloperidol withdrawal in schizophrenia [van Kammen] 673 (Au)
Considering neuroleptic maintenance and taper on a continuum: need for individual rather than dogmatic approach [Jeste] 209 (Mr)
Early course of schizophrenia and long-term maintenance neuroleptic therapy [Nuechterlein] 203 (Mr)
Long-term treatment for lifetime disorders? [Greden] 197 (Mr)
Multiple-family groups and psychoeducation in the treatment of schizophrenia [McFarlane] 679 (Au)
Neuroleptic withdrawal in schizophrenic patients [Baldessarini] 189 (Mr)
Neuroleptic withdrawal in schizophrenic patients: a review of the literature [Gilbert] 173 (Mr)
Neuroleptic withdrawal in schizophrenic patients: an idea whose time has come [Meltzer] 200 (Mr)
Risks of withdrawing antipsychotic medications [Wyatt] 205 (Mr)
Signs and symptoms: what can they tell us about the clinical course and pathophysiologic processes of schizophrenia? [Lieberman] 361 (My)

Referral and Consultation
Trial of the effect of a standardized psychiatric consultation on health outcomes and costs in somatizing patients [Smith] 238 (Mr)

Regional Blood Flow
Positron emission tomographic study of simple phobic symptom provocation [Rauch] 20 (Ja)
Reciprocal lateralization of frontal lobe functions (letter) [Goldberg] (reply) [Rauch] 159 (Fe)

Relapse see Recurrence

Relaxation Techniques
Critical review of psychosocial interventions in cancer care [Fawzy] 100 (Fe)

Reliability and Validity see Reproducibility of Results

Reproducibility of Results
More reliable outcome measures can reduce sample size requirements [Leon] 867 (Oc)
Test-retest reliability of the Diagnostic Interview Schedule for Children (DISC 2.1): parent, child, and combined algorithms [Jensen] 61 (Ja); correction, 312 (Ap)

Research
Between the past and the future of psychotherapy research [Akhtar] 642 (Au)
Child and adolescent mental disorders and the search for an NIMH director: quo vadis? [Barchas] 873 (Oc)
Personality: psychodynamic perspectives [Shapiro] 651 (Au)
Role-relationship model configurations: a summation [Horowitz] 654 (Au)
Role-relationship models: are they useful for research and practice? [Jones] 646 (Au)
Some thoughts about the *Archives* [Barchas] 313 (Ap)

Response Time see Reaction Time

Reviewers
Reviewers for 1995 [Abdul-Jalil] 990 (De)

Risk Factors
Family-environment risk factors for attention-deficit hyperactivity disorder: a test of Rutter's indicators of adversity [Biederman] 464 (Je)
Structure of the genetic and environmental risk factors for six major psychiatric disorders in women: phobia, generalized anxiety disorder, panic disorder, bulimia, major depression, and alcoholism [Kendler] 374 (My)

RNA, Messenger
Gene expression for glutamic acid decarboxylase is reduced without loss of neurons in prefrontal cortex of schizophrenics [Akbarian] 258 (Ap)
In reply [Akbarian] 277 (Ap)
Neural circuitry of the prefrontal cortex in schizophrenia [Lewis] 269 (Ap)
Reduced inhibitory capacity in prefrontal cortex of schizophrenics [Lee] 267 (Ap)

Robins, Eli (1921-1994)
Eli Robins, MD, February 22, 1921, to December 21, 1994 [Hudgens] 1080 (De)

Role
Are case formulations useful for outcomes research? [Clarkin] 645 (Au)
Diagnosis, assessment, and individual complexity [Emde] 637 (Au)
Personality: psychodynamic perspectives [Shapiro] 651 (Au)
Personality theory: clinical practice, social development, and the biology of individual differences [Reiss] 633 (Au)
Progress on case formulation [Crits-Christoph] 639 (Au)
'Richly complex' but needs an emotion theory [Dahl] 649 (Au)
Role-relationship model configurations: a summation [Horowitz] 654 (Au)
Role-relationship models: are they useful for research and practice? [Jones] 646 (Au)
Role-relationship models for case formulation [Horowitz] 625 (Au)

Romano, John (1908-1995)
John Romano, MD, November 20, 1908 to June 19, 1995 [Joynt] 1076 (De)

Roscommon Family Study
Schizotypal symptoms and signs in the Roscommon Family Study: their factor structure and familial relationship with psychotic and affective disorders [Kendler] 296 (Ap)

S

Safety
Double-blind parallel comparison of three dosages of sertraline and placebo in outpatients with obsessive-compulsive disorder [Greist] 289 (Ap)

Sample Size
More reliable outcome measures can reduce sample size requirements [Leon] 867 (Oc)

Schizoaffective Disorder see Psychotic Disorders

Schizophrenia
Abnormal excitatory neurotransmitter metabolism in schizophrenic brains [Tsai] 829 (Oc)
Abnormally high neuronal density in the schizophrenic cortex: a morphometric analysis of prefrontal area 9 and occipital area 17 [Selemon] 805 (Oc)
Altered glutamatergic and GABAergic mechanisms in the cingulate cortex of the schizophrenic brain [Benes] 1015 (De)

Behavioral vs biochemical prediction of clinical stability following haloperidol withdrawal in schizophrenia [van Kammen] 673 (Au)
Clozapine therapy and increases in homovanillic acid (letter) [Risch] 244 (Mr)
Clozapine-induced increase in plasma levels of soluble interleukin-2 receptors (letter) [Pollmächer] 877 (reply) [Ganguli] 878 (Oc)
Considering neuroleptic maintenance and taper on a continuum: need for individual rather than dogmatic approach [Jeste] 209 (Mr)
Constraints on concepts of pathogenesis: language and the speciation process as the key to the etiology of schizophrenia [Crow] 1011 (De)
Developmental brain abnormalities in schizophrenia: contributions of genetic and perinatal factors (letter) [Vita] (reply) [Cannon] 157 (Fe)
Early course of schizophrenia and long-term maintenance neuroleptic therapy [Nuechterlein] 203 (Mr)
Event-related potentials in the study of psychiatric disorders [Pfefferbaum] 559 (Jy)
Frontal and temporal lobe brain volumes in schizophrenia: relationship to symptoms and clinical subtype [Turetsky] 1061 (De)
Gene expression for glutamic acid decarboxylase is reduced without loss of neurons in prefrontal cortex of schizophrenics [Akbarian] 258 (Ap)
Glutamate receptor dysfunction and schizophrenia [Olney] 998 (De)
Impaired mismatch negativity generation reflects widespread dysfunction of working memory in schizophrenia [Javitt] 550 (Jy)
In pursuit of the molecular neuropathology of schizophrenia [Trojanowski] 274 (Ap)
In quest of identifying vulnerability markers for psychiatric disorders by all-night polysomnography [Lauer] 145 (Fe)
In reply [Akbarian] 277 (Ap)
In vivo D_2 dopamine receptor density in psychotic and nonpsychotic patients with bipolar disorder [Pearlson] 471 (Je)
In vivo study of the prefrontal cortex of schizophrenic patients at different stages of illness via phosphorus magnetic resonance spectroscopy [Stanley] 399 (My); correction, 799 (Oc)
Increased rate of P300 latency prolongation with age in schizophrenia: electrophysiological evidence for a neurodegenerative process [O'Donnell] 544 (Jy)
Longitudinal study of symptom dimensions in schizophrenia: prediction and patterns of change [Arndt] 352 (My)
Long-term treatment for lifetime disorders? [Greden] 197 (Mr)
Low levels of pertussis toxin adenosine diphosphate ribosylation in the schizophrenic brain (letter) [Okada] 319 (Ap)
Meta-analyses of studies of ventricular enlargement and cortical sulcal prominence in mood disorders: comparisons with controls or patients with schizophrenia [Elkis] 735 (Se)
Mitogen-stimulated interleukin-2 production in never-medicated, first-episode schizophrenic patients: the influence of age at onset and negative symptoms [Ganguli] 668 (Au)
Multiple-family groups and psychoeducation in the treatment of schizophrenia [McFarlane] 679 (Au)
Neocortical abnormalities in schizophrenia [Watson] 819 (Oc)
Neural circuitry of the prefrontal cortex in schizophrenia [Lewis] 269 (Ap)
Neuroleptic withdrawal in schizophrenic patients [Baldessarini] 189 (Mr)
Neuroleptic withdrawal in schizophrenic patients: a review of the literature [Gilbert] 173 (Mr)
Neuroleptic withdrawal in schizophrenic patients: an idea whose time has come [Meltzer] 200 (Mr)
New York High-Risk Project: psychoses and cluster A personality disorders in offspring of schizophrenic parents at 23 years of follow-up [Erlenmeyer-Kimling] 857 (Oc)
Pharmacotherapy of impaired affect in recovering schizophrenic patients [Hogarty] 29 (Ja)
Plasma haloperidol levels and clinical effects in schizophrenia and schizoaffective disorder [Volavka] 837 (Oc)
Prefrontal cortex and schizophrenia: a quantitative magnetic resonance imaging study [Wible] 279 (Ap)
Prevalence of schizophrenia in Ireland: readdressing the enigma (letter) [Waddington] (reply) [Walsh] 509 (Je)
Reduced inhibitory capacity in prefrontal cortex of schizophrenics [Lee] 267 (Ap)
Response to commentaries and to the challenge of building a perfect theory to explain schizophrenia: response to Dr Benes' commentary [Olney] 1019 (De)
Resting cerebral glucose metabolism in first-episode and previously treated patients with schizophrenia relates to clinical features [Gur] 657 (Au)
Risks of withdrawing antipsychotic medications [Wyatt] 205 (Mr)
Schizotypal symptoms and signs in the Roscommon Family Study: their factor structure and familial relationship with psychotic and affective disorders [Kendler] 296 (Ap)
Signs and symptoms: what can they tell us about the clinical course and pathophysiologic processes of schizophrenia? [Lieberman] 361 (My)
Spatial working memory deficits in the relatives of schizophrenic patients [Park] 821 (Oc)
Structure and course of positive and negative symptoms in schizophrenia [Eaton] 127 (Fe)
Symptoms of schizophrenia: methods, meanings, and mechanisms [Andreasen] 341 (My)
Why neuroleptic withdrawal in schizophrenia? [Carpenter] 192 (Mr)

Schizophrenia, Disorganized
Longitudinal study of symptom dimensions in schizophrenia: prediction and patterns of change [Arndt] 352 (My)
Signs and symptoms: what can they tell us about the clinical course and pathophysiologic processes of schizophrenia? [Lieberman] 361 (My)

Schizotypal Personality Disorder
Schizotypal symptoms and signs in the Roscommon Family Study: their factor structure and familial relationship with psychotic and affective disorders [Kendler] 296 (Ap)

Seasons
Seasonal variation in plasma L-tryptophan availability in healthy volunteers: relationships to violent suicide occurrence [Maes] 937 (No)

Selegiline
Role of methylphenidate in psychiatry [Klein] 429 (Je)

Self Mutilation
Failure of naltrexone hydrochloride to reduce self-injurious and autistic behavior in mentally retarded adults: double-blind placebo-controlled studies [Willemsen-Swinkels] 766 (Se)

Sensitivity and Specificity
Relationship of panic disorder to posttraumatic stress disorder (letter) [Safadi] 76 (reply) [Southwick] 77 (Ja)

Serotonin
Efficacy and tolerability of serotonin transport inhibitors in obsessive-compulsive disorder: a meta-analysis [Greist] 53 (Ja)
Pindolol, 5-hydroxytryptamine, and antidepressant augmentation (letter) [Artigas] 969 (No)
Suicidal behaviors and the tryptophan hydroxylase gene [Abbar] 846 (Oc)
Tryptophan depletion in stable lithium-treated patients with bipolar disorder in remission (letter) [Benkelfat] 154 (reply) [Delgado] 155 (Fe)

Serotonin Reuptake Inhibitors see Serotonin Uptake Inhibitors

Serotonin Uptake Inhibitors
Biochemical effects of antidepressant augmentation (letter) [Howland] 156 (Fe)
Double-blind parallel comparison of three dosages of sertraline and placebo in outpatients with obsessive-compulsive disorder [Greist] 289 (Ap)
Interactions of serotonin reuptake inhibitors with tricyclic antidepressants (letter) [Harvey] 783 (reply) [Popli] 784 (Se)

Sertraline Hydrochloride
Double-blind parallel comparison of three dosages of sertraline and placebo in outpatients with obsessive-compulsive disorder [Greist] 289 (Ap)
Efficacy and tolerability of serotonin transport inhibitors in obsessive-compulsive disorder: a meta-analysis [Greist] 53 (Ja)

Sex
Prevalence and correlates of drug use and dependence in the United States: results from the National Comorbidity Survey [Warner] 219 (Mr)
Reciprocal lateralization of frontal lobe functions (letter) [Goldberg] (reply) [Rauch] 159 (Fe)

Signal Transduction
Signal transduction pathways: molecular targets for lithium's actions [Manji] 531 (Jy)

Sleep
Effects of the menstrual cycle on dependent variables in mood disorder research [Leibenluft] **51**:761 (Oc); correction, **52**:144 (Fe)

Sleep Disorders
In quest of identifying vulnerability markers for psychiatric disorders by all-night polysomnography [Lauer] 145 (Fe)
Neuroleptic withdrawal in schizophrenic patients: a review of the literature [Gilbert] 173 (Mr)

Social Behavior Disorders
Structure and course of positive and negative symptoms in schizophrenia [Eaton] 127 (Fe)

Social Class
Family-environment risk factors for attention-deficit hyperactivity disorder: a test of Rutter's indicators of adversity [Biederman] 464 (Je)
Role of methylphenidate in psychiatry [Klein] 429 (Je)

Social Isolation
Schizotypal symptoms and signs in the Roscommon Family Study: their factor structure and familial relationship with psychotic and affective disorders [Kendler] 296 (Ap)

Socioeconomic Status see Social Class

Somatization Disorder see Somatoform Disorders

Somatoform Disorders
Trial of the effect of a standardized psychiatric consultation on health outcomes and costs in somatizing patients [Smith] 238 (Mr)

Somatosensory Cortex
Positron emission tomographic study of simple phobic symptom provocation [Rauch] 20 (Ja)

Spatial Behavior
Spatial working memory deficits in the relatives of schizophrenic patients [Park] 821 (Oc)

Spinal Puncture
Behavioral vs biochemical prediction of clinical stability following haloperidol withdrawal in schizophrenia [van Kammen] 673 (Au)

Statistics
More reliable outcome measures can reduce sample size requirements [Leon] 867 (Oc)

Stress Disorders, Posttraumatic
Dose-response changes in plasma cortisol and lymphocyte glucocorticoid receptors following dexamethasone administration in combat veterans with and without posttraumatic stress disorder [Yehuda] 583 (Jy)
Posttraumatic stress disorder in the National Comorbidity Survey [Kessler] 1048 (De)
Relationship of panic disorder to posttraumatic stress disorder (letter) [Safadi] 76 (reply) [Southwick] 77 (Ja)

Stress, Psychological
Critical review of psychosocial interventions in cancer care [Fawzy] 100 (Fe)
Is hyperarousal essential to obsessive-compulsive disorder? diminished physiologic flexibility, but not hyperarousal, characterizes patients with obsessive-compulsive disorder [Hoehn-Saric] 688 (Au)

Substance Abuse
Adoption study demonstrating two genetic pathways to drug abuse [Cadoret] 42 (Ja)
Mental illness and suicide: a case-control study in east Taiwan [Cheng] 594 (Jy)
Prevalence and correlates of drug use and dependence in the United States: results from the National Comorbidity Survey [Warner] 219 (Mr)
Suicidal behaviors and the tryptophan hydroxylase gene [Abbar] 846 (Oc)

Substance Dependence
Dose-response changes in plasma cortisol and lymphocyte glucocorticoid receptors following dexamethasone administration in combat veterans with and without posttraumatic stress disorder [Yehuda] 583 (Jy)
Prevalence and correlates of drug use and dependence in the United States: results from the National Comorbidity Survey [Warner] 219 (Mr)

Substance Withdrawal Syndrome
Behavioral vs biochemical prediction of clinical stability following haloperidol withdrawal in schizophrenia [van Kammen] 673 (Au)
Complicating factors in the analysis of acute drug-induced akathisia (letter) [Rosebush] 878 (reply) [Sachdev] 879 (Oc)
Considering neuroleptic maintenance and taper on a continuum: need for individual rather than dogmatic approach [Jeste] 209 (Mr)
Early course of schizophrenia and long-term maintenance neuroleptic therapy [Nuechterlein] 203 (Mr)
Long-term treatment for lifetime disorders? [Greden] 197 (Mr)
Neuroleptic withdrawal in schizophrenic patients [Baldessarini] 189 (Mr)
Neuroleptic withdrawal in schizophrenic patients: a review of the literature [Gilbert] 173 (Mr)
Neuroleptic withdrawal in schizophrenic patients: an idea whose time has come [Meltzer] 200 (Mr)
Risks of withdrawing antipsychotic medications [Wyatt] 205 (Mr)
Why neuroleptic withdrawal in schizophrenia? [Carpenter] 192 (Mr)

Suicide
Comments on the report card from a services research perspective [Kruesi] 727 (Se)
Mental illness and suicide: a case-control study in east Taiwan [Cheng] 594 (Jy)
Seasonal variation in plasma L-tryptophan availability in healthy volunteers: relationships to violent suicide occurrence [Maes] 937 (No)

Suicide, Attempted
Suicidal behaviors and the tryptophan hydroxylase gene [Abbar] 846 (Oc)

T

Taiwan
Mental illness and suicide: a case-control study in east Taiwan [Cheng] 594 (Jy)

Temperament
Switching from 'unipolar' to bipolar II: an 11-year prospective study of clinical and temperamental predictors in 559 patients [Akiskal] 114 (Fe)

Temporal Lobe
Frontal and temporal lobe brain volumes in schizophrenia: relationship to symptoms and clinical subtype [Turetsky] 1061 (De)
Impaired mismatch negativity generation reflects widespread dysfunction of working memory in schizophrenia [Javitt] 550 (Jy)

In pursuit of the molecular neuropathology of schizophrenia [Trojanowski] 274 (Ap)
Prefrontal cortex and schizophrenia: a quantitative magnetic resonance imaging study [Wible] 279 (Ap)
Terminology see Nomenclature
Tetragastrin
Premenstrual dysphoric disorder and response to cholecystokinin-tetrapeptide (letter) [Le Melledo] 605 (Jy)
Premenstrual dysphoric disorders, anxiety, and depressions: vulnerability traits or comorbidity (letter) [Halbreich] 606 (Jy)
THIS MONTH IN *ARCHIVES OF GENERAL PSYCHIATRY*
253 (Ap), 339 (My), 422 (Je), 525 (Jy), 619 (Au), 713 (Se), 798 (Oc), 893 (No), 989 (De)
Thymoleptics see Antidepressive Agents
Thyrotropin
Effects of the menstrual cycle on dependent variables in mood disorder research [Leibenluft] 51:761 (Oc); correction, 52:144 (Fe)
Tic
Efficacy of methylphenidate for attention-deficit hyperactivity disorder in children with tic disorder [Gadow] 444 (Je); correction, 836 (Oc)
Role of methylphenidate in psychiatry [Klein] 429 (Je)
Tomography, Emission-Computed
In vivo D_2 dopamine receptor density in psychotic and nonpsychotic patients with bipolar disorder [Pearlson] 471 (Je)
Is methylphenidate like cocaine? studies on their pharmacokinetics and distribution in the human brain [Volkow] 456 (Je)
Positron emission tomographic study of simple phobic symptom provocation [Rauch] 20 (Ja)
Reciprocal lateralization of frontal lobe functions (letter) [Goldberg] (reply) [Rauch] 159 (Fe)
Resting cerebral glucose metabolism in first-episode and previously treated patients with schizophrenia relates to clinical features [Gur] 657 (Au)
Tourette Syndrome
Reciprocal lateralization of frontal lobe functions (letter) [Goldberg] (reply) [Rauch] 159 (Fe)
Transference (Psychology)
Personality theory: clinical practice, social development, and the biology of individual differences [Reiss] 633 (Au)
Tryptophan
Seasonal variation in plasma L-tryptophan availability in healthy volunteers: relationships to violent suicide occurrence [Maes] 937 (No)
Tryptophan depletion in stable lithium-treated patients with bipolar disorder in remission (letter) [Benkelfat] 154 (reply) [Delgado] 155 (Fe)
Tryptophan Hydroxylase
Suicidal behaviors and the tryptophan hydroxylase gene [Abbar] 846 (Oc)
Twin Studies
Developmental brain abnormalities in schizophrenia: contributions of genetic and perinatal factors (letter) [Vita] (reply) [Cannon] 157 (Fe)
Structure of the genetic and environmental risk factors for six major psychiatric disorders in women: phobia, generalized anxiety disorder, panic disorder, bulimia, major depression, and alcoholism [Kendler] 374 (My)

U

Unipolar Depression see Depressive Disorder
United States
Prevalence and correlates of drug use and dependence in the United States: results from the National Comorbidity Survey [Warner] 219 (Mr)

V

Veterans
Dose-response changes in plasma cortisol and lymphocyte glucocorticoid receptors following dexamethasone administration in combat veterans with and without posttraumatic stress disorder [Yehuda] 583 (Jy)
Relationship of panic disorder to posttraumatic stress disorder (letter) [Safadi] 76 (reply) [Southwick] 77 (Ja)
Volition
Longitudinal study of symptom dimensions in schizophrenia: prediction and patterns of change [Arndt] 352 (My)
Symptoms of schizophrenia: methods, meanings, and mechanisms [Andreasen] 341 (My)

W

Water Intoxication
Why neuroleptic withdrawal in schizophrenia? [Carpenter] 192 (Mr)
Withdrawal Symptoms see Substance Withdrawal Syndrome
Women
Structure of the genetic and environmental risk factors for six major psychiatric disorders in women: phobia, generalized anxiety disorder, panic disorder, bulimia, major depression, and alcoholism [Kendler] 374 (My)
Wortis, Joseph (1906-1995)
Joseph Wortis, MD October 2, 1906, to February 22, 1995 [Halmi] 1077 (De)

Y

Yohimbine
Effects of Alzheimer's disease and normal aging on cerebrospinal fluid norepinephrine responses to yohimbine and clonidine [Peskind] 774 (Se)
Relationship of panic disorder to posttraumatic stress disorder (letter) [Safadi] 76 (reply) [Southwick] 77 (Ja)